INFERTILITY

Evaluation and Treatment

INFERTILITY
Evaluation and Treatment

WILLIAM R. KEYE, JR., M.D.

Chief, Division of Reproductive Endocrinology
Department of Obstetrics and Gynecology
William Beaumont Hospital
Royal Oak, Michigan

Associate Clinical Professor
Department of Obstetrics and Gynecology
University of Michigan School of Medicine
Ann Arbor, Michigan

R. JEFFREY CHANG, M.D.

Professor and Chair
Department of Obstetrics and Gynecology
University of California, Davis, School of Medicine
Davis, California

ROBERT W. REBAR, M.D.

Professor and Chair
Department of Obstetrics and Gynecology
University of Cincinnati College of Medicine
Cincinnati, Ohio

MICHAEL R. SOULES, M.D.

Professor and Director, Division of Reproductive
   Endocrinology and Infertility
Department of Obstetrics and Gynecology
University of Washington School of Medicine
Seattle, Washington

Illustrated by
Theodore G. Huff

W.B. SAUNDERS COMPANY
A Division of Harcourt Brace & Company

Philadelphia   London   Toronto   Montreal   Sydney   Tokyo

W.B. SAUNDERS COMPANY
A Division of
Harcourt Brace & Company

The Curtis Center
Independence Square West
Philadelphia, Pennsylvania 19106

Library of Congress Cataloging-in-Publication Data

Infertility: evaluation and treatment / [edited by] William R. Keye . . . [et al.].

   p.   cm.

Includes bibliographical references.

ISBN 0-7216-3970-4

1. Infertility.   I. Keye, William R., 1943–

RC889.I5625   1995

618.1'78—dc   93-48748

Infertility: Evaluation and Treatment   ISBN 0–7216–3970–4

Printed in the United States of America.

Last digit is the print number: 9   8   7   6   5   4   3   2   1

TO THE PATIENTS, MENTORS, AND COLLEAGUES FROM WHOM
WE HAVE GAINED OUR EXPERIENCE AND KNOWLEDGE
AND TO THE FUTURE STUDENTS
WHO WE HOPE WILL BENEFIT FROM THIS BOOK

To Gwen and Harry for their intellectual stimulation;
To Hans and Sharon and their family for their friendship;
To Bob Jaffe for being a model
of personal and professional excellence;
To Margaret Kulmann for her dedicated effort and loyalty;
To Sue, Debbie, and Jeff for their encouragement and support.

WILLIAM R. KEYE, JR., M.D.

To my parents, Elsie and Ray,
for their faithful support, generous love, and
inherent gift of character and courage;
To my wife, Carol, for all her
understanding, enthusiasm, and encouragement.

R. JEFFREY CHANG, M.D.

To Griff Ross (deceased), Rees Midgley, and Sam Yen
for serving as inspiring mentors and role models;
To Marianne Niehaus and Elizabeth Bourne
for their dedication and concerted efforts;
To Margo, Bryan, Jeannette, and Darren
for their patience and understanding.

ROBERT W. REBAR, M.D.

To Chuck Hammond for being an exemplary model;
To Robert Steiner, Bill Bremner, and Don Clifton
for being friends and noncompromising research partners;
To Nancy Canino (Cohen) and Gretchen Davis as two of the
finest research coordinators anywhere;
To Melissa and Ryan, my two wonderful children who
still don't quite understand what their dad does for a living;
and finally and most importantly
To my wife, Diane,
for her encouragement and understanding about
extra projects such as this book.

MICHAEL R. SOULES, M.D.

Contributors

G. David Adamson, M.D.
Clinical Associate Professor, Stanford University School of Medicine, Stanford; Associate Clinical Professor, University of California, San Francisco; Active Staff, Good Samaritan Hospital of Santa Clara Valley and Stanford University Hospital, Palo Alto, California.
Principles of Surgical Management of the Infertile Female

Linda D. Applegarth, Ed.D.
Clinical Assistant Professor of Psychology, Departments of Obstetrics and Gynecology, and Psychiatry, Cornell University Medical College; Program Psychologist, Center for Reproductive Medicine and Infertility, Department of Obstetrics and Gynecology, New York Hospital–Cornell Medical Center, New York, New York.
The Psychological Aspects of Infertility

Ricardo M. Asch, M.D.
Professor, Department of Obstetrics and Gynecology; Director, Center for Reproductive Health; and Assistant Dean, University of California, Irvine, College of Medicine, Irvine; Staff, Saddleback Center for Reproductive Health, Laguna Hills, California.
Gamete Intrafallopian Transfer

Jose P. Balmaceda, M.D.
Professor, Department of Obstetrics and Gynecology; Director, Division of Reproductive Endocrinology and Infertility, University of California, Irvine, Orange; Medical Director, Saddleback Center for Reproductive Health, Laguna Hills, California.
Gamete Intrafallopian Transfer

Robert L. Barbieri, M.D.
Kate Macy Ladd Professor of Obstetrics, Gynecology and Reproductive Biology, Harvard Medical School; Chief, Department of Obstetrics and Gynecology, Brigham and Women's Hospital, Boston, Massachusetts.
Endometriosis: Medical Therapy

Richard E. Berger, M.D.
Professor of Urology, University of Washington Affiliated Hospitals, Seattle, Washington.
Infection and Male Infertility

Stephen P. Boyers, M.D.
Associate Professor and Chief, Division of Reproductive Biology and Medicine, Department of Obstetrics and Gynecology, University of California, Davis, School of Medicine; Associate Professor, Department of Obstetrics and Gynecology, University of California, Davis, Medical Center, Sacramento, California.
Evaluation and Treatment of Disorders of the Cervix

D. Ware Branch, M.D.
Associate Professor, Department of Obstetrics and Gynecology, University of Utah Medical Center, Salt Lake City, Utah.
Evaluation and Treatment of Recurrent Miscarriages

William Byrd, M.D.
Associate Professor, Department of Obstetrics and Gynecology, University of Texas Southwestern Medical Center, Dallas, Texas.
Sperm Penetration and Homologous Insemination

Sandra A. Carson, M.D.
Associate Professor, Department of Obstetrics and Gynecology, Baylor College of Medicine, Houston, Texas.
Management of Early Pregnancy and Pregnancy Outcome in Assisted Reproductive Technologies

Marcelle Cedars, M.D.
Associate Professor, University of Cincinnati School of Medicine, Cincinnati, Ohio.
Prediction, Detection, and Evaluation of Ovulation

R. Jeffrey Chang, M.D.
Professor and Chair, Department of Obstetrics and Gynecology, University of California, Davis, School of Medicine, Davis, California.

Jacques Cohen, M.D.
Associate Professor of Embryology in Gynecology and Obstetrics and Scientific Director, The Center for Reproductive Medicine and Infertility, The New York Hospital–Cornell Medical Center, New York, New York.
Micromanipulation of Human Gametes, Zygotes, and Embryos

John A. Collins, M.D., F.R.C.S.(C)
Professor, Department of Obstetrics and Gynecology, Faculty of Health Sciences, McMaster University; Active Staff and Chief, Department of Obstetrics and Gynecology, Chedoke-McMaster Hospitals; Associate Staff, Hamilton Civic Hospitals and St. Joseph's Hospital, Hamilton, Ontario, Canada.
Unexplained Infertility

Alan B. Copperman, M.D.
Martin J. Clyman Fellow, Division of Reproductive Endocrinology, Department of Obstetrics and Gynecology,

Mount Sinai School of Medicine; Staff, Mount Sinai Medical Center and Elmhurst Hospital Center, New York, New York.
Treatment of Disorders of the Fallopian Tube

Owen K. Davis, M.D.
Associate Professor of Obstetrics and Gynecology, Cornell University Medical College; Assistant Attending Obstetrician-Gynecologist, The New York Hospital–Cornell Medical Center, New York, New York.
In Vitro Fertilization

Russell O. Davis, M.D.
Assistant Professor, Division of Reproductive Biology and Medicine, Department of Obstetrics and Gynecology, University of California, Davis, School of Medicine, Davis, California.
Methods and Interpretation of Semen Analysis

A. H. DeCherney, M.D.
Professor and Chairman, Department of Obstetrics and Gynecology, Tufts University School of Medicine and New England Medical Center, Boston, Massachusetts.
Infertility: A Historical Perspective
Management of the Ectopic Pregnancy

Michael P. Diamond, M.D.
Associate Professor, Departments of Obstetrics and Gynecology, Surgery, and Molecular Physiology and Biophysics, Vanderbilt University School of Medicine, Nashville, Tennessee.
Treatment of Disorders of the Fallopian Tube

Joseph Feste, M.D.
Clinical Associate Professor, Department of Obstetrics and Gynecology, Baylor College of Medicine and University of Texas Health Science Center; Staff, Woman's Hospital of Texas, The Methodist Hospital, Texas Childrens Hospital, and Ben Taub General Hospital, Houston, Texas.
Operative Instrumentation for Infertility Surgery

Bettina G. Fleige-Zahradka, M.B., Ch.B., F.R.C.S.(C)
Research Fellow, University of British Columbia; Active Staff, Duncan Hospital, Vancouver, British Columbia, Canada.
The Fallopian Tube: Pathophysiology

Robert H. Glass, M.D.
Professor, Obstetrics, Gynecology, and Reproductive Sciences, University of California, San Francisco, School of Medicine, San Francisco, California.
Female Infertility

Victor Gomel, M.D., F.R.C.S.(C), F.R.C.O.G.
Professor of Obstetrics and Gynecology, University of British Columbia, Faculty of Medicine; Chair Emeritus, University of British Columbia Department of Obstetrics and Gynecology; Staff, Department of Obstetrics and Gynecology, Vancouver Hospital and Health Sciences Centre and Grace Hospital, Vancouver, British Columbia, Canada.
Diagnostic Laparoscopy in Infertility

John E. Gould, M.D., Ph.D.
Associate Professor, Department of Urology, University of California, Davis, Medical Center, Sacramento, California.
Immunology of Spermatozoa

Jouko Halme, M.D., Ph.D.
Associate Professor, University of North Carolina at Chapel Hill; Staff, North Carolina Center for Reproductive Medicine, Cary, North Carolina.
Endometriosis: Pathophysiology and Presentation

Mary G. Hammond, M.D.
Director of Clinical Services, North Carolina Center for Reproductive Medicine; Staff, Western Wake Hospital, Cary, North Carolina.
Pharmacology of Ovulation-Inducing Drugs

Alan H. Handyside, Ph.D.
Senior Lecturer, Institute of Obstetrics and Gynaecology, Human Embryology Laboratory, Royal Postgraduate Medical School, Hammersmith Hospital, London, England.
In Vitro Fertilization and Preimplantation Genetic Diagnosis for Prevention of Inherited Disease

A. F. Haney, M.D.
Roy T. Parker Professor of Obstetrics and Gynecology, Duke University School of Medicine; Director, Division of Reproductive Endocrinology and Infertility, Department of Obstetrics and Gynecology, Duke University Medical Center, Durham, North Carolina.
Controlled Ovarian Hyperstimulation and Intrauterine Insemination

Stanton C. Honig, M.D.
Fellow, Male Reproductive Medicine and Surgery Program, Scott Department of Urology, Baylor College of Medicine, Houston, Texas.
Sexual and Ejaculatory Dysfunction as a Cause of Male Infertility

Ami S. Jaeger, J.D., M.A.
Consultant to the Ethical, Legal, and Social Implications (ELSI) Branch of the National Center for Human Genome Research, National Institutes of Health, Washington, D.C.
Legal and Ethical Challenges of Medically Assisted Reproduction

Patricia Irwin Johnston, A.B., M.S.
Infertility and Adoption Educator, Perspectives Press, Indianapolis, Indiana.
Infertility: A Patient's Perspective

Howard W. Jones, Jr., M.D.
Professor, Obstetrics and Gynecology, Eastern Virginia Medical School, Norfolk, Virginia; Professor Emeritus, Obstetrics and Gynecology, Johns Hopkins University School of Medicine, Baltimore, Maryland; Visiting Gynecologist, Norfolk General Hospital, Norfolk, Virginia.
History of In Vitro Fertilization

John F. Kerin, M.D., Ph.D.
Professor, Department of Reproductive Medicine, The Flinders University of South Australia; Director, Reproductive Medicine Programme, Flinders Medical Centre, Bedford Park, South Australia.
Tubal Microendoscopy: Salpingoscopy and Falloposcopy
Extended Techniques in Assisted Reproductive Technologies

Bruce Kessel, M.D.
Assistant Professor, Department of Obstetrics, Gynecology, and Reproductive Biology, Harvard Medical School, Boston, Massachusetts.
Practical Evaluation of Amenorrhea and Abnormal Uterine Bleeding

William R. Keye, Jr., M.D.
Associate Clinical Professor, Department of Obstetrics and Gynecology, University of Michigan School of Medicine, Ann Arbor; Director, Division of Reproductive Endocrinology, Infertility, and In Vitro Fertilization, Department of Obstetrics and Gynecology, William Beaumont Hospital, Royal Oak, Michigan.
Initial Approach to the Infertile Couple

Stephen R. Lincoln, M.D.
Assistant Professor of Obstetrics and Gynecology and Active
Staff, University of Mississippi Medical Center, Jackson,
Mississippi.
Surgical Treatment of Diseases of the Ovary

Larry I. Lipshultz, M.D.
Professor of Urology, Scott Department of Urology, Baylor
College of Medicine, Houston, Texas.
Sexual and Ejaculatory Dysfunction as a Cause of Male Infertility

James H. Liu, M.D.
Associate Professor and Head, Division of Reproductive
Endocrinology and Infertility, Department of Obstetrics and
Gynecology, University of Cincinnati College of Medicine;
Attending Staff, University Hospital and The Christ Hospital,
Cincinnati, Ohio.
*Practical Evaluation of Amenorrhea and Abnormal Uterine Bleeding
Hypothalamic-Pituitary Disorders*

Rogerio A. Lobo, M.D.
Professor of Obstetrics and Gynecology, University of
Southern California School of Medicine, Los Angeles; Chief,
Division of Reproductive Endocrinology and Infertility,
Department of Obstetrics and Gynecology, Los Angeles
County–University of Southern California Medical Center,
Los Angeles, California.
*Chronic Anovulation and Polycystic Ovary Syndrome: Treatment for
Infertility*

Laurence A. Mack, M.D.
Professor of Radiology, University of Washington School of
Medicine; Director of Ultrasound, University of Washington
Medical Center, Seattle, Washington.
*Imaging of the Reproductive Tract in Infertile Women:
Hysterosalpingography, Ultrasonography, and Magnetic Resonance
Imaging*

Alejandro Manzur, M.D.
Research Fellow in Reproductive Endocrinology and
Infertility, Center for Reproductive Health, University of
California, Irvine, Orange, California.
Gamete Intrafallopian Transfer

Sanford M. Markham, M.D.
Vice Chairman and Assistant Professor, Division of
Reproductive Endocrinology, Department of Obstetrics and
Gynecology; Attending Obstetrician-Gynecologist,
Georgetown University Medical Center, Washington, D.C.
Developmental Anomalies of the Reproductive Tract

Alvin M. Matsumoto, M.D.
Associate Professor, Department of Medicine, Division of
Gerontology and Geriatric Medicine, University of
Washington School of Medicine; Chief, Gerontology;
Associate Director, Gerontology Research, Education and
Clinical Center; Associate Chief of Staff for Geriatrics and
Extended Care; Veterans Administration Medical Center,
Seattle, Washington.
Pathophysiology of Male Infertility

R. Dale McClure, M.D., F.R.C.S.(C)
Associate Clinical Professor of Urology, University of
Washington School of Medicine; Director, Male Infertility
and Microsurgery, Virginia Mason Medical Center, Seattle,
Washington.
Male Infertility

Peter F. McComb, M.B., B.S., F.R.C.S.(C)
Professor, Department of Obstetrics and Gynaecology,
University of British Columbia; Active Staff, Vancouver
Hospital and Health Sciences Center, Vancouver, British
Columbia, Canada.
The Fallopian Tube: Pathophysiology

David R. Meldrum, M.D.
Clinical Professor, Department of Obstetrics and Gynecology,
University of California, Los Angeles, School of Medicine,
Los Angeles; Staff, Little Company Hospital and South Bay
Hospital, Redondo Beach, California.
*Assisted Reproductive Technology: Choice of Patient, Program, and
Procedure*

Arlene J. Morales, M.D.
Assistant Professor, University of California, San Diego,
School of Medicine; Attending Physician, University of
California, San Diego, Medical Center and Thornton
Hospital, San Diego, California.
Endometriosis: Surgical Therapy

Ana A. Murphy, M.D.
Associate Professor, Department of Obstetrics and
Gynecology, Emory University School of Medicine; Active
Staff, Emory University Hospital and Crawford Long
Hospital, Atlanta, Georgia.
Endometriosis: Surgical Therapy

Harris M. Nagler, M.D.
Professor of Urology, Albert Einstein College of Medicine of
Yeshiva University; Chairman, Department of Urology, Beth
Israel Medical Center, New York, New York.
Surgical Treatment of Male Infertility

David L. Olive, M.D.
Associate Professor and Chief, Reproductive Endocrinology
and Infertility, Department of Obstetrics and Gynecology,
Yale University School of Medicine; Director of Repro-
ductive Endocrinology, Yale–New Haven Hospital and
Hospital of Saint Raphael, New Haven, Connecticut.
Evaluating the Infertility Literature

James W. Overstreet, M.D.
Professor, Department of Obstetrics and Gynecology,
University of California, Davis, School of Medicine, Davis,
California.
Methods and Interpretation of Semen Analysis

Tim H. Parmley, M.D.
Professor of Obstetrics and Gynecology and Pathology,
University of Arkansas for Medical Sciences, Little Rock,
Arkansas.
The Endometrial Biopsy

Anthony J. Pearlstone, M.D.
Instructor, Clinical Obstetrics and Gynecology, Washington
University School of Medicine, St. Louis; Staff, Division of
Reproductive Endocrinology and Infertility, Department of
Obstetrics and Gynecology, St. Luke's Hospital, Chesterfield,
Missouri.
Tubal Microendoscopy: Salpingoscopy and Falloposcopy

Patrick Quinn, Ph.D.
Laboratory Director, San Fernando Valley Fertility and
Reproductive Center and Encino-Tarzana Regional Medical
Center, Tarzana, California.
Cryopreservation of Embryos and Oocytes

Robert W. Rebar, M.D.
Professor and Director, Department of Obstetrics and Gynecology, University of Cincinnati College of Medicine; Chief of Obstetrics and Gynecology, University Hospital, Cincinnati, Ohio.
The Normal Menstrual Cycle

John A. Rock, M.D.
Professor and Chairman, Department of Obstetrics and Gynecology, Emory University School of Medicine; Chief of Service, Emory University Hospital, Crawford W. Long Hospital, and Grady Memorial Hospital, Atlanta, Georgia.
Developmental Anomalies of the Reproductive Tract

Zev Rosenwaks, M.D.
The Revlon Distinguished Professor of Reproductive Medicine in Obstetrics and Gynecology; Professor, Obstetrics and Gynecology, Cornell University Medical College; Attending Obstetrician-Gynecologist and Director, The Center for Reproductive Medicine and Infertility, The New York Hospital–Cornell Medical Center, New York, New York.
In Vitro Fertilization

Vicken Sahakian, M.D.
Fellow, Reproductive Endocrinology, University of North Carolina at Chapel Hill, North Carolina.
Endometriosis: Pathophysiology and Presentation

Joseph S. Sanfilippo, M.D.
Professor of Obstetrics and Gynecology, University of Louisville School of Medicine; President, Medical Staff, Alliant Adult Health Services; Active Staff, University Hospital; and Chief of Gynecology, Kosair Childrens Hospital, Louisville, Kentucky.
Surgical Treatment of Diseases of the Ovary

Cecilia L. Schmidt-Sarosi, M.D.
Professor of Obstetrics and Gynecology and Director of Reproductive Endocrinology and Infertility, New York University School of Medicine; Director of Reproductive Endocrinology and Infertility, Tisch Hospital, New York, New York.
In Vitro Fertilization with Donor Oocytes

Lisa Barrie Schwartz, M.D.
Assistant Professor of Reproductive Endocrinology, New York University Medical Center, New York, New York.
Management of the Ectopic Pregnancy

James R. Scott, M.D.
Professor and Chairman, Department of Obstetrics and Gynecology, University of Utah Medical Center; Chief, Department of Obstetrics and Gynecology, University of Utah Hospital, Salt Lake City, Utah.
Evaluation and Treatment of Recurrent Miscarriages

F. N. Shamma, M.D.
Assistant Professor, Michigan State University College of Human Medicine, East Lansing; Staff, Ann Arbor Reproductive Medicine Associates, Ypsilanti; St. Joseph Hospital, Ann Arbor; Chelsea Hospital, Chelsea, Michigan.
Infertility: A Historical Perspective

Sander S. Shapiro, M.D.
Professor, Department of Obstetrics and Gynecology, University of Wisconsin Medical School; Director, Reproductive Endocrine Service, University Hospital, University of Wisconsin, Madison, Wisconsin.
Therapeutic Donor Insemination

Alfred Shtainer, M.D.
Clinical Instructor, Albert Einstein School of Medicine and Beth Israel Medical Center; Voluntary Attending Staff, Cabrini Medical Center, New York, New York.
Surgical Treatment of Male Infertility

Michael R. Soules, M.D.
Professor and Director, Division of Reproductive Endocrinology and Infertility, Department of Obstetrics and Gynecology, University of Washington School of Medicine; Director, Fertility and Endocrine Center, University of Washington Medical Center, Seattle, Washington.
Luteal Phase Deficiency: A Subtle Abnormality of Ovulation
Imaging of the Reproductive Tract in Infertile Women: Hysterosalpingography, Ultrasonography and Magnetic Resonance Imaging
Glossary of Terminology for Assisted Reproductive Technologies and Early Embryonic Development

Ronald C. Strickler, M.D., F.R.C.S.(C), M.B.A.
Virginia S. Lang Professor of Obstetrics and Gynecology, Washington University School of Medicine; Chief, Obstetrics and Gynecology, The Jewish Hospital of St. Louis; Staff, Barnes Hospital and Regional Medical Center, St. Louis, Missouri.
Factors Influencing Fertility

Eric S. Surrey, M.D.
Assistant Clinical Professor, Department of Obstetrics and Gynecology, University of California, Los Angeles, School of Medicine, Los Angeles; Medical Director, Center for Reproductive Medicine and Surgery, Beverly Hills, California.
Hyperstimulation Syndrome
Tubal Microendoscopy: Salpingoscopy and Falloposcopy
Extended Techniques in Assisted Reproductive Technologies

Ronald S. Swerdloff, M.D.
Professor of Medicine, University of California, Los Angeles, School of Medicine, Los Angeles; Chief, Division of Endocrinology, Harbor-UCLA Medical Center, Torrance, California.
Medical Treatment of Male Infertility

Patrick J. Taylor, M.D., F.R.C.S.(C), F.R.C.O.G.
Professor of Obstetrics and Gynecology, University of British Columbia, Faculty of Medicine; Chairman, Department of Obstetrics and Gynecology, St. Paul's Hospital, Vancouver, British Columbia, Canada.
Diagnostic Laparoscopy in Infertility

Samuel T. Thompson, M.D.
Fellow, Male Reproductive Medicine and Surgery Program, Scott Department of Urology, Baylor College of Medicine, Houston, Texas.
Sexual and Ejaculatory Dysfunction as a Cause of Male Infertility

Ronald L. Urry, M.D.
Professor of Surgery (Urology), Obstetrics and Gynecology, and Physiology, University of Utah School of Medicine, Salt Lake City, Utah.
Tests of Sperm Function

Rafael F. Valle, M.D.
Associate Professor, Department of Obstetrics and Gynecology, Northwestern University Medical School; Attending Physician, Prentice Women's Hospital and Maternity Center of Northwestern Memorial Hospital, Chicago, Illinois.
Diagnostic Hysteroscopy

Lucinda L. Veeck, M.L.T., D.Sc.(hon)
Lecturer, Department of Obstetrics and Gynecology, Eastern Virginia Medical School, Norfolk, Virginia.
The Gamete Laboratory: Design, Management, and Techniques

Christina Wang, M.D.
Professor of Medicine, University of California, Los Angeles, School of Medicine, Los Angeles; Director, Clinical Study Center, Harbor-UCLA Medical Center, Torrance, California.
Medical Treatment of Male Infertility

Gerson Weiss, M.D.
Professor and Chairman, Department of Obstetrics and Gynecology; Chief of Obstetrics and Gynecology, University Hospital, University of Medicine and Dentistry of New Jersey, Newark, New Jersey.
Management of Uterine Myomata

Craig A. Winkel, M.D.
Professor of Obstetrics and Gynecology, Jefferson Medical College; Staff, Thomas Jefferson University Hospital, Philadelphia, Pennsylvania.
Lesions Affecting the Uterine Cavity

Don P. Wolf, Ph.D.
Professor, Departments of Obstetrics and Gynecology, and Physiology; Director, Andrology/Embryology Laboratory, Oregon Health Sciences University, Portland, Oregon.
Sperm Cryopreservation

Preface

Nearly 20 years ago, four young physicians began their journey into the field of reproductive endocrinology. Under the guidance of some of this country's premier reproductive endocrinologists, these fledgling physicians began to acquire knowledge and experience in the diagnosis and management of couples with infertility. From Michigan, California, North Carolina, and the National Institutes of Health, they went off to begin their academic careers. Early in their careers, their research activities often brought them together at regional and national meetings where ideas and projects were shared and lifelong friendships were developed. Now, some two decades later, these same physicians have come together to attempt to construct a major work, a comprehensive textbook devoted to the diagnosis and treatment of infertility.

These four clinicians and teachers have witnessed and participated in the dramatic changes in the science and clinical management of infertility that have occurred in the past two decades. Assisted reproductive technologies, lasers, oocyte donation, operative laparoscopy and hysteroscopy, and in vitro sperm enhancement all have been developed and become common procedures during the last decade. Obstetricians/gynecologists, urologists, andrologists, laboratory scientists, psychologists, and other health care providers have joined together to form teams to care for infertile couples. Unfortunately, as scientific knowledge has grown and as clinical practices have changed, there has been no comprehensive resource for students, residents, fellows, and practitioners who wish to learn about infertility. Many books are devoted solely to individual topics, including those listed above. There are books that survey the recent developments or address new questions and controversies. However, no current book can stand alone as a complete resource for the student of reproductive medicine who wishes to consider all aspects of the scientific basis and clinical practice of infertility.

To this end, we have asked experts in the science and practice of infertility to help us create what we believe will become a valued resource for many. We have set out to discuss the modern practice of infertility in as concise, complete, and unbiased a manner as possible. Therefore, our contributors have provided practical information and solid science in a format that can be appreciated and understood by a broad range of readers. As a result of these efforts, this book is directed to all those who care for couples with impaired fertility. It includes pertinent discussions of topics that relate to infertility from the perspective of the patient as well as the physician, the psychologist, the social worker, the laboratory scientist, and the technician. It is designed to appeal to the medical student as well as to the resident, the fellow, and the seasoned practitioner. It is also our belief and our hope that this text can serve as a solid foundation for the future.

We, the editors, gratefully acknowledge the stimulation provided by our initial editor, Martin Wonsiewicz; the enthusiasm and nurturing of our final editor, Avé McCracken; and the staff at W.B. Saunders.

WILLIAM R. KEYE, JR., M.D.

R. JEFFREY CHANG, M.D.

ROBERT W. REBAR, M.D.

MICHAEL R. SOULES, M.D.

Contents

SECTION ONE

The Problems of Infertility

WILLIAM R. KEYE, Jr.

CHAPTER 1

Infertility: A Historical Perspective

F. N. SHAMMA and A. H. DeCHERNEY

Seeds spring from seeds, and beauty breedeth beauty;
Thou wast begot; to get it is thy duty.

Venus and Adonis 167
—SHAKESPEARE

Throughout history human societies were preoccupied by the process of procreation. They attempted to describe the details of this process through art and religion. However, the early civilizations were unable to grasp the details of such a complicated process and thus encompassed it with divine and magical interpretations. They were at a marked disadvantage. To link even the act of intercourse with pregnancy entailed an unbelievable and outstanding achievement in view of the long interval between such an act and birth or even the first sign of pregnancy. Such an achievement was facilitated by observations of animals and made easier when livestock were domesticated. The second difficulty in linking the acts of mating with giving birth was the inequality in number between such acts and pregnancy. Despite these difficulties, the association between intercourse and birth has been made since the early civilizations, including the Egyptians, Greeks, and Babylonians.

Despite the limitations of their observations of the process of procreation, early humans tried not only to understand but also to manipulate and change the outcome of procreation. Throughout this chapter a brief description of human understanding, interpretation, and manipulation of infertility throughout the ages is presented. It certainly falls short in elucidating the thinking and practices of every early civilization concerning one of the major aspects of maintaining survival and perpetuation of the human race. In view of the entwined nature between sexuality, morality, and reproduction, fertility played a pivotal role in almost all religions on this earth. Such association is presented in the context of the progression of the human thought throughout the history of mainly the near eastern and western world.

INFERTILITY AND THE EGYPTIANS

The first written understanding of infertility dates back to the Egyptians in the form of several papyri.[1] The translation of these remarkable documents was made possible by the discovery by Boussard in 1799 of the Rosetta Stone, which included hieroglyphic and Greek inscriptions. The Kahoun papyrus, dating back to 2200 to 1950 B.C., is the earliest known written document involving various aspects of infertility and fertility. It was deciphered by F. L. Griffith in 1893.[2, 3] Other papyri, known as the *Ebers,* the *Calsburg,* the *Edwin Smith,* and the *Berlin* papyri, dealt with various aspects of gynecologic disorders. Among all these papyri, the Kahoun, which was found in a fragmentary state and pieced together, and the Ebers, written by a scribe around 1550 B.C. and discovered in a very preserved state in a tomb at Thebes, are the most informative. The Ebers papyrus constituted a review of medical and gynecologic information as handed down from many earlier generations.[4] In all those writings, the mythical was merged with the factual. The papyri dealt with various aspects of diagnosis and treatment of infertility, the latter attributed to the woman in almost all instances.

The papyri described the use of various tampons and suppositories in the management of pelvic disorders. Uterine prolapse was also recognized and treated.

The methods suggested for testing fertility were clearly useless. Although they were ineffectual, they lacked any religious or magical incantations in most instances.

The diagnosis of infertility was based on the concept of continuity, or free passage, of the external genitalia and the vagina with the rest of the body. If the odor of garlic placed in the vagina was detected in a women's breath, this meant she was fertile; otherwise, barrenness was assumed.

Watermelon, which was pounded and mixed with the milk of a woman who had given birth to a male child, was administered orally to a woman suspected to be infertile. If she vomited, she was considered able to achieve pregnancy. If she simply eructated, she was considered infertile. Another diagnostic test involved the "growth-promoting effects" of the urine of women suspected to be sterile. If wheat and spelt were watered by the woman's urine and neither grew, the patient would not be able to bear children. If the wheat grew, the patient would bear a boy. If the spelt grew, she would have a girl. It is not clear as to the sex of the child if both grew! Another diagnostic method involved the use of hippopotamus dung. If the woman was fumigated intravaginally with this material and she then defecated, urinated, or passed flatus, she was considered fertile; if not, she was not thought to be able to bear a child.

The Egyptians described the use of various ointments, herbs, and fruit medications derived from the excrement of animals and humans in the therapy of various gynecologic disorders. Amenorrhea, described in the Edwin Smith papyrus, was attributed to a disease of the upper part of the vulva. Ointment consisting of oil, eye paint, and lepnent was applied to the vulva. In addition, the patient had to cook wanu grease and sweet beer and drink the mixture for several days. Menstrual irregularities were also discussed in the various papyri. To regulate menstrual periods, the patient was advised to use douches of wine and garlic. If these failed, honey and sweet beer were similarly used. As noted earlier, for the treatment of infertility natural substances such as beer, wine, oil, cow's milk, and dates were frequently recommended. However, the offensive nature of some of these substances is striking. The quantities of drugs used were sometimes specified exactly and other times left to the discretion of the practitioner.

The papyri also described various therapies for difficulties in lactation, leukorrhea, diseases of the breasts and the genitalia, induction of abortion, and enhancement of labor.[5, 6]

INFERTILITY AND BIBLICAL REFERENCES

". . . Be fruitful, and multiply, and replenish the earth and subdue it . . . ."[7] As noted in this biblical statement, fertility and procreation were the cornerstone of early Jewish life and beliefs. The inability to conceive was considered the ultimate curse, as quoted of the Lord, ". . . Write ye this man childless . . . ."[8] As a result, infertility was viewed as the punishment for wrongdoing, with the Lord being a source of fertility and infertility. The Lord was able to close the wombs of Sarah,[9] Michal,[10] and Hannah.[11] He also made others fertile, including Leah[12] and Rachel.[13] As such, therapy involved mostly prayers.

What was known about the process of procreation included understanding that conception is limited to a certain interval during the female menstrual cycle. The best time for conception, according to Jewish beliefs, was the 7 days after the clearing bath—the mikva—that the woman took after completion of her menses.[6]

Infertility, dominated by divine interpretations, was thought to have a significant impact on the personality of women. This was illustrated in the Bible.[14] Mehal was described as sweet, calm, and loving. However, she was the only wife of David, who could not bear children. As a result, her personality was depicted to change. She was the one that chastised David publicly during his celebration of the return of the Ark of the Covenant.

The medical system of the early Jewish people was not as elaborate as that of the Egyptians. The emphasis on sanitation took the place of elaborate recipes of diagnosis and therapy.

Fertility occupied a pivotal role in the life of these early cultures. Infertility as a problem not only was most often attributed to the female partner but was carried further in pressuring the wife to provide a suitable fertile partner. This was illustrated when Sarah, who was barren, told Abraham to have a child from her housemaid, Hagar. In fact, the inability to conceive was considered grounds for divorce.[7]

INFERTILITY IN THE BABYLONIAN-ASSYRIAN CIVILIZATION

Knowledge of Babylonian-Assyrian medicine is derived almost exclusively from clay tablets found in Nineveh in what was the palace of the Assyrian King Ashurbanapal (668 to 626 B.C.). The tablets included knowledge accumulated from the remote past. The study of infertility in particular and gynecology in general was primitive. All diseases of women were regarded as secondary to demons who controlled the female body. As a result of these beliefs, elaborate religious and magical rituals, including distasteful and noxious herbs and ointments, were used to "drive" the demons away and restore the well-being of the female patient.[1]

INFERTILITY AND THE GREEKS

The Greeks carried forward much of the knowledge of the Egyptians, elaborating various aspects of gynecologic disorders and infertility. Early Greek medicine, in addition to relying on the Egyptians' pharmacologic and therapeutic armamentarium, mixed in religious beliefs.

Hippocrates (460 to 370 B.C.) was the first author of various medical works dealing with Greek gynecology. It is unclear, however, if the six treatises that deal with reproduction—On Airs, Waters and Places; On Sterile Women; On Semen; On Development of the Child; On Diseases of Women; and On Disease of Young Girls—were actually written by Hippocrates. It is as likely that these and other Hippocratic treatises were written by various scholars of the time and attributed to Hippocrates. Regardless of the true author, these works reflect the medical views around 400 B.C. The works involved discussion of the process of procreation, the etiology of various disorders related to infertility, and diagnostic and therapeutic options.

According to Hippocrates, semen was considered as a concentrate from every part of the male body. This concentrate was thought to travel through conduits that finally made their way to the penis. Various injuries interrupting this flow were thought to result in male sterility. Castration resulted in sterility. This belief was not due, however, to knowledge of the importance of the testis in the production of semen but to the mistaken belief that sterility was due to the interruption of the semen channels that were believed to pass through the testis. It was also believed that women produced a similar "semen concentrate" that condensed from various parts of the body into the uterus. If pregnancy was to occur, the semen concentrate had to be retained in the uterus. If pregnancy did not occur, the female semen concentrate was discharged. Regular coitus was also deemed to be important. Conception, according to Hippocrates, resulted from the combination and retention of the male and female semen within the uterine cavity. Menstrual flow was regarded as necessary for fetal development and nutrition, being retained during pregnancy and otherwise discharged regularly. The necessity of entry of the penis into the uterine cavity was considered imperative for conception to occur. As such, the early Greeks believed that fertility was most likely to be achieved immediately after menses, when the cervix was dilated. This is similar to the Jewish beliefs. In addition, it is clear how malpositions of uterus, including prolapse and retroversion, cervical stenosis, and cervicitis, were thought to lead to infertility by interrupting the entry of the penis into the uterus.

Retention of blood in the uterine cavity was believed to occur in some cases of amenorrhea that resulted in sterility, because blood coagulated within the uterus created an obstacle to the entry of the semen. The Hippocratic treatises described also the role of obesity in subfertility. In *On Airs, Waters and Places,* the subfertility of the Scythian people was discussed. Obesity was considered of equal importance in men and women. In men, obesity caused a decrease in desire. In women, the uterus could not accommodate the semen with the mouth of the womb obstructed by fat. Hippocrates also noted that obesity was associated with scanty menses at longer intervals.

The Hippocratic writings also discussed diagnostic tests to evaluate infertility. These tests were in accordance with the Egyptians' beliefs pertaining to the connection between the vagina and the rest of the body. A woman was wrapped with a blanket and fumigated. If the scent appeared on her breath, infertility was dismissed.

Therapeutic options for the male included eating substantial foods, drinking strong wine, and avoiding hot baths. Such a reference to hot baths may be the earliest observation leading to the now-established association between scrotal temperature and spermatogenesis. As for women, cervical dilation as well as intrauterine douching was performed to enhance fertility.

In the *Prognostics* Hippocrates described pseudocyesis in accurate detail. He noted that these women had an increase in their abdominal girth with movement in it. They might complain of headache and some watery breast discharge. He also described cases of chronic breast discharge referring to galactorrhea. He noted that these women complained of headaches and at times some "dimness of sight." Such case reports suggest the occurrence of macroadenomas with optic nerve compression.[1, 7, 15]

Aristotle of Stagira (384 to 322 B.C.), one of the greatest Greek-Alexandrian philosophers, was also one of the greatest zoologists and naturalists of antiquity. Although not a physician, he discussed many issues relating to reproduction in his thesis, "Generation of Animals." Aristotle gave to medicine certain fundamentals such as comparative anatomy and embryology. He emphasized the role of obesity, and he reiterated that the best time for conception was immediately after the menses ceased. He considered that males and females both produce residues in terms of semen and menstrual fluid. He emphasized the role of intercourse and ejaculation in the process of procreation. Aristotle did not believe that orgasm in the female was necessary for conception. However, he considered it helpful, for he thought it would dilate the cervix.[16–18]

INFERTILITY AND THE ROMANS

Decreased fertility was an important issue in ancient Rome probably related to three main factors: lead poisoning, widespread promiscuous sexual practices by the various classes of society, and the use of hot baths. During that time, various aspects of medical and surgical gynecology flourished.

In the first century, Aulus Cornelius Celsus (27 B.C. to 50 A.D. [?]) was a physician and an author of a major medical textbook in Latin. The textbook was not considered seriously by the medical establishment of that time, and it soon was neglected. However, it resurfaced in the fifteenth century as a major reference of medicine. Celsus adhered to Hippocratic and Alexandrian principles of medicine. His book, *De Medicina,* described the condition of amenorrhea. He noted that some of the women with amenorrhea had headaches. He prescribed for amenorrhea a pessary composed of either cavnean figs and soda, crushed garlic seeds with myrrh, and sasine lily ointment or pulp of a wild cucumber mixed with human milk. He also suggested phlebotomy for others. Lion's fat softened with rose oil was recommended for sterility.[19]

Soranus, who lived in the second century, is considered the father of gynecology. The barest facts of his life are known. Born in Asia Minor, he was considered the greatest authority in the field of gynecology and obstetrics of ancient times. He lived in the times of Trajan (98 to 117 A.D.) and Hadrian (117 to 138 A.D.), practicing in both Alexandria and Rome. Soranus, who did not belong to either the "dogmatic school" relying on scientific investigations as the basis of medicine or the "empirical school" relying on experience, was a "methodist." Such a school of thought was based on observations of the disease process itself. Among his works, *Gynecology* was the major reference in the field for centuries. He is to be commended for his fight against superstitions and mysticism in medicine.

Soranus believed that failure of conception was secondary to improper timing of sexual intercourse. The best period for conception was believed to be at the end of menstruation because "the body is not oppressed by intoxication." He emphasized the role of an adequate desire for intercourse in enhancing conception. He also believed in moderation, advocating avoidance of excessive food or drink. Based on observation, he challenged some of the established ideas of his forebearers. Obesity, according to Soranus, was not always associated with infertility. He also discredited the well-established diagnostic test using fumigation and vaginal suppositories with subsequent detection of the odor in a woman's breath. He recognized the role of hot baths in causing widespread subfertility among the Romans of the time.[20]

INFERTILITY IN ARABIAN MEDICINE

Arabian medicine flourished during the period of the seventh to the twelfth century. This coincided with domination of the Arabic Moslem culture in the middle eastern part of the Mediterranean, the northern part of Africa, and the Iberian Peninsula, including all the major cities in Spain. The value of Arabian medicine lay not in its originality but in its more or less faithful preservation of the Greek culture during the darkest centuries of European civilization. During that period superb medical schools and hospitals were erected by the Umayyad and Abbassid Caliphs of Baghdad. The Arabian physicians depended on clinical observation and carried this method of medicine to commendable limits far beyond those of their Greek and Roman predecessors. While the Greeks argued philosophically about diseases, the Arabian physicians taught at the bedside. Their interest in herbs allowed the introduction of larger numbers of drugs, many of which are still used. They introduced a new specialty in medicine called *pharmacology.* However the Arabian contribution to gynecology is scattered throughout their large medical manuals, and the search for these data is tedious. This might have been part of the hesitancy of the Arabian physicians to invade the realm of female medicine owing to cultural beliefs. Rhazes (850 to 923 A.D.), one of the greatest Arabian physicians and an author of 130 medical treatises included in his book, *Al Kawi,* a resume of all previously published gynecologic practices. For sterility in obese women, regulation of the diet and exercise were recommended. However, tampons of honey and oil and venesection were also prescribed. For an imperforate hymen, he advised incision followed by daily coitus to keep the orifice open. Avicenna (980 to 1037 A.D.), an author of 20 medical treatises, also wrote *The Canon,* a systematic compendium of assimilated clinical knowledge and experience. It was one of the most popular medical books in the universities of the Middle Ages for more than five centuries. Concerning infertility, he believed that sterility is due to causes involving the male and female. Avicenna believed that if the semen floats in water, it is defective. He reasserted earlier views concerning vaginal fumigation for the diagnosis of female infertility.[1]

INFERTILITY IN THE MIDDLE AGES

Very few advances occurred in the study of infertility in the Middle Ages. The church played an important role in surrounding the process of conception and procreation with unsurmountable myths and beliefs not subject to investigation or interpretation. Infertility was viewed as a result of anatomic incompatibility between the size of the vagina and the penis.

INFERTILITY SINCE THE RENAISSANCE

Although many beliefs continued to be propagated, the sixteenth century marked the beginning of the age when scientific observations resulted in a marked contribution to the development of science in general and medicine in particular.

In 1538, Andreas Vesalius (1514 to 1564) contributed an accurate description of the entire female genital system, including ligaments, tubes, and blood supply. He was the first to use the words *pelvis* and *decidua.* One of his many distinguished pupils, Gabriele Fallopio of Modena (1523 to 1562),

made one of the most significant anatomic contributions to the study of female infertility. His name was permanently connected to that part of the genital system known as the fallopian tube, although the tube had been previously described by Soranus and Vesalius. He also named the clitoris, the vagina, and the placenta and attempted to describe their functions. Matteo Colombo (1516 to 1559), another pupil of Vesalius, not only used the term *labia* for the first time but also described the first case of congenital absence of the uterus and vagina. Reijnier de Graaf (1641 to 1673) in 1672 in his treatise "De Mulerum Organis Generationi Inservientibus," described the role played by the ovary and specifically the graafian follicle—which he assumed to be the female egg itself—in the process of conception. Marcello Malpighi (1628 to 1694) in 1668 named the *corpus luteum.* Despite these phenomenal anatomic advances, none of these men made suggestions pertaining to the process of fertilization.

During the eighteenth century, the scientific method was used to understand various concepts in the process of conception. The discovery of spermatozoa is credited to both Anton van Leeuwenhoek (1632 to 1723) and Johannes Ham (1651 to 1730). The former, noted for his work with the microscope, showed the existence of spermatozoa in the ejaculate and suggested their contribution in the process of fertilization.

Lazzaro Spallanzani of Scandiamo (1729 to 1799), an intellectual and a lawyer, was the first to describe the process of fertilization in his work, *Fecondazione Artificiale.* In 1780, he showed that conception was achieved as a result of contact between eggs and sperm. He succeeded in fertilizing frog eggs (detached from the aminal) by placing them in immediate contact with the secretions expressed from the testicles of the male. He dispelled the belief that semen produced vapors that resulted in the fertilization of eggs. In addition to being the first to describe artificial insemination in dogs, John Hunter (1728 to 1793) was the first to perform successful insemination in the human depositing the semen of a male with hypospadias in the vagina of a woman.[1, 21, 22]

The nineteenth and twentieth centuries carried gynecology from the realm of a descriptive anatomic practice to a scientific field capable of advancement. Marion Sims (1813 to 1883) is considered the father of American Gynecology. In his "Clinical Notes on Uterine Surgery with Special Reference to the Management of the Sterile Condition," he advocated almost wholly radical surgical procedures for the cure of infertility. Infertility was considered mainly a cervical factor to be treated with either dilation, with the use of a bougie, or excision of the entire cervix. He also emphasized manual and surgical corrections of malpositions of the uterus in the management of infertility. Sims played an important role in establishing the role of cervical secretions in affecting sperm survival in the genital tract. On that basis, Max Hühner (1873 to 1947), in his book *Sterility in the Male and Female,* introduced in 1913 the postcoital test as a reliable means to study male factor infertility.[23]

August Martin, a guest from Berlin at the fourteenth Annual Meeting of American Gynecologic Society in 1889, finally exonerated retroversion as a cause of infertility. He emphasized the role of the uterus, fallopian tubes, and ovaries in conception without overlooking the male's role in the process.[23]

The role of endocrinology in infertility first started with

the discovery of the presence, and then understanding some biologic effects, of ovarian and testicular secretions. The endocrine function of the testicles was first documented by Arnold Adolph Berthold (1803 to 1861). He transplanted testes into castrated roosters, avoiding the manifestations of hypoandrogenism.

Adolf Butenandt in 1931 was the first to extract androsterone, and Ernest Laqueur (1880 to 1947) in 1935 isolated testosterone. Robert Morris (1857 to 1945), Joseph Halban (1870 to 1937), and Herman Rubinstein (1871 to 1955) first documented the endocrine function of the ovaries by showing that ovarian tissue transplanted into castrated females prevented uterine atrophy. The function of the corpus luteum in the maintenance of early pregnancy was first ascertained by the early leutectomy experiments of Ludwig Fraenkel (1870 to 1953) and Vilhelm Magnus (1871 to 1929).[24]

After the development of reliable bioassays for the assessment of the biologic effects of ovarian and testicular extracts, the isolation of the various gonadal steroids progressed rapidly. Edward Doisy isolated estrone in 1929. George Corner and Willard Allen's work led to the discovery and isolation of progesterone in 1934 by several investigators simultaneously.[24] Subsequently, the pituitary hormones were discovered, and the control of the ovarian secretions by hypothalamic pituitary regulators was ascertained.[24] Bernhard Zondek (1891 to 1966) and Selmar Aschheim (1878 to 1965) demonstrated the presence of prolan A and B, now known as *follicle-stimulating hormone* and *luteinizing hormone*.[24]

The development of tubal surgery for pelvic adhesive disease was pioneered by Alwin Mackenrodt (1859 to 1925), who reported the first successful tubal surgeries in 1894. To evaluate tubal patency, Isidor Rubin (1883 to 1958) introduced in 1920 a test later named after him, using oxygen as a test medium. Rubin later used carbon dioxide as an insufflating medium because it was reabsorbed more rapidly, caused less discomfort, and avoided the danger of embolism. This test is considered by some authors as the most important achievement in the clinical evaluation of infertility in the first half of the twentieth century.[23]

The development of endoscopy has added to the progress in the evaluation and management of tuboperitoneal disease. Kelling in 1901 was the first to perform the procedure in a dog. Laparoscopy was later introduced to the United States during the 1920s. Progress in the field of infertility continued with the manipulation and augmentation of ovulation owing to the introduction of clomiphene citrate and human menopausal gonadotropins. These developments have culminated in the development of in vitro fertilization and various other assisted reproductive technologies. In 1978, the birth of Louise Brown (the first product of in vitro fertilization) in a small town in northwestern England was the culmination of a dream pioneered by Patrick Steptoe and Robert Edwards. With the advances in genetic biotechnology and molecular biology and physiology, the study and management of infertility will be carried to realms yet to be imagined.

REFERENCES

1. Ricci JV. The Gynealogy of Gynecology. Philadelphia: Blakiston, 1943.
2. Griffith FL. The Petrie (Kahoun) Papyrus. London, 1898.
3. Griffith FL. A Medical Papyrus from Egypt. Br Med J 1893; 1:1172–1174.
4. Bryan PC. The Papyrus Ebers. London, 1930.
5. Guttmacher AF. Past attitudes, especially towards female infertility. In: Fertility Disturbances in Men and Women. Basel: Karger, 1971:317–327.
6. DeCherney AH, Harris TC. The barren woman through history. In: Reproductive Failure. New York: Churchill Livingstone, 1986.
7. Genesis 1:28.
8. Jeremiah 22:30.
9. Genesis 16:2.
10. II Samuel 6:23.
11. I Samuel 1:6.
12. Genesis 24:31.
13. Genesis 30:22.
14. I Samuel 6:16.
15. Adams F (translator): The Genuine Works of Hippocrates. New York: William Wood, 1849.
16. Peck AL (translator). Aristotle. Generation of Animals. Cambridge, MA: Harvard University Press, 1943.
17. Cianfrani T. A short history of obstetrics and gynecology. Springfield, IL: Charles C Thomas, 1960.
18. McKay WJS. History of Gynaecology. London: Balliere, Tindall and Cox, 1901.
19. Spencer WG (translator). Celsus' De Medicina. Cambridge MA: Harvard University Press, 1938.
20. Temkin O (translator). Soranus' Gynecology. Baltimore: Johns Hopkins Press, 1956.
21. Effler LR. The Eponyms of Anatomy. Toledo, OH: McManus-Troup, 1935.
22. Speert H. Obstetric and Gynecologic Milestones: Essays in Eponymy. New York: Macmillan, 1958.
23. Speert H. Obstetrics and Gynecology in America: A History. Baltimore: Waverly Press, 1980.
24. Zander J. History of Human Reproduction Science. In: Human Reproduction: Current Status, Future Prospect. New York: Elsevier, 1988.

CHAPTER 2

Factors Influencing Fertility

RONALD C. STRICKLER

Fertility is defined in dictionaries as the state or quality of being capable of reproducing. Infertility in a couple is generally defined as the inability to achieve conception after 1 year of frequent, unprotected intercourse. This definition takes into account two factors, time and frequency of coitus, that influence the likelihood of becoming pregnant. This chapter addresses factors that modify the efficiency of establishing pregnancy, for it is against this background that the effectiveness of therapies is judged and a prognosis is provided for patients.

PREVALENCE OF INFERTILITY

Among married couples aged 15 to 44 years who lived in the United States and were not surgically sterile, 13.3% self-reported that they were infertile in the 1965 National Survey of Family Growth (NSFG) and 13.9% said they were infertile in the 1982 NSFG.[1] Although these summary statistics reveal no increase in the prevalence of couples who identify themselves as having been attempting pregnancy longer than 1 year, subsets within the data did change. From 1965 to 1982, the number of childless infertile couples doubled from 500,000 to 1 million and among 20- to 24-year-old couples, infertility increased from 3.6% to 10.6%. It is these statistics that have been the fodder of popular titles proclaiming an infertility epidemic. Certainly, the "sexual revolution," the small number of adoptable newborns consequent to the availability of abortion and societal acceptance of single parents, and the proclamation that infertility is a medical condition rather than a social shame contributed to the growing demand for infertility services. However, the major explanation for growing demand is population demographics: the first of the Baby Boom generation (the population born between 1946 and 1964) came of "reproductive age" during the years between the two surveys. This explanation is supported by analysis of the 1988 NSFG: 8450 women of all marital status, aged 15 to 44 years, were interviewed, and the rate of impaired fecundity remained unchanged from the earlier surveys.[2] Stratification of the 1988 data identified more infertile 25- to 44-year-old women because the Baby Boom genera-

tion, who have delayed childbearing into this age group, is now aged 27 to 45 years.

In 1982, the risk of infertility in black couples was 1.5 times that for white couples.[3] No data explain this observation, but speculation is that an increased rate of tubal disease arises from the socioeconomic forces that contribute to contraceptive choices, the prevalence of sexually transmitted diseases (STD), and the rate of infection after childbirth and abortion in blacks. These speculations are consistent with an examination of factors influencing a fertility decline in black women living in the Mississippi Delta between 1880 and 1930.[4] STD played the major role, facilitated by nutritional and other health problems, in causing infertility.

Among the married women in rural areas of nineteenth century Sweden, infertility and subfertility were found in 13.6%.[5] In a recent survey of pregnant Danish women, 13% reported longer than 1 year of delay in conception.[6] A postal questionnaire survey of 766 randomly selected 46- to 50-year-old women who had completed their families identified an overall prevalence of infertility of 14% in Aberdeen, Scotland.[7] Canadian statistics from the turn of the century show a stable prevalence of infertility.[8, 9] Thus, international summary data are accordant with the American observations and show no trend to increased infertility in developed countries (Table 2–1). In contrast, the prevalence rate of infertility in rural Nigeria increases from 12.9% for primary infertility to 54.1% for secondary infertility.[10] Puerperal sepsis is still a major public health problem for the developing world.

TIME TO CONCEPTION IN FERTILE WOMEN

Guttmacher[11] assessed the number of months of exposure before conception occurred in 5574 English and American women who all achieved pregnancy from 1946 to 1956 (Fig. 2–1). More than one half of these women were pregnant by 3 months; 72% and 85% had conceived within 6 and 12 months, respectively. During 1984 to 1987, Olsen[6] administered a survey questionnaire to all women at the 36th week of pregnancy in Odense and Aalborg, Denmark. In the

TABLE 2–1. Childlessness in Developed Countries

Country	Year(s)	Prevalence (%)
Canada	1896–1901*	14.6
	1911–1916	14
	1926–1931	8.4
	1951–1956	15.4
	1961†	13.5
	1971	16.3
	1981	21.5
Denmark	1984–1987‡	13
Scotland	1945–1988*	14
Sweden	1810–1870*	13.6
United States	1965‡	13.3
	1982	13.9
	1988	8.4

*Lifetime observation in a population sample.
†Census data: may include women currently electing childless lifestyle.
‡Prevalence data based on population sample.

11,888 responses, 5% of pregnancies occurred despite contraception; 73% of women conceived within 6 months, and 82% within 1 year. Women who conceive by insemination with donor sperm provide another measure of human fecundity: the women have generally been screened or treated for factors that diminish fertility and the semen samples, selected from healthy young males, have normal parameters. In women treated using fresh donated sperm between 1971 and 1974 in St. Louis, 63% of conceptions were achieved by 3 months, and 86% of the women were pregnant by 6 months (see Fig. 2–1).[12] No conceptions occurred after 12 treatment cycles in the small number of women who continued treatment; patients were discouraged by the continuing expense and declined further participation in the program. A decade later, 47% of women in New England who achieved pregnancy after donor insemination did so within three cycles.[13] A third study population to gauge time to conception was composed of women who discontinued contraception. Tietze[14] observed 611 women, most of whom had borne a child and were using contraception for family spacing, after they had an intrauterine contraceptive device removed. The different populations summarized in Figure 2–1 have almost identical fecundability. Thus, the 1-year period inherent in

the definition of infertility is soundly based on observations that 85% of women will have achieved conception within this time. There has been no change in the efficiency of reproduction over two generations.

COITAL FREQUENCY

MacLeod and Gold's 1953 report[15] is the only study that directly addressed a correlation between coital frequency and fertility. The rate of conception within 6 months for all 428 couples was 48%, a slower rate than shown in Figure 2–1. This likely reflects data that were not corrected for age of the partners or length of marriage, important variables addressed later in this chapter. Nonetheless, the trend shown in Table 2–2 indicates that intercourse more than three times per week gives the best efficiency for conception. These data are consistent with a window of conception that opens 3 days before ovulation and closes the day following ovulation.[12, 16] Equally, sperm concentration and ejaculate volume decrease with daily emission.[17] Finally, it is generally stated that human ova can be fertilized in the 12 to 24 hours after release, and sperm in the fallopian tube retain the capacity to fertilize an egg for 48 hours.[18] Coital frequency contributes to reproductive efficiency and is an appropriate part of the infertility definition. However, "frequent" needs to be quantified: intercourse every other day provides excellent efficiency for conception.

AGE OF WOMAN

The concept that fertility decreases as a woman ages is not new. In nineteenth century Sweden, fecundity of 35- to 39-year-old women was 42% less than fecundity of 20- to 24-year-old women.[5] Guttmacher[11] made a parallel observation during the 1950s in the United States: the median time for conception nearly doubled in the 20-year interval between ages 15 to 24 and 35 to 44. Among 470 Canadian women, mean age (±SE) 30.1 (±0.2) years, with unexplained infertility longer than 3 years, variables to explain infertility were examined using a proportional hazards analysis. Each addi-

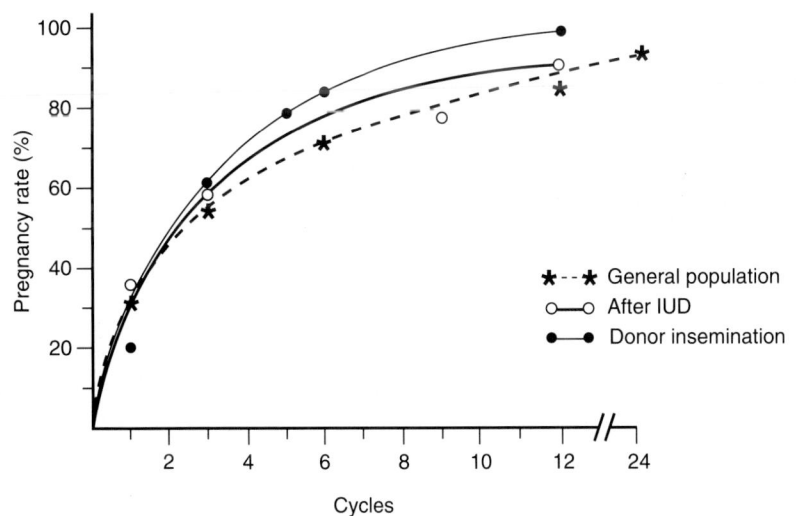

FIGURE 2–1. Time to pregnancy in three study groups. The near identity of the curves argues that these data fairly represent the fecundity of a normal population. (Data on *general population* from Guttmacher AF. Factors affecting normal expectancy of conception. JAMA 1956;161:855–860; *population after discontinuing intrauterine device contraception* from Tietze C. Fertility after discontinuation of intrauterine and oral contraception. Int J Fertil 1968;13:385–389; and *therapeutic donor insemination population* from Strickler RC, Keller DW, Warren JC. Artificial insemination with fresh donor semen. N Engl J Med 1975;293:848–853.)

tional year in age of the female partner reduced the outlook for conception by 9%.[19] Inherent in these and many other observations are possible biases: as examples, couples tend to be of similar age; coital frequency decreases with years of marriage; and systemic illness is more common with aging.

Donor insemination can control for variables such as frequency and timing of exposure and the age of partner. The Federation des Centres d'Etude et de Conservation du Sperme Humain (CECOS) reported results in 2193 nulliparous French women presumed normally fecund on the basis of history, physical examination, hysterosalpingography, ovulatory basal temperature records, and cervical mucus examination, and treated with donor insemination.[20] The cumulative success rates over 12 cycles, stratified in 5-year groups, unequivocally documented the statistically significant decline in female fertility with age (Fig. 2–2). Data from 751 donor insemination cycles in 210 women with a negative infertility evaluation were projected by life table analysis.[21] The mean ($\pm$SD) monthly fecundability was 0.19 ($\pm$0.13) for women younger than 35 years and 0.1 ($\pm$0.12) for women 35 years and older. A woman's 35th birthday marks a watershed that irreversibly lowers the effectiveness of reproduction in her life. A generation of women have accepted the increased probability of chromosomal anomalies in children conceived after age 35 years. Environmental assaults on the fixed complement of ova arrested in the first meiotic division is a popular explanation. Perhaps infertility and chromosomal nondysjunction are merely different faces of the same fall-off in reproduction with age.

AGE OF MAN

There are no data that isolate the role of advancing age in the male partner. MacLeod and Gold's observations[15] from the 1950s showed that 75% of men younger than 25 years of age impregnated their partners within six cycles, whereas only 25% of men older than 35 years of age had achieved a conception within six cycles. Because the age of the female partner is such a strong variable that was uncontrolled, these widely cited data are unreliable.

In vitro fertilization using donor eggs from women younger than 30 years of age and sperm from "older" husbands will answer whether there is a decline in male fertility with age.

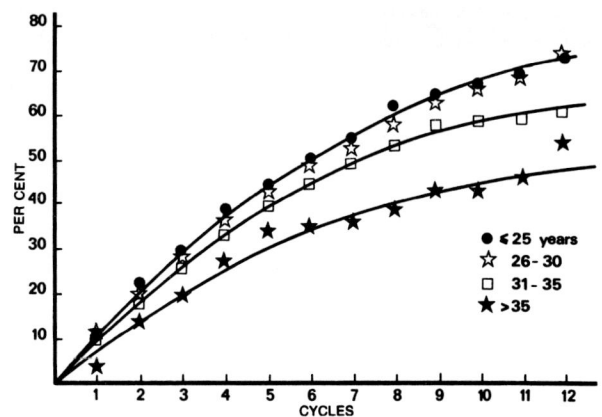

FIGURE 2–2. Effect of age on the theoretical cumulative pregnancy rate in a donor insemination program. Because the curves of the two youngest groups were similar, they are represented by a single tracing. These curves differ significantly from those of the two older groups ($P < 0.03$ for those 30 to 35 and $P < 0.001$ for those older than 35 years). (Reprinted with permission from the *New England Journal of Medicine*, 306:404–406, 1982.)

DURATION OF INFERTILITY

To clarify the contributions of clinical factors to the prognosis of unexplained infertility, Collins and Rowe[19] isolated duration of infertility, age of the female partner, and other factors using proportional hazards analysis. The 470 unexplained infertile patients were 22% of couples registered in 12 Canadian infertility clinics between 1984 and 1987. The duration of infertility was a significant independent predictor of prognosis: the expected pregnancy rate was lowered by 2% for each month of infertility beyond 40 $\pm$ 1.2 (mean $\pm$ SE) months, which was the average duration of infertility in all couples.

TIME TO PREGNANCY IN INFERTILE COUPLES

Katayama and associates[22] analyzed data from 636 patients with primary infertility seen at Johns Hopkins Hospital. Reasoning that pregnancy rate is a function of the time for which patients were followed, they calculated a pregnancy rate that assumed infinite duration of observation. The cumulative pregnancy rate for all patients was 64% after 6 years with no appreciable increase thereafter. Because the effectiveness of therapy is not uniform for all causes of infertility, the Baltimore group stratified 459 patients with only one diagnosis and projected the infinite followup pregnancy rate (Table 2–3).

Much of the infertility literature is anecdotal because there are no control couples for comparison. The importance of a control population is clear from the work of Collins and coworkers,[23] who followed 1145 couples for as long as 7 years to determine the frequency of pregnancy occurring independent of treatment. Pregnancy, which occurred in 191 untreated couples, in couples more than 3 months after the last medical treatment, and more than 12 months after adnexal surgery, was considered treatment independent. They accounted for 61% of all pregnancies; for 44% of the women with ovulation defects; for 61% of tubal problems, male fac-

TABLE 2–2. Conception as a Function of Coital Frequency	
Weekly Frequency of Coitus	**Conception Within 6 Months (%)**
<1	17
1–2	32
2–3	46
3–4	51
>4	83

From MacLeod J, Gold RZ. The male factor in fertility and infertility: VI. Semen quality and certain other factors in relation to ease of conception. Fertil Steril 1953; 44:10–33. Reproduced with permission of the publisher, The American Fertility Society.

	Patients		Pregnancy Rate	
Factor	*Number*	*Percentage*	*Observed*	*At Infinity*
Endometriosis	114	25	31	52
Male factor	82	18	38	74
Anovulation I*	61	13	44	79
Anovulation II†	9	2	67	83
Tubal factor	55	12	26	48
Luteal phase defect	33	7	46	58
Cervical factor	23	5	26	45
Uterine factor	9	2	33	38
Ovarian factor	6	1	33	33
Unspecified	67	15	55	70

TABLE 2–3. Expectation of Pregnancy in 459 Women with Primary Infertility

*Hypothalamic-pituitary; polycystic ovary syndrome; psychosis.
†Thyroid or adrenal dysfunction; weight related.
Adapted from Katayama KP, Ju K-S, Manuel M, et al. Computer analysis of etiology and pregnancy rate in 636 cases of primary infertility. Am J Obstet Gynecol 1979; 135:207–214.

tors, and endometriosis; and for 96% of conceptions in couples with cervical factor and unexplained infertility. The pregnancy efficiency over a 48-month period was identical for the 171 couples with treatment-related and the 266 couples with treatment-independent pregnancies. These unique Canadian data emphasize the importance of a control population to judge the benefits, if any, of infertility therapies.

There is remarkable similarity in the cumulative pregnancy rate projected by the Baltimore group and that observed by the Canadian investigators. Moreover, comparison of the cumulative pregnancy curves for normal populations and infertile couples show that they have the same shape and only a different scale on the horizontal time axis. This argues that treatments do not resolve infertility; rather, at best, management changes the efficiency curve such that patients conceive in a shorter time. Helping couples to achieve their life reproductive goals in a time-acceptable way is a valuable medical service. It is, however, a different service from curing infertility. This difference should cause infertility physicians to reconsider, rather than take pride in, their therapies and success rates. The treatment-independent pregnancy rate observed by Collins and coworkers[23] is an even more sobering reason for infertility physicians to challenge beliefs in their treatments and outcomes: more controlled, prospective studies must be demanded.

ANALYSIS OF INFERTILITY DATA

The infertility literature is rich with case reports and uncontrolled observations. Understanding will be greatly enhanced by studies that delineate pregnancy rates that are disease specific and controlled for treatment-related and treatment-independent conceptions. Next, those rates need to be adjusted for at least the age of the female partner and perhaps other variables that may confound the efficiency of becoming pregnant. Third, there is need for a standard measure of infertility. Adoption of one standard statistic that incorporates duration of infertility and length of followup will facilitate comparison among treatments and across studies.

Figure 2–1 contains fertility rates described in two different ways. The general population data are a raw fertility rate: the number of conceptions divided by the number of cou-

ples. The data do not include the cycles in which a couple may have had "exposure" before declaring their intention to conceive. The curve has not reached a plateau and therefore describes childlessness so far rather than a true prevalence of infertility. The donor insemination curve reflects only women who conceived; thus, 100% of the population achieve pregnancy at 12 months. In the study, only 57% of all women treated and only 77% of those undergoing six cycles of therapy conceived. All the data in Figure 2–1 are enriched in the early cycles by women who conceive quickly and underrepresent the total effectiveness of therapy or the passage of time by lumping dropouts with nonresponders.

Figure 2–2 is a theoretical cumulative success rate calculated after 12 cycles. A cumulative success rate uses life table analysis to assume life-long followup. The curves are "theoretical" because an assumption made is that no patient would abandon or be lost from treatment. Data such as shown in Table 2–3 were used by Katayama and colleagues[22] to develop a model that assumed infinite followup of patients (Fig. 2–3A). They also showed that cumulative rates could be represented as expected outcomes (Fig. 2–3B).

Keller and associates[24] introduced the plotting of expectancy data on a semilogarithmic graph (ordinate, logarithm of the percentage of patients remaining nonpregnant; abscissa, time on a linear scale). This presentation converts hyperbolic-curved data, as shown in Figure 2–3B, to a linear trend that is intuitive for physician and patient (Figure 2–4A). A linear projection clearly shows the concept of a half-time. Over five cycles, one half of nulligravid couples achieve pregnancy. Of the remaining 50%, half of them conceive during the next five cycles and so forth. When treatment data are represented this way, the likelihood for conception is equally obvious. For example, among couples whose primary infertility was 2 years or longer and unexplained by ovulation, luteal phase, sperm survival in cervical mucus, semen analysis, and endoscopy studies, a physician should expect one half to achieve treatment-independent pregnancy during the subsequent 6 years (Fig. 2–4B).

There is no standard to measure infertility. We infertility physicians cannot tell a couple how much a given diagnosis contributes to pregnancy delay. We do not know a prognosis, quantified as likelihood for conception, for our treatments. Clinicians and patients will revel when we have data, analyzed in an easy-to-understand form, that answers two ques-

Primary Infertility
ALL FACTORS

$$E = R_1 + \sum_{i=1}^{\infty} R_{i+1} \prod_{j=1}^{i} (1-R_j)$$

A

CUMULATIVE RATE OF PREGNANCY (%)

MONTHS AFTER TREATMENT

ALL FACTORS

B

EXPECTANCY OF PREGNANCY (%)

MONTHS AFTER TREATMENT

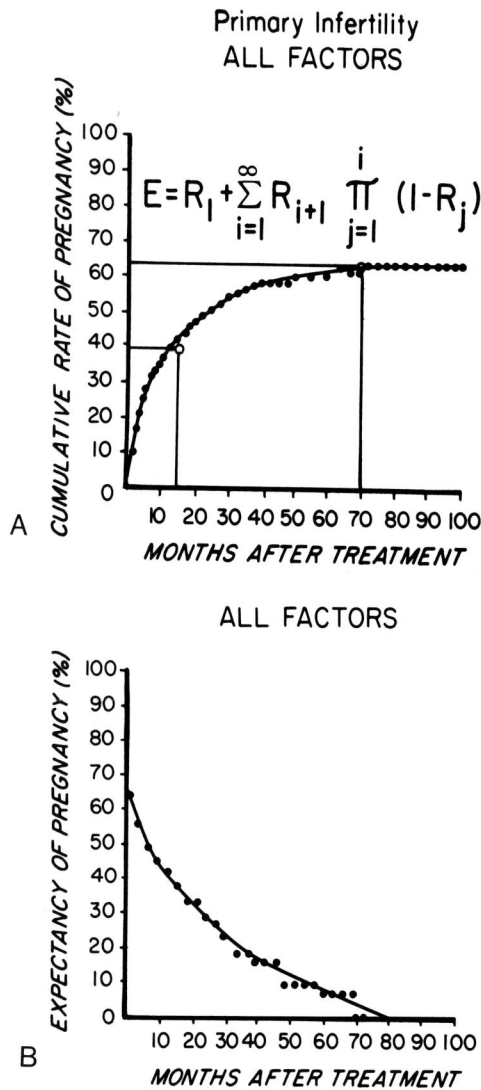

FIGURE 2–3. *A,* Cumulative rate of pregnancy over months after treatment for 636 patients with primary infertility. The formula calculates E, the ultimate rate of pregnancy, in I, the infinite month of followup. The graphed results from the formula calculation predict that when couples have not conceived during 70 months of treatment that corrects any recognized causes of infertility, pregnancy will not occur. *B,* Expectancy of pregnancy (y axis) for patients who did not conceive after X months, based on the assumption of infinite followup as shown in *A.* As an example, when a patient has passed 20 months from beginning treatment without pregnancy, there remains a 35% probability that conception will occur in the next 50 months. After 70 months, there is zero expectancy for pregnancy. (*A* and *B* from Katayama KP, Ju K-S, Manuel M, et al. Computer analysis of etiology and pregnancy rate in 636 cases of primary infertility. Am J Obstet Gynecol 1979;135:207–214.)

tions: What is the likelihood this couple can conceive? When should this couple focus on other treatments or options?

CIGARETTE SMOKING

An extensive literature, which was recently reviewed in a multiauthor volume,[25] has associated cigarette smoking with impaired fertility, ectopic pregnancy, spontaneous abortion, earlier age of menopause, poorer pregnancy outcomes, and cervical cancer. Smoke from one cigarette increases the tone and amplitude of peristalsis in fallopian tubes of humans and rhesus monkeys. Cigarette smoke suppresses the function of both the humoral and immune systems and causes the destruction of rodent oocytes-follicles leading to an earlier loss of reproductive function. Effects of nicotine on ovulation mechanisms and granulosa cell function have been shown in vitro. The question of which mechanisms contribute to the strong association between smoking and decreased fecundity and fertility in women remains unclear.

In a retrospective study of 678 pregnant women, there was a dose-response relationship to infertility in those women who smoked fewer than 20 cigarettes per day compared to more than one-pack-a-day smokers.[26] Baird and Wilcox[26] concluded that women who smoked cigarettes were 3.4 times more likely to experience longer than a 1-year delay in conception compared with nonsmokers (Fig. 2–5). Decreased fertility with increased numbers of cigarettes smoked each day was observed in the Oxford Family Planning Association Study.[27] Table 2–4 summarizes the Oxford data and shows that in each year of attempts for pregnancy, a larger percentage of women who smoke more than 15 cigarettes per day are infertile. Interviews at 20 weeks' gestation of 2198 women living in Tampere, Finland, showed a dose dependence for delay of conception in cigarette smokers.[28] The odds ratio of conception delay in these soon-to-be mothers, if they were smokers, was 1.5 (nonsmokers versus smokers, 95% confidence limits, 1.3 to 1.8). The odds ratio for a conception delay when fathers were smokers was 1.3 (95% confidence interval, 1.2 to 1.4). This observation suggests that there may be a fertility-related effect of side-stream and second-hand smoke. Tubal factor infertility has been linked to cigarette smoking.[29] Cigarette smoking is a predictor for chlamydial isolation from cervical culture, and animal studies show nicotine effects on tubal motility.[30] It is therefore no surprise that cigarette smoking is associated with a relative risk of 3.1 for ectopic pregnancy compared with control pregnant women.

Cigarette smoking decreases the weight of newborns, an effect that supports the transplacental passage of chemicals such as carbon monoxide to the fetus. Weinberg and coworkers[31] sought a relation between exposure in utero to cigarette smoke inhaled by the mother and fecundability when the child becomes an adult in data from a prospective study of 221 offspring stopping oral contraceptives. Prenatal exposure to mother's smoke reduced fecundability by one half (95% confidence limits, 0.4 to 0.8) after adjustment for age, coital

TABLE 2–4. Smoking and the Percentage of Women Remaining Undelivered

Cigarettes (no./d)	Months Attempting Conception			
	12	24	48	60
Never smoked	41.0	12.5	6.2	5.4
Ex-smoker	41.3	12.8	6.3	5.5
1–5	41.1	12.6	6.2	5.4
6–10	42.3	13.5	6.8	6.0
11–15	43.8	14.5	7.5	6.6
16–20	50.4	20.0	11.5	10.4
>20	50.9	20.5	11.9	10.7

From Howe G, Westhoff C, Vessey M, Yeate D. Effects of age, cigarette smoking, and other factors on fertility: findings in a large prospective study. Br Med J 1985; 290:1697–1700.

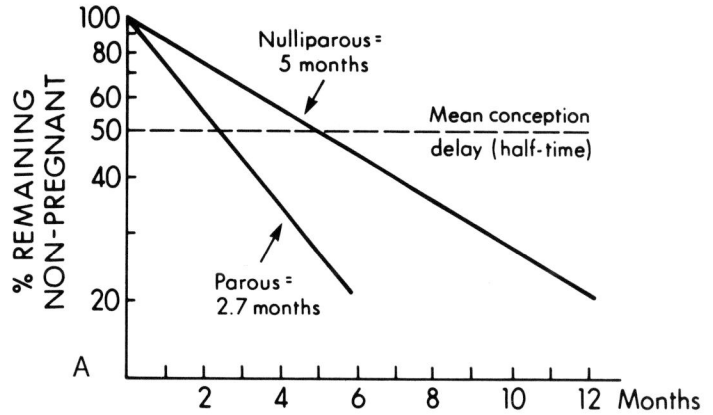

FIGURE 2–4. *A*, Expectancy for pregnancy over months in an unse-lected population. Half of the nulliparous patients achieve pregnancy within the first 5 months. In each subsequent 5-month interval, half of those who were not pregnant at the onset of that period will achieve pregnancy. In parous patients, the expected half-time to pregnancy is 2.7 months. Thus, if we begin with 100 parous (secondary infertility) women, 50 couples are pregnant within 3 months; 25, half of the remainder, conceive in the next 3 months, and so forth. After 12 months, which is four half-times, 93 patients have conceived. *B*, Ex-pectancy for pregnancy over years in a population with 2 years of infertility and a negative workup. The half-time to pregnancy is 6 years for the nulligravid couples whose primary infertility is unexplained. For couples who have previously had a term pregnancy and whose current secondary infertility is unexplained, half become pregnant in 2.5 years. The logarithm of the percentage of patients remaining non-pregnant is the ordinate, and time is a linear scale on the abscissa. (*A* and *B* from Keller DW, Strickler RC, Warren JC. Clinical Infertility. Norwalk, CT: Appleton-Century-Crofts, 1984.)

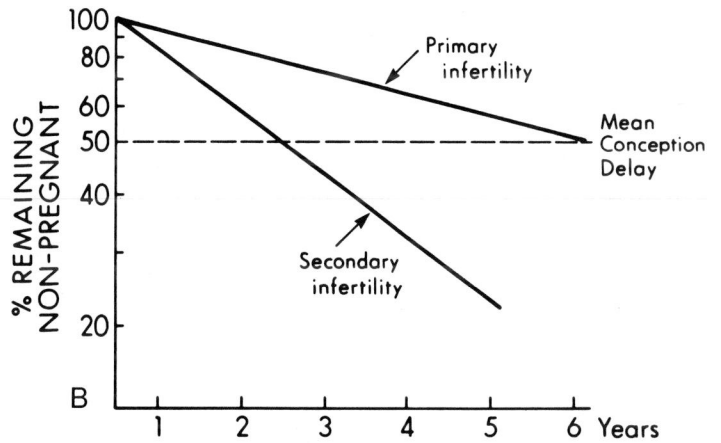

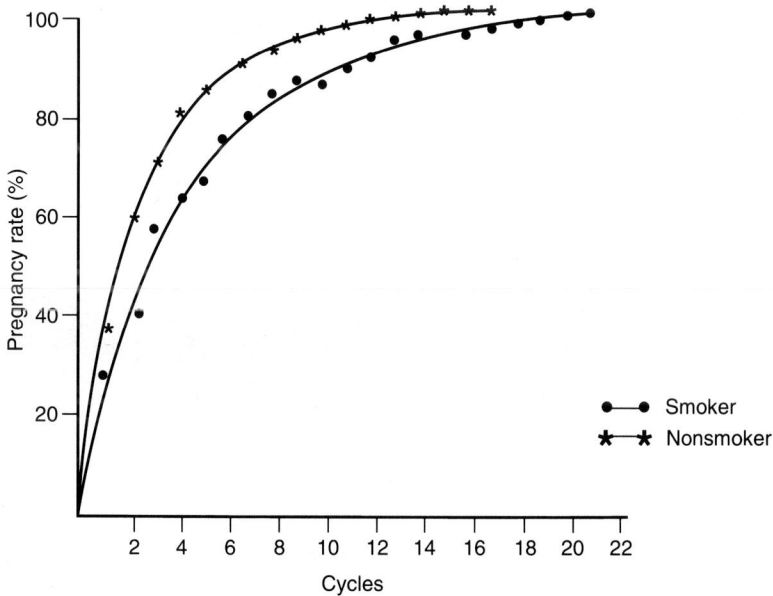

FIGURE 2–5. Time to conception for smokers and non-smokers. Cigarette smokers take approximately one third longer than do nonsmokers to achieve pregnancy. (Adapted from Baird DD, Wilcox AJ. Cigarette smoking associated with delayed conception. JAMA 1985;253:2979–2983. Copyright 1985, American Medical Association.)

frequency, current smoking, and passive smoke exposure as a child.

A Canadian study of 362 consecutive couples undergoing in vitro fertilization treatment in early 1991 included 53 women who continued smoking.[32] Smoking at the time of treatment was associated with retardation of embryo cleavage and a reduced likelihood, 0.75 (95% confidence interval, 0.54 to 1.0), of transferring four or more embryos compared with nonsmokers. Women who smoked 15 cigarettes or more per day were 63% as likely to receive four or more embryos as a nonsmoker. The ongoing pregnancy rate in nonsmokers, 9.7%, was marginally different from a 6.5% rate in current smokers ($P = 0.47$).

There has been no association between cigarette smoking, impairment of the semen profile, or altered male fertility.[26] However, in a study of 546 men seen at the University of North Carolina infertility clinic between 1978 and 1982, those who drank more than 4 cups of coffee per day and smoked more than 20 cigarettes per day had a lower percentage of motile sperm. Coffee intake, alcohol consumption, and cigarette smoking, as independent variables, did not impact on sperm motility.[33] Makler and colleagues[34] streamed cigarette smoke into a sealed chamber containing samples of washed sperm. They observed a dose-response relationship between the amount of smoke, a decline in motility of sperm, and the time to immobilization of sperm. Thus, crude cigarette smoke, in vitro, is harmful to sperm motility and survival.

Young women are the only group of cigarette smokers whose number is growing. Cardiovascular risk, osteoporosis, and cancer, known risks of cigarette use, seem to be meaningless diseases of old people when one is young and healthy. Perhaps stressing the association of tobacco, tubal damage, and impaired fertility will give some young couples a reason, which has meaning today, to stop smoking. Unfortunately, youth is an age when we believe that we are invincible and "it" only happens to someone else.

There is little information on infertility in prior cigarette smokers. The reversal of cardiovascular risk and the reduced likelihood for lung cancer in reformed smokers could be viewed as a hopeful sign that reproductive system effects also can recover. However, tubal cilia impaired by cigarette smoke toxins and further damaged by opportunistic infection may not regenerate. Oocytes that are destroyed by cigarette smoke cannot be replaced. Until the important mechanisms that impair fertility are clear, the prognosis after discontinuing smoking cannot be deduced.

EXERCISE, DIET, AND WEIGHT CHANGE

Exercise physiology and the impact of exercise on reproductive function are subjects of a multiauthor review.[35] Exercise has become associated with menstrual irregularity. Usable questionnaire data was provided by 330 of the 1841 women who entered the New York City Marathon in 1979. The mean age was 32.1 years, with a range of 16 to 53 years.[36] Regular menses prior to training were reported by 80% of women and by 77% of women during training. Only 10% of responders claimed an inability to conceive, but the duration of attempting pregnancy was not questioned.

Schwartz and associates[37] emphasized that amenorrheic runners were more likely to have had irregular menses before exercise, to have lost more weight since beginning exercise, and to be leaner and lighter than other runners who achieve comparable levels of training without menstrual dysfunction (Fig. 2–6). Bullen and coworkers[38] prospectively studied 28 untrained college women who began a program of 3½ hours of moderate-intensity sports each day. Only 5 of 53 cycles were normal during the exercise period, and these occurred in four subjects, three of whom maintained their weight. Thus, it appears that weight change rather than exercise alone is required for menstrual change in most women. In a subsequent report,[39] 20 cycles, out of 53 total, showed a luteal phase defect defined as a reduced total area under the curve of measured urinary progesterone. The mechanisms that lead to these diet-and-exercise-associated changes are unknown, but most speculation is toward a neuroendocrine rather than an ovarian dysfunction.

The association between exercise and menstrual irregularity has prompted comment that exercise could be a contributor to infertility. No study has provided data to support such speculation. Similarly, studies in men have observed changes in semen parameters that are the grist of speculation, but no data support a link between exercise and male infertility.[40]

Deficiency of vitamin B_{12}[41] and pernicious anemia in a woman with vitiligo[42] have been separately linked to infertility. Bringer and colleagues[43] implicated a vegetarian low-calorie diet with short luteal phase, and associated slimness with disturbed pulsatile release of gonadotropins. Hypercarotinemia produces a sallow skin and "golden ovaries," which were endoscopically diagnosed in women with infertility.[44]

Ovulation dysfunction is more common in obese women, especially those who put on weight rapidly. Associated hormonal changes include reduced sex hormone-binding globulin, increased ovarian and adrenal androgen production, increased aromatization of androgens to estrogens, altered pulsatile secretion of gonadotropins, and hyperinsulinemia due to insulin resistance.[43] The relative importance of these factors in the genesis of anovulation and the reduced efficiency of ovulation-promoting therapies is unknown. Green and associates[45] used a case control design in women with ovulatory dysfunction. In 204 nulligravid women, body weight for height 85% or less than the Metropolitan Life Insurance table ideal was associated with a 4.7-fold increased risk of infertility (95% confidence interval, 1.5 to 14.7). Nulligravid women who were 120% or more above their ideal weight had a relative risk for ovulatory dysfunction–infertility of 2.1 (95% confidence interval, 1.0 to 4.3). These observations blend with two reports from Bates and coworkers[46, 47]: fertility was restored to 73% of women 15% or more below ideal body weight who regained pounds, and to 10 of 13 obese women who lost more than 15% of their body weight.

Although there are data to support a window of weight for height that maximizes the efficiency of reproduction (Fig. 2–7), the application of these observations to individual patients is difficult. The birth rate in malnourished, third world populations and the uninhibited fertility of overweight, fast food–fed Americans argue that weight is a cofactor rather than a cause of infertility. The mechanisms that link exercise, weight, and menstrual function are an enigma.

WEIGHT LOSS AFTER ONSET OF RUNNING

POUNDS

24   34   12
MDR   LDR   AR

A

PAST CYCLE IRREGULARITY

PERCENT

15   24   34   11
NC   MDR   LDR   AR

B

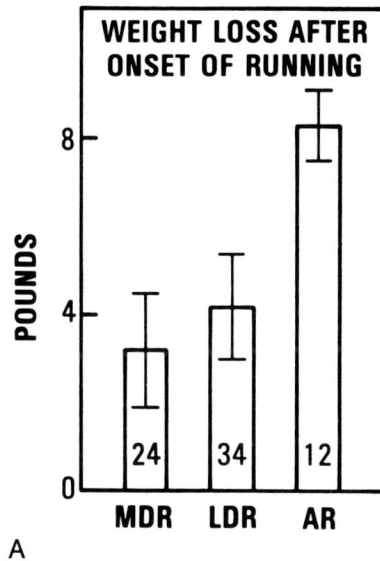

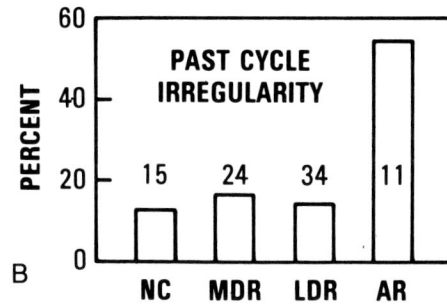

FIGURE 2–6. *A,* Mean (± SE) weight loss after the onset of running. *B,* Percentage of patients who reported a history of menstrual cycle irregularity. NC, nonrunning, eumenorrheic control subjects. MDR, eumenorrheic middle distance runners (5 to 30 miles per week). LDR, eumenorrheic long distance runners (>30 miles per week). AR, amenorrheic runners. (*A* and *B* from Schwartz B, Cumming DC, Riordan E, et al. Exercise-associated amenorrhea: a distinct entity? Am J Obstet Gynecol 1981;141:662–670.)

PSYCHOEMOTIONAL FACTORS
(see also Chapter 4)

Stress has become such a part of our culture that our vocabulary is almost casual in describing home, family, occupation, and recreation as contributors to or treatment for the distress in our lives. Advertising bombards us with the headache pain or the gastrointestinal irritability caused by stress. Women are told that stress stops menses or contributes to irregular bleeding. It is therefore logical that couples and physicians assume that stress can contribute to infertility. Anecdotes of couples who "relaxed," "adopted," or "came to grips with their emotions" and soon thereafter became pregnant are common. However, current data does not support a causal relationship between emotion and infertility.

Paulson and colleagues[48] compared 50 women with infertility and 50 control women who were of similar age and duration of marriage. Test scores on 41 psychological variables did not differ between groups and indicated that emotional maladjustment in women with infertility had a similar prevalence to that in the general population. Downey and associates[49] prospectively followed 59 couples with infertility from the time of diagnosis and a comparison group of 35 women seeking routine gynecologic care. The psychometric observations defined no psychiatric or sexual aberrations and no diminished self-esteem in the infertile group.

Patients undergoing diagnosis and treatment in infertility clinics show significantly higher levels of emotional distress than do control groups.[49, 50] Infertile women score more distress on scales of anxiety, depression, hostility, cognitive disturbance, stress, and self-esteem than do their male partners.[50] Marital discord and sexual dysfunction are not increased in infertile couples. Nonetheless, infertility couples clearly need emotional understanding. Physicians and their office staff must be empathetic listeners, sensitive to the frustration, disappointment, and anger that infertility can evoke. Husbands and wives are mutually supportive, one sign of a strong relationship. However, some couples need more: a minister, social worker, support group such as RESOLVE, psychologist, or psychiatrist. Open communication is the goal that must be achieved: hearing by both the patient and the caregiver is the mechanism that makes them partners in the selection of treatments and equal participants in the decision to stop therapy.

MEDICAL AND SURGICAL ILLNESSES

Pelvic adhesions that interfere with access of the fallopian tubes to the ovaries are a significant cause for infertility. In a study of 273 women undergoing laparoscopy, the only historical predictor of adhesive disease was previous pelvic surgery.[51] Using life table analysis on 69 women whose periadnexal adhesions were treated by laparotomy and 78 patients who were not treated, the 24-month cumulative pregnancy rates were 45% and 16%, respectively. An exception to the rule that pelvic surgery causes adhesions, as many obstetricians will attest, is cesarean section.[52]

Pelvic adhesions are not solely the result of gynecologic surgery. Among 71 women who had a proctocolectomy for ulcerative colitis or Crohn's disease, 72% had been able to conceive before surgery, and only 37% who desired fertility had a postoperative pregnancy.[53] These data are muted because one cannot account for the fertility inhibition of chronic illness before surgery and the health improvement

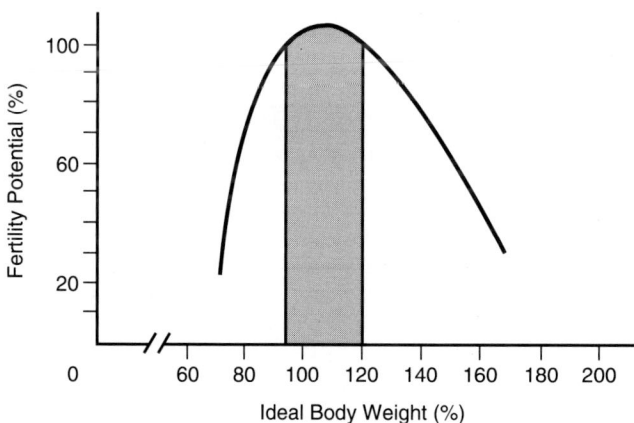

Fertility Potential (%)

100

60

20

0   60   80   100   120   140   160   180   200
Ideal Body Weight (%)

FIGURE 2–7. Schematic representation of fertility potential and ideal body weight.

brought about by the surgical treatment. For example, among 54 women, aged 16 to 62 years, with newly diagnosed celiac sprue, 38.8% complained of amenorrhea.[54] Five patients had experienced repeated abortion. In men, inflammatory bowel disease, Crohn's disease, and ulcerative colitis do not diminish overall reproductive capacity.[55]

Mueller and coworkers[56] studied a history of appendectomy for appendicitis in 279 women with surgically diagnosed tubal infertility. No excess risk of tubal infertility was found after a simple appendectomy without rupture. However, when the operation was reported for appendiceal rupture, the relative risk of tubal infertility was 4.8 (95% confidence, 1.5 to 14.9). In a retrospective analysis of patients coming to pelviscopy in Germany, 55% of the patients with periovarian and peritubal adhesions were infertile after appendectomy.[57] Ruptured appendix in children may have a different prognosis. A case review[58] of 181 girls operated on between 1957 and 1975 when they were 10 months to 13 years of age found 82% of the married women and 11% of unmarried women had one or more children. Of 18 women without living children, 1 had bilateral tubal disease consistent with pelvic inflammatory disease and 1 had an ectopic pregnancy.

DRUGS AND CHEMICALS

Additives in food and water, emissions to the environment, medications, and pollutants from home and factory contribute to the increasing chemical assault every person experiences every day. It began before birth, from the transplacental passage of agents to which mothers were exposed. The impact that these biologically foreign compounds may be having on reproduction is the basis of speculation and sounding for caution, but there is little of substance to guide clinicians.

In a widely reported survey of 104 women who had been attempting pregnancy for 3 months, those who drank 1 cup of coffee per day had one half the per-cycle fertility of women who drank less coffee.[59] A response study of 2817 women who had recently delivered a liveborn child investigated consumption of coffee, tea, and cola beverages.[60] No differences in the efficiency of conception were observed among women who drank less than 1 cup of coffee-equivalent to those who drank more than 2 cups per day. Further, comparison of 1818 infertile women and their primiparous controls did not identify coffee as a risk for infertility.[60]

Herbst and colleagues[61] reported that prenatal exposure to diethylstilbestrol (DES) impaired fertility, whereas Barnes and associates[62] found that most DES daughters were able to conceive. In men exposed prenatally to DES, maldescent of the testes, epididymal cysts, and abnormal semen parameters may be seen, but a risk of infertility has not been demonstrated.[63] Chemotherapeutic agents directly damage the gonads, and the likelihood of diminished fertility is directly related to the degree of gonadal activity at the time of treatment.[64, 65] Ataya and coworkers' studies[66] showing protection against chemotherapy-induced gonadal failure using gonadotropin-releasing hormone agonist in a rat model charted an opportunity to protect reproductive function in patients. However, there are no published data regarding the protective effect of ovarian suppression at this time.

Recreational drug use impairs fertility.[67] Women who had used marijuana in the year before conceiving had a 2.1 relative risk of infertility (95% confidence interval, 1.1 to 4.0) compared with a matched control group.[68] Cocaine users have an increased risk for tubal factor infertility.[68] Cocaine use was twice as common among men with sperm concentrations lower than 20 million/mL.[69] At Washington University, Yazigi and colleagues[70] have observed specific binding of cocaine to sperm, and in our in vitro fertilization laboratory, the sperm from men who have used codeine in the previous 2 weeks had slow, nondirectional motility.

Giacoia[71] surveyed reproductive hazards in the workplace, and Field and associates[72] reviewed the potential reproductive toxicities of environmental compounds. Testicular atrophy with azoospermia followed occupational exposure to the soil fumigant, 1,2-dibromo-3-chloropropane (Nemagon, Fumazone, DBCP).[73] Welding mild steel (steel with a low carbon content and no alloys), but not stainless steel (chromium alloy steel), was associated with reduced fertility in Danish metal workers.[74] Nitrous oxide, a widely used inhalation analgesic-anesthetic, came under suspicion as a reproductive toxin in the 1970s. Rowland and coworkers[75] analyzed survey information from 459 female California dental assistants, ages 18 to 39 years. In 19 women who worked 5 or more hours per week in a room where nitrous oxide gas was unscavenged, the probability of conception was 0.41 (0.23 to 0.74, 95% confidence interval, $P < 0.003$) compared with unexposed women. Thus, exposure to high levels of nitrous oxide can impair fertility in women.

Medications suspected to contribute to infertility include antihistamines, which can decrease vaginal lubrication; antihypertensives, which impair erection; barbiturates, which can inhibit gonadotropin release; and nonsteroidal anti-inflammatory drugs, which can block egg release. Lists of chemicals mention heavy metals such as lead and mercury, which are enzyme poisons; cytotoxins such as polycyclic hydrocarbons; or hormone look-a-likes such as the plant phytoestrogens. Such lists (Table 2–5) spawn speculation, media reports, and questions from concerned patients. By law, employers are required to make readily available to employees Material Safety Data Sheets on any hazardous substance used at the work site. The sheets give the names of all product ingredients, toxicologic information, and contact information on manufacturers. The Reproductive Toxicology Center maintains a database, REPROTOX, that summarizes the reproductive effects of industrial chemicals. Many states have pregnancy hotlines to address questions about workplace hazards.

TABLE 2–5. Drugs and Chemicals That May Alter Male Reproduction	
Classification	**Drug or Chemical**
Recreational	Narcotics, marijuana, androgens, tobacco, alcohol
Occupational	Dibromochloropropane, benzene, carbon disulfide, lead, anesthetic gases
Medical	Chemotherapy agents (cyclophosphamide, mustargen), diethylstilbestrol (in utero), sulfasalazine, spironolactone, ketoconazole, cyproterone acetate, cimetidine, antihypertensives (methyldopa, reserpine, clonidine), antidepressants (tricyclic, monoamine oxidase inhibitors), antipsychotics (phenothiazines, lithium)

TABLE 2–6. Factors Associated with Tubal Infertility

Number of sexual partners
Cigarette smoking
Intrauterine device
Sexually transmitted disease
Septic abortion
Ruptured appendix
Pelvic surgery

PELVIC INFECTION

Sexually transmitted disease (STD) is a leading contributor to infertility in women, and the "sexual revolution" has energized an epidemic. Teenage women in the United States average 4.5 sexual partners per adolescent.[76] One million women annually are diagnosed as having acute salpingitis, and pelvic inflammatory disease (PID) is twice as common among adolescents and young women compared with all women aged 15 to 44 years. In the 1982 National Survey of Family Growth, 20% of women in their early 30s volunteered a history of PID.[77] One episode of laparoscopy-proven, aggressively treated PID in a Scandinavian population left 13% with tubal infertility.[78] Second and third infections caused sterility in 36% and 75% of women, respectively. The frequency of ectopic pregnancy increases 10-fold in women with a history of acute salpingitis.[79]

Because even the aggressive treatment of acute PID carries a one-in-eight risk of tubal infertility, prevention becomes far more important than earlier diagnosis. (Table 2–6 lists the factors associated with tubal infertility.) Reversing current sexual freedom, even if possible, will be an education process requiring a generation to complete. The promotion of "safe sex" to minimize STD transmission is a pragmatic, immediately achievable goal. Women who had ever used barrier methods of contraception have a significantly decreased (0.6 relative risk) of tubal infertility (95% confidence limits, 0.5 to 0.8) after controlling for age, religion, education, smoking, number of partners, geography, age at menarche, and use of other contraceptives.[80, 81] When spermicides are combined with diaphragm or condom, the protection is greater than with the barrier alone. Oral contraceptives do not prevent exposure to STDs, but they may lessen the likelihood of spread to the upper reproductive system and consequent infertility. Finally, effective contraception prevents unwanted pregnancy and therefore avoids the small risk of infection and tubal damage after a medical interruption of early pregnancy.

SUMMARY

The efficiency of conception clearly decreases as the age of the woman increases beyond 25 years and as the frequency of intercourse decreases below three times per week. Smoking 15 or more cigarettes per day is a third, well-documented contributor to impaired fertility. The total number of conceptions in a population is a function of time allowed for followup. In the 20- to 30-year-old age group, one half of women achieve pregnancy within six cycles. By age 35 years, the half-time has doubled. After age 40, the average time for conception has tripled and is rising exponentially. As we evaluate management protocols, control groups must be studied because the rate of treatment-independent conceptions is large. It is only against these normative data that we can scientifically weigh the factors that influence the likelihood for conception and honestly promote the treatments that assist the infertile couple.

REFERENCES

1. Mosher WD. Infertility: why business is booming. Am Demogr 1987;9:42–43.
2. Mosher WD, Pratt WF. Fecundity and infertility in the United States: incidence and trends. Fertil Steril 1991;56:192–193.
3. United States Congress, Office of Technology Assessment. Infertility: Medical and Social Choices [OTA-BA-358]. Washington DC: US Government Printing Office, May 1988:51.
4. Wright P. An examination of factors influencing black fertility decline in the Mississippi Delta, 1880–1930. Soc Biol 1989;36:213–239.
5. Hogberg U, Akerman S. Reproductive pattern among women in 19th century Sweden. J Biosoc Sci 1990;22:13–18.
6. Olsen J. Subfecundity according to the age of the mother and father. Dan Med Bull 1990;37:281–282.
7. Templeton A, Fraser C, Thompson B. The epidemiology of infertility in Aberdeen. Br Med J 1990;301:148–152.
8. Needleman L. Canadian fertility trends in perspective. J Biosoc Sci 1986;18:43–56.
9. Ram B. The Canadian family in transition. J Biosoc Sci 1988;20:19–30.
10. Ebomoyi E, Adetoro OO. Socio-biological factors influencing infertility in a rural Nigerian community. Int J Gynaecol Obstet 1990;33:41–47.
11. Guttmacher AF. Factors affecting normal expectancy of conception. JAMA 1956;161:855–860.
12. Strickler RC, Keller DW, Warren JC. Artificial insemination with fresh donor semen. N Engl J Med 1975;283:848–853.
13. Yeh J, Seibel MM. Artificial insemination with donor sperm: a review of 108 patients. Obstet Gynecol 1987;70:313–316.
14. Tietze C. Fertility after discontinuation of intrauterine and oral contraception. Int J Fertil 1968;13:385–389.
15. MacLeod JM, Gold RZ. The male factor in fertility and infertility: VI. Semen quality and certain other factors in relation to ease of conception. Fertil Steril 1953;4:10–33.
16. Ogino K. Histological studies on corpora lutea, period of ovulation, relation between corpora lutea and cyclic changes in uterine mucous membrane, and the period of fertilization. Int Rev Natur Family Plan 1978;2:92–95. [Translation reprinted from The Japan Medical World, 1978.]
17. Levin RM, Latimore J, Wein AJ, Van Arsdalen KN. Correlation of sperm count with frequency of ejaculation. Fertil Steril 1986;45:732–734.
18. Edwards RG. Conception in the Human Female. London: Academic Press, 1980:559.
19. Collins JA, Rowe TC. Age of the female partner is a prognostic factor in prolonged unexplained infertility: a multicenter study. Fertil Steril 1989;52:15–20.
20. Schwartz D, Mayaux MJ. Female fecundity as a function of age: results of artificial insemination in 2193 nulliparous women with azoospermic husbands. N Engl J Med 1982;307:404–406.
21. Stovall DW, Toma SK, Hammond MG, Talbert LM. The effect of age on female fecundity. Obstet Gynecol 1991;77:33–36.
22. Katayama KP, Ju K-S, Manuel M, et al. Computer analysis of etiology and pregnancy rate in 636 cases of primary infertility. Am J Obstet Gynecol 1979;135:207–214.
23. Collins JA, Wrixon W, Janes LB, Wilson EH. Treatment-independent pregnancy among infertile couples. N Engl J Med 1983;309:1201–1206.
24. Keller DW, Strickler RC, Warren JC. Clinical Infertility. Norwalk, CT: Appleton-Century-Crofts, 1984.
25. Stillman RJ (editor). Smoking and reproductive health. Semin Reprod Endocrinol 1989;7:291–348.
26. Baird DD, Wilcox AJ. Cigarette smoking associated with delayed conception. JAMA 1985;253:2979–2983.
27. Howe G, Westhoff C, Vessey M, Yeate D. Effects of age, cigarette smoking, and other factors on fertility: findings in a large prospective study. Br Med J 1985;290:1697–1700.
28. Suonio S, Saarikoski S, Kauhanen O, et al. Smoking does affect fecundity. Eur J Obstet Gynecol Reprod Biol 1990;34:89–95.

29. Daling JR, Weiss NS, Metch BJ, Chow WH. Primary tubal infertility in relation to the use of an intrauterine device. N Engl J Med 1985;312:937–941.

30. Weathersbee PS. Nicotine and its influence on the female reproductive system. J Reprod Med 1980;25:243–250.

31. Weinberg CR, Wilcox AJ, Baird DD. Reduced fecundability in women with prenatal exposure to cigarette smoking. Am J Epidemiol 1989;129:1072–1080.

32. Hughes EG, YoungLai EV, Ward SM. Cigarette smoking and IVF outcome: results of an ongoing prospective study [Abstract FP84]. Presented at the Annual Meeting, Canadian Fertility and Andrology Society, Quebec City, September 1991.

33. Marshburn PB, Sloan CS, Hammond MG. Semen quality and association with coffee drinking, cigarette smoking, and ethanol consumption. Fertil Steril 1989;52:162–165.

34. Makler A, Blumenfeld Z, Reiss J, et al. Use of a sealed minichamber for direct observation and evaluation of the in vitro effect of cigarette smoke on sperm motility. Fertil Steril 1993;59:645–651.

35. Rebar RW (editor). Exercise and reproduction. Semin Reprod Endocrin 1983;3:1–88.

36. Shangold MM, Levine HS. The effect of marathon training upon menstrual function. Am J Obstet Gynecol 1982;143:862–869.

37. Schwartz B, Cumming DC, Riordan E, et al. Exercise-associated amenorrhea: a distinct entity? Am J Obstet Gynecol 1981;141:662–670.

38. Bullen BA, Skrinar GS, Beitins IZ, et al. Induction of menstrual disorders by strenuous exercise in untrained women. N Engl J Med 1985;312:1349–1353.

39. Beitins IZ, McArthur JW, Turnbull BA, et al. Exercise induces two types of human luteal dysfunction: confirmation by urinary free progesterone. J Clin Endocrin Metab 1991;72:1350–1358.

40. Schinfeld JS. Effects of athletics on male reproduction and sexuality. Med Aspects Hum Sex 1989;23:67–70.

41. Sanfilippo JS, Liu YK. Vitamin B_{12} deficiency and infertility: report of a case. Int J Fertil 1991;36:36–38.

42. Gulden KD. Pernicious anemia, vitiligo, and infertility. J Am Board Fam Pract 1990;3:217–220.

43. Bringer J, Hedon B, Giner B, et al. Influence of abnormal weight and imbalanced diet on female fertility. Presse Med 1990;19:1456–1459.

44. Page SW. Golden ovaries. Aust NZ J Obstet Gynecol 1971;11:32–36.

45. Green BB, Weiss NS, Daling JR. Risk of ovulatory infertility in relation to body weight. Fertil Steril 1988;50:721–726.

46. Bates GW, Bates SR, Whitworth NS. Reproductive failure in women who practice weight control. Fertil Steril 1982;37:373–378.

47. Bates GW, Whitworth NS. Effect of body weight reduction on plasma androgens in obese, infertile women. Fertil Steril 1982;38:406–409.

48. Paulson JD, Haarmann BS, Salerno RL, Asmar P. An investigation of the relationship between emotional maladjustment and infertility. Fertil Steril 1988;49:258–262.

49. Downey J, Yingling S, McKinney M, Husami N. Mood disorders, psychiatric symptoms and distress in women presenting for infertility evaluation. Fertil Steril 1989;52:425–432.

50. Wright J, Duchesne C, Sabourin S, et al. Psychosocial distress and infertility: men and women respond differently. Fertil Steril 1991;55:100–108.

51. Tulandi T, Collins JA, Burrows E, et al. Treatment-dependent and treatment-independent pregnancy among women with periadnexal adhesions. Am J Obstet Gynecol 1990;162:354–357.

52. Wolf ME, Daling JR, Voigt LF. Prior cesarean delivery in women with secondary tubal infertility. Am J Public Health 1990;80:1382–1383.

53. Wilkland M, Jansson I, Asztiely M, et al. Gynaecological problems related to anatomical changes after conventional proctocolectomy and ileostomy. Int J Colorect Dis 1990;5:49–52.

54. Molteni N, Bardella MT, Bianchi PA. Obstetric and gynecological problems in women with untreated celiac sprue. J Clin Gastroenterol 1990;12:37–39.

55. Narendranathan M, Sandler RS, Suchindran CM. Male infertility in inflammatory bowel disease. J Clin Gastroenterol 1989;11:403–406.

56. Mueller BA, Daling JR, Moore DE, et al. Appendectomy and the risk of tubal infertility. N Engl J Med 1986;315:1506–1508.

57. Lehmann-Willenbrock E, Mecke H, Riedel HH. Sequelae of appendectomy, with special reference to intra-abdominal adhesions, chronic abdominal pain, and infertility. Gynecol Obstet Invest 1990;29:241–245.

58. Puri P, McGuinness EPJ, Guiney EJ. Fertility following perforated appendicitis in girls. J Pediatr Surg 1989;24:547–549.

59. Wilcox A, Weinberg C, Baird D. Caffeinated beverages and decreased fertility. Lancet 1988;2:1453–1456.

60. Joesoef MR, Beral V, Rolfs RT, et al. Are caffeinated beverages risk factors for delayed conception? Lancet 1990;335:136–137.

61. Herbst AL, Hubby MM, Blough RR, Azizi F. A comparison of pregnancy experience in DES-exposed and DES-unexposed daughters. J Reprod Med 1980;24:62–69.

62. Barnes AB, Colton T, Gundersen J, et al. Fertility and outcome of pregnancy on women exposed in utero to diethylstilbestrol. N Engl J Med 1980;302:609–613.

63. Stenchever MA, Williamson RA, Leonard J, et al. Possible relationship between in utero diethylstilbestrol exposure and male fertility. Am J Obstet Gynecol 1981;140:186–191.

64. Averette HE, Boike GM, Jarrell MA. Effects of cancer chemotherapy on gonadal function and reproductive capacity. CA 1990;40:199–210.

65. Rivkees SA, Crawford JD. The relationship of gonadal activity and chemotherapy-induced gonadal damage. JAMA 1988;259:2123–2125.

66. Ataya KM, McKanna JA, Weintraub AM, Clark MR. A luteinizing hormone-releasing hormone agonist for the prevention of chemotherapy-induced ovarian follicular loss in rats. Cancer Res 1985;45:3651–3656.

67. Smith CG, Smith MT. Substance abuse and reproduction. Semin Reprod Endocrinol 1990;8:55–64.

68. Mueller BA, Daling JR, Weiss NS, Moore DE. Recreational drug use and the risk of primary infertility. Epidemiology 1990;1:195–200.

69. Bracken MB, Eskenazi B, Sachse K, et al. Association of cocaine use with sperm concentration, motility, and morphology. Fertil Steril 1990;53:315–322.

70. Yazigi RA, Odem RR, Polakoski KL. Demonstration of specific binding of cocaine to human spermatozoa. JAMA 1991;266:1956–1959.

71. Giacoia GP. Reproductive hazards in the workplace. Obstet Gynecol Surv 1992;47:679–687.

72. Field B, Selub M, Hughes CL. Reproductive effects of environmental agents. Semin Reprod Endocrinol 1990;8:44–54.

73. Olsen GW, Lanham JM, Bodner KM, et al. Determinants of spermatogenesis recovery among workers exposed to 1,2-dibromo-3-chloropropane. J Occup Med 1990;32:979–984.

74. Bonde JP, Hansen KS, Levine RJ. Fertility among Danish male welders. Scand J Work Environ Health 1990;16:315–322.

75. Rowland AS, Baird DD, Weinberg CR, et al. Reduced fertility among women employed as dental assistants exposed to high levels of nitrous oxide. N Engl J Med 1992;327:993–997.

76. Hofferth SL, Kahn JR, Baldwin W. Premarital sexual activity among US teenage women over the past three decades. Fam Plan Perspect 1987;19:46–53.

77. Aral SO, Mosher D, Cates W. Self-reported pelvic inflammatory disease in the US: a common occurrence. Am J Public Health 1985;75:1216–1219.

78. Westrom L. Incidence, prevalence, and trends of acute pelvic inflammatory disease and its consequences in industrialized countries. Am J Obstet Gynecol 1980;138:880–892.

79. World Health Organization. Task force on intrauterine devices for fertility regulation: a multinational case-control study of ectopic pregnancy. Clin Reprod Fertil 1985;3:131–143.

80. Cramer DW, Goldman MB, Schiff I, Belisle S, et al. The relationship of tubal infertility to barrier method and oral contraceptive use. JAMA 1987;257:2446–2450.

81. Cramer DW, Schiff I, Schoenbaum SC, Gibson M. Tubal infertility and intrauterine device. N Engl J Med 1985;312:941–947.

CHAPTER 3

Infertility: A Patient's Perspective

PATRICIA IRWIN JOHNSTON

Two images from my childhood resurface and merge. The first, a plastic toy—child height, air filled, weighted at the bottom with sand and adorned with grinning face—whose purpose was to be punched and to bounce back grinning, to be punched again. The second, Lucy and Ethel trying to fill boxes with chocolates at a candy factory, at the mercy of an out-of-control conveyor belt.

For many of the 16 years it took us to build our family of three children (battling infertility issues all the way), my husband Dave and I were a pair of those grinning, air-filled toys bobbling down an out-of-control conveyor belt. We stepped onto the track together—young, optimistic members of the first birth control generation, and thus expecting (unlike our parents' generation) to have full control over our reproductive lives. Like so many of our peers, we naively expected to be able to plan our first child's arrival right down to the month. When, having dispensed with the pills and attempted to become pregnant, that did not happen, we reached out for help.

With little preparation we found ourselves carried along infertility's conveyor belt, moving at breakneck speed from physician to lab to physician to pharmacy to physician to hospital to lab to physician to adoption agency. At each position along the way, new diagnoses or new options came at us like swing-arm gates at a railway crossing, swooping down to knock us slightly off balance as we wobbled down the moving belt.

Despite our love for and commitment to one another, the two of us were different: raised in different towns, schools, churches—each with slightly different values, slightly different expectations, slightly different needs. So every time we were knocked askew we each careened wildly in different directions before bouncing back to center, only occasionally accidentally bumping together to steady one another.

Several human beings were stationed at each of those swing-arm gates, but each was so busy doing his or her own job that no one really *saw* us as we lurched along; no one ever noticed that the belt was moving out of control; no one ever suggested that the belt be stopped so that we could get off, reevaluate, and decide whether or not to try again. Each

caregiver had assumed that we had gotten on the belt that passed before him or her on purpose, so that we were assumed to be in control of it.

As reproductive health professionals, when are you successful? Only when you are able to use your education and training to help a couple achieve a pregnancy? When is a couple successful in resolving infertility? Only when they conceive and give birth to a jointly conceived child? These are the questions dealt with in this chapter.

INFERTILITY AS AN INTERGENERATIONAL JOURNEY

Our family has faced infertility in two successive generations, so that it colors yet a third generation. Dave's parents, Perry and Helen, dealt with infertility in the 1930s and 1940s. Although they certainly mourned the loss of several babies to miscarriages, his parents' acceptance of medical fragility and an inability to control fertility as "the way things were" has always seemed hard for Dave and me to understand. Raised in an era of "country doctors" and home remedies, they had relatively low expectations about medical options. Furthermore, conservative social mores made family building by adoption a relatively quick and inexpensive—and expected—alternative.

But the profile of post–birth-control generation couples hoping to conceive has changed dramatically from that of couples of a generation and a half ago. Raised to feel empowered in so many areas of life, couples today become frustrated, angry, and depressed when faced for the first time with the loss of control over a part of life that our peers take very much for granted, and yet soon find that in facing a fertility impairment, we have lost control not only of our reproductive lives but also of many other aspects of our lives. Social calendars and vacation schedules fall victim to the menstrual cycle and treatment regimens. Decisions about housing (condo or house? suburbs or city?) and even auto purchases (two-seater sports car or minivan?) are difficult to make when one is not sure whether one will be a parent

19

soon—or ever. Commitments to continuing education or to job transfers and promotions can be colored by the projected impact on treatment options, insurance coverage, how moves might influence the length of a "wait" on the list of an in vitro fertilization clinic or an adoption agency, and so forth. Even underwear purchases can be dictated by infertility!

Today's couples live in an environment in which daily exposure to chemicals, pollutants, medications, and "recreational" drugs and a more relaxed attitude about sexual experimentation has put each partner at increased risk of fertility impairment. A variety of sociologic shifts may have led us to delay marriage and childbearing until our naturally less fertile thirties. At the same time we *expect* to be fertile or to be able to do something about fertility impairment. In a North American culture that has for generations embraced a "you can do anything if you try hard enough" philosophy and has led the cutting edge of medical research, have we ever before had such an opportunity to feel in control of our reproductive lives? Unlike previous generations, we are informed and often demanding medical consumers.

And yet there is still much about which we are uninformed. Friends and family, more concerned about uncontrolled fertility than they are aware of impaired fertility, rush to feed our initial denial. We are trying too hard. We just need to relax, take a vacation, or have a glass of wine before bedtime. Perhaps it is God's will for our lives or punishment for a past indiscretion, but perhaps we should light a candle. Everyone's second cousin's physician is a world-renowned expert. Everyone who ever adopted subsequently became pregnant. Grocery lines are filled with 11-month's pregnant women pushing newborn infants in carts while toddlers whine at their knees. Mailboxes overflow with birth announcements and baby shower invitations. Family events always include Aunt Gladys asking us when we are going to make our poor parents grandparents. Brother-in-law Charlie leeringly wants to know whether we need a little advice on how it is done. It is all something slightly off color, not to be taken too seriously, certainly not something important enough to grant us the privilege of raining on pregnant cousin Janice's parade. And so we tend to isolate ourselves from others—whether they are well meaning or not—and to begin to build defenses around our rapidly deflating egos (Table 3–1).

In today's age of rapidly changing technologic and pharmacologic advancements in the area of infertility, many presume that the infertile couple is living in the best of all possible times to be infertile. After all, diagnosis of infertility is conclusive in more than 90% of cases, and with appropriate medical care, successful treatment that results in the birth of a healthy child genetically related to both of its parents is probable for more than 50% of fertility-impaired couples. Research in this area is at an all-time high, and new treatments are being announced with astonishing frequency.

But making decisions about testing and treatment has never been more complicated. Testing has become more sophisticated and more invasive. The simple temperature graph of a generation ago has given way to complex blood studies, ultrasonography, and other monitoring. More than one approach may be taken to deal with various reproductive problems. Surgical options include microsurgery and laser surgery. Drugs can be administered by mouth, by hypodermic sy-

ringe, by pump. Sperm can be centrifuged, washed, zona drilled. Assisted reproductive technologies can involve donor gametes for one or both partners. An alphabet soup of drugs and ART techniques and diagnostic procedures from hCG to hMG to GnRH, from IVF to GIFT to ZIFT to PROST, from HSG to CVS to SPA boggles the most well-informed and sophisticated mind!

How could the infertile couple of the 1990s not be optimistic about their chances for conception and birth? Yet for many couples, it is this very one-more-chance milieu that has made this the worst of all possible times to be infertile! The amount of information we must process, the ethical ramifications of the options open to us, can be staggering. Where do we stop, and when?

Each professional we meet is justifiably optimistic about our chances of succeeding under his or her care. When one is dealing with a problem such as infertility, which has a tendency to dent self-esteem, when operating in a communication vacuum so common to male-female relationships, it can often seem so much easier to simply abdicate control to the professionals. After all, if the professional can just fix it, it will all be better. The columnist Anna Quindlen, in a *New York Times* article about a controversial book in the medical field, summarized it well. "When you become a patient," she wrote, "often you cease to be an actor and become an acted upon."

And so the conveyor belt moves forward, carrying us numbly on. Far too often, as we move from station to fruitless station, a mounting sense of desperation builds. We would, we too often think, do *anything* to have a baby—swallow rat poison, make love in the town square at noon and stand on our heads for an hour, pay ridiculous sums of money. And, more realistically, we *do* do almost anything—have intercourse (it is no longer making love) according to schedule whether we even like each other today, beg for just a little higher dose or just one more cycle of a drug that causes miserable side effects and unpromising results, plead with our insurers or our bankers to help us fund just one more assisted reproductive technology attempt.

HOW MEDICAL CARE PROVIDERS CAN HELP

Sensitive health practitioners can help infertile couples with more than medicine (Table 3–2). Often unmentioned is the need for a pause for reflection and clear decision making that is colored only by the values of the couple themselves. In suggesting such a time out, uncolored by their own personal values, physicians, nurses, and mental health professionals can help desperate couples ensure that the decisions they make in the face of what for many is a first life crisis will create contentment and strength that will last them a lifetime.

Even though each professional should rightfully take great pride in his or her credentials and experience, it is also important that professionals acknowledge that they bring personal values and expectations to their relationships with patients or clients. Fascinated enough by the conception and birth process and by the value of genetic connection between parent and child to have made it a career, reproductive med-

TABLE 3-1. Common Reactions to Fertility Impairment from Family and Friends

You're probably trying too hard, so. . .
   relax
   take a vacation
   have a glass of wine before bedtime
   buy some sexy nightwear
It's probably God's will, so. . .
   light a candle
   accept this punishment
There's always adoption! But. . .
   how would any decent person ever give up their very own flesh and blood?
   bad blood will out
   too bad there will be no children of "your own"
   aren't you people wonderful! I know that I couldn't love "someone else's child"
   then you'll get pregnant! They ALWAYS do after adopting!

icine professionals are, in many instances, hard put to consider that one who has once sought a pregnancy would later choose to live childfree or to embrace adoption as a positive option in family building.

It will take a conscientious effort to create a nurturing yet value-neutral environment that supports the empowerment of patients to make decisions that are their own. This may be easier said than done. To date, full-spectrum services have rarely been linked. Emotional support is often a missing component of a medical practice, and in too many instances mutual support groups such as RESOLVE in the United States or the Infertility Awareness Association of Canada are perceived as a threat by the general obstetrician-gynecologist who devotes only a part of his or her practice to infertility. Counseling focused on making decisions about options, including those outside of medical treatment, is a rare component in the infertility clinic. Donor insemination is likened to a drug that will cure infertility rather than presented as an option that produces a quasi-adoption. Adoption information is unavailable or reluctantly offered only as a last-chance option to those leaving the practice with no more medical hope. The option of building a childfree (as opposed to childless) lifestyle is rarely mentioned at all.

But creating such a program produces results that are worth the effort. Careful evaluation of options can help couples regain some sense of their lost control. By choosing to

TABLE 3-2. Empowering Patients: Suggestions for the Reproductive Health Care Practitioner

1. Offer a model of broadly focused decision making as an alternative to the common style of crisis management from test to test.
   a. Establish a stepped program of evaluation, and have it available in written form on first visit.
   b. As early as possible in the evaluation process, lay out *all* possible treatment and lifestyle options.
   c. Provide resources and information about both medical and nonmedical options in an unbiased manner.
2. Offer assistance in developing needed communications skills.
   a. Help the couple understand each of the losses they are experiencing as a result of infertility.
   b. Help the couple to understand their own and their spouse's values and goals and how to reach consensus and compromise in making decisions.

analyze their treatment and lifestyle alternatives as they move along, setting measurable goals and objectives that reflect clear understanding of their limited resources—time, money, emotional energy, and physical capacity—couples can be reempowered.

The process is best accomplished in stages. Early on, patients need clear information about what lies ahead for them. An orientation session should outline the steps in and a realistically condensed timeline for a basic workup and should acknowledge from the outset the likelihood of the development of stress in one or both partners.

Among the most stressful parts of infertility treatment is the roller coaster ride of monthly hope and despair. Therefore, a schedule that moves as quickly as possible through the diagnostic process without stopping to treat identified problems until everything has been checked usually causes less stress than a plan that tests and treats, tests some more, and tries something new. Because people in crisis tend not to hear much of what is said to them, it is important to provide as much material as possible in written form, so that the information can be referred to again and again.

Once the workup has been completed, another meeting between patients and physician should lay out treatment and lifestyle alternatives and offer the couple as much information as they need to create their own game plan. Practitioners should never presume to know what course a patient may wish to pursue. Because nearly all treatment-related decisions involve changed expectations, coping successfully with the psychosocial pressures of infertility includes a need to step off the conveyor belt at this point, and possibly at other subsequent points, to reevaluate that first decision to become pregnant.

The couple needs to ask themselves several questions: What were our initial expectations about beginning to try to start a family? How have they changed in light of our experience with a fertility impairment? Supportive caregivers not only will encourage this pause for reflection but also will have gathered material to be used as information in this process: clear information about risks, costs, benefits, statistical odds of success of various treatments; ready referral for a second opinion or for more specialized care; referral for information about medically assisted adoption alternatives from donor insemination to surrogacy to embryo transfer; up-to-date information about a local or national adoption advocacy group for information about domestic and international, agency, and private adoption; a list of suggested reading; and a referral to a local support group or counselor. With this material in hand, a couple is ready to explore their thoughts and feelings about what lies ahead for them.

DEALING WITH LOSS: MORE THAN A DREAM CHILD

A series of potential losses accompany infertility, each of which may have significantly different importance to any two people or any two couples (Table 3-3). At the same time, we deal with limited resources—we have just so much time, just so much money, just so much physical capacity, and just so much emotional energy. Understanding what it is we want most to have from our fertility and what we want most to

Loss of control over multiple aspects of life
Loss of individual genetic continuity
Loss of the dream of a jointly conceived child
Loss of the physical gratifications of the pregnancy/impregnating experience
Loss of emotional expectations about the pregnancy/birth experience
Loss of opportunity to parent

avoid in our infertility can help us communicate more effectively with spouses, think logically and carefully about our alternatives, and compromise when needed to make choices with which we can live for a lifetime.

We begin by exploring our feelings about six major losses that may accompany the infertility experience.

1. A loss of control over many facets of life. Here in the late twentieth century, empowerment is expected. The feeling of having no control can become a major stressor.

2. The loss of individual genetic continuity—our personal linkage with our families of birth from the past to the future. Avoiding such a loss may be of particular importance to those raised in cultures heavily invested in the value of blood ties.

3. The loss of the romantic dream of a jointly conceived child—the child with good and bad traits from both families, the one about whom we fantasized as we first seriously considered building a family with a particular partner. For many, this jointly conceived child appears to be the ultimate gift of commitment couples can give to one another.

4. The loss of the physical gratifications of impregnating and becoming pregnant—seen by many as a final "proof" of adulthood and the ultimate expression of maleness or femaleness.

5. The loss of the emotional expectations of the pregnancy and birth experience, with its often unrealistically idealized components of jointly attended prepared childbirth classes, perfectly coordinated circumstances and control throughout the birth process, and mystical expectations about a delivery room moment of never-otherwise-replicable "bonding" as a kind of superglue that will ensure a family a proper start.

6. The loss of the opportunity to parent, a major life goal for most adults, and, according to the renowned developmental psychologist Erik Erikson, one of the most important stages in human psychological growth.

Our reactions to the possibility, probability, or actuality of these losses and their importance to us are uniquely our own. Partners rarely rank them identically. Yet when couples are encouraged to examine the prospective losses individually and then to share their responses honestly with their partners, they can more rationally address their options and communicate with one another about potential compromises that will create win-win decisions for them as a couple even out of individual losses.

REGAINING CONTROL: INDIVIDUAL NEEDS, DIFFERING SOLUTIONS

Even couples facing what seem, on the surface, to be similar fertility impairments and medical diagnoses may make entirely different decisions about how to proceed based on their individual and jointly shared values (Table 3–4). Some examples of couples who have worked through the decision-making process I outline in my workshops include the following:

Karen and Randy have been stymied by Karen's premature ovarian failure. Both want desperately to parent, but Randy is finding the idea of adoption particularly difficult because of his myth-filled but firmly held convictions (not shared by Karen, who is ready to adopt!) that bonding can be achieved only through the process of birth. Because Karen cannot ovulate, they can see no hope, and their relationship has become increasingly pressured by their blaming of one another for their joint failure to become parents. Almost serendipitously they approach their pastor, who has recently met just the right counselor—a woman well versed in infertility issues. After spending several sessions with the counselor, working through their reactions to their individual and joint losses and mourning those lost expectations, Karen and Randy find open windows not even seen before: surrogacy (finding a woman willing to donate both egg and the gestational use of her uterus) and the use of donor oocytes (also called *adoptive embryo transfer,* which involves implanting a fertilized egg from another woman into Karen's uterus). They seriously consider both, find medical and legal advisors to answer their questions about each, and decide to pursue as first choice adoptive embryo transfer. If successful, this option will allow the two of them to experience the pregnancy and birth together. If not, and if they decide on surrogacy, Randy will have his genetic connection and Karen her child to love and nurture. There will be winners all around!

Sara and Matt are the owners and operators of a family farm. Together they are clear about their major interest—to become parents. They have pursued all the least-invasive medical treatments they can to try to prod Sara's stubbornly uncooperative ovaries. She responded best to a cycle of Pergonal—expensive for this uninsured couple with limited financial resources. The reproductive endocrinologist working with them at a major medical center sees GIFT as a promising treatment and has provided them with a great deal of literature, encouraging statistics of success for couples who try three cycles at the center's clinic, and a promise to work them into the waiting list quickly. Their physician is convincing. It is tempting, and, frankly, they are having trouble letting this very nice physician down, but they really do not see how they afford up to three cycles of GIFT. Sara and Matt more or less disappear from the clinic—not formally ending treatment but just not coming back. Through their church, they learn of a young woman in another community who is parenting one child alone and is pregnant again. Within months they are the parents of two children—a toddler and a

Encourage couples to take a management-by-objectives approach to their treatment, suggesting that they examine their medical and lifestyle options, determining their reactions to losses (see Table 3–3), gathering data concerning pro's and con's, expense, and odds of success and then charting a course that includes budgeting their four limited resources:

   Time
   Money
   Physical capacity
   Emotional reserves

newborn—in an open adoption. The birthmother's employer has covered all medical expenses of the birth, the local department of social services provided their home study, and their total expenses involved minimal legal fees of an attorney who is also a member of their congregation.

John and Mary consider the losses of infertility and identify what they each wanted most from their original decision to become pregnant. For Mary, the need was to experience a pregnancy as well as to be a parent, yet she also mourns the loss of sharing a pregnancy and then a child with John. For John, on the other hand, individual continuity is just not important. John's dreams are of parenting—reading bedtime stories, coaching athletic teams. For this couple the carefully discussed choice to use donor insemination will be an attractive one—offering each the opportunity to achieve their dreams and avoid infertility's most painful losses. If this option is successful for them, each wins what he or she wants most. Both, however, agree that their highest priority is shared parenthood, so that should donor insemination prove unsuccessful, John and Mary are ready to embrace adoption as an equally attractive way to build a family. They have begun to gather information about international adoption just in case.

Mark and Amy acknowledge different needs. The grandchild of Holocaust victims and survivors, Mark mourns deeply his inability to provide another generation for his family. He is willing to go to dramatic lengths to improve his sperm count and to enhance his chances of impregnating his wife. Amy, too, wants a genetic connection, and initially sees clearly that she can have it, if only she can convince Mark to agree to donor insemination. Their physician, too, has endorsed this choice, reminding Mark that no one need ever know that Amy's child is not his by blood. With the help of a skilled facilitator, each comes to see that for Mark to accede to such a demand from Amy would create a win-lose situation in the balance of their relationship and could impair his ability to relate positively to the child to whom Amy would give birth, because the child would serve as a daily reminder that Mark had lost what both wanted most—genetic continuity—while Amy had achieved it! Additionally, for this couple, the interest in parenting is simply not strong enough in the face of their powerful interest in genetic linkage for either to consider that there could be a win-win after loss-loss in the compromise option of adoption. After careful reflection and a reaffirmation of their primary commitment to one another and to their marriage, this couple decides that their interest in a jointly conceived child is strong enough for them to spend significant amounts of time, money, and energy researching and seeking out the clinics in the world with the highest rate of success in treating Mark's problem. After surgery, medications, and several courses of in vitro fertilization have not helped them to achieve a pregnancy, this couple chooses to embrace a child-*free* lifestyle.

Each of these couples considers themselves successful in resolving infertility issues and making family-building decisions. Their carefully considered choices were right for each couple. Each was ultimately nurtured by a caring, helpful professional who accepted their personal needs, limitations, and values and was able to feel personal success reflected in their joy. There could be more Mark and Amy's, Karen and Randy's, Sara and Matt's, and John and Mary's and fewer drifting, disappointed infertile people if all the professionals working with fertility-impaired people would make it a part of their practice to link services and provide a full spectrum of information and care for their patients and clients.

Helen Keller, a woman intimately familiar with profound loss, may have said it best, "When one door of happiness closes, another opens. But often we spend so much time looking at the closed doors that we cannot see the doors that have opened for us. We must all find these doors, and, if we do, we will make ourselves and our lives as beautiful as God intended." The infertile couple comes to a medical professional seeking the key to a locked door. Although the professional may not have the key that has been requested, by helping this couple look through many doors the professional can assist them in finding a good door. In the patient's success professionals find their own success, no matter what the ultimate outcome.

SUGGESTED READING

Andrews LB. New Conceptions: A Consumer's Guide to the Newest Infertility Treatments. New York: St. Martin's Press, 1984. (An attorney specializing in reproductive law and ethics looks at new technology and offers consumers issues to consider in their decision making.)

Carter JW, Carter M. Sweet Grapes: How to Stop Being Infertile and Start Living Again. Indianapolis: Perspectives Press, 1989. (An infertile couple—she an ob/gyn and he a professor—share the process of decision making that led them to end treatment and embrace a childfree lifestyle.)

Johnston PI. Adopting After Infertility. Indianapolis: Perspectives Press, 1992. (A decision-making tool looking at the adoption option as a lifelong experience as examined through the eyes of the infertile couple.)

Johnston PI. Taking Charge of Infertility. Indianapolis: Perspectives Press, 1994. (A management-by-objectives approach to making decisions about infertility treatment options, family-building alternatives, and lifestyle choices.)

Johnston PI. Understanding: A Guide to Impaired Fertility for Family and Friends. Indianapolis: Perspectives Press, 1983. (A booklet explaining infertility's psychosocial impact to caring others.)

Menning BE. Infertility: A Guide for the Childless Couple. Revised edition. New York: Prentice-Hall, 1988. (The psychosocial impact of infertility as presented by the founder of RESOLVE; the classic in the field.)

Tannen D. You Just Don't Understand: Women and Men in Conversation. New York: Balantine Books, 1990. (Clearly points out the differences in communication styles and interpretations between men and women, offering manageable techniques for improving communication between opposite-sexed partners.)

Zoldbrod AP. Getting Around the Boulder in the Road: Using Imagery to Cope with Fertility Problems. Lexington, MA: Center for Reproductive Problems, 1990. (A booklet that offers professionals and consumers practical tools for using imagery to deal with the stresses of infertility.)

Organizational resources offering services to consumers and assistance to professionals:

RESOLVE, Inc, 1310 Broadway, Somerville, MA 02144, is the 20-year-old national network of more than 50 chapters serving 70+ cities and a membership of more than 15,000. Offering monthly meetings, periodic seminars, advocacy services on insurance and other issues, national and local newsletters, professionally facilitated support groups, fact sheets and other up-to-date literature, current referral to alternative resources, and more, RESOLVE is a first line of support, information, and referral for anyone dealing with fertility impairment on either a personal or professional level.

Infertility Awareness Association of Canada, 206-2378 Holly Lane, Ottawa, Ontario K1V7P1 is RESOLVE's counterpart in Canada. Now in its third year, IAAC is working under a Canadian federal grant to build a network of local mutual support groups throughout Canada during 1992–1993.

The Organization of Parents Through Surrogacy (OPTS), 7054 Quito Ct., Camarillo, CA 93012, is a national nonprofit, volunteer organization whose purpose is mutual support, networking, and the dissemination of information regarding surrogate parenting, egg donation, sperm donation as well as assisted reproductive technology including in vitro fertilization and GIFT. OPTS publishes a quarterly newsletter, holds annual meetings, has a telephone support network, and actively lobbies for legislation concerning surrogacy.

Adoptive Families of America, 3333 Highway 100 North, Minneapolis, MN 55422, is a 20+-year-old network of more than 15,000 families built by or interested in adoption. Local affiliate groups number more than 250. AFA publishes a bimonthly award-winning magazine, *OURS,* and provides information and referral on all kinds of adoption (agency and private, domestic and international, infant and older child) to couples and singles interested in family building through adoption. An annual national conference for prospective parents and those parenting in adoption rotates throughout four geographic areas of the United States. AFA's Parent Resources store offers an extensive list of culturally sensitive books, games, and toys. As an active lobbyist, AFA is a respected presence in Washington.

CHAPTER 4

The Psychological Aspects of Infertility

LINDA D. APPLEGARTH

INFERTILITY AS A LIFE CRISIS

To maximize our understanding of infertility, it is imperative that we also understand the psychological factors of this condition. Infertility not only has significant impact on the psychological status of the individual, but also places stress on the relationship between husband and wife.

For many individuals and couples, the ability to conceive and give birth to a child is paramount to one's lifelong notions of femininity and masculinity, to gender identity, and ultimately to the meaning of life. Bearing children and parenting is often one of the foundations around which a couple builds a relationship.

Möller and Fällström[1] note that men and women, as social and sexual beings, have historically attempted to plan their reproduction. It is not only frustrating, but also devastating, to many couples who want to have children but cannot. Becker[2] points out that "parenthood is a pivotal stage of the human life cycle" and that it, more than marriage, symbolizes full responsibility as an adult. How one views parenting, Becker adds, is key to the way in which one sees life itself. Parenting, in fact, is a bond that seals the generations together, and the opportunity to pass along life experiences to the next generation is what, for many, gives life its meaning. Erikson[3] describes that important stage of the life cycle as *generativity*. For many infertile people, the goal of having children is therefore profoundly intertwined with higher level goals of fulfillment and happiness in life (Fig. 4–1).[4]

Despite advances in the feminist movement, there are still clearly cultural and social factors that influence women's and men's views of themselves as parents. Wright and associates[5] found, for example, that there are clear gender differences in psychological responses to infertility, with infertile women showing higher distress than their partners on a global measure of stress and self-esteem. In general, women are raised with expectations that they will be caregivers—mothers. Despite other life goals and expectations, the message has always been clear: Motherhood is the primary job in a woman's life. For men, the expectations regarding fatherhood and family have been more ambiguous. They may, in fact, not con-template having a family except generally until it becomes an issue in a relationship. Because women tend to accept primary responsibility for continuing the family life cycle, infertility becomes a major life crisis of adulthood for them (Table 4–1). From an emotional standpoint, a number of studies have supported the notion that women are more often adversely affected by infertility than men.[6–8]

In psychoanalytic thinking, maternal identification provides a background for parenting, and infertility disrupts the opportunity to recapitulate this relationship or make reparation for early maternal failures.[9] When pregnancy, childbirth, and parenting are thwarted by infertility, Klempner[9] noted that identifications with the maternal object are disrupted for many women, thereby altering self and object representations. Notman and Lester[10] added that a woman's knowledge that she is able to bear children is essential for the development of a notion of femininity, gender identity, and self-esteem. Because motherhood is usually a primary goal of adulthood for most women, infertility can be interpreted as an important interruption of a primary developmental stage. Thus, infertility represents a psychological loss of tremendous magnitude.

The literature suggests repeatedly that infertility is a life crisis.[11–14] The inability to conceive or give birth to a healthy infant clearly threatens gender identity, places one's values and motivations for parenthood in question, and forces the couple to re-evaluate the meaning of their relationship. The couple is thrust into a state of emotional disequilibrium.

As such, a crisis requires maximum adjustment (coping), and if one can learn appropriate responses and coping mechanisms, the crisis usually leads to emotional growth and development.[1] Many infertile couples discover, however, that infertility is the first major life crisis that they have confronted as individuals and as a partnership. They describe infertility as akin to the death of a loved one or a divorce. As a result, many find that their coping mechanisms are insufficient to manage the devastating impact of infertility. Self-esteem and self-confidence often plummet, and the relationship can suffer from blame, guilt, frustration, and disappointment.

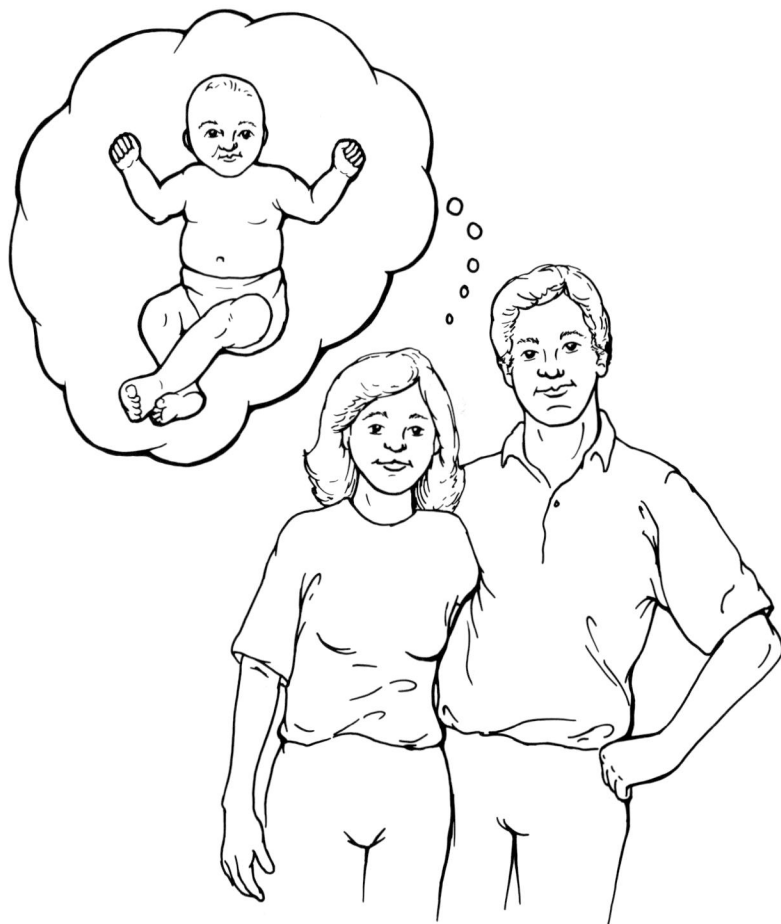

FIGURE 4–1. Most couples expect to have a child together.

EMOTIONAL RESPONSES TO INFERTILITY

Lalos and colleagues[15] found that, during formal interviews with infertility patients, most symptoms can be generally categorized as depression, guilt, and isolation. They also in-

dicate that women are more likely than men to manifest depressive responses to infertility. Men, by contrast, tend to suppress or deny emotional reactions.[15] In addition to the emotional responses of depression, guilt, and isolation, anger can be a significant component in the infertility experience (Table 4–2).

Guilt

Women tend to assume, before the infertility investigation, that they are the cause of the infertility. If the assumptions prove true, they suffer from guilt feelings and decreased self-confidence. Often women diagnosed with infertility begin (often fruitlessly) to search for a cause: They reproach themselves for a past legal abortion, for having had several partners before marriage, for using intrauterine devices (IUDs) or oral contraceptives, and so on. Some women even offer to divorce their husbands so as to free them for the opportunity to have children with other women.

The attempt to determine how and why the infertility happened can take on an obsessional quality. As the condition persists, many patients feel increasingly out of control or powerless. In an effort to dissipate the tremendous anxiety that results from fruitless efforts to conceive, many develop an obsessional defense as an adaptive (albeit unsatisfactory) device to deal with these feelings. These ruminations are such that they can think of little else but the infertility.

Because infertility threatens identity at such a primary

TABLE 4–1. Some Gender Differences and the Infertility Experience	
Men	**Women**
Expectations regarding fatherhood and family may be ambiguous	See motherhood as primary goal of adulthood
Men often initially assume that they are not the cause of the infertility	Women often initially assume that they are the cause of the infertility
In male factor infertility, men may experience strong guilt feelings but are reluctant to express these feelings. They may undergo treatments or move forward with parenting alternatives prematurely	In female factor infertility, women search endlessly for a cause and may reproach themselves for past "misdeeds"
Men often perceive their role as the optimist during the infertility crisis	Women become pessimistic regarding outcomes in an effort to protect themselves from disappointments
Workplace is seen by men as a distraction from the infertility crisis	Infertility often distracts women from efforts to be productive in the workplace
Express anger and irritation toward medical personnel	Feel depressed and helpless

TABLE 4–2. Common Emotional Responses to Infertility*
Guilt
One or both partners assume blame for the infertility. Self-reproach increases and self-esteem decreases
Depression
One or both partners develop a sense of hopelessness, loss and despair, tearfulness, fatigue, anxiety, sleep or eating disturbances, or an inability to concentrate. The onset of menses can often trigger a depression in many infertile couples
Anger
The infertile couple often feels that life has treated them unfairly. They may feel out-of-control, resentful, and angry with others, including family, friends, and medical personnel
Isolation
A sense of social separateness or feeling "left out" of the mainstream of life. Emotional and social isolation negatively impact self-confidence and self-esteem

*The manifestation of these responses may differ significantly between men and women.

level, women have also described themselves as experiencing inferiority or as feeling inferior to the marital relationship. Similarly, the crisis of infertility can also result in a spiritual or religious crisis.[16] The guilt becomes translated into a belief that God is punishing them for past misdeeds and that He is withholding the one thing that they value most—a child.

Men may also experience guilt feelings, particularly if they have a diagnosed male infertility factor.[8] They often are reluctant, however, to express these feelings as well as those of disappointment or grief to their partner. Their reasoning behind this restraint may rest in the notion that they will only contribute further to the emotional distress that the couple already experiences. Problematically they may agree to undergo treatments or move ahead with alternatives, such as donor insemination or adoption, out of guilt or denial rather than as the result of an emotional resolution of the problem.

Men often perceive their roles during the infertility crisis as being the "optimist" during difficult periods when their partners are distraught, discouraged, or depressed. The dynamic seems to occur regardless of which partner carries the diagnosis and may be grounded in sociocultural factors that dictate male behavior. An infertility patient, however, poignantly describes the emotional price that he has paid in being unable to talk about his feelings:

> It is not part of my experience as a male to talk openly of my feelings about failure. Even after 6 years—on and off—of dealing with infertility, it is still difficult for me to allow my feelings to surface. I take refuge in numbness. Numbness allows me to deny my pain, anger, and confusion as my hopes routinely drown in the wake of my wife's menstrual cycle. This denial system has a deadening effect on joy, love, and hope. By losing contact with my own feelings, I also lose contact with the people to whom I am close . . . . I had to confront the code of silence with which men traditionally surround themselves when dealing with infertility. For it is our fear of expressing our feelings on this subject that distances us from ourselves and others.[17]

Feelings of guilt as well as a general sense of inferiority may be exacerbated by the overt and covert demands and expectations of family and friends. The infertile couple may experience overwhelming guilt and sorrow about disappointing or denying grandparents-to-be or potential aunts and uncles. Additionally the couple may be consumed with guilt

about fulfilling their duties and responsibilities related to "carrying on the family name" or providing an heir. Family pressures on the infertile couple may or may not be real. It is not uncommon for those suffering from the emotional anguish of infertility to project their own desires and needs onto others with whom they are emotionally close.

Depression

The depression resulting from infertility may manifest itself in a variety of ways. Women and men describe feelings of sadness and despair, tearfulness, persistent fatigue, sleep or eating disturbances, anxiety or irritability, and pessimism, which are all indications of a depressive state. Lalos and colleagues[15] found that although several infertile women experienced long periods of profound depression, most more commonly described short but recurrent episodes often precipitated by the onset of menses; social events such as baby showers, family holidays, and reunions; or the announcement of a friend's or family member's pregnancy.

Certainly depression is a normal response to the emotional pain and loss engendered by infertility; however, severe, ongoing depression can develop resulting in feelings of hopelessness, an inability to function in daily living, severe anxiety or agitation as well as suicidal ideation or behavior. Clearly this condition requires immediate mental health intervention.

Because depression is frequently a response to loss, it is important to point out ways in which loss is inherent in the condition of infertility. Mahlstedt[12] points to research that has categorized the losses occurring in adulthood that are of greatest clinical significance as factors causing depression. These include real or potential losses of a relationship, health, status or prestige, self-esteem, and self-confidence; the loss of a fantasy or the hope of fulfilling an important fantasy; and the loss of something or someone of great symbolic value. The author delineates how the experience of infertility involves each of these losses.

The loss of a sense of control over one's life and life plans is probably the one factor that significantly underscores the *life crisis* component of infertility. The inability to have a child—something that everyone else seems to do with ease—leaves one feeling intensely vulnerable and helpless (Fig. 4–2). No matter how many physicians with whom the couple consults, no matter how many treatments they undertake, and no matter what they do, there are no certainties or guarantees that they will conceive or give birth to a child. This feeling of powerlessness and loss of control is foreign to many people confronting infertility. Despite their efforts, this problem may not be solved. In addition to the loss of control over the infertility, a loss of control over one's body, one's emotional health, and one's future happiness may also be experienced by one or both partners.

Anger

Most men and women who experience infertility describe feelings of anger, often at life because it has treated them unfairly. This generalized anger and feeling of helplessness, however, can be displaced onto the self (resulting in depres-

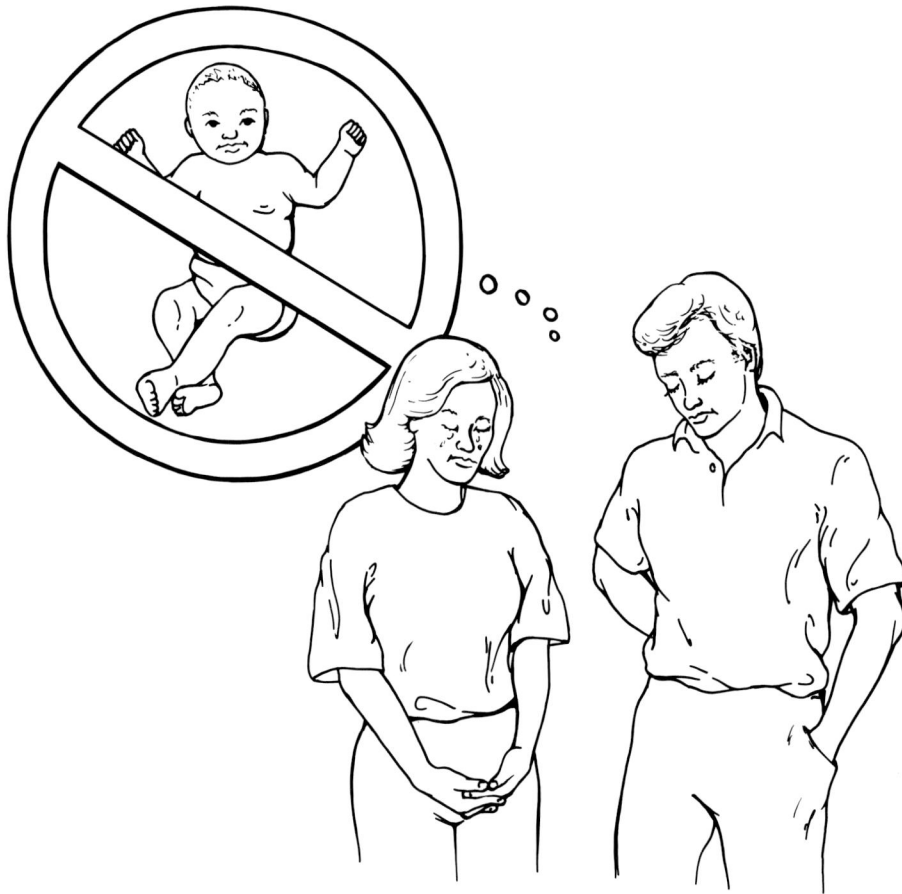

FIGURE 4–2. Infertility leaves the couple feeling sad, helpless, and emotionally vulnerable.

sion), onto one's partner, onto family members and friends, and onto the medical staff or adoption agency.

Anger can be directed at family and friends because they cannot comprehend the pain that infertility creates and they are insensitive to it. Individually these friends and family members, who under other circumstances provide an important source of emotional support, may withdraw or distance themselves so as to avoid uncomfortable moments. When the anger is directed at one's partner, it can be particularly destructive to the relationship. The need to assign blame for causing the infertility or to accuse one's partner of not caring enough or not understanding can have long-term detrimental effects.

Physicians, nurses, and other medical personnel may find themselves working with infertile men and women who are particularly angry or demanding. Although these patients are especially difficult to deal with, it is important to know that these individuals' feelings and behavior usually mask anxiety, fear, and emotional anguish. In addition, the medical staff is sometimes viewed by the couple as exercising control or power over them.

Infertility patients may also develop more irrational targets for their angry feelings. They may become enraged at every pregnant woman they see or at other couples who exhibit happiness and hopefulness about the future. Not infrequently, anger is expressed as belligerence and oppositionalism, and the individual may be unaware that this behavior stems from resentment at life as well as from sorrow and frustration about the infertility.

Problems can also arise with patients who are unable to express their anger in any way or even acknowledge this powerful feeling. They may refrain from doing so because they fear negative repercussions from its expression: a negative pregnancy outcome or rejection and abandonment by one's spouse, family, friends, and medical personnel. They may even fantasize that if they vent their anger, they might lose control over it (and themselves) indefinitely. The inability to express anger and work it through appropriately can potentially result in passive-aggressive or other self-destructive behaviors.

Isolation

Because infertility is inherently sexual and is often considered a "private" problem, many infertile couples find it exceedingly difficult to discuss their problem openly with others. They (often correctly) assume that no one else can understand the extent of the emotional pain, longing, and turmoil that it brings.

Feelings of isolation and social separateness begin to develop when the couple realizes that others around them conceive and bear children effortlessly—that others easily accomplish this life goal. This sense of isolation may develop when the couple is continuously questioned or teased about their childlessness. The need to insulate oneself from the emotional pain brought on by curiosity and by social celebrations such as baby showers, christenings, and family events involving children is acute. These and other events leave the couple feeling "left out" of the mainstream of life (Fig. 4–3).

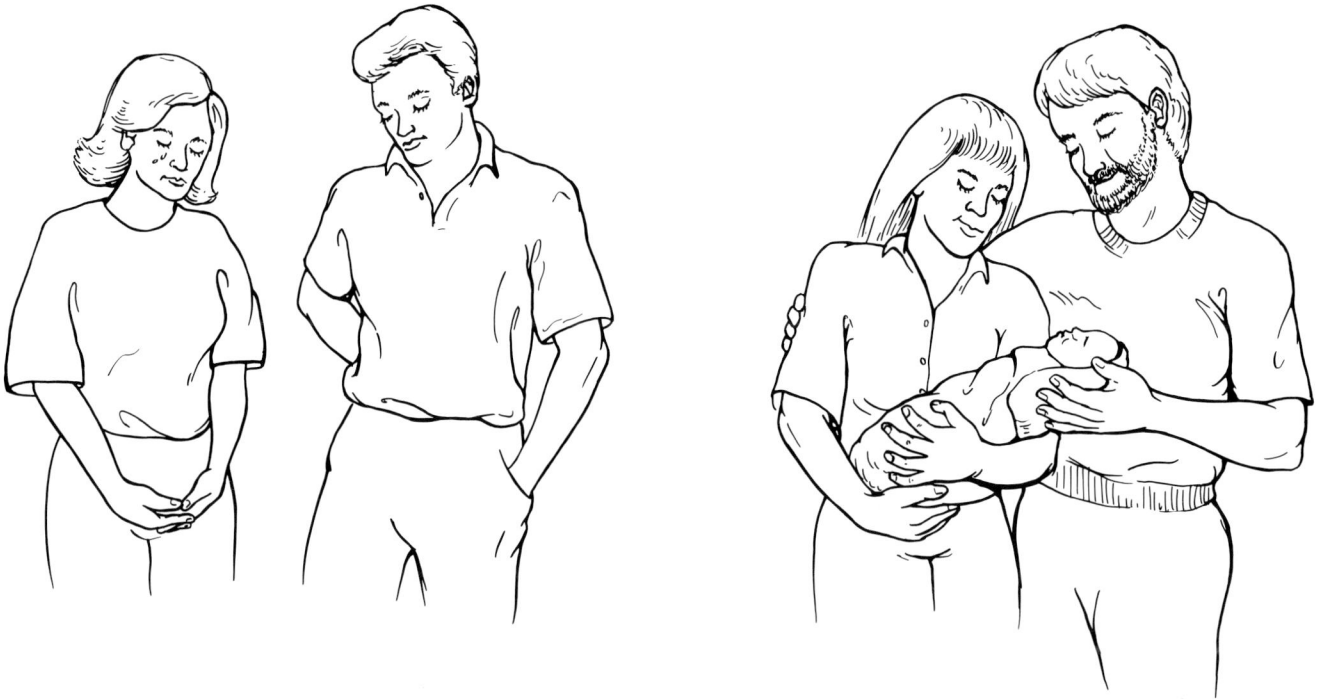

FIGURE 4–3. Infertile couples feel "left out" of the mainstream of life.

Infertility can also sometimes be experienced as shame and embarrassment depending on one's social and cultural environment. Emotional and social isolation has an impact on self-confidence and self-esteem. Infertility can make the couple feel estranged from others, impaired, and prohibited from being a part of a larger social context. A number of authors have underscored the importance of obtaining social support as a means of coping more effectively with the isolation of infertility.[11, 18–20]

IMPACT OF INFERTILITY ON THE COUPLE'S RELATIONSHIP

Infertility not only has significant psychological ramifications for the individual, but also it can deal a powerful blow to the solidity of a marriage. In addition to falling in love with one another, many couples marry because they expect to have children together. When this important life accomplishment is denied them, husbands and wives not only question the meaning of their lives, but also the meaning of their relationship. The powerful feelings surrounding infertility often threaten the one thing that couples need and value most in their relationship: intimacy and emotional closeness.[21]

Because the crisis of infertility is also a crisis in the marriage, many couples are ill-prepared to cope with the uncertainties, fears, and potential losses that infertility encompasses. Infertility can disrupt the intimate marital relationship and create a fear, real or potential, that the marriage will never survive the overwhelming medical and emotional ordeal.

As the infertility crisis heightens, so then does the couple's need for emotional support and nurturance. Difficulties arise between partners because each may be suffering emotionally

and is helpless to change the situation. Partners cannot give one another what they want and need, and they respond to this disappointment by distancing themselves from each other. This occurs despite the clear knowledge that the couple is working toward the same ultimate goal and both partners are willing to undergo significant emotional and medical hardships to achieve it (Table 4–3).

Frequently there are expectations on the part of one partner as to how the other should react to a stressful circumstance. A husband may see his role during the infertility crisis as one of consoling and comforting his wife. Women tend to react to the infertility with significant emotional expression, and they may not understand why their husbands do not behave in an equally distressed manner. Thus, as a husband responds to his partner with calm, reason, and optimism (in an effort to console and comfort), his wife may accuse him of not caring enough about the infertility or of not truly being invested in having a child. As efforts to have a child go unrewarded, thoughts about the infertility can reach obsessional proportions so that many women feel a need to talk about the problem continuously. As the obsession grows, a wife may resent her husband's ability to function effectively at work and distract himself from the problem for longer periods of time. She becomes angry because she is needy, unhappy, and emotional; he is distressed because his wife is

---

TABLE 4–3. The Infertile Couple's Search for Intimacy

1. When the lifelong goal of conceiving a child goes unmet, the couple may feel angry, anxious, and fearful
2. Infertility may be the first life crisis that the couple has faced together, and they may be ill-prepared to cope effectively
3. Husband and wife may view their roles quite differently throughout the infertility experience yet each may feel misunderstood or uncared for
4. Because of fear, anxiety, and emotional neediness, the infertile couple may be unable to communicate with one another

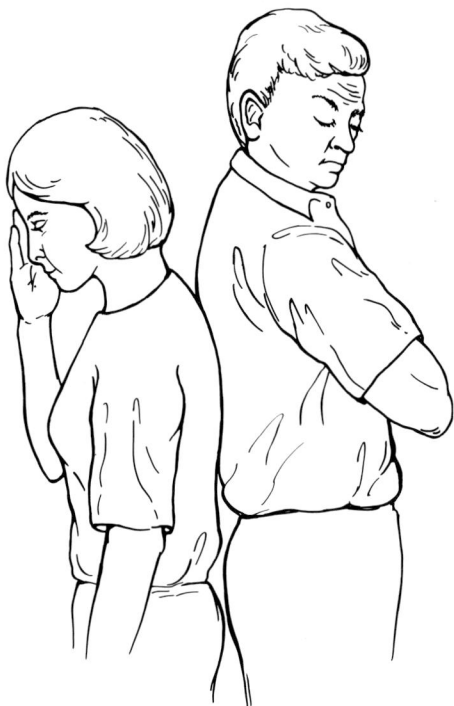

FIGURE 4–4. As infertility persists, the couple may emotionally withdraw from one another, feeling unable to communicate.

inconsolable. As both partners feel enormously helpless, they may withdraw from one another, feeling tense, angry, and alone (Fig. 4–4).

The other dynamic experienced by some infertile couples is usually more difficult to manage. These are the couples who are unable to talk at all with one another about the infertility. Undoubtedly these couples are concerned and worry often about the problem. Yet the infertility is so emotionally painful that to talk about it can be excruciatingly difficult. In an effort to hide their feelings and protect their partners, these couples seldom discuss the infertility or their feelings about it with one another. Even while undergoing medical diagnosis and treatment, neither partner is willing or able to risk breaking their unspoken code of silence. Men and women may also visit physicians alone so as not to "trouble" or "inconvenience" their partners with the medical details. Husband and wife therefore suffer silently, sometimes resentfully, behaving as strangers around this deeply powerful issue in their lives.

In either of these two cases, the support and caring normally experienced by married couples can be significantly restricted at a time when they need it more than ever before. Certainly if a couple has a healthy relationship before the onset of the infertility crisis, their chances of overcoming the many emotional hurdles inherent in the diagnosis and treatment process are good. Many couples, in fact, openly state that their marriages have grown stronger and closer as a result of this unexpected, unwelcome life circumstance.[11] Couples who generally have had a problematic or dysfunctional relationship are likely to find that difficulties intensify with the stress of infertility procedures.

When help is sought from a mental health professional, it is more likely that the woman in the infertile couple will see

herself as needing assistance in coping with the problem. Not infrequently, women present without their spouses to counseling or psychotherapy by stating that "He [husband] is doing fine with the infertility, but I'm having a terrible time dealing with it." Although it is generally not inappropriate for one or the other partner of the couple to seek individual help from a mental health professional, they should be reminded that infertility is always an issue that affects and involves the *couple* and not only the individual with the diagnosed medical problem. The relationship between husband and wife is inevitably affected by the ongoing stresses and strains brought on by medical interventions, social and family pressures, sexual demands, and the reawakening of old conflicts and issues regarding self-image and competence.

Certainly there are partners among whom there are different degrees of interest and motivation to have a child. One may be ambivalent about becoming a parent and unwilling to undergo extensive medical treatment, whereas the other is consumed with the idea of having a child. This basic difference in long-term goals can obviously lead to significant problems in the marital relationship. Ultimately open and effective communication will be key to enabling the couple to withstand and resolve the infertility crisis (Fig. 4–5).

INFERTILITY AND THE SEXUAL RELATIONSHIP

Infertility often has a profound impact on the couple's sexual relationship.[22, 23] Under these circumstances, sex can become disappointing and emotionally painful because it has ceased to be the pleasurable, spontaneous vehicle for bringing a child into the world. Thus, sexual intercourse, no longer "love-making," instead becomes routine, mechanized,

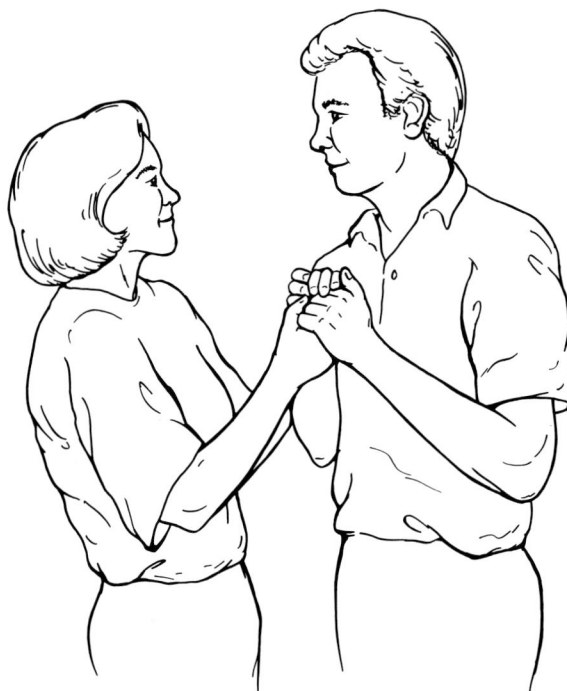

FIGURE 4–5. As the infertile couple begins to develop more effective coping strategies and communication skills, the relationship becomes stronger.

and precisely timed. It becomes, by necessity, "sex on demand." Shapiro[24] points out that the sources of stress and strain the infertility brings into a sexual relationship are primarily threefold:

1. The recognition that procreation rather than sexual pleasure is the goal of most efforts at lovemaking.
2. The stress of the imagined presence of others (medical professionals) in the bedroom.
3. The demise of self-esteem as infertility persists.

Again because fertility is so intimately tied in most people's minds to sexuality and identity as a sexual being, it is not surprising that some infertility patients begin to think of themselves as inadequate as well as sexually undesirable. With the loss of self-esteem may also come a loss of sexual desire or capacity for orgasm. In women who are infertile, the most common sexual complaints by far are frigidity and changes in orgasmic achievement. Vaginismus is also a frequent complaint, which lends itself to therapy directed toward relaxation and reassurance.[25] Partners may find themselves becoming more and more distant and isolated from one another in the one place they have felt closest and most intimate—the bedroom. Sexuality then takes on a new definition: failure and despair. The bedroom becomes a painful reminder, a place to avoid.

As a couple's sexual relationship becomes impaired, it can also impair medical treatment. For example, temporary impotence may commonly occur when a Huhner or postcoital test is scheduled. The need to have intercourse to produce a semen sample under pressure can be extremely difficult if not impossible for some men. Their partners, in turn, may feel angry and resentful or accept responsibility for the husband's failure to perform.[25]

Sexual difficulties or dysfunction may be long-standing problems that existed before the infertility crisis. Burns[26] suggests that past traumatic sexual experience, inadequate or inappropriate sexual information, feelings of inadequacy or confusion about one's psychosexual role, depression, or poor self-image may contribute significantly to the impaired sexual relationship. In these cases, infertility may act as a catalyst in bringing sexual difficulties to the surface. Under the best of circumstances, the infertility crisis can ultimately enable the couple to improve their sexual relationship, often with the help of an informed, sensitive physician or sex therapist.

It is not surprising that infertility patients cannot feel positive about themselves as healthy, "normal" people. Shapiro[24] points out that those working in the health and mental health professions cannot protect couples from all the threats that infertility presents to a satisfying, fulfilling sexual relationship, but there are efforts that can be made to assist the couple in coming to terms with their "bedroom demons." These include

1. Helping the couple bring sexual issues into the open. Many may need the professional's reassurance that they are not sexually maladjusted but are responding normally to the strains that infertility puts on sex.
2. Encouraging the couple to be innovative about their sexual practices so as to counteract the sexual routinization and monotony that arises from such purposeful lovemaking.
3. Assessing adequately the extent of depression that an individual or couple is experiencing as well as underlying

feelings of helplessness. These factors can interfere significantly with libido.

Once a couple is given a final diagnosis of infertility or told that they are no longer appropriate candidates for the assisted reproductive technologies (ART), or once highly sought-after pregnancy is achieved, the couple may also find further complicating factors to re-establishing a satisfying sexual relationship. First, with the final word that a couple will not be able to have a biologic child together, a period of intense mourning also takes its toll on a sexual relationship.[24] Feelings of apathy and depression or a desire to avoid sex altogether is not uncommon at such an emotionally difficult time. Infertile couples who do achieve pregnancy often avoid sexual intercourse indefinitely for fear that they will cause a miscarriage or damage the fetus. Rather than "sex on schedule," the modus operandi is "no sex" despite the obstetrician's reassurances.

In either case, it becomes the work of health and mental health professionals to help couples acknowledge the loss of a healthy, satisfying sexual relationship and assist them in the work of renewal. As with other psychological factors of infertility, couples need to be made aware that their sexual relationships will take time to heal. The healing process takes differing amounts of time depending on the individual and on the couple. These patients may need assistance in learning to be more imaginative and creative with their sexuality. For those couples who at one time enjoyed an active, mutually pleasurable, and spontaneous sex life, a return to that relationship can be difficult and time-consuming, but it can be done, and it must be done if they are to recover appropriately from the chronic and emotionally painful circumstances of infertility.

PREGNANCY LOSS

The loss of a pregnancy can have complex psychological ramifications for a couple.[27] Many women who have been able to conceive tend to view themselves as failures because of the inability of their bodies to carry a healthy child to term.[28] Often those who have suffered a pregnancy loss feel personally responsible for the loss and thus experience overwhelming guilt and fear. A pregnancy loss is mourned regardless of whether the loss was early in the pregnancy or after birth, and the initial expression of grief may be as great with a miscarriage as with a stillbirth. The intensity and the duration of the grief, however, tend to be less in a miscarriage.[29]

Clearly there has been increased interest in the psychological aspects of losing a pregnancy, although some authors believe that more emphasis has been placed on changing attitudes toward those who have experienced stillbirth and neonatal death rather than those who experience miscarriage.[30–33] As a result, the professional as well as the lay community still tends to regard miscarriage as a relatively insignificant event from which a woman can quickly recover with no lasting psychological effects on either the woman or her partner.[30] With pregnancy loss in general, there has been cultural denial with respect to its impact on the couple and a tendency not to define miscarriage or stillbirth as a legitimate source of grief.[34] Those who usually provide emotional support, such as family members and friends, often are not completely informed of the situation or are too uncomfortable to ask about it. Additionally a woman may not be encouraged to cry, grieve, or talk about the loss. As a result, there is a sense on the part of the couple that their feelings are unjustified, and they may try to deny them—even to themselves. Medical personnel can perpetuate these feelings of isolation by tending to minimize the emotional and psychological effects of the pregnancy loss.

For couples who experience grief and bereavement after pregnancy loss, there is often a lack of community support either because the loss is regarded with little importance or because the loss is generally not spoken of. For example, there has historically been an absence of rites and rituals, which denies the couple emotional comfort and legitimizes the grieving process. Often if a woman is not given an opportunity to deal with her grief, there may be continuing feelings of sadness, inadequacy, and fearfulness as well as impairment in the relationships with her partner and children.[35]

Men as well as women can experience a profound emotional reaction to a pregnancy loss, although the degree of a father's grief tends to correlate more closely to the gestational age of the fetus.[36] Fathers, in fact, are most often forgotten in a family bereaved by a pregnancy loss. The husband's concern for the physical and emotional well-being of his wife often overrides his own feelings of sadness and grief. His role becomes that of comforter and emotional caretaker of the woman.[30]

As with the inability to conceive, stress within the couple's relationship may occur after the loss. Frequently this is because the man and woman go through the grieving process in different ways and at varying rates.

Although it has been found that there is no significant difference between perinatal grief reactions in women suffering miscarriage, stillbirth, or neonatal death, Greenfeld and Walther[33] point out that there are important considerations that must be made to understand fully the psychological implications for women who suffer recurrent pregnancy loss. Their findings suggest that "both the cumulative grief and the increasing ambivalence associated with the recurrent difficulty cause ongoing emotional problems for couples in this group." Women in this group may, with each pregnancy, begin the grieving process and separation from the pregnancy before the actual loss occurs simply in anticipation of another failure. Men also indicate feelings of helplessness, lack of control, anger, guilt, and acute loss of self-esteem. It is recommended that couples who experience recurrent pregnancy loss be provided with reassurance, clear statements about prognosis, and psychological support throughout the medical investigation and subsequent pregnancy.[32]

Couples who are able to conceive after infertility treatment and subsequently suffer a pregnancy loss, in all likelihood, experience this loss differently than couples who have had no difficulty with conception. In addition to the feeling that there is something innately defective about them, women who lose a pregnancy after prolonged attempts to conceive may suffer from a severe grief reaction.[33] In this case, the couple experiences a dual loss—the loss of a much longed-for fantasy child as well as the real loss of the pregnancy.[37]

Several authors[30, 33, 36] have described factors that are important in coping with a pregnancy loss and that influence the couple's adjustment to the loss. These include

1. Obtaining emotional support from family and friends.

2. Obtaining supportive and sensitive responses from professionals during the loss.

3. Obtaining information from professionals concerning the possibility of loss as well as about the loss itself.

4. Obtaining community recognition and ritualization of the loss.

5. Obtaining support from others who have also experienced pregnancy loss (support groups).

6. Obtaining treatment from a mental health professional in cases of severe depression or pathologic grief reactions or in cases of severe anxiety regarding subsequent pregnancies.

Medical facilities have begun to establish bereavement care for couples who have miscarried or suffered a stillbirth. The purpose of such care is to attempt to make the loss a reality, to provide immediate emotional support and preparation for the grieving process, and to impart information on community resources to help the families once they leave the hospital or clinic.[34] Followup care after a pregnancy loss can be of great significance to the couple in light of the often prolonged emotional aftermath. Wells[31] stresses, in fact, that the physician can play a valuable role in alleviating the patient's feelings of guilt, grief, and frustration.

SECONDARY INFERTILITY

The emotional impact of secondary infertility can, for some couples, be no less severe than for those who have never conceived nor borne a child. Couples with secondary infertility experience great sadness, longing, anxiety, and pain. They describe the joy of parenthood and feel profoundly deprived because it now eludes them.

For those who had difficulty having a child in the past, they are now faced with reliving their infertility and its painful implications again. For couples who had no difficulty conceiving or carrying a pregnancy, the initial reaction to the news of their infertility is that of confusion and disbelief. Some, in fact, may deny the possibility of infertility and delay the medical investigation. Even after having sought treatment, denial may continue.

Similarly, people with only one child find themselves in the paradoxical position of being a biologic parent and being infertile. For many, it is a confusing state. Although maintaining an active parenting role, these individuals feel different and apart from the "normal" family. Bound to all of these emotional dynamics is the societal pressure to produce more than one child.

Similar to the childless couple, those with secondary infertility can develop and use coping skills to deal with their emotional pain and frustration. It is first important to recognize that this is a real problem fraught with feelings of guilt, depression, and frustration. Some may tell a couple to "just relax," but a thorough medical evaluation is crucial. As a couple begins to explore and undergo medical treatment, they may also have to consider and decide on another alternative to having a biologic child. Support from RESOLVE or help from a trained mental health professional can be useful to couples who may need assistance in sorting through the many complex issues and feelings that arise during the difficult struggle with secondary infertility.

INFERTILITY AND MIDLIFE

Many women in their late 30s and early 40s have postponed marriage or childbearing to obtain their educations, establish themselves in careers, and become financially secure. These aspirations frequently have worked against the decision to have children.[38] The passage of time, however, alters the way many women feel about motherhood by changing their perceptions about themselves as well as about the world around them. Additionally these changes may also have to do with having a new sense of maturity as well as a feeling of accomplishment. Thus, as women—and men—feel more sure about themselves, their feelings and ideas about children and parenthood may also change.

As a couple moves into midlife, they must also begin recognizing and coming to terms with their own immortality.[2] For many, parenthood is a part of successfully completing an important stage in life. As couples begin to see and understand the passage of their own lives, the need to pass along life experiences to new generations enhances the meaning of life.

Men and women in midlife who have made the decision to have children are frequently thwarted by the inability to conceive or by recurrent miscarriages. For women, the realities of the biologic clock cannot be overlooked. At this point, many couples are faced with *dual crises*—infertility as well as the developmental life changes that normally occur in the middle years.

As women reach menopause, they begin to realize that the option of conceiving and bearing a child is closed to them. Just as the array of other life choices begins to narrow, the loss of this ability to choose to have a child can result in sadness and deep disappointment. The realization of this "missed opportunity" can also lead to self-recrimination and depression. Occasionally this painful emotional circumstance can lead to the need for mental health intervention.

EMOTIONAL FACTORS AS A CAUSE OF INFERTILITY

Although the psychological consequences of infertility are well substantiated, it is less clear what impact psychological disturbances may have on fertility. As recently as the late 1960s, it was commonly believed that reproductive failure was the result of psychological and emotional factors. Psychogenic infertility occurred because of unconscious anxiety about sexual feelings,[39] ambivalence toward motherhood, unresolved Oedipal conflict,[40, 41] or conflicts of gender identity.[42, 43] Cases of idiopathic infertility were most certainly seen as the obvious result of psychological and emotional disturbances.

Advances in reproductive endocrinology and medical technology as well as in psychological research have de-emphasized the significance of psychopathology as the basis of infertility. There has, in turn, been greater empiric concentration on the psychological sequelae and their impact on gender identity, social functioning, and sexuality.

Several authors indicate that sexual dysfunctions may result in the inability to conceive.[44, 45] Because reproduction and sexuality are so closely intertwined, marital and sexual problems may be hidden under the guise of infertility.[46] A

fear of parenthood, for example, can lead to anxiety and sexual dysfunction and consequently to infertility. Similarly, amenorrhea as well as other types of endocrine and reproductive dysfunction has sometimes been shown to be stress induced and may occur throughout a woman's reproductive life.[47] Others have hypothesized that social factors may be a significant component of the overall psychological distress syndrome, which appears to be a causal part of infertility.[48]

Although the notion of a psychogenic basis for infertility is not an entirely unreasonable one, most current research has found no strong empiric evidence behind this theory.[49] There is overwhelming evidence that infertility can cause stress and that stress can have an adverse effect on physiologic function, thereby affecting fertility outcomes. Möller and Fällström's[50] study indicates that an obsession with or a *fixation* on the desire to have a child and the resulting stress from that wish can decrease the chances of having a child. Their model of causes and consequences of infertility (Fig. 4–6) also suggests that stress can be a contributing factor to infertility. It is also *increased* as a result of the infertile condition, creating a vicious cycle, which may then further impair the couple's ability to conceive.

Despite the circular aspects of stress and infertility, it appears, however, that the effects of stress on men and women seem not to be so deleterious to the body as they are to the psyche. Domar and colleagues[51, 52] have hypothesized that stress reduction, based on the elicitation of the relaxation response, increases the potential for conception. Their studies also clearly demonstrated that in women with idiopathic infertility, the eliciting of the relaxation response was capable of reducing anxiety, depression, anger, and fatigue, while increasing a sense of well-being. Domar's group behavioral treatment program for many patients, including those who had not conceived, reported significant subjective improvements, such as increased feelings of control and coping strategies for feeling better.

PSYCHOLOGICAL FACTORS INHERENT IN ASSISTED REPRODUCTIVE TECHNOLOGIES

Many couples who seek treatment via the ART have faced chronic infertility. As a result, they bring with them a number of significant psychological issues and concerns on presentation to a program. These may include exaggerated and uncomfortable dependency needs, generalized feelings of loss, and a lack of a sense of control over life decisions (helplessness). Such powerful issues create anxiety and stress, often leading to emotional regression.

Similar to other infertility patients, couples in the ART are in crisis, and their difficulties are manifested in a variety of ways depending on the particular personality structure and coping mechanisms of the patient. The medical team often describes individual patients in a variety of ways:

- Angry and demanding
- Passive and compliant
- Cavalier
- Depressed and guilt-ridden
- Fatigued
- Hopeless or inappropriately optimistic

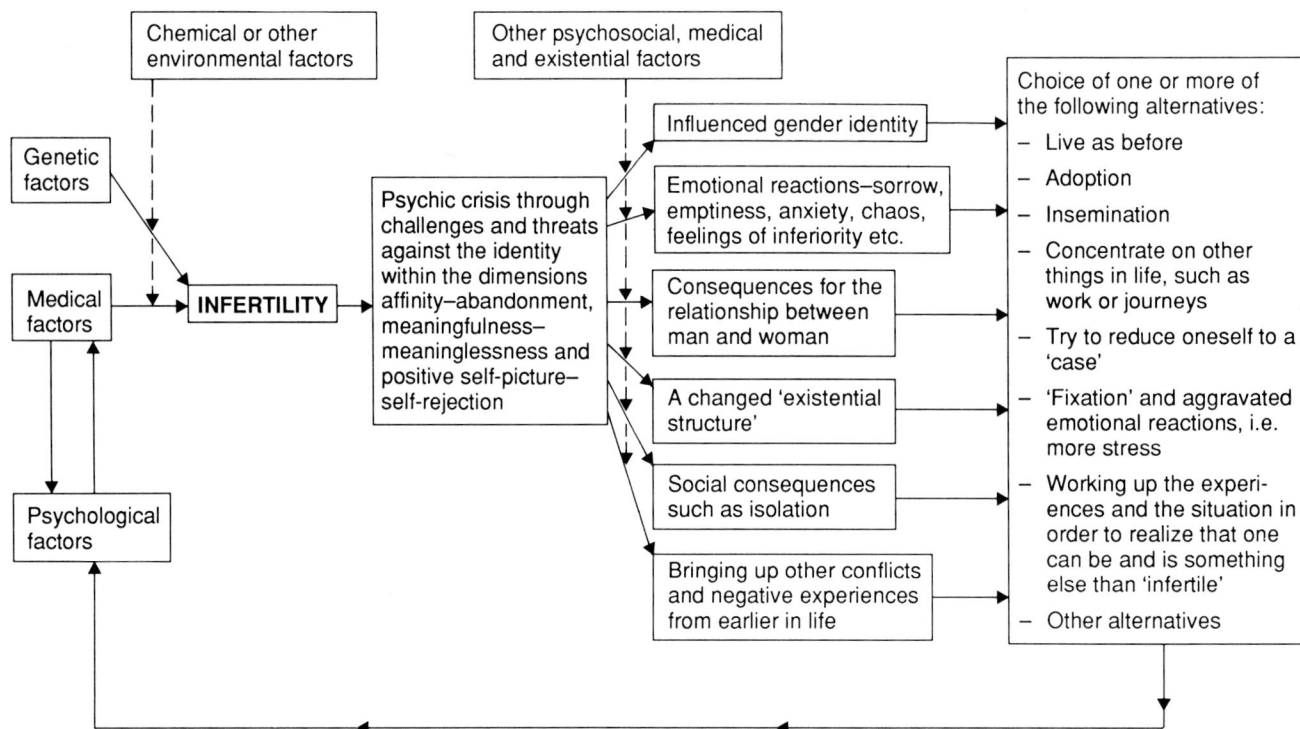

FIGURE 4–6. Schematic model of causes and consequences of infertility. (From Möller A, Fällström K. Psychological consequences of infertility: a longitudinal study. J Psychosom Obstet Gynaecol 1991; 12:241.)

- Expressing somatic complaints
- Demonstrating exaggerated fears regarding various aspects of the procedures, e.g., injections, ultrasound scans, and egg retrieval and transfer

Although these are only descriptive categories, the psychological reality for these couples goes deeper than the above-listed simple adjectives. It is a reality that health professionals need to be aware of to look beyond the infertile couples' presenting behaviors.

By the time most couples undertake an advanced reproductive technology, they have depended on physicians, nurses, and other medical personnel to help them reach an illusive goal: to conceive and bear a child. That dependency can be an uncomfortable one for many patients. Their psychological stress can be exacerbated by inconsistent communication, inadequate patient education, and poor coordination of medical strategies on the part of medical personnel involved in the couple's treatment.[53] Many of these couples, in fact, have suffered a deep narcissistic injury from which many never fully recover, although most learn to cope with it.

Thus, health professionals in the ART meet with patients who not only require help with medical problems, but also who are emotionally and psychologically wounded. Although one might anticipate that these patients are in a state of moderate-to-severe psychopathology, it is this author's impression that many find their patients surprisingly well integrated, with sometimes surprising inner resources for coping with what most patients consider to be the greatest crisis of their lives. A number of studies have corroborated this as well.[54, 55] What is seen instead are frequently normal responses to that which is viewed as an abnormal situation—chronic and unrelenting infertility.[56]

Most clinicians working in the area of the ART see the goal of such treatments as the achievement of pregnancy or, better, an "ongoing" pregnancy. That, too, is obviously the goal of the couple. In fact, that goal is so powerful and compelling for them that *not* to achieve pregnancy on any given cycle not only indicates a failure to conceive, but also may imply to couples that they have failed as human beings—as competent, capable people. Thus, at the end of a failed cycle, at any point in the procedure, the loss is magnified—the loss of a dream child and the chipping away of another piece of self-esteem. As one patient put it, "I feel like a disabled person, and I can't seem to get that idea out of my mind."

Most couples entering into in vitro fertilization/gamete intrafallopian transfer (IVF/GIFT) programs focus anxiously on one primary concern: *failure of the procedure.* To compound this anxiety, couples usually enter this treatment correctly sensing that any control they have over the outcome of this is relatively superficial.

To gain a better sense of control, couples who undertake a procedure in the ART need to feel prepared for both the medical and the emotional processes that lie before them. Their understanding of the stresses involved can be expanded beyond the fear of failure, and their goals for undergoing these taxing procedures need to be broadened beyond that of achieving pregnancy. Couples in the ART cannot control the outcome of the procedure, but they can be helped to control their responses to the various phases of the process and to the overall outcome.[51, 53]

To assist patients in expanding their goals, health care providers in the ART also must clarify and expand their own goals for the patient. The medical team may then be doing themselves service as well as the infertile couple. They become less likely to fall victim to meeting couples' compelling, inexhaustible needs to conceive through these procedures. Instead it may be that the couple's and the medical team's goals can be multifaceted and almost as significant as achieving pregnancy. These goals might include

1. Obtaining a definitive diagnosis.
2. Helping the couple end treatment.
3. Assisting the couple to feel that they have done the best they could.

If these goals can be integrated more firmly into the medical staff's way of thinking, they can also become real and acceptable goals for the couple as well.

Perhaps not surprisingly, IVF/GIFT can lead to closure for many couples who do not achieve pregnancy.[53] They feel that they have tried everything and now can begin to face the painful reality that they will not be able to have a child together. Couples sometimes come to this resolution after one attempt; others may be unwilling to leave treatment even after six or more trials.

In addition to the above-mentioned goals, there is another, which has to do with confidence-building in patients. That goal is to assist them in feeling that they can manage—or cope—with any outcome, at any state along the way. They may not like that outcome—they may be grief-stricken, angry, sad, or disappointed, but they must be helped to believe that they can and will manage.

How can this be done? First, it is of primary importance that medical personnel truly try to understand each couple's struggles, fears, and vulnerabilities. That understanding, in turn, provides an opportunity to establish a relationship with the couple. It is that *relationship*—one that conveys genuine caring and concern, one that demonstrates *respect* for the couple—that helps to rebuild and maintain self-esteem. In addition, most studies regarding psychological characteristics of IVF participants uniformly indicate that although psychopathologic conditions do exist, the majority of couples entering a program do present with normal personality functioning.[54, 55] Therefore, it seems appropriate that health and mental health providers should focus on assisting couples with the stresses that they encounter through the various stages of the procedure.

Because so many aspects of the ART are unpredictable (e.g., response to medication, oocyte retrieval, fertilization, and outcome of ovum transfer), it is probable that many of these couples find themselves in a situation that is clearly *not* complementary to their inherent personality needs. To address this discrepancy, programs in the ART can provide specific strategies for coping during each phase of the process. Merari and coworkers[57] support this notion by suggesting that success in IVF treatment may depend, in part, on differential modes of coping with anxiety and depression, also involving hormonal or endorphin mediation. Some coping strategies for managing the ART procedure are noted on Table 4–4.[53]

The decision to end treatment can be a heart-wrenching one for couples who had hoped—or perhaps assumed—that medical technology would ultimately reward them a biologic child. Many couples cling to the fantasy that "one more try" would have resulted in a healthy pregnancy; as a result, the

TABLE 4–4. Assisted Reproductive Technologies: Strategies for Coping
Before Procedure
Accurate and adequate information about medical, financial, emotional, and logistical aspects of the procedure
Consultation with the nurse coordinator or other nursing personnel
Support groups or meetings with mental health professional
Information and referrals regarding options other than assisted reproductive technologies
During Procedure
In vitro fertilization telephone support
Support and access to mental health professional
Printed recommendations for managing free time
Encouraging open communication between partners and between patients and staff. Staff accessibility
After Procedure
Followup calls or appointments with couples
Access to and direct referrals to mental health professionals when necessary
Support groups
Evaluation and feedback from couples

decision to end treatment seems like "giving up" or a lack of an ability to persevere and beat the odds.[24] Often these couples have lived a lifetime with the notion that if they try hard enough, they will succeed. Many patients may need to examine whether it is a baby they want, or proof of their fertility, or affirmation of their gender identity after so many sad disappointments. Some seem to lose sight of their ultimate goals—to become parents—and instead become obsessively caught up in the importance of conception. Mental health professionals may need to explore this and other issues with couples if decision making and resolution are to occur.[53]

Lastly couples often enter treatment in the ART with a profound ability to deny the reality of the odds against them. The literature indicates that they leave after one or two attempts for two main reasons: (1) The financial burden is too great, and (2) the stress of the procedure creates too much anxiety, depression, disruption, and strain.[58] Nonetheless, it appears that the vast majority of individuals do believe that trying an ART procedure is worth the effort.

PSYCHOLOGICAL CONSIDERATIONS SURROUNDING THE USE OF DONOR GAMETES

Although the use of donated oocytes or sperm appears to be a quick and "reasonable" solution to some couples' infertility problems, it is a decision that is fraught with long-term psychosocial and emotional implications. The use of donor gametes is not, in fact, another "treatment" or "cure" for infertility. The physician's recommendation that a couple consider donation as a potential means of providing them with a child brings with it a number of important concerns.

First, this recommendation in all likelihood follows a statement to the couple that there are no medical treatments available that will enable them to have a child that is completely genetically theirs. The finality of the couple's infertility must then be accepted, and the accompanying losses must be grieved for. In the midst of their profound grief, therefore, the couple is confronted with an option that feels either completely untenable or is seen as a "quick fix" to a seemingly unbearable pain. Even for couples pursuing treatment via the ART, the option of *donor sperm backup* is frequently provided for couples when there is a significant male factor. Under these difficult, uncertain circumstances, the couple may agree to gamete donation before they are truly emotionally ready to do so. Couples need time to grieve over the finality of their infertility, and they need time to consider the other options that lead to parenthood. For example, it has been recommended that couples should wait at least 6 months after learning of the definitiveness of their infertility before moving ahead with the use of donor gametes. As well as giving couples time to grieve, this time period also provides an opportunity to consider many psychosocial issues inherent in the donor alternative and to prepare for emotional demands of this procedure.[59, 60]

Second, infertile couples and medical professionals alike need to acknowledge that gamete donation is dramatically different than having a child using the couple's own gametes. The couple initially set out to have their genetic child, and when this goal cannot be obtained, the couple must come to terms with the long-term ramifications of donor conception. The decision to use donor gametes has an impact on the marriage, and it most assuredly has an impact on the child.[59, 61]

Specifically the writings of Edelmann[59] and those of Mahlstedt and Greenfeld[60] point to several issues that need to be examined so couples can feel prepared and comfortable with having a child by donor conception. These issues include the following.

IMPACT OF THE DONATION ON THE COUPLE

A diagnosis of infertility can be damaging to a man or woman's self-esteem and gender identity. A recommendation of gamete donation in no way mitigates the loss of one's fertility. Couples should be encouraged to voice their fears and concerns about this alternative and to explore their fantasies about their future lives as a family. Psychological counseling and support enable couples to consider issues as they relate to individual values and self-esteem, to the marriage, and to the potential child. In confronting the impact of the donation on the couple, some couples may feel that this alternative is not the solution to their childlessness, whereas others may come to feel that it is the best option for them.

SECRECY

Secrecy about gamete donation has been the "modus operandi" for most couples and medical professionals. It is important, however, that the reasons behind the need for secrecy be explored carefully. Does it have to do with the need to protect the man or woman from the stigma of infertility? Does it have to do with a fear that the nongenetic parent will be less loved by the child or that the child will only be "burdened" by the information? Does it have to do with the fact that the child will be deemed "unacceptable" by family and friends?

Keeping family secrets tends to imply that there is something "bad" or "wrong" within the family. Is that, in fact, how the couple truly feels about the donor conception? Most certainly the decision to maintain secrecy "places a lie at the center of the most basic of relationships, the one between parent and child."[36] As a child becomes increasingly integrated into the couple's life, this deception may become a greater and greater hardship for the couple.

Whether secrecy is harmful to the child is a debatable issue, particularly in light of the lack of research data on this subject. If secrecy is not maintained, what are the effects on the child? Most certainly in cases of sister oocyte donation as well as with other known gamete donors, the maintenance of secrecy should be openly discouraged. The risks of the secret being shared inappropriately with the child or being overheard by the child may be great and could be potentially destructive to the child's self-esteem and family relationships.

Couples who choose to maintain secrecy should be assisted in anticipating (1) the many questions that will require lying, (2) the burden that secrecy will place on the marital relationship, (3) the possibility that one partner will change his or her mind about maintaining the secret, and (4) the possibility that extenuating circumstances might require sharing the secret. For those who do wish to inform their offspring regarding their donor conception, Probasco[63] posits that sharing the information can be seen as a "building block process," which spans a number of childhood developmental stages. She adds that underscoring the decision to tell is an unconditional love and acceptance of the child.

With the ongoing use of donor gametes in reproductive health and especially in the ART, the need to investigate parents' adaptation to having a donor child should not be understated. There is also a need to know more about the possible deleterious effects of both providing information and maintaining secrecy on the child and the family.[60]

DONOR ANONYMITY

We are told that one reason the practice of donor anonymity came about in the United States was because of a lack of legal protection for social fathers and donors.[64] Presumably this is also the case for the use of anonymous oocyte donors. For many, donor anonymity is considered crucial for maintaining secrecy around this parenting option.

The question has been raised as to whether donor procedures should be more anonymous than current adoption procedures.[62] As in adoption, having extensive social, medical, and education information about donors' backgrounds may be extremely helpful to couples who plan to tell their children about their donor origins and who wish to develop positive, comfortable feelings about the circumstances of the conception, not only for the child, but also for themselves.

Donors themselves may also be less concerned about anonymity than has been thought. Mahlstedt and Probasco's[64] investigation of sperm donors indicates that not only are they willing to provide extensive psychosocial information, but also these donors believe that potential parents and children have a right to this information.[64]

SOCIAL ATTITUDES

Because of the wide range of social attitudes regarding the use of sperm and oocyte donation for conception, it is important that infertile couples explore carefully their own sensitivities and vulnerabilities to public opinion regarding this procedure. Religious prohibitions must also be considered by those whose religious faith plays an active part in their lives.

In this case, conception does not involve the conjugal act. Fears on the part of the couple that they will be rejected by their religious community or that the child will be shunned by family members, especially grandparents, often underpin the couple's decision to maintain secrecy. These fears should be appreciated and addressed, and couples may need to learn how to feel comfortable in defending themselves against negative social attitudes.

RELATIONSHIP BETWEEN THE INFERTILE COUPLE AND THE MEDICAL STAFF

As noted previously, not only the inability to conceive, but also the resulting medical evaluation and treatment can be highly emotionally charged and stressful for the infertile couple. The medical staff, physicians, nurses, and other professional and administrative personnel can have a profound impact on the couple's sense of well-being and can either significantly increase or reduce the psychological stress that the couple experiences.

Contacting a physician for an initial infertility consultation can be especially anxiety producing for a couple. They are often in a state of disbelief and denial about the mere possibility of infertility. The couple neither feels nor looks ill, and the inability to conceive is virtually incomprehensible for these people, especially in light of all the years of conscientious birth control.

The infertile couple is also frightened about seeing a physician. Many openly express fears about potential medical tests and procedures. Others fear that they will be told that they will never be able to have a child, that they will fail.

Seemingly by its very nature, the inability to conceive or bear a child arouses feelings of shock, anxiety, and concern.

As couples embark on the journey of medical diagnosis and treatment, they must often face difficult decisions regarding treatment options, when to end treatment, and when to consider other parenting alternatives. Many sensitive and vulnerable couples need help with these decisions. Most often, they turn to their physicians for advice and guidance (Fig. 4–7).

Physicians and other medical personnel, however, although trained to manage physiologic and medical considerations, treatment protocols, and office procedures, may not be especially well equipped to help patients and couples address their many psychological concerns. Möller and Fällström[1] comment that "the medical care system takes a great responsibility on itself when intervening in situations that, like infertility . . . are existentially loaded." Appleton[65] also stresses that infertility is a health care problem that has clear physiologic, psychological, and social implications. Medical care therefore must go beyond the patient's physical treatments. Emotional stresses must be a concern, and health care professionals must be careful not to add additional stress to the infertile couple's existing problems.[65]

Nothing can be more frustrating, painful, or humiliating for infertility patients, for example, than having to wait several hours beyond the scheduled appointment time to meet with the physician and not be given an explanation or an apology. Nothing is more irritating than meeting with a new physician who is ignorant of the couple's medical history despite the fact that the couple was required to send all medical records weeks or even months in advance of the appointment. The simple failure on the part of the physician or nurse to introduce himself or herself properly to new patients is also disrespectful and demeaning. Even minor "oversights" on the part of the physician or medical staff can have great significance to couples who are emotionally wounded and rendered powerless by their infertility.

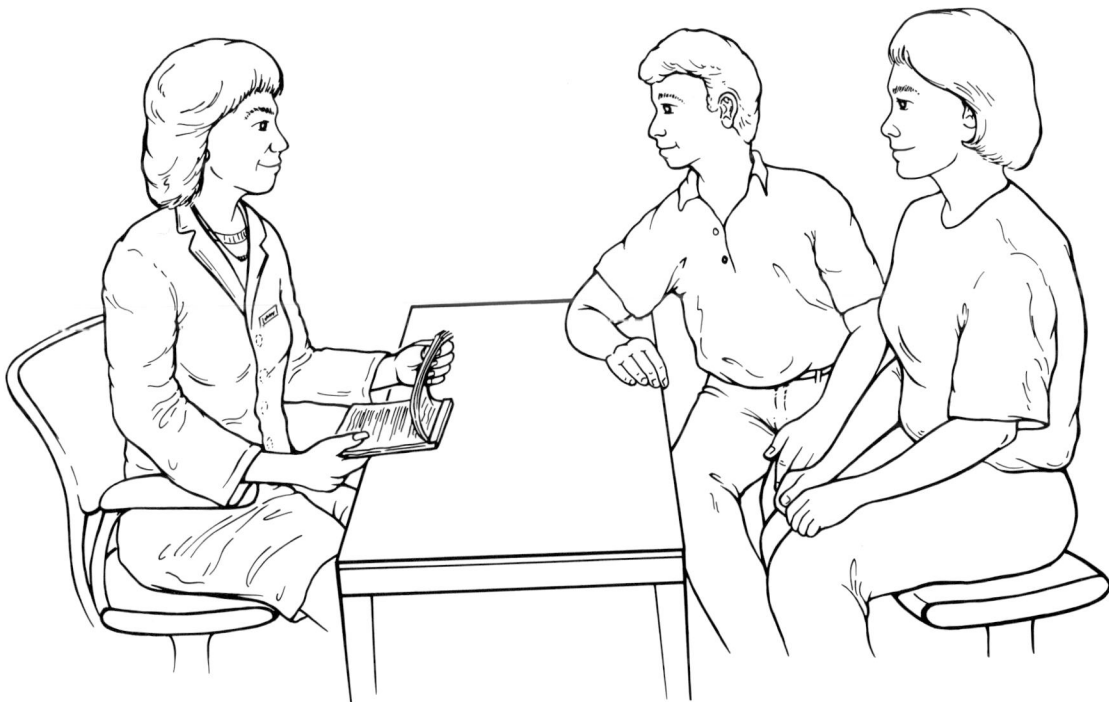

FIGURE 4–7. The physician's role is extremely important in helping the couple cope with the emotional side of infertility.

A number of authors have established guidelines for medical professionals working with infertility patients.[1, 11, 66] There are several important steps that health care personnel can take along with patients to minimize stress for the infertile couple and maximize their self-esteem and ability to tolerate the fertility investigation and treatment (Table 4–5).

Although it is often extremely difficult for both patients and medical professionals to confront the fact that "enough is enough," this sad reality must be faced, especially when treatment options have significantly diminished, when the marital relationship is deteriorating, or when the prolonged infertility is seriously threatening one's psychological equilibrium and ability to function productively in other areas of life. As the likelihood of having a biologic offspring becomes less and less promising, it is imperative not to push medical treatment on those who do not have the emotional stamina to withstand it. At this moment, ideas and thoughts about other parenting alternatives can be carefully and sensitively introduced to the couple. Clearly the data suggest that the suffering experienced by infertile individuals is real and that those in reproductive health care need to remind themselves regularly that they are treating "people who are infertile" rather than "infertility."[65]

ROLE OF THE MENTAL HEALTH PROFESSIONAL IN THE MEDICAL PRACTICE

Mental health clinicians as well as infertile couples have emphasized the need for psychological services in the areas of infertility.[68, 69] Previous sections of this chapter point to a number of psychological factors inherent in infertility, which may lead to individual or marital distress. Those who seek infertility services frequently confront protracted, expensive procedures. These can lead to ongoing anxiety and depression, which in turn can result in social and occupational dysfunction. Daniluk[70] indicates that 97% of couples supported a need for psychological services in their initial contacts with an infertility clinic, and more than 50% stated that they would use these services during the infertility investigation and treatment if they were available.

If the mental health professional (e.g., psychologist, psychiatrist, social worker) is included as part of the delivery of comprehensive fertility services, his or her role can be determined in a variety of ways.[71] This role, in any case, is seldom clear primarily because historically few nonpsychiatric medical practices or teams have had a need routinely to include a mental health professional in the group. As a result, the members of an infertility practice may feel ambivalent or uncertain as to how to integrate this type of professional expertise into the work of the medical group. Additionally the mental health practitioner often does not have a professional background in reproductive medicine. This lack of a similar frame of reference can sometimes lead to further difficulties in role definition. Both the mental health professional and the infertility clinician may be left unclear as to how mental health services can be provided. As the dimensions of the ART have broadened, however, especially regarding gamete and embryo donation as well as gestational carrier programs, the need for psychological screening and intervention with all involved parties has increased dramatically.

Specifically the functions in which the mental health professional can serve in relation to the infertility practice might include, but are not limited to, the following.

The Mental Health Professional as a Group or Team Member

This role is one of direct involvement with patients and staff. For example, the mental health professional might meet briefly with all new infertility patients to obtain psychosocial information and to inform them of areas of potential stress

---

TABLE 4–5. Guidelines for Medical Personnel Working with the Infertile Couple

1. Infertility should be seen as a couple's problem. Both partners should be encouraged to participate all the time, regardless of who has the diagnosed medical problem
2. Establish a clear testing and treatment plan with the couple. Discussions can then focus on the order of the investigative procedures, effects of medications, options for treatment, prognoses, costs, and time schedules. For most couples, time is pressing, physically and psychologically
3. Information is crucial to the emotional well-being of the couple. It should be given voluntarily and continually. Couples should also be encouraged to ask questions. Information not only increases feelings of effectiveness, but also it demonstrates respect for the couple and promotes a more positive self-image. For example, it is often helpful to have relevant brochures and articles available in the waiting room
4. Develop a knowledge and understanding of the emotional components of infertility. Be observant of the individual's and couple's psychological status, especially as the investigation becomes protracted. Empathy, understanding, and accessibility are of great importance
5. It should be made clear at the commencement of the infertility investigation that there is always a risk that the couple may not successfully conceive and give birth to a child despite everyone's best efforts. It should be stated that the investigation cannot continue forever. At the same time, couples should be allowed to end treatment or seek a second opinion without "losing face" or feeling guilty or embarrassed
6. Before meeting new patients, review their medical records carefully. Infertile couples often become distressed and indignant when physicians are ignorant of their medical situation, particularly when they are told that the physician will not meet with them unless the records are sent well in advance of the designated appointment
7. It is important to meet with new infertility couples for the first time in the office rather than in an examination room. Patients feel infantilized meeting the physician when undressed or lying or sitting on an examination table
8. Describe in advance what the various medical procedures entail and what potential side effects may be experienced from the medications. When patients know what to expect, they tend to respond more calmly and with less fear or confusion. The importance of the physician's role as educator to the patient cannot be underestimated[67]
9. Acknowledge to the couple that the infertility is a life crisis and that there is always someone to talk with about the situation. Be sure to have available the name(s) of a mental health professional who is trained to work with infertility patients so referrals can be made readily of those who are having difficulty coping with this crisis. Provide information about RESOLVE or other infertility support organizations, and make these resources readily available
10. Treat the infertile man and woman respectfully both as individuals and as a couple. The infertile couple is usually in great need of positive regard

during the medical workup.[37] Patients are therefore made aware of the availability of clearly stated and direct channels for emotional support. Similarly, to expedite the counseling and support process, medical staff and the mental health professionals communicate with one another regarding particular issues that a couple must confront during various procedures. General feedback is provided to medical personnel from the mental health professional regarding areas of potential concern or areas of need for additional support. Maintaining a balance between honoring patient confidentiality and building an effective support system within the context of the treatment program is also paramount.

Some individuals or couples may elect to establish a short-term supportive counseling relationship or undergo longer term psychotherapy. Not all patients want or require mental health intervention. Others may find it to be indicated after an unexpected event occurs during treatment, for example, several failed cycles, pregnancy loss, or unexpected diagnoses.

When the mental health professional is part of an ART team, he or she may also be called on to provide psychological screening for potential gamete donors or to meet with all potential donor gamete recipient couples. This can be a critical function, which not only assists the medical team in determining appropriate gamete donors, but also enables recipient couples to be more aware of and prepared for the decision to become parents through this alternative.[60]

Some infertility facilities may be unable to incorporate the services of a mental health professional into the team because of a lack of necessary resources, such as financial constraints, available space, or qualified or experienced mental health personnel. In these cases, as the need for a mental health professional arises, the role of such an individual professional may be that of an outside referral source.

The Mental Health Professional as an Outside Referral Source

As an outside referral source, the mental health professional does not function as a team member. Instead he or she is available to the IVF couple who may be in need of mental health intervention. The IVF team may believe that the couple is in need of additional emotional support beyond that which the nurse, physician, or team members can provide. Similarly, the IVF patient or couple may feel that they are having difficulty coping with the procedure, are having marital difficulties, or are unable to make important decisions regarding treatment. It is important that if an ART program does not provide on-site mental health services adequate resources are available.

There are several advantages to having the mental health professional as an outside referral source. These include the following:

1. There are patients who feel more comfortable confiding in someone not directly involved with the infertility practice.
2. For the mental health professional, it can be helpful not to be directly intertwined with the dynamics of the team. In this case, the mental health practitioner maintains a different perspective and may be less likely to become involved with emotional issues that are related to particular group dynamics or individual differences within the team.

Disadvantages may include the following:

1. There can be lack of understanding on the part of the mental health professional of existing group dynamics within the team.
2. There can be difficulty with patient and medical personnel followup.
3. Patients often prefer the convenience of having the mental health professional on site and believe that he or she has a better understanding of all aspects of their individual infertility treatment.

The Mental Health Professional as Consultant to the Team

Technically when the mental health professional is brought on as a consultant, he or she does not work directly with the patient population. Instead that individual might advise nursing, physician, and other support personnel as to how they might work with especially difficult patients or establish a more supportive environment.

Another role of the mental health consultant might be to analyze the psychodynamics of the medical group itself and offer suggestions and strategies for how the team might more effectively work together. Issues that might often interfere with effective team functioning include the individual need to control, scapegoating, competitive behavior, or power struggles that may exist around professional role definitions.

Research

The mental health professional may work independently or in conjunction with other team members in developing research projects that consider the psychosocial/physiologic aspects of issues such as reproductive health, infertility, and pregnancy loss.

SUMMARY

Infertility treatments and the new reproductive technologies have provided dramatic opportunities for thousands of infertile men and women. Intrinsic to infertility, its diagnosis, treatment, and outcome, however, are significant psychological factors that should be understood and appreciated to provide the highest quality medical care.

For most couples, the desire to have children has roots deeply imbedded in our biosociocultural histories. The meanings of fertility for a man and woman may differ, but ultimately most of those who experience prolonged infertility confront a variety of feelings and thoughts, such as anger, guilt, isolation, and depression. The infertile couple is also often forced to undertake an in-depth examination of their relationship as well as their personal values, beliefs, and goals concerning parenthood.

This chapter has addressed a variety of psychological aspects of infertility and discussed specific topics that are intended to provide further insight regarding ways in which these emotional factors can be better understood and attended to with sensitivity by the health care professional.

Infertility diagnosis and treatment, including the ART, presents continuing challenges to health and mental health professionals. The social changes of the past 25 years have clearly precipitated shifts in family configurations and lifestyles, and many couples have therefore delayed having children. Some have encountered infertility. In light of the chronicity of many infertility conditions, it would seem imperative that there be greater emphasis on helping couples enhance their coping strategies and reduce the toll taken by the problem, so those affected can minimize the damage to their self-esteem as well as to their relationships with one another and their families.

REFERENCES

1. Möller A, Fällström K. Psychological consequences of infertility: a longitudinal study. J Psychosom Obstet Gynaecol 1991; 12:27.
2. Becker G. Healing the Infertile Family. New York: Bantam Books, 1990.
3. Erikson E. Childhood and Society. New York: WW Norton & Co, 1950.
4. Clark LF, Henry SM, Taylor DM. Cognitive examination of motivation for childbearing as a factor in adjustment to infertility. In: Stanton AL, Dunkel-Schetter C, editors. Infertility: Prospectives from Stress and Coping Research. New York: Plenum Press, 1991: 157–180.
5. Wright JD, Duchesne C, Sabourin S, et al. Psychosocial distress and infertility: men and women respond differently. Fertil Steril 1991; 55:100.
6. Greil AL, Leitko TA, Porter KL. Infertility: his and hers. Gend Soc 1988; 2:172.
7. Raval H, Slade P, Buck P, Lieberman BE. The impact of infertility on emotions and the marital and sexual relationship. J Reprod Infant Psych 1987; 55:221.
8. Nachtigall RD, Becker G, Wozny M. The effects of gender-specific diagnosis on men's and women's response to infertility. Fertil Steril 1992; 57:113.
9. Klempner L. Infertility: identification and disruptions with the maternal object. Clin Soc Work J 1992; 20:193.
10. Notman MT, Lester EP. Pregnancy: theoretical consideration. Psychanalytic Inq 1988; 8:139.
11. Salzer LP. Surviving Infertility: A Compassionate Guide Through the Emotional Crisis of Infertility. New York: Harper Perennial, 1991.
12. Mahlstedt PP. The psychological component of infertility. Fertil Steril 1985; 43:335.
13. Cook EP. Characteristics of the biopsycho-social crisis of infertility. J Counsel Dev 1987; 65:465.
14. Forest L, Gilbert MS. Infertility: an unanticipated and prolonged life crisis. Special issue: Women and health. J Ment Health Couns 1992; 14:42.
15. Lalos A, Lalos O, Jacobsson L, Von Schoultz B. Depression, guilt and isolation among infertile women and their partners. Psychosom Obstet Gynecol 1986; 5:197.
16. Stephenson LR. Give Us a Child: Coping with the Personal Crisis of Infertility. San Francisco: Harper & Row, 1987.
17. Knipper C, editor. Person to person: Bob's story. Conceive: The Magazine of Infertility Issues 1990; 2:26.
18. Abbey A, Andrews FM, Haldman LJ. The importance of social relationships for infertile couples' well-being. In: Stanton AL, Dunkel-Schetter C, editors. Infertility: Perspectives from Stress and Coping Research. New York: Plenum Press, 1991:61.
19. Mahlstedt PP, Johnson PT. Support to persons experiencing infertility: family and friends can help. Journal of Social Work and Human Sexuality 1987; 6:65.
20. Woollett A. Childlessness: strategies for coping with infertility. Special issue: development of self in lifespan perspective. Int J Behav Dev 1985; 8:473.
21. Applegarth LD. Communication. Conceive: The Magazine of Infertility Issues 1990; 2:7.
22. Berg B, Wilson JF. Psychological functioning across stages of treatment for infertility. J Behav Med 1991; 14:11.
23. Keye WR. Psychosexual responses to infertility. Clin Obstet Gynecol 1984; 27:760.
24. Shapiro CH. Infertility and Pregnancy Loss: A Guide for Helping Professionals. San Francisco: Jossey-Bass, Inc, 1988.
25. Walker HE. Psychiatric aspects of infertility. Symposium on male infertility. Urol Clin North Am 1978; 5:481.
26. Burns LH. Sexual dysfunction and the infertile couple: diagnosis and treatment. Personal communication.
27. Conway P, Valentine D. Reproductive losses and grieving. Journal of Social Work and Human Sexuality 1987; 6:43.
28. Garner CH. Pregnancy after infertility. J Obstet Gynecol Neonat Nursing 1985; 14:58.
29. Peppers LG, Knapp RJ. Maternal reactions to involuntary fetal/infant death. Psychiatry 1980; 43:155.
30. Conway K. Miscarriage. J Psychosom Obstet Gynaecol 1991; 12:121.
31. Wells RG. Managing miscarriage. The need for more than medical mechanics. Postgrad Med 1991; 89:207.
32. Stirrat GM. Recurrent miscarriage: clinical associations, causes, and management. Lancet 1990; 1:728.
33. Greenfeld D, Walther V. Psychological aspects of recurrent pregnancy loss. Infert Reprod Med Clin North Am 1991; 2:235.
34. Layne LL. Motherhood lost: cultural dimensions of miscarriage and stillbirth in America. Women and Health 1990; 16:69.
35. Stirtzinger R, Robinson GE. The psychologic effects of spontaneous abortion. Can Med Assoc J 1989; 140:799.
36. Covington SN. Pregnancy loss. Paper presented at Pacific Coast Fertility Society Annual Meeting; Indian Wells, CA, 1991.
37. Covington SN, Valentine D, editor. Psychosocial evaluation of the infertile couple: implications for social work practice. In: Infertility and Adoption: A Guide for Social Work Practice. Binghamton, NY: Haworth Press, 1988:21.
38. McKaughan M. The Biological Clock: Balancing Miscarriage, Motherhood, and Career. New York: Penguin Books, 1987.
39. Deutch H. The Psychology of Women. Vol II. New York: Grune & Stratton, 1945.
40. Benedek T. Infertility as a psychosomatic defense. Fertil Steril 1952; 3:257.
41. Sandler B. Infertility of emotional origin. J Obstet Gynaecol Br Emp 1961; 68:809.
42. Mai FM, Munday RN, Rump EE. Psychosomatic and behavioral mechanisms in psychogenic infertility. Br J Psychiatr 1972; 120:199.
43. Kipper DA, Ziegler-Shani Z, Serr DM, Insler V. Psychogenic infertility, neuroticism and the feminine role: a methodological inquiry. J Psychosom Res 1975; 21:353.
44. Berger DM. The role of the psychiatrist in a reproductive biology clinic. Fertil Steril 1977; 28:141.
45. Palti Z. Psychogenic male infertility. Psychosom Med 1969; 31:326.
46. Elstein M. Effect of infertility on psychosexual function. BMJ 1975; 2:296.
47. Barnea ER, Tal J. Stress-related reproductive failure. J In Vit Emb Trans 1991; 8:15.
48. Wasser SK, Sewall G, Soules MR. Psychosocial stress as a cause of infertility. Fertil Steril 1993; 59:685.
49. Seibel M, Taymor M. Emotional aspects of infertility. Fertil Steril 1982; 37:137.
50. Möller A, Fällström K. Psychological factors in the etiology of infertility: a longitudinal study. J Psychosom Obstet Gynaecol 1991; 12:13.
51. Domar AD, Seibel MM, Benson H. The mind/body program for infertility: a new behavioral treatment approach for women with infertility. Fertil Steril 1990; 53:246.
52. Domar AD, Zuttermeister PC, Seibel M, Benson H. Psychological improvement in infertile women after behavioral treatment: a replication. Fertil Steril 1992; 58:144.
53. Applegarth LD, Mahlstedt PP. The psychological issues of in-vitro fertilization: coping and control. Paper presented at the Second Annual Conference for IVF Nurse Coordinators (Serono Symposia USA), Norfolk, VA, 1987.
54. Reading AE, Chang LIC, Kerin JF. Psychological state and coping styles across an IVF treatment cycle. Special issue: psychology and infertility. J Repro Infant Psychol 1989; 7:95.
55. Mazure CM, Greenfeld DA. Psychological studies of in-vitro fertilization/embryo transfer participants. J In Vit Emb Trans 1989; 6:242.
56. Berg BJ, Wilson JF. Psychiatric morbidity in the infertile population: a reconceptualization. Fertil Steril 1990; 53:654.
57. Merari D, Feldberg D, Elizur A, Goldman J, Modan B. Psychological and hormonal changes in the course of in-vitro fertilization. J Assist Reprod Genet 1992; 9:161.
58. Lasker JN, Borg S. In Search of Parenthood: Coping with Infertility and High-Tech Reproduction. Boston: Beacon Press, 1987.
59. Edelmann RJ. Psychological aspects of artificial insemination by donor. J Psychosom Obstet Gynaecol 1989; 10:3.

60. Mahlstedt PP, Greenfeld DA. Assisted reproductive technology with donor gametes: the need for patient preparation. Fertil Steril 1989; 52:908.

61. de Parseval GD. Clinical remarks concerning parents (potential and real) after different "treatments" for the sterility of couples. J Psychosom Obstet Gynaecol 1992; 13:21.

62. Mahlstedt PP. The use of donor gametes in conception: the decision making process. National Newsletter of Resolve Inc, Somerville, MA 1991; 16:1.

63. Probasco KA. Discussion with children about their donor conception. In: Insights into Infertility. Serono Symposia USA, Norwell, MA, 1992.

64. Mahlstedt PP, Probasco KA. Sperm donors: their attitudes toward providing medical and psychosocial information for recipient couples and donor offspring. Fertil Steril 1991; 56:747.

65. Appleton T. Counselling, care in infertility: the ethnic of care. Br Med Bull 1990; 46:842.

66. Feldman PR, Covington SN. The perfect patient. Newsletter of Resolve of Metro-Washington, DC, 1986; 3:1.

67. Rodning CB, Dasco CC. Realistic expectations of a patient-physician encounter. South Med J 1987; 70:1208.

68. Reading AE, Kevin J. Psychologic aspects of providing infertility services. J Reprod Med 1989; 34:861.

69. Klock SC, Maier D. Guidelines for the provision of psychological evaluations for infertile patients at the University of Connecticut Health Center. Fertil Steril 1991; 56:680.

70. Daniluk JC. Infertility: intrapersonal and interpersonal impact. Fertil Steril 1988; 49:982.

71. English ME, Applegarth LD, Holman T. Psychological support for the IVF patient: the collaborative role of the nurse and the mental health professional. Paper presented at the 4th Annual Conference of IVF Nurse Coordinators and Support Personnel (Serono Symposia USA), St. Petersburg, FL, 1990.

CHAPTER 5

Evaluating the Infertility Literature

DAVID L. OLIVE

The infertility-related literature, similar to the medical literature in general, is proliferating at a staggering rate. The task of the clinician to remain current in the face of this increasing body of knowledge is becoming progressively more difficult. All too often the temptation is to skim the abstracts of the latest journals, trusting that the peer review process has ferreted out those manuscripts with faulty methodology or illogical conclusions.

Unfortunately such blind faith in the review process frequently proves inadequate. The art of medicine is to apply that which is published, frequently under sharply controlled circumstances, to the uncontrolled situation of the patient facing you from across the desk. To do this requires more than simply a knowledge of what the literature says; it requires an *understanding* of the literature, including its assets and limitations.

This chapter strives to provide the clinician with the tools necessary to evaluate the infertility literature critically. It focuses on two areas. The first, evaluation of diagnostic tests, provides the information necessary to sort through the available diagnostic modalities and determine what is truly required for evaluation. The second, evaluation of treatment trials, clarifies those issues necessary to place such studies in their proper perspective.

EVALUATING DIAGNOSTIC TESTS

A large number of diagnostic tests are used in the traditional infertility evaluation, and an even larger number are regularly proposed as adjunctive tests for this process. Danger exists, however, in blindly accepting the relative importance of test results without first understanding the limitations and applicability of the method. This section reviews the features of a test that should be known and understood by the critical reviewer.

What Is Normal?

The problem of establishing the concept of normal and demarcating its range is complex, for *normal* can be defined in different ways. For our purposes, however, two categories suffice: correlated normality and isolated normality.

Using the correlated approach, the normal test result must be associated with the ability to achieve a desired state of health. Conversely, the abnormal state is one that results in varying degrees of inability to attain the desired health level. For diagnostic tests in infertility, the desired state would generally be the attainment of pregnancy and the abnormal state a persistence of reproductive failure.

Although a correlated definition of normal and abnormal is optimal, there are several problems inherent to this approach. One difficulty in establishing a correlated normality is the vast amount of additional data that must be considered simultaneously. A thorough examination of all other known modifiers of the conception rate must be performed and the results considered. Although this multivariate approach can often be expressed as a statistical model, the complexity of such an expression is often quite cumbersome. An additional problem with correlated normality is that many test results are changed by the outcome. For example, pregnancy alters the length of a luteal phase, making it unusable as a test for luteal phase defect.[1]

Much less complex is the definition of isolated normality, a univariate concept emergent from boundaries set on values of a single variable.[2] These boundaries define the *usual* and are frequently determined statistically. A common method is the selection of the central 95% of the population as *normal;* an alternative, for a population with a gaussian distribution, is to delineate the limits of normal as the mean ± 2 standard deviations (Fig. 5–1). The option certainly exists, however, to set more stringent or lax boundaries, as may be warranted or desired.

Although commonly used, isolated normality has several characteristics critical to understanding its limitations. First, because the limits of normal are arbitrarily (albeit statistically) chosen, the rate of abnormality in the population is predetermined rather than being based on the clinical demonstration of the dysfunction. Second, because no outcome is correlated, the reference population used to determine normal must be carefully chosen to be applicable to the clinical question involved. For this reason, male prolactin levels

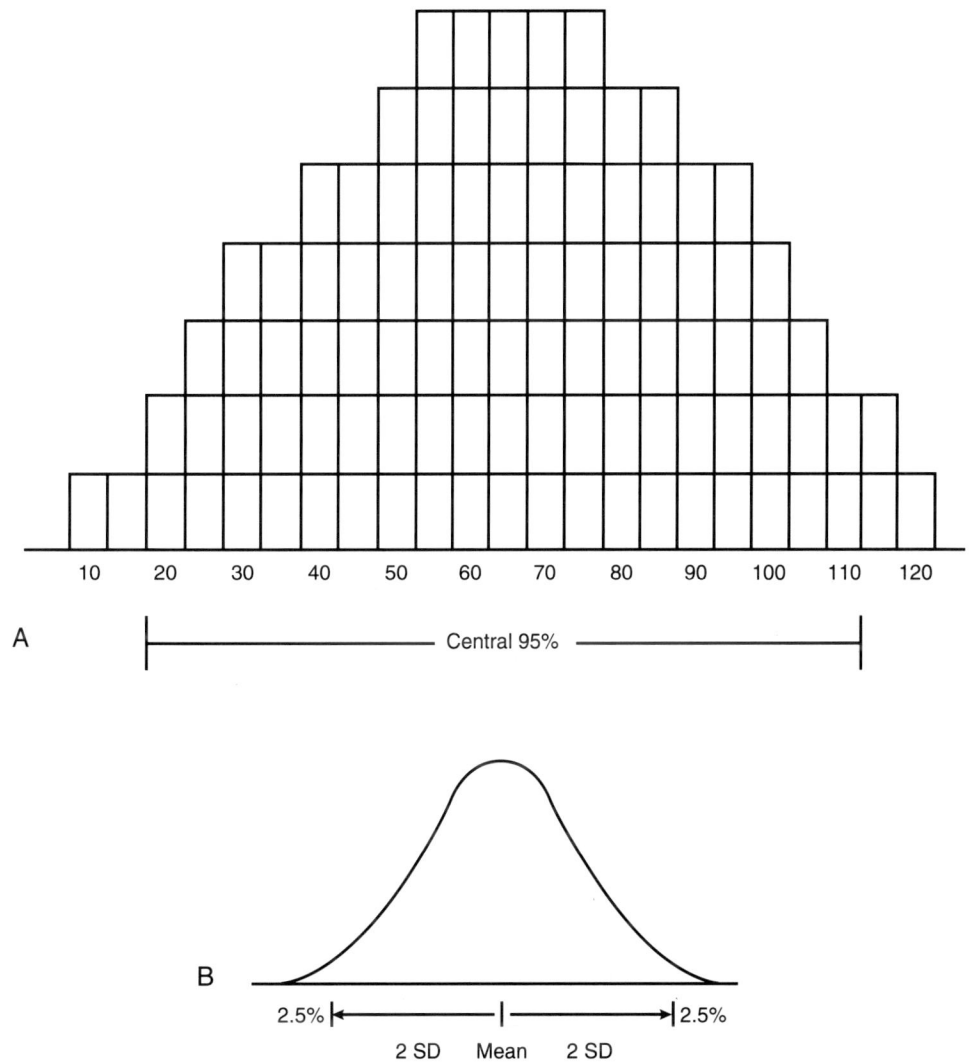

10   20   30   40   50   60   70   80   90   100   110   120

A |———————————— Central 95% ————————————|

B   2.5% |←————————|————————→| 2.5%

2 SD   Mean   2 SD

FIGURE 5–1. Two methods to determine "normal" from a population distribution. *A,* 95% confidence limits: the central 95% of the values are deemed to be the range of normal. *B,* Mean ±2 SD; with a gaussian distribution, these limits encompass 95% of the values.

should never be used to determine the normal range for the female, and infertile women should not be used to create standards for the endometrial biopsy as a tool for diagnosing luteal insufficiency.

Variability of a Test

A perfect test would produce the same results each time it was performed and would exactly reflect the true value of the tested sample. In other words, it would be completely reproducible (precise) and completely accurate. Unfortunately this situation is not practical in the real world. Nevertheless, all too often we neglect to consider this when evaluating a test. Numerically assessing the precision and accuracy of a test can have a major impact on its clinical utility.[3]

Test precision can vary owing to test conditions or test interpretation. Test conditions should be identical with each determination; if they are not, variation results. A laboratory assay for a steroid hormone might vary if a slightly different amount of serum is placed in each of two duplicate test tubes. Such fluctuations are termed intra-assay variability. Similarly, conditions may not be exactly duplicated the fol-

lowing day when the test is again performed: This illustrates interassay variability.

Analysis of tests can vary similarly when interpretation is involved. Differences in conclusions by the same individual on the same sample is termed intraobserver variation, whereas different physicians assessing a single test sample exhibit interobserver variability.

Given that tests show varying degrees of precision, some method of quantification is needed to judge if the amount of variation is tolerable. This measure is termed the *coefficient of variation* (CV), defined as the standard deviation divided by the mean for a set of measurements. A CV can be determined for each of the aforementioned types of variations; the larger the value, the less precise the test under the specified conditions.

Precision is not to be confused with accuracy or the ability of a test to come close to the "true" value. Although accuracy is a required property of a good test, the assessment of accuracy requires comparing the test to a gold standard of measurement. An example can be found in the radioimmunoassay (RIA) for estradiol. If a known amount of estradiol (200 pg/mL) is assayed by RIA, the degree to which the result approaches 200 pg/mL represents the accuracy of the test. If, however, the RIA result is 600 pg/mL each of three separate times, the test is quite precise but not terribly accurate. Unfortunately many tests do not have a gold standard on which to compare but merely a "best test" that has been deemed the standard after lengthy experience with its use. Thus, it may not be easy to determine the absolute accuracy of a test, only the comparative accuracy versus other "best tests" evaluating the same sample.

Variability in a Population

As alluded to earlier, not all "normal" individuals produce the same result for a test; this variation is the basis for selecting a normal range. This range of acceptable values is graphically illustrated as a distribution of possible normal results. Frequently the distribution is gaussian in nature and is referred to as a *normal distribution*. Nongaussian distributions can frequently be transformed into gaussian (normal) bell-shaped curves by mathematical manipulation. By the same token, the abnormal population has a range of test values. If there is no overlap between the normal and abnormal subjects, interpretation of the test is easy. When overlap occurs, however, certain quantitative measures are needed to help us identify the discriminative capacity of a test in a clinical situation (Fig. 5–2).

How Good Is a Test?

From the preceding discussion, it is clear that few tests are perfect in their ability to separate diseased (infertile) from nondiseased (normal) subjects. The measures of the diagnostic ability of a test to separate these groups are called *sensitivity* and *specificity*. Sensitivity measures the proportion of those with disease who are correctly identified as such by the test in use. Specificity is the proportion of those who do not have

the disease whom the test identifies as disease-free. Of importance is the fact that neither measure changes with the frequency of disease in the population studied; in other words, they are characteristics inherent to the test. Neither can predict, however, the actual number of subjects correctly categorized (this depends on the rate of disease in the population under study). Thus, these measures evaluate the test, not the population on which the test is performed.

Two clinically relevant questions cannot be answered by sensitivity and specificity: (1) If the test is positive, how likely is it that the individual is diseased? (2) If the test is negative, how likely is it that the individual is disease-free? To answer these queries requires two different measures. The *positive predictive value* answers the first question, and the *negative predictive value* answers the second. Predictive values differ from sensitivity and specificity in that predictive values vary considerably depending on the rate of disease in the study population. Thus, these values are specific for particular clinical settings, and the clinician should take care not to extrapolate freely from one situation to another. For example, a test useful for confirming a diagnosis may be worthless as a screening test.

The calculations for sensitivity, specificity, positive predictive value, and negative predictive value are shown in Figure 5–3.

Role of Diagnostic Tests

Diagnostic tests are usually designed for one of three purposes: discovery, exclusion, and confirmation.[2] Tests to discover disease in a population are generally called screening tests and are used when the disease is silent in an unsuspecting group being screened. Because a discovery test should be able to detect the disease whenever present, it should be designed to have a high sensitivity. The specificity must be reasonably high too, to prevent an avalanche of false-positive

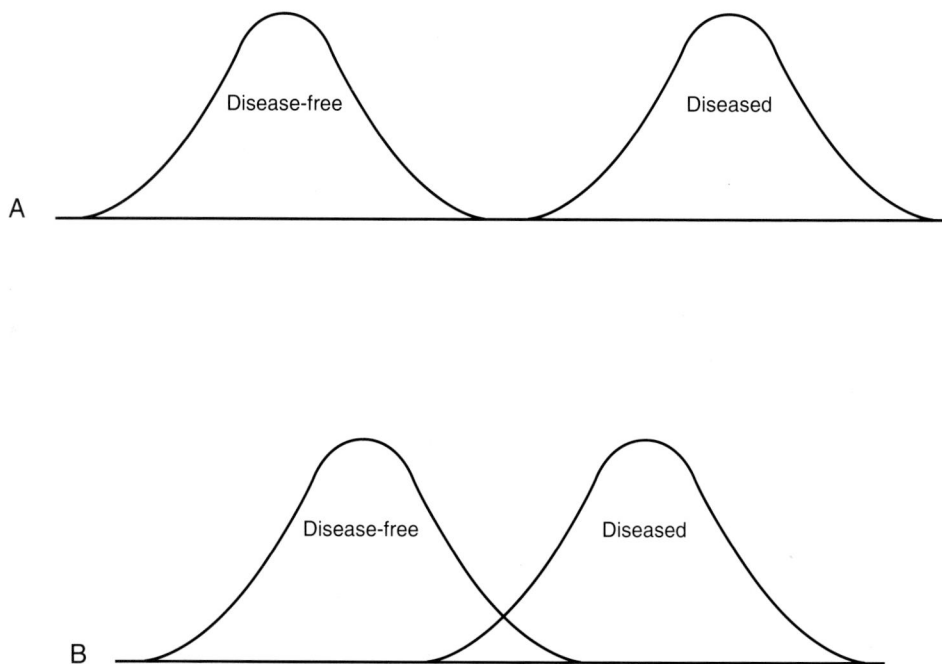

FIGURE 5–2. Possible relationships between test values of normal and abnormal subjects. *A*, No overlap between distributions. *B*, Partial overlap between distributions.

TEST | GOLD STANDARD DISEASED | GOLD STANDARD DISEASE-FREE

	GOLD STANDARD DISEASED	GOLD STANDARD DISEASE-FREE	
Positive	a = Number of individuals diseased and positive	b = Number of individuals disease-free and positive	a + b = Total number of positives
Negative	c = Number of individuals diseased and negative	d = Number of individuals disease-free and negative	c + d = Total number of negatives
	a + c = Total number of diseased individuals	b + d = Total number of disease-free individuals	

$$\text{Sensitivity} = \frac{a}{a + c} = \text{The proportion of the diseased labeled positive by the test}$$

$$\text{Specificity} = \frac{d}{b + d} = \text{The proportion of the disease-free labeled negative by the test}$$

$$\text{Predictive value of a positive test} = \frac{a}{a + b} = \text{Proportion of those with a positive test who actually have the disease as measured by the gold standard}$$

$$\text{Predictive value of a negative test} = \frac{d}{c + d} = \text{Proportion of those with a negative test who actually are free of the disease as measured by the gold standard}$$

FIGURE 5–3. Calculation of sensitivity, specificity, predictive value of a positive test (positive predictive value), and predictive value of a negative test (negative predictive value).

patients, but the value need not be as high as the sensitivity, particularly if a good confirmation test is available to follow. An example of such a discovery test is mammography to screen for breast cancer. Although there is certainly a high sensitivity for this test, the specificity is modest; the goal is to detect women who might need breast biopsies, not to make a definitive diagnosis by the test alone.

A confirmation test is used when the disease is strongly suspected of being present. In this clinical situation, we want to be sure that the disease is present when the test is positive, whereas occasional false-negative results are acceptable. An example is peritoneal biopsy for endometriosis at laparoscopy. If characteristic histologic changes indicative of endometriosis are seen in the biopsy, the disease is confirmed. Failure to see such findings on biopsy does not exclude the disease, however, and the possibility of its existence must still be a consideration. Thus, a high positive predictive value is imperative for a confirmation test, usually in combination with a high specificity.

Tests of exclusion are performed to rule out a disease being considered in the differential diagnosis. Because the need is to be confident that a negative test result excludes the disease, a high negative predictive value is critical. To enhance the value of the test further, a high sensitivity is valued. Doppler flow ultrasound studies of ovarian cysts are an example. If the value of the resistance index (RI) is above 0.46, ovarian cancer is absolutely excluded. If the RI is below 0.46,

however, the possibility of cancer still exists, and further diagnostic studies are required.

When Should a Test Be Repeated?

Because a wide range of values can be considered either normal or abnormal when they fall into the area of overlapping distributions, a need arises to determine somehow if the patient is truly normal or not. To help sort this out, a convenient statistical property referred to as *regression toward the mean* can be used.[4] Briefly this means that members of a normal distribution are randomly strewn throughout the gaussian curve. If a normal patient's test is at an extreme of this bell-shaped curve, chances are that a second test will be closer to the normal mean. Conversely, if the patient was initially abnormal, the second test will move toward the abnormal mean test value (Fig. 5–4). Thus, whenever a test value falls into the gray zone that does not allow easy discrimination between normal and abnormal, a repeat test value can help clarify the issue. If the initial test is clearly normal or abnormal, however, there is no reason to repeat testing (unless the result seems at odds with clinical impressions; in this situation you are repeating the test to rule out gross laboratory error).

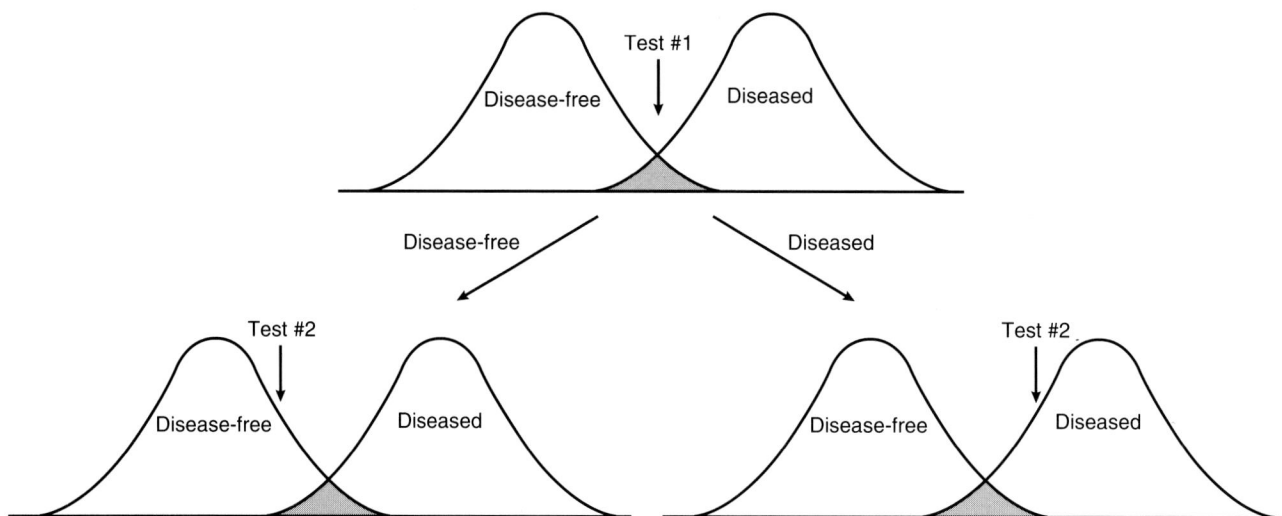

FIGURE 5-4. Use of repeat testing to determine if the subject is normal or abnormal. Odds favor a second test value closer to the mean of the true distribution of which the subject is a member.

Comparing Tests—the Receiver-Operating-Characteristic Curve

Numerous diagnostic tests may be developed for a single diagnosis, and it is our responsibility to be able to determine which test is the best of the lot. It is for this purpose that receiver-operating-characteristic (ROC) curves have been used in the medical literature.[5-7] These curves offer comparisons when use of the dichotomous indices of sensitivity and specificity proves difficult.

An ROC curve is calculated by first choosing a set of potential thresholds that might distinguish a positive test result from a negative result. The sensitivity and specificity can then be calculated for each of the threshold values. The results are plotted, with the ordinate being *sensitivity* and the abscissa being *1-specificity*. Tests may be compared by calculating the area under the ROC curve: the greater the value, the better the test. One such curve is illustrated in Figure 5-5.

Handling Uncertainty

Try as we might, absolute diagnostic certainty is usually unattainable. Our task is not to attain certainty but to reduce the level of diagnostic uncertainty enough to be able to make optimal therapeutic decisions. As the cost of infertility care spirals upward, we as clinicians are frequently confronted with the dilemma of containing patient expenditures while still making the "correct" diagnosis.

How should we handle this uncertainty? To a large degree, the level of diagnostic certainty needed in a clinical decision is a function of the characteristics of the next step in the process.[8] When a specific therapy for a given diagnosis is high in effectiveness and low in risk, one can handle substantial diagnostic uncertainty. Few tests need be performed, and their quality need not even be especially good, if the treatment works in those with the disorder yet causes little harm to those that do not have the disease. Any therapy that combines low efficacy with high risk requires substantial

diagnostic certainty: Multiple additional tests might be justified in such a situation.

Just as reproductive medicine will never be reduced to a series of flow charts, the employment of diagnostic tests is medicine as an art form. A thorough understanding of each test, its assets and liabilities, and its consequences is required for optimal application. Only then can the quality of infertil-

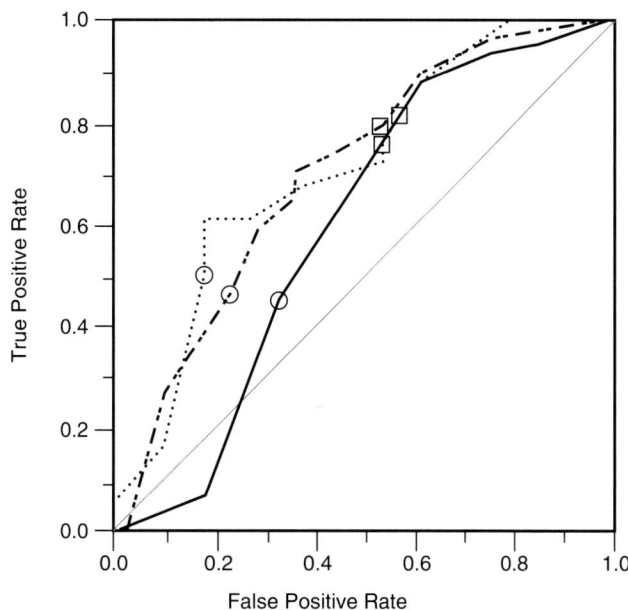

FIGURE 5-5. Receiver-operating-characteristic curves for serum progesterone (P) levels as a predictor of consecutive out-of-phase endometrial biopsies. Lines shown represent curves for a single random P (——), a single morning P (——●●——), and three pooled morning P samples (●●●). *Circles* designate the points on each curve representing a diagnostic threshold of 10 ng/mL P. *Squares* designate the points on each curve representing a diagnostic threshold of 15 ng/mL P. (From Olive DL, Thomford PJ, Torres SE, Lambert TS, Rosen GF. Twenty-four-hour progesterone and luteinizing hormone profiles in the midluteal phase of the infertile patient: correlation with other indicators of luteal phase insufficiency. Fertil Steril 1989;51:587-592. Reproduced with permission of the publisher.)

Type	Real-Time Events Occur	Research Direction	Example
Experimental (RCT) Observational survey	Current	Antecedent to outcome	Treatments compared; random assignment
Prospective	Current	Antecedent to outcome	Clomiphene-treated patients enrolled with diagnosis of ovulatory dysfunction; endpoint is pregnancy
Retrospective	Past	Antecedent to outcome (cohort)	Chart review determining pregnancy rate among women diagnosed with endometriosis
		Outcome to antecedent (trohoc)	Chart review determining types of ovulation dysfunction in women pregnant following clomiphene treatment

TABLE 5–1. Types of Clinical Trials

RCT, randomized clinical trial.

ity diagnosis rise above the cookbook as a dynamic, scientific practice.

EVALUATING INFERTILITY TREATMENTS

Treating infertility involves a large series of options that range from the simplistic to ultra-high technology. Treatments may be medical, surgical, or expectant in nature, and the risks may be virtually nonexistent or quite substantial. The clinician must sort through this morass of techniques with each couple presenting for infertility treatment.

To aid the clinician in his or her search for optimal therapy is a medical literature replete with suggestions, each purporting to prove the value of the technique discussed. It is the clinician's responsibility to evaluate these studies carefully and determine the optimal approach for a given patient. Unfortunately this is no easy task because to do so requires being equipped with a firm foundation in study design, data reporting, and data comparison. This section reviews these topics in an attempt to provide the critical reader with the tools necessary to evaluate the therapeutic literature.

Trial Design

TYPES OF CLINICAL TRIALS

Research design is often divided into two major categories: descriptive and analytic. Descriptive studies are those that have no basic hypothesis being tested but rather attempt to quantify what happens over the course of a disease. Analytic studies are designed to investigate a specific hypothesis, generally involving a cause-and-effect relationship. The analytic study is the type generally used to evaluate therapeutic maneuvers in infertile patients.

Analytic studies also comprise two types. A design is termed *experimental* if patients are assigned in an unbiased way to each of the study groups. If the treatment is determined for each subject because of physician preference, the study is referred to as *observational*.[9]

Observational surveys can be further divided by the date on which the data were collected in relation to the present (real-time relationship). Studies with data accumulation in the past are called *retrospective*, whereas those with data ac-

cumulation after the study was conceived are termed *prospective*.[10]

Another method of subclassifying observational studies is by research pursuit direction; that is, were the subjects enrolled in a study because of their starting diagnosis and followed to observe an outcome (antecedent-to-outcome), or was the enrollment criterion a known outcome and records were reviewed to determine the initial diagnosis (outcome-to-antecedent)? The former design is commonly referred to as a *cohort study*, and the latter is termed a *trohoc design*. These analytic study types are summarized in Table 5–1.

Retrospective Versus Prospective. Retrospective observation is generally used as a means of broadly evaluating an issue to form one or several testable hypotheses; it is inferior to prospective observation, however, in terms of hypothesis testing. Data are generally gleaned from medical records or patient recall; both can be unreliable to the point of severely prejudicing the conclusions. In addition, when medical records are reviewed, the study is limited to those data recorded in the chart, regardless of how well the recorded information addresses the question being asked. When a retrospective analysis of infertility treatment is carried out, these issues must be carefully considered: What qualified the patient for inclusion in the study, and were these criteria uniformly applied? Were all women followed and evaluated in the same manner, or were some more closely followed than others? Inconsistencies in these areas substantially decrease the value of the study, and information extracted from such investigation should be considered preliminary and in need of prospective confirmation. Thus, although retrospective study is a good place to begin an inquiry, it is a poor way to complete one.

A prospective observational study is not without potential pitfalls, however. When subjects are not randomly allocated to study groups, care must be taken in evaluating the distribution of known confounding factors among the various treatments. Furthermore, because treatment assignments were made for a reason, careful consideration must be given to whether the reason will affect results.

Control Groups. To determine the value of a therapeutic maneuver on fertility status, it must be clear what would have happened had the therapy not been administered. This concept, the determination of baseline values as a source of comparison, is termed *control*.[11] The observational survey may be controlled or uncontrolled. If it is controlled, the comparison group may consist of data collected simultaneously to the experimental group (concurrent nonrandomized controls) or as a group of patients previously accumulated (historical controls). Observational surveys, by their very nature, cannot have a randomized control group.

Uncontrolled studies are treatment results without any direct comparison to another treatment (or no treatment). This may be appropriate if the disorder in question produces absolute sterility, such as azoospermia. In such an instance, it would be pointless to have a control group for comparison because all pregnancies following treatment are a direct result of that treatment and not a chance event. If the disorder produces a relative decrease in fertility, however, any pregnancies following treatment must be shown to occur at greater frequency than in untreated patients.[12] This cannot be done with uncontrolled trials.

A common remedy for this situation is the use of historical controls. Such control patients are from the group of patients seen and treated previously and have been treated with no therapeutic maneuver or standard historical therapy. The major difficulty with historical controls is ensuring that the comparison is fair. If, for instance, the treatment and control groups differ with respect to important prognostic factors or if the two groups were assessed for pregnancy in drastically different manners, an apparent improvement in fertility rate may be due to these variations in protocol rather than to the new treatment. Generally the problems inherent to the use of historical controls merely compound those already noted for retrospective studies; the results are usually trials of suspect validity.

When investigators wish to have concurrent controls without randomization, they often assign subjects to treatment groups based on "clinical judgment." Unfortunately such an approach can result in considerable bias.[13] For instance, in a study comparing embryo transfer to the fallopian tube via laparoscopy versus intrauterine transfer, a physician may determine that the patient with fewer embryos should not undergo the expense and risk of laparoscopy, thereby placing her in the intrauterine group. Thus, patients proceeding to tubal transfer represent those with uniformly good chances of conception, whereas all with a poor prognosis are shunted into the intrauterine transfer group. A poorer result with intrauterine transfer is indicative of how the subjects were assigned, not the technique itself. When such an approach of nonrandomized assignment is used, it is imperative to evaluate carefully the reasoning behind the choice of treatment groups to see if such decision making could affect the validity of the results.

Confounding Variables. Patient characteristics known to affect reproductive success can have substantial impact on results of a fertility trial. These characteristics include such items as a woman's age and a couple's duration of infertility, both of which are known to affect therapeutic results. Furthermore, the presence of additional problems contributing to infertility often lowers the success rate of a therapeutic intervention. To understand the impact of these confounding variables, at the very least they should be compared for each of the groups in the study. Matching the study groups for particular characteristics may help reduce the influence of confounding variables.[14] If this is insufficient or not possible, specific statistical methods can be applied to the analysis to ensure that such a maldistribution does not unduly affect results.

Randomized Clinical Trial. The randomized clinical trial (RCT) differs from the aforementioned prospective surveys in that a true experimental situation is developed: Patients are randomly allocated to either an experimental or a control group. This approach removes several sources of bias.[15] First, it is the only known safeguard against selection bias: The physician does not know the treatment assignment for a given patient, and the assignment is maximally unpredictable. Second, randomization is an insurance against substantial accidental bias between treatment groups with respect to some important patient variable. Any such important prognostic factors affecting outcome should be expected to distribute randomly between the groups. Finally, the logical foundation for many statistical tests is the premise that each patient could have received any one of the treatments being compared.

Although this study design is generally preferable to those previously discussed, there are specific caveats with this type of approach. Random allocation does not necessarily mean equal allocation, and with random assignment of patients to control or treatment, a prognostic factor may be found disproportionately in one of the two.[16] This chance occurrence is analogous to "the luck of the draw" in a poker game: Although the chances of being dealt four aces is unlikely, it certainly can happen. To guard against the possibility, careful assessment of the distribution of known prognostic factors must be undertaken at the conclusion of the study.

A second potential flaw in the RCT is variation in observation after treatment intervention. For instance, in a study analyzing the ovulation rate in oligo-ovulatory women with two dosage schedules of clomiphene citrate, the value of randomization is negated if the experimental group is followed with basal body temperatures, luteal phase progesterone levels, endometrial biopsy, and ultrasound scans, and the controls are evaluated by temperature alone. Care must always be taken to provide equivalent followup of each study subject.

A third danger in RCTs is the use of the wrong control. This does not invalidate the results, but it alters the conclusions drawn from the study. An example would be a RCT evaluating conservative surgery versus danazol in the enhancement of fertility in women with mild endometriosis. To demonstrate danazol to be more effective than surgery in promoting fertility would be interesting, but it would not demonstrate efficacy because neither therapy has been proved effective when compared with expectant management. The principle is a simple one: Although it is valid to use a control group receiving standard therapy (rather than no therapy), to state that an experimental modality is of value requires the prior demonstration that the standard therapy was in fact efficacious.

When randomization is to be undertaken, it can be accomplished in a variety of ways. Tables of random numbers or computer-generated random assignments are preferable owing to their lack of predictability. Methods such as even/odd social security numbers for assignment, or even alternating assignment, are suboptimal owing to the potential predictability: The physician may know before enrollment into which group the patient will be placed, thus potentially biasing the vigor with which enrollment is pursued. Simple randomization has significant disadvantages, however, in three circumstances: if the size of the trial is less than 100 patients, if the trial is multicenter, or if interim analyses are planned.[17] In these situations, a method known as restricted randomization is recommended to ensure that the numbers of patients allocated to each treatment are approximately equal in the trial as a whole or in important subgroups of patients. Such methods, in order of increasing complexity, include random permuted blocks, stratified randomization, and minimization. These methods are reviewed in detail elsewhere.[18, 19]

In infertility treatment trials, the RCT may be particularly difficult to accomplish. Patients presenting for infertility treatment are generally electively seeking care and thus seek to participate as intelligent consumers in the choice for their therapy. It may frequently be difficult to persuade patients to accept the possibility of being assigned to a nontreatment arm of a study. If a true clinical equipoise exists, however, and the clinician is convinced of this, he or she should be able to express this to the infertile couple. Nevertheless, many couples may find such arguments less than convincing, and enrollment may suffer for this reason. The shortage of RCTs in the infertility literature may more reflect this generalized preference for treatment, any treatment, by the patient than the failure of researchers to understand the value of such a study design.

RCTs may be structured in a variety of ways when applied to an infertility issue. Patients may be randomized initially, and their assignment remains unchanged thereafter. A common alternative is to randomize initially, then switch the patient to the alternate treatment in the next menstrual cycle. This switching, referred to as a crossover design, continues until the study is concluded or pregnancy is achieved. Such a design is appropriate only when a specific treatment interval, such as a menstrual cycle, can be specified. Finally, patients could conceivably be *randomized* to treatments with each menstrual cycle; such a technique is administratively difficult but significantly adds to the unpredictability of patient assignment.

Daya[20] has stated that the crossover design should be avoided in clinical infertility trials. He reasons that the advantages routinely presented by crossing over are lost owing to the nature of the disease process. For example, one advantage generally recognized for crossover trials is the ability for the patient to act as her own control, thus requiring fewer patients than usual for adequate power.[21] This is lost in infertility treatment trials because the outcome of interest (pregnancy) is a terminal event, and the patient may not have the opportunity to be her own control. This does not mean, however, that the crossover design is without value in infertility studies. Olive and colleagues[22] have shown that the sample size required is unchanged for routine randomization or randomization with crossover, thus demonstrating that crossover design does not place the investigator at a disadvantage. Moreover, many patients find the idea of alternating treatments more acceptable than being limited to a single treatment, thus increasing enrollment and reducing the time required for study completion. When contemplating a study design, these issues (and others) must be carefully considered so the optimal approach can be used for the question at hand.

Surgery and the Randomized Clinical Trial. RCTs have gained widespread acceptance in the evaluation of medical therapy, yet there has been resistance to such designs in the surgical community. The reason for this is that the RCT for surgical procedures has a number of inherent pitfalls that must be dealt with.[23, 24]

In contrast to the administration of a medication, performing an operation requires technical skill and experience. This skill in turn affects the treatment itself. In surgical trials, the treatment varies greatly with the participating surgeons' operative skill and experience. Thus, identically structured trials with different surgeons may give drastically different results.[23]

A second problem with the surgical RCT is the fact that new or innovative surgical techniques require training. New operations are introduced tentatively with uncertain indications and high risk. Techniques are then refined, and results improve, often dramatically. A RCT conducted during such an evolutionary phase often presents an unfairly pessimistic view. Such studies are usually invalidated even before completion, owing to evolution of techniques and results.

A design that attempts to cope with these unique problems is the random order operations trial.[23] In this type of study, an envelope is opened when the operation has reached a certain stage, and the surgeon then proceeds as indicated by the contents of the envelope. Unfortunately this design has a systematic bias that favors both methods currently in wide use and technically simple procedures. To avoid this, a prerandomization period is needed during which the surgeons can practice the experimental technique with carefully selected patients, with the ability to "bail out" when the degree of difficulty becomes excessive.

The aforementioned caveats are not to discourage the use of RCT for surgical innovations; indeed, the RCT can be of tremendous value in this area. Given the built-in hazards noted, however, considerable care should be exercised in the design and implementation of such studies.

Noncomparative Data Reporting

When controlled trials report success rates for treatment interventions, there are a variety of tools available to convey the data. Each has its assets, but there are limitations inherent to each method.

SIMPLE PREGNANCY RATES

The most common calculation in infertility treatment trials is the simple pregnancy rate. This value is defined as the number of pregnancies divided by the number of patients treated. It is among the easiest of analyses to perform, yet there are a number of major drawbacks.

First, this approach does not adjust for sample bias—that is, confounding variables that may affect fertility. An example is testing a treatment for ovulation dysfunction among all women with infertility and disordered ovulation. If the purpose of the study is to determine the value of the drug in producing pregnancy, a different picture might emerge if couples with male factor contributions were eliminated from the calculation. Second, the simple pregnancy rate depends on length of followup study. Women treated successfully for anovulation each month are clearly more likely to conceive the longer they attempt conception; thus, six monthly attempts at conception with successful ovulation induction are more likely to result in pregnancy than merely following the couple for one monthly attempt.

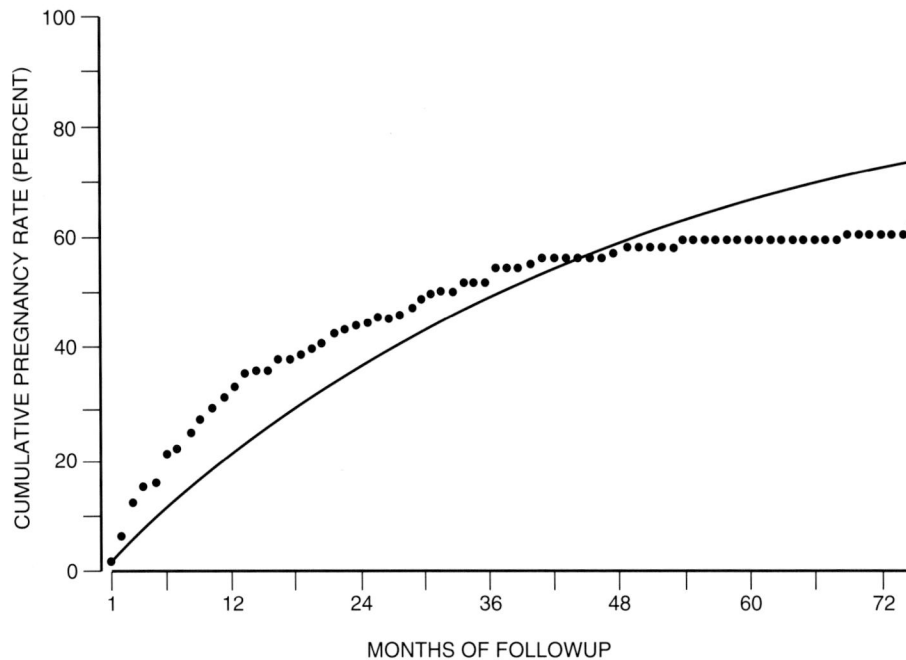

FIGURE 5–6. Comparison of the observed cumulative pregnancy curve (*darkened circles*) following conservative surgery for endometriosis with that predicted by monthly fecundity rate. Note the initial underestimation by the model, followed later by overestimation of pregnancy rate. (From Guzick DS, Rock JA. Estimation of a model of cumulative pregnancy following infertility therapy. Am J Obstet Gynecol 1981; 140:573–578.)

In the infertility treatment trial in which all patients enroll for the entire investigative period and none are lost to followup, the simple pregnancy rate may provide a rapid means of comparing study groups. For analyzing data with censored patients (women not completing the full followup period), however, or comparing groups with variable duration of followup, the simple pregnancy rate is a poor standard.

CORRECTED PREGNANCY RATES

Corrected pregnancy rates are calculated similarly to simple pregnancy rates except that couples with additional infertility factors are excluded from the statistics. In this way, a more homogeneous patient population is obtained for study. The same problems with variable followup seen with crude pregnancy rates, however, make this analytic approach of little value to the clinical investigator. Furthermore, there is an additional difficulty: a lack of standardization among researchers as to what defines a confounding factor in the infertile couple. The phrase "corrected for additional infertility factors" can have different meanings with different researchers, making it virtually impossible to draw generalizable conclusions from such studies.

CYCLE FECUNDITY RATES

Although simple or corrected pregnancy rates over a prolonged treatment interval have serious methodologic drawbacks, if one shortens the interval to a single, universal unit, many of these flaws can be eliminated. For treatments that are effective only in the menstrual cycle used (such as ovulation induction agents or donor inseminations), this unit is the treatment cycle itself. Thus, calculating the pregnancy rate per treatment cycle gives equal weight to each attempt at pregnancy by each study patient. This statistic is called the *cycle fecundity rate* (CFR). Advantages include the simplicity to calculate the CFR, its confidence limits, and statistical comparisons.[25] Furthermore, it approximates the expected chance of conception with each attempt at pregnancy, a clinically relevant figure to convey to patients.

The single serious problem with the CFR lies in its inherent assumption: All cycles have equal probability to result in a pregnancy. This assumption may not be true under two circumstances. First, patients may have a variety of confounding factors that make lumping patients into a single cohort inappropriate. To remedy this complexity, stratification of the patient population is required.

Second and more important, it is infrequent that each subsequent attempt at conception in a woman carries the same rate of success as its preceding cycle. For this to be the case, the assumption is that given an infinite number of induction cycles, the pregnancy rate will approach 100%. Although the reasoning approximates the situation with parous women seeking therapeutic donor insemination,[26] it rarely holds for other infertile women. Such a model initially underestimates the chance of conception but eventually overestimates the probability of conception (Fig. 5–6). This principle has been well illustrated in previous publications.[27, 28]

MONTHLY FECUNDITY RATES

When patients undergo a one-time treatment (usually surgical), it is rarely practical to measure the followup in terms of menstrual cycles. Instead the unit of time is a month, and the calculation appropriate in this situation is the *monthly fecundity rate* (MFR). This value is determined by taking the total number of pregnancies achieved during followup divided by the total number of months of followup for all study subjects.

As with the CFR, the MFR has the advantage of being easy to calculate. Furthermore, it gives the patient a rough idea what the chances of conception are each month after treatment. It also maintains, however, the same disadvantage of the CFR: that each month following surgery is deemed to be of equal likelihood to result in pregnancy. Should a treatment modality cause a brief, limited effect on fertility enhancement or even no initial success followed by delayed conceptions, this model is probably inappropriate unless limited to a specific time interval for followup.

LIFE-TABLE ANALYSIS

A method to deal with variable length of followup or treatment is to produce a graphic display of the cumulative rate of pregnancy as treatment duration increases.[29–32] This technique is commonly referred to as the *life table*. This method has the advantage of identifying the rate of conception at any particular time after initiation of treatment; it thus does not suffer from any assumptions of uniformity of success from month to month. Life tables are best applied to treatments in which single interventions produce long-term results; an example would be pregnancy rates following tubal anastomosis. Life-table calculations also compensate for variable followup after treatment. If patients drop out of the study without conceiving, these "censored" patients can be mathematically corrected for, to give an estimate of what would have happened if all patients continued in the trial.

With large patient numbers, the life table often takes on the appearance of a relatively smooth curve. As the number of patients decreases with increasing length of followup, the variance for each data point increases.

Although the life table represents a tremendous improvement over the simple calculation of pregnancy rates, there is one potentially misleading aspect of the technique. Women who are lost to followup are assumed to be identical to those who continue to be followed up. Unfortunately this premise is frequently untrue. Often the woman lost to followup has circumstances different from those remaining in the study. An example would be ovulation induction with gonadotropin, in which those women who stop trying are those with poor responses following high doses. In this case, the patients continuing in the study have a better prognosis than those dropping out; the ultimate pregnancy rate of those remaining is not indicative of the rate to be expected among the entire group starting the study.

TWO-PARAMETER EXPONENTIAL MODELS

Mathematical models of cumulative pregnancy curves have been developed in which the entire curve is expressed as a concise parametric equation, one that summarizes the characteristics of the curve by capturing its key features. Two-parameter exponential models have been designed to describe the cumulative pregnancy curve.[27, 33] The underlying assumption of these models is that the observed cumulative pregnancy curve is really a weighted average of two curves, one for patients who will eventually conceive (cured) and the other for those who will never conceive (not cured). In the latter instance, the curve is a horizontal line at 0%. As time advances and women from the cured group achieve pregnancy, the uncured group represents a larger and larger population of those remaining in the study; thus, the cumulative pregnancy curve appears to plateau well before 100% conception is achieved. Two clinically meaningful parameters describe this model: the *cure rate*, which represents the percentage of women who conceive given an infinite length of followup, and the *monthly probability of pregnancy* (MPP) for

those who achieve conception. This model appears to correspond well to empiric data generated in fertility trials.

In some situations, it may be appropriate to consider a population consisting of more than two groups. An example is seen in women undergoing donor insemination for male factor infertility, in which the prognosis for success is inversely proportional to the severity of the abnormality in the male. Groupings might consist of (1) women with azoospermic husbands, (2) women with severely oligospermic husbands, and (3) women with mildly oligospermic husbands, with each group having a subgroup of patients eventually "cured" and a subgroup that will never conceive. Thus, six groups rather than two must be considered. In this case, multiparameter exponential models can be devised to describe the pregnancy rates for such a heterogeneous patient population.[33]

REGRESSION MODELS

Many studies investigate the association of a number of different confounding variables on the outcome of ovulation induction. Regression models are frequently used in such multifactor situations. These models take a variety of forms, but their common aim is to study the individual and joint effect of a number of different factors on an outcome variable.

When the outcome is binary (pregnant versus not pregnant) at a specifically defined time point without censoring of patients, multiple logistic regression modeling is the appropriate method used.[34] By performing logistic regression for a number of predictor variables, the effect of each on the chance of achieving pregnancy can be determined. Furthermore, interactions between predictor variables can be assessed and their magnitudes determined.[35] Thus, this method is the desired approach when attempting to sort out the value of a treatment in the face of multiple confounding factors.

More often, however, the situation is such that the outcome is not a simple yes or no at a specified time point but rather a cumulative pregnancy curve across a wide span of time. In this situation, the Cox proportional hazards model[36] (an analog of multiple linear regression) corrects for confounding variables yet takes into account the overall structure of the pregnancy curve.[37] The major advantages of this technique include the ability to correct for confounding influences and independence from traditional exponential models of life tables. A major disadvantage of the technique is a greater sensitivity to rate of pregnancy rather than to ultimate cure rate.

DANGERS OF STATISTICAL MODELS

Although many well-known physical equations provide an exact description, statistical models use equations quite differently. The equation for a statistical model is not expected to be exactly true; instead it represents a useful framework within which the statistician is able to study relationships that are of interest.[38] There are often no biologically plausible reasons supporting statistical models; in general, they should be regarded simply as an attempt to provide an empiric summary of observed data. Whenever such modeling is to be attempted, it is suggested that consultation with a statistician is appropriate to ensure proper handling and interpretation.

Comparing Data

Frequently a study is designed to compare the effects of two different interventions on the rate of conception. Several methods exist to accomplish this task.

CATEGORICAL COMPARISONS

With pregnancy (yes/no), methods used to compare two treatment groups must deal with this categorical type of outcome. Categorical comparisons are appropriate for simple and corrected pregnancy rates, CFRs, and MFRs. In each case, the outcome may be expressed as falling into one of two categories. Two tests appropriate for comparing treatments with these end points include Fisher's test and the chi-squared test.

Fisher's test is limited to data that can be summarized in a 2×2 table.[39] Thus, no more than two groups can be compared, and no more than two outcomes can be possible. Such a test is appropriate in a situation such as the following: In women with polycystic ovarian disease, treatment with clomiphene citrate, 50 mg daily for 5 days versus 8 days, is tested. The outcome observed is pregnant versus not pregnant. Based on the values for each of the four combinations of treatment and outcome, specific calculations can be made to determine if the distribution among categories is random or not (Table 5–2).

Fisher's test is commonly referred to as Fisher's exact test because it calculates the exact significance level of the null hypothesis that the probability of success is the same in two distinct groups. In the past, studies with large numbers made calculations for the test quite formidable. Today, however, with the advent of the microcomputers for statistical analysis, it is clear that any 2×2 categorical comparison should be analyzed by Fisher's test rather than the chi-squared test with continuity correction. If, however, the comparison involves a grid larger than 2×2, chi-squared testing is indicated. For instance, if four medical treatments were used to attempt ovulation induction in women with hyperprolactinemia (outcome is ovulation/no ovulation), a 4×2 grid is designed, and chi-squared testing is appropriate.

With either of the preceding tests, there are two important assumptions. One is that the probability of success entering the study is the same for each subject in a group. Second, the outcome of the experiment for any subject may not influence the outcome for any member of either group. When these requirements are overlooked or ignored, such analyses could mask important effects or generate spurious ones.

TABLE 5–2. Categorical Data from a Two-Treatment Trial*			
	Pregnant	**Nonpregnant**	**Total**
5-day treatment	13	27	40
8-day treatment	25	17	42
Total	38	44	82

*This is a 2×2 table. Significance testing is best accomplished by use of Fisher's test. Treatment compared is the use of clomiphene citrate for 5 days vs. 8 days for ovulation induction in anovulatory women.

COMPARING CUMULATIVE PREGNANCY CURVES

When cumulative pregnancy curves are generated for two groups in a treatment trial, it becomes desirable to compare them with one another. One test, called the log-rank or Mantel-Haenszel test,[40, 41] is frequently used to compare cumulative rates of two or more populations. The log-rank test is designed specifically to detect a difference between cumulative pregnancy curves that results when the pregnancy rate in one group is consistently higher than the corresponding rate in a second group, and the ratio of these two rates is constant over time; that is, the pregnancy rate for treatment *A* may be 5% per month, and that of treatment *B* may be 15% per month. In this case, the ratio is 1:3 for each month of observation, and the log-rank test would seem particularly appropriate.

Another method of comparing these curves is the Breslow formulation of the Kruskal-Wallis test.[42] This test is similar to the log-rank test, but its particular strength is in weighing points along the cumulative pregnancy curve. Thus, if a study contains large numbers of censored patients, the Breslow test may be optimal.

These tests are but two of many designed to compare cumulative curves. Under particular circumstances, more specialized testing may be required.

TWO-PARAMETER EXPONENTIAL MODEL COMPARISON

A likelihood ratio test has been devised to allow easy comparison of two populations modeled via the two-parameter exponential method described previously.[43] In this test, the cure rate and monthly probability of pregnancy (MPP) are estimated under varying assumptions about these parameters in the two curves, corresponding to four "models."

- Model 1: Cure rates and MPP are both different.
- Model 2: Cure rates are the same, but MPPs are different.
- Model 3: Cure rates are different, but MPPs are the same.
- Model 4: Both cure rates and MPPs are the same.

For each model, the maximized value of the likelihood function is computed. The hypothesis that one or both of the parameters differ between groups is tested by comparison of pairs of each of the models under consideration, with the comparison statistic providing a chi-squared distribution.

COMPARISON VIA REGRESSION

Logistic regression modeling can allow comparison of treatment modalities by making one of the predictor variables equal to treatment. If two treatments were attempted, the determination can be made as to whether a change in treatment influences the outcome variable (pregnancy). If a significant relationship is determined, it can be concluded that one of the treatments is superior to the other in producing the desired outcome.

SEQUENTIAL CHANGES IN TREATMENT STATUS

The evaluation of comparative pregnancy data is subject to a variety of biases. One bias commonly encountered is analysis of patients who transfer from one treatment group to another or even back and forth between two or more treatment groups.

The Mantel-Byars analysis method, an approach for constructing and comparing modified life tables and reflecting sequential changes of treatment status, is applicable to just these types of situations.[44] The method can compensate for patient transfer from one comparison group to another (or even back and forth between groups).

SIGNIFICANCE AND POWER

When comparing the results of two treatments (or one treatment versus no therapy) on pregnancy, absolutely conclusive results are not attainable. Instead one must "play the odds" when trying to decide if success rates differ. The key to determining this is *statistical significance,* a concept that states that, given the available data, the odds overwhelmingly favor there being a real difference between two groups. Generally statistical significance requires that, given an observed difference between two treatments, it will in fact be a real difference (rather than just a statistical fluke) at least 95% of the time.

Occasionally a study suggests a difference in success between treatments, yet in reality there is not one. This is called type I statistical error. The rate for a type I error in a given experiment is termed the *alpha value* and is generally set at not more than 5%.

Some studies suggest no difference in pregnancy rates between treatments. When this occurs, the reader must discern between two alternative possibilities: Either there is truly no difference in outcome between the groups, or the study failed to detect an actual difference. The occurrence of the latter is called a type II statistical error.[45–47] The rate for a type II error in a given experiment is termed the *beta value,* and a maximum chance is generally set at no more than 20%. In such a situation, the statistical *power* to avoid a type II error is 1-beta (usually at least 80%). Statistical tables and computer programs are available to compute power for a given sample size and study design. Such calculations can be performed either a priori (in an attempt to estimate the sample size necessary when planning a study) or post hoc (to determine a study's risk of a false-negative conclusion). The power calculations for these two situations, interestingly, are often quite disparate.[48]

Significance and power are two critical concepts that must be clearly delineated in a treatment trial. If a study presumes to show a difference between treatments, it is imperative to know whether statistical significance was achieved and if so what the preset alpha value was. If the authors claim no difference, one must ask if the study achieved reasonable power to avoid a type II error given its sample size and significance threshold. It is all too often the case that a poorly conceived study fails to demonstrate a significant difference between treatments yet is not of sufficient power to exclude with reasonable certainty that such a difference exists. These investigations are of little value to anyone and generally serve only to muddle the literature. This failure highlights the importance of thoroughly planning an investigation before its initiation, again emphasizing the inherent value of the prospective approach.

META-ANALYSIS

A technique of statistical manipulation has appeared in the medical literature that attempts to evaluate and combine the results of previous studies.[49, 50] This technique, termed meta-analysis, is useful for the following purposes: (1) to increase statistical power for primary end points and for subgroups, (2) to resolve uncertainty when reports disagree, (3) to improve estimates of effect size, and (4) to answer questions not posed at the start of individual trials. This method is used nearly exclusively to pool RCTs.

There are five areas of importance in assessing the quality of a meta-analysis: study design, combinability, control of bias, statistical analysis, and problems of applicability.[50] Study design must be rigorous and well defined; details of the literature search should be spelled out and should be comprehensive. All trials analyzed and accepted or rejected for inclusion should be listed. Finally, criteria for inclusion/exclusion should be clearly stated.

Combinability of studies is always an important premise. The meta-analysis should note any differences in the combined studies and explain how these differences affect the conclusion. If there seems to be significant between-study variability, tests of homogeneity help determine the degree of caution with which pooled results should be interpreted.

As with any scientific study, a meta-analysis should be controlled for potential sources of bias. A major potential source in these studies is publication bias—the tendency for a study showing a difference in treatment to be more readily published than a "negative" study showing no difference.[51] Care must be taken to search out all studies performed, whether published or not.

Statistical analysis should include a recognized method for evaluating pooled data, such as the Mantel-Haenszel test. Confidence limits, types I and II error rates, and relevant subgroup analyses should be included. Finally, a sensitivity analysis should show how results of the meta-analysis vary depending on different assumptions and criteria for inclusion.

Once the results are obtained, a meta-analysis must consider their value in addressing the initial hypothesis. Are the conclusions definitive or merely suggestive? By giving quantitative estimates of the weight of available evidence, meta-analyses can be quite useful in making clinical decisions. Such analyses, however, are only as good as the studies they combine. If meta-analyses are to provide meaningful clinical information, they must be conducted scientifically and written thoroughly. The reader should remain skeptical of sketchy reports combining studies.

ROLE OF THE LITERATURE IN CLINICAL DECISIONS

The infertility literature is filled with research studies investigating nearly every aspect of clinical care. Despite this, there remains significant variation in the way clinicians approach patients. This is as it should be. The purpose of clinical research is not to provide definitive guidelines for clinical practice; rather each study addresses a specific problem from a particular, often unique, viewpoint. Answers may be clear-cut for a cohort of women fitting a long list of narrow inclusion and exclusion criteria. Our patients, however, rarely fit neatly into these defined categories.

Clinical medicine is a messy business, filled with considerable guesswork and gambling. To be most successful, a good clinician (like a good gambler) must combine a thorough knowledge of the "odds" with a keen intuition for the situation at hand. The literature represents the former, the best source of facts poised for application. An outstanding physician never swears by these facts, but rather uses such guidance, along with experience, to optimize individual patient care. This role, as suggestion box rather than bible, is the true utility of the medical literature in clinical decisions.

REFERENCES

1. Olive DL. The prevalence and epidemiology of luteal-phase deficiency in normal and infertile women. Clin Obstet Gynecol 1991; 34:157–166.
2. Feinstein AR. Clinical Epidemiology: The Architecture of Clinical Research. Philadelphia: WB Saunders, 1985.
3. Riegelman RK. Studying a Study and Testing a Test: How to Read the Medical Literature. Boston: Little, Brown & Co, 1981.
4. Galton F. Regression toward mediocrity in hereditary stature. J Anthropological Institute 1886; 15:246–263.
5. Metz CE, Goodenough DJ, Rossman K. Evaluation of receiver operating characteristic curve data in terms of information theory, with applications in radiography. Radiology 1973; 109:297–303.
6. Hanley JA, McNeil BJ. The meaning and use of the area under a Receiver Operating Characteristic (ROC) curve. Radiology 1982; 143:29–36.
7. McNeil BJ, Hanley JA. Statistical approaches to the analysis of Receiver Operating Characteristic (ROC) curves. Med Decis Making 1984; 4:137–150.
8. Kassirer JP. Our stubborn quest for diagnostic certainty: a cause of excessive testing. N Engl J Med 1989; 320:1489–1491.
9. Feinstein AR. Clinical biostatistics. XLIV. A survey of the research architecture used for publications in general medical journals. Clin Pharmacol Ther 1978; 24:117–125.
10. Feinstein AR. Clinical biostatistics. XLVIII. Efficacy of different research structures in preventing bias in the analysis of causation. Clin Pharmacol Ther 1979; 26:129–141.
11. Feinstein AR. Clinical biostatistics. LVIII. A glossary of neologisms in quantitative clinical science. Clin Pharmacol Ther 1981; 30:564–577.
12. Leridon H, Spira A. Problems in measuring the effectiveness of infertility therapy. Fertil Steril 1984; 41:580–586.
13. Student. The Lenarkshire milk experiment. Biometrika 1931; 23:398.
14. Cates W Jr, Ory HW. What matching achieves. Contemp Ob Gyn 1983; 21:171–175.
15. Gore SM. Assessing clinical trials—why randomise? BMJ 1981; 282:1958–1960.
16. Feinstein AR. Clinical biostatistics. XXII. The role of randomization in sampling, testing, allocation, and credulous idolatry (Part I). Clin Pharmacol Ther 1973; 14:601–615.
17. Gore SM. Assessing clinical trials—simple randomisation. BMJ 1981; 282:2036–2039.
18. Gore SM. Assessing clinical trials—restricted randomisation. BMJ 1981; 282:2114–2117.
19. Zelen M. The randomisation and stratification of patients to clinical trials. J Chron Dis 1974; 27:365–375.
20. Daya S. Is there a place for the crossover design in infertility trials? Fertil Steril 1993; 59:6–7.
21. Louis TA, Lavori PW, Bailar JC, Polansky M. Crossover and self-controlled designs in clinical research. N Engl J Med 1984; 310:24–31.
22. Olive DL, Doody M, Silverberg KM, Klein NA, Burns WN. A comparison of study design methods for cycle-specific treatments of infertility. Abstract #0-068. Presented at the 48th Annual Meeting of the American Fertility Society, New Orleans, 1992.
23. vander Linden W. Pitfalls in randomized surgical trials. Surgery 1980; 87:258–262.
24. Bonchek LI. The role of the randomized clinical trial in the evaluation of new operations. Surg Clin North Am 1982; 62:761–769.
25. Cramer DW, Walker AM, Schiff I. Statistical methods in evaluating the outcome of infertility therapy. Fertil Steril 1979; 32:80–86.
26. Peek JC, Godfrey B, Matthews CD. Estimation of fertility and fecundity in women receiving artificial insemination by donor semen and in normal fertile women. Br J Obstet Gynaecol 1984; 91:1019–1024.
27. Guzick DS, Rock JA. Estimation of a model of cumulative pregnancy following infertility therapy. Am J Obstet Gynecol 1981; 140:573–578.
28. Olive DL. How to evaluate reports of infertility treatment. In: Hammond MG, Talbert LM, editors. Infertility, A Practical Guide for the Physician. 3rd edition. Boston: Blackwell Scientific, 1992:279–299.
29. Berkson J, Gage RP. Calculation of survival rates for cancer. Mayo Clin Proc 1950; 25:270.
30. Cutler SJ, Ederer F. Maximum utilization of the life-table method of analyzing survival. J Chron Dis 1958; 8:699–712.
31. Katayama KP. A method of analyzing data with incomplete follow-up. Am J Obstet Gynecol 1975; 123:214–215.
32. Lamb EJ, Cruz AL. Data collection and analysis in an infertility practice. Fertil Steril 1972; 23:310–319.
33. Hershlag A, Kaplan EH, Loy RA, DeCherney AH, Lavy G. Heterogenicity in patient populations explains differences in in vitro fertilization programs. Fertil Steril 1991; 56:913–917.
34. Matthews DE, Farewell VT. Binary logistic regression. In: Using and Understanding Medical Statistics. 2nd edition. New York: Karger, 1988:141–154.
35. Gunst RF, Mason RL. Regression Analysis and Its Applications. New York: Marcel Dekker, 1980.
36. Cox DR. Regression models and life tables. J R Stat Soc (B) 1972; 34:187.
37. Lee KL, McNeer JF, Starmer CF, Harris PJ, Rosati RA. Clinical judgement and statistics: lessons from a simulated randomized trial in coronary artery disease. Circulation 1980; 61:508–515.
38. Matthews DE, Farewell VT. Linear regression models for medical data. In: Using and Understanding Medical Statistics. 2nd edition. New York, Karger, 1988, pp 124–140.
39. Brown GW. 2×2 tables. Am J Dis Child 1985; 139:410–416.
40. Mantel N. Evaluation of survival data and two new rank order statistics arising in its consideration. Cancer Chemother Rep 1966; 50:163–170.
41. Peto R, Pike MC, Armitage P, et al. Design and analysis of randomized clinical trials requiring prolonged observation of each patient. II. Analysis and examples. Br J Cancer 1977; 35:1–39.
42. Kruskal WH, Wallis WA. Use of ranks in one-criterion variance analysis. Am J Stat Assoc 1952; 47:583.
43. Guzick DS, Bross DS, Rock JA. A parametric method for comparing cumulative pregnancy curves following infertility therapy. Fertil Steril 1982; 37:503–507.
44. Mantel N, Byars DP. Evaluation of response-time data involving transient states: an illustration using heart-transplant data. Am J Stat Assoc 1974; 69:81.
45. Kraemer HC. Sample size: when is enough enough? Am J Med Sci 1988; 296:360–363.
46. Javitt JC. When does the failure to find a difference mean that there is none? Arch Ophthalmol 1989; 107:1034–1040.
47. Young MJ, Bresnitz EA, Strom BL. Sample size nomograms for interpreting negative clinical studies. Ann Int Med 1983; 99:248–251.
48. Detsky AS, Sackett DL. When was a 'negative' clinical trial big enough? How many patients you needed depends on what you found. Arch Int Med 1985; 145:709–712.
49. Hughes EG. Meta-analysis and the critical appraisal of infertility literature. Fertil Steril 1992; 57:275–277.
50. Sacks HS, Berrier J, Reitman D, Ancona-Berk VA, Chalmers TC. Meta-analysis of randomized controlled trials. N Engl J Med 1987; 316:450–455.
51. Dickersin K, Chan S, Chalmers TC, Sacks HS, Smith H Jr. Publication bias and clinical trials. Contr Clin Trials 1987; 8:343–353.

SECTION TWO

Evaluation of the Infertile Couple

WILLIAM R. KEYE, Jr.

CHAPTER 6

Female Infertility

ROBERT H. GLASS

Women are the ones most likely to seek help for infertility, and thus it is incumbent on the gynecologist to provide some coherence in the investigation and treatment. This requires not only mastery of the medical aspects of infertility, but also a logical approach to the problem. The cornerstone of all interactions should be a dialogue between physician and patient. The physician should be willing to inform, to allow participation in decision making by the individual or couple seeking help, and to have periodic consultations designed to update the status of the investigation and to provide a long-term outlook.

From the onset, it should be made clear that infertility is not an exact science. Almost every aspect of diagnosis and treatment is subject to some controversy. In addition, there is a spontaneous cure-rate with almost every problem in infertility, and in some cases, nature may provide a chance equal to that accomplished with active therapy. Because infertility and its medical care can be psychologically and financially draining, the physician and staff should be supportive during all interactions and should be ready to refer to support groups or to mental health professionals when appropriate.

No review of current infertility practice can avoid consideration of the effects of age on fertility. Many women are delaying childbearing even into their 40s as they concentrate energies on advancing their careers or seek financial stability before starting a family. Although there may be disagreements over the absolute figures, there is little to dispute the decline of fertility that starts in the middle thirties and becomes marked after age 40. Studies of Hutterite women published in 1957 indicated that in this highly fertile population, which at the time did not use contraception, only 16% of women retained their fertility at age 44 and only 66% at age 39.[1] A similar trend was noted in French women who were artificially inseminated with frozen semen.[2] Even the newer reproductive technologies cannot eliminate the biologic effects of age on oocyte potential. The United States Registry of In Vitro Fertilization (IVF) reported the age-related clinical pregnancy rates per transfer following IVF in 1989 (Table 6–1).[3] The spontaneous abortion rate in the 40+ group was approximately twice that seen with younger women.

It is difficult to decide at what age therapy is likely to be nonproductive. Many women want to pursue all avenues of treatment even into their midforties. With the exception of the ovum donor technique discussed elsewhere in this book and realizing that spontaneous pregnancies do occur in women well into their forties, it should be recognized that aggressive therapy for women older than 42 is difficult to justify. For the woman approaching or just past 40, measurement of follicle-stimulating hormone (FSH) on cycle day 3 of the menstrual cycle can be a useful screen, with values less than 15 mIu/mL suggesting normally responsive ovaries and values greater than 25 mIu/mL suggestive of impending cessation of ovarian function. At FSH levels between 15 and 25 mIu/mL, there is increasing difficulty in stimulating the ovaries. FSH values, however, can vary from cycle to cycle.

A health history is important for pinpointing problems that may have impact on infertility as well as those that may adversely affect general health. The couple's desire for fertility can provide a spur to change adverse behavior, such as cigarette smoking, excess alcohol intake, and drug use. Historical information can influence the approach to diagnosis and treatment. For example, a history of a severe pelvic infection not only raises a suspicion of tubal disease but also provides a warning not to do a hysterosalpingogram, which has the potential for reactivating tubal infection.

Similarly, the health practitioner should do a general examination, including measurements of blood pressure, breast examination, auscultation of the heart, and abdominal examination as well as the pelvic examination. Concentration on the problem of infertility should not obscure the possibility that other illnesses can coexist and that this may be the woman's only current interaction with a physician. Although completeness of the history and physical examination is stressed, a more selective approach to laboratory testing is

TABLE 6–1. Clinical Pregnancy Rates per Transfer After In Vitro Fertilization	
Age (yr)	Pregnancies/Embryo Transfer (%)
<25	35
25–29	23
30–34	21
35–39	19
40+	12

Data from in vitro fertilization–embryo transfer (IVF-ET) in the United States: 1989 results from the IVF-ET registry. Fertil Steril 1991; 55:14.

recommended. Routine ordering of gonadotropin assays and thyroid function tests in the woman who has regular cycles is unlikely to aid in diagnosis or in treatment. Serial monitoring of follicle growth and disappearance (ovulation) throughout a cycle to diagnose the luteinized unruptured follicle (LUF) syndrome should be reserved for those women in whom no obvious cause for infertility is found. The diagnosis of LUF syndrome (discussed elsewhere in this chapter) is not easy to establish even with serial ultrasound monitoring.

Preovulatory measurements of estradiol levels to determine if there is defective follicle formation are both expensive and unlikely to provide a firm diagnosis because of a wide range of normal values. In all matters of testing, there should be a clear idea of what impact a specific test will have on diagnosis and treatment and how remote the possibility is of obtaining a positive finding. Routine ordering of thyroid function tests rarely produces an unexpected abnormal result. Although positive tests for *Mycoplasma* are common in infertile women, the usefulness of routine treatment of this organism in the infertile couple has not been proved.

Although this chapter concerns female infertility, it should be kept in mind that infertility often involves both partners. In addition, current therapy may use simultaneous treatment of both partners, for example, in those cases in which sperm separation and intrauterine insemination are performed in conjunction with superovulation of the female.

The focus of this chapter is on those areas of diagnosis and treatment that can be performed in an office setting. An approach that stresses performing the basic tests within 2 to 3 months is emphasized in an effort to prevent undue delay in initiating proper therapy. If there are no evident causes for the failure to conceive, we usually assess the semen first and then proceed from least invasive to more invasive tests (Table 6–2). Consideration is given to the controversies surrounding each diagnostic test and some of the therapies.

TESTS FOR OVULATION

If a woman's periods occur at 26- to 36-day intervals, she is, in all likelihood, ovulatory, but confirmatory evidence can be obtained in a number of ways. Least expensive is the monitoring of the basal body temperature. Charting throughout just one cycle to identify the biphasic pattern associated with ovulation is sufficient. Confirmatory evidence of ovulation can be obtained by measuring a serum progesterone level 1 week after presumptive ovulation or by doing an endometrial biopsy 10 to 12 days after ovulation. Pinpointing

ovulation can best be done by self-monitoring of the luteinizing hormone (LH) surge with one of a variety of urinary LH kits that are available as over-the-counter products. Similar over-the-counter kits for measuring the progesterone metabolite, pregnanediol, are also available to confirm ovulation.[4] This qualitative assay, however, does not provide the more quantifiable information available from measured progesterone levels or from dating the endometrial biopsy. These latter tests allow assessment of the adequacy of the luteal phase as well as confirming the presence or absence of ovulation. An inadequate luteal phase diagnosed by lower than normal serum progesterone levels or by an out-of-phase endometrial biopsy is thought to play a role in infertility and recurrent pregnancy loss. This view has not been uniformly accepted because many women with normal fertility have evidence on biopsy of an inadequate luteal phase. In one study, the prevalence of the abnormality in a group of fertile women was not different from that found in an infertile population.[5] Despite this finding, much attention has been concentrated on making this diagnosis. The defect can arise because of a hormone deficiency during the proliferative phase of the menstrual cycle, an improper LH surge, or defective steroidogenesis in the corpus luteum, all of which can lower progesterone levels.

The diagnosis of inadequate luteal phase too often is established based on limited information. A single progesterone assay is insufficient to establish the diagnosis, especially if the timing is suspect. As noted, use of urinary LH kits allows good timing for scheduling a serum progesterone test 6 to 7 days after ovulation or an endometrial biopsy 10 to 12 days after ovulation.[6] Because of the pulsatile nature of progesterone release, it is hard to accept one value as definitive. If the value is equal to or greater than 15 ng/mL, however, the endometrial biopsy can be delayed while other diagnoses are pursued. Values between 10 and 15 ng/mL are in a gray zone and worthy of repetition. A value between 3 and 10 ng/mL is highly suspicious for luteal phase deficiency; a value less than 3 ng/mL indicates anovulation.

Although the endometrial biopsy is thought to provide a better assessment of progestational output during the luteal phase, its drawbacks include pain, expense, the somewhat subjective criteria involved in dating the endometrium, and the suspicion that it may not be a gold standard.[7] Premedication with a prostaglandin inhibitor to alleviate pain and use of flexible biopsy instruments such as the Pipelle lessen the degree of discomfort. More than one abnormal biopsy result is required to establish a diagnosis of an inadequate luteal phase because a biopsy result showing a lag greater than 2 days in not uncommonly found in random cycles of individuals with normal fertility.[5] This poses a dilemma for the physician and the patient who may be reluctant to undergo a second biopsy. A solution might be to accept a combination of a lower than normal serum progesterone level in one cycle and a biopsy result that lags more than 2 days behind the expected day in another cycle as evidence of a luteal phase deficiency. Treatment is varied and includes clomiphene citrate stimulation (although this drug has been implicated as a cause of an inadequate luteal phase); progesterone vaginal suppositories, 25 mg twice a day starting 2 to 3 days after ovulation; or human chorionic gonadotropin, 1500 or 2500 IU every 3 days for three to four doses during the luteal

TABLE 6–2. Testing in Unexplained Infertility	
Test	**Time in Cycle**
Semen analysis	—
Basal temperature chart	Throughout one cycle
Postcoital test	Periovulatory
Hysterosalpingography	3–5 days after cessation of menses
Serum progesterone	Midluteal phase
Endometrial biopsy	2–4 days before menses
Sperm antibodies	—
Hamster penetration assay and/or human zona assay	—
Laparoscopy/hysteroscopy	Proliferative phase

phase of the cycle. If pregnancy occurs, supplementation with progesterone is continued through the first 8 to 12 weeks of pregnancy. Clomiphene citrate has been shown to be effective especially in cases in which there is a marked (5 days or more) lag in the endometrial biopsy result.[8] Because of the "softness" of the diagnosis and the lack of good controlled studies, the efficacy of diagnosing and treating the inadequate luteal phase remains uncertain.

On occasion, an oocyte becomes entrapped in a follicle, and it is not extruded at ovulation (LUF syndrome). In all likelihood, this is a sporadic event, and the intensive, sequential ultrasound monitoring needed to make the diagnosis can be both expensive and misleading.[9] Failure of the follicle to collapse and continued growth of the follicle after the presumptive time of ovulation is thought to establish the diagnosis of LUF syndrome. More frequent than daily monitoring may be necessary, however, to catch the collapse of the follicle, and "growth" after ovulation could result from formation of a corpus luteum. Moreover, even if the diagnosis is entertained, the usual therapy in the form of clomiphene citrate or human menopausal gonadotropin stimulation is frequently offered as empiric treatment to infertile women, perhaps in conjunction with intrauterine insemination, even if LUF is not found. Thus, with current practice, making the diagnosis may have little impact on therapy.

It has been suggested that ovulation from a smaller than normal follicle (less than 16 mm in diameter) also may be an infertility factor. Here, too, treatment with ovulation-inducing drugs has been proposed, but the experience is too limited to know whether the diagnosis is important and whether the therapy is useful.

POSTCOITAL TEST

Vaginal ultrasound has become an important tool in the management of infertility. It can be used for assessing uterine contour, but its more vital role is in the monitoring of ovarian follicle development in response to stimulation with clomiphene citrate, human menopausal gonadotropins, or gonadotropin-releasing hormone. It also can be used to ensure proper timing for a postcoital test (PCT). An ultrasound examination is scheduled for 2 to 3 days before expected ovulation and measurement made of the preovulatory follicle. Because ovulation usually occurs when the follicle is between 17 and 25 mm in diameter in an unstimulated cycle and follicles usually grow 2 to 3 mm a day, the PCT can be scheduled for a day close to the anticipated time of ovulation and 2 to 8 hours after intercourse. If poor mucus is found in a cycle not monitored with ultrasound, a single ultrasound scan immediately after the PCT may show a preovulatory follicle, which should be associated with ample cervical mucus. Conversely, visualization of a small follicle is an indication to schedule a repeat PCT a few days later.

The finding of scant or absent mucus on two well-timed PCTs is an indication for treatment by intrauterine inseminations. In the past, reliance was placed on estrogen treatment of poor mucus, but success is sporadic, especially when poor mucus follows use of clomiphene citrate.[10] The finding of nonmotile, shaking, or absent sperm in the face of good mucus and a normal sperm count can indicate an abnormal pH in the mucus, an immunologic abnormality, presence of

infection, or rarely some failure of coital technique. Couples should be cautioned that lubricants such as K-Y Jelly and Surgilube have a spermicidal effect and should not be used.

The pH of the mucus should be 7.0 or higher at the time of ovulation.[11] More acidic pHs can be treated with precoital douches composed of 1 tablespoon of sodium bicarbonate in a quart of warm water.[12] Immunologic infertility is considered later in this chapter.

What constitutes the lower limit of normal for the number of motile sperm/hpf? In a number of studies, the eventual pregnancy rate bore little relationship to numbers of sperm found in the PCT.[13, 14] In addition, in another study, approximately 20% of *fertile* women had either no sperm or less than 1 sperm/hpf in the PCT.[15] One group, however, found that intrauterine inseminations enhanced the chances for pregnancy when there were 3 or fewer sperm/hpf but not when there were 5 or more sperm/hpf.[16] Thus, a PCT can be valuable in determining appropriate therapy. Moreover, the results of the PCT may indicate the need for other testing. For example, a test for sperm antibodies should be ordered if the sperm in the PCT are shaking in place, dead, or absent. In addition, the PCT may provide prognostic information. Individuals with few sperm took longer to achieve pregnancy than those with higher numbers of sperm in the PCT.[17] The PCT should not be considered a substitute for the semen analysis. Only if there are more than 20 motile sperm/hpf can it be assumed that the sperm count is normal. With less than 20, the sperm count can be either normal or abnormal.

TUBAL FUNCTION

Assessment of the fallopian tubes by hysterosalpingography (HSG) has its own methodologic shortcomings, including limitations in assessing peritoneal disease (e.g., adhesions). In addition, although patency or nonpatency of the tubes can be assessed, subtle damage to the tubal epithelium cannot. Nor is it possible to diagnose dysfunction of the tubal musculature. The introduction of falloposcopy into clinical practice gives promise that intratubal pathology will be diagnosable in the near future. Similarly, now that the tubal ostium can be cannulated through the uterus, it is not difficult to imagine the introduction of pressure gauges to measure tubal muscle contractility.

Presently the major techniques for assessing the fallopian tubes are HSG and direct visualization of the pelvis by laparoscopy.

Although some would relegate the HSG to the scrap heap and rely only on laparoscopy, the HSG is valuable as a nonsurgical initial test for tubal patency. Although laparoscopy is important for diagnosing pelvic adhesions and endometriosis, a normal HSG result is followed by conception within 6 months in 30% to 50% of cases.[18] Therefore, a good part of the infertility population is able to avoid laparoscopy if given a reasonable chance to attain pregnancy on their own.

Patient screening is important to minimize the risk of pelvic inflammatory disease with HSG. In a population at high risk, severe infection can occur in approximately 3% of women having an HSG, almost exclusively in those having occluded tubes on HSG.[19] Thus, women who have had a pelvic infection in the past are candidates for laparoscopy, not HSG. This is also true of women with known distal tubal occlusion or significant pelvic adhesions. In a population at low risk for pelvic infection, the risk of initiating infection is probably under 1%. If dilated tubes are found on HSG, the woman should be treated with 7 days of doxycycline, 200 mg/day.[20] HSG is performed 3 to 5 days after cessation of the menstrual flow. Premedication with a prostaglandin inhibitor is helpful to prevent or lessen the uterine contractions that occasionally accompany the injection of radiopaque media. The radiopaque media can be injected using a classic Jarcho cannula after the injection of a local anesthetic into the anterior lip of the cervix and the application of a single-tooth tenaculum. More common techniques use a suction apparatus appended to the cervix with a small cannula leading into the cervical canal through which radiopaque media can be injected or a pediatric Foley catheter threaded through the cervix into the uterus. The latter technique may obscure abnormalities of the uterine contour, such as those found after intrauterine exposure to diethylstilbestrol.

Use of image intensification fluoroscopy with limited exposure and only three to four spot films should limit radiation exposure to less than 1 rad. The taking of 8 to 10 spot films, a not uncommon practice, is usually of no diagnostic value, and it unnecessarily increases radiation exposure.

The diagnosis of an incompetent cervix should not be routinely attempted by HSG, but an abnormally wide cervix can sometimes be visualized. Defects in the uterine cavity indicative of myoma, polyps, and synechiae should be looked for. Occasionally a single (or multiple) relatively sharp, narrow, uniform line transects the uterine cavity either transversely or longitudinally. This is usually a normal variant and may reflect muscle spasm. These transecting lines often disappear in a subsequent HSG study. A small, straight line transecting the tube at the uterotubal junction is also a physiologic phenomenon. Pathology at the proximal portion of the tubes can include speckling of radiopaque media outside the tubal lumen (salpingitis isthmica nodosa) or a filling defect within the tube (polyp). The former suggests both damage to the tube and an increased risk of ectopic pregnancy. Because of limited experience, it is uncertain whether tubal polyps require surgical excision to enhance fertility. When a water-based radiopaque medium is used for HSG, an assessment can be made of tubal rugae. If present, they are a good prognostic factor in cases in which tubal surgery is needed. Conversely, a ballooning of the ends without spill of radiopaque media on HSG is a sign of extensive damage and an indication of only limited possibilities of success with tubal surgery. The spread of radiopaque media uniformly throughout the pelvis on a postinjection delay film is usually associated with normal anatomy. It should be recognized, however, that a normal HSG scan should be supplemented by a laparoscopy if pregnancy does not occur within the 6 to 9 months following the study.

There is now reasonable evidence that HSG performed with an oil-based radiopaque medium (Ethiodol) has a greater fertility-enhancing effect for 4 to 9 months compared with HSG done with a water-based radiopaque medium.[20] This beneficial effect is seen when there is no evidence of tubal pathology because injection of radiopaque medium does not overcome tubal closure. In a prospective study, the cumulative pregnancy rate at 9 months post-HSG in the Ethiodol group was 33% compared with 12%, 17.6%, and 20.8% achieved with three different types of water-soluble

contrast media.[21] The reason for the beneficial effect on fertility produced by the oil radiopaque media is unknown, although it has been shown that Ethiodol may decrease peritoneal macrophage activity. Thus, the macrophages may be less likely to ingest sperm. Whatever the reason, the fertility-enhancing effect of Ethiodol (only seen with normal tubes) makes it our radiopaque medium of choice.

Oil radiopaque medium has the disadvantage of potentially long-term (years) sequestration of radiopaque media if it is injected into a hydrosalpinx. The medium is iodine containing and may affect thyroid function tests during the time it remains in the body. In addition to the risk of infection mentioned earlier, there also may be, with both types of radiopaque media, embolization. Viewing with image intensification fluoroscopy allows early identification of lymphatic or venous intravasation, a signal to stop the injection of radiopaque media. Fortunately major complications of HSG are rare.[22] There is less peritoneal discomfort associated with Ethiodol compared with the water-soluble radiopaque media. Among the latter, Hypaque is extremely irritating.

The major tests for assessing infertility—the semen analysis, PCT, tests of ovulation, and HSG—can be completed within a few cycles. After an appropriate interval, these can be followed by laparoscopy, possibly combined with hysteroscopy. There are, however, a few other tests that may be helpful before moving on to the endoscopic procedures. Specifically to be discussed here is testing for sperm antibodies; the hamster penetration assay is considered in Chapter 7.

SPERM ANTIBODIES

It has long been known that antibodies to sperm can arise in both males and females. In the male, this occurs most commonly in response to vas ligation or trauma. Less obvious is the precise role of antibodies in infertility and secondarily what test for antibodies is best suited to the clinical situation. Opinions range from one suggesting that all infertile couples should be tested for antibody to the opinion that holds antibody testing to be a useless activity. The prevalence of sperm antibodies in infertility has been estimated to be approximately 10% for males and slightly lower for females. A high percentage of positive sperm antibody tests are associated with poor PCT results, and it would seem to be cost-effective to screen initially for antibodies only in individuals whose PCT shows no sperm, all dead sperm, or a high percentage of sperm shaking in place. More arbitrary is defining abnormal PCT results as having less than 3 sperm/hpf or having less than 5 or even less than 1 as the cutoff value for doing a sperm antibody test.

Current technology for antisperm antibody tests uses polyacrylamide beads with attached anti-IgG, anti-IgA, or anti-IgM. When evaluating the male partner, his sperm are incubated with the beads and attachment assessed with a light microscope. The anatomic sites of attachment, that is, head or tail, can be noted as well as the percentage of sperm that are bound by immunobeads. Antibody attached to the main piece of the tail can interfere with sperm transport, whereas head-directed antibodies can interfere with sperm/egg fusion. Antibody attached only to the tip of the tail does not seem to be significant. In one study, if more than 50% of sperm were antibody-bound, the subsequent pregnancy rate was 15.3%, whereas if less than 50% of sperm had attached antibodies, the pregnancy rate was 66.7%.[23] In the female, it is the serum that must be evaluated after it is used to incubate control, nonantibody-bearing sperm. A clear-cut value for positivity or negativity has not been established for the female. Moreover, a report by Critser and colleagues[24] showed that levels of sperm antibodies in serum were similar in fertile and infertile individuals. Therefore, testing the serum may not be of value. There are also spontaneous fluctuations in antibody levels. Haas and Manganiello[25] reported that 58% of males receiving placebo treatment showed a decrease in sperm-bound immunoglobulins.

Treatment with corticosteroids has been advocated, especially if antibodies are found in the male. High doses, however, are associated with significant side effects, and the efficacy of this treatment is still disputed. For males with sperm antibodies, Hendry and coworkers[26] prescribed prednisolone, 20 mg twice a day from day 1 to 10 of their partner's cycle, followed by 5 mg on days 11 and 12. The dose was increased if the antibody titer did not fall in 3 months. The partners of 9 of 29 men who received prednisolone achieved pregnancy, whereas only 1 of 20 who received placebo was successful. The advantage for prednisolone was not seen until after 5 months of treatment.

Treatment for the female with antisperm antibodies is uncertain. The most popular current therapy is intrauterine inseminations with washed sperm in conjunction with controlled ovarian hyperstimulation using human menopausal gonadotropins. The same treatment also has been used for positive antibodies in the males with the added technique of having the male ejaculate into culture medium to dilute out antibodies in seminal fluid. No control study has been performed to evaluate the value of this therapy.

Finally, IVF has been used for antibodies found in both males and females. If the female is antibody positive, her serum is not used to culture the oocytes and the sperm.

Although the past decade has seen a major emphasis on the advanced reproductive technologies, most individuals with infertility do not need or cannot afford them. The physician working in an office setting can still provide diagnosis and management for the majority of his or her infertility patients. The testing as outlined in Table 6–2 is adequate for most cases of unexplained infertility. Additional testing of the male with the hamster penetration assay or human hemizona binding assay may be appropriate. Throughout the investigation, periodic consultation (perhaps every 3 to 4 months) should provide a forum to assess progress, to clarify ambiguities where possible, and to outline with the couple timetables and guidelines for future treatment. In some cases, this may involve a recommendation to discontinue therapy when all reasonable possibilities have been tried or the individuals are emotionally or physically ready to discontinue. The physician can be a wise counselor by suggesting options, such as adoption, or, for others, support groups that discuss childless living. In all cases, the physician should be guided by the needs of the individuals and should avoid unwarranted therapy.

REFERENCES

1. Tietze C. Reproductive span and rate of reproduction among Hutterite women. Fertil Steril 1957; 8:89.
2. Federation CECOS, Schwartz D, Mayaux MJ. Female fecundity as a function of age. N Engl J Med 1982; 306:404.
3. In vitro fertilization–embryo transfer (IVF-ET) in the United States: 1989 results from the IVF-ET registry. Fertil Steril 1991; 55:14.
4. Ammirati E, Fraser C, Hay-Kaufman M, et al. Clinical evaluation of a new home test for confirmation of ovulation. Program of the 47th Annual Meeting of the American Fertility Society. 1991; 56:S115.
5. Davis OK, Berkeley AS, Naus GJ, et al. The incidence of luteal phase defect in normal, fertile women, determined by serial endometrial biopsies. Fertil Steril 1989; 51:582.
6. Shoupe D, Mishell DR Jr, Lacarra M, et al. Correlation of endometrial maturation with four methods of estimating day of ovulation. Obstet Gynecol 1989; 73:88.
7. Davidson BJ, Thrasher TV, Seraj IM. An analysis of endometrial biopsies performed for infertility. Fertil Steril 1987; 48:770.
8. Downs KA, Gibson M. Clomiphene citrate therapy for luteal phase defect. Fertil Steril 1983; 39:34.
9. Kerin JF, Kirby C, Morris D. Incidence of luteinized unruptured follicle phenomenon in cycling women. Fertil Steril 1983; 40:620.
10. Bateman BG, Nunley WC Jr, Kolp LA. Exogenous estrogen therapy for the treatment of clomiphene citrate-induced cervical mucus abnormalities: is it effective? Fertil Steril 1990; 54:577.
11. Eggert-Kruse W, Köhler A, Rohr G, Runnebaum B. The pH as an important determinant of sperm-mucus interaction. Fertil Steril 1993; 59:617.
12. Ansari AH, Gould KG, Ansari VM. Sodium bicarbonate douching for improvement of the postcoital test. Fertil Steril 1980; 33:608.
13. Jette NT, Glass RH. Prognostic value of the postcoital test. Fertil Steril 1972; 23:29.
14. Collins JA, So Y, Wilson EH, et al. The postcoital test as a predictor of pregnancy among 355 infertile couples. Fertil Steril 1984; 41:703.
15. Kovacs GT, Newman GB, Henson GL. The postcoital test: what is normal? BMJ 1978; 1:818.
16. Quagliarello J, Arny M. Intracervical versus intrauterine insemination: correlation of outcome with antecedent postcoital testing. Fertil Steril 1986; 46:870.
17. Hull MGR, Savage PE, Bromham DR. Prognostic value of the post coital test: prospective study based on time-specific conception rates. Br J Obstet Gynaecol 1982; 89:299.
18. Mackey RA, Glass RH, Olson LE, Vaidya RA. Pregnancy following hysterosalpingography with oil and water soluble dye. Fertil Steril 1971; 22:504.
19. Stumpf PG, March CM. Febrile morbidity following hysterosalpingography: identification of risk factors and recommendations for prophylaxis. Fertil Steril 1980; 33:487.
20. Pittaway DE, Winfield AC, Maxson W, et al. Prevention of acute pelvic inflammatory disease after hysterosalpingography: efficacy of doxycycline prophylaxis. Am J Obstet Gynecol 1983; 147:623.
21. Rasmussen F, Lindequist S, Larsen C, Justesen P. Therapeutic effect of hysterosalpingography: oil versus water soluble contrast media—a randomized prospective study. Radiology 1991; 179:75.
22. Bateman BG, Nunley WC Jr, Kitchin JD. Intravasation during hysterosalpingography using oil-base contrast media. Fertil Steril 1980; 34:439.
23. Ayvaliotis B, Bronson R, Rosenfeld D, Cooper G. Conception rates in couples where autoimmunity to sperm is detected. Fertil Steril 1986; 44:739.
24. Critser JK, Villines PM, Coulam CB, Critser ES. Evaluation of circulating anti-sperm antibodies in fertile and patient populations. Am J Reprod Immunol 1989; 21:137.
25. Haas GG Jr, Manganiello P. A double-blind placebo-controlled study of the use of methylprednisolone in infertile men with sperm-associated immunoglobulins. Fertil Steril 1987; 47:295.
26. Hendry WF, Hughes L, Scammell G, et al. Comparison of prednisolone and placebo in subfertile men with antibodies to spermatozoa. Lancet 1990; 335:85.

CHAPTER 7

Male Infertility

R. DALE McCLURE

Reproductive difficulties encountered by couples are receiving increasing attention both in the news media and in public discussion. Several factors are responsible for this. The large baby boom generation, born 1946 through 1964, has been delaying childbearing into the ages when their reproductive potential has decreased. Also discoveries in biology have now led to major advances in reproductive techniques that are giving new avenues of hope for the infertile couple. Fortunately there are more physicians being trained to deal with this increasing demand for infertility services.

In the last decade, investigations have found significant pathology related to the male alone in approximately one-third of infertility cases, and in 20%, abnormalities are found in both the man and the woman.[1] Because the male factor is so prominent, ideally the initial screening evaluation of the male should be performed early in the infertility workup.

The couple should be considered as a unit and evaluated in a parallel manner until a significant problem is uncovered. Although the partners are often being cared for by different physicians, they should be interviewed together during the initial visit. This allows the physician to gain information regarding their dynamics as a couple and individual motivation and helps alleviate the stress that the infertility investigation tends to elicit. At all times during the infertility evaluation, the couple should feel free to question the indications, rationale, and outcomes of various diagnostic procedures. An explanation of the fundamental aspects of male reproductive biology and fertility, whether this be by information pamphlets, charts, or diagrams (Fig. 7–1), helps this goal to be accomplished.

The diagnostic evaluation of the male should proceed in a logical, cost-effective sequence to elucidate possible causes of the infertility (Table 7–1).[2] Cooperation and communication with the female's physician allows both an efficient and appropriate workup and avoids unnecessary tests and procedures. In an ideal situation, the male's physician and the female's physician should hold a "joint fertility clinic."

HISTORY

The cornerstone of the workup of the infertile male is a careful history and physical examination. An infertility workup sheet that addresses most of the pertinent historical points is extremely useful (Table 7–2). Documentation should be made of the duration of unprotected coitus with this or other partners as well as whether the male has fathered children in the past. Notation should be made of the male's previous infertility evaluation, including semen analysis, hormones, and the more sophisticated tests, such as sperm antibody and sperm penetration assays. Determining whether these tests were performed in a physician's office or in a reproductive laboratory helps one assess the reliability of these investigations. There are actually three levels of quality: a physician's office; a general hospital laboratory, and a gamete laboratory. Analyses performed in a physician's office and in many general hospital laboratories often fail to match the quality, reliability, and reproducibility of a reproductive laboratory.

Because the couple should be considered a unit and be evaluated in a parallel manner, it is important for the physician investigating the male to be aware of the status of his partner's workup. The presence of the wife or the availability of her detailed records during the initial visit helps better elucidate the investigations and diagnostic conclusions to date. The following are historical details that are important to the andrologist in terms of the female's history: her previous fertility, including spontaneous or induced abortions; use of contraceptives; and duration of past exposure to pregnancy. Previous episodes of genital tract infections or acute salpingitis may have led to reproductive tract obstruction. Ovulation may have been assessed by a variety of methods, including menstrual history, basal body temperature, urinary luteinizing hormone (LH) kits, as well as serum progesterone. Luteal phase adequacy may have been determined by endometrial biopsy or serum progesterone. Tubal patency and assessment of uterine cavity are usually carried out with a hysterosalpingogram. A properly timed postcoital test evaluates the cervical mucus, the delivery of the semen sample, and the survival of sperm within the cervical mucus. Pelvic pathology, including adnexal adhesions, endometriosis, leiomyomata uteri, and tubal pathology, may be identified by laparoscopy.[1]

Documentation of developmental abnormalities in the male are the next step in the investigation. Timing of puberty is important because precocious puberty may indicate the presence of adrenal-genital syndrome, whereas delayed puberty may indicate Klinefelter's syndrome or idiopathic hy-

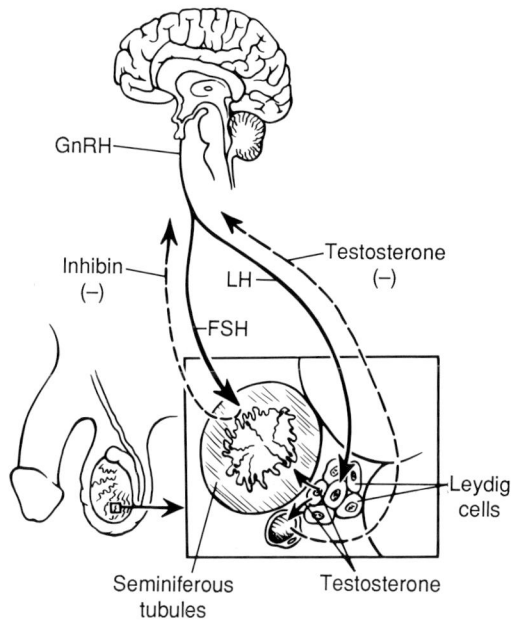

FIGURE 7–1. Male reproductive axis (hypothalamic-pituitary-gonadal axis). GnRH, gonadotropin-releasing hormone; LH, luteinizing hormone; FSH, follicle-stimulating hormone. Testosterone or its conversion to dihydrotestosterone or estradiol may have an inhibitory effect on the hypothalamic-pituitary axis. Inhibin specifically inhibits serum FSH levels.

pogonadism. Similarly, gynecomastia may indicate an endocrine abnormality. Specific childhood illnesses should be sought, including cryptorchidism,[3, 4] postpubertal mumps orchitis,[5] and testicular trauma or pain (torsion).[6] Approximately 50% of men with a history of bilateral cryptorchidism and 30% of men with unilateral cryptorchidism may have sperm counts below normal.[3] Whether or not the early morphologic alterations seen in the cryptorchid testes are reversed by early orchidopexy is still unknown. Trauma or torsion may result in testicular atrophy or, if occurring after the time of puberty, may be related to the presence of sperm antibodies.[6, 7] Approximately 10% of individuals who develop mumps orchitis bilaterally postpubertally may end up with severe testicular damage.[5]

Previous surgical procedures, such as bladder neck operations (Y-V plasty) or retroperitoneal lymph node dissection for testicular cancer, may cause retrograde ejaculation or absent emission. Similarly, diabetic neuropathy may result in either retrograde ejaculation or impotence. Both the vas deferens and the testicular blood supply can easily be injured during a hernia repair or during scrotal surgery.

Recurrent respiratory infections and infertility may be associated with the immotile cilia syndrome, in which the sperm count is normal, but spermatozoa are completely nonmotile owing to ultrastructural defects.[8] Kartagener's syndrome, a variant of immotile cilia syndrome, consists of chronic bronchiectasis, sinusitis, situs inversus, and immotile spermatozoa. In Young's syndrome, also associated with pulmonary disease, the cilia ultrastructure is normal, but the epididymis is obstructed owing to inspissated material, and these patients present with azoospermia (absence of spermatozoa).[9] Many males with cystic fibrosis have congenital absence of the vas deferens and seminal vesicles.[10] These individuals present with low semen volume, failure of the semen to coagulate, and azoospermia.

Inflammatory processes that involve either the lower urinary tract or the reproductive tract may result in scarring and obstruction of the reproductive ducts or damage to the secondary sex organs. A generalized febrile illness can impair spermatogenesis. In 1941, MacLeod and Hotchkiss,[11] by increasing intratesticular temperature, produced oligospermia within 3 weeks that lasted approximately 50 days. More recently, Buch and Havlovec[12] found that 6 to 7 weeks following a febrile illness (temperature 101°F), both sperm density and percent penetration (sperm penetration assay) decreased. The ejaculate, however, may not be affected for 3 months after the event because spermatogenesis takes about 74 days from initiation to the appearance of mature spermatozoa, and there is also a varied transport time in the ducts.[13] Therefore, events that have occurred in the previous 3 to 6 months are extremely important.

A variety of gonadotoxins, whether occupational, environmental, or therapeutic, may have detrimental effects on fertility.[14] Cancer chemotherapy has a dose-dependent, potentially devastating effect on the testicular germinal epithelium and may also compromise Leydig cell function.[15] The alkalinating agents, cyclophosphamide, mustargen, and chlorambucil, are particularly damaging. Exposure to x-rays, neutrons, and radioactive materials may also affect spermatogenesis. Radiation effects depend on the total dose received and the developmental stage of the germ cell during exposure.[15] Permanent sterility generally occurs after a single field dose of radiation of 600 to 800 rads. Semen cryopreservation is recommended for men before either chemotherapy or radiotherapy. Although numerous chemicals are known to affect the male reproductive tract, few have been extensively studied. Dibromochloropropane (DBCP) is a nematocide used widely in agriculture, and it appears to be a testicular toxin.[14, 16] Likewise, lead, known to be a reproductive toxin since the Roman Empire, affects the hypothalamic-pituitary-testicular axis resulting in suppression of serum testosterone.[17]

Both cigarette smoking and marijuana have been associated with infertility.[18, 19] Some studies have shown an impairment of sperm density, motility, and morphology among male smokers, whereas other authors have found no statistically significant effect of smoking.[1, 19] Individual susceptibility may

---

TABLE 7–1. Differential Diagnosis of Male Infertility

Treatable Causes
Varicocele
Obstruction (acquired, congenital)
Infection
Ejaculatory dysfunction
Hypogonadotropic hypogonadism
Immunologic problem
Sexual dysfunction
Hyperprolactinemia
Potentially Treatable Causes
Idiopathic
Cryptorchidism
Vasal agenesis
Gonadotoxins (drugs, radiation)
Untreatable Causes
Bilateral anorchism
Germinal cell aplasia
Primary testicular failure
Chromosomal anomalies
Immotile cilia syndrome

TABLE 7–2. Male Infertility History	
Male Reproductive History ■ Duration of unprotected coitus ■ Previous marital/extramarital offspring ■ Previous infertility evaluation (hormones/semen analysis/sperm antibodies/sperm penetration assay) ■ Other tests/investigation ■ Diagnostic conclusions and previous therapy **Female Reproductive History** ■ Age ■ Gravida ■ Para ■ Ovulation (technique to assess) ■ Corpus luteal function (technique to assess) ■ Hysterosalpingography ■ Postcoital test ■ Laparoscopy (findings) ■ Previous therapy ■ Diagnostic conclusions **Personal History** Developmental ■ Onset of puberty (precocious/normal/delayed) ■ Undescended testes ■ Gynecomastia Surgical ■ Retroperitoneal surgery ■ Pelvic (Y-V plasty bladder neck, transurethral surgery) ■ Inguinal (herniorrhaphy, orchidopexy) ■ Scrotal (trauma/torsion/vasectomy/hydrocele) Medical ■ Systemic illnesses and therapy (diabetes mellitus/ulcerative colitis/respiratory infections/cystic fibrosis) ■ Mumps orchitis ■ History of venereal disease/urethritis/epididymitis/orchitis/prostatitis ■ Recent (3–6 months) febrile/viral illness	Gonadotoxins (occupational/environmental) ■ Occupation(s) (past/present) ■ Thermal exposure (work/saunas/baths/bikini tights) ■ Radiation (work/diagnostic/therapeutic) ■ Chemical exposure (work/insecticides/therapeutic) ■ Smoking (amount/duration) ■ Alcohol (amount/duration) Sexual history ■ Potency/libido ■ Coital technique ■ Timing and frequency of intercourse ■ Lubricants **Medications** ■ Personal (past/present) ■ Maternal (diethylstilbestrol) ■ Recreational drugs (marijuana/cocaine) **Family History** ■ Hypogonadism/congenital midline defects ■ Cystic fibrosis ■ Androgen receptor deficiency (undermasculinization) **Endocrine History** Hypothalamic-pituitary ■ Headaches/visual changes/polydipsia/impaired ability to smell ■ Excessive growth of jaw, hands, feet Thyroid ■ Heat or cold intolerance ■ Change in bowel movements ■ Increased appetite with weight loss ■ Palpitations Adrenal ■ Muscle weakness/anorexia/purpura ■ Postural hypotension/hyperpigmentation Gonadal ■ Retardation of hair growth (facial/body) ■ Breast changes

be responsible for this difference. Human studies have shown that with marijuana usage, there is a lowering serum testosterone and a temporary decrease in sperm counts and motility.[18, 20] Among abusers of alcohol, there is a reduction in sperm density, motility, and the number of normal-appearing sperm.[21] Independent of its effect on the liver, alcohol reduces testosterone levels both acutely and chronically. The liver disease concomitant with chronic alcoholism leads to changes in androgen metabolism and may result in sexual dysfunction.[22] Opiate abuse also inhibits gonadotropin secretion, lowering serum testosterone.[23]

Although many people believe that boxer shorts, as compared with briefs, should be worn by individuals with suboptimal semen quality, little data support this. Early studies in the 1960s with the application of excessive heat to men did show, with time, altered sperm density.[24] The higher than normal scrotal temperature in men with cryptorchidism and varicocele may explain their abnormal spermatogenesis. It is therefore recommended that one discontinue using saunas, hot tubs, or tight nylon bikinis because the elevated temperature may impair sperm production.

Sexual habits, including frequency of intercourse, type of ejaculation (antegrade/retrograde), use of coital lubricants (spermicidals), and the patient's understanding of the ovulatory cycle, should be discussed. Decreased coital frequency may be related to decreased libido, marital difficulties, or work-related absences from the home as well as religious practices, such as the Mikveh among orthodox Jews.[25] Caution must be used when using lubricants. Lubricants such as K-Y Jelly, Lubrifax, and Keri lotion as well as saliva have been shown to cause a deterioration of sperm motility when tested in vitro. Raw egg white, peanut oil, vegetable oil, and petroleum jelly do not appear to impair in vitro motility.[17] The optimal timing of intercourse is still not understood by many couples. Because sperm survival within the cervical mucus and the cervical crypts is approximately 48 hours, intercourse is most effective every 48 hours around the time of ovulatory peak. This allows viable sperm to be available within the 12- to 24-hour period when the egg is within the fallopian tube and capable of being fertilized.

A variety of therapeutic medications may also affect reproductive function. Prenatal exposure to diethylstilbestrol (DES) may cause an increased incidence of epididymal cysts and slightly increased frequency of cryptorchidism and may in some individuals affect semen quality.[26] Sulfasalazine, a drug commonly used in the treatment of ulcerative colitis, has been associated with a drop in sperm motility and density, which may be reversed on stopping therapy.[27] A variety of drugs are also known to inhibit androgen production. These antiandrogen drugs include spironolactone, cyproterone, ketoconazole (an antifungal agent), and cimetidine.[28] These all may significantly affect fertility. During short-term therapy, tetracycline lowers serum testosterone about 20%.[28] Nitrofurantoin depresses spermatogenesis and therefore should be avoided. Other antimicrobial agents (e.g., erythromycin and gentamicin) may also impair spermatozoal function and spermatogenesis.[29] Low-dose androgens, given by some physicians for male infertility, may also affect sperm

TABLE 7–3. Infertility Physical Examination		

Height
Span
Weight
Skin (wrinkles/pigmentation)
Hair
   Pubic
   Axillary
   Chest
Virilization
Visual fields
Sense of smell
Breasts (gynecomastia/galactorrhea)
Abdomen (hepatomegaly/previous surgical scars)
Penis (length/meatus/deformities)
Prostate (size/consistency/tenderness)

Testes	Right	Left
Size (length × width or volume by Prader)		
Consistency		
Vas deferens		
Epididymis		
Varicocele (grade I–III)		

TABLE 7–4. Features of Eunuchoidism

Eunuchoid Skeletal Proportions
   Upper body to lower body ratio below 1
   Arm span more than 2 inches greater than height
Lack of Male Hair Distribution
   Sparse axillary, pubic, and body hair
   Lack of temporal hair recession
Infantile Genitalia
   Small penis, testes, and prostate
Diminished Muscular Development and Mass

production by inhibiting gonadotropin secretion. Anabolic steroids, used by many professional and amateur athletes, also depress gonadotropin secretion, acting as a "male contraceptive."[30] This effect on spermatogenesis appears to be temporary and should be reversible after discontinuing steroids.

Symptoms of other endocrine gland abnormalities (pituitary, thyroid, and adrenal) should be elucidated (see Table 7–2). Unless testicular damage is severe or sufficient time has elapsed to regression of male secondary sex characteristics, Leydig cell failure occurring after puberty is difficult to diagnose clinically. Complaints of decreasing libido and poor erections associated with the decreased testicular function may precede changes in shaving pattern, loss of pubic and axillary hair, and development of gynecomastia. Hot flashes may occasionally be seen in men with declining testicular function. A rapid loss of beard and body hair (over 6 to 12 months) should make one suspicious of concomitant adrenal insufficiency.[31]

PHYSICAL EXAMINATION

A carefully performed physical examination on the initial visit may delineate abnormalities causing male factor infertility (Table 7–3). Particular attention should be given to discerning the features of hypogonadism, if present; poorly developed secondary sexual characteristics; eunuchoidal skeletal proportion (arm span 2 inches greater than height); ratio of upper body segment (crown to pubis) to lower body segment (pubis to floor) less than 1; and lack of normal male hair distribution (sparse axillary, pubic, facial, and body hair) and lack of temporal hair recession (Table 7–4).[31–33] Headache, visual field defects, galactorrhea, and signs of other tropic hormone deficiency may point to a secondary (hypothalamic-pituitary) cause.[34] A man with congenital hypogonadism may have associated midline defects, such as anosmia, color blindness, cerebellar ataxia, harelip, and cleft palate.[35]

Gynecomastia is a consistent finding of a feminizing state. Its presence may be a clue to testicular dysfunction, whether the failure is primary testicular or secondary to disease in the hypothalamic-pituitary axis. Palpation with the flat of the hand with the patient supine may fail to detect minimal breast enlargement. Gynecomastia may be more easily found by examining the patient when sitting, using the fingers to grasp the glandular tissue.

Particular emphasis should be placed on the male's genitalia. Testicular size correlates well with semen quality and fertility. Seminiferous tubules account for approximately 95% of testicular volume. The normal adult testis averages 4.6 cm in length (range, 3.6 to 5.5 cm) and 2.6 cm in width (2.1 to 3.2 cm) with a mean volume of 18.6 ± 4.8 (SD) mL (Fig. 7–2).[31, 36] The lower limit of normal length and width for a mature testis is approximately 4 cm × 2.5 cm, which is equivalent to a testicular volume of 15 mL. A ruler, caliper, or Prader orchidometer may be used to measure testicular size (Fig. 7–3). When the seminiferous tubules are damaged before puberty, the testes are small and firm; with postpubertal damage, they are usually soft and small. The finding of a unilateral smaller testis may indicate the presence of a varicocele or a previous inflammatory or vascular injury to that testis.

Irregularities in the epididymis or vas may suggest a previous infection and possible obstruction. Examination may reveal a small prostate in men with androgen deficiency or slight tenderness (bogginess) in those with prostatic infection. The penis should be at least 5 cm in length when stretched. Any penile abnormality (hypospadias, abnormal curvature, phimosis) should be looked for. These problems may interfere with the deposition of the ejaculate in the

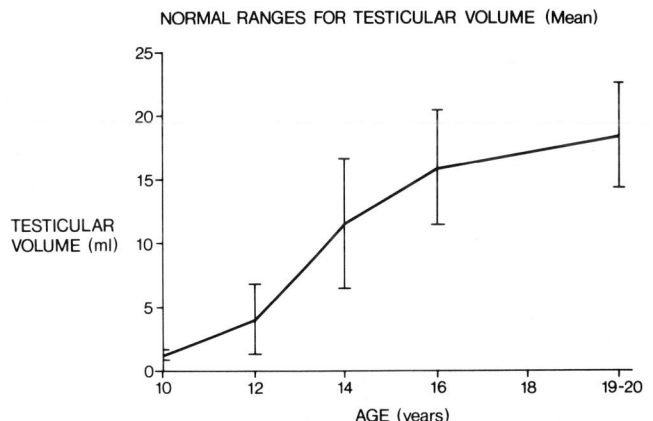

FIGURE 7–2. Normal values for testicular volume in relation to age. (Modified from Zachmann M, Prader A, Kind HP, et al. Testicular volume during adolescence: cross sectional and long term studies. Helv Paediatr Acta 1974;29:61.)

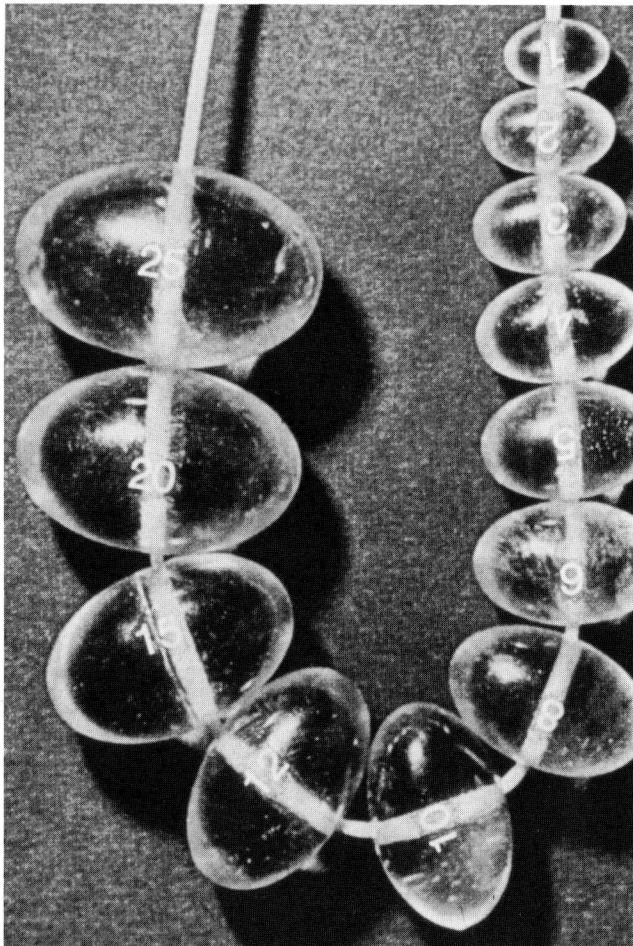

FIGURE 7–3. A Prader orchidometer for measuring testicular volume.

vagina. Both vasa should be palpated because 2% of infertile men have congenital absence of the vasa and seminal vesicles.

Because varicocele is the most common diagnosis made in the infertile male, it should be carefully searched for.[37] The patient should be examined in a warm environment, both in the supine and the standing position, with and without the Valsalva maneuver. Spermatic cord structures from both sides are palpated and compared. With the patient performing the Valsalva maneuver, the examiner compares the cord between index fingers and thumb. An increase in the thickness of the cord during this maneuver or a discrete pulse wave, indicative of a venous reflex, indicates the presence of a varicocele. On occasion, the cremasteric muscle contracts, foreshortening the cord and leading to an erroneous positive diagnosis. A smaller left testis and a boggy feeling in the surrounding scrotal tissue (bag of worms) even in the supine position should make one suspicious that a varicocele is present.

The examination should not be complete without a thorough physical examination to rule out chronic or unsuspected systemic disease that may contribute to infertility. Proper neck examination rules out thyromegaly, a bruit, or nodularity associated with thyroid disease. Liver disease may represent undiagnosed cirrhosis, and lymphadenopathy may be an early symptom of Hodgkin's disease. Although previously undiagnosed systemic disease is usually unlikely in the workup of an infertile male, correction of this illness may improve the male's overall health and improve his semen quality.

LABORATORY INVESTIGATION AND INTERPRETATION

Semen Analysis

A carefully performed semen analysis provides important information concerning the male reproductive hormonal cycle, spermatogenesis, and the patency of the reproductive tract. The World Health Organization (WHO) laboratory manual for the examination of human semen and semen-cervical mucus is highly recommended for normal values and proper techniques of testing.[38] A past history of paternity or an adequate postcoital test does not eliminate the need for semen analysis, which may reveal subtle but important abnormalities.

The standard techniques of analysis allow variations of up to 20% between laboratories. Besides laboratory error, there are variations in sperm density, motility, and morphology among multiple samples from a given man (Fig. 7–4).[39] Abstinence intervals give a large source of variability. With each day of abstinence (up to 1 week), semen volume increases by 0.4 mL, sperm concentration by 10 to 15 million per mL, and total sperm count by 50 to 90 million. Sperm motility and morphology appear unaffected by 5 to 7 days of abstinence, but longer periods lead to impaired motility.[40]

Interpretation of semen analysis must take into consideration the variations between samples that exist in individuals. The minimum number of specimens to define good or poor quality of semen is three samples over a 2-month period with a consistent period of abstinence (48 to 72 hours). In a longitudinal analysis of semen from both fertile and infertile men, Sherins and associates[41] found that 97% of men with initial good sperm concentration would continue to show good density after as many as three to six specimens. Those rated poor at the first specimen also remained poor at the third and sixth specimens. For those rated equivocal, the first specimen was of little value, and at least three specimens were needed to obtain stability. Conventional semen analysis is an indirect assessment of fertility potential. Pregnancy is the only irrefutable proof of sperm's capability to fertilize. Despite its limitation, semen analysis is a simple, inexpensive screening test.

Recommendations, therefore, are that if the first analysis is normal, one should at least repeat the analysis for confirmation. If, however, the first one is abnormal, one should get at least three analyses to document abnormalities.

NORMAL VALUES

Semen specimens should be regarded as abnormal if the following values with these different characteristics persist: volume, less than 2.0 mL; sperm concentration, less than 20×10^6 per mL; total sperm number of fewer than 40 million; sperm motility of less than 50% of cells with forward progression and quality graded below 2 (scale 0 to 4); and sperm morphology of less than 30% normal forms (Table 7–5).[38, 42] The terms *oligospermia, asthenospermia,* and *teratospermia* re-

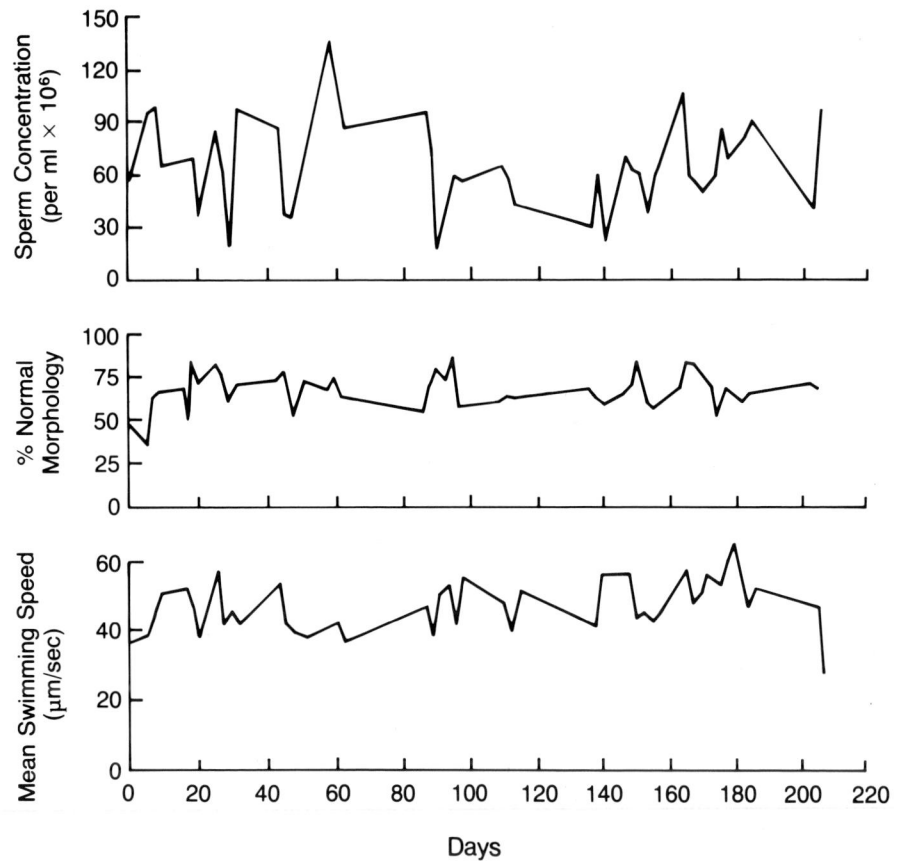

FIGURE 7–4. Day-to-day variation in semen quality in a fertile man over a 200-day period of observation. (Modified from Overstreet JW. Assessment of disorders of spermatogenesis. In: Lockey JE, editor. Reproduction: The New Frontier in Occupational and Environmental Health Research. New York: Alan R. Liss, 1984:282. © 1984, Wiley-Liss. Reprinted by permission of Wiley-Liss, a division of John Wiley and Sons, Inc.)

fer to individual semen samples with abnormalities in sperm numbers, motility, or morphology.

FRUCTOSE

Fructose is androgen dependent and is produced in the seminal vesicles. Fructose levels should be determined in any patient with azoospermia and especially in those whose ejaculate volume is less than 1 mL, suggesting seminal vesicle obstruction or atresia or ejaculatory tract duct obstruction. Absence of fructose, low semen volume, and failure of the semen to coagulate indicate either congenital absence of the vas deferens and seminal vesicles or obstruction of the ejaculatory duct.

ADDITIONAL CRITERIA

Semen from normal men coagulates and then, over the next 5 to 20 minutes, liquefies. Delayed liquefaction of the

semen (greater than 60 minutes) may indicate disorders of accessory gland function. If spermatozoa are capable of reaching the cervical mucus, problems of semen liquefaction are not clinically relevant.

Increased semen viscosity, which is unrelated to the coagulation-liquefaction phenomenon, also signifies accessory gland function and may affect accuracy of assessment of both sperm density and motility. It is only clinically relevant when there are very few sperm in the postcoital test (PCT). Occasional clumps of agglutinated sperm are not infrequent in semen samples, but increased clumpings suggest an inflammatory or immunologic process.

A leukocyte count greater than 1 million per mL is considered abnormal on a semen analysis. The laboratory must carefully differentiate between white blood cells and immature germinal cells.

COMPUTER-ASSISTED SEMEN ANALYSIS

Subjective measures of standard semen analysis are now being replaced by objective measures from stored, digitalized sperm images. Computer-assisted semen analysis (CASA) systems couple video technology and sophisticated microcomputers for automated image digitalization and processing.[43] Measurements of sperm concentration as well as curvilinear velocity (VCL), straight line velocity (VSL), linearity (LIN), and amplitude of lateral head (ALH) displacements are commonly reported.[44]

There are still some problems with the CASA system's ability to measure the traditional semen analysis parameters. A comparison study between manual semen analysis and

TABLE 7–5. Semen Analysis: Normal Values	
Ejaculate volume	≥ 2.0 mL
Sperm concentration	≥ 20 million/mL
Total sperm count	≥ 40 million
Motility	≥ 50% with forward progression
Rapid progression	≥ 25%
Morphology	> 30% normal forms

Data from World Health Organization. Laboratory Manual for the Examination of Human Semen and Semen-Cervical Mucus Interaction. Cambridge: Cambridge University Press, 1992.

OLIGOSPERMIA/AZOOSPERMIA

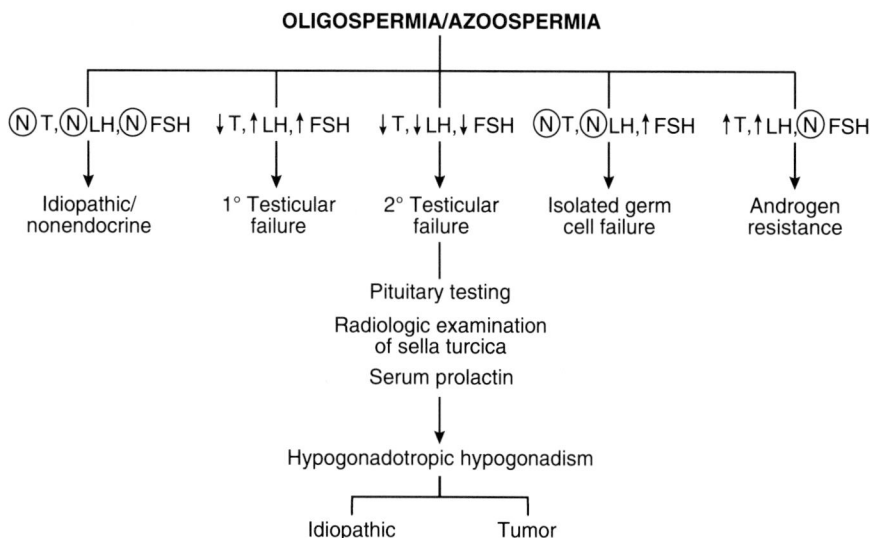

FIGURE 7–5. Algorithm for the diagnosis of male infertility. (Adapted from Swerdloff RS, Boyers SP. Evaluation of the male partner of an infertile couple: an algorithmic approach. JAMA 1982; 247:2418–2427. Copyright 1982, American Medical Association.)

CASA showed an overestimation of sperm concentration by 30% by CASA.[45] In a review of 17 azoospermic patients, CASA misinterpreted particles in the seminal fluid for sperm and gave an average sperm density of 2.2 million per mL.[45] The CASA system also tends to underestimate percent motility at high sperm concentrations. The data generated also depend on the parameter settings as well as other operator-dependent variables. CASA does allow an objective determination of a wide variety of sperm movement parameters that cannot be measured by manual techniques.[43]

CASA's full potential will be realized once a number of technical issues are resolved and the methods and measures are standardized.[46] As yet, both the biologic and clinical relevance of the data generated remains unclear.

Hormone Evaluation

Most cases of male infertility are nonendocrine in origin. Routine hormonal evaluation is not warranted unless sperm density is extremely low or one has clinical suspicion of an endocrinopathy. The incidence of primary endocrine defects in infertile men is less than 3% and is rare in men with sperm concentrations greater than 5×10^6 per mL. When an endocrinopathy is discovered, however, specific hormonal therapy is often successful.[33] Individuals with a history of birth anomalies, delayed or premature sexual maturation, erectile difficulties, or libido loss may need hormonal evaluation. Small testicular volumes, features of eunuchoidism, and the presence of gynecomastia on physical examination are highly suggestive of endocrine disease. Because the majority of the ejaculate fluid arises from the prostate and seminal vesicles, which are androgen dependent, a decreased ejaculate volume may also indicate hypogonadism.

Understanding reproductive physiology is pivotal in the evaluation of endocrine causes of male infertility (see Fig. 7–1). The two testicular functions (spermatogenesis and steroid hormone production) are intimately related. Testosterone synthesis is required not only for sperm production, but also for the development of secondary sexual characteristics and normal sexual behavior. The anterior pituitary controls both these functions through the secretion of the gonadotropins

LH and follicle-stimulating hormone (FSH). In turn, the anterior pituitary is regulated by the hypothalamic secretion of gonadotropin-releasing hormone (GnRH). Production of FSH in the pituitary is regulated in part by the negative feedback inhibition of inhibin, a protein produced in the Sertoli cells. The hypothalamic-pituitary-gonadal axis consists of a closed-loop feedback control mechanism directed at maintaining normal reproductive function.[31–33]

The algorithm presented in Figure 7–5 demonstrates common patterns of serum gonadotropins and testosterone by which a diagnosis may be made.[47]

Because of the episodic nature of LH secretion and its short half-life, a single LH determination has an accuracy of ± 50%. Similarly, testosterone is secreted episodically in response to the LH pulses and has a diurnal pattern with an early morning peak.[31] To overcome these sampling inaccuracies, three blood samples should be drawn at least 15 to 20 minutes apart and an equal volume of serum from each pooled for a single determination.[48] Because LH should be interpreted in light of serum testosterone, levels of both should be assessed from the pooled samples. Serum FSH has a longer half-life, and these fluctuations are less obvious.

A low serum testosterone level is one of the best indicators of hypogonadism of hypothalamic or pituitary origin. Mean serum LH and FSH concentrations are significantly lower in hypogonadotropic patients than in normal men, although in some individuals, they can overlap with the lower limits of normal. Low LH and FSH values concurrent with low serum testosterone indicate hypogonadotropic hypogonadism, which may also be apparent clinically.

Elevated serum FSH and LH values help to distinguish primary testicular failure (hypergonadotropic hypogonadism) from secondary testicular failure (hypogonadotropic hypogonadism). Most patients with primary hypogonadism usually have severe, irreversible testicular defects. Secondary hypogonadism has a hypothalamic or pituitary origin, and in these patients, infertility may be correctable.

Numerous animal and human studies have demonstrated that a nonsteroidal Sertoli cell factor, inhibin, is extremely important in the feedback regulation of FSH. Decreases in spermatogenesis are generally accompanied by decreases in inhibin production, and this reduction in negative feedback is associated with a reciprocal elevation of FSH levels.[49] Elevated FSH is usually a reliable indicator of germinal epithelial damage and is usually associated with azoospermia or severe oligospermia (less than 5×10^6 per mL), indicative of significant, usually irreversible germ cell damage. In azoospermic and severely oligospermic patients with normal FSH, primary spermatogenic defects cannot be distinguished from obstructive lesions by normal investigation alone; scrotal exploration, testicular biopsy, and vasography should be considered. An elevated serum FSH associated with small atrophic testes implies irreversible infertility, and biopsy is not warranted.

Hyperprolactinemia has been reported to cause oligospermia, but the diagnostic value of routine prolactin measurements is extremely low in men with semen abnormalities, unless these are associated with decreased libido, impotence, and evidence of hypogonadism.[34, 50] Prolactin measurement is warranted in patients with low serum testosterone without an associated increase in serum LH. In individuals with hyperprolactinemia and testosterone deficiency, serum LH levels are inappropriately low, indicating that the hypothalamic-pituitary axis fails to respond to the reduced testosterone level.[34] Individuals with gynecomastia or suspected androgen resistance (elevated serum testosterone and LH levels with undermasculinization) should have a serum estradiol determination.[32]

Individuals with a rapid loss of secondary sex characteristics implying both testicular and adrenal failure (adrenal androgens) should undergo investigation of adrenal function. In men with a history of precocious puberty, one should consider congenital adrenal hyperplasia.[51] In the common variant (21-hydroxylase deficiency), serum levels of 17-hydroxyprogesterone are elevated, as is urinary pregnanetriol. With 11-hydroxylase deficiency, serum 11-deoxycortisol is elevated.[31]

In patients with hypogonadotropic hypogonadism, the pituitary hormones other than LH and FSH should also be assessed (adrenocorticotropic hormone [ACTH], thyroid-stimulating hormone [TSH], and growth hormone). Thyroid dysfunction is such a rare cause of infertility that routine screening for thyroid function abnormality should be discouraged.

In addition to the standard radioimmunoassay for LH, bioassays have been developed to measure the response of mouse Leydig cells to LH in serum. Rarely a patient may be infertile owing to immunologically active but biologically inactive LH.[52]

Testicular Biopsy, Seminal Vesiculography, and Vasography

In azoospermic patients with normal FSH, primary spermatogenic defects cannot be distinguished from obstructive lesions by hormonal investigation alone, and testicular biopsy and vasography should be considered.[53, 54] When patients have azoospermia or severe oligospermia and markedly shrunken testes, the physician should determine the serum FSH level. If it is elevated (more than two times normal), testicular biopsy can be avoided. Such a patient almost always has irreversible germ cell damage. The exception is the patient who has undergone chemotherapy, in whom the elevated FSH may normalize with return of spermatogenesis.

Rarely, testicular biopsy is warranted in men with severe oligospermia to rule out partial obstruction. This is so uncommon, however, that routine biopsy for severe oligospermia is not indicated.[53]

Before biopsy, obvious causes of azoospermia should be eliminated, and at least two semen analyses should reveal azoospermia. Retrograde ejaculation should be ruled out by examining the postejaculatory urine. In men with acidic semen (pH <7.0) and a volume of less than 1 mL, suspect ejaculatory obstruction or congenital absence of the seminal vesicles and vas deferens. For confirmation, seminal fructose levels should be determined. The presence of fructose rules out bilateral obstruction or atresia of the ejaculatory ducts but does not verify total ductal patency. Historically, vasography has been the best method of imaging the seminal vesicles and ejaculatory ducts. Presently, transrectal ultrasonography is a new diagnostic modality that provides valuable information about these structures and may be used instead to identify obstruction or congenital abnormalities of the ejaculatory ducts and seminal vesicles.[55]

Only when there is a clinical suggestion of different pathologic conditions on each side are bilateral biopsies indicated.[56] The samples of testicular tissue should be placed immediately into containers with Bouin's, Zenker's, or Conroy's solution. Formalin should be avoided because it distorts the distinctive architecture.

When vasography is performed, the radiopaque medium should be injected in the distal direction (toward the penis) (Fig. 7–6A). If the radiopaque medium is injected in a proximal direction (toward the testes), it is extremely difficult to interpret images of the epididymal anatomy, and there is a significant risk of rupturing the delicate epididymal tubule (Fig. 7–6B). An excellent book by Boreau[57] gives an exhaustive study of seminal vesiculography and vasography.

Sperm Function Tests

SPERM–CERVICAL MUCUS TESTS

Aspects of sperm function related to transport in the female may be assessed by evaluating the interaction of sperm with cervical mucus. The PCT assesses the quality of cervical mucus at ovulation time, whether sperm are properly deposited, and the survival of sperm within the cervix (human sperm reservoir).[58] The PCT involves the microscopic examination of the cervical mucus 2 to 18 hours after intercourse at the time of expected ovulation. Although the PCT is an integral part of the infertility workup, controversy still exists concerning its proper technique, interpretation, and correlation to pregnancy.[1] In the male, it is indicated in individuals with hyperviscous semen, normal semen (unexplained infertility), low ejaculatory volume, and abnormal penile anatomy. A normal or positive test result is often defined as one in which there are more than 5 to 10 motile, forward progressing sperm per hpf ($20\times$ objective). A positive result implies good semen and mucus, whereas poor results in an individual with normal semen parameters imply a cervical factor, improper timing of the PCT, presence of sperm antibodies, or male factor infertility.

If the PCT appears abnormal, a semen-mucus cross-penetration test may be performed in a four-way comparison with

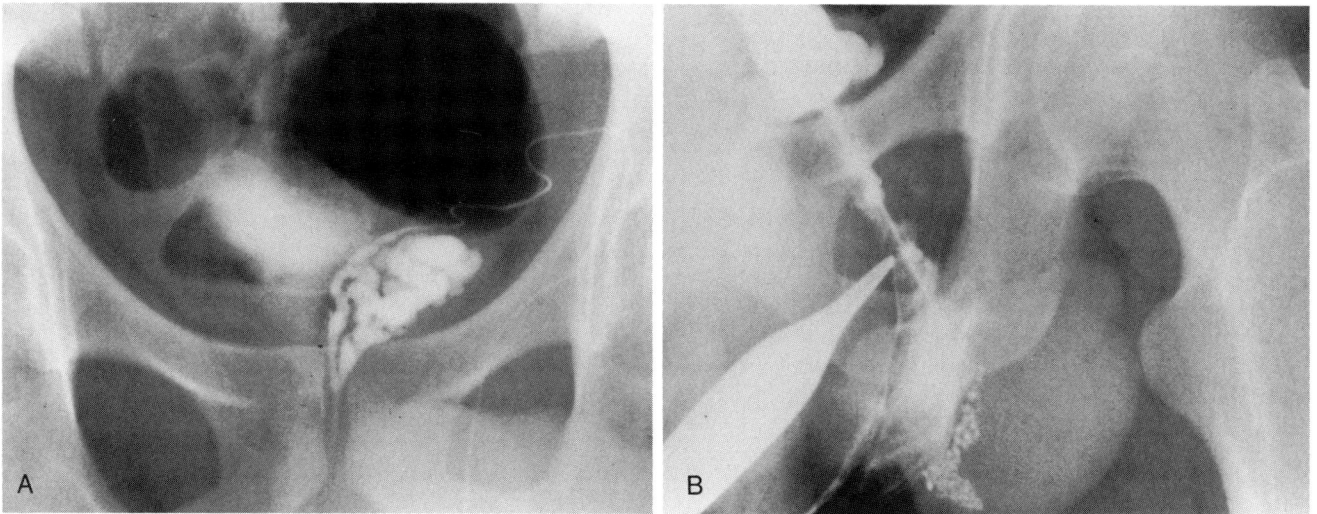

FIGURE 7–6. Seminal vasography. *A*, Normal-appearing vas in seminal vesicles with normal reflux into the bladder verifying distal patency. *B*, Extravasation demonstrating the difficulty in determining a point of epididymal obstruction with proximal vasography.

semen and cervical mucus from fertile donors. This allows one to determine whether the abnormality is in the husband's semen or the wife's mucus.

SPERM PENETRATION ASSAY

The zona-free hamster egg penetration, often called the sperm penetration assay (SPA), measures the ability of the sperm to undergo capacitation and the acrosome reaction and to fuse with the oocytes.[59–61] This surrogate human egg system evaluates the fertilizing capacity of human sperm directly. As such, it has been used as a bioassay of human sperm fertilizing function.

Although the SPA has been used clinically for more than 10 years, a number of problems still persist despite its widespread use. In particular, the SPA remains inadequately standardized, making it sometimes difficult to compare results between laboratories. Therefore, this test is most effectively used in laboratories with long-standing, established protocols in which the test results can be interpreted in the context of internal controls.

Many investigators have shown that fertile and subfertile populations can be differentiated by the SPA and that it is superior to routine seminal fluid analysis in discriminatory ability. Although variations do exist between laboratories, there appears to be general agreement that less than 10% of ova penetrated is evidence of sperm dysfunction and male infertility.[60]

For the clinician, the most significant outcome of the SPA is a repeated 0% penetration score. Because this result profoundly influences the couple's management, the SPA has significant prognostic value. In a 2.3-year followup of 68 patients with unexplained infertility, Aitken et al[62] found that none of four individuals with 0% penetration scores initiated pregnancy. Although 5 of 25 with scores of 1% to 10% were successful in this respect, the pregnancy rate was significantly lower than in the remaining population with an SPA score greater than 10%.[62] Clearly penetration scores less than 10% are not incompatible with pregnancy, but fertility is significantly reduced. Interestingly in the same series, the frequency

of conception in wives of patients with penetration scores above 75% was also reduced. This could be explained by the emergence of a female factor or impaired sperm transport.

Although most studies show some correlation of the SPA to conventional semen parameters (particularly motility), the principal advantage of the SPA is its ability to detect defects in sperm function that are not assessable by conventional semen analysis. In a group of 443 men with 0% SPA, 16.3% had no readily detectable abnormality on routine semen analysis.[60]

The SPA has also proved valuable in screening patients with varicocele to identify those with an accompanying sperm defect. Of 194 men in whom the SPA was performed before and after varicocelectomy, men whose penetration rates were greater than 10% before surgery did not achieve paternity postoperatively. There appears, therefore, to be a group of individuals who will not benefit from surgical repair, and unnecessary surgery may be avoided. Those varicocele patients who converted from negative to positive postoperatively had a 70% pregnancy rate.[63]

With the high cost and low success associated with in vitro fertilization (IVF) and embryo transfer, the SPA has been a common method for screening men before entry into these programs. Variable results have been obtained from correlating SPA and IVF outcome in those couples in whom the male has a "normal" semen analysis. In general, most studies have found that in males with both normal semen parameters and SPA, the results are predictive of successful IVF. A negative SPA score with a normal semen analysis suggests a lessened chance of successful IVF.

To overcome the limitations of SPA, in particular in those individuals with oligospermia or asthenospermia samples, several techniques have been used to optimize the assay. Both TES and Tris (TEST)–yolk buffer systems have been used to improve sperm function and the accuracy of the SPA.[64] Female reproductive tract secretions and ovulatory products, which could play an essential role in the events leading to gamete fusion, are missing in the SPA. McClure and colleagues[65] modified the SPA by the addition of human follicular fluid to induce the acrosome reaction in an attempt to improve the false-negative rates of the conventional SPA technique. In 26 patients with negative results, the findings became positive in 20 with human follicular fluid. Comparing the results of the conventional and the modified assays with the outcome of IVF, the false-positive rate was the same, but the false-negative rate was reduced from 40% to 7% with this new technique.[65]

The SPA does not measure sperm motility and transport in the female reproductive tract, nor does it evaluate events that occur after fertilization or ability of sperm to bind to the zona. Positive results simply mean that the sperm functions tested are intact. A 0% penetration rate is particularly useful because it indicates that the sperm are dysfunctional, and fertilization is unlikely to occur. The SPA is expensive, and it cannot replace the standard semen analysis in the evaluation of the infertile couple. When repeated routine semen analyses are neither clearly normal nor clearly abnormal, an SPA should be performed.

HEMI-ZONA ASSAY

Because sperm–zona pellucida binding is an important step in fertilization, the hemi-zona assay (HZA) is an additional assessment of sperm-fertilizing ability. This test uses the zona pellucida from nonfertilizable, nonliving human oocytes.[66] The zona pellucida is divided in half using micromanipulation techniques, and then each half is incubated with either fertile donor sperm or the patient's sperm. The number of sperm bound to each half is determined, and a ratio, the *hemi-zona index*, is calculated by dividing the number of bound sperm from the patient by the number of bound sperm from the fertile donor.

In the initial report, 95% of patients achieving no fertilization with IVF were found to have HZA of less than 62%.[66] Subsequent studies have shown fertilization was predicted in 26 of 28 cases, using the HZA ratio.[67]

Further studies with other groups and larger number of patients will help delineate the role of this new assay. One shortcoming of this assay (similar to that of the SPA) is that a minimal number of motile sperm must be present for adequate binding. That minimum number has not been defined as yet. The HZA also requires an IVF program supplying human ova as well as expertise in micromanipulation.

HYPO-OSMOTIC SWELLING TEST

Because the SPA is both labor intensive and expensive, scientists have turned their attention to develop functional assays that are both simpler and more economical. One such assay, the hypo-osmotic swelling (HOS) test, was developed by Jeyendran and associates[68] to assess the functional activity of the spermatozoal membrane. It is based on the assumption that an intact, functional sperm membrane is required for successful union of sperm and oocyte. Under hypo-osmotic conditions, spermatozoa swell with the influx of water and expansion of the membrane. Around the tail fibers, the plasma membrane is more loosely attached and is particularly susceptible to hypo-osmotic conditions. The swelling of the sperm tail, visible under phase contrast microscopy, signifies that water is being transported across the membrane normally and implies sperm integrity and normal functional activity.

The usefulness of the HOS test as an adjunct to standard semen analysis is controversial. Although Jeyendran and associates found a good correlation between the HOS test and the SPA, their study population comprised men with either demonstrated fertility or normal semen parameters.[68] Chan and colleagues[69] looked at the HOS test as an indicator of infertility in a much larger, heterogeneous group of men and found it unreliable.

Other innovative tests of sperm function, which include sperm nuclear maturity testing, the acrosome, and acrosome reaction, are currently still research tools.[70]

HYPERACTIVITY TESTS

Yanagimachi[71] described in hamster sperm a type of sperm motility attained after capacitation in which there were large-amplitude movements of the head and tail of sperm, often coupled with slow or nonprogressive motility. This motility was called *hyperactivity*. In human sperm, Burkman[72] reported hyperactivity pattern in only 0.4% in fertile human donors, but the percentage increased to 22% after capacitation. Only 8.4% of capacitated sperm from oligospermic patients showed this hyperactivity movement.[72] Further clinical research using CASA needs to be carried out to evaluate the usefulness of this hyperactivity movement.

Immunologic Studies

Sperm antibodies have been reported in 3% to 7% of infertile men and may be a relative cause of infertility.[1, 7] One must recognize clinical parameters that may be associated with antibody-mediated infertility in men. A history of inflammation of the genitourinary tract, testicular injury or torsion, and a previous vasectomy may lead to the development of sperm antibodies.[7, 73]

Although the majority of infertile men with sperm immunity have normal findings on semen analysis, the presence of a spontaneous agglutination or poor motility should alert the clinician to the possibility of antibodies. Often spermagglutination is nonspecific and may be related to the presence of bacteria or cellular debris and may not reflect an immunologic problem. Postcoital testing provides an excellent means to screen for antisperm antibodies. If fewer than 5 motile sperm per field are seen in a well-estrogenized mucus sample or if the sperm are seen to shake or vibrate, sperm antibody testing should be performed.

Most reproductive biology laboratories have attempted to identify antibodies to spermatozoa using one of four types of serologic tests: spermagglutination, complement-dependent sperm immobilization, indirect immunofluorescence, and the enzyme-linked immunosorbent assay (ELISA). The standard immunologic tests have frequently been insensitive, nonspecific, or both.[65]

Sperm antibodies can be found in the circulation, in the seminal plasma, or directly on the sperm surface. Several studies have shown a discordance between results of sperm antibody tests in matched serum and sperm samples. Humoral antibodies may be detected in blood but not in sperm, and conversely locally secreted antisperm antibodies within the genital tract may be detected on sperm with no evidence in the blood. In 166 of 856 matched samples, Bronson[73] found humoral antibodies in blood but not on sperm. Conversely, he found antibodies in the genital tract with no evidence in the serum in 14% of cases.[73] The presence of humoral antibodies directed against sperm is not relevant to fertility, unless these circulating antibodies are also present within the reproductive tract. Therefore, the convenience of assaying blood for antisperm antibodies is outweighed by the lack of clinical relevance of these measurements in comparison with assays that identify immunoglobulins directly on the sperm's surface. Similarly, seminal plasma antisperm antibodies are not attached to the sperm's surface and are probably of little clinical significance because seminal plasma components do not ascend past the vagina. It appears, therefore, that tests capable of detecting immunoglobulins on living sperm retrieved from the ejaculate are the most direct way to determine whether significant autoimmunity to sperm exists.

Over the last several years, there have been several useful assays developed to detect immunoglobulins present on the surface of motile spermatozoa. They include the mixed antiglobulin reaction (MAR), the radiolabeled antiglobulin test (RAT), and the immunobead test (IBT). Each of these tests can be used either as a *direct test* for detecting immunoglobulins already bound to patients' spermatozoa or as an *indirect test*.[7, 65, 74] In the indirect test, passive antibody is transferred to donor sperm (previously tested and found to be negative) from any body fluid (e.g., serum, seminal plasma, cervical mucus, or follicular fluid).

The IBT or the immunobead rosette test is one of the most informative and specific of all assays currently available to detect antisperm antibodies bound to the surface of sperm. The assay is performed with immunobeads, which are polyacrylamide spheres to which rabbit antihuman antibodies have been linked. These antiglobulins are specific for human antibodies of IgA, IgG, or IgM class. This test determines the isotope of immunoglobulin bound and the percentage of sperm bound with antibody. More importantly, in contrast to the radiolabeled antiglobulin assay and the MAR assay, it determines the region of sperm to which specific antibodies are bound. The significance of this lies in the effect that antibodies bound to different areas of sperm have on various sperm functions, such as motility, survival, and fertilization.[65]

Bacteriologic Studies

Obviously any symptomatic genital tract infection should be treated to prevent injury to the seminiferous tubules or obstruction to the epididymis. Epididymitis in young men under the age of 35 is usually secondary to *Neisseria gonorrhoeae* or *Chlamydia trachomatis.* Although asymptomatic *C. trachomatis* salpingitis may lead to tubal disease in women, there is no evidence of this organism causing a silent epididymal obstruction in men.

The investigation and therapy of individuals with asymptomatic genital tract infection is controversial.[75, 76] The common sexually transmitted organisms, such as *C. trachomatis, Mycoplasma hominis,* and *Ureaplasma urealyticum,* have been implicated, but not proved, as causes of male infertility. In a study comparing a fertile and nonfertile group of males, colonization rates for genital *Mycoplasma* (*Mycoplasma hominis* and *Ureaplasma*) were not significantly different for men with

normal or abnormal semen analysis.[77] The serologic evidence of recent or remote *Chlamydia* infection was found to be equally common among these groups. Genital *Mycoplasma* organisms are commonly isolated from urethral cultures of normal males, and the incidence appears to be related to the number of sexual partners. Gram-positive aerobic bacteria, primary *Staphylococcus epidermidis,* diphtheroids, and streptococcal species frequently colonize the male urethra. The ubiquitous nature of the gram-positive bacteria is responsible for urethral contamination of the ejaculate during semen cultures. Aerobic enterobacteria (gram-negative coliforms and enterococcus) are pathogens of the urethra and should be treated accordingly. The findings of greater than 5 white blood cells per hpf on the first voided 10 mL of urine (VB 1) are abnormal and indicative of urethral inflammation.[76, 77] This should lead to appropriate intervention and treatment of the organisms, including treatment of the female partner, if sexually transmitted.

In any evaluation of semen for pyospermia, one must properly differentiate leukocytes from immature sperm cells. This can be carried out with stains, such as the Bryan-Leishman stain or Papanicolaou's stain.[38] Without proper staining, immature sperm cells are often misidentified as leukocytes. Leukocytes may be a normal constituent of both seminal and prostatic fluid. The mean concentration of leukocytes in the seminal fluid of normal males is between 1 and 3.3×10^6 per mL.[76] Increases in seminal leukocytes (pyospermia) are associated with decreased sperm motility, a decrease in sperm density, and a decreased fertilization capacity as measured by the SPA.[78, 79]

There is still little evidence to suggest that asymptomatic genital tract infections are a significant cause of male infertility. Therefore, there is little justification for empiric antibiotic therapy. Treatment of symptomatic infection, in particular *Chlamydia,* is warranted. If on the first voided 10 mL there are greater than 5 white blood cells per hpf or greater than 2×10^6 leukocytes per mL in the semen, one must do appropriate cultures and institute therapy.

Chromosome Analysis

A variety of somatic chromosomal abnormalities are associated with male infertility, and the prevalence increases as the sperm count decreases. In his study of 1263 infertile couples, Kjessler[80] found the incidence of chromosome abnormalities in the male to be 6.2%. The incidence rose in this group to 11% in those whose count was less than 10 million per mL, and in azoospermic subjects, it was 21%.[80] In only isolated cases has infertility been documented in association with a specific chromosome abnormality, but subtle genetic studies should be considered in men with severe oligospermia and azoospermia to look for both autosomal and sex chromosome abnormalities. The diagnostic yield is greatest in men with small testes, azoospermia, and elevated FSH levels. The most consistent chromosomal disorder associated with abnormal testicular function and severe hypogonadism is Klinefelter's syndrome (47, xxy).[31]

Radiologic Investigation

SCROTAL ULTRASONOGRAPHY

Both clinical and laboratory investigations have provided convincing evidence that varicoceles are detrimental to sper-

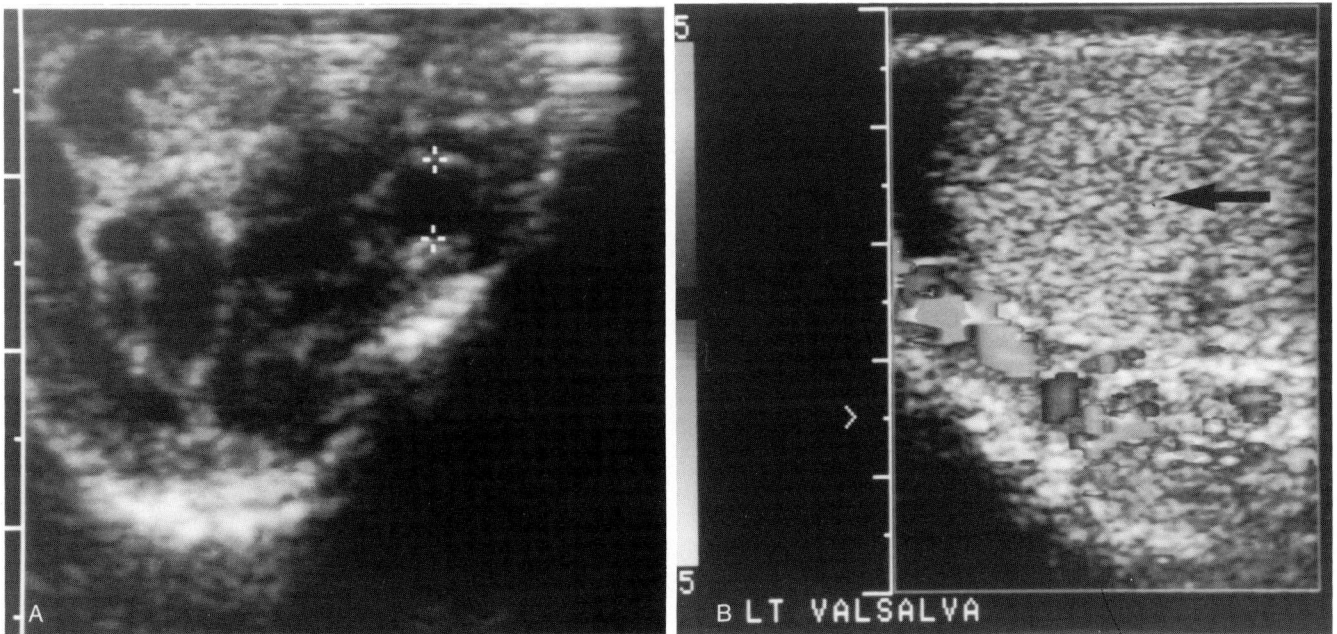

FIGURE 7–7. Scrotal ultrasonography. *A,* A transverse scan using a 7.5 MHz transducer demonstrating dilated spermatic veins (varicocele) as echo-free structures. The electronic marker measures the vein diameter as 51 mm. *B,* Testis in longitudinal axis showing normal echogenicity (*arrow*). During a Valsalva maneuver, incompetent valves in the spermatic vein allow for retrograde flow rapid enough for color Doppler detection.

matogenesis in some men.[37] Dubin and Amelar[81] reported that improvement in semen quality after varicocelectomy bears no relation to the palpable size of the varicocele. Because small but clinically significant varicoceles may be missed, even on careful physical examination, several diagnostic techniques have been tried. The Doppler pencil-probe stethoscope is one of the earliest techniques. Questionable regurgitant sounds are a drawback with the Doppler stethoscope, and unequivocal answers cannot be obtained in cases of questionable varicoceles. Another diagnostic technique is scrotal thermography; however, in patients with a single or atrophic testicle or bilateral varicoceles, this test is inadequate because diagnosis relies on the temperature difference between the two sides of the scrotum. Scrotal ultrasonography is a readily available noninvasive method that can detect many intrascrotal abnormalities and has a unique ability to visualize both the testes and the surrounding structures. It is useful in documenting the size of the varicosities as well as documenting reflux (Fig. 7–7A and B).[82] High-resolution color Doppler ultrasonography is an additional useful technique. It can simultaneously display blood flow superimposed on detailed gray scale anatomic images.

VENOGRAPHY

This technique seems to be the most specific method of identification of varicoceles, but it is invasive, is associated with some morbidity, requires specialized skills and equipment, and is expensive. It should be reserved for use in recurrent varicoceles for postoperative detection of aberrant veins. The advantage of using venography to look for recurrent varicoceles is that if these vessels are discovered, either coils or balloons may be used to occlude these vessels at that time.

TRANSRECTAL ULTRASONOGRAPHY

The routine evaluation of individuals with azoospermia, or low ejaculate volume, has included endocrine testing, postejaculate urinalysis, seminal fructose with subsequent vasography, and testicular biopsy. Historically, vasography has been the best technique of imaging the seminal vesicles and ejaculatory ducts. Transrectal ultrasonography is a new diagnostic modality that provides valuable information about these structures and may be used in place of vasography to identify obstruction or congenital anomalies of the ejaculatory ducts or seminal vesicles. It is accurate, noninvasive, and readily available.[55]

REFERENCES

1. Jaffe SB, Jewelewicz R. The basic infertility investigation. Fertil Steril 1991; 56:599–613.
2. McClure RD. Evaluation of the infertile male. Prob Urol 1987; 1:443–460.
3. Kogan SJ. Cryptorchidism. In: Kelalis PP, King LR, Belman AB, editors. Clinical Pediatric Urology. Philadelphia: WB Saunders, 1985:864–887.
4. Lipshultz LI, Caminos-Torres R, Greenspan CS, et al. Testicular function after unilateral orchiopexy for unilaterally undescended testis. N Engl J Med 1976; 295:15–18.
5. Werner CA. Mumps orchitis and testicular atrophy. Ann Intern Med 1950; 32:1066.
6. Nagler HM, Deitch AD, de Vere White R. Testicular torsion: temporal considerations. Fertil Steril 1984; 42:257–262.
7. Bronson R, Cooper G, Rosenfeld D. Sperm antibodies: their role in infertility. Fertil Steril 1984; 42:171–183.
8. Zamboni L. The ultrastructural pathology of the spermatozoon as a cause of infertility: the role of electron microscopy in the evaluation of semen quality. Fertil Steril 1987; 48:711–734.
9. Handelsman DJ, Conway AJ, Boylan LM, Turtle JR. Young's syndrome: obstructive azoospermia and chronic sinopulmonary infections. N Engl J Med 1984; 310:3–9.
10. Kaplan E, Shwachman H, Perlmutter AD, et al. Reproductive failure in males with cystic fibrosis. N Engl J Med 1968; 279:65–69.

11. MacLeod J, Hotchkiss RS. The effects of hyperpyrexia on spermatozoa counts in men. Endocrinology 1941; 28:780.

12. Buch JP, Havlovec SK. Variation in sperm penetration assay related to viral illness. Fertil Steril 1991; 55:844–846.

13. Heller CG, Clermont Y. Kinetics of the germinal epithelium in man. Rec Prog Horm Res 1964; 20:545.

14. Whorton MD. Male occupational reproductive hazards. West J Med 1982; 137:521–524.

15. Oates RD, Lipshultz LI. Fertility and testicular function in patients after chemotherapy and radiotherapy. In: Lytton B, editor. Advances in Urology. Vol. 2. Chicago: Year Book Medical Publishers, 1989:63.

16. Lipshultz LI, Ross CE, Whorton D, et al. Dibromochloropropane and its effect on testicular function in man. J Urol 1980; 124:464–468.

17. Sigman M, Lipshultz LI, Howards SS. Evaluation of the subfertile male. In: Lipshultz L, Howards SS, editors. Infertility in the Male. St. Louis: Mosby-Year Book, 1991:179–210.

18. Kolodny RC, Masters WH, Kolodner RM, et al. Depression of plasma testosterone levels after chronic intensive marihuana use. N Engl J Med 1974; 290:872–874.

19. Stillman RJ, Rosenberg MJ, Sachs BP. Smoking and reproduction. Fertil Steril 1986; 46:545–546.

20. Mendelson JH, Kuehnle J, Ellingboe J, et al. Plasma testosterone levels before, during, and after chronic marihuana smoking. N Engl J Med 1974; 291:1051–1055.

21. Smith CG, Asch RH. Drug abuse and reproduction. Fertil Steril 1987; 48:355–373.

22. Van Thiel DH, Lester R, Sherins RJ. Hypogonadism in alcoholic liver disease: evidence for a double defect. Gastroenterology 1974; 67:1188–1199.

23. Berul CI, Harclerode JE. Effects of cocaine hydrochloride on the male reproductive system. Life Sci 1989; 45:91–95.

24. Rock J, Robinson D. Effect of induced intrascrotal hyperthermia on testicular function in man. Am J Obstet Gynecol 1965; 93:793–801.

25. Feldman P. Sexuality, birth control and childbirth in orthodox Jewish tradition. Can Med Assoc J 1992; 146:29–33.

26. Whitehead ED, Leiter E. Genital abnormalities and abnormal semen analyses in male patients exposed to diethylstilbestrol in utero. J Urol 1981; 125:47–50.

27. Toth A. Reversible toxic effect of salicylazosulfapyridine on semen quality. Fertil Steril 1979; 31:538–540.

28. Griffin JE, Wilson JD. Disorders of the testes and male reproductive tract. In: Wilson JD, Foster DW, editors. Textbook of Endocrinology. 7th edition. Philadelphia: WB Saunders, 1986:259–311.

29. Schlegel PN, Chang TSK, Marshall FF. Antibiotics: potential hazards to male fertility. Fertil Steril 1991; 55:235.

30. Swerdloff RS, Palacios A, McClure RD, et al. Male contraception: clinical assessment of chronic administration of testosterone enanthate. In: Hansson V, editor. Endocrine Approach to Male Contraception. Copenhagen: Scriptor, 1978:731–747.

31. Bardin CW, Paulsen CA. The testes. In: Wilson JD, Foster DW, editors. Textbook of Endocrinology. 6th edition. Philadelphia: WB Saunders, 1981:293–354.

32. Griffin JE, Wilson JD. The syndromes of androgen resistance. N Engl J Med 1980; 302:198–209.

33. McClure RD. Endocrine investigation and therapy. Urol Clin North Am 1987; 14:471–488.

34. Carter JN, Tyson JE, Tolis G, et al. Prolactin-secreting tumors and hypogonadism in 22 men. N Engl J Med 1978; 299:847–852.

35. Lieblich JM, Rogol AD, White BJ, et al. Syndrome of anosmia with hypogonadotropic hypogonadism (Kallmann syndrome): clinical and laboratory studies in 23 cases. Am J Med 1982; 73:506–519.

36. Zachmann M, Prader A, Kind HP, et al. Testicular volume during adolescence. Cross-sectional and longitudinal studies. Helv Paediatr Acta 1974; 29:61–72.

37. Pryor JL, Howards SS. Varicocele. Urol Clin North Am 1987; 14:499–513.

38. World Health Organization. Laboratory Manual for the Examination of Human Semen and Semen-Cervical Mucus Interaction. Cambridge: Cambridge University Press, 1992.

39. Overstreet JW. Assessment of disorders of spermatogenesis. In: Lockey JE, editor. Reproduction: The New Frontier in Occupational and Environmental Health Research. New York: Alan Liss, 1984:275–292.

40. Clark RV, Sherins RJ. Use of semen analysis in the evaluation of the infertile couple. In: Santen RJ, Swerdloff RS, editors. Male Reproductive Dysfunction. New York: Marcel Dekker, 1986:253–266.

41. Sherins RJ, Brightwell D, Sternthal PM. Longitudinal analysis of semen

of fertile and infertile men. In: Troen P, Nankin HR, editors. The Testis in Normal and Infertile Men. New York: Raven Press, 1977:473–488.

42. MacLeod J, Gold RZ. The male factor in fertility and infertility. J Urol 1951; 66:436.

43. Boyers SP, Davis RO, Katz DF. Automated semen analysis. Curr Probl Obstet Gynecol Fertil 1989; 12:165.

44. Overstreet JW, Katz DF. Semen analysis. Urol Clin North Am 1987; 14:441–449.

45. Vantman D, Koukoulis G, Dennison L, et al. Computer-assisted semen analysis: evaluation of method and assessment of the influence of sperm concentration on linear velocity determination. Fertil Steril 1988; 49:510–515.

46. Davis RO, Katz DF. Computer-aided sperm analysis: technology at a crossroads. Fertil Steril 1993; 59:953–955.

47. Swerdloff RS, Boyers SP. Evaluation of the male partner of an infertile couple: an algorithmic approach. JAMA 1982; 247:2418–2422.

48. Goldzieher JW, Dozier TS, Smith KD, et al. Improving the diagnostic reliability of rapidly fluctuating plasma hormone levels by optimized multiple-sampling techniques. J Clin Endocrinol Metab 1976; 43:824–830.

49. Rosen SW, Weintraub BD. Monotropic increase of serum FSH correlated with low sperm count in young men with oligospermia and aspermia. J Clin Endocrinol Metab 1971; 32:410–416.

50. Segal S, Polishuk WZ, Ben-David M. Hyperprolactinemic male infertility. Fertil Steril 1976; 27:1425–1427.

51. Urban MD, Lee PA, Migeon CJ. Adult height and fertility in men with congenital virilizing adrenal hyperplasia. N Engl J Med 1978; 299:1392–1396.

52. Beitins IZ, Axelrod L, Ostrea T, et al. Hypogonadism in a male with an immunologically active luteinizing hormone: characterization of the abnormal hormone. J Clin Endocrinol Metab 1981; 52:1143–1149.

53. Lipshultz LI, Howards SS, McClure RD, Nagler HM. When and how to do a testis biopsy and vasogram. Contemp Urol 1990; 2:45.

54. McClure RD. Azoospermia. In: Rajfer J, editor. Current Problems in Infertility and Impotence. Chicago: Year Book Medical Publishers, 1990:31–36.

55. Patterson L, Jarow JP. Transrectal ultrasonography in the evaluation of the infertile man: a report of 3 cases. J Urol 1990; 44:1469–1471.

56. Posinovec J. The necessity of bilateral biopsy in oligo- and azoospermia. Int J Fertil 1975; 21:189–191.

57. Boreau J. Images of the seminal tracts. New York: Karger, 1974.

58. Overstreet JW. Evaluation of sperm-cervical mucus interaction. Fertil Steril 1986; 45:324–326.

59. Aitken RJ. Use of sperm-ova penetration tests to evaluate the infertile couple. In: Santen RJ, Swerdloff RS, editors. Male Reproductive Dysfunction. New York: Marcel Dekker, 1986:267–294.

60. Rogers BJ. The sperm penetration assay: its usefulness reevaluated. Fertil Steril 1985; 43:821–840.

61. Yanagimachi R. Mechanisms of fertilization in mammals. In: Mastroianni L, Biggers JD Jr, editors. Fertilization and Embryonic Development In Vitro. New York: Plenum Publishing, 1981:81–183.

62. Aitken RJ, Best FS, Warner P, Templeton A. A prospective study of the relationship between semen quality and fertility in cases of unexplained infertility. J Androl 1984; 5:297–303.

63. Rogers BJ, Mygatt GG, Soderdahl DW, Hale RW. Monitoring of suspected infertile men with varicocele by the sperm penetration assay. Fertil Steril 1985; 44:800–805.

64. Veeck LL. TES and Tris (TEST)–yolk buffer systems, sperm function testing, and in vitro fertilization. Fertil Steril 1992; 58:484–486.

65. McClure RD, Tom RA, Watkins M, et al. SpermCheck: a simplified screening assay for immunological infertility. Fertil Steril 1989; 52:650–654.

66. Burkman LJ, Coddington CC, Franken DR, et al. The hemizona assay (HZA): development of a diagnostic test for the binding of human spermatozoa to the human hemizona pellucida to predict fertilization potential. Fertil Steril 1988; 49:688–697.

67. Oehninger S, Coddington CC, Scott R, et al. Hemizona assay: assessment of sperm dysfunction and prediction of in vitro fertilization outcome. Fertil Steril 1989; 51:665–670.

68. Jeyendran RS, Van der Ven HH, Perez-Pelaez M, et al. Development of an assay to assess the functional integrity of the human sperm membrane and its relationship to other semen characteristics. J Reprod Fertil 1984; 70:219–228.

69. Chan SY, Fox EJ, Chan MM, et al. The relationship between the human sperm hypoosmotic, routine semen analysis, and the human sperm zona-free hamster ovum penetration assay. Fertil Steril 1985; 44:668–672.

70. Liu DY, Baker HWG. Tests of human sperm function and fertilization in vitro. Fertil Steril 1992; 58:465–483.

71. Yanagimachi R. The movement of golden hamster spermatozoa before and after capacitation. J Reprod Fertil 1970; 23:193–196.

72. Burkman JL. Characterization of hyperactivated motility by human spermatozoa during capacitation: comparison of fertile and oligozoospermic sperm populations. Arch Androl 1984; 13:153–165.

73. Bronson RA. Current concepts on the relation of antisperm antibodies and infertility. Semin Reprod Endocrinol 1988; 6:364.

74. Haas GG Jr. How should sperm antibody tests be used clinically? Am J Reprod Immunol Microbiol 1987; 15:106.

75. Fowler JE Jr. Genital tract infection. In: Lipshultz L, Howards SS, editors. Infertility in the Male. St. Louis: Mosby-Year Book, 1991:297–312.

76. McConnell JC. The role of infection in male infertility. Prob Urol 1987; 1:467–475.

77. Hellstrom WJ, Schachter J, Sweet RL, McClure RD. Is there a role for *Chlamydia trachomatis* and genital *Mycoplasma* in male infertility? Fertil Steril 1987; 48:337–339.

78. Berger RE, Smith WD, Critchlow CW, et al. Improvement in the sperm penetration (hamster ova) assay (SPA) results after doxycycline treatment of infertile men. J Androl 1983; 4:126–130.

79. Wolff H, Politch JA, Martinez A, et al. Leukocytospermia is associated with poor semen quality. Fertil Steril 1990; 53:528.

80. Kjessler B. Facteurs genetiques dans la subfertile male humaine. In: Thibault C, editor. Fécondité et Stérilité du Male: acquisitions récentes. Paris: Masson et Cie, 1972.

81. Dubin L, Amelar RD. Varicocele size and results of varicocelectomy in selected subfertile men with varicocele. Fertil Steril 1970; 21:606–609.

82. McClure RD, Hricak H. Scrotal ultrasound in the infertile man: detection of subclinical unilateral and bilateral varicoceles. J Urol 1986; 135:711–715.

CHAPTER 8

Initial Approach to the Infertile Couple

WILLIAM R. KEYE, Jr.

The success of medical care of a couple with infertility can be measured in many ways. The most obvious measure of success is whether the couple is able to achieve a pregnancy that is carried to term with the delivery of a healthy infant. However, there are other ways in which couples measure the success of their infertility care. For example, it may be as important for a member of an infertile couple to know whether or not he or she is solely or partially responsible for the infertility. For others it may be learning whether or not they, individually or as a couple, even have a potential for fertility. Yet for others it may be important to learn whether past medical (e.g., an induced abortion) or lifestyle practices (e.g., multiple sexual partners) have impaired their fertility. Still other couples feel successful when their medical team has been supportive of their decision to explore other ways to build a family or to choose to live childfree. As a result, the health care team providing care for the infertile couple must be sensitive to the individual needs of their infertile patients and be able and willing to design a program to meet those needs. In addition, it is important for the infertility team to provide care in a warm, supportive, and nonthreatening environment. To meet all of these objectives, it is necessary that the initial meeting with an infertile couple deal with medical, psychological, and social aspects of the couple and their infertility problem. The initial visit establishes a foundation for subsequent visits. The ability of the team to respond to the needs of the couple and the ability and willingness of the couple to follow through with the programs set up by the medical care team are established largely at the time of the initial evaluation. Furthermore, the sense of confidence and trust that the patient has in the health care team and the belief of the infertile couple that they will be able to communicate effectively with a sensitive, responsive health care team will be established at the initial visit.

SCHEDULING THE INITIAL VISIT

The initial visit to discuss infertility may occur at any time in the course of the couple's attempts to conceive. Although most clinicians consider a couple to be infertile when they have not achieved a pregnancy after 1 year of unprotected intercourse, many couples are now seeking advice regarding fertility even before their initial attempts to conceive. For example, persons with long-standing medical diseases or a family history of genetic diseases may seek preconceptual counseling. Couples may seek help conceiving soon after their marriage if one of the couples has had a previous history of an infection and surgery of the reproductive organs, or if the wife does not have regular menstrual periods. In addition, those couples who first attempt to conceive after the age of 35 years may want information regarding age-related factors and the best method of conceiving in the shortest period. Finally, couples who have been attempting to conceive for periods as short as 3 to 6 months may become impatient and seek advice from the physician regarding their attempts to conceive. Thus, the classic definition of infertility should not always be interpreted literally nor used to discourage couples without a year of infertility from seeking information about conception and infertility. Because the particular motives behind the visit will vary from couple to couple, the request for care or advice regarding fertility should be all that is necessary for a couple to receive an appointment with a physician.

PREPARATION FOR THE FIRST VISIT

The initial visit to discuss fertility is often enhanced if the physician has access to previous records of medical care, including the radiologic films such as a hysterosalpingogram and pelvic ultrasonography and a videotape of any previous surgery. The office staff can often arrange for those records and films to be forwarded at the time that the patient makes the initial appointment. It is helpful to ask patients to call back to the office approximately 1 week before their scheduled visit to be sure that the records have arrived prior to the scheduled office visit. At the time the patient calls to make her initial appointment, an infertility questionnaire can be mailed to the couple. Each member of the couple is asked to complete the questionnaire and bring it with them to their visit. A review of the appropriate records and radiologic tests at or before the patient's first visit often aids and facilitates the efficient gathering of data at the first visit. However, reviewing the records with the patient at the first visit is also important.

At the time the initial appointment is made, the office staff should also establish how and when to contact the couple. Because of the sensitive nature of infertility, some individuals or couples may not want family, friends, or coworkers to know about their medical care. Therefore, specific guidelines regarding phone calls and messages for the patient from the office should be discussed with the patient.

Although there may be circumstances in which only one member of the couple wishes to be interviewed and evaluated, the couple usually should be encouraged to attend together. To see the couple together often helps the physician understand the dynamics of their relationship. By interviewing the couple together, one can see how they interact and how they communicate with regard to reproduction, an inherently sensitive and personal subject. However, it is advantageous on occasion to interview each member of the couple without his or her spouse in addition to the joint interview. In some instances there may be aspects of the person's past medical or personal life that they do not wish to divulge to his or her partner. In addition, each member of the couple may feel more free to discuss their motives and psychosexual responses to infertility when interviewed alone as opposed to discussing these sensitive issues in front of the partner. When husband or wife are interviewed separately, he or she also may discuss more freely a personal sense of responsibility or perceived fault for the infertility. They may not feel as free to do this when interviewed in front of their partner. The female partner can be interviewed alone in the examination room, and the male partner can be interviewed alone while his wife is in the examination room, changing into or out of her clothes. However, the main principle guiding the infertility evaluation and treatment is that it is a couple's problem and is handled most efficiently and effectively when both members are involved. Seeing a couple together may also provide the physician with an opportunity to uncover and dispel various myths and misunderstandings that may be a source of friction between them. Finally, a joint interview gives both members of the couple a sense that they have an advocate and that their opinions and voices carry equal weight. The husband who is included by the health care team is usually more cooperative and enthusiastic in carrying out the infertility evaluation and treatment than a husband who is not included in the planning.

In most practices the first visit typically is scheduled on weekdays between the hours of 8:00 and 4:00. However, there are many women and men who find these conventional times inconvenient. Because the visit usually is more efficient and effective if both husband and wife are present, it may be beneficial to offer the couple new to infertility a visit in either the evening or on a weekend day. In addition, the initial appointment typically requires 45 minutes of the physician's time and should be scheduled appropriately.

Finally, it is important that the couple have adequate time allotted for their visit so the psychosocial and psychosexual aspects of their infertility problem can be discussed as well as the pure medical aspects. Because many couples with infertility find it difficult to be around pregnant women, it is often helpful if infertility couples are scheduled when there are no obstetric patients in the office. Furthermore, infertility couples greatly resent the fact that a physician may be called away from their visit to deliver a baby. Therefore, if it is at all possible, it is desirable to schedule infertility visits with the physician at a time when the physician does not have responsibility for obstetric call. Most couples will also appreciate having magazines other than *American Baby* or *Parents* available in the waiting room.

THE INITIAL VISIT

Determining the Reason for the Clinic Visit

It is important to inquire of the couple why they have decided to seek medical care for their infertility problem at the present time. For some it may be the fact that they have just passed a milestone birthday (age 30 or 35). For others it may be that a close friend or relative has just conceived or delivered a baby. Yet for others it may be because their opportunities for a change in lifestyle or a new job or a move requires making a decision whether or not to pursue attempts to conceive. The couple is often seeking information about their potential for fertility and may make the decision about lifestyle changes based on the physician's best estimate of whether or not they stand a likely chance of conceiving within a certain period. The physician may also ask why the couple has sought care in his or her office. The dialogue that ensues will often provide information about the expectations of the couple. For some patients it may be simply a matter of convenience in terms of office location or appointment times. For others it may be the result of a detailed search of the infertility resources within the community, perhaps in consultation with a national support organization such as RE-SOLVE. Such a discussion may also allow the couple to discuss any interaction they have had with other physicians with respect to their infertility care. An in-depth discussion of the things that the couple liked or disliked about the previous medical care may allow the physician to avoid repetition of any discomfort or unhappiness. Because there is no single office practice style that meets with the approval of each and every patient, it is often helpful to know the specific aspects of medical care that particularly distress each couple or individual. If it is not possible to design the office practice in such a way as to meet the demands or requests of a specific couple, it is useful to discuss these difficulties with them at the initial visit. They have the choice then of leaving the office and seeking care elsewhere or of modifying their expectations and demands.

Infertility and Medical History

At the time of the initial visit the medical records and questionnaire can be reviewed with the couple. Because many couples are confused and, at times, overwhelmed by medical terminology, it is important to be sure that they understand what tests have been done and the results. It is also important to be sure that the validity of their answers is established if they have completed a questionnaire. For example, many patients will confuse the infusion of dye into their fallopian tubes at the time of laparoscopy with a hysterosalpingogram. Other couples may not understand the difference between a laparoscopy and a hysteroscopy. A list of the items that should be covered in the initial interview with infertility couples is noted in Table 8–1. In addition to general medical information, the questionnaire should include information about menstrual periods, previous preg-

nancies, birth control methods used, previous pelvic surgeries that have been performed, and prior infertility tests. Additional specific information that should be elicited includes the duration of their relationship; how long the couple or individual has been attempting to conceive; and whether the husband has fathered any children or the wife has achieved a pregnancy in a prior relationship. These questions are usually best asked at the time of separate interviews.

TABLE 8–1. Infertility History

1. Identifying Information
    Woman: Name, age, how to contact patient, occupation
    Man: Name, age, how to contact patient, occupation
2. Reason for Visit
    Infertility? Repeated pregnancy loss? To establish ability to conceive or father a child in the future? To determine impact of previous medical or surgical procedures or lifestyles on fertility?
3. Infertility History
    Menstrual history: menarche, frequency, duration, intensity, pain, premenstrual symptoms
    Duration of attempts to conceive
    Previous medical care for infertility: results of tests and treatments
    Children from previous relationships or marriages
    Details regarding infertility prior to previous pregnancies
    Previous obstetric and gynecologic history
    Contraceptive agents used in the past
4. General Medical History
    Hospital admissions
    Current problems
    Use of vitamins (folic acid) or nutritional supplements
    Medications
5. Surgical History
    Pelvic surgery: Dilation and curettage; cesarean section, ovarian cystectomy, cervical conization, myomectomy, ablation, fallopian tube surgery, ectopic pregnancy
    Nonpelvic surgery: appendectomy
6. Sexual History
    Frequency and timing of coitus?
    Use of lubricants?
    Ejaculation? Leakage of semen from vagina after coitus?
    Discomfort?
    Postcoital douching?
7. Lifestyle
    Occupation? exposure to toxins or radiation?
    Alcohol use? Smoking? Recreational drugs?
    Exercise? frequency, duration, intensity?
    Dietary habits? Eating disorders?
    Hot tubs and saunas?
8. Assessing Beliefs
    "Why do you think you have not achieved a pregnancy?"
9. Assessing Motives
    To experience a pregnancy
    To raise a child
    To pass on family name
    To pass on family genes
    To save a troubled marriage
10. Assessing Psychosocial Environment
    Pressure to have children from family or friends
    Impact of pregnancy on career
    Cultural factors
    Marital stability
    Reactions of others to the couple's childlessness or infertility
11. Assessing Psychosexual Responses to Infertility
    Depression, anxiety, anger, impact on self-esteem, body image, sexuality
    Impact on relationship with husband, wife, family, friends, job, church
    Reaction
    Use or awareness of peer support groups (e.g., RESOLVE)
12. Personal, Ethical, and Moral Concerns
    Acceptance of donor insemination? In vitro fertilization, assisted reproductive technologies? Gamete intrafallopian transfer? Egg donation? Adoption?

Surgical History

The past surgical history of each member of the infertile couple is important. In the female it may uncover a past history of appendicitis, pelvic surgery, or pelvic infection. It may also uncover use of an intrauterine device that may be associated with an increased risk of developing pelvic adhesions even in the absence of a clinical pelvic infection. Previous surgical procedures may significantly influence fertility. A postpartum dilation and curettage or abortion may result in intrauterine adhesions. Previous cryosurgery or conization of the cervix may have caused cervical stenosis or damage to cervical glands with a decreased ability to produce cervical mucus. Uterine surgery for fibroids or ovarian surgery for cysts may result in significant pelvic adhesions. In the male a history of surgery of the bladder neck during childhood may alert the physician to the possibility of retrograde ejaculation on the part of the male.

Sexual History

A sexual history should include the frequency and timing of intercourse throughout the menstrual cycle. The couple should also be asked if the infertility has affected coital frequency and encounters. In addition, they should be questioned about the use of coital lubricants and whether or not there is leakage of semen out of the vagina following intercourse. The absence of semen discharge suggests retrograde ejaculation. The presence or absence of pain may also provide a useful clue to the possibility of endometriosis or pelvic adhesions. In addition, both may be asked about unprotected intercourse in other relationships that had the potential for fertility. This question is often best asked of each individual member of the couple when seen separately.

Lifestyle

The lifestyle of each couple should also be reviewed. This should include a work history with attention to possible exposure to environmental agents that may interfere with fertility. In addition, the use of alcohol and prescription or street drugs is important. Other features of their lifestyle that are important include their dietary pattern and caloric intake as well as the extent of stress and exercise in their lives and whether they have recently experienced any marked weight loss or weight gain.

Assessing the Couple's Beliefs

After reviewing in detail the medical, surgical, social, and sexual aspects of the couple, it is helpful to ask the couple why they think conception has not occurred. This may elicit significant additional information about medical factors that have not been uncovered in the standard questionnaire. Women may relate the fact that their mother had taken diethylstilbestrol during their pregnancy. Men may talk about the infrequency or poor timing of intercourse due to a heavy work schedule or the demands of job-related travel. In addition, the interview may uncover significant new information that pertains to their failure to conceive.

Occasionally, women will discuss their concern that they have not conceived because of the presence of an "infantile uterus." Occasionally, these messages have been left with the patient from previous physicians. The woman may also be concerned that her retroverted or tipped uterus may be contributing to her infertility. By seeking this information from the couple, the physician may be provided with an opportunity to dispel myths or misunderstandings and to allay fears that the patient or couple may have regarding these real or imagined infertility factors.

Assessing Motives

It is helpful also to inquire about the motivations for seeking infertility care. This is best done with the couple together on one occasion and separately on another. For some the motivation to seek infertility care is simply to dispel the fear that some past life or medical event has rendered them subfertile and to regain control of their reproductive lives. For others it may be to experience a shared pregnancy. Yet for others it may be to experience the pregnancy and birth process. For some it may be to pass on the family name or the genes of the family to the next generation. Finally, for some it is the opportunity to raise a child. Understanding the motives will aid the physician in determining the order, sequence, and content of an infertility evaluation. It also helps the physician understand which treatment options will be most acceptable to a patient or couple. If, for example, the main motivation of one or both members of the couple is to share the conception of a child or to pass on the genetic make-up of the individuals to the next generation, adoption will not be an acceptable alternative. In this situation, the use of donor sperm also may not be acceptable. Gathering this information at the initial visit often avoids uncomfortable and distressing confrontation with the couple in the future when inappropriate suggestions for treatment for them may be offered by the physician. When the motives for seeking infertility care differ significantly between the members of the couple, it may be important for the couple to spend time in conversation or counseling before any medical evaluation has even commenced. This is particularly useful when one member of the couple is highly motivated to achieve a biologic pregnancy and the other member of the couple is simply doing it as a favor to his or her spouse. Often this situation occurs when a person who has had several pregnancies or children marries someone who has never had a child.

Assessing the Psychosocial Environment

The physician should also ask the couple about any social pressures that they are experiencing. Family and friends may be placing pressure on the couple to have children, perhaps at a time when it is less than ideal for the couple. In addition, one member of the couple may be putting significant pressure on his or her spouse to achieve a pregnancy. Finally, the concerns of increasing age or the need to make a decision regarding a job opportunity or move may be pressuring the couple to seek medical care. Sometimes alternatives to infertility care may be appropriately offered or suggested. The woman who believes that she will experience greater difficulty conceiving because she has reached 30 years of age may be relieved to know that she still has many good years of reproduction left. As a result, she may decide to defer the workup and to pursue a new job or educational opportunity and plan to come back to the infertility evaluation at a later time. Finally, it is important to understand the cultural background of a couple. There are times when cultural pressures and expectations are great and may be driving the couple to seek infertility care before they actually wish to conceive. In some situations, the expectation that the marriage will lead to the birth of a biologic child and that the failure to do so may lead to divorce and rejection by the culture and the family may be a great source of stress as well as a motivating factor. It is important for the physician to realize the pressure under which the couple or individuals may be functioning so that they may understand the intense and sometimes irrational behavior of the couple. The woman who fears that she may be divorced by her husband if she does not conceive within a short period may feel resentful and angry about this and direct that resentment and anger toward the medical care staff. By understanding these factors and forces at the beginning of the infertility evaluation and treatment process, the office staff can provide appropriate support and referral.

Assessing Psychosexual Responses to Infertility

It is also useful to ask the couple about their responses to the stress of infertility. Like any chronic illness, infertility can have a profound effect on one's self image. As discussed elsewhere in this text, people experiencing infertility may have a loss of self-esteem and a poor body image and develop a sense of inadequacy. In addition, emotions such as depression, anger, anxiety, paranoia, and hopelessness may develop. Finally, infertility may also have an impact on the way the couple is perceived by friends and family. Often infertile couples who wish not to discuss their infertility with their family may be viewed by family members as being selfish and more interested in career or jobs or money than in having children. They may be rejected or excluded from family or church or social events, which may lead to a feeling of isolation. To avoid these negative feelings and rejection, they may withdraw from social circles and isolate themselves. By obtaining this information at the initial visit, a couple may be directed to a local peer support group or other self-help group, where they may find other people who can counsel or share the pain and discomfort of their infertility. They will usually find people who are supportive and understand the emotional trauma that they are experiencing. A social worker or psychologist trained and experienced in counseling infertile couples may be a valuable resource under certain circumstances (Table 8–2).

PLANNING THE INFERTILITY EVALUATION

In planning the infertility evaluation, many individual factors must be taken into account. Although there is a standard approach to the order or timing of testing that considers expense and risk, individual factors should be taken into account. What is appropriate for one couple is not necessarily appropriate for another. The principles that guide an infertility evaluation, however, are essentially the same for all couples. These principles include the following:

1. Evaluate the man as well as the woman.
2. Consider the possibility that there may be more than one factor responsible for the infertility. This means that once an abnormality is found the workup should not necessarily come to a halt. Depending on the age of the patient and the timetable established by the couple for the evaluation, it is usually appropriate to continue to complete all the testing despite the fact that a significant fertility factor has been demonstrated.
3. The infertility evaluation should be designed not only to uncover reasons for infertility but also to answer significant questions that the patient and her partner may have regarding their overall health as well as their reproductive capacity.
4. The infertility evaluation should take into account the resources of the couple. These resources include not only financial resources but also resources of time, physical energy, and emotional energy. Limited resources may influence the order or timing of tests.
5. The rate at which the tests are performed and the timetable for the performance of the tests should be negotiated with the couple and take into account both their motivations and their resources. A complete infertility evaluation may take as short a time as 1 month or as long as a year or longer.
6. The plan for the evaluation of the infertile couple

should be clearly spelled out for the couple so they know not only which tests will be performed but the order of the tests. This plan should be written down and given to the couple. People under stress tend to forget or misunderstand complex technical, and often unfamiliar, details. Without this written information the couple may argue over the details when they "remember differently."
7. Procedures should be performed after thoroughly educating the couple and assuring them that the procedures will be performed with attention paid to their comfort as well as the technical aspects of the tests.

Because, ideally, the first visit includes both partners, their respective roles in the infertility evaluation should be discussed. The infertile couple usually comes to the first visit expecting that the woman will undergo a series of tests. They do not usually expect a semen analysis to be among the first tests performed. When this request is made, some men will argue that because they have fathered a child in the past they do not need to undergo fertility testing. A brief explanation of the frequency with which male infertility occurs will usually convince the man that a semen analysis is warranted. The man also can be invited to attend any of the testing procedures that involve the woman and vice versa. This will provide the opportunity to include the man in the discussion of the results and to discuss the next step in the evaluation. Some men enjoy the opportunity to look underneath the microscope at a postcoital examination or to look at the films of a hysterosalpingogram.

It is also important to include in the "game plan" a consideration of the couple's concerns and questions. As discussed earlier, many couples come with many questions and issues. These include not only overcoming their infertility but also learning whether any previous medical care or lifestyles may have influenced their reproductive capacity. Some infertile people also may be concerned that they may have cancer or some other serious disease accounting for their infertility and have a need to be reassured through appropriate testing that they are in good health. It is therefore important to ask the couple about other issues they may have or any other questions they want answered so that the infertility evaluation can include appropriate ancillary tests in addition to the standard infertility tests.

Not all couples come to the infertility evaluation with the same resources. The selection of tests and the order of tests may be altered depending on the resources that the couple possess. The cost of various procedures can be discussed with the couple so that they have the opportunity to decline the performance of expensive tests such as the sperm penetration assay. In the case of a couple with recurrent pregnancy losses, they may decide against performing karyotypes on the man and the woman. For those couples who must travel a great distance and therefore have limited resources with respect to time, it may be possible to combine one or more tests at a single visit. Couples who perceive their advanced age to be an important factor and time a limited resource may wish to proceed rapidly. By discussing these issues with the couple, one may combine a semen analysis and a hysterosalpingogram or even an endometrial biopsy and a laparoscopy at the same visit. A properly timed visit could even allow the performance of a hysterosalpingogram, postcoital test, laparoscopy, and semen analysis within a 3-day period. This strategy

---

TABLE 8–2. Indications for Referral to Social Workers or Psychologists

1. Marital problems or conflicts
2. Sexual problems
3. Substance abuse or alcoholism
4. Disagreement regarding pursuing versus ending treatment
5. Psychological-emotional problems, e.g., depressive reactions, anxiety attacks
6. Assessment regarding decisions to adopt versus continuing treatment*
7. Couples considering using sperm donation or an egg donor program*
8. Adoption information or consultation*
9. Supportive counseling regarding coping with infertility and treatment (individually or as a couple)
10. Bereavement-grief counseling after a pregnancy loss (stillbirth, miscarriage, or ectopic pregnancy) or after an unsuccessful in vitro fertilization cycle or infertility treatment
11. Severe premenstrual symptoms

*Appropriate counseling usually requires that the social worker or psychologist specialize in these areas.

is helpful for couples undergoing their evaluation after traveling from a foreign country.

One also should consider the emotional resources and reserves of the couple. For some who have been through a number of previous tests and evaluations, the thought of undergoing a battery of tests over a several-month period may be overwhelming or discouraging. In this case it may be advantageous to do a rapid workup so that within a 6- to 8-week period all of the necessary tests have been performed and an assessment of the factors responsible for the infertility determined. Therefore, the couple can proceed with the therapy soon after their initial evaluation. Finally, some people have a limited ability to tolerate physical stress or discomfort, and it may be necessary to combine a hysterosalpingogram and a laparoscopy, or an endometrial biopsy and a laparoscopy, so that the procedures can be performed under general anesthesia. Because general anesthesia may influence ovarian steroid secretion and the onset of the next menstrual period, the validity of such a biopsy may be uncertain.

The sequence and rate at which the tests are performed also should be negotiated with the couple. Offering couples the opportunity to control as much as possible their evaluation and treatment is almost always desirable. They often have a personal timetable established in their own mind as to how rapidly they wish to undergo their fertility testing. The most common complaint of couples seeking care in the practice of a reproductive endocrinologist who specializes in infertility is that the generalist they have seen has not been as aggressive as they would have liked. An honest discussion with the couple regarding their sense of urgency and personal timetable will make it clear to the physician how quickly to proceed with the evaluation. As noted earlier, practical considerations also will determine how fast the evaluation is performed.

CONCLUDING THE INITIAL VISIT

Finally, at the conclusion of the initial visit, this game plan should be established and clearly communicated to the couple. As noted earlier, it is helpful to actually write the game plan down, spelling out the order of tests and the timing of these tests to increase compliance and decrease conflict. Sometimes a decision tree can be drawn so that the couple knows how the results of a test may influence the next step in the evaluation process. Also, it is helpful to discuss with the couple the relative odds of success given the tentative diagnosis made on the basis of the history and physical examination performed at the time of the initial evaluation. It also might be helpful to discuss with the couple the possible options of artificial insemination by donor sperm, an assisted reproductive technology, or even adoption. When given an honest and objective evaluation of their problem based on history and physical examination, some couples may choose not to pursue the evaluation because of the low chance of success and the high cost of the procedures outlined.

SUMMARY

The bulk of the initial evaluation often involves education and preparation of the patients for the many decisions that they will have to make as they move into their infertility evaluation and treatment. In addition, it provides an opportunity for the physician to assess the psychosocial and marital health of the couple and to determine whether an evaluation by a mental health professional familiar with infertility will be helpful. It may be necessary for the couple to discuss some important and basic issues surrounding their infertility before the evaluation of it begins. The initial evaluation carried out along the lines described will ensure that the care of the couple is appropriate as well as effective. A physician who empowers his or her patients to feel in control of their evaluation, treatment, and choices and appears genuinely to support choices other than medical treatment helps his or her patients to successfully resolve the impact of infertility on their lives.

SECTION THREE

Medical Management of the Infertile Female

ROBERT W. REBAR

PART A

EVALUATION OF THE MENSTRUAL CYCLE

CHAPTER 9

The Normal Menstrual Cycle

ROBERT W. REBAR

CHARACTERISTICS OF THE NORMAL MENSTRUAL CYCLE

Ovulatory menstrual cycles are characterized by regular, cyclic menstruation at predictable intervals and occur only in response to closely coordinated interactions involving the hypothalamus, pituitary gland, and ovaries to produce cyclic changes in the target tissues (endometrium, cervix, and vagina) of the reproductive tract. The purpose of the menstrual cycle may be viewed as setting in motion those physiologic processes in the woman necessary for perpetuation of the species.

By convention, each menstrual cycle begins with the first day of genital bleeding (day 1) and ends just prior to the onset of the subsequent menstrual cycle (Fig. 9–1). Median menstrual cycle length is 28 days, but normal ovulatory menstrual cycles may range from about 21 to 40 days in length.[1] The length of the menstrual cycle varies most in the years immediately following menarche and in the years immediately preceding menopause, mostly because of an increase in anovulatory cycles (Fig. 9–2). Irregular menstrual cycles also may be caused by sudden changes in diet, exercise, and environment; emotional disturbances; and following delivery and abortion. Menstrual cycles are least variable in length between the ages of 20 and 30 years. The menstrual cycle is commonly divided into the follicular phase and the luteal phase, with ovulation separating the two. The luteal phase of the menstrual cycle is more constant, approximating 14 ± 2

days in length. In contrast, the follicular phase may be as short as 7 days or more than 3 weeks in length.

Follicular Phase

Although the name *follicular phase* implies that follicular growth, or folliculogenesis, is what occurs in the first portion of each menstrual cycle, folliculogenesis actually is initiated in the last few days of the luteal phase of the preceding cycle. It is more appropriate to think of menstrual cycles as waves of follicular development and ovulation occurring in continuous succession.

A small increase in circulating follicle-stimulating hormone (FSH) levels begins in the preceding luteal phase, continues into the early follicular phase, and initiates *recruitment* and growth and development of a small group, or cohort, of 3 to 30 follicles.[2] Thus, several morphologically identical follicles may be observed within the ovary prior to cycle days 5 to 7 (Fig. 9–3). Destruction of any one of these follicles does not delay ovulation. From this cohort, one follicle is selected for ovulation, but the process of *selection* is not yet understood. This one follicle, from which the oocyte will be extruded and which will form the corpus luteum, is the *dominant follicle*. Destruction of the dominant follicle, such as by selective cautery, delays ovulation by approximately the number of days that have passed from cycle onset to follicle destruction. Once the dominant follicle is selected, *dominance* cannot be

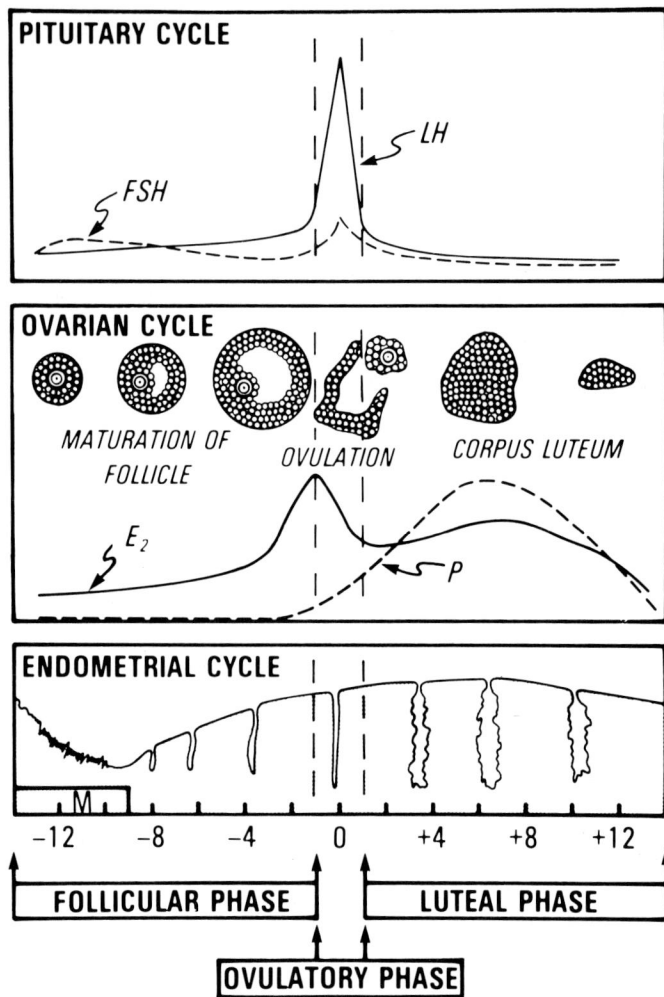

FIGURE 9–1. Idealized cyclic changes observed in the pituitary gonadotropins, follicle-stimulating hormone (FSH) and luteinizing hormone (LH), estradiol (E₂), progesterone (P), ovarian follicles, and uterine endometrium during the normal menstrual cycle. The data are centered around the day of the peak LH surge (day 0). Days of menstrual bleeding are indicated by M. (From Rebar RW. Normal physiology of the reproductive system. Endocrinology and Metabolism Continuing Education Program, American Association for Clinical Chemistry, Arlington, VA, November 1982.)

FIGURE 9–2. Median menstrual cycle lengths (*solid line*) throughout the reproductive life of women from menarche (year 0) to menopause (year 40). Ninety per cent of all cycles fall within the upper and lower *dashed lines.* (From Treloar AE, Boynton RE, Benn BG, Brown BW. Variation of human menstrual cycle through reproductive life. Int J Fertil 1967;12:77.)

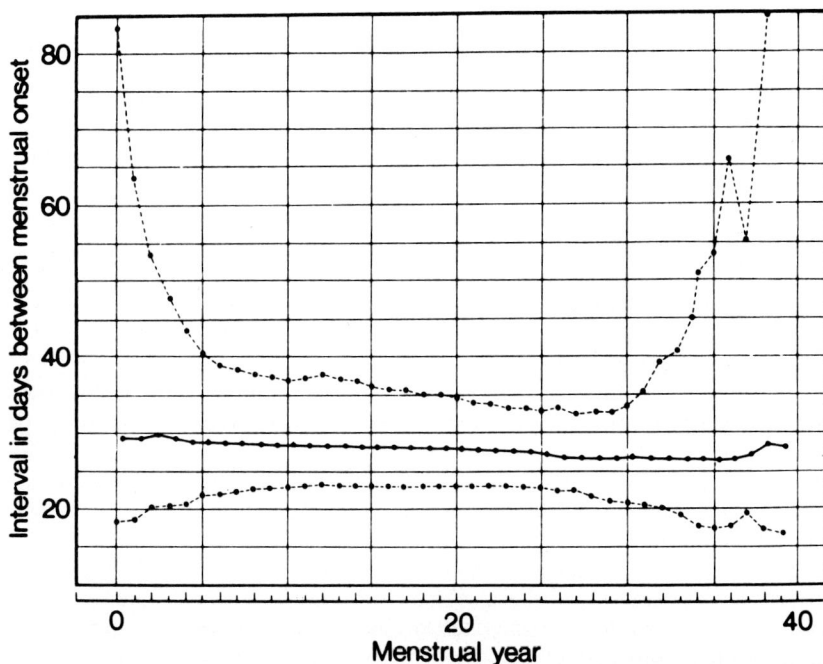

SELECTION AND MATURATION OF THE DOMINANT FOLLICLE

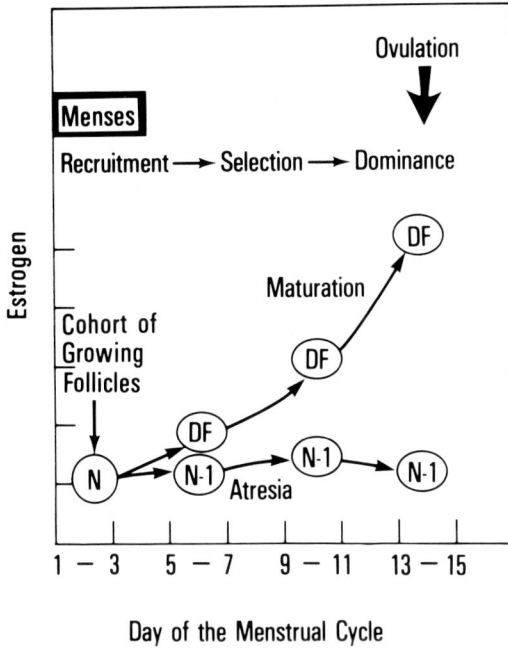

FIGURE 9–3. Time course for recruitment, selection, and ovulation of the dominant ovarian follicle (DF), with the onset of atresia among all other follicles of the cohort (N-1) in the normal menstrual cycle. (From Hodgen GD. The dominant ovarian follicle. Fertil Steril 1982;38:281–300. Reproduced with permission of the publisher, The American Fertility Society.)

transferred. On selection of the single dominant follicle, all other follicles in the cohort become destined to degenerate, that is, to undergo *atresia*. Data from ultrasonographic studies of normal women indicate that the site of ovulation occurs randomly in consecutive cycles and does not alternate between the two ovaries.[3] With removal of one ovary, ovulation will occur in the single remaining ovary each month. There is no evidence that removal of one ovary (and even a small portion of the second) decreases the number of ovulatory menstrual cycles the average woman has during her reproductive years.

Circulating luteinizing hormone (LH) levels increase slowly during the follicular phase, but FSH levels decrease after the early follicular phase increase in response to the negative feedback of estradiol (E_2) and possibly inhibin secreted by the developing follicle.[4] E_2 levels increase during the follicular phase as a result of increased numbers of granulosa cells contained within the enlarging dominant follicle (Fig. 9–4; see also Fig. 9–1).

The early increase in FSH leads to an increase in FSH receptors, which are located only on granulosa cells; by binding to these receptors, it is FSH that initiates the increased secretion of E_2 by the granulosa cells in the follicular phase. In the presence of E_2, FSH induces the formation of LH receptors on granulosa cells late in the follicular phase. With the development of LH receptors, the preovulatory granulosa cells begin to secrete small quantities of progesterone and 17-hydroxyprogesterone. Together with the positive feedback effect of E_2 on estrogen-primed gonadotropes in the anterior pituitary gland, progesterone appears to play a role in induc-

ing the midcycle surge of LH. The rising LH levels in the follicular phase also stimulate theca cells, which contain LH receptors, to secrete androgens. These androgens are aromatized to estrogens in granulosa cells under the stimulus of FSH.

Until recently it was generally believed that E_2 played a central role in feedback to the central nervous system and in preparing the endometrium for implantation as well as within the ovary, especially the developing dominant ovarian follicle itself, in maturing the oocyte for ovulation. This concept was derived from experiments using cells obtained from a rat model in vitro and is subject to refinement based on findings in women. Nuclear estrogen (and progesterone) receptors apparently cannot be identified in human granulosa cells of the dominant follicle until just before the LH surge,[5, 6] and

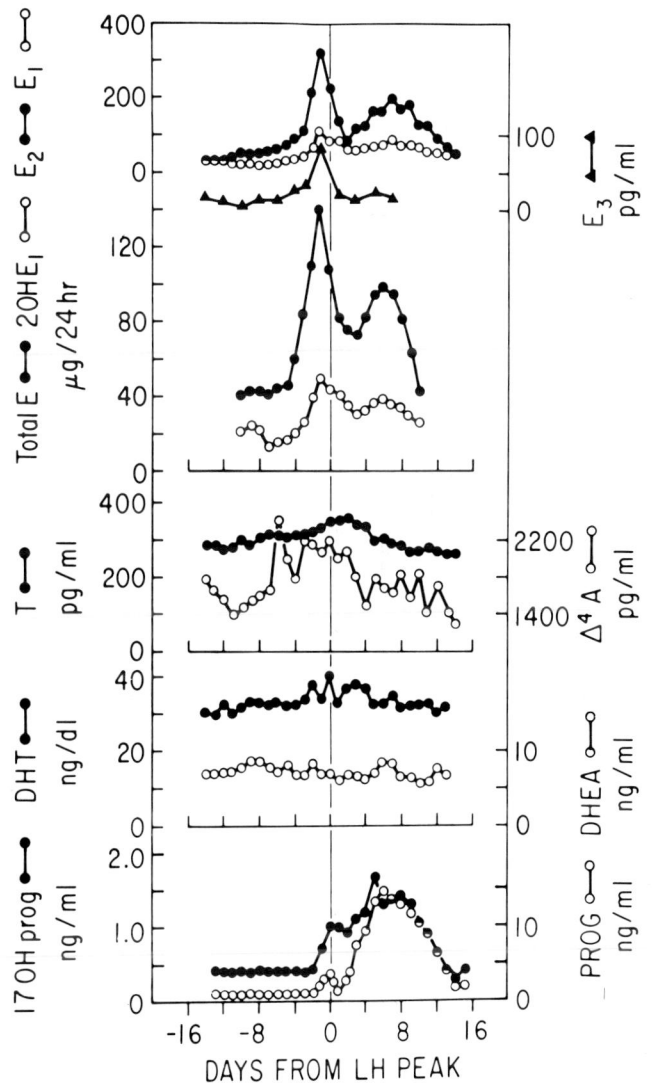

FIGURE 9–4. Steroid patterns during the menstrual cycle. All changes are those observed in the circulation except for total estrogens (Total E) and 2-hydroxyestrone (2OHE₁), for which changes in 24-hour urinary excretion are shown. E_1, estrone; E_2, estradiol; E_3, estriol; T, testosterone; Δ⁴ A, Δ⁴-androstenedione; DHT, dihydrotestosterone; DHEA, dehydroepiandrosterone; 17OH prog, 17-hydroxyprogesterone; PROG, progesterone. (From Rebar RW, Yen SSC. Endocrine rhythms in gonadotropins and ovarian steroids with reference to reproductive processes. In: Krieger DT, editor. Endocrine Rhythms. New York: Raven Press, 1979:259.)

androgen receptors do not appear in both granulosa and theca cells until the secondary stage of development.[6] If these findings, consistent with those reported for the nonhuman primate,[7] are confirmed, many of the concepts previously held will require modification. Support for the concept that androgens and estrogens are not essential for maturation of the oocyte is provided by the startling observation that normal follicular growth and development with successful fertilization in vitro were achieved using exogenous gonadotropins in a woman with 17α-hydroxylase deficiency who therefore had no ability to synthesize androgens or estrogens.[8] However, the "two-cell" theory emphasizing the importance of granulosa cells in synthesizing estrogen and theca cells in synthesizing androgen, both necessary for pregnancy, still is valid.

If estrogen is not required for follicular growth and development, however, then what factors are important for ovulation in women? Several peptides are secreted by granulosa cells, most, if not all, in response to FSH. These include inhibin and the structurally similar activin, insulin-like growth factors (IGF) I and II, a series of IGF-binding proteins (IGF-BP-1 to -6), epidermal growth factor, fibroblast growth factor, transforming growth factor-β (which is structurally similar to müllerian inhibiting hormone), follistatin, and growth hormone–binding proteins among others. Based on in vitro studies involving primate granulosa and theca cells, it has been determined that these growth factors may play important modulatory roles in follicular development.[9] Initially, FSH stimulates activin and inhibin synthesis by granulosa cells. In immature granulosa cells, activin augments FSH action, especially FSH receptor expression and aromatase activity.[10] Inhibin appears to enhance LH stimulation of androgen synthesis in theca cells to serve as the substrate for aromatization to estrogen in the granulosa cells. As noted, inhibin inhibits FSH secretion centrally at the level of the gonadotrope. In the luteinized granulosa cells of the dominant follicle just before ovulation, inhibin synthesis appears to come under the control of LH. IGF-I and IGF-II also stimulate a number of activities in both theca and granulosa cells in conjunction with FSH, and their effects are modulated by various IGF-BPs.[11–13] The other growth factors appear to have modulatory effects on follicular development as well. These findings have made it clear that follicular development in women is not as clearly understood as was believed previously and is far more complex than was theorized from animal studies in vitro. New concepts may well emerge that impact on ovulation induction in anovulatory and infertile women.

Ovulation

The ovum is released from the mature graafian follicle 32 to 34 hours after the onset of the preovulatory surge of LH. In normal ovulatory cycles, the mean interval from the late follicular phase peak of estradiol to the peak LH level approximates 24 hours (Fig. 9–5). Ovulation follows about 9 hours later, for a total interval of about 33 hours.[14] As peak LH levels are reached, E_2 levels decrease, but progesterone levels continue to increase. In in vitro fertilization cycles, using human menopausal gonadotropin (hMG) to stimulate follicular development and human chorionic gonadotropin (hCG)

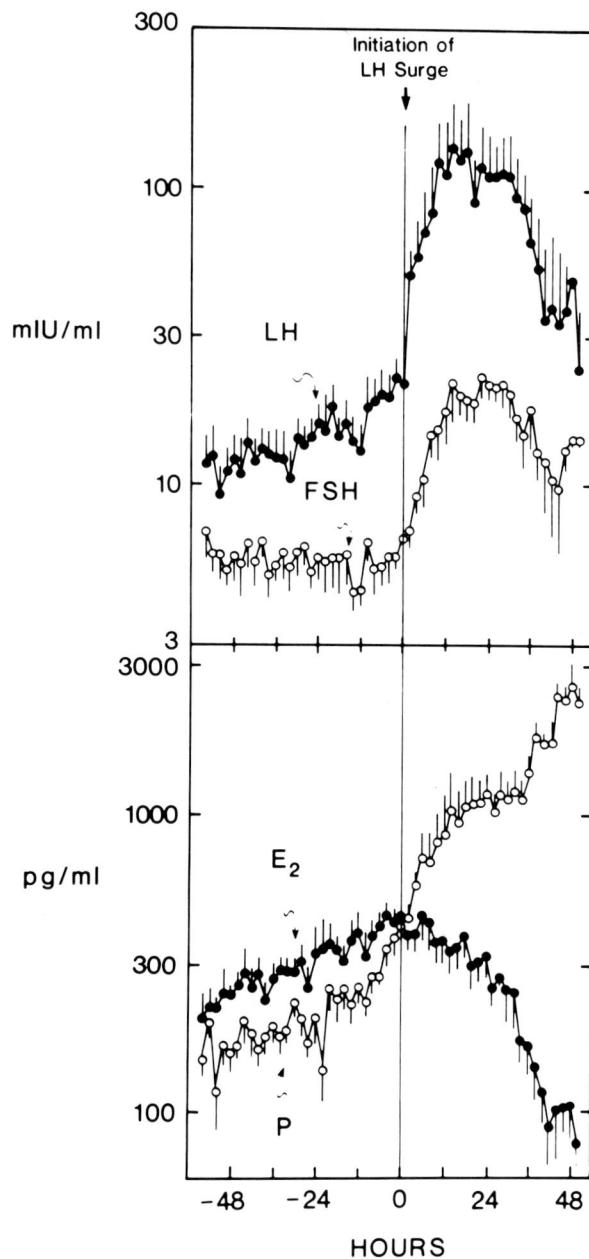

FIGURE 9–5. Mean (±SE) luteinizing hormone (LH), follicle-stimulating hormone (FSH), estradiol (E_2), and progesterone (P) concentrations in five women, measured at 2-hour intervals for 5 days at midcycle. The initiation of the LH surge has been used as the reference point (at time 0) from which data have been compiled. The hormone concentrations have been plotted on a logarithmic scale. (From Hoff JD, Quigley ME, Yen SSC. Hormonal dynamics at midcycle: a reevaluation. J Clin Endocrinol Metab 57:792–796, 1983; © The Endocrine Society.)

to trigger ovulation, follicular rupture seldom occurs until 36 hours after hCG administration. Similarly, ovulation seldom occurs until 34 or more hours after treatment with clomiphene citrate and hCG.

For convenience in summarizing hormonal data, the day of maximal LH secretion is commonly referred to as day 0, and hormonal events are centered around the LH surge (see Fig. 9–1). Days before the surge are numbered negatively, and days following the surge are numbered positively away from 0. Some women experience dull, unilateral pain around the time of ovulation that lasts from a few minutes to a few hours and has been termed *mittelschmerz*. The temporal association of this pain with ovulation is unknown, as is its cause. Mittelschmerz may occur before or following follicular rupture or not at all in ovulatory cycles and may be due to sudden follicular expansion before ovulation or to leakage of follicular fluid and associated blood into the abdominal cavity at ovulation.

The actual events that result in the expulsion of the oocyte in either spontaneous or induced cycles are incompletely characterized. Before ovulation, the follicle becomes extensively vascularized. The stigma, a small protrusion on the follicular wall representing the site of rupture, is evident well in advance of ovulation even though release of the ovum itself takes only a few minutes.

Several factors have been implicated in extrusion of the oocyte and the adherent granulosa cells immediately surrounding it (known as the *oocyte-cumulus complex*). Granulosa cells produce large quantities of plasminogen activator, apparently in response to gonadotropins.[15] Because plasminogen is present in follicular fluid and because plasmin has the ability to weaken follicle wall strips in vitro, LH-mediated enzymatic digestion of the follicle wall may be important in ovulation. Second, based on experiments in mice, FSH-dependent deposition of a glycosaminoglycan by granulosa cells may be necessary for ovulation.[16] The glycosaminoglycan appears to be necessary for cumulus expansion, an event that occurs with maturation of the oocyte-cumulus complex before its detachment from the other granulosa cells of the follicle wall. This complex becomes detached before actual follicular rupture. Third, LH-stimulated prostaglandin $F_2\alpha$ ($PGF_2\alpha$) may play a role in stimulating contractions of the smooth muscle of the follicle wall to aid with oocyte extrusion.[17] Fourth, a possible role for an angiogenic factor present in follicular fluid[18] remains to be assessed. It is now believed that this angiogenic factor plays an important role in ensuring delivery of gonadotropins to the developing dominant follicle.

Abnormalities in the process of follicular rupture and oocyte extrusion appear to cause the infrequent luteinized unruptured follicle syndrome. It has been suggested that women taking large quantities of prostaglandin synthetase inhibitors such as indomethacin are especially apt to develop unruptured follicles, further implicating prostaglandins in ovulation.[19, 20] As a consequence, women desiring pregnancy should be advised to avoid the use of drugs inhibiting prostaglandin before ovulation.

Luteal Phase

The luteal, or postovulatory, phase begins with the expulsion of the oocyte. The luteinized granulosa cells, as well as the theca interna and externa, together form the corpus luteum ("yellow body"), which supports the released ovum by secreting progesterone and prepares the endometrium to accept the fertilized ovum. Progesterone secretion generally increases to peak 6 to 8 days after the LH surge. Parallel but smaller increases in 17-hydroxyprogesterone, estrone (E_1), and E_2 also occur. If the oocyte is not fertilized, progesterone levels then decrease until menses, and the corpus luteum degenerates in a process termed *luteolysis* and ultimately can be identified only as a fibrous streak, the corpus albicans.

The control of steroid secretion by the corpus luteum is incompletely understood, but several factors clearly are important. That LH is the most important luteotropic hormone has been established by studies documenting that the amount of progesterone secreted is dependent on the amount of LH administered to hypophysectomized women[21] and by observations that exogenous LH or hCG can extend the functional life of the corpus luteum and secretion of progesterone for as long as 2 weeks in the absence of pregnancy.[22] As is true for almost all hormones, progesterone is secreted in a pulsatile fashion, with the peaks in the circulation following those observed for LH.[23]

The roles of other luteotropic factors aside from LH are not clear. Although luteal dysfunction may exist in women with hyperprolactinemia and in those in whom prolactin levels are suppressed by bromocriptine,[24, 25] prolactin itself does not appear to have a luteotropic effect in women. Prostaglandin E_2 stimulates both progesterone and cyclic adenosine monophosphate (cAMP) secretion in isolated human corpus luteum in vitro.[26] Inhibin, oxytocin, and relaxin, which are secreted by the corpus luteum and which may modulate its function, do not appear important in the maintenance of the corpus luteum and of early pregnancy because agonadal women who receive donor embryos require only estrogen and progesterone in the first trimester.

Although luteolysis begins 9 to 11 days after ovulation in the absence of fertilization of the ovum, little is known about this process involving the demise of the corpus luteum. $PGF_2\alpha$ is apparently luteolytic in women.[27, 28] Although it appears that exogenous estrogen is also luteolytic,[29] observations in nonhuman primates indicate that antiestrogens and aromatase inhibitors, which might then be expected to increase the length of the luteal phase, fail to do so.[30] In addition, both oxytocin and vasopressin appear to be secreted by and may have luteolytic effects on the corpus luteum.[24, 31] Finally, LH has the capacity to induce downregulation of its own receptor, and LH receptor number declines toward the end of the luteal phase.

Typically, serum progesterone levels exceed 3 ng/mL during the midluteal phase of regularly menstruating (i.e., ovulatory) women.[32] Moreover, midluteal progesterone levels of at least 10 ng/mL have been noted in the midluteal phase of spontaneous conception cycles.[33, 34] Because progestins increase basal morning body temperature, a "thermogenic shift" of more than 0.3°C occurring after a temperature nadir is a presumptive sign of ovulation and progesterone secretion. The precise relationships of the temperature nadir and increase to the LH peak and ovulation vary among patients.[35] Unfortunately, taking basal temperatures on a daily basis can be tedious and subject to error.

CYCLIC CHANGES IN TARGET ORGANS

Ovary

EARLY DEVELOPMENT

Before about 6 weeks of fetal age, the gonads are paired, undifferentiated gonadal ridges. By the sixth week, the primordial germ cells have migrated to these gonadal ridges. Over the next few weeks, the ovaries rapidly differentiate, and the number of germ cells, at this point termed *oogonia,* increases by mitosis to a maximum of 6 million to 7 million by 20 to 24 weeks' gestation (Fig. 9–6).[36-38] By the seventh month of gestation, the germ cells (now termed *oocytes*) all have undergone meiosis to become arrested in meiotic prophase. Although the oocyte of the dominant follicle remains arrested in meiosis until the LH surge, follicles begin development and then undergo degeneration, or atresia, throughout life. Thus, from midgestation onward, the number of oocytes decreases progressively until menopause, by which time virtually no oocytes remain. No further oocytes are generated in the woman. By birth only 2 million to 4 million oocytes remain, and by menarche there are only 200,000 to 400,000 oocytes remaining. In a normal reproductive life span in the absence of pregnancy, only 300 to 400 oocytes will ever be ovulated. All the rest—more than 99.9%—undergo atresia. Even if one ovary is removed surgically, there are sufficient excess oocytes such that reproductive life span is not shortened. Much more is known about follicular development than about atresia.

THE ADULT OVARY

The adult ovary is composed of a central medulla surrounded by a larger outer cortex (Fig. 9–7). The entire ovary is bounded by a single cell layer known as the *germinal epithelium.* The medulla contains the blood vessels and nerves as well as nests of steroid-secreting hilus cells. The cortex contains the follicles, each composed of an oocyte, granulosa cells, and theca cells. Definite changes occur during follicle growth and differentiation.[39, 40] Interactions among the follicular components give rise to the oocyte and to the estrogens

and progestins necessary for establishing and maintaining early pregnancy following fertilization of the oocyte.

Follicles exist in two major categories: growing and nongrowing. At any given time during reproductive life, 90% to 95% of follicles are nongrowing or primordial. Each primordial follicle contains a small oocyte arrested in meiotic prophase, surrounded by a single layer of squamous cells that become granulosa cells. These cells are surrounded by a basement membrane that allows some solute through to the granulosa cells and oocyte. This complex is surrounded by the stroma, containing the steroid-secreting theca interstitial cells, blood vessels, connective tissue cells, and contractile cells. Primordial follicles are recruited in turn to become growing follicles and pass through primary, secondary, and tertiary (or graafian) phases. As noted, atresia may occur in any phase.

The individual small primordial follicle with a diameter of 50 μm is transformed into a mature graafian follicle 1 to 2 cm in diameter in two distinct steps.[41] In the first step, the follicle grows to form a *primary follicle,* apparently independent of gonadotropin control (Fig. 9–8). The oocyte itself increases 10-fold in diameter, from 15 to 150 μm in diameter, and becomes surrounded by the zona pellucida, a translucent "shell" composed of glycoproteins. The single layer of cells surrounding the oocyte becomes cuboidal and takes on the characteristics of granulosa cells. In the second step, which is dependent on gonadotropin and sex steroid stimulation, the follicle matures through several steps into a *graafian follicle.*

The tertiary graafian follicle contains a fluid-filled cavity, or antrum, and increases from 200 μm to 1 to 2 cm in diameter, primarily because of the increasing accumulation of follicular fluid. Contained within the follicular fluid are many substances that are found in higher concentrations there than in blood. These include the mucopolysaccharides, chondroitin sulfate, hyaluronic acid, and heparin sulfate. Their synthesis by granulosa cells is stimulated by FSH.[42] The concentrations of chondroitin sulfate and heparin sulfate decrease, whereas hyaluronic acid increases with follicular maturation. Concentrations of ovarian steroids in follicular fluid markedly exceed those in blood. In large developing follicles, concentrations of estrogen are high, whereas those of androgen are relatively low; the opposite is true in small and atretic follicles.[39, 43] Progesterone levels are relatively low and constant and are increased only in preovulatory follicles. Measurable quantities of FSH, LH, and prolactin also are present in preovulatory follicles, with LH undetectable until just before ovulation.[40] Follicular fluid also contains a number of other substances in high concentrations, including, among others, PGE_2 and $PGF_2\alpha$, oxytocin, and vasopressin. Moreover, the fluid contains several distinctive proteins apparently important in the control of oocyte maturation and follicular development, including inhibin, activin, an oocyte maturation inhibitor (OMI), a luteinization inhibitor, and a luteinization stimulator.[44] These observations indicate that follicles control their own environment and are important in determining follicular maturation and atresia. Substances secreted by the cells of the dominant follicle may play roles in inducing atresia in the other follicles of the cohort.

As noted, under normal physiologic conditions approximately 2 weeks are needed for the presumptive preovulatory follicle to complete its final growth and release a mature

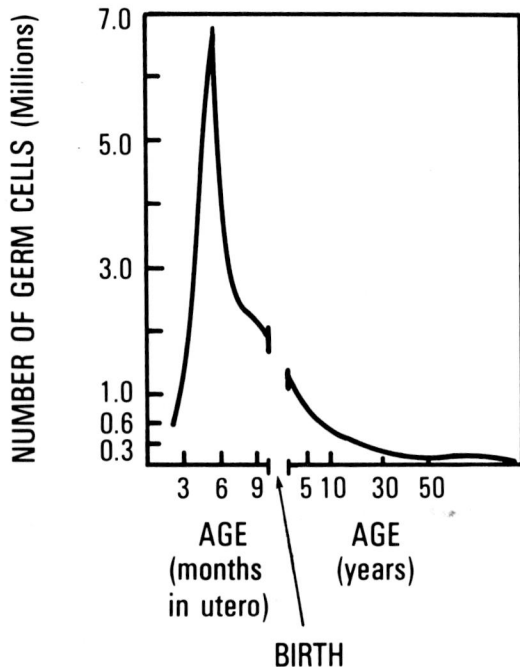

FIGURE 9–6. Changes in the total population of germ cells within the human ovary with increasing age. (Data from Baker TG. Oogenesis and ovulation. In: Austin CR, Short RV, editors. Reproduction in Mammals. Volume 1: Germ Cells and Fertilization. London: Cambridge University Press, 1972:14.)

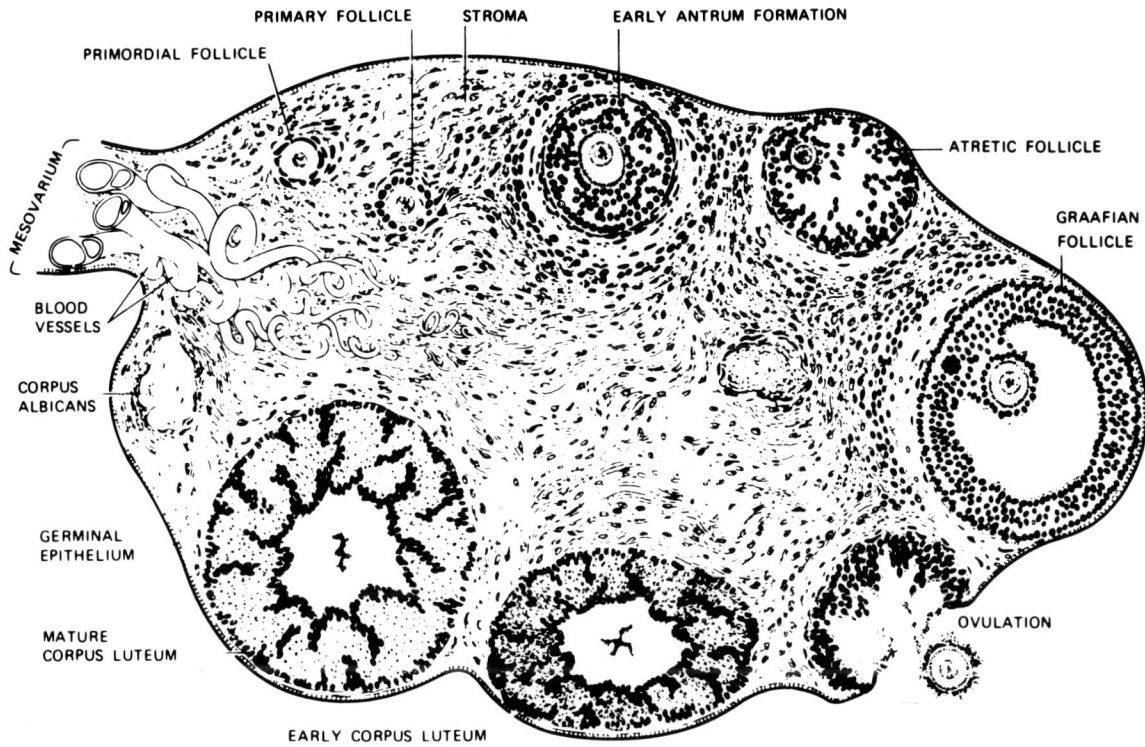

FIGURE 9–7. Idealized adult human ovary showing the life cycle of follicular structures. (Modified from Ham AW, Leeson TS. Histology. 4th edition. Philadelphia: JB Lippincott, 1968.)

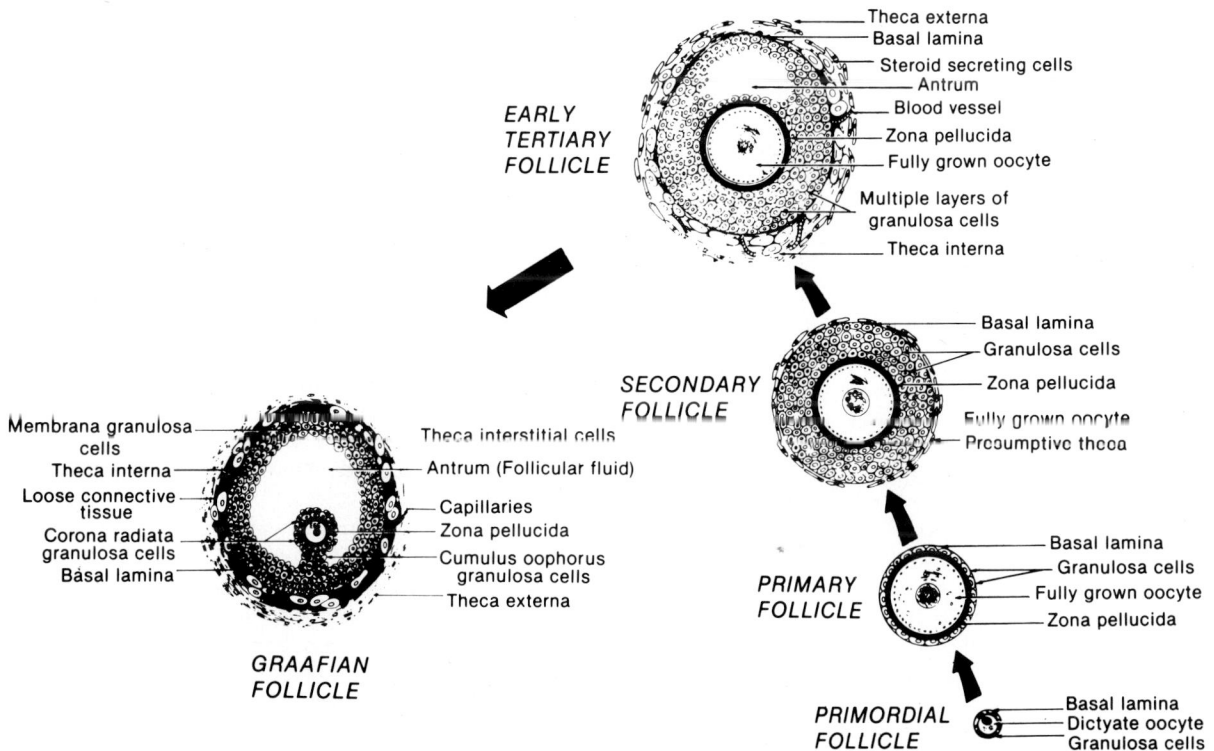

FIGURE 9–8. Architecture and classification of ovarian follicles during development. Recruitment occurs from the pool of primordial follicles. Selection of the dominant preovulatory follicle occurs between the early tertiary and graafian stages. (From Erickson GF, Magoffin DA, Dyer CA, Hofeditz C. The ovarian androgen-producing cells: a review of structure/function relationships. Endocr Rev 6:371–399, 1985; © The Endocrine Society.)

oocyte at ovulation. It appears that the oocyte is inhibited from resuming maturation by granulosa cell–oocyte interaction and by an OMI until following the LH/FSH surge.[45] Within 36 hours of the onset of the surge, the oocyte completes the first meiotic division (reducing to 22 + X chromosomes), and the first polar body (containing the other 23 chromosomes) is extruded. The second meiotic division occurs only if the oocyte is fertilized by a spermatozoon. It is now clear that if fertilization occurs, hCG, which is structurally similar to LH, is secreted by the developing blastocyst even before implantation and helps support the corpus luteum by stimulating it to secrete progesterone until the fetoplacental unit produces sufficient progesterone to support itself.[46]

The Endometrium

During the menstrual cycle, as detailed in Chapter 12, the endometrium undergoes a number of histologic changes culminating with menstrual bleeding as the corpus luteum regresses and progesterone secretion decreases (see Fig. 9–1).[47, 48] Of the three layers of the endometrium, only the basal layer is not shed at menstruation. This basal layer in turn regenerates the superficial layer of compact epithelial cells lining the uterine cavity and an intermediate layer of spongiosa early in the follicular phase under the influence of increasing estrogen secretion. The endometrial glands continue to proliferate throughout the follicular phase in response to estrogen. In the luteal phase, the glands become coiled and secretory, with increased vascularity and edema of the stroma, under the influence of progesterone. As both estrogen and progesterone secretion decrease in the late luteal phase, the stroma becomes increasingly edematous, glandular and endothelial necrosis occurs, and endometrial bleeding begins. Local release of prostaglandins appears to initiate vasospasm and ischemic necrosis in the endometrium and the uterine contractions (resulting in cramping) that accompany menstruation.[49] For this reason, prostaglandin synthetase inhibitors are effective in relieving dysmenorrhea.[50] Fibrinolytic activity in the endometrium also peaks at the time of menstruation, explaining the noncoagulability of menstrual blood.[51] As described in Chapter 12, endometrial biopsies can be used to confirm ovulation, to date the stage of the menstrual cycle, and to assess the adequacy of the endometrial response to gonadal steroids.[47, 48]

Cervix and Cervical Mucus

The cervix and cervical mucus are influenced by gonadal steroids.[52, 53] Under the influence of increasing quantities of estrogen in the follicular phase of the menstrual cycle, cervical vascularity and edema increase. The external cervical os opens to a diameter of 3 mm at ovulation and then decreases to 1 mm thereafter. Cervical mucus increases 10- to 30-fold in quantity as it becomes clear, and its elasticity (spinnbarkeit) increases as well (Fig. 9–9). So-called "palm leaf" arborization ("ferning") becomes marked just before ovulation owing to increased sodium chloride content of the mucus and can be demonstrated by allowing mucus to dry thickly on a glass slide and examining it microscopically. Under the influ-

ence of progesterone in the luteal phase, cervical mucus thickens, becomes opaque, and loses its elasticity and ability to fern. These characteristics of the cervix and cervical mucus may be used clinically to aid in assessing estrogen status in amenorrheic women and the stage of the menstrual cycle in spontaneous and induced cycles.[54]

Vagina

In the early follicular phase, the vaginal epithelium of the normal woman in her reproductive years is, relatively speaking, thin and pale owing to the low circulating estrogen levels.[55] As estrogen levels increase, the epithelium thickens and becomes more dusky, and the number of mature cornified epithelial cells increases. In the luteal phase the percentage of cornified cells decreases, and the numbers of precornified intermediate epithelial cells and polymorphonuclear cells increase in response to progesterone. Progesterone also leads to increased cellular debris and clumping of shed desquamated cells.

The histologic changes observed in the vaginal epithelium, as well as the changes in the cervix and cervical mucus, are the most sensitive indicators of estrogen's effects in the body. However, the reliability of these parameters as "bioassays" of estrogen status depends on the absence of vaginal infection. Moreover, any exogenous steroid will influence the findings.

OVARIAN STEROIDOGENESIS

As has been noted, the follicular complexes within the ovaries synthesize and secrete sex steroids (estrogens, androgens, and progestins), which play important roles in ovulation and in the preparation of the endometrium to receive the fertilized ovum.[56, 57] Two separate but interrelated pathways exist for synthesizing these steroids: (1) the Δ^5 pathway, in which 17α-hydroxypregnenolone and dehydroepiandrosterone with double bonds between carbon atoms 5 and 6 are intermediates, and (2) the Δ^4 pathway, in which pregnenolone is converted to progesterone and in which 17α-hydroxyprogesterone and androstenedione with double bonds between carbon atoms 4 and 5 are the intermediate steroids (Fig. 9–10). Cholesterol is used as the substrate for steroid synthesis and is obtained from circulating low-density lipoproteins even though the ovaries have the capacity to synthesize steroids from 2-carbon fragments.

Different structures and cells within the ovary synthesize different steroids, in part because of different gonadotropin receptors. Gonadotropin binding to its cell surface receptor activates adenylate cyclase and stimulates cAMP production. The cAMP in turn activates various protein kinases to catalyze phosphorylation of proteins to mediate the cellular effects of the gonadotropin. LH acts primarily to regulate the conversion of cholesterol to pregnenolone, the first major step in steroid biosynthesis. FSH acts to convert ("aromatize") androgens to estrogens. Thus, LH is important to ensure the presence of steroid intermediates ("substrate") and for the synthesis of androgens or progesterone, or both. In the absence of LH, FSH action is decreased because of reduced substrate for aromatization.

Androgens, primarily androstenedione and testosterone, are

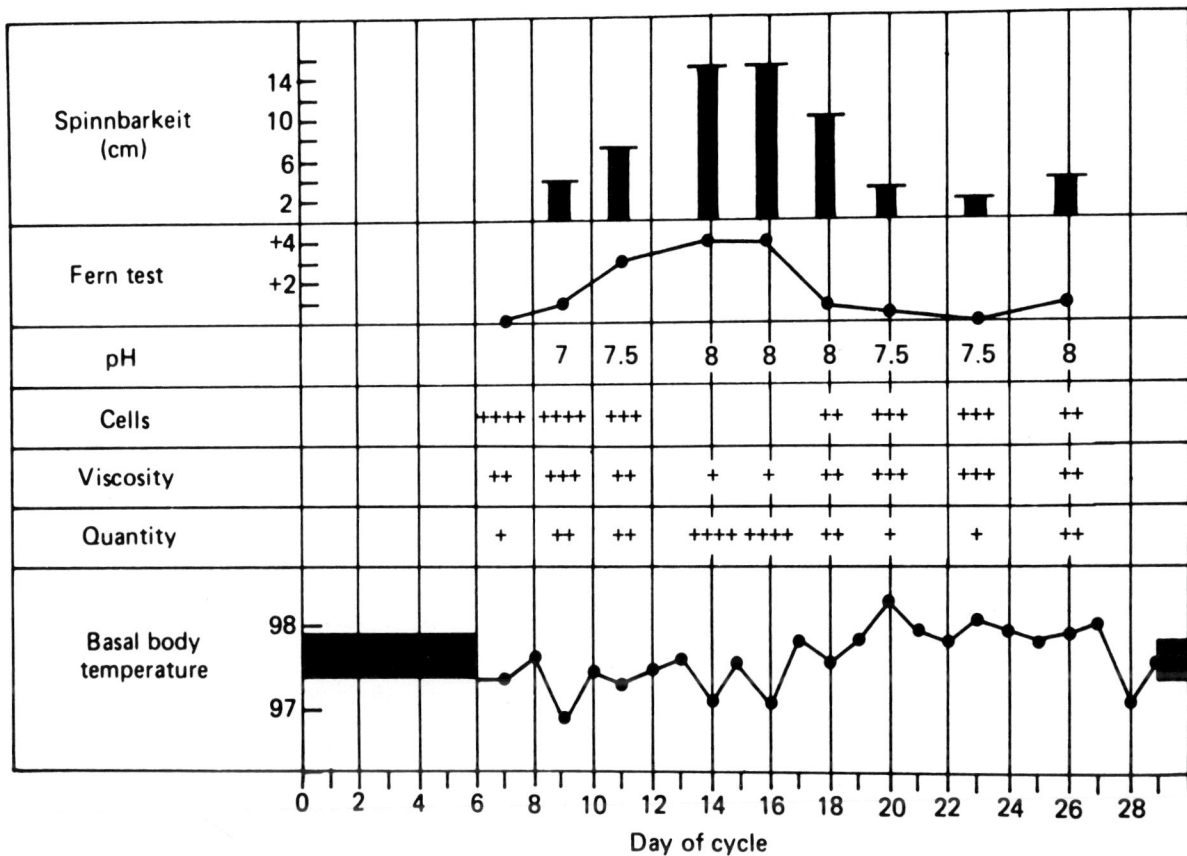

FIGURE 9–9. Changes in the composition and properties of cervical mucus during the menstrual cycle. (From Moghissi KS, Neuhaus OW. Cyclic changes of cervical mucus proteins. Am J Obstet Gynecol 1966; 96:91–95.)

19-carbon steroids secreted by the interstitial and theca cells and serve as substrate for the granulosa cells in which aromatization to estrogens occurs (Table 9–1). Androstenedione, the major ovarian androgen, also can be converted to testosterone and estrogens in peripheral tissues such as fat and skin. When ovarian androgen synthesis is increased, as in ovarian androgen-secreting neoplasms, or when aromatization of androgen to estrogen in the ovary is decreased, as in polycystic ovary syndrome (see Chapter 16), hirsutism may result. Testosterone, the most potent of the androgens produced by the ovary, is bound tightly to sex hormone–binding globulin (sometimes called *testosterone-estradiol binding globulin*) so that in normal women only about 1% of circulating testosterone is free and biologically active.

Estrogens are produced almost exclusively by granulosa cells by aromatization of the A ring of androgens that diffuse into the cells from the theca cells. Estrogens contain 18 carbon atoms and, by definition, stimulate proliferation of the endometrium. The amount of estrogen secretion depends on the phase of the menstrual cycle. In the early follicular phase, 60 to 170 μg of both E_2 and E_1 are secreted each day. As the dominant follicle is selected and enlarges, E_2 secretion becomes far greater than E_1 secretion and may reach 800 μg/day. Almost all E_2 is produced by the granulosa cells of the dominant follicle. After ovulation, the corpus luteum continues to produce significant quantities of E_2. In the late follicular and luteal phases, E_1 secretion is about one fourth as great as E_2. Although E_1 is of relatively minor importance in the ovulating woman, its secretion is often greater in the anovulatory woman and is always greater in the postmeno-

Steroid	Menstrual Cycle Phase	Production Rate (mg/24 h)	Serum Concentration (ng/mL)
Estradiol	F	0.08–0.95	0.03–0.35
	L	0.10–0.80	0.05–0.29
Estrone	F	0.11–0.66	0.02–0.10
	L	0.15–0.70	0.03–0.14
Progesterone	F	1.5–3.0	0.15–0.60
	ML	20.0–30.0	5.0–27.0
Testosterone		0.19–0.26	0.30–0.55
Androstenedione		3.2	0.4–2.3

TABLE 9–1. Production Rates and Serum Concentrations of Major Ovarian Steroid Hormones

F, follicular; L, luteal; ML, midluteal.

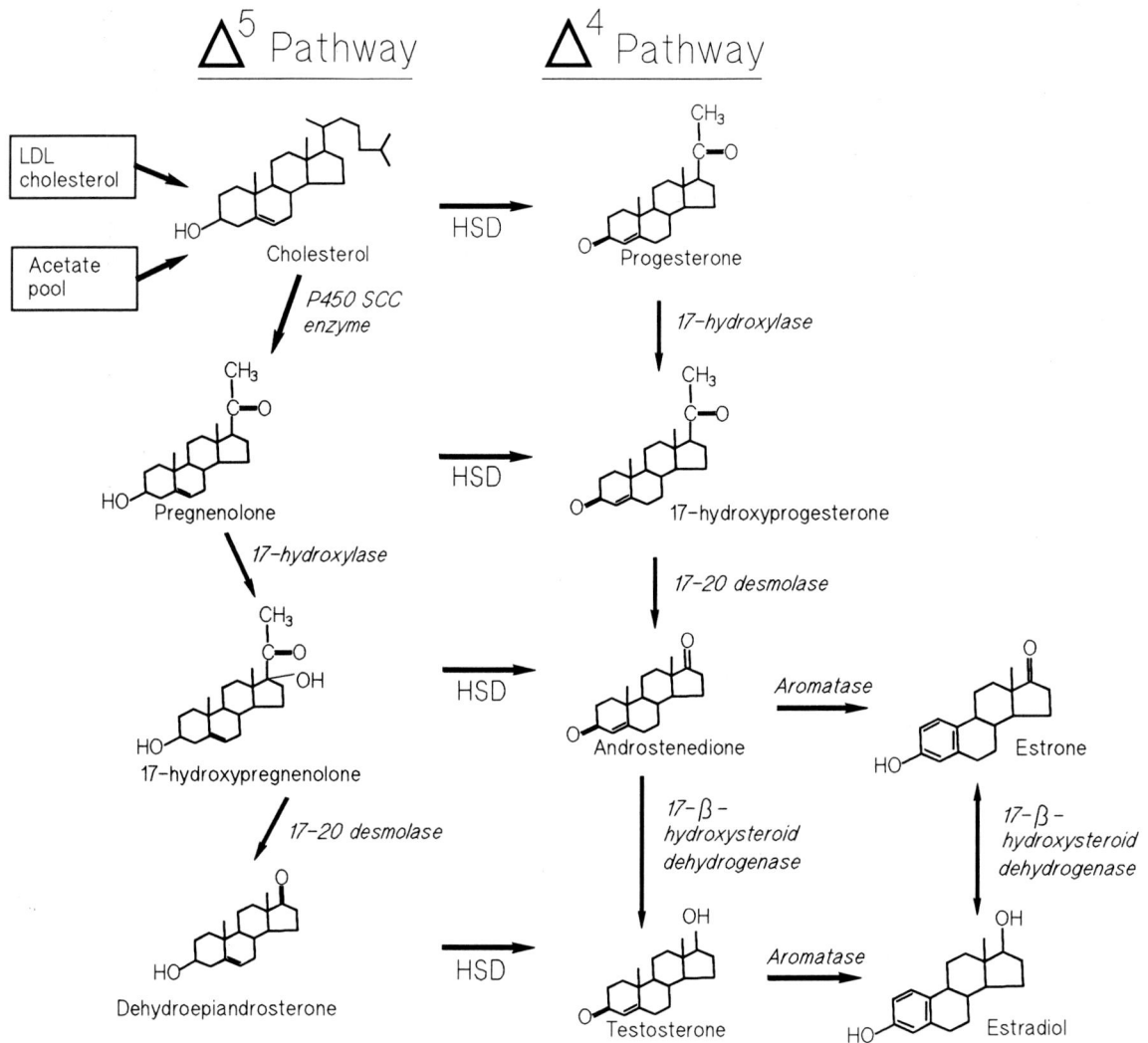

FIGURE 9–10. The two major pathways of ovarian steroidogenesis: the Δ^5 and the Δ^4 pathways. LDL, low-density lipoprotein; HSD, $\Delta^{4,5}$ 3β-hydroxysteroid dehydrogenase.

pausal woman. In the postmenopausal woman, most of the E_1 is synthesized by peripheral conversion of adrenal (and ovarian) androgens, especially androstenedione.

Progesterone synthesis is relatively low in the follicular phase (about 2 to 3 mg/day), is increased approximately 10-fold in the midluteal phase (25 to 30 mg/day), and is increased another 10-fold in pregnancy at term (250 to 300 mg/day). It is clear that LH stimulation is required for progesterone production by the corpus luteum. The clinical corollary is that gonadotropin stimulation must be provided in the luteal phase to women who have no pituitary function in whom ovulation is induced by exogenous gonadotropins.

CENTRAL AND FEEDBACK CONTROL OF OVULATION

Hypothalamic Signals

As is true for virtually all hormones, the gonadotropins (especially LH) are secreted in a pulsatile manner, with intervals of 1 to 4 hours between pulses, depending on the phase of the menstrual cycle (Fig. 9–11A and B). LH pulse frequency is least during the luteal phase of the menstrual cycle, apparently because of the effects of progesterone.[58]

Appropriate pulsatile secretion of the decapeptide gonadotropin-releasing hormone (GnRH) is required for normal pulsatile secretion of LH and FSH by the anterior pituitary gland.[59, 60] The absolute requirement for pulsatile secretion of GnRH was proved when monkeys without any GnRH secretion were induced to ovulate only when exogenous GnRH was given for 6 minutes at 60-minute intervals.[59] The synthesis, secretion, and clinical usefulness of GnRH are considered in greater detail in Chapters 13 and 15.

Classic neurotransmitters, including norepinephrine, dopamine, and serotonin, as well as several neuromodulators, including endogenous opiates and PGs, appear to influence GnRH secretion from the hypothalamus.[60–68] Norepinephrine appears to stimulate GnRH release, whereas dopamine and possibly serotonin exert inhibitory effects. The endogenous opiates suppress hypothalamic secretion of GnRH and thus also inhibit gonadotropin secretion. Furthermore, both androgens and estrogens bind to neurons within the hypothalamus and the anterior pituitary,[69] and progestins[70] bind to

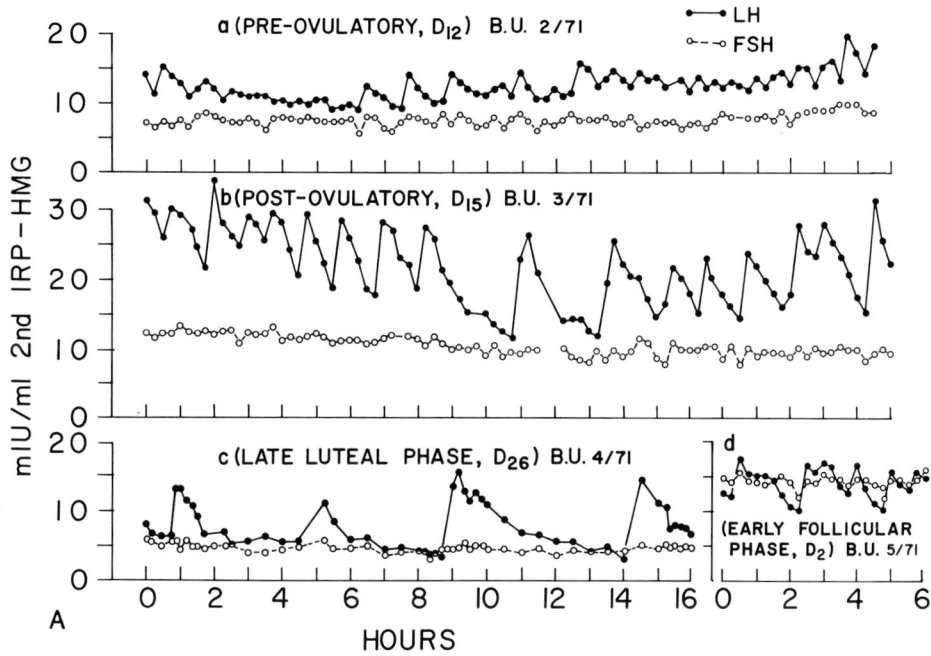

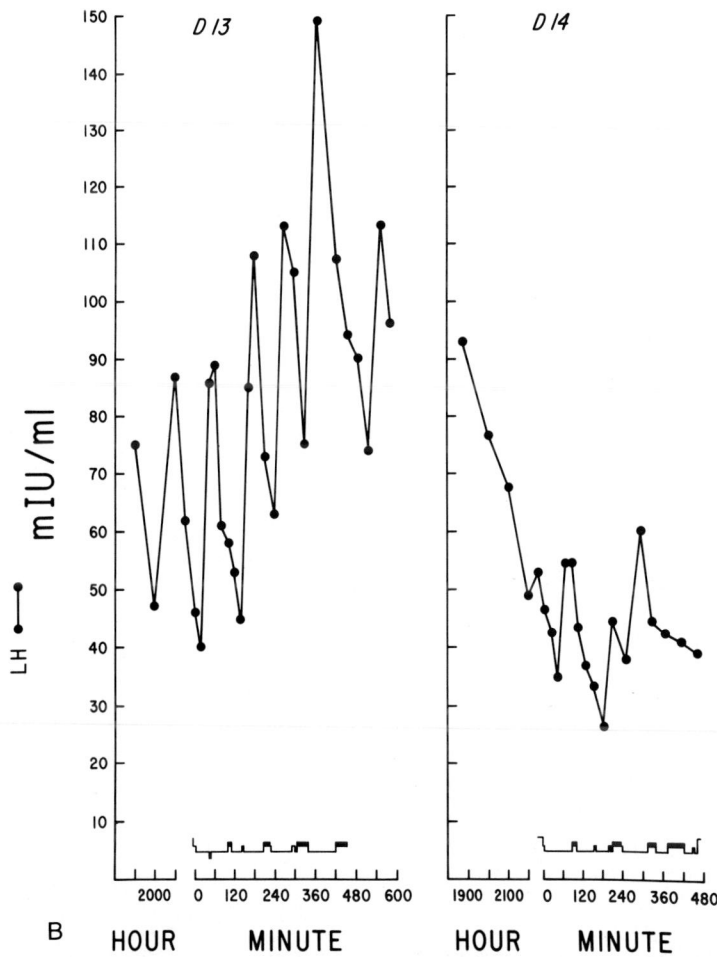

FIGURE 9–11. *A,* Variations in the frequency and amplitude of pulsatile patterns of circulating luteinizing hormone (LH) and follicle-stimulating hormone (FSH) during different phases of the menstrual cycle. Day 1 is the first day of menstrual bleeding. Results are presented in terms of the Second International Reference Preparation for Human Menopausal Gonadotropin (2nd IRP-HMG). *B,* LH and FSH concentrations associated with the stage of sleep during the midcycle surge. (*A* and *B* from Yen SSC, Rebar R, Vandenberg G, et al. Pituitary gonadotropin responsiveness to synthetic LRF in subjects with normal and abnormal hypothalamic-pituitary-gonadal axis. J Reprod Fertil Suppl 1973;20:137–161.)

neurons within the hypothalamus and can modulate secretion of GnRH and gonadotropins. Other peptide factors, including some, like inhibin, from the ovary, may modulate gonadotropin secretion.

Gonadal Steroid Feedback

Gonadal steroids can exert both negative and positive feedback effects on gonadotropin secretion. Among ovarian steroids, E_2 is the most potent inhibitor of gonadotropin secretion. Thus, ovariectomy results in a rapid increase in gonadotropin secretion,[71] and infusion of exogenous E_2 into hypoestrogenic women leads to almost immediate decreases in both LH and FSH.[72] Although low concentrations of E_2 inhibit gonadotropin secretion from the gonadotropes, E_2 also stimulates synthesis and storage of gonadotropin so that the intracellular content of LH and FSH increases.

For ovulation to occur, E_2 must have the ability to stimulate (positive feedback) as well as to inhibit (negative feedback) gonadotropin secretion.[73, 74] The development of a positive feedback effect by E_2 is known to require increasing quantities of E_2 over a defined interval.[75] The high concentrations of E_2 present in the late follicular phase stimulate synthesis and storage of gonadotropin and also augment the effect of GnRH in eliciting release of gonadotropin.[76, 77] Thus, in the normal menstrual cycle, the positive feedback action of E_2 is preceded by several days in which lower E_2 levels are present with their negative feedback effects.

Presumed Mechanism for the LH Surge

The basic secretory activity of the pituitary gonadotropes is determined by the direct input of GnRH but is modulated by the feedback effects of gonadal steroids, primarily E_2. Early in the follicular phase E_2 stimulates synthesis and storage of gonadotropins while inhibiting secretion. As E_2 levels increase, the gonadotropes, filled with LH and FSH, finally become sufficiently sensitive such that the midcycle gonadotropin surge occurs.[77] The surge also occurs because of what has been called the "self-priming effect" of E_2 on the ability of gonadotropes to release gonadotropin in response to GnRH. A second pulse of GnRH will elicit greater release of gonadotropin than the first pulse in the estrogen-primed state.[78]

It is unknown if GnRH secretion itself is increased at midcycle. Experimental studies have documented that the midcycle surge can occur without any increase in GnRH release.[59, 79, 80] The midcycle surge may reflect only a rapid increase in the number of GnRH receptors on each gonadotrope and the attainment of maximal capacity by gonadotropes.

Exogenous E_2 alone can induce an LH surge in monkeys and women.[81] This surge, however, is not identical to that observed at midcycle. The characteristics of the induced surge appear much more similar to the physiologic midcycle surge if (as occurs at midcycle) a small quantity of exogenous progesterone is administered with the E_2 after several hours in which E_2 alone is administered.[82]

REFERENCES

1. Treloar AE, Boynton RE, Benn BG, Brown BW. Variation of human menstrual cycle through reproductive life. Int J Fertil 1967; 12:77–81.
2. di Zerega GS, Hodgen GD. Folliculogenesis in the primate ovarian cycle. Endocr Rev 1981; 2:27–49.
3. Baird DT. A model for follicular selection and ovulation: lessons from superovulation. J Steroid Biochem 1987; 27:15–23.
4. McNeilly AS, Tsonis CG, Baird DT. Inhibin. Hum Reprod 1988; 3:45–52.
5. Iwai T, Nanbu Y, Iwai M, et al. Immunohistochemical localization of oestrogen receptors and progesterone receptors in the human ovary throughout the menstrual cycle. Virchows Arch A Pathol Anat Histopathol 1990; 417:369–375.
6. Horie K, Takakura K, Fujiwara H, et al. Immunohistochemical localization of androgen receptor in the human ovary throughout the menstrual cycle in relation to oestrogen and progesterone receptor expression. Hum Reprod 1992; 7:184–190.
7. Hild-Petito S, Stouffer RL, Brenner RM. Immunocytochemical localization of estradiol and progesterone receptors in the monkey ovary throughout the menstrual cycle. Endocrinology 1988; 123:2896–2905.
8. Rabinovici J, Blankstein J, Goldman B, et al. In vitro fertilization and primary embryonic cleavage are possible in 17α-hydroxylase deficiency despite extremely low intrafollicular 17β-estradiol. J Clin Endocrinol Metab 1989; 68:693–697.
9. Hillier SG. Paracrine control of follicular estrogen synthesis. Semin Reprod Endocrinol 1991; 9:332–340.
10. Miro F, Hillier SG. Relative effects of activin and inhibin on steroid hormone synthesis in primate granulosa cells. J Clin Endocrinol Metab 1992; 75:1556–1561.
11. Giudice LC. Insulin-like growth factors and ovarian follicular development. Endocr Rev 1992; 13:641–669.
12. Hernandez ER, Hurwitz A, Vera A, et al. Expression of the genes encoding the insulin-like growth factors and their receptors in the human ovary. J Clin Endocrinol Metab 1992; 74:419–425.
13. Dor J, Costritsci N, Pariente C, et al. Insulin-like growth factor-I and follicle-stimulating hormone suppress insulin-like growth factor binding protein-1 secretion by human granulosa–luteal cells. J Clin Endocrinol Metab 1992; 75:969–971.
14. Pauerstein CJ, Eddy CA, Croxatto HD, et al. Temporal relationships of estrogen, progesterone, and luteinizing hormone levels to ovulation in women and infrahuman primates. Am J Obstet Gynecol 1978; 130:876–886.
15. Strickland S, Beers WH. Studies on the role of plasminogen activator in ovulation: In vitro response of granulosa cells to gonadotropins, cyclic nucleotides, and prostaglandins. J Biol Chem 1976; 251:5694–5702.
16. Eppig JJ. Regulation of cumulus oophorus expansion by gonadotropins in vivo and in vitro. Biol Reprod 1980; 23:545–552.
17. Wallach EE, Wright KH, Hamada Y. Investigation of mammalian ovulation with an in vitro perfused rabbit ovary preparation. Am J Obstet Gynecol 1978; 132:728–738.
18. Frederick JL, Shimanuki T, di Zerega GS. Initiation of angiogenesis by human follicular fluid. Science 1984; 224:389–390.
19. Killick S, Elstein M. Pharmacologic production of luteinized unruptured follicles by prostaglandin synthetase inhibitors. Fertil Steril 1987; 47:773–777.
20. Murdoch WJ, Cavender JL. Effect of indomethacin on the vascular architecture of preovulatory ovine follicles: possible implications in the luteinized unruptured follicle syndrome. Fertil Steril 1989; 51:153–155.
21. Vande Wiele RL, Bogumil RJ, Dyrenfurth I, et al. Mechanisms regulating the menstrual cycle in women. Recent Prog Horm Res 1970; 26:63–103.
22. Segaloff A, Sternberg WH, Gaskill CJ. Effect of luteotrophic doses of chorionic gonadotropin in women. J Clin Endocrinol Metab 1951; 11:936–944.
23. Filicori M, Butler JP, Crowley WF Jr. Neuroendocrine regulation of the corpus luteum in the human. J Clin Invest 1984; 73:1638–1647.
24. Auletta FJ, Flint AFP. Mechanisms controlling corpus luteum function in sheep, cows, nonhuman primates, and women especially in relation to the time of luteolysis. Endocr Rev 1988; 9:88–105.
25. Schulz KD, Geiger W, Del Poso E, Kunzig HJ. Pattern of sexual steroids, prolactin, and gonadotropic hormones during prolactin inhibition in normal cycling women. Am J Obstet Gynecol 1978; 132:561–566.
26. Hahlin M, Dennefors B, Johanson C, Hamberger L. Luteotropic effects of prostaglandin E_2 on the human corpus luteum of the menstrual cycle and early pregnancy. J Clin Endocrinol Metab 1988; 66:909–914.

27. Wentz AC, Jones GS. Transient luteolytic effects of prostaglandin $F_2\alpha$ in the human. Obstet Gynecol 1973; 42:172–181.

28. Auletta FJ. The role of prostaglandin $F_2\alpha$ in human luteolysis. Contemp Ob-Gyn 1987; 30:119–123.

29. Gore BA, Caldwell BV, Speroff L. Estrogen-induced human luteolysis. J Clin Endocrinol Metab 1973; 36:615–617.

30. Ellinwood WE, Resko JA. Effect of inhibition of estrogen synthesis during the luteal phase on function of the corpus luteum in rhesus monkeys. Biol Reprod 1983; 28:636–644.

31. Khan-Dawood FS, Huang JC, Dawood MY. Baboon corpus luteum oxytocin: an intragonadal peptide modulator on luteal function. Am J Obstet Gynecol 1988; 158:882–891.

32. Israel R, Mishell DR, Stone SC, et al. Single luteal phase serum progesterone assay as an indicator of ovulation. Am J Obstet Gynecol 1972; 112:1043–1046.

33. Swyer GI, Radwanska E, McGarrigle HH. Plasma estradiol and progesterone estimation for the monitoring of induction of ovulation with clomiphene and chorionic gonadotrophin. Br J Obstet Gynaecol 1975; 82:794–804.

34. Hull MG, Savage PE, Bromham DR, et al. Value of a single serum progesterone measurement in the midluteal phase as a criterion of a potentially fertile cycle derived from treated and untreated conception cycles. Fertil Steril 1982; 37:355–360.

35. Bauman JE. Basal body temperature: unreliable method of ovulation detection. Fertil Steril 1981; 36:729–733.

36. Block E. Quantitative morphological investigations of the follicular system in women: variations at different ages. Acta Anat 1952; 14:108–123.

37. Block E. A quantitative morphological investigation of the follicular system in newborn female infants. Acta Anat 1953; 17:201–206.

38. Baker TG, Sum OW. Development of the ovary and oogenesis. Clin Obstet Gynaecol 1976; 3:3–26.

39. Erickson GF, Magoffin DA, Dyer CA, Hofeditz C. The ovarian androgen-producing cells: a review of structure/function relationships. Endocr Rev 1985; 6:371–399.

40. Hisaw FL. Development of the graafian follicle and ovulation. Physiol Rev 1947; 27:95–119.

41. Erickson GF. An analysis of follicle development and ovum maturation. Semin Reprod Endocrinol 1986; 4:233–254.

42. Ax RL, Ryan RJ. FSH stimulation of ^{3}H-glucosamine-incorporation into proteoglycans by porcine granulosa cells in vitro. J Clin Endocrinol Metab 1979; 49:646–651.

43. Erickson GF, Yen SSC. New data on follicle cells in polycystic ovaries: a proposed mechanism for the genesis of cystic follicles. Semin Reprod Endocrinol 1984; 2:231–243.

44. Eppig JJ, Downs SM. Chemical signals that regulate mammalian oocyte maturation. Biol Reprod 1984; 30:1–11.

45. Edwards RG. Maturation in vitro of mouse, sheep, cow, pig, rhesus monkey, and human oocytes. Nature 1965; 208:349–351.

46. Fishel SB, Edwards RG, Evans CJ. Human chorionic gonadotropin secreted by preimplantation embryos cultured in vitro. Science 1984; 223:816–818.

47. Noyes RW, Hertig AT, Rock J. Dating the endometrial biopsy. Fertil Steril 1950; 1:3–25.

48. Tredway DR, Mishell DR Jr, Moyer DL. Correlation of endometrial dating with luteinizing hormone peak. Am J Obstet Gynecol 1973; 117:1030–1033.

49. Henzl MR, Smith RE, Boost G, Tyler ET. Lysosomal concept of menstrual bleeding in humans. J Clin Endocrinol Metab 1972; 34:860–875.

50. Ylikorkala O, Dawood MY. New concepts in dysmenorrhea. Am J Obstet Gynecol 1978; 130:833–847.

51. Todd AS. Localization of fibrinolytic activity in tissues. Br Med Bull 1964; 20:210–212.

52. Moghissi KS, Syner FN, Evans TN. A composite picture of the menstrual cycle. Am J Obstet Gynecol 1972; 114:405–418.

53. Moghissi KS. Composition and function of cervical secretion. In: Greep RO, editor. Handbook of Physiology, Endocrinology, volume II, part 2. Washington, DC: American Physiological Society, 1973:25–48.

54. Billings EL, Billings JJ, Brown JB, Burger HG. Symptoms and hormonal changes accompanying ovulation. Lancet 1972; 1:282–284.

55. Rakoff AE. Hormonal cytology in gynecology. Clin Obstet Gynecol 1961; 4:1045–1061.

56. O'Malley BW, Strott CA. Steroid hormones: metabolism and mechanism of action. In: Yen SSC, Jaffe RB, editors. Reproductive Endocrinology: Physiology, Pathophysiology and Clinical Management. 3rd edition. Philadelphia: WB Saunders, 1991:156–180.

57. Lloyd CW, Lobotsky J, Baird DT, et al. Concentration of unconjugated estrogens, androgens and gestagens in ovarian and peripheral venous plasma of women: the normal menstrual cycle. J Clin Endocrinol Metab 1971; 32:155–166.

58. Filicori M, Butler JP, Crowley WF Jr. Neuroendocrine regulation of the corpus luteum in the human: evidence for pulsatile progesterone secretion. J Clin Invest 1984; 73:1638–1647.

59. Knobil E. The neuroendocrine control of the menstrual cycle. Recent Prog Horm Res 1980; 36:53–88.

60. Halász B. Hypothalamic mechanisms controlling pituitary function. Prog Brain Res 1972; 38:97–122.

61. Pohl CR, Knobil E. The role of the central nervous system in the control of ovarian function in higher primates. Annu Rev Physiol 1982; 44:583–593.

62. Fink G. Neuroendocrine control of gonadotropin secretion. Br Med Bull 1979; 35:155–160.

63. Gallo RV. Neuroendocrine control of pulsatile luteinizing hormone release in the rat. Neuroendocrinology 1980; 30:122–131.

64. Barraclough CA, Wise PM. The role of catecholamines in the regulation of pituitary luteinizing hormone and follicle-stimulating hormone secretion. Endocr Rev 1982; 3:91–119.

65. Ropert JF, Quigley ME, Yen SSC. The dopaminergic inhibition of LH secretion during the menstrual cycle. Life Sci 1984; 34:2067–2073.

66. Eskay RL, Warbert J, Mical RS, Porter JC. Prostaglandin E_2-induced release of LHRH into hypophysial portal blood. Endocrinology 1975; 97:816–824.

67. Quigley ME, Yen SSC. The role of endogenous opiates on LH secretion during the menstrual cycle. J Clin Endocrinol Metab 1980; 51:179–181.

68. Ropert JF, Quigley ME, Yen SSC. Endogenous opiates modulate pulsatile luteinizing hormone release in humans. J Clin Endocrinol Metab 1981; 52:583–585.

69. Stumpf WE, Sar M, Keeper DA. Anatomical distribution of estrogen in the CNS of mouse, rat, tree shrew and squirrel monkey. In: Raspe G, Bernhard A, editors. Central Actions of Estrogenic Hormones (Advances in the Biosciences, volume 15). Oxford: Pergamon Press, 1975:77.

70. Sar M, Stumpf WE. Neurons of the hypothalamus concentrate (^{3}H) progesterone or its metabolites. Science 1973; 182(suppl):1266–1268.

71. Yen SSC, Tsai CC. The effect of ovariectomy on gonadotropin release. J Clin Invest 1971; 50:1149–1153.

72. Yen SSC, Tsai CC, Vanden Berg G, Rebar RW. Gonadotropin dynamics in patients with gonadal dysgenesis: a model for the study of gonadotropin regulation. J Clin Endocrinol Metab 1972; 35:897–904.

73. Tsai CC, Yen SSC. Acute effects of intravenous infusion of 17β-estradiol on gonadotropin release in pre- and post-menopausal women. J Clin Endocrinol Metab 1971; 32:766–771.

74. Tsai CC, Yen SSC. The effect of ethinyl estradiol administration during early follicular phase of the cycle on the gonadotropin levels and ovarian function. J Clin Endocrinol Metab 1972; 33:917–923.

75. Lasley BL, Wang CF, Yen SSC. The effects of estrogen and progesterone on the functional capacity of the gonadotrophs. J Clin Endocrinol Metab 1975; 41:820–826.

76. Yen SSC, Lein A. The apparent paradox of the negative and positive feedback control system on gonadotropin secretion. Am J Obstet Gynecol 1976; 126:942–954.

77. Hoff JD, Lasley BL, Wang CF, Yen SSC. The two pools of pituitary gonadotropin: regulation during the menstrual cycle. J Clin Endocrinol Metab 1977; 44:302–312.

78. Hoff JD, Lasley BL, Yen SSC. The functional relationship between priming and releasing actions of LRF. J Clin Endocrinol Metab 1979; 49:8–11.

79. Crowley WF Jr, McArthur JW. Stimulation of the normal menstrual cycle in Kallmann's syndrome by pulsatile administration of luteinizing hormone-releasing hormone (LHRH). J Clin Endocrinol Metab 1980; 51:173–175.

80. Miller DS, Reid RR, Cetel NS, et al. Pulsatile administration of low-dose gonadotropin-releasing hormone: ovulation and pregnancy in women with hypothalamic amenorrhea. JAMA 1983; 250:2937–2941.

81. Hoff JD, Quigley ME, Yen SSC. Hormonal dynamics at midcycle: a reevaluation. J Clin Endocrinol Metab 1983; 57:792–796.

82. Liu JH, Yen SSC. Induction of midcycle gonadotropin surge by ovarian steroids in women: a critical evaluation. J Clin Endocrinol Metab 1983; 57:797–802.

CHAPTER 10

Practical Evaluation of Amenorrhea and Abnormal Uterine Bleeding

JAMES H. LIU and BRUCE KESSEL

PRACTICAL EVALUATION OF AMENORRHEA

Amenorrhea denotes the absence of menstruation and is an extremely important sign in the evaluation of the infertile female. From a physiologic perspective, amenorrhea represents a failure of the reproductive axis to function in a coordinated manner to achieve ovulation and induce endometrial growth and shedding. Traditionally, amenorrhea has been designated as either primary or secondary. *Primary amenorrhea* is defined as the absence of menstruation by age 16 years. *Secondary amenorrhea* refers to absence of menstruation for more than 3 months in women with prior menses. Regardless of classification, amenorrhea may indicate potential abnormalities at various levels in the hypothalamic-pituitary-ovarian-endometrial axis; therefore, the evaluation should not be influenced by whether the amenorrhea is primary or secondary.

Although the workup of amenorrhea may seem to be fairly complex, a detailed history and a carefully performed physical examination should permit the clinician to narrow the diagnostic possibilities and help define which levels in the reproductive system may be involved.

For most patients with amenorrhea, dysfunction of the reproductive axis can arise from (1) abnormalities in stimulatory input from the higher centers (hypothalamic-pituitary function); (2) abnormalities in sex steroid production (ovarian function); or (3) abnormalities in the reproductive outflow tract (uterovaginal function). During the evaluation, it is important for the clinician to recognize that the patient should serve as the bioassay for exposure to estrogens and androgens. The clinical classification of amenorrhea is shown in Table 10–1. Once the defects are identified, a tentative diagnosis can be established, and detailed testing can be carried out to confirm the cause. This clinical approach, summarized in Figure 10–1, reduces unnecessary testing and shortens the overall evaluation.

Clinical History: Essential Elements

The history should initially exclude possible physiologic conditions associated with amenorrhea such as *pregnancy, prepuberty, lactation-associated amenorrhea,* and *early menopause.* Pubertal milestones such as age of thelarche, pubarche, and menarche should be reviewed. In general, the evaluation should proceed if there is no evidence of secondary sex characteristics by the age of 13 years; if there are no menses by age 16; or there is a disruption in the normal sequence of pubertal maturation, that is, it has been longer than 5 years from the onset of pubertal changes without menarche.

Areas of the history that are often inadequately reviewed are the lifestyle and environmental circumstances relating to the patient. Patients should be questioned regarding exercise (type, duration, frequency); eating habits (vegetarian, amounts, frequency), weight changes, their concept of ideal weight, and possible eating disorders (bulimia, use of laxatives); recent changes in social relationships, work or school stresses; sleep habits; and prior psychological disturbances. These lifestyle variables have emerged as major factors for hypothalamic amenorrhea and are helpful for screening of abnormalities related to the central nervous system–hypothalamic-pituitary compartment (see Table 10–1).

Information on the menstrual history, sexual activity, and contraceptive practices is important to exclude pregnancy and pregnancy-associated causes. It is also important to inquire about signs of increased endogenous androgen secretion such as hirsutism (increase in midline, facial, and body hair), acne, temporal balding, voice changes, decrease in breast size, and increased muscle mass. These latter signs of

TABLE 10–1. Classification of Amenorrhea

Physiologic Anovulation
  Prepubertal phase
  Pregnancy
  Postpartum lactational phase
  Postmenopause
Disorders Associated with CNS-Hypothalamic-Pituitary
  Dysfunction
  Functional hypothalamic amenorrhea
    Psychogenic or stress factors
    Nutritional factors
    Exercise-related factors
  Pharmacologic-associated anovulation
    Dopaminergic antagonist
    Opiate agonist
    Other CNS-active medications
  Psychiatric-associated disorders
    Anorexia nervosa
    Pseudocyesis
  Organic defects of the hypothalamic-pituitary unit
    Isolated gonadotropin deficiency
    Kallmann's syndrome
    Pituitary tumors
    Sheehan's syndrome
    Pituitary apoplexy
    Empty sella syndrome
    Head trauma
    Inappropriate prolactin secretion
    Infection (HIV, tuberculosis)
    Postradiation effects
Disorders Associated with Ovarian Dysfunction
  Premature ovarian failure
  Gonadal dysgenesis
  Ovarian hyperandrogenism
    Polycystic ovary syndrome
    Thecoma
    Granulosa cell tumor
Disorders Associated with the Genital Outflow Tract
  Asherman's syndrome
  Müllerian agenesis or dysgenesis
  Male pseudohermaphroditism (androgen insensitivity)

CNS, central nervous system; HIV, human immunodeficiency virus.

masculinization warrant an assessment of circulating androgen levels. In a few patients, these changes may be rapidly progressive and suggest androgen-producing neoplasms of the ovary or adrenal gland. A history of menstrual irregularity from the time of menarche may suggest polycystic ovary disease or nonclassic late-onset 21-hydroxylase deficiency.

A prior history of pregnancy-associated dilation and curettage (D & C) or cervical cryocautery may suggest Asherman's syndrome[1] or cervical stenosis as the cause of amenorrhea. This situation is often evident in patients who fail to menstruate when taking oral contraceptives after an elective abortion.

Patients should be evaluated for hypoestrogenism and other endocrinopathies. The presence of hot flushes and vaginal dryness may suggest premature ovarian failure. Other symptoms such as hyperactivity, palpitations, nervousness, and weight loss may indicate hyperthyroidism. The clinician should also ask about characteristic symptoms of thyroid or adrenal insufficiency and other systemic illnesses.

All amenorrheal patients should be questioned regarding the presence of breast discharge. Galactorrhea is often associated with ingestion of psychotropic and antihypertensive agents. Galactorrhea also may be caused by hypothyroidism,[2] excessive nipple stimulation, or a prolactin (PRL)-secreting pituitary tumor.[3]

Physical Examination: The Patient as a Bioassay for Endocrine Abnormalities

A carefully conducted physical examination in combination with the history often allows formulation of a working diagnosis and reduces the extent of laboratory testing. The examination should focus on characteristic physical changes that may take place in response to the overall hormonal environment. In addition to a general examination, four special aspects should be assessed: (1) body habitus and distribution of body fat; (2) breast development and secretion; (3) skin and body hair distribution; and (4) genital outflow tract function.

The height, weight, and arm span of every patient should be determined. The arm span of most patients does not exceed the height by more than 2 in. In patients with delayed closure of the bony epiphyses due to low estrogen-androgen secretion (eunuchoid habitus), the arm span is significantly greater than the height.

The overall distribution of body fat should be assessed with the patient fully unclothed. In an appropriately estrogenized postpubertal female, fat deposition should be localized mainly to the breast and hips. In the virilized patient, fat is more evenly distributed over the truncal areas, and there is increased muscle mass most noticeably in the upper shoulder girdle and upper arms. In hypercortisolism, the fat deposition is centripetal, with a prominent supraclavicular fat pad and a moon-shaped face.

In very thin patients, such as those with anorexia nervosa, the skin has a sallow appearance with fine, lanugo-type hair over the extremities. Unusual pigmentation of the skin, such as in acanthosis nigricans (thickened, darker-pigmented, keratinized skin) localized to the skin folds, typically at the posterior neck, between the breasts, and in the intertriginous areas of the thighs, can be associated with androgen excess, polycystic ovary syndrome, and insulin-resistant diabetes mellitus.[4]

The presence of acne, oily skin, and dark, terminal-type hair in the facial and midline truncal areas indicates increased androgen secretion, most commonly from the ovaries. The extent of hirsutism can be quantitated most practically on the face using the criteria described by Bardin and Lipsett.[5] A score of 1+ is assigned for excess terminal hair on the upper lip, chin, and sideburn areas, whereas 4+ is given for a full beard. On the lower trunk, a male-type escutcheon indicates an increased androgen effect. The increased sensitivity of midline tissue to circulating androgens is due in part to the increased 5α-reductase activity localized in these areas.[6] This type of hair distribution is different from increased vellus hair on the extremities (termed *hypertrichosis*), which is not specifically associated with androgen excess.

The thyroid gland should be examined and carefully palpated for size, consistency, and mobility. Enlargement of the thyroid in association with bradycardia, coarse skin, and lower extremity edema suggests hypothyroidism.

The breasts should be carefully evaluated for stage of development according to criteria established by Marshall and Tanner (Table 10–2).[7] To assess for breast secretion, the patient should be upright, and the examiner should be positioned behind the patient so that pressure can be applied to the breast from the base, gradually working toward the nip-

History
    Puberty milestones
        Thelarche, pubarche, menarche
    Chronic illness
        Thyroid, renal, diabetes, sarcoid
    Exercise
        Activity type, duration, frequency
    Nutritional status
        Bulimia, anorexia, weight changes

Headaches, head trauma, visual disturbances
Medications
    Hormones, antidepressants, anxiolytics
Hot flushes, vaginal dryness
Breast discharge or lactation
Hirsutism or acne
Irradiation
Uterine instrumentation

Physical Examination

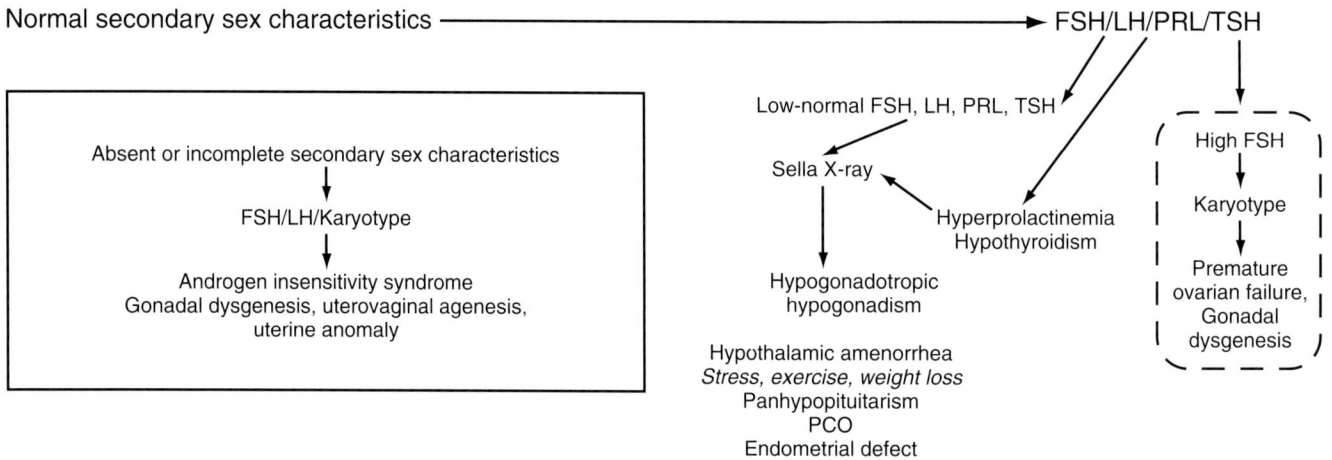

Normal secondary sex characteristics ⟶ FSH/LH/PRL/TSH

Absent or incomplete secondary sex characteristics
↓
FSH/LH/Karyotype
↓
Androgen insensitivity syndrome
Gonadal dysgenesis, uterovaginal agenesis,
uterine anomaly

Low-normal FSH, LH, PRL, TSH

Sella X-ray

Hyperprolactinemia
Hypothyroidism

Hypogonadotropic
hypogonadism

Hypothalamic amenorrhea
Stress, exercise, weight loss
Panhypopituitarism
PCO
Endometrial defect

High FSH
↓
Karyotype
↓
Premature
ovarian failure,
Gonadal
dysgenesis

FIGURE 10–1. Diagnostic flow diagram for the evaluation of amenorrhea. FSH, follicle-stimulating hormone; LH, luteinizing hormone; PRL, prolactin; TSH, thyroid-stimulating hormone; PCO, polycystic ovary syndrome.

ple. Any secretions obtained should be examined microscopically for the presence of fat globules, which is characteristic of galactorrhea.

The type of escutcheon and stage of pubic hair development (see Table 10–2) should be noted before examination of the female genitalia. The presence of labial fusion may suggest prenatal androgen exposure, present in conditions

such as congenital adrenal hyperplasia. Clitoral size should be evaluated. Clitoromegaly is arbitrarily defined as enlargement of the clitoral shaft diameter to 1 cm or larger when measured at the base. This finding is consistent with virilization if it is associated with other signs of androgen excess.[8] Isolated clitoromegaly can be a result of excessive masturbation. Other genital anomalies such as imperforate hymen, vaginal agenesis, vaginal septum, and didelphic uterus should be evident on careful speculum inspection and bimanual examination.

The vaginal mucosa should have a characteristic moist, pinkish-gray, rugated appearance in women of reproductive age. In women with prolonged hypoestrogenism, the mucosal folds are flattened and appear pale-pink and dry. The cervical mucus can serve as a bioassay and should be assessed for the "ferning" pattern, which is indicative of recent estrogen exposure and the absence of significant progesterone effect.

Traditionally, a progestin challenge test is carried out to confirm that the genital outflow tract is patent and to serve as a bioassay for estrogen-primed endometrium. In this test, medroxyprogesterone acetate, 5 to 10 mg/day orally for 5 to 10 days, or progesterone in oil, 100 to 200 mg intramuscularly, is administered. Vaginal bleeding should occur within 10 days of progestin administration. If the cervical mucus demonstrates a ferning pattern, most women will have some amount of vaginal bleeding in response to the progestin challenge. For women with negative test results, any combination

TABLE 10–2. Tanner Staging of Breast and Pubic Hair Development		
Tanner Stage	**Breast Changes**	**Pubic Hair Changes**
1	Papillary elevation	Lanugo-type hair
2	Elevation of breast bud and papilla	Dark, terminal hair on labia majora
3	Further enlargement of breast tissue and papilla	Terminal hair covering the labia majora and spreading to the mons pubis
4	Elevation of the papilla and areola unit from the breast; papilla is at or above the equator of the breast	Terminal hair covering the labia majora and mons pubis fully
5	Areola is recessed into the breast and/or papilla is below the equator of the breast	Terminal hair covering the labia majora, mons pubis, and inner thighs

oral contraceptive containing 35 μg of ethinyl estradiol can be given to determine if the genital outflow tract is intact.

Laboratory Assessment: Essential Screening Tests

After exclusion of pregnancy-related conditions, basal levels of PRL, thyroid-stimulating hormone (TSH), and follicle-stimulating hormone (FSH) should be determined to confirm the working diagnosis in amenorrheic women. These three determinations should serve as the key hormonal markers in the diagnostic evaluation of amenorrhea (see Fig. 10–1). The measurement of luteinizing hormone (LH) should be considered optional but can assist in making a definitive diagnosis.

PRL levels have been reported to be elevated in as many as one third of patients presenting with amenorrhea.[9] The upper limit of the normal range for PRL in most laboratories is between 20 and 25 ng/mL. Because PRL levels may also be elevated under various physiologic conditions, such as during sleep,[10] food ingestion, and stress,[11] any modest increases in PRL levels should be repeated before expanding the workup. Patients should also be questioned regarding drug intake, a frequent cause of hyperprolactinemia. If galactorrhea or hyperprolactinemia is present, primary hypothyroidism should be excluded because, in this latter condition, increased secretion of thyrotropin-releasing hormone also stimulates increased secretion of PRL by the pituitary lactotropes. A normal TSH level (≤5 μU/mL) essentially excludes hypothyroidism. For patients with persistent hyperprolactinemia, radiographic evaluation, such as computed tomography (CT) with contrast and magnetic resonance imaging (MRI), of the sella turcica is warranted.

In the patient with normal physical findings, four different profiles of LH and FSH secretion may be present. Elevated levels of both FSH (>30 mIU/mL) and LH (>20 mIU/mL) suggest ovarian failure.[12] In a young woman (<30 years of age), a karyotype should be obtained because of the increased incidence of chromosomal abnormalities associated with gonadal dysfunction, that is, gonadal dysgenesis. If a Y chromosome is detected, bilateral gonadectomy is indicated because of the malignant potential of the gonads.[13] In older women, an elevation in FSH levels reflects decreased ovarian output of estradiol and inhibin and incipient ovarian failure.

For women with an elevation of LH (>20 mIU/mL) and an exaggerated ratio of LH:FSH (>2:1), chronic anovulation associated with polycystic ovary syndrome is the most likely diagnosis.[14] Other less common conditions that may result in this pattern of gonadotropin secretion include the midcycle gonadotropin surge (menses occurs 2 weeks after testing) and, rarely, testicular feminization.

In women with hypothalamic amenorrhea[15] or chronic anovulation (including polycystic ovary syndrome), LH and FSH levels can be in the normal range (7 to 20 mIU/mL), and thus the clinician must place greater weight on the history and physical examination. Low LH and FSH levels (usually <10 mIU/mL) are typically associated with hypothalamic amenorrhea, isolated gonadotropin deficiency, Kallmann's syndrome, anorexia nervosa, and panhypopituitary disorders. These patients also generally have lower levels of PRL as well. To exclude the rare instance of an occult central nervous system lesion in patients with the diagnosis of hypothalamic

amenorrhea, radiographic evaluation of the sella turcica region should be performed.

For the patient who is hirsute or virilized on physical examination, serum levels of total testosterone and dehydroepiandrosterone sulfate (DHEAS) should also be obtained. In general, an elevation in serum testosterone level greater than 200 ng/dL suggests the possibility of an androgen-producing tumor either from an ovarian or an adrenal site, although the ovarian neoplasm is much more common. Elevations in the DHEAS levels (>700 μg/dL) suggests adrenal hyperfunction or adrenal neoplasia. In these latter conditions, the stigmata of Cushing's syndrome (hypertension, centripetal obesity, "buffalo hump," pigmented striae) should be evident on physical examination. The DHEAS levels also can be elevated in patients with nonclassic congenital adrenal hyperplasia, sometimes termed *cryptic 21-hydroxylase deficiency*.[16] In this condition, there is a relative deficiency of the 21-hydroxylase enzyme and an accumulation of the 17-hydroxyprogesterone intermediate product in the cortisol biosynthetic pathway. Most patients with this diagnosis provide a strong family history of hirsutism or irregular cycles at menarche, or both, and have elevations in basal 17-hydroxyprogesterone levels. The diagnosis should be confirmed by adrenocorticotropic hormone stimulation testing.[17]

CLINICAL APPROACH TO ABNORMAL UTERINE BLEEDING

Abnormal uterine bleeding (AUB) is a common gynecologic disorder and may account for as many as 15% of outpatient visits and 25% of gynecologic operations. AUB may be manifested by excessive bleeding at the time of expected menses or too frequent or irregular bleeding episodes. Commonly used terms for patterns of abnormal bleeding are listed in Table 10–3. The causes of AUB can be broadly divided into two groups: (1) AUB secondary to an organic cause and (2) AUB secondary to anovulation, also called *dysfunctional uterine bleeding* (DUB). The clinical assessment, therefore, centers around an evaluation of organic causes and the determination of ovulatory status. Because the incidence of ovulatory cycles varies with age and the incidence of many organic causes of AUB increases with age, the history, physical examination, and testing are more easily understood when placed in the framework of the age of the patient.

TABLE 10–3. Common Terminologies Used to Describe Uterine Bleeding Patterns	
Terminology	**Uterine Bleeding Pattern**
Intermenstrual bleeding	Bleeding occurring between regular menstrual cycles
Menorrhagia (hypermenorrhea)	Excessive bleeding occurring at regular intervals
Metrorrhagia	Bleeding at irregular and frequent intervals
Menometrorrhagia	Prolonged and irregular bleeding
Polymenorrhea	Regular bleeding at <21-d intervals
Postmenopausal bleeding	Bleeding occurring >1 yr after menopause

The Endometrium and Menstrual Bleeding

Normal average menstrual cycle length is 28 days, with a range of 21 to 35 days. The average duration of menstrual flow is 4 days. The average blood loss during menses is approximately 35 mL, with a range of 20 to 80 mL. Menses of more than 8 days' duration or when there is more than 80 mL of menstrual blood loss (MBL) should be considered abnormal.

Following menstruation, only the basalis layer of the endometrium remains, and the endometrium is thin, usually less than 0.5-mm thick. With estrogenic stimulation during the follicular phase, the endometrial epithelium undergoes rapid mitotic activity to achieve a thickness of approximately 5 to 7 mm over a 7-day period. After ovulation, under the influence of progesterone, the endometrium progressively differentiates with little further increase in height but with well-characterized histologic changes that correlate with the number of days of progesterone exposure.[18] If conception does not occur, the corpus luteum spontaneously undergoes luteolysis, a process that is associated with a decrease in estradiol and progesterone levels and endometrial breakdown.

The physiology of normal endometrial growth and shedding is incompletely understood. The demonstration of estrogen and progesterone receptors in endometrium and changes in receptor content throughout the menstrual cycle provide direct evidence for sex steroid–induced endometrial changes.[19] The current concept suggests that the following biochemical events take place prior to the onset of menstrual flow: (1) a decline in progesterone levels; (2) a destabilization of endometrial cell lysosomal membranes; (3) an increase in tissue levels of prostaglandin (PG) precursors and $PGF_{2\alpha}$ levels; (4) vasospasm of the adjacent spiral artery; and (5) release of proteolytic enzymes (collagenases and plasminogen activators), which degrade endometrial stroma.[20] Menstrual flow is self-limiting due to the rapid regeneration of endometrial glands and stroma from the basalis layer under the influence of estrogen from the new dominant follicle.

Etiology of Abnormal Uterine Bleeding

Causes of AUB, aside from anovulation, are listed in Table 10–4. All patients of reproductive age need to be evaluated for a pregnancy-related event resulting in AUB. As many as 20% of all patients with clinical pregnancies experience abnormal bleeding. This percentage increases to more than 50% when chemical pregnancies are also included. The differential diagnosis in the patient with AUB during early pregnancy should include threatened or incomplete spontaneous abortion, ectopic pregnancy, and, more rarely, gestational trophoblastic neoplasm.

Pelvic infections such as vaginitis, cervicitis, and endometritis can be associated with AUB. In most instances, this diagnosis is evident during the pelvic examination, although the diagnosis of endometritis usually requires an endometrial biopsy.

AUB also may be the first sign of a pelvic neoplasm. The most common benign uterine neoplasms include endometrial polyps, endometrial hyperplasia, and leiomyomata. Although uterine myomas are associated with abnormal bleeding (in

TABLE 10–4. Possible Causes (other than anovulation) of Abnormal Uterine Bleeding

Pregnancy-Related Events
Spontaneous abortion
Incomplete or threatened abortion
Ectopic pregnancy
Gestational trophoblastic disease
Genital Tract Infection
Vaginitis
Cervicitis
Endometritis
Genital Tract Neoplasms
Cervical dysplasia
Cervical carcinoma
Endometrial hyperplasia
Endometrial carcinoma
Uterine leiomyoma
Fallopian tube carcinoma
Ovarian estrogen-producing tumors
Systemic Illness
Coagulation disorders
Thyroid disease
Liver disease
Iatrogenic Causes
Oral contraceptives
Progestin-only contraceptives
Intrauterine contraceptive device

approximately 30% of patients with myomas), the mechanism is unknown. Possible explanations for this phenomenon include (1) abnormalities in the endometrium overlying a submucous myoma; (2) an overall increase in the endometrial surface area; (3) interference with the normal uterine contractile mechanism necessary for hemostasis; and (4) compression of the venous plexus in adjacent endometrium and myometrium leading to increased local venous pressure.[21] Estrogen-secreting ovarian tumors can cause bleeding by stimulating the endometrium.

In the perimenarcheal patient, coagulopathies constitute an important part of the differential diagnosis for AUB. Leukemia, which can be associated with coagulation disorders, may also result in AUB. Other systemic illnesses that should be considered include thyroid dysfunction and severe liver disease.

The diagnosis of DUB is made after exclusion of organic causes. Based on the clinical presentation, this diagnosis should focus on the cause of anovulation. From an acute treatment standpoint, it is not always necessary to find the cause of DUB if a careful history and physical examination are performed and if premalignant and malignant conditions are excluded.

With regard to the causes of DUB, several theories have been proposed. During an anovulatory cycle, the endometrium is exposed to prolonged estrogen stimulation unopposed by progesterone. There is overgrowth of the endometrium, unsupported by sufficient stroma, thus predisposing this tissue to structural instability and breakdown. Alternatively, there may be an increase in endometrial PGE receptors or in PGE_2 or prostacyclin levels that can increase local vasodilation and decrease platelet aggregation. Myometrial PGE receptor concentrations have been reported to be significantly higher in patients with menorrhagia in comparison with those who have normal measured MBL.[22]

AUB secondary to hormonal therapies is quite common.

An understanding of the endometrial response to various hormonal regimens often provides insight into modifying the hormonal treatment. With the increased use of progestin-only contraception (Norplant and Depo-Provera), the incidence of progestin breakthrough bleeding will continue to increase.[23]

Evaluation of Abnormal Uterine Bleeding

In the evaluation of AUB, it is important to perform a focused history and physical examination, with emphasis on the pattern and quantity of bleeding. During the course of the history and examination, organic causes of AUB should be eliminated, and an assessment of ovulatory status aids in the diagnosis of suspected DUB. In general, anovulation occurs at the highest frequency at both extremes of reproductive age and constitutes the most common abnormality. Figure 10–2 provides a general schema and differential diagnosis for the evaluation of AUB. In the absence of another identifiable cause, DUB is likely.

HISTORY AND PHYSICAL EXAMINATION

Historical assessment of the amount of MBL is usually inaccurate. Common questions, such as the number of days of flow and number of pads or tampons used per day, do not correlate with measured MBL. Objective measurement of blood loss in 92 women with regular but heavy periods showed that in 30% of patients reporting light menses, there was more than 80 mL of blood loss, whereas in 47% of patients describing heavy menses, the flow was objectively light.[24] In the assessment of MBL, it is important to determine any change from the patient's prior menstrual pattern. The regular occurrence of menstrual flow accompanied by premenstrual molimina is suggestive of ovulation, whereas completely irregular, noncyclic bleeding is indicative of anovulation. The normal average MBL is reported to be 35 mL, whereas an MBL greater than 80 mL appears to be associated with anemia and changes in red blood cell indices.[25] To aid in the evaluation of AUB, all patients should be asked to keep a prospective menstrual calendar in which the pattern and the severity of bleeding are recorded. The findings must be interpreted in the light of the age of the patient.

Prepubertal Females. During the first several months following birth, it is not uncommon for a female infant to experience scant vaginal bleeding. This is secondary to placental estrogenic stimulation of the endometrium. In the infant, adnexal masses are easily palpable abdominally.

Between the ages of 1 and 10 years, vaginal bleeding is uncommon and often secondary to nonendocrine-related problems, including vaginal foreign objects, vaginitis, or genital trauma. If there are no other signs of secondary sexual development in addition to the bleeding, attention should focus on examination of the genitalia. External evidence of trauma and infection should be sought. Evaluation of the vagina may reveal foreign objects. Often, such an evaluation may require general anesthesia and use of a hysteroscope or urethroscope. In rare instances, this type of bleeding is due to malignancies, such as botryoid sarcoma.

If AUB is associated with any signs of estrogen activity (breast development or increase in height), an ovarian source of estrogen must be excluded. Possible abnormalities include a benign ovarian cyst or, more rarely, a malignant neoplasm. In the presence of secondary sexual characteristics, any of the causes of precocious puberty also should be considered. A careful abdominal examination for masses should be performed.

In a selected population of children 10 years of age and younger seen at a secondary referral center, 21% were found to have malignant genital tract tumors, 21% to have precocious puberty, and 54% to have local lesions of unknown

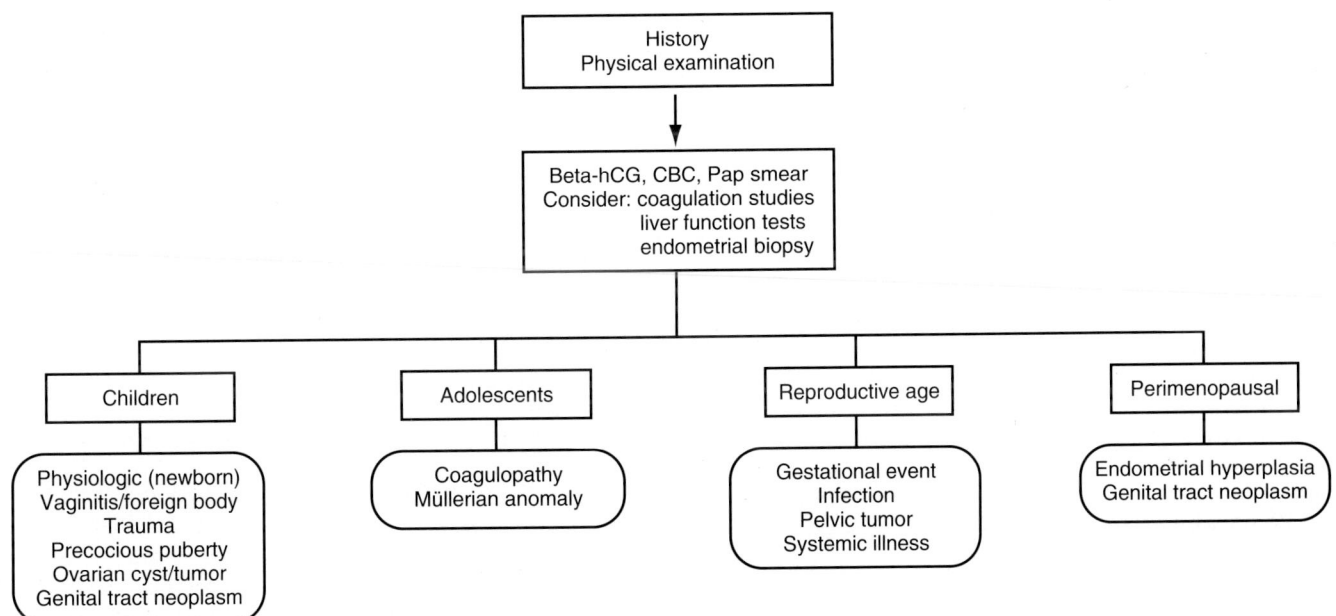

FIGURE 10–2. Flow diagram and differential diagnoses for the evaluation of abnormal uterine bleeding. Beta-HCG, β-human chorionic gonadotropin; CBC, complete blood count.

etiology.[26] It is likely that the percentages of patients with tumors and precocious puberty are higher in this study as a consequence of the referral pattern to this center.

Perimenarcheal Females. The menstrual history of perimenarcheal females should include a review of the pubertal milestones as well as provide an assessment of menstrual cycle characteristics. Pubertal landmarks such as breast development, growth spurt, and menarche are ovarian estrogen dependent, whereas pubic and axillary hair development are adrenal androgen dependent. These events normally take place in the following order: growth spurt, breast budding, pubic hair, peak growth velocity, and menarche. Ovarian steroid–mediated and adrenal steroid–mediated pubertal changes are independent, and one can occur without the other.

In the perimenarcheal female, the incidence of anovulation is high. During the first year following menarche, as many as 50% of bleeding episodes are anovulatory. Serum levels of estrone and 17β-estradiol are in the normal range; thus, the cause of anovulation is not inadequate ovarian estrogen production but rather the inability of the hypothalamic-pituitary axis to respond appropriately to positive estrogen feedback with an LH surge.[27, 28]

In the adolescent, AUB may be the first sign of an underlying coagulation disorder. In these patients, there may be a history of gum bleeding, easy bruisability, and prolonged bleeding after minor cuts. In a study by Claessens and Cowell,[29] 19% of all teenagers admitted for AUB were found to have a coagulation disorder. If the hemoglobin level was less than 10 g/dL at presentation, the incidence increased to 25%. In those patients who were hospitalized during menarche, the incidence was as high as 50%. The types of coagulation disorders found included von Willebrand's disease, idiopathic thrombocytopenia purpura, Glanzmann's disease, thalassemia major, and Fanconi's anemia.

The physical examination should include Tanner staging (see Table 10–2). Height and weight should be plotted on standard percentile charts, and the ratio of lower body to trunk and arm span to height should be determined. The pelvic examination may reveal the presence of infantile external genitalia, the degree of estrogen effect on the vaginal mucosa, cervical lesions, or an adnexal mass.

Women of Reproductive Age. In women of reproductive age, regular menses (at intervals between 24 and 36 days) with the association of premenstrual molimina are indicative of ovulatory cycles. The history should focus on prior episodes of AUB, pelvic infection, sexually transmitted disease, prior D & C of the uterus, and gestational events. A history related to anovulation can be most helpful. The onset of anovulation can often be linked to the initiation of strenuous exercise, psychological stress, weight loss, eating disorders, or significant weight gain.

A careful pelvic examination may reveal vaginal or cervical lesions or an enlarged, irregular uterus suggestive of leiomyomata. Concomitant findings of obesity, hirsutism, or acanthosis nigricans may suggest polycystic ovary disease.

Perimenopausal Women. Perimenopausal women have an increased incidence of anovulatory cycles because of the natural decline in ovarian responsiveness. During the perimenopausal period, estrone and 17β-estradiol levels can fluctuate significantly.[30] Many perimenopausal women experience intermittent hypoestrogenic symptoms, such as hot flushes,

mood changes, and vaginal dryness. The physical examination should focus on the presence of lymphadenopathy, evidence of ascites, pelvic masses, and signs of hypoestrogenism.

LABORATORY EVALUATION

Laboratory testing should include a complete blood count, β-human chorionic gonadotropin determination, and Papanicolaou smear. In the adolescent patient, coagulation screening tests should include a bleeding time, prothrombin time, partial thromboplastin time, and a platelet count. The clinical history or physical examination may also suggest the need for tests of thyroid or liver function.

An endometrial biopsy should be performed in all patients older than 35 years of age and in younger patients at increased risk for unopposed estrogen stimulation, such as in polycystic ovary syndrome, estrogen hormone treatment, and chronic anovulation associated with obesity. Historically, the "gold standard" for endometrial sampling has been D & C of the uterus. This has been replaced in large part by office endometrial biopsy. The rationale for this approach is the increased operative risk and medical costs of a formal D & C. Moreover, recent studies have suggested that the accuracy of office biopsies and D & C is equal.[31] In one study comparing D & C, Vabra aspiration, and the Novak curette with hysterectomy specimens, there were only 30 instances in 619 patients (4.8%) in which blind sampling failed to identify correctly endometrial hyperplasia or carcinoma.[32] More important, there was no difference in accuracy among the three sampling techniques. Flexible plastic suction curettes (2 to 3 mm in diameter) are now used increasingly for office endometrial biopsies. These devices appear to offer a greater safety margin. Most studies indicate a decrease in patient discomfort when compared with the Novak curette or Vabra aspiration. Office biopsies comparing these instruments with Vabra aspiration have found no difference in the ability to obtain the correct diagnosis.[33]

Routine imaging studies are unnecessary in most patients presenting with AUB. However, ultrasonography can be helpful in patients who have AUB associated with ovulatory cycles (such as secretory endometrium) or who are refractory to medical management.

Hysterosalpingograms are most useful in the evaluation of müllerian anomalies but may be less accurate in the diagnosis of submucous myomas and endometrial polyps. Several studies suggest that direct visualization of the endometrial cavity by hysteroscopy offers the most accuracy. Of 553 patients with abnormal bleeding, hysteroscopy was able to establish the diagnosis in 352 patients.[34] In one study comparing hysteroscopic-directed biopsy with D & C, hysteroscopy was equal to curettage in 223 patients (81%) and revealed more information than curettage in 44 patients (16%), whereas curettage revealed more information than hysteroscopy in 9 patients (3%).[35]

The guidelines for the use of ultrasonography, CT, or MRI in the assessment of various aspects of AUB and DUB remain to be established. Ultrasonography appears to be 75% to 80% accurate in detecting uterine myomas when the criteria of contour irregularity, altered echogenic pattern, and uterine enlargement are considered.[36] Ultrasonography is also of benefit in evaluating ovarian cysts. More controversial is the routine use of ultrasonography for the evaluation of endometrial thickness with regard to the cause of abnormal bleeding. Early studies suggest that endometrial thickness greater than 20 mm is associated with endometrial hyperplasia, carcinoma, and polyps, whereas an endometrial thickness less than 5 mm is rarely associated with endometrial hyperplasia.[37] Although increased endometrial thickness alone is not a definitive test for endometrial cancer, an endometrial thickness less than 5 mm can be reassuring. Concomitant estrogen replacement therapy also alters endometrial thickness, with a higher percentage of these women having an endometrial thickness greater than 5 mm. Preliminary studies suggest that assessment of the pulsatility index with color-flow Doppler ultrasonography may be more accurate in detecting the presence of endometrial carcinoma.[38] Owing to the high cost and limited information made available, the use of CT or MRI should be confined to investigational studies.

Treatment of Abnormal Uterine Bleeding

The initial goal of medical therapy for AUB should be to stabilize the endometrium. Acute control of AUB with any combination oral contraceptive (with 35 μg of ethinyl estradiol combined with 1 mg of norethindrone being one reasonable choice) can be achieved by a variety of regimens (such as one tablet three times a day for 7 days, followed by a short 5-day withdrawal bleed and two standard pill cycles). Estrogens can also be given intravenously as 25 mg of conjugated estrogens every 4 hours, or orally.[39] In the latter case, a concomitant progestin (medroxyprogesterone acetate, 10 mg, twice daily) should also be administered. Androgens also have been successfully used to treat menorrhagia; however, use of danazol (Danocrine) should be limited because of its androgenic side effects and expense.[40]

For chronic management of AUB secondary to anovulation, periodic administration of a progestin such as medroxyprogesterone acetate at a dosage of 10 mg for 10 days each month may be effective. In addition, the concomitant administration of PG synthase inhibitors during menses can reduce mean blood loss by 30%. Both mefenamic acid (500 mg three times a day for 3 days) and naproxen (250 mg three times a day for 3 days) have been shown to be effective in this regard.[41]

Gonadotropin-releasing hormone (GnRH) agonists can be useful adjuncts in the short-term management of AUB, particularly for bleeding secondary to uterine myomas. After medically induced hypoestrogenism, there is a rapid decrease in uterine size, a cessation in bleeding, and an increase in hematocrit levels.[42] Myomas, however, return to their pretreatment size within 6 months after discontinuation of GnRH agonist therapy.[43] Long-term GnRH agonist use may be associated with osteopenia. Studies are in progress that examine the long-term use of GnRH agonists in combination with hormone replacement to protect against bone loss.[44]

A variety of minor surgical procedures are commonly used in the management of AUB. D & C can be effective in the acute control of AUB and provides a histopathologic diagnosis, but the procedure is inadequate therapy for long-term management. In a study of 630 patients, 65% had a recurrence of abnormal bleeding within 3 months of the D & C.[45]

Thus, there is little use for curettage in the treatment of abnormal bleeding.

Hysteroscopic resection of submucous myomas and endometrial polyps is effective in the treatment of AUB without permanently compromising uterine function. Several studies report a high incidence (71%) of amenorrhea or hypomenorrhea following endometrial ablation with the neodymium:YAG laser or electrosurgical techniques.[46] This approach should be considered in patients who are unresponsive to endocrine manipulation and are at high risk for other surgical procedures.[47] The long-term effectiveness of endometrial ablation remains to be established. Hysterectomy remains the standard therapy for persistent AUB.

Health Care Impact

AUB has a significant impact on the quality of life and the health care costs of women. Progressive anemia associated with more than 80 mL of blood loss per cycle can lead to fatigue and decreased productivity. In addition, in women with heavy irregular bleeding, both work and social activities may be curtailed owing to the possibility of unexpected bleeding episodes.

Uterine leiomyomata account for about 30%, and DUB for about 20%, of hysterectomies. Hysterectomies are the second most common major operation performed in the United States. There are approximately 590,000 hysterectomies performed annually, with the annual costs exceeding $5 billion. There are significant variations in hysterectomy rates by country and within regions in a country. Indications for hysterectomy continue to evolve, and additional research is necessary to determine outcomes of hysterectomy and alternative medical and surgical treatments.[48]

SUMMARY

AUB is a common gynecologic complaint. The goal of the evaluation for AUB is to exclude organic causes, including gestational events, infection, benign and malignant pelvic pathology, and systemic diseases. The clinical approach relies on a thorough history and physical examination with limited laboratory evaluation. Treatment of organic lesions is directed at the specific diagnosis. Most patients with DUB should respond to hormonal therapy. In instances when AUB is either unresponsive to medical therapy or occurs in an ovulatory patient, hysteroscopic evaluation should be considered. The efficacy of other diagnostic modalities such as ultrasonographic measurement of endometrial thickness, color-flow Doppler imaging, and CT and MRI scanning remains to be defined. Similarly, experimental treatment modalities, including the use of GnRH analog therapy in combination with estrogen addback and endometrial ablative techniques, need additional study.

REFERENCES

1. Asherman JG. Amenorrhea traumatica (atretica). J Obstet Gynaecol Br Emp 1948;55:23–30.
2. Thomas DJB, Touzel R, Charlesworth M, et al. Hyperprolactinaemia and microadenomas in primary hypothyroidism. Clin Endocrinol 1987;27:289–295.

3. Herman TN, Molitch ME. Bromocriptine: indications and use in patients with endocrine disease. Hosp Formulary 1984;19:784–791.

4. Dunaif A, Graf M, Mandeli J, et al. Characterization of groups of hyper-androgenic women with acanthosis nigricans, impaired glucose tolerance, and/or hyperinsulinemia. J Clin Endocrinol Metab 1987;65:499–507.

5. Bardin CW, Lipsett MB. Testosterone and androstenedione blood production rates in normal women and women with idiopathic hirsutism or polycystic ovaries. J Clin Invest 1967;46:891–902.

6. Ehrmann DA, Rosenfield RL. Clinical Review 10: An endocrinologic approach to the patient with hirsutism. J Clin Endocrinol Metab 1990;71:1–4.

7. Marshall WA, Tanner JM. Variations in the pattern of pubertal changes in girls. Arch Dis Child 1969;44:291–303.

8. Tagatz GE, Kopher RA, Nagel TC, Okagaki T. The clitoral index: a bioassay of androgenic stimulation. Obstet Gynecol 1979;54:562–564.

9. Molitch ME, Reichlin S. Hyperprolactinemic disorders. Dis Mon 1982;28:1–58.

10. Ehara Y, Siler T, Vandenberg G, et al. Circulating prolactin levels during the menstrual cycle: episodic release and diurnal variation. Am J Obstet Gynecol 1973;117:962–970.

11. Noel GL, Suh HK, Stone JG, Frantz AG. Human prolactin and growth hormone release during surgery and other conditions of stress. J Clin Endocrinol Metab 1972;35:840–851.

12. Rebar RW, Erickson GF, Yen SSC. Idiopathic premature ovarian failure: clinical and endocrine characteristics. Fertil Steril 1982;37:35–41.

13. Manuel M, Katayama KP, Jones HW Jr. The age of occurrence of gonadal tumors in intersex patients with a Y chromosome. Am J Obstet Gynecol 1976;124:293–300.

14. Rebar RW, Judd HL, Yen SSC, et al. Characterization of the inappropriate gonadotropin secretion in polycystic ovary syndrome. J Clin Invest 1976;57:1320–1329.

15. Liu JH. Hypothalamic amenorrhea: clinical perspectives, pathophysiology, and management. Am J Obstet Gynecol 1990;163:1732–1736.

16. Levine LS, Dupont B, Lorenzen F, et al. Genetic and hormonal characterization of cryptic 21-hydroxylase deficiency. J Clin Endocrinol Metab 1981;53:1192–1198.

17. New MI. Polycystic ovarian disease and congenital and late-onset adrenal hyperplasia. Endocrinol Metab Clin North Am 1988;17:637–648.

18. Noyes RW, Hertig AT, Rock J. Dating the endometrial biopsy. Fertil Steril 1950;1:3–25.

19. Beaulieu EE. In: Diczfalusy E, Fraser IS, Webb FTG, editors. WHO Symposium on Steroid Contraception and Endometrial Bleeding. England: Pitman Press, 1980.

20. Abel MH, Kelly RW. Differential production of prostaglandins within the human uterus. Prostaglandins 1979;18:821–828.

21. Buttram VC Jr, Reiter RC. Uterine leiomyomata: etiology, symptomatology, and management. Fertil Steril 1981;36:433–445.

22. Adelantado JM, Rees MCP, Bernal AL. Increased uterine prostaglandin E receptors in menorrhagic women. Br J Obstet Gynaecol 1988;95:162–165.

23. Shoupe D, Mishell DR, Bopp BL. The significance of bleeding patterns in Norplant implant users. Obstet Gynecol 1991;77:256–260.

24. Chimbira TH, Anderson ABM, Turnbull AC. Relation between menstrual blood loss and patient's subjective assessment of loss, duration of bleeding, number of sanitary towels used, uterine weight, and endometrial surface area. Br J Obstet Gynaecol 1980;87:603–609.

25. Hallberg L, Hogdahl A, Nilsson L, Rybo G. Menstrual blood loss—a population study. Acta Obstet Gynecol Scand 1966;45:320–351.

26. Hill NCW, Oppenheimer LW, Morton KE. The aetiology of vaginal bleeding in children: a 20-year review. Br J Obstet Gynaecol 1989;96:467–470.

27. Winter JSD, Faiman C. The development of cyclic pituitary-gonadal function in adolescent females. J Clin Endocrinol Metab 1973;37:714–718.

28. Fraser IS, Michie EA, Wide L, Baird DT. Pituitary gonadotropins and ovarian function in adolescent dysfunctional uterine bleeding. J Clin Endocrinol Metab 1973;37:407–414.

29. Claessens EA, Cowell CA. Acute adolescent menorrhagia. Am J Obstet Gynecol 1981;139:277–280.

30. Sherman BM, West JH, Korenman SG. The menopausal transition: analysis of LH, FSH, estradiol, and progesterone concentrations during the menstrual cycles of older women. J Clin Endocrinol Metab 1976;42:629–636.

31. Grimes DA. Diagnostic dilation and curettage: a reappraisal. Am J Obstet Gynecol 1982;142:1–6.

32. Stovall TG, Soloman SK, Ling FW. Endometrial sampling prior to hysterectomy. Am J Obstet Gynecol 1989;73:405–409.

33. Kaunitz AM, Masciello A, Ostrowski M, Rovira EZ. Comparison of endometrial biopsy with the endometrial pipelle and Vabra aspirator. J Reprod Med 1988;33:427–431.

34. Valle RF. Hysteroscopic evaluation of patients with abnormal uterine bleeding. Surg Gynecol Obstet 1981;153:521–526.

35. Gimpelson RJ, Rappol HO. A comparative study between panoramic hysteroscopy with directed biopsies and dilatation and curettage. Am J Obstet Gynecol 1988;158:489–492.

36. Gross BH, Silver TM, Jaffe MH. Sonographic features of uterine leiomyomas: analysis of 41 proven cases. J Ultrasound Med 1983;2:401–406.

37. Granberg S, Wikland M, Karlsson B. Endometrial thickness as measured by endovaginal ultrasonography for identifying endometrial abnormality. Am J Obstet Gynecol 1991;164:47–53.

38. Bourne TH, Campbell S, Steer CV, et al. Detection of endometrial cancer by transvaginal ultrasonography with color flow imaging and blood flow analysis: a preliminary report. Gynecol Oncol 1991;40:253–258.

39. DeVore GR, Owens O, Kase N. Use of intravenous Premarin in the treatment of dysfunctional uterine bleeding—a double-blind randomized control study. J Obstet Gynecol 1982;59:285–291.

40. Dockeray CJ, Sheppard BL, Bonnar J. Comparison between mefenamic acid and danazol in the treatment of established menorrhagia. Br J Obstet Gynaecol 1989;96:840–844.

41. Cameron I, Hainging R, Lumsden M, et al. The effects of mefenamic acid and norethisterone on measured menstrual blood loss. Obstet Gynecol 1990;76:85–88.

42. Kessel B, Liu J, Mortola J, et al. Treatment of uterine fibroids with agonist analogs of gonadotropin-releasing hormone. Fertil Steril 1988;49:538–541.

43. Friedman A, Harrison-Atlas D, Barbieri R, et al. A randomized, placebo-controlled, double-blind study evaluating the efficacy of leuprolide acetate depot in the treatment of uterine leiomyomata. Fertil Steril 1989;51:251–256.

44. Friedman AJ, Daly M, Juneau-Norcross M, et al. A prospective, randomized trial of gonadotropin-releasing hormone agonist plus estrogen-progestin or progestin "add-back" regimens for women with leiomyomata uteri. J Clin Endocrinol Metab 1993;76:1439–1445.

45. Haynes PJ, Hodgson H, Anderson ABM. Measurement of menstrual blood loss in patients complaining of menorrhagia. Br J Obstet Gynaecol 1977;84:763–768.

46. Davies J. Hysteroscopic endometrial ablation with the neodymium:YAG laser. Br J Obstet Gynaecol 1989;96:928–932.

47. Lockwood M, Magos AL, Baumann R, Turnbull AC. Endometrial resection when hysterectomy is undesirable, dangerous, or impossible. Br J Obstet Gynaecol 1990;97:656–658.

48. Carlson KJ, Nichols DH, Schiff I. Indications for hysterectomy. N Engl J Med 1993;328:856–860.

CHAPTER 11

Prediction, Detection, and Evaluation of Ovulation

MARCELLE CEDARS

Ovulation appears to be a precisely timed event that is preceded and followed by multiple functional and morphologic changes involving the ovary, the hypothalamic-pituitary-ovarian axis, and the associated target organs. Documentation of ovulation becomes important in (1) evaluation of infertility, when as many as 20% to 25% of all infertile couples have an abnormality in ovulation; (2) treatment of infertility, when documentation of ovulation is needed to improve timing for insemination; and (3) natural family planning to avoid conception. The only definitive proof of ovulation is the occurrence of pregnancy or the recovery of the ovum from the fallopian tube. These "proofs" are obviously of limited usefulness clinically because a predictive method is desired. Presumptive evidence of ovulation may be obtained by taking advantage of those changes that occur in concert with ovulation. These changes can be primarily divided into two categories: clinical and hormonal. To be able to detect ovulation, it is essential to have an understanding of the normal menstrual cycle, as detailed in Chapter 9.

The hypothalamus, pituitary gland, ovary, and endometrium all function as coordinated elements in the cyclic reproductive system of the female mammal (Fig. 11–1) Any of the hormonal parameters or functional changes that occur during the normal menstrual cycle can be used as guides for the detection of ovulation.

TESTS BASED ON CLINICAL CHANGES

Clinical History

A careful history can be one of the best "tests" for the detection of ovulation. A history of *regular* (bleeding the same number of days ±2 each cycle), *cyclic* (interval the same number of days ±2 each cycle), and *predictable* (moliminal symptoms present) menses indicates ovulation is present in almost 98% of women.[1] As history-taking should be part of an initial visit, this simple task should not be overlooked.

However, as with most tests to detect ovulation, the history does not assess the adequacy of ovulation or luteal function.

Basal Body Temperature

The basal body temperature (BBT) undergoes a sustained rise of 0.3° to 0.5°F during the luteal phase. This shift in BBT is secondary to the thermoregulatory effect of progesterone at the hypothalamus and is associated with progesterone levels of 4 ng/mL or higher. For this reason the BBT follows the ovulatory peak of LH by approximately 2 days[1] and is employed by many clinicians as an inexpensive and easy method to detect ovulation. In most women, the biphasic pattern of BBT is indicative of ovulation (Fig. 11–2). However, there may be instances when ovulatory women exhibit a monophasic BBT chart.[2]

Practically speaking, obtaining an interpretable temperature chart may not be so easy. The woman must take her oral or rectal temperature for 5 minutes with a basal thermometer every morning on awakening before any physical activity. Six to eight hours of uninterrupted sleep is deemed necessary before the temperature is obtained. These restrictions, as well as the added stress placed on the infertile patient, make this "test" unappealing to some. When used for coital timing, it must be emphasized to patients that ovulation occurs prior to the elevation of temperature. Thus, BBT charts may be used only retrospectively to determine if ovulation occurred.

Adequacy of ovulation cannot be assessed solely by the BBT chart. However, the duration of temperature elevation has been used in an attempt to evaluate luteal phase function. Downs and Gibson[3] compared BBT charts of 20 infertile patients with biopsy-proven luteal phase defects (LPDs) with those of 20 patients with biopsy-confirmed normal luteal phases. None of the women with normal biopsy results had luteal phase lengths of less than 11 days. Only six of the patients with LPD, diagnosed by endometrial biopsy, had luteal lengths of less than 11 days. The investigators con-

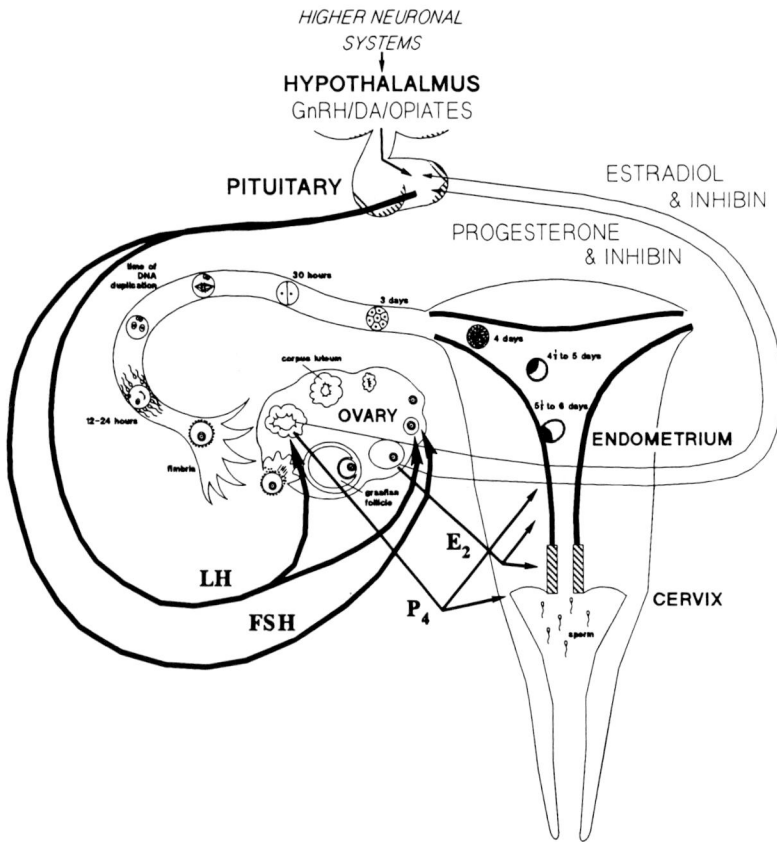

FIGURE 11–1. Diagrammatic scheme of the elements required for normal cyclic reproductive function. GnRH, gonadotropin-releasing hormone; DA, dopamine; LH, luteinizing hormone; FSH, follicle-stimulating hormone; E$_2$, estradiol; P$_4$, progesterone.

cluded that the duration of the temperature rise was not correlated with the presence of LPD. This information is consistent with the conclusion that either the BBT chart is not a sensitive indicator of luteal phase function or that there are two types of luteal phase inadequacy, one associated with a short luteal phase and one associated with a luteal phase of adequate length but inadequate function (see Chapter 17). In either instance, it is clear that the BBT chart cannot be used as the only test for luteal phase adequacy.

Cervical Mucus

The normal changes in cervical mucus quality and quantity have been used as part of natural family planning for many years. Estrogen stimulates the production of large amounts of

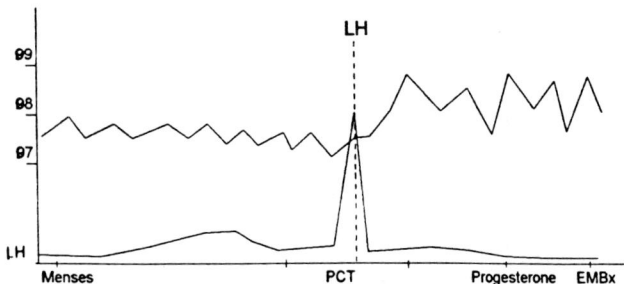

FIGURE 11–2. Diagrammatic representation of a normal menstrual cycle based on measurement of basal body temperature. The *dotted line* represents the peak of LH. LH, luteinizing hormone; PCT, postcoital test; EMBx, endometrial biopsy.

thin, watery, acellular, alkaline cervical mucus with ferning and spinnbarkeit (threadlike stretchability). Progesterone, on the other hand, inhibits the secretory activity of the cervical glands, resulting in thick, viscous mucus with low spinnbarkeit and absence of ferning. In 1972, Billings and associates[4] attempted to correlate changes in cervical mucus, as detected by the woman, with changes in gonadotropins and urinary estrogens and pregnanediol. Clear, "lubricative" mucus correlated closely with the day of ovulation as estimated from the hormonal measurements. The changes, however, occurred over several days and rarely coincided exactly with the surge of LH (see Fig. 11–2) Therefore, to determine the time of ovulation by assessing cervical mucus, serial examinations must be made at midcycle. The preovulatory peak in estrogen coincides with cervical mucorrhea. As progesterone levels increase, the mucus becomes scant and viscous. Testing should begin 1 to 3 days before expected ovulation. There may not always be adequate secretion of progesterone, as assessed by urinary pregnanediol, in the face of ovulatory mucus, again suggesting that this clinical symptom reveals more about estrogen secretion than adequacy of luteal function.

Knowledge of the composition of cervical mucus and the finding of a significant decrease in certain soluble proteins such as albumin,[5] α-antitrypsin,[6] and immunoglobulins[7] coincident with the time of peak cervical mucus changes and with ovulation have led to efforts to develop more sophisticated methods to evaluate cervical mucus and detect ovulation. For example, using laser nephelometry, a technique based on principles of light scattering, rapid measurement of immunoglobulins is possible. Mucus specimens, combined with 0.9% sodium chloride, are centrifuged for 15 minutes following a 30- to 45-second vortexing. Aliquots of the resultant mix may then be subjected to nephelometry. Cervical mucus in patients with normal ovulation contained predictable minima and maxima of both extractable immunoglobulins G and A, with the minimum amount of immunoglobulin being present at midcycle.[7] It has been suggested that this prospective method of determining ovulation may be advantageous in timing of intercourse or insemination, but confirmatory studies are needed.

Enzymes, such as alkaline phosphatase, esterase, aminopeptidase, amylase, lactate dehydrogenase, guaiacol peroxidase, and components of the fibrinolytic system, have been found in cervical mucus and appear to show cyclic variations coincident with ovulation.[8-11] The ability to develop simple dipstick-type assays for these enzymes may yield simple assays for home or office detection of ovulation in the future.

Endometrial Biopsy

The histologic determination of endometrial maturation according to the criteria of Noyes and colleagues[12] yields an integrated assessment of the effect of estrogen and progesterone on the endometrium (see Chapter 12). This test has been considered the gold standard in determining adequacy of luteal function and therefore the occurrence of normal ovulation. However, in one large, classic study, only 3% of the infertile population was found to have LPDs by this technique.[13] Therefore, the usage of this test to routinely assess luteal function in infertile women is considered overzealous and unnecessary by some clinicians. Also, the diagnosis of inadequate luteal phase cannot be made on the basis of a single biopsy, because 20% of fertile patients have a single out-of-phase biopsy, whereas only 3% have two consecutive endometrial biopsies out of phase and thus can be diagnosed as having a luteal phase abnormality.[14] The use of the endometrial biopsy to diagnose LPD remains the standard against which other tests are measured.

Interpretation of endometrial samples is hampered by variability in interpretation of the endometrial response. Shoupe and coworkers[15] demonstrated that endometrial dating correlates best with midcycle events, particularly with ultrasound documentation of maximal follicular diameter and less so with the LH surge and the rise in BBT charts. All these midcycle events resulted in better correlations with the findings on endometrial biopsy than did the onset of the next menstrual period. Excellent correlation has been noted between home urinary LH testing and ultrasonography or serum LH levels.[16] As a result, home self-testing of LH may provide an easy method of accurately dating the endometrial histology.

Endometrial sampling should occur approximately 12 days after the surge of LH is detected in the urine. If couples have not abstained from sexual relations, a sensitive test for human chorionic gonadotropin may be obtained prior to the biopsy even though the risk to an ongoing pregnancy of a single anterior wall biopsy is small. A small polypropylene cannula, which causes less discomfort, may be used, but it is important to note that a single study documented a significant difference in endometrial maturation when such a catheter was compared with a Novak curette.[17] Which instrument yields the most accurate results is not known, and a subsequent study[18] found no difference in results using the same two instruments.

Endometrial histology provides a useful bioassay of the effect of estrogen and progesterone during the menstrual cycle. The glands and stroma of the endometrium undergo predictable cyclic changes that demonstrate the influence of estrogen alone or estrogen and progesterone. The histologic findings are outlined in detail in Chapter 12. Any given endometrial biopsy can be assigned or "dated to" a certain day of the menstrual cycle based on these histologic changes.[12] Only changes more than 2 days behind those predicted are considered significant. Treatment should be considered only in those patients with repetitive delays in endometrial development.

Ultrasonography

Only in the last decade has the use of ultrasonography, particularly vaginal probe ultrasonography, become readily available to the gynecologist. The close proximity of the ovaries and uterus to the vaginal wall allows for the use of high-frequency vaginal probes, thus increasing the discriminatory ability of ultrasound. As a result, the gynecologist is able to obtain an accurate picture of the function, both physiologic and pathologic, of the ovary.

During the past decade, ultrasonography has been used to follow normal follicular growth patterns. Hackeloer and associates[19] were the first to demonstrate a positive correlation between follicular size and mean estradiol level. Renaud and colleagues[20] studied 18 spontaneous cycles and noted approximately 3 mm of growth per day in the preovulatory phase. Queenan and coworkers[21] found a rapid exponential growth in follicular diameter during the last 24 hours before ovulation. O'Herlihy and associates[22] described good correlation between ultrasonographic and laparoscopic measurements and noted a mean follicular diameter of 17 to 25 mm at the time of ovulation.

Using parameters of follicular development derived from the studies discussed earlier, Bryce and colleagues[23] showed that a maximal mean diameter of 20 mm was the best predictor of ovulation when compared with serum measurements of FSH, LH, and estradiol. They again noted the linear correlation between estradiol levels and follicular size before ovulation. A well-designed study, using couples at an artificial insemination clinic, suggested that a minimum diameter of 18 mm is required for conception, with most pregnancies occurring with a diameter of 20 mm or larger.[24]

The use of ultrasonography to assess the ovulatory process requires serial examinations to document normal follicular growth and subsequent disappearance of the follicle with the formation of a corpus luteum (Fig. 11-3). As a result, it may be of benefit to those patients with unexplained infertility or documented LPD. For routine ovulation detection, this form of testing is not only inconvenient for the patient but also expensive.

As early as 1983, Geisthövel and coworkers[25] demonstrated smaller maximal diameters for the dominant follicles in "insufficient" cycles. More recently, Ying and coworkers[26] evaluated patients with luteal phase inadequacy before and after treatment. They detected a spectrum of disorders in

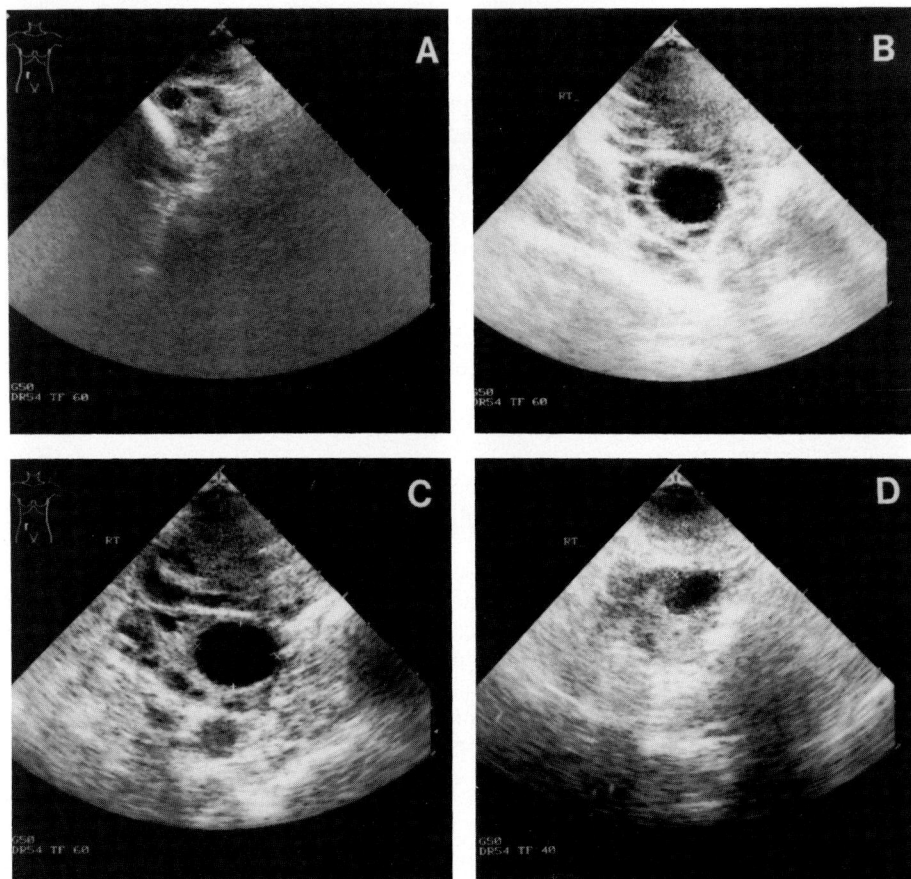

FIGURE 11–3. Sequential views obtained by transvaginal ultrasound of a follicle's development and collapse following ovulation during a normal menstrual cycle. *A*, 6 days before ovulation; follicle measured 16 × 14 mm. *B*, 3 days before ovulation; follicle measured 21 × 18 mm. *C*, 1 day before ovulation; follicle measured 23 × 21 mm. *D*, Follicular collapse indicating ovulation (day 0).

follicular development and rupture associated with LPD, consistent with the conclusion that some luteal disorders are the result of inadequate follicular phase development. Hamilton and colleagues,[27] in comparing patients with unexplained infertility to normal volunteers, found a smaller maximal follicle diameter on day −1 (relative to the LH surge) and a greater likelihood for luteal phase cyst formation in the patients with unexplained infertility. None of the subjects underwent an endometrial biopsy, but the ultrasound changes noted, minimal as they were, correlated with lower progesterone production and other indices suggestive of LPD (see Chapter 17).

The introduction of color-flow Doppler into vaginal ultrasonography has allowed the study of changes in intrafollicular morphology and blood flow during the periovulatory period.[28, 29] Changes in blood flow to the follicle are visible and correlate with the surge of LH. Although clearly a research tool at this time, this information allows for noninvasive documentation of previously described morphologic changes in the ovary coincident with the normal process of ovulation.

When using ultrasonography to assess ovulatory function, serial examinations should begin 3 or 4 days before the expected day of ovulation. Evaluation should be repeated every 2 days until a mean follicular diameter of 15 mm is noted, after which daily scanning should be performed until evidence of ovulation. Ovulation is documented by at least two of the following: (1) a decrease in follicular diameter; (2) blurring of the follicular border; (3) presence of internal echoes; and (4) free fluid in the cul-de-sac. Follicular diameter is expected to be at least 18 mm before normal ovulation.

Recently, ultrasonography also has been used to assess endometrial adequacy noninvasively. Available evidence, most of which has been obtained during cycles with controlled ovarian hyperstimulation, only supports a requirement for a minimum thickness of 9 mm at ovulation for pregnancy to occur and suggests an increase in spontaneous pregnancy loss with a thickness of more than 13 mm.[30] Further studies are needed to correlate endometrial thickness with endometrial biopsy in the natural cycle and to determine the variability inherent in the measurement of endometrial thickness.

TESTS BASED ON HORMONAL ASSAYS

Based on knowledge of the normal menstrual cycle, useful hormonal determinations include measurement of estrogens, LH, and progesterone. These hormones or their metabolites can be measured in serum, urine, or saliva, and each of these are considered independently. A composite illustration of the temporal pattern of secretion of each hormone is seen in Figure 11–4.[31] Figure 11–5 illustrates changes in follicular diameter and endometrial thickness correlated with urinary metabolites of estrogen and progesterone.

Estrogens

Serum estradiol levels exhibit a progressive rise throughout the follicular phase, reaching a peak coincident with the

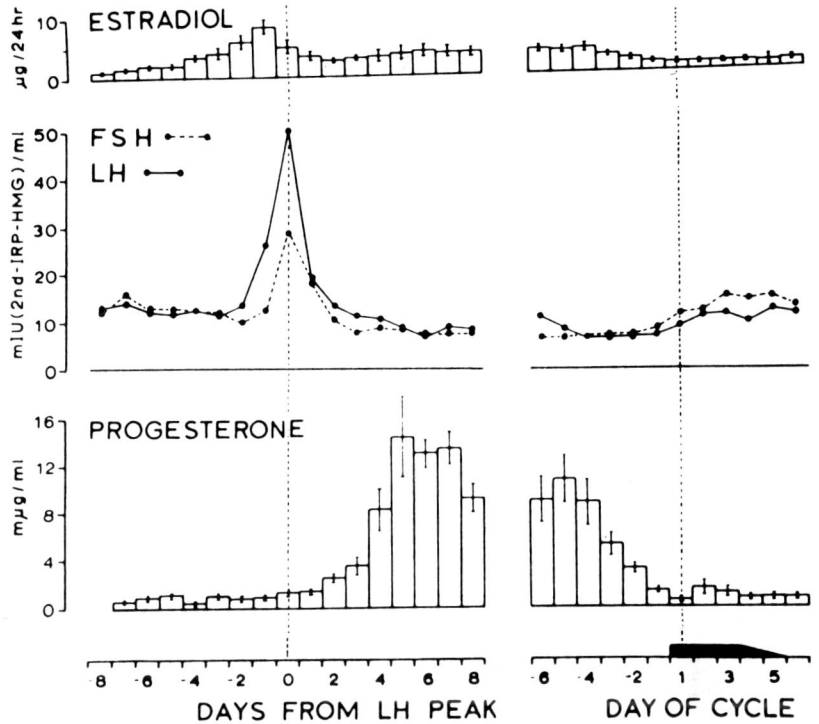

FIGURE 11–4. Levels of ovarian estrogen and progesterone in relation to pituitary hormones during the normal menstrual cycle. (From Ross GT, et al. Pituitary and gonadal hormones in women during spontaneous and induced ovulatory cycles. Recent Prog Horm Res 1970; 26:1.)

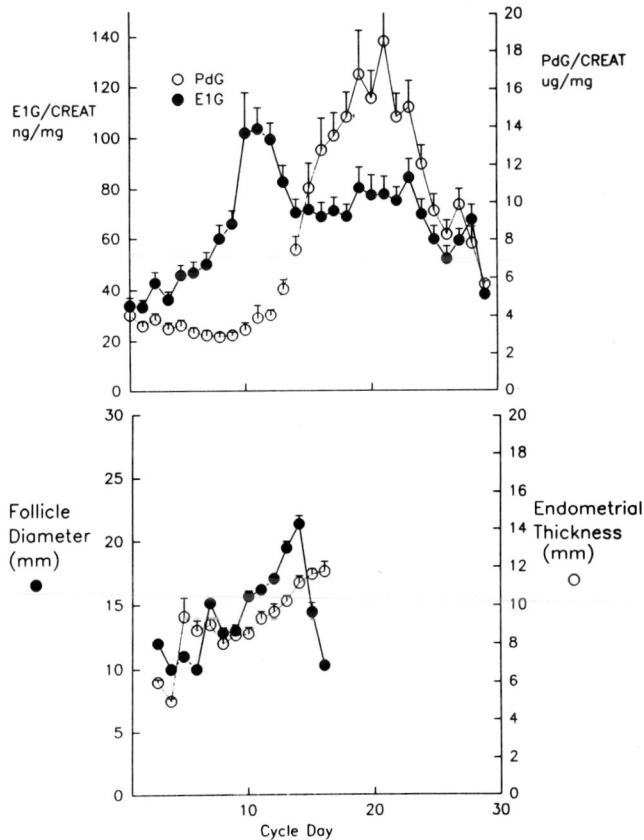

FIGURE 11–5. Concentrations of estrone glucuronide (E_1G) and pregnanediol glucuronide (PdG) in early-morning urine samples from 45 normally cycling women over an entire menstrual cycle. Ultrasound documentation of follicular growth and collapse, along with endometrial thickness, is shown in the lower panel. CREAT, creatinine. (Cedars M and Liu J, unpublished data.)

abrupt onset of the LH surge and 36 hours before ovulation (see Fig. 11–4). Daily blood sampling can therefore yield some idea of the time of ovulation. This monitoring is obviously cumbersome and expensive. However, the ability to measure estradiol metabolites in the *urine* has allowed the assessment of this hormonal endpoint to achieve some clinical applicability. Great interest has been directed in this area with particular reference to natural family planning and the avoidance of "fertile" periods. Clearly, an accurate diagnostic test also would be applicable to those seeking to achieve pregnancy.

In 1980, Stanczyk and colleagues[32] performed direct radioimmunoassay using specific antisera of urinary estrogen metabolites, including estrone glucuronide (E_1G), estradiol-3-glucuronide (E_2-3G), estradiol-17β-glucuronide (E_2-17G), estriol-3-glucuronide (E_3-3G), and estriol-16β-glucuronide (E_3-16G). Excretion of E_2-17G exhibited the earliest and steepest ascending slope for the preovulatory estrogen surge and correlated best with serum estradiol levels. Urinary excretion of E_1G, E_2-3G, and E_3-16G also showed early and steep preovulatory rises. These findings were consistent regardless of whether 24-hour or simple overnight urinary samples were used in the assays. Correlation with serum levels was improved by measuring creatinine levels in all samples. However, the correlation of even overnight specimens was sufficiently high so as to allow assessment without the need for this correction.

In an effort to facilitate steroid hormone determination, a simple, nonradiometric assay, the enzyme immunoassay (EIA), has been developed for the measurement of urinary steroid metabolites.[33, 34] In an attempt to further develop the EIA to be used in a nonlaboratory environment, a noninstrumented EIA for urinary estrone conjugates has been adapted from the instrumented microliter plate technique.[35] Parallel profiles were found between serum and urinary levels. As shown in Figure 11–5, urinary estrogen metabolites peak approximately 36 to 48 hours before the ovulatory collapse of the dominant follicle.

Progesterone

One of the most widely used diagnostic techniques for the detection of ovulation is the measurement of progesterone. *Serum* progesterone levels higher than 4 ng/mL are consistent with the presumptive diagnosis of ovulation.[36] This value yields little information about the adequacy of the luteal phase. Although it is true that inadequate production of progesterone by the corpus luteum results in LPD, there has been great controversy about the reliability of a single determination to make this diagnosis. A progesterone level of approximately 10 ng/mL has been suggested to be representative of a potentially fertile cycle and thus "normal" ovulation.[37] However, many authors have questioned the acceptability of such a single, simple cutoff value. Daya and Ward[38] found very low sensitivity and specificity for a single midluteal serum progesterone level in the prediction of LPD as diagnosed by endometrial biopsy. Daya[39] subsequently suggested that improved sensitivity and specificity could be achieved with measurement of late luteal phase (day 25 to 26) progesterone levels. One of the most compelling reasons to avoid the use of a single random sample of progesterone is the presence of documented circadian and ultradian rhythms in progesterone secretion.[40–43] Another confounding element is the inherent variability of the progesterone assay itself.

The inability of a single serum progesterone value to yield predictive results with respect to luteal phase adequacy has led some authors to suggest obtaining serial progesterone determinations. Abraham and coworkers[44] noted that the sum of three progesterone levels, obtained every other day during the midluteal phase, was never less than 15 ng/mL in the face of normal ovulation. Multiple daily serum levels of progesterone with calculation of an integrated value appears to be an accurate indicator of luteal function,[45] although the logistical problems of inconvenience and cost may be prohibitive. Daily or more frequent sampling may serve as a research tool but is not practical for routine patient management.

The measurement of *urinary metabolites* of progesterone obviates the need for frequent patient office visits and provides an integrated measurement via the collection of 24-hour or overnight urinary specimens. A simple radioimmunoassay for pregnanediol using ^{3}H-20α-hydroxy-4-pregnen-3-one as the radioligand and applied to a single morning voided specimen was first developed by Chatterton and colleagues[46] in 1982 and validated in normal cycling women. Subsequent use of this assay in women with known LPD revealed no difference in total excretion of pregnanediol when compared with women with normal endometrial findings.[47] However, significantly less pregnanediol was excreted by the LPD group during the first 5 days of the luteal phase, suggesting a delay in progesterone secretion in these women. Nonradiometric assays, as described for urinary estrogens, also have been developed for urinary progesterone metabolites.[34]

Although the rise in E_1G correlates best with follicular growth and the peak with the ovulatory surge and the fertile period, it is the decrease in E_1G and subsequent rapid increase in pregnanediol that heralds the luteal phase. These known parameters and their predictable sequence allow for improved natural family planning,[48] but their usefulness in routine detection of ovulation, or evaluation or treatment of infertility, remains to be seen.

Salivary concentrations of steroids reflect the free fraction in plasma and appear to correlate well with serum levels. Salivary measurements have the advantages of easier collection, presumed independence from flow rate, and the possibility that secretory peaks noted in serum are absent. Concentrations of steroids in the saliva are only 1% to 3% of those noted in serum, but the advent of sensitive assay systems has made salivary steroid measurement an attractive alternative.[49]

Daily measurement of salivary progesterone during the luteal phase appears to yield a threshold level above which normal luteal function can be predicted. Using serum progesterone levels and BBT charts[50] or morphometric studies of the endometrium[51] for the diagnosis of LPD, two studies were able to separate those patients with presumed normal ovulatory function from those with defective luteal function by measurement of salivary progesterone. Both studies however, found the evaluation of salivary progesterone levels adequate only to detect gross defects in ovulatory function.

More recently, a study evaluating salivary progesterone levels in women with unexplained infertility found a variety of disturbances, including lower overall secretion of or a preovulatory rise in progesterone, falls in progesterone secretion during the luteal phase, and abnormal elevations at the beginning of menstruation.[52] Seventy percent of the cycles in patients with unexplained infertility in this study had some abnormality in the progesterone profile compared with only 15% of the control cycles. This finding again suggests that there may be a high incidence of LPD in women otherwise diagnosed as having unexplained infertility. However, given the presence of abnormal endometrial development in women in the presence of normal progesterone profiles,[51] further studies are needed before routine application of this assay for infertility management.

Luteinizing Hormone

Radioimmunoassay of LH in the *serum* has been possible since the late 1960s. Daily measurement accurately predicts the timing of ovulation but is clearly burdensome for patients and requires considerable laboratory time and equipment. Even more precise distinctions can be made about luteal phase adequacy by frequent sampling and LH measurement. Abnormal patterns of LH pulsatility,[53] as well as a subnormal midcycle surge and abnormal levels of bioactive LH during the luteal phase,[54] may be detected and perhaps give some clue as to the cause of the luteal phase inadequacy. Clearly, however, these tools remain in the realm of the research environment.

Measurement of *urinary* LH offers a practical alternative to daily serum sampling and diminishes the effect of episodic LH secretion. The development of nonradiometric EIAs has allowed for the simple, rapid determination of urinary LH

TABLE 11–1. Methods of Detecting Ovulation

Fertility
Ovulatory status
  Clinical history
  Midluteal progesterone level
  LH surge (urinary)
  Ultrasound follicular dynamics
  BBT
  Cervical mucus changes
Timing of intervention
  LH surge (urinary)
  Ultrasound follicular dynamics
Assessment of "adequacy" of ovulation (endometrial receptivity)
  Endometrial biopsy
  Future directions
    PEP
    Ultrasound assessment of endometrium
Fertility Control
  Urinary metabolites
  Cervical mucus changes
  BBT

LH, luteinizing hormone; BBT, basal body temperature; PEP, progestogen-associated endometrial protein.

secretion. Dipstick-type test kits are available for home use. These test kits, when used once or twice a day, are accurate in more than 85% of cycles in determining the timing and occurrence of ovulation.[16] The predictive ability of different test methods may vary, and patients need to be made aware and directed toward those with the best correlations with ovulation. Although these kits predict the time of ovulation with relative accuracy, their efficacy relative to an improvement in fecundity rates is still doubtful.[55]

Urinary LH testing was originally intended for use every 2 to 4 hours around the clock to detect the peak of the LH surge. This is obviously impractical. We now have patients test every 24 hours at the same time of the day. Testing should begin 3 or 4 days before the expected day of ovulation. During the midcycle surge, the increase of LH appearing in the urine follows that occurring in the blood by about 12 hours. Daily testing therefore allows detection of the LH surge within 12 to 24 hours after its onset. A clear color change in the urinary dipstick indicates ovulation will occur 12 to 24 hours in the future and thus allows fertility intervention to be performed on a prospective basis.

Alternative Assays

PROGESTOGEN-ASSOCIATED ENDOMETRIAL PROTEIN

Joshi[56] demonstrated in 1983 that gestational-phase endometrium synthesizes and secretes a specific glycoprotein designated *progestogen-associated endometrial protein* (PEP). More recently, Joshi's group[57] measured serum concentrations of PEP in an attempt to noninvasively identify patients with inadequacies of endometrial function. They found serum levels of PEP reflected the stage of endometrial maturation as determined by histologic evaluation. Furthermore, 83% of women with inadequate endometrium by standard criteria had serum PEP levels below the 95% confidence interval compared with only 16% of those women with adequate endometrium. More data are needed to determine if this

technique will adequately replace established methods of ovulation detection and diagnosis of LPD.

SUMMARY

A knowledge of the hormonal and physical characteristics of the menstrual cycle has led to the development of many tests for the detection of ovulation and the possibility for assessing ovulatory "adequacy." As discussed in the introduction, the applicability of any method is determined by its expected application and its ease of use.

Table 11–1 lists the available methods for the detection of ovulation and the role each may play in patient management. Some couples may ultimately require more than one of these detection methods.

The best currently available techniques for conception avoidance appear to involve the measurement of urinary metabolites of estrogen and progesterone. For those physicians working with couples attempting to achieve pregnancy, the options are more varied and the selection less clear. For the simple separation of those patients who ovulate from those who do not, a careful history may be the most efficient and certainly the least expensive. For timing of ovulatory events such as inseminations, the usage of home urinary LH testing, perhaps with the addition of judicial usage of ultrasonography, may be most appropriate.

Determination of luteal phase adequacy represents a much greater challenge. Continued research in this area will assess if endometrial biopsy remains the gold standard or may be replaced by less invasive alternatives.

REFERENCES

1. Magyar DM, Boyers SP, Marshall JR, Abraham GE. Regular menstrual cycles and premenstrual molimina as indicators of ovulation. Obstet Gynecol 1979;53:411.
2. Johansson EDB, Larsson-Cohn U, Gemzell C. Monophasic basal body temperature in ovulatory menstrual cycles. Am J Obstet Gynecol 1972;113:933.
3. Downs KA, Gibson M. Basal body temperature graph and the luteal phase defect. Fertil Steril 1983;40:466.
4. Billings EL, Brown JB, Billings JJ, Burger HG. Symptoms and hormonal changes accompanying ovulation. Lancet 1972;1:282.
5. Moghissi KS. Cyclic changes of cervical mucus in normal and progestin-treated women. Fertil Steril 1966;17:663.
6. Schumacher GFB, Yang SL. Cyclic changes of immunoglobulins and specific antibodies in human and rhesus monkey cervical mucus. In: Insler V, Bettendorf G, editors. The Uterine Cervix in Reproduction. Stuttgart: Thieme, 1977:187.
7. Davis KP, Maciulla GJ, Yannone ME, et al. Cervical mucus immunoglobulins as an indicator of ovulation. Obstet Gynecol 1983;62:388.
8. Trefes C, Vincenzini MT, Vanni P, et al. Changes in enzyme levels in human cervical mucus during the menstrual cycle. Int J Fertil 1986;3:59.
9. Moghissi KS, Syner FN, Borin B. Cyclic changes of cervical mucus enzymes related to the time of ovulation: I. Alkaline phosphatase. Am J Obstet Gynecol 1976;125:1044.
10. Moghissi KS, Syner FN, Borin B. Cyclic changes of cervical mucus enzymes related to the time of ovulation: II. Aminopeptidase and esterase. Obstet Gynecol 1976;48:347.
11. Takehisa T. Lactate dehydrogenase in human cervical mucus: correlation with ovulation, influence of ovarian steroid hormones, and isozyme pattern. Fertil Steril 1980;33:135.
12. Noyes RW, Hertig AT, Rock J. Dating the endometrial biopsy. Fertil Steril 1950;1:3.
13. Jones GES, Pourmand K. An evaluation of etiologic factors and therapy in 555 private patients with primary infertility. Fertil Steril 1962;13:398.

14. Rosenberg SM, Luciano AA, Riddick DH. The luteal phase defect: the relative frequency of, and encouraging response to, treatment with vaginal progesterone. Fertil Steril 1980;34:17.

15. Shoupe D, Mishell DR Jr, LaCarra M et al. Correlation of endometrial maturation with four methods of estimating day of ovulation. Obstet Gynecol 1989;73:88.

16. Vermesh M, Kletzky OA, Davajan V, et al. Monitoring techniques to predict and detect ovulation. Fertil Steril 1987;46:259.

17. Honore LH, Cumming DC, Fahmy N. Significant difference in the frequency of out-of-phase biopsies depending on the use of the Novak curette or the flexible polypropylene endometrial biopsy cannula ("Pipelle"). Gynecol Obstet Invest 1988;26:338.

18. Hill GA, Herbert CM, Parker RA, Wentz AC. Comparison of late luteal phase endometrial biopsies using the Novak curette or Pipelle endometrial suction curette. Obstet Gynecol 1989;73:443.

19. Hackeloer BJ, Fleming R, Robinson JP, et al. Correlation of ultrasonic and endocrinologic assessment of human follicular development. Am J Obstet Gynecol 1979;135:122.

20. Renaud RL, Macler J, Dervain I, et al. Echographic study of follicular maturation and ovulation during the normal menstrual cycle. Fertil Steril 1980;33:272.

21. Queenan JT, O'Brien GD, Bains LM, et al. Ultrasound scanning of ovaries to detect ovulation in women. Fertil Steril 1980;34:99.

22. O'Herlihy C, de Crespigny LCH, Lopata A, et al. Preovulatory follicular size: a comparison of ultrasound and laparoscopic measurements. Fertil Steril 1980;34:24.

23. Bryce RL, Shuter B, Sinosich JF, et al. The value of ultrasound, gonadotropin, and estradiol measurements for precise ovulation prediction. Fertil Steril 1982;37:42.

24. Marinho AO, Hassan N, Goessens KV, et al. Real-time pelvic ultrasonography during the peri-ovulatory period of patients attending an artificial insemination clinic. Fertil Steril 1982;37:633.

25. Geisthövel F, Skubsch U, Zabel G, et al. Ultrasonographic and hormonal studies in physiologic and insufficient menstrual cycles. Fertil Steril 1983;39:277.

26. Ying K, Daly D, Randolph RF, et al. Ultrasonographic monitoring of follicular growth for luteal phase defects. Fertil Steril 1987;48:433.

27. Hamilton MPR, Fleming R, Coutts JRT, et al. Luteal phase deficiency: ultrasonic and biochemical insights into pathogenesis. Br J Obstet Gynaecol 1990;97:569.

28. Collins WP, Jurkovic D, Bourne T, et al. Ovarian morphology, endocrine function, and intrafollicular blood flow during the periovulatory period. Hum Reprod 1991;6:319.

29. Bourne TH, Jurkovic D, Waterstone J, et al. Intrafollicular blood flow during human ovulation. Ultrasound Obstet Gynecol 1991;1:63.

30. Dickey RP, Olar TT, Curole DN, et al. Endometrial pattern and thickness associated with pregnancy outcome after assisted reproduction. Hum Reprod 1992;7:418.

31. Ross GT, Cargille CM, Lipsett MB, et al. Pituitary and gonadal hormones in women during spontaneous and induced ovulatory cycles: Gregory Pincus Memorial Lecture. Recent Prog Horm Res 1970;26:1.

32. Stanczyk FZ, Miyakawa I, Goebelsmann U. Direct radioimmunoassay of urinary estrogen and pregnanediol glucuronides during the menstrual cycle. Am J Obstet Gynecol 1980;137:443.

33. Czekala NM, Galluser S, Meier J, Lasley BL. The development and application of and enzyme assay for estrone conjugates. Zool Biol 1986;6:1.

34. Munro CJ, Stabenfeldt GH, Cragun JR, et al. Relationship of serum estradiol and progesterone concentrations to the excretion profiles of their major urinary metabolites as measured by enzyme immunoassay and radioimmunoassay. Clin Chem 1991;37:838.

35. Lasley BL, Shideler SE, Munro CJ. A prototype for ovulation detection: pros and cons. Am J Obstet Gynecol 1991;165:2003.

36. Israel R, Mishell DR, Stone SC, et al. Single luteal phase serum progesterone assay as an indicator of ovulation. Am J Obstet Gynecol 1972;112:1043.

37. Hull MGR, Savage PE, Bromham DR, et al. The value of a single serum progesterone measurement in the midluteal phase as a criterion of a potentially fertile cycle ("ovulation") derived from treated and untreated conception cycles. Fertil Steril 1982;37:355.

38. Daya S, Ward S. Diagnostic test properties of serum progesterone in the evaluation of luteal phase defects. Fertil Steril 1988;49:168.

39. Daya S. Optimal time in the menstrual cycle for serum progesterone measurement to diagnose luteal phase defects. Am J Obstet Gynecol 161;1009, 1989.

40. Filicori M, Butler JP, Crowley WF. Neuroendocrine regulation of the corpus luteum in the human: evidence for pulsatile progesterone secretion. J Clin Invest 1984;73:1638.

41. Syrop CH, Hammond MG. Diurnal variations in midluteal serum progesterone measurements. Fertil Steril 1987;47:67.

42. Veldhuis JD, Christiansen E, Evans WS, et al. Physiological profiles of episodic progesterone release during the midluteal phase of the human menstrual cycle: analysis of circadian and ultradian rhythms, discrete pulse properties, and correlations with simultaneous luteinizing hormone release. J Clin Endocrinol Metab 1988;66:414.

43. Fujimoto VY, Clifton DK, Cohen NL, Soules MR. Variability of serum prolactin and progesterone levels in normal women: the relevance of single hormone measurements in the clinical setting. Obstet Gynecol 1990;76:71.

44. Abraham GE, Maroulis GB, Marshall JR. Evaluation of ovulation and corpus luteum function using measurements of plasma progesterone. Obstet Gynecol 1974;44:522.

45. Wu CH, Minassian SS. The integrated luteal progesterone: an assessment of luteal function. Fertil Steril 1987;48:937.

46. Chatterton RT, Haan JN, Jenco JM, Cheesman KL. Radioimmunoassay of pregnanediol concentrations in early morning urine specimens for assessment of luteal function in women. Fertil Steril 1982;37:361.

47. Miller MM, Hoffman DI, Creinin M, et al. Comparison of endometrial biopsy and urinary pregnanediol glucuronide concentration in the diagnosis of luteal phase defect. Fertil Steril 1990;54:1008.

48. Brown JB, Blackwell LF, Holmes J, Smyth K. New assays for identifying the fertile period. Int J Gynecol Obstet 1989;19Suppl):111.

49. Riad-Fahmy D, Read GF, Walker RF, Griffiths K. Steroids in saliva for assessing endocrine function. Endocr Rev 1982;3:367.

50. Walker RF, Wilson DW, Truran PL, et al. Characterization of profiles of salivary progesterone concentrations during the luteal phase of fertile and subfertile women. J Endocrinol 1985;104:441.

51. Li TC, Lenton EA, Dockery P, et al. The relation between daily salivary progesterone profile and endometrial development in the luteal phase of fertile and infertile women. Br J Obstet Gynaecol 1989;96:445.

52. Vuorento T, Hovatta O, Kurunmaki H, et al. Measurements of salivary progesterone concentrations throughout the menstrual cycle in women suffering from unexplained infertility reveal high frequency of luteal phase defects. Fertil Steril 1990;54:211.

53. Soules MR, Steiner RA, Clifton DK, et al. Abnormal patterns of pulsatile luteinizing hormone in women with luteal phase deficiency. Obstet Gynecol 1984;63:626.

54. Soules MR, McLachlan RI, Ek M, et al. Luteal phase deficiency: characterization of reproductive hormones over the menstrual cycle. J Clin Endocrinol Metab 1989;69:804.

55. Corson GH, Ghazi D, Kemmann E. Home urinary luteinizing hormone immunoassays: clinical applications. Fertil Steril 1990;53:591.

56. Joshi SG. Progestin-regulated proteins of the human endometrium. Semin Reprod Endocrinol 1983;1:221.

57. Joshi SG, Rao R, Henriques EE, et al. Luteal phase concentrations of a progestogen-associated endometrial protein (PEP) in the serum of cycling women with adequate or inadequate endometrium. J Clin Endocrinol 1986;63:1247.

CHAPTER 12

The Endometrial Biopsy

TIM H. PARMLEY

The endometrium of infertile women has been "dated" since 1937[1] and used to diagnose luteal phase defects since 1949.[2] Both the clinical entity and the practice of dating the endometrium have been controversial for the entire time. Of the many sources of this controversy, at least four relate directly to the endometrial biopsy and are the subject of this chapter. They are

1. The technical requirements for an adequate biopsy specimen.
2. The accuracy with which an adequate biopsy specimen can be interpreted.
3. The clinical meaning of an accurately interpreted biopsy specimen.
4. The observer's definition of the word *accurate*.

While exploring these controversies, this chapter also reviews the pertinent history of each.

TECHNICAL REQUIREMENTS FOR AN ADEQUATE ENDOMETRIAL BIOPSY SPECIMEN

Biopsy specimens should be taken from functional endometrium. Maximal physiologic development of the endometrium takes place over the middle of the anterior and posterior walls of the uterus. The lower uterine segment, the sides of the cavity, and the top of the fundus may possess endometrial surfaces that are less well developed at any given point in the cycle. Under normal circumstances, the lower uterine segment is probably the only one of the less well developed sites sampled by a biopsy instrument.

Although a complete transverse section of a secretory endometrium routinely reveals that the anterior and posterior walls are better developed than the sides, this point is not the least of the controversies surrounding this issue. Noyes[3] wrote that uniformity of the secretory endometrium was a basic assumption in dating endometrial biopsy specimens that needed to be studied. He interpreted biopsy specimens obtained from four sites in 100 patients and reported that secretory endometrium displayed uniform development. His data, however, reveal that uniformity is a matter of definition. Using one of the four biopsy specimens as a standard and

computing the standard deviations (SDs) of the other three specimens, he found that

1. About 30% of the time, the SD was greater than half a day.
2. About 45% of the time, it was no greater than 1 day.
3. Close to 20% of the time, the SD was no greater than 1.5 days.
4. About 5% of the time, it was greater than 1.5 days.

If 2 SDs is the normal limit of variation, 25% of the time biopsy specimens from one area of the endometrium differ from specimens taken elsewhere by 2 days. Such differences are, of course, clinically significant. Noyes recognized that some readers might find these differences outside their own definition of uniform, and he pointed out that "What is demonstrated here is relative uniformity. In a biologic system absolute uniformity is not to be expected."[3]

Operator technique is important. Pathologists learn that good biopsy specimens are consistently sent to the laboratory by some operators and not by others. Errors in interpretation occur when a biopsy specimen does not contain sufficient intact tissue for the pathologist to distinguish a surface and deeper portions of the endometrium's functional zone.

As soon and as atraumatically as possible, biopsy specimens should be transferred to fixative. The endometrium is soft, and any technique that involves scraping or poking the tissue crushes it. Instruments such as the Pipelle Endometrial Suction Curette (Unimar, Wilton, CT) can provide good biopsy specimens, not only because they obtain adequate tissue samples to begin with, but also because they eliminate much operator handling in the transfer of the tissue.[4]

The fixative used can alter results. Details of cellular morphology are important in interpreting the epithelial changes that accompany the early secretory phase as well as in interpreting the stromal changes that characterize the late secretory phase. Both are more difficult to interpret with fixatives such as formalin, which produce cytoplasmic shrinkage of decidual cells, condensation of mitoses, or clumping of secretory products. For the endometrium, Bouin's solution is the fixative of choice, but most laboratories rely on buffered formalin for economic reasons. When routine hematoxylin and eosin sections are prepared from paraffin blocks, the tissue should be sectioned thinly enough to allow for the interpretation of individual cells.

When the histologic sections are examined, the basics are most commonly omitted.

1. Is the biopsy specimen large enough, intact enough, and free enough of artifact to be interpretable?

2. Is the biopsy specimen from a reactive portion of the endometrium?

3. Are both a zona compacta and a zona spongiosa present?

4. Does the tissue lack obvious abnormalities, such as inflammation or focal areas of nonresponse suggesting polyps? (See Fig. 12–1.)

If the answer is not yes to all these questions, the biopsy specimen cannot be satisfactorily interpreted, and attempts to do so may result in errors. Failure to take these basic factors into account has been a persistent problem. Noyes[3] gave detailed examples to illustrate that much of the reported variation in his study of endometrial uniformity could be attributed to errors in interpretation, caused by these factors. Scott and associates[5] demonstrated anew that this problem persists. Among the factors perpetuating such errors is that when the uninterpretable nature of a particular biopsy specimen is communicated to the clinician, the most frequent response is a request for "the best estimate you can give me." Such a request is a clinical error because even if the pathologist responds, the estimate is meaningless.

INTERPRETATION

Interpretation is based on the description of Noyes and colleagues.[6] A summary follows.

In the immediate postmenstrual phase, the endometrium is repairing itself. The basalis contains simple glands lined with pseudostratified, columnar epithelium. These glands are embedded in a cellular stroma of mononuclear and fibroblas-

tic cells. Stromal tissue nearer the surface contains a few fragments of clumped necrotic cells and an associated inflammatory infiltrate. The epithelium lining some of the superficial glands is secretory, reflecting the previous cycle. The surface epithelium may be composed of flattened metaplastic cells with abundant eosinophilic cytoplasm. This is new or repairing epithelium. Old epithelium may reveal apoptosis. This state of repair is quickly transformed into a truly proliferating endometrium. The necrotic fragments of stroma, as well as the secretory and repairing epithelia, are all removed.

Proliferative endometrium displays the histology of simple growth. The cells, of all types, consist of nuclei with minimal cytoplasm (Fig. 12–2). Mitoses are frequent in the developing upper portion of the glands and stroma. Straight tubular glands embedded in a loose matrix result from this growth (Fig. 12–3). Glandular epithelium is pseudostratified and columnar. Fibroblasts and mononuclear cells make up the stroma. Occasionally, small subnuclear vacuoles appear in the epithelial cells of endometrium that has been stimulated only by estrogen, but they are small and sharply angulated. There is some increase in stromal edema in the midproliferative phase, but this observation is not a reliable microscopic feature.

With ovulation and rising progesterone levels, epithelial cells in the most reactive portion of the endometrium begin to accumulate subnuclear glycogen (Fig. 12–4). The most reactive portion of the endometrium is the middle portion of the tubular glands in the middle of the anterior and posterior walls of the uterine cavity. The basal portion of the glands does not respond, and the most superficial portion tends to respond slowly.

On the second postovulatory day, day 16 of the 28-day cycle, subnuclear vacuoles are widespread in the epithelium of the glands. By day 17, these vacuoles form a consistent subnuclear layer, uniformly elevating the nuclei to the middle of the cell (Fig. 12–5). On day 18, the vacuoles slip past the

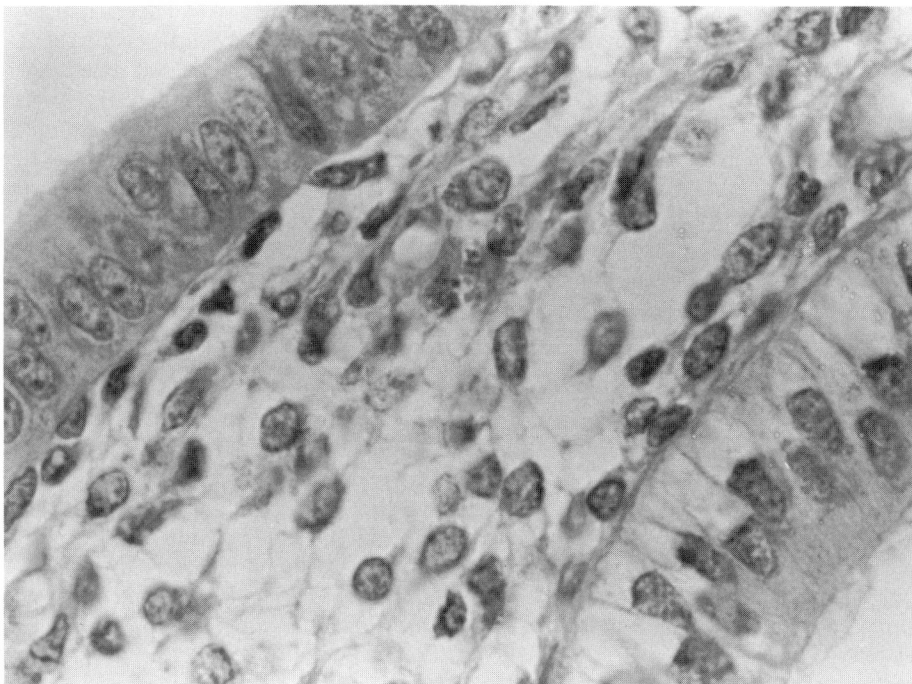

FIGURE 12–1. Well-developed secretory epithelium lines the gland below. However, the gland above is unresponsive and has not undergone any secretory change.

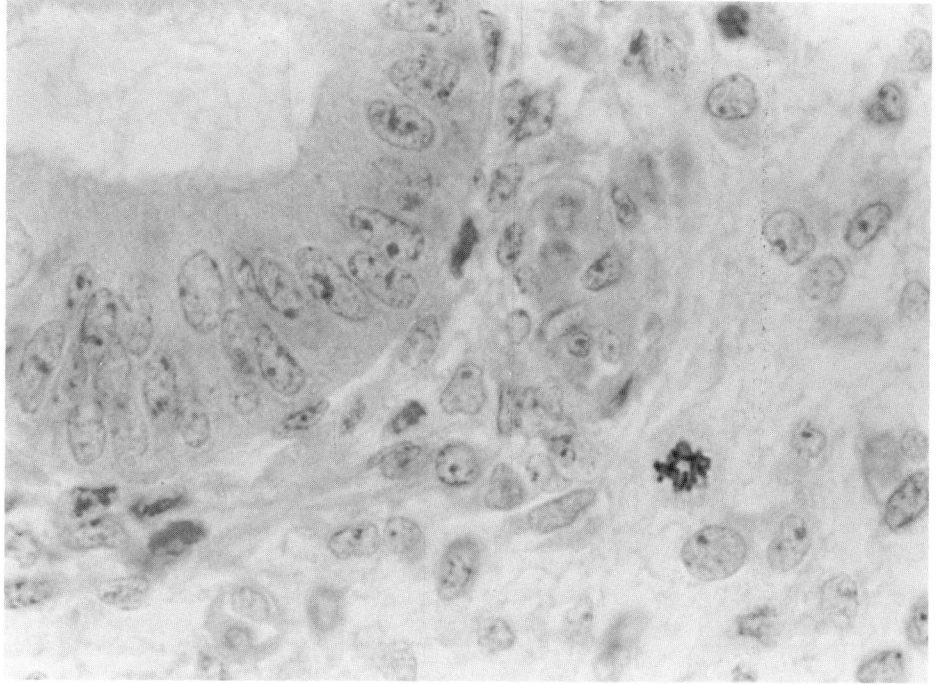

FIGURE 12–2. The gland cells are largely undifferentiated with large nucleus:cytoplasm ratios. The epithelium is pseudostratified. The stromal cells are also largely undifferentiated and most are spindle shaped. A mitosis is present.

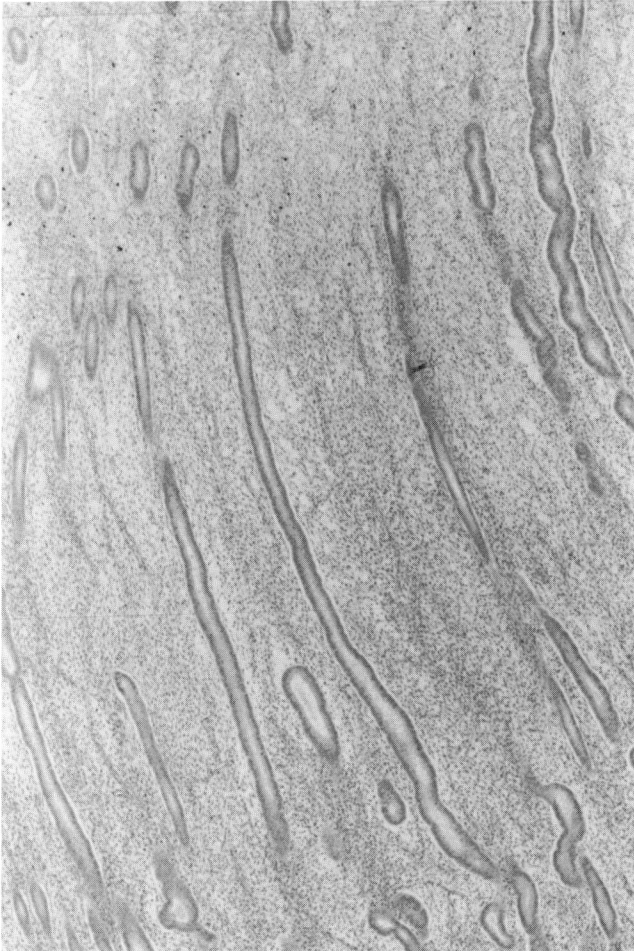

FIGURE 12–3. Long tubular glands extend from the basalis to the new surface. The stroma is loose.

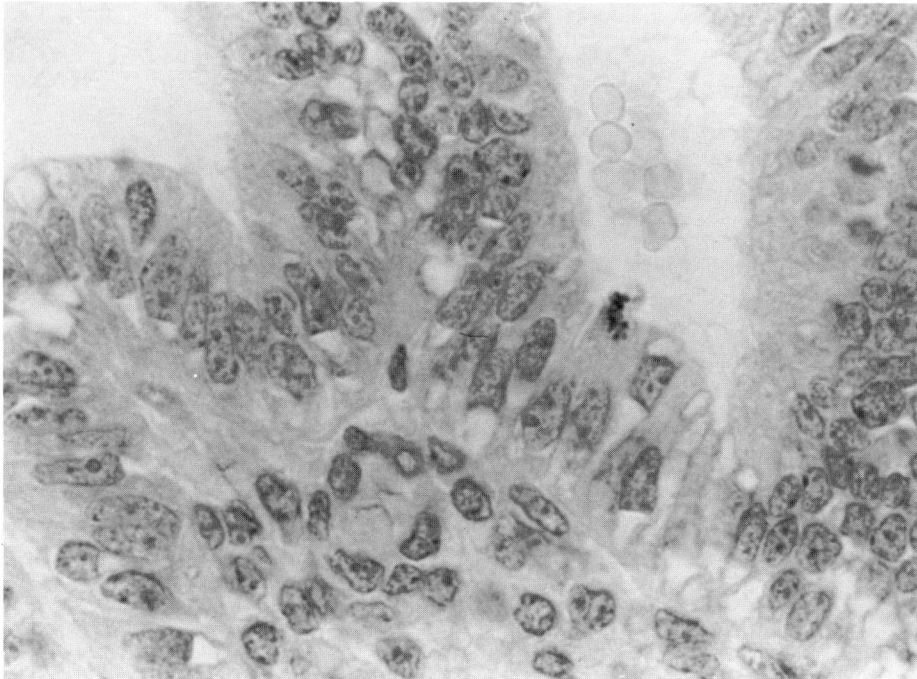

FIGURE 12–4. Subnuclear vacuoles are widespread but are not yet large and uniform. A mitotic figure is seen at the luminal edge of the gland on the right.

nuclei, and on day 19, they reach the cell's luminal pole. Subsequently they are secreted by an apocrine mechanism into the lumen of the glands (Fig. 12–6). Histologically this activity peaks on days 19, 20, and 21. The apocrine secretory mechanism produces intact secretory vacuoles in the lumen of the glands. On about day 21, the secretion begins to form a dense inspissated core within the glands' lumen, and in a nonconception cycle, secretion begins to abate (Fig. 12–7).

The epithelial events described take place in the middle or spongiosa layer of the functioning endometrium. The more superficial epithelium in the upper portions of the glands lags behind, and even late in the secretory phase of the cycle, vacuoles are subnuclear in these sites. Therefore to date an endometrial biopsy specimen appropriately, the pathologist must have a piece of tissue large enough and sufficiently intact to determine that the glands are some distance removed from the endometrial surface.

In the middle to late secretory phase, the reactive portion of the glands becomes quite tortuous. This gives the middle zone of the endometrium its name, the zona spongiosa. The

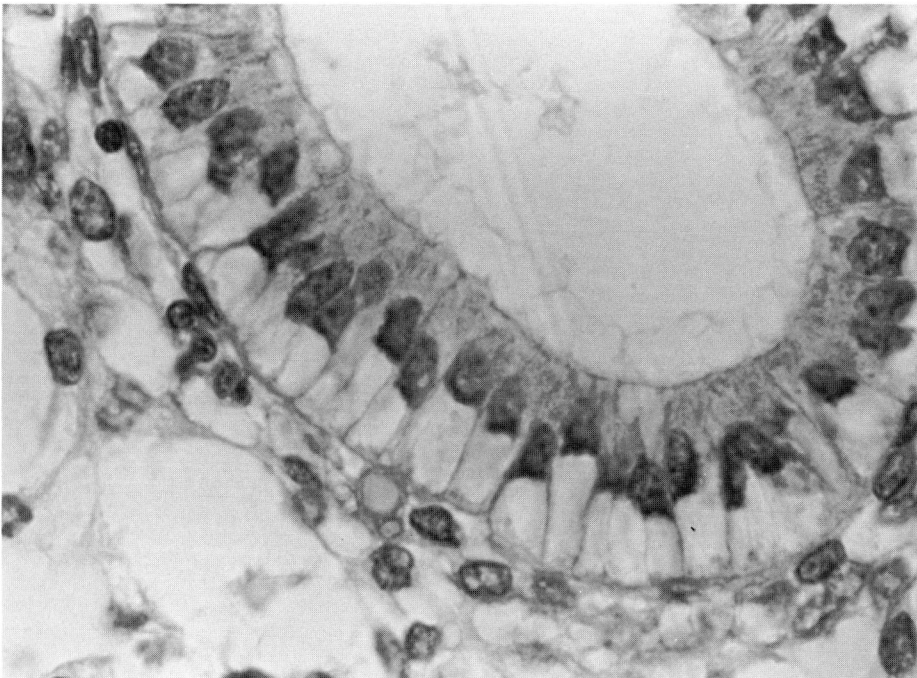

FIGURE 12–5. Uniformly subnuclear vacuoles elevate the nuclei to a position midway between the base and the apex of the secretory cell. (Day 17.)

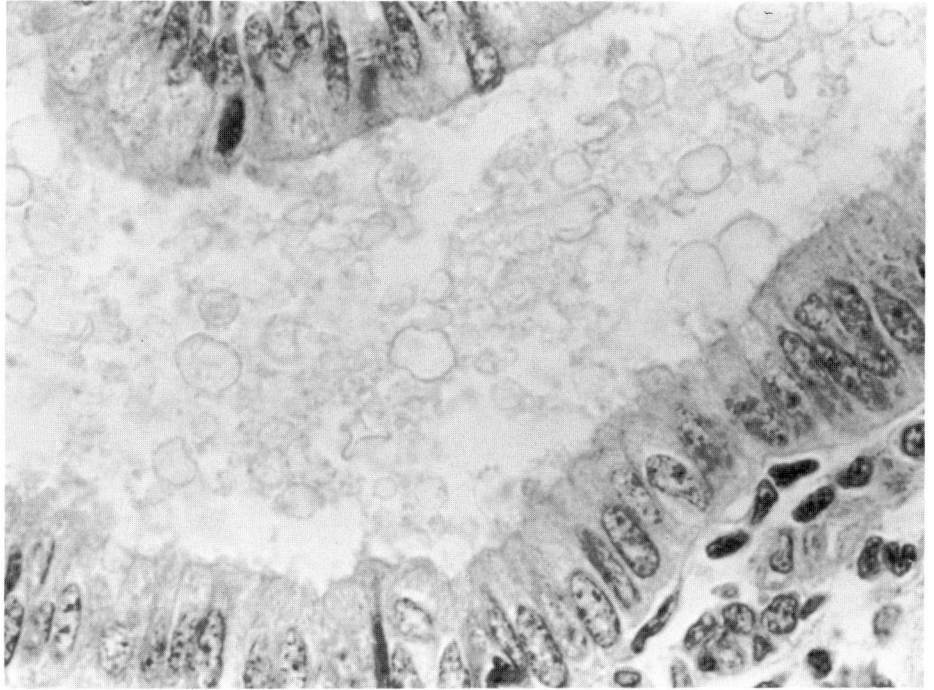

FIGURE 12–6. Multiple secretory vacuoles fill the lumen of this gland. Some are being extruded from the surface of the secretory cells, which mostly look "fuzzy." (Day 18.)

development of the zona compacta, the third and most superficial layer in the classic description, is a feature of the last week of the cycle.

In the 28-day cycle, implantation tends to occur on day 20 or 21. Coincident with this potential occurrence is a relatively acute increase in intercellular fluid or stromal edema in the functional portion of the endometrium. This specifically stromal event heralds a shift in emphasis from the epithelium of the glands, which has been used to date the endometrium to this point, to the stroma. Subsequent datable events occur in the stroma and result in the production of the zona compacta.

About day 23, the spiral arterioles high in the interglandular spaces begin to exhibit perivascular cuffs of stromal cells that are accumulating cytoplasm (Fig. 12–8). This constitutes a process of differentiation induced by progesterone. The cells are becoming decidualized, and when fully differentiated, they become decidual cells. The term *pseudodecidual*

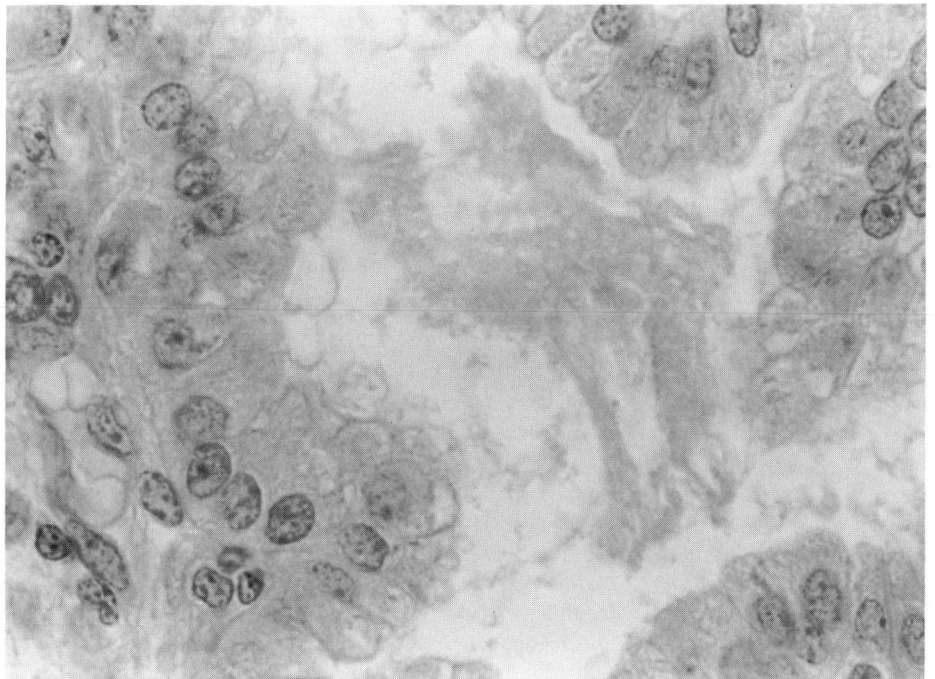

FIGURE 12–7. A central core of inspissated secretion fills the lumen of this gland, which is collapsing around it. A few secretory vacuoles persist. (About day 21.)

stroma that extend from the spongiosa to the surface (Fig. 12–12). Here they spread laterally and produce the so-called zona compacta. This process is generalized on day 27. In association with it, the endometrial granulocytes become more prominent (Fig. 12–13). These cells, thought to be of bone marrow origin, are not decidualized.[7] Small round cells with oval, often indented nuclei, the granulocytes possess eosinophilic cytoplasmic granules visible under the light microscope. Although they have been present throughout the cycle, they are more visible when their neighbors become decidualized. Polymorphonuclear leukocytes also become frequent. The glandular epithelium in the gland necks in the zona compacta still resembles early secretory epithelium with intracellular vacuoles.

The most superficial portion of the endometrium is required for evaluating the last week of the cycle. A biopsy specimen in which only the spongiosa can be visualized does not demonstrate extensive decidualization. The adequacy of the material presented for evaluation is complicated by the fact that the zona compacta does not develop well in nonreactive portions of the endometrial cavity. The glandular epithelium in the gland necks in the zona compacta still resembles early secretory epithelium with intracellular vacuoles, and so as not to be misled by this phenomenon, the pathologist must have a biopsy specimen that allows for making the determination that the gland epithelium is superficial.

One of Noyes and associates'[6] original criteria for evaluating the late luteal phase, the number of leukocytes, has been re-examined. Endometrial granulocytes, which are normal constituents of the endometrium throughout the cycle, along with polymorphonuclear leukocytes, increase in the late luteal phase. This increase has been quantitated by Daly and colleagues,[8] who found that this histologic criterion correlated more closely with the next menses than it did with other criteria of endometrial maturity. Thus, it occurred earlier in the cycle in patients with luteal phase defects than in those without. They interpret this to mean that the infiltrate is related to the impending breakdown of the endometrium.

The first signs of endometrial breakdown occur superficially. They consist of small foci where stromal cells have clumped and become much more basophilic. The overlying epithelium is elevated. There may be slight hemorrhage or a fibrin thrombus in an adjacent capillary. Both the stromal and epithelial processes become generalized and involve most of the zona compacta and spongiosa. Epithelial repair begins immediately and frequently occurs simultaneously with tissue loss. The repairing epithelial cells have abundant eosinophilic cytoplasm, which has led to their being interpreted as squamous.

In a conception cycle, this sequence is altered beginning as early as day 24. The cycling endometrium demonstrates peak secretion on days 20 to 21, peak edema on days 21 to 22, and peak decidualization in the immediate premenstrual phase. When conception occurs, the edema persists, and secretion begins again on about day 24. This resumption of function produces enlargement of the glands that now contain light fluffy new secretion around a more dense eosinophilic core of old secretion (Fig. 12–14). The epithelium becomes newly vacuolated, and the enlarged clear cells are called hypersecretory. The combination of marked decidualization, persistent edema, and hypersecretory glands has been

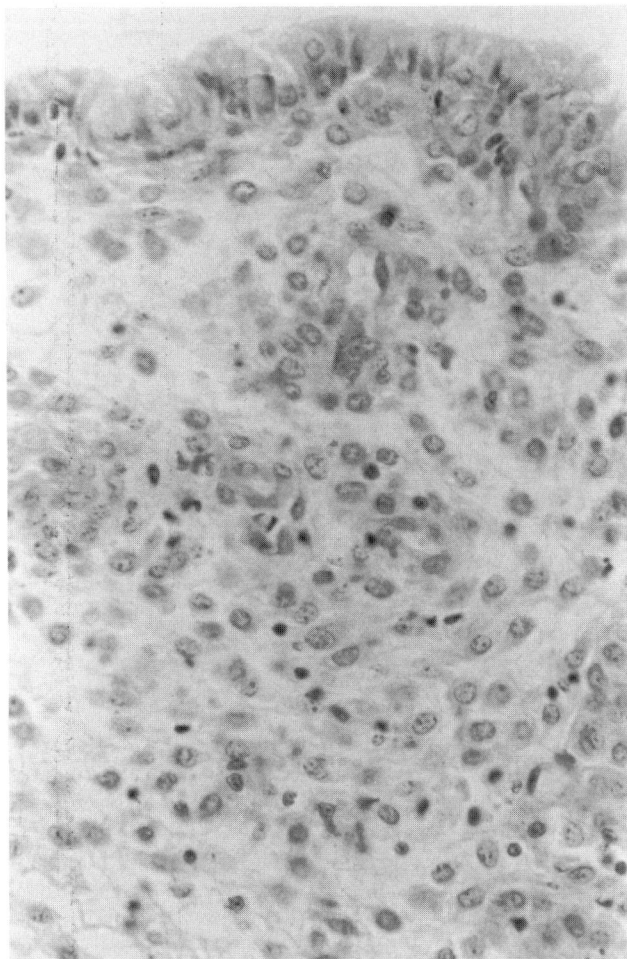

FIGURE 12–8. A "blush" appears around these vessels produced by stromal cells with expanded cytoplasm. (About day 23.)

is misleading, but it refers to less than complete decidualization of endometrial stromal cells. The latter usually requires the hormonal stimulation of pregnancy.

Because decidualization of the stromal cell involves the circumnuclear accumulation of cytoplasm, the spindle-shaped stromal cells are converted into polyhedral cells. The increase in cytoplasm and the relative decrease of intercellular space make the stroma look dense.

This appearance can be simulated, which leads to diagnostic error. Dense stromal proliferation associated only with estrogen may result in apparent decidualization because of increased cellularity and thus increased cytoplasm. The cells, however, remain spindle shaped. Similarly, increased intercellular matrix, such as the scarring that may occur in polyps, has been misinterpreted as decidua. For day 23 to be accurately indicated by the biopsy specimen, the perivascular cuff must be composed of decidual-type cells (Fig. 12–9). Occasionally stromal edema that leaves only structural cells around a vessel creates a picture that simulates a cuff; however, the stromal cells remain spindle shaped.

On day 24 of the cycle, spiral arterioles possess well-developed cuffs composed of decidualized cells (Fig. 12–10). By day 25, foci of decidualized cells appear underneath the surface epithelium (Fig. 12–11). On day 26, many spiral arterioles are contained within columns of decidualized

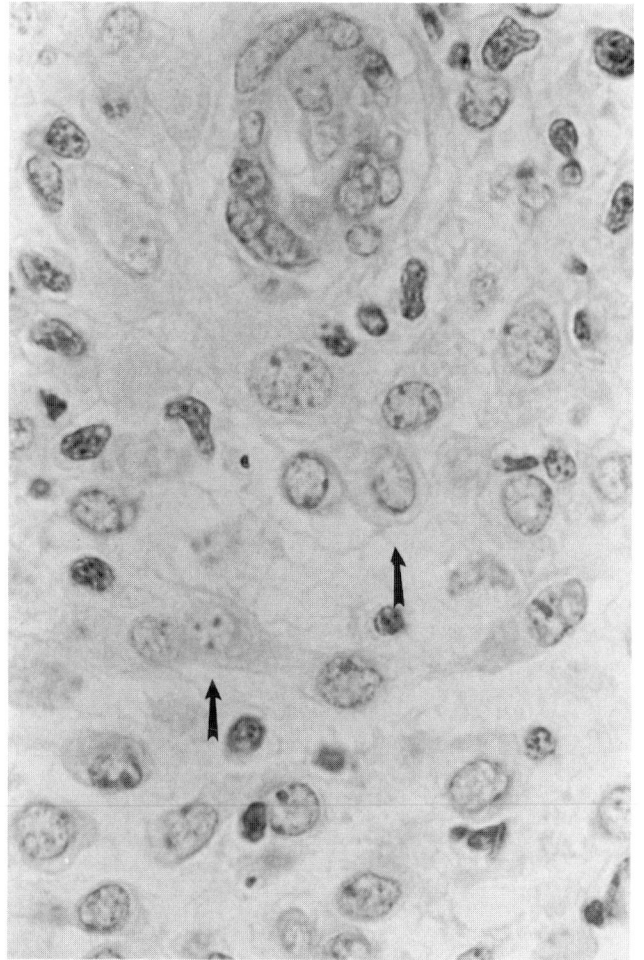

FIGURE 12–9. A small vessel is surrounded by stromal cells that are no longer spindle shaped. Their cytoplasm is expanded, and cell borders are becoming visible (arrows). (Day 23.)

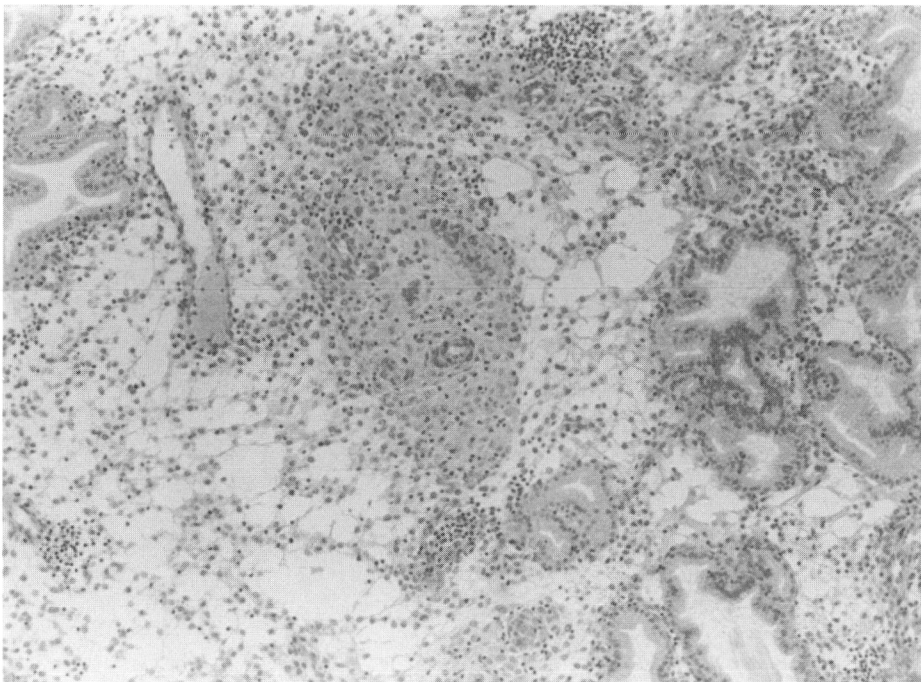

FIGURE 12–10. A spiral arteriole is entirely contained by a population of decidualized cells. (Day 24.)

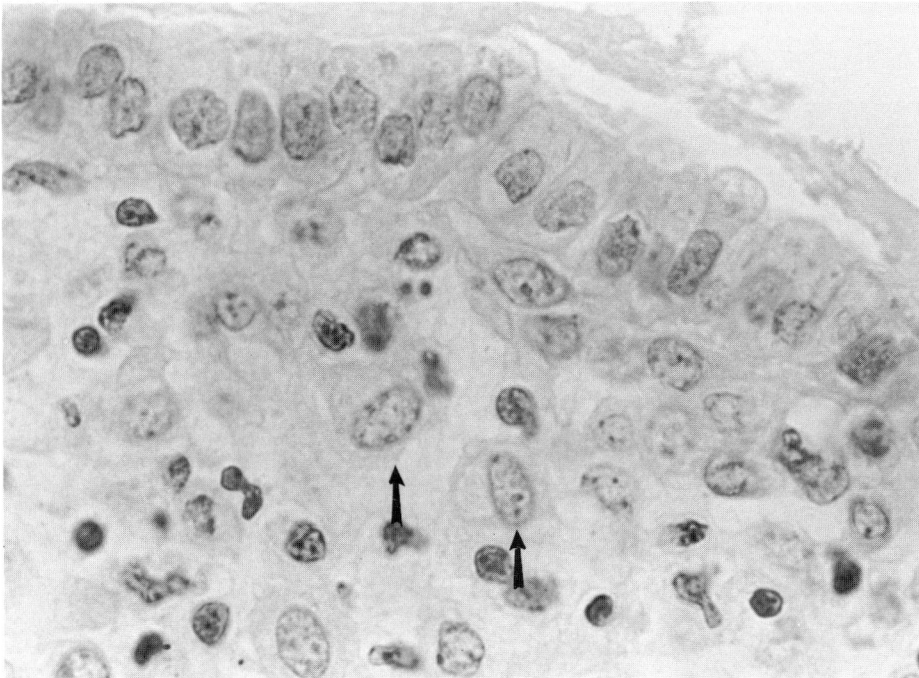

FIGURE 12–11. True decidualization is indicated by the conversion of these endometrial stromal cells to polyhedral cells (*arrows*). The surface is above. (Day 25.)

termed *gestational hyperplasia* by Hertig.[9] It precedes more complete decidualization as pregnancy progresses.

ACCURACY OF HISTOLOGIC INTERPRETATIONS

The histology of the normally cycling endometrium has been studied since the nineteenth century. These observations culminated in the work of Hitschmann and Adler,[10] who collected the endometria of 58 women in whom surgery was done at a known time in their cycle. Because the material encompassed the cycle, they were able to describe the sequential changes in the endometrium as the cycle progressed. They described postmenstrual, interval, premenstrual, and menstrual phases. Both in humans and in other primates, their basic descriptions remain valid.

Rock and Bartlett,[1] however, first described the use of endometrial biopsies to "date" the endometrium in the current sense. Their series of valuable observations remains pertinent. For instance, one observation was that the location from which the biopsy specimen is taken makes a difference:

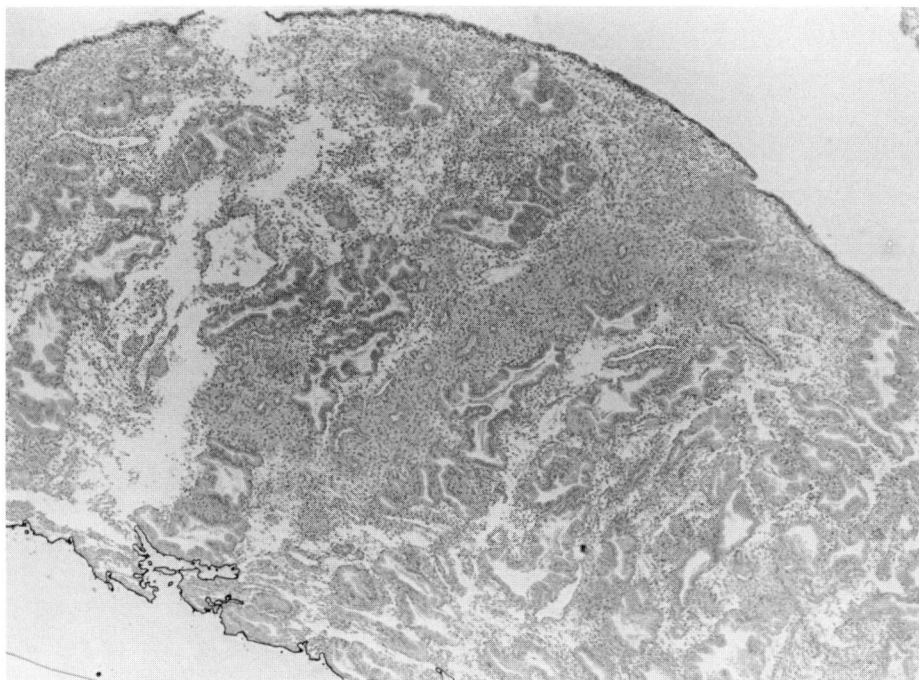

FIGURE 12–12. Lateral to the glands, a column of decidualized stromal cells contains a spiral arteriole. Decidualization extends to the surface and spreads laterally, forming an incipient zona compacta. (Day 26.)

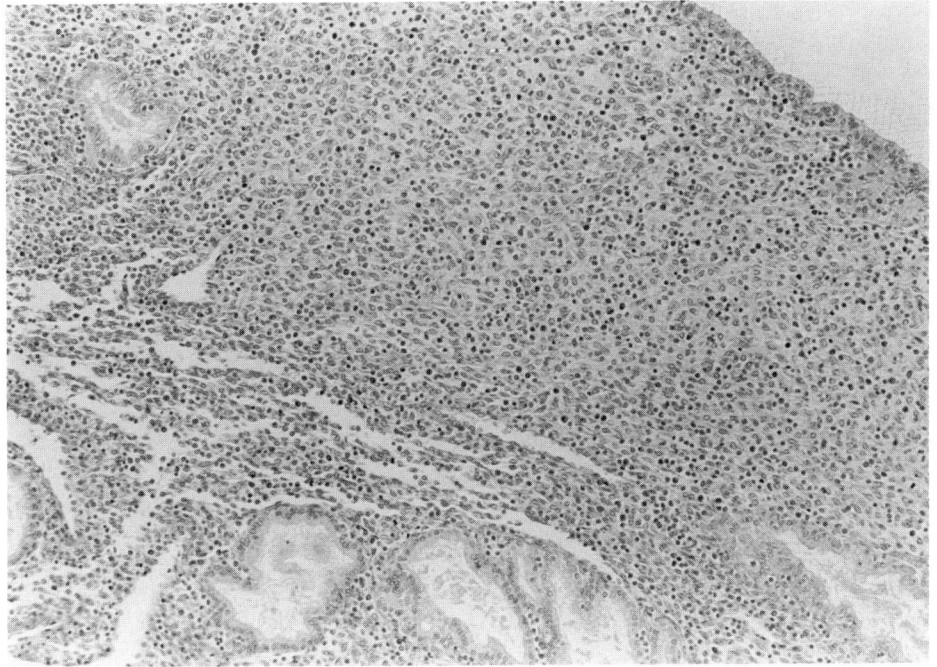

FIGURE 12–13. The zona compacta found by a sheet of decidualized cells lies between the surface epithelium above and the glands, in the spongiosa, below. It is sprinkled with endometrial granulocytes and polymorphonuclear leukocytes, indicating impending breakdown. (Day 27.)

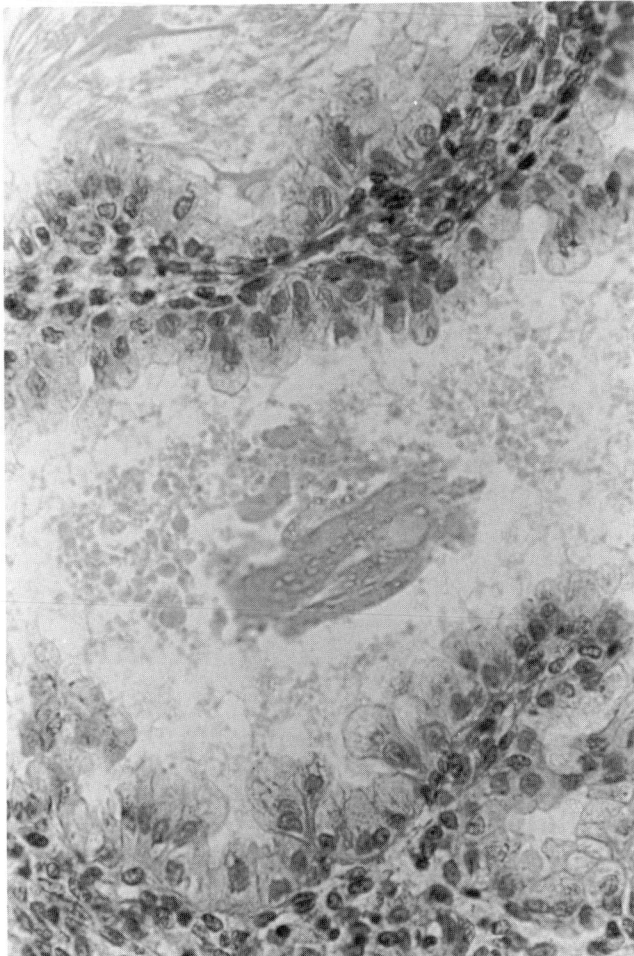

FIGURE 12–14. A central core of inspissated secretion is surrounded by lighter, less dense secretion. The gland is dilated, and most of the epithelial cells possess secretory "domes" that they are preparing to secrete.

High on the anterior or posterior wall is the appropriate site. Another observation was that the biopsy specimen should be evaluated to determine if it was taken from an appropriate site before being interpreted. They pointed out that proliferative phase endometrium could not be assigned to any given day, and they described the day-by-day changes that may be observed in secretory phase endometrium. They discussed the limits of accuracy inherent in the method, they anticipated most of the issues, and they pointed out the variation to be expected. Subsequently Rock collaborated with Noyes and Hertig in the 1950 publication of probably the most widely quoted paper in gynecology.[6] This article emphasized using the most advanced date ascertainable from any given biopsy specimen and was supported by detailed pictures. The authors discussed the limits of accuracy and made the point that when it is possible to do so, the method correlates better with the known time of ovulation than it does with the next menstrual period. This point recurs in subsequent literature. In their case, they used the basal body temperature chart to achieve better correlation than they achieved with the next menstrual period.

From the inception of endometrial dating, its accuracy has been both criticized and defended. It therefore comes as a surprise to find that most authors have, in fact, made similar observations. In the original publication, Rock and Bartlett[1] repeatedly emphasized that they were making no claims of "exact accuracy." Indeed, they predicted the exact date of menstruation only 16% of the time and were within ±2 days 70% of the time. Noyes and colleagues'[6] landmark article reported that a dozen different observers who dated 300 biopsy specimens were able to pick the day of menstruation only 14% of the time and were within ±1 day 38% of the time; overall, the range of error was from 12 days early to 8 days late. Suspecting interobserver variation, Noyes personally reviewed the 300 biopsy specimens, and using the most advanced area in them, he predicted the day of menstruation only 20% of the time and was within ±1 day 60% of the time; overall, his range of error was from 6 days early to 10 days late.

Novak, among others, criticized these initial publications.[11] Although Novak produced no data to support his stance, his eminent stature provoked a response. Noyes and Haman[12] published more than 1000 cases, independently read by the two of them, in which the endometrial biopsy results were correlated with those predicted by the basal body temperature record and the date of the next menstrual period. Haman used the initial criteria of Rock and Bartlett,[1] and Noyes used the modification of these that he published with Hertig and Rock.[6] The modification was primarily to use the most advanced date observed in the tissue rather than an overall average. Noyes's dates might therefore have been expected to be consistently advanced with respect to those of Haman. All their data suggest that this conclusion holds true early in the cycle, but the reverse is true after day 24. In any case, the two observers agreed on the exact date of menstruation 29% of the time, within 1 day 62% of the time, and within 2 days 81% of the time. In individual cases, however, they disagreed as much as 12 days in either direction, with the greatest deviation occurring early and late in the secretory phase. Obviously if an endometrial biopsy specimen is dated in the middle of the secretory phase, there is room for only 7 days of deviation on either side. The length of the phase and the closeness of the chosen date to either cyclic endpoint limits possible deviation, which Noyes and Haman pointed out. In view of this individual variation, the authors' data do not support the idea that the modified criteria are more accurate than the original ones. They were able to predict the exact date of menstruation about 25% of the time; they were within a day about 60% of the time and within 2 days about 80% of the time.

There have been several subsequent attempts to improve or to document the accuracy or inaccuracy of endometrial dating. Tredway and coworkers[13] obtained biopsy specimens from patients in cycles monitored with daily luteinizing hormone (LH) determinations. The correlation between the day of ovulation, LH peak plus 1 day, and the day of the endometrial biopsy was 0.79. Only one pathologist was involved in this study. Five of 11 patients had endometrial biopsy dates 2 days behind the date predicted by the LH peak, and 3 had dates 2 or 3 days beyond the date predicted by the LH peak. These cases are of interest, with 1 standard deviation around the mean of luteal phase cycle length being 1.9 days, but the numbers are too small for comparison with previous studies.

Lundy and associates[14] published the best correlations between the endometrial histologic date and the LH peak ($r = 0.97$); this was the result of having two pathologists review the material and then using the most advanced date given. This does provide some support for the common dictum about endometrial dating being best based on the most advanced date. The correlation between the two pathologists in this study was $r = 0.85$.

Koninckx and associates[15] also correlated biopsies with LH peaks and demonstrated accuracy similar to that achieved by others. The standard deviation of their correlations was 1.2 and 1.3 days in two groups of women.

Johannisson and associates[16] quantitated several histologic criteria and correlated them with the LH surge and with daily estradiol and progesterone levels. Again they were able to agree within a day with the LH surge in 64% of cases and within 2 days in 81%. Despite the authors' attempts to be quantitative, the spread in their data was similar to that of others. These authors also attempted to take biopsy specimens from both lateral walls and from the anterior wall of the cavity, and they could demonstrate no differences in these specimens. Because complete transverse sections of the endometrium repeatedly demonstrate that the endometrium of the lateral walls does not respond as consistently to progesterone as does the anterior and posterior walls, these biopsy specimens, presumably taken from the lateral walls, could not, in fact, have sampled that site. When admonitions are here given about making sure the tissue is from the correct site, this means that the histology should be assayed, not the operator's intention.

Balasch and coworkers[17] further documented variability of results by pointing out that subsequent biopsy specimens tend to reverse the initial impression, but of the 17 patients whose first two biopsy specimens documented a luteal phase defect, only one had a normal specimen with a third biopsy. This is of interest because two successive biopsy specimens demonstrating a deficiency is a common clinical criterion for a luteal phase defect. In contrast, 83 of 172 patients whose initial biopsy specimens suggested a deficiency were normal when a second biopsy was done.

Li and colleagues[18] obtained a correlation of $r = 0.70$ between two observers, and each of these observers got better results with the LH surge ($r = 0.65$; $r = 0.75$) than with the next menstrual period ($r = 0.28$; $r = 0.41$). These authors also noticed a tendency to err toward the center of the cycle.

Subsequently Li and colleagues,[19] using morphometric methods, demonstrated that they could achieve a correlation of $r = 0.98$ with the LH surge. This compared with a correlation of $r = 0.88$ using conventional dating criteria. Although 17 morphometric measurements were made, multiple regression analysis demonstrated that only 5 were required to achieve this result. These were the number of mitoses per 1000 gland cells, the amount of secretion in gland lumina, the volume fraction of gland occupied by gland cells, the amount of pseudostratification of gland cells, and the amount of predecidual reaction. Of these, the volume fraction of gland occupied by gland cells alone achieved a correlation of $r = 0.91$. Although the methods used in this study may not be universally applicable, they demonstrate that endometrial histology bears a close relationship to ovarian function.

Scott and colleagues[5] have looked at interobserver variation in a group of pathologists not specifically interested in gynecologic pathology. Five different pathologists examined the same material in a blinded fashion. Their results were remarkably good in that interobserver variation was less than previously reported by Noyes and Haman.[12] The mean variation in days between two observers was 0.96 days, as compared with 1.46 days by Noyes and Haman. Using a single-day diagnosis, as opposed to a 2-day range, all five pathologists agreed on the same date 55% of the time, and four of five agreed an additional 25% of the time. Despite this superior performance, it was demonstrated that the chance that the diagnosis of the presence or absence of a luteal phase defect would be altered by having a biopsy specimen reexamined was close to 40%. Of particular note in this study was the fact that they retrieved cases from their files that had previously been assigned a date but had to discard a large number of them because the tissue sections were not adequate.

Shoupe and associates[20] have re-emphasized that endometrial biopsies correlate better with ovulation than with the next menses. In 25 of 26 patients, two observers were within 2 days of the day of ovulation as determined by ultrasonography. Li and coworkers,[21] using conventional methods, demonstrated that between-cycle variation in the same woman was substantially greater than intraobserver variation, and they concluded that the result of endometrial dating in a cycle was not a reliable predictor of a subsequent cycle. Gibson and associates[22] used a design that allowed them to calculate the relative importance of several sources of imprecision in endometrial dating. They found that 65% of the variability in endometrial dating was due to interobserver variation, 27% was due to intraobserver variation, and 8% was due to regional differences in endometrial histology. They concluded that the overall error rate contributed to a substantial risk of a false-positive diagnosis of luteal phase defect.

CLINICAL MEANING OF AN ACCURATELY INTERPRETED BIOPSY SPECIMEN

If all the technical factors are discounted, and if accurate dating is assumed, a third source of controversy remains, and there are much less data with which to discuss it. What does the biopsy mean? There appears to be minimal consensus that it relates to the amount of progesterone that has been produced since ovulation. Shoupe and colleagues[20] found a significant correlation between endometrial histology and the area under the progesterone curve since ovulation was determined by ultrasound scanning. Miller and coworkers[23] compared patients with and without biopsy-diagnosed luteal phase defects and found that in the first 5 days of a defective luteal phase, patients excreted significantly less pregnanediol glucuronide than did controls. Hecht and associates[24] treated ovulatory women with clomiphene citrate, and in only 1 out of 29 cycles in 10 women did the endometrium suggest a luteal phase defect. That was also the only case in which integrated progesterone output after the LH surge was reduced.

What does the biopsy mean in terms of clinical outcome for the patient? Perhaps the most disturbing result quoted is the one of Scott and coworkers,[5] in which it was shown that despite relatively low interobserver variation, the chance that a biopsy specimen read in or out of phase would be reversed by a subsequent reading was as high as 40%. This alarming figure is reflected in some clinical observations and not in others. Driessen and colleagues[25] described a heterogeneous group of infertility patients in which the diagnosis of luteal phase defect by biopsy had no effect on prognosis. This study is flawed by the facts, however, that if the authors treated the defect, this is not recorded, and that the patient population is heterogeneous. Many patients with luteal phase defect had other possible contributing factors to their infertility. Nevertheless, the authors concluded that endometrial biopsies meant nothing useful.

Daly and colleagues[26] obtained a different result. Not only did endometrial biopsy specimens suggesting a luteal phase defect respond to specific treatment in most cases, but the correction of the histologic abnormality, documented by additional biopsy, was associated with pregnancy leading to viable infants. Using morphometric methods, Li and colleagues[27] demonstrated that 20% of infertile women had retarded endometrial development as compared with only 3% of fertile women. In this paper, the morphologic features that varied between the two groups were the amount of secretion in the gland lumen, the volume fraction of gland occupied by gland cells, the volume fraction of gland cell occupied by the nucleus, the number of subnuclear vacuoles per 100 gland cells, and the amount of pseudostratification of gland cells. In contrast to Driessen and associates, the last two groups of authors think that endometrial biopsies mean a lot, which brings us to the fourth source of controversy.

DIFFERENT VIEWPOINTS

From a careful review of the literature on the endometrial biopsy, it is apparent that the controversies surrounding this topic are not so much a matter of numbers as a matter of differing points of view. Many arguments develop because two different observers have different definitions of the word *accurate*. Although this point may seem trivial, no small part of the literature on endometrial biopsies cited here, or of the literature on luteal phase defects not cited here, has been generated by semantic disagreements.

REFERENCES

1. Rock J, Bartlett MK. Biopsy studies of human endometrium: criteria of dating and information about amenorrhea, menorrhagia and time of ovulation. JAMA 1937; 108:2022–2028.
2. Jones GS. Some newer aspects of the management of infertility. JAMA 1949; 141:1123–1129.
3. Noyes RW. Uniformity of secretory endometrium: study of multiple sections from 100 uteri removed at operation. Fertil Steril 1956; 7:103–109.
4. Hill GA, Herbert CM III, Parker RA, Wentz AC. Comparison of late luteal phase endometrial biopsies using the Novak curette or Pipelle endometrial suction curette. Obstet Gynecol 1988; 73:443–445.
5. Scott RT, Snyder RR, Strickland DM, et al. The effect of interobserver variation in dating endometrial histology on the diagnosis of luteal phase defects. Fertil Steril 1988; 50:888–892.
6. Noyes RW, Hertig AT, Rock J. Dating the endometrial biopsy. Fertil Steril 1950; 1:3–25.
7. Bulmer JN, Sunderland CA. Bone marrow origin of endometrial granulocytes in the early human placental bed. J Reprod Immunol 1983; 5:383–387.
8. Daly DC, Tohan N, Doney TJ, et al. The significance of lymphocytic-leukocytic infiltrates in interpreting late luteal phase endometrial biopsies. Fertil Steril 1982; 37:786–791.
9. Hertig AT. Gestational hyperplasia of the endometrium. Lab Invest 1964; 13:1153.
10. Hitschmann F, Adler L. Der bau der uterusschleimhaut des geschlechtsreifen weibes mit besonderer berucksichtigung der menstruation. In: Monatsschrif fur geburtshulfe u. gynakologie. Bd XXVI, Heft 1, 1908.
11. Novak E. Editorial. Obstet Gynecol Surv 1950; 5:564.
12. Noyes RW, Haman JO. Accuracy of endometrial dating: correlation of endometrial dating with basal body temperature and menses. Fertil Steril 1953; 4:504–517.
13. Tredway DR, Mishell DR, Moyer DL. Correlation of endometrial dating with luteinizing hormone peak. Am J Obstet Gynecol 1973; 117:1030–1033.

14. Lundy LE, Lee SG, Levy W, et al. The ovulatory cycle: a histologic, thermal, steroid, and gonadotropin correlation. Obstet Gynecol 1974; 44:14–25.

15. Koninckx PR, Goddeeris PG, Lauweryns JM, et al. Accuracy of endometrial biopsy dating in relation to the midcycle luteinizing hormone peak. Fertil Steril 1977; 28:443–445.

16. Johannisson E, Parker RA, Landgren BM, Diczfalusy E. Morphometric analysis of the human endometrium in relation to peripheral hormone levels. Fertil Steril 1982; 38:564–571.

17. Balasch J, Vanrell JA, Creus M, et al. The endometrial biopsy for diagnosis of luteal phase deficiency. Fertil Steril 1985; 44:699–701.

18. Li TC, Rogers AW, Lenton EA, et al. A comparison between two methods of chronological dating of human endometrial biopsies during the luteal phase, and their correlation with histologic dating. Fertil Steril 1987; 48:928–932.

19. Li TC, Rogers AW, Dockery P, et al. A new method of histologic dating of human endometrium in the luteal phase. Fertil Steril 1988; 50:52–60.

20. Shoupe D, Mishell DR, Lacarra M, et al. Correlation of endometrial maturation with four methods of estimating day of ovulation. Obstet Gynecol 1989; 73:88–92.

21. Li TC, Dockery P, Rogers AW, Cooke ID. How precise is histologic dating of endometrium using the standard dating criteria? Fertil Steril 1989; 51:759–763.

22. Gibson M, Badger GJ, Byrn F, et al. Error in histologic dating of secretory endometrium: variance component analysis. Fertil Steril 1991; 56:242–247.

23. Miller MM, Hoffman DI, Creinin M, et al. Comparison of endometrial biopsy and urinary pregnanediol glucuronide concentration in the diagnosis of luteal phase defect. Fertil Steril 1990; 54:1008–1011.

24. Hecht BR, Bardawil WA, Khan-Dawood FS, Dawood MY. Luteal insufficiency: correlation between endometrial dating and integrated progesterone output in clomiphene citrate–induced cycles. Am J Obstet Gynecol 1990; 163:1986–1991.

25. Driessen F, Holwerda PJ, Putte SCJ vd, Kremer J. The significance of dating an endometrial biopsy for the prognosis of the infertile couple. Int J Fertil 1980; 25:112–116.

26. Daly DC, Walters CA, Soto-Albors CE, Riddick DH. Endometrial biopsy during treatment of luteal phase defects is predictive of therapeutic outcome. Fertil Steril 1983; 40:305–310.

27. Li TC, Dockery P, Rogers AW, Cooke ID. A quantitative study of endometrial development in the luteal phase: comparison between women with unexplained infertility and normal fertility. Br J Obstet Gynaecol 1990; 97:576–582.

PART B

TREATMENT OF OVULATORY DISORDERS

CHAPTER 13

Pharmacology of Ovulation-Inducing Drugs

MARY G. HAMMOND

Several factors have altered the practice of ovulation induction since the initial reports of conceptions following ovulation induction with human menopausal gonadotropin (hMG) in 1958 and clomiphene citrate in 1961. Success rates of 15% to 30% per cycle have become routine in uncomplicated ovulation induction therapy owing in part to increased understanding of the treatment cycle and improved patient management as a result of widespread availability of hormone radioimmunoassay and pelvic ultrasonography.

The development of portable intermittent pumps for the administration of gonadotropin-releasing hormone (GnRH) and the availability of bromocriptine have provided more specific therapy for patients with severe hypothalamic dysfunction and hyperprolactinemia.

New indications for ovulation-inducing drugs have led to the extension of their use to women with normal ovulation. As a consequence, the drugs are now used by a significantly larger group of physicians and patients.

This chapter addresses the pretreatment evaluation of women with ovulatory dysfunction, the mechanism of action and metabolism of the commonly used drugs, the selection of appropriate therapy, and the methods available to confirm normal ovulatory response. Expected pregnancy rates and complications of therapy are also discussed.

MANAGEMENT OF THE PATIENT WITH OVULATORY DYSFUNCTION

Appropriate candidates for ovulation induction include women with amenorrhea and those who have oligomenorrhea (irregular cycles >35 days) or luteal phase dysfunction who have failed to conceive after 1 year of unprotected intercourse. Because of the association of ovulatory dysfunction with systemic disease (see Chapter 10) and the improved pregnancy rates after specific therapy, the causes of anovulation should be determined before therapy is initiated, and other fertility factors should be evaluated and corrected when possible.

Evaluation of Abnormal Factors

The evaluation of the patient with menstrual dysfunction is described in detail in Chapter 10. In brief, abnormal ovarian function may result from irregularities in the hypothalamic-pituitary axis or from primary ovarian dysfunction. If the patient is amenorrheic, a thorough evaluation including a history and physical examination (emphasizing neurologic symptoms and signs, metabolic disturbances, hirsutism, and galactorrhea) should be performed. Recent changes in weight, activity, or body contour are significant. The possibility of pregnancy should always be excluded. Laboratory studies including follicle-stimulating hormone (FSH) and prolactin are essential. Thyroid function or adrenal and ovarian androgen levels (dehydroepiandrosterone sulfate [DHEAS], testosterone) should be assessed if symptoms or signs of thyroid disease or hyperandrogenism are present. Computed tomography or magnetic resonance imaging of the pituitary is indicated in many patients before ovulation is induced, especially in those with hyperprolactinemia, hypoestrogenism, or both.

Patients with oligomenorrhea should be evaluated with history and physical examination as well as determination of FSH, prolactin, and testosterone levels. These studies may aid in the selection of appropriate treatment and serve to exclude patients with impending ovarian failure.

Demonstration of anovulation by extensive basal body temperature (BBT) charting, endometrial biopsy, or study of serum progesterone levels is not essential in the oligomenorrheic patient. These tests may be useful, however, in the eumenorrheic infertile patient to diagnose anovulation or luteal phase dysfunction. Low serum progesterone levels (<10 ng/mL on menstrual days − 10 to − 5) or endometrial biopsies that are out of phase by more than 2 days in two cycles confirm luteal phase dysfunction.

Evaluation of Other Factors Affecting Fertility

Additional fertility factors should be investigated. Evaluation of the male and documentation of tubal patency are advised prior to ovulation induction, although some centers defer hysterosalpingography (HSG) until three ovulatory cycles have been completed without conception. In our center, we prefer a motile sperm count of at least 20 million motile sperm per ejaculate and at least one patent fallopian tube. We defer postcoital testing to assess cervical factor until normal ovulatory cycles have been established. Usually this is performed in the third ovulatory cycle.

Tailoring Drug Selection to the Individual Patient

Patients with FSH levels of 30 mIU/mL or higher have absent or resistant ovarian follicles and should not be treated by ovulation induction without extensive counseling regarding poor success rates.

Patients with a demonstrable endocrine abnormality, such as hypothyroidism and congenital adrenal hyperplasia (CAH), should receive appropriate therapy. Patients with hyperprolactinemia who have been judged suitable for ovulation induction are treated with bromocriptine. Patients who remain anovulatory after several months of appropriate hormonal management can be treated with clomiphene as the primary drug of choice.

There has been extensive discussion of the appropriate initial therapy for amenorrheic patients, especially because patients with severe hypothalamic dysfunction will not respond to clomiphene. Several investigators have recommended a series of simple or more sophisticated tests to guide therapy, including withdrawal to progestin, GnRH stimulation tests, and assessment of positive feedback with an estradiol (E$_2$) bolus.[1] A trial of clomiphene to assess the response of the hypothalamic-pituitary axis before the initiation of other drugs such as GnRH and gonadotropins is reasonable in patients without severe hypothalamic or pituitary disorders such as panhypopituitarism, Kallmann's syndrome, and specific gonadotropin deficiency. Patients with Kallmann's syndrome respond to GnRH. Patients with pituitary disease generally require gonadotropins for induction of ovulation.

The treatment of patients with oligomenorrhea is less controversial: clomiphene is the initial drug of choice. However, some authors have recommended bromocriptine in patients with polycystic ovary syndrome (PCO) to reduce luteinizing hormone (LH) values and induce normal ovulation. The latter therapy is still investigational and should not be used routinely.

Considerable controversy surrounds the diagnosis and therapy of luteal phase dysfunction (see Chapter 17). Timed endometrial biopsies and serum progesterone determinations may be required to assess the luteal phase. Clomiphene citrate, progesterone suppositories, and human chorionic gonadotropin (hCG) have been used to correct luteal phase abnormalities. Bromocriptine is appropriate if prolactin levels are increased.

Confirmation of Ovulation

The ability to confirm ovulation and assess luteal phase function is important in the management of ovulatory drugs. These techniques are discussed in detail in Chapters 11, 12, and 17.

METHODS BASED ON PROGESTERONE PRODUCTION BY THE CORPUS LUTEUM

Until recently, only methods based on progesterone secretion by the corpus luteum have been available. Technically, these methods only confirm luteinization of the follicle but not follicle rupture or ovum release.

The three primary methods are BBT, endometrial biopsy, and measurement of serum progesterone levels.

BBT is useful to pinpoint the approximate time of ovulation and to assess crudely the length of the luteal phase. It does not confirm adequate luteal phase function. The exact relationship of the temperature nadir and rise to LH peak and ovum release varies among patients.[2]

Endometrial biopsy for confirmation of ovulation has been widely used in the past. However, the technique is a painful and expensive means to confirm ovulation and may lead to reduced conception rates in biopsied cycles.[3] Endometrial biopsies are necessary for thorough evaluation of the luteal phase in apparently ovulatory patients who do not conceive. Biopsies should be obtained 2 or 3 days before expected menses and should be dated by an experienced pathologist or clinician. The use of a soft plastic curette reduces discomfort and gives adequate samples.[4] Newer methods of endometrial dating bases analysis on the time from LH surge rather than retrospectively from the subsequent onset of menses. Fewer false-positive results are obtained using this method.[5] The measurement of luteal phase serum progesterone levels to confirm ovulation is quite common. Physician visits are not required, and numeric values are reproducible from laboratory to laboratory. Serum progesterone levels of at least 3 ng/mL have been reported during the midluteal phase of regularly cycling women by Israel and coworkers.[6] In contrast, midluteal progesterone levels of at least 10 ng/mL have been measured in spontaneous conception cycles monitored in the midluteal phase by several authors.[7–9] Higher progesterone levels (we use 15 ng/mL) are required in clomiphene or hMG cycles. We obtain progesterone on day 21 of clomiphene cycles or 1 week post-hCG in clomiphene/hCG or hMG/hCG therapy cycles. Alternatively, the samples can be obtained 7 days after BBT shift or LH surge, or 5 to 10 days before menses.

Studies have demonstrated the pulsatile secretion of progesterone.[10] The pulsatility is significantly dampened in the midluteal phase, and diurnal variation becomes more evident.[11] However, the serum values continue to be useful to confirm ovulation during drug therapy.

PHYSICAL TECHNIQUES

Ultrasonography is useful to detect both follicle rupture and luteinization of the unruptured ovarian follicle in spontaneous cycles.[12] Ultrasonography is used to monitor growth of follicles in clomiphene and hMG-induced cycles and to time hCG administration. In addition, collapse of the follicle appears to confirm ovulation. Ultrasonographic studies alone, however, do not provide adequate evaluation of follicular maturation or luteal function. Currently, pregnancy and visualization of an ovarian stigma at laparoscopy provide the most reliable evidence of ovum release, and either serum progesterone determination or endometrial biopsy is superior for assessment of the luteal phase.

Effect of Other Fertility Factors on Conception

Life table analyses of series of patients using clomiphene and other fertility drugs suggest that fecundability rates of 12% to 30% per cycle are expected in ovulating patients. Thus, 35% to 65% should be pregnant by 3 months, and 60% to 85% by 6 months.[13] Monthly fecundability remains constant up to 10 ovulatory cycles in women with no other factors affecting fertility. As patients undergo multiple ovulatory treatment cycles without pregnancy, the likelihood of coexisting abnormal fertility factors increases.

Consequently, we reevaluate our ovulatory patients at 3-month intervals, repeating the postcoital test and measurement of serum progesterone. If HSG has been deferred, it should be performed after three ovulatory cycles. Abnormal mucus, which is common with clomiphene, is treated with high-dose estrogen (2.5 mg conjugated estrogen days 8 through 15) or intrauterine insemination by some clinicians. Others believe that cervical mucus in clomiphene cycles does not impair fertility. If the progesterone level is low, drug dosages are adjusted.

If serum testosterone is 90 ng/dL or higher, prednisone 5 mg at bedtime may be initiated and testosterone levels re-

evaluated.[14] After six cycles of therapy, diagnostic laparoscopy should be performed if it was not evaluated previously.

If the results of all the studies are normal, ovulation induction may be continued for 1 year. GnRH or hMG may be discontinued earlier (after six to eight cycles) because of time or financial limitations. Obviously, in the absence of pregnancy the number of cycles depends in part on the desires of the infertile couple.

Poor mucus, male factor, or peritubal adhesions may reduce fecundability, and longer periods may be required to achieve pregnancy in patients with these problems. If these factors cannot be corrected, treatment periods longer than 1 year may be used.[15]

MANAGEMENT WITH SPECIFIC DRUGS

Clomiphene Citrate

INDICATIONS AND MODE OF ACTION

Clomiphene citrate (Clomid, Serophene) is the drug of choice for ovulation induction in anovulatory patients with intact pituitary function and is useful in the management of those with luteal phase dysfunction. Clomiphene is a nonsteroidal estrogen that is readily absorbed orally; it is cleared by the liver and excreted in feces. The body half-life of clomiphene has been reported to be 48 hours after intravenous injection in monkeys; 83% to 90% is excreted in 6.3 days.[16] Recent studies suggest significant individual variation in clearance rates, and some patients may accumulate the drug.[17] The tendency to accumulate the drug may be responsible for apparent drug resistance, poor mucus, and endometrial atrophy.

The mode of action of clomiphene remains speculative. Administration of the drug leads to increased circulating levels of LH and FSH presumed secondary to hypothalamic release of GnRH. Clomiphene is presumed to interfere with hypothalamic or pituitary estrogen receptor binding or replenishment, blocking estrogen feedback and leading to increasing levels of serum gonadotropins.[18] These receptors are present in high concentrations in the periventricular area and arcuate nucleus of the hypothalamus. Clomiphene administration leads to increased LH pulse frequency, but not amplitude, supporting a hypothalamic site of action.[19] Opiate neurons do not appear to mediate this effect.[20]

An alternative proposal is that clomiphene has a direct effect on ovarian steroidogenesis, reducing steroid levels and leading to increasing gonadotropin levels.[21] This effect on folliculogenesis was confirmed in the monkey, when very-high-dose clomiphene administered in the follicular phase produced a marked decline in E_2 production.[22]

In anovulatory estrogenized patients, clomiphene administration leads to a rise in LH and FSH levels and follicle recruitment. Most patients develop a positive midcycle gonadotropin surge, progesterone secretion, and normal corpus luteal function (Fig. 13–1).[18] Some patients require hCG injection at midcycle to initiate follicle rupture. Recruitment of multiple follicles is extremely common. Indeed, one proposed mechanism of action in the treatment of luteal phase dysfunction is multiple follicle recruitment and corpus luteum formation to account for the increased progesterone production observed with clomiphene administration.[23]

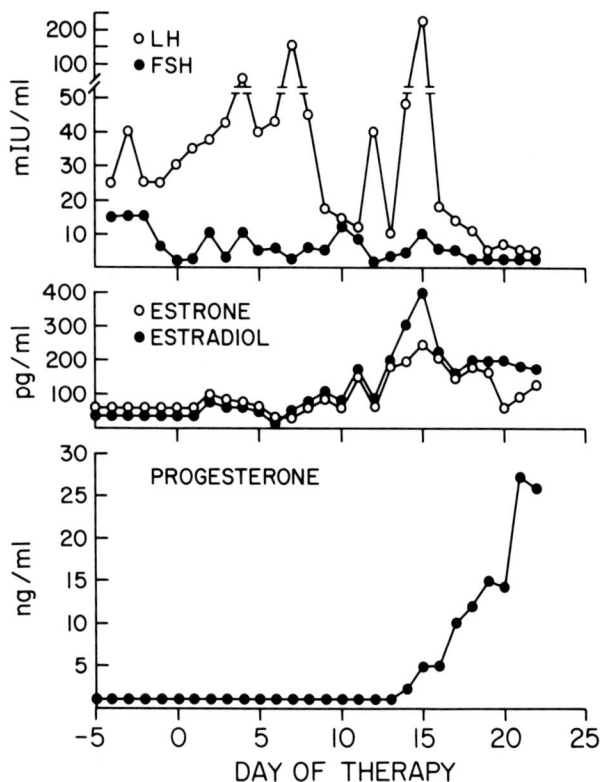

FIGURE 13–1. Serum hormone levels during an ovulatory clomiphene cycle (200 mg/day for 5 days). LH, luteinizing hormone; FSH, follicle-stimulating hormone. (From Hammond MG. Monitoring techniques for improved pregnancy rates during clomiphene ovulation induction. Fertil Steril 1984;42:501. Reproduced with permission of the publisher, The American Fertility Society.)

METHOD OF ADMINISTRATION

Clomiphene is administered orally beginning on the third to fifth day after the onset of spontaneous menses or progestin-induced withdrawal bleeding. Therapy is typically initiated at 50 mg/day for 5 days; an ovulatory response may be confirmed by BBT, serum progesterone determination, or endometrial biopsy during the luteal phase. If ovulation does not occur or the luteal phase is inadequate, the dosage is generally increased to 100 mg daily for 5 days in the subsequent cycle. Dosage may be increased in this fashion to a total of 200 to 250 mg/day.[24]

The addition of 10,000 IU of hCG administered intramuscularly on day 14 or 15 of the cycle may improve ovulation rates.[9] This drug may prove useful in the few patients who develop adequate folliculogenesis but develop no spontaneous midcycle LH surge.[1] A second injection of hCG (5000 IU) 1 week later may stimulate the corpus luteum and sustain the luteal phase. Ultrasonographic monitoring of follicle diameter may be used to time the hCG injection,[25] which is generally administered when the leading follicle has a mean diameter of 18 to 20 mm.

It is our practice to monitor for ovulation using day 21 progesterone levels. We increase our dose from 50 to 100 mg if the patient is anovulatory. We add hCG at the next treatment cycle if she remains anovulatory. We rarely exceed a dose of 150 mg, with hCG added on day 14 or 15.

Approximately 10% to 20% of patients treated with clo-miphene in doses as high as 250 mg/day for 5 days will not ovulate. Several alterations in the treatment plan have been identified. Lobo and coworkers[26] reported the use of 250 mg/day for 8 days. Except in obese patients,[27] increasing the dosage of clomiphene much higher than 150 to 200 mg/day may lead to significant antiestrogenic effects and abnormal folliculogenesis.[28] Patients who metabolize the drug abnormally may benefit from every-other-month therapy.

RESULTS OF THERAPY

Because the criteria to confirm ovulation and the pretreatment evaluation vary from one series to another, there are large variations in reported ovulation and conception rates. Interpretation of conception rates represents a significant problem because only raw conception rates and not per-cycle rates are often reported. Historically, rates of 25% to 49% have been noted.[24, 28–33] Recent studies have reported 80% to 90% ovulation rates, with uncorrected pregnancy rates of 40% to 45% after about six cycles of therapy.

The discrepancy between ovulation rates and pregnancy rates is frequently mentioned as suggesting that ovulation in response to clomiphene is abnormal, but if pregnancy rates are evaluated by the life table method that corrects for patients who discontinue therapy, monthly pregnancy rates in ovulating patients are comparable with those of patients undergoing artificial insemination by donor semen or normal couples discontinuing contraception (Fig. 13–2).[28, 33, 34] In our series, patients ovulating on clomiphene had a monthly fecundability of 15.7% compared with 24.7% for patients terminating diaphragm contraception. The fecundability rate in anovulatory patients with no other infertility factors was 22%.[28] Patients being treated with clomiphene for the correction of luteal phase defects have a reported fecundability of 12%[35] to 16%.[33]

SIDE EFFECTS

Antiestrogenic effects are important. Considerable debate surrounds the effect of clomiphene on the quality of cervical mucus. Van Campenhout and colleagues[36] reported that clomiphene, 25 or 50 mg/day, partially blocked or eliminated the increase in spinnbarkeit of cervical mucus induced in postmenopausal women by 50 μg of ethinyl estradiol (EE_2).

These findings have been confirmed in anovulatory patients by several authors.[28, 37] In our series of clomiphene-treated patients, 50% of those evaluated had poor-quality mucus during therapy. This is in contrast with the study of Gysler and associates,[30] in which only 15% of cervical mucus evaluations were abnormal. When abnormal mucus is found, conjugated estrogen, 0.625 to 2.5 mg/day,[28, 38] EE_2, 75 to 150 μg/day,[39] or diethylstilbestrol (DES), 0.1 mg on days 8 to 15, has been suggested to overcome this effect. Conjugated estrogen, 7.5 mg/day, or EE_2, 150 μg/day, has been demonstrated to have no effect on ovulation in cycles induced with 100 mg of clomiphene.[38] No study has documented that exogenous estrogen increases the conception rate in clomiphene-treated cycles.

An alternative explanation for the poor mucus has been suggested. Some patients with poor mucus may have developed a premature LH surge, producing progesterone, which reduces cervical mucus.

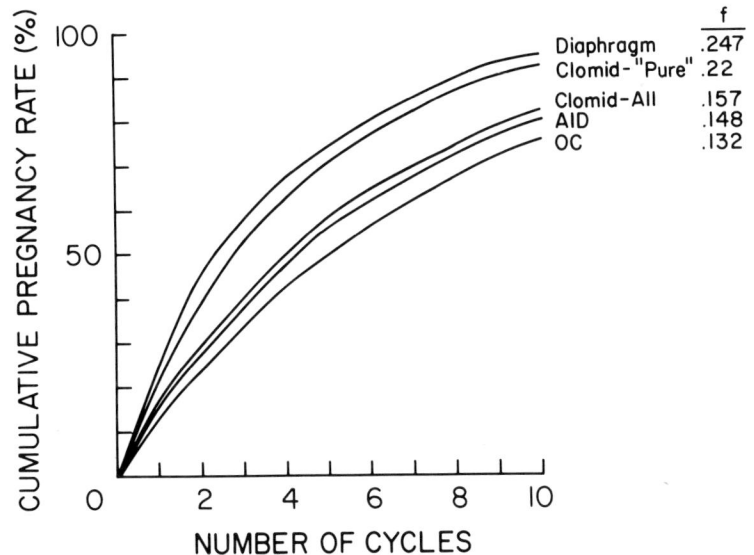

FIGURE 13–2. Cumulative pregnancy rates in patients undergoing ovulation induction compared with women discontinuing contraception to conceive and patients treated by artificial donor insemination (AID). "Pure"—no other cause of infertility; All—all patients treated with Clomid; OC—oral contraceptives. (From Hammond MG. Monitoring techniques for improved pregnancy rates during clomiphene ovulation induction. Fertil Steril 1984;42:503. Reproduced with permission of the publisher, The American Fertility Society.)

Endometrial atrophy also has been suggested as an antiestrogenic effect of the drug. However, studies of estrogen and progesterone receptor levels in the peri-implantation period showed no reduction in numbers or binding properties.[40]

Gonen and associates[29] and Dickey and colleagues[41] demonstrated a positive correlation between endometrial thickness on vaginal sonography at midcycle and fecundity in in vitro fertilization and ovulation induction. The endometrial thickness was less during clomiphene treatment as compared with hMG treatment.

Vasomotor flushes were reported by 10.4% of patients in the original studies. These are most common at higher doses. Pelvic discomfort, nausea, or breast pain are reported by 2% to 5% of patients.

Visual symptoms occur in approximately 1.5% of women using clomiphene. The condition, called *palinopsia,* is due to an effect of the drug on the visual cortex, not the eye. Women experiencing palinopsia commonly experience afterimages and streaks of bright light, especially after dark. Although visual field examinations and electroretinograms are normal, the symptoms are distressing enough to warrant discontinuance of the medication.

Headaches may occur in a small percentage of women taking clomiphene and often justify discontinuing the medicine.

COMPLICATIONS

Ovarian Hyperstimulation. Ovarian enlargement was reported in 13.6% of patients in early series, but true ovarian hyperstimulation occurs infrequently with clomiphene therapy and is usually restricted to patients with PCO. Ultrasonographic and estrogen monitoring of clomiphene cycles reveal multiple follicle development and mean E_2 levels similar to hMG cycles, suggesting that caution should be used, particularly if the practitioner increases dosages in ovulating patients. Some clinicians recommend that patients be examined before the next clomiphene dose until ovulation is achieved. If no cysts are noted and no pain is reported, examinations can be discontinued. Other clinicians believe that examina-

tions or ultrasonography is required only when high doses of clomiphene are used.

Multiple Gestations. Because of multiple follicular development, the risk for multiple pregnancies is increased. Twins occur in 6.9% of pregnancies, triplets in 0.5%, quadruplets in 0.3%, and quintuplets in 0.13%.[16, 42]

Birth Defects. Animals given large doses of clomiphene in utero have a dose-dependent increase in congenital anomalies.[16] In particular, adenosis of the vagina similar to that correlated with DES has been noted in the offspring of rodents receiving high doses throughout pregnancy.[43] Of 158 children whose mothers received clomiphene in the first 6 weeks after conception, only 8 had birth defects; this represents a rate of 44 in 1000, as compared with 23 in 1000 for pregnancies in which clomiphene was given before conception. Neither of these birth defect rates is increased more than that reported for the normal U.S. population. No increase in any specific anomalies were noted in a large series.[44] Malformation rates from several series are shown in Table 13–1.

Abortion Rate. Rates of spontaneous abortion as high as 35% were reported in early studies of clomiphene-induced pregnancies and were believed to be increased compared with the rate in spontaneous conception.[31, 32, 49] Some authors postulated that this is due to an increased incidence (83%) of chromosomal anomalies in abortuses in induced cycles versus 60% in spontaneous pregnancies or to endocrine abnormalities in the clomiphene treatment cycle.[32] It was not

TABLE 13–1. Malformation Rates after Clomiphene Therapy				
			Malformations	
Author	**Country**	**No.**	*Major*	*Minor*
Hack and Lunenfeld[45]	Israel	344	14.5/1000	32/1000
Gysler et al[30]	United States	193	10.0/1000	5/1000
Correy et al[46]	Tasmania	156	12.8/1000	19/1000
Ahlgren et al[47]	Sweden	148	54.0/1000	54/1000
Adashi et al[48]	United States	86	23.0/1000	—
Normal population[45]	United States	50,282	30–65/1000	—

believed to be an inherent defect in the infertile couple,[49] because abortion rates following donor insemination, bromocriptine, or therapy for endometriosis reportedly range between 9.3% and 11.8%. More recent reports suggest that the early studies may have overestimated the abortion rate (perhaps because of increased surveillance) or that improved methods of therapy may have decreased it. In most recent studies, pregnancy losses approach those of the normal population (10.1% to 15%).[28, 30, 46, 47] The largest study, of 1034 patients, reported a frequency of 14.2%.[49]

Effect of In Vitro Clomiphene on Granulosa Cells and Developing Embryos. In vitro studies suggest that clomiphene may reduce progesterone secretion by granulosa cells, an effect that can be reversed by hCG.[50] Decreased embryo growth rates and increased embryo degeneration rates are seen in mouse embryos exposed to clomiphene in vitro.[51] The role of these findings is unclear if clomiphene is cleared before fertilization and corpus luteum formation; however, if the drug persists, this may be more important clinically.

Tamoxifen

Tamoxifen is a nonsteroidal antiestrogen similar in structure to DES and clomiphene. It has been used for ovulation induction since 1971.[52] The drug has a similar mode of action to clomiphene[53] and is equally effective in ovulation induction.[54] Patients are begun at 20 mg daily for 5 days, and doses are increased in 20 mg increments to 80 mg/day maximum. No advantage of the drug over clomiphene has been demonstrated for simple ovulation induction. However, some reports have suggested benefit for therapy of corpus luteal defect[55] and abnormal cervical mucus.[55a] One group reported higher ovulation rates and better-quality cervical mucus cycles compared with those in clomiphene treatment.[56]

Human Menopausal Gonadotropins

INDICATIONS AND MODE OF ACTION

Gonadotropins are the primary method of inducing ovulation in patients with pituitary abnormalities such as panhypopituitarism, hypophysectomy, pituitary necrosis or tumor, and significant hypothalamic dysfunction or failure. Severe hypothalamic dysfunction or failure is characterized by failure to withdraw to progestins and by failure of LH and FSH to increase in response to an intravenous bolus of GnRH (100 μg). In addition, gonadotropins can be used to treat anovulatory patients or those with an abnormal luteal phase who fail to ovulate in response to clomiphene or develop resistance to the drug or poor cervical mucus. Clinicians also commonly use hMG in patients who fail to conceive in response to clomiphene and together with intrauterine insemination in couples with unexplained infertility.

hMG acts by direct stimulation of ovarian follicles. FSH stimulates recruitment and development of primary follicles.[57] LH may be required for the development of the preovulatory follicle as well as for the normal function of the corpus luteum. Injection of hCG is required for follicle rupture and ovum maturation. Doses from 3000 to 10,000 IU have been used. A second dose of 5000 to 6000 IU of hCG

has been recommended 1 week later to improve luteal function, particularly in gonadotropin-deficient women.[58, 59]

hMG is available in the United States as Pergonal and in Europe as Humegon. It is supplied in lyophilized form, with 75 IU of FSH and 75 IU of LH per vial. The preparation contains partially degraded FSH and LH extracted from the urine of menopausal women. A newer formulation, a partially purified FSH (Metrodin), is also available. A major problem with the various formulations is the heterogeneity of the glycoprotein preparations. A variety of gonadotropin species are present in each batch, with differing radioimmunoassay and bioassay potency.[60] Although this has not been a major problem in induction of ovulation, with the advent of in vitro fertilization, new interest has been focused on the extent of lot variation. Recent studies suggested that biopotency of FSH varies most significantly.[61]

Recently, work has begun on the production of pure gonadotropins using recombinant deoxyribonucleic acid technology. An LH product has been tested and found to induce follicle rupture and provide support of the corpus luteum.[62]

MONITORING THE TREATMENT CYCLE

Monitoring has three objectives: (1) to determine the dosage and length of therapy; (2) to determine when or whether to administer hCG; and (3) to ensure an adequate ovulatory response and to avoid hyperstimulation. Three techniques of monitoring are used: clinical, chemical, and ultrasonic.[63]

Clinical Techniques. Before the development of readily available estrogen assays and ultrasonography, vaginal cytology, cervical mucus quality, and ovarian size were used extensively to follow patients undergoing ovulation induction.[64]

Chemical Techniques. Serum E_2 measurement to assess the progression of follicle maturation is the currently preferred method of monitoring. Therapeutic "windows" for the administration of hCG have been reported by several authors (Table 13–2). In their hospitals, these levels confirm adequate follicular development and predict a low incidence of hyperstimulation. The period from the last hMG injection to hCG varies from 24 to 72 hours.

Ultrasonic Monitoring. Ultrasonic monitoring of follicle development in spontaneous cycles has permitted more accurate assessment of follicle size than has clinical examination.[7] Preovulatory follicles just before ovulation in spontaneous cycles range from 14 to 28 mm in diameter. Sonography has been applied extensively to patients undergoing gonadotropin ovulation induction.[69] Follicle growth is more rapid, but preovulatory follicle size, at 17 to 25 mm, is similar to that seen in spontaneous cycles. HCG is usually adminis-

TABLE 13–2. Acceptable Estradiol Ranges for Adequate Follicular Development in Human Menopausal Gonadotropin Therapy

Author	Serum Estradiol (pg/mL)
Gemzell[65]	600–800
Schwartz et al[66]	500–1500
Radwanska et al[67]	300–1500
Haning et al[68]	1000–2000

tered when the largest follicles are 16 to 18 mm in mean diameter.

Sonography permits the early detection of hyperstimulation based on follicle number and size. In particular, it appears that large numbers of small-sized (<9-mm) follicles contribute most significantly to hyperstimulation.[70] Ultrasonography is the first technique available to predict the number of preovulatory follicles and maximum number of possible ova for fertilization.

PRACTICAL REGIMENS FOR GONADOTROPIN USE

Patients with evidence of reduced endogenous estrogenic activity are given two ampules daily at the outset.[71] Patients with normal endogenous estrogen levels are given one ampule initially. The dosage is administered daily, and serum estrogen levels are evaluated. If no response occurs in 4 or 5 days, the dose is increased by one ampule. When a response occurs, that dose is continued until the serum estrogen levels reach the therapeutic window. Ideally, this should occur over 8 to 10 days. Ultrasonographic examinations also can be used to follow follicle growth. When the estrogen is in the ideal range and the largest follicles are 16 to 18 mm in mean diameter, 3,000 to 10,000 IU of hCG is given. Several authors have suggested that a second dose of hCG 1 week later prolongs the luteal phase[59] and increases pregnancy rates in hyperestrogenic patients.[58] Subsequent treatment cycles are initiated at the dosage that stimulated the initial response.

RESULTS OF THERAPY

Since the first pregnancy with gonadotropin therapy was reported in 1958, several treatment series have been reported. Ovulation rates have varied from 73% to 97%. Pregnancy rates have been somewhat lower, with a range of 23% to 82%. Because smaller numbers of treatment cycles are used in hMG treatment, data are easier to interpret. Several studies suggested that cycle fecundity can approach 30%.

Lunenfeld and Eshkol,[72] analyzing more than 12,000 treatment cycles, reported an overall pregnancy rate of 42.9%. These authors included an analysis of a group of 1002 of their own patients who received 3234 treatment cycles. The results, evaluated by life table analysis, more closely approached results reported in the general fertile population. In the hypoestrogenic patient group, the cumulative pregnancy rate was 91.2% after six cycles. Healy and coworkers[73] also reported similar cumulative pregnancy rates when multiple cycles of therapy were used.

Several series have reported lower cumulative pregnancy rates in patients with oligomenorrhea or other indications of endogenous estrogen activity. Unsatisfactory results with the use of hMG in patients with PCO who failed to ovulate in response to clomiphene are common. The lower pregnancy rates may be associated with specific effects of hyperandrogenism or with the variable responses that patients with PCO have to exogenous gonadotropin.

In both hypoestrogenic patients and those with estrogenic activity, 90% who became pregnant conceived within the first four treatment cycles. The mean number of hMG ampules per treatment cycle in hypoestrogenic patients was 40.2 as compared with 18.2 ampules for patients with estrogenic

activity. Multiple pregnancy rates with hMG treatment have varied over the years. Although a reduction was achieved with the introduction of estrogen monitoring, multiple gestations still occur in 10% to 35% of pregnancies. It is unclear if sonographic studies have affected multiple pregnancy rates. Twin and triplet gestations are a frequent result of therapy; therefore, ultrasonography early in pregnancy is recommended.

An abortion rate of 20% to 30% appears to be fairly uniform across all studies[44] and appears to be higher than that occurring after spontaneous conception. Early detection of pregnancy and multiple pregnancy may create the impression of increased rates of abortion, although these rates are not seen in closely monitored patients receiving clomiphene therapy. Abnormalities of ovulation or inadequate luteal phase function have been suggested as the cause. There may be a higher risk of subsequent abortion after a single first-trimester loss.[74] No increase in malformation rates is noted. The incidence of major malformations was 21.6 in 1000 and minor, 32.7 in 1000 in a recent study (Table 13–3).[44]

COMPLICATIONS

Occasional patients have a febrile response to menotropins, perhaps because of allergy to the drug or its vehicle.

Ovarian hyperstimulation has been the major complication reported with hMG. Symptoms range from mild ovarian enlargement to large cysts, ascites, and coagulation defects. Severe hyperstimulation is usually noted only in patients who ovulate and conceive after treatment. The extent of hyperstimulation correlates well with serum estrogen levels,[72] and hCG should be withheld if estrogen levels exceed the therapeutic window established in each center. Ovarian hyperstimulation usually does not occur in the absence of ovulation,[51] but we have seen a severe case in a patient with PCO with an elevation of LH levels in whom hCG was withheld.

The management of hyperstimulation syndrome is discussed in detail in Chapter 14. Hyperstimulation usually becomes apparent 3 to 7 days after hCG is administered. Mild hyperstimulation can be managed without hospital ad-

TABLE 13–3. Malformation Rates after hMG-hCG Therapy

Author	No.	Malformations	
		Major	Minor
Hack et al[75a]	122	4	2
Spadoni[75b]	32	2	—
Harlap[75c]	66	1	5
Caspi et al[75d]	157	4	11
Schwartz et al[75e]	132	2	—
Kurachi et al[75f]	132	3	—
Lunenfeld et al[75g]	312	9	20
TOTAL	1160	25 (21.6/1000)	38 (32.7/1000)
Normal Population[45]	50,282	(30–65/1000)	

hMG, human menopausal gonadotropin; hCG, human chorionic gonadotropin

From Shoham Z, Zosmer A, Insler V. Early miscarriage and fetal malformations after induction of ovulation (by clomiphene citrate and/or human menotropins), in vitro fertilization, and gamete intrafallopian transfer. Fertil Steril 1991; 55:1–11. Reproduced with permission of the publisher, The American Fertility Society.

mission. Intercourse and strenuous activity should be avoided. In the absence of pregnancy, symptoms will resolve after menses; however, if pregnancy occurs, symptoms may persist for as long as 6 to 8 weeks.

In patients with more severe forms of hyperstimulation, hospitalization is necessary. Massive fluid shifts occur, and hematocrit, coagulation, and electrolyte values should be followed. Fluid intake, urine output, weight, and abdominal girth should be monitored carefully. Cautious fluid and electrolyte replacement should be initiated. The role of plasma expanders and paracentesis and the monitoring of arterial and venous pressure is currently unsettled,[75, 76] but aspiration of ascitic fluid may speed recovery.[77]

Symptoms are usually transitory; surgical exploration is indicated only when there is evidence of intraperitoneal hemorrhage or ovarian torsion or when another abdominal emergency, such as acute appendicitis, is suspected.

Clomiphene and Gonadotropins

INDICATIONS AND MODE OF ACTION

The combination of clomiphene and hMG has been recommended for women with some endogenous estrogenic activity who respond poorly to clomiphene alone. This method is intended to reduce the amount of menotropins required per cycle. A modification of this method is used in several centers for follicle recruitment for in vitro fertilization (see Chapter 52).

The apparent mechanism of action is to increase endogenous FSH and LH levels, leading to decreased requirements for hMG needed to promote follicular maturation.

METHOD OF ADMINISTRATION

Clomiphene, 100 to 200 mg, is administered days 5 through 9, with daily injection of hMG initiated in either an overlapping or sequential fashion. Daily monitoring of estrogen and ultrasonography are used. HCG is given 24 to 48 hours after adequate stimulation is obtained using the same criteria as for hMG alone.

RESULTS OF THERAPY

Jarrell and coworkers[78] reported an increase in the ovulation rate with the clomiphene and hMG regimen but no increase in pregnancy rates. They confirm the results of others who report a 50% reduction in hMG requirements.[79]

Growth Hormone and Gonadotropins

Growth factors have been implicated as autocrine regulators of granulosa cell function. Synthesis of insulin-like growth factor-1, a major growth factor, is stimulated by growth hormone. Homburg and coworkers[80] reported the results of a randomized, double-blind, placebo-controlled study of biosynthetic growth hormone (24 IU every other day) and placebo in combination with hMG. Statistically significant reductions in ampules of hMG (37.4 versus 24.2), days of treatment (17.7 versus 13.3), and daily dose (3.1

versus 2.5) were reported. Growth hormone apparently acts to augment hMG in ovulation induction. However, growth hormone is quite expensive, and the feasibility of its use now seems questionable unless more specific improvement in quality of ovulation is noted.

Follicle-Stimulating Hormone

INDICATIONS AND MODE OF ACTION

"Pure" FSH (Metrodin) has been approved for the management of PCO patients who fail to ovulate when taking clomiphene. It is prepared from hMG by immunochromatography, producing a preparation containing 75 IU of FSH and less than 1 IU of LH activity per vial.

FSH injections lead to correction of the abnormal LH:FSH ratio in PCO and result in follicle recruitment.[81] Patients may develop an endogenous LH surge, although hCG is usually given to induce ovulation. FSH is not effective in inducing ovulation in hypoestrogenic patients or those with hypothalamic dysfunction.[82, 82a] After intramuscular injection, FSH concentrations peak in 6 to 18 hours and are still elevated 72 hours after injection.[83]

METHOD OF ADMINISTRATION

A variety of administration schedules have been reported, including long-term low-dose therapy (one ampule or less per day) and step-up and step-down regimens.[82, 84] The usual treatment is to start at one ampule daily and increase by increments every 7 days. Increments as small as one third of an ampule may be effective. Very sensitive patients may be treated with one half an ampule daily. Criteria for hCG administration are similar to hMG, although the quantity of E_2 produced by each follicle seems to be less. There is no evidence that this preparation is more effective than cruder hMG.

Gonadotropin-Releasing Hormone

INDICATIONS AND MODE OF ACTION

GnRH treatment is indicated primarily for patients with amenorrhea and intact pituitary function who fail to respond to clomiphene. It has the advantage of being more physiologic in patients with hypothalamic dysfunction. GnRH stimulates endogenous pituitary release of LH and FSH and subsequent folliculogenesis. Normal negative and positive feedback by gonadal steroids at the pituitary level is expected; thus, there is a significant reduction in the incidence of hyperstimulation syndrome compared with that with hMG.

A number of administration systems are available for the required pulsatile administration of the drug. GnRH is available as Factrel (100- and 500-μg vials) and Lutrepulse (800- and 3200-μg vials). It is a synthetic decapeptide that is identical to the naturally occurring hypothalamic hormone that stimulates gonadotropin release by the pituitary gland.

METHOD OF ADMINISTRATION

Schally and associates reviewed the results of ovulation induction with GnRH in 1975.[85] At that point, several centers had confirmed that follicular development and occasional ovulation could be obtained with intermittent (usually three times daily) GnRH therapy. Of 80 women treated, 32.5% ovulated and 12.5% conceived.

Nillius and Wide[25] reported success with induction of ovulation in amenorrheic women with anorexia nervosa. GnRH, 500 μg subcutaneously, was self-administered every 8 hours. A normal 28-day cycle resulted. During the course of therapy, as estrogen levels began to increase, FSH responses decreased. This pattern of responsiveness was believed to represent an advantage over hMG, because it might prevent the development of multiple follicles and hyperstimulation. High doses of GnRH were required, and either GnRH had to be continued beyond ovulation or hCG was required in the luteal phase for normal luteal phase function.

Subsequent to these clinical trials, Knobil and colleagues[86] documented that pulsatile administration is necessary for normal gonadotropin release in female rhesus monkeys made GnRH deficient.

Leyendecker and Wildt[87] reported inducing ovulation in women with hypothalamic amenorrhea using pulsatile GnRH. Reports from a series of other centers have followed. Most series have involved intravenous administration of 5 to 10 μg of GnRH every 90 to 120 minutes. Increases in FSH and LH occur, followed by a rise in serum E_2, resulting in a midcycle LH peak and ovulation (Fig. 13–3).

GnRH is now administered with the use of an automatic portable infusion pump with a pulsatile mechanism. Several models are available commercially, including products from Autosyringe, Inc. (Hookset, NJ), Lutrepulse, from Ortho Pharmaceuticals (Raritan, NJ), and the Zyklomat, made by Ferring GmbH (Kiel, Germany). The microchip-controlled peristaltic pumps offer several choices of dosage and pulse frequency. The pumps are commonly worn on a belt around the waist. The activity of the reconstituted drug is stable for as long as 4 weeks at room temperature.[88] GnRH also can be injected by the patient under sterile conditions through a heparin lock at 2-hour intervals nine times a day from 7 A.M. until 11 P.M. Subcutaneous needle placement and drug administration is also possible, thus eliminating the problem of intravenous needle maintenance.[89]

There is considerable variation in the metabolism of the drug based on the method of administration. The intravenous bolus results in circulating GnRH levels (and thus presumably pituitary levels) that most closely approximate what is believed to be the physiologic response (Fig. 13–4).[90]

Dosages ranging from 1 to 20 μg/pulse at 90- to 120-minute intervals have been used. Some individualization of doses probably is required. Generally, subcutaneous doses of 10 to 20 μg/pulse seem to be adequate for patients with secondary amenorrhea. Smaller doses (5 to 10 μg) are used for intravenous therapy. Considerable debate surrounds the concept that higher doses may contribute to hyperstimulation.[91] Little human research has been done to determine the optimal pulse frequency. Pulse intervals of 90 or 120 minutes have been used with good results. GnRH pulses may be continued at 4-hour intervals in the luteal phase, or hCG, 1000 to 2000 IU, may be given at 3- to 4-day intervals after the temperature shift to maintain corpus luteum function. Studies have also demonstrated that progesterone given intramuscularly or by suppository may be administered in the luteal phase with good results.

RESULTS OF THERAPY

Results of therapy with pulsatile subcutaneous or intravenous administration of GnRH are accumulating. The first

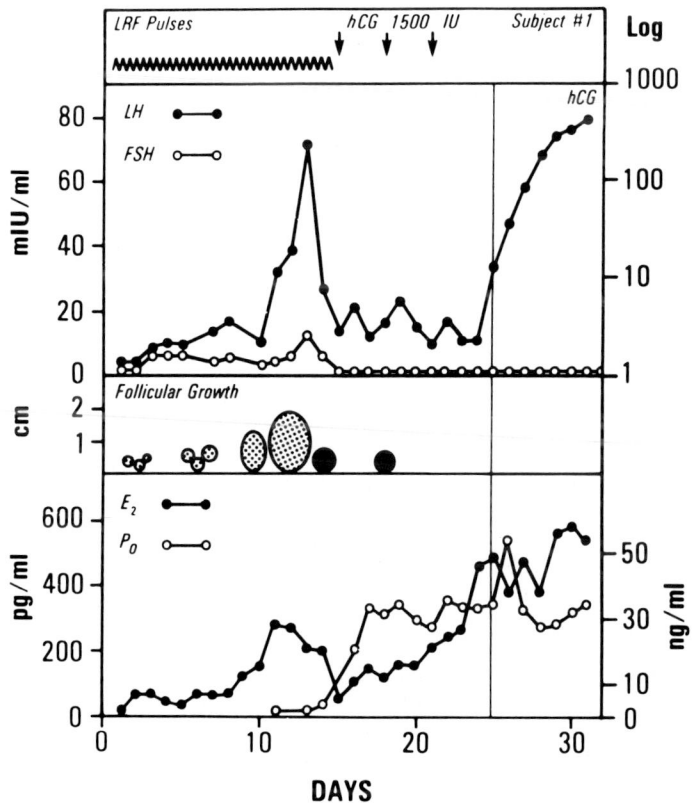

FIGURE 13–3. Endocrine and ovarian follicular changes during ovulation induction with 5 μg of intravenous gonadotropin-releasing hormone at 120-minute intervals. LRF, luteinizing hormone-releasing factor; hCG, human chorionic gonadotropin, E_2, estradiol, P_0, progesterone. (From Reid RL, Leopold GR, Yen SSC. Induction of ovulation and pregnancy with pulsatile luteinizing hormone releasing factor: dosage and mode of delivery. Fertil Steril 1981;36:556. Reproduced with permission of the publisher, The American Fertility Society.)

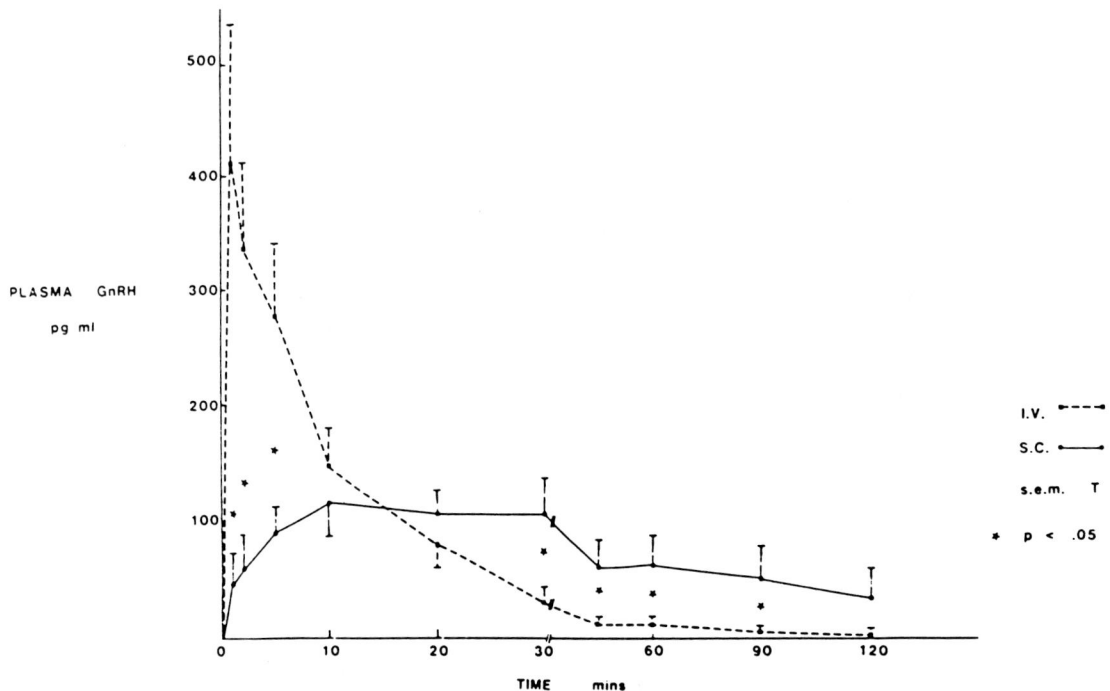

FIGURE 13–4. Mean (±SEM) plasma gonadotropin-releasing hormone (GnRH) levels in six hypogonadotropic patients after a single 5-μg intravenous (IV) dose or the mean of three single subcutaneous (SC) doses of 5 μg. (From Handelsman DJ, Jansen RPS, Boylan LM, et al. Pharmacokinetics of gonadotropin releasing hormone: comparison of intravenous and subcutaneous routes. J Clin Endocrinol Metab 1984;59[4]:739–746. © The Endocrine Society.)

series reported was that of Leyendecker and Wildt,[87] who induced ovulation in 15 patients with primary and secondary hypothalamic amenorrhea; 6 of these patients became pregnant. Shoemaker and associates[92] treated six hypogonadotropic patients for 16 cycles. Fifteen cycles were ovulatory, and five of the patients conceived. Coelingh-Bennink,[93] Seibel and associates (subcutaneous injection),[94] Hurley and co-workers,[95] and Goerzen and colleagues[96] published series suggesting high ovulation and pregnancy rates with this therapy in patients with hypothalamic amenorrhea. Santoro[96a] reported a multicenter study of 109 patients with hypothalamic amenorrhea. Of these, 94% ovulated and 60% conceived. Depending on the luteal support, a 24% to 32% abortion rate was noted. Most studies report higher rates of ovulation with intravenous as compared with subcutaneous administration.

Results in patients with PCO have been less rewarding. A literature review reported an ovulation rate of 89% and a pregnancy rate per cycle of 27% in 273 hypothalamic amenorrhea patients versus 43% ovulation and 12% pregnancy rates in 51 patients with PCO.[97]

SIDE EFFECTS AND COMPLICATIONS

No serious complications of GnRH therapy have been reported, except for localized phlebitis[92] and one case of bacteremia that resolved after removal of a heparin lock. These appear to be the most significant problems associated with intravenous administration of GnRH.

Multiple pregnancies and hyperstimulation are rare. Ultrasonographic studies have revealed two large follicles in 10% and three large follicles in 5% of cycles. Eleven percent twins and 1% triplets were reported in one review.[76]

Animal studies have revealed the drug to be essentially devoid of acute toxicity. No symptoms were recorded when GnRH was administered to mice in dosages of 100 μg/kg and in rats in dosages as high as 150 μg/kg. Continuous therapy in rats failed to reveal any change in survival, biochemical parameters, physical examination data, or postmortem gross and microscopic observations. No adverse effects were noted in either the fetus or maternal parent after administration of GnRH to pregnant mice. Litter size, sex distribution, fetal length, and weight were comparable between the treatment and control groups. No congenital anomalies were noted.[98]

Bromocriptine

INDICATIONS AND MODE OF ACTION

Syndromes of amenorrhea-galactorrhea have been recognized for many years. A variety of ovulation-inducing agents have been used with variable results. Since the identification of discrete adenomas, surgical therapy also has been used.

Hyperprolactinemia is present in 14% to 20% of women with secondary amenorrhea and less frequently in those with primary amenorrhea. Eumenorrheic patients with elevated prolactin levels and luteal phase defects have been reported. It is postulated that elevated prolactin levels may disrupt the normal menstrual cycle at the hypothalamic, pituitary, and ovarian levels. Lowering the serum prolactin level by surgical, radiologic, or medical means usually restores normal function. The most common medical approach to therapy is to reduce serum prolactin levels with dopamine agonists such as bromocriptine.

Bromocriptine (Parlodel) is rapidly and completely absorbed. Peak plasma levels are achieved in 2 to 3 hours and remain detectable in the serum as long as 24 hours.[99] Bromocriptine interacts with dopamine receptors in the central nervous system and the anterior pituitary gland, and it inhibits prolactin release.[100] It is supplied in 2.5-mg tablets and is indicated in the therapy of amenorrhea-galactorrhea to restore normal menstrual cycles, to inhibit lactation, and to induce ovulation in infertile women.

Bromocriptine is rapidly absorbed orally, with peak serum levels noted at 3 hours. Although the effect of bromocriptine continues for as long as 11 hours, serum levels of drug reach half-maximum levels after 8 hours, and the ideal dosing is at 8-hour intervals (Fig. 13–5).[101] Bromocriptine is also absorbed readily from vaginal mucosa (Fig. 13–6).[101a] Bromo-

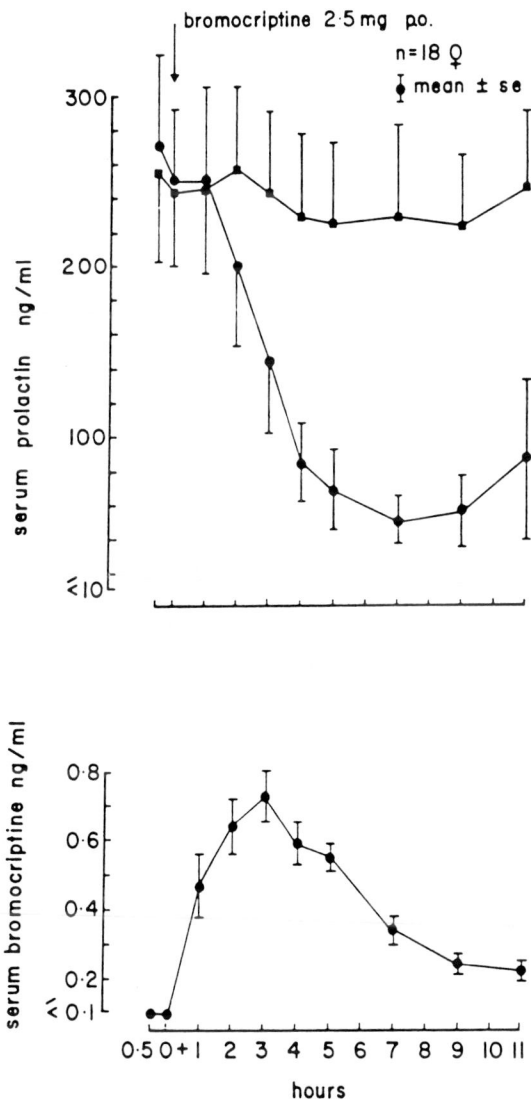

FIGURE 13–6. Mean (±SEM) plasma levels of bromocriptine and prolactin after vaginal administration of 2.5 mg of bromocriptine. (From Vermesh M, Fossum GT, Kletzky OA. Vaginal bromocriptine: pharmacology and effect on serum prolactin in normal women. Obstet Gynecol 1988;72:694. Reprinted with permission from The American College of Obstetricians and Gynecologists.)

criptine is a semisynthetic ergot alkaloid and dopamine receptor agonist. It restores normal prolactin secretion by inhibiting prolactin gene transcription and messenger ribonucleic acid accumulation in pituitary cells.[102]

SELECTION OF PATIENTS FOR THERAPY

The pros and cons of medical and surgical management of pituitary microadenomas have been reviewed extensively.[103] Medical management is now favored, although prepregnancy surgical reduction is occasionally recommended in large macroadenomas. For all patients with disorders of ovulation, serum prolactin levels should be determined, and abnormal values should be repeated to confirm that an actual elevation does exist. Drugs that cause hyperprolactinemia should be discontinued if feasible. Serum levels of thyroid-stimulating hormone (TSH) and thyroxine levels should be measured. If the TSH level is elevated, thyroid replacement therapy should be instituted until thyroid function returns to normal. If prolactin levels are still elevated after 3 months of replacement therapy, treatment with bromocriptine may be indicated.

In patients with persistent hyperprolactinemia, radiographic assessment of the sella turcica should be performed. If a pituitary macroadenoma is identified, baseline visual field evaluation should be performed and the integrity of other functions regulated by pituitary hormones determined. A multidisciplinary team should be involved in deciding if surgical or medical management is warranted.

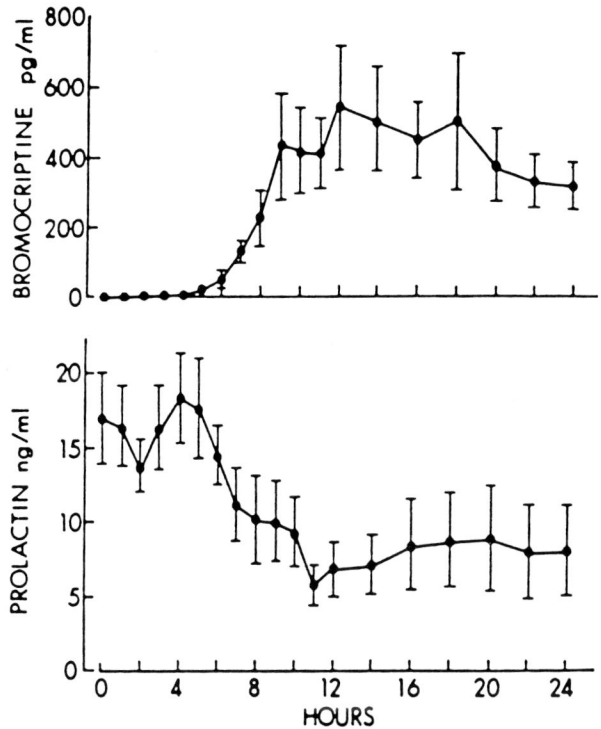

FIGURE 13–5. Mean (±SEM) prolactin and bromocriptine levels in 18 hyperprolactinemic patients during control study and after bromocriptine (2.5 mg orally at 0 hours). In the *upper panel,* the top line represents control data, and the bottom line, the treatment data. (From Thorner MO, Schran HF, Evans WS, et al. A broad spectrum of prolactin suppression by bromocriptine in hyperprolactinemic women: a study of serum prolactin and bromocriptine levels after acute and chronic administration of bromocriptine. J Clin Endocrinol Metab 1980;50[6]:1026–1033. © The Endocrine Society.)

METHOD OF ADMINISTRATION

Therapy is begun at 1.25 mg daily for 1 to 2 weeks to reduce side effects. Administering the drug with the evening meal initially may decrease gastrointestinal upset. If tolerated, the dosage is increased to one and then two tablets daily. BBT charts may be maintained to determine whether ovulation has occurred. The prolactin level should be reevaluated every 2 to 3 weeks; if it is elevated, bromocriptine should be increased by one tablet (2.5 mg) until the prolactin level is less than 20 mg/ml. If prolactin levels are less than 5 ng/mL, the dose should be reduced. Ovulation can be monitored by BBT and serum progesterone levels. The occurrence of regular menses will provide presumptive evidence of ovulation. The medication may be discontinued as soon as pregnancy is confirmed, unless required for size reduction in macroadenomas.

For patients who do not tolerate oral doses because of nausea or other gastrointestinal symptoms, vaginal therapy can be used. A single tablet (2.5 mg) daily placed high in the vagina gave adequate suppression in 13 of 15 women studied.[104]

RESULTS OF THERAPY

The manufacturer reported that 66% of 492 hyperprolactinemic patients conceived on medication.[105] More data are available in patients treated for amenorrhea-galactorrhea,[105] of whom 80% resumed menses with a mean of 5.7 weeks; 76% had decreased galactorrhea in a mean of 6.4 weeks. Maximum reduction in prolactin occurred within 4 weeks. In patients with no other causes of infertility who resume ovulation, normal rates of conception are anticipated.

A prospective, multicenter study by Molitch and coworkers[103] demonstrated the value of bromocriptine as primary therapy for prolactin-secreting macroadenomas. Prolactin levels were reduced to normal during therapy in 18 of 27 patients, and 46% of patients had a reduction in tumor size of more than 50%. Reexpansion of the tumor was noted in several patients when the drug was withdrawn.

SIDE EFFECTS

In 226 patients evaluated in clinical trials,[105] 14% developed significant reductions in blood pressure. A variety of other reactions, including nausea, headache, fatigue, and nasal congestion, have been reported. At least one adverse reaction was noted by 68% of patients, and 6% withdrew because of symptoms.

A single study reported two cases of myocardial infarction in postpartum women who received bromocriptine for lactation suppression.[106] No similar reports have been noted in anovulatory patients.

PREGNANCY OUTCOMES AND COMPLICATIONS

The outcomes of 1410 pregnancies of women taking bromocriptine have been reported.[107] Of these patients, 50% took the drug less than 4 weeks during pregnancy, and 77% discontinued the drug within 6 weeks of conception. Although progesterone levels were significantly depressed from 9 to 12 weeks of pregnancy by hyperprolactinemia, abortion rates (11.1%) were not increased. Normal rates of ectopic gestations and twinning were noted. There were 25 in 1000 minor and 10 in 1000 major anomalies, which are not increased compared with the incidence in the normal population.

Gemzell and Wang[108] reviewed 217 pregnancies in 187 patients with radiologically demonstrable pituitary tumors. Of these, 65 with prolactin-secreting microadenomas were treated with bromocriptine. One developed headache and another diabetes insipidus. Both were managed conservatively and delivered at term.

Of 21 patients with untreated prolactin-producing macroadenomas who conceived on bromocriptine, one developed headaches; three developed headaches and visual field defects and were treated during pregnancy. One was treated with bromocriptine, and two were subjected to hypophysectomy.

On the basis of small series, the relative risks of complications during pregnancy following bromocriptine therapy are approximately 3% for microadenomas versus 19% for macroadenomas. There have been no reports of tumor expansion in pregnant patients with normal radiographic studies prior to pregnancy.[109]

USE DURING PREGNANCY

Patients with hyperprolactinemia require close followup during pregnancy. Patients with evidence of tumor should have a monthly reevaluation of visual fields and be questioned regarding headaches. Patients with no evidence of prior tumor can be followed symptomatically.

Pregnant patients who develop symptoms of tumor expansion (such as visual field changes and diabetes insipidus) can be managed with bromocriptine, which reduces tumor size in most patients while also inhibiting the pregnancy-induced rise in maternal prolactin levels and reducing fetal prolactin levels. Fetal development, however, is normal.

Other Dopamine Agonists

A variety of new drugs similar to bromocriptine but with longer half-lives and fewer side effects have been introduced. Pergolide, 25 μg daily,[110] cabergoline, weekly or twice a week,[111] and hydergine, 2 mg three times a day,[112] all have been used to correct hyperprolactinemia in amenorrheic patients, but extensive pregnancy data have not been collected in the United States, and bromocriptine appears to remain the drug of choice for ovulation induction.

However, a new dopamine agonist, CV 205-502, is under investigation and may find use in selected patients for ovulation induction. After a dose of 0.06 mg, prolactin levels are suppressed at 24 hours and single daily-dose administration is used.[113] In a prospective, randomized, double-blind study, van der Heijden and associates[114] noted equal success in reduction of prolactin levels and resumption of cyclic menses in comparison with bromocriptine, but adverse side effects were judged to be less severe in patients receiving CV 205-502. Shoham and colleagues[113] reported 20 patients treated with CV 205-502 and noted four pregnancies with drug treatment with normal fetal development.

GnRH Agonists in Ovulation Induction

A variety of GnRH agonists are available for use. These include a daily subcutaneous injectable (Lupron), a three-times-daily inhalant (Synarel), and depot products (Depo-Lupron and Zoladex). These drugs have found a number of uses in infertility therapy.

A major problem in ovulation induction with hMG is occurrence of a premature LH surge[115] at a time when conception is not optimal. This is more common in normally ovulating women undergoing controlled hyperstimulation and can be prevented if GnRH agonists are begun several weeks before hMG is begun.[116] The agonists down-regulate the pituitary and deplete LH stores. GnRH agonists also may be useful in reducing LH levels in patients with PCO[117] and, in a combined so-called flare protocol, may reduce hMG dosage in certain patients in whom ovulation induction is difficult.[118]

METHOD OF ADMINISTRATION

Two different approaches are used with GnRH agonist–hMG therapy. One involves down-regulation of the pituitary for 2 to 3 weeks followed by hMG therapy. The other involves beginning the GnRH agonist and hMG concurrently.

In the first protocol, leuprolide 1 mg subcutaneously daily is given, and E_2 levels are monitored. When E_2 is less than 50 pg/mL, the dosage of agonist may be reduced to 0.5 mg daily and administration of two to four ampules of hMG daily may be begun. Monitoring is performed by the usual methods.

When the drugs are begun simultaneously, leuprolide, 0.75 mg, is begun on day 3 of the cycle, and hMG, two to four ampules, is initiated on day 5. This so-called flare approach is based on the fact that GnRH agonists initially increase gonadotropin and gonadal steroid secretion for 1 to 2 weeks before down-regulation occurs. Luteal phase support is required.

Few studies exist in patients undergoing ovulation induction to support the benefits of these treatments. Currently, data are limited to patients with PCO and older oligo-ovulatory patients, or to patients in assisted reproductive technology programs.

SIDE EFFECTS AND COMPLICATIONS

Use of GnRH agonists leads to hot flashes, irritability, and some memory disturbances during therapy. The quantity of hMG used for ovulation induction is increased significantly.

Use of Glucocorticoids in Anovulatory Women

INDICATIONS AND MODE OF ACTION

Before clomiphene citrate became available, glucocorticoids were used to induce ovulation in some circumstances; however, the results were poor. The best outcomes were achieved in patients with adrenal disorders such as CAH of neonatal or adult onset[119, 120] and hypoadrenalism. Suppression of serum androgen levels during clomiphene therapy in patients with hyperandrogenism may increase the success of therapy.[121]

Elevated levels of serum androgens may suppress gonadotropins at the hypothalamic level either directly or as a result of peripheral or local conversion to estrogens. In addition, positive feedback of estrone (a peripheral conversion product of androstenedione) on the hypothalamic-pituitary unit may lead to chronic anovulation. In patients with either severe or mild CAH, reduced cortisol synthesis leads to increased secretion of adrenocorticotropic hormone (ACTH) and accumulation of androgens. Glucocorticoids suppress ACTH and ACTH-dependent adrenal androgen synthesis.

In patients with elevated dehydroepiandrosterone sulfate in association with a PCO-like syndrome, glucocorticoid suppresses adrenal androgen secretion and may break the cycle of chronic anovulation. As an adjunct to clomiphene therapy, glucocorticoids suppress adrenal function and cause a reduction in androstenedione and testosterone production and, consequently, the circulating testosterone level.[14, 121] Such changes may increase either the central response to clomiphene or the ovarian response to gonadotropins.

METHOD OF ADMINISTRATION

The highest ACTH levels occur in the early morning hours; therefore, in patients with CAH and PCO, suppressive doses should be administered at bedtime. If increased dosage is required, supplements are given in the morning.

Glucocorticoid dosages recommended by various authors include the following: prednisone—5 mg at bedtime, 2.5 mg in the morning[119]; cortisone acetate—25 mg three times daily[122]; and dexamethasone—0.25 to 0.75 mg twice daily.[122] Patients should be followed by measuring serial testosterone or 17-hydroxyprogesterone levels to confirm adequate suppression. Richards and coworkers[122] suggested that for regulation of menstrual function, serum testosterone levels are more predictive than 17-hydroxyprogesterone. If testosterone levels remain elevated, dosages are increased. If patients fail to ovulate normally after 3 months, clomiphene citrate should be used.

RESULTS OF THERAPY

A number of small series reporting pregnancy rates of 50% to 100% were reviewed by Kotz and Herrmann.[123] Jefferies[124] used small doses of cortisone (5 mg three times a day) and reported 67% pregnancy rates. Klingensmith and associates[125] reported results of fertility in patients with CAH. Of 18 patients treated since infancy, 55% conceived. Birnbaum and Rose reported a 64% pregnancy rate in patients with partial CAH[119] or 93% when corrected for other fertility factors. Raj and colleagues[120] reported that 65% of PCO patients with elevated adrenal androgen levels resumed ovulation on prednisone alone and 17% conceived.

COMPLICATIONS

Use of glucocorticoids in low dosages or replacement levels rarely leads to clinical cushingoid changes. Adrenal suppression is transient, and dosages can be discontinued without tapering. Decreased adrenal reserve has been reported but probably is not of clinical significance. Although rare, aseptic necrosis of the hip can occur. The use of a low-dose corticoid in the first half of pregnancy did not result in any increase in fetal complications.[126]

Progesterone for Therapy of Luteal Phase Dysfunction

INDICATIONS AND MODE OF ACTION

The use of progesterone for the treatment of luteal phase defects was first suggested by Jones.[127] Patients diagnosed by two out-of-phase endometrial biopsies may be treated with progesterone supplementation by vaginal suppository or intramuscular injection to correct a postulated abnormal response of endometrium to normal progesterone or to supplement abnormal corpus luteal function.

The use of progesterone in luteal phase dysfunction is discussed further in Chapter 17.

METHODS OF ADMINISTRATION

Progesterone given orally is poorly absorbed and rapidly metabolized. However, recent studies suggest micronized preparations may be useful. Usually, transmucosal absorption per vagina or rectum is necessary, or intramuscular injection may be used. Synthetic progestins are generally avoided.

Therapy is generally begun 3 days after the BBT temperature shift and is continued until menses. If pregnancy occurs, supplementation is continued to approximately 10 weeks' gestation. 17-Hydroxyprogesterone caproate 250 mg weekly can be substituted at 6 weeks' gestation.[128]

Either progesterone suppositories (25 mg twice a day) or progesterone in oil (12.5 mg/day intramuscularly) may be used. Rarely, the onset of menstruation is delayed by the medication. If pregnancy testing results are negative, the drug should be discontinued and menses should ensue. The drug is then reinstituted after the next ovulation.

Therapy may be monitored by endometrial biopsy during the treatment cycle, and dosages may be increased until the defect is corrected. Therapy is then continued for six cycles.

RESULTS

Many small, uncontrolled series have been reported with uncorrected pregnancy rates of about 50%. A recent study of 54 women by Maxson and coworkers reported a 43% pregnancy rate.[129] One study using life table analysis has reported per-cycle pregnancy rates of approximately 10%.[130] The mean cycle of conception in another study was 2.4 months.[131] Whether such treatment actually increases pregnancy rates has never been established.

SPECIAL PROBLEMS IN OVULATION INDUCTION

Polycystic Ovary Syndrome

Anovulation in hyperandrogenic women can be extremely difficult to treat effectively. These patients tend to be more resistant to clomiphene and more sensitive to hyperstimulation with gonadotropins. Even when ovulation occurs, pregnancy rates are reduced and abortion and multiple pregnancy rates are increased.

Many approaches have been tried in an effort to optimize the response of these patients to ovulation induction. These include use of glucocorticoids, bromocriptine, and GnRH agonists alone or together with other agents for ovulation induction. There is no indication that these newer approaches lead to higher delivery rates.[82]

EVALUATION OF THE ANOVULATORY HIRSUTE PATIENT

Many clinicians believe that before ovulation induction, hirsute patients should have serum levels of testosterone, DHEAS, early morning 17-hydroxyprogesterone, LH, FSH, and prolactin determined. Patients with elevated adrenal androgen levels, in particular those with 17-hydroxyprogesterone levels higher than 5 ng/dL[132] or those with an ethnic background associated with high rates of CAH, should have an ACTH stimulation test performed to rule out nonclassic adult-onset forms of CAH (see Chapter 16).

DRUGS TO INDUCE OVULATION IN PATIENTS WITH PCO

Clomiphene Citrate. Treatment with clomiphene citrate is the initial therapy for induction of ovulation in patients with PCO. Although clomiphene increases LH secretion, the LH:FSH ratio in PCO decreases during therapy, perhaps related to the longer plasma half-life of FSH.

One of the most important concepts in the use of clomiphene in PCO is the need to adequately monitor cycles. Patients with PCO are theoretically at greater risk for ovarian cyst formation and hyperstimulation, although this is rarely seen.

If the hyperandrogenic patient fails to ovulate in response to clomiphene, prednisone 5 mg at bedtime and 2.5 mg in the morning or dexamethasone 0.5 mg at bedtime can be instituted. This approach usually reduces testosterone levels approximately 30%, and some patients ovulate with such treatment, particularly if DHEAS levels are elevated.[14, 121]

Human Gonadotropins. For patients with PCO who fail to respond to clomiphene, the second-line treatment is human gonadotropins.

Patients with PCO appear to be more sensitive to hMG. Daily therapy is begun with one ampule and increased to two ampules if E_2 levels have not increased in 5 days. Once estrogen levels increase, determinations are repeated at 1- or 2-day intervals, and vaginal sonographic examination is done at appropriate intervals. Patients with PCO tend to respond to hMG by developing large numbers of follicles with high estrogen levels. Consequently, the usual criteria for acceptable stimulation may need to be modified. Large numbers of small- and medium-sized follicles are associated with a high incidence of hyperstimulation syndrome following hCG administration.

Purified human FSH was initially recommended to increase FSH without increasing LH levels in patients with PCO. Although early experience suggested the pregnancy rate and the incidence of ovarian hyperstimulation were similar to those in women treated with hMG, newer studies show promise of improved treatment outcome.[16] The issue remains unresolved.

Although amenorrheic patients with low E_2 and gonadotropin levels have been shown to be excellent candidates for pulsatile GnRH therapy, patients with hyperandrogenism often have poor responses to such therapy. The theoretical advantage of pulsatile GnRH therapy is that it reduces the risks of hyperstimulation and multiple pregnancy compared with hMG and may reduce costs of both monitoring and medication. Obese patients and those with high LH:FSH ratios are particularly difficult to induce with this treatment. Ovulation and pregnancy rates are low compared with those in patients with hypothalamic amenorrhea.[134]

Use of Adjuvant Therapies to Correct Postulated Hypothalamic-Pituitary Defects. Two drugs have been used in an attempt to correct presumptive abnormalities of hypothalamic-pituitary gonadotropin secretion. Bromocriptine has been used to increase dopaminergic tone and reduce LH levels. Studies have suggested decreased dopaminergic activity in patients with PCO.[89] Ovulation and pregnancies have occurred in treated euprolactinemic and hyperprolactinemic patients with PCO.[89] There are no controlled studies to document the effectiveness of bromocriptine in this group of patients.

Recent studies have suggested the use of GnRH analogs to reduce serum LH and androgen levels before hMG is initiated.[134] Other investigators followed GnRH analog treatment with GnRH therapy.[135] Ovulation and pregnancy rates with these stimulation regimens have not been greatly increased.

Ovulation Induction in Older Patients or Those with Elevated FSH Levels

Frequently, patients with amenorrhea or oligomenorrhea have significantly elevated but variable serum FSH concentrations. Multiple studies indicated that elevated basal FSH values are predictive of poor ovulatory response.[136] Levels of FSH are generally obtained on day 3 of the menstrual cycle; values greater than 20 mIU/mL indicate a particularly poor prognosis.

Suppression of serum FSH levels with EE_2 or leuprolide acetate followed by subsequent induction of ovulation with hMG may be effective. Check and coworkers[137] treated 100 patients and reported ovulation in 19% of cycles in women with FSH levels higher than 35 mIU/mL and 5.2% pregnancies per cycle, with 2.2% viable pregnancies per cycle. Surrey and Cedars[138] treated 20 patients and reported only one ovulation (5%). These results may be no higher than spontaneous pregnancy rates in perimenopausal women and in those with ovarian failure. Patients should be counseled about the low success rates and the much higher pregnancy rates (more than 30% per cycle) in donor oocyte programs.

SUMMARY

Many drugs are available for treating the anovulatory woman. The widespread use of steroid hormone assays and vaginal ultrasonography has increased our ability to adequately monitor treatment cycles and permits us to confirm ovulatory response and adjust dosages in attempting to re-

duce the incidence of hyperstimulation and multiple pregnancy.

Therapy for ovulatory dysfunction can lead to satisfying results for the patient and the physician if a rational approach is taken in pretreatment evaluation, cycle monitoring, and persistent treatment for at least six to nine cycles of therapy. Ovulation induction in anovulatory women is more likely to result in pregnancy than any other infertility treatment for any other cause of infertility.

REFERENCES

1. Shaw RW, Butt WR, London DR, et al. The oestrogen provocation test: a method of assessing the hypothalamic pituitary axis in patients with amenorrhea. Clin Endocrinol (Oxf) 1975;4:267.
2. Bauman JE. Basal body temperature: unreliable method of ovulation detection. Fertil Steril 1981;36:729.
3. Jacobson A, Marshall JR. Detrimental effect of endometrial biopsies on pregnancy rate following hMG/hCG induced ovulation. Fertil Steril 1980;33:602.
4. Hill GA, Herbert CM, Parker PA, Wentz AL. Comparison of late luteal endometrial biopsy using Novak or pipelle curette. Obstet Gynecol 1989;73:443.
5. Shoupe D, Mishell DR, Lacarra M, et al. Correlation of endometrial maturation with four methods of estimating day of ovulation. Obstet Gynecol 1989;73:88.
6. Israel R, Mishell DR, Stone SC, et al. Single luteal phase serum progesterone assay as an indicator of ovulation. Am J Obstet Gynecol 1972;112:1043.
7. Haning RV Jr, Austin CW, Carlson IH, et al. Plasma estradiol is superior to ultrasound and urinary estriol glucuronide as a predictor of ovarian hyperstimulation during induction of ovulation with menotropins. Fertil Steril 1983;40:31.
8. Hull MG, Savage PE, Bromham DR, et al. Value of a single serum progesterone measurement in the midluteal phase as a criterion of a potentially fertile cycle derived from treated and untreated conception cycles. Fertil Steril 1982;37:355.
9. Swyer GI, Radwanska E, McGarrigle HH. Plasma estradiol and progesterone estimation for the monitoring of induction of ovulation with clomiphene and chorionic gonadotropin. Br J Obstet Gynecol 1975;82:794.
10. Filicori M, Butler JP, Crowley W Jr. Neuroendocrine regulation of the corpus luteum in the human: evidence for pulsatile progesterone secretion. J Clin Invest 1984;73:1638.
11. Syrop CH, Hammond MG. Diurnal variations in midluteal serum progesterone measurements. Fertil Steril 1987;47:67.
12. Coulam CB, Hill LM, Breckle R. Ultrasonic evidence for luteinization of unruptured preovulatory follicles. Fertil Steril 1982;37:524.
13. Cramer DW, Walker AM, Schiff I. Statistical methods in evaluating the outcome of infertility therapy. Fertil Steril 1979;32:80.
14. Radwanska E, Sloan C. Serum testosterone levels in infertile women. Int J Fertil 1979;24:176.
15. Hammond MG. Monitoring techniques for improved pregnancy rates during clomiphene ovulation induction. Fertil Steril 1984;42:499.
16. Product information brochure. Merrell Dow Company, Cincinnati, OH, 1972.
17. Mikkelson TJ, Kroboth PD, Cameron WJ. Single-dose pharmacokinetics of clomiphene citrate in normal volunteers. Fertil Steril 1986;46:392.
18. Wu CH, Prazak LM. Endocrine basis for ovulation induction. Clin Obstet Gynecol 1974;17:65.
19. Kerin JF, Liu JH, Phillipou G, Yen SSC. Evidence for a hypothalamic site of action of clomiphene in women. J Clin Endocrinol Metab 1985;61:265.
20. Judd, SJ, Alderman J, Bowden I, Micharlov L. Evidence against the involvement of opiate neurons in mediating the effect of clomiphene citrate on gonadotropin-releasing hormone neurons. Fertil Steril 1987;47:574.
21. Hammerstein J. Mode of action of clomiphene: I. Inhibitory effect of clomiphene citrate on the formation of progesterone from acetate-1-^{14}C by human corpus luteum slices in vitro. Acta Endocrinol 1969;60:635.
22. Marut EL, Hodgen DG. Antiestrogenic action of high-dose clomiphene

in primates: pituitary augmentation with ovarian attenuation. Fertil Steril 1982;38:100.

23. Guzick DS, Zeleznik A. Efficacy of clomiphene citrate in the treatment of luteal phase deficiency: quantity versus quality of preovulatory follicles. Fertil Steril 1990;54:205.

24. Rust LA, Israel R, Mishell DR. An individualized graduated therapeutic regimen for clomiphene citrate. Am J Obstet Gynecol 1974;120:785.

25. Nillius SJ, Wide L. GnRH treatment for induction of follicular maturation and ovulation in amenorrheic women with anorexia nervosa. Br Med J 1975;3:405.

26. Lobo RA, Granger LR, Davijan V, et al. An extended regimen of clomiphene in women unresponsive to standard therapy. Fertil Steril 1982;37:762.

27. Shepard MK, Balmaceda JP, Leija CG. Relationship of weight to successful induction of ovulation with clomiphene citrate. Fertil Steril 1979;32:641.

28. Hammond MG, Halme JK, Talbert LM. Factors affecting the pregnancy rate in clomiphene citrate induction in ovulation. Obstet Gynecol 1983;62:196.

28a. Gorlitsky GA, Kase NG, Speroff L. Ovulation and pregnancy rates with clomiphene citrate. Obstet Gynecol 1978;51:265.

29. Gonen Y, Casper RF, Jacobsen W, Blankier J. Endometrial thickness and growth during ovarian stimulation: a possible predictor of implantation in in vitro fertilization. Fertil Steril 1989;52:446.

30. Gysler M, March LM, Mishell DR, et al. A decade's experience with an individualized clomiphene treatment regimen, including its effect on the postcoital test. Fertil Steril 1982;37:161.

31. MacGregor AH, Johnson JE, Bunde CA. Further clinical experience with clomiphene citrate. Fertil Steril 1979;32:641.

32. O'Herlihy C, Pepperell RJ, Robinson HP. Ultrasound timing of hCG administration in clomiphene-stimulated cycles. Obstet Gynecol 1982;59:40.

33. Downs KA, Gibson M. Clomiphene citrate therapy for luteal phase defect. Fertil Steril 1983;39:34.

34. Lamb EJ, Colliflower WW, Williams JW. Endometrial histology and conception rates after clomiphene citrate. Obstet Gynecol 1972;39:389.

35. Hammond MG, Talbert LM. Clomiphene citrate therapy of infertile women with low luteal phase progesterone levels. Obstet Gynecol 1982;59:275.

36. Van Campenhout J, Simard R, Leduc B. Antiestrogenic effect of clomiphene in the human being. Fertil Steril 1968;19:700.

37. Lamb EJ, Guderian AM. Clinical effects of clomiphene in anovulation. Obstet Gynecol 1966;28:505.

38. Taubert HD, Dericks-Tan JS. High doses of estrogens do not interfere with the ovulation-inducing effect of clomiphene. Fertil Steril 1976;27:375.

39. Insler V, Zakut H, Serr DM. Cycle pattern and pregnancy rate following combined clomiphene-estrogen therapy. Obstet Gynecol 1973;41:602.

40. Hecht BR, Khan-Dawood FS, Dawood MY. Peri-implantation phase endometrial estrogen and progesterone receptors: effect of ovulation induction with clomiphene citrate. Am J Obstet Gynecol 1989;161:1688.

41. Dickey RP, Olar TT, Taylor SN, et al. Relationship of endometrial thickness and pattern to fecundity in ovulation induction cycles: effect of clomiphene citrate alone and with human menopausal gonadotropin. Fertil Steril 1993;59:756.

42. Schenker JG, Jarkoni S, Granat M. Multiple pregnancies following induction of ovulation. Fertil Steril 1981;35:105.

43. McCormack S, Clark JH. Clomid administration to pregnant rats causes abnormalities of the reproductive tracts in offspring and mothers. Science 1979;204:629.

44. Shoham Z, Zosmer A, Insler V. Early miscarriage and fetal malformations after induction of ovulation (by clomiphene citrate and/or human menotropins), in vitro fertilization, and gamete intrafallopian transfer. Fertil Steril 1991;55:1.

45. Hack M, Lunenfeld B. Influence of hormone induction of ovulation on the fetus and newborn. Pediatr Adolesc Endocrinol 1979;5:191.

46. Correy JF, Marsden DE, Schokman FC. The outcome of pregnancy resulting from clomiphene-induced ovulation. Aust NZ J Obstet Gynaecol 1982;22:18.

47. Ahlgren M, Kallen B, Rannevik G. Outcome of pregnancy after clomiphene therapy. Acta Obstet Gynecol Scand 1976;55:371.

48. Adashi EY, Rock JA, Sapp KC, et al. Gestational outcome of clomiphene-related conceptions. Fertil Steril 1979;31:620.

49. Jansen RP. Spontaneous abortion incidence in the treatment of infertility. Am J Obstet Gynecol 1982;143:451.

50. Yuen BH, Mari N, Duleba AJ, Moon YS. Direct effects of clomiphene citrate on the steroidogenic capability of human granulosa cells. Fertil Steril 1988;49:626.

51. Schmidt GE, Sites C, Mansour R, et al. Embryo toxicity of clomiphene citrate on mouse embryos fertilized in vitro and in vivo. Am J Obstet Gynecol 1985;153:679.

52. Klopper A, Hall M. A new synthetic agent for the induction of ovulation: preliminary trials in women. Br Med J 1971;1:152.

53. Tajima C, Fukushima T. Endocrine profiles in tamoxifen-induced ovulatory cycles. Fertil Steril 1983;40:23.

54. Messinis IE, Nillius SJ. Comparison between tamoxifen and clomiphene for induction of ovulation. Acta Obstet Gynecol Scand 1982;61:377.

55. Fukushima T, Tajima C, Fukuma K, Maeyama M. Tamoxifen in the treatment of infertility associated with luteal phase deficiency. Fertil Steril 1982;37:755.

55a. Roumen MEF, Doesburg HW, Roland R. Treatment of infertile women with a deficient postcoital test with two anti-estrogens: clomiphene and tamoxifen. Fertil Steril 1984;41:237.

56. Bounstein R, Shoham Z, Vermini M, et al. Tamoxifen treatment in women with failure of clomiphene citrate therapy. Aust NZ J Obstet Gynaecol 1989;29:173.

57. Vermesh M, Kletzky OA. Follicle-stimulating hormone is the main determinant of follicular recruitment and development in ovulation induction with human menopausal gonadotropin. Am J Obstet Gynecol 1987;157:1397.

58. Messinis IE, Bergh T, Wide L. The importance of human chorionic gonadotropin support of the corpus luteum during human gonadotropin therapy in women with anovulatory infertility. Fertil Steril 1988;50:31.

59. Grazi RV, Taney FH, Gagliardi LL, et al. The luteal phase during gonadotropin therapy: effect of two human chorionic gonadotropin regimens. Fertil Steril 1991;55:1088.

60. Diczfalusy E, Harlin J. Clinical-pharmacologic studies on human menopausal gonadotropins. Hum Reprod 1988;3:21.

61. Cook AS, Webster BW, Terranova PF, Keel VA. Variation in the biologic and biochemical characteristics of human menopausal gonadotropins. Fertil Steril 1988;49:704.

62. Simon JA, Danforth DR, Hutchison JS, Hodgen GD. Characterization of recombinant DNA–derived human luteinizing hormone in vitro and in vivo. JAMA 1988;259:3290.

63. March CM. Improved pregnancy rate with monitoring of gonadotropin therapy by three modalities. Am J Obstet Gynecol 1987;156:1473.

64. Taymor ML, Sturgis SH, Lieberman BL, et al. Induction of ovulation with human postmenopausal gonadotropin. Fertil Steril 1966;17:731.

65. Gemzell CA. Experience with the induction of ovulation. J Reprod Med 1978;21:205.

66. Schwartz M, Jewelewicz R, Dyrenfurth I, et al. Use of hMG/hCG for induction of ovulation: sixteen years' experience at the Sloan Hospital for Women. Am J Obstet Gynecol 1980;138:801.

67. Radwanska E, Hammond J, Hammond M, et al. Current experience with a standardized method of hMG/hCG administration. Fertil Steril 1980;33:510.

68. Haning RV, Levin RM, Berhman HR, et al. Plasma estradiol window and urinary estriol glucuronide determinations for monitoring menotropin induction of ovulation. Obstet Gynecol 1979;54:442.

69. O'Herlihy C, Evans JH, Brown JB, et al. Use of ultrasound in monitoring ovulation induction with human pituitary gonadotropin. Obstet Gynecol 1982;60:577.

70. Blankstein J, Shalen J, Saadon T, et al. Ovarian hyperstimulation syndrome: prediction by number and size of preovulatory ovarian follicles. Fertil Steril 1987;47:597.

71. Schwartz M, Jewelewicz R. Use of gonadotropins for induction of ovulation. Fertil Steril 1981;35:3.

72. Lunenfeld B, Eshkol A. Induction of ovulation with gonadotropin. In: Rolland R, van Hall EV, Hillier SG, editors. Follicular Maturation and Ovulation. Amsterdam: Excerpta Medica, 1982:361.

73. Healy DL, Kovacs GT, Pepperell RJ, et al. A normal cumulative conception rate after HPG. Fertil Steril 1980;34:341.

74. Corsan GH, Kemmann E. Risk of a second consecutive first-trimester spontaneous abortion in women who conceive on menotropins. Fertil Steril 1990;53:817.

75. Borenstein R, Elhalah U, Lunenfeld B, et al. Severe ovarian hyperstimulation syndrome: a re-evaluated therapeutic approach. Fertil Steril 1989;51:791.

75a. Hack M, Brish M, Seer DM, et al. Outcome of pregnancy after induced ovulation: followup of pregnancies and children born after gonadotropin therapy. JAMA 1970;211:791.

75b. Spadoni LR, Cox DW, Smith DC. Use of human menopausal gonadotropin for the induction of ovulation. Am J Obstet Gynecol 1974;120:988.

75c. Harlap S. Ovulation induction and congenital malformation. Lancet 1976;1:962.

75d. Caspi E, Ronen J, Schreyer P, Goldberg MD. The outcome of pregnancy after gonadotropin therapy. Br J Obstet Gynaecol 1976;83:967.

75e. Schwartz M, Jewelewicz R, Dyrenfurth I, et al. The use of human menopausal and chorionic gonadotropins for induction of ovulation. Am J Obstet Gynecol 1980;138:801.

75f. Kurachi K, Aono T, Minagawa J, Miyake A. Congenital malformations of newborn infants after clomiphene-induced ovulation. Fertil Steril 1983;40:187.

75g. Lunenfeld B, Blankstein J, Kotev-Emet S, et al. Drugs used in ovulation induction: safety of patients and offspring. Hum Reprod 1986;1:435.

76. Schenker JG, Weinstein D. Ovarian hyperstimulation syndrome: a current survey. Fertil Steril 1978;30:255.

77. Aboulghar MA, Mansour RT, Serour GI, Amin Y. Ultrasonically guided vaginal aspiration of ascites in the treatment of severe ovarian hyperstimulation syndrome. Fertil Steril 1990;53:933.

78. Jarrell J, McInnes R, Crooke R, et al. Observations on the combination of clomiphene citrate–hMG/hCG in the management of anovulation. Fertil Steril 1981;35:634.

79. March CM, Tredway DR, Mishell DR. Effect of clomiphene on amount and duration of hMG therapy. Am J Obstet Gynecol 1976;125:699.

80. Homburg R, West C, Torresani T, Jacobs HS. Cotreatment with human growth hormone and gonadotropins for induction of ovulation: a controlled clinical trial. Fertil Steril 1990;53:254.

81. Anderson RE, Cragun JM, Chang RI, et al. Pharmacodynamic comparison of human urinary follicle-stimulating hormone and human menopausal gonadotropin in normal women and polycystic ovary syndrome. Fertil Steril 1989;52:216.

82. Meldrum DR. Low-dose follicle-stimulating hormone therapy for polycystic ovarian disease. Fertil Steril 1991;55:1039.

82a. Shoham Z, Balen A, Patel A, Jacobs HS. Results of ovulation induction using human menopausal gonadotropin or purified follicle-stimulating hormone in hypogonadotropic hypogonadism patients. Fertil Steril 1991;56:1048.

83. Sharma V, Williams J, Collins M, et al. Studies on the measurement and pharmacodynamics of human follicle-stimulating hormone. Fertil Steril 1987;47:244.

84. Shoham Z, Patel A, Jacobs HS. Polycystic ovarian syndrome: safety and effectiveness of stepwise and low-dose administration of purified follicle-stimulating hormone. Fertil Steril 1991;55:1051.

85. Schally AV, Kastin AJ, Arimura A. The hypothalamus and reproduction. Am J Obstet Gynecol 1975;122:857.

86. Knobil E, Plant TM, Wildt L, et al. Control of the rhesus monkey menstrual cycle: permissive role of hypothalamic gonadotropin-releasing hormone. Science 1980;207:1371.

87. Leyendecker G, Wildt L. Induction of ovulation with chronic intermittent (pulsatile) administration of GnRH in women with hypothalamic amenorrhea. J Reprod Fertil 1983;69:397.

88. Hahn PM, Van Vugt DA, Reid RL. The stability of synthetic gonadotropin-releasing hormone in solution. Fertil Steril 1987;48:155.

89. Seibel MM, Oskowitz S, Kamrana M, et al. Bromocriptine response in normoprolactinemic patients with polycystic ovary disease: a preliminary report. Obstet Gynecol 1984;64:213.

90. Handelman DJ, Jansen RPS, Boylan LM, et al. Pharmacokinetics of gonadotropin-releasing hormone: comparison of subcutaneous and intravenous routes. J Clin Endocrinol Metab 1984;59:739.

91. Bratt DDM, Shoemaker J. Endocrinology of gonadotropin-releasing hormone–induced cycles in hypothalamic amenorrhea: the role of the pulse dose. Fertil Steril 1991;56:1054.

92. Shoemaker J, Simons AHM, Burger CM, et al. Induction of ovulation with LHRH. In: Rolland R, van Hall EV, Hillier SG, editors. Follicular Maturation and Ovulation. Amsterdam: Excerpta Medica, 1982:373.

93. Coelingh-Benninck HJT. Induction of ovulation by pulsatile intravenous administration of GnRH in hypothalamic amenorrhea. Fertil Steril 1984;41:67S.

94. Seibel MM, Kamrava M, McArdle C, et al. Ovulation induction and conception using subcutaneous LHRH. Obstet Gynecol 1983;61:292.

95. Hurley DM, Brian R, Dutch K, et al. Induction of ovulation and fertility in amenorrheic women by pulsatile low-dose GnRH. N Engl J Med 1984;310:1069.

96. Goerzen J, Corenblum B, Wiseman D, et al. Ovulation induction and pregnancy in hypothalamic amenorrhea using self-administered intravenous GnRH. Fertil Steril 1984;41:319.

96a. Santoro N. Efficacy and safety of intravenous pulsatile gonadotropin-releasing hormone: Lutrepulse for injection. Am J Obstet Gynecol 1990;163:1959.

97. Filicori M, Flamigni C, Meriggiola MC, et al. Ovulation induction with pulsatile gonadotropin-releasing hormone: technical modalities and clinical perspectives. Fertil Steril 1991;56:1.

98. HRF Ayerst product brochure, Ayerst International, 1976.

99. Mehta AE, Tolis G. Pharmacology of bromocriptine in health and disease. Drugs 1979;17:313.

100. Hausler A, Rohr HP, Marbach P, et al. Changes in prolactin secretion in lactating rats assessed by correlative morphometric and biochemical methods. J Ultrastruct Res 1978;64:74.

101. Thorner MO, Schran HF, Evans WS, et al. A broad spectrum of prolactin suppression by bromocriptine in hyperprolactinemic women: a study of serum prolactin and bromocriptine levels after acute and chronic administration of bromocriptine. J Clin Endocrinol Metab 1980;50:1026.

101a. Vermesh M, Fossum GT, Kletzky OA. Vaginal bromocriptine: pharmacology and effect on serum prolactin in normal women. Obstet Gynecol 1988;72:693.

102. Maurer RA. Transcriptional regulation of the prolactin gene by ergocryptine and cyclic AMP. Nature 1981;294:94.

103. Molitch ME, Elton RL, Blackwell RE, et al. Bromocriptine as primary therapy for prolactin-secreting macroadenomas: results of a prospective multicenter study. J Clin Endocrinol Metab 1985;60:698.

104. Kletsky OA, Vermesh M. Effectiveness of vaginal bromocriptine in treating women with hyperprolactinemia. Fertil Steril 1989;51:269.

105. Cuellar FG. Bromocriptine mesylate (Parlodel) in the management of amenorrhea/galactorrhea associated with hyperprolactinemia. Obstet Gynecol 1980;55:278.

106. Iffy L, Ten Hove W, Frisoli G. Acute myocardial infarction in the puerperium in patients receiving bromocriptine. Am J Obstet Gynecol 1986;155:371.

107. Turkalj I, Baun P, Krupp P. Surveillance of bromocriptine in pregnancy. JAMA 1982;247:1589.

108. Gemzell C, Wang CF. Outcome of pregnancy in women with pituitary adenoma. Fertil Steril 1979;31:363.

109. Pepperell RJ. Prolactin and reproduction. Fertil Steril 1981;35:267.

110. Kletzky OA, Borenstein R, Mileikowsky GN. Pergolide and bromocriptine for treatment of patients with hyperprolactinemia. Am J Obstet Gynecol 1986;154:431.

111. Ciccarelli E, Giusti M, Miola C, et al. Effectiveness and tolerability of long-term treatment with cabergoline, a new long-lasting ergolise derivative, in hyperprolactinemic patients. J Can Endocrinol Metab 1989;69:725.

112. Tamura T, Satoh T, Minakami H, Tamala T. Effect of hydergine in hyperprolactinemia. J Clin Endocrinol Metab 1989;69:470.

113. Shoham Z, Homburg R, Jacobs HS. CV 205-502—effectiveness, tolerability, and safety over 24-month study. Fertil Steril 1991;55:501.

114. van der Heijden PFM, de Wit W, Brownell J, et al. CV 205-502, a new dopamine agonist, versus bromocriptine in the treatment of hyperprolactinaemia. Eur J Obstet Gynecol Reprod Biol 1991;40:111.

115. Talbert LM. Endogenous luteinizing hormone surge and superovulation. Fertil Steril 1988;49:24.

116. Serafini P, Stone B, Kerin J, et al. An alternative approach to controlled ovarian hyperstimulation in poor responders. Fertil Steril 1988;49:90.

117. Dodson WC, Hughes CL, Whitesides DB, Haney AF. The effect of leuprolide acetate on ovulation induction with human menopausal gonadotropins in polycystic ovary syndrome. J Clin Endocrinol Metab 1987;65:95.

118. Garcia JE, Padilla SL, Bayati J, Baramki TA. Follicular-phase gonadotropin-releasing hormone agonist and human gonadotropins: a better alternative for ovulation induction in in vitro fertilization. Fertil Steril 1990;53:302.

119. Birnbaum MD, Rose LI. Late-onset adrenocortical hydroxylase deficiencies associated with menstrual dysfunction. Obstet Gynecol 1984;63:445.

120. Raj SG, Thompson IE, Berger MJ, et al. Clinical aspects of the polycystic ovary syndrome. Obstet Gynecol 1977;49:552.

121. Daly DC, Walters CA, Soto-Albors CE, et al. Randomized study of dexamethasone in ovulation induction with clomiphene citrate. Fertil Steril 1984;41:844.

122. Richards GE, Grumbach MM, Kaplan SL, et al. The effect of long-

acting glucocorticoids on menstrual abnormalities in patients with virilizing congenital adrenal hyperplasia. J Clin Endocrinol Metab 1978;47:1208.

123. Kotz HL, Herrmann W. A review of the endocrine induction of human ovulation: IV. Cortisone. Fertil Steril 1961;12:299.

124. Jefferies WM. Further experience with small doses of cortisone and related steroids in infertility associated with ovarian dysfunction. Fertil Steril 1960;11:100.

125. Klingensmith GJ, Garcia SC, Jones JW, et al. Glucocorticoid treatment of girls with congenital adrenal hyperplasia: effects on height, sexual maturation, and fertility. J Pediatr 1977;90:996.

126. Lee F, Nelson N, Faiman C. Low-dose corticoid therapy for anovulation: effect upon fetal weight. Obstet Gynecol 1982;60:314.

127. Jones GES. Luteal phase insufficiency. Clin Obstet Gynecol 1973;16:255.

128. Johnson JWC, Austin KL, Jones GS. Efficacy of 17-hydroxyprogesterone caproate in the prevention of premature labor. N Engl J Med 1975;293:675.

129. Maxson WS, Wentz AC, Herbert CM. Outcome of progesterone therapy of luteal phase inadequacy. Fertil Steril 1984;41:195.

130. Huang K. The primary treatment of luteal phase inadequacy: progesterone versus clomiphene citrate. Am J Obstet Gynecol 1986;155:824.

131. Daly DC, Walters CA, Soto-Albors C, et al. Multiple therapeutic modalities improve pregnancy rates in luteal phase defects. Fertil Steril 1982;39:393a.

132. Dewailly D, Vantyghem-Haudiquet M-C, et al. Clinical and biological phenotypes in late-onset 21-hydroxylase deficiency 1986;63(2):418.

133. Jansen PRS, Handelsman DJ, Boylan LM, et al. Intravenous GnRH for ovulation induction in infertile women: II. Analysis of follicular and luteal phase responses. Fertil Steril 1987;48:39.

134. Steingold KA, Judd HL, Nieberg RK, et al. Treatment of severe androgen excess due to ovarian hyperthecosis with a long-acting gonadotropin-releasing hormone agonist. Am J Obstet Gynecol 1986;154:1241.

135. Surrey ES, deZiegler D, Lu JKH, et al. Effects of gonadotropin-releasing hormone (GnRH) agonist in pituitary and ovarian responses to pulsatile GnRH therapy in polycystic ovarian disease. Fertil Steril 1989;52:547.

136. Toner JP, Philput CB, Jones GS, Muasher SJ. Basal follicle-stimulating hormone level is a better predictor of in vitro fertilization performance than age. Fertil Steril 1991;55:784.

137. Check JH, Nowloozi K, Chase JS, et al. Ovulation induction and pregnancies in 100 consecutive women with hypergonadotropic amenorrhea. Fertil Steril 1990;53:811.

138. Surrey ES, Cedars MI. The effect of gonadotropin suppression on the induction of ovulation in premature ovarian failure patients. Fertil Steril 1989;52:36.

CHAPTER 14

Hyperstimulation Syndrome

ERIC S. SURREY

The refinement of controlled ovarian hyperstimulation techniques has increased the effectiveness of ovulation induction and enhanced the ability to recruit multiple mature oocytes for use in conjunction with the assisted reproductive technologies. However, the administration of the medications associated with these techniques is not without its risks. Ovarian hyperstimulation syndrome (OHSS) represents a significant complication with protean manifestations. The pathogenesis and presentation, as well as options for prevention and management of this disorder, are reviewed in this chapter.

CLASSIFICATION

OHSS does not represent a single pathologic entity but rather forms a spectrum of disorders ranging from a benign inconvenience to a life-threatening condition. Two fundamental pathologic changes are characteristic: ovarian enlargement with underlying stromal edema and multiple hemorrhagic luteinized cysts coupled with a dramatic shift of fluid from the intravascular spaces into the peritoneal, pleural, and pericardial cavities.[1]

Several classification systems for OHSS have been developed. In 1967, Rabau and coworkers suggested three overall clinical categories for this disorder—mild, moderate, and severe—with six grades based on laboratory findings and the severity of symptoms.[2] The enhanced sensitivity provided by new sonographic techniques has allowed for more accurate assessments of ovarian size than by physical examination alone. Similarly, measurements of cervical mucus and total urinary estrogen and pregnanediol levels have been replaced by rapid radioimmunoassay techniques that more accurately reflect circulating ovarian hormone levels.

Golan and associates presented a revised classification system that is extremely useful given currently employed diagnostic techniques and is shown in Table 14–1.[3] Mild OHSS is marked by abdominal distention and sonographic evidence of ovarian enlargement and can be associated with gastrointestinal symptoms such as nausea, vomiting, and diarrhea. If sonographic evidence of ascites is present as well, the patient

has moderate OHSS. Severe OHSS encompasses the features of moderate disease with the addition of one or more of the following: clinically evident ascites, hydrothorax, dyspnea, hypercoagulable states, severe dehydration, and compromised renal perfusion and function. Adult respiratory distress syndrome has been described in association with severe OHSS.[4] Evidence of hemoconcentration and subsequent enhanced blood viscosity can lead to thrombotic events. We have reported a case of internal jugular vein thrombosis extending into the superior vena cava resulting from severe hemoconcentration in the absence of other significant symptoms associated with this disorder (Fig. 14–1).[5] Others have described carotid artery thrombosis and cerebral artery occlusion.[6, 7] Increases in coagulation factor V and fibrinogen levels with concomitant decrements in partial thromboplastin time and antithrombin III have been reported.[8, 9] Transient abnormalities in liver function have also been described, although the causation is not clear.[10]

INCIDENCE

The incidence of severe OHSS in patients treated with clomiphene citrate is relatively rare, with most of the publications represented by individual case reports.[11, 12] In one large series of 200 treatment cycles, Polishuk and Schenker reported a 2.5% incidence of hyperstimulation after clomiphene administration.[13] Ito and coworkers noted a higher incidence (5.9%) in patients with polycystic ovary syndrome (PCO).[14]

The use of human menopausal gonadotropins (hMGs) for controlled ovarian hyperstimulation is associated with a somewhat higher incidence of OHSS. A representative selection of results from reported series is depicted in Table 14–2. The incidence of mild disease varies from 2.8% to 23%, whereas that of moderate disease ranges from 2.9% to 16.25% in the series presented. Severe OHSS ranges from being unreported in some series to a peak incidence of 7.1%. Koyama and colleagues reported that increases in the ratio of follicle-stimulating hormone (FSH) to luteinizing hormone (LH) in hMG preparations is associated with a greater inci-

TABLE 14–1. Revised Classification of OHSS

Classification of OHSS	Criteria
Mild	
Grade 1	Abdominal distention and discomfort
Grade 2	Features of grade 1 plus nausea, vomiting, and/or diarrhea
Moderate	Ovarian enlargement: 5–12 cm
Grade 3	Features of mild OHSS + sonographic evidence of ascites
Severe	
Grade 4	Features of moderate OHSS + clinical evidence of ascites and/or hydrothorax or respiratory compromise
Grade 5	All of the above + hypovolemia, hemoconcentration, coagulation abnormalities, or diminished renal perfusion and function

OHSS, ovarian hyperstimulation syndrome.
Modified from Golan A, Ron-El R, Herman A, et al. Ovarian hyperstimulation syndrome: an update review. Obstet Gynecol Surv 44:430–440. © by Williams & Wilkins, 1989.

TABLE 14–2. Incidence of OHSS in hMG-Stimulated Cycles

Reference	Cycles (N)	Classification of OHSS Mild (%)	Moderate and Severe (%)
Lunenfeld and Insler[15]	1405	8.4	0.8
Navot et al[16]	1822	1	1.95
McArdle et al[17]	80	11.25	20
Haning et al[18]	70	11.4	10
Tulandi et al[19]	89	23	9
Tal et al[20]	36	11.4	6.8
Kurachi et al[21]	6069	—	5.3*
Buvat et al[22]	65	27.7	7.7
Wang and Gemzell[23]	77	—	11.7
Dodson et al[24]	25	—	8
Schwartz et al[25]	67	—	6.3*
Oelsner et al[26]	1897	—	4.62*

*Overall (all grades).
OHSS, ovarian hyperstimulation syndrome; hMG, human menopausal gonadotropin.

dence of OHSS.[27] McArdle and coworkers reported that with the use of sonographic examinations to detect ovarian enlargement, the overall incidence of OHSS was 44%.[17] Thus, with modern sonographic techniques, it may be concluded that milder forms of OHSS, which may not be clinically relevant, are extremely common after gonadotropin administration. Combining clomiphene with hMGs is associated with a lower incidence of OHSS than has been described with the use of gonadotropins alone.[20]

Check and coworkers described a 5.3% incidence of severe OHSS and a 23% overall incidence of OHSS with the use of purified urinary FSH.[28] More recently, others have presented information to suggest that use of "slow," prolonged treatment protocols for patients with PCO may reduce the risk of OHSS engendered by conventional FSH or hMG regimens.[22]

It has been suggested that despite the need for larger doses of hMG over longer periods of stimulation, the incidence of OHSS is lower in anovulatory patients who are hypogonadotropic and hypoestrogenic than in those with relatively normal gonadotropin levels associated with evidence of endogenous estrogen activity (e.g., PCO).[21, 29] This enhanced risk of hyperstimulation in patients with PCO may be due to increased recruitment of follicles in varying maturational states associated with pathologic gonadotropin and steroid hormone responses to exogenous stimulation.[30] In contrast, Oelsner and coworkers reported that the occurrence rates of OHSS were similar between these two groups of anovulatory women.[26]

The suppression of endogenous pituitary gonadotropin secretion and ovarian sex steroid hormone production with

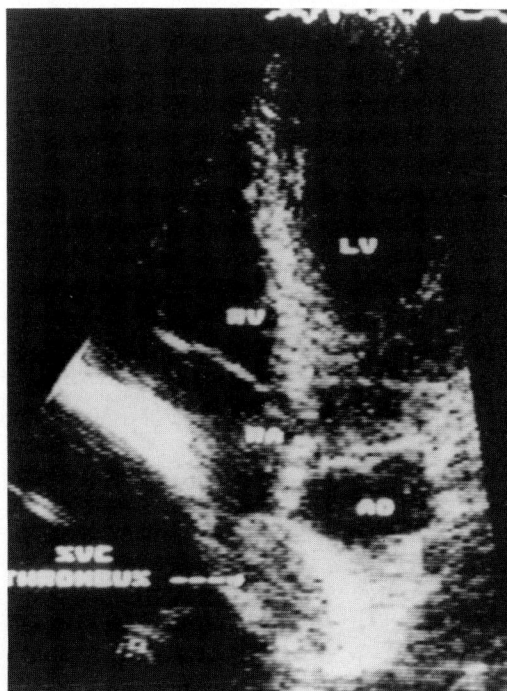

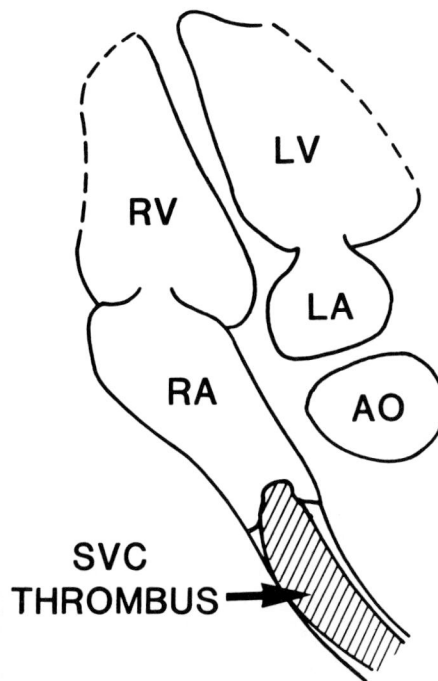

FIGURE 14–1. Superior vena cava (SVC) thrombosis associated with severe ovarian hyperstimulation syndrome. Echocardiographic appearance is shown on the *left,* and a diagrammatic representation is shown on the *right.* LV, left ventricle; RV, right ventricle; LA, left atrium; RA, right atrium; AO, aorta. (From Fournet N, Surrey E, Kerin J. Internal jugular vein thrombosis after ovulation induction with gonadotropins. Fertil Steril 1991;56:355. Reprinted with permission of the publisher, The American Fertility Society.)

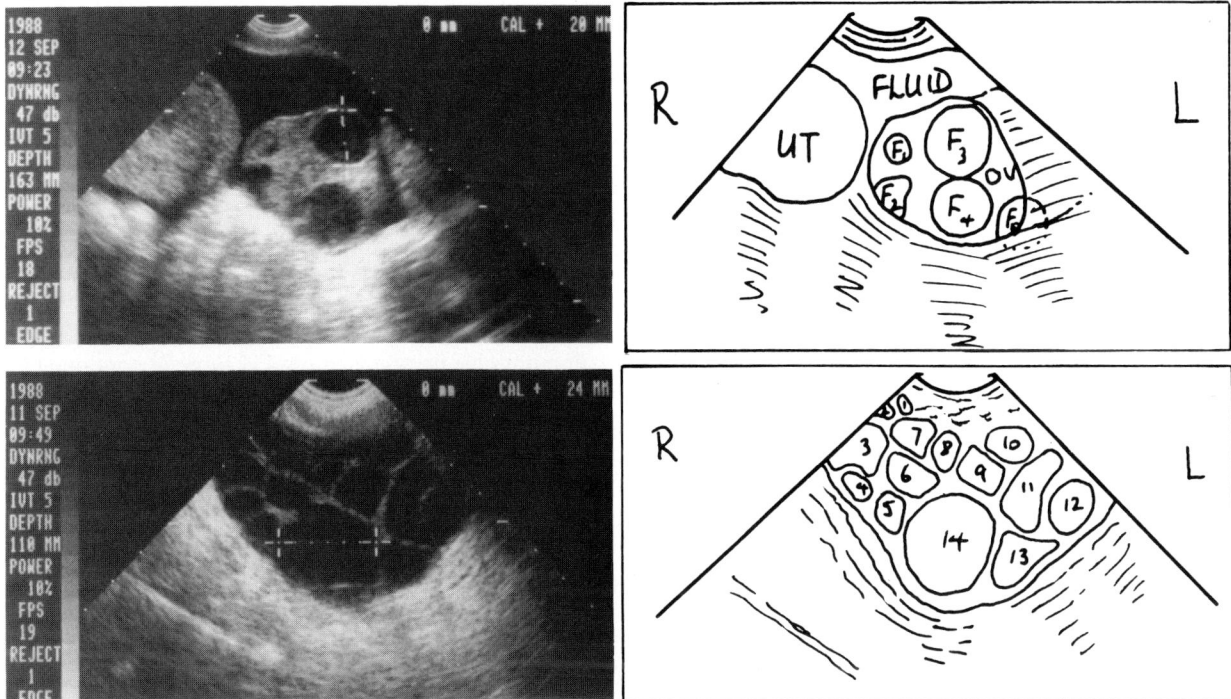

FIGURE 14–2. *Upper,* Transverse sonographic view (left) and diagrammatic representation (right) of uterus and multicystic left ovary 5 days after human menopausal gonadotropin/human chorionic gonadotropin (hMG/hCG)–controlled ovarian hyperstimulation. This patient presented with abdominal pain and fullness with grade 2 ovarian hyperstimulation syndrome (OHSS) that resolved spontaneously. Note the echogenic hemorrhagic ovarian cysts and ascitic fluid. *Lower,* Multiple intermediate-sized follicles noted on transvaginal ultrasound examination of the right ovary in a patient administered gonadotropin for controlled ovarian hyperstimulation. A similar pattern occurred in the left ovary. The patient's blood estradiol level reached 4500 pg/mL. Because the risk of OHSS was considered to be very likely, hCG was withheld. The cysts regressed spontaneously without incident over a 4-week period. (From Kerin JF, Surrey ES. Transvaginal imaging and the infertility patient. Obstet Gynecol Clin North Am 1991;18:770.)

the use of highly potent gonadotropin-releasing hormone (GnRH) agonists has been well documented.[31] It was hypothesized that pretreatment of PCO patients with GnRH agonists prior to gonadotropin stimulation would result in a hypogonadotropic hypoestrogenic state, thus decreasing the risk of OHSS. However, in a randomized study, Dodson and associates could find no significant difference in the incidence of OHSS between PCO patients pretreated with GnRH agonists prior to hMG and those treated with hMG alone.[24] Others have in fact demonstrated a heightened incidence of all grades of OHSS in patients treated with GnRH agonists.[32, 33] Charbonnel and coworkers reported a 6% incidence of severe OHSS and a 40% incidence of moderate OHSS in PCO patients treated during 33 GnRH agonist–hMG cycles.[34] A case of OHSS associated with the sole use of the GnRH agonist leuprolide acetate in the absence of hMG has been recently reported.[35] Golan and colleagues have hypothesized that the abolition of premature luteinization with GnRH agonists may enhance the likelihood of OHSS.[36]

It had been assumed that follicular aspiration during in vitro fertilization (IVF) or gamete intrafallopian transfer (GIFT) cycles would significantly decrease the incidence of hyperstimulation despite recruitment of multiple oocytes by administration of extremely high doses of hMG.[37] Smitz and coworkers described only a 0.6% incidence of severe OHSS in 1673 cycles of IVF, GIFT, or zygote intrafallopian transfer preceded by administration of the GnRH agonist buserelin and hMG.[38] In another series, however, Golan and coworkers reported an 8.4% incidence of OHSS in 143 IVF cycles.

Seven of these 12 cases were severe in nature despite pretreatment with a GnRH agonist and subsequent follicular aspiration.[36]

The more physiologic approach of inducing ovulation with intravenous or subcutaneous pulsatile GnRH theoretically should reduce the potential for ovarian hyperstimulation. Although no studies of sufficient size are available to assess the true incidence of OHSS with this form of therapy, several case reports suggest that this complication is not entirely eliminated even in the absence of human chorionic gonadotropin (hCG) administration.[39–41]

PATHOGENESIS

As previously described, OHSS is marked by massive bilateral cystic ovarian enlargement. The ovaries are noted to have a significant degree of stromal edema interspersed with multiple hemorrhagic follicular and theca-lutein cysts, areas of cortical necrosis, and neovascularization.[42] The second pathologic phenomenon is that of a significant third-space loss by shifts in intravascular volume. This can result in marked ascites, pleural and pericardial effusions, peripheral edema, and anasarca. The typical sonographic appearance of ascites and ovarian cystic enlargement is demonstrated in Figure 14–2 *(upper panel).* Rare cases of secondary pulmonary edema with concomitant adult respiratory distress syndrome have been reported.[4] These fluid shifts are believed to be the result of enhanced capillary permeability. Conflicting evidence based on measurements of protein and electrolyte concentrations has been presented as to whether this fluid represents a transudate or an exudate.[43-45]

The nature of the inciting vasoactive agent remains controversial. A direct relationship between total gonadotropin dose administered and development of ovarian enlargement and ascites was noted by Polishuk and Schenker employing a rabbit model.[13] These investigators suggested that the inciting factor for OHSS was of ovarian origin by demonstrating that this syndrome could be induced with gonadotropins administered to female rabbits that had undergone hysterectomy and ovarian extraperitonealization, but not to males.[13] Rabau and associates, however, could find no such correlation in humans administered exogenous gonadotropins for ovulation induction.[2]

High levels of circulating estrogens were initially implicated as the primary inciting factor for the development of this syndrome. In animal models, estrogens have been shown to have some relationship to increases in capillary permeability.[46, 47] Investigators have shown that mean serum estradiol (E_2) levels were higher in patients who experienced OHSS despite having been administered similar doses of hMG as those who failed to develop this disorder.[36, 48] In contrast, others have demonstrated that estrogen levels alone were not predictive of the onset of OHSS.[20, 49, 50] In the animal model, direct administration of high doses of exogenous estrogens did not induce the changes characteristic of OHSS.[51]

Elevations in serum prolactin levels have also been reported in patients with OHSS.[52] A correlation between elevated local prolactin concentrations and enhanced membrane permeability has been shown to influence amniotic fluid circulation.[53] An association between pathologic elevations of this hormone and abnormal capillary permeability has been hypothesized. Leung and coworkers demonstrated that ascites production was significantly greater in rabbits treated with hMG and purified ovine prolactin than those receiving hMG alone.[54] Prolactin played no role in the induction of ovarian enlargement in this model. This causal relationship has not been demonstrated in humans.

Increases in LH have been shown to enhance follicular biosynthesis of prostaglandins.[55-57] Schenker and Polishuk showed that ascites was minimized by administration of indomethacin, an inhibitor of prostaglandin synthesis, to rabbits with gonadotropin-induced OHSS.[58] Using a similar model, Pride and coworkers were unable to reproduce these findings.[59] In fact, they noted that elevated prostaglandin F levels apparently derived from ovarian sources appeared to correlate with amelioration of ascites.[59] These findings call into question the role of prostaglandins as the critical vasoactive agent in the development of OHSS.

Histamine has a well-established role in the inflammatory response as a vasoactive substance acting to significantly enhance vascular permeability. In addition, it has been shown to play a role in prolactin release, potentially acting via serotonergic pathways.[60] In an effort to establish the role of histamines in OHSS, several investigators have demonstrated that antihistamines can markedly reduce formation of ascites[61-63]; however, these data could not be confirmed in subsequent studies employing an animal model. No differences in peripheral histamine levels were noted between rabbits with OHSS and control subjects.[64] One could certainly argue, however, that peripheral levels do not accurately reflect local ovarian activity. Nevertheless, Zaidise and associates were unable to demonstrate that either serotonergic antagonists or H_1 receptor blockers had any clear effect on the resolution of ascites in rabbits with OHSS, although the former did somewhat inhibit ovarian enlargement.[65]

One of the weaknesses of the animal models that have been employed for the investigation of OHSS is their failure to explain the strictly postovulatory phenomenon of OHSS in humans. Gonadotropin administration alone to the rabbit in the absence of ovulation can result in ovarian enlargement and ascites formation.[42] However, OHSS can be prevented in the human by withholding hCG.[66] This would imply that a supraphysiologic preovulatory LH surge or continued stimulus in the luteal phase may trigger release of some critical vasoactive substance. The most likely candidate is a product of the intrinsic ovarian renin-angiotensin system, the nature of which has been extensively reviewed elsewhere.[67] The active peptide of this system, angiotensin II, plays a key role in fluid and electrolyte balance and may potentially play a role in local increases in vascular permeability, neovascularization, and prostaglandin release.[68, 69] The activity of this pathway appears to peak at the time of the LH surge in unstimulated cycles as reflected by increased levels of prorenin, the inactive renin precursor.[68] Itskovitz and associates demonstrated that prorenin levels are significantly higher in stimulated cycles, peaking several days after hCG administration.[70] These rises in prorenin levels were significantly enhanced by conception, failing to resolve until the hCG was systemically cleared. Such patterns parallel the clinical picture of OHSS, a syndrome that does not present until several days after hCG administration and is exacerbated with pregnancy. Indirect confirmatory evidence has been provided by two sets of investigators. Haning and coworkers noted a marked increase in plasma renin activity, aldosterone, and antidiuretic hormone in patients experiencing OHSS.[71] More recently, Navot and colleagues reported that plasma renin activity directly correlated with the severity of OHSS.[72] The lack of a strict correlation between circulating aldosterone levels and the severity of the disorder suggests the role of an extrarenal source for this detectable renin activity.

PREVENTION

As with any pathologic disorder, the ideal means of treating hyperstimulation syndrome lies in its prevention. OHSS is a strictly postovulatory event in humans. As previously mentioned, withholding hCG during hMG cycles can lead to prevention of this disorder in virtually all cases.[66] One must therefore have a means of appropriately selecting those patients who are at particularly high risk so that hCG can be withheld without unnecessarily cancelling cycles.

Early techniques of assessing ovarian response to exogenous gonadotropin stimulation such as vaginal cytology, cervical scores, and measurements of urinary estrogen levels have been replaced by accurate quantification of serum E_2 by rapid radioimmunoassay.[3, 43, 73] Relatively higher E_2 levels have been noted in patients experiencing OHSS receiving hMG/hCG before both intrauterine insemination and IVF.[19, 36] Several investigators have attempted to provide threshold levels of serum E_2 beyond which hCG should be withheld. Schenker and Weinstein recommended a limit of 800 pg/

OVARIAN HYPERSTIMULATION
Mean number of follicles on day of HCG administration

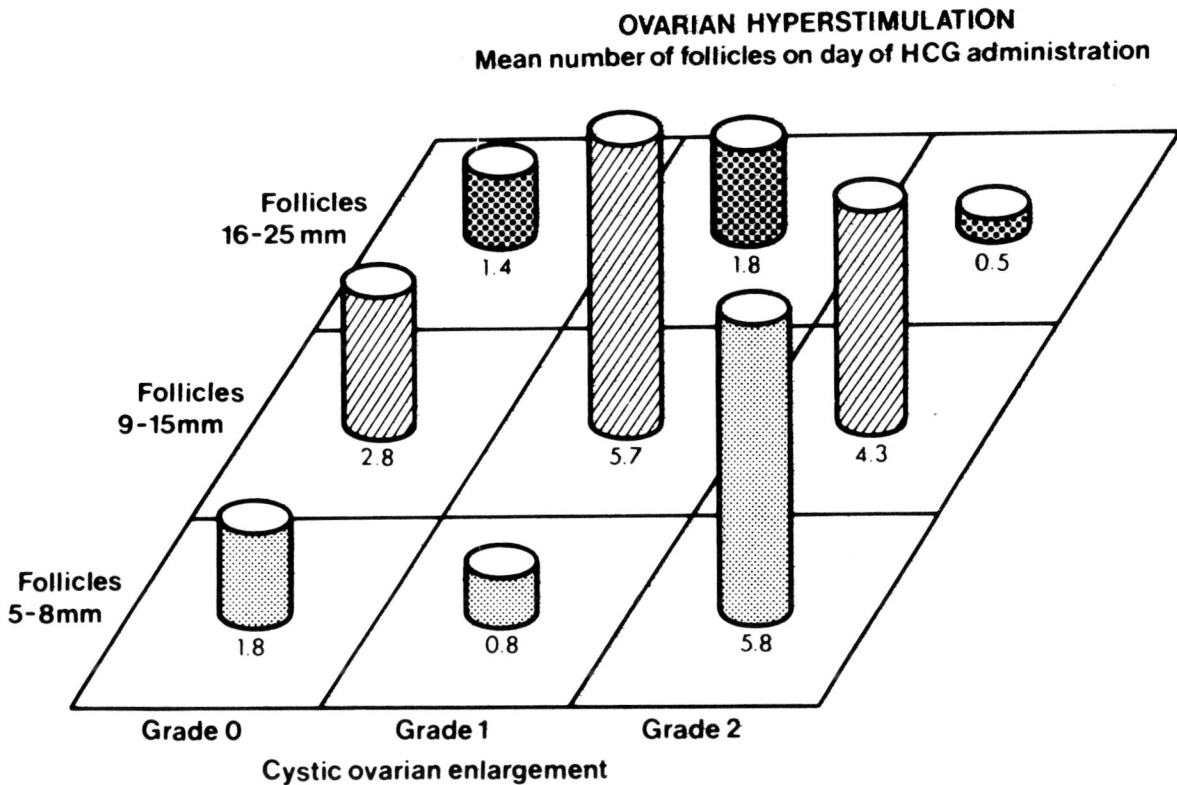

FIGURE 14–3. Schematic representation of follicular size on day of human chorionic gonadotropin (hCG) administration in relation to severity of ovarian hyperstimulation syndrome. (From Blankstein J, Shalev J, Saadon T, et al. Ovarian hyperstimulation syndrome: prediction by number and size of preovulatory ovarian follicles. Fertil Steril 1987;47:600. Reprinted with permission of the publisher, The American Fertility Society.)

mL.[43] Schwartz and coworkers believed that an ideal range of E_2 to achieve optimal follicular development while avoiding OHSS was 500 to 1500 pg/mL.[25] In contrast, McArdle and associates suggested that mild and moderate grades of OHSS failed to correlate with E_2 levels.[17] Hancock and coworkers believed that an enhanced rate of increase was of greater concern than maximal absolute values in predicting hyperstimulation.[66] Haning and coworkers compared maximal serum E_2 values to both the maximal number of follicles measured sonographically as well as to peak urinary excretion of estriol glucuronide to determine the best single predictor for development of OHSS during induction of ovulation with hMGs in 70 cycles.[18] They noted that serum E_2 peaked 8 to 10 hours after an injection of hMG. Plasma E_2 was the best single predictor of OHSS in this study, with levels lower than 4000 pg/mL believed to be associated with a decreased risk of developing hyperstimulation.

Given earlier data suggesting that E_2 levels correlated with total follicular volume and not the size of the dominant follicle,[74, 75] it is illogical to rely solely on serum levels to predict OHSS. The relative contribution of stimulated granulosa cells from a varying number of individual follicles to the pool of circulating E_2 must play a role. Indeed, Leya and coworkers demonstrated that although serum E_2 levels were higher in patients who experienced hyperstimulation during GIFT and IVF cycles, E_2 levels measured from follicular fluid of dominant follicles were similar in patients with or without OHSS.[48] However, E_2 levels were significantly higher from follicles less than 15-mm mean diameter in patients who developed OHSS. This corroborates an earlier report by Tal

and associates suggesting that the presence of three or more secondary follicles 14 to 16 mm in diameter was associated with a significantly increased incidence of OHSS.[20] In a review of 65 hMG/hCG cycles, Blankstein and coworkers clearly correlated an enhanced number of small (5 to 8 mm) and intermediate (9 to 15 mm) sized follicles with enhanced risk of hyperstimulation (Fig. 14–3).[76] An example of this ominous sonographic pattern is displayed in Figure 14–2 (lower panel).

Others have attempted to salvage treatment cycles in the face of incipient OHSS. Itskovitz and coworkers described 14 patients desiring IVF with exaggerated E_2 responses to gonadotropins believed to be at high risk for hyperstimulation.[77] The GnRH agonist buserelin was administered in place of hCG to induce final oocyte maturation by taking advantage of the short-acting agonist effect of this agent on endogenous gonadotropin release. No evidence of OHSS was noted. This was believed to be a result of induction of a more physiologic LH surge rather than the heightened and prolonged pharmacologic stimulus provided by hCG. This interesting approach has not yet been corroborated in larger series. Others have withheld administration of hCG in potential IVF cycles with high risk for development of OHSS and continued GnRH agonist therapy alone until pituitary desensitization was achieved before restarting ovarian stimulation.[78] In an effort to inhibit luteinization in similar high-risk cycles, Amso and colleagues administered hCG, aspirated oocytes, cryopreserved resultant embryos, and continued GnRH agonist therapy during the luteal phase with some success.[79] As previously discussed, some controversy exists as to whether follicular aspiration decreases the incidence of OHSS.[37, 80] An uncontrolled series reported a decreased incidence of OHSS in high-risk anovulatory patients scheduled to undergo intrauterine insemination after gonadotropin stimulation who were treated instead with follicular aspiration and subsequent IVF.[81]

Careful patient selection and conservative gonadotropin dosage regimens cannot eliminate OHSS entirely. Meticulous monitoring of the rate of E_2 rise as well as absolute levels achieved, along with assessment of sonographic patterns of follicular development, all are crucial factors that should be considered to decrease the incidence of this disorder. Newer techniques employing GnRH agonists to either substitute for hCG or suppress luteinization after embryos have been cryopreserved await corroboration in larger controlled series to determine their true value.

MANAGEMENT

Symptoms of OHSS may commence 24 to 96 hours after hCG administration, and, in the absence of pregnancy, tend to resolve within 7 to 14 days, although cystic ovarian enlargement may dissipate more slowly. The clinical course is more protracted in patients who conceive.[2, 43] Some have suggested that the likelihood of pregnancy is higher in the face of OHSS, although this has not been consistently demonstrated.[19] Rare cases of nonovulatory OHSS secondary to hypothyroidism or GnRH agonist administration alone have been described.[35, 82] A case report of ovarian carcinoma masquerading as OHSS in a patient receiving clomiphene led one set of investigators to advise careful assessment of cystic ovarian enlargement that fails to resolve after 4 weeks. The presence of solid components is of particular concern.[83]

The management of this syndrome is primarily supportive and medical in nature. Given the hemorrhagic nature of the multiple theca-lutein cysts, surgery should be avoided if at all possible. Surgical intervention should be undertaken only in the event of hemoperitoneum resulting from cyst rupture or torsion. Mashiach and coworkers reported that of 201 cases of OHSS, ovarian torsion occurred in 16% of conception cycles but in only 2.3% of nonconception cycles.[84] Adnexectomy was required in only one of those cases, with others managed more conservatively by unwinding of the ovary, cystectomy, or suture of the ruptured cortex.

Although milder grades of hyperstimulation can be managed with bed rest, avoiding hospitalization, all patients must be carefully evaluated. Pregnancy should be diagnosed as expeditiously as possible by sensitive serum radioimmunoassay. Pelvic sonographic evaluation can afford an accurate measure of the extent of ovarian enlargement and ascites formation. Patients should be instructed to record their weight twice daily and remain relatively sedentary. Criteria for hospitalization include severe abdominal pain, intraperitoneal hemorrhage, ovarian torsion, peritonitis, respiratory compromise, rapid weight gain and accumulation of ascites, severe hemoconcentration, electrolyte imbalances, compromise of renal function, presyncopal or syncopal episodes, or evidence of pleural or pericardial effusion.

Potential metabolic alterations associated with OHSS are summarized in Table 14–3. Initial laboratory assessment on admission must include a complete blood count; serum elec-

TABLE 14–3. Metabolic Alterations Associated with OHSS
Volume Status
Hypovolemia
Hemoconcentration
Renal Perfusion
Increased blood urea nitrogen, creatinine levels
Increased aldosterone level, plasma renin activity, antidiuretic hormone
Electrolyte Imbalance
Hyperkalemia
Hyponatremia
Coagulation Factors
Increased factor V, fibrinogen
Decreased antithrombin III, partial thromboplastin
Liver Function
Increased serum glutamic-oxalocetic transaminase and serum glutamic-pyruvic transaminase levels

OHSS, ovarian hyperstimulation syndrome.

trolyte, creatinine, and urea nitrogen measurement; liver function tests; and albumin, total protein, coagulation profile, and β-hCG determinations. Chest radiography and arterial blood gas determinations should be performed as indicated. Careful monitoring of daily weights and fluid balance is vital. Placement of a Foley catheter can be particularly helpful during more severe stages.

The most crucial phase of management is that of correction of hypovolemia. Hemoconcentration as reflected by hematocrit level on hospital admission has been shown to best correlate with the severity of the syndrome.[42] Patients with OHSS experience a decrease in effective intravascular volume due to third-space loss. The administration of diuretics is therefore relatively contraindicated owing to the risk of further depletion of an already compromised effective arterial blood volume that may result in intravascular collapse. Intravenous access for fluid management is therefore critical. The use of invasive hemodynamic monitoring to assess central venous or pulmonary artery pressures by placement of a central venous line or Swan-Ganz catheter may be necessary in extreme circumstances. Although sodium and water restriction was initially recommended as a means of combating third-space loss,[85] Thaler and coworkers failed to demonstrate any clinical improvement with this approach.[86] It is preferable to replace fluids judiciously with a balanced salt solution such as Ringer's lactate. Severe oliguria is managed by administering volume expanders such as 25% albumin and dextran. Severe hyperkalemia may require administration of cation exchange resins.

Before the resolution of symptoms, patients undergo a rather massive diuresis. Intravascular volume depletion can rapidly be transformed into volume overload as the ascites is mobilized. Similarly, hypokalemia can result. Thus, meticulous attention to rapidly shifting fluid and electrolyte status is vital to patient well-being.

The combination of hemoconcentration with the previously described coagulation factor abnormalities can predispose patients to developing life-threatening thromboembolic phenomena.[5-9] Prophylactic use of low-dose subcutaneous heparin should be considered in chronically hemoconcentrated patients or those with massive ascites leading to compromised venous return. Patients with evidence of thromboembolic phenomena or clear coagulation abnormalities should undergo complete anticoagulation.

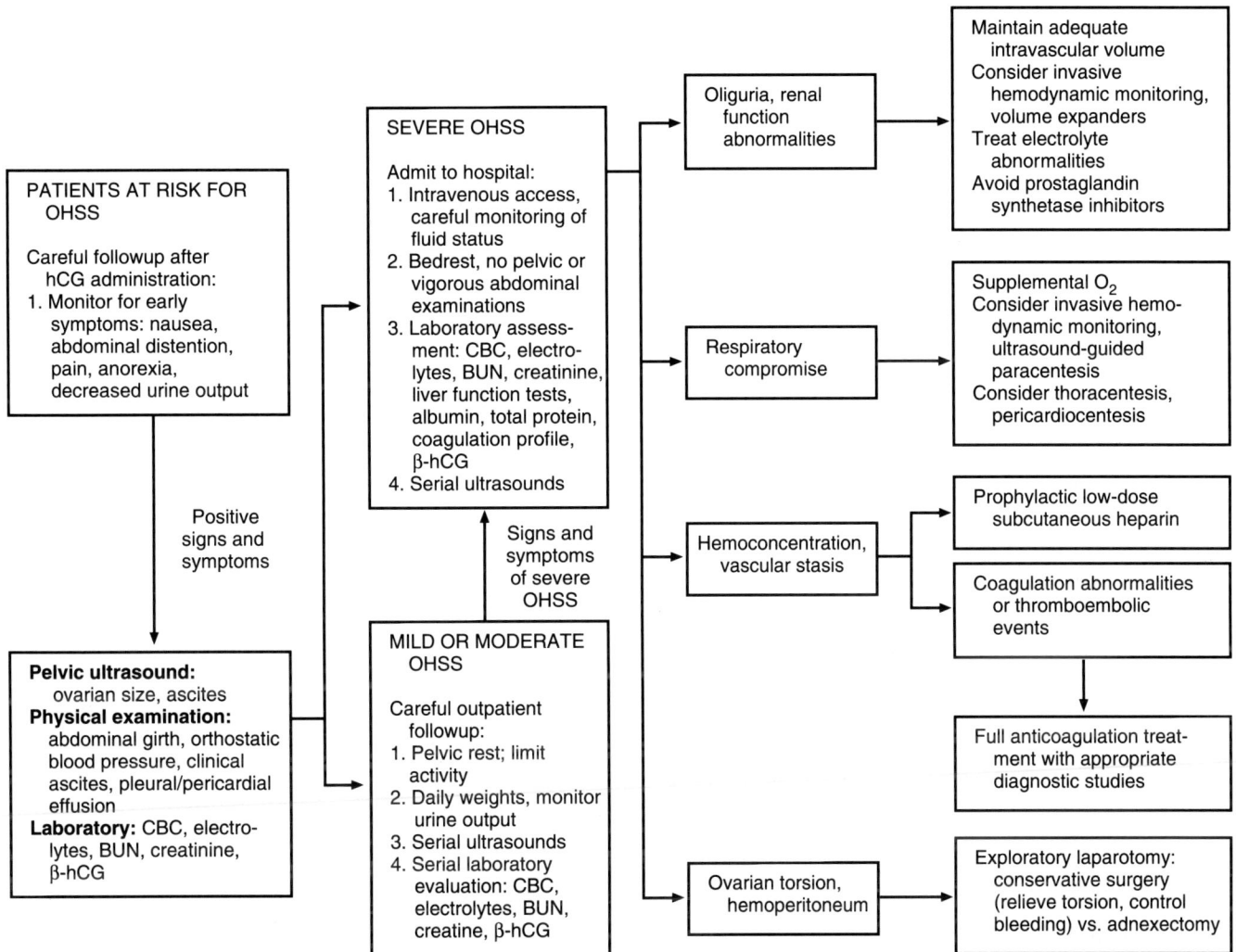

PATIENTS AT RISK FOR OHSS

Careful followup after hCG administration:
1. Monitor for early symptoms: nausea, abdominal distention, pain, anorexia, decreased urine output

Pelvic ultrasound:
  ovarian size, ascites
Physical examination:
  abdominal girth, orthostatic blood pressure, clinical ascites, pleural/pericardial effusion
Laboratory: CBC, electrolytes, BUN, creatinine, β-hCG

Positive signs and symptoms

SEVERE OHSS

Admit to hospital:
1. Intravenous access, careful monitoring of fluid status
2. Bedrest, no pelvic or vigorous abdominal examinations
3. Laboratory assessment: CBC, electrolytes, BUN, creatinine, liver function tests, albumin, total protein, coagulation profile, β-hCG
4. Serial ultrasounds

Signs and symptoms of severe OHSS

MILD OR MODERATE OHSS

Careful outpatient followup:
1. Pelvic rest; limit activity
2. Daily weights, monitor urine output
3. Serial ultrasounds
4. Serial laboratory evaluation: CBC, electrolytes, BUN, creatine, β-hCG

Oliguria, renal function abnormalities

Maintain adequate intravascular volume
Consider invasive hemodynamic monitoring, volume expanders
Treat electrolyte abnormalities
Avoid prostaglandin synthetase inhibitors

Respiratory compromise

Supplemental O₂
Consider invasive hemodynamic monitoring, ultrasound-guided paracentesis
Consider thoracentesis, pericardiocentesis

Hemoconcentration, vascular stasis

Prophylactic low-dose subcutaneous heparin

Coagulation abnormalities or thromboembolic events

Full anticoagulation treatment with appropriate diagnostic studies

Ovarian torsion, hemoperitoneum

Exploratory laparotomy: conservative surgery (relieve torsion, control bleeding) vs. adnexectomy

FIGURE 14–4. A proposed schematic for management of ovarian hyperstimulation syndrome (OHSS). hCG, human chorionic gonadotropin; CBC, complete blood count; BUN, blood urea nitrogen.

Respiratory compromise induced by severe ascites, pulmonary effusions, or enhanced pulmonary capillary permeability should be managed aggressively. Supplemental oxygen, thoracentesis, and invasive cardiovascular monitoring all should be considered. Pericardial effusions may also require aspiration if symptoms develop.

The issue of paracentesis for aspiration of ascitic fluid is a controversial one. The risk of inducing intraperitoneal hemorrhage by puncturing enlarged, friable cystic ovaries makes "blind" paracentesis a contraindicated procedure. A second concern is that the removal of large volumes of ascitic fluid may simply create an osmotic draw leading to rapid reaccumulation of peritoneal fluid and further depletion of intravascular volume. In the face of secondary respiratory compromise and incapacitating distention due to massive ascites, controlled paracentesis may become necessary. The use of sonographic guidance to avoid ovarian puncture has greatly increased the safety of this procedure.[86–89] This procedure should not be performed routinely but only when made unavoidable by the clinical situation. Vascular access for fluid resuscitation should be established in the event of rapid fluid shifts. A proposed management scheme for severe OHSS as described by Borenstein and coworkers is depicted in Figure 14–4.[89]

Other medical approaches to management of severe OHSS have been employed. The use of prolonged administration of GnRH agonists during the luteal phase has been discussed previously. There is little conclusive evidence to support the routine therapeutic use of these agents. GnRH agonist administration clearly precludes pregnancy during the treatment cycle in question. Given the initial support of the role of enhanced levels of prostaglandins as inciting factors in the cause of this disorder, the therapeutic role of antiprostaglandin agents has been investigated. As previously discussed, Schenker and Polishuk successfully inhibited ascites formation in the rabbit by administration of indomethacin, a finding that has not been consistently reproduced.[58] Measuring the effectiveness of this agent in arresting ascites formation in humans has produced conflicting results.[89, 90] Data implicating an association between histamine release and OHSS led Kirshon and coworkers to administer the antihistamine chlorpheniramine maleate intravenously in an effort to arrest severe OHSS.[45] Third-space loss in the form of ascites and pleural effusions was stabilized in this case report. A controlled clinical trial clearly is warranted to assess the efficacy of this approach before its use can be routinely recommended.

SUMMARY

In this chapter, the clinical manifestations, pathogenesis, and management of OHSS have been reviewed. This almost exclusively iatrogenic disorder can be best treated by its prevention. Meticulous management of controlled ovarian stimulation techniques helps reduce the incidence of the protean and life-threatening manifestations of this process.

REFERENCES

1. Schenker JG, Polishuk WZ. Ovarian hyperstimulation syndrome: clinical and experimental data. Excerpta Med Int Congr Ser 1976;396:204.
2. Rabau E, Serr DM, David A, et al. Human menopausal gonadotropin for anovulation and sterility. Am J Obstet Gynecol 1967;96:92.
3. Golan A, Ron-El R, Herman A, et al. Ovarian hyperstimulation syndrome: an update review. Obstet Gynecol Surv 1989;44:430.
4. Zosner A, Katz Z, Lancet M, et al. Adult respiratory distress syndrome complicating ovarian hyperstimulation syndrome. Fertil Steril 1987;47:524.
5. Fournet N, Surrey E, Kerin J. Internal jugular vein thrombosis after ovulation induction with gonadotropins. Fertil Steril 1991;56:354.
6. Mozes M, Bogokowsky H, Antebi E, et al. Thromboembolic phenomenon after ovarian stimulation with human gonadotropins. Lancet 1965;2:1213.
7. Rizk B, Meagher S, Fisher AM. Severe ovarian hyperstimulation syndrome and cerebrovascular accidents. Hum Reprod 1990;5:697.
8. Philipps LL, Gladstone W, Van de Wiele R. Studies of the coagulation and fibrinolytic systems in hyperstimulation syndrome after administration of gonadotropins. J Reprod Med 1975;14:138.
9. Kaaja R, Siegberg R, Tiitinen A, Koskimies A. Severe ovarian hyperstimulation syndrome and deep venous thrombosis. Lancet 1989;2:1043.
10. Younis JS, Zeevi D, Rabinowitz R, et al. Transient liver function tests: abnormalities in ovarian hyperstimulation syndrome. Fertil Steril 1988;50:176.
11. Holtz G, Kling OR, Miller DD, Wilson DA. Ovarian hyperstimulation syndrome caused by clomiphene citrate. S Med J 1982;75:368.
12. Chow KK, Choo HT. Ovarian hyperstimulation syndrome with clomiphene citrate: case report. Br J Obstet Gynecol 1984;91:1051.
13. Polishuk WZ, Schenker JG. Ovarian overstimulation syndrome. Fertil Steril 1969;20:443.
14. Ito T, Michioka T, Kobayashi M, et al. A study on follicle stimulation and ovulation induction in polycystic ovary syndrome (PCOS). Horm Res 1990;33(suppl 2):32.
15. Lunenfeld B, Insler V. Classification of amenorrheic states and their treatment by ovulation induction. Clin Endocrinol 1974;3:223.
16. Navot D, Relou A, Birkenfeld A, et al. Risk factors and prognostic variables in ovarian hyperstimulation syndrome. Am J Obstet Gynecol 1988;159:210.
17. McArdle C, Seibel M, Hann LE, et al. The diagnosis of ovarian hyperstimulation (OHS): the impact of ultrasound. Fertil Steril 1983;39:464.
18. Haning RV, Austin CW, Carlson IH, et al. Plasma estradiol is superior to ultrasound and urinary estriol glucuronide as a predictor of ovarian hyperstimulation during induction of ovulation with menotropins. Fertil Steril 1983;40:31.
19. Tulandi T, McInnes RA, Arronet GH. Ovarian hyperstimulation syndrome following ovulation induction with human menopausal gonadotropin. Int J Fertil 1984;29:113.
20. Tal J, Paz B, Samberg I, et al. Ultrasonographic and clinical correlates of menotropins versus sequential clomiphene citrate: menotropin therapy for induction of ovulation. Fertil Steril 1985;44:342.
21. Kurachi K, Aono T, Suzuki M, et al. Results of hMG (Humegon)-hCG therapy in 6096 treatment cycles of 2166 Japanese women with anovulatory infertility. Eur J Obstet Gynecol Reprod Biol 1985;19:43.
22. Buvat J, Buvat-Herbaut M, Marcolin G, et al. Purified follicle-stimulating hormone in polycystic ovary syndrome: slow administration is safer and more effective. Fertil Steril 1989;52:553.
23. Wang CF, Gemzell C. The use of human gonadotropins for the induction of ovulation in women with polycystic ovarian disease. Fertil Steril 1980;33:479.
24. Dodson WC, Hughes CL Jr, Yancy SE, et al. Clinical characteristics of ovulation induction with human menopausal gonadotropins with and without leuprolide acetate in polycystic ovary syndrome. Fertil Steril 1989;52:915.
25. Schwartz M, Jewelewicz R, Dyrenfurth I, et al. The use of human menopausal and chorionic gonadotropins for induction of ovulation. Am J Obstet Gynecol 1980;138:801.
26. Oelsner G, Serr DM, Mashiach S, et al. The study of induction of ovulation with menotropins: analysis of results of 1897 treatment cycles. Fertil Steril 1978;30:538.
27. Koyama T, Kamata S, Kubota T, et al. Ovarian response and induction of ovulation with human menopausal gonadotropin of different ratio of FSH to LH content in women with ovarian insufficiency. Acta Obstet Gynaecol Jpn 1988;40:445.
28. Check JH, Wu C-H, Gocial B, Adelson HG. Severe ovarian hyperstimulation syndrome from treatment with urinary follicle-stimulating hormone: two cases. Fertil Steril 1985;43:317.
29. Jewelewicz R, Dyrenfurth I, Warren MP, Van de Wiele RL. Ovarian hyperstimulation syndrome. In: Rosenberg E, editor. Gonadotropin Therapy in Female Infertility. Amsterdam: Excerpta Medica, 1973:217.
30. Surrey ES, DeZiegler D, Lu JKH, et al. Effects of gonadotropin-releasing hormone (GnRH) agonist on pituitary and ovarian responses to pulsatile GnRH therapy in polycystic ovarian disease. Fertil Steril 1989;52:547.
31. Chang RJ, Laufer LR, Meldrum DR, et al. Steroid secretion in polycystic ovarian disease after ovarian suppression by a long-acting gonadotropin-releasing hormone agonist. J Clin Endocrinol Metab 1983;56:897.
32. Lindner C, Braendle W, Kohler S, Bettendorf G. Increased incidence of ovarian hyperstimulation syndrome following combined GnRH agonist/hMG therapy. Geburtshilfe Frauenheilkd 1989;49:337.
33. Caspi E, Ron-El R, Golan A, et al. Results of in vitro fertilization and embryo transfer by combined long-acting gonadotropin-releasing hormone analog D-Trp-6-luteinizing hormone–releasing hormone and gonadotropins. Fertil Steril 1989;51:95.
34. Charbonnel B, Kraupf M, Blanchard P, et al. Induction of ovulation in polycystic ovary syndrome with a combination of luteinizing hormone–releasing analog and exogenous gonadotropins. Fertil Steril 1987;47:920.
35. Yeh J, Barbieri RL, Ravnikar VA. Ovarian hyperstimulation associated with the sole use of leuprolide acetate. J In Vitro Fertil Embryo Transfer 1989;6:261.
36. Golan A, Ron-El R, Herman A, et al. Ovarian hyperstimulation syndrome following D-Trp-6 luteinizing hormone–releasing hormone microcapsules and menotropins for in vitro fertilization. Fertil Steril 1988;50:912.
37. Rabinowitz R, Laufer N, Lewin A, et al. Rate of ovarian hyperstimulation syndrome after high-dose hMG for induction of ovulation in IVF cycles (Abstract). Proceedings of the Third Meeting of the European Society of Human Reproduction and Embryology, Cambridge, UK, June 28–July 1, 1987. Oxford: IRL Press, 1987:18.
38. Smitz J, Camus M, Devroey P, et al. Incidence of severe ovarian hyperstimulation syndrome after GnRH agonist/hMG superovulation for in vitro fertilization. Hum Reprod 1990;5:933.
39. Schweditsch M, Keller P, Floersheim Y, Mohr E. Ovarian hyperstimulation during chronic pulsatile GnRH therapy. Gynecol Obstet Invest 1984;17:276.
40. Geisthovel F, Peters F, Breckwoldt M. Ovarian hyperstimulation due to long-term pulsatile intravenous GnRH treatment. Arch Gynaekol 1985;236:255.
41. Corenblum B, Wiseman D. Ovarian hyperstimulation with exogenous pulsatile gonadotropin-releasing hormone therapy. J Ultrasound Med 1985;4:405.
42. Pride SM, James C St J, Ho Yuen B. The ovarian hyperstimulation syndrome. Semin Reprod Endocrinol 1990;8:247.
43. Schenker JG, Weinstein D. Ovarian hyperstimulation syndrome: a current syndrome. Fertil Steril 1978;30:255.
44. Schenker JG, Polishuk WZ. Ovarian hyperstimulation syndrome. Obstet Gynecol 1975;46:23.
45. Kirshon B, Doody MC, Cotton DB, Gibbons W. Management of ovarian hyperstimulation syndrome with chlorpheniramine maleate, mannitol, and invasive hemodynamic monitoring. Obstet Gynecol 1988;71:485.
46. Pappas GD, Blanchette EJ. Transport of colloidal particles from small blood vessels correlated with cyclic changes in permeability. Invest Ophthalmol 1965;4:1026.

47. Davis JS. Hormonal control of plasma and erythrocyte volume of rat uterus. Am J Physiol 1960;199:841.

48. Leya J, Molo MW, Olson D, Radwanska E. Serum and follicular fluid (FF) estradiol (E$_2$) levels in ovarian hyperstimulation syndrome (OHSS) during in vitro fertilization (IVF) and gamete intrafallopian transfer (GIFT) conception cycles after pituitary suppression. J In Vitro Fertil Embryo Transfer 1991;8:137.

49. Brown JB, Evans JH, Adey FD, et al. Factors involved in clinical induction of fertile ovulation with human gonadotropins. J Obstet Gynaecol Br Common 1969;76:289.

50. O'Herlihy C, Evans JH, Brown JB, et al. Use of ultrasound in monitoring ovulation induction with human pituitary gonadotropins. Obstet Gynecol 1982;60:577.

51. Schenker JG, Polishuk WZ. An experimental model of ovarian hyperstimulation syndrome. In: Proceedings of the International Congress on Animal Reproduction, Krakow, Drukarnia Nankova, 1976;4:635.

52. Yuen B, McComb P, Sy L, et al. Plasma prolactin, human chorionic gonadotropin, estradiol, testosterone and progesterone in the ovarian hyperstimulation syndrome. Am J Obstet Gynecol 1979;133:316.

53. Manka MS, Mtabaji JP, Horrobin DT. Effect of cortisol, prolactin, and ADH on the amniotic membrane. Nature 1975;258:78.

54. Leung P, Ho Yuen B, Moon YS. Effect of prolactin in an experimental model of the ovarian hyperstimulation syndrome. Am J Obstet Gynecol 1983;145:847.

55. Bauminger S, Linder HR. Periovulatory changes in ovarian prostaglandin formation and their hormonal control in the rat. Prostaglandins 1975;9:737.

56. Armstrong DT, Grinwich DL. Blockage of spontaneous and LH-induced ovulation in rats by indomethacin, an inhibitor of prostaglandin synthesis. Prostaglandins 1972;1:21.

57. Tsafriri A, Linder HR, Zor U, Lamprecht SA. Physiological role of prostaglandins in the induction of ovulation. Prostaglandins 1972;2:1.

58. Schenker JG, Polishuk WZ. The role of prostaglandins in ovarian hyperstimulation syndrome. Eur J Obstet Gynecol Reprod Biol 1976;6:47.

59. Pride SM, Ho Yuen B, Moon YS, Leung PCS. Relationship of GnRH, danazol and prostaglandin blockade to ovarian enlargement and ascites formation of the ovarian hyperstimulation syndrome in the rabbit. Am J Obstet Gynecol 1986;154:1155.

60. Knigge U, Sleimann I, Matzen S, Warberg J. Histaminergic regulation of prolactin secretion: involvement of serotonergic neurons. Neuroendocrinology 1988;48:527.

61. Pride SM, Ho Yuen B, Moon YS. Clinical, endocrinological and intraovarian prostaglandin-F response to H-1 receptor blockade in the ovarian hyperstimulation syndrome. Am J Obstet Gynecol 1984;148:670.

62. Knox GE. Antihistamine blockade of the ovarian hyperstimulation syndrome. Am J Obstet Gynecol 1974;118:992.

63. Gergly RZ, Paldi E, Erlik Y, Makler A. Treatment of ovarian hyperstimulation syndrome by antihistamine. Obstet Gynecol 1976;47:83.

64. Erlik Y, Naot Y, Friedman M, et al. Histamine levels in ovarian hyperstimulation syndrome. Obstet Gynecol 1978;53:580.

65. Zaidise I, Friedman M, Lindenbaum, et al. Serotonin and the ovarian hyperstimulation syndrome. Eur J Obstet Gynecol Reprod Biol 1983;15:55.

66. Hancock KW, Stitch SR, Oakey RE, et al. Ovulation stimulation: problems of prediction of response to gonadotropins. Lancet 1970;2:482.

67. Lightman A, Palumbo A, DeCherney AH, Naftolin F. The ovarian renin-angiotensin system. Semin Reprod Endocrinol 1989;7:79.

68. Robertson AL, Khairallah PA. Effects of angiotensin II and some analogues on vascular permeability in the rabbit. Circ Res 1972;31:923.

69. Alexander RW, Gimbrone MA Jr. Prostaglandin production by vascular smooth muscle in tissue culture. Proc Natl Acad Sci USA 1976;73:1617.

70. Itskovitz J, Sealey J, Glorioso W, et al. Plasma prorenin response to human chorionic gonadotropin in ovarian hyperstimulated women: correlation with the number of ovarian follicles and steroid hormone concentrations. Proc Natl Acad Sci USA 1987;84:7285.

71. Haning RV Jr, Strawn EY, Nolten WE. Pathophysiology of the ovarian hyperstimulation syndrome. Obstet Gynecol 1985;66:220.

72. Navot D, Margalioth EJ, Laufer N, et al. Direct correlation between plasma renin activity and severity of the ovarian hyperstimulation syndrome. Fertil Steril 1987;48:57.

73. Diamond MP, Wentz AC. Ovulation induction with human menopausal gonadotropins. Obstet Gynecol Surv 1986;41:480.

74. Itull ME, Moglussi KS, Magyar DM, et al. Correlation of serum estradiol levels and ultrasound monitoring to assess follicular maturation. Fertil Steril 1986;46:42.

75. Marrs RP, Vargyas JM, March CM. Correlation of ultrasonic and endocrinologic measurements in human menopausal gonadotropin therapy. Am J Obstet Gynecol 1983;145:417.

76. Blankstein J, Skalev J, Saadon T, et al. Ovarian hyperstimulation syndrome: prediction by number and size of preovulatory ovarian follicles. Fertil Steril 1987;47:597.

77. Itskovitz J, Boldes R, Levron J, et al. Induction of preovulatory luteinizing hormone surge and prevention of ovarian hyperstimulation syndrome by gonadotropin-releasing hormone agonist. Fertil Steril 1991;56:213.

78. Forman RG, Frydman R, Egan D, et al. Severe ovarian hyperstimulation syndrome using agonists of gonadotropin-releasing hormone for in vitro fertilization: a European series and a proposal for prevention. Fertil Steril 1990;53:502.

79. Amso NN, Ahuja KK, Morris N, Shaw RW. The management of predicted ovarian hyperstimulation involving gonadotropin-releasing hormone analog with elective cryopreservation of all pre-embryos. Fertil Steril 1990;53:1087.

80. Friedman CI, Schmidt GE, Chang FE, Kim MH. Severe ovarian hyperstimulation following follicular aspiration. Am J Obstet Gynecol 1984;150:436.

81. Lessing JB, Amit A, Libal Y, et al. Avoidance of cancellation of potential hyperstimulation cycles by conversion to in vitro fertilization–embryo transfer. Fertil Steril 1991;56:75.

82. Rotmensch S, Scommegna A. Spontaneous ovarian hyperstimulation syndrome associated with hypothyroidism. Am J Obstet Gynecol 1989;160:1220.

83. Ben-Hur H, Dgani R, Lancet M, et al. Ovarian carcinoma masquerading as ovarian hyperstimulation. Acta Obstet Gynecol Scand 1986;65:813.

84. Mashiach S, Bider D, Moran O, et al. Adnexal torsion of hyperstimulation ovaries in pregnancies after gonadotropin therapy. Fertil Steril 1990;53:76.

85. Shapiro AG, Thomas T, Epstein M. Management of hyperstimulation syndrome. Fertil Steril 1977;28:237.

86. Thaler I, Yoffe N, Kaftory JK, Brandes JM. Treatment of ovarian hyperstimulation syndrome: the physiologic basis for a modified approach. Fertil Steril 1981;36:110.

87. Padilla SL, Zamaria S, Baramki T, Garcia JE. Abdominal paracentesis for the ovarian hyperstimulation syndrome with severe pulmonary compromise. Fertil Steril 1990;53:365.

88. Aboulghar MA, Mansour RT, Serour GI, Amin Y. Ultrasonically guided vaginal aspiration of ascites in the treatment of severe ovarian hyperstimulation syndrome. Fertil Steril 1990;53:933.

89. Borenstein R, Elhalah U, Lunenfeld R, Schwartz ZS. Severe ovarian hyperstimulation syndrome: a reevaluated therapeutic approach. Fertil Steril 1989;51:791.

90. Katz Z, Lancet M, Borenstein R, Chemke J. Absence of teratogenicity of indomethacin in ovarian hyperstimulation syndrome. Int J Fertil 1984;29:186.

CHAPTER 15

Hypothalamic-Pituitary Disorders

JAMES H. LIU

The functional role of the hypothalamic-pituitary unit in the control of ovulation and regulation of the menstrual cycle is well established.[1] In humans, the pulsatile secretion of gonadotropin-releasing hormone (GnRH) from neurons in the hypothalamus is responsible for maintaining pituitary gonadotropin secretion.

Disorders of the hypothalamic-pituitary axis can lead to disruption of the normal pulsatile secretion from the hypothalamus and the tightly coupled secretion of luteinizing hormone (LH) and follicle-stimulating hormone (FSH). These disorders can be commonly classified into disorders that are associated with organic disease such as hyperprolactinemia, central nervous system (CNS) tumors, pituitary tumors, isolated gonadotropin deficiency, head trauma, Sheehan's syndrome, pituitary apoplexy, and radiation effects; and disorders that are associated with normal neuroanatomic findings and characterized by changes in lifestyle, such as excessive exercise, excessive weight changes, and psychogenic stress. A classification scheme is shown in Table 15–1. Irrespective of etiology, the final common pathway is the disruption of episodic GnRH and gonadotropin secretion leading to ovulatory abnormalities.

OVERVIEW OF THE HYPOTHALAMIC-PITUITARY AXIS

The GnRH neuronal system has been localized to the medial basal hypothalamus, primarily to the arcuate nucleus (Fig. 15–1), which contains the highest concentration of GnRH neurons.[2] GnRH neuronal cell bodies project toward and terminate in the median eminence.[2] GnRH and other peptides from hypothalamic neurons are transported from the median eminence by the pituitary portal capillary bed to the anterior pituitary. Unlike other capillaries in the brain, this capillary network is lined by fenestrated endothelium, which allows diffusion of larger molecules into the vascular space.[3] Because these portal vessels are also able to carry secretions from the pituitary toward the brain, the portal capillary bed may serve as an ultra-short feedback loop mechanism.

Electrophysiologic studies in lower primates indicate that these GnRH neurons depolarize and release GnRH in a synchronous fashion at a characteristic frequency between 60 and 120 minutes[4, 5] and stimulate the episodic secretion of LH.[6] Studies of pulsatile LH secretion in humans show a similar episodic pattern of secretion.[7] When the frequency of GnRH-LH secretion is shifted from this frequency window, pituitary gonadotropin release is altered, and there is disruption of the normal ovulatory cycle. In addition to GnRH neurons, other neuronal networks are also present in the arcuate nucleus. These networks consist of neurons that can secrete β-endorphin, dopamine, and norepinephrine. Because each system has synaptic contacts or interneuronal connections with GnRH neurons, these neurotransmitters can modify GnRH neurosecretion. For example, activation of the opioidergic system inhibits GnRH activity,[8, 9] whereas activation of the noradrenergic pathways can augment GnRH release (Fig. 15–2).[1, 10]

The anterior pituitary gland is composed of cells that are capable of synthesizing and releasing LH, FSH, prolactin (PRL), corticotropin (adrenocorticotropic hormone [ACTH]), thyroid-stimulating hormone (TSH), human chorionic gonadotropin (hCG), and growth hormone (GH). The LH/FSH secreting cells (gonadotropes) are scattered throughout the gland. The gland is richly supplied by the superior, middle, and inferior hypophyseal arteries.[3] Secretion of LH and FSH requires regular intermittent exposure to "pulses" of GnRH. The relative amounts of LH and FSH released are dependent on the amount of GnRH exposure. Low levels of GnRH exposure (decreased GnRH pulse frequency) lead to preferential transcription of β-subunit FSH messenger ribonucleic acid with preferential release of FSH (such as in mid-puberty), whereas normal GnRH pulse frequencies stimulate release of nearly equal amounts of LH and FSH.[11–13] If GnRH pulses occur more frequently than at intervals of 45 to 60 minutes, an exaggerated LH:FSH ratio (such as seen in some patients with polycystic ovary syndrome) can result.[11, 12]

The PRL-producing cells (lactotropes) are concentrated in the lateral wings of the gland. Release of PRL is regulated primarily by hypothalamic dopamine secretion.[14] Administration of dopamine receptor antagonists such as metoclopra-

TABLE 15–1. Classification of Ovulatory Dysfunction Secondary to Hypothalamic-Pituitary Disorders

Functional Hypothalamic Amenorrhea
  Psychogenic or stress factors
  Nutritional factors
  Exercise-associated factors
Pharmacologic-Induced Anovulation
  Dopaminergic antagonists (antipsychotics)
  Opiate agonists
Psychiatric Disorders
  Anorexia nervosa
  Bulimia
  Pseudocyesis
Organic Defects of the Hypothalamic-Pituitary Unit
  Hypothalamic lesions
    Craniopharyngioma
    Pinealoma
    Entodermal sinus tumors
    Infections (human immunodeficiency virus, tuberculosis)
    Infiltrative diseases (histiocytosis X, sarcoidosis)
  Isolated gonadotropin deficiency (Kallmann's syndrome)
  Pituitary tumors
  Sheehan's syndrome
  Pituitary apoplexy/aneurysm
  Empty sella syndrome
  Head trauma
  Inappropriate prolactin secretion
  Postirradiation effects

Modified from Liu JH. Hypothalamic amenorrhea: Clinical perspectives, pathophysiology, and management. Am J Obstet Gynecol 1990;163:1732–1736.

mide and haloperidol promptly increases PRL secretion sixfold to tenfold. Administration of thyrotropin-releasing hormone (TRH) also stimulates PRL release because lactotropes contain TRH receptors.[15]

HYPOTHALAMIC AMENORRHEA SECONDARY TO FUNCTIONAL FACTORS

Functional hypothalamic amenorrhea (HA) can be defined as the lack of menstrual cycles for more than 6 months in the absence of anatomic or organic abnormalities. The first description of anovulation attributed to hypothalamic factors was by Klinefelter and associates in 1943.[16] These investigators coined the term *hypothalamic hypoestrinism* to describe patients with anovulation and hypoestrogenism associated with psychological stress factors. They believed that this type of disorder was caused by the "failure of the hypothalamic-pituitary nervous pathways to release LH from the anterior pituitary." Many recent clinical studies have confirmed this notion.[17–20] These studies show that the common underlying defect is a slowing in the pulsatile secretion of LH, which is probably a reflection of decreased endogenous GnRH secretion.[21]

Careful and thorough interviews of many of these patients reveal common environmental problems or lifestyle changes that seem to coincide with onset of the ovulatory dysfunction. Many of these patients provide a history of increasing psychogenic stress related to their job or school, the death of a close friend or relative, divorce, marital strife, or sexual abuse. Other patients may provide a history of lifestyle changes with respect to diet, exercise pattern, and sleep hab-

its. Because our current culture places emphasis on a youthful appearance, exercise, and slenderness, the incidence of HA appears to have increased.

Chronic exposure to stress can disrupt reproductive function in both animals and humans.[22–24] In women with HA, there is convincing evidence linking environmental or endogenous "stressors" to chronic activation of the hypothalamic-pituitary-adrenal (HPA) axis. The stress response is associated with an increased secretion of corticotropin-releasing hormone (CRH) at the hypothalamic level, ACTH, cortisol, PRL, oxytocin, vasopressin, epinephrine, and norepinephrine.[25] The HPA axis in these patients is at a higher set point and is characterized by higher elevations in daytime cortisol levels, a delay or absent response in ACTH or cortisol during the noon meal, and a blunted response to CRH.[26] Because increased levels of CRH, ACTH, and cortisol have been shown to inhibit GnRH and LH secretion,[27] we now have direct evidence linking environmental stresses to the development of ovulatory dysfunction and amenorrhea.

Clinical Evaluation of Hypothalamic Amenorrhea

The diagnosis of functional HA is considered a diagnosis of exclusion. The history and physical examination must focus on exclusion of more serious organic disorders that may mimic HA (e.g., hyperprolactinemia and isolated gonadotropin deficiency).

Patients who present with HA are usually intelligent, highly motivated, and thin or of normal body weight. Most patients have a history of a normal onset of menarche. There is usually a transition from regular menstrual cycles to intermenstrual spotting, then decreased menstrual flow, followed by amenorrhea. A more complete list of features is provided in Table 15–2.

The structured interview should focus on lifestyle variables (diet, exercise), weight changes, use of sedatives or hypnotics, and emotional crises or stressful events preceding the onset of amenorrhea. Additional environmental or interpersonal factors that may be present include academic pressure, social maladjustment, and psychosexual problems.

Complete physical examination should be carried out to exclude evidence of excessive androgen secretion, thyroid enlargement, and galactorrhea. Pelvic examination may reveal evidence of long-standing hypoestrogenism, including a thinned, pale vaginal mucosa, absent cervical mucus, and a small- or normal-sized uterus. Although estradiol levels in these patients are in the menopausal range (<35 pg/mL),

TABLE 15–2. Common Clinical Features of Women with Hypothalamic Amenorrhea

1. Single marital status
2. Involved in professional occupations
3. Highly intelligent
4. Obsessive-compulsive habits
5. History of antecedent stressful life events
6. Tendency to use sedatives or hypnotic drugs
7. Normal or slightly underweight
8. History of prior menstrual irregularity
9. Increased incidence of sexual abuse

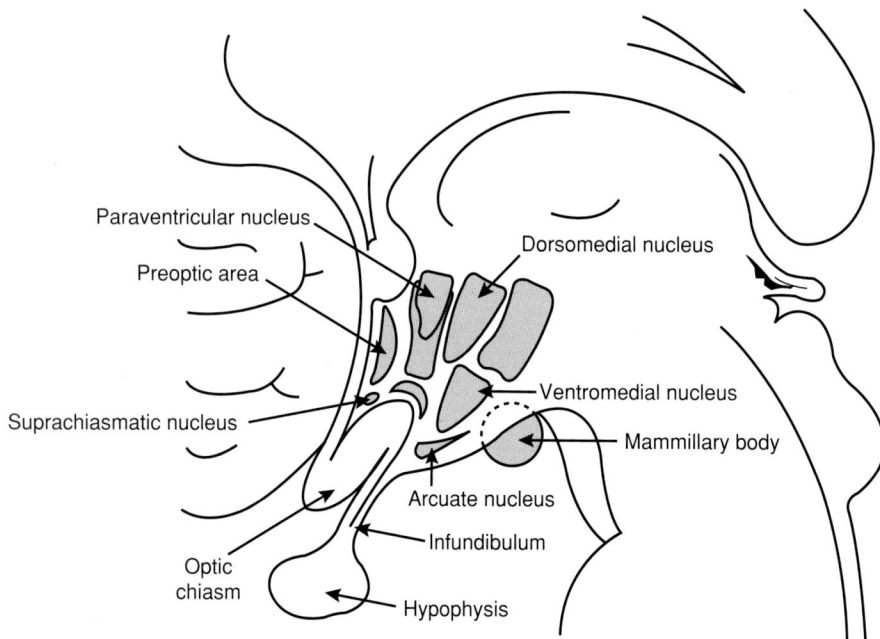

FIGURE 15–1. Sagittal view of the neuroanatomic relationships among the arcuate nucleus, the median eminence (infundibulum), the adjacent hypothalamic nuclei, and the pituitary gland (hypophysis).

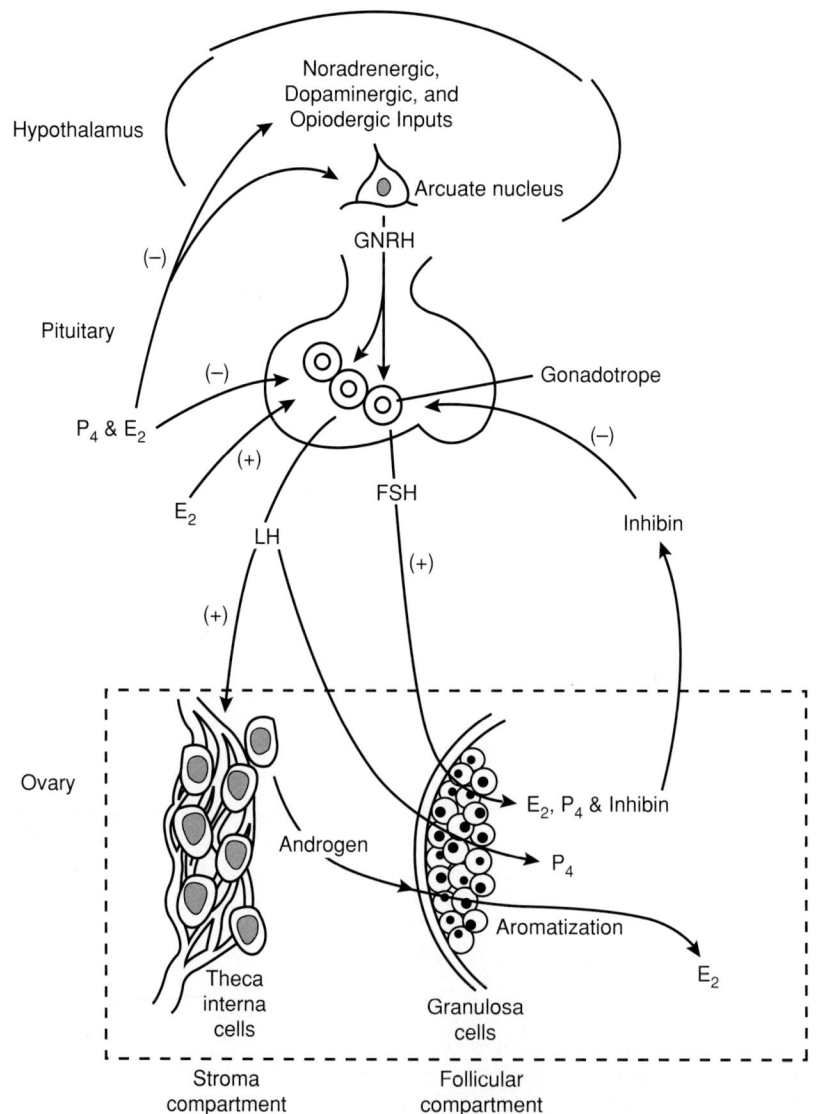

FIGURE 15–2. Schematic representation of the hypothalamic-pituitary-ovarian axis and the feedback regulation of gonadotropin-releasing hormone (GnRH) neuronal activity. E_2, estradiol; P_4, progesterone; LH, luteinizing hormone; FSH, follicle-stimulating hormone.

these patients typically will not have vasomotor symptoms (hot flushes).

Laboratory tests should include FSH, PRL, and TSH. In general, other pituitary hormone levels are in the normal range (Table 15–3). The progestin challenge test (100 mg of progesterone in oil intramuscularly [IM] or 10 mg of medroxyprogesterone acetate for 7 to 10 days) shows an absence of withdrawal endometrial bleeding in most patients. To exclude an occult pituitary or hypothalamic lesion, it is important to perform radiographic imaging (lateral coned view, computed tomography [CT], or magnetic resonance imaging [MRI]) of the sella turcica and adjacent structures. In isolated instances, a hypothalamic tumor such as a craniopharyngioma may be clinically silent and present with normal PRL, FSH, and TSH levels.

The pituitary gland's ability to release gonadotropins does not appear to be compromised in HA patients. Stimulation with GnRH shows a variable response in HA such that LH and FSH responses can be absent, normal, or exaggerated.[17, 28] These gonadotropin responses can be normalized by exogenous pulsatile GnRH administration for 7 to 10 days.[20] Thus, routine use of the GnRH stimulation test is usually not helpful.

Exercise-Induced Hypothalamic Amenorrhea

For millions of young women, regular strenuous exercise has become part of their lifestyle. This evolution has led to an increase in the incidence of menstrual abnormalities, oligo-ovulation, and secondary amenorrhea.[29] Women who participate in gymnastics or ballet dancing are especially vulnerable. In serious ballet dancers, the pubertal progress and onset of menarche can be delayed in as many as 30% of girls and occurs at a mean age of 15 years (normal 12.8 years). Advancement of pubertal stages and return of menstrual cycles seem to coincide with times of prolonged rest or following recovery from injury.[30]

Activities that are associated with an increased frequency of reproductive dysfunction are those that favor a slimmer, lower-body-weight physique such as middle and long distance running, ballet dancing, and gymnastics.[31] Swimmers and bicyclists appear to have lower rates of amenorrhea despite comparable training intensities. Those people at increased risk for amenorrhea include runners whose training schedule exceeds 30 miles/week; people with low body fat content (<20%) or who are 10% below ideal body weight; women younger than the age of 20; and women with a prior history of menstrual cycle irregularity. These types of observations have led Frisch and others to postulate that there is a critical threshold in body fat composition that is required for normal menstrual function.[32, 33] In addition, the psychological stress of competition may also play a significant role, because the incidence of amenorrhea is higher in competitive athletes.

In untrained women who underwent a program of strenuous aerobic exercise (running 4 to 10 miles/day) combined with caloric restriction, Bullen and coworkers were able to experimentally induce menstrual dysfunction.[29] The spectrum of abnormalities that can be seen in many of these women include luteal phase dysfunction, loss of the midcycle LH surge, prolonged menstrual cycles, altered patterns of gonadotropin secretion, and amenorrhea.

Many amenorrheic athletes are not concerned about their menstrual status and often welcome the onset of amenorrhea. However, significant osteopenia, usually affecting trabecular bone, has been reported in these women.[34] Many athletes are unaware that the loss in bone density secondary to hypoestrogenism nullifies the beneficial effects of weight-bearing exercise in strengthening and remodeling bone.[35] These women remain at risk for stress fractures, particularly in the weight-bearing lower extremities. These people should be counseled to either decrease their exercise intensity, alter the type of exercise, increase their calcium intake (1200 mg/day), or gain weight. If these lifestyle changes are unacceptable, serious consideration should be given to long-term hormone replacement.

Treatment of Hypothalamic Amenorrhea

For many patients, spontaneous recovery of menstrual function takes place after a modification in lifestyle, psychological counseling, or accommodation to environmental stress. For these reasons, it is prudent to manage these patients on an individualized, expectant basis. In patients who remain amenorrheic, periodic assessment of reproductive status (e.g., every 6 months) is recommended. Assessment should include bioassays suggesting return to a euestrogenic state, such as presence of cervical mucus and a normal vaginal maturation index. Determinations of gonadotropin or estradiol levels are unlikely to be helpful. If the interval of

TABLE 15–3. Serum Hormone Concentrations in Hypothalamic Amenorrhea

Hormone	Hypothalamic Amenorrhea	Early Follicular Phase
LH (IU/L)	8.5 ± 1.1*	11.6 ± 1.2
FSH (IU/L)	9.3 ± 0.5*	12.1 ± 1.0
PRL (ng/mL)	12.2 ± 0.8†	17.1 ± 1.4
TSH (μU/mL)	1.05 ± 0.33	1.33 ± 0.26
Estradiol		
(pmol/L)	142 ± 15	156 ± 10
(pg/mL)	38.7 ± 4	42.5 ± 2.7
ACTH		
(pmol/L)	1.2 ± 0.2	1.3 ± 0.2
(pg/mL)	5.4 ± 0.9	5.9 ± 0.9
Cortisol		
(nmol/L)	230 ± 10†	170 ± 10
(ng/mL)	83 ± 3.6†	61.6 ± 3.6
Testosterone		
(nmol/L)	1.1 ± 0.2	0.9 ± 0.1
(pg/mL)	291 ± 58	262 ± 29
T_3		
(nmol/L)	1.19 ± 0.07*	1.48 ± 0.09
(ng/dL)	7.7 ± 0.4*	9.6 ± 0.6
T_4		
(nmol/L)	59.2 ± 4.4*	79.8 ± 5.1
(μg/dL)	4.6 ± 0.3*	6.2 ± 0.4

*$P < 0.05$.
†$P < 0.01$.
See text for abbreviations; mean ± SEM shown.
Data from Berga S, Mortola J, Gierton L, et al. Neuroendocrine aberrations in women with functional hypothalamic amenorrhea. J Clin Endocrinol Metab 1989;68:301–308; and Suh BY, Liu JH, Berga S, et al. Hypercortisolism in patients with functional hypothalamic amenorrhea. J Clin Endocrinol Metab 1988;66:733–739.

anovulation is longer than 1 year, a major concern is the long-term effect of hypoestrogenism on bone mineral content. Based on studies in ovariectomized women or those who have undergone treatment with GnRH agonists for endometriosis, bone density would be expected to decrease between 5% and 10% per year during the first 3 years of amenorrhea.[36] Because many of these patients are usually reluctant to take medications, bone density measurements may be necessary to justify estrogen replacement therapy. The minimal estrogen replacement doses required to maintain bone density (0.625 mg of conjugated equine estrogen, 1 mg of micronized estradiol, 50 μg of transdermal estradiol) have been established in postmenopausal women. Estrogen should be used in combination with a progestin (e.g., 5 to 10 mg of medroxyprogesterone acetate) for 12 to 14 days to ensure adequate shedding of the endometrium. The recommended calcium intake in these women should be 1200 mg/day.

For those desiring fertility, and those who remain amenorrheic with lifestyle changes, a trial of clomiphene citrate is warranted. Because of the hypoestrogenic environment in these people, lower doses of clomiphene (25 mg/day for 5 days) can be effective. The clomiphene dosage should be increased in 25- to 50-mg increments every 2 months. Because clomiphene also has weak estrogenic properties, higher doses (>100 mg/day) are unlikely to stimulate ovulation and may exert a paradoxical effect and suppress gonadotropin secretion. Sonographic assessment of follicular development at higher clomiphene doses may be helpful. If follicular development is present, but there is an absence of a urinary LH surge, hCG administration (5000 IU IM) can be administered once the dominant follicle or follicles have achieved a mean diameter of 18 mm or larger. There is no evidence that the addition of hCG increases the likelihood of conception.

For patients who fail clomiphene, use of pulsatile GnRH or human menopausal gonadotropins (hMGs) is the next step. Because the primary underlying defect in HA is decreased endogenous GnRH secretion, pulsatile GnRH can be viewed as "physiologic" replacement therapy. This latter approach has the therapeutic advantages of a decreased requirement for ultrasonographic and estradiol monitoring, reduced frequency of multiple pregnancies, and a virtual absence of ovarian hyperstimulation. A starting intravenous dose of GnRH of 5 μg/90 minutes has been shown to be effective.[37] After ovulation is detected by urinary LH testing, the corpus luteum can be supported either by continuation of pulsatile GnRH or by hCG (1500 IU IM every 3 days for four doses). In patients with HA, ovulation rates of 90% and conception rates of 30% per ovulatory cycle should be expected.[38] For a detailed discussion of ovulation induction with GnRH and hMG, see Chapter 13.

In those patients who have resumed normal menstrual cycles but remain infertile, a careful assessment of the quality of ovulation should be performed. A timed endometrial biopsy 10 to 12 days after the urinary LH surge can be performed to exclude luteal phase dysfunction. If a lag greater than 2 days in endometrial maturation is present in two biopsies, progesterone supplementation (e.g., progesterone suppositories, 25 mg, twice daily) may be appropriate. Alternatively, clomiphene may be administered in low doses early in the follicular phase (beginning days 1 to 3) to stimulate increased FSH secretion and more appropriate follicular development.

Bulimia and Anorexia Nervosa

Bulimia is an eating disorder characterized by alternating episodes of binge eating (consumption of large amounts of food at a sitting) followed by periods of food restriction, self-induced vomiting, or excessive use of laxatives or diuretics.[39] Anorexia nervosa is a related psychosomatic disorder characterized by the triad of extreme weight loss (>25% of ideal body weight), body image disturbance, and an intense fear of becoming obese.[39]

Demographically, 90% to 95% of bulimic and anorectic patients are white females from middle-income or upper-income families. Bulimic behavior is fairly common, with an estimated incidence ranging from 4.5% to 18% among high school and college students. *Bulimia nervosa,* as defined by the *Diagnostic and Statistical Manual of Mental Disorders (Third Edition—Revised)* criteria, is much less frequent and is present in approximately 1% to 2% of the female population.[40] Bulimia usually begins between the ages of 17 and 25 years.

The incidence of anorexia has been estimated to range from 0.64 in 100,000 to 1.12 in 100,000.[39] Patients with anorexia are usually between the ages of 12 and 35 years, with bimodal ages of onset at 13 to 14 years and 17 to 18 years. The mortality rate associated with anorexia has been reported to be as high as 9%. Generally, death is secondary to cardiac arrhythmias precipitated by electrolyte abnormalities and diminished heart muscle mass.[41] These patients show signs of depression with a reported suicide rate of 2% to 5%. Because of the seriousness of this life-threatening disorder in a young patient, it is important for the clinician to recognize early signs of these disorders (Tables 15–4 and 15–5) so that prompt intervention and appropriate treatment can be instituted.

Gonadotropin secretion in anorectic patients exhibits a prepubertal pattern (Fig. 15–3) that is similar to other forms of severe HA. As anorectic patients improve and regain weight, gonadotropin levels will increase and responses to GnRH may be normal or supranormal. Despite their recovery to normal body weight, as many as 50% of anorectic patients remain anovulatory.

Both bulimic and anorectic patients exhibit hyperactivation of the HPA axis with persistent hypersecretion of cortisol throughout the day.[42, 43] This characteristic, which is similar to other forms of HA, suggests that hyperactivation of the HPA axis may be the common mechanism that accounts for inhibition of GnRH and gonadotropin secretion. The increased cortisol production in anorectic patients is not associated with peripheral effects or manifestations of hypercortisolism because there is a concomitant reduction in intracellular glucocorticoid receptors.[44] Adrenal dehydroepiandrosterone concentrations are reduced and resemble those of prepubertal children.

In the face of reduced caloric intake, metabolic homeosta-

TABLE 15–4. Clinical Features of Bulimia

1. Menstrual irregularity
2. Parotid gland enlargement
3. Hypokalemia
4. Dental enamel erosion
5. Esophageal scarring

TABLE 15–5. Clinical Characteristics of Anorexia Nervosa

1. Amenorrhea
2. Constipation, decreased gastric emptying
3. Preoccupation with handling of food
4. Hyperactivity
5. Distortion of body self-image
6. Obsessive-compulsive personality
7. Increased incidence of past sexual abuse
8. Bulimic behavior
9. Coarse, dry skin
10. Soft lanugo-type hair
11. Osteopenia
12. Increased serum beta-carotene levels
13. Elevated hepatic enzymes
14. Anemia, leukopenia
15. Elevated corticotropin-releasing hormone levels in cerebrospinal fluid
16. Hypotension
17. Hypokalemia secondary to diurectic or laxative abuse
18. Hypothermia

sis is maintained by decreased peripheral conversion of thyroxine (T_4) to triiodothyronine (T_3).[45] Instead, T_4 is converted via an alternative pathway to reverse T_3, a relatively inactive isoform. These metabolic changes are similar to those seen in severely ill patients and during starvation. Anorectic patients also have partial diabetes insipidus and are unable to appropriately concentrate urine owing to impaired secretion of vasopressin.[46] Table 15–5 summarizes the clinical and endocrine manifestations of anorexia nervosa.

Treatment. Current treatment modalities for bulimia and anorexia nervosa have low success rates. Suggested therapeutic approaches include individual and group psychotherapy and behavioral modification.[47, 48] There are no large controlled studies that compare the efficacy of these treatments. Because these disorders can become life threatening, it is important that a team of clinicians with special expertise in eating disorders assist in the differential diagnosis and treatment planning.

Significant clinical consequences that should be addressed by the gynecologist include estrogen deficiency, associated osteoporosis, and generalized effects of malnutrition. In patients who weigh less than 75% of their ideal body weight, in-hospital treatment should be instituted. In chronic anorectic-bulimic patients, long-term estrogen replacement therapy is indicated. At least one study has suggested that exogenous estrogen may permit more rapid weight gain in anorectic patients.

Pseudocyesis

Pseudocyesis is a classic example of a psychoneuroendocrine disorder that disrupts the menstrual cycle. This word is derived from the Greek terms *pseudes,* meaning false, and *kyesis,* meaning pregnancy. This uncommon disorder is characterized by subjective symptoms of pregnancy, including amenorrhea or oligomenorrhea, morning sickness, an increase in abdominal girth secondary to fat deposition or intestinal gas, breast enlargement, nipple pigmentation and areolar enlargement, galactorrhea, and softening of the cervix. More detailed biochemical characterization in a few patients

includes evidence of hyperprolactinemia, elevated LH levels, and reduced FSH levels.[49]

When the diagnosis is revealed to the patient, this psychogenic disorder will spontaneously resolve with fairly rapid recovery of hormonal changes toward the normal values. It is important to obtain psychiatric consultation because there is often a significant underlying emotional problem with depression. This can be associated with multiple suicide attempts.

ANATOMIC HYPOTHALAMIC-PITUITARY LESIONS

The presence of tumors or lesions in the hypothalamus or the pituitary can disrupt GnRH and gonadotropin secretion owing to compression effects destroying surrounding functional tissue (suprasellar meningiomas) or, more rarely, direct invasion into normal tissue (gliomas). Because of the central location of these tumors, there may be an associated "parachiasmal syndrome" characterized by generalized headaches, visual defects, diabetes insipidus, hypogonadism, and hypopituitarism. In some instances, these parachiasmal lesions are clinically silent, leading to a delay in diagnosis. Rarely, the only initial presenting complaint may be infertility associated with oligo-ovulation and reproductive dysfunction.

HYPOTHALAMIC LESIONS

Tumors and Other Lesions

Tumors arising from surrounding neural tissue in the hypothalamus are extremely uncommon. Many of these lesions are developmental tumors derived from vestigial embryologic remnants such as craniopharyngiomas, dysgerminomas (pinealomas), teratomas, choriocarcinomas, and entodermal sinus tumors. The hypothalamus also may be a site for metastatic tumors, most commonly from primary carcinomas of the lung and breast.

Craniopharyngiomas are one of the more common developmental tumors and arise from epidermoid remnants of Rathke's pouch. These tumors can have both solid and cystic components and may contain calcified necrotic tissue and cholesterol crystals. Although these lesions are usually quiescent until they have achieved large size (>2 cm), initial presenting symptoms include visual field deficits, signs of intracranial pressure, and occasional endocrine dysfunction (menstrual disturbances). On CT scan, these lesions have characteristic calcifications and a cystic pattern (Fig. 15–4). Because these lesions are often diagnosed after intracranial compression symptoms develop, surgical therapy with radical excision is usually the primary treatment. In many instances, owing to tumor location or to the size of the lesion, total excision is impossible, and postoperative adjunctive radiation therapy must be administered. Posttreatment hypopituitarism is fairly common so that long-term endocrine replacement therapy is often necessary.

Dysgerminomas, also known as *ectopic pinealomas* or *atypical teratomas,* and entodermal sinus tumors may arise from vestigial embryologic cell rests at the base of the third ventricle. These rare tumors are detected after they exert midline

Variations in Pulsatile LH Secretion

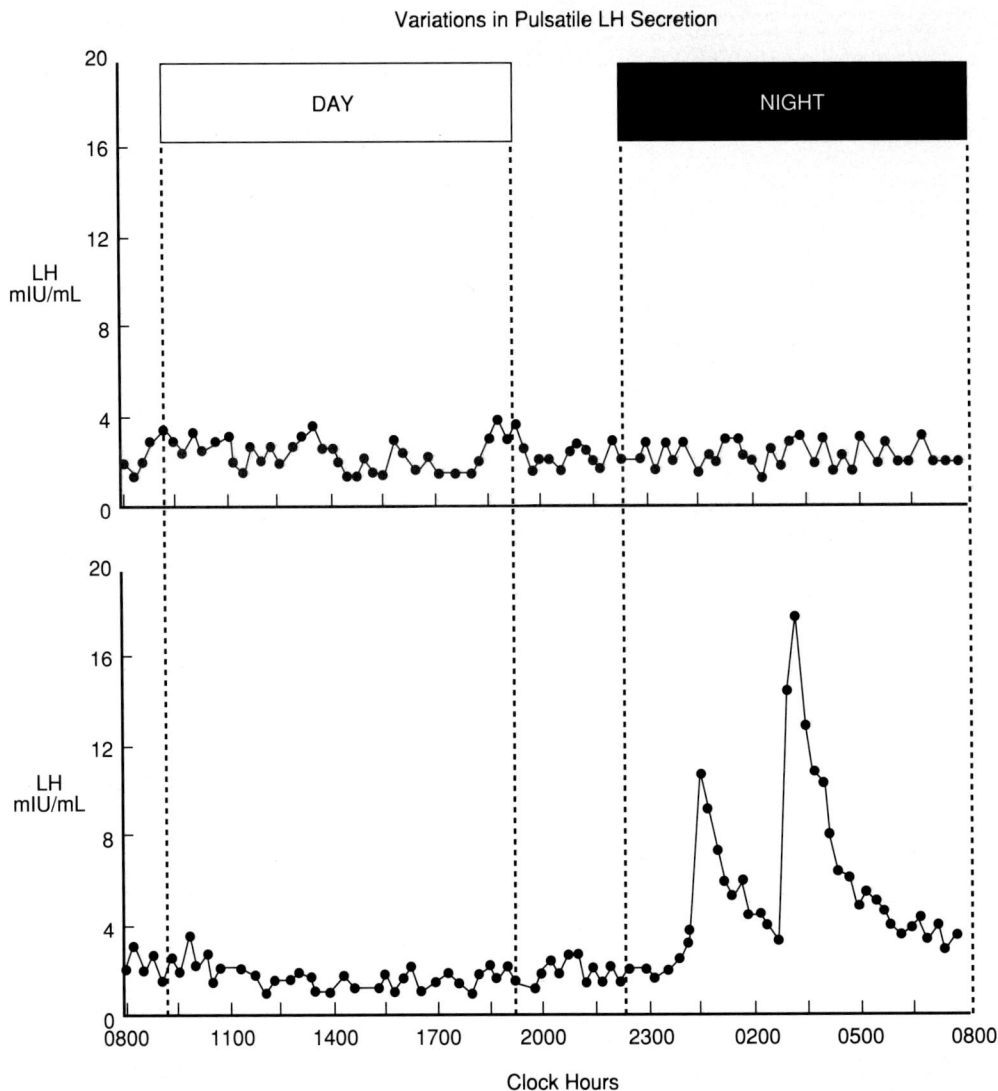

FIGURE 15–3. Examples of varying pulsatile patterns of luteinizing hormone (LH) secretion in a woman with hypothalamic amenorrhea. In the *upper panel,* LH secretion is apulsatile, reflecting decreased endogenous gonadotropin-releasing hormone release that is similar to the prepubertal state. During the recovery phase *(lower panel),* LH secretion increases during the night, as is seen during pubertal maturation. (Modified from Khoury, SA, Reame NE, Kelch RP, Marshall JC. Diurnal patterns of pulsatile luteinizing hormone secretion in hypothalamic amenorrhea: reproducibility and responses to opiate blockade and an alpha₂-adrenergic agonist. J Clin Endocrinol Metab 1987;64(4):755–762. © The Endocrine Society.)

suprasellar compression effects, including diabetes insipidus, visual field loss, and hypopituitarism. These lesions are usually identified on MRI and may secrete hCG (dysgerminomas) or alpha-fetoprotein (entodermal sinus tumors) into the cerebrospinal fluid (CSF). In general, dysgerminomas are radiosensitive, and cure or long-term palliation is possible with radiation therapy. In contrast, entodermal sinus tumors are resistant to radiation, and responses to chemotherapy have been discouraging. Both types of tumors may metastasize via the subarachnoid space.

Infiltrative diseases due to either infectious or granulomatous processes can be associated with hypopituitarism. These relatively rare disorders may be associated with systemic diseases such as tuberculosis and sarcoidosis. Other disorders such as histiocytosis X (also known as *eosinophilic granuloma, Hand-Schüller-Christian disease,* or *Letterer-Siwe disease*) are characterized by eosinophilic or histiocytic infiltrates in the hypothalamic or pituitary stalk area. The cause of this process

is unknown. Treatment should be tailored to the underlying disease process. For histiocytosis X, a combination of glucocorticoids and antimetabolites (i.e., methotrexate) appears to be effective.

Other disorders that can compromise hypothalamic function include (1) arachnoid cysts arising in the parachiasmal area that may cause compressive symptoms characterized by hypopituitarism, headache, and visual loss and (2) aneurysms or infarction of vessels originating from the internal carotid artery that may cause focal hemorrhages and ischemic necrosis of hypothalamic tissue. Treatment of these lesions is based on the location and the specific process.

Isolated Gonadotropin Deficiency (Kallmann's Syndrome)

One disorder that shares many of the biochemical features with functional HA is Kallmann's syndrome, or isolated go-

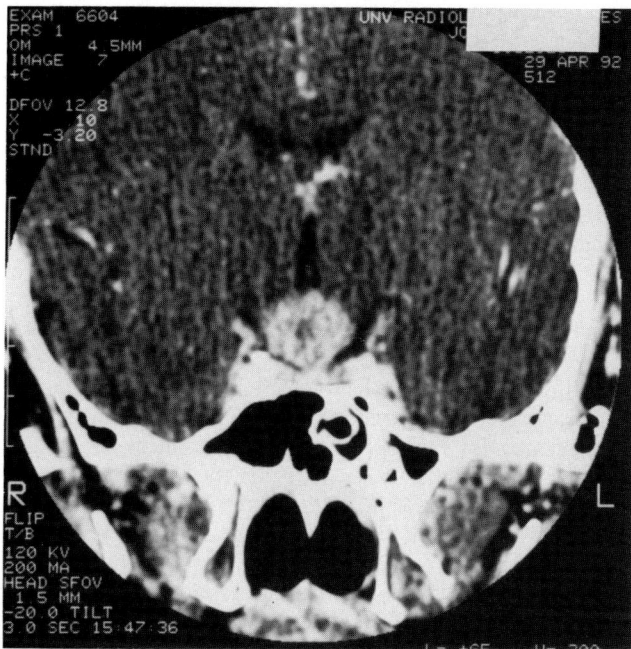

FIGURE 15–4. Computed tomography scan of a patient presenting with a craniopharyngioma with suprasellar involvement.

nadotropin deficiency (IGD). IGD is characterized by a decrease or absence of secretion of endogenous GnRH leading to hypogonadotropic hypogonadism, eunuchoid features, incomplete development of secondary sexual characteristics, primary amenorrhea, and in some instances, anosmia.[50, 51] This disorder can be transmitted in an autosomal dominant pattern.[50] Although Kallman's syndrome was originally described in men, it is clear that it is found in women as well. The defect is due to a failure of GnRH neurons to form completely in the medial olfactory placode of the developing nose[52] or failure of GnRH neurons to migrate from the olfactory bulb to the medial basal hypothalamus during embryogenesis. In some patients with this disorder, anosmia or hyposmia is associated with structural defects of the olfactory bulbs that can be seen on MRI scans.[53] Structurally, this disorder forms a continuum with other midline defects, with septo-optic dysplasia representing the most extreme disorder.

Baseline gonadotropin levels in this disorder are in the low or normal range and are similar to those in patients with other forms of HA. Levels of other pituitary hormones such as GH, TSH, PRL, and ACTH are also in the normal range. Because these patients fail to undergo pubertal maturation, closure of the epiphyseal plates of the long bones is delayed, resulting in a eunuchoid habitus (i.e., the patient's arm span is longer than the height). Not uncommonly, patients will have been treated with exogenous sex steroids such as birth control pills prior to diagnosis. This will lead to partial or complete development of secondary sex characteristics; however, breast development is usually incomplete (Tanner stage III) and may be delayed in comparison to pubic hair development (Tanner stage IV or V). Provocative testing with GnRH yields highly variable LH and FSH responses, dependent on the degree of endogenous GnRH deficiency.[54, 55] However, if pulsatile GnRH is given for 7 to 10 days intravenously, gonadotropin responses will become similar to those

of eumenorrheic women owing to the priming effect of the exogenous GnRH.

The treatment goals in patients with IGD is to induce the completion of pubertal development and provide continued estrogen replacement until pregnancy is desired. Estrogen treatment should be started at lower doses (i.e., 100 ng/kg of ethinyl estradiol daily). Patients should be followed at 2- or 3-month intervals to assess rates of growth and development. The addition of a progestin such as medroxyprogesterone acetate 5 to 10 mg daily for 12 days should be instituted after 3 to 6 months of continuous estrogen administration to stabilize and shed the endometrium. Once secondary sexual characteristics are completely developed, maintenance doses of estrogen (2 mg of micronized estradiol or 0.625 to 1.25 mg of conjugated estrogens given daily) with 12 days of progestin can be given. If fertility is desired, ovulation induction with pulsatile GnRH is the most physiologic choice. Although hMGs are equally efficacious, this latter approach exposes the patient to the unnecessary risk of multiple births and ovarian hyperstimulation syndrome.

PITUITARY LESIONS

Tumors

Pituitary tumors constitute the most common intracranial neoplasms in the general population. Most pituitary adenomas originate from the anterior lobe and are usually asymptomatic. In a postmortem assessment of 120 patients who died from other causes, there was a 27% incidence of microadenomas. Prolactinomas were the most common, constituting 41% of these adenomas. Pituitary tumors can be divided into those that are functional and those that are nonfunctional. In general, nonfunctional tumors are diagnosed when tumor enlargement has compressed adjacent structures, leading to the parachiasmal syndrome as discussed previously. Patients with functional pituitary tumors tend to have endocrine manifestations that are associated with excess hormonal production (e.g., PRL and galactorrhea). Except for prolactinomas that can be treated uniquely with dopamine agonists, as discussed subsequently, ovulation can be induced once the neoplasm has been treated. Patients with hypopituitarism require hMGs, as discussed in Chapter 13.

Prolactinomas and Prolactin Disorders

The basal secretion of PRL is tightly regulated by the hypothalamus within a very small range, that is, between 5 and 25 ng/mL. Irrespective of the etiology, modest elevations of PRL above this level (40 to 100 ng/mL) can be associated with abnormal folliculogenesis, luteal phase dysfunction, galactorrhea, and amenorrhea. The incidence of hyperprolactinemia in an infertile population has been reported to be as high as 20%. Such patients almost always have defects in ovulation and menstrual aberrations. In patients with amenorrhea and galactorrhea, the incidence of hyperprolactinemia is approximately 80%.

PRL secretion is primarily under tonic inhibitory control of dopamine, the principal prolactin-inhibiting factor. The secretion of dopamine is in turn regulated by the basal hypothalamus and the tuberoinfundibular neurons. This dopaminergic system is sensitive to changes within the CNS. For example, any CNS lesions or drugs that impair or alter dopamine secretion affect circulating PRL levels. Thus, PRL levels can serve as a valuable index for perturbations in hypothalamic function.

Evaluation. A variety of physiologic events can stimulate an increase in serum PRL levels. PRL concentrations increase above the normal basal range during sleep, coitus, increased exercise, acute stress, and with food intake (especially lunch). Thus, it is important to obtain PRL levels in the fasting state during the morning hours. PRL levels are elevated more than 10-fold during late pregnancy and lactation.[56] In patients with modest increases in PRL (<100 ng/mL), it is also important to confirm that the levels are abnormally elevated by repeated measurements. A basal TSH level should also be obtained: serum PRL levels can be elevated in primary hypothyroidism because TRH stimulates secretion of both TSH and PRL. The history should focus on potential causes for hyperprolactinemia (Table 15–6). Concomitant medications are a common cause of hyperprolactinemia. On physical examination, thyroid gland size should be determined, and the presence of galactorrhea should be sought. The pelvic examination may provide an estimate of the severity and duration of the hypoestrogenism that commonly accompanies hyperprolactinemia.

The most important test is the radiologic assessment of the pituitary sella and suprasellar regions. In this regard, lateral skull films and sellar tomography are inadequate. CT scanning with contrast enhancement or nuclear MRI appears to be superior in the detection of small adenomas. CT scans provide better detail in evaluation of bony erosion of the sella, whereas MRI scans are more useful in characterizing suprasellar masses. Pituitary microadenomas are defined as lesions smaller than 10 mm in diameter, whereas macroadenomas are 10 mm or larger.

In patients with macroadenomas, basal and dynamic pituitary testing are necessary to monitor and document the extent of pituitary compromise. Formal visual fields testing (Goldman perimetry) should be performed to assess for optic chiasmatic compression. This test serves as a baseline, as well as indicates early optic nerve compromise (loss of red color visual acuity), in cases of suprasellar extension. The diagnosis of idiopathic hyperprolactinemia is made only in the absence of a detectable lesion and exclusion of other causes for PRL elevation.

Treatment. The natural history of prolactinomas is that of a slow-growing tumor. Observational studies suggest that with expectant management, as many as 37% of patients will have a gradual increase in PRL levels, whereas 30% to 55% will experience a decline in levels. In most patients with microadenomas managed expectantly, most will have a benign course, and fewer than 5% will progress to macroadenomas.[57]

Surgical resection of microadenomas via a transphenoidal approach has been successful in the past in normalizing PRL levels; however, long-term followup in these patients suggests a recurrence rate of approximately 39% during the first 5 years.[58, 59] These results strongly suggest that the basic hypothalamic abnormality leading to prolactinoma formation remains uncorrected, and hypertrophy and hyperplasia of the lactotrope population would be expected. Thus, despite low surgical morbidity, the high recurrence rates indicate that this should not be the primary therapeutic approach.

Surgical treatment for macroadenomas is even less successful, with fewer than 46% of patients achieving normal PRL levels. The success rates appear to be inversely correlated with macroadenoma size. In patients who are symptomatic (e.g., those with pituitary stalk compression), a combination of preoperative treatment with bromocriptine to achieve size reduction with subsequent surgical resection appears to be the most effective approach. However, no prospective studies have critically examined this therapeutic regimen. For patients who are asymptomatic, medical treatment of macroadenomas remains a viable option.[60]

Medical suppression of PRL secretion with dopamine receptor agonists (bromocriptine or pergolide) is the most common therapy for hyperprolactinemia and microadenomas.[57] This approach is effective in reducing the size of prolactinomas and is considered the primary treatment. Bromocriptine achieves serum levels rapidly after oral dosing and has a duration of action between 10 and 12 hours. Side effects of dopamine agonists include nausea, vomiting, hypotension, and nasal congestion. To reduce side effects, the starting dose should be 1.25 mg at bedtime. After 1 week, a morning dose (1.25 mg) can be added. If nausea is particularly severe, the vaginal route of administration can be used. To assess the level of PRL suppression, a serum PRL level should be obtained 4 weeks after beginning the medication. If the PRL levels have not decreased to the normal range, the dose should be increased by 1.25 to 2.5 mg, and PRL levels should

---

TABLE 15–6. Conditions Associated with Hyperprolactinemia

Hypothalamic
Tumors—craniopharyngiomas, gliomas, pinealoma, hamartomas
Infiltrative diseases—histiocytosis X, sarcoidosis, tuberculosis
Pituitary
Tumors—prolactinoma, GH-secreting tumors, ACTH-secreting tumors, nonfunctional tumors
Pituitary stalk transection or compression
Empty sella syndrome
Medications
Antipsychotics—phenothiazines, butyrophenones
Antidepressants
Anxiolytics
CNS-acting antihypertensives—α-methyldopa, clonidine, reserpine
Dopamine receptor antagonists—metaclopramide
H₁ blocker—cimetidine
Endocrine
Primary hypothyroidism
Ectopic tumor production
Polycystic ovary syndrome
Physiologic
Sleep
Nipple stimulation
Food intake
Acute stress
Exercise
Coitus
Pregnancy
Lactation
Miscellaneous
Head trauma
Encephalitis
Herpes zoster
Neurofibromatosis

GH, growth hormone; ACTH, corticotropin; CNS, central nervous system.

be checked again in 4 weeks.[61] The therapeutic dose range for bromocriptine is between 2.5 and 7.5 mg.[60] For pergolide, a longer-acting dopamine agonist than bromocriptine, the dose range is between 0.025 mg and 0.1 mg/day.[62] Medical therapy will be successful in suppressing PRL levels and will allow resumption of ovulatory cycles in approximately 80% of patients.

Although prolactinomas appear to decrease in size with dopamine agonist treatment, it is not established if long-term treatment will result in a "cure." For this reason, one has the option to stop dopamine suppression after 2 years of treatment and monitor PRL levels and menstrual cycle regularity. In most patients, PRL levels rapidly rebound to pretreatment levels within 2 months, and medical therapy will need to be continued.[63] In some patients, the prolactinoma appears to resolve.[57, 64]

Regular menstrual cycles may continue in a few patients with hyperprolactinemia. If infertility or hypoestrogenism is not a factor, these patients can be managed expectantly with semiannual monitoring of PRL levels. For most patients with elevated PRL levels and amenorrhea, expectant management is not an appropriate long-term option because of hypoestrogenism. The related decrease in bone density necessitates either beginning dopamine agonist suppression or hormone replacement therapy. Because high levels of estrogen (e.g., pregnancy) may increase tumor growth, the use of estrogen-progestin combinations in patients not receiving dopamine agonists must be carefully monitored. However, the low likelihood of microadenomas progressing to macroadenomas has led clinicians to view replacement estrogen as a viable option for patients with hyperprolactinemia.

Long-term management of patients with microprolactinomas, irrespective of initial treatment modality, should be expectant owing to the slow-growing behavior of these lesions.[65] Serum PRL levels should be obtained at 6- to 12-month intervals along with careful inquiry regarding headaches or visual disturbances. Repeat radiographic examination should be performed periodically (i.e., at years 2 and 5). If no change in lesion size is documented, additional imaging studies are unnecessary unless symptoms or PRL elevations warrant repeat studies.

Prolactinomas in Pregnancy. During pregnancy, the higher levels of estrogen and progesterone normally induce a twofold to threefold increase in pituitary gland size. The increase in size and number of lactotropes accounts for most of the pituitary enlargement. Despite these physiologic changes, most women with microadenomas can be managed expectantly. In patients who conceive during dopamine agonist treatment, the medication should be discontinued once pregnancy has been confirmed. Pregnant patients should be followed carefully for development of headaches and visual disturbances. The risk of symptomatic enlargement is less than 2% in patients with microadenomas and less than 16% in those with macroadenomas.[66, 67] Baseline visual fields should be performed and repeated if symptoms warrant. For those with symptomatic enlargement, reinitiation of dopamine agonist suppression is often effective in rapidly reducing tumor size, with improvement in visual symptoms beginning in a few days. No long-term side effects on the fetus have been reported after bromocriptine administration. With adenomas in pregnancy, there is an increased risk of pituitary apoplexy, a rare but life-threatening disorder characterized by

an abrupt increase in adenoma volume owing to hemorrhage, swelling, and necrosis. Clinical signs and symptoms include severe frontal headaches, a rapid decrease in visual acuity, nose bleed, and CSF rhinorrhea. There can be a rapid deterioration in consciousness. Treatment should include corticosteroid therapy to reduce edema and either expectant medical management or transphenoidal decompression, depending on the severity of the process.

During pregnancy, serial measurements of PRL are not helpful because PRL levels are already elevated and increase to 10- to 20-fold above the normal nonpregnant range at term. Although breast-feeding increases PRL levels, there is no contraindication to breast-feeding in these patients.

Growth Hormone–Secreting Adenomas of the Pituitary

Excess GH secretion leading to acromegaly is insidious and may not be recognized until late in the disease process when irreversible clinical changes in connective tissue and bone are prominent. The classic acromegalic features include enlargement of the jaw, nose, and supraorbital ridges; tufting of the bone and overgrowth of soft tissue of the phalanges; enlargement of the tongue; vocal cord thickening; carpal tunnel syndrome; hypertension; and diabetes mellitus (Fig. 15–5). Because of the difficulty in early detection in this disorder, large adenomas with suprasellar expansion are not uncommon. Both serum GH and insulin-like growth factor-1 (IGF-1) levels are elevated in these patients, with IGF-1 levels being the more discriminating test. Mean levels of IGF-1 are approximately 10-fold higher than controls with almost no overlap. Failure of GH to suppress in response to exogenous glucose challenge is the classic diagnostic test for excess GH secretion.[68]

Most centers favor a primary surgical approach for treatment of this tumor. In instances in which the tumor is only partially resectable or inoperable, radiation therapy also can be effective. However, the response to radiation therapy is slow to arrest the progressive changes in connective tissue and bone. Medical suppression of this tumor with bromocriptine or somatostatin analogs is successful in some patients.[69] Hypopituitarism is often a complication of surgery or radiation therapy.

ACTH-Secreting Adenomas of the Pituitary

Pituitary hypersecretion of ACTH (also known as *Cushing's disease*) leads to peripheral hypercortisolism (Cushing's syndrome) and adrenal hyperplasia. This tumor accounts for approximately 60% of all patients with Cushing's syndrome. Because of the profound peripheral manifestations of hypercortisolism (including centripetal obesity, hypertension, pink abdominal striae, and muscle wasting), the diagnosis is usually made before there is significant adenoma enlargement (Fig. 15–6). Even when diagnosed early, osteoporosis may be a significant problem. Most of these tumors are microadenomas (<10 mm in diameter) that can be removed by transphenoidal resection. Approximately 75% of patients with Cushing's syndrome have amenorrhea or irregular menstrual cycles. The disruption of menstrual cycles is probably in part

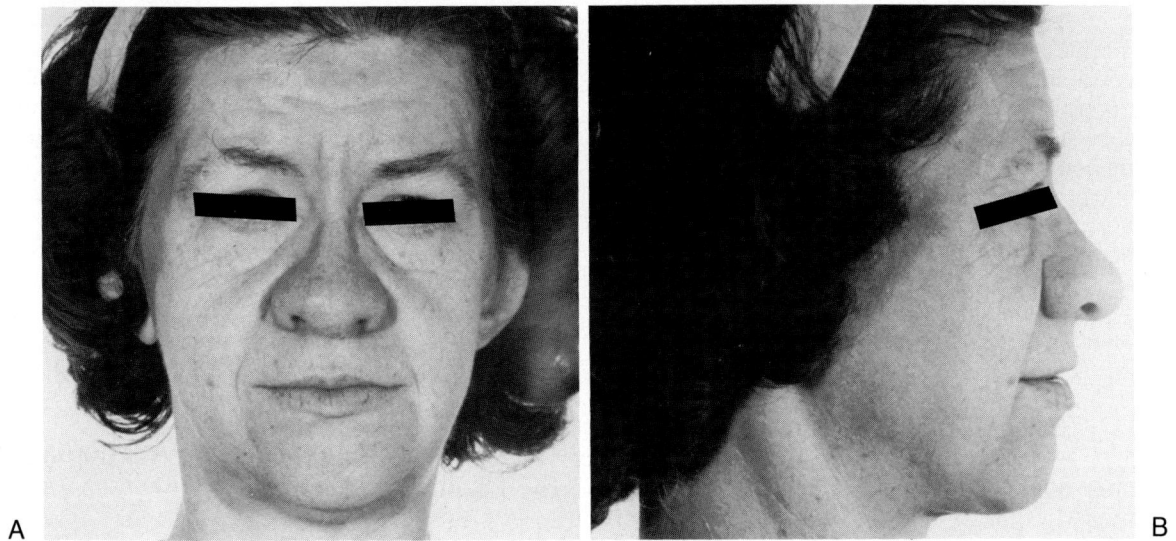

FIGURE 15–5. *A* and *B.* Example of a 43-year-old woman presenting with excess growth hormone secretion. Note the overgrowth of facial bones, including enlargement of the jaw, nose, and supraorbital ridges. The coarsening of the facial features occurred slowly over several years. (Courtesy of R. Rebar and D. L. Loriaux.)

a result of excess cortisol secretion, which has been shown to suppress GnRH-gonadotropin secretion. The increased secretion of adrenal androgens may contribute to anovulation as well.

To screen for Cushing's syndrome, a rapid overnight dexamethasone suppression test (1 mg dexamethasone at 11 P.M.) should be performed. If this test is abnormal (8 A.M. cortisol > 5 μg/dL), a 24-hour urine for measurement of urinary free cortisol should be obtained. The diagnosis of Cushing's syndrome is based on increased production of cortisol and an abnormal suppression of serum cortisol by formal dexamethasone testing.[70] The screening test is often abnormal in obese persons, those with endogenous depression, and those who do not experience sufficient sleep on the night prior to testing.

Gonadotrope Adenomas of the Pituitary

Pituitary tumors that produce gonadotropins are quite rare and have been reported to occur primarily in men. Most of these adenomas secrete FSH or an excess of α subunit. More recently, LH-producing tumors have been reported.[71] Because these tumors may be clinically silent, the diagnosis is usually made after symptomatic enlargement or hypopituitarism becomes evident.

Empty Sella Syndrome

The sella turcica is a bony space that surrounds the pituitary gland. The main body of the pituitary is separated from the base of the brain and the subarachnoid-CSF space by a membrane called the *diaphragm sella*. In some patients, there is incomplete development of the diaphragm sella, which allows CSF pressure to be transmitted directly to the sella turcica, essentially allowing the subarachnoid space to extend to surround the pituitary gland. Eventually, the increased CSF

pressure on the pituitary can cause the gland to shift upward (still attached to the pituitary stalk) above the sella turcica toward the base of the brain. Thus, the term *empty sella syndrome* was coined.[72] Symptoms associated with this syndrome include headaches, visual field deficits, hypopituitarism, and occasionally CSF rhinorrhea. In two thirds of patients, normal pituitary function is maintained, and the empty sella is discovered serendipitously after routine radiologic studies. The remaining one third of patients may demonstrate selective pituitary deficits, moderate elevation in PRL, or abnormal gonadotropin secretion. The empty sella syndrome can also be found in patients following pituitary surgery or radiation therapy. It is most common in young obese women.

Hypothalamic-Pituitary Trauma

In patients who sustain significant injury following an incident in which there is sudden deceleration (e.g., head-on collision), traumatic injury to the hypothalamus and pituitary stalk structures may occur. Often, the abrupt deceleration will cause a whiplash effect on soft and delicate tissue structures because of the surrounding unyielding skull and may lead to tearing of the pituitary stalk, focal hemorrhages, and surrounding tissue edema. These patients present with diabetes insipidus, acute PRL elevations, and partial or complete loss of anterior pituitary function. It is important to institute glucocorticoid and vasopressin replacement in these patients. In some cases, partial recovery of pituitary function can occur once tissue edema has subsided. It is important to evaluate and document pituitary deficits with pituitary function testing and institute appropriate replacement therapy. If pregnancy is desired, these patients will require ovulation induction with gonadotropins.

Sheehan's Syndrome

The onset of postpartum pituitary necrosis (Sheehan's syndrome) constitutes a potentially life-threatening endocrine

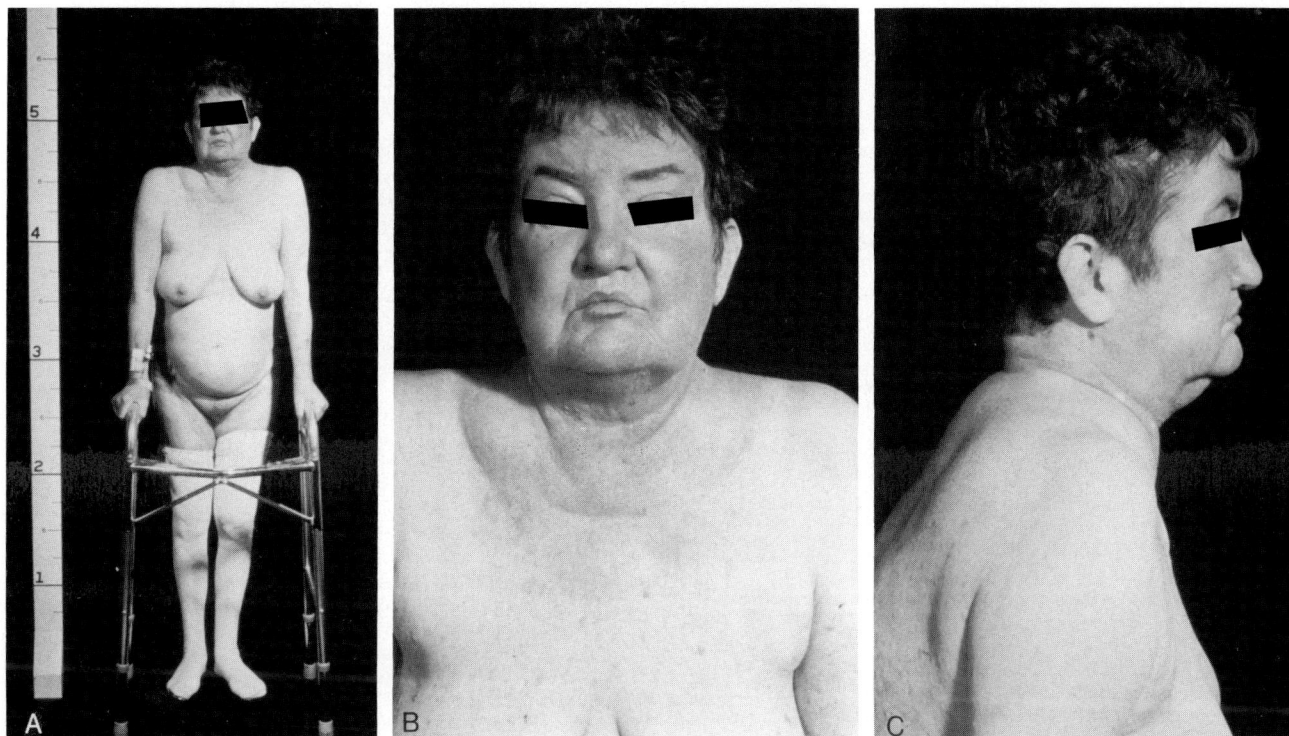

FIGURE 15-6. *A* to *C*. Clinical features of a patient presenting with Cushing's syndrome, including proximal muscle weakness, centripetal obesity, moon facies, plethora, and abdominal striae.

emergency. Autopsy studies of obstetric patients who died between 12 hours to 35 days following delivery revealed that approximately 25% had necrosis of the anterior pituitary.[73] The most complete characterization of this entity was by Sheehan, although Simmonds first described the disorder in 1914.[74, 75]

In almost all instances, pituitary necrosis is preceded by a history of massive obstetric hemorrhage resulting in severe circulatory collapse, hypotension, and shock. Because the pituitary gland increases in size during pregnancy, severe hypotension predisposes the pituitary to ischemia. Sheehan hypothesized that this leads to occlusive spasm of the arteries that supply the anterior pituitary and the stalk. When arteriospasm relaxes, blood flows into the damaged vessels, resulting in stasis and thrombosis.[73] The exact pathogenesis, however, remains unclear.

Autopsy studies reveal a variable degree of pituitary necrosis; thus, the spectrum of clinical manifestations may range from partial deficiency of one or two pituitary hormones to panhypopituitarism.[76] The posterior pituitary is usually not compromised because its blood supply is less dependent on portal vasculature. In most patients, the most common clinical feature is absence of postpartum breast engorgement and failure to initiate lactation because of deficient PRL secretion. More severe damage to the anterior pituitary may result in hypocortisolism and is characterized by hypotension, nausea, vomiting, lethargy, and asthenia. Patients may also report the loss of pubic and axillary hair. Later, signs of hypothyroidism may appear with a failure to resume normal menstrual cycles. Because of the variable extent of pituitary necrosis, isolated case reports have documented return of normal fertility in some instances.[77] In most instances, these patients require ovulation induction with menotropins.

REFERENCES

1. Knobil F. The neuroendocrine control of the menstrual cycle. Rec Prog Horm Res 1980;36:53–88.
2. Silverman AJ, Antunes JL, Abrams GM, et al. The luteinizing hormone–releasing hormone pathways in rhesus (*Macaca mulatta*) and pigtailed (*Macaca nemestrina*) monkeys: new observations in thick, unembedded sections. J Comp Neurol 1982;211:309–317.
3. Bergland RM, Page RB. Can the pituitary secrete directly to the brain? (affirmative anatomical evidence). Endocrinology 1978;102:1325–1338.
4. Kesner JS, Kaufman J, Wilson RC, et al. On the short-loop feedback regulation of the hypothalamic luteinizing hormone–releasing hormone "pulse generator" in the rhesus monkey. Neuroendocrinology 1986;42:109–111.
5. Williams C, Thalabard J, Hotchkiss J, et al. The duration of phasic electrical activity of the hypothalamic gonadotropin-releasing hormone (GnRH) pulse generator and its influence on resultant LH pulse dynamics (Abstract). Program and Abstracts of the 71st Annual Meeting of the Endocrine Society 1989;71:256.
6. Wildt L, Hausler A, Marshall G, et al. Frequency and amplitude of gonadotropin-releasing hormone stimulation and gonadotropin secretion in the rhesus monkey. Endocrinology 1981;109:376–385.
7. Filicori M, Santoro N, Merriam GR, Crowley WF. Characterization of the physiological pattern of episodic gonadotropin secretion throughout the human menstrual cycle. J Clin Endocrinol Metab 1986;62:1136–1144.
8. Williams CL, Nishihara M, Thalabard JC, et al. Duration and frequency of multiunit electrical activity associated with the hypothalamic gonadotropin-releasing hormone pulse generator in the rhesus monkey: differential effects of morphine. Neuroendocrinology 1990;52:225–228.
9. Ferin M, Van Vugt D, Wardlaw S. The hypothalamic control of the menstrual cycle and the role of endogenous opioid peptides. Rec Prog Horm Res 1984;40:441–485.
10. Khoury SA, Reame NE, Kelch RP, Marshall JC. Diurnal patterns of pulsatile luteinizing hormone secretion in hypothalamic amenorrhea: reproducibility and responses to opiate blockade and an alpha₂-adrenergic agonist. J Clin Endocrinol Metab 1987;64(4):755–762.
11. Katt J, Duncan J, Herbon L, et al. The frequency of gonadotropin-releasing hormone stimulation determines the number of pituitary gonadotropin-releasing hormone receptors. Endocrinology 1985;116:2113.

12. Dalkin A, Haisenleder D, Ortolano G, et al. The frequency of gonadotropin-releasing hormone stimulation differentially regulates gonadotropin subunit messenger ribonucleic acid expression. Endocrinology 1989;125:917–924.

13. Christman GM, Randolph JF, Kelch RP, Marshall JC. Reduction of gonadotropin-releasing hormone pulse frequency is associated with subsequent selective follicle-stimulating hormone secretion in women with polycystic ovarian disease. J Clin Endocrinol Metab 1991;72:1278–1285.

14. Judd SJ, Rigg LA, Yen SSC. The effects of ovariectomy and estrogen treatment on the dopamine inhibition of gonadotropin and prolactin release. J Clin Endocrinol Metab 1979;49:182–184.

15. O'Brien RC, Cooper ME, Murray RML, et al. Comparison of sequential cyproterone acetate/estrogen versus spironolactone/oral contraceptive in the treatment of hirsutism. J Clin Endocrinol Metab 1991;72:1008–1013.

16. Klinefelter HF Jr, Albright F, Griswold GC. Experience with a quantitative test for normal or decreased amounts of follicle-stimulating hormone in urine in endocrinological diagnosis. J Clin Endocrinol Metab 1943;3:529–547.

17. Yen SSC, Rebar RW, Vandenberg G. Hypothalamic amenorrhea and hypogonadotropism: responses to synthetic LRF. J Clin Endocrinol Metab 1973;36:811–816.

18. Lachelin GCL, Yen SSC. Hypothalamic chronic anovulation. Am J Obstet Gynecol 1978;130:825–831.

19. Sanborn CF, Martin BJ, Wagner WW. Is athletic amenorrhea specific to runners? Am J Obstet Gynecol 1982;143:859–861.

20. Liu JH. Hypothalamic amenorrhea: clinical perspectives, pathophysiology, and management. Am J Obstet Gynecol 1990;163:1732–1736.

21. Berga SL, Loucks AB, Rossmanith WG, et al. Acceleration of luteinizing hormone pulse frequency in functional hypothalamic amenorrhea by dopaminergic blockade. J Clin Endocrinol Metab 1991;72:151–156.

22. Selye H. The stress syndrome. Nature 1936;138:32.

23. Kalin NH, Carnes M, Barksdale CM, et al. Effects of acute behavioral stress on plasma and cerebrospinal fluid ACTH and β-endorphin in rhesus monkeys. Neuroendocrinology 1985;40:97–101.

24. Rivier C, Vale W. Diminished responsiveness of the hypothalamic-pituitary-adrenal axis of the rat during exposure to prolonged stress: a pituitary-mediated mechanism. Endocrinology 1987;121:1320–1328.

25. Gibbs DM. Dissociation of oxytocin, vasopressin, and corticotropin secretion during different types of stress. Life Sci 1984;35:487–491.

26. Chrousos GP, Gold PW. The concepts of stress and stress system disorders. JAMA 1992;267:1244–1252.

27. Xiao E, Luckhaus J, Niemann W, Ferin M. Acute inhibition of gonadotropin secretion by corticotropin-releasing hormone in the primate: are the adrenal glands involved? Endocrinology 1989;124:1632–1637.

28. Rebar RW, Harman SM, Vaitukaitis JL. Differential responsiveness for LRF after estrogen therapy in women with hypothalamic amenorrhea. J Clin Endocrinol Metab 1978;46:48–54.

29. Bullen BA, Skriinar GS, Beitins IZ, et al. Induction of menstrual disorders by strenuous exercise in untrained women. N Engl J Med 1985;312:1349–1345.

30. Warren MP. Effect of exercise and physical training on menarche. Semin Reprod Endocrinol 1985;3:17–26.

31. Frisch RE, Gotz-Webergen AV, McArthur JW, et al. Delayed menarche and amenorrhea of college athletes in relation to age of onset of training. JAMA 1981;246:1559–1563.

32. Frisch RE, McArthur JW. Menstrual cycles: fatness as a determinant of minimum weight for height necessary for their maintenance or onset. Science 1974;185:949–953.

33. Frisch RE. Body fat, menarche, and reproductive ability. Semin Reprod Endocrinol 1985;3:45–54.

34. Drinkwater BL, Nilson K, Chestnut CH III, et al. Bone mineral content of amenorrheic and eumenorrheic athletes. N Engl J Med 1984;311:277–281.

35. Marcus R, Cann C, Madvig P, et al. Menstrual function and bone mass in elite women distance runners. Ann Intern Med 1985;102:158–163.

36. Johansen JS, Riis BJ, Hassager C, et al. The effect of a gonadotropin-releasing hormone agonist analog (nafarelin) on bone metabolism. J Clin Endocrinol Metab 1988;67:701–706.

37. Liu JH, Yen SSC. The use of gonadotropin-releasing hormone for the induction of ovulation. Clin Obstet Gynecol 1984;27:975–982.

38. Martin K, Santoro N, Hall J, et al. Management of ovulatory disorders with pulsatile gonadotropin-releasing hormone. J Clin Endocrinol Metab 1990;71:1081A.

39. Herzog DB, Copeland MD. Eating disorders. N Engl J Med 1986;313:295–303.

40. Pyle RL, Mitchell JE, Eckert ED, et al. The incidence of bulimia in freshman college students. Int J Eat Disord 1983;2:75–85.

41. Patton G. Mortality in eating disorders. Psychol Med 1988;18:947–951.

42. Gold PW, Gwirtsman H, Avgerinos PC, et al. Abnormal hypothalamic-pituitary-adrenal function in anorexia nervosa. N Engl J Med 1986;314:1335–1342.

43. Boyar RM, Hellman LD, Roffwarg H, et al. Cortisol secretion and metabolism in anorexia nervosa. N Engl J Med 1977;296:190–193.

44. Kontula K, Anderson LC, Huttumen M, Pelkonen R. Reduced level of cellular glucocorticoid receptors in patients with anorexia nervosa. Horm Metab Res 1982;14:619–620.

45. Moshang T Jr, Utiger R. Low triiodothyronine euthyroidism in anorexia nervosa. In: Vigersky RA, editor. Anorexia Nervosa. New York: Raven Press, 1977:263–270.

46. Vigersky RA, Loriaux D, Andersen AE, Lipsett MR. Anorexia nervosa: behavioral and hypothalamic aspects. Clin Endocrinol Metab 1976;5:517–535.

47. Schwartz DM, Thompson M. Do anorectics get well?: Current research and future needs. Am J Psychiatry 1981;138:319–323.

48. Swift WJ. The long-term outcome of early-onset anorexia nervosa: a critical review. J Am Acad Child Psychiatry 1982;21:38–46.

49. Yen SSC, Rebar RW, Quesenberry W. Pituitary function in pseudocyesis. J Clin Endocrinol Metab 1976;43:132–136.

50. Kallmann F, Schonfeld WA, Barrera SW. Genetic aspects of primary eunuchoidism. Am J Ment Defic 1944;48:203–236.

51. Lieblich JM, Rogol AD, White BT, Rosen SW. Syndrome of anosmia with hypogonadotropic hypogonadism (Kallmann's syndrome). Am J Med 1981;73:506–519.

52. Schwanzel-Fukuda M, Pfaff DW. Origin of luteinizing hormone–releasing hormone neurons. Nature 1989;338:161–164.

53. Klingmuller D, Dewes W, Krahe T, et al. Magnetic resonance imaging of the brain in patients with anosmia and hypothalamic hypogonadism (Kallmann's Syndrome). J Clin Endocrinol Metab 1987;65:581–584.

54. Weinstein RL, Reitz RE. Pituitary-testicular responsiveness in male hypogonadotropic hypogonadism. J Clin Invest 1974;53:408–415.

55. Yeh J, Rebar RW, Liu JH, Yen SSC. Pituitary function in isolated gonadotropin deficiency. Clin Endocrinol 1989;31:375–387.

56. Nunley WC, Urban RJ, Kitchin JD, et al. Dynamics of pulsatile prolactin release during the postpartum lactational period. J Clin Endocrinol Metab 1991;71:287–293.

57. Serri O, Beauregard H, Lesage J, et al. Long-term treatment with CV 205-502 in patients with prolactin-secreting pituitary macroadenomas. J Clin Endocrinol Metab 1990;71:682–687.

58. Dominque JN, Richmond IL, Wilson CB. Results of surgery in 114 patients with prolactin-secreting adenomas. Am J Obstet Gynecol 1980;137:102.

59. Serri O, Rasio E, Beauregard H, et al. Recurrence of hyperprolactinemia after selective transphenoidal adenectomy in women with prolactinoma. N Engl J Med 1983;309:280.

60. Herman TN, Molitch ME. Bromocriptine: indications and use in patients with endocrine disease. Hosp Formulary 1984;19:784–791.

61. Thorner MO, Schran HF, Evans WS, et al. A broad spectrum of prolactin suppression by bromocriptine in hyperprolactinemic women: a study of serum prolactin and bromocriptine levels after acute and chronic administration of bromocriptine. J Clin Endocrinol Metab 1980;50:1026–1033.

62. Lamberts S, Quik R. A comparison of the efficacy and safety of pergolide and bromocriptine in the treatment of hyperprolactinemia. J Clin Endocrinol Metab 1991;72:3:635.

63. Wang V, Lam KSL, Ma JTC, et al. Long-term treatment of hyperprolactinaemia with bromocriptine: effect of drug withdrawal. Clin Endocrinol 1987;27:363–371.

64. Moriondo P, Travaglini P, Nissim M, et al. Bromocriptine treatment of microprolactinomas: evidence of stable prolactin decrease after withdrawal. J Clin Endocrinol Metab 1985;60:764.

65. Schlechte J, Dolan K, Sherman B, et al. The natural history of untreated hyperprolactinemia: a prospective analysis. J Clin Endocrinol Metab 1989;68:412–430.

66. Ruiz-Velasco V, Tolis G. Pregnancy in hyperprolactinemic women. Fertil Steril 1984;41:793–805.

67. Molitch ME. Pregnancy and the hyperprolactinemic woman. N Engl J Med 1985;312:1364–1379.

68. Cryer PE, Daughaday WH. Regulation of growth hormone secretion in acromegaly. J Clin Endocrinol Metab 1969;29:386.

69. Williams TC, Kelijman M, Crelin WC, et al. Differential effects of somatostatin (SRIH) and a SRIH analog, SMS 201-995, on the secretion

of growth hormone and thyroid-stimulating hormone in man. J Clin Endocrinol Metab 1988;66:39–45.

70. Liddle GW, Estep HL, Kendall JW Jr, et al. Clinical approach of a new test of pituitary reserve. J Clin Endocrinol Metab 1959;19:875.

71. Synder PJ. Gonadotroph cell adenomas of the pituitary. Endocr Rev 1985;6:552.

72. Kaufman B. The turcica—a manifestation of the intrasellar subarachnoid space. Endocrinology 1968;90:931.

73. Sheehan HL, Davis JC. Pituitary necrosis. Br Med Bull 1968;24:59.

74. Sheehan HL. Postpartum necrosis of the anterior pituitary. J Pathol Bacteriol 1937;45:189–213.

75. Rosner B. Fundamentals of biostatistics. Boston: Duxbury Press, 1982:251.

76. Sheehan HL. Atypical hypopituitarism. Proc Roy Soc Med 1961;54:43–48.

77. Jackson IMD, Whyte WG, Garrey MM. Pituitary function following uncomplicated pregnancy in Sheehan's syndrome. J Clin Endocrinol Metab 1969;29:315–318.

78. Berga S, Mortola J, Gierton L, et al. Neuroendocrine aberrations in women with functional hypothalamic amenorrhea. J Clin Endocrinol Metab 1989;68:301–308.

79. Suh BY, Liu JH, Berga SL, et al. Hypercortisolism in patients with functional hypothalamic amenorrhea. J Clin Endocrinol Metab 1988;66:733–739.

CHAPTER 16

Chronic Anovulation and Polycystic Ovary Syndrome: Treatment for Infertility

ROGERIO A. LOBO

The focus of this chapter is the treatment of women with chronic anovulation and polycystic ovary syndrome (PCO). For women with these disorders who are desirous of fertility, induction of ovulation is necessary. Although all women with chronic anovulation occasionally may ovulate, any ovulations are sporadic and unpredictable. Even women who report regular cycles but at frequencies of greater than 35 days benefit from induction of ovulation to increase their reproductive efficiency.

Before a discussion of the treatment of women with chronic anovulation in PCO, it is important to give a brief overview of the differential diagnosis of women presenting with hyperandrogenism. Not all hyperandrogenic women exhibit hirsutism or other manifestations of androgen excess. These signs are largely determined by skin sensitivity in addition to elevated androgen levels. Hirsutism, however, remains a common manifestation of androgen excess in women, and the differential diagnosis may be found in Table 16–1.

PCO (described subsequently) and idiopathic hirsutism are the most common disorders resulting in hirsutism. Idiopathic hirsutism is diagnosed in women who have normal ovulatory menses and normal levels of both adrenal and ovarian androgens. The disorder is the result of increased skin sensitivity to androgens and in most women may be explained by enhanced 5α-reductase activity. Ovarian and adrenal tumors are characterized by a history of the rapid onset of manifestations of androgen excess, including virilization in many circumstances. High levels of testosterone or dehydroepiandrosterone sulfate under these circumstances warrant further investigation by obtaining scans of the ovary or adrenal. A more detailed diagnostic approach may be found in another review.[1] Adult-onset or nonclassic congenital adrenal hyperplasia occurs rarely, and the prevalence of this disorder is determined by the ethnic background of the patient. In some racial groups (Eskimos and Ashkenazi Jews), the prevalence is high, and screening for this disorder in these and other racial groups by measuring 17-hydroxyprogesterone may be indicated.[1]

PCO is a heterogeneous clinical disorder for which there is no consensus regarding appropriate diagnostic criteria.[2] A majority of women with chronic anovulation are found to have PCO. The syndrome includes a variety of clinical presentations, mixed glandular hyperandrogenism, and a spectrum of biochemical and ovarian morphologic changes. For these reasons, we have argued that it may be appropriate to rename the syndrome and to include in its name only the two cardinal features of the disorder, hyperandrogenism and chronic anovulation (HCA).[3]

In one study,[4] we found that these two cardinal features do not exhibit ethnic diversity. In addition, similar incidences of adrenal androgen excess and insulin resistance were identified among women in the United States, Italy, and Japan (Fig.

TABLE 16–1. Differential Diagnosis of Hirsutism and Virilization*

Source	Diagnosis
Nonspecific	Exogenous/iatrogenic
	Abnormal gonadal or sexual development
Peripheral	Idiopathic hirsutism
Ovarian	Polycystic ovary syndrome
	Stromal hyperthecosis
	Ovarian tumors
Adrenal	Adrenal tumors
	Cushing's syndrome
	Adult-onset congenital adrenal hyperplasia (nonclassic)

*Idiopathic hirsutism and polycystic ovary syndrome do not present with virilization.

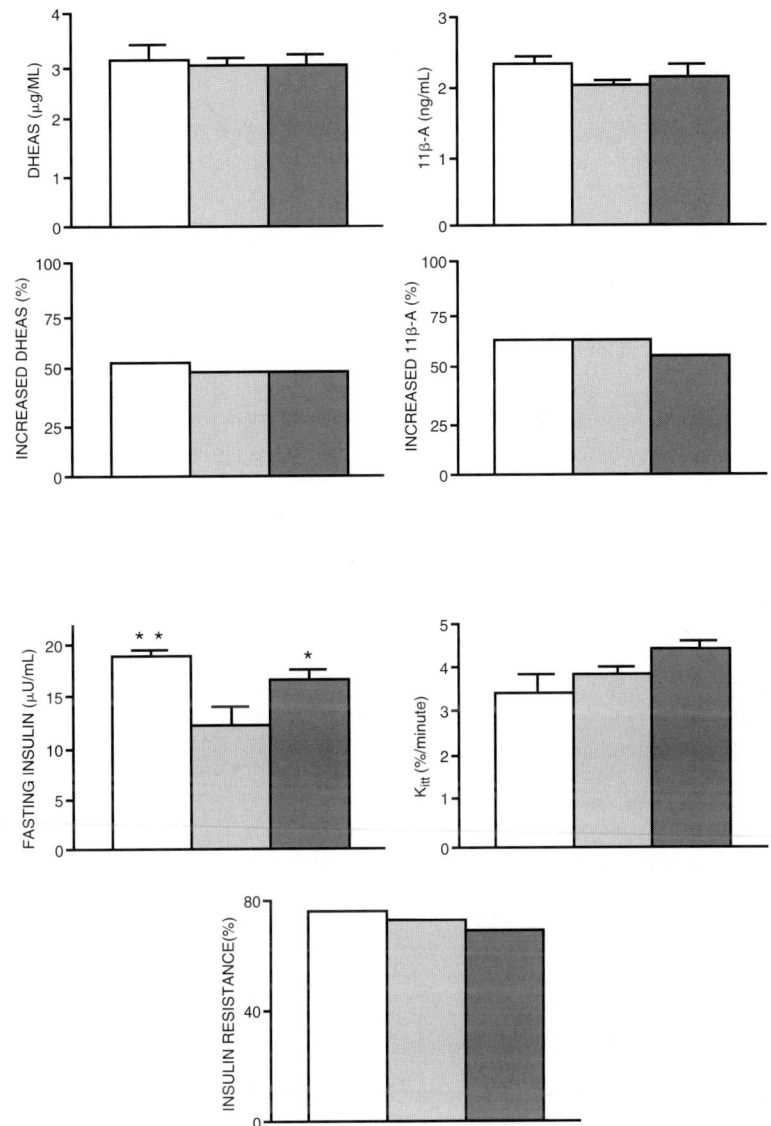

FIGURE 16–1. Adrenal androgen and fasting insulin measurements and excess in three ethnic groups: United States (*open bars*), Japan (*light gray bars*), and Italy (*black bars*). Fasting insulin is significantly different in Japanese women versus U.S. and Italian women. *$P < 0.05$; **$P < 0.01$; DHEAS, dehydroepiandrosterone sulfate; 11β-A, 11-β-hydroxyandrostenedione; K_{itt}, dissociation constant of insulin tolerance test. (From Carmina E, Koyama T, Chang L, et al. Does ethnicity influence the prevalence of adrenal hyperandrogenism and insulin resistance in polycystic ovary syndrome? Am J Obstet Gynecol 1992; 167:1807–1812.)

16–1). The finding of cystic ovaries, diagnosed to be consistent with PCO, occurred in 60% of patients in each group.

This common finding of polycystic ovaries on ultrasound studies has been the primary diagnostic criterion for some investigators. Alternatively, we have preferred to use the term HCA and then to subcategorize patients into those with cystic ovaries (the majority) and those without the classic ovarian morphologic features. In a study of Arabian women,[5] cystic ovaries were found in 65% of women with PCO, in 50% of women with hyperprolactinemia, in 100% of women with congenital adrenal hyperplasia, and in 16% of normal women. The finding of cystic ovaries in some "normal" women has also been our experience.[3] Polycystic changes were also found in almost a quarter of women with hypothalamic anovulation. Thus, we do not view the morphologic appearance of the ovary as a primary diagnostic criterion but as an important observation that has bearing on treatment and potentially also in the genetic or endocrinologic aspects of the syndrome. We suggest that the diagnosis of PCO should not be based on ovarian morphology alone.

Women with chronic anovulation who have no evidence

of hyperandrogenism should not be considered as having HCA/PCO. As reviewed previously,[5] however, these women may have "cystic" ovaries. In this setting, chronic anovulation is usually the result of other disorders. These include hypothyroidism and hyperprolactinemia, which should be sought. Other causes include drug exposure, strenuous (perhaps excessive) exercise, and systemic disease. By exclusion, all other patients fall into a category of idiopathic hypothalamic anovulation for which a specific cause cannot be identified. Psychogenic or neurotransmitter defects may be implicated but are difficult to diagnose. From a practical viewpoint, if an offending cause, such as hypothyroidism, is not found, induction of ovulation is carried out in a routine fashion. Clomiphene citrate is the drug of choice except for hypoestrogenic women with amenorrhea. In these patients, gonadotropin therapy or pulsatile gonadotropin-releasing hormone (GnRH) may be chosen, as discussed in Chapter 13.

In the hyperandrogenic patients with HCA/PCO, hirsutism may be a complaint. Treatment for hirsutism is largely directed at suppressing the abnormal source(s) of hyperandrogenism or blocking skin androgen action.[6, 7] Usually, however, this treatment is not carried out in conjunction with induction of ovulation. The chronic anovulation in HCA, which is characteristically of perimenarcheal onset, may result in dysfunctional uterine bleeding. In women not desirous of fertility, progestin suppression of the endometrium is necessary to prevent abnormal bleeding episodes and because of the concern of endometrial hyperplasia. In this chapter, the focus is on the treatment of women desirous of fertility. Specific details on suppressive therapy for hyperandrogenism and for dysfunctional bleeding may be found elsewhere.[8, 9]

INDUCTION OF OVULATION

In this section, we are considering ovulation induction for anovulatory women with and without hyperandrogenism but who do not have other specific diagnoses after initial evaluation. Clomiphene citrate, a synthetic estrogen antagonist, is the mainstay of therapy for ovulation induction. Clomiphene acts in competition with endogenous estrogens for estrogen binding sites in the hypothalamus or pituitary.[10, 11] The inhibition of the normal negative feedback of estrogen results in an increase in GnRH pulse frequency and an increase in follicle-stimulating hormone (FSH) and luteinizing hormone (LH). Clomiphene may also directly affect ovarian steroidogenesis.

In our previous studies of patients with clomiphene resistance, virtually all such patients exhibited biochemical features compatible with PCO.[12] More recently, we found that in "resistant" patients, clomiphene evoked the anticipated increase in LH pulse frequency, which was similar in responders and nonresponders, but that estradiol production was not commensurate with gonadotropin production in resistant women.[13] These data are compatible with the concept that it is ovarian hyporesponsiveness that is responsible for clomiphene resistance in PCO. This conclusion is similar to that reached earlier by others.[14]

In analyzing results of clomiphene treatment, a discrepancy seemingly exists between ovulatory responses and pregnancy rates. Although ovulation rates of approximately 80% are common, unadjusted pregnancy rates have been reported to be only 40%. More recent data using life-table analyses suggest that this figure is artificially low and should be approximately 70% at 6 months, thus closing the gap somewhat between ovulation rates and pregnancy rates.[15]

In our experience, the overall pregnancy rate for PCO (66.7%)[16] was similar to that of other anovulatory patients without PCO. A discussion of potential factors influencing reproductive performance in PCO follows later.

In treating women with clomiphene, although we have used doses of up to 250 mg for 5 days, most clinicians would argue that patients requiring doses in excess of 150 mg/day should be considered to be clomiphene resistant. In these patients, we have achieved success in terms of both ovulation and pregnancy with the adjunctive use of dexamethasone[17] or by extending the days of administration.[18] Nevertheless, our preference for treatment in these clomiphene-resistant patients is to administer gonadotropins.

If a patient is found to be clomiphene resistant or if pregnancy does not occur after several cycles with clomiphene in women who have had other infertility factors ruled out, gonadotropin therapy may be considered. A life-table analysis

of pregnancy rates in patients receiving gonadotropin therapy is shown in Figure 16–2.[19] Comparing anovulatory patients with clomiphene resistance (typically those with PCO) with those with hypogonadotropic amenorrhea shows that clomiphene-resistant patients had much lower pregnancy rates. After six cycles, a pregnancy rate of only 40% was observed compared with a rate of 95% in hypogonadotropic patients and a rate of 60% in an anovulatory nulliparous population.

A review of 16 years of experience using human menopausal gonadotropins (hMG) at our institution showed results that are more encouraging in that pregnancy rates increased substantially merely with the advent of ultrasound monitoring.[20] When looking specifically at oligomenorrheic patients, a pregnancy rate of 71.1% was observed. These rates, however, are still lower than those observed in amenorrheic hypogonadotropic patients.

The use of "pure" FSH instead of hMG (LH and FSH) in women with PCO is attractive from a physiologic standpoint. It has been argued that because patients with PCO have higher endogenous levels of LH, the additional LH in hMG may not be needed and may instead aggravate the gonadotropin imbalance. We have shown that intramuscular urinary FSH administration reduces serum immunoreactive LH[21] (Fig. 16–3). This effect, together with the increase in serum FSH from urinary FSH administration, resulted in significantly lowered LH:FSH ratios. Based on the pharmacokinetic profiles, the use of "pure" FSH appears to have theoretical advantages. These advantages, however, have not been confirmed clinically. Garcea and colleagues[22] treated 18 PCO patients with Metrodin ("pure" FSH) for induction of ovulation. Ovulation was achieved in 91% of the cycles attempted, but only 50% of these patients conceived. In studies comparing hMG with "pure" FSH, significant advantages of one therapeutic regimen over the other could not be demonstrated.[23–29]

Several investigators have advocated the use of a GnRH agonist before gonadotropin treatment. A doubling of pregnancy rates has been proposed to result with combined GnRH agonist/gonadotropin therapy[30] (Fig. 16–4). This con-

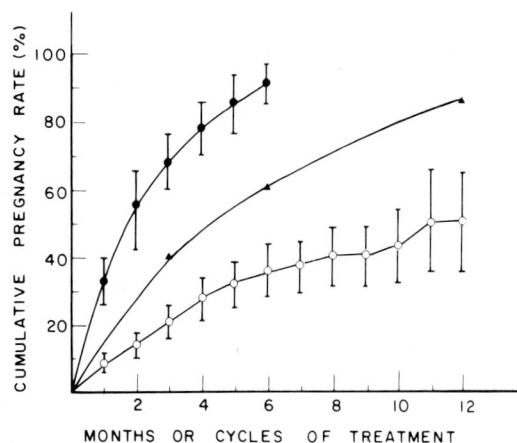

FIGURE 16–2. Cumulative pregnancy rates in women receiving human menopausal gonadotropin for ovulation induction. Hypogonadotropic patients (*solid circles*), anovulatory patients resistant to clomiphene (*open circles*), and normal nulliparous population (*triangles*). (From Dor J, Itzkowic DJ, Mashiach S, et al. Cumulative conception rates following gonadotropin therapy. Am J Obstet Gynecol 1980;136:102–105.)

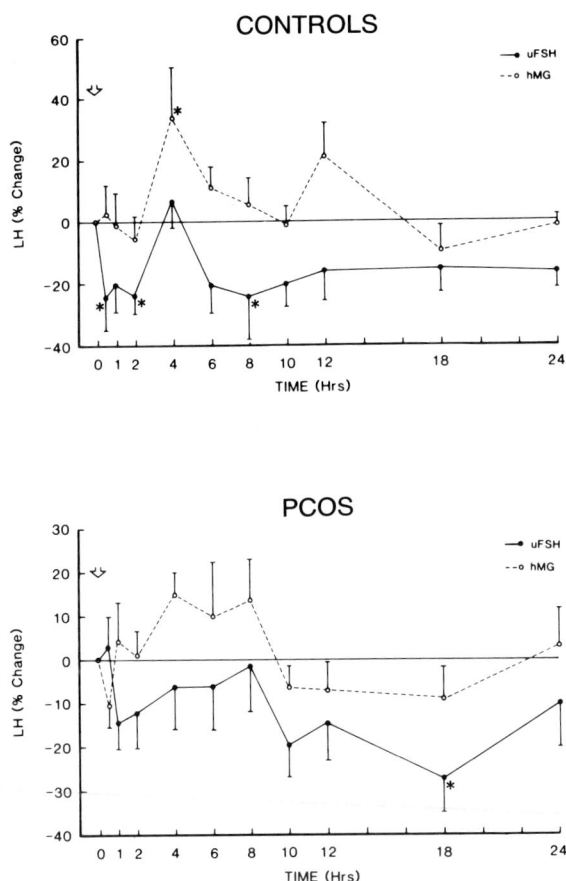

FIGURE 16–3. Percentage of change in serum luteinizing hormone (LH) after an intramuscular injection (*arrow*) of either human urinary follicle-stimulating hormone (UFSH) or human menopausal gonadotropin (hMG) (150 IU) in normal ovulatory controls (*upper panel*) and patients with polycystic ovary syndrome (PCO) (*lower panel*). In controls, significant decreases were observed at 30 minutes, 2 hours, and 8 hours after UFSH. A significant increase was observed at 4 hours after hMG. In patients with PCO, a significant decrease was observed at 18 hours after UFSH. *$P < 0.05$ compared with baseline levels of LH. (From Anderson RE, Cragun JM, Chang RJ, et al. A pharmacodynamic comparison of human urinary follicle-stimulating hormone and human menopausal gonadotropin in normal women and polycystic ovary syndrome. Fertil Steril 1989;52:216–220. Reproduced with permission of the publisher, The American Fertility Society.)

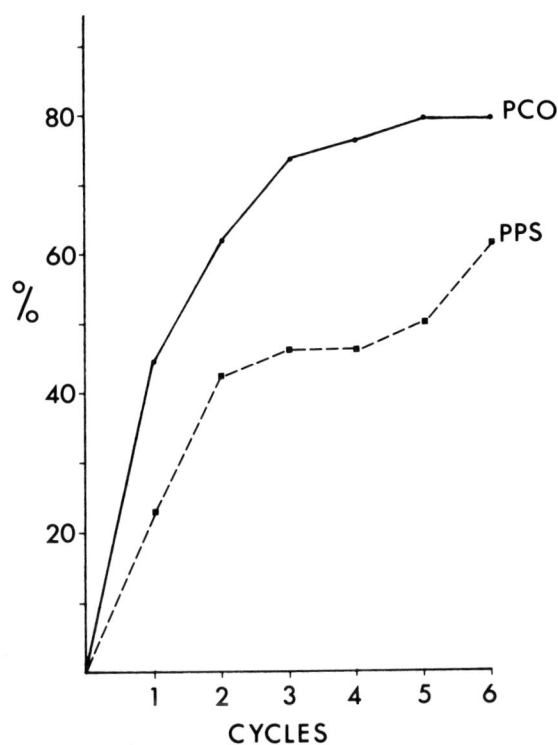

FIGURE 16–4. Cumulative pregnancy rates (percentage of total group) in patients with polycystic ovarian syndrome (PCO) and poor progesterone surge (PPS) receiving combined gonadotropin-releasing hormone agonist and human menopausal gonadotropin therapy. (From Fleming R, Haxton MJ, Hamilton MPR, et al. Combined gonadotropin-releasing hormone analog and exogenous gonadotropins for ovulation induction in infertile women: efficacy related to ovarian function assessment. Am J Obstet Gynecol 1988;159:376–381.)

cept, however, has not been universally accepted, and similar pregnancy rates have been reported with and without adjunctive GnRH agonist use in prospective, randomized trials.[28, 29] The theoretical benefit of lowering LH and androgen levels before gonadotropin stimulation may be offset by the variable responses of an enlarged ovary having an intrinsically abnormal local endocrine milieu. In addition, some concern has been raised that prior GnRH agonist treatment may increase the risk of hyperstimulation. Although not universally accepted, a consensus view is that in PCO, prior treatment with the GnRH agonist either has little effect on the rate of hyperstimulation or may increase it.[28, 31, 32] There may be, however, other benefits to using the GnRH agonist in PCO, as discussed subsequently.

To avoid hyperstimulation and improve success rates, several regimens have been proposed for gonadotropin administration. The most popular and widely used of these regimens is the low-dose regimen, in which small increments of gonadotropins (37.5 IU/day) are given at 7-day intervals.[33–38]

This treatment has been shown to be more effective than conventional therapy (Table 16–2). With this regimen, equal success rates have been reported in a randomized trial using either hMG or FSH and either intramuscular or subcutaneous routes of administration.[38] A similar approach has been proposed by Schoemaker drawing from the general principles of Brown.[33] A threshold dose of FSH is determined for each patient by measuring levels of serum FSH achieved and the minimal dose at which follicles are recruited. It has been suggested for normal women that this threshold is a serum level of 8 mIU/mL.[39] In PCO, however, the range is predictably much wider, and responses have been noted in the range of 6 to 10 mIU/mL.

TABLE 16–2. Comparison of the Low-Dose Protocol Compared With the Conventional Protocol for Follicle-Stimulating Hormone Administration in Polycystic Ovary Syndrome

	Low Dose	Conventional
Follicles	1.5 ± 3	$4.4 \pm 1, p < 0.0002$
Estradiol (pmol/L)	1539	$4050, p < 0.04$
Pregnancy	5/8	0/6

Adapted from Shoham Z, Patel A, Jacobs HS. Polycystic ovarian syndrome: safety and effectiveness of stepwise and low-dose administration of purified follicle-stimulating hormone. Fertil Steril 1991; 55:1051–56. Reproduced with permission of the publisher, The American Fertility Society.

The other regimen that has been suggested is a step-down regimen, in which an initial high dose of 225 IU/day is used for 2 days followed by a step-down to 75 IU/day.[40] Although no improvement in pregnancy rates has been demonstrated, a significant decrease in the rate of hyperstimulation was reported. The potential success of this approach has been confirmed by a decrease in the recruitment of midsized follicles.[41]

The use of intravenous pulsatile GnRH alone, although extremely effective in the hypogonadotropic patient, is generally ineffective in our experience for inducing ovulation in patients with PCO. In one of several studies, patients given this regimen were noted to have elevated LH and testosterone levels.[42] Luteal phase progesterone was reduced, and low ovulatory responses of 38% were observed with a pregnancy rate of only 8%.[42] In combination with a GnRH agonist, however, pretreatment with the agonist rendered significantly improved ovulatory and pregnancy rates.[42, 43] Serum androgen levels and LH remain suppressed once the GnRH agonist has been stopped and pulsatile GnRH is begun (Fig. 16–5).

Another regimen that is gaining popularity for clomiphene-resistant patients is ovarian cautery. Before the development of improved medical therapy for the induction of ovulation, ovarian wedge resection was advocated. This, however, has been abandoned and should not be carried out because significant adhesion formation can occur. Currently new modifications on this technique using laparoscopic ovarian cautery or laser vaporization have been developed,[26, 44–52]

which perhaps allow more liberal indications for this procedure. Serum LH, FSH, androstenedione, and testosterone levels have been reported to decrease immediately after these procedures. The bioactivity and amplitude of LH are decreased,[50, 51] but LH pulse frequency is not affected.[51] Spontaneous ovulation in one series was shown to be as great as 53% after surgery, with an additional 32% of patients responding to low-dose clomiphene therapy. Fifty-six percent of these patients conceived within 6 months of surgery.[49] Although the results appear dramatic, long-term effects are as yet unknown, and adhesion formation still occurs, although perhaps to a lesser extent than with the older wedge techniques at laparotomy. At a conference on the treatment of PCO, an adhesion formation rate of 25% was suggested to occur.[53]

REASONS FOR POOR REPRODUCTIVE OUTCOME IN POLYCYSTIC OVARY SYNDROME

Although not firmly established, it is generally accepted that even with the more ideal regimens of ovulation induction in PCO, pregnancy rates are reduced. Also, the spontaneous abortion rate is increased, to some degree, in virtually all series reported. Although an average figure of more than 25% for the miscarriage rate of various treatments in PCO

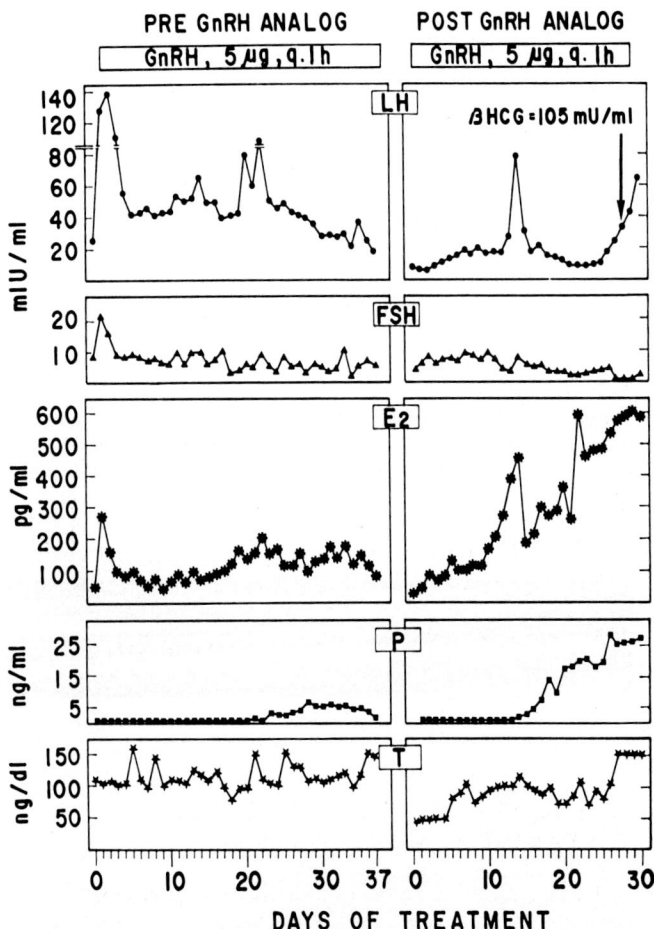

FIGURE 16–5. Daily serum luteinizing hormone (LH), follicle-stimulating hormone (FSH), and sex steroid levels (estradiol [E_2], progesterone [P], and testosterone [T]) during induction of ovulation with pulsatile gonadotropin-releasing hormone (GnRH) before (*left*) and after (*right*) GnRH agonist administration in a patient with polycystic ovarian syndrome. (From Filicori M, Campaniello E, Michelacci L, et al. Gonadotropin-releasing hormone (GnRH) analog suppression renders polycystic ovarian disease patients more susceptible to ovulation induction with pulsatile GnRH. J Clin Endocrinol Metab 1988;66:327–333; © The Endocrine Society.)

has been suggested,[54] the range is extremely great and varies from 22% to 66%. Probably a more consistent figure for the miscarriage rate is 30%, which means that up to a third of all pregnancies might be anticipated to be lost. Some of the presumed reasons for this poor reproductive outcome are listed in Table 16–3. A substantial literature is emerging indicating that high levels of LH (as found in PCO) may be detrimental.[55–61] In one study with clomiphene use,[61] a subgroup of patients with PCO demonstrated an abnormal LH response and a poor outcome (Fig. 16–6). In another study involving the use of a GnRH agonist,[62] the miscarriage rate was not reduced. Although others have suggested that agonist therapy reduces the miscarriage rate,[63, 64] the effect of the agonist has not been studied prospectively in a randomized trial. Nevertheless, because miscarriage in women with PCO is a significant problem, the GnRH agonist may offer some promise for treatment.

The endocrine milieu surrounding developing oocytes in PCO is clearly abnormal and may or may not be altered by pretreatment with a GnRH agonist. The milieu of the oocytes may be responsible, at least in part, for the poor reproductive outcome. The oocytes per se, however, are probably not abnormal, and mature oocytes, when taken out of their environment, have been shown to result in fertilization rates equal to those of other patients during in vitro fertilization.[65]

The endometrium of many patients may be abnormal, and this includes women who have endometrial hyperplasia. Although abnormal endometrial prostaglandin production in PCO has been suggested,[66] whether or not this explains the poor reproductive performance remains unclear. The endometrium as a potential factor for poor reproductive performance has not been adequately studied.

Obesity has been thought to be a significant negative factor as well. We showed some time ago that once the patient is ovulatory, obesity per se does not influence outcome.[12] Nevertheless, others have found that obesity, independent of LH levels, increases the miscarriage rate.[67]

Regardless of whether obesity does or does not influence prognosis, weight reduction is obviously beneficial for overall health concerns. Weight reduction in obese women may lead to resumption of ovulation and regular menstrual cycles. This may occur, in part, as a result of an increase in sex hormone–binding globulin (SHBG) levels, a decrease in free androgens, a decrease in fasting insulin, and an increase in insulin-like growth factor–binding protein (Fig. 16–7).[68] Therefore, weight loss should be advocated and used in combination with medical therapy.

Review of the papers examining ovarian cautery in PCO has also suggested that the miscarriage rate may be slightly reduced (15% to 21%) in pregnancies resulting after such therapy. Although these data need to be confirmed, the specific mechanisms for this reduced rate have not been explained in that many factors, including LH, androgens, and ovarian size, are affected by this surgery.

TABLE 16–3. Potential Factors Influencing Poor Reproductive Outcome in Polycystic Ovary Syndrome

High levels of luteinizing hormone
Ovarian factor
Oocyte quality
Endometrium
Obesity
Combination of factors

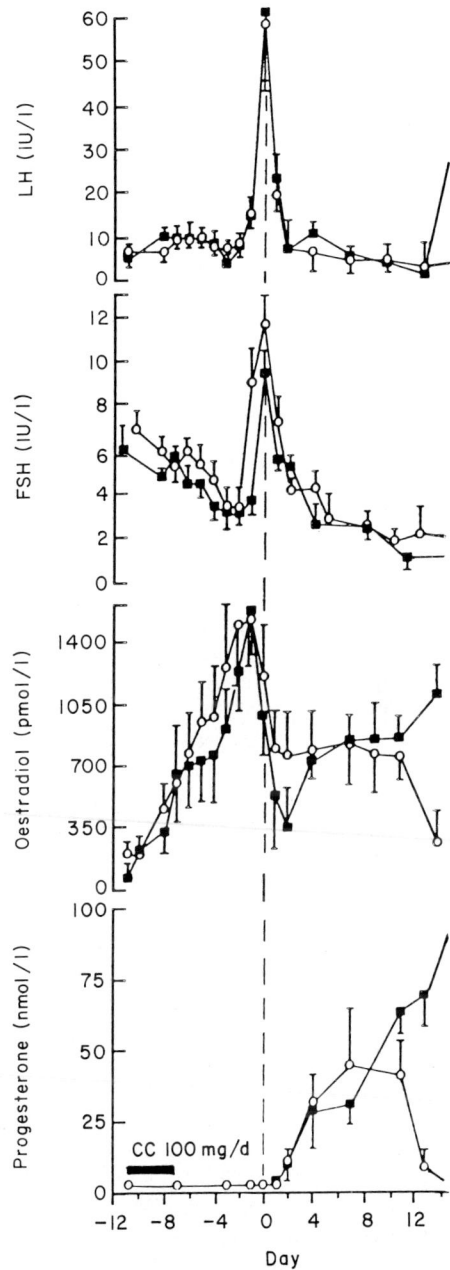

FIGURE 16–6. Patterns of hormonal secretion in patients exhibiting normal response (*solid square*) and abnormal response (*open circle*) to clomiphene citrate (CC) therapy. For luteinizing hormone (LH) levels: $P < 0.05$ on days -8 to -2; $P < 0.02$ on day 0. For follicle-stimulating hormone (FSH) levels: $P < 0.05$ on days -1 and 0. For oestradiol levels: $P < 0.01$ on days -10 to -4; $P < 0.001$ on days -3 to 0 and on days 4 to 10. For progesterone levels: $P < 0.05$ on days 0 to 10. (From Shoham Z, Borenstein R, Lunenfeld B, Pariente C. Hormonal profiles following clomiphene citrate therapy in conception and nonconception cycles. Clin Endocrinol 1990;33:271–278.)

ADJUNCTS TO TREATMENT AND PRETREATMENT EVALUATION

The addition of dexamethasone to hMG therapy has also been shown to improve ovulation rates in patients resistant

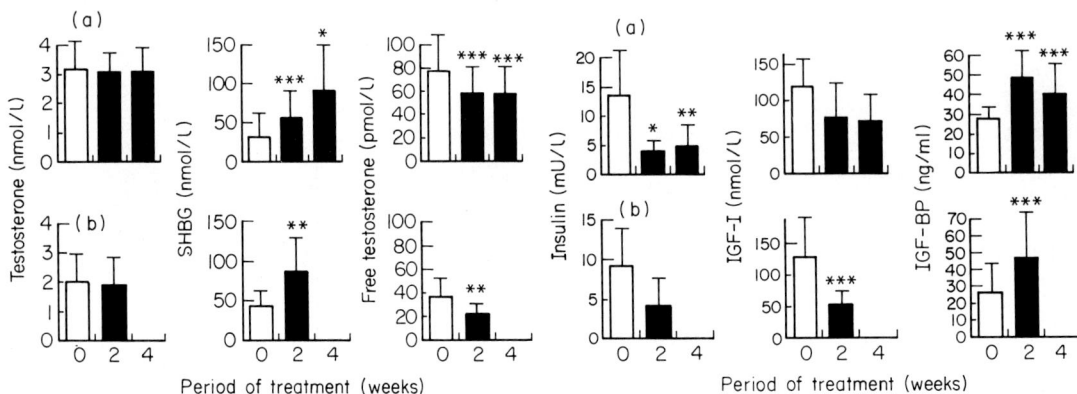

FIGURE 16–7. Women with polycystic (*a*) or normal (*b*) ovaries studied before (*open bars*) or after (*solid bars*) 2 (or 4) weeks of a low-calorie diet. *Left group:* Serum concentrations (mean ± SD) of testosterone, sex hormone–binding globulin, and free testosterone. *Right group:* Serum concentrations (mean ± SD) of insulin, insulin-like growth factor-1 (IGF-I), and IGF binding protein (IGF-BP). Significant changes in posttreatment as compared with pretreatment results: *$P < 0.05$, **$P < 0.02$, and ***$P < 0.01$ by Student's paired *t* test. (From Kiddy DS, Hamilton-Fairley D, Seppala M, et al. Diet-induced changes in sex hormone binding globulin and free testosterone in women with normal or polycystic ovaries: correlation with serum insulin and insulin-like growth factor-1. Clin Endocrinol 1989;31:757–763.)

to standard therapy. An ovulation rate of 81% resulting in a conception rate of 75%[69] in otherwise nonresponders was seen with the addition of dexamethasone. Although these data have not been confirmed, the results are consistent with the notion that lowering androgens is beneficial for inducing ovulation.

Antiandrogens, such as spironolactone, have been used to lower androgen levels and inhibit androgen action. The use of spironolactone in combination with clomiphene or bromocriptine has been found to induce ovulation in otherwise clomiphene-resistant patients.[70] To date, however, there are no large prospective, randomized studies on the efficacy of this combination therapy. On a theoretical basis, blockade of androgen action in PCO should be beneficial. Potential detrimental effects of antiandrogens on fetal sexual differentiation would seem to make this approach to ovulation induction unwise.

Bromocriptine has also been used in patients with elevated prolactin levels. Although bromocriptine may be effective in inducing ovulation in those patients with elevated prolactin levels, in patients with normal prolactin levels, there is probably no additional benefit.

Before treatment, factors to consider include obesity, androgen status, endometrial thickness, ovarian morphology, and glucose intolerance. Weight reduction is important, and patients should attempt to achieve pregnancy only if and when they are euglycemic. Although ovarian size before treatment affords some prognostic significance, routine pretreatment suppression cannot be advocated at present. Clearly, however, a hyperplastic endometrium should be shed before ovulation induction. If adrenal androgen levels are extremely high (see later), we have routinely used dexamethasone. The true benefit of suppressing LH and ovarian androgens with a GnRH agonist deserves further study.

CHOICE OF THERAPY

Clomiphene should be the starting point for ovulation induction in PCO. In all patients, attention should be paid to (1) weight loss, (2) normalizing the endometrium, and (3)

instituting androgen suppression if adrenal androgen levels are extremely high (e.g., dehydroepiandrosterone sulfate >6 µg/mL). Ovarian morphology on ultrasound studies should be used as a guide to assess the prognosis of the response and to suggest the need for laparoscopic cautery if poor clomiphene responses (low progesterone levels) or resistance ensues. It is important to re-emphasize here that the diagnosis of HCA/PCO is not based on ovarian morphology but that polycystic ovaries as seen on ultrasound studies are often found in HCA/PCO and other ovulatory disorders. In one study, ovarian morphology on ultrasound studies was shown to predict the response to gonadotropins, whether or not the patient had endocrinologic features of PCO (Fig. 16–8).[71]

In clomiphene-resistant patients, a randomized study

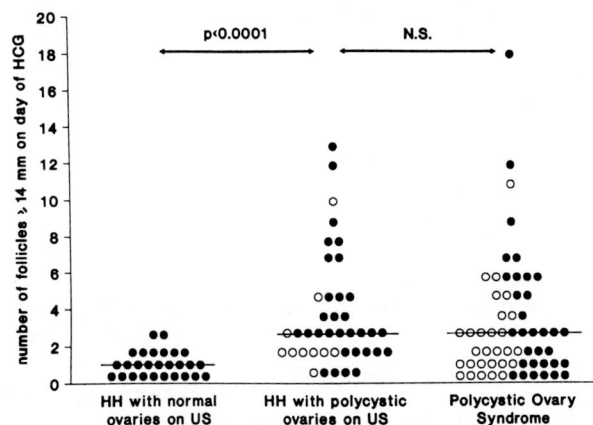

FIGURE 16–8. The number of follicles ≥ 14 mm in diameter that developed in three different groups of patients after ovulation induction with human menopausal gonadotropin with either the conventional protocol (*solid circles*) or the low-dose protocol (*open circles*) are shown. No significant difference was noted comparing multifollicular development in patients with hypogonadotropic hypogonadism (HH) with normal and polycystic ovaries on ultrasound (US) with polycystic ovary patients. (From Shoham Z, Conway GS, Patel A, Jacobs HS. Polycystic ovaries in patients with hypogonadotropic hypogonadism: similarity of ovarian response to gonadotropin stimulation in patients with polycystic ovarian syndrome. Fertil Steril 1992;58:37–45. Reprinted with permission from the publisher, The American Fertility Society.)

Infertility: Induction of ovulation

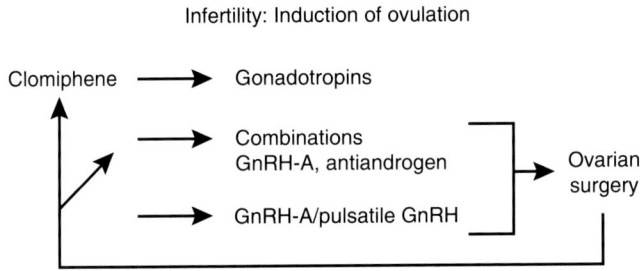

FIGURE 16–9. Proposed schematic for inducing ovulation in a clomiphene-resistant patient with polycystic ovary syndrome. GnRH, gonadotropin-releasing hormone; GnRH-A, GnRH agonist.

showed equal efficiency of hMG, FSH, and ovarian cautery.[26] Figure 16–9 shows a proposed scheme for choosing therapy in resistant patients. Although pretreatment with a GnRH agonist and GnRH pulsatile therapy should not be regarded as first choices, they may be used selectively or according to patient preference. The pregnancy rates in general with a GnRH agonist and pulsatile GnRH appear to be lower overall.[72] In general, patients benefit most from a low-dose regimen of hMG or FSH, the latter being more often preferred, even in the absence of data showing its superiority over hMG. If the response is poor, ovarian cautery can be carried out. In other clomiphene-resistant patients, if a need for laparoscopy exists, even before hMG or FSH, ovarian cautery may be considered earlier. In patients not responding well to one or the other regimen, pretreatment with a GnRH agonist also may be considered. It should be obvious that substantial clinical and biochemical heterogeneity exists in patients with PCO and that not all patients respond to the various regimens outlined here. As a result, the clinician has to be flexible in considering an approach to ovulation induction in PCO.

CONGENITAL ADRENAL HYPERPLASIA

In the rare patient with adult-onset congenital adrenal hyperplasia, induction of ovulation may be achieved by adrenal suppression. Although corticosteroid suppression has been found not to be necessary for treatment of hirsutism in congenital adrenal hyperplasia,[73] adrenal suppression is necessary for normal ovulatory menstrual function. The goal of such therapy should be the suppression of the C21 progestins (progesterone and 17-hydroxyprogesterone) rather than the androgens (dehydroepiandrosterone sulfate, androstenedione, and testosterone).[74] Indeed a higher dose of dexamethasone is usually required to suppress the C21 progestins than is needed for androgen suppression. After 3 months of suppression, if spontaneous ovulation does not ensue, it is reasonable to add clomiphene citrate. In our experience, however, this is usually not necessary. Once pregnancy has been established, we have continued corticosteroid therapy (usually switching to hydrocortisone) through the first trimester of pregnancy.

REFERENCES

1. Lobo RA. Androgen excess. *In:* Mishell DR Jr, Davajan V, Lobo RA, editors. Infertility, Contraception and Reproductive Endocrinology. 3rd edition. Cambridge, MA: Blackwell Scientific Publications, 1991:422–446.
2. Lobo RA. Androgen secretion in the syndrome of hyperandrogenic chronic anovulation. *In:* Dunaif A, Givens JR, Haseltine FP, Merriam GR, editors. Polycystic Ovary Syndrome. Cambridge, MA: Blackwell Scientific Publications, 1992:319–332.
3. Lobo RA. The syndrome of hyperandrogenic chronic anovulation. *In:* Mishell DR Jr, Davajan V, Lobo RA, editors. Infertility, Contraception and Reproductive Endocrinology. 3rd edition. Cambridge, MA: Blackwell Scientific Publications, 1991:447–487.
4. Carmina E, Koyama T, Chang L, et al. Does ethnicity influence the prevalence of adrenal hyperandrogenism and insulin resistance in polycystic ovary syndrome? Am J Obstet Gynecol 1992; 167:1807–1812.
5. Gadir AA, Khatim MS, Mowafi RS, et al. Implications of ultrasonically diagnosed polycystic ovaries. I. Correlations with basal hormonal profiles. Hum Reprod 1992; 7:453–457.
6. Lobo RA, Goebelsmann U, Horton R. Evidence for the importance of peripheral tissue events in the development of hirsutism in polycystic ovary syndrome. J Clin Endocrinol Metab 1983; 57:393–397.
7. Matteri RK, Stanczyk FZ, Gentzschein EE, et al. Androgen sulfate and glucuronide conjugates in nonhirsute and hirsute women with polycystic ovarian syndrome. Am J Obstet Gynecol 1989; 161:1704–1709.
8. Lobo RA. Endocrine therapy of hyperandrogenism. *In:* Barbieri RL, Schiff I, editors. Reproductive Endocrine Therapeutics. New York: Alan R. Liss, 1988:101–126.
9. March CM. Dysfunctional uterine bleeding. *In:* Mishell DR Jr, Davajan V, Lobo RA, editors. Infertility, Contraception and Reproductive Endocrinology. 3rd edition. Cambridge, MA: Blackwell Scientific Publications, 1991:488–502.
10. Adashi EY. Clomiphene citrate: mechanism(s) and site(s) of action—a hypothesis revised. Fertil Steril 1984; 42:331–344.
11. Kerin JF, Liu JH, Phillipou G, Yen SSC. Evidence for a hypothalamic site of action of clomiphene citrate in women. J Clin Endocrinol Metab 1985; 61:265–268.
12. Lobo RA, Gysler M, March CM, et al. Clinical and laboratory predictors of clomiphene response. Fertil Steril 1982; 37:168–174.
13. Levin JH, Hickey MJ, Lobo RA. Mechanisms of clomiphene citrate (CC) resistance in polycystic ovary syndrome (PCO) (abstr. #44). Presented at the 37th Annual Meeting of the Society for Gynecologic Investigation, St. Louis, 1990.
14. Polson DW, Kiddy DS, Mason HD, Franks S. Induction of ovulation with clomiphene citrate in women with polycystic ovary syndrome: the difference between responders and nonresponders. Fertil Steril 1989; 51:30–34.
15. Hammond MG. Monitoring techniques for improving pregnancy rates during clomiphene ovulation induction. Fertil Steril 1984; 42:499–509.
16. Gysler M, March CM, Mishell DR Jr, Bailey EJ. A decade's experience with an individualized clomiphene treatment regimen including its effect on the postcoital test. Fertil Steril 1982; 37:161–167.
17. Lobo RA, Paul W, March CM, et al. Clomiphene and dexamethasone in women unresponsive to clomiphene alone. Obstet Gynecol 1982; 60:497–501.
18. Lobo RA, Granger LR, Davajan V, Mishell DR Jr. An extended regimen of clomiphene citrate in women unresponsive to standard therapy. Fertil Steril 1982; 37:762–766.
19. Dor J, Itzkowic DJ, Mashiach S, et al. Cumulative conception rates following gonadotropin therapy. Am J Obstet Gynecol 1980; 136:102–105.
20. March CM. Improved pregnancy rate with monitoring of gonadotropin therapy by three modalities. Am J Obstet Gynecol 1987; 156:1473–1479.
21. Anderson RE, Cragun JM, Chang RJ, et al. A pharmacodynamic comparison of human urinary follicle-stimulating hormone and human menopausal gonadotropin in normal women and polycystic ovary syndrome. Fertil Steril 1989; 52:216–220.
22. Garcea N, Campo S, Panetta V, et al. Induction of ovulation with purified urinary follicle-stimulating hormone in patients with polycystic ovarian syndrome. Am J Obstet Gynecol 1985; 151:635–640.
23. Hoffman DI, Lobo, RA, Campeau JD, et al. Ovulation induction in clomiphene-resistant anovulatory women: differential follicular response to purified urinary follicle-stimulating hormone (FSH) versus purified urinary FSH and luteinizing hormone. J Clin Endocrinol Metab 1985; 60:922–927.
24. Venturoli S, Paradisi R, Fabbri R, et al. Comparison between human urinary follicle-stimulating hormone and human menopausal gonadotropin treatment in polycystic ovary. Obstet Gynecol 1984; 63:6–11.

25. Tanbo T, Dale PO, Kjekshus E, et al. Stimulation with human menopausal gonadotropin versus follicle-stimulating hormone after pituitary suppression in polycystic ovarian syndrome. Fertil Steril 1990; 53:798–803.

26. Gadir AA, Mowafi RS, Alnaser HMI, et al. Ovarian electrocautery versus human menopausal gonadotropin and pure follicle-stimulating hormone therapy in the treatment of patients with polycystic ovarian disease. Clin Endocrinol 1990; 33:585–592.

27. Larsen T, Bostofte E, Larsen JF, et al. Comparison of urinary human follicle-stimulating hormone and human menopausal gonadotropin for ovarian stimulation in polycystic ovarian syndrome. Fertil Steril 1990; 53:426–431.

28. Homburg R, Eshel A, Kilborn J, et al. Combined luteinizing hormone releasing hormone analogue and exogenous gonadotrophins for the treatment of infertility associated with polycystic ovaries. Hum Reprod 1990; 5:32–35.

29. Sagle MA, Hamilton-Fairley D, Kiddy DS, Franks S. A comparative, randomized study of low-dose human menopausal gonadotropin and follicle-stimulating hormone in women with polycystic ovarian syndrome. Fertil Steril 1991; 55:56–60.

30. Fleming R, Haxton MJ, Hamilton MPR, et al. Combined gonadotropin-releasing hormone analog and exogenous gonadotropins for ovulation induction in infertile women: efficacy related to ovarian function assessment. Am J Obstet Gynecol 1988; 159:376–381.

31. Buckler HM, McLachlan RI, MacLachlan VB, et al. Serum inhibin levels in polycystic ovary syndrome: basal levels and response to luteinizing hormone-releasing hormone agonist and exogenous gonadotropin administration. J Clin Endocrinol Metab 1988; 66:798–803.

32. Charbonnel B, Krempf M, Blanchard P, et al. Induction of ovulation in polycystic ovary syndrome with a combination of a luteinizing hormone-releasing hormone analog and exogenous gonadotropins. Fertil Steril 1987; 47:920–924.

33. Brown JB. Pituitary control of ovarian function—concepts derived from gonadotrophin therapy. Aust N Z J Obstet Gynecol 1978; 18:47–54.

34. Kamrava MM, Seibel MM, Berger MJ, et al. Reversal of persistent anovulation in polycystic ovarian disease by administration of chronic low-dose follicle stimulating hormone. Fertil Steril 1982; 37:520–523.

35. Seibel MM, McArdle C, Smith D, Taymor ML. Ovulation induction in polycystic ovary syndrome with urinary follicle-stimulating hormone or human menopausal gonadotropins. Fertil Steril 1985; 43:703–708.

36. Polson DW, Mason HD, Saldahna MBY, Franks S. Ovulation of a single dominant follicle during treatment with low-dose pulsatile follicle-stimulating hormone in women with polycystic ovary syndrome. Clin Endocrinol 1987; 26:205–212.

37. Buvat J, Buvat-Herbaut M, Marcolin G, et al. Purified follicle-stimulating hormone in polycystic ovary syndrome: slow administration is safer and more effective. Fertil Steril 1989; 52:553–559.

38. Polson DW, Mason HD, Kiddy DS. Low-dose follicle-stimulating hormone in the treatment of polycystic ovary syndrome: a comparison of pulsatile subcutaneous with daily intramuscular therapy. Br J Obstet Gynaecol 1989; 96:746–748.

39. Van Weissenbruch MM. Gonadotrophins for induction of ovulation. Thesis. Vrije Universiteit Amsterdam, The Netherlands, 1990.

40. Mizunuma H, Takagi T, Honjyo S, et al. Clinical pharmacodynamics of urinary follicle-stimulating hormone and its application for pharmacokinetic stimulation program. Fertil Steril 1990; 53:440–445.

41. Schoot DC, Pache TD, Hop WC, et al. Growth patterns of ovarian follicles during induction of ovulation with decreasing doses of human menopausal gonadotropin following presumed selection of polycystic ovary syndrome. Fertil Steril 1992; 57:1117–1120.

42. Filicori M, Campaniello E, Michelacci L, et al. Gonadotropin-releasing hormone (GnRH) analog suppression renders polycystic ovarian disease patients more susceptible to ovulation induction with pulsatile GnRH. J Clin Endocrinol Metab 1988; 66:327–333.

43. Filicori M, Flamigni C, Campaniello E, et al. The abnormal response of polycystic ovarian disease patients to exogenous pulsatile gonadotropin-releasing hormone: characterization and management. J Clin Endocrinol Metab 1989; 69:825–831.

44. Gjonnaess H. Polycystic ovarian syndrome treated by ovarian electrocautery through the laparoscope. Fertil Steril 1984; 41:20–25.

45. Aakvaag A, Gjonnaess H. Hormonal response to electrocautery of the ovary in patients with polycystic ovary disease. Br J Obstet Gynaecol 1985; 92:1258–1264.

46. Gjonnaess H, Norman N. Endocrine effects of ovarian electrocautery in patients with polycystic ovarian disease. Br J Obstet Gynaecol 1987; 94:779–783.

47. Greenblatt E, Casper RF. Endocrine changes after laparoscopic ovarian cautery in polycystic ovarian syndrome. Am J Obstet Gynecol 1987; 156:279–285.

48. Sumioki H, Utsunomiya T, Matsuoka K, et al. The effect of laparoscopic multiple punch resection of the ovary on hypothalamo-pituitary axis in polycystic ovary syndrome. Fertil Steril 1988; 50:567–572.

49. Daniell JF, Miller W. Polycystic ovaries treated by laparoscopic laser vaporization. Fertil Steril 1989; 51:232–236.

50. Skata M, Tasaka K, Kurachi H, et al. Changes of bioactive luteinizing hormone after laparoscopic ovarian cautery in patients with polycystic ovarian syndrome. Fertil Steril 1990; 53: 610–613.

51. Rossmanith WG, Keckstein J, Spatzier K, Lauritzen C. The impact of ovarian laser surgery on the gonadotrophin secretion in women with polycystic ovarian disease. Clin Endocrinol 1991; 34:223–230.

52. Armar NA, McGarrigle HHG, Honour J, et al. Laparoscopic ovarian diathermy in the management of anovulatory infertility in women with polycystic ovaries: endocrine changes and clinical outcome. Fertil Steril 1990; 53:45–49.

53. Personal communication. Intraovarian regulations and polycystic ovarian syndrome: recent progress on clinical and therapeutic aspects. Athens, Greece, 1992.

54. Wiegerinck MAHM. Early pregnancy loss in chronic hyperandrogenic anovulation. In: Coelingh Bennink HJT, Vemer HM, van Keep PA, editors. Chronic Hyperandrogenic Anovulation. Carnforth, UK: The Parthenon Publishing Group Ltd, 1991:169–174.

55. Stanger JD, Yovich JL. Reduced in-vitro fertilization of human oocytes from patients with raised basal luteinizing hormone levels during the follicular phase. Br J Obstet Gynaecol 1985; 92:385–393.

56. Howles CM, Macnamee MC, Edwards RG, et al. Effect of high tonic levels of luteinising hormone on outcome of in-vitro fertilisation. Lancet 1986; 2:521–522.

57. Homburg R, Armar NA, Eshel A, et al. Influence of serum luteinizing hormone concentrations on ovulation, conception, and early pregnancy loss in polycystic ovary syndrome. BMJ 1988; 297:1024–1026.

58. Punnonen R, Ashorn R, Vilja P, et al. Spontaneous luteinizing hormone surge and cleavage of in vitro fertilized embryos. Fertil Steril 1988; 49:479–482.

59. Watson H, Hamilton-Fairley D, Kiddy D, et al. Abnormalities of follicular phase LH secretion in women with recurrent early miscarriage (abstr. no. 25). J Endocrinol 1989;123(suppl).

60. Regan L, Owen EJ, Jacobs HS. Hypersecretion of luteinising hormone, infertility, and miscarriage. Lancet 1990; 336:1141–1144.

61. Shoham Z, Borenstein R, Lunenfeld B, Pariente C. Hormonal profiles following clomiphene citrate therapy in conception and nonconception cycles. Clin Endocrinol 1990; 33:271–278.

62. Fleming R. Induction of ovulation with GnRH analogs and gonadotropins in polycystic ovary syndrome. In: Coelingh Bennink HJT, Vemer HM, van Keep PA, editors. Chronic Hyperandrogenic Anovulation. Carnforth, UK: The Parthenon Publishing Group Ltd, 1991:109–116.

63. Johnson P, Pearce JM. Recurrent spontaneous abortion and polycystic ovarian disease: comparison of two regimens to induce ovulation. BMJ 1990; 300:154–156.

64. Homburg R. Personal communication. Intraovarian regulations and polycystic ovarian syndrome: recent progress on clinical and therapeutic aspects. Athens, Greece, 1992.

65. Urman B, Fluker MR, Yuen BH, et al. The outcome of in vitro fertilization and embryo transfer in women with polycystic ovary syndrome failing to conceive after ovulation induction with exogenous gonadotropins. Fertil Steril 1992; 57:1269–1273.

66. Bonney RC, Franks S. The endocrinology of implantation and early pregnancy. Baillieres Clin Endocrinol Metab 1990; 4:207–231.

67. Hamilton-Fairley D, Kiddy D, Watson H, et al. Association of moderate obesity with a poor pregnancy outcome in women with polycystic ovary syndrome treated with low dose gonadotrophin. Br J Obstet Gynaecol 1992; 99:128–131.

68. Kiddy DS, Hamilton-Fairley D, Seppala M, et al. Diet-induced changes in sex hormone binding globulin and free testosterone in women with normal or polycystic ovaries: correlation with serum insulin and insulin-like growth factor-1. Clin Endocrinol 1989; 31:757–763.

69. Evron S, Navot D, Laufer N, Diamant YZ. Induction of ovulation with combined human gonadotropins and dexamethasone in women with polycystic ovarian disease. Fertil Steril 1983; 40:183–186.

70. Blum I, Bruhis S, Kaufman H. Clinical evaluation of the effects of combined treatment with bromocriptine and spironolactone in two women with the polycystic ovary syndrome. Fertil Steril 1981; 35:629–633.

71. Shoham Z, Conway GS, Patel A, Jacobs HS. Polycystic ovaries in patients with hypogonadotropic hypogonadism: similarity of ovarian response to gonadotropin stimulation in patients with polcystic ovarian syndrome. Fertil Steril 1992; 58:37–45.

72. Filicori M, Flamigni C, Campaniello E, et al. The abnormal response of polycystic ovarian disease patients to exogenous pulsatile gonadotropin-releasing hormone: characterization and management. J Clin Endocrinol Metab 1989; 69:825–831.

73. Spritzer P, Billaud L, Thalabard J-C, et al. Cyproterone acetate versus hydrocortisone treatment in late-onset adrenal hyperplasia. J Clin Endocrinol Metab 1990; 70:642–646.

74. Burstein S, Turkington E, Rosenfield RL. Elevated progesterone (P) in congenital adrenal hyperplasia (CAH) alters LH secretory dynamics (abstr. no. 336). Presented at the 7th International Congress of Endocrinology, Quebec, 1984.

CHAPTER 17

Luteal Phase Deficiency: A Subtle Abnormality of Ovulation

MICHAEL R. SOULES

Luteal dysfunction refers to a clinical disease entity in women when there is a recurrent deficiency in the secretion or effect of progesterone (P) that is thought to be a direct cause of infertility and recurrent miscarriage. In the medical literature, this entity has many synonyms, such as *luteal phase dysfunction* and *corpus luteum inadequacy*. It may appear that these names refer to variations of pathophysiology, but they all refer to the same ubiquitous entity. In this chapter, it is referred to as *luteal phase deficiency* (LPD).

There are few diseases that are new; most are merely newly discovered. LPD fits into the latter category because it was first described in 1949.[1] This study by Jones at Johns Hopkins Medical Center in Baltimore included 255 menstrual cycles in 98 women with endocrine infertility (tubal obstruction and male factor had been excluded). Each subject was evaluated with basal body temperature (BBT) charts, a 48-hour midluteal urinary pregnanediol measurement, and a premenstrual endometrial biopsy. Evaluation of the BBT charts found that 13% of the cycles demonstrated inadequate luteal function (short luteal duration or poor temperature rise, or both). The pregnanediol measurements found that 34.3% of the cycles were luteal phase deficient, whereas the endometrial biopsy samples were considered ovulatory but abnormal in 50% of the cycles. (Although the three methods showed these discrepancies in identifying LPD, they agreed within 2% in identifying ovulatory versus nonovulatory cycles.) Jones concluded that the BBT chart was the most sensitive indicator of ovulation and that an endometrial biopsy was the most quantitative test of corpus luteum (CL) function. This study proposed the endometrial biopsy as the standard for the diagnosis of LPD; however, some questions remain regarding the conclusions of this study.[1] It is improper to assume that the diagnostic method that yields the highest prevalence (endometrial biopsy) is a priori the most accurate. Some other problems with the first clinical description of LPD were (1) the criteria for normal control subjects were not presented; (2) it is uncertain whether the control women were subjected to all three diagnostic tests; and (3) the endo-

metrial biopsies were quantified only as being nonsecretory, interval, or premenstrual. Nevertheless, this original description of LPD is a classic article, and Jones deserves much credit for the recognition of this disease entity.

Luteal dysfunction is a general concept that refers to endocrine abnormalities in the latter part of the menstrual cycle. These abnormalities may consist of alterations in hormonal secretion from the CL or defects in hormonal action. There are a number of hormones secreted by the CL in the luteal phase, including P, estradiol, 17-OH P, relaxin, and inhibin. In terms of physiologic and clinical relevance, the focus has been on P secretion and effect. In most women with true or alleged luteal dysfunction, the primary problem is inadequate quantity or duration of P secretion. A few cases of luteal dysfunction are problems of P effect, primarily on the endometrium. There is a case report of absent P receptors in the endometrium and a confusing complex of several studies that have reported both increases and decreases in endometrial steroid receptors in women with luteal dysfunction.[2–5] An established cause of inadequate P effect on the endometrium is inflammation secondary to endometritis (i.e., *Chlamydia* infection). For current practical clinical purposes, LPD should be considered a disease of decreased P secretion from the CL. There are no interpretable tests or clinical treatments for decreased P effect in current clinical practice except for the obvious treatment of endometritis with antibiotics.

NORMAL CORPUS LUTEUM PHYSIOLOGY

The CL is a complex and fascinating segment of the ovary. Even though most scientific and clinical attention has been focused on ovarian follicular development and function, the CL is also of critical importance to normal menstrual function and conception. Actually, the follicle is the precursor to the CL: (1) interference with follicular development leads to abnormal CL function; (2) granulosa cells become luteinized

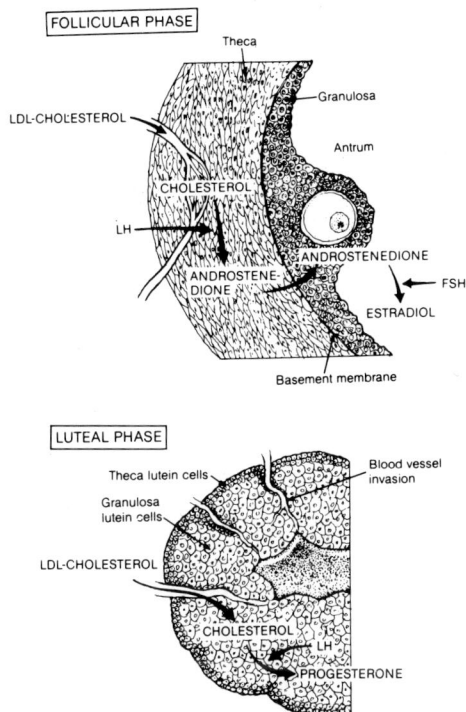

FIGURE 17–1. In the follicular phase, a basement membrane separates the theca layer from the granulosa layer. After ovulation, the basement membrane breaks down, and angiogenesis occurs. Therefore, in the luteal phase cholesterol can be delivered directly to the luteinized cells. (From Carr BR, MacDonald PC, Simpson ER. The role of lipoproteins in the regulation of progesterone secretion by the human corpus luteum. Fertil Steril 1982;38:303–311. Reproduced with permission of the publisher, The American Fertility Society.)

and become the so-called large cells of the CL; and (3) theca cells also become luteinized and become the so-called small cells of the CL. The CL forms after ovulation when the basement membrane between the theca and granulosa layers breaks down.[6] After basement membrane breakdown, angiogenesis occurs rapidly (over 2 to 4 days), thereby allowing the direct vascular delivery of cholesterol (via circulating low-density lipoprotein) to luteinized cells that use cholesterol as the primary precursor for the formation of P (Fig. 17–1). The normal life span of the human CL in a nonconceptive cycle is 12 to 16 days. In the life span of the normal CL, an equilibrium evolves between luteotropic and luteolytic factors (Fig. 17–2). Initially, luteotropic factors (i.e., luteinizing hormone [LH]) are dominant; later, luteolytic factors (i.e., prostaglandins) become dominant. The presence of human chorionic gonadotropin (hCG) (due to pregnancy or after exogenous administration) temporarily overrides luteolysis and gives the CL an extension on its life span. The principal secretory products from the CL are P, estradiol, inhibin, and relaxin. The steroids P and estradiol have as their primary function the maturation of the endometrium to enhance nidation. The possible primary role of inhibin is to suppress follicle-stimulating hormone (FSH) and folliculogenesis during the early and midluteal phases, but steroids are also necessary for this endocrine function. However, the primary role of inhibin in relation to the CL may be as a paracrine growth factor. Relaxin has no known role in the luteal phase; rather, its secretion is pertinent after conception and throughout pregnancy.

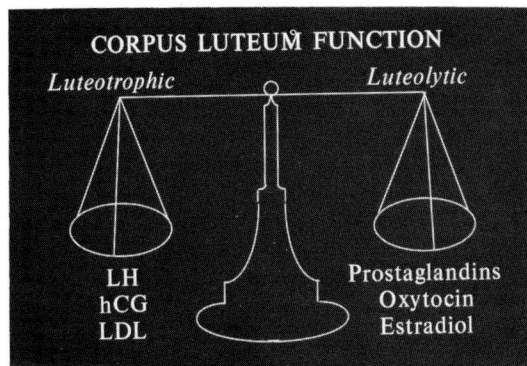

FIGURE 17–2. Corpus luteum function represents a balance between luteotropic and luteolytic factors.

P is the principal secretory product of the CL in terms of the clinical practice of reproductive medicine. P is secreted in a pulsatile pattern in synchrony with LH. The luteal phase pulsatile LH pattern determines the timing and quantity of P secretion by the CL (Fig. 17–3). If daily levels of P are determined, a bell-shaped curve is noted in normal cycling women with a rather sharp peak in the midluteal phase (Fig. 17–4). It is apparent on examination of the shape of this curve that certain quantitative thresholds that are used clinically for P are very dependent on the cycle day selected for sampling. In other words, a sample is valid only if it is obtained within a known interval.

Figure 17–4 illustrates the daily average P levels over the luteal phase for a group of normal women. This curve is presumed to be normal because the volunteers were selected for being normal women (aged 18 to 35 years) who had never experienced any infertility or pregnancy wastage. However, these P levels are from nonconceptive cycles and therefore have not been confirmed as physiologically normal. (Note that P levels in conceptive cycles are altered by hCG.) Considering the variation in the P curve in Figure 17–4, as represented by the shaded area indicating two standard de-

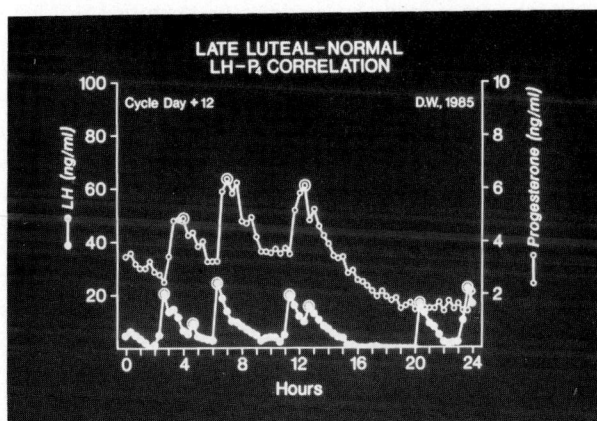

FIGURE 17–3. The simultaneous pulsatile luteinizing hormone (LH) and pulsatile progesterone levels are illustrated over 24 hours in the late luteal phase of a normal woman's cycle. The points on the LH and progesterone secretion curves that have been identified as indicating secretory events (pulses) are indicated by a circle around that data point. It can be appreciated that there is a progesterone secretory event (pulse) following most, but not all, of the LH secretory events.

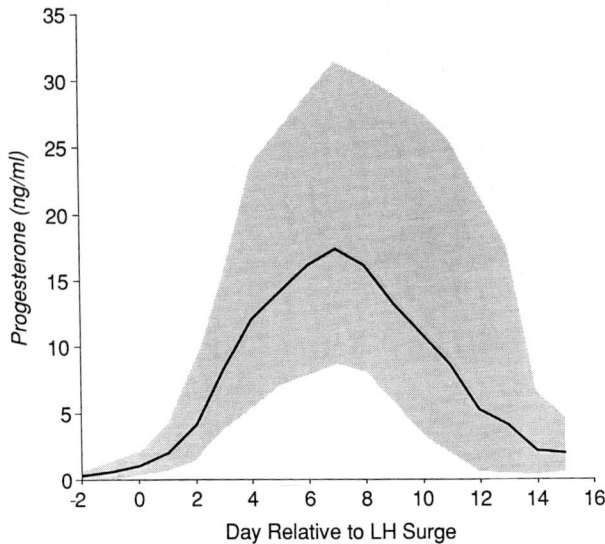

FIGURE 17–4. The average daily progesterone levels for 15 normal women are indicated by the *solid line* over the duration of a 14-day luteal phase. The *shaded area* represents plus or minus 2 SDs from this average curve. Day 0 is the day of the luteinizing hormone (LH) surge.

viations, a moderate amount of variation is noted. This variation among normal women is caused primarily by pulsatile secretion and biologic variation among normal volunteers; minor causes for the variation are the circadian rhythm in P secretion and assay variation.[7] From inspecting this normal curve, it can be appreciated that the lower limit of normal P in the midluteal phase is 8 to 10 ng/mL. When the area under the curve for an entire luteal phase is calculated for research purposes, the lower limit of normal for integrated P is 80 to 100 ng/mL/day.

A CONTROVERSIAL DIAGNOSIS: DOES LUTEAL PHASE DEFICIENCY REALLY EXIST?

For the purposes of this section, the definition of LPD is decreased P secretion over the luteal phase as determined by daily serum P levels. Using this method to define LPD (which is practical only in a research setting), an investigator determines P secretion over the entire secretory phase of the menstrual cycle. This definition is considered quite valid and is generally accepted as indicating an endocrine deficiency in the CL. A number of studies that approach the question of CL deficiency in different settings are examined for the purpose of gaining a perspective on this controversial entity. Note that these settings are descriptions of LPD in women who were not experiencing infertility or recurrent miscarriage. By and large, the women in these studies were not currently testing their fertility potential.

Subnormal luteal phase serum P levels were reported in rhesus monkeys in 1976.[8] Low P secretion was discovered in a subgroup of these animals (n = 5) when a group of mature rhesus monkeys that had normal cycle duration were studied. The P levels in this subgroup were significantly less than in the other monkeys over the duration of their respective luteal phases. This finding in rhesus monkeys is similar to a

description of a subgroup of normal women who had low P and short luteal phases as described by Sherman and associates.[9] Therefore, in both women and in female monkeys, a significant minority had spontaneous menstrual cycles with significant decreases in luteal phase P levels. The persistence of LPD in subsequent cycles was not addressed in these studies. In these instances, LPD was noted to occur spontaneously.

Other studies have focused on the occurrence of LPD in normal women under certain physiologic and social circumstances. LPD as demonstrated by low daily P levels has been noted to be more frequent in women as normal reproductive function is initiated and declines.[10] Immediately after the menarche, when most girls go through a period with anovulation, it is common for the first few ovulatory cycles to be associated with low P levels. Also, as women approach menopause, they are more likely to experience variations in their menstrual cycles, and one of these variations is LPD. Even the occurrence of postpartum resumption of menstrual cyclicity is associated with a high prevalence of LPD. Gray and coworkers[11] studied 22 postpartum, non–breast-feeding women as they resumed menstrual cyclicity. They reported that during their first ovulatory cycles, 73% had abnormally low luteal phase pregnanediol secretion.[11] In the second and subsequent cycles, there was a progressive increase in luteal pregnanediol secretion until most resumed normal function.[11] These series of studies would indicate that as menstrual cyclicity is starting or ending under normal age or physiologic circumstances, LPD is a common occurrence.

Another situation in which LPD is thought to be common is in association with the physical stress of exercise. A number of studies have reported low P levels in the luteal phase of otherwise normal women undergoing moderate to high levels of exercise. The first several studies that mentioned this problem were cross-sectional studies in which luteal phase length was noted to be short or there were low midluteal P levels in exercising women compared with sedentary control subjects.[12–14] A subsequent study noted that most normal women who undertook a demanding exercise program had degeneration of their cycles proceeding from normal to LPD to amenorrheic cycles.[15] In 1989, Loucks and colleagues[16] reported that 3 of 9 athletic women had low luteal phase pregnanediol levels compared with control subjects. Prior and associates[17] reported that 16 of 32 ovulatory cycles in women who were training for marathons had shortening of the luteal phase. Another social circumstance that has been associated with LPD is weight changes and dieting. Pirke and coworkers[18] performed a number of studies on dieting and weight restriction in regard to menstrual function. Most healthy women of normal weight who were subjected to a 1000-calorie diet over a menstrual cycle had LPD.[18] Those who received their calories from a vegetarian diet were more prone to LPD. Furthermore, when 22 healthy women were studied based on their questionnaire scores regarding cognitive dietary restraint, those who were classified as restrained eaters demonstrated LPD.[19] Note that these women were of normal weight and without any recognized eating disorders such as anorexia nervosa and bulimia. It appears that rather subtle changes in lifestyle can be associated with subtle but real disturbances of the menstrual cycle, such as LPD (Fig. 17–5).

Another approach to the existence of LPD would be epi-

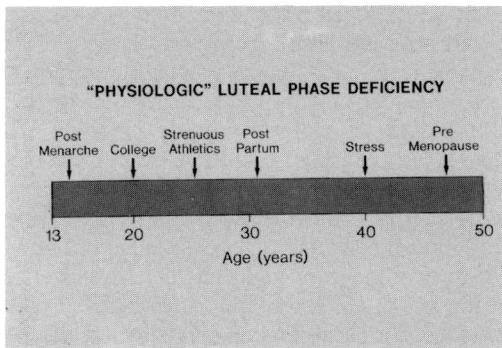

FIGURE 17–5. Luteal phase deficiency (LPD) can occur sporadically throughout the reproductive life span of a normal woman. This figure illustrates some common occurrences that have been shown to be associated with LPD. For instance, when the menstrual cycle is either maturing or aging, intermittent LPD cycles are more common, such as during the postmenarchal and premenopausal periods. Both physical (e.g., athletic) and psychosocial (e.g., occupational) stress has also been associated with intermittent LPD. Most of the time when LPD occurs in association with such life events, there are no clinical sequelae unless the woman is attempting to conceive.

demiologic studies that assess the prevalence of LPD in a defined population. There has been a paucity of such studies, in general, especially studies that have used strict criteria for the diagnosis of LPD. In 1984, Lenton and colleagues[10] published a report in which they studied 335 ovulatory cycles from women aged 18 to 50 years. This study focused on luteal phase length as determined by daily blood samples, which accurately identified the day of the LH surge. They found that 5.2% of the population has short luteal phases that were 9 days or less. They also reported a significant increase in short luteal phases in younger women (aged 10 to 24 years) and older women (aged 45 to 50 years). Although P levels were not reported, there is a strong presumption that these short luteal phases would be associated with low integrated P levels. In 1991, Li and associates[20] reported the prevalence of LPD in various types of infertility, including a control group of 68 women with normal fertility. The diagnosis of LPD in this study was defined as an endometrial biopsy specimen greater than 2 days retarded when dated according to the midcycle LH surge. They reported a 4.4% prevalence of LPD in normal fertile women and 2.9% in those with tubal infertility, whereas couples with unexplained infertility had a 21% prevalence of LPD. Another study examined the prevalence of LPD in five regularly menstruating women of proven fertility by endometrial biopsies that were considered out of phase when the lag was 3 or more days.[21] These five women underwent sequential biopsies in consecutive cycles. It was reported that the incidence of single and sequential out-of-phase endometrial biopsies was 31% and 7% in this group of women.

The prevalence of LPD in older women in the fifth decade who remain ovulatory has become controversial. As originally reported by Sherman and coworkers in 1976,[9] it appeared that older women tended to have lower levels of P and a higher incidence of LPD. Later studies, notably those of Lee[22] and Metcalf and colleagues,[23] examined this question of LPD in older women in more detail and found no increased prevalence of LPD as determined by daily P levels and urinary pregnanediol.

Another set of studies that support the existence of LPD are those that induced low postovulatory P levels by interference with follicular development. Stouffer and Hodgen[24] first reported inadequate development of the CL in monkeys as determined by weight and stimulated P production in vitro in animals treated in the follicular phase with follicular fluid. This follicular fluid treatment temporarily suppressed follicular development. Subsequent studies examined the effects of interference with follicular development in women. A gonadotropin-releasing hormone (GnRH) agonist administered for 3 successive days in the early follicular phase of normal cycling women induced a shortened luteal phase with significantly decreased levels of P.[25] Returning to the monkey model, DiZerega and Hodgen[26] demonstrated that exogenous gonadotropin treatment in monkeys with suppressed folliculogenesis would prevent the occurrence of LPD.

Another set of experiments that studied LPD by daily P levels are those that examined gonadotropin support of the CL. At one time, it was unclear whether the CL was dependent on LH for P secretion, but various studies have demonstrated that LH secretion is necessary and vital for CL function. For instance, in 1985, Hutchison and Zeleznik[27] reported that rhesus monkeys who had received lesions in their arcuate nucleus were entirely dependent on exogenous GnRH for CL function. The CL could be turned off and on with the intermittent pulsatile secretion of GnRH. This physiologic concept was confirmed when it was reported that a GnRH antagonist administered in the luteal phase was capable of acutely decreasing P secretion and causing luteolysis.[28] Besides P, a subsequent study using a GnRH antagonist demonstrated that both P and inhibin secretion were decreased when LH secretion was acutely suppressed.[29] When LH was suppressed with RU486, this induced luteolysis as well.[30] In these settings, induced luteolysis is essentially LPD in that there are significant decreases in integrated P levels.

Another way to approach the question regarding the existence and relevance of LPD is to examine studies that relate to other aspects of CL function. A series of studies by Daly and colleagues[31] reported on the production of prolactin by explants of late secretory endometrium in an in vitro culture system. They discovered that the production of prolactin by these explants correlated with the degree of histologic decidualization of both normal and LPD endometria.[31] Those women with LPD, as diagnosed by endometrial biopsy, were noted to have normal in vitro prolactin secretion based on the histologic but not the menstrual dates. This defect in in vitro prolactin secretion was corrected when LPD was treated.[32] These data document an end organ defect in LPD women and thereby further substantiate LPD as a significant entity. Noting that the CL produces hormones other than P, it is pertinent to examine whether other CL hormones are deficient in spontaneous or induced LPD. Certainly, in induced LPD (GnRH antagonist–induced luteolysis), other CL hormones (estradiol and inhibin) have been demonstrated to be acutely suppressed.[29] In spontaneous LPD in infertile women, Soules and coworkers[33] have demonstrated decreased inhibin and estradiol levels in association with decreased integrated P levels. Relaxin has been reported to be decreased along with P levels in spontaneous LPD. Therefore, in terms of physiologic significance, LPD is primarily a problem of decreased P levels, but physiologically this deficiency appears to involve all hormones known to be secreted by the CL.

The studies described in this section certainly document that LPD exists as a biologic phenomenon. In certain populations at particular ages and under particular treatments and conditions, decreased P levels in the luteal phase clearly occur. Therefore, the correct question is not "Does LPD really exist?" because it has clearly been shown to be present in certain research settings. Most of the research studies described have used daily P levels as their criteria for LPD, and therefore the presence of LPD has been clearly established in these instances. The more relevant question in regard to LPD is to inquire whether it exists in a clinical setting to the degree that it poses a health problem for reproductive-age women. The primary clinical problems that have been ascribed to LPD are infertility and recurrent miscarriage. It is clear that deficient CL function has the potential to prevent or disrupt a pregnancy. What is not clear from the medical literature is the prevalence of LPD among infertile women or those experiencing recurrent miscarriage. At one extreme, LPD could be viewed as a variation of the menstrual cycle wherein women intermittently have cycles demonstrating low P and other hormone secretion in the luteal phase that rarely, if ever, persists. If LPD occurs in this sporadic and inconsistent manner, then it has minor importance as a disease entity. At the other extreme, LPD could be viewed as a common problem in reproductive medicine that is frequently overlooked and underdiagnosed. If it is truly quite prevalent among different populations of women and potentially caused by a number of factors, it may occur to an extent that makes it a relatively common cause of infertility and miscarriage. It would be necessary to have a sensitive and specific test for LPD that would be practical in the clinical setting to reliably discern the true status of LPD in clinical reproductive medicine. Such a test does not currently exist. Considering all the evidence, a current consensus in reproductive medicine is that LPD is a relatively uncommon but significant cause of infertility and recurrent pregnancy loss. It is estimated that 5% to 10% of women in a referral reproductive medical practice experience LPD in most, if not all, of their menstrual cycles. Studies have been published that indicate the prevalence of LPD may be 30% to 60% in an infertile population. Some of these studies examined only one menstrual cycle in the population under study.[34–36] Altogether, these studies with a high prevalence appear to be flawed and are grossly overestimating the prevalence. It appears that LPD is overlooked and underdiagnosed in many gynecologic practices. In other practice settings, it appears to be overdiagnosed. The current recommendation is to remain aware of LPD as a potential cause of infertility or recurrent miscarriage in a given patient. Whether single or multiple tests are used for the diagnosis of LPD, these tests should be applied as rigorously as possible and within more than one menstrual cycle in a given patient.

PATHOPHYSIOLOGY OF LUTEAL PHASE DEFICIENCY

LPD is a heterogeneous disease that has been found in both the research and clinical settings. The final common pathway is an inadequate quantity or duration (or both) of P secretion. Although many factors have been found to be associated with LPD in some women (e.g., altered gonadotro-pin ratio in the follicular phase, small-size preovulatory follicle, elevated prolactin level), few studies have addressed the pathophysiology of LPD. There may be a single common pathway for inadequate P secretion by the CL, or there may be multiple pathophysiologic pathways. Pathophysiologic mechanisms may be extrinsic to the CL, such as support by gonadotropic hormones, or the abnormality may be intrinsic to the CL, such as inadequate LH-hCG receptor concentrations in the luteal cells themselves. CL function represents a balance between luteotropic and luteolytic factors that compete during a normal luteal phase. LPD may result from inadequate luteotropic factors or excessive luteolytic factors. Treatment studies do not appropriately address the question of the pathophysiology of LPD because increased P levels and possibly pregnancy that result from treatment do not necessarily indicate that the therapeutic intervention specifically addressed the physiologic abnormality. For instance, P supplementation simply corrects the hormone deficit and does not change endogenous CL function.

In some diseases in reproductive medicine, there is a well-defined pool of patients available for study (e.g., polycystic ovary disease). Comparatively speaking, LPD is difficult to study because there are relatively few patients with persistent spontaneous LPD available for pathophysiologic studies. Hypothalamic-pituitary-ovarian function in each menstrual cycle is a dynamic and ongoing process; just because LPD was present in a previous cycle does not mean that it is present in the current cycle under study. Studies on the pathophysiology of LPD are significantly more relevant if it was documented that LPD occurred in the cycle under investigation. As noted, the diagnostic methodology for LPD is controversial. To be considered seriously, a study that investigates the pathophysiology of LPD should have as strong a diagnosis of LPD as possible (which usually means low integrated levels of P over the extent of the luteal phase). Considering all of these difficulties, there have been few studies that have addressed the pathophysiology of LPD. The remainder of this section discusses two pathophysiologic concepts in regard to LPD. The first concept examines the pathophysiology of LPD from the perspective of exogenous CL control mechanisms, such as LH. The second concept explores the pathophysiology of LPD from an endogenous (paracrine, autocrine) perspective.

There are good indications that interference with folliculogenesis can lead to LPD. It makes intuitive sense if the precursor to the CL does not form normally that the CL itself will not be able to function adequately. Several studies have reported abnormal FSH levels in women with LPD.[37–39] These studies found either low absolute FSH levels or low FSH:LH ratios in daily samples from women who subsequently demonstrated either low P levels or out-of-phase endometrial biopsies. When Soules and coworkers[33] reported on daily reproductive hormone levels in 10 women with LPD (out-of-phase endometrial biopsy and low integrated P levels), however, they found no evidence of inadequate follicular development. They also found no abnormalities in follicular phase levels of immunoactive or bioactive FSH, in follicular phase duration, in peak or integrated follicular phase estradiol levels, or in ultrasound-determined follicle size (Figs. 17–6 and 17–7). In the same group of women studied by this investigative team, they performed frequent sampling studies with samples obtained every 10 minutes to determine the pulsatile

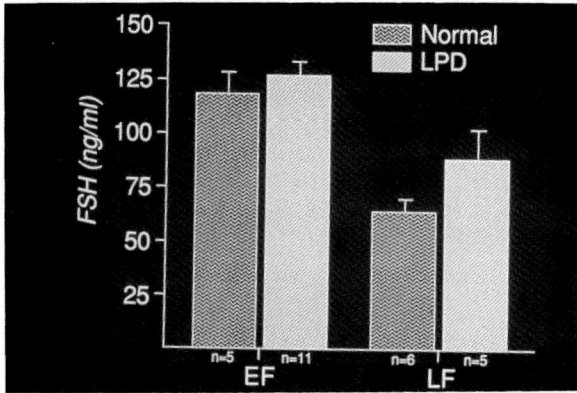

FIGURE 17–6. The mean follicle-stimulating hormone (FSH) level was calculated for both normal women and women with luteal phase deficiency (LPD) during an admission when frequent blood samples were obtained every 10 minutes over 12 hours. There were no differences in the mean FSH level between normal women and those with LPD in either the early (EF) or late (LF) follicular phases of their cycles.

ing of the LH secretion pattern in the luteal phase is the result of P feedback on the GnRH pulse generator, which is mediated by endogenous opioid peptides.[41] P secretion by the CL is pulsatile as well and has been shown to be coupled with LH pulses in the midluteal and late luteal phases.[42] LH appears to be required in both a permissive and a quantitative manner for normal P secretion by the CL.[42] Significant abnormalities in the hypothalamic-pituitary-ovarian axis in women with LPD have been reported by the research team of Soules and coworkers.[33, 40] These subjects had an increased LH pulse frequency in the early follicular phase, decreased mean LH levels during the LH surge, decreased bioactive LH levels in the midluteal and late luteal phases, and decreased P pulse amplitude in the luteal phase, accounting for their low integrated P levels.[40] In addition, these women also had low integrated estradiol and inhibin levels in the luteal phase. Their LH pulse frequency was significantly higher in the early follicular phase (12.8 versus 8.2 pulses per 12 hours), but there was no difference in LH pulse frequency between LPD and normal women in the late follicular phase (Fig. 17–8).[40] Therefore, women with LPD appeared to have a rapid LH secretion pattern throughout the follicular phase. In a separate study, LPD was induced in normal women by causing a supraphysiologic LH pulse frequency during the follicular phase.[43] This supraphysiologic frequency was induced with

pattern of LH.[40] As part of these studies, they determined the mean serum FSH levels over 12 hours in both the early and late follicular phases. No difference in mean FSH levels between normal women and those with LPD was found. Therefore, although it is accepted that impaired folliculogenesis is likely to lead to LPD, inadequate follicular development does not appear to be a common cause of spontaneous LPD. Other clinical studies continue to report a few patients diagnosed with LPD as having small follicle size before ovulation. (If small follicle size was documented in two or more luteal-deficient cycles, inadequate follicular development could well be the cause in that particular patient, and ovulation induction would be a reasonable therapy.)

There is a complex relationship between the hypothalamic-pituitary unit and the CL in women. A well-described shift in LH pulse frequency and amplitude occurs from the follicular to the luteal phase, with fewer LH pulses of higher amplitude present in the second half of the cycle. This slow-

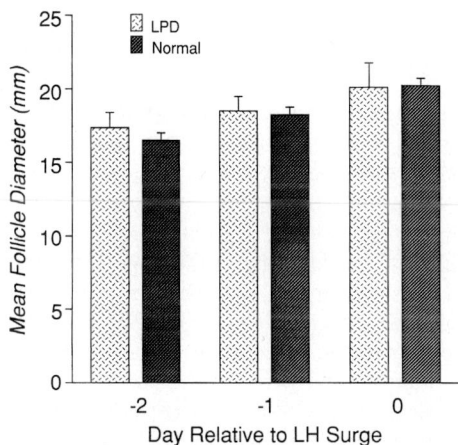

FIGURE 17–7. Leading up to ovulation, the mean follicle diameter was determined for both normal women and women with luteal phase deficiency (LPD). The maximum mean follicle size was approximately 20 mm and occurred on the day 0—the day prior to follicle disappearance (ovulation). There was no difference in follicle size between the two groups of women. LH, luteinizing hormone.

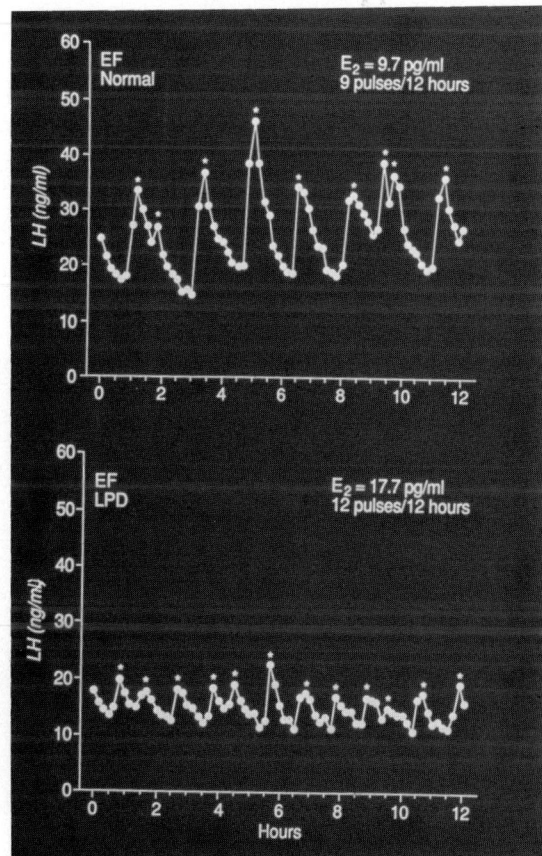

FIGURE 17–8. A 12-hour luteinizing hormone (LH) secretory pattern is illustrated for a normal woman (top graph) and a woman with luteal phase deficiency (LPD) (bottom graph). Increases in LH that were determined to be secretory events (pulses) are indicated by an asterisk. Note that the LH secretory pattern in the woman with LPD is more rapid, and the LH pulses are of lower amplitude.

intravenous GnRH administered every 30 minutes at a dose of 25 ng/kg. With this rapid pulse pattern, most of the volunteers developed two or more follicles and supraphysiologic preovulatory estradiol levels. After a spontaneous LH surge followed by ovulation and removal of the GnRH pump, however, these women had an average luteal-phase length of 9 days and a significant decrease in their integrated luteal P levels (152 ng/mL/day versus 66 ng/mL/day) in cycle 1 versus cycle 2 (Fig. 17–9). Therefore, the rapid early follicular LH pulse pattern appeared to be a key element in the pathogenesis of LPD because it was found to occur spontaneously in women with LPD and could be induced in normal women with LPD as the result. Other investigators have found abnormalities (both rapid and slow) in early follicular LH pulse frequency in LPD as well. The report by Suh and Betz[44] on 14 infertile women with LPD noted a significant increase in the early follicular phase LH pulse frequency. Schweiger and associates[45] studied a different group of patients—relatively younger women whose LPD appeared to be related to exercise or dieting, or both. The study by Loucks and colleagues[16] also found abnormal (slower) LH pulse frequency in the follicular phase in athletes with short luteal phases and low P levels. Different methods of pulse analysis were used in these various studies. It is interesting that all groups found an abnormal gonadotropin secretion pattern in the same cycle phase—early follicular. Perhaps a change in either direction (fast or slow) in the LH secretion rate in the early part of the menstrual cycle can lead to LPD.

Previous isolated observations of some individual LPD cycles have noted what appeared to be an attenuated midcycle LH surge. In a study of 10 women with LPD, the midcycle LH surge was deficient in both LH immunoassays and bioassays.[33] For instance, the integrated immunoassay LH surge was 482 versus 672 ng/mL in normal subjects. Perhaps the preceding rapid follicular-phase LH secretion pattern evokes a relatively small LH surge, but there are no studies to support or refute this hypothesis. When women with LPD were

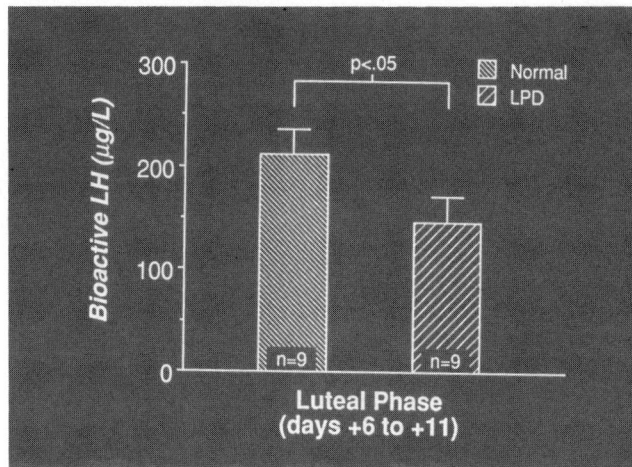

FIGURE 17–10. The bar graphs illustrate that the average daily levels of bioactive luteinizing hormone (LH) were lower over the latter part of the luteal phase in women with luteal phase deficiency (LPD).

studied in the luteal phase, no abnormalities in LH pulse secretion were found, but there were abnormalities in P secretion (decreased P pulse amplitude of 2.5 versus 5 ng/mL), and the mean serum P level was decreased (6.3 versus 13.8 ng/mL).[40] Approximately half of these women with LPD had coupling of their LH-P secretion patterns, which was similar to the degree of coupling that had been noted in normal women. Insufficient LH support of the CL was documented in these women with LPD. The daily LH immunoassay levels over the luteal phase were not different between women with LPD and normal women during the latter part of the luteal phase. On days +6 to +11, both the normal women and the women with LPD had daily LH immunoassay levels that bordered on the lower level of assay sensitivity.[33] When these same daily serum samples on days +6 to +11 were compared by LH bioassay, there was a significant decrease (146 versus 212 μg/L) in the LPD group compared with normal values (Fig. 17–10). Because low LH bioassay levels in the luteal phase were noted in the normal women in whom a supraphysiologic follicular phase LH pulse frequency had been induced,[43] it seemed reasonable to assume that the rapid follicular phase pulse pattern could lead to low luteal phase LH bioassay levels. In a subsequent study by Soules and coworkers,[46] the following hypothesis was entertained: Decreased P secretion in a given luteal phase could result in an excessively rapid gonadotropin pulse pattern in the subsequent follicular phase that, in turn, would lead to LPD in that and future cycles. This hypothesis takes into account the fact that luteal P levels suppress the hypothalamus and slow the GnRH pulse generator. If there were inadequate P levels in a given luteal phase, it was hypothesized that the GnRH pulse generator would be released sooner from this negative feedback influence and increase the pulse frequency sooner and perhaps to a greater degree than is found in a normal cycle. Therefore, a study was designed and performed in which LPD was induced in normal women with a GnRH antagonist (premature luteolysis), and the subsequent cycle was monitored in terms of the follicular LH secretion pattern and CL function.[46] LPD was induced in six normal women, with their integrated P levels decreasing from 137 to 81 ng/

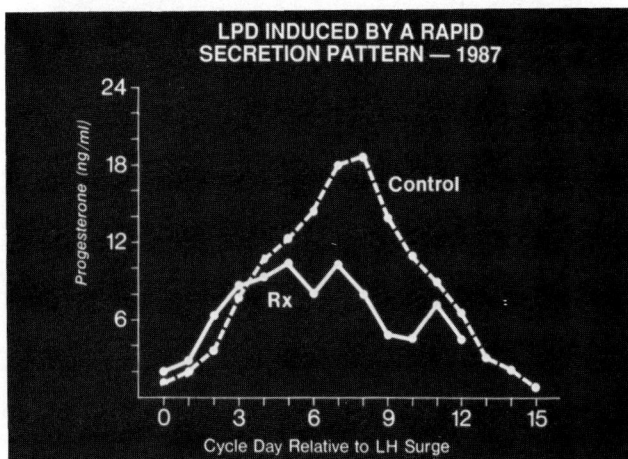

FIGURE 17–9. A control curve of progesterone levels comprised of mean daily levels is illustrated over the duration of a luteal phase in normal women. The curve indicated as *Rx* represents the daily progesterone levels after normal women were exposed to a superphysiologic (rapid) gonadotropin-releasing hormone stimulation rate in the preceding follicular phase. Note that the progesterone levels following an ultrarapid gonadotropin secretion pattern in the follicular phase are lower than normal and the luteal phase is shorter in length. LH, luteinizing hormone.

mL/day between the control and treatment cycles. The LH pulse pattern in the early follicular phase of the posttreatment cycle was indistinguishable from the control cycle in terms of LH pulse frequency, pulse amplitude, and mean LH level (Fig. 17–11). Further, the integrated P level in that posttreatment cycle was indistinguishable from the control cycle as well. Therefore, inducing LPD in one cycle did not perpetuate the problem into the subsequent cycles. Assuming that an altered follicular phase GnRH pulse generator is a key to understanding the pathophysiology of LPD, and realizing that this alteration does not appear to be secondary to P feedback effects, it is necessary to look at other modulators of the GnRH pulse generator to understand these phenomena. There are many examples of suprahypothalamic influences (neurotransmitters) on the GnRH pulse generator that have profound effects on the menstrual cycle. Conditions such as anorexia nervosa, bulimia, hypothalamic amenorrhea, heavy exercise, and dieting all have in common psychological or physical stress, abnormal gonadotropin secretion patterns, and menstrual dysfunction. It is postulated that LPD, as a mild and subtle cause of menstrual dysfunction, commonly occurs because of stress-induced alterations in the GnRH pulse generator, as mediated by neurotransmitters.

CLs of all mammalian species examined so far, including humans, consist of at least two different steroidogenic cell types: (1) the so-called small luteal cells, which are derived from follicular theca cells, and (2) the large luteal cells, which are derived from granulosa cells.[47] In the human CL, the large-cell subgroup is 20 to 30 μm in diameter and the small cell is considered to be 5 to 20 μm in diameter. Each cell type also has distinct ultrastructural characteristics. In humans, the large luteal cells have a homogeneous electron-lucent nuclear matrix, abundant smooth endoplasmic reticulum, extensive Golgi complexes, nonextractable lipid droplets, and prominent gap junctions. Large luteal cells are primarily responsible for the basal (LH independent) secre-

Cell Type	Progesterone	Estradiol	Androgens
Small (thecal)	–hCG ↑	—	–Basal –hCG ↑
Large (granulosa)	–Basal	–Basal –FSH ↑	—

FIGURE 17–12. Small luteal cells are derived from theca cells, and large luteal cells are derived from granulosa cells. It is the small luteal cells that are particularly responsive to human chorionic gonadotropin (hCG) in terms of progesterone secretion. The large luteal cells demonstrate a relatively greater level of basal progesterone secretion than the small cells. There also appear to be inherent differences in the cell types in terms of their ability to secrete estradiol and androgens. FSH, follicle-stimulating hormone. (Adapted from Ohara A, Mori T, Taii S, et al. Functional differentiation in steroidogenesis of two types of luteal cells isolated from mature human corpora lutea of menstrual cycle. J Clin Endocrinol Metab 1987;65:1192–1200; © The Endocrine Society.)

tion of P throughout the luteal phase. These large luteal cells were also identified as the primary source of estrogens.[48] When stimulated with hCG, small luteal cells responded with significant increases in P, androstenedione, and testosterone, but large cells did not. Therefore, in women, there are two distinct cell types in the human CL that can be distinguished both anatomically and functionally.

To generalize, it appears that large luteal cells secrete P at a constant level during the luteal phase, whereas small luteal cells add to the total amount of P secreted when there is an LH pulse or hCG is secreted (Fig. 17–12). Considering that LPD could occur from endogenous defects within the CL, there are a number of areas in which changes in this complex system could lead to deficient P secretion. Wuttke and associates[49] recently presented a preliminary report that describes three types of LPD. They studied 15 women with LPD as determined by serum levels of P being lower than 8 ng/mL on three occasions. The LH secretion pattern and corresponding P secretion pattern were studied in these women in the luteal phase. It was reported that 7 of the 15 women had depressed LH secretory episodes, with basal P levels at 5.6 ng/mL. These women were classified as having hypothalamic LPD secondary to inadequate LH secretion. Four of the 15 subjects had a normal luteal LH secretion pattern and demonstrated a normal increase in P secretion to an LH secretory episode but overall had low basal P levels of 6.2 ng/mL. This group of patients was classified as having large luteal cell defects in that their basal steady-state P secretion was deficient but their small cells could response to LH in a normal manner. Another 4 of the 15 patients had relatively low basal P levels of 3.1 ng/mL and a subnormal response in terms of P secretion to a normal number and amplitude of LH episodes. This last group was classified as having small luteal cell defects in that they did not display any LH response capability. It remains to be seen whether these findings are corroborated by other investigators.

Another concept in relation to the pathophysiology of LPD that considers the two functional cell types is a so-called two-phase model of luteal inadequacy.[50] This concept originates from the evaluation of endometrial histology from two endometrial biopsies performed in the same luteal phase. In a study of 85 women who had two endometrial biopsies in the same luteal phase, 32% (27 of 85) of midluteal endometrial biopsy specimens showed a deficiency in endometrial maturation. Of these 27 subjects, 14 (52%) had normal biopsies

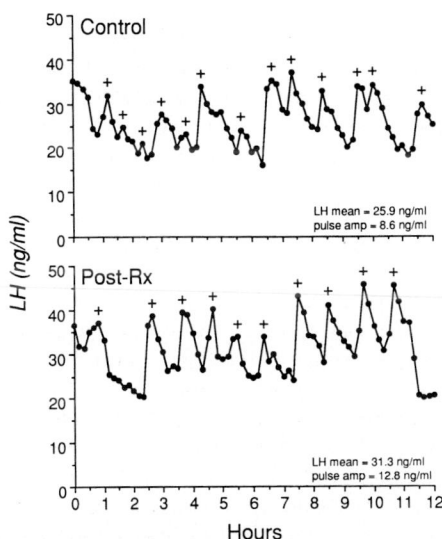

FIGURE 17–11. The luteinizing hormone (LH) secretion pattern over 12 hours is illustrated for a normal woman in the early follicular phase of a control cycle (upper panel) and the early follicular phase of a subsequent cycle that had been immediately preceded by luteolysis (lower panel). There were no changes in the LH secretion pattern in normal women following induced luteal phase deficiency.

when late luteal phase specimens were obtained. It would appear from these data that midluteal phase progesterone deficiency can be overcome by events that act to mature the endometrium, which is presumed to be increased P secretion. The early luteal to midluteal phase P deficiency causing a midluteal lag in endometrial development may be due to defects in large luteal cells. In some women, this type of LPD (large luteal cell derived) can be corrected when small luteal cells can respond appropriately to LH or hCG and make up the P deficiency.

Another set of in vitro experiments has been performed with intact CLs that take into account the different functional capabilities of the small and large cells. In a series of experiments in sow and human CLs, a research group has identified paracrine effects between large and small luteal cells that have relevance in the context of the pathophysiology of LPD.[51] These experiments in intact CLs have investigated the interaction between large and small cells as well as the differential effects of compounds known to modulate CL function. These compounds are primarily prostaglandin (PG) $F_2\alpha$ and oxytocin. Only the large luteal cells are believed to produce oxytocin, whereas the small luteal cells lack the capability of peptide production. In the young CL (early luteal and midluteal phases), the large and small cell types interact in a paracrine fashion with each other. Oxytocin released by large luteal cells reduces small luteal cell P release but increases estradiol release in both cell types. In the young CL, estrogens are strong luteotropic hormones that act primarily on small luteal cells to stimulate P production. Furthermore, PG $F_2\alpha$ also acts to increase estradiol production in small and large luteal cells. At the same time, PG $F_2\alpha$ reduces P release from both small and large cell types. The overall net effect, primarily from the increased intraluteal estradiol concentrations, is a stimulation of total CL P production. In the older CL, the stimulatory effects on estrogen by PG $F_2\alpha$ and oxytocin are diminished, and the direct suppressive effect on P secretion is dominant. This is a description of the physiology of luteolysis as seen by these investigators. Certainly, such a complex system could develop intrinsic abnormalities that would result in decreased P secretion and LPD. At this time, however, there is no evidence that LPD occurs in the clinical setting because of intrinsic abnormalities within the CL.

CLINICAL ISSUES

P is the principal secretory product of the CL in terms of physiologic reproductive relevance. Nidation and the maintenance of early pregnancy are dependent on P. The principal human study to demonstrate this dependence was published in 1972.[52] Women who were scheduled for therapeutic abortion underwent luteectomy between 7 and 9 weeks' gestation (menstrual age). Postluteectomy P levels were determined daily, and the status of the pregnancy was followed. At 7 weeks' gestation, the P levels fell and all aborted (n = 6); at 9 weeks, the P levels only transiently decreased and none aborted (n = 3). In a subsequent study, when serum P levels were maintained with exogenous P after luteectomy at 7 weeks' gestation, the subjects did not abort.[53] Although the placenta begins to produce P at about 5 weeks' gestation, it appears that the levels become sufficient to maintain pregnancy at 8 to 9 weeks.

The recent data from oocyte donation pregnancies (in vitro fertilization in women with ovarian failure) confirm the role of P and the timing of the shift from an ovarian to a placental source of P. Early pregnancy after oocyte donation can be maintained only with P and estradiol.[54-56] When serial serum P levels were followed in nine women who were receiving a fixed dose of exogenous P during early pregnancy after oocyte donation, there was a significant increase in P at the 7th week of gestation.[56] These data corroborate the luteectomy studies.

Considering what is known about P (that it is necessary for implantation in animal models and during early human pregnancy), the claim that an endogenous deficiency in P (LPD) is capable of causing infertility and spontaneous abortions seems reasonable. When a "new" disease is described,[1] studies generally follow that are designed to ascertain the most accurate diagnostic method(s) that are clinically relevant (i.e., cost effective, tolerable risk, limited pain). Treatment studies usually follow in which patients, in whom the disease in question has been clearly diagnosed, are randomized into treatment and control groups and the outcomes carefully examined. Since LPD was first described in 1949 until the present, neither of these standard validations have completely occurred for various and complex reasons. That LPD causes infertility and recurrent miscarriage by interfering with implantation remains a reasonable speculation that is still unproved.

Diagnostic Tests Not Completely Validated

As noted, several diagnostic tests were proposed in conjunction with the original description of LPD. In addition to BBT charts, a urinary pregnanediol determination, and an endometrial biopsy, a number of other diagnostic tests have been proposed and used for LPD: single and multiple serum P levels drawn in the luteal phase, measurement of salivary free P levels, plasma endometrial protein levels, assessment of preovulatory follicle size, endometrial thickness by ultrasound, assay of serum prolactin, and measurement of serum levels of proteins emanating from the CL (relaxin and inhibin). Each of these methods, when proposed, seemed reasonable because they were based on an understanding of the physiology of the CL. For true accuracy and clinical validity, however, each and every one of these diagnostic methods needed to be validated in a clinical population that was determined to have LPD by a recognized gold standard. When it comes to LPD, the absence of a recognized gold standard presents a major problem for both clinicians and researchers. The total quantity of P produced over the luteal phase in normal women is the logical gold standard. Such a gold standard needs to be validated by physiologic relevance—in this instance, the support of an ongoing and normal pregnancy. hCG emanating from the placenta, however, alters and changes the CL of the menstrual cycle and precludes the determination of normal P secretion in the luteal phase of a menstrual cycle in which conception occurs. Therefore, there has never been a gold standard for the diagnosis of LPD that is based on solid physiologic grounds. This gold standard problem has clouded most attempts in the medical literature to identify a clinically relevant diagnostic test for LPD. In general, what has occurred are attempts at validating one clinical diagnostic test by referring to another (earlier) diagnostic test (e.g., endometrial biopsy "validated by" BBT chart data) (Fig. 17–13). Currently, there are no completely validated diagnostic tests for LPD that are practical in the clinical setting. (In the research setting, an integrated luteal phase P level is considered to be a more valid gold standard, but it is not practical in the clinical setting.) Investigators who have studied LPD in the clinical setting have remained frustrated that there are no clearly established diagnostic tests that are both accurate and sensitive. Therefore, when treatment studies have been performed and reported, the results are always questionable because the diagnosis of the treated patients is questionable.

Lack of Proper Treatment Trials

Another aspect of the LPD validation problem is the lack of controlled treatment trials for LPD reported in the medical literature. Each newly described disease should be validated by altering or curing the disease in a treatment compared with a control group. Although various therapies have been used for LPD, only one small randomized trial in women who have been diagnosed with this problem has been published.[57] The absence of properly conducted clinical trials is common in the infertility literature because it is difficult to obtain patient consent to withhold therapy. When a couple understands that they may have a treatable problem (e.g., LPD) causing their infertility, they are reluctant to participate in a trial in which they may not receive any treatment (placebo). In the case of LPD, it is still important to pursue the validation of both the diagnostic methods and the treatment of this entity.

Current Clinical Consensus of Luteal Phase Deficiency

Considering the validation difficulties in LPD, it would be reasonable to question the status of this diagnosis in clinical

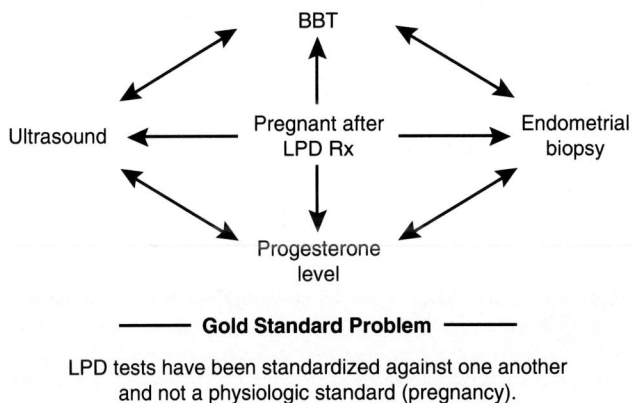

FIGURE 17–13. The various tests that have been promoted for use in the diagnosis of luteal phase deficiency (LPD) require validation. Examination of the pertinent medical literature reveals that these tests have been validated one against another and not against a gold standard. Other studies have attempted to validate these tests by pregnancies that occurred after treatment. A claim then arises that the diagnosis based on a particular test was correct if the patient achieved pregnancy. However, pregnancy may have occurred regardless and is not a valid claim for test validation. BBT, basal body temperature.

reproductive medicine. The clinical diagnosis, pathophysiology, treatment, and other aspects of LPD in the clinical setting were the subject of a recent symposium.[58] A brief summary follows here.

LPD in the clinical setting is believed to occur in 3% to 10% of infertile women who are evaluated in a referral (subspecialty) setting. Although normal women can have occasional cycles with inadequate P secretion, the infertile woman with LPD has inadequate P secretion in most, but not necessarily all, of her spontaneous menstrual cycles. This quantitative deficiency in the duration or quantity of P secretion is believed to preclude implantation in most instances but occasionally can transiently support a pregnancy before the deficiency leads to a spontaneous abortion. Therefore, most women with this problem appear to have normal ovulatory function, and many have been diagnosed as having unexplained infertility. The tests that are commonly used for the diagnosis of LPD in the clinical setting are late luteal phase endometrial biopsies dated according to the criteria of Noyes and colleagues[59] or P levels obtained in the midluteal phase.[60] These midluteal P determinations can be from single or several samples. There is a consensus that the diagnosis of LPD should be made in two or more cycles to preclude a false-positive diagnosis in normal ovulatory women who happen to have low P levels in the cycle in which the test was performed. Therefore, a modern infertility evaluation often includes a routine test for the diagnosis of LPD. If not performed as a routine diagnostic evaluation, tests for LPD should be performed in couples who appear to have unexplained infertility. Once a diagnosis of LPD has been made in two or more cycles, a presumption is made that LPD is present in most, if not all, of a particular woman's cycles.

DIAGNOSIS

Two primary approaches have been taken in evaluating the adequacy of P secretion in the luteal phase: (1) direct measurement of P levels, and (2) inferential assessment of P by a bioassay, an endometrial biopsy.

Direct measurement of P is theoretically most appealing because of its apparent simplicity. However, close examination reveals several difficulties. It appears that, like other hormones, P is secreted in a pulsatile manner correlating with the pulsatile secretion of LH (see Fig. 17–3).[61] Because the half-life of P is 20 to 30 minutes and the pulse frequency of LH in the luteal phase is between 2 and 3 1/2 hours, nearly all the P released with each pulse will have been cleared from circulation by the next pulse.[62, 63] Thus, single serum samples may not be representative of the average P concentration present in the circulation. At a minimum, multiple serum samples in a single day or over several days are required to always make a reliable diagnosis.[33, 61] In addition, as already noted, "normal" values in known fertile women have never been defined precisely in normal conceptive cycles, but statistical means have been used in attempts to separate normal fertile women from those with LPD. More recently, both urinary pregnanediol glucuronide[64] and salivary progesterone[65] levels have been used. Salivary progesterone levels also appear to be affected by the pulsatile release of progesterone,[66] and pregnanediol values overlap in normal fertile women and in infertile women with presumptive LPD.[64]

In some women with apparent LPD, peak serum P levels in the midluteal phase remain below 10 ng/mL. Several studies have reported that maximum luteal phase P levels are consistently above 10 ng/mL in menstrual cycles in which conception occurs.[67] A recent publication revisited the question regarding the efficacy of serum P levels for the diagnosis of LPD.[68] The standard for determining whether single or multiple serum P levels were accurate in identifying LPD was integrated P levels as calculated over the duration of the luteal phase. An integrated P level lower than 80 ng/mL/day was used as diagnostic of LPD and is supportable from the literature. A single serum P level lower than 10 ng/mL obtained between days 5 and 9 after the LH surge (midluteal) had a sensitivity of 86% for the diagnosis of LPD; if the sum of three serum P determinations obtained in the same interval was lower than 30 ng/mL, the sensitivity was 100%.

Because late luteal phase endometrial biopsy reflects the biologic action of P on the endometrium, it has been regarded as the gold standard for the diagnosis of LPD. As already noted, however, there is difficulty in histologically assessing the CL function. The correlation between endometrial histology and peak serum P levels is often poor.[69] The criteria as described originally by Noyes and coworkers[59] are subject to considerable differences in interpretation by different individuals[70] and may lead to a significant incidence of both false-positive and false-negative diagnoses. Although the requirement to document an abnormality in two separate cycles to establish the diagnosis of LPD will decrease the false-positive incidence, it may actually increase the false-negative rate.

It is clear that, in using biopsies to date endometrial samples, it is important to adhere to several strict guidelines, many originally proposed by Noyes and associates,[59] as follows:

1. Each sample must be obtained from the anterior fundal wall of the uterus. A sample obtained from the lower uterine segment is uninterpretable.
2. Ideally, biopsies should be obtained 11 to 13 days after ovulation (2 to 3 days prior to expected menses).
3. Specimens may be accurately evaluated in relation to either ovulation events or the subsequent menses.[71, 72]
4. A "lag" of 3 or more days should be considered abnormal.
5. A luteal phase of less than 11 days should be considered abnormal.
6. The diagnosis of LPD should be based on abnormal findings in at least two cycles.

The use of BBT charts to diagnose LPD is not recommended. Simply stated, the BBT charts are not reflective of any specific serum P level. A maximal increase in BBT may occur with as little as 3 ng/mL of P in serum.[73]

There is no clearly superior diagnostic test for LPD that is practical in the clinic setting at this time. It is recommended that the diagnosis of LPD be based on abnormal findings in at least two spontaneous cycles. Either of the following tests and criteria is recommended:

1. Serum P level(s): a single level lower than 10 ng/mL or the sum of three levels lower than 30 ng/mL obtained between days 5 and 9 after the LH surge. A determination of a urinary LH level is sufficient to identify the LH surge.

2. Endometrial biopsy: obtained in a proper manner from the uterine fundus, dated according to the criteria of Noyes and associates,[59] and found to be more than 2 days out of phase according to midcycle events or the next menstrual period.

RECOMMENDATIONS FOR TREATMENT

Recurrent Pregnancy Loss

Women with recurrent pregnancy loss and abnormal endometrial biopsies are the patients originally described as having LPD. Because pregnancies do occur in these women, it has been presumed that any defect must reside in P synthesis or in the response of the endometrium to P. A series of studies have suggested that the incidence of LPD in women with a history of recurrent pregnancy loss, as based on diagnoses established by endometrial biopsies, ranges from 23% to 40%.[74–78] Before initiating any therapy in such women, it is important to rule out thyroid, prolactin, or adrenal dysfunction, which may be found in 10% to 15% of affected patients. In uncontrolled trials, exogenous P has been reported to be successful in 80% to 91% of patients when the underlying endometrial defect, as documented by repeat biopsy, is corrected.[74, 75, 79] Furthermore, it is rare to identify a patient whose biopsy is not corrected by P therapy, even though a few patients appear to have P-resistant endometrium (Table 17–1).

Because none of these studies was conducted in a prospective, randomized manner, and because couples with two prior spontaneous abortions have a 60% or greater likelihood of having a normal child with their next pregnancy, it is a legitimate criticism that the efficacy of P therapy is unproved. The best data, though far from ideal, to refute this criticism may be in the report of Tho and colleagues.[74] Sixty patients with recurrent pregnancy losses were defined either as having LPD based on abnormal findings (n = 23) or as believed to be normal (n = 37). (The study predates immunologic evaluation of patients with recurrent pregnancy losses.) All 23 patients with LPD were administered P suppositories in the luteal phase. Of those 37 women considered normal, 15 received no treatment and the remaining 22 were treated empirically with both tetracycline and P suppositories in the luteal phase. Chi-square analysis of the results (not performed in the original article) reveals that the LPD group treated with P had a significantly higher rate of successful

TABLE 17–1. Progesterone Treatment of Luteal Phase Deficiency (LPD) in Patients with Recurrent Miscarriage					
Authors	LPD Patients	Treatment Biopsy	Corrected Biopsy	Pregnancy	Percentage Viable
Tho et al[74]	23	NA	NA	23	91
Wentz et al[77]	17	11	11	10†	80
Daya et al[79]	26	26	26*	16	81

*Two of three nontreatment pregnancies miscarried.
†A "few" patients required double dosage.
NA, not available.

TABLE 17–2. Progesterone Treatment in Luteal Phase Deficient (LPD) and Non-LPD Patients with Recurrent Miscarriage

Protocol	Pregnancy			
	Patients	Success	Miscarriage	Percentage
LPD/Prog supp	23*,†	21	2	91
Unknown—total	37*	23	14	62
Unknown—Tx	22†	16	6	73
Unknown—no Tx	15†	7	8	47

*Chi-square with Yates correction $\chi^2 = 4.66$ $df = 1$ $P < .05$.
†Chi-square with Yates correction $\chi^2 = 7.06$ $df = 2$ $P < .05$.
Prog supp, treatment with progesterone suppositories; Tx, treatment with progesterone suppositories and tetracycline.

Adapted from Tho PT, Byrd JR, McDonough PG. Etiologies and subsequent reproductive performance of 100 couples with recurrent abortion. Fertil Steril 1979;32:389–395. Reproduced with permission of the publisher, The American Fertility Society.

pregnancy than either of the "normal" groups (Table 17–2). The untreated "normal" women had the lowest pregnancy rate, raising the possibility that the empirically treated "normal" group may have contained some undiagnosed women with P deficiency.

Infertility

Most of the controversy in the treatment of infertility associated with LPD revolves directly or indirectly around whether exogenous P supplementation in the luteal phase or clomiphene citrate in the follicular phase is the therapy of choice. Other modalities, including FSH,[80] hCG,[81] and GnRH,[82] have been used as well, either as therapeutic trials to lend credence to a suggested cause of LPD or as a last line of treatment in couples with unexplained infertility. Although concern persists as to whether there is even any "defect" to treat based on the data published to date,[83] one recent report of the long-term followup of patients with subtle abnormalities diagnosed by endometrial biopsy indicated that those with abnormalities who are left untreated have a lower probability of pregnancies than those without abnormalities on biopsy.[84]

As is true for women with recurrent abortion and LPD, infertile women with suspected LPD should have thyroid dysfunction, hyperprolactinemia, and adrenal dysfunction excluded by measuring basal values of serum prolactin, thyroid-stimulating hormone (TSH), and dehydroepiandroster-

one sulfate in the early follicular phase. If an abnormality is found, definitive treatment should be instituted but should not be assumed to be adequate. Confirmation of correction of the defect is warranted if pregnancy does not occur promptly.

The initial use of P to correct infertility due to LPD was based on uncontrolled reports of success in a series of patients.[85, 86] Successful pregnancies have been reported in 47% to 80% of patients, with the mean of several uncontrolled series approaching 50% (Table 17–3).[77, 85–88] However, the lack of significant followup of these patients when they were not on progestational therapy adds further uncertainty to the efficacy of therapy.

Initial reports documenting the use of clomiphene citrate were even less convincing than for P supplementation. In one of these studies, 7 of 9 patients with a 2- to 3-day lag on endometrial biopsy who failed to conceive on clomiphene citrate responded to P supplementation with pregnancy.[89] Conversely, in one series of 8 patients with luteal phases of 10 days or less, 7 conceived in response to clomiphene.[90] In another larger series involving 25 patients, of the 12 patients found to have a 5-day or greater lag on endometrial biopsy, 9 conceived with clomiphene citrate[91]; yet in the 13 patients with a less dramatic lag of 3 to 4 days, only 1 conceived with clomiphene. One interpretation of the results with clomiphene is that the closer the dysfunctional ovulation is to anovulation, the more likely the patient is to respond to clomiphene. Moreover, in all of these studies, clomiphene citrate was administered on cycle days 5 to 9. In view of the present understanding of follicular recruitment and development, it may be more appropriate to administer the clomiphene citrate earlier in the menstrual cycle (e.g., on days 3 to 7).

Comparative and Sequential Studies

Two studies using exogenous P and clomiphene citrate are worthy of detailed discussion. Although not randomized prospective studies, they address critical issues pertaining to the adequacy and selection of therapy. Moreover, because both use life table analysis and calculate treatment fecundity, they diffuse much of the criticism leveled at other treatment studies. In a sequential study performed before the routine use of ultrasonography, Daly and colleagues[92] treated 33 women with LPD diagnosed by endometrial biopsy with P suppositories in the luteal phases of six consecutive menstrual cycles. The 17 patients whose biopsies normalized with therapy had

TABLE 17–3. Treatment of Luteal Phase Deficient (LPD) Patients with Infertility with Progesterone Suppositories

Authors	No. of Patients	No. of Viable Preg	No. of Viable Preg—Tx	No. of Viable Preg—no Tx	Percentage of Viable Preg
Wentz et al[77]	37	14	12	2	38
Jones and Pourmand[85]	16	12	12	0	80
Rosenberg et al[86]	13	7	7	0	54
Soules et al[87]	15	7	7	0	47
Katayama et al[88]	33	15	13	2	46
Total	116	55	51	4	47

Preg, pregnancy; Tx, treatment with progesterone suppositories.

normal fecundity, with 15 viable conceptions (Fig. 17–14A and B). In contrast, the 16 women whose biopsies remained uncorrected by P failed to have a single successful conception. These women with treatment failures were then treated for six cycles with clomiphene citrate, administered from days 5 to 9 of each cycle. If the endometrial biopsy was not corrected by the clomiphene, successful pregnancy did not occur. In total, 81% of patients successfully conceived, but clomiphene citrate appeared to be less effective because of the low biopsy correction rate. However, the patients who did not respond to P also may have been those most difficult to treat. In any event, if correction of the biopsy occurred, fecundity was normal.

Murray and associates[93] reported results of a comparative study in which patients with LPD received either vaginal P in the luteal phase or clomiphene citrate on days 2 to 6 of the cycle. Patients were continued on therapy if their endometrial biopsy was corrected. The fecundity of the patients approached normal, with 31 of 35 patients receiving P suppositories and 23 of 25 patients on clomiphene citrate conceiving (Fig. 17–15A and B). Correction of the biopsy findings correlated with pregnancy. In both studies, the fecundity of the successfully treated patients was improved statistically over that projected from life table analysis,[94] indicating a real effect of therapy provided.

Specific Recommendations

It is clear that it is important to exclude any underlying causes of LPD. In principle, this can be accomplished by measuring basal serum prolactin concentrations to rule out hyperprolactinemia and TSH to exclude primary hypothyroidism or hyperthyroidism. Known risk factors for LPD such as heavy exercise, dieting, and occupational stress should be identified and addressed.

The diagnosis of LPD should be made by either a midluteal serum P level(s) or by timed endometrial biopsy. Two abnormal cycles need to be demonstrated to establish a diagnosis.

In general, four different types of therapy have been recommended for patients with LPD. As already indicated, the ideal approach to therapy depends, insofar as possible, on identifying the specific cause and planning appropriate therapy. The use of bromocriptine for documented hyperprolactinemia in association with LPD is the prime example of therapy directed to a specific etiology. However, most women with LPD have normal prolactin levels. Therefore, it is usually a case of physician preference combined with patient choice that leads to the selection of either P supplementation or clomiphene citrate as the initial therapy for LPD. Occasionally, some additional information or factors that pertain to a particular patient will point toward clomiphene citrate being a better initial drug for LPD, as follows:

1. If a patient is oligo-ovulatory and has LPD, clomiphene would be the recommended first choice.
2. If a particular patient has undergone ultrasound or estradiol monitoring, or both, of ovulation for indications other than LPD and has been demonstrated to ovulate from a small follicle (<18 mm mean diameter) or achieved a preovulatory maximum serum estradiol of less than 200 pg/mL, then clo-

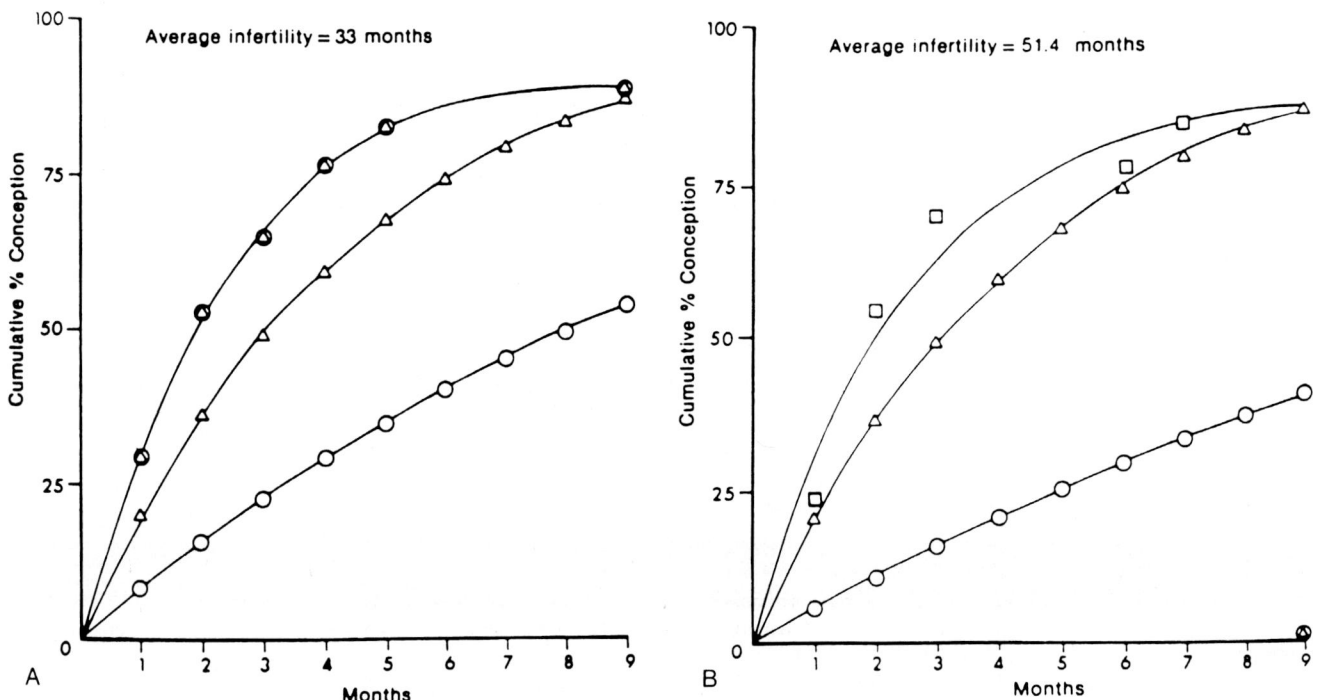

FIGURE 17–14. A, In patients with dysfunctional ovulation, the 95% upper confidence limit for fecundity (f) projected from life table calculations in patients with an average duration of infertility of 33 months is f = 0.08 (open circles) and is easily exceeded by patients with corrected biopsies on progesterone suppositories (triangles in circles). In fact, their f is nearly identical to that projected for a normal population (f = 0.20; open triangles). B, Likewise, patients with corrected biopsies on clomiphene (after failing to correct or conceive on progesterone suppositories) have a normalized f (open squares) compared with the normal population projection (open triangles) or the upper 95% f projection for a population with an average duration of infertility of 51.4 months (f = 0.06; open circles). (A and B from Daly DC, Walters CA, Soto-Albors CE, Riddick DH. Endometrial biopsy during treatment of luteal phase defects is predictive of therapeutic outcome. Fertil Steril 1983; 40:305–310. Reproduced with permission of the publisher, The American Fertility Society.)

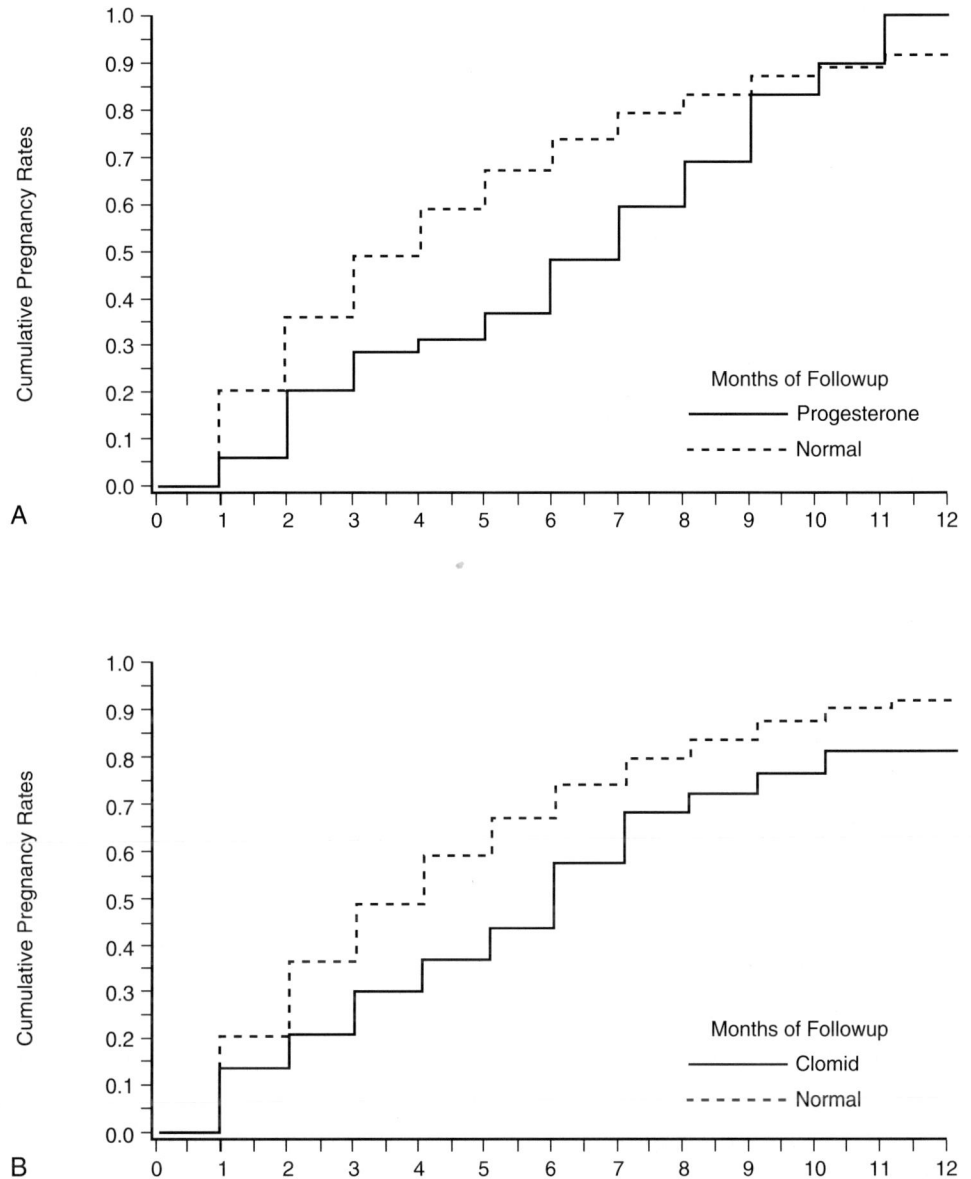

FIGURE 17–15. Patients with corrected biopsies on progesterone (*A*) or clomiphene (*B*) conceived with a fecundity rate that approached that of an idealized normal population, indicating that treatment was therapeutic if it corrected the underlying endometrial abnormality. (*A* and *B* from Murray DL, Reich L, Adashi EY. Oral clomiphene citrate and vaginal progesterone in the treatment of luteal phase dysfunction: a comparative study. Fertil Steril 1989; 51:35–41. Reproduced with permission of the publisher, The American Fertility Society.)

miphene would be an appropriate first-line medication for LPD in these cases.

3. If a particular patient cannot time P supplementation properly (cannot keep an interpretable BBT chart or her LH surge does not register on a urine LH test), then clomiphene would be the first choice.

Other than these considerations, there is no established superiority to initially treating LPD with either P supplementation or clomiphene.

PROGESTERONE

One 25-mg P suppository is inserted into the vagina or rectum twice a day during the luteal phase, either beginning with the 3rd day of rise in BBT or the 4th day following the LH surge. Unfortunately, P suppositories are not available commercially and must be prepared locally by a pharmacist. Suppositories are made by combining 25 mg of P powder in

a water-soluble base of 60% polyethylene glycol 400, USP, and 40% polyethylene glycol 6000, USP, in a mold for rectal suppositories. Alternatively, 12.5 to 25 mg of P in oil can be given intramuscularly daily. Another popular alternative is the use of oral micronized P. The initial supplemental dose is 100 mg three times per day. The absorption is superior when the oral P capsules are taken with food. These capsules yield peak serum P levels at 2 hours after ingestion and have a 6-hour duration of action (Fig. 17–16). P capsules are available from a number of large regional pharmacies; however, no manufacturer produces them and therefore local pharmacies cannot simply order a supply.

If pregnancy results, progesterone treatment should be continued until approximately the 12th week of pregnancy, after the luteoplacental shift in P production has occurred. The luteoplacental shift occurs at 5 to 9 weeks—treating until 12 weeks allows for a margin of safety. To ensure adequate P effect in the enhanced P environment of pregnancy,

PROGESTERONE CAPSULES DOSE STUDY

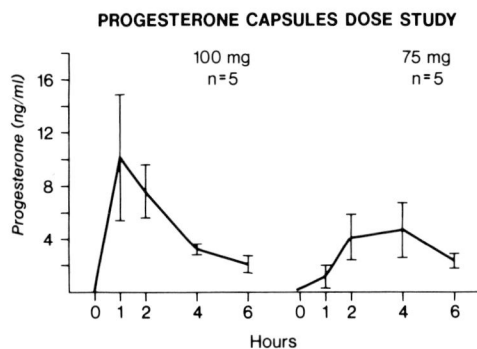

FIGURE 17–16. Serum progesterone levels are indicated over a 6-hour interval after five normal women ingested either 100 mg *(left panel)* or 75 mg *(right panel)* of oral micronized progesterone capsules at 0 hours. It can be seen that the progesterone levels tend to peak at 2 hours after ingestion.

250 mg of 17-OH P caproate administered intramuscularly one time per week also has been recommended.

CLOMIPHENE THERAPY

Although clomiphene citrate has itself been implicated in inducing ovulatory cycles with LPD, it is also advocated for therapy. The presumed mechanism of action is by increasing FSH secretion in the follicular phase. Because patients with short luteal phases often have reduced levels of serum FSH in the early follicular phase, as detailed previously, clomiphene should be particularly effective in such women. Clomiphene citrate should be administered early in the follicular phase, beginning on cycle days 3 to 5 at a dose of 50 mg for 5 days. No more than 100 mg per day should be administered to correct LPD. P supplementation in the first trimester of pregnancy is unnecessary when the conception has occurred during clomiphene treatment.

HUMAN CHORIONIC GONADOTROPIN

hCG also has been advocated for the treatment of LPD, but one older study reported that it is less effective than P in reversing the defect.[81] Different dosage regimens have been advocated by different clinicians. A dose of 2500 to 5000 IU given at 3-day intervals in the luteal phase should be more than sufficient. However, if this form of therapy is used, qualitative pregnancy tests using hCG cannot be used to confirm a pregnancy. Quantitative tests documenting serial increases consistent with a normal intrauterine pregnancy or ultrasound documentation of a viable intrauterine pregnancy are required instead. As a consequence, hCG is seldom used to treat LPD. P supplementation in the first trimester of pregnancy is unnecessary when the conception has occurred during hCG treatment.

BROMOCRIPTINE

Therapy with bromocriptine is indicated only in patients with LPD and hyperprolactinemia. Older studies indicate that such therapy is effective in this specific circumstance.[95, 96] A daily dose of bromocriptine (1.25 mg twice daily) administered orally is usually effective in correcting LPD. During bromocriptine treatment, a repeat prolactin level should be obtained to verify that it is now in the normal range. P supplementation in the first trimester of pregnancy is not necessary when the conception has occurred during bromocriptine treatment.

Treatment Failures and Duration

Whichever treatment approach is selected, the clinician should verify the adequacy of the treatment. An endometrial biopsy should be performed in an early treatment cycle and dated according to the standard criteria of Noyes and associates.[59] This biopsy should be performed in the late luteal phase (1 to 3 days prior to the expected next menstrual period). To avoid disrupting an early pregnancy (theoretically possible but practically unlikely), the couple should either use barrier contraception during the cycle when the biopsy is performed, or the clinician could obtain a negative quantitative serum pregnancy test on the day of the scheduled biopsy. An endometrial biopsy is recommended for verification of adequate treatment because serum P levels are less reliable in this setting. Most of the recommended treatments alter the pharmacodynamics of circulating P; in this setting, a serum P level is difficult to interpret. For instance, if a woman with LPD is receiving supplemental oral P treatment, the serum P level obtained could vary considerably, whether it was obtained 1 hour before or 1 hour after the ingestion of a micronized P capsule.

When the current treatment of LPD is determined to be inadequate (by out-of-phase biopsy), the clinician has two alternatives, either of which is valid: (1) increase the dose of the current medication, or (2) empirically switch to another treatment modality (e.g., if on P supplementation, switch to clomiphene). Once again, the modified treatment regimen needs to be verified with a late luteal phase endometrial biopsy. If the repeat biopsy remains abnormal (>2 days out of phase), then a more potent treatment regimen would be the next step. A regimen of small doses (75 to 150 IU) of hMG administered daily beginning on cycle day 3 would be recommended for persistent treatment failures. For hMG treatment, standard monitoring of ovulation induction would be required (daily estradiol levels and intermittent ultrasound scans). Once again, in the patient with LPD, the adequacy of hMG treatment needs to be verified with yet another endometrial biopsy.

Once the initial or modified treatment regimen has been verified as adequate, the couple can proceed to attempt conception in subsequent cycles. A reasonable duration of treatment in which most conceptions in women with LPD will be realized is six treated menstrual cycles. If no pregnancy occurs after six treated cycles following treatment verification, then the entire evaluation of a particular couple should be reviewed. In some instances, further tests would be indicated; in other couples, more accelerated treatment (e.g., controlled ovarian hyperstimulation with intrauterine insemination) would be appropriate; and still others may wish to forego further treatment. It would not be unreasonable to resume further LPD treatment if those considerations have been reviewed and the couple and physician are in agreement. However, if a couple has received adequate LPD treatment for a total of 10 to 12 cycles, a change in direction would definitely be in order.

CONCLUSIONS

LPD is a subtle entity and probably the most common abnormality of the menstrual cycle. When it persists in a woman of reproductive age who wishes to conceive, it may cause infertility or recurrent spontaneous pregnancy loss. The presence of such subtle defects should be sought in couples with infertility who have no other obvious causes for the infertility (i.e., unexplained). Adherence to strict diagnostic criteria and careful consideration of therapeutic options should provide good clinical results in carefully selected patients.

REFERENCES

1. Jones GES. Some newer aspects of the management of infertility. JAMA 1949;141:1123–1129.
2. Keller DW, Wiest WG, Askin FB, et al. Pseudocorpus luteum insufficiency: a local defect of progesterone action on endometrial stroma. J Clin Endocrinol Metab 1979;48:127–132.
3. Gautray JP, DeBrux J, Tajchner G, et al. Clinical investigation of the menstrual cycle: III. clinical, endometrial, and endocrine aspects of luteal defect. Fertil Steril 1981;35:296–303.
4. Spirtos NJ, Yurewicz EC, Moghissi KS, et al. Pseudocorpus luteum insufficiency: a study of cytosol progesterone receptors in human endometrium. Obstet Gynecol 1985;65:535–540.
5. Saracoglu OF, Aksel S, Yeoman RR, Wiebe RH. Endometrial estradiol and progesterone receptors in patients with luteal phase defects and endometriosis. Fertil Steril 1985;43:851–855.
6. Carr BR, MacDonald PC, Simpson ER. The role of lipoproteins in the regulation of progesterone secretion by the human corpus luteum. Fertil Steril 1982;38:303–311.
7. Fujimoto V, Clifton DK, Cohen NL, Soules MR. Variability of serum prolactin and progesterone levels in normal women: the relevance of single hormone measurements in the clinical setting. Obstet Gynecol 1990;76:71–78.
8. Wilks JW, Hodgen GD, Ross GT. Luteal phase defects in the rhesus monkey: the significance of serum FSH:LH ratios. J Clin Endocrinol Metab 1976;43:1261–1267.
9. Sherman BM, West JH, Korenman SG. The menopausal transition: analysis of LH, FSH, estradiol and progesterone concentrations during menstrual cycles of older women. J Clin Endocrinol Metab 1976;42:629–636.
10. Lenton EA, Landgren B-M, Sexton L. Normal variation in the length of the luteal phase of the menstrual cycle: identification of the short luteal phase. Br J Obstet Gynaecol 1984;91:685–689.
11. Gray RH, Campbell OM, Zacur HA, et al. Postpartum return of ovarian activity in non–breast-feeding women monitored by urinary assays. J Clin Endocrinol Metab 1987;64:645–650.
12. Dale E, Gerlach DH, Wilhite AL. Menstrual dysfunction in distance runners. Obstet Gynecol 1979;54:47–53.
13. Bonen A, Belcastro AN, Simpson AA. Profiles of menstrual cycle hormones in teenage athletes. J Appl Physiol 1981;50:545–551.
14. Ronkainen HR, Pakarinen AJ, Kirkinen P, Kauppila AJ. Physical exercise–induced changes and season-associated differences in the pituitary-ovarian function of runners and joggers. J Clin Endocrinol Metab 1985;60:416–422.
15. Bullen BA, Skrinar GS, Beitins IZ, et al. Induction of menstrual disorders by strenuous exercise in untrained women. N Engl J Med 1985;312:1349–1353.
16. Loucks AB, Mortola JF, Girton L, Yen SSC. Alterations in the hypothalamic-pituitary-ovarian and the hypothalamic-pituitary-adrenal axes in athletic women. J Clin Endocrinol Metab 1989;68:402–411.
17. Prior JC, Cameron K, Ho Yuen B, Thomas J. Menstrual cycle changes with marathon training: anovulation and short luteal phase. Can J Sport Sci 1982;7:173–177.
18. Pirke KM, Schweiger U, Strowitzki T, et al. Dieting causes menstrual irregularities in normal weight young women through impairment of episodic luteinizing hormone secretion. Fertil Steril 1988;51:263–268.
19. Schweiger U, Tuschl RJ, Platte P, et al. Everyday eating behavior and menstrual function in young women. Fertil Steril 1992;57:771–775.
20. Li TC, Dockery P, Cooke ID. Endometrial development in the luteal phase of women with various types of infertility: comparison with women of normal fertility. Hum Reprod 1991;6:325–330.
21. Davis OK, Berkeley AS, Naus GJ, et al. The incidence of luteal phase defect in normal, fertile women determined by serial endometrial biopsies. Fertil Steril 1989;51:582–586.
22. Lee SJ, Lenton EA, Sexton L, Cooke ID. The effect of age on the cyclical patterns of plasma LH, FSH, oestradiol and progesterone in women with regular menstrual cycles. Hum Reprod 1988;3:851–855.
23. Metcalf MG, Livesey JH. Gonadotropin excretion in fertile women: effect of age and the onset of the menopausal transition. J Endocrinol 1985;105:357–362.
24. Stouffer RL, Hodgen GD. Induction of luteal phase defects in rhesus monkeys by follicular fluid administration at the onset of the menstrual cycle. J Clin Endocrinol Metab 1980;51:669–671.
25. Sheehan KL, Casper RF, Yen SSC. Luteal phase defects induced by an agonist of luteinizing hormone–releasing factor: a model for fertility control. Science 1982;215:170–172.
26. DiZerega GS, Hodgen GD. Luteal phase dysfunction infertility: a sequel to aberrant folliculogenesis. Fertil Steril 1981;35:489–499.
27. Hutchison J, Zeleznik AJ. The corpus luteum of the primate menstrual cycle is capable of recovering from a transient withdrawal of pituitary gonadotropin support. Endocrinology 1985;117:1043–1049.
28. Mais V, Kazer RR, Cetel NS, et al. The dependency of folliculogenesis and corpus luteum function on pulsatile gonadotropin secretion in cycling women using a gonadotropin-releasing hormone antagonist as a probe. J Clin Endocrinol Metab 1986;62:1250–1255.
29. McLachlan RI, Cohen NL, Vale WW, et al. The importance of luteinizing hormone in the control of inhibin and progesterone secretion by the human corpus luteum. J Clin Endocrinol Metab 1989;68:1078–1085.
30. Garzo VG, Liu J, Ulmann A, et al. Effects of an antiprogesterone (RU486) on the hypothalamic-hypophyseal-ovarian-endometrial axis during the luteal phase of the menstrual cycle. J Clin Endocrinol Metab 1988;66:508–517.
31. Daly DC, Maslar IA, Rosenberg SM, et al. Prolactin production by luteal phase defect endometrium. Am J Obstet Gynecol 1981;140:587–591.
32. Ying Y-K, Walters CA, Kuslis S, et al. Prolactin production by explants of normal, luteal phase defective, and corrected luteal phase defective late secretory endometrium. Am J Obstet Gynecol 1985;151:801–804.
33. Soules MR, McLachlan RI, Ek M, et al. Luteal phase deficiency: characterization of reproductive hormones over the menstrual cycle. J Clin Endocrinol Metab 1989;69:804–812.
34. Grant A, McBride WG, Moyes JM. Luteal phase defects in abortion. Int J Fertil 1959;4:323–329.
35. Huang K-E. The primary treatment of luteal phase inadequacy: progesterone versus clomiphene citrate. Am J Obstet Gynecol 1986;155:824–828.
36. Zhang Y, Ji H, Han M, et al. Luteal function in patients with endometriosis. Proc Chin Acad Med Sci 1989;4:96–101.
37. Strott CA, Cargille CM, Ross GT, Lipsett MB. The short luteal phase. J Clin Endocrinol 1970;30:246–251.
38. Sherman BM, Korenman SG. Measurement of plasma LH, FSH, estradiol, and progesterone in disorders of the human menstrual cycle: the short luteal phase. J Clin Endocrinol Metab 1974;38:89–93.
39. Cook CL, Rao CV, Yussman MA. Plasma gonadotropin and sex steroid hormone levels during early, midfollicular, and midluteal phases of women with luteal phase defects. Fertil Steril 1983;40:45–48.
40. Soules MR, Clifton DK, Cohen NL, et al. Luteal phase deficiency: abnormal gonadotropin and progesterone secretion patterns. J Clin Endocrinol Metab 1989;69:813–820.
41. Soules MR, Steiner RA, Clifton DK, et al. Progesterone modulation of pulsatile luteinizing hormone secretion in normal women. J Clin Endocrinol Metab 1984;58:378–383.
42. Soules MR, Clifton DK, Steiner RA, et al. The corpus luteum: determinants of progesterone secretion in the normal menstrual cycle. Obstet Gynecol 1988;71:659–666.
43. Soules MR, Clifton DK, Bremner WJ, Steiner RA. Corpus luteum insufficiency induced by a rapid gonadotropin-releasing hormone–induced gonadotropin secretion pattern in the follicular phase. J Clin Endocrinol Metab 1987;65:457–464.
44. Suh BY, Betz G. Altered luteinizing hormone pulse frequency in the early follicular phase of the menstrual cycle with luteal phase defect patients in women. Fertil Steril 1993;60:800–805.
45. Schweiger U, Laessle RG, Tuschl RJ, et al. Decreased follicular phase gonadotropin secretion is associated with impaired estradiol and progesterone secretion during the follicular and luteal phases in normally menstruating women. J Clin Endocrinol 1989;68:888–892.

46. Soules MR, Bremner WJ, Dahl KD, et al. The induction of premature luteolysis in normal women: follicular phase luteinizing hormone secretion and corpus luteum function in the subsequent cycle. Am J Obstet Gynecol 1991;164:989–996.

47. Fritz MA, Fitz TA. The functional microscopic anatomy of the corpus luteum: the "small cell"–"large cell" controversy. Clin Obstet Gynecol 1991;34:144–156.

48. Ohara A, Mori T, Taii S, et al. Functional differentiation in steroidogenesis of two types of luteal cells isolated from mature human corpora lutea of menstrual cycle. J Clin Endocrinol Metab 1987;65:1192–1200.

49. Wuttke W, Hinney B, Imse V, et al. Differentiation of three types of luteal insufficiencies [Abstract 30]. Presented at the Second International Capri Conference, May 22–26, 1992, Capri, Italy.

50. Kusunda M, Nakamura G, Matsukuma K, Kurano A. Corpus luteum insufficiency as a cause of nidatory failure. Acta Obstet Gynecol Scand 1983;62:199–205.

51. Maas S, Jarry H, Teichmann A, et al. Paracrine actions of oxytocin, prostaglandin $F_2\alpha$, and estradiol within the human corpus luteum. J Clin Endocrinol Metab 1992;74:306–312.

52. Csapo AI, Pulkkinen MO, Ruttner B. The significance of the human corpus luteum in pregnancy maintenance: I. preliminary studies. Am J Obstet Gynecol 1972;112:1061–1067.

53. Csapo AI, Pulkkinen MO, Wiest WG. Effect of luteectomy and early progesterone replacement therapy in early pregnant patients. Am J Obstet Gynecol 1973;115:759–765.

54. Navot D, Laufer N, Kopolovic J. Artificially induced endometrial cycles and establishment of pregnancies in the absence of ovaries. N Engl J Med 1986;314:806–811.

55. Sauer MV, Paulson RJ. Understanding the current status of oocyte donation in the United States: what's really going on out there? Fertil Steril 1992;58:16–18.

56. Scott R, Navot D, Liu H-C, Rosenwaks Z. A human in vivo model for luteoplacental shift. Fertil Steril 1991;56:481–484.

57. Balasch J, Vanrell JA, Marquez M, et al. Dydrogesterone versus vaginal progesterone in the treatment of the endometrial luteal phase deficiency. Fertil Steril 1982;37:751–754.

58. Soules MR, editor. Luteal phase deficiency. Clin Obstet Gynecol 1991;34:1.

59. Noyes RW, Hertig AT, Rock J. Dating the endometrial biopsy. Fertil Steril 1950;1:3–25.

60. McNeely MJ, Soules MR. The diagnosis of luteal phase deficiency: a critical review. Fertil Steril 1988;50:1–15.

61. Filicori M, Butler JP, Crowley WF Jr. Neuroendocrine regulation of the corpus luteum in the human: evidence for pulsatile progesterone secretion. J Clin Invest 1984;73:1638–1647.

62. Healy DL, Schenken RS, Lynch A, et al. Pulsatile progesterone secretion: its relevance to clinical evaluation of corpus luteal function. Fertil Steril 1984;41:114–121.

63. Rosenfeld DL, Chudow S, Bronson RA. Diagnosis of luteal phase inadequacy. Obstet Gynecol 1988;56:193–196.

64. Miller MM, Hoffman DI, Creinin M, et al. Comparison of endometrial biopsy and urinary pregnanediol concentration in the diagnosis of luteal phase deficiency. Fertil Steril 1990;54:1008–1011.

65. Vining RF, McGinley RA. The measurement of hormones in saliva: possibilities and pitfalls. J Steroid Biochem 1987;27:81–89.

66. O'Rourke MT, Ellison PT. Salivary measurement of episodic progesterone release. Am J Phys Anthropol 1990;81:423.

67. Hull MGR, Savage PE, Bromham DR, et al. The value of a single serum progesterone measurement in the midluteal phase as a criterion of a potentially fertile cycle ("ovulation") derived from treated and untreated conception cycles. Fertil Steril 1982;37:355–360.

68. Jordan J, Craig K, Clifton DK, Soules MR. Luteal phase deficiency: the sensitivity and specificity of diagnostic methods in common clinical use. Fertil Steril, 1994;62:54–62.

69. Shangold M, Berkeley A, Gray J. Both midluteal serum progesterone levels and late luteal endometrial histology should be assessed in all infertile women. Fertil Steril 1983;40:627–630.

70. Scott RT, Snyder RR, Stricklin DM, et al. The effect of interobserver variation in dating endometrial histology on the diagnosis of luteal phase defects. Fertil Steril 1988;50:888–892.

71. Shoupe D, Mishell DR Jr, Lacarra M, et al. Correlation of endometrial maturation with four methods of estimating day of ovulation. Obstet Gynecol 1989;73:88–92.

72. Daly DC, Tohan N, Doney TJ, et al. The significance of lymphocytic-leukocytic infiltrates in interpreting late luteal phase endometrial biopsies. Fertil Steril 1982;37:786–791.

73. Israel R, Mishell DR Jr, Stone SC, et al. Single luteal phase progesterone assay as an indicator of ovulation. Am J Obstet Gynecol 1972;112: 1043–1046.

74. Tho PT, Byrd JR, McDonough PG. Etiologies and subsequent reproductive performance of 100 couples with recurrent abortion. Fertil Steril 1979;32:389–395.

75. Jones GS, Delfs E. Endocrine patterns in term pregnancies following abortion. JAMA 1951;146:1212–1218.

76. Botella-Llusia J. The endometrium in repeated abortion. Int J Fertil 1962;7:147–154.

77. Wentz AC, Herbert CM, Maxson WS, Garner CH. Outcome of progesterone treatment of luteal phase inadequacy. Fertil Steril 1984;41:856–862.

78. Varnell JA, Balasch J. Luteal phase defects in repeated abortion. Int J Gynaecol Obstet 1986;24:111–115.

79. Daya S, Ward S, Burrows E. Progesterone profiles in luteal phase defect cycles and outcome of progesterone treatment in patients with recurrent spontaneous abortion. Am J Obstet Gynecol 1988;158:225–232.

80. Huang KE, Muechler EK, Bonfiglio TA. Follicular phase treatment of luteal phase defect with follicle-stimulating hormone in infertile women. Obstet Gynecol 1984;64:32–36.

81. Jones GS, Aksel S, Wentz AC. Serum progesterone values in the luteal phase defects: effect of chorionic gonadotropin. Obstet Gynecol 1974;44:26–34.

82. Loucopoules A, Ferin M. The treatment of luteal phase defects with pulsatile gonadotropin-releasing hormone. Fertil Steril 1987;48:933–936.

83. Karamardian LM, Grimes DA. Luteal phase deficiency: effect of treatment on pregnancy rates. Am J Obstet Gynecol 1992;167:1391–1398.

84. Klentzeris LD, Li T-C, Dockery P, Cooke ID. The endometrial biopsy as a predictive factor of pregnancy rate in women with unexplained infertility. Eur J Obstet Gynecol Reprod Biol 1992;45:119–124.

85. Jones GS, Pourmand K. An evaluation of etiologic factors and therapy in 555 private patients with primary infertility. Fertil Steril 1962;13:398–410.

86. Rosenberg SM, Luciano AA, Riddick DH. The luteal phase defect: the relative pregnancy of, and encouraging response to, treatment with vaginal progesterone. Fertil Steril 1980;34:17–20.

87. Soules MR, Wiebe RH, Aksel S, Hammond CB. The diagnosis and therapy of luteal phase deficiency. Fertil Steril 1977;28:1033–1037.

88. Katayama KP, Ju KS, Manuel M, et al. Computer analysis of etiology and pregnancy rate in 636 cases of primary infertility. Am J Obstet Gynecol 1979;135:207–214.

89. Garcia J, Jones GS, Wentz AC. The use of clomiphene citrate. Fertil Steril 1977;28:707–717.

90. Quagliarello J, Weiss G. Clomiphene citrate in the management of infertility associated with shortened luteal phase. Fertil Steril 1979;31:373–377.

91. Downs KA, Gibson MA. Clomiphene citrate therapy for luteal phase defect. Fertil Steril 1983;39:34–38.

92. Daly DC, Walters CA, Soto-Albora CE, Riddick DH. Endometrial biopsy during treatment of luteal phase defects is predictive of therapeutic outcome. Fertil Steril 1983;40:305–310.

93. Murray DL, Reich L, Adashi EY. Oral clomiphene citrate and vaginal progesterone in the treatment of luteal phase dysfunction: a comparative study. Fertil Steril 1989;51:35–41.

94. Cramer DW, Walker AM, Schaff I. Statistical methods in evaluating the outcome of infertility therapy. Fertil Steril 1979;32:80–86.

95. Muhlenstadt D, Bohnet HG, Hanker JP, et al. Short luteal phase and prolactin. Int J Fertil 1978;23:213–218.

96. Andersen AN, Larsen JF, Eskildsen PC, et al. Treatment of hyperprolactinemic luteal insufficiency with bromocriptine. Acta Obstet Gynecol Scand 1979;58:379–383.

PART C

OTHER MEDICAL CONDITIONS

CHAPTER 18

Evaluation and Treatment of Disorders of the Cervix

STEPHEN P. BOYERS

To treat sterility, we must ascertain if the spermatozoa go into the cervix uteri. Also, we must treat the cervix until the discharge fails to kill the spermatozoa.

—J. MARION SIMS (1865)[1]

The concept of cervical infertility is time-honored, but significant controversies about its diagnosis and treatment remain. In some mammals, like the horse and the pig, semen is ejaculated directly into the uterus. In humans, however, as well as in ruminants, rabbits, and nonhuman primates, semen is deposited in the vagina, and the cervix is thought to play an important role in reproduction. A number of functions have been ascribed to the cervix, including (1) receptivity to sperm penetration at or near ovulation and inhibition of sperm entry at other times; (2) protection of sperm from the hostile environment of the vagina; (3) support of the energy requirements for sperm motion; (4) filtration of morphologically abnormal sperm; (5) storage of normal sperm for sustained release to the upper reproductive tract; and (6) participation in the process of sperm capacitation.[2, 3] In the simplest terms, the human cervix has been viewed as a biologic valve[3] that, at alternate times during the menstrual cycle, either prevents or promotes the entry of sperm into the uterus and the upper reproductive tract. The regulation of sperm transport through the cervix and the interactions between spermatozoa and cervical mucus have been widely studied, with important implications for fertility control. Much is known, but much remains controversial. Although there is general support for the concept of a cervical factor in infertility, and intuitive acceptance of the common tests to evaluate sperm–cervical mucus interaction, there is disagreement about the performance, interpretation, and prognostic significance of these tests, about the incidence of cervical infertility and the factors that cause it, and about their treatment.

In this chapter, we review the physiology of human cervical mucus and sperm–cervical mucus interaction and the mechanisms of sperm passage through the cervical canal. We review the tests used to diagnose cervical factor and show that the postcoital test (PCT) remains important to the infertility investigation. We discuss the limitations of the PCT and the corroborative value of in vitro sperm–cervical mucus testing and present a plan to investigate the causes of sperm–cervical mucus dysfunction. Finally, we examine the causes of cervical infertility and discuss options for therapy.

BIOLOGY OF THE CERVIX AND PHYSIOLOGY OF SPERM–CERVICAL MUCUS INTERACTION

One of the most remarkable odysseys in reproductive biology is the perilous journey of spermatozoa from the vagina through the cervix to the upper reproductive tract and the site of fertilization. Even in normal, fertile matings, 99.9% of inseminated sperm perish before reaching the relative sanctuary of the cervix, and fewer still ever confront an oocyte.[4] There are a number of excellent reviews of the biology of the cervix in reproduction, emphasizing its gross and microscopic anatomy[5–9]; cervical mucus production, biochemistry, and biophysical properties[10–13]; sperm–cervical mucus interaction; and sperm transport through the normal female reproductive tract.[3, 14–18] In this section, we briefly review information that is basic to understanding the role of the cervix in infertility.

The Vagina

In humans and a number of other mammals, the vagina is the site of insemination. Although its role in sperm transport has yet to be fully understood, the vagina is generally viewed as a hostile domain from which sperm must escape to survive. In the normal vagina, pH ranges between 3.5 and 4.0.[19] In contrast, the optimal pH for sperm survival is more alkaline, between 7.0 and 8.5,[20–23] and motility is sharply inhibited below a pH of 6.0.[24–26] Several factors work at the time of insemination to neutralize vaginal acidity. The production of vaginal-lubricating fluids during sexual stimulation has a modest but measurable effect, raising pH to 4.2 to 4.5.[19] More important, seminal fluid itself is alkaline, with a mean pH about 7.5.[27] Using radiotelemetry to monitor vaginal pH, Fox and colleagues[28] reported an increase to pH 7.0 within 8 seconds of ejaculation, confirming work by Masters and Johnson,[19] who measured vaginal pH serially after coitus and showed that vaginal pH stayed above 6.0 for as long as 2 hours.

In keeping with these observations, sperm rapidly lose their motility in the vagina,[29, 30] making a vaginal sperm storage mechanism unlikely. The precise length of time during which functionally competent sperm are able to migrate from the vagina to the cervix is unknown.

The Cervix

In all species studied, sperm have been found in cervical mucus within minutes of mating. In humans, motile sperm were found in both endocervical and exocervical mucus 1.5 to 3 minutes after ejaculation.[31] If the vaginal sperm population in rabbits was destroyed by sodium dodecyl sulfate 2 minutes after mating, only 25% had fertilized oocytes, whereas 93% had fertilized if the interval was 5 minutes.[32] These experiments indicate that, at least in the rabbit, functionally competent sperm colonize the cervix within 5 minutes.

In contrast with the vagina, the pH of normal cervical mucus is alkaline throughout the menstrual cycle,[21, 26, 33] with peak pH (8.4) occurring on the day of the luteinizing hormone (LH) surge, coincident with peak sperm penetrability. In this section, we review cervical anatomy as it pertains to cervical mucus production, as well as to the composition and biophysical structure of cervical mucus and its changes during the menstrual cycle. We then discuss the major aspects of sperm–cervical mucus interaction, including the mechanism and significance of rapid sperm transport and the role of the cervix in sperm selection, storage, and capacitation.

CERVICAL ANATOMY

The anatomy of the human cervix as it pertains to reproduction and cervical mucus production has been thoroughly reviewed elsewhere.[5–9] In brief, the endocervical canal ranges in length from 18 to 35 mm (mean 27 mm), with a widest diameter of about 7 mm. It receives an abundant vascular supply, both from the uterine artery and from ascending branches of the vaginal artery, and an extensive network of autonomic nerves. The endocervix is lined with tall columnar epithelium composed of two primary cell types: nonciliated secretory and kinociliated (Fig. 18–1). Although commonly referred to as *endocervical glands,* the human cervix has no true glandular component but rather a mucosa in an intricate system of clefts and folds (Fig. 18–2) that form crypts branching from the central canal, likened to the "trunk and branches of a tree."[34, 35] The secretory cells contain glycoproteins and stain prominently with periodic acid–Schiff (PAS); they are covered with many short microvilli, about 2 μ long $\times$ 0.2 μ in diameter. The ciliated cells display kinocilia that have been shown in vitro to beat toward the vagina.[6] It has been postulated that provaginal ciliary currents serve to orient cervical mucus into low-viscosity channels or strings that lead from a mucus secretory unit to the cervical canal and external cervical os,[8, 36, 37] ensuring clearance and replenishment of cervical mucus and perhaps providing a system of low-resistance pathways that facilitate sperm migration and

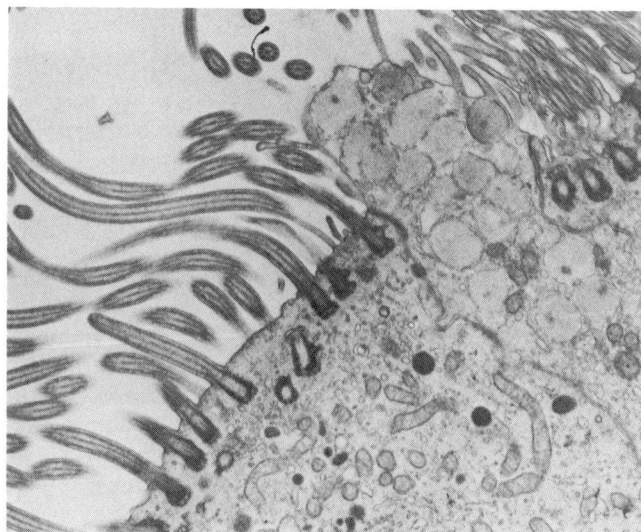

FIGURE 18–1. Electron micrograph showing the ciliated and secretory cells of the cervical epithelium. (From Blandau RJ. Sperm transport through the mammalian cervix: Comparative aspects. In: Blandau RJ, Moghissi K, editors. The Biology of the Cervix. Chicago: University of Chicago Press, 1973:285–304.)

CERVIX

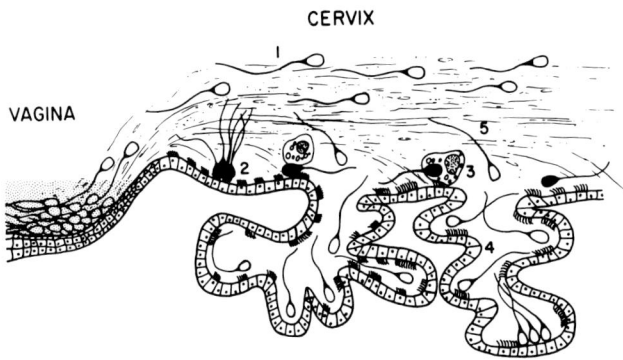

FIGURE 18–2. Diagrammatic illustration of the relationship of sperm motility to cilial beat and movement to mucin in the cervix uteri. Macromolecules of cervical mucin are arranged in channels in filament-like micelles against the direction of the cilia beat. Nonviable sperm (2) are not transported to the uterine cavity and may undergo phagocytosis by the leukocytes (3). An intricate biophysical and biochemical relationship may exist between the micelle (5) and the sperm. The cervical cilia are of importance for the directional flow of the cervical mucin from the narrow crypts (4) to the cervical lumen (1). (Modified from Hafez ESE. Histology and microstructure of the cervical epithelial secretory system. In: Elstein M, Moghissi KS, Borth R, editors. Cervical Mucus in Human Reproduction. Copenhagen: Scriptor, 1973:23–32.)

storage. There remains some disagreement regarding the number of secretory units in the normal cervix, with estimates differing by two orders of magnitude, from about 100[38] to more than 10,000.[39, 40]

CERVICAL MUCUS

Cervical mucus is produced by the nonciliated cells of the cervical epithelium by the mechanism of merocrine secretion, which leaves the secreting cells intact. These cells contain large numbers of PAS-positive cytoplasmic granules that appear to displace the cell nucleus basally. The granules, about 1 μ in diameter, are discharged by exocytosis into the lumen of the cervical crypt, where they coalesce to form cervical mucus. It is unclear whether mucus is secreted with both gel and aqueous phases fully developed and hydrated or primarily as the mucin molecule, which forms a network that acquires its aqueous phase as a serum transudate, like a sponge. The production of cervical mucus is clearly under hormonal control. Estrogenic (type E) cervical mucus is abundant in amount, watery and thin in consistency, clear, acellular, and supportive of sperm penetration and survival. Gestagenic (type G) cervical mucus is scant, thick, opaque, cellular, and inhibitive of sperm penetration.[13, 33] Figure 18–3 illustrates the changes in cervical mucus throughout the menstrual cycle, centered around day 0 (day of the serum LH peak) in 10 normal young women. The peak in cervical mucus quantity and spinnbarkeit occurred 1 day before the LH surge, and the nadir of cervical mucus viscosity and cellularity and the peak of ferning, pH, and sperm penetration occurred on the day of the LH surge. The amount of mucus secreted is a function of both hormonal stimulation and the number of responsive secretory units and varies from 60 mg/day in the early follicular phase to 700 mg/day at midcycle.[6] There are a number of excellent reviews of the biophysical and biochemical properties of cervical mucus, but understanding of the interaction between spermatozoa and either the insoluble

or soluble components of cervical secretions remains rudimentary. Research in this area has applications to contraception as well as to cervical infertility.

Biophysical Properties. Cervical mucus is a hydrogel—a heterogeneous, two-phase fluid with both high-viscosity and low-viscosity components. The high-viscosity, insoluble gel phase consists of a network or mesh of filamentous glycoproteins known as *mucin*. This macromolecule has a peptide core that is rich in hydroxyl amino acids; the core accounts for about 20% of mucin's molecular weight. Attached to this backbone are numerous carbohydrate side chains (80% of the molecular weight). The organization of mucin molecules has been studied by a variety of techniques, including transmission and scanning electron microscopy,[41, 42] nuclear magnetic resonance,[38] and laser light-scattering spectroscopy.[43] In general the filamentous mucin macromolecules are thought to form a network of interconnected micelles, either linked by disulfide bridges or randomly coiled, forming a three-dimensional mesh (Fig. 18–4) whose intermicellar spaces support an aqueous phase. The size of the aqueous space varies with the degree of hydration or bridging, or both, between micelles, which, in turn, is determined by hormonal signals. In the periovulatory phase of the cycle, when mucus is thin and watery, the intermicellar space is large enough to allow sperm penetration. Under the influence of progesterone, hydration decreases and the intermicellar space narrows, restricting sperm penetration.

Biochemical Properties. The water content of cervical mucus varies between 85% and 92% in the luteal phase and between 95% and 98% at midcycle. The aqueous phase contains a variety of dissolved electrolytes and trace elements, primarily sodium chloride, but including potassium, calcium, magnesium, zinc, copper, and iron (see review in reference 13). It remains isotonic throughout the cycle. Low-molecular-weight organic compounds are also present, including glucose, maltose, and mannose. Lipids (phospholipids, cholesterol, cholesterol esters, monoglycerides, diglycerides, triglycerides, and free fatty acids) have been identified, as well as cyclic adenosine monophosphate, glycogen, and a variety of free amino acids. A variety of both serum-type and non-serum-type soluble proteins, enzymes, and enzyme inhibitors have also been identified in cervical mucus.[44] The functional roles that these compounds play in sperm transport is unclear. Many fluctuate during the menstrual cycle and have been investigated as possible markers of ovulation. Some may serve as substrates for sperm metabolism,[45, 46] although the data remain contradictory.[47–50] Many of the soluble proteins, including the immunoglobulins (Fig. 18–5), show a pronounced nadir in the periovulatory portion of the cycle.[44] Whether these changes represent a simple dilutional effect, owing to increased hydration of cervical mucus, or another mechanism remains unclear, but they have implications for therapy, as discussed later.

Rapid Sperm Transport

Considering the optimal pH for sperm survival, the difference in pH between the vagina (3.5 to 4.0) and midcycle cervical mucus (8.0), and the evanescent buffering effect of seminal fluid, it is not surprising that few sperm survive in the vagina longer than 30 minutes. The rapid entry of sperm

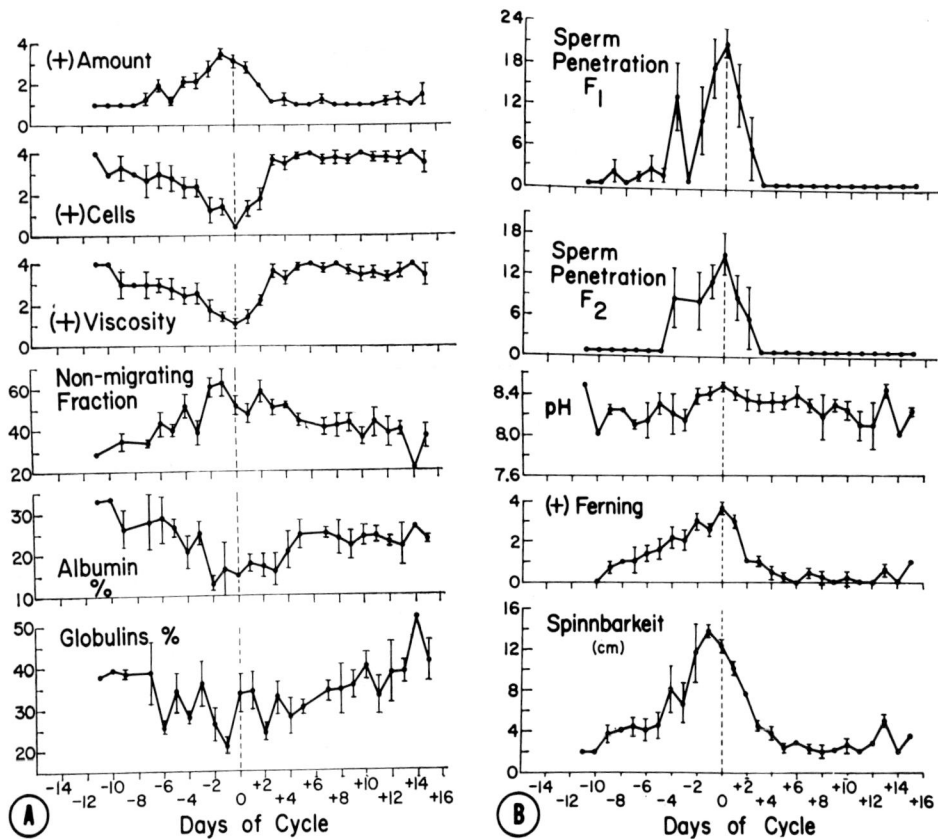

FIGURE 18–3. Changes in various properties of cervical mucus throughout the menstrual cycle. Day 0 = day of luteinizing hormone peak (*dotted line*). F_1 and F_2 indicate the number of spermatozoa in first and second microscopic fields (×200) from interface in in vitro sperm–cervical mucus penetration test. *Vertical bars* represent 1 SEM. NMF, nonmigrating fraction that contains principally the high-molecular-weight glycoproteins or mucin of cervical mucus. (From Moghissi KS, Syner FN, Evans TN. A composite picture of the menstrual cycle. Am J Obstet Gynecol 1972;114:405–418.)

into cervical mucus is necessary to ensure the survival of a motile subpopulation. More unexpected, however, is the rapidity with which sperm populate the upper female reproductive tract. The mechanism and possible biologic significance of rapid sperm transport have implications for the clinical evaluation of cervical infertility and disordered sperm transport.

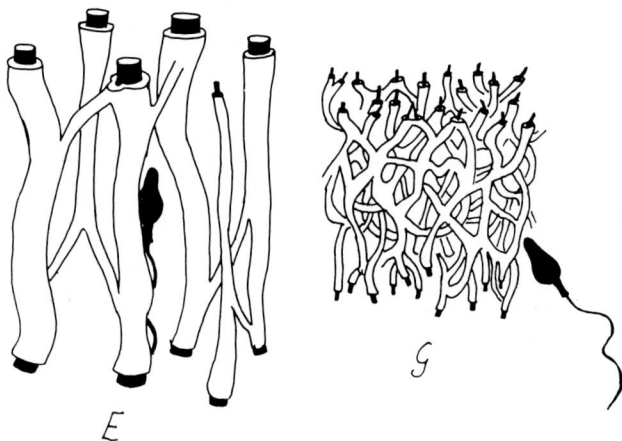

FIGURE 18–4. Schematic three-dimensional view of the structure of mucus types E (estrogenic) and G (gestagenic). The macromolecular cores (consisting of several long molecules side by side) are shown in black, together with the surrounding hydration cells (white). A spermatozoon moving in the cervical plasma between the micelles of type E and a noninvading spermatozoon outside type G are also shown. (From Odeblad E. Biophysical techniques of assessing cervical mucus and microstructure of cervical epithelium. In: Elstein M, Moghissi KS, Borth R, editors. Cervical mucus in human reproduction. Copenhagen: Scriptor, 1973:58–74.)

In a classic study of normal human sperm transport,[4] eight fertile women who agreed to bilateral salpingectomy for surgical tubal sterilization were recruited. All were ovulatory, and the preovulatory serum estradiol peak was identified by serial estradiol assays. All subjects were restricted from coitus for 11 to 14 days preoperatively, and daily cervical mucus and vaginal examinations confirmed the absence of sperm. Each patient was inseminated with fresh whole donor semen by intravaginal technique. The interval between insemination and salpingectomy varied from zero to 45 minutes. Total sperm numbers, percentage and grade of motility, and percentage of morphologically normal sperm were known for each inseminate. Before salpingectomy, each tube was clamped at the tubouterine, the isthmoampullary, and the ampullofimbrial junctions, isolating the isthmic, ampullary, and fimbrial segments. Total sperm numbers for each segment were evaluated and compared with the number inseminated. Endocervical mucus and uterine washings were also studied.

The authors reported that sperm were present in the fallopian tubes by 5 minutes after insemination; that the total number of tubal sperm was directly related to the number inseminated; and that the population of tubal sperm plateaued after 15 minutes. At steady-state, 1 in every 2000 inseminated sperm was in cervical mucus and 1 in 14 million was in the oviduct. Earlier studies had also reported rapid transport in humans[51, 52] but failed to control for important variables, using infertile (rather than fertile) subjects, coitus rather than artificial insemination (precluding full characterization of sperm parameters), imprecise periovulatory timing, and surgical techniques that did not preclude redistribution of spermatozoa by manipulation.

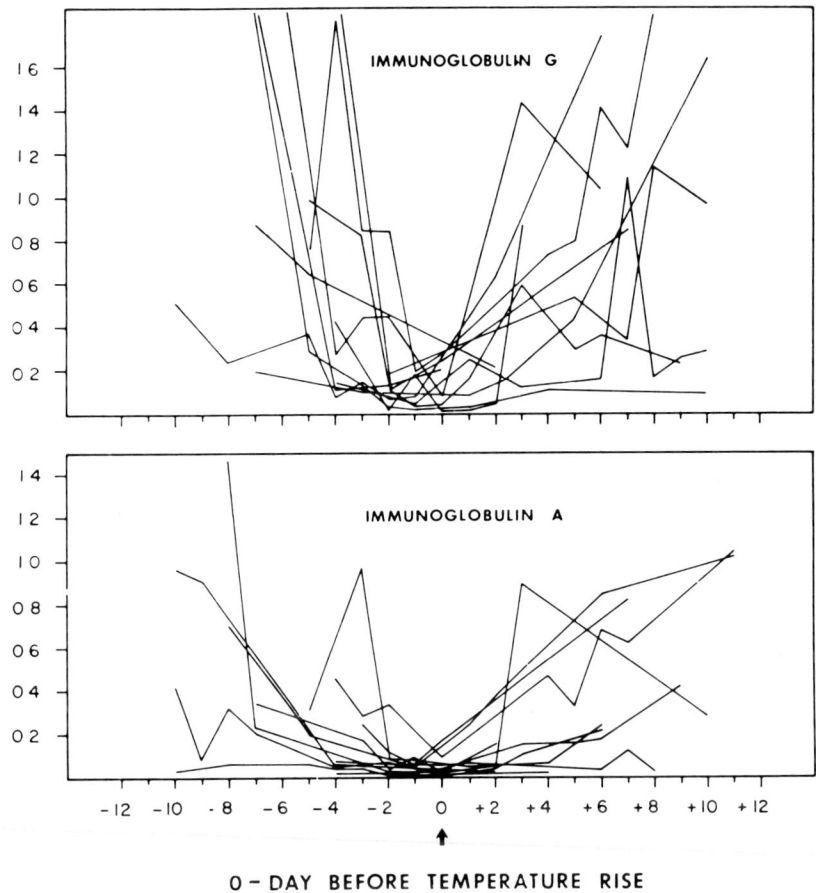

FIGURE 18–5. Immunoglobulins G and A in cervical mucus during 10 presumably ovulatory cycles. The last day of low basal body temperature was designated as day 0. The curves were arranged accordingly. The results were obtained by microradial immunodiffusion techniques. (Modified from Schumacher GFB. Soluble proteins of human cervical mucus. In: Elstein M, Moghissi KS, Borth R, editors. Cervical Mucus in Human Reproduction. Copenhagen: Scriptor, 1973:93–113.)

The mechanism of rapid sperm transport has been debated, but a passive phenomenon rather than active migration is conceded to play the primary role.[17] Several lines of evidence support this conclusion. Carbon particles placed in the vagina[53] have been found in the fallopian tubes in short order. Radiolabeled inert particles display a similar migration pattern.[54] In fact, radionuclide hysterosalpingoscintigraphy has been proposed as a test of functional tubal patency.[55, 56] In a number of animals, including the rabbit and the pig, even dead sperm exhibit rapid transport into the fallopian tube.[57, 58]

Although the concept of passive transport has been challenged because of experiments that failed to demonstrate the passage of radiographic contrast fluid through the cervix from a cervical cap,[59, 60] it has been pointed out that substantial biomechanical differences exist between small particles and a radiocontrast liquid.[18] Failure of contrast liquid to enter the uterus does not negate the evidence that supports the passive transport theory. Furthermore, unless the velocity of sperm in vivo is much greater than in vitro,[61] sperm are simply incapable of migrating unaided over such distances in the observed time.

The mechanism that best explains passive transport is thought to be coordinated contractions of the vagina, uterus, and fallopian tubes. Such contractions are well documented at orgasm. Seminal prostaglandins or other substances such as endothelin, a 21–amino acid peptide with potent smooth muscle–stimulating activity, may also play a role.[62] In keeping with this hypothesis, double mating in rabbits enhances early

sperm transport, even when the second coital stimulus is from a vasectomized male. The destruction of vaginal sperm 2 minutes after a single mating resulted in a 25% fertilization rate. The same experiment performed after a double mating resulted in 90% fertilization.[32]

Although rapid sperm transport clearly occurs, the biologic significance of this phenomenon remains obscure. There is evidence that the first sperm to enter the reproductive tract may not be functional. In rabbits,[63] sheep,[64] and hamsters,[65] all species that demonstrate rapid sperm transport, postcoital tubal ligation prevents fertility. In addition, capacitation is required to modify the sperm head membrane so it is capable of undergoing the acrosome reaction, and capacitation is a process that requires time—hours rather than the minutes reported for rapid sperm transport.[66] In the rabbit model at least, most of the sperm observed in the fallopian tube after rapid transport are disrupted, immotile, and nonviable.[67]

Delayed Transport and the Sperm Reservoir

The arguments in support of the sperm reservoir hypothesis are several. Within hours of deposition, sperm that remain in the vagina perish, and it is unlikely that the human vagina performs a sperm storage function. At the same time, normal midcycle cervical mucus is alkaline, and sperm that gain access to the endocervical canal remain viable for many hours,[68–70] perhaps for as long as 7 days.[71] A number of sperm reach the fallopian tube quickly,[4] but they may not be competent to fertilize an oocyte. The fertilizing spermatozoa probably reach the fallopian tubes later, after capacitation has had time to occur. Motile sperm have been seen in the human oviduct in hysterectomy specimens as long as 50 hours after insemination,[52] 85 hours after intercourse,[72] and in the peritoneal cavity 36 hours after coitus.[73] Because vaginal sperm are quickly rendered nonviable, motile sperm in the upper reproductive tract must come from another reservoir. It is unclear whether that reservoir is the cervix or a site higher in the reproductive tract, and the reservoir may be different in different species.[74] In the rabbit model, for instance, the isthmus of the fallopian tube probably serves as a sperm reservoir.[75] The mechanisms of tubal sperm retention and release in the rabbit have been reviewed[17] and probably include adherence of sperm to epithelial surfaces and a reversible suppression of motility, perhaps mediated by changes in potassium ion concentrations.[75]

Several lines of evidence are seen as favoring a cervical storage site, including the configuration of the endocervical epithelium, with its multiple clefts and crypts. In ruminants, sperm are observed unevenly distributed in the cervical canal, aggregated near the mucosa.[76] There is also evidence of depressed sperm motility at these sites and of adherence to mucosal surfaces. In vitro, sperm enter human cervical mucus readily when it is stretched, and human cervical mucus stretched on a slide is seen to form channels.[36, 77] Although there has been no direct observation of such an organization in vivo, it has been postulated that the flow of cervical mucus from endocervical cells to the vagina causes a similar linear alignment of macromolecules, creating low-resistance channels that guide sperm to cervical crypts.[77, 78] It has not been established, however, that sperm in cervical crypts or adherent to cervical mucosa are able to leave and migrate to the fallopian tubes. It may be that sperm in cervical mucus remain there and represent an excluded population, trapped in the lower reproductive tract.

It is clear, however, that human sperm in cervical mucus retain their functional capacity for at least several days. Clinically, there is a correlation between fertility and the number of sperm seen in cervical mucus 48 hours after artificial insemination with fresh donor spermatozoa.[79] Sperm recovered from cervical mucus as long as 80 hours after artificial insemination are capable of penetrating the human zona pellucida, and sperm recovered as long as 120 hours after artificial insemination are motile and have swimming speeds comparable with freshly capacitated sperm.[80–82] Almost 100% of viable sperm recovered from cervical mucus as long as 3 days after artificial insemination have an intact acrosome, and these sperm are able to undergo an acrosome reaction in response to a biologic stimulus.[83]

Capacitation

The cervix and cervical mucus are important not only to sperm transport but also to the regulation of sperm physiology. Capacitation is one clear example. Several excellent reviews are available.[84, 85]

The mature human oocyte has a number of investing layers that must be penetrated for fertilization to occur. The sperm, in turn, has a number of enzymes designed to assist in oocyte penetration, including hyaluronidase, corona-penetrating enzyme, and acrosin. These enzymes are found in a caplike region of the sperm nucleus that is known as the *acrosome*. The acrosome reaction is a process that involves the localized fusion of sections of the double-layered acrosomal membrane, lysis of these fused areas, vesiculation, and dispersal and release of the acrosomal contents. A prerequisite for the acrosome reaction is capacitation. Capacitation involves modification of the sperm head membrane so it is capable of undergoing the acrosome reaction. It is important that the acrosome reaction occur in the immediate vicinity of the oocyte, and to that end seminal fluid has been shown to contain a high-molecular-weight decapacitation factor that is thought to coat or otherwise alter the sperm head membrane to prevent the acrosome reaction from occurring prematurely. Seminal spermatozoa are incapable of penetrating the human zona pellucida or of fusing with the zona-free hamster oocyte.[82] Capacitation can be accomplished in vitro over 5 to 7 hours,[86] making in vitro fertilization possible. In vivo, capacitation occurs during residence in the female reproductive tract, and cervical mucus appears to be involved in that process. Sperm recovered from cervical mucus demonstrate capacitation by their ability to acrosome react and penetrate the human zona pellucida even when recovered as long as 80 hours after insemination, demonstrating not only that capacitation has occurred but also that the capacitated state can be maintained over time.[80–82] Electron-microscopic observations of acrosomal status[83, 87] are consistent. Collectively, these data support the concept of a cervical sperm reservoir.

The mechanism of capacitation remains unclear. The process is reversible, whereas the acrosome reaction is not. There are no apparent structural changes associated with the capacitated state, consistent with its reversibility. Capacitated sperm reincubated in seminal plasma become decapacitated, losing their ability to penetrate oocyte investments.[88] Physiologic changes are clearly associated with the capacitated state, as reflected by hyperactivated sperm motility.[89] Seminal fluid and cervical mucus enzymes may be involved. The corona-penetrating enzyme, for example, is thought to be an esterase, and seminal plasma has esterase inhibitor activity. The removal or modification of such inhibitors by counterregulatory enzymes in cervical mucus or by biomechanical shearing as sperm push through the meshwork of mucin filaments[15] may be involved in capacitation.

Sperm Selection

Periovulatory human cervical mucus selectively restricts the migration of morphologically abnormal human spermatozoa. The proportion of morphologically normal spermatozoa in cervical mucus[29, 52, 90–93] and in uterine fluid[1] after intercourse is much higher (80% to 90%) than is typically seen in semen (50%). These observations have been confirmed following artificial insemination[29, 94] when the parameters of the inseminate have been characterized and sperm morphology in cervical mucus and semen can be more accurately compared. These differences can be seen as early as 1 hour after insemination, suggesting that morphologically abnormal spermatozoa are culled, at least in part, by a process of restricted entry. In vitro studies support these findings.[95]

The mechanism of sperm selection is not entirely clear but is probably the result of both intrinsic sperm properties and sperm–cervical mucus interaction. Simultaneous analysis of human sperm motility and morphology in semen shows that morphologically abnormal sperm are less likely to be motile and swim with a lower velocity than normal cells.[96, 97] Sperm migration through simple culture medium in a capillary tube also selects a morphologically enriched population (74% normal), an effect best explained by intrinsic differences in sperm motility, but the proportion of morphologically normal sperm is significantly higher (91%) after the same ejaculate migrates through a cervical mucus column,[98] suggesting that mucus also plays a role. Katz and associates[99] used videomicrography to simultaneously analyze sperm motility and morphology in human cervical mucus in vitro. Morphologically normal sperm swam faster but flagellar beat frequencies and amplitudes were not different for normal versus abnormal sperm, suggesting that morphologically abnormal sperm meet greater resistance from mucus and that this difference, rather than decreased intrinsic sperm vigor, is responsible for the exclusion of abnormal cells.

Summary

In summary, the normal cervix behaves like a biologic valve, alternately supporting or preventing the transport of spermatozoa from the vagina to the upper reproductive tract. The mucus-secreting cells of the endocervical epithelium respond to changes in circulating estrogen and progesterone. The preovulatory increase in estrogen stimulates these cells to produce an abundant, thin cervical mucus with maximal volume, pH, spinnbarkeit and ferning, and minimal viscosity and cellularity on the day before or the day of the serum LH peak. (These characteristics have been graded in a semiquantitative manner, known as the *cervical mucus score* [Table 18–

TABLE 18–1. The Cervical Mucus Score

A. Volume
　0: 0 mL
　1: 0.1 mL
　2: 0.2 mL
　3: 0.3 mL or more

B. Consistency
　0: Thick, highly "viscous," premenstrual mucus
　1: Mucus of intermediate "viscosity"
　2: Mildly "viscous" mucus
　3: Watery, minimally "viscous," midcycle (preovulatory) mucus

C. Ferning
　0: No crystallization
　1: Atypical fern formation
　2: Primary and secondary stem ferning
　3: Tertiary and quaternary stem ferning

D. Spinnbarkeit
　0: <1 cm
　1: 1–4 cm
　2: 5–8 cm
　3: 9 cm or more

E. Cellularity
　0: >20 cells per hpf
　1: 11–20 cells per hpf
　2: 1–10 cells per hpf
　3: 0 cells

hpf, high-power field.

1].[100–102]) In normal midcycle cervical mucus, some sperm are rapidly transported to the upper reproductive tract, whereas a selected group with normal morphology populates the cervical crypts where they may be stored and periodically released, ensuring a continuous supply of capacitated, acrosome-intact sperm capable of fertilization.

CERVICAL FACTOR INFERTILITY: DEFINITION AND DIAGNOSTIC TESTS

Definitions

Cervical abnormalities associated with infertility can be defined as (1) failure to produce optimal cervical mucus as judged by the cervical mucus score (in which case poor sperm penetration and survival are expected) or (2) failure of sperm penetration and survival despite apparently optimal periovulatory mucus (the unexpected poor PCT). Because either anovulation or poor timing may result in a suboptimal cervical score, the cervical factor cannot be judged fairly without knowledge of the patient's ovulatory status and of the relationship between postcoital testing and the time of ovulation. Similarly, disorders that prevent the intravaginal deposition of an ejaculate (e.g., severe dyspareunia, impotence, severe hypospadias) or an abnormality of sperm number, motility, or morphology (e.g., classic male factor infertility) may result in abnormal sperm penetration and survival. The cervical factor cannot be judged fairly without documentation that coitus and intravaginal ejaculation occurred or without an independent evaluation of semen parameters. The latter is particularly important, because the relationship between semen quality and the number of motile sperm in periovulatory cervical mucus after either coitus or artificial insemination has been well documented (Fig. 18–6).[29, 103–106] In the absence of an independent assessment of semen quality, poor sperm penetration and survival with a normal cervical score should be presumed secondary to male rather than cervical factors.

Table 18–2 classifies the possible causes of an abnormal PCT.

Diagnostic Tests

There are two broad components to the clinical evaluation of cervical function: (1) a semiquantitative assessment of cervical anatomy and cervical mucus production at midcycle (the cervical or cervical mucus score[100–102]) and (2) an assessment of sperm–cervical mucus interaction, under in vivo or in vitro circumstances, by counting the number, motility, and movement quality of sperm in cervical mucus. The cervical mucus score has been variously described. The World Health Organization (WHO) version totals 15; 10 or more points defines normal. The in vivo test has been practiced for more than a century and is known as the *Sims-Huhner test*, or PCT.[107–110]

THE POSTCOITAL TEST

The Controversy. Despite its longtime use, the PCT remains the subject of heated contemporary debate. Accepted

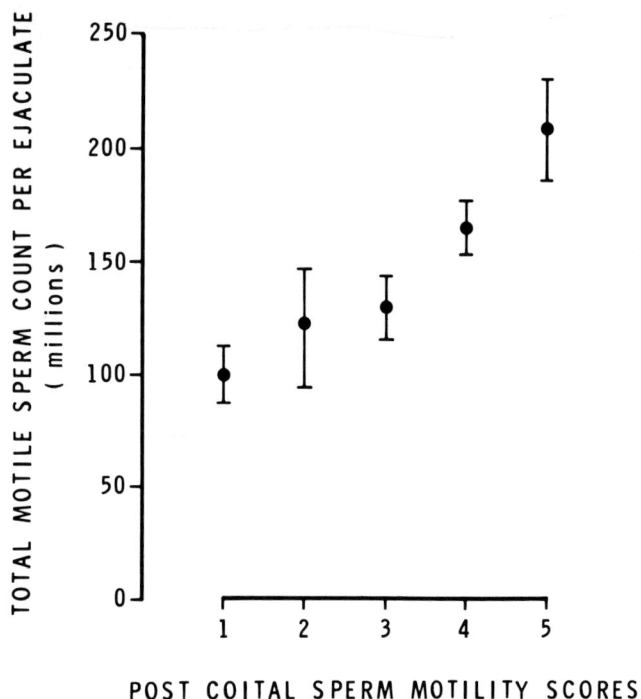

POST COITAL SPERM MOTILITY SCORES

FIGURE 18–6. Total motile sperm count per ejaculate as determined by semen analysis and postcoital sperm motility scores. Postcoital sperm motility groups are as follows: 1, no sperm seen; 2, no motile sperm; 3, 1 to 5 motile sperm per high-power field (hpf); 4, 6 to 10 motile sperm per hpf; and 5, 11 or more motile sperm per hpf. Analysis of variance: F = 5.38, P < 0.001. (From Collins JA, So Y, Wilson EH, Wrixon W, Casper RF. The postcoital test as a predictor of pregnancy among 355 infertile couples. Fertil Steril 1984; 41:703–708. Reproduced with permission of the publisher, The American Fertility Society.)

as an essential component of the infertility investigation by the American College of Obstetricians and Gynecologists,[111] the American Fertility Society,[112] WHO,[102] and most modern texts[113–117] and reviews,[118] it has been alternately described as "an unnecessary and cumbersome process"[119] with little value in predicting infertility, and "a clear and useful means of predicting the chance of conception."[120] A recent review provocatively concludes:

Despite performance of millions on millions of postcoital tests during the past century, the validity of the test has never been established. The limited available literature suggests that its validity is poor. The lack of standard technique, the absence of population-based norms, and the large effect of biologic variation render the existing literature nearly uninterpretable.[119]

There has been considerable skepticism about the negative and positive predictive value of postcoital testing—the ability of a normal (negative) test to exclude a cervical factor and identify couples who will conceive, and the ability of an abnormal (positive) test to identify a cervical factor and couples who will not conceive. That skepticism is based on several lines of evidence, including several reports (Table 18–3) that noted a poor correlation between PCT results and the ability to recover sperm from the upper reproductive tract, either the uterine fundus[1] or the peritoneal cavity, after intercourse[121, 122, 124, 125] or after artificial insemination.[123] The fact that sperm were recovered from the peritoneal cavity in 44%

to 86% of patients who had a poor PCT suggests that the PCT is a poor predictor of sperm transport and, by inference, fertility. The observation that patients with a positive peritoneal sperm recovery test had a significantly higher crude pregnancy rate than those with no peritoneal sperm (46.2% versus 9.5%, respectively)[124] lends credence to that argument. In addition, there are many reports of a poor correlation between either cervical mucus quality or postcoital sperm penetration and survival and a couple's ability to conceive (Table 18–4). Crude pregnancy rates between 37% and 39% were reported for infertile women with poor-quality cervical mucus, whereas only 43% to 54% of patients with good-quality mucus conceived.[126, 127] The 24-month cumulative pregnancy rates in subjects with poor versus good mucus scores were 41.4% and 47.0%, respectively.[103] Poor-quality cervical mucus is even reported in 17% to 18% of conception cycles (Table 18–5).[126, 130, 131]

The high false-positive and false-negative rates for PCT scores are equally apparent (see Table 18–4). When there were no sperm or only rare sperm at postcoital testing, crude pregnancy rates were still 32% to 42%,[126, 127] the per cycle conception rate was 25%,[128] and the 24-month cumulative pregnancy rate was 36%.[103] With normal test results, crude pregnancy rates were 49% to 56%,[126, 127] the per cycle conception rate was 22%,[128] and the 24-month cumulative pregnancy rate was only 44%.[103] Poor sperm penetration and survival (no sperm or only rare motile sperm) were also reported in 12% to 25% of conception cycles[126, 130, 131] and in 23% of women who conceived within 3 months of the PCT.[1]

Arguments for the Validity of Postcoital Testing. There are, however, several problems with these data. First, none of the studies in Table 18–3 conclusively proved that the spermatozoa found in peritoneal fluid at the time of laparoscopy were not there from a preceding coital event, when sperm–cervical mucus interaction was presumably more normal. Stone[125] did not specify the abstinence interval; Templeton

TABLE 18–2. The Abnormal Postcoital Test: Classification of Possible Causes

A. Repeated failure to produce normal periovulatory cervical mucus
1. Inadequate number of normal mucus-producing endocervical cells
  a. Acquired
    (1) Destruction of endocervical cells by surgery
    (2) Destruction of endocervical cells by infection
  b. Congenital
    (1) Isolated cervical agenesis or aplasia
    (2) Diethylstilbestrol-associated anomalies
    (3) Cystic fibrosis
2. Inadequate response of normal numbers of mucus-producing endocervical cells to an estrogen stimulus
  a. Receptor blocked by antiestrogen
  b. Primary receptor disorder
  c. Cervical infection
3. Inadequate estrogen stimulus
B. Repeated failure of normal periovulatory cervical mucus to support sperm penetration and survival
1. Overlooked male factor
  a. Coital problem
  b. Abnormal semen parameters
  c. Sperm-bound antisperm antibodies
2. Vaginal factor
3. Normal male factor, hostile cervical mucus
  a. Abnormal cervical mucus pH
  b. Cervical mucus antisperm antibodies
4. Idiopathic hostile cervical mucus

TABLE 18–3. Postcoital Testing: Sperm in Cervical Mucus Versus Uterine or Peritoneal Sperm

Author	Study Variables	Study Population	No. of Subjects	Covariables	PCT Definition	Study Outcome	
						PCT Result	*Percentage with Uterine or Peritoneal Sperm (%)*
Grant, 1958[1]	PCT vs. fundal sperm	Infertile with positive fundal test	368	Not specified	Poor: none progressively motile	Poor	10
Asch, 1976 and 1978[121, 122]	PCT vs. peritoneal sperm	Infertile with three poor PCT in 18 mo	14	All ovulatory, NL mucus, NL SE, NL HSG, NL cervical anatomy	Neg: no sperm Poor: no motile sperm	Neg Poor	80 100
Templeton and Mortimer, 1980[123]	PCT (after AIH) vs. peritoneal sperm	Infertile ≥2 yr	24	All ovulatory, NL SE, NL HSG, NL laparoscopy	Poor: no motile sperm Good: any number motile sperm	Poor Good	71 59
Templeton and Mortimer, 1982[124]	PCT (after AIH or coitus) vs. peritoneal sperm	Infertile ≥2 yr	47	All ovulatory, NL SE, NL HSG, NL laparoscopy	Poor: no motile sperm Good: any number motile sperm	Poor (AIH) Poor (PCT) Good (AIH) Good (PCT)	80 44 50 62
Templeton and Mortimer, 1982[124]	Peritoneal sperm vs. pregnancy	Infertile ≥2 yr	47	All ovulatory, NL SE, NL HSG, NL laparoscopy	Neg: no peritoneal sperm	Neg Pos	9.5 (pregnant) 46.2 (pregnant)
Stone, 1983[125]	PCT vs. peritoneal sperm	"Normal infertile"	40	"Comprehensive evaluation revealed no other factor" and NL laparoscopy	Poor: no motile sperm Good: any number motile sperm	Poor Good	56.1 53.3

NL, normal; Neg, negative; Pos, positive; PCT, post coital test; AIH, artificial insemination with husband's sperm; SE, semen evaluation; HSG, hysterosalpingogram.

and Mortimer[124] and Asch[121, 122] reported 3 and 4 days of abstinence, respectively, and it is possible that sperm from a more remote coital event might have remained. There was no convincing effort to verify abstinence by daily vaginal and cervical examinations.

More important, it is a misconception to think that the presence of sperm in the peritoneal cavity reflects physiologic sperm transport. As reviewed earlier, the phenomenon of rapid sperm transport has been clearly documented. Rapid transport is primarily passive, probably mediated by smooth muscle contractions in the female reproductive tract. The functional importance of rapidly transported sperm is in doubt both because of the requirement for capacitation and because rapidly transported sperm frequently appear disrupted. Given these facts, a correlation between sperm in the peritoneal cavity and sperm in cervical mucus is not necessarily expected. Currently, there is no direct information about the functional competence of sperm isolated from the peritoneal cavity. The significantly higher pregnancy rate in couples with positive peritoneal sperm recovery is interesting, but none of those subjects, nor the four reported by Asch,[122] conceived in the cycle of testing, so the physiologic significance of these studies remains unclear.

For the most part, the high false-positive and false-negative rates illustrated in Table 18–4 can be explained by failure to recognize the narrowness of the periovulatory window of normal sperm penetration, poor PCT timing, the inappropriate use of crude rather than cumulative pregnancy rates,[132, 133] and poorly defined infertile populations whose success or

failure versus PCT results is confounded by unrecognized covariables. There is now abundant evidence that (1) the window of optimal cervical mucus, especially for sperm penetration, is narrow, making timing critical; (2) optimal timing is difficult—a single PCT planned on clinical grounds for the predicted periovulatory phase has a high probability of falling outside of the optimal window; and (3) the most common cause of an abnormal PCT (in couples with normal semen parameters) is poor timing. In an extension of Moghissi and associates' classic work,[33] Kerin and colleagues[134] collected and stored daily cervical mucus samples over 5 or 6 periovulatory days in 47 cycles in 23 women with azoospermic partners. Mucus samples were tested with a single-donor ejaculate, eliminating sperm parameters as a variable. The maximum cervical score was noted on day 0 (day of the serum LH peak) and the day before. Optimal in vitro linear sperm migration was also seen on day 0 and day −1 (Fig. 18–7), with significantly reduced sperm penetration on day −2 versus day −1, and day +1 versus day 0. The day-to-day changes in mucus quality and sperm penetration within subjects were considerable, and the authors concluded that "even within the periovulatory window, the use of any sperm-mucus test must . . . be timed critically."[134]

There is similar data from normospermic couples when daily midcycle cervical mucus samples were stored at 4°C and tested in vitro with a single ejaculate.[135] There was no apparent change in physicochemical properties of cervical mucus, or in its penetrability, after storage for as long as 14 days. Many of the samples were suboptimal, and the best day

			No. of Subjects with Poor	No. (and Percentage) of Subjects Who
Author(s)	No. of Subjects	Definitions for PCT/Mucus Results	vs. Good Result	Conceived
Buxton and Southam, 1958[126]	726	Mucus		
		Poor: thick, tenacious, cellular	201	79 (39.3)
		Good: clear, abundant to moderate, acellular	525	226 (43.0)
		Sperm		
		Poor: no sperm or rare motile sperm	171	54 (31.6)
		Good: > rare motile sperm	354	172 (48.9)
Jette and Glass, 1972[127]	205	Mucus		
		Poor: thick, tenacious, cloudy, loaded with WBCs	73	27 (37.0)
		Good: clear, watery, no WBC	132	71 (53.8)
		Sperm		
		Good CM: 0 sperm	27	12 (45)
		Good CM: any number of sperm	105	59 (56)
		Good CM: >20 sperm	32	25 (78)
Giner et al, 1974[128]	107 (cycles)	Poor: no sperm or no motile sperm	40	10 (25 per cycle)
		Good: 1 or more, motility grade 3	67	15 (22 per cycle)
Taymor, 1978[129]	569	Poor: <5 active sperm/hpf	168	47 (28)
		Equivocal: 5–9	233	77 (33)
		Good: >10	168	79 (47)
Collins et al, 1984[103]	355	Mucus		
		Score 0–3	—	41.4% at 24 mo
		Score 7–9	—	47.0% at 24 mo
		Sperm		
		Poor: no sperm	—	35.5% at 24 mo
		Poor: none motile	—	28.5% at 24 mo
		Good: 1–5	—	30.7% at 24 mo
		Good: 6–10	—	47.9% at 24 mo
		Good: >10	—	44.4% at 24 mo

PCT, postcoital test; WBC, White blood cell; CM, cervical mucus; hpf, high-power field.

for sperm penetration could be determined only after testing serial samples. A number of the normal tests would not have been seen if testing had been performed only once, and half of the patients who had previously demonstrated negative PCTs had normal penetration when tested in vitro over several mucus samples. These studies provide clear evidence that, even around midcycle, cervical mucus varies significantly and the cause of infertility should not be said to be cervical unless based on repeated tests when optimal timing has been ensured.

Serial postcoital testing is the exception, not the rule. The nine studies profiled in Table 18–6 are representative of more than 20 reviewed and are compared with current WHO recommendations for postcoital testing. For each study, the table lists the method by which the PCT was timed; whether single or repeated tests were performed; and a number of other variables of test performance, including the period of abstinence prior to testing, the interval between coitus and postcoital testing, and the source and method of collection of cervical mucus. Only one study[120] verified an abnormal result by repeat testing, and all gauged midcycle by the usual clinical criteria: cycle length, basal body temperature (BBT) pattern, and cervical mucus score. In stimulated cycles, a single human chorionic gonadotropin (hCG)-timed PCT may suffice,[136] but BBT nadir and serum LH peak are coincident or within 1 day of one another in only 65% of cycles,[137] and PCTs timed by BBT frequently fall outside of the narrow window of optimal sperm penetration. The relationship between the cervical score and the serum LH peak is debated. In one study,[137] the peak mucus score and the LH peak were coincident or within 1 day of one another in 93% of 171 cycles in which both were identified. In another,[138] timing based on cervical mucus parameters resulted in postcoital testing over a 6-day window, extending from 3 days before to 2 days after the serum LH peak. Because the serum LH peak generally precedes the urinary LH surge by 12 hours,[139] even a PCT planned for the day after the urinary LH surge may be late, and planning PCTs for the day of the surge would be logistically difficult for both patients and physicians. Given these difficulties, the practical solution is serial testing and the verification of abnormal tests by repetition in a separate cycle. Under these conditions, the predictive value of postcoital testing has been convincingly demonstrated. The best example is the report by Hull and coworkers.[120]

					Proportion with Poor vs. Good Result in Conception Cycle	
Author(s)	**Study Variables**	**Study Subjects**	**No. of Subjects**	**Definitions for PCT/Mucus**	*No. of Poor (%)*	*No. of Good (%)*

Buxton and Southam, 1958[126]	Mucus quality in conception cycles	Infertile women, not otherwise defined	70	Mucus
				  Poor: thick, tenacious, cellular
				  Good to fair: clear, abundant, acellular
					12/70 (17.1)	58/70 (82.9)

Danezis et al, 1962[130]	Mucus quality in conception cycles	Infertile women, ovulatory by BBT	33	Mucus
				  Poor: scanty, opaque, viscous, cellular, poor spinn
				  Good: abundant. clear, watery, acellular, spinn >10 cm
					6/33 (18)	27/33 (82)

Buxton and Southam, 1958[126]	Sperm migration in conception cycles	Infertile women, not otherwise defined	70	PCT
				  Poor: no sperm or rare motile sperm
				  Good: more than rare motile sperm
					10/40 (25) (of those with good mucus)	30/40 (75) (of those with good mucus)

Danezis et al, 1962[130]	PCT in conception cycles	Infertile women ovulatory by BBT	33	PCT
				  Poor: no sperm or none motile
				  Good: any motile sperm, grade 3 or better
					4/33 (12)	29/33 (88)

TABLE 18–5. Postcoital Testing: Results in Conception Cycles

PCT, postcoital test; BBT, basal body temperature; spinn, spinnbarkeit.

Their study group consisted of 80 patients with at least 12 months of infertility, all with normal male factor and confirmed ovulatory cycles. Patients who never produced good-quality cervical mucus were excluded, as were those with bilateral tubal or peritubal disease at laparoscopy or a significant uterine anomaly. The PCT was planned for 14 to 16 days before expected menses and endocervical mucus was aspirated 6 to 18 hours after coitus. Strict criteria were used to define a negative test. At least three microscopic fields in separate parts of the mucus sample were examined to count the number of progressively motile sperm, and an extensive search was made when none could be found. A negative test was defined as either no sperm or no progressively motile sperm, and an initial negative test was accepted as valid only

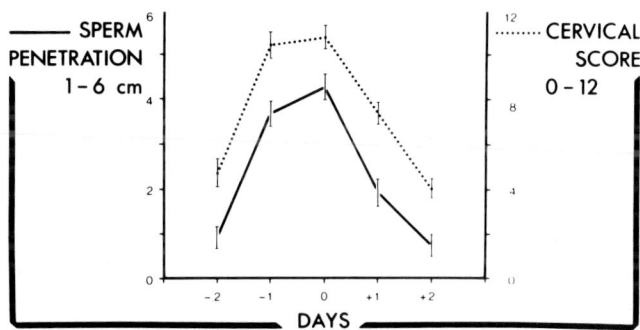

FIGURE 18–7. Relationships between cervical mucus score and linear sperm migration in 47 cycles. Day 0 is the day of the serum luteinizing hormone peak. (Modified from Kerin JF, Matthews CD, Svigos JM, Makin AE, Symons RG, Smeaton TC. Linear and quantitative migration of stored sperm through cervical mucus during the periovular period. Fertil Steril 1976;27:1054–1058. Reproduced with permission of the publisher, The American Fertility Society.)

if (1) the cervical mucus score was normal, and (2) the same result was obtained on repeat testing in another menstrual cycle. Time-specific cumulative conception rates were calculated by life table analysis and were compared for patients with negative versus positive PCTs. The 24-month cumulative conception rates in those two groups were significantly different, at 16% and 84%, respectively (Fig. 18–8). The authors concluded that, when confounding infertility factors are excluded and strict criteria are used to define a negative PCT, the test "provides a clear-cut and useful prognosis for fertility."[120]

Standards for Postcoital Testing: Time and Sampling Variables. Beyond the problems of poor timing, inadequately defined study populations, and invalid outcome measures, postcoital testing has long suffered from the lack of standardized performance criteria. Table 18–6 also profiles representative inconsistencies in abstinence interval, the coitus-to-PCT interval, and mucus sampling techniques.

Abstinence Interval. The number of sperm available for ejaculation (the extragonadal reserve [EGR]) is a function of the rate of sperm production by the testes, sperm resorption by the epididymides, and sperm removal from the EGR by ejaculation.[140] Men have a small EGR, and ejaculate volume, sperm concentration, and total motile sperm numbers decline as ejaculation frequency increases.[140–146] Because 2 days of abstinence is sufficient to restore the EGR[147] and sperm motility peaks after 3 days of abstinence,[144] a 2- to 3-day abstinence interval is commonly recommended to precede formal semen evaluation.[102] Despite these data and the clear link between ejaculate quality and the number of sperm in cervical mucus after coitus, there is no direct information about the effect of varying abstinence intervals on PCT results in couples with either normal or abnormal semen parameters. The current WHO recommendation is that 2 days of

TABLE 18–6. Postcoital Testing: Time and Sampling Variables							
Author(s)	**Time in Cycle**	**Midcycle Gauged by:**	**Single or Repeated Test**	**No. of Days of Abstinence**	**No. of Hours— Coitus to PCT**	**Mucus Source**	**Sampling Instrument**
Grant, 1958[1]	Approximate time when ovulation was expected	BBT	Single	NS	2–8	Cervical	NS
Danezis et al, 1962[130]	−48 to +24 h from thermal shift	BBT	Single	NS	1–8 (82% 1–4)	Endocervical	TB syringe, no needle
Glass and Mroueh, 1967[104]	At midcycle	NS	Single	NS	10–16	Endocervical	Nasal polyp forceps
Giner et al, 1974[128]	During the ovulatory period	BBT	Single	NS	2–8	Cervical	Papanicolaou pipette
Asch, 1976[121]	At midcycle	Cycle day 12–16, good cervical score	Single	4	3–8	Cervical	TB syringe
Tredway et al, 1978[106]	At midcycle	Spinn >6 cm	Single	2	2	Endocervical, fractional method	3-mm polyethylene catheter and syringe
Skaf and Kemmann, 1982[136]	Day hCG was given or day before	hMG/hCG cycle; daily E₂	Single	NS	8–12	Endocervical	No. 18 polyethylene tube
Hull et al, 1982[120]	14–16 days before expected menses	Cycle length, mucus score	Repeated	NS	6–18	Endocervical	10-cm 1-mL syringe, no needle
Collins et al, 1984[103]	Preovulatory phase	NS	Repeated when no mucus obtained	NS	2–12	Endocervical	By suction
World Health Organization, 1992[102]	As closely as possible to the time of ovulation	Clinical criteria and, when available, E₂ assay, ultrasonography	Repeated if negative or abnormal	2	9–24	Endocervical	TB syringe, pipette, or polyethylene tube

NS, not specified; BBT, basal body temperature; TB, tuberculin; Spinn, Spinnbarkeit; hMG, human menopausal gonadotropin; hCG, human chorionic gonadotropin; E₂, estradiol.

abstinence precede postcoital testing.[102] Longer or shorter intervals may influence test results and should at least be noted.

Coitus-to-PCT Interval. Immediately after intercourse, the population of spermatozoa in cervical mucus increases as sperm escape from the vagina to survive. In the absence of a vaginal sperm reservoir, the population of cervical spermato-

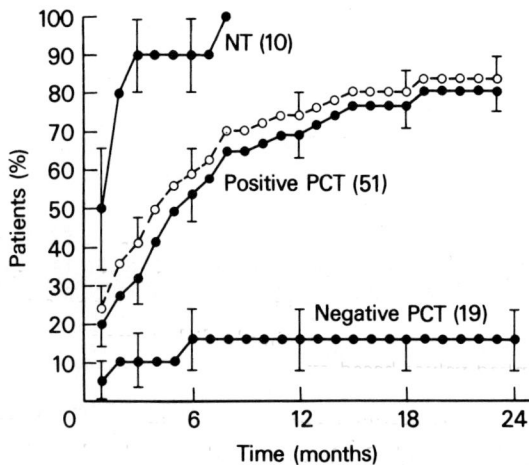

FIGURE 18–8. Cumulative conception rates related to the result of the postcoital test (PCT). NT, not tested. The *open circles* represent a subgroup from pooling of NT and positive PCT groups. SE bars are shown. (Modified from Hull MGR, Savage PE, Bromham DR. Prognostic value of the postcoital test: prospective study based on time-specific conception rates. Br J Obstet Gynecol 1982;89:299–305.)

zoa stabilizes early[148] and remains stable for at least the next 24 hours.[69] Postcoital testing has usually been done within 24 hours of intercourse, but the interval has not been standardized and is the subject of some controversy (see reference 149 for a review.) An early test (1 to 3 hours after intercourse), a standard test (6 to 10 hours after intercourse), and a delayed test (18 to 24 hours after intercourse) all have been described.[112] There is little direct evidence that one interval is better than another, although an early test is intuitively the least desirable of the three. The prescription of a short interval between coitus and testing presents obvious practical problems for many couples, including anxiety and nonperformance. In addition, the physiologic significance of short-term sperm survival is debatable. Given the concept of a cervical sperm reservoir, the demonstration of survival beyond 3 hours would appear to be more reassuring.

The distinction between standard and delayed tests appears less clear, considering that the number of sperm in cervical mucus is constant over the first 24 hours. One may postulate that couples with the longest period of sperm survival have the best chance to conceive, but there are no direct data to support that hypothesis. In practical terms, a protocol that minimizes stress is recommended. In keeping with current WHO guidelines,[102] we suggest that coitus take place sometime the night before the day of postcoital testing, allowing whatever flexibility best suits a couple's schedule.

Source of Cervical Mucus. Sperm survival in cervical mucus is affected by mucus pH. Within the cervical canal there is a pH gradient; exocervical mucus has a lower pH than mucus found in the more protected confines of the upper endocervical canal.[12, 20] As a consequence, the upper and

TABLE 18–7. Postcoital Testing: Classification of Test Results						
Author(s)	**Classification System**					
Grant, 1958[1]	None	None progressing	Any number progressing	—	—	—
Danezis et al, 1962[130]	None	None motile	1–5 grade 3	6–15 grade 3	>15 grade 3	—
Glass and Mroueh, 1967[104]	None	1–2 progressive	3–5	6–10	11–20	>20
Giner et al, 1974[128]	None	None motile	1–5 grade 3	6–10 grade 3	>10 grade 3	—
Asch, 1976[121]	None	None motile	1–4 actively motile	≥ 5 active	—	—
Tredway et al, 1978[106]	—	—	<5 motile	5–9	10–15	>15
Skaf and Kemmann, 1982[136]	—	None motile	1–4 motile	5–9	10–19	>20
Hull et al, 1982[120]	None	None motile	1–5 forward moving	6–20	>20	—
Collins et al, 1984[103]	None	None motile	1–5 motile	6–10	≥11	—
World Health Organization, 1992[102]	<500/mm^3 with directional motility			>500/mm^2 with directional motility		

lower canals differ in their sperm population dynamics. Within 2 or 3 hours after intercourse, sperm are found in large numbers in both the lower and upper canal. After 4 hours, however, the population of sperm in the lower canal decreases, whereas that in the upper canal remains constant over 24 hours.[148] The source of cervical mucus is clearly a variable that may influence PCT results.

The collection of cervical mucus has not been standardized, and much of the literature about postcoital testing is vague with regard to mucus source. A variety of collection devices have been described (see Table 18–6), including nasal polyp forceps, syringes with or without needles attached, and flexible plastic cannulas of different materials and construction, with obvious differences in their ability to sample mucus from the upper cervical canal. The fractional PCT was an effort to standardize cervical mucus collection.[150] A 3-mm polyethylene catheter was slowly advanced from the external to internal cervical os while gently aspirating a mucus column. Cervical mucus at the tip of the catheter was thought to represent a sample from the upper canal, whereas mucus closest to the syringe represented a sample from the lower cervix. The fractional technique was never validated, either clinically[151] or methodologically, and has since been largely abandoned. In fact, this technique contaminated mucus in the upper canal with material from the lower cervix.[152] The simple precaution of removing exocervical mucus with a forceps or a cotton swab is a more practical approach and ensures recovery of an uncontaminated endocervical sample. The primary requirement of the collection device itself is that it be able to aspirate from within the canal; no particular instrument has been designated as the standard.[102]

Standards for Postcoital Testing: Assessment of Sperm in Cervical Mucus

Microscope. Variables such as specimen preparation, optical configuration, and image-processing algorithms are now recognized as critical factors in computer-aided sperm analysis (CASA),[153] and standards have been promulgated to enhance the accuracy and reproducibility of CASA measures.[154] Little has been done, however, to standardize the microscopic assessment of sperm in cervical mucus. The length of time between specimen collection and microscopic examination, ambient temperature and temperature of the optical stage, and sample volume and pH stability all are factors that may affect sperm survival. The thickness of the cervical mucus preparation (the distance between the microscope slide and the coverslip), the degree of magnification, and the number

and location of optical fields surveyed affect the number of motile sperm seen and classification of the test as normal or abnormal. My review of more than 20 studies published between 1958 and 1987 indicates that most of these variables are usually ignored.[1, 29, 69, 103, 104, 106, 120, 121, 123, 125–130, 136, 138, 155–157] Only six studies specified the degree of magnification,[106, 120, 128, 130, 155, 157] and only six indicated that more than one optical field was surveyed.[120, 123, 126, 128, 129, 136] None used any systematic approach, such as a grid, to ensure that representative, nonoverlapping fields were examined. Some progress has been made. WHO's revised *Laboratory Manual for the Examination of Human Semen and Semen–Cervical Mucus Interaction*[102] recommended that slides be examined at 400×. For the first time, there was also a recommendation for standardization of the depth of the mucus sample by supporting the coverslip with silicone grease impregnated with 100-μ glass microspheres. When the slide-to-coverslip distance is constant, a known volume of cervical mucus is examined in each microscopic field of view, and a sperm concentration can be calculated. Much of the variability in the microscopic portion of the PCT can be controlled by such spacers.[158]

Classification Systems. As currently practiced, the PCT is at best a semiquantitative measure of cervical mucus quality and sperm–cervical mucus interaction. In even its strictest form, the cervical mucus score (see Table 18–1)[100, 101] is largely a subjective measure, where cervical mucus volume, consistency, ferning, spinnbarkeit, and cellularity each are graded on a scale of zero to three. Sperm–cervical mucus interaction is typically judged by microscopic assessment of sperm in the mucus sample, but a formal count of the number and motility of sperm per average microscopic field has limited meaning considering the uncontrolled nature of the microscopic examination, the subjective terms used to grade motility, and the general lack of standards for PCT performance. A variety of classification schemes have been published to express PCT results—Table 18–7 outlines 10 of the most common. They vary from simple dichotomous assessments to ranked values based on sperm number and motility. Most count only motile sperm but differ in the subjective terms used to grade motility: active, progressive, forward moving, grade 2, and grade 3. Most are overly complex, because there is little evidence of a significant correlation between the conception rate and the number of motile sperm per field. It is clear from a number of studies[103, 120, 127–129] that the most important determinant is simply the presence or absence of any forward-moving spermatozoa. A PCT that reveals no sperm or only nonmotile sperm in cervical mucus is clearly not reassuring and should be repeated; the presence of any progressively motile spermatozoa makes cervical infertility unlikely and dictates completion of the workup for other causes.

Summary. In summary, the information about postcoital testing is confusing but not uninterpretable. The positive relationship between the number of motile sperm in the ejaculate and the numbers seen in cervical mucus seems well established, making it essential to independently evaluate semen quality. There is also general recognition of the dependence of cervical mucus characteristics on hormonal changes in the ovulatory cycle and the importance of periovulatory timing, but the narrowness of the window of optimal sperm penetration and the need to repeat nonreassuring tests have often been overlooked. Many of the reports about the validity of postcoital testing suffer from faults common to much of the infertility literature—incomplete and varying lengths of followup not corrected by life table methods, poorly characterized populations and failure to consider important covariables, and limited information about norms for fertile couples, who generally escape testing. In addition, the lack of strict standards for the test itself compounds the difficulty of comparing study outcomes. Standards have been developed by WHO,[102] and these should be the guide for test performance. Despite its shortcomings, postcoital testing is and should remain an important part of the basic infertility investigation.

IN VITRO TESTS

In vivo (postcoital) and in vitro tests of sperm–cervical mucus interaction are complementary. A normal PCT is reassuring and makes a cervical factor unlikely. In couples with normal semen parameters, abnormal PCTs usually reflect suboptimal timing. Nonreassuring PCTs must be repeated. Repeatedly abnormal PCT results in the face of normal semen parameters and estrogenic cervical mucus are puzzling. Timing and coital performance are always suspect, and either sperm or cervical mucus may be the cause of poor sperm penetration. These issues usually can be resolved with in vitro testing. The advantages are several. The ejaculate can be studied, and the testing of one or more mucus samples with a single well-characterized ejaculate eliminates the performance variables that cannot be accounted for in vivo. The collection of daily mucus samples ensures that cervical mucus is being evaluated during its period of optimal sperm penetrability, eliminating the abnormal PCTs caused by imprecise timing.[134, 135] Also, when done in the context of a crossed format, with sperm and cervical mucus from both donors and patients, in vitro tests both verify abnormal sperm–cervical mucus interaction and separate sperm from cervical mucus causes. Although lacking uniform standards, in vitro tests have generally been performed in two ways: on a flat microscope slide or in a capillary tube filled with estrogenic cervical mucus.

The most widely used modification of the original slide test is called the *sperm–cervical mucus contact* (SCMC) *test.*[159] A drop of semen and a drop of cervical mucus are placed next to one another on a glass microscope slide, thoroughly mixed, and covered with a coverslip. A second drop of semen (without mucus) is placed on the same slide. Sperm motility

is evaluated both with and without cervical mucus, usually in a crossed design that includes donor samples. A positive (abnormal) test result is defined as a change from progressive to nonprogressive or "shaking" motility by more than 25% of the spermatozoa. This peculiar motility pattern is thought to represent an interaction between the network of gel-phase glycoprotein molecules in cervical mucus and antisperm antibody (ASAB)-coated spermatozoa[160] because a portion of antibody "sticks" to glycoprotein filaments. The SCMC test is a valuable screen for ASABs. There is a good correlation between the proportion of sperm that exhibit shaking motility in the SCMC test and the proportion that are shown to be antibody bound by the immunoglobulin A (IgA) mixed-agglutination reaction (MAR) test (Fig. 18–9).[160]

The most widely used version of the capillary tube test (Fig. 18–10) was originally described by Kremer.[161] It is also semiquantitative. The endpoint is an assessment of the distance traveled by the vanguard spermatozoa over a given period of observation. At 2 hours, normal sperm should travel the full length of the column of cervical mucus, and the concentration of sperm at both ends of the capillary tube should be roughly equivalent, with most sperm progressively motile. There have been several modifications of the original sperm penetration meter,[161] seeking to improve the test's reproducibility,[162, 163] but no universal standard has been adopted, and the various forms of sperm–cervical mucus penetration (SCMP) tests remain subjective and semiquantitative. Nonetheless, there appears to be a significant correlation between the SCMP tests and both MAR-IgA and SCMC testing.[160, 164] Both capillary tube and slide tests are usually performed in a crossed format, testing sperm–cervical mucus interaction in a four-block design: donor sperm and donor

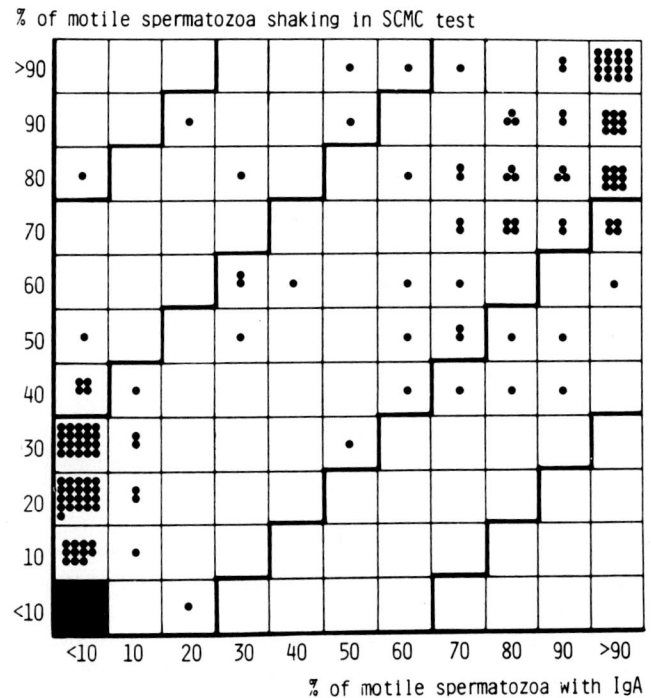

FIGURE 18–9. Agreement between the results of the mixed agglutination reaction immunoglobulin A (IgA) test and the sperm–cervical mucus contact (SCMC) test. (From Kremer J, Jager S. Sperm–cervical mucus interaction, in particular in the presence of antispermatozoal antibodies. Hum Reprod 1988;3:69–73; by permission of Oxford University Press.)

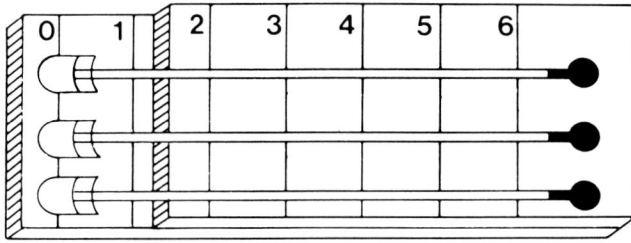

FIGURE 18–10. Sperm penetration meter (SPM). The flat capillary tubes are filled with cervical mucus. One end is closed with modeling clay, and the other end is placed in a small semen reservoir. The capillary tubes are on a higher level than the reservoirs to prevent the formation of a thin cleft into which semen is drawn by capillary force. The SPM is as large as a microscope slide. (From Kremer J, Jager S. Sperm–cervical mucus interaction, in particular in the presence of antispermatozoal antibodies. Hum Reprod 1988;3:69–73; by permission of Oxford University Press.)

mucus, donor sperm and patient's mucus, husband's sperm and donor mucus, and husband's sperm and patient's mucus.[157, 159, 161, 162, 165, 166] When abnormal sperm–cervical mucus interaction has been verified in vitro, and sperm or mucus causes identified by crossed testing, immunologic testing can be completed by either the MAR or immunobead methods.

The MAR test was adapted for ASAB testing by Jager and associates.[167] A drop of fresh semen, a drop of monospecific anti-IgA (or IgG) antiserum, and a drop of IgA (or IgG)-coated latex beads or erythrocytes are mixed on a glass slide. The test is rapid and simple, with no need for sperm washing or prolonged incubation. The endpoint—mixed agglutination—occurs when IgA (or IgG) antibody–bound sperm and test particles adhere. The percentage of motile sperm that are involved in mixed agglutinates is the percentage that are antibody bound.

The immunobead test[168] is more involved but provides additional specific information. Sperm are washed free of seminal plasma, resuspended in buffer, and mixed with a suspension of micronized polyacrylamide beads to which rabbit antihuman antibodies specific for IgA, IgG, or IgM are attached. As sperm swim among these beads, those that carry ASABs of the various isotypes adhere to the beads. The visual endpoint is assessed microscopically. The pattern of binding allows determination of the site of antibody attachment (head, tail, tail tip) as well as the isotype and proportion of sperm involved. Direct tests, either MAR or immunobead, detect sperm-bound antibodies. Indirect tests measure serum or cervical mucus antibodies by preincubating donor sperm in the fluids to be analyzed, allowing sperm cells to be coated.

HUMAN CERVICAL MUCUS SUBSTITUTES

Donor human cervical mucus is not always available. Estrous bovine and human midcycle cervical mucus are similar in molecular structure, and bovine cervical mucus (BCM) allows rapid penetration by human sperm.[169, 170] It has been suggested that BCM, which can be collected in large quantities and stored, might serve as a more standardized test medium than human cervical mucus,[170] and a commercial test (Penetrak, Syva Company, Palo Alto, CA) has been developed. Unfortunately, BCM does not appear capable of identi-

fying poor sperm penetration associated with sperm-bound ASABs.[168, 171] Other cervical mucus substitutes, such as fresh hen's egg white, also discriminate poorly.[164] Crossed tests of sperm–cervical mucus interaction should use human donor mucus rather than a human mucus substitute.

INCIDENCE AND CAUSES OF CERVICAL FACTOR INFERTILITY

Incidence

Estimates of the incidence of a cervical factor in infertile couples range from less than 5%[172] to 40%,[173] a reflection of the disagreements about diagnostic criteria, differences in the extent of the infertility investigation, and true differences in the infertile populations studied by different investigators. Most modern textbooks and reviews estimate the incidence at 5% to 10%.[111, 114, 117, 174–176]

Causes

The causes of cervical factor infertility may be subdivided into two major groups: (1) those presenting with persistently poor-quality cervical mucus, and (2) those with normal mucus but poor sperm penetration and survival (see Table 18–2).

REPEATED FAILURE TO PRODUCE NORMAL PERIOVULATORY CERVICAL MUCUS

Inadequate Number of Normal Mucus-Producing Endocervical Cells

Acquired Defects. Endocervical cells may be destroyed by cervical infection (discussed later in the chapter) or by surgery.

Sturmdorf[177] popularized the procedure known commonly as *cervical conization*, emphasizing "complete excision of the entire cervical mucosa to the internal os [in which the endocervix was] cored out of its muscular bed as a hollow cone." For many years there has been concern that this procedure and its many modifications may eliminate the functional continuity of the cervical canal and produce intractable sterility. Despite these concerns and the widespread practice of cervical conization, there are no reliable data on the relationship of conization to cervical infertility. The focus instead has been on its long-term efficacy in the diagnosis and treatment of cervical intraepithelial neoplasia.

Cervical conization is generally regarded as the most common cause of cervical stenosis. Table 18–8 summarizes 11 studies, totaling 4005 conizations, that address this issue. The average rate of stenosis is 3.1%; the incidence ranges from zero to 7.1%. A single study,[184] accounting for almost half of the patients followed, reported a stenosis rate of 2.7%. The variations in stenosis rates reflect differences in surgical technique, patient populations, followup protocols, and definitions of stenosis. Rates are higher for larger cones,[189] for postmenopausal[187] and diethylstilbestrol (DES)-exposed women,[190] for suture versus no-suture,[183, 191] and for cold-knife versus laser techniques.[187] It has been suggested that sounding after the first postcone menses and one or more

TABLE 18–8. Cervical Conization: Cervical Stenosis Rates

Author (s)	Year	No. of Cones	No. Stenotic	Percentage
Hester and Read[178]	1960	155	11	7.1
Doran and Shier[179]	1964	95	2	2.1
Kern et al[180]	1967	165	6	3.4
Krieger and McCormak[181]	1968	418	23	5.5
Davis et al[182]	1972	400	0	0
Jonas[183]	1973	51	3	5.9
Bjerre et al[184]	1976	1833	49	2.7
Jones and Buller[185]	1980	114	6	5.3
Holdt et al[186]	1982	271	0	0
Larsson et al[187]	1983	428	20	4.7
Salat-Baroux et al*[188]	1988	125	4	3.2
Total		4005	124	3.1

*Electrosurgical/carbon dioxide laser.

times in the next 3 months should be a routine part of aftercare[192] and that such a regimen decreases the incidence of cervical stenosis.[193] Such efforts seem prudent, especially in young women who may desire future fertility.

The incidence of *cervical infertility after conization* is less clear. There is not a single study that adequately addresses the issue. Despite conclusions such as "conization with our technique does not impair fertility"[184] and "fertility and pregnancy outcome did not seem to be affected by cone biopsy in our small series,"[185] the data are inadequate to decide. Table 18–9 summarizes seven studies that have been frequently cited as providing information about fertility after cervical conization. Crude pregnancy rates vary from 28% to 84%, but a critical analysis reveals a number of deficiencies that obscure the true impact of cervical conization on the ability to conceive. These include retrospective data collection with poorly characterized populations, lack of information about covariates in patients who fail to conceive, and incomplete followup; the use of crude rather than adjusted pregnancy rates; an inappropriate denominator, often taken simply as the number of patients who underwent conization rather than the number actually trying to conceive; and the equation of failure to conceive with cervical infertility without a formal assessment of either cervical mucus quality or sperm–cervical mucus interaction. Only one study[200] prospectively evaluated the cervical score both before and after treatment, but the therapy was diathermocoagulation, a primarily exocervical therapy that is not comparable with cold-knife conization. The authors reported a significant decrease in cervical score 60 days post-therapy but a return to pre-treatment scores by 1 year. Postcoital testing was not reported, and fertility was not evaluated.

With the widespread adoption of colposcopy, the indications for cold-knife cervical conization have decreased, and more patients, especially those in their reproductive years, can be treated by *cryosurgery, carbon dioxide (CO_2) laser vaporization, or electrocautery.* For the most part, these women have exocervical lesions. Intuitively, the risk for impaired cervical mucus production would seem linked to the degree to which the procedure destroys endocervical mucus-producing endothelium. When the squamocolumnar junction can be delineated colposcopically, it might be anticipated that therapy would have less impact on the endocervical epithelium and cervical mucus production. However, few investi-

gators have adequately addressed this question. Problems with study design exist much as for the literature on cold-knife cervical conization. Although one study[187] reported a significantly lower incidence of cervical stenosis for CO_2 laser compared with cold-knife methods (0.4% and 4.7%, respectively), others report stenosis rates in the 3% to 6% range for CO_2 laser,[201] cryotherapy,[201] and combined electrocautery and CO_2 laser,[188] not different from the mean for cold-knife conization (see Table 18–8). In most studies, the issue of fertility has been neglected.[188, 201–207] When fertility has been considered, it has usually been as an afterthought, with the familiar spectrum of methodologic problems. Crude pregnancy rates of 76%[196] and 89%[208] have been reported after electrocoagulation diathermy and 15% to 42% following cryotherapy,[209–212] but none of these studies adequately addressed the problem, and there is certainly nothing in the literature to document the common claim that these procedures do not interfere with fertility.[203]

In reference to the *Lash procedure,* it has also been stated that it "may cause infertility and has no place in the management of cervical incompetence,"[213] but supporting evidence is elusive. Stillman and associates[214] did report a single patient who had 3 years of infertility, a persistent purulent, nonestrogenic cervical mucus, and poor PCTs following a Lash procedure. Permanent sutures were visible in the endocervical canal. After hysteroscopic removal of these foreign bodies, cervical mucus quality dramatically improved, the PCT became normal, and the patient conceived.

Cervical injury is also a recognized complication of legally *induced abortion,* with an incidence between 0.18 and 0.96 in 100 procedures.[215] Injury typically occurs during mechanical cervical dilation. The result may be cervical synechia and stenosis,[216] although there is "no convincing evidence that legal abortion produces clinical infertility."[215]

In summary, although there is legitimate concern about the reproductive consequences of any procedure that potentially destroys endocervical mucus–producing cells, little definitive information is available on the actual effects of those procedures on cervical function or fertility. There is clearly a risk (about 3%) of cervical stenosis after conization, and after cervical cryotherapy or laser vaporization as well, but the impact of these procedures on cervical mucus production and fertility has not been adequately assessed. Crude pregnancy rates range widely from 29% to 84% and probably reflect differences in surgical technique and characteristics of the patient population. It is encouraging to note that crude

TABLE 18–9. Cervical Conization: Crude Conception Rates

Author (s)	Year	No. at Risk	No. Pregnant	Percentage
Boyd et al[194]	1962	56	16	28.6
Green[195]	1966	116	50	43.1
Kern et al[180]	1967	37	31	83.8
MacVicar and Willocks*[196]	1968	203	155	76.4
Kullander and Sjöberg[197]	1971	66	55	83.3
McLaren et al[198]	1974	112	50	44.6
Buller and Jones[199]	1982	100	61	61.0
Total		690	418	60.6

*Electrosurgical.

pregnancy rates higher than 75% have been reported by three centers[180, 196, 197] with a combined population of more than 300 at-risk subjects, but appropriate prospective trials are needed to accurately identify the impact of these procedures on cervical fertility.

Congenital Defects. Congenital defects that may contribute to a reduction in the number of mucus-producing endocervical cells include (1) isolated cervical agenesis or aplasia, (2) DES-associated anomalies, and (3) cystic fibrosis (CF).

Complete müllerian agenesis, with absence of the uterus, cervix, and upper portion of the vagina is incompatible with fertility.[217] Although it is possible to have a normal uterine body and normal vagina with an isolated absence of the uterine cervix (so-called type IB defect), such a lesion is exceedingly rare.[218]

In terms of *DES-associated anomalies,* although both epithelial and fibromuscular abnormalities of the cervix and vagina are present in a large proportion of DES-exposed daughters, it is unclear whether these abnormalities translate into cervical infertility or whether DES exposure affects fertility at all. The evidence has been reviewed.[190, 219] In the vagina, in utero DES exposure causes persistence of müllerian-derived columnar epithelium (vaginal adenosis). On the cervix these changes appear as an exaggerated eversion of the columnar endocervical epithelium (cervical ectropion). Collectively, these findings have been termed *vaginal epithelial changes* and were observed in 34% of the 1275 DES-exposed women who have been followed in the national cooperative DES adenosis (DESAD) project.[220] DES also affects the embryologic development of fibromuscular elements in the cervix and vagina, causing characteristic ridgelike structural malformations. On the cervix these have been called "cocks-combs," collars, hoods, and pseudopolyps. In the vagina they appear as septae, bands, annular rings, and forniceal obliteration. A hypoplastic cervical canal has been described by planimetry,[221] and upper reproductive tract changes, including T-shaped uterus,[222] uterine hypoplasia, and abnormal fallopian tubes have been identified by radiography and endoscopy.[223]

This spectrum of well-characterized epithelial and structural abnormalities may be expected to cause infertility, but the functional significance of these anomalies remains controversial,[224] with very little evidence of either impaired cervical mucus production or impaired sperm transport. The DESAD project, a case control study of 618 pairs of sexually active DES-exposed and unexposed women, reported no significant difference between case and control groups in the percentages who became pregnant (47% versus 50%), the distribution of ages at which first pregnancy occurred, or the number of pregnancies achieved, even after adjustment for variables other than DES exposure.[220] A University of California at San Diego study reached similar conclusions even for the subgroup of DES-exposed subjects with gross cervicovaginal changes. Forty-six percent of the group with gross changes and 46% of the control patients had been pregnant at least once.[225]

The University of Chicago studies differ in both design and conclusions. Although the DESAD study was a case control model, the University of Chicago study followed the exposed and unexposed daughters of mothers who had participated in the original double-blind, controlled DES clinical trial. In the most recent analysis, which focused on married women who were not using contraception and who were actively trying to conceive, more DES-exposed women than control subjects experienced primary infertility (33% versus 14%).[226] The cause of infertility in these subjects, however, is more likely tubal than cervical. An increased incidence of both pelvic inflammatory disease and tubal ectopic pregnancy has been reported in this DES-exposed population,[227] and tubal abnormalities were found by hysterosalpingogram in 42% of the exposed and none of the unexposed women.[226] When patients with cervical stenosis were included, more DES-exposed (63%) than unexposed (25%) women were said to have a cervical factor, but the difference was not statistically significant, the number of patients tested by PCT was small, and abnormal PCTs were not strictly defined by repeat testing. The only other data about cervical factor come from 20 DES-exposed women who underwent serial postcoital testing in single cycles.[228] Fifteen of 20 (75%) had abnormal tests despite normal semen parameters. It is not known whether these findings are representative of the at-large population of DES-exposed women. Considering the number of women estimated to have been DES-exposed and the prevalence of cervicovaginal abnormalities, it is unfortunate that there has been no effort to thoroughly evaluate cervical mucus characteristics and sperm–cervical mucus interaction in these patients.

CF is a genetic disorder characterized by abnormal exocrine glandular secretion, including abnormally viscous secretions from mucus-producing glands (mucoviscidosis). The major clinical manifestations are chronic obstructive pulmonary disease, pancreatic exocrine insufficiency, intestinal malabsorption and obstruction, chronic sinusitis, and nasal polyps.[229, 230] CF is transmitted as an autosomal recessive trait. Major advances in the study of CF have been made possible by the mapping and partial characterization of the CF gene, located on chromosome 7. About 1 in 25 of the white North American population carries a CF mutation, and the incidence of homozygosity is about 1 in 2000 births, making CF "probably the most common semilethal genetic disease of the white population in the United States."[230] Heterozygotes may have no obvious clinical manifestations, and both sexes are affected with equal frequency.

In the male, classic CF is associated with a high incidence of azoospermia and sterility due to absent or rudimentary vasa deferentia.[231] Recently, Anguiano and colleagues[232] reported that 64% of 25 otherwise healthy azoospermic men with congenital bilateral absence of the vas deferens had at least one detectable CF mutation and postulated the existence of a primarily genital CF phenotype.

Less is known about the effects of CF on the female reproductive tract or about the incidence of CF gene mutations in otherwise healthy but infertile women. Pregnancy is clearly possible. A number of young women with CF have conceived, but it is reasonable to postulate that mutations of the CF gene in some women might result in abnormal cervical mucus production and cervical infertility. Only sketchy data are available. Oppenheimer and Esterly[233] performed autopsies on 26 children who died from CF complications. Most had not reached reproductive age, but the authors noted "excessive" mucus in endocervical glands in 50% of cases compared with only 5 (16%) of 32 non-CF control subjects. There is also a case report that described an endocervical polyp and a "viscid cervical mucus plug" in a 22-year-old woman who had CF. There was no assessment of time in the menstrual cycle or even whether the patient was ovulatory.[234] It is an area for future study.

Inadequate Response of Normal Numbers of Mucus-Producing Endocervical Cells to an Estrogen Stimulus

Receptor Blocked by Antiestrogen. Clomiphene citrate is widely used to induce ovulation in infertile women who are anovulatory in the setting of chronic unopposed estrogen. In this setting, clomiphene citrate is thought to function as an antiestrogen, binding to estrogen receptors in the hypothalamus and pituitary, interfering with the negative feedback effect of endogenous estrogens, and leading to a gonadotropin surge and a new round of folliculogenesis. Although 85% of patients ovulate in response to clomiphene citrate, only 50% conceive.[235, 236] A popular hypothesis is that this discrepancy is best explained by poor-quality cervical mucus and impaired sperm penetration caused by binding of clomiphene citrate to cervical estrogen receptors. The hypothesis is partially correct.

During administration, clomiphene clearly has antiestrogenic effects, inducing vasomotor symptoms,[237] a decrease in the karyopyknotic index of vaginal epithelial cells,[237, 238] a shift to nonestrogenic cervical mucus,[237, 239, 240] and an inhibition of sperm penetration.[240] These studies are often cited as evidence of clomiphene's adverse effect on cervical function, but they have limited relevance to clomiphene's clinical use, when the purpose is to induce follicular maturation. When that occurs, the antiestrogenic effects of clomiphene are largely reversed, and cervical mucus becomes estrogenic and supportive of sperm penetration.[237, 239, 240]

A number of investigators have evaluated cervical mucus quality in ovulatory clomiphene citrate cycles.[235, 236, 241, 242] As a group, these studies have many of the same deficiencies that cloud the interpretation of postcoital testing in spontaneous cycles, confounded further by differences in the dose, timing, and duration of clomiphene citrate administration. They consistently show, however, that most women who ovulate in response to clomiphene citrate have normal cervical mucus and sperm transport. The reported incidence of poor-quality cervical mucus ranges from 15%[235] to 52%,[242] but these figures are overestimates because postcoital testing has been generally reserved for patients who do not conceive in the first few cycles of ovulation induction. If it is assumed that patients who conceive in clomiphene-induced cycles have normal sperm transport, and those subjects are included in the denominator, the incidence of poor-quality mucus in these uncontrolled studies decreases to between 10% and 25%.

To determine if clomiphene citrate is causally linked to a deterioration in cervical mucus quality, three separate studies[243–245] compared periovulatory cervical mucus scores and serum estradiol concentrations in a total of 119 spontaneously ovulating women and 144 subjects induced to ovulate with 100 to 150 mg of clomiphene citrate. All reported significantly higher mean estradiol levels and significantly reduced cervical mucus scores in clomiphene-induced cycles. One[243] also measured serum progesterone concentration and found mean periovulatory levels increased as well. None of the three studies assessed sperm penetration, but their findings have been supported and extended by an elegant study that used spontaneously ovulating subjects as its controls.[246] In a prospective, paired-cycles design, cervical mucus score

and in vitro sperm–cervical mucus penetration were analyzed in both spontaneous and clomiphene-induced cycles in 22 couples with unexplained infertility. Precise periovulatory timing was facilitated by daily transvaginal ultrasonography, serum estradiol determination, and LH monitoring. Despite significantly elevated mean serum estradiol levels in clomiphene-induced cycles, mean scores for both cervical mucus and in vitro sperm–cervical mucus penetration were significantly reduced.

With a smaller clomiphene dose (50 mg/day) given early in the cycle (days 2 to 6), some have found no deterioration in cervical mucus score or sperm penetration in vivo or in vitro,[247, 248] but most of the evidence supports the hypothesis that clomiphene citrate impairs cervical mucus quality. The mechanism may be through estrogen receptor binding or an increase in periovulatory progesterone concentration, or both. The impact of a reduced cervical mucus score on the conception rate in clomiphene-induced cycles, however, is probably small, and this effect alone does not explain the large discrepancy between ovulation and crude conception rates reported by many investigators. The incidence of frankly poor-quality cervical mucus in clomiphene-induced cycles is modest (10% to 25%); at least one normal cervical mucus score can be found by serial testing in 83% of clomiphene-induced cycles[243]; and the conception rate in a selected population of women with pure anovulatory infertility is 88%.[235] The most common cause of an abnormal PCT in clomiphene-induced as well as spontaneous cycles is poor timing, and failure to conceive despite ovulation is frequently the result of coexisting problems other than a cervical factor.

Primary Receptor Disorder. In the absence of infection, antiestrogens (clomiphene citrate, tamoxifen), or a history of cervical surgery (conization, cryotherapy) that may have ablated endocervical cells, the cause of persistently poor-quality cervical mucus in ovulatory women is unknown. The mucus-producing cells of the endocervix are estrogen responsive, and this response appears to be receptor mediated. Unoccupied estrogen receptors have been localized to the nuclei of target cells.[249, 250] Nuclear binding of estrogen to columnar cervical epithelium has been demonstrated by autoradiography,[251] and the inhibition of normal estrogen–estrogen receptor interaction by clomiphene citrate can impair cervical mucus production. It has been postulated that idiopathic poor-quality mucus might be due to deficient or abnormal estrogen receptors or to a postreceptor defect, but only limited experimental data are available to support that hypothesis. A deficiency of cytosol estrogen receptor in endocervical cells was demonstrated in a small group of infertile women with persistently poor-quality preovulatory cervical mucus,[252] but there is no information about nuclear estrogen receptors in these patients. The use of cloned complementary deoxyribonucleic acid and genes for the estrogen receptor promise to provide new insight into this problem. Patients who fail to respond to an estrogen challenge and those who have poor-quality cervical mucus despite normal circulating estradiol levels would appear to be good candidates for study.

Cervical Infection. Forty years ago, it was commonly presumed that poor-quality cervical mucus and a poor PCT were caused by cervical infection.[253] The cervices of infertile women were reported to harbor potentially pathogenic bacteria, including several strains capable of inhibiting sperm motility, and there were anecdotal reports of improved PCTs and conception following treatment with antibiotics.[253] *Ureaplasma urealyticum* has received the most attention,[254-256] but other micro-organisms have been implicated as well. Cell-free supernatants from cultures of *Escherichia coli, Pseudomonas aeruginosa,* and *Bacillus subtilis* were reported to be spermicidal,[257] and a role for bacterially elaborated elastase has been proposed.[258]

Although colonization of the cervix by a variety of micro-organisms appears to be common, most evidence suggests that true cervical infection is uncommon. There is little correlation between the bacteriology of cervical mucus and the cervical mucus score, sperm penetrability, or fertility.[259-261] A recent study screened 1000 randomly selected infertile couples. Microbial testing was done on both semen and cervical mucus coincident with an in vitro SCMP test. Polymicrobial colonization was the rule, and a variety of organisms were isolated (Table 18–10). Despite these organisms, there were few leukocytes in either cervical smears or semen. There was also no correlation between the micro-organisms isolated and cervical mucus score, PCT, or in vitro sperm–cervical mucus penetration. A subset of couples (n = 263) was enrolled in a prospective, randomized trial of specific antibiotic therapy. There was no significant difference in 6-month cumulative pregnancy rates between treated and nontreated groups.

Initial interest in *U. urealyticum* was sparked by reports of large-scale differences in isolation rates for *T-mycoplasma* (now primarily *U. urealyticum*) in infertile women (89%) versus both female (23%) and male (26%) control subjects[255, 256] and of high conception rates in *T-mycoplasma* carriers who were treated with doxycycline.[254] In the last 20 years, however, most epidemiologic studies have failed to confirm a role for *U. urealyticum* in infertility. The topic has been thoroughly reviewed,[262-266] with much of the confusion attributed to "an exasperating . . . failure in study design."[265] Among the prob-lems are poorly characterized infertile populations and failure to control for sexual activity, despite clear evidence that *U. urealyticum* colonization increases dramatically with the number of sexual partners.[267] Although *U. urealyticum* is present in a significant proportion of normal, sexually active couples, cervical isolation rates for *U. urealyticum* in fertile and infertile couples[268-270] and conception rates in untreated culture-positive and culture-negative populations[270] are not different. Treatment with doxycycline, although efficiently eradicating the organism, has not been associated with an improved rate of conception in either retrospective, nonrandomized studies[271-274] or in prospective, randomized, controlled clinical trials.[275, 276] There is also no apparent correlation between the presence of cervical *U. urealyticum* and the quality of cervical mucus, PCT results, or in vitro sperm penetration and survival.[259-261, 272, 276-278]

These data do not support the concept of cervical screening for *U. urealyticum* in either infertile patients in general or in those with abnormal cervical mucus or poor PCTs. There is also little rationale for the antibiotic treatment of culture-positive patients, although the bacteriology of cervical mucus in the subset of women with strictly defined cervical infertility has yet to be examined. It is possible that adverse effects may be limited to specific *U. urealyticum* serotypes.[279] That concept warrants further investigation.

Chlamydia trachomatis is another cervical isolate that has been linked to the number of sexual partners. The relationships between *Chlamydia* and infertility have been extensively studied, and there are several excellent reviews.[280-283] *Chlamydia* is a common etiologic agent in acute salpingitis,[284] and the adverse economic and reproductive consequences of both *Chlamydia* and *Neisseria gonorrhoeae* are enormous. Although *Chlamydia* can produce a mucopurulent cervical discharge and clinical signs of cervicitis,[285, 286] it can also be recovered from asymptomatic women with clinically normal cervices.[287, 288] Epidemiologic studies find *Chlamydia* in infertile women more often than in age and socioeconomic status–matched fertile control groups (26.3% versus 12.5%),[289] but the mechanism of infertility appears to be tubal rather than cervical. When adjusted for diagnosis, 49.3% of infertile women with tubal factor were *Chlamydia* positive, whereas the incidence of *Chlamydia* in nontubal infertility (13.4%) was no different than in fertile control groups. *Chlamydia* is rarely isolated from women with poor PCTs[290, 291]; as noted, most abnormal PCTs are explained by poor timing. As for *Ureaplasma* and other micro-organisms, there is no correlation between *Chlamydia* isolation and either cervical mucus quality or sperm–cervical mucus interaction. Antichlamydial antibodies, although highly correlated with tubal infertility, bear no relation to ASAB status, PCT, or in vitro sperm–cervical mucus penetration test results,[292] making it unlikely that a past chlamydial infection might impair cervical function.

In summary, there is little evidence that any particular microbiologic agent is causally linked to cervical infertility, and cervical findings should not influence the decision to culture the endocervical canal. Considering the high asymptomatic carrier rates and the economic and reproductive consequences of pelvic inflammatory disease, routine cervical screening for *N. gonorrhoeae* and *Chlamydia* is justified for all infertile couples, regardless of cervical findings. Screening for other microbiologic agents, including *U. urealyticum,* is not

TABLE 18–10. Results of Cervical Microbial Screening in 1000 Infertile Women		
	Cervix	
Microorganisms*	*Percentage*	*No. Positive/No. Total*
Mycoplasmas (total)	11.8	117/995
Mycoplasma hominis	1.7	17/995
Ureaplasma urealyticum	10.7	106/995
Staphylococcus epidermidis	20.1	196/973
Enterococcus spp.	17.1	166/973
Streptococcus pyogenes (group A)	10.2	99/973
Streptococcus agalactiae (group B)	9.9	96/973
Escherichia coli	7.8	76/973
Proteus spp.	0.8	8/973
Corynebacterium, Diphtheroids	5.7	55/973
Gardnerella vaginalis	3.6	34/935
Bacteroides spp.	2.8	26/935
Peptostreptococcus spp.	0.9	8/935
Lactobacillus spp.	56.8	531/935
Yeasts (total)†	9.9	99/1000
Candida albicans	7.7	77/1000
Torulopsis glabrata	2.2	22/1000
Trichomonas vaginalis†	0.1	1/900
Herpes simplex virus	4.5	40/888

*Not including many others with a lower prevalence.
†From posterior vaginal fornix.
Modified from Eggert-Kruse W, Pohl S, Naher H, et al. Microbial colonization and sperm-mucus interaction: results in 1000 infertile couples. Hum Reprod 1992;7:612–620; by permission of Oxford University Press.

currently indicated, and there is no rationale for empiric antibiotic therapy in infertile couples with a suspected cervical etiology.

Inadequate Estrogen Stimulus. There are two subgroups of patients with poor-quality cervical mucus in clomiphene-induced ovulatory cycles: those with estradiol levels lower than 600 pg/mL and those with estradiol levels higher than 600 pg/mL. The former group responds to exogenous estrogen with an improvement in mucus quality, whereas the latter do not.[293] It has been suggested that a similar phenomenon occurs in spontaneous cycles. Supporting data are limited. Sher and Katz[294] reported plasma estradiol levels lower than 100 pg/mL in three of four women whose infertility was unexplained except for scant or absent cervical mucus in ovulatory cycles. All were treated with human menopausal gonadotropins (hMGs); two of three responded with an improvement in cervical mucus quality, presumably the result of higher circulating estradiol levels. Both conceived, but the small sample size, lack of control groups, and incomplete hormonal profiles severely limited conclusions.

Roumen and coworkers[295] have also been cited as supporting this concept, but their patients had normal cervical scores and unexplained poor sperm penetration. Compared with fertile control groups, the group with poor PCTs had lower mean preovulatory serum estradiol levels (200 versus 260 pg/mL). The authors assumed that the changes in cervical mucus penetrability were due to lower estradiol levels, but they did not attempt to alter PCT results by either estrogen or gonadotropin therapy, and none of their subjects were tested for ASABs. The concept deserves further investigation. Women who demonstrate a significant improvement in cervical mucus score in response to estrogen might benefit from a trial of either estrogen or gonadotropin therapy.

REPEATED FAILURE OF NORMAL PERIOVULATORY CERVICAL MUCUS TO SUPPORT SPERM PENETRATION AND SURVIVAL

Overlooked Male Factor. When cervical mucus is optimal, the most common causes of persistent poor sperm penetration are male factor in origin: coital problems or ejaculatory dysfunction, abnormal semen parameters, or sperm-bound ASABs. The focus of this chapter is cervical infertility, but it is important to remember that cervical factors cannot be evaluated without accurate, up-to-date information about the male. The unexplained poor PCT result should immediately trigger concern for an overlooked male factor. The first thought should be to performance problems; the vaginal pool should be examined to confirm that intravaginal ejaculation actually occurred. Previous semen evaluations should be reviewed and normal semen parameters verified. An in vitro test of sperm–cervical mucus interaction should be conducted to confirm postcoital findings; a crossover design can distinguish whether sperm or cervical mucus factors are responsible for poor sperm penetration. Sperm-bound ASABs can be assessed by either direct immunobead or MAR testing.

Vaginal Factor. Vaginal factor can be defined as the combination of (1) repeated failure of optimal cervical mucus to demonstrate postcoital sperm penetration and survival; (2) normal semen parameters; (3) apparently normal ejaculation (sperm identified in the vagina); (4) normal sperm–cervical mucus interaction by in vitro testing; and (5) normal sperm

penetration and survival in cervical mucus following cup artificial insemination with husband's sperm (AIH/cup).

Those findings point to a sperm transport problem that is corrected either by ensuring an adequate interface between the ejaculate and cervical mucus or by protecting the ejaculate-mucus interface from the putatively hostile vaginal milieu. Vaginal factor is probably a misnomer, because the most likely explanation for such findings is low ejaculate volume. Low volume may hamper sperm transport by its decreased buffering capacity, by a decrease in total sperm number, or by a decreased opportunity for seminal fluid–cervical mucus interface. AIH/cup maximizes sperm–cervical mucus contact and sequesters the ejaculate, prolonging its buffering capacity and protecting sperm from the low vaginal pH, vaginal lubricants, or other as yet unknown vaginal factors.

Normal Male Factor, Hostile Cervical Mucus

Abnormal Cervical Mucus pH. The concept of cervical mucus hyperacidity is an old one. Huhner wrote in 1942:

If we find the vaginal or cervical secretions markedly acid in the case under consideration, and suspect that hyperacidity is the cause of the death of the spermatozoa, we should order a bicarbonate of soda douche to be taken before coitus and then make another test.[109]

Low pH is frequently offered as an explanation for the unexplained poor PCT, when sperm penetration is limited despite estrogenic cervical mucus and a normal semen evaluation.[116, 176]

The low pH of the normal vagina and the importance of seminal fluid buffering and a reservoir of alkaline cervical mucus to sperm survival have been reviewed.[20, 27] Although it is clear that sperm survival is poor when cervical mucus has a pH lower than 6.0,[20, 25 26] there are no studies that measure cervical mucus pH in well-defined populations of couples with unexplained poor PCTs. The *WHO Laboratory Manual for the Examination of Human Semen and Sperm–Cervical Mucus Interaction* has recommended pH testing of cervical mucus since its first edition (1980), but pH has rarely been measured in clinical studies, with conflicting results. Giner and associates[128] measured cervical mucus pH in conjunction with postcoital testing in 107 ovulatory cycles in which the PCT was the only coital event. Eighty-three percent had a pH of 7.0 or higher; pH was less than 6.0 in only one subject. The conception rates per cycle were similar when pH was 6.0 to 6.9 (25%), 7.0 to 7.9 (24%), and 8.0 or higher (22%). In other studies, cervical mucus pH has been below 6.0 in 19% to 27% of PCTs,[25, 26] but one study sampled exocervical mucus,[26] and these measurements were done in unselected infertile couples in single tests with the usual questions about optimal timing. The incidence of low cervical mucus pH in strictly defined unexplained poor PCTs remains unknown.

The measurement of cervical mucus pH should become part of the routine for evaluating couples with unexplained poor PCTs. The technology is available. There is a good correlation between the pH of cervical mucus in vivo and in vitro, using the appropriate pH paper,[25] and a good correlation between pH measurements made with paper versus a minielectrode.

WHO Recommendations (1992).[102] The WHO revised recommendations include the following:

The pH of cervical mucus should be obtained with pH paper, range 6.4–8.0, in situ or immediately following collection. If the pH is measured in situ, care should be taken to measure it correctly, since the pH of exocervical mucus is always lower than that of mucus in the endocervical canal. Care should also be taken to avoid contamination with secretions of the vagina, which have an acidic pH.

Spermatozoa are susceptible to changes in pH of the cervical mucus. Acid mucus immobilizes sperm, whereas alkaline mucus may enhance motility. Excessive alkalinity of the cervical mucus (pH >8.5) may, however, adversely affect the viability of spermatozoa. The optimum pH value for sperm migration and survival in the cervical mucus is between 7.0 and 8.5, which represents the pH range of normal, mid-cycle cervical mucus. However, a pH value of between 6.0 and 7.0 may still be compatible with sperm penetration.[120]

Cervical Mucus Antisperm Antibodies. There are a number of excellent reviews that detail the pathophysiology of ASABs and the evolving concept of immunologic infertility.[160, 168, 296–302] Spermatozoa possess antigens that are capable of eliciting an immune response in either the male (autoimmunization) or the female (isoimmunization). Autoimmunization is thought to occur because of a breakdown in the normal blood–seminiferous tubule barrier, and ASABs in the male can be found both in the circulation and bound to sperm cells. The genesis of isoimmunization is less clear; ASABs appear in the circulation and in the female reproductive tract.

ASABs are thought to cause infertility by interfering with sperm transport or sperm-ovum interaction. Several mechanisms may be involved in antibody-associated sperm transport failure: (1) ASAB may impair the ability of spermatozoa to penetrate cervical mucus; (2) ASAB binding may subject sperm to complement-mediated cell lysis; and (3) ASAB may activate phagocytosis of sperm by macrophages (a process known as *opsonization*). The relative importance of these mechanisms is unclear, but most of the evidence points to an inability of sperm to penetrate cervical mucus. The aqueous phase of normal cervical mucus contains immunoglobulins. Both IgG and IgA (but not IgM) have been detected by microradial immunodiffusion in daily cervical mucus samples, with a midcycle nadir.[302] IgM, which makes up 10% of circulating immunoglobulins, is a very large molecule (molecular weight about 900,000) and does not diffuse into cervical mucus. IgA can be produced locally in the female tract as well as systemically. IgG comprises 75% of circulating immunoglobulins and is small enough (about 200,000) to reach cervical mucus by diffusion. Because IgG is complement dependent, however, and complement activity in human cervical mucus is low,[303] IgG-mediated complement-dependent sperm immobilization is an unlikely cause of poor sperm penetration. IgA-class ASABs are noncomplement fixing, are produced locally, and are viewed as primarily responsible for impaired sperm penetration in cervical mucus.[301, 304] It has been postulated that the mechanism involves an interaction between the Fc portion of the immunoglobulin molecule and gel-phase components of cervical mucus.[159, 160]

Most of the evidence for antibody-induced sperm transport failure comes from studying sperm-bound ASABs. The proportion of sperm bound by ASAB, as judged by immunobead testing, has been shown to correlate with the number of motile sperm in cervical mucus at postcoital testing.[168, 171] High levels of sperm-bound ASAB completely prevent the entry of sperm into cervical mucus. Experimentally, the transfer of ASAB to the sperm surface by incubation in antibody-positive serum causes normal spermatozoa to lose their ability to penetrate cervical mucus[167] and induces the phenomenon of shaking sperm motility, an abnormal pattern of nonprogressive motion believed to be caused by antibody–cervical mucus interaction.[159, 305] In addition, the site of bound antibody and the isotype affect results; head-directed ASABs impair cervical mucus penetration more than those bound to the tail tip,[171, 306] and IgA class ASABs have more of an adverse effect than IgG.[306]

The primary indications for immunologic testing are (1) an unexplained poor PCT result or (2) an abnormal pattern of sperm motion in cervical mucus (shaking motility). The presence of IgA in cervical mucus is essentially excluded if many forward-moving spermatozoa are seen 8 to 12 hours after coitus,[301] and a severe disturbance of sperm–cervical mucus interaction is unlikely if even one or more forward-moving sperm are seen. In vitro testing, with either the SCMC or the SCMP test, or both, can confirm abnormal postcoital findings, and a crossover design helps distinguish sperm from cervical mucus causes. Early epidemiologic studies about ASABs and infertility used nonspecific tests and focused on serum rather than sperm-bound or cervical mucus antibodies. Because there is a poor correlation between ASABs in the circulation and those in either cervical mucus[160, 307, 308] or bound to sperm,[296] the focus must instead be local. Immunologic tests should be directed at sperm and cervical mucus rather than serum.

Idiopathic Hostile Cervical Mucus

It is not known to what extent sperm survival and motility in cervical mucus are influenced by the amount of utilizable carbohydrates or other sperm nutrients present in cervical secretions.[157]

Cervical mucus is complex in both its biophysical and biochemical properties. The metabolic changes that occur during sperm transport, capacitation, storage, and release are poorly defined. Little is known about the relationships between mucus chemical composition and sperm–cervical mucus interaction, or the differences, if any, in cervical mucus composition between fertile women and those with cervical infertility. Glucose, for example, and other reducing substances, are present in cervical mucus, and it has been postulated that "saccharopenia" may explain poor sperm penetration.[309] A decrease in cervical mucus glucose concentration in infertile women has been reported,[48] but there is normally a periovulatory nadir in the cervical mucus glucose level that mirrors the increase in hydration, suggesting that these changes may be dilutional in nature.[12, 45] Considering the few sperm that enter cervical mucus and its large volume and rapid turnover at midcycle, energy substrates may be nonlimiting.

It is well known that many vaginally administered compounds, such as vaginal lubricants, have spermaticidal effects and should be avoided in couples who are trying to conceive.[310] It is less known that toxicants may enter cervicovaginal fluids systemically. D-Propranolol, a pharmacologic compound with β-receptor–blocking activity, inhibits sperm motility in vitro,[311] and the maximum mean concentration of

D-propranolol in cervical mucus is more than four times the serum peak after an 80-mg oral dose.[312] More than 2500 chemicals have been identified in tobacco smoke, the best known being nicotine and carbon monoxide.[313] Nicotine and other compounds in cigarette smoke are ciliary toxins and may be sperm toxic as well.[314] High levels of nicotine and its major metabolite, cotinine, have been found in the cervical mucus of female smokers.[315] Nicotine has also been found in the uterine and oviductal fluid of pregnant rabbits in concentrations 10-fold higher than in plasma.[316] A recent epidemiologic study[317] reported a specific association between both cervical and tubal infertility and the use of cigarettes. Although the data are preliminary, nicotine, cotinine, and other environmental toxicants in cervical mucus may play a role in unexplained cervical mucus hostility. All of these issues warrant further investigation.

TREATMENT OF CERVICAL FACTOR INFERTILITY

Poor-Quality Cervical Mucus and Abnormal Cervical Anatomy

Anatomic cervical factor infertility may be the easiest cause of cervical infertility to diagnose but the most difficult to treat.[318] The stenotic cervix that results from cervical conization or other procedures that destroy endocervical epithelium usually resists attempts to restore cervical mucus production. There are anecdotal reports of estrogen therapy and efforts to dilate the cervical canal, with no improvement in cervical mucus.[318] An estrogen challenge may be useful to identify the occasional patient who could benefit from this approach, but there is no information about the proportion who might be expected to respond, and the challenge has never been standardized. Several protocols have been published, including conjugated estrogens 5 mg daily, cycle days 2 to 15[319]; ethinyl estradiol 40 μg daily, cycle days 2 to 15[319]; ethinyl estradiol 100 μg daily for 4 days, then 150 μg daily for 4 days[113]; and ethinyl estradiol 50 to 75 μg daily, cycle days 5 to 26, with the PCT repeated after 7 to 14 days of estrogen.[118] Failure to make estrogenic cervical mucus during this test would seem to bode poorly for either estrogen or gonadotropin therapy. A few patients with endocervical varicosities and a fragile, bleeding epithelium have been treated by cryotherapy; a normal PCT was restored in one patient, who conceived.[318]

Therapy for this condition usually consists of intrauterine insemination (IUI) with washed husband's sperm (AIH/IUI), but it may be necessary to reestablish a cervical canal by cervical dilation to permit passage of the IUI catheter. It may not be possible to identify the endocervical canal and overcome severe stenosis in the office setting. Pittaway and colleagues[320] reported a successful pregnancy following the combined vaginal-abdominal reconstruction of the cervical canal in a young DES-exposed daughter who developed severe cervical stenosis after cervical conization. The cervical canal was impossible to identify vaginally but could be located and cannulated through a uterine fundal incision at laparotomy. The canal was dilated and a Foley catheter left in place for 7 days, and the patient received conjugated estrogens, 2.5 mg twice daily.

Poor-Quality Cervical Mucus and Normal Cervical Anatomy

ESTROGENS

Estrogen therapy has been widely mentioned[20, 113–115, 117, 118, 174, 176, 319, 321] for both clomiphene-associated and idiopathic poor-quality cervical mucus, but its efficacy has never been demonstrated in controlled clinical trials.

The rationale for treating clomiphene-associated poor-quality cervical mucus with exogenous estrogens has not been clearly articulated, considering that mean periovulatory serum estradiol concentrations in clomiphene-induced cycles range from 600 to 1250 pg/mL, levels that are threefold to fourfold higher than serum estradiol concentrations in unstimulated control subjects.[243–247] Nonetheless, a variety of estrogen preparations and dosing protocols have been reported in patients receiving an equally varied assortment of clomiphene regimens (Table 18–11). The seven studies listed include more than 500 treatment cycles but give conflicting testimony about the efficacy of estrogen supplementation. Most are uncontrolled and simply report the addition of estrogen to clomiphene citrate regimens in patients who had poor-quality cervical mucus in response to clomiphene alone.[235, 322, 323, 325] There were no apparent differences in ovulation rates in clomiphene-induced cycles with or without estrogen supplementation. One study[325] noted no improvement in cervical mucus quality after the addition of estrogen, but three others[235, 322, 323] reported improved cervical mucus quality in most (68% to 83%) of the subjects treated. Crude pregnancy rates of 20%[322] and 24%[323] were reported following the addition of estrogen to clomiphene citrate in patients who failed to conceive on clomiphene alone. Again, these studies lacked suitable control groups.

The double-blind, randomized addition of placebo, micronized estradiol, or conjugated estrogens to 12 subjects who demonstrated persistently poor-quality cervical mucus during clomiphene-induced cycles failed to show a difference in periovulatory cervical mucus scores.[326] And in a larger, unselected group of 192 women, there was no significant difference in conception rates among those randomly assigned to clomiphene citrate alone (35%), clomiphene citrate and hCG (41%), or clomiphene citrate, hCG, and estrogen supplementation (45%).[242]

The reports concerning low-dose estrogen therapy for idiopathic poor-quality cervical mucus in natural cycles are equally unclear. Table 18–12 summarizes nine studies published between 1966 and 1990. The principal criteria for treatment was poor-quality midcycle cervical mucus and a poor PCT. None of these subjects had received clomiphene citrate, and all had partners with normal semen parameters. The rate of cervical mucus "improvement" (poorly defined) ranged from 15% to 100%, but these results should be skeptically viewed. The number of subjects was small, and the study populations were incompletely characterized. The estrogen preparations, dosages, and days of administration were varied, and there was little documentation of PCT timing vis-à-vis ovulation in either the index or treatment cycles. All lacked suitable controls, and none adequately evaluated fertility (as opposed to cervical mucus quality) as an outcome.

Although these data failed to demonstrate efficacy for es-

TABLE 18–11. Estrogen Supplementation Regimens in Clomiphene Citrate (CC) Cycles

Author(s)	Year	Estrogen Regimen	CC Regimen	No. of Cycles
Sharf et al[322]	1971	Quinestrol 50 µg daily, cycle days 6–16	50–100 mg daily, cycle days 5–9	41
Poliak et al[242]	1973	Conjugated estrogens 0.625 mg daily, cycle days 10–20	50 mg daily, cycle days 5–9	236
Insler et al[323]	1973	Ethinyl estradiol 75–150 µg daily, cycle day 7 to ovulation	100 mg daily, cycle days 5–9	100
Taubert and Dericks-Tan[324]	1976	Ethinyl estradiol 180 µg daily, cycle days 10–16	100 mg daily, cycle days 5–9	29
		Conjugated estrogens 7.5 mg daily, cycle days 10–16	100 mg daily, cycle days 5–9	29
Van der Merwe[325]	1981	Conjugated estrogens 2.5 mg daily, cycle days 10–17	50–100 mg daily, cycle days 5–9	39
Gysler et al[235]	1982	Diethylstilbestrol 0.1 mg daily, cycle day 10 to ovulation	50–250 mg daily, cycle days 5–9	6
Bateman et al[326]	1990	Micronized estradiol 2 mg daily, cycle days 9–15	50–150 mg daily, cycle days 5–9	12
		Conjugated estrogens 5 mg daily, cycle days 9–15	50–150 mg daily, cycle days 5–9	12

trogen supplementation in patients with poor-quality cervical mucus, the definitive studies have not yet been done. There may be a subgroup of women who have poor-quality mucus associated with low preovulatory estrogen levels when estrogen therapy might be of benefit. A small group (n = 6) of subjects with estradiol levels lower than 600 pg/mL during clomiphene-induced cycles showed a significant improvement in cervical mucus score after estrogen supplementation, whereas those (n = 6) with estradiol levels higher than 600 pg/mL showed no improvement.[293] The data are preliminary, but estrogen therapy may be warranted for a small group of

patients. For the remainder, poor-quality mucus may be treated by either hMGs or IUI.

GONADOTROPINS

hMGs (Pergonal) have been used in a variety of circumstances to treat poor-quality periovulatory cervical mucus. All of the data are anecdotal and uncontrolled and fail to separate the drug's effect on cervical mucus from its ability to induce superovulation. For example, Pergonal was used to induce ovulation in four patients who had poor cervical mu-

TABLE 18–12. Estrogen Supplementation Regimens in Natural Cycles

Author(s)	Year	Study Population	No. of Subjects	Therapy	No. Improved (%)	No. Pregnant	Comments
Cohen[327]	1967	Infertile; only abnormality was poor mucus and poor PCT	19	Quinestrol 50 µg/d, days 5–24	18 (94.7)	NS	Uncontrolled
Roland[328]	1967	Oligomucorrhea and poor PCT	14	Quinestrol 50 µg/d, days 6–16	8 (57.1)	NS	Uncontrolled
Skerlavay et al[329]	1969	Ovulatory but consistently scanty, poor-quality mucus	3	Conjugated estrogens 1.25 mg/d, days 6–15	3 (100)	NS	Uncontrolled
Cohen et al[330]	1970	Infertile, ovulatory but poor-quality mucus	6	Intracervical estrogen Silastic capsule	1 (16.7)	NS	Uncontrolled
Moran et al[151]	1974	Abnormal fractional PCT	16	DES 0.1 mg/d	6 (37.5)	3	Uncontrolled
Scott et al[318]	1977	Infertile; only abnormality was poor-quality mucus	28	DES 0.1–0.2 mg/d, days 5–20	11 (39.2)	6	Uncontrolled
		Infertile; only abnormality was very-low-quantity mucus	35	DES 0.1–0.2 mg/d, days 5–20	18 (51.4)	5	Uncontrolled
Rezai et al[331]	1979	Cervical factor infertility	10	Estriol 0.25 mg/d × 10 days	6 (60)	2	Uncontrolled
Krzeminski et al[332]	1988	Infertile; only abnormality was "pathologic mucus" and poor PCT	28	Mestranol 50 µg/d, days 5–14, then 100 µg/d, days 15–20	11 (39.2)	6	Uncontrolled
	1988	Infertile; only abnormality was "small amount" cervical mucus	35	Mestranol 50 µg/d, days 5–14, then 100 µg/d, days 15–20	18 (51.4)	5	Uncontrolled
Check et al[333]	1990	Unexplained poor PCT (normal mucus and NL SE, poor PCT)	30	Conjugated estrogens 5 mg/d, days 5–13	8 (26.7)	4	Uncontrolled

NS, not specified; PCT, postcoital test; DES, diethylstilbestrol; NL SE, normal semen evaluation.

cus scores in clomiphene-induced cycles and failed to improve with the addition of ethinyl estradiol. All four conceived.[236] Similar results were reported in four patients who had unexplained infertility except for poor cervical mucus scores and low estradiol levels in natural ovulatory cycles. Cervical mucus score improved and PCTs became normal in three patients, and all three conceived.[294] There is a series of anecdotal reports on the combined use of hMG and high-dose exogenous estrogens.[334–338] Conjugated estrogens given 2.5 to 5 mg/day and hMG improved cervical mucus quality and PCT results in 28 of 34 women (82%) who had idiopathic poor-quality cervical mucus in natural ovulatory cycles.[336] Nineteen women conceived. About one third of those who benefited had previously failed to improve with Pergonal alone. The combination of ethinyl estradiol 50 to 100 µg/day and Pergonal produced similar results: 50 of 70 patients (71%) improved mucus scores and 37 conceived. The best results have been reported in the subgroup of patients who have isolated idiopathic poor-quality mucus and respond favorably to an estrogen challenge.[339] In these highly selected patients, a limited trial of Pergonal seems reasonable, although the efficacy of this therapy has not yet been evaluated in an adequately controlled trial.

EXPECTORANTS AND MUCOLYTICS

Expectorants and mucolytic agents are commonly used in cough remedies and as adjuvant therapy for patients with abnormally viscous bronchopulmonary secretions; they have been extensively reviewed.[340–342] Although their modes of action in the respiratory tract are not clearly understood, their effect is to increase the volume and decrease the viscosity of respiratory tract secretions. At least part of the mechanism may be through vagal pathways. Anticholinergic agents clearly decrease the volume of respiratory tract secretions. The effects of guaifenesin (glyceryl guaiacolate) and saturated solutions of potassium iodide are reported to depend on intact vagal innervation. In addition, the iodides are rapidly excreted into bronchial secretions, where they may stimulate ciliary activity to enhance mucus clearance. An increase in the secretory activity of lacrimal and nasal glands has been reported as well. Mucolytic agents such as acetylcysteine contain sulfhydryl groups that can reduce disulfide bonds and work by depolymerizing respiratory tract mucoproteins.

It is not known whether the respiratory tract effects of any of these agents are duplicated in the cervix, and their abilities to enhance cervical mucus volume or decrease its viscosity and improve sperm penetrability have never been adequately studied. Because guaifenesin and estrogens both have an aromatic ring, it has been postulated that guaifenesin may have an estrogen-like effect on endocervical cells.[252] Guaifenesin was given orally from cycle day 5 until the BBT shift to 40 women who had ill-defined poor-quality cervical mucus and abnormal PCTs despite normal semen parameters. The PCT improved in 23 (58%), and 15 of these conceived.[343] The study was uncontrolled. Although there are a number of publications that mention guaifenesin therapy in this context,[336, 337, 344] claims for its efficacy remain unsubstantiated.

CERVICAL CURETTAGE AND CRYOTHERAPY

The persistence of nonestrogenic cervical mucus despite antibiotic or high-dose estrogen therapy has been called "absolute" dysmucorrhea.[113, 345] In these patients, poor-quality mucus is commonly attributed to chronic cervicitis.[116, 118, 176, 319, 321] The fact that such mucus is not associated with an identifiable bacteriologic agent[77] and resists conventional antibiotic therapy has been ascribed to involvement of cells deep within endocervical crypts. Histologic evaluation of cells obtained by endocervical curettage has been advocated as a diagnostic test.[346]

By definition, absolute dysmucorrhea is seldom reversed, but several therapies have been proposed, including endocervical curettage combined with antibiotics[346, 347] and cervical cryotherapy.[117, 176, 321] The hypothesis has been that these treatments ablate cells that harbor deep-seated chronic infection and stimulate the regeneration of normal endocervical epithelium.[347] Considering the lack of information documenting efficacy, the potential for cryotherapy to cause cervical stenosis, and the availability of IUI, these potentially destructive procedures have limited, if any, roles in the treatment of cervical infertility.

DONOR CERVICAL MUCUS

Before the development of techniques for sperm washing and the popularization of IUI, there was interest in donor cervical mucus and human mucus substitutes to support sperm transport in infertile women who had absent cervical mucus. Check and Rakoff[348] reported three couples who conceived following intracervical insemination (ICI) with a mixture of 0.5 mL of the husband's semen and an equal volume of human donor mucus. All three subjects had been refractory to more conventional therapies, including low-dose and high-dose estrogens and even hMGs. The donor mucus had been collected at midcycle and stored frozen for less than 10 days. A fourth case was reported by Segal and Sherer,[349] using donor mucus and AIH/cap. The discovery that BCM is similar in composition to human cervical mucus,[169] that it supports penetration by human spermatozoa,[170] and that it can also be stored frozen without deterioration of penetrability or viscoelastic properties[350] prompted the suggestion that BCM might serve as a clinically useful substitute.[170, 351] There have been no clinical trials to evaluate its safety or usefulness, and concern about the transmission of infectious agents has precluded further use of human donor or bovine mucus. Other potential substitutes, including dextrose 5% and Ringer's lactate[352] and methylcellulose[351] have been mentioned but not studied clinically.

Good-Quality Cervical Mucus and Poor Sperm Penetration and Survival

ALKALINIZATION OF CERVICAL MUCUS

Although there is little information about the distribution of cervical mucus pH values in infertile couples with strictly defined unexplained poor PCTs, vaginal irrigation with a sodium bicarbonate solution effectively increases pH in the vagina and in cervical mucus,[20] and this treatment has often been mentioned as an effective therapy in infertile couples.[109, 117, 118, 175, 176] Clinical data, however, are limited. In a frequently cited but uncontrolled study, 35 women with poor PCTs despite normal semen parameters and abundant clear cervical mucus were treated with a precoital alkaline douche. Individual pH measurements were not reported either before or after therapy, but PCT results improved in 29 of 35 subjects (83%), and 16 conceived. Success was attributed to "alteration of the cervical mucus pH from acid to alkaline."[353] A recent prospective, double-blind, randomized trial comparing the effects of sodium bicarbonate and sodium chloride douches on sperm penetration in vivo and in vitro demonstrated significantly improved penetration with bicarbonate therapy, but cervical mucus pH was not measured, and improvement correlated with a reduction in cervical mucus viscoelasticity, suggesting a mechanism other than alkalinization.[354] The study population was small (25 patients); two conceived, both during sodium bicarbonate therapy, but the data are preliminary and inadequate to prove clinical efficacy.

INTRAUTERINE INSEMINATION

The rationale for IUI in couples with cervical infertility is largely intuitive. It is based on the hypothesis that placement of spermatozoa beyond the cervix increases the number of sperm in the upper reproductive tract and increases the pregnancy rate in women with a cervical barrier to normal sperm transport. Despite the popularity of IUI, this hypothesis remains unsupported. Most studies are anecdotal, uncontrolled, and poorly designed. Controlled trials are few, and their results are contradictory. In addition, this hypothesis ignores much of what is currently understood about normal cervical physiology and sperm–cervical mucus interaction, including the cervical reservoir concept and the role cervical mucus may play in sperm selection, capacitation, and metabolism. Pregnancy is clearly possible after IUI. The question is whether pregnancy occurs more often with IUI than with comparably timed intercourse or ICI.

Simple AIH for cervical infertility appears to be ineffective.[355] The crude pregnancy rate in a collected series of 192 subjects (12%) was not better than the spontaneous pregnancy rate in noninseminated patients (14%). In 1985, a collection of five small, uncontrolled studies suggested that IUI was more effective, with 60% of 58 couples conceiving.[356] The procedure was simplified by the adaptation of sperm-washing techniques,[357] and a host of reports followed touting its role in treating unexplained and male factor as well as cervical infertility. As the popularity of IUI has grown, however, so has the debate about its clinical efficacy.

Table 18–13 adds 21 uncontrolled studies to Allen's original review. At face value, the collection records 252 pregnancies in 927 patients who were treated by IUI for cervical infertility, a crude pregnancy rate of 27%. It also documents 1544 IUI cycles, of which 171 (11.1%) resulted in pregnancy. None of these studies, however, proves the hypothesis that IUI increases the chance to conceive in couples with cervical infertility. All were uncontrolled, and most had major flaws in design and execution. Analyzed individually, however, several reports do provide an estimate of the efficacy of IUI, information that is helpful in evaluating controlled trials.

The studies in Table 18–13 reported a wide range of results: crude pregnancy rates range from zero to 68%, and fecundities from zero to 31%. Comparisons are difficult. Sample size ranged from 4[364, 376] to 276 subjects.[369] There were major differences in the definition of cervical infertility

and in the thoroughness with which potentially confounding infertility factors were eliminated. Most excluded couples with abnormal semen parameters, but few[368] required laparoscopy of every woman or systematically identified couples with ASABs.[361, 365, 371, 377] Only five conducted IUI in natural cycles[360, 361, 365, 366, 375]; the rest induced ovulation, introducing another variable. The conduct of IUI also varied greatly, with differences in the techniques for sperm preparation and insemination timing, the number and frequency of inseminations per treatment cycle, and the technique for placement of the inseminate.

By discounting publications with fewer than 10 subjects, with only crude pregnancy rates, or with poorly characterized patients or insemination protocols, 18 of the 22 studies listed in Table 18–13 can be eliminated. Three of the four remaining studied IUI in natural cycles.[360, 365, 375] Conception rates per cycle varied from 8.8% to 20.6%. Collectively, there were 55 pregnancies in 438 cycles (12.6% per cycle).

Table 18–14 lists six controlled clinical trials. Two[378, 380] compared IUI with ICI, primarily in natural cycles. Their results are contradictory: the larger trial[380] reported identical conception rates for the two insemination techniques, whereas the other[378] reported success only with IUI. Three studies compared IUI with intercourse in natural cycles. One of the studies[379] should probably be discounted because the technique of "high AIH" involved ICI rather than true IUI as currently practiced. The remaining two studies also presented contradictory results. Both reported fecundities for IUI that were in the range of those reported by the most credible uncontrolled trials (15.9% and 12.1%); however, one observed no success with coitus,[381] whereas the other[382] reported a fecundity of 8% after intercourse, not significantly different than for IUI. The combination of IUI and controlled ovarian hyperstimulation may be more effective than IUI alone, but the per cycle conception rates for IUI in stimulated cycles in uncontrolled trials (11% to 20%)[339, 370, 374] are not obviously different than for uncontrolled studies without hMG. Only one study compares hMG-IUI to IUI alone and to hMG-coitus,[383] with a significant advantage going to the hMG-IUI group, but the study suffers from its retrospective, nonrandomized design, leaving the question open to further investigation. If a trial of IUI is elected, it should be limited to four treatment cycles; most conceptions occur early, and the probability of conception falls dramatically after the fourth cycle.[375]

The treatment of infertility caused by ASABs is controversial and beyond the scope of this review. Neither condoms nor glucocorticoids are unequivocally effective. By default, IUI has been commonly used with the intention of bypassing ASABs in cervical mucus. That concept may be naive considering the lack of data about the relationship between ASAB in the cervix and ASAB higher in the reproductive tract. Because the concentrations of immunoglobulins in cervical mucus are lowest at midcycle and mirror the estrogen peak, controlled ovarian hyperstimulation has been proposed as an adjunct to IUI in these patients in the hope that ASAB in cervical mucus might decrease. A pregnancy rate of 11% per cycle was reported in 28 women who had circulating ASAB and were treated with hMG/IUI. The study was not controlled, and cervical mucus ASAB were not measured.[384] Because the major histocompatibility antigens are not expressed on human sperm,[385] ASABs appear to be generic, eliminating

TABLE 18–13. Intrauterine Insemination for Cervical Infertility: Uncontrolled Studies

Author(s)	Year	No. of Subjects	No. of Cycles	Treatment(s)	No. Pregnant	Crude Pregnancy Rate (%)	Per Cycle Rate (%)	Comments
Allen et al[356]	1985	58	—	IUI	35	60.3	—	Collected series
Toffle et al[358]	1985	10	—	IUI	2	20.0	—	—
Hewitt et al[359]	1985	30	59	IUI	2	7.0	3.0	All CC
		18	21	IVF	8	44.0	38.0	All CC/hMG
Confino et al[360]	1986	19	63	IUI	13	68.4	20.6	All natural
Hull et al[361]	1986	19	65	IUI	3	15.8	4.6	All natural
Yovich and Matson[362]	1986	—	155	IUI	20	—	12.9	Mixture of regimens
			58	GIFT	18	—	31.0	
Arny and Quagliarello[363]	1987	25	—	IUI	8	32.0	—	Mixture of regimens
Dodson et al[364]	1987	4	7	IUI	2	50.0	28.6	All hMG
Byrd et al[365]	1987	29	113	IUI	10	34.5	8.8	All natural
Makler[366]	1987	110	431	IUI	44	40.0	10.2	All natural
Pardo et al[367]	1988	17	—	IUI	5	29.4	—	Mixture of regimens
Sunde et al[368]	1988	5	7	IUI	0.0	0.0	0.0	All CC/hMG
Yovich and Matson[339]	1988	(1)45	106	IUI	5	11.1	4.7	(1) Poor Mucus
		(2)88	171	IUI	27	30.7	15.8	(2) Negative PCT All CC/hMG
Horvath et al[369]	1989	(3)121	—	IUI	14	11.6	—	(3)Cervical factor
		(4)155	—	IUI	22	14.2	—	(4)Poor PCT All CC/hMG
Corson et al[370]	1989	100	127	hMG-IUI	14	—	11.0	Retrospective,
			180	IUI	9	—	5.0	nonrandom
Francavilla et al[371]	1990	18	76	IUI	7	38.9	10.5	Mixture of regimens
Tredway et al[372]	1990	31	—	IUI	6	19.4	—	Mixture of regimens
Galle et al[373]	1990	28	—	IUI	7	25.0	—	Mixture of regimens
Dodson and Haney[374]	1991	—	25	IUI	5	—	20.0	All hMG
Friedman et al[375]	1991	91	262	IUI	32	35.2	12.2	All natural
Tarlatzis et al[376]	1991	4	4	IUI	1	25.0	25.0	Mixture of regimens
Karlstrom et al[377]	1991	20	—	IUI	7	35.0	—	All CC

IUI, intrauterine insemination; IVF, in vitro fertilization; GIFT, gamete intrafallopian transfer; CC, clomiphene citrate; hMG, human menopausal gonadotropin; PCT, postcoital test.

TABLE 18–14. Intrauterine Insemination for Cervical Infertility: Controlled Studies

Author(s)	Year	No. of Subjects	No. of Cycles	Treatment(s)	No. Pregnant	Crude Pregnancy Rate (%)	Per Cycle Rate (%)	Comments
Quagliarello and Arny[378]	1986	20	72	IUI	6	30.0	8.3	CC in 6/20 subjects
			66	ICI	0	0.0	0.0	
Glazener et al[379]	1987	43	223	"High AIH"	2	4.3	0.9	All natural cycles
		46	252	Coitus	3	6.5	1.2	
Friedman et al[380]	1989	54	113	IUI	7	13.0	6.2	All natural cycles
			113	ICI	7	13.0	6.2	
Te Velde et al[381]	1989	27	82	IUI	13	48.1	15.9	All natural cycles
			61	Coitus	0	0.0	0.0	
Kirby et al[382]	1991	24	58	IUI	7	29.1	12.1	All natural cycles
			52	Coitus	4	16.7	7.8	
Chaffkin et al[383]	1991	—	58	LH-IUI	3	—	5.1	Retrospective,
			91	hMG-IUI	24	—	26.2	nonrandomized
			76	hMG-coitus	6	—	7.9	

IUI, intrauterine insemination; ICI, intracervical insemination; CC, clomiphene citrate; AIH, artificial insemination with husband's sperm; LH, luteinizing hormone; hMG, human menopausal gonadotropin.

SERIAL PERIOVULATORY POSTCOITAL TESTS

CERVICAL MUCUS SCORE

Abnormal — Normal

EVALUATE CERVICAL COMPONENT

EVALUATE SPERM IN CERVICAL MUCUS

ESTROGEN CHALLENGE TEST

Progressively motile sperm | No progressively motile sperm | No sperm

Mucus improves | No change

EVALUATE SPERM IN VAGINA

Consider estrogen or hMG | Consider IUI

REPEAT PCT

NORMAL

Sperm present | Sperm absent

REPEAT PCT

No change

REPEAT PCT

Coital problem or ejaculatory dysfunction

REPEAT PCT

CONTINUE INFERTILITY TESTING

IN VITRO CROSSED SPERM-CERVICAL MUCUS PENETRATION TEST

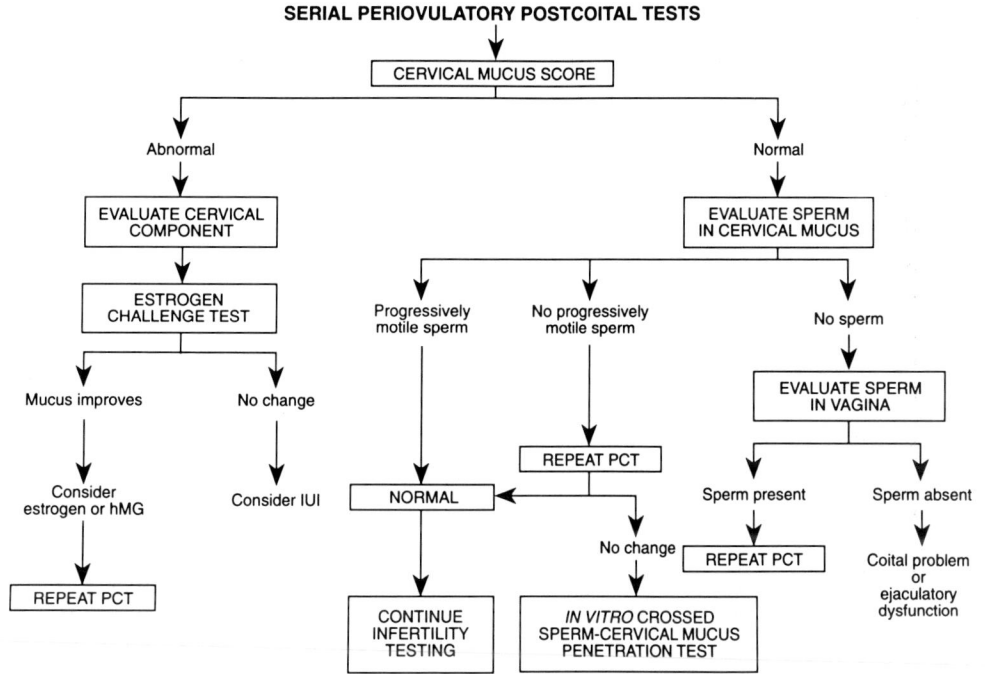

FIGURE 18–11. Algorithm for the management of postcoital test results. hMG, human menopausal gonadotropin; PCT, postcoital test; IUI, intrauterine insemination.

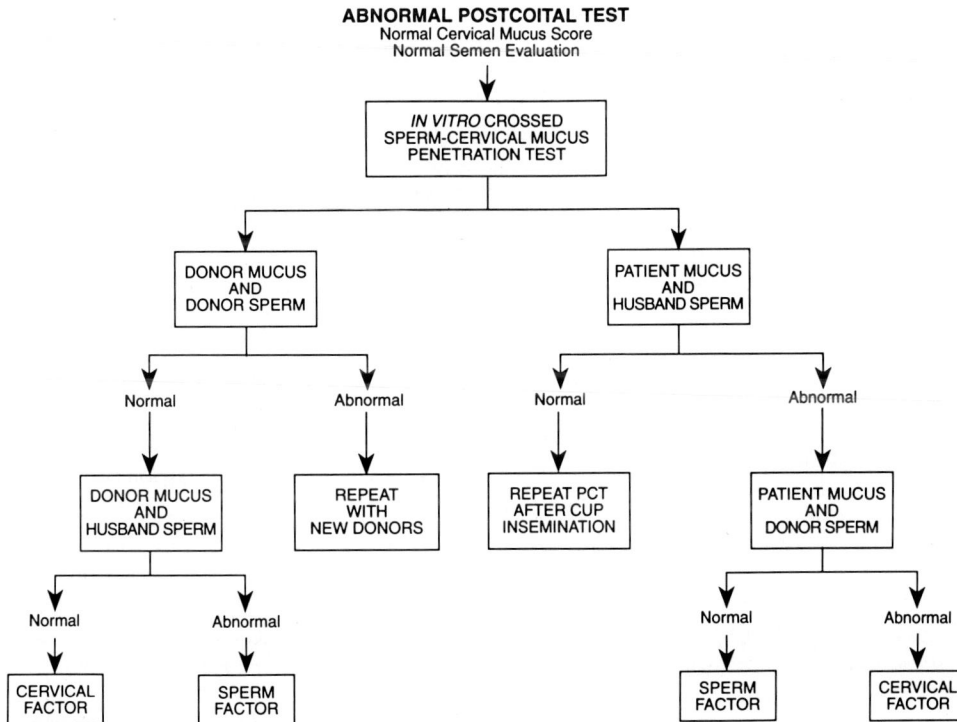

ABNORMAL POSTCOITAL TEST
Normal Cervical Mucus Score
Normal Semen Evaluation

IN VITRO CROSSED SPERM-CERVICAL MUCUS PENETRATION TEST

DONOR MUCUS AND DONOR SPERM

PATIENT MUCUS AND HUSBAND SPERM

Normal | Abnormal

Normal | Abnormal

DONOR MUCUS AND HUSBAND SPERM

REPEAT WITH NEW DONORS

REPEAT PCT AFTER CUP INSEMINATION

PATIENT MUCUS AND DONOR SPERM

Normal | Abnormal

Normal | Abnormal

CERVICAL FACTOR

SPERM FACTOR

SPERM FACTOR

CERVICAL FACTOR

FIGURE 18–12. Algorithm for the conduct of an in vitro crossed sperm–cervical mucus penetration test.

donor insemination as an option. Much more work needs to be done to develop an effective therapy for cervical mucus ASAB.

Summary: An Algorithm for the Evaluation and Treatment of Cervical Infertility

The mainstay of the clinical evaluation of cervical mucus and sperm–cervical mucus interaction is the PCT (Fig. 18–11), supported by semen evaluation and in vitro sperm–cervical mucus penetration testing. The PCT and semen evaluation are complementary. It is not possible to diagnose a cervical cause for abnormal sperm–cervical mucus interaction without knowledge of sperm parameters. A common cause of poor sperm penetration after intercourse is male factor.

The window of cervical mucus receptivity for sperm penetration is narrow, and the peak in cervical mucus quality is closely tied to periovulatory events. It is important to know the patient's ovulatory status and the relation of the PCT to midcycle. A single PCT timed by clinical criteria has a high probability of falling outside the optimal window, and the most common error in postcoital testing is poor timing. A single normal PCT result is reassuring, but the diagnosis of poor-quality cervical mucus or abnormal sperm–cervical mucus interaction should never be based on a single PCT result or on postcoital testing in a single cycle.

A repeatedly abnormal cervical mucus score despite periovulatory timing most commonly occurs in women with a history of cervical surgery. Couples who are culture positive for *N. gonorrhoeae* or *Chlamydia* should be treated according to Centers for Disease Control and Prevention guidelines, but empiric antibiotic therapy in women who are culture negative is of questionable value. An estrogen challenge test (80 μg of ethinyl estradiol daily for 7 to 10 days) may identify a subgroup of patients in whom estrogen or hMG therapy should be considered. Patients who fail to produce an estrogenic cervical mucus despite an estrogen challenge are unlikely to benefit and may elect a trial of IUI. There is little rationale for the use of expectorants, mucolytics, donor cervical mucus, or mucus substitutes in these couples. When poor-quality mucus occurs in clomiphene-induced cycles, the options include a reduction in clomiphene citrate dose; the addition of exogenous estrogen; a change to hMG therapy; or the addition of IUI.

A repeatedly abnormal PCT result despite a normal cervical mucus score and normal semen parameters cannot distinguish male from cervical factors. When there are no sperm in cervical mucus, the first thought should be to performance problems, and vaginal fluid should be examined. The absence of sperm suggests a coital problem or ejaculatory dysfunction. When sperm are present in the vagina but absent from cervical mucus, the PCT should be repeated. If there are no sperm or no progressively motile sperm in cervical mucus despite a normal cervical score, normal semen evaluation, and sperm in the vagina, an in vitro crossed sperm–cervical mucus penetration test (Fig. 18–12) should be performed. This test has the following two controls: First, the patient's mucus versus the partner's sperm should confirm the poor sperm penetration that was previously seen in vivo. A normal in vitro test requires an evaluation for vaginal factor. If there is normal sperm penetration after AIH/cup, a trial of that therapy is warranted. Second, donor mucus versus donor sperm should demonstrate normal sperm penetration and survival as a quality control. A sperm factor should be suspected when husband's sperm do poorly in both donor and patient mucus, and the patient's mucus supports normal penetration by donor sperm. A cervical mucus factor should be suspected when both husband and donor sperm do poorly in the patient's mucus and penetrate donor mucus normally.

Sperm-bound or cervical mucus ASABs can be evaluated by immunobead or MAR testing, as appropriate. IUI is often prescribed in either instance, but documentation of ASAB status is important in outlining long-term therapeutic options. Superovulation with hMG may be reasonable in patients with antibodies in cervical mucus, and the response to therapy can be quantitated.

REFERENCES

1. Grant A. Cervical hostility: incidence, diagnosis and prognosis. Fertil Steril 1958;9:321–333.
2. Moghissi KS. Sperm migration through the human cervix. In: Blandau RJ, Moghissi K, editors. The Biology of the Cervix. Chicago: University of Chicago Press, 1973:305–327.
3. Moghissi KS. Sperm migration through the human cervix. In: Elstein M, Moghissi KS, Borth R, editors. Cervical Mucus in Human Reproduction. Copenhagen: Scriptor, 1973:128–152.
4. Settlage DSF, Motoshima M, Tredway DR. Sperm transport from the external cervical os to the fallopian tubes in women: a time and quantitation study. Fertil Steril 1973;24:655–661.
5. Ferenczy A, Winkler B. Anatomy and histology of the cervix. In: Kurman RJ, editor. Blaustein's Pathology of the Female Genital Tract. 3rd edition. New York: Springer–Verlag, 1987:141–157.
6. Hafez ESE. Histology and microstructure of the cervical epithelial secretory system. In: Elstein M, Moghissi KS, Borth R, editors. Cervical Mucus in Human Reproduction. Copenhagen: Scriptor, 1973:23–32.
7. Hafez ESE. The comparative anatomy of the mammalian cervix. In: Blandau RJ, Moghissi K, editors. The Biology of the Cervix. Chicago: University of Chicago Press, 1973:23–56.
8. Hafez ESE. Functional anatomy of uterine cervix. In: Insler V, Lunenfeld B, editors. Infertility: Male and Female. Edinburgh: Churchill Livingstone, 1986:3–25.
9. Krantz KE. The anatomy of the human cervix, gross and microscopic. In: Blandau RJ, Moghissi K, editors. The Biology of the Cervix. Chicago: University of Chicago Press, 1973:57–69.
10. Mann T. Energy requirements of spermatozoa and the cervical environment. In: Blandau RJ, Moghissi K, editors. The Biology of the Cervix. Chicago: University of Chicago Press, 1973:329–338.
11. Odeblad E, Rudolfsson C. Types of cervical secretions: biophysical characteristics. In: Blandau RJ, Moghissi K, editors. The Biology of the Cervix. Chicago: University of Chicago Press, 1973:267–283.
12. Pommerenke WT. Some biochemical aspects of the cervical secretions. Ann NY Acad Sci 1962;97:581–590.
13. Schumacher GFB. Biochemistry of cervical mucus. Fertil Steril 1970;21:697–705.
14. Blandau RJ. Sperm transport through the mammalian cervix: comparative aspects. In: Blandau RJ, Moghissi K, editors. The Biology of the Cervix. Chicago: University of Chicago Press, 1973:285–304.
15. Katz DF, Drobnis EZ, Overstreet JW. Factors regulating mammalian sperm migration through the female reproductive tract and oocyte vestments. Gamete Res 1989;22:443–469.
16. Mastroianni L Jr, Zausner-Guelman B, Go KJ. Sperm transport in the female reproductive tract. In: Behrman SJ, Kistner RW, Patton GW, editors. Progress in Infertility. 3rd edition. Boston: Little, Brown, 1988:663–672.
17. Overstreet JW. Transport of gametes in the reproductive tract of the female mammal. In: Hartmann JF, editor. Mechanism and Control of Animal Fertilization. New York: Academic Press, 1983:499–543.
18. Overstreet JW, Katz DF. Sperm transport and capacitation. In: Sciarra JJ, Simpson JL, Speroff L, editors. Gynecology and Obstetrics. 5th edition. Philadelphia: Harper & Row, 1987:1–10.

19. Masters WH, Johnson VE. Human Sexual Response. Boston: Little, Brown, 1966:68–100.
20. Kroeks MVAM, Kremer J. Sperm migration. In: Insler V, Bettendorf G, editors. The Uterine Cervix in Reproduction. Stuttgart: Georg Thieme, 1977:109–118.
21. Moghissi KS. Cyclic changes of cervical mucus in normal and progestin-treated women. Fertil Steril 1966;17:663–675.
22. Moghissi KS, Dabich D, Levine J, Neuhaus OW. Mechanism of sperm migration. Fertil Steril 1964;15:15–23.
23. Tampion D, Gibbons RA. Effect of pH on the swimming rate of bull spermatozoa. J Reprod Fertil 1963;5:249–258.
24. Makler A, David R, Blumenfeld Z, Better OS. Sperm viability as affected by change of pH and osmolality of semen and urine specimens. Fertil Steril 1981;36:507–511.
25. Peek JC, Matthews CD. The pH of cervical mucus, quality of semen, and outcome of the postcoital test. Clin Reprod Fertil 1986;4:217–225.
26. Zavos PM, Cohen MR. The pH of cervical mucus and the postcoital test. Fertil Steril 1980;34:234–238.
27. Wolters-Everhardt E, Dony JMJ, Lemmens WAJG, et al. Buffering capacity of human semen. Fertil Steril 1986;46:114–119.
28. Fox CA, Meldrum SJ, Watson BW. Continuous measurement by radiotelemetry of vaginal pH during human coitus. J Reprod Fertil 1973;33:69–75.
29. MacLeod J, Martens F, Silberman C, Sobrero AJ. The postcoital and post-insemination cervical mucus and semen quality. Stud Fertil 1959;10:41–51.
30. Wallace-Haagens MJ, Duffy BJ, Holtrop HR. Recovery of spermatozoa from human vaginal washings. Fertil Steril 1975;26:175–179.
31. Sobrero AJ, MacLeod J. The immediate post-coital test. Fertil Steril 1962;13:184–189.
32. Bedford JM. The rate of sperm passage into the cervix after coitus in the rabbit. J Reprod Fertil 1971;25:211–218.
33. Moghissi KS, Syner FN, Evans TN. A composite picture of the menstrual cycle. Am J Obstet Gynecol 1972;114:405–418.
34. Fluhmann CF. The Cervix Uteri and Its Disease. Philadelphia: WB Saunders, 1961.
35. Fluhmann CF, Dickmann Z. The basic pattern of the glandular structures of the cervix uteri. Obstet Gynecol 1958;11:543–555.
36. Davajan V. Nakamura RM. The in vitro sperm–cervical mucus testing. In: Elstein M, Moghissi KS, Borth R, editors. Cervical Mucus in Human Reproduction. Copenhagen: Scriptor, 1973:153–161.
37. Moghissi KS. Inflammatory and traumatic conditions of the cervix. In: Gondos B, Riddick DH, editors. Pathology of Infertility. New York: Thieme Medical, 1987:1–11.
38. Odeblad E. Biophysical techniques of assessing cervical mucus and microstructure of cervical epithelium. In: Elstein M, Moghissi KS, Borth R, editors. Cervical Mucus in Human Reproduction. Copenhagen: Scriptor, 1973:58–74.
39. Bernstein D, Glezerman M, Zeidel L, Insler V. Quantitative study of the number and size of cervical crypts. In: Insler V, Bettendorf G, editors. The Uterine Cervix in Reproduction. Stuttgart: Georg Thieme, 1977:14–21.
40. Insler V, Glezerman M, Bernstein D, et al. Cervical crypts and their role in storing spermatozoa. In: Insler V, Bettendorf G, Geissler K-H, editors. Advances in Diagnosis and Treatment of Infertility. New York: Elsevier/North Holland, 1981:195–211.
41. Chretien FC, Gernigon C, David G, Psychoyos A. The ultrastructure of human cervical mucus under scanning electron microscopy. Fertil Steril 1973;24:746–757.
42. Elstein M, Daunter B. The electron microscopy of human cervical mucus in the normal menstrual cycle and the first trimester of pregnancy. In: Insler V, Bettendorf G, editors. The Uterine Cervix in Reproduction. Stuttgart: Georg Thieme, 1977:52–62.
43. Lee WI, Verdugo P, Blandau RJ, Gaddum-Rosse P. Molecular arrangement of cervical mucus: a reevaluation based on laser light–scattering spectroscopy. Gynecol Invest 1977;8:254–266.
44. Schumacher GFB. Soluble proteins of human cervical mucus. In: Elstein M, Moghissi KS, Borth R, editors. Cervical Mucus in Human Reproduction. Copenhagen: Scriptor, 1973:93–113.
45. Pommerenke WT. Cyclic changes in the physical and chemical properties of cervical mucus: Am J Obstet Gynecol 1946;52:1023–1031.
46. Pommerenke WT, Viergiver E. Comparison of rates of penetration of unwashed and washed spermatozoa in cervical mucus. Proc Soc Exp Biol (NY) 1947;66:161–163.
47. Breckenridge MAB, Pommerenke WT. Analysis of carbohydrates in human cervical mucus. Fertil Steril 1951;2:29–44.
48. Kellerman AS, Weed JC. Sperm motility and survival in relation to glucose concentration: an in vitro study. Fertil Steril 1970;11:802–805.
49. Van der Linden PJQ, Kets M, Gimpel JA, Wiegerinck MAHM. Cyclic changes in the concentration of glucose and fructose in human cervical mucus. Fertil Steril 1992;57:573–577.
50. Weed JC, Carrera AE. Glucose content of cervical mucus. Fertil Steril 1970;21:866–872.
51. Brown RL. Rate of transport of spermia in human uterus and tubes. Am J Obstet Gynecol 1944;47:407–411.
52. Rubenstein BB, Strauss H, Lazarus ML, Hankin H. Sperm survival in woman: motile sperm in the fundus and tubes of surgical cases. Fertil Steril 1951;2:15–19.
53. Egli GE, Newton M. The transport of carbon particles in the human female reproductive tract. Fertil Steril 1961;12:151–155.
54. Steck T, Wurfel W, Becker W, Albert PJ. Serial scintigraphic imaging for visualization of passive transport processes in the human fallopian tube. Hum Reprod 1991;6:1186–1191.
55. Brundin J, Dahlborn M, Ahlberg-Are E, Lundberg HJ. Radionuclide hysterosalpingography for measurement of human oviductal function. Int J Gynecol Obstet 1989;28:53–59.
56. Stone SC, McCalley M, Braunstein P, Egbert R. Radionuclide evaluation of tubal function. Fertil Steril 1985;43:757–760.
57. First NL, Short RF, Peters JB, Stratman FW. Transport of boar spermatozoa in estrual and luteal sows. J Anim Sci 1968;27:1032–1036.
58. Overstreet JW, Tom RA. Experimental studies of rapid sperm transport in rabbits. J Reprod Fertil 1982;66:601–606.
59. Masters WH. The sexual response of the human female: I. Gross anatomic considerations. West J Surg 1960;68:57–72.
60. Sobrero AJ. Sperm migration in the human female. In: Westin B, Wiqvist N, editors. Fertility and Sterility. Proceedings of the Fifth World Congress. Amsterdam: Excerpta Medica Foundation, 1967:701–703.
61. Katz DF, Overstreet JW. Mammalian sperm movement in the secretions of the male and female genital tracts. In: Steinberger A, Steinberger E, editors. Testicular Development, Structure, and Function. New York: Raven Press, 1980:481–489.
62. Casey ML, Byrd W, MacDonald PC. Massive amounts of immunoreactive endothelin in human seminal fluid. J Clin Endocrinol Metab 1992;74:223–225.
63. Adams CE. A study of fertilization in the rabbit: the effect of post-coital ligation of the fallopian tube or uterine horn. J Endocrinol 1956;13:296–308.
64. Hunter RF, Nichol R, Crabtree SM. Transport of spermatozoa in the ewe: timing of the establishment of a functional population in the oviduct. Reprod Nutr Dev 1980;20:1869–1875.
65. Yanagimachi R, Chang MC. Sperm ascent through the oviduct of the hamster and rabbit in relation to the time of ovulation. J Reprod Fertil 1963;6:413–420.
66. Bedford JM. Sperm capacitation and fertilization in mammals. Biol Reprod 1970;2(Suppl):128–158.
67. Overstreet JW, Cooper GW. Sperm transport in the reproductive tract of the female rabbit: I. The rapid transit phase of transport. Biol Reprod 1978;19:101–114.
68. Frenkel DA. Sperm migration and survival in the endometrial cavity. Int J Fertil 1961;6:285–290.
69. Gibor Y, Garcia CJ, Cohen MR, Scommegna A. The cyclical changes in the physical properties of the cervical mucus and the results of the postcoital test. Fertil Steril 1970;21:20–27.
70. Nicholson R. Vitality of spermatozoa in the endocervical canal. Fertil Steril 1965;16:758–764.
71. Perloff WH, Steinberger E. In vivo survival of spermatozoa in cervical mucus. Am J Obstet Gynecol 1964;88:439–442.
72. Ahlgren M. Sperm transport to and survival in the human fallopian tube. Gynecol Invest 1975;6:206–214.
73. Horne HW Jr, Audet C. Spider cells, a new inhabitant of peritoneal fluid. Obstet Gynec 1958;11:421–423.
74. Hunter RHF. Human fertilization in vivo, with special reference to progression, storage and release of competent spermatozoa. Hum Reprod 1987;2:329–332.
75. Overstreet JW, Cooper GW, Katz DF. Sperm transport in the reproductive tract of the female rabbit: II. The sustained phase of transport. Biol Reprod 1978;19:115–132.
76. Mattner PE. The cervix and its secretions in relation to fertility in ruminants. In: Blandau RJ, Moghissi K, editors. The Biology of the Cervix. Chicago: University of Chicago Press, 1973:339–350.

77. Davajan V, Nakamura RM. The cervical factor. In: Behrman SJ, Kistner RW, editors. Progress in Infertility. 2nd edition. Boston: Little, Brown, 1975:17–46.

78. Gibbons RA, Mattner P. Some aspects of the chemistry of cervical mucus. Int J Fertil 1966;11:366.

79. Hanson FW, Overstreet JW, Katz DF. A study of the relationship of motile sperm numbers in cervical mucus 48 hours after artificial insemination with subsequent fertility. Am J Obstet Gynecol 1982;143:85–90.

80. Gould JE, Overstreet JW, Hanson FW. Assessment of human sperm function after recovery from the female reproductive tract. Biol Reprod 1984;31:888–894.

81. Gould JE, Overstreet JW, Hanson FW. Interaction of human spermatozoa with the human zona pellucida and zona-free hamster oocyte following capacitation by exposure to human cervical mucus. Gamete Res 1984;12:47–54.

82. Lambert H, Overstreet JW, Morales P, et al. Sperm capacitation in the human female reproductive tract. Fertil Steril 1985;43:325–327.

83. Zinaman M, Drobnis EZ, Morales P, et al. The physiology of sperm recovered from the human cervix: acrosomal status and response to inducers of the acrosome reaction. Biol Reprod 1989;41:790–797.

84. Dukelow WR, Williams WL. Capacitation of sperm. In: Behrman SJ, Kistner RW, Patton GW, editors. Progress in Infertility. 3rd edition. Boston: Little, Brown, 1988:673–687.

85. Zaneveld LJD, De Jonge DJ, Anderson RA, Mack SR. Human sperm capacitation and the acrosome reaction. Hum Reprod 1991;6:1265–1274.

86. Soupart P, Strong PA. Ultrastructural observations on human oocytes fertilized in vitro. Fertil Steril 1974;25:11–44.

87. Barros C, Jedlicki A, Fuenzalida I, et al. Human sperm–cervical mucus interaction and the ability of spermatozoa to fuse with zona-free hamster oocytes. J Reprod Fertil 1988;82:477–484.

88. Chang MC. A detrimental effect of seminal plasma on the fertilizing capacity of sperm. Nature 1957;179:258–259.

89. Burkman LJ. Characterization of hyperactivated motility by human spermatozoa during capacitation: comparison of fertile and oligozoospermic sperm populations. Arch Androl 1984;13:153–165.

90. Cohen MR, Stein IF. Sperm survival at estimated ovulation time—comparative morphology: relative male infertility. Fertil Steril 1951;2:20–28.

91. Fredricsson B, Bjork G. Morphology of postcoital spermatozoa in the cervical secretion and its clinical significance. Fertil Steril 1977;28:841–845.

92. Gonzales J, Jezequel F. Influence of the quality of the cervical mucus on sperm penetration: comparison of the morphologic features of spermatozoa in 101 postcoital tests with those in the semen of the husband. Fertil Steril 1985;44:796–799.

93. Pretorius E, Franken DR, De Wet J, Grobler S. Sperm selection capacity of cervical mucus. Arch Androl 1984;12:5–7.

94. Hanson FW, Overstreet JW. The interaction of human spermatozoa with cervical mucus in vivo. Am J Obstet Gynecol 1981;140:173–178.

95. Perry G, Glezerman M, Insler V. Selective filtration of abnormal spermatozoa by the cervical mucus in vitro. In: Insler V, Bettendorf G, editors. The Uterine Cervix in Reproduction. Stuttgart: Georg Thieme, 1977:118–128.

96. Katz DF, Diel L, Overstreet JW. Differences in the movement of morphologically normal and abnormal human seminal spermatozoa. Biol Reprod 1982;26:566–570.

97. Morales P, Katz DF, Overstreet JW, et al. The relationship between the motility and morphology of spermatozoa in human semen. J Androl 1988;9:241–247.

98. Barros C, Vigil P, Herrera E, et al. Selection of morphologically abnormal sperm by human cervical mucus. Arch Androl 1984;12(Suppl):95–107.

99. Katz DF, Morales P, Samuels SJ, Overstreet JW. Mechanisms of filtration of morphologically abnormal human sperm by cervical mucus. Fertil Steril 1990;54:513–516.

100. Insler V, Melmed H, Eichenbrenner I, et al. The cervical score. Int J Gynecol Obstet 1972;10:223–228.

101. Moghissi KS. Significance and prognostic value of postcoital test. In: Insler V, Bettendorf G, editors. The Uterine Cervix in Reproduction. Stuttgart: Georg Thieme, 1977:231–238.

102. World Health Organization. WHO Laboratory Manual for the Examination of Human Semen and Sperm–Cervical Mucus Interaction. 3rd edition. New York: Cambridge University Press, 1992.

103. Collins JA, So Y, Wilson EH, et al. The postcoital test as a predictor of pregnancy among 355 infertile couples. Fertil Steril 1984;41:703–708.

104. Glass RH, Mroueh A. The postcoital test and semen analysis. Fertil Steril 1967;18:314–317.

105. Tredway DR. The interpretation and significance of the fractional postcoital test. Am J Obstet Gynecol 1976;124:352–355.

106. Tredway DR, Buchanan GC, Drake TS. Comparison of the fractional postcoital test and semen analysis. Am J Obstet Gynecol 1978;130:647–652.

107. Huhner M. Sterility in the male and female and its treatment. New York: Robman, 1913.

108. Huhner M. Importance of Huhner test in cases of necrospermia. J Obstet Gynaecol Br Emp 1937;44:334–336.

109. Huhner M. The diagnosis and treatment of sexual disorders in the male and female including sterility and impotence. Philadelphia: FA Davis, 1942:62.

110. Sims JM. Clinical notes of uterine surgery with special reference to the management of the sterile condition. New York: William Wood, 1869.

111. American College of Obstetricians and Gynecologists: Infertility. ACOG Technical Bulletin No. 125. Washington, DC: ACOG, 1989.

112. American Fertility Society, Investigation of the Infertile Couple, Birmingham, AL, 1986:29.

113. Blankstein J, Mashiach S, Lunenfeld B. Ovulation induction and in vitro fertilization. Chicago: Year Book Medical, 1986:61–76.

114. Davajan V. Postcoital testing: The cervical factor as a cause of infertility. In: Mishell DR Jr, Davajan V, Lobo RA, editors. Infertility, Contraception and Reproductive Endocrinology. 3rd edition. Boston: Blackwell Scientific, 1991:599–611.

115. Glass RH. Infertility. In: Yen SSC, Jaffe RB, editors. Reproductive Endocrinology. 3rd edition. Philadelphia: WB Saunders, 1991:689–709.

116. Moghissi KS. Diagnosis and classification of disturbed sperm–cervical mucus interaction. In: Insler V, Lunenfeld B, editors. Infertility: Male and Female. Edinburgh: Churchill Livingstone, 1986:299–314.

117. Speroff L, Glass RH, Kase NG. Clinical Gynecologic Endocrinology and Infertility. 4th edition. Baltimore: Williams & Wilkins, 1989:513–546.

118. Moghissi KS. Evaluation and management of cervical hostility. Semin Reprod Endocrinol 1986;4:343–355.

119. Griffith CS, Grimes DA. The validity of the postcoital test. Am J Obstet Gynecol 1990;162:615–620.

120. Hull MGR, Savage PE, Bromham DR. Prognostic value of the postcoital test: prospective study based on time-specific conception rates. Br J Obstet Gynecol 1982;89:299–305.

121. Asch RH. Laparoscopic recovery of sperm from peritoneal fluid in patients with negative or poor Sims-Huhner test. Fertil Steril 1976;27:1111–1114.

122. Asch RH. Sperm recovery in peritoneal aspirate after negative Sims-Huhner test. Int J Fertil 1978;23:57–60.

123. Templeton AA, Mortimer D. Laparoscopic sperm recovery in infertile women. Br J Obstet Gynaecol 1980;87:1128–1131.

124. Templeton AA, Mortimer D. The development of a clinical test of sperm migration to the site of fertilization. Fertil Steril 1982;37:410–415.

125. Stone SC. Peritoneal recovery of sperm in patients with infertility associated with inadequate cervical mucus. Fertil Steril 1983;40:802–804.

126. Buxton L, Southam AL. Human Infertility. New York: Hoeber-Harper, 1958:184–195.

127. Jette NT, Glass RH. Prognostic value of the postcoital test. Fertil Steril 1972;23:29–32.

128. Giner J, Merino G, Luna J, Aznar R. Evaluation of the Sims-Huhner postcoital test in fertile couples. Fertil Steril 1974;25:145–148.

129. Taymor ML. Infertility. New York: Grune and Stratton, 1978:46–55.

130. Danezis J, Sujan S, Sobrero AJ. Evaluation of the postcoital test. Fertil Steril 1962;13:559–574.

131. Southam AL, Buxton L. Seventy postcoital tests made during the conception cycle. Fertil Steril 1956;7:133–140.

132. Cramer DW, Walker AM, Schiff I. Statistical methods in evaluating the outcome of infertility therapy. Fertil Steril 1979;32:80–86.

133. Olive DL. Analysis of clinical fertility trials: A methodologic review. Fertil Steril 1986;45:157–170.

134. Kerin JF, Matthews CD, Svigos JM, et al. Linear and quantitative migration of stored sperm through cervical mucus during the periovular period. Fertil Steril 1976;27:1054–1058.

135. Makler A. New method for evaluating cervical penetrability using daily aspirated and stored cervical mucus. Fertil Steril 1976;27:533–540.

136. Skaf RA, Kemmann E. Postcoital testing in women during menotropin therapy. Fertil Steril 1982;37:514–519.

137. Templeton AA, Penney GC, Lees MM. Relation between the luteinizing

hormone peak, the nadir of the basal body temperature, and the cervical mucus score. Br J Obstet Gynecol 1982;89:985–988.

138. Zegers F, Lenton EA, Sulaimann R, Cooke ID. The cervical factor in patients with ovulatory infertility. Br J Obstet Gynecol 1981;88:537–542.

139. Nulsen J, Wheeler C, Ausmanas M, Blasco L. Cervical mucus changes in relationship to urinary luteinizing hormone. Fertil Steril 1987;48:783–786.

140. Freund M. Effect of frequency of emission on semen output and an estimate of daily sperm production in man. J Reprod Fertil 1963;6:269–286.

141. Lampe EH, Masters WH. Problem of male fertility: II. Effect of frequent ejaculation. Fertil Steril 1956;7:123–127.

142. Levin RM, Latimore J, Wein AJ, Van Arsdalen KN. Correlation of sperm count with frequency of ejaculation. Fertil Steril 1986;45:732–734.

143. Matilsky M, Battino S, Ben-Ami M, et al. The effect of ejaculatory frequency on semen characteristics of normozoospermic and oligozoospermic men from an infertile population. Hum Reprod 1993;8:71–73.

144. Mortimer D, Templeton AA, Lenton EA, Coleman RA. Influence of abstinence and ejaculation-to-analysis delay on semen analysis parameters of suspected infertile men. Arch Androl 1982;8:251–256.

145. Poland ML, Moghissi KS, Giblin PT, et al. Variation of semen measures within normal men. Fertil Steril 1985;44:396–400.

146. Schwartz D, Laplanche A, Jouannet P, David G. Within-subject variability of human semen in regard to sperm count, volume, total number of spermatozoa and length of abstinence. J Reprod Fertil 1979;57:391–395.

147. Johnson L. A reevaluation of daily sperm output of men. Fertil Steril 1982;37:811–816.

148. Tredway DR, Settlage DSF, Nakamura RM, et al. Significance of timing for the post-coital evaluation of cervical mucus. Am J Obstet Gynecol 1975;121:387–393.

149. Taymor ML, Overstreet JW. Some thoughts on the postcoital test. Fertil Steril 1988;50:702–703.

150. Davajan V, Kunitake GM. Fractional in vivo and in vitro examination of postcoital cervical mucus in the human. Fertil Steril 1969;20:197–210.

151. Moran J, Davajan V, Nakamura R. Comparison of the fractional postcoital test with the Sims-Huhner post-coital test. Int J Fertil 1974;19:93–96.

152. Versteegh LR, Shade AR. The fractional postcoital test: a reappraisal. Fertil Steril 1979;31:40–44.

153. Boyers SP, Davis RO, Katz DF. Automated semen analysis. Curr Prob Obstet Gynecol Fertil 1989;12:165–200.

154. Davis RO, Katz DF. Operational standards for CASA instruments. J Androl 1993;14:385–394.

155. Harrison RF. The diagnostic and therapeutic potential of the postcoital test. Fertil Steril 1981;36:71–75.

156. Kovacs GT, Newman GB, Henson GL. The postcoital test: What is normal? Br Med J 1978;1:818.

157. Moghissi KS. Postcoital test: physiologic basis, technique, and interpretation. Fertil Steril 1976;27:117–129.

158. Doody MC, Good MC. The postcoital test: a quantitative method. J Androl 1993;14:149–154.

159. Kremer J, Jager S. The sperm–cervical mucus contact test: a preliminary report. Fertil Steril 1976;27:335–340.

160. Kremer J, Jager S. Sperm–cervical mucus interaction, in particular in the presence of antispermatozoal antibodies. Hum Reprod 1988;3:69–73.

161. Kremer J. A simple sperm penetration test. Int J Fertil 1965;10:209–215.

162. Katz DF, Overstreet JW, Hanson FW. A new quantitative test for sperm penetration into cervical mucus. Fertil Steril 1980;33:179–186.

163. Pandya IJ, Mortimer D, Sawers RS. A standardized approach for evaluating the penetration of human spermatozoa into cervical mucus in vitro. Fertil Steril 1986;45:357–365.

164. Eggert-Kruse W, Hofsass A, Haury E, et al. Relationship between local antisperm antibodies and sperm–mucus interaction in vitro and in vivo. Hum Reprod 1991;6:267–276.

165. Eggert-Kruse W, Gerhard I, Tilgen W, Runnebaum B. Clinical significance of crossed in vitro sperm–cervical mucus penetration test in infertility investigation. Fertil Steril 1989;52:1032–1040.

166. Kunitake G, Davajan V. A new method of evaluating infertility due to cervical mucus–spermatozoa incompatibility. Fertil Steril 1970;21:706–714.

167. Jager S, Kremer J, Kuiken J, Van Slochteren-Draaïsma T. Immunoglobulin class of antispermatozoal antibodies from infertile men and inhibition of in vitro sperm penetration in cervical mucus. Int J Androl 1980;3:1–14.

168. Bronson RA, Cooper GW, Rosenfeld DL. Sperm antibodies: their role in infertility. Fertil Steril 1984;42:171–183.

169. Gaddum-Rosse P, Blandau RJ, Lee WI. Sperm penetration into cervical mucus in vitro: I. Comparative studies. Fertil Steril 1980;33:636–643.

170. Gaddum-Rosse P, Blandau RJ, Lee WI. Sperm penetration into cervical mucus in vitro: II. Human spermatozoa in bovine mucus. Fertil Steril 1980;33:644–648.

171. Bronson RA, Cooper GW, Rosenfeld DL. Autoimmunity to spermatozoa: effect on sperm penetration of cervical mucus as reflected by postcoital testing. Fertil Steril 1984;41:609–614.

172. Hull MGR, Glazener CMA, Kelly NJ, et al. Population study of causes, treatment and outcome of infertility. Br Med J 1985;291:1693–1697.

173. Simmons FA. Human Infertility. N Engl J Med 1956;255:1140–1146; 1186–1192.

174. Marrs RP. Evaluation of the infertile female. In: DeCherney AH, editor. Reproductive Failure. New York: Churchill Livingstone, 1986:41–49.

175. Moghissi KS. The cervix in infertility. Clin Obstet Gynecol 1979;22:27–42.

176. Tredway DR. The postcoital test. In: Sciarra JJ, Simpson JL, Speroff L, editors. Gynecology and Obstetrics. 5th edition. Philadelphia: Harper & Row, 1987:1–7.

177. Sturmdorf A. Tracheloplastic methods and results. Surg Gynecol Obstet 1916;16:390–400.

178. Hester LL Jr, Read RA. An evaluation of cervical conization. Am J Obstet Gynecol 1960;80:715–721.

179. Doran TA, Shier CB. Conization of the cervix. Am J Obstet Gynecol 1964;88:367–374.

180. Kern G, Aslani A, Kern-Bontke E, Grafin zu Eulenburg H. The consequences of conization of the uterine cervix. Geburtsh Frauenheilk 1967;27:879.

181. Krieger JS, McCormack LJ. Graded treatment for in situ carcinoma of the uterine cervix. Am J Obstet Gynecol 1968;101:171–182.

182. Davis RM, Cooke JK, Kirk RF. Cervical conization: an experience with 400 patients. Obstet Gynecol 1972;40:23–27.

183. Jonas AG. Cervical cone biopsies with the use of a solution of vasopressin and oxidized gauze packing. Am J Obstet Gynecol 1973;117:188–193.

184. Bjerre B, Eliasson G, Linell F, et al. Conization as only treatment of carcinoma in situ of the uterine cervix. Am J Obstet Gynecol 1976;125:143–152.

185. Jones HW III, Buller RE. The treatment of cervical intraepithelial neoplasia by cone biopsy. Am J Obstet Gynecol 1980;137:882–886.

186. Holdt DG, Jacobs AJ, Scott JC Jr, Adam GM. Diagnostic significance and sequelae of cone biopsy. Am J Obstet Gynecol 1982;143:312–318.

187. Larsson G, Gullberg B, Grundsell H. A comparison of complications of laser and cold-knife conization. Obstet Gynecol 1983;62:213–217.

188. Salat-Baroux J, Antoine JM, Hamou J, Mergui JL. Cervical surgery in infertility. Hum Reprod 1988;3:193–196.

189. Claman AD, Lee N. Factors that relate to complications of cone biopsy. Am J Obstet Gynecol 1974;120:124–128.

190. Stillman RJ, Hershlag A. Pathology of infertility and adverse pregnancy outcome after in utero exposure to diethylstilbestrol. In: Gondos B, Riddick DH, editors. Pathology of Infertility: Clinical Correlations in the Male and Female. New York: Thieme Medical, 1987:41–55.

191. Gilbert L, Saunders NJ, Stringer R, Sharp F. Hemostasis and cold-knife cone biopsy: a prospective randomized trial comparing a suture versus non-suture technique. Obstet Gynecol 1989;74:640–643.

192. Tovell HMM, Newton M, Barber HRK. Cone biopsy of the cervix. Clin Obstet Gynecol 1976;19:2–20.

193. Champion PK, Thompson NJ. Effect of conization of the cervix on subsequent pregnancy. Am J Obstet Gynecol 1951;62:1321–1326.

194. Boyd JR, Royle D, Fidler HK, Boyes DA. Conservative management of in situ carcinoma of the cervix. Am J Obstet Gynecol 1962;85:322–327.

195. Green GH. Pregnancy following cervical carcinoma in situ. J Obstet Gynaec Br Common 1966;73:897–902.

196. MacVicar J, Willocks J. The effect of diathermy conization of the cervix on subsequent fertility, pregnancy and delivery. J Obstet Gynaecol Br Common 1968;75:355–356.

197. Kullander S, Sjöberg N-O. Treatment of carcinoma in situ of the cervix uteri by conization. Acta Obstet Gynaecol Scand 1971;50:153–157.

198. McLaren HC, Jordan JA, Glover M, Attwod ME. Pregnancy after cone

biopsy of the cervix. J Obstet Gynaecol Br Common 1974;81:383–384.

199. Buller RE, Jones HW. Pregnancy following cervical conization. Am J Obstet Gynecol 1982;142:506–512.

200. Ragni G, Goisis F, Wyssling H, et al. Changes in cervical mucus after diathermocoagulation of the cervix. Int J Fertil 1988;33:36–39.

201. Berget A, Andreasson B, Bock JE, et al. Outpatient treatment of cervical intraepithelial neoplasia. Acta Obstet Gynecol Scand 1987;66:531–536.

202. Bryson SCP, Lenehan P, Lickrish GM. The treatment of grade 3 cervical intraepithelial neoplasia with cryotherapy: an 11-year experience. Obstet Gynecol 1985;151:201–206.

203. Ferenczy A. Comparison of cryo- and carbon dioxide laser therapy for cervical intraepithelial neoplasia. Obstet Gynecol 1985;66:793–798.

204. Hemmingsson E, Stendahl U, Stenson S. Cryosurgical treatment of cervical intraepithelial neoplasia with follow-up of five to eight years. Am J Obstet Gynecol 1981;139:144–147.

205. Richart RM, Townsend DE, Crisp W, et al. An analysis of "long term" follow-up results in patients with cervical intraepithelial neoplasia treated by cryotherapy. Am J Obstet Gynecol 1980;137:823–826.

206. Townsend DE, Ostergard DR. Cryocauterization for preinvasive cervical neoplasia. J Reprod Med 1971;6:55–60.

207. Townsend DE, Richart RM. Cryotherapy and carbon dioxide laser management of cervical intraepithelial neoplasia: a controlled comparison. Obstet Gynecol 1983;61:75–78.

208. Hollyock VE, Chanen W, Wein R. Cervical function following treatment of intraepithelial neoplasia by electrocoagulation diathermy. Obstet Gynecol 1983;61:79–81.

209. Collins RJ, Pappas HJ. Cryosurgery for benign cervicitis with follow-up of six-and-a-half years. Am J Obstet Gynecol 1972;113:744–750.

210. Einerth Y. Cryosurgical treatment of CIN: I–III. Acta Obstet Gynaecol Scand 1988;67:627–630.

211. Monaghan JM, Kirkup W, Davis JA, Edington PT. Treatment of cervical intraepithelial neoplasia by colposcopically directed cryosurgery and subsequent pregnancy experience. Br J Obstet Gynaecol 1982;89:387–392.

212. Weed JC Jr, Curry SL, Duncan ID, et al. Fertility after cryosurgery of the cervix. Obstet Gynecol 1978;52:245–246.

213. Pritchard JA, MacDonald PC, editors. Williams Obstetrics. 16th edition. New York: Appleton-Century-Crofts, 1980:587–621.

214. Stillman RJ, Schinfeld J, Schiff I. Use of the operating hysteroscope in the treatment of infertility caused by a cervical foreign body. Fertil Steril 1980;33:335–336.

215. Grimes DA, Cates W Jr. Complications from legally induced abortion: a review. Obstet Gynecol Surv 1979;34:177–191.

216. Hakim-Elahi E. Post-abortal amenorrhea due to cervical stenosis. Obstet Gynecol 1976;48:723–724.

217. Buttram VC, Gibbons WE. Müllerian anomalies: a proposed classification (an analysis of 144 cases). Fertil Steril 1979;32:40–46.

218. Farber M, Marchant DJ. Congenital absence of the uterine cervix. Am J Obstet Gynecol 1975;121:414–417.

219. Stillman RJ. In utero exposure to diethylstilbestrol: adverse effects on the reproductive performance in male and female offspring. Am J Obstet Gynecol 1982;142:905–921.

220. Barnes AB, Colton T, Gundersen J, et al. Fertility and outcome of pregnancy in women exposed in utero to diethylstilbestrol. N Engl J Med 1980;302:609–613.

221. Haney AF, Hammond CB, Soules MR, Creasman WT. Diethylstilbestrol-induced upper genital tract abnormalities. Fertil Steril 1979;31:142–146.

222. Kaufman RH, Binder GL, Grau PM Jr, Adam E. Upper genital tract changes associated with exposure in utero to diethylstilbestrol. Am J Obstet Gynecol 1977;128:51–59.

223. DeCherney AH, Cholst I, Naftolin F. Structure and function of the fallopian tubes following exposure to diethylstilbestrol (DES) during gestation. Fertil Steril 1981;36:741–745.

224. American College of Obstetricians and Gynecologists, ACOG Committee Opinion No. 131, Washington, DC, December 1993.

225. Cousins L, Karp W, Lacey C, Lucas WE. Reproductive outcome of women exposed to diethylstilbestrol in utero. Obstet Gynecol 1980;56:70–76.

226. Senekjian EK, Potkul RK, Frey K, Herbst AL. Infertility among daughters either exposed or not exposed to diethylstilbestrol. Am J Obstet Gynecol 1988;158:493–498.

227. Herbst AL, Hubby MM, Azizi F, Makii MM. Reproductive and gynecologic surgical experience in diethylstilbestrol-exposed daughters. Am J Obstet Gynecol 1981;141:1019–1028.

228. Rosenfeld DL, Bronson RA. Reproductive problems in the DES-exposed female. Obstet Gynecol 1980;55:453–456.

229. Doerschuk CF, Boat TF. Cystic fibrosis. In: Behrman RE, Vaughan VC, Nelson WE, editors. Nelson Textbook of Pediatrics. 13th edition. Philadelphia: WB Saunders, 1987:926–935.

230. Finegold SM. Cystic fibrosis. In: Wyngaarden JB, Smith LH Jr, editors. Cecil Textbook of Medicine. Philadelphia, WB Saunders, 1982:387–388.

231. Kaplan E, Schwachman H, Perlmutter AD, et al. Reproductive failure in males with cystic fibrosis. N Engl J Med 1968;279:65–69.

232. Anguiano A, Oates RD, Amos JA, et al. Congenital bilateral absence of the vas deferens. JAMA 1992;267:1794–1797.

233. Oppenheimer EH, Esterly JR. Observations on cystic fibrosis of the pancreas: VI. The uterine cervix. J Pediatr 1970;77:991–995.

234. Oppenheimer EA, Case AL, Esterly JR, Rothberg RM. Cervical mucus in cystic fibrosis: a possible cause of infertility. Am J Obstet Gynecol 1970;108:673–674.

235. Gysler M, March CM, Mishell DR Jr, Bailey EJ. A decade's experience with an individualized clomiphene treatment regimen including its effect on the postcoital test. Fertil Steril 1982;37:161–167.

236. Hammond MG, Halme JK, Talbert LM. Factors affecting the pregnancy rate in clomiphene citrate induction of ovulation. Obstet Gynecol 1983;62:196–202.

237. Lamb EJ, Guderian AM. Clinical effects of clomiphene in anovulation. Obstet Gynecol 1966;28:505–512.

238. Riley GM, Evans TN. Effects of clomiphene citrate on anovulatory ovarian function. Am J Obstet Gynecol 1964:89:97–110.

239. Cohen MR, Perez-Pelaez M. The effect of norethindrone acetate–ethinyl estradiol, clomiphene citrate, and dydrogesterone on spinnbarkeit. Fertil Steril 1965;16:141–150.

240. Ruiz-Velasco V, Uriza RB, Conde BI, Salas E. Changes during clomiphene citrate therapy. Fertil Steril 1969;20:829–839.

241. Graff G. Suppression of cervical mucus during clomiphene therapy. Fertil Steril 1971;22:209–212.

242. Poliak A, Smith JJ, Romney SL. Clinical evaluation of clomiphene; clomiphene and human chorionic gonadotropin; and clomiphene, human chorionic gonadotropin, and estrogens in anovulatory cycles. Fertil Steril 1973;24:921–925.

243. Fedele L, Brioschi D, Marchini M, et al. Enhanced preovulatory progesterone levels in clomiphene citrate–induced cycles. J Clin Endocrinol Metab 1989;69:681–683.

244. Marchini M, Dorta M, Bombelli F, et al. Effects of clomiphene citrate on cervical mucus: analysis of some influencing factors. Int J Fertil 1989;34:154–159.

245. Maxson WS, Pittaway DE, Herbert CM, et al. Antiestrogenic effect of clomiphene citrate: correlation with serum estradiol concentrations. Fertil Steril 1984;42:356–359.

246. Randall JM, Templeton A. Cervical mucus score and in vitro sperm mucus interaction in spontaneous and clomiphene citrate cycles. Fertil Steril 1991;56:465–468.

247. Asaad M, Abdulla U, Hipkin L, Diver M. The effect of clomiphene citrate treatment on cervical mucus and plasma estradiol and progesterone levels. Fertil Steril 1993;59:539–543.

248. Thompson LA, Barratt CLR, Thornton SJ, et al. The effects of clomiphene citrate and cyclofenil on cervical mucus volume and receptivity over the preovulatory period. Fertil Steril 1993;59:125–129.

249. King WJ, Greene GL. Monoclonal antibodies localize oestrogen receptor in the nuclei of target cells. Nature 1984;307:745–746.

250. Welshons WV, Lieberman ME, Gorski J. Nuclear localization of unoccupied oestrogen receptors. Nature 1984;307:747.

251. Gould SF, Shannon JM, Cunha GR. The autoradiographic demonstration of estrogen binding in normal human cervix and vagina during the menstrual cycle, pregnancy, and the menopause. Am J Anat 1983;168:229.

252. Abuzeid MI, Weibe RH, Askel S, et al. Evidence for a possible cytosol estrogen receptor deficiency in endocervical glands of infertile women with poor cervical mucus. Fertil Steril 1987;47:101–107.

253. Matthews CS, Buxton CL. Bacteriology of the cervix in cases of infertility. Fertil Steril 1951;2:45–52.

254. Friberg J, Gnarpe H. *Mycoplasma* and human reproductive failure: III. Pregnancies in "infertile" couples treated with doxycycline for *T-mycoplasmas*. Am J Obstet Gynecol 1973;116:23–26.

255. Gnarpe H, Friberg J. *Mycoplasma* and human reproductive failure. Am J Obstet Gynecol 1972;114:727–731.

256. Gnarpe H, Friberg J. *T-mycoplasma* as a possible cause for reproductive failure. Nature 1973;242:120–121.

257. Kaur M, Tripathi KK, Bansal MR, et al. Bacteriology of cervix in cases of infertility: effect on human sperm. Am J Reprod Immunol 1986;12:21–24.

258. Kaur M, Tripathi KK, Bansal MR, et al. Bacteriology of the cervix in cases of infertility: effect on human and animal spermatozoes and role of elastase. Am J Reprod Immunol 1988;17:14–17.

259. Eggert-Kruse W, Gerhard I, Hofmann H, et al. Influence of microbial colonization on sperm-mucus interaction in vivo and in vitro. Hum Reprod 1987;2:301–308.

260. Eggert-Kruse W, Hofmann H, Gerhard I, et al. Effects of antimicrobial therapy on sperm-mucus interaction. Hum Reprod 1988;3:861–869.

261. Eggert-Kruse W, Pohl S, Naher H, et al. Microbial colonization and sperm-mucus interaction: results in 1000 infertile couples. Hum Reprod 1992;7:612–620.

262. Bernstein GS. Occult genital infection and infertility. In: Mishell DR Jr, Davajan V, Lobo R, editors. Infertility, Contraception, and Reproductive Endocrinology. 3rd edition. Boston: Blackwell Scientific, 1991:769–775.

263. Cassell GH, Cole BC. Mycoplasmas as agents of human disease. N Engl J Med 1981;304:80–89.

264. Friberg J. Mycoplasmas and Ureaplasmas in infertility and abortion. Fertil Steril 1980;33:351–359.

265. Styler M, Shapiro SS. Mollicutes (mycoplasma) in infertility. Fertil Steril 1985;44:1–12.

266. Taylor-Robinson D, McCormack WM. The genital mycoplasmas: I. N Engl J Med 1980;302:1003–1067.

267. McCormack WM, Almeida PC, Bailey PE, et al. Sexual activity and vaginal colonization with genital mycoplasmas. JAMA 1972;221:1375–1377.

268. Cassell GH, Younger JB, Brown MB, et al. Microbiologic study of infertile women at the time of diagnostic laparoscopy. N Engl J Med 1983;308:501–505.

269. de Louvois J, Harrison RF, Blades M, Hurley R. Frequency of mycoplasma in fertile and infertile couples. Lancet 1974;1:1073–1075.

270. Nagata Y, Iwasaka T, Wada T-mycoplasma infection and infertility. Fertil Steril 1979;31:392–395.

271. Matthews CD, Clapp KH, Tansing JA, Cox LW. T-mycoplasma genital infection: the effect of doxycycline therapy on human unexplained infertility. Fertil Steril 1978;30:98–99.

272. Rehewy MSE, Jaszczak S, Hafez ESE, et al. Ureaplasma urealyticum (T-mycoplasma) in vaginal fluid and cervical mucus from fertile and infertile women. Fertil Steril 1978;30:297–300.

273. Stray-Pedersen B, Bruu A-L, Molne K. Infertility and uterine colonization with Ureaplasma urealyticum. Acta Obstet Gynecol Scand 1982;61:21–24.

274. Upadhyaya M, Hibbard BM, Walker SM. The role of mycoplasmas in reproduction. Fertil Steril 1983;39:814–818.

275. Harrison RF, Blades M, de Louvois J, Hurley R. Doxycycline treatment and human infertility. Lancet 1975;1:605–607.

276. Hinton RA, Egdell LM, Andrews BE, et al. A double-blind cross-over study of the effect of doxycycline on mycoplasma infection and infertility. Br J Obstet Gynaecol 1979;86:379–383.

277. Gump DW, Gibson M, Ashikaga T. Lack of association between genital mycoplasmas and infertility. N Engl J Med 1984;310:937–941.

278. Tredway DR, Wortham JWE, Condon-Mahony M, et al. Correlation of postcoital evaluation with in vitro sperm–cervical mucus determinations and Ureaplasma cultures. Fertil Steril 1985;43:286–289.

279. Busolo F, Zanchetta R. The effect of Mycoplasma hominis and Ureaplasma urealyticum on hamster egg in vitro penetration by human spermatozoa. Fertil Steril 1985;43:110–114.

280. Schachter J. Chlamydial infections: I. N Engl J Med 1978;298:428–434.

281. Schachter J. Chlamydial infections: II. N Engl J Med 1978;298:490–495.

282. Schachter J. Chlamydial infections: III. N Engl J Med 1978;298:540–548.

283. Paavonen J, Wolner-Hanssen P. Chlamydia trachomatis: a major threat to reproduction. Hum Reprod 1989;4:111–124.

284. Mardh P-A, Ripa T, Svensson L, Westrom L. Chlamydia trachomatis infection in patients with acute salpingitis. N Engl J Med 1977;296:1377–1379.

285. Brunham RB, Paavonen J, Stevens CE, et al. Mucopurulent cervicitis: the ignored counterpart of urethritis in the male. N Engl J Med 1984;311:1–6.

286. Harrison HR, Phil D, Costin M, et al. Cervical Chlamydia trachomatis infection in university women: relationship to history, contraception, ectopy, and cervicitis. Am J Obstet Gynecol 1985;153:244–252.

287. Campbell WF, Dodson MG. Clindamycin therapy for Chlamydia trachomatis in women. Am J Obstet Gynecol 1990;162:343–347.

288. Paavonen JA, Saikku P, Vesterinen E, Lehtovirta P. Infertility and cervical Chlamydia trachomatis infections. Acta Obstet Gynecol Scand 1979;58:301–303.

289. Soong Y-K, Kao S-M, Lee C-J, et al. Endocervical chlamydial deoxyribonucleic acid in infertile women. Fertil Steril 1990;54:815–818.

290. Battin DA, Barnes RB, Hoffman DI, et al. Chlamydia trachomatis is not an important cause of abnormal postcoital test in ovulating patients. Fertil Steril 1984;42:233–236.

291. Ruijs GJ, Kauer FM, Jager S, et al. Further details on sequelae at the cervical and tubal level of Chlamydia trachomatis infection in infertile women. Fertil Steril 1991;56:20–26.

292. Eggert-Kruse W, Gerhard I, Naher H, et al. Chlamydial infection: a female and/or male infertility factor? Fertil Steril 1990;53:1037–1043.

293. Kokia E, Bider D, Lunenfeld B, et al. Addition of exogenous estrogens to improve cervical mucus following clomiphene citrate medication. Acta Obstet Gynecol Scand 1990;69:139–142.

294. Sher G, Katz M. Inadequate cervical mucus: a cause of "idiopathic" infertility. Fertil Steril 1976;27:886–891.

295. Roumen FJME, Doesburg WH, Rolland R. Hormonal patterns in infertile women with a deficient postcoital test. Fertil Steril 1982;38:42–47.

296. Bronson RA. Immunologic abnormalities of the female reproductive tract. In: Gondos B, Riddick DH, editors. Pathology of Infertility. New York: Thieme Medical, 1987:13–28.

297. Bronson RA. Current concepts on the relation of antisperm antibodies and infertility. Semin Reprod Endocrinol 1988;6:363–368.

298. Bronson RA, Cooper GW, Rosenfeld DL. Factors affecting the population of the female reproductive tract by spermatozoa: their diagnosis and treatment. Semin Reprod Endocrinol 1986;4:371–381.

299. Haas GG Jr. The uterine cervix as an immune organ. Semin Reprod Endocrinol 1986;4:357–370.

300. Haas GG Jr. Immunologic factors in recurrent abortion and infertility. In: Garcia C-R, Mastroianni L Jr, Amelar RD, Dubin L, editors. Current Therapy of Infertility. 3rd edition. Toronto: BC Decker, 1988:44–46.

301. Kremer J, Jager S. The significance of antisperm antibodies for sperm–cervical mucus interaction. Hum Reprod 1992;7:781–784.

302. Schumacher GFB. Immunology of spermatozoa and cervical mucus. Hum Reprod 1988;3:289–300.

303. Price RJ, Boettcher B. The presence of complement in human cervical mucus and its possible relevance to infertility in women with complement-dependent sperm immobilizing antibodies. Fertil Steril 1979;32:61–66.

304. Jager S, Kremer J, de Wilde-Janssen IW. Are sperm-immobilizing antibodies in cervical mucus an explanation for a poor postcoital test? Am J Reprod Immunol 1984;5:56–60.

305. Jager S, Kremer J, Kuiken J, et al. Induction of the shaking phenomenon by pretreatment of spermatozoa with sera containing antispermatozoal antibodies. Fertil Steril 1981;36:784–791.

306. Wang C, Baker HWG, Jennings MG, et al. Interaction between human cervical mucus and sperm surface antibodies. Fertil Steril 1985;44:484–488.

307. Friberg J. Postcoital testing in relation to circulating sperm-agglutinating antibodies in women. Am J Obstet Gynecol 1981;139:587–591.

308. Moghissi KS, Sacco AG, Borin K. Immunologic Infertility: I. Cervical mucus antibodies and postcoital test. Am J Obstet Gynecol 1980;136:941–950.

309. Steinberg W. Cervical aspects in sterility and infertility. Fertil Steril 1955;6:169–179.

310. Boyers SP, Corrales MD, Huszar G, DeCherney AH. The effects of Lubrin on sperm motility in vitro. Fertil Steril 1987;47:882–884.

311. Hong CY, Chaput de Saintonage DM, Turner P. The inhibitory action of procaine, (+)propranolol, and (±)propranolol on human sperm motility: antagonism by caffeine. Br J Clin Pharmacol 1981;12:751–753.

312. Pearson RM, Ridgway EJ, Johnston A, Vadukul J. Concentration of D-propranolol in cervicovaginal mucus. Lancet 1984;2:1480.

313. American College of Obstetricians and Gynecologists, ACOG Technical Bulletin No. 180: Smoking and Reproductive Health. Washington, DC: ACOG, May 1993.

314. Mattison DR. The effects of smoking on fertility from gametogenesis to implantation. Environ Res 1982;28:410–433.

315. Sasson IM, Haley NJ, Hoffman D, et al. Cigarette smoking and neoplasia of the uterine cervix: smoke constituents in cervical mucus. N Engl J Med 1985;312:315–316.

316. McLachlan JA, Dames NM, Sieber SM, Fabro S. Accumulation of nicotine in the uterine fluid of the six-day-pregnant rabbit. Fertil Steril 1976;27:1204.

317. Phipps WR, Cramer DW, Schiff I, et al. The association between smoking and female infertility as influenced by cause of infertility. Fertil Steril 1987;48:377–382.

318. Scott JZ, Nakamura RM, Mutch J, Davajan V. The cervical factor in infertility: diagnosis and treatment. Fertil Steril 1977;28:1289–1294.

319. Keller DW, Strickler RC, Warren JC. Clinical Infertility. Norwalk, CT: Appleton-Century-Crofts, 1984:89–98.

320. Pittaway DE, Daniell J, Maxson W, Boehm F. Reconstruction of the cervical canal after complete postconization obstruction. J Reprod Med 1984;29:339–340.

321. Beck WW Jr. The cervical factor. In: Garcia C-R, Mastroianni L, Amelar RD, Dubin L, editors. Current Therapy of Infertility. 3rd edition. Toronto: BC Decker, 1988:118–120.

322. Sharf M, Graff G, Kuzminsky T. Quinestrol therapy in hypomucorrhea due to clomiphene. Am J Obstet Gynecol 1971;110:423–424.

323. Insler V, Zakut H, Serr DM. Cycle pattern and pregnancy rate following combined clomiphene-estrogen therapy. Obstet Gynecol 1973;41:602–607.

324. Taubert H-D, Dericks-Tan JSE. High doses of estrogens do not interfere with the ovulation-inducing effect of clomiphene citrate. Fertil Steril 1976;27:375–382.

325. Van der Merwe JV. The effect of clomiphene and conjugated estrogens on cervical mucus. S Afr Med J 1981;60:347–349.

326. Bateman BG, Nunley WC Jr, Kolp LA. Exogenous estrogen therapy for treatment of clomiphene citrate–induced cervical mucus abnormalities: is it effective? Fertil Steril 1990;54:577–579.

327. Cohen MR. Quinestrol therapy in functional infertility. Fertil Steril 1967;17:541–546.

328. Roland M. Effects of quinestrol on cervical mucus and sperm penetration in patients with cervical hostility. Int J Fertil 1967;12:251–254.

329. Skerlavay M, Epstein JA, Sobrero AJ. The comparative effects of estrogens on amylase levels of cervical mucus. Fertil Steril 1969;20:581–589.

330. Cohen MR, Pandya GN, Scommegna A. The effects of an intracervical steroid-releasing device on the cervical mucus. Fertil Steril 1970;21:715–723.

331. Rezai P, Dmowski WP, Auletta F, Scommegna A. Effect of oral estradiol on cervical secretions and on ovulatory response in infertile women. Fertil Steril 1979;31:627–633.

332. Krzemenski A, Sikorski R, Bokiniec M. Sperm penetration through cervical mucus in infertile couples in relation to selected cervical factors. Hum Reprod 1988;3:353–355.

333. Check JH, Nowroozi K, Adelson HG, et al. An in vivo technique for screening immunologic factors in the etiology of the unexplained poor postcoital test. Int J Fertil 1990;35:215–221.

334. Balasch J, Vanrell JA. Further data on the usefulness of combined high-dose estrogen and human menopausal gonadotropins for cervical factor. Int J Fertil 1986;31:263–271.

335. Check JH. Treatment of cervical factor with combined high-dose estrogen and human menopausal gonadotropins. Fertil Steril 1980;33:562–563.

336. Check JH, Adelson HG. Improvement of cervical factor by high-dose estrogen and human menopausal gonadotropin therapy with ultrasound monitoring. Obstet Gynecol 1984;63:179–181.

337. Check JH, Wu CH, Dietterich C, et al. The treatment of cervical factor with ethinyl estradiol and human menopausal gonadotropins. Int J Fertil 1986;31:148–152.

338. Check JH, Wu CH, Kurtz A, et al. Combined high-dose estrogen and human menopausal gonadotropins for cervical factor: improvement with pelvic ultrasound. Infertility 1982:5:117–125.

339. Yovich JL, Matson PL. The treatment of infertility by the high intrauterine insemination of husband's washed spermatozoa. Hum Reprod 1988;3:939–943.

340. Clark WG, Brater DC, Johnson AR. Goth's Medical Pharmacology. 12th edition. St. Louis: CV Mosby, 1988:506–517.

341. Lish PM, Salem H. Expectorants. In: Salem H, Aviado DM, editors. Antitussive Agents: International Encyclopedia of Pharmacology and Therapeutics, section 27. New York: Pergamon Press, 1970; vol. 3:759–784.

342. Sheffner AL, Lish PM. Acetylcysteine and other mucolytic agents. In: Salem H, Aviado DM, editors. Antitussive Agents: International Encyclopedia of Pharmacology and Therapeutics, section 27. New York: Pergamon Press, 1970; vol. 3:785–833.

343. Check JH, Adelson HG, Wu C-H. Improvement of cervical factor with guaifenesin. Fertil Steril 1982;37:707–708.

344. Check JH, Dietterich C, Lauer C, Liss J. Ovulation-inducing drugs versus specific mucus therapy for cervical factor. Int J Fertil 1991;36:108–112.

345. Zondek B, Rozin S. Cervical mucus arborization: its use in the determination of corpus luteum function. Obstet Gynecol 1954;3:463–470.

346. Kremer J. Treatment of disturbed sperm–cervical mucus interaction. In: Insler V, Lunenfeld B, editors. Infertility: Male and Female. Edinburgh: Churchill Livingstone, 1986:521–529.

347. Sadovsky E, Aboulafia Y. Organic dysmucorrhea treated by endocervical curettage. Int J Fertil 1965;10:307–310.

348. Check JH, Rakoff AE. Treatment of cervical factor by donor mucus insemination. Fertil Steril 1977;28:113–114.

349. Segal S, Sherer M. The use of donor mucus and insemination for cervical factor. Int J Fertil 1979;24:291–292.

350. Lee WI, Gaddum-Rosse P, Blandau RJ. Sperm penetration into cervical mucus in vitro: III. Effect of freezing on estrous bovine cervical mucus. Fertil Steril 1981;36:209–213.

351. Blandau RJ, Gaddum-Rosse P, Lee WI. Letter to the editor. Fertil Steril 1978;29:707.

352. Kantor HI. Letter to the editor. Fertil Steril 1977:28:781.

353. Ansari AH, Gould KG, Ansari VM. Sodium bicarbonate douching for improvement of the postcoital test. Fertil Steril 1980;33:608–612.

354. Everhardt E, Dony JMJ, Jansen H, et al. Improvement of cervical mucus viscoelasticity and sperm penetration with sodium bicarbonate douching. Hum Reprod 1990;5:133–137.

355. Nachtigall RD, Faure N, Glass RH. Artificial insemination of husband's sperm. Fertil Steril 1979;32:141–144.

356. Allen NC, Herbert CM, Maxson WS, et al. Intrauterine insemination: a critical review. Fertil Steril 1985;44:569–580.

357. Marrs RP, Vargyas JM, Saito H, et al. Clinical applications of techniques used in human in vitro fertilization research. Am J Obstet Gynecol 1983;146:477–481.

358. Toffle RC, Nagel TC, Tagatz GE, et al. Intrauterine insemination: the University of Minnesota experience. Fertil Steril 1985;43:743–747.

359. Hewitt J, Cohen J, Krishnaswamy V, et al. Treatment of idiopathic infertility, cervical mucus hostility, and male infertility: artificial insemination with husband's semen or in vitro fertilization. Fertil Steril 1985;44:350–355.

360. Confino E, Friberg J, Dudkiewicz AB, Gleicher N. Intrauterine inseminations with washed human spermatozoa. Fertil Steril 1986;46:55–60.

361. Hull ME, Magyar DM, Vasquez JM, et al. Experience with intrauterine insemination for cervical factor and oligospermia. Am J Obstet Gynecol 1986;154:1333–1338.

362. Yovich JL, Matson PL. Pregnancy rates after high intrauterine insemination of husband's spermatozoa or gamete intrafallopian transfer. Lancet 1986;2:1287.

363. Arny M, Quagliarello J. Semen quality before and after processing by a swim-up method: relation to outcome of intrauterine insemination. Fertil Steril 1987;48:643–648.

364. Dodson WC, Whitesides DB, Hughes CL, et al. Superovulation with intrauterine insemination in the treatment of infertility: a possible alternative to gamete intrafallopian transfer and in vitro fertilization. Fertil Steril 1987;48:441–445.

365. Byrd W, Ackerman GE, Carr BR, et al. Treatment of refractory infertility by transcervical intrauterine insemination of washed spermatozoa. Fertil Steril 1987;48:921–927.

366. Makler A. Washed intrauterine insemination in the treatment of idiopathic infertility. Semin Reprod Endocrinol 1987;5:35–43.

367. Pardo M, Barri PN, Bancells N, et al. Spermatozoa selection in discontinuous Percoll gradients for use in artificial insemination. Fertil Steril 1988;49:505–509.

368. Sunde A, Kahn J, Molne K. Intrauterine insemination. Hum Reprod 1988;3:97–99.

369. Horvath PM, Bohrer M, Shelden RM, Kemmann E. The relationship of sperm parameters to cycle fecundity in superovulated women undergoing intrauterine insemination. Fertil Steril 1989;52:288–294.

370. Corson SL, Batzer FR, Gocial B, Maislin G. Intrauterine insemination and ovulation stimulation as treatment of infertility. J Reprod Med 1989;34:397–406.

371. Francavilla F, Romano R, Santucci R, Poccia G. Effect of sperm morphology and motile sperm count on outcome of intrauterine insemination in oligozoospermia and/or asthenozoospermia. Fertil Steril 1990;53:892–897.

372. Tredway DR, Chan P, Henig I, et al. Effectiveness of stimulated men-

strual cycles and Percoll sperm preparation in intrauterine insemination. J Reprod Med 1990;35:103–108.

373. Galle PC, McRae MA, Colliver JA, Alexander JS. Sperm washing and intrauterine insemination for cervical factor, oligospermia, immunologic infertility, and unexplained infertility. J Reprod Med 1990;35:116–122.

374. Dodson WC, Haney AF. Controlled ovarian hyperstimulation and intrauterine insemination for treatment of infertility. Fertil Steril 1991;55:457–467.

375. Friedman AJ, Juneau-Norcross M, Sedensky B, et al. Life table analysis of intrauterine insemination pregnancy rates for couples with cervical factor, male factor, and idiopathic infertility. Fertil Steril 1991;55:1005–1007.

376. Tarlatzis BC, Bontis J, Koblibianakis EM, et al. Evaluation of intrauterine insemination with washed spermatozoa from the husband in the treatment of infertility. Hum Reprod 1991;6:1241–1246.

377. Karlstrom P-O, Bakos O, Bergh T, Lundkvist O. Intrauterine insemination and comparison of two methods of sperm preparation. Hum Reprod 1991;6:390–395.

378. Quagliarello J, Arny M. Intracervical versus intrauterine insemination: correlation of outcome with antecedent postcoital testing. Fertil Steril 1986;46:870–875.

379. Glazener CMA, Coulson C, Lambert PA, et al. The value of artificial insemination with husband's semen in infertility due to failure of postcoital sperm–mucus penetration: controlled trial of treatment. Br J Obstet Gynaecol 1987;94:774–778.

380. Friedman A, Haas S, Kredentser J, et al. A controlled trial of intrauterine insemination for cervical factor and male factor: a preliminary report. Int J Fertil 1989;34:199–203.

381. Te Velde ER, van Kooy RJ, Waterreus JJH. Intrauterine insemination of washed husband's spermatozoa: a controlled study. Fertil Steril 1989;51:182–185.

382. Kirby CA, Flaherty SP, Godfrey BM, et al. A prospective trial of intrauterine insemination of motile spermatozoa versus timed intercourse. Fertil Steril 1991;56:102–107.

383. Chaffkin LM, Nulsen JC, Luciano AA, Metzger DA. A comparative analysis of the cycle fecundity rates associated with combined human menopausal gonadotropin (hMG) and intrauterine insemination (IUI) versus either hMG or IUI alone. Fertil Steril 1991;55:252–257.

384. Margalloth EJ, Sauter E, Bronson RA, et al. Intrauterine insemination as treatment for antisperm antibodies in the female. Fertil Steril 1988;50:441–446.

385. Anderson DL, Bach DL, Yunis EJ, DeWolf WC. Major histocompatibility antigens are not expressed on human epididymal sperm. J Immunol 1982;129:452–454.

CHAPTER 19

Evaluation and Treatment of Recurrent Miscarriages

JAMES R. SCOTT and D. WARE BRANCH

Recurrent miscarriages are frustrating and discouraging for both the physician and the patient. A variety of diagnostic tests and treatments have been recommended and are widely publicized in both the medical and lay literature. Few, however, have been adequately tested with properly designed studies. The purpose of this chapter is to evaluate objectively the evidence available regarding the cause and appropriate management of recurrent miscarriages, also referred to as repetitive pregnancy loss (RPL). The intent is to incorporate scientifically sound guidelines into a practical approach for the physician who is confronted with this important clinical problem. Nonimmunologic factors are discussed to the extent not covered in other chapters and as they relate specifically to RPL.

Miscarriage is the most common complication of pregnancy. The frequency in clinically recognized pregnancies is 15% to 20%, and undetected postimplantation embryonic loss is almost four times higher. A commonly accepted definition for recurrent miscarriage is the occurrence of three or more consecutive first-trimester spontaneous miscarriages. RPL may be classified as primary or secondary. Primary RPL is sometimes defined as that occurring in women who have never had a successful pregnancy, and secondary RPL as repetitive miscarriages following a live birth. There is presently no specific classification for those women who have multiple spontaneous miscarriages interspersed with normal pregnancies. It is also unclear whether previously unrecognized or occult early miscarriages now diagnosed by sensitive human chorionic gonadotropin (hCG) tests are significant and should be included in these definitions. Although the term *recurrent miscarriage* has usually referred to those losses occurring in the first trimester, this time limit is somewhat arbitrary and does not take into account a variety of potential underlying causes that may result in fetal death anytime during the first half of gestation. With the development of ultrasonography, we believe that it is clinically more relevant to consider a classification based on whether a live fetus was present or not.[1]

Previous reports suggest that the chance of a successful pregnancy in an untreated patient following three consecutive first-trimester miscarriages and no live births is in the range of 30% to 50%.[2, 3] If a woman has had even one normal pregnancy in addition to the recurrent miscarriages, the chance of delivering a live infant in the next pregnancy without treatment approaches 60% to 70%.[2–4] Our own data indicate a somewhat lower chance that the next pregnancy will be successful in these situations, but almost 70% eventually achieve a live birth in subsequent pregnancies without treatment. Unfortunately, an accurate success rate in untreated patients is difficult to ascertain from the literature, even though this information is urgently needed to evaluate the efficacy of any diagnostic or therapeutic maneuvers that are recommended.

The following is a discussion of the contemporary evaluation and management of patients with RPL, which has been divided into six major clinical categories. The prevalence of each in patients seen at the University of Utah is shown in Table 19–1.

GENETIC FACTORS

Today genetic problems can be categorized as either (1) cytogenetic, involving a karyotypic abnormality of the genome detectable by cytogenetic preparation of the chromosomes, or (2) molecular, involving a defect in one or more genes detectable by DNA analytic techniques. Cytogenetic abnormalities of the conceptus are a well-recognized cause of pregnancy loss. In some couples, the cytogenetic abnormalities in the conceptus result from structural chromosomal abnormalities in one parent (e.g., a balanced translocation). In contrast, aneuploidy in the conceptus (not found in one parent) appears to be responsible for a large proportion of sporadic miscarriages, but a link between aneuploidy and recurrent miscarriage is not yet obvious. With the coming age of DNA analysis, attention will focus on the possibility that inherited or spontaneous molecular abnormalities may cause RPL.

Cytogenetic Abnormalities

NUMERICAL CHROMOSOME ABNORMALITIES

Table 19–2 shows the types of chromosome abnormalities found in first-trimester abortuses in several large series.[5] The

TABLE 19–1. Cause of Recurrent Miscarriages*

Miscarriage	Anatomic	Endocrine	Genetic	Autoimmune	Multiple†	Idiopathic
Primary (n = 116)	11 (9.5%)	8 (6.9%)	5 (4.3%)	3 (2.6%)	9 (7.8%)	80 (69.0%)
Secondary (n = 36)	1 (2.8%)	5 (13.9%)	1 (2.8%)	1 (2.8%)	2 (5.5%)	26 (72.2%)
Totals (n = 152)	12 (7.9%)	13 (8.6%)	6 (3.9%)	4 (2.6%)	11 (7.2%)	106 (69.7%)

*More than 400 patients have been evaluated at the University of Utah during the past 10 years for RPL. This table represents those for whom complete data are available, including results of hysterosalpingograms, late luteal phase endometrial biopsies, parental chromosome analyses, and antiphospholipid antibodies.

†More than one abnormality present.

majority are numerical in nature and consist of either (1) a multiple of the haploid number of chromosomes (polyploidy) or (2) the presence of one too many or one too few chromosomes (aneuploidy). These abnormalities are the result of a chromosomal accident of parental meiosis at the time of fertilization or early cell division in the zygote. Note that the data shown in Table 19–2 are taken from series of patients with sporadic, not recurrent, spontaneous miscarriage.

Polyploidy may result from (1) double fertilization of the ovum (dispermy) or (2) abnormal cell division of the ovum or sperm. In either case, the resulting conceptus has a multiple of the haploid number of chromosomes. The most commonly encountered polyploidies are triploidy (69 chromosomes) and tetraploidy (92 chromosomes). Triploidy occurs in about 7% to 8% and tetraploidy in about 2% to 3% of

TABLE 19–2. Frequency of Chromosomal Complements in First-Trimester Spontaneous Miscarriages

Abnormality	Chromosomal Complement	Percentage	Total Frequency (%)
Normal karyotype	46,XX;46,XY		54.1
Autosomal trisomy			22.3
	+16	7.3	
	+22	2.3	
	+21	2.1	
	+15	1.7	
	+18	1.2	
	+2	1.1	
	+13	1.1	
	+7	0.9	
	+14	0.8	
	Others	4.0	
Monosomy X	45X		8.6
Triploidy			7.7
	69,XXY	4.0	
	69,XXX	2.7	
	69,XYY	0.2	
	Other	0.8	
Tetraploidy			2.6
	92,XXX	1.5	
	92,XXYY	0.6	
	Other	0.5	
Structural abnormalities			1.5
Sex chromosome polysomy			0.2
	47,XXY	0.15	
	47,XXX	0.05	
Other abnormalities			3

Data modified from Simpson JL. Fetal wastage. In: Gabbe SG, Niebyl JR, Simpson JL, editors. Obstetrics. Normal and problem pregnancies. New York; Churchill Livingston, 1991:783.

sporadic spontaneous miscarriages.[6] Triploid miscarriages are often anembryonic,[7] but triploid gestations may also present as a "partial" mole.[8] The majority of triploid conceptions have a 69,XXY karyotype, and the extra set of chromosomes are paternal in origin.[9] It appears that tetraploid abortions are virtually always anembryonic.

Aneuploidy usually arises by nondisjunction, wherein both chromosomes of a pair segregate into one cell, leaving the other cell lacking. Thus, one cell has one chromosome too many (trisomy), and the other cell has one chromosome too few (monosomy). Nondisjunction may occur either in meiosis or in mitosis. Autosomal trisomies make up the largest single group of cytogenetically abnormal sporadic spontaneous miscarriages (more than 50%). The most common trisomy complement among abortuses is trisomy 16. Other frequently encountered trisomy karyotypes include trisomy 13, 15, 18, 21, and 22. Most trisomies result from nondisjunction during maternal meiosis I.[10–12] In part, this may account for the increased rate of spontaneous miscarriage seen with increasing maternal age (most pronounced after the mid-30s).[13]

The single most frequent chromosome abnormality among spontaneous miscarriages is monosomy X. Monosomy X conceptions occur because of paternal sex chromosome loss.[14] Most conceptuses are lost in the first trimester. Fetal losses (after 10 to 12 weeks' gestation), however, also occur, and in these cases, the anomalies characteristic of Turner's syndrome may be found.[15]

To what extent do recurrent numerical chromosome abnormalities of the abortus (in parents with normal karyotypes) contribute to RPL? The answer to this question is not clear because of the scant data on the abortus karyotypes from series of women with RPL. One investigator analyzed cases in which karyotypes were obtained on two consecutive abortus specimens.[16] Hassold found that if the complement of the first abortus was abnormal, the complement of the second abortus was also abnormal in 80% of cases. Contrariwise, if the complement of the first abortus was normal the complement of the second abortus was abnormal in only 30% of cases. In a second analysis of 273 women, if the complement of the first abortus was normal, the complement of the second abortus was also normal in 57% of cases (65 of 114).[17] If the complement of the first abortus was normal, the complement of the second abortus was abnormal in only 20% of cases (35 of 177). The findings in these studies suggest that recurrent numerical chromosome abnormalities may occur as a nonrandom event in couples predisposed toward such an event, although not all experts agree.[17] If recurrent aneuploidic miscarriage does occur, there are four possible sources of the error: (1) paternal meiosis I, (2) paternal meiosis II, (3) maternal meiosis I, or (4) maternal meiosis II. Each has a different implication for management and future treatment.

STRUCTURAL CHROMOSOME ABNORMALITIES

Translocations. Structural chromosome abnormalities are found in 1% to 2% of sporadic spontaneous miscarriages. Similar to numerical abnormalities, structural abnormalities may arise during gametogenesis. Of more importance to the issue of RPL, however, structural chromosome abnormalities may be inherited from a parent with a balanced translocation or inversion. Translocations, which account for the largest percentage of chromosome abnormalities in couples with RPL, are of two types: reciprocal and robertsonian. In reciprocal translocations, chromatin is exchanged between two nonhomologous chromosomes. In robertsonian translocations, two acrocentric chromosomes (chromosomes 13–15 and 21–22) fuse at the centromeric region and lose their heterochromatic short arms. Both types of balanced translocations are compatible with a normal adult phenotype.

Genetically balanced translocations are found in about 0.2% of the normal adult population. However, in as many as 5% of couples with RPL, one or the other partner will have a balanced translocation.[18] Simpson and colleagues[19] indicated that translocations are relatively infrequent among couples with RPL and do not result in other adverse perinatal outcomes (e.g., stillborns, anomalous infants). Interestingly, pooled data show that the frequency of translocations is twice as high in the female partner.[19] At present, no historical factor allows the clinician to determine unequivocally which couples should undergo parental karyotype analysis.

A reciprocal translocation in one parent can theoretically result in a large number (nearly 100) of different gamete complements, depending on the segregation of chromosomes during meiosis I, the effects of crossover in meiosis I, and the possibility of nondisjunction in meiosis II (Fig. 19–1). In turn, if these abnormal gametes participate in fertilization, they result in abnormal conceptuses with a high probability of spontaneous miscarriages. Because only two of the possible gamete complements can result in phenotypically normal conceptuses, a high theoretical risk exists that an individual carrying a reciprocal translocation will produce a pregnancy that results in either a spontaneous miscarriage or an unbalanced fetus. Fortunately, however, the observed risk of miscarriage or an unbalanced fetus is not as high. It is likely that some abnormal chromosome complements are selected against during gametogenesis and hence are never available to participate in fertilization. Many, if not most, grossly chromosomally abnormal conceptuses are lost before a clinical pregnancy is evident (these are usually not considered recurrent pregnancy losses). It is generally accepted that factors such as the size of the translocation affect the pregnancy outcome.

Heterologous robertsonian translocations may also be found among couples with RPL. Figure 19–2 shows the theoretical gamete complements for a heterologous robertsonian translocation.

Unfortunately, no data are available to show the risk of recurrence for spontaneous miscarriage in a couple in whom a balanced translocation is the cause of RPL. Data derived from prenatal genetics studies, however, provide circumstan-

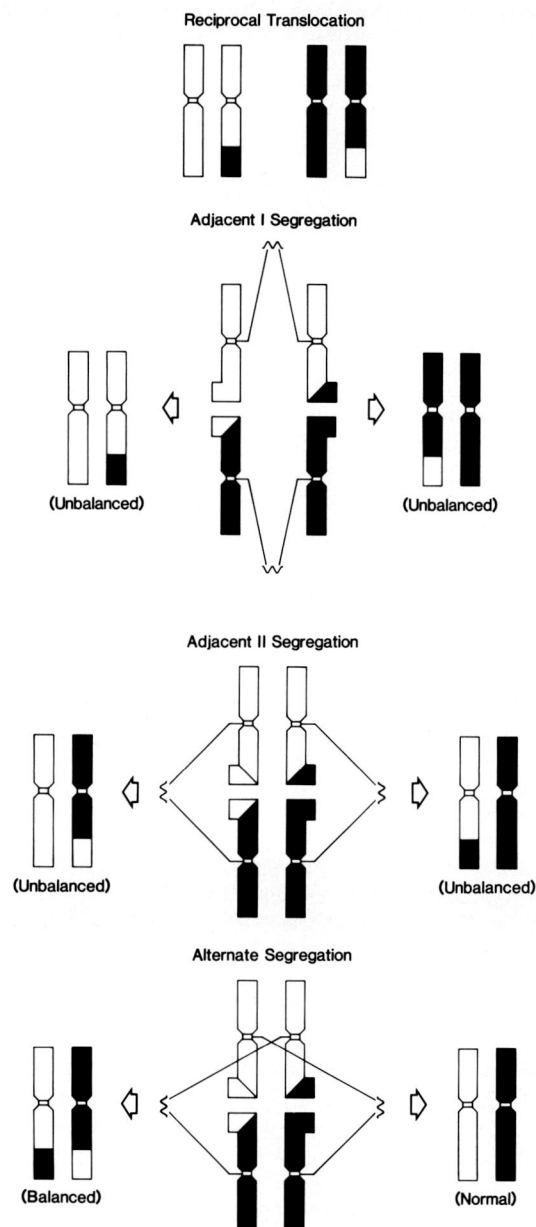

FIGURE 19–1. Possible effects of segregation in meiosis I on chromosome complement of gametes. For most reciprocal translocations, pairing involves two pairs of chromosomes (instead of one pair), shown here as hypothetical chromosomes. Depending on how the chromosomes are aligned on the equatorial plane in metaphase I, a large number of possible gametes are formed. The three most common types of segregation and their gametes are schematically represented.

tial evidence and insight. Boue and Gallano[20] compiled data from genetic amniocenteses performed because of a reciprocal translocation in one parent. If parental translocation was identified because of spontaneous miscarriages, the frequency of an abnormal (unbalanced) karyotype at amniocentesis was 3.4% (7 of 205). Overall, the pooled data indicated that the frequency of an unbalanced fetal karyotype did not differ according to which parent carried the reciprocal translocation. One might guess that the frequency of an unbalanced translocation in the first-trimester conceptus is higher; this prediction was supported by the chorionic villus sampling (CVS) data of Mikkelson.[21] Nearly 39% (7 of 19) of the CVS

Robertsonian Translocation

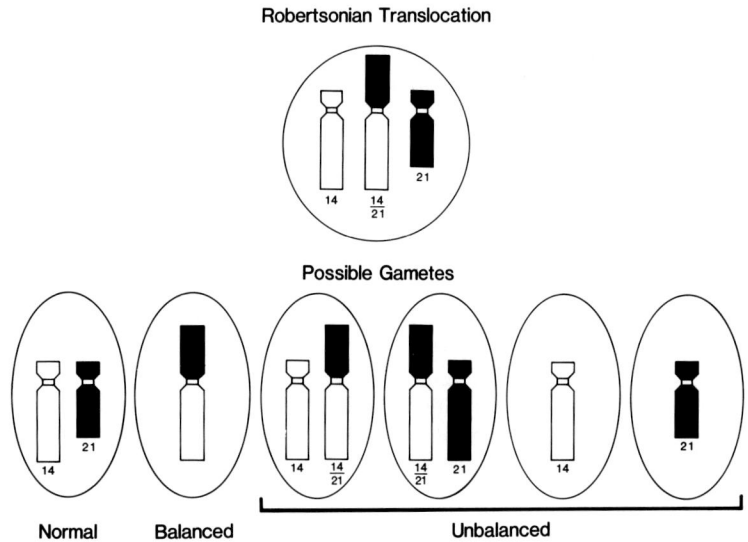

Possible Gametes

FIGURE 19–2. Possible chromosome complements of gametes for heterozygous robertsonian translocation involving chromosomes 14 and 21.

Normal   Balanced   Unbalanced

samples taken from a pregnancy in which one parent had a reciprocal translocation also had an unbalanced karyotype. If one considers the data sets from these two studies to be comparable, more than a quarter of conceptuses with an unbalanced karyotype are lost as miscarriages between the time of CVS (about 9 to 12 weeks' gestation) and amniocentesis (about 15 to 20 weeks' gestation). This figure, however, does not account for pregnancies lost before CVS.

The data of Boue and Gallano[20] indicate that nearly 10% of fetuses of women with a heterologous robertsonian translocation (pooled data) are chromosomally abnormal at the time of amniocentesis. As with reciprocal translocations, CVS data indicate a much higher frequency of chromosome abnormalities (about 30%).[21] Again this suggests that about 20% of conceptions are lost as abortions between the time of CVS and amniocentesis. In contrast to the situation with reciprocal translocations, the risk of an unbalanced offspring for couples in which the male partner carries the heterologous robertsonian translocation is substantially lower than if the female partner carries the translocation. Indeed, both amniocentesis and CVS data indicate a negligible risk of an unbalanced karyotype in the conceptus if the carrier is the male partner,[20, 21] suggesting selection against chromosomally abnormal sperm.

Homologous robertsonian translocations, in either the female or male partner, are incompatible with a normal conceptus. Although this type of translocation is rare, the hopeless nature of the situation is a strong argument for karyotypes in couples with RPL and no previous live births.

Inversions. A chromosome inversion occurs when a segment of a chromosome is reinserted "upside-down," or in the reverse order after breakage of the chromosome. Pericentric inversions involve the centromere (i.e., the break points are on opposite sides of the centromere). Paracentric inversions do not involve the centromere (i.e., the break points are on the same side of the centromere). In general, there is no net loss of genetic material, and the individual carrying the inversion is phenotypically normal. Because of abnormal pairing of the homologous chromosomes, however, inversions lead to pregnancy loss (or abnormal liveborns). During the pachytene stage of meiosis I, homologous chromosomes pair with each other at one or more alleles and exchange genetic ma-

terial in a process referred to as *crossing-over.* In the normal situation, this exchange of material leaves chromatids with a normal amount and orientation of genetic material. With chromosome inversions, however, the inverted chromosome pairs with the normal homologue only by forming a loop structure. If the inversion is paracentric and a single crossover occurs, the result is (1) a normal chromatid, (2) an inverted chromatid, and (3) two unstable chromatids (one with no centromere and one with two centromeres). The fragment with no centromere cannot participate in cell divisions and is presumably lost. The chromatid with two centromeres carries duplications and deletions. According to Thompson and Thompson,[22] the dicentric chromatid is also unstable and does not participate in gamete formation. Nevertheless, paracentric inversions are rarely if ever identified as causes of spontaneous abortion or RPL.

Pericentric inversions may lead to stable abnormal gametes and consequently to a spontaneous miscarriage or an unbalanced fetus. If the inversion is pericentric and a single crossover occurs, the result is (1) a normal chromatid, (2) an inverted chromatid, and (3) two recombinant chromatids, each with genetic deficiencies and duplications. The genetic imbalances occur outside the region of the inversion. Small inversions lead to large deficiencies and duplications, whereas large inversions lead to small deficiencies and duplications. This point is clinically relevant because large chromosome abnormalities are not likely to result in functioning, viable gametes or conceptuses and because small abnormalities may be clinically insignificant. It is the pericentric inversion of intermediate length that poses the biggest clinical problem and is most likely to result in a recognized problem, such as pregnancy loss.

The recurrence risk for miscarriages among couples in which one partner has an inversion is not precisely known. As with translocations, the empiric risks appear to be lower than the theoretical risks. Among couples identified because of a previous abnormal live-born infant, the risk of an unbalanced fetus detected at midtrimester amniocentesis is about 7.5% if the mother is the carrier of the inversion and about 4% if the father is the carrier of the inversion.[20] Unfortunately, these numbers are too small to determine specific risk figures for the spontaneous miscarriage per se or for the recurrence risk among couples ascertained because of RPL. If a balanced translocation is identified in either the man or woman, the clinician is obligated to counsel the couple regarding the need for fetal chromosome analysis.

Clinical Recommendations Regarding Chromosome Analysis

The expense of parental chromosome analysis, the relatively low yield among couples with RPL, and the inability to correct an abnormal karyotype have discouraged clinicians and patients from obtaining chromosome studies in some couples with RPL. A strong argument can be made, however, for parental chromosome analysis in all couples with three or more consecutive pregnancy losses based on the following points:

1. The causative nature of chromosome abnormalities in RPL is well established. In contrast, some other causes of RPL (e.g., luteal phase defect, certain immunologic abnormalities, and infection) are controversial and possibly misleading.
2. There is considerable emotional satisfaction and relief for the couple in identifying the cause of RPL, even if the problem cannot be corrected.
3. Having identified a chromosome abnormality, many couples find further attempts at pregnancy emotionally easier because aborted conceptions are probably chromosomally abnormal and, in most situations, repeated attempts at pregnancy are likely to lead eventually to success.
4. Couples who seek consultation regarding RPL usually want the satisfaction of a completed evaluation, including chromosome analysis. If a couple believes their evaluation is somehow incomplete, they are likely to seek the advice of other physicians and spend even more time and money.
5. Although rare, one member of a couple with RPL and no live births might have a chromosome abnormality incompatible with a successful pregnancy (e.g., a homologous robertsonian translocation). Such couples can then be counseled not to attempt further pregnancy.

If for some reason a couple under evaluation for RPL has not had a chromosome analysis and the woman aborts again, a karyotype of the products of conception is useful. In our experience, this is best done by performing a curettage when an impending or incomplete miscarriage is found. The abortus material should be collected using sterile technique, placed in a sterile container with a small amount of sterile saline or culture medium, and transported promptly to the cytogenetic laboratory. The finding of a chromosomally normal abortus weighs against a parental cytogenetic abnormality as the cause of the couple's RPL and provides guidance for further evaluation or counseling.

Molecular Mutation

In the last decade, the importance of single-gene mutations as a cause for a wide variety of human diseases has been brought to light by the development of techniques for DNA analysis. The question of whether molecular mutations may cause RPL has never been more obvious, and it is anticipated that the literature in this area will blossom over the next

decade. The potential mechanisms by which such a defect might result in pregnancy loss are seemingly innumerable. For example, a defect in the maternal gene that codes for human chorionic gonadotropin (hCG) receptors in the ovary could lead to inadequate corpus luteum support in early pregnancy. Also, a defect in the genes of the conceptus that code for syncytiotrophoblastic invasion proteins or cell adhesion molecules could preclude successful implantation or development.

There are literally thousands of other possible scenarios, but is there any evidence that such a mutation might exist? In animal models, the answer is clearly "yes." The *t* gene complex on chromosome 17 of the mouse contains mutations that are lethal for the homozygous conceptus.[23] One of the mutations is recognizable among heterozygotes as the brachyury (*T*), or short-tail mutation. Embryos homozygous for the *T* mutation are lost in midpregnancy, apparently because of severe developmental abnormalities detectable morphologically by day 9 of murine pregnancy. There are many other *t* complex genes that are lethal to the embryo or fetus when present in the homozygous state that cause embryonic or fetal death between 3.5 and 17 days of gestation. In the rat, the *grc* gene may represent a "semilethal" gene.[24] Homozygotes are underrepresented among offspring, suggesting that many homozygous zygotes are lost before implantation. Unfortunately, the nature of the gene products of the *t* and *grc* complexes is unknown at this time.

Despite these fascinating observations in rodents, no gene mutation that causes early pregnancy loss in humans (repetitive or sporadic) has been described. With the application of molecular genetic techniques to human disease, however, it seems likely that molecular genetics may provide some crucial answers in future investigations of RPL.

ENDOCRINE ABNORMALITIES

Disorders of thyroid function and overt clinical diabetes, at least when untreated or poorly controlled, have been associated with a higher risk of fetal loss. Series of recurrent miscarriages, however, have failed to demonstrate either condition as a significant etiologic factor.[25, 26] Because there is little evidence that undetected diabetes mellitus or subclinical thyroid disorders are implicated, there is no need to order laboratory tests, such as glucose tolerance tests or thyroid function tests, in the general evaluation of recurrent miscarriage.

The most commonly diagnosed endocrinopathy in recurrent miscarriage patients is luteal phase inadequacy. Still there is no concensus regarding the pathophysiology, the method of diagnosis, or its proper treatment (see Chapter 17). Luteal phase defects (LPD) are believed to result from multifactorial neuroendocrine causes, such as hypothalamic-pituitary, ovarian, and endometrial dysfunction and inadequate endometrial receptors.[27, 28] Inadequate progesterone production by the corpus luteum during the luteal phase may result in endometrial development that is unable to support an early pregnancy. The specific physiologic action of progesterone at the cellular level, however, remains poorly understood. Progesterone converts the estrogen-primed endometrium of the proliferative phase to a secretory endometrium that produces abundant proteins, most of which are of unknown function.

Nevertheless, the late secretory endometrial pattern reflects the total effect of the endocrine events of the cycle and the endometrial response to cyclic hormonal stimuli.

Progesterone, perhaps mediated through endometrial prostaglandin production, has also been implicated as a local immunosuppressive factor in the survival of the fetoplacental allograft. Whatever the mechanism, it is clear that adequate progesterone is a prerequisite for both nidation and the normal progress of early pregnancy. Surgical removal of the corpus luteum before the seventh week of gestation is promptly followed by a continuous fall in plasma progesterone and eventual miscarriage; however, miscarriage in these luteectomized women may be prevented by exogenous administration of progesterone.[27, 29] In recurrent miscarriage patients, luteal phase progesterone levels are lower than those of normal women.[30] These levels are often lower during pregnancies that eventually miscarry as compared with normal pregnancies, but this may be a result rather than a cause of spontaneous miscarriages.

Diagnosis

The extremes of reproductive age, hyperprolactinemia, regular strenuous exercise, elevated circulating androgens, follicular phase elevated luteinizing hormone (LH) levels, oligoovulation, and treatment with ovulation-inducing agents have been linked to luteal inadequacy.[25, 31] The disorder is also seen after discontinuation of suppressive medical therapies and after termination of pregnancy. If these underlying conditions are suspected from the history and physical examination, they can be further evaluated by appropriate laboratory tests.

Debate about how to establish the diagnosis of LPD has centered around the unreliability of cycle length, slow or irregular temperature rise on basal body temperature records, and wide variations in serum progesterone levels. Therefore, endometrial biopsy remains the standard diagnostic method accepted by most investigators and is at present the most practical test for physicians to use. Specimens obtained with small flexible plastic catheters such as the Pipelle have been found to be accurate and have made the procedure much less painful and more acceptable to patients. An endometrial biopsy is taken in the late luteal phase of the cycle 12 to 13 days after ovulation and within 1 to 3 days of subsequent menses in a nonconception cycle. The biopsy specimen is histologically dated according to the established criteria of Noyes and associates.[32] Timing of the biopsy is more reliable if the day of ovulation is determined by means of the basal body temperature chart, midcycle transvaginal ultrasonography, or urine LH determinations. Histologic dating that shows a lag of greater than 2 days documents the presence of LPD in that cycle. Two abnormal biopsy specimens are required to diagnose persistent LPD for which treatment is indicated because delayed endometrial histology occurs sporadically in up to 20% of women with no reproductive problems.

The use of the endometrial biopsy to diagnose an inadequate luteal phase is not without problems. The proper acquisition of endometrial tissue and its accurate interpretation are subject to a number of pitfalls, including poor timing, insufficient tissue for histologic evaluation, a nonfundal site of biopsy, an inexperienced interpreter, and mistaken estimation of the onset of subsequent menses.

Treatment

If LPD exists in a recurrent miscarriage patient, it presumably follows inadequate progesterone synthesis in the luteal phase or inability of the corpus luteum to respond to hCG with progesterone synthesis during early pregnancy. The most commonly advocated treatment is supplementation with either 25-mg progesterone suppositories (inserted into the vagina twice a day) or oral micronized progesterone (100 mg four times a day) beginning on the fourth day of basal body temperature rise and continuing until menses begin or through the first 10 weeks of pregnancy. Adequate correction of this defect demonstrated by repeat biopsy reveals successful pregnancy rates of 80% to 90%.[33–36] No study, however, has been done in a randomized, prospective manner. In our experience, this treatment has been unsuccessful in many recurrent miscarriage patients. Moreover, several small studies suggest no beneficial effect with the use of progesterone.[37, 38] Because of the questionable efficacy of progesterone therapy in recurrent miscarriage/LPD patients, enthusiasm for this regimen should be tempered by the risk of producing a missed abortion.

Clomiphene citrate has been recommended as treatment for LPD but has also been incriminated as inducing an inadequate luteal phase.[25] Most investigators, however, have studied this differential in infertility patients rather than in recurrent miscarriage patients. This is also true for other suggested treatments, such as hCG, human menopausal gonadotropin (hMG), and bromocriptine.

ANATOMIC DEFECTS

The incidence and classification of uterine abnormalities and the extent of associated reproductive failure and its management are far from clear. For example, intrauterine synechiae (Asherman's syndrome) and submucous uterine myomas are occasionally responsible for first-trimester spontaneous miscarriages, although they represent only a small percentage of the total RPL problem associated with anatomic defects. The diagnosis of either condition is usually not a problem; to establish either as the actual cause of RPL in an individual patient, however, requires that all other potential factors are ruled out. The hysteroscopic excision of intrauterine synechiae and techniques for myomectomy are straightforward and well known to most gynecologists (see Chapters 28 and 29). In women with repetitive spontaneous miscarriages, live birth rates of 53% to 79% have been reported after treatment for Asherman's syndrome and are even higher after surgical removal of leiomyomata.[39]

Incompetent Cervix

Little progress has been made in understanding the pathophysiology of the incompetent cervix since the concept was introduced 35 years ago, but three major causes are usually suggested: trauma, congenital, and hormonal. Although most obstetricians believe that cervical cerclage can prolong pregnancy in a patient with classic midtrimester signs and symptoms, no proof of its efficacy exists for patients with recurrent first-trimester miscarriages or fetal death.

A variety of methods for diagnosis have been suggested, but cervical incompetence remains a diagnosis of exclusion based primarily on features of previous pregnancies. The typical history is one of successive second-trimester pregnancy losses characterized by premature rupture of membranes with no preceding painful uterine contractions. Delivery of the fetus occurs after a short, relatively painless labor, and the fetus is typically alive at presentation.

In modern obstetrics, virtually all elective cerclage procedures are performed after conception and generally toward the end of the first trimester after an ultrasound study that demonstrates a normal fetus with cardiac activity. In the midtrimester, cerclage is performed only in the case of unanticipated cervical effacement and dilatation. The greatest experience is with the Shirodkar and McDonald procedures. When these procedures are performed before cervical effacement and dilatation, postoperative fetal survival rates are in the range of 75% to 85%; after these changes occur, the rates are somewhat lower.[40] In a patient whose cervix is markedly foreshortened, deeply lacerated, or infected, a transabdominal cervicoisthmic cerclage may be useful. Although this approach is as effective as transvaginal cerclage, intraoperative complication rates are higher, and the infant must be delivered by cesarean section. With any cerclage procedure, there is no evidence that specific perioperative measures (e.g., prophylactic antibiotics, uterine relaxants, or hormones) are of any benefit. Furthermore, cervical cerclage is not benign; it carries a significant risk of perioperative morbidity and a 2% risk of pregnancy loss.[40]

Uterine Malformations

The prevalence of nonobstructive müllerian anomalies is estimated to occur in about 1 in 700 women.[41] These congenital abnormalities of the uterus are widely recognized and accepted by most physicians as a definite cause of RPL. Some estimates suggest that the loss is as high as 50% to 75% with these anatomic defects.[39] This clinical impression is supported by evidence that müllerian abnormalities are more common in women with recurrent miscarriages (10% to 27%) than in women with normal pregnancies.[42, 43] The spectrum is wide, however: Septate uteri are associated with the highest incidence of spontaneous miscarriage, whereas other anomalies reveal lesser degrees of association, and the arcuate uterus has no proven relationship (Table 19–3). Structural changes in the upper genital tract of diethylstilbestrol (DES)-exposed women are also associated with higher first-trimester and second-trimester spontaneous miscarriage rates (18% to 48%).[39]

The pathogenesis of RPL with uterine abnormalities is incompletely understood. The most plausible explanation is poor vascularization of the septal endometrium and myometrium, which results in compromised implantation and decidual and placental growth. Despite the increased risk of early pregnancy loss, some pregnancies are successful (particularly when implantation occurs in the lateral uterine wall) in untreated patients with all anomalies. In one large series

TABLE 19–3. Miscarriage Rate with Various Types of Uterine Anomalies before Therapy

Uterine Anomaly	Number of Patients	Rate of Spontaneous Miscarriages
Unicornuate	220	35%
Didelphis	31	29%
Bicornuate	154	33%
Septate	113	53%
Diethylstilbestrol	472	28%

Modified and reprinted with permission from Seminars in Reproductive Endocrinology, vol. 6, 217–233, 1988, Thieme Medical Publishers, Inc.

of women with septate uteri with no surgical treatment, the spontaneous miscarriage rate was only 22%.[44] Many müllerian malformations are never detected because no clinical symptoms are demonstrated.

DIAGNOSIS

Classification systems for uterine anomalies are typically cumbersome and sometimes even contradictory (see Chapter 27). The only practical way for the physician to establish the relationship between early pregnancy loss and a müllerian abnormality is to rely on a patient's previous pregnancy history.[45] Moreover, the diagnosis of RPL secondary to a uterine anomaly always involves exclusion of other causes.

Uterine anomalies are detected by hysterosalpingography or hysteroscopy. The hysterosalpingogram (HSG) is widely available and is the most commonly used diagnostic test (see Chapter 23). It should be carefully performed by initially instilling only a small amount of contrast material so intrauterine defects are not missed. Filling defects and septa are more readily detected when using a cannula technique with traction on the cervix to straighten the uterine axis for a perpendicular view of the uterine cavity. Because differentiation of a septate from a bicornuate uterus by HSG or hysteroscopy can be misleading, direct visualization of the fundus at laparoscopy is recommended. What appears on HSG to be a unicornuate configuration may represent a didelphic uterus with only one side filled with contrast material; similar errors may occur with hysteroscopy. Structural changes are seen on HSG in 42% to 69% of DES-exposed women and include T-shaped, widened lower uterine segments; midfundal constrictions; filling defects; and irregular margins.[46]

Sonography, which is reportedly diagnostic in only 28% of patients, is actually incorrect in 12% when used to evaluate potential reproductive tract anomalies.[47] Magnetic resonance imaging (MRI), however, has been shown to differentiate reliably between various classes of congenital uterine abnormalities.[48] It is a noninvasive procedure that does not use ionizing radiation and provides information about both the internal and the external uterine contour. Therefore, it may eventually replace laparoscopy in the workup of women with uterine anomalies.

MANAGEMENT

Most, but not all, uterine anomalies are amenable to surgical correction after all other causes of recurrent miscarriage are excluded. No surgical reconstruction can enlarge a uni-

TABLE 19–4. Comparison of Treatment Results After Hysteroscopic and Tompkins Metroplasty for Septate Uterus					
	Patients	**Pregnancies**	**Miscarriage**	**Full-Term**	**Fetal Survival**
Hysteroscopic resection					
Before	19	21	90%	0%	0%
After	19	16	13%	87%	87%
Tompkins metroplasty					
Before	14	36	83%	0%	0%
After	14	10	20%	70%	70%

Data from Fayez JA. Comparison between abdominal and hysteroscopic metroplasty. Obstet Gynecol 1986; 68:399–432.

cornuate uterus, and none is usually indicated for a didelphic uterus. In patients with uterine anomalies, the incidence of an incompetent cervix is increased. Although the use of cervical cerclage is controversial in this situation, it is reportedly effective, particularly when metroplasty is not an option.[39] Rarely is surgery indicated in a patient with a previous live birth in the third trimester because of a tendency for subsequent pregnancies to progress further in gestation. There are no controlled studies, and the effectiveness of surgery for müllerian defects in recurrent miscarriage patients is based on miscarriage and live birth rates before and after reconstruction in the same patients. Reported postsurgical successful pregnancy rates are in the range of 70% to 90%.[45]

Traditionally candidates for metroplasty include women with septa who have had repeated first-trimester losses, a single second-trimester loss, or a history of premature births. These indications and guidelines, however, are no longer as clear-cut as in the past. Many women now attempt pregnancy later in life, and the costs of neonatal units and the morbidity associated with prematurity are high. Therefore, surgical indications have been gradually liberalized because it no longer seems reasonable to require repetitive poor pregnancy outcomes in every patient before correcting a uterine defect. Nevertheless, the sole indication for uterine reconstruction or septal incision is a poor reproductive performance when RPL is thought to occur as the result of the anomaly.

Abdominal procedures such as Tompkins or Strassman metroplasties are still sometimes necessary in patients with true bicornuate or didelphic uteri. The most important surgical principles include meticulous hemostasis with careful apposition of layers and the use of fine sutures in the serosal layer to decrease the incidence of adhesions and postoperative infertility. The disadvantage of abdominal procedures is that the majority of pregnancies are delivered by cesarean section to avoid uterine rupture.

Most recurrent miscarriage patients with uterine anomalies have septate uteri, which are amenable to hysteroscopic surgery. Hysteroscopically directed removal of septa by scissors, electrocautery, or laser now achieves anatomic results and live birth rates similar to those reported with abdominal metroplasty (Table 19–4).[49] Concomitant laparoscopy is advisable to reduce the incidence of uterine perforation. Operative hysteroscopy is best carried out in the follicular phase using a standard distending medium. The fibrous, relatively avascular septum is transected in its midportion and retracts into the uterine wall as the incision is continued up to the vascular fundus. Postoperatively the incised area becomes covered with endometrium. Although prophylactic antibiotics may be indicated, intrauterine devices and postoperative estrogen are not necessary. Advantages to the hysteroscopic

approach (which can often be done on an outpatient basis) include safety, less operating time and expense, fewer problems with adhesions and infertility, and the ability to deliver vaginally.

AUTOIMMUNE CAUSES

Interest in possible autoimmune causes of RPL have increased within the last decade. Two autoimmune syndromes linked to RPL have emerged. One is the antiphospholipid syndrome (APS), in which RPL (or other clinical features) occur in a patient with antiphospholipid antibodies (aPL). The other, less well-accepted, syndrome is subclinical autoimmunity, in which positive autoantibody tests are found in patients with no other explanation for RPL.

Antiphospholipid Syndrome

OVERVIEW

APS is a recently described autoimmune condition characterized by the production of moderate-to-high levels of aPL and certain clinical features (Table 19–5). Most authorities now agree that the most specific features are thrombotic phenomena (venous or arterial, including stroke), autoimmune thrombocytopenia, and pregnancy loss.[50] More debatable clinical features include livedo reticularis,[51, 52] Coombs'

TABLE 19–5. Clinical and Laboratory Criteria for the Antiphospholipid Syndrome	
Clinical Features	**Laboratory Features**
Pregnancy loss	Lupus anticoagulant
Fetal death	
Recurrent pregnancy loss	
Thrombosis	Anticardiolipin antibodies
Venous	IgG, medium or high-positive
Arterial, including stroke	
Autoimmune thrombocytopenia	
Other	Anticardiolipin antibodies
Coombs' positive hemolytic	IgM, medium or high-positive and
anemia	lupus anticoagulant
Livedo reticularis	

*Patients with antiphospholipid syndrome should have at least one clinical and one laboratory feature at some time in the course of their disease. Laboratory tests should be positive on at least two occasions more than 8 weeks apart.
Data from Abir R, Zusman I, Ben Hur H, et al. The effects of serum from women with miscarriages on the in vitro development of mouse pre-implantation embryos. Acta Obstet Gynecol Scand 1990; 69:27–33.

positive hemolytic anemia,[51] and cardiac valvular lesions.[53] APS probably occurs most commonly in patients with other underlying autoimmune diseases, such as systemic lupus erythematosus (SLE). In this setting, the syndrome is known as *secondary* APS. The condition, however, is also diagnosed in women with no other recognizable autoimmune disease. This expression of the syndrome is known as *primary* APS and is what obstetrician-gynecologists encounter most frequently. To be classified as having APS, the patient must have at least one clinical feature of the syndrome along with moderate-to-high levels of aPL.

LABORATORY DETECTION OF ANTIPHOSPHOLIPID ANTIBODIES

Unfortunately, laboratory testing for aPL remains somewhat difficult and confusing because of the limited number of laboratories that perform high-quality testing. Even for experienced investigators, aPL is modestly difficult to perform. Undoubtedly many of the problems related to aPL testing will be resolved over time. Therefore, the best advice for the clinician is to identify and use a reliable laboratory with a special interest in aPL testing.

There are three aPL tests for which well-established assays are available: (1) the biologic false-positive test for syphilis (BF-STS), (2) the test for lupus anticoagulant (LA), and (3) the test for anticardiolipin antibody (aCL). All of these tests bind moieties on negatively charged phospholipids or the moieties formed by the interaction of negatively charged phospholipids with other lipids and proteins. Both BF-STS and aCL are detected by conventional immunoassay methods. The assay for aCL is standardized using sera obtainable from the Antiphospholipid Standardization Laboratory in Louisville, Kentucky. Results are calibrated against these standards and determined as "GPL" (IgG aCL) or "MPL" (IgM aCL) units. Results should be reported in semiquantitative terms as negative, low-positive, medium-positive, or high-positive.[54] Low-positive results and isolated IgM aCL results (LA negative, IgG aCL negative) are of questionable clinical significance and should be carefully interpreted in light of the clinical situation. LA is detected in plasma by phospholipid-dependent clotting assays, such as the activated partial thromboplastin time (aPTT), dilute Russell viper venom time, or kaolin clotting time. Because LA binds to the phospholipid portion of the clotting tests, the clotting time is prolonged (even though the patients have a thrombotic, not a bleeding, tendency). More than one clotting assay is required to determine that the prolonged clotting time is due to LA, but the clinician needs to know only whether the test is positive or negative. One should also recognize that the sensitivity of the assays for LA varies considerably. For this reason, the clinician should use a laboratory known to perform reliable and sensitive LA testing.

At least two groups of investigators identify that LA and aCL may be separated in the laboratory, suggesting that they are different immunoglobulins.[55, 56] Others believe that LA and aCL are the same immunoglobulin detected by different methods. This controversy notwithstanding, LA and aCL are associated with the same set of clinical problems and therefore seem likely to be members of the same "family." The majority of patients with APS have LA and IgG aCL. Given, however, the state of the controversy about whether LA and aCL are the same immunoglobulin and the wide variety of assays that have been used in the past to detect LA or aCL, it is not surprising that many studies have found some patients with APS to have either aCL or LA but not both. When considering the diagnosis of APS, both tests should definitely be obtained. The relative contribution of the BF-STS to APS is unclear at this time. Tests for other aPL are done in the research setting, but they should not be used for the diagnosis of APS or related clinical decision making.

ANTIPHOSPHOLIPID SYNDROME AND PREGNANCY LOSS

Early case reports focused attention on a possible relationship between aPL and pregnancy loss.[57–59] We confirmed this relationship by studying the obstetric history of women with LA detected in the coagulation laboratory of the University of Utah.[60] In particular, fetal death (death of the conceptus after 10 to 12 weeks' gestation) appeared to be specific for aPL-related pregnancy loss. A summary of our data showed that more than 90% of women with APS who presented with pregnancy loss had suffered at least one fetal death.[61] It is uncommon, although not unheard of, for APS to present with recurrent first-trimester pregnancy loss.

Most studies linking aPL to pregnancy loss have found aPL in highly selected patients with underlying autoimmune disease, fetal death(s), or thrombosis. Studies of less highly selected populations have identified the emergence of two important facts. First, significant levels of aPL are infrequently found in otherwise normal women. In the best study of more than 1000 unselected obstetric patients, fewer than 2% had IgG aCL and 4% had IgM aCL.[62] More than 80% of the positive results were in the low-positive range, with only 0.2% of IgG results and 0.7% of IgM results in the medium or high-positive range. Other studies have also demonstrated a relatively small proportion of positive results in unselected obstetric patients.[63–65] Only one investigation has found pregnancy complications in patients with positive aPL results.[64] In that study, 2 of 723 (0.3%) unselected patients were found to have LA; both suffered a second-trimester fetal death. Overall, aPL testing in the general population as a screening test for pregnancy loss or complications seems unwarranted.

The second important finding is that APS is not a common "cause" of RPL. Table 19–6 summarizes five studies[66–70] that determined the frequency of aPL in women with RPL. The median frequency of LA or aCL IgG in women with RPL was 11% (versus 2.5% for controls). The studies by Petri and colleagues[70] and Parke and associates[68] found that women with predominantly recurrent first-trimester losses were not statistically more likely than controls to have LA and/or aCL. The other three studies in Table 19–6 found aPL to be statistically more frequent among women with RPL than among controls. Given that APS is not a common cause of RPL, only larger series (e.g., Parazzini and coworkers[69]) are likely to test statistical significance. Only the study of Out and coworkers[67] compared the frequency of positive tests for LA or aCL in patients with fetal death (>12 weeks' gestation) to patients with only first-trimester miscarriages. Although a trend was found, the figures were not statistically different from each other in this small study. Finally, one study identified a statistically higher prevalence of aPL in women with three or more pregnancy losses compared with those with less than three

Author (Reference)	Anticoagulant or Anticardiolipin IgG	
	RPL	*Controls*
Petri (70)*	7/44 (16%)	1/40 (2%)
Barbul (66)†	7/49 (14%)	0/141 (0%)
Parazzini (69)‡	10/99 (10%)	4/157 (3%)
Parke (68)§	8/81 (10%)	4.88 (5%)
Out (67)‖	11/102 (11%)	NA
Median	11%	2.5%

*RPL defined as ≥3 consecutive pregnancy losses. Other causes of RPL evaluated but did not exclude patients from the study.

†RPL defined as ≥2 consecutive pregnancy losses. Other causes of RPL excluded.

‡RPL defined as ≥2 consecutive pregnancy losses. Other causes of RPL excluded.

§RPL defined as ≥3 consecutive pregnancy losses. Evaluation for other causes of RPL incomplete in some cases.

‖RPL defined as ≥3 consecutive first-trimester losses or at least one unexplained fetal death >12 weeks' gestation. Not all patients had other causes of RPL excluded.

pregnancy losses,[71] again indicating the importance of patient selection. In our own experience, between 4% and 5% of patients with three or more consecutive pregnancy losses and no more than one live birth have APS.[61]

Infrequently, sporadic miscarriage or fetal death is due to aPL, a finding that is not surprising given the infrequency of APS. Haddow and associates[72] found only one medium-to-high positive IgG aCL among 309 cases of sporadic second-trimester or third-trimester fetal deaths (all after 14 weeks' gestation). Tests for LA were not done. Another study of 331 women with first pregnancy losses found no relationship between aPL and miscarriage when results were compared with 993 controls.[73] Only 86 patients could be determined to have had a fetal death. These two studies suggest that APS, similar to parental karyotype abnormalities or uterine malformations, is not the cause of pregnancy loss in a large proportion of unselected cases. Restated another way, most human pregnancy loss is unexplained by currently available evaluations, a fact that experienced practitioners intuitively understand. The importance of identifying APS lies not in its prevalence but in its implications for the patient and the fact that it is a potentially treatable cause of pregnancy loss.

TREATMENT OF ANTIPHOSPHOLIPID SYNDROME DURING PREGNANCY

Since 1983, investigators have suggested that women with APS and previous pregnancy loss could be treated during pregnancy to improve the chance of delivering a live infant. The initial reports used prednisone and low-dose aspirin (PRED/LDA).[74, 75] Table 19–7 summarizes the larger series[76–82] of APS pregnancies treated with this regimen. Although none of the series included appropriately selected controls, the majority of authors concluded that PRED/LDA was beneficial. The single exception was the study of Lockshin and coworkers,[79] in which the outcome of PRED/LDA–treated pregnancies was poor. Unfortunately, direct comparison of these studies is virtually impossible owing to the nature of the

Author and Year (Reference)	Number of Pregnancies	Spontaneous Abortions	Fetal Deaths*	Live Births
Lubbe, 1988 (80)	18	NA	NA	15 (78%)
Gatenby, 1989 (78)	27	NA	NA	17 (63%)
Ordi, 1989 (81)	9	0	2 (22%)	7 (78%)
Lockshin, 1989 (79)	11	3 (27%)	6 (55%)	2 (18%)
Cowchock, 1992 (77)	19	NA	NA	13 (68%)
Reece, 1991 (82)	18	3 (17%)	1 (5%)	14 (78%)
Branch, 1992 (76)†	39	8 (21%)	8 (21%)	23 (59%)‡

*Fetal deaths defined as intrauterine death of a fetus proved to be alive after 10 weeks' gestation.

†These figures are slightly different than previously reported.[61] The series was recently updated, adding one new patient and two new pregnancies. Two patients and two pregnancies were removed because the patients were found to be taking heparin as well as prednisone.

‡Includes two neonates that subsequently succumbed to complications of prematurity.

patients (e.g., SLE versus no SLE; numbers of previous fetal deaths), their diagnoses (e.g., LA and aCL versus LA alone or aCL alone), and the use of different treatments (e.g., dose of corticosteroids). Treatment with corticosteroids was potentially complicated by numerous minor and several serious adverse effects. In addition, gestational diabetes was rather common among women treated with high doses of corticosteroids.

The most attractive alternative to corticosteroids and low-dose aspirin is subcutaneous heparin treatment, with or without low-dose aspirin (Table 19–8). The first published series was that of Rosove and colleagues.[83] Using a mean dose of 24,700 units of heparin daily beginning in the first trimester, 14 of 15 pregnancies (93%) were successful. Cowchock and colleagues[77] have completed a randomized trial comparing treatment with corticosteroids to treatment with heparin. The mean dose of heparin was 17,000 units daily. Although only 20 patients were randomized, the results suggested that the two treatments were of similar efficacy in achieving a successful pregnancy. Moreover, treatment with corticosteroids was associated with an increased neonatal morbidity (preterm delivery and low birth weight) and maternal morbidity (gestational diabetes and pregnancy-induced hypertension).

In our experience, we treated patients with heparin and low-dose aspirin therapy. One low-dose aspirin was taken daily throughout pregnancy. As soon as a normal platelet count was ascertained in the first trimester, patients were

Author and Year (Reference)	Number of Pregnancies	Spontaneous Miscarriages	Fetal Deaths*	Live Births
Rosove, 1990 (83)	15	NA	NA	14 (93%)
Cowchock, 1992 (77)	8	NA	NA	6 (75%)
Branch, 1992 (76)	19	1 (5%)	2 (11%)	16 (84%)†

*Fetal deaths defined as intrauterine death of a fetus proved to be alive after 10 weeks' gestation.

†Includes two neonates that subsequently succumbed to complications of prematurity.

injected subcutaneously with 15,000 units of heparin daily. In the second trimester, a median dose of 20,000 units per day was used. Of the 19 pregnancies, 16 were successful; however, two infants died of complications of prematurity. In our current management scheme, heparin is not started until the patient has an ultrasound study demonstrating a live embryo (usually 5 to 7 weeks' gestation); this eliminates early first-trimester losses and anembryonic pregnancies. We continue to use low-dose aspirin in the treatment regimen because it may prevent or ameliorate preeclampsia in patients at risk.[84, 85]

Heparin treatment is by no means benign. The most common significant risk is heparin-induced osteoporosis. In an attempt to avoid severe osteoporosis, we advise patients treated with either corticosteroids or heparin to take at least 1 g of calcium daily (vitamin D is contained in prenatal vitamins) and to walk for 1 hour daily. Heparin is also associated with an uncommon idiosyncratic thrombocytopenia. This phenomenon is independent of the route of administration or dose and may have its onset from several days to several weeks after starting heparin. The frequency is difficult to determine but probably occurs in fewer than 5% of patients treated with heparin. In its most severe form, heparin-induced thrombocytopenia is associated with antibodies directed against vascular endothelial cells. Occasionally thromboembolic events or disseminated intravascular coagulation accompanies the thrombocytopenia and may be fatal. This complication of heparin may be less frequent in pregnant patients, but formal data are not available.

We believe that the concomitant use of corticosteroids and heparin should be avoided at present because the combination of these two medications has not been shown to be better than either alone in achieving a live infant. Several cases of severe osteoporosis with fractures have occurred in women with APS treated with a combination regimen.

The use of high-dose intravenous immune globulin has generated interest because of anecdotal reports of successful pregnancy outcomes. In our experience, three women with APS were treated with immune globulin and corticosteroids. One had a successful pregnancy, and two had fetal losses despite treatment. This suggests that immune globulin may not be better than other regimens.

The chance of a successful pregnancy outcome for women who undergo treatment for APS partially depends on the number of pregnancy losses suffered in the past.[76] For physicians involved in the evaluation and treatment of women with RL, these observations come as no surprise. Regardless of cause, the more consecutive pregnancy losses, the worse the prognosis is for future pregnancies. The reason(s) is unknown, but the observation may influence a patient's decision to attempt a treated pregnancy. Some patients with APS have successfully achieved pregnancy without specific medical therapy. This has focused attention on the medical necessity of treatment for APS patients. One might argue that the recognition of fetal risk in APS pregnancies has resulted in increased attention to the fetus and improved outcome by means of timely delivery. A report by Trudinger and colleagues[86] supports this view. The authors successfully managed six untreated pregnancies in women with APS using close fetal surveillance with Doppler velocimetry. Although close fetal surveillance is an obvious key to successful pregnancy, the relative contribution of fetal surveillance (versus

treatment) is yet to be determined. Even careful, frequent fetal surveillance cannot prevent fetal or neonatal death before 22 to 24 weeks' gestation.

Do patients with APS but no history of fetal loss need medical therapy during pregnancy? Too few data are available from which to draw conclusions. As suggested previously, some women with APS may have a live birth with close obstetric observation and fetal surveillance. There is no way, however, to identify patients prospectively, and in many cases, instituting treatment after the recognition of fetal compromise would probably not save a pregnancy.

Because APS is clearly associated with venous and arterial thrombosis, concern is raised regarding the risks to the mother during an untreated pregnancy. Is it safe to allow patients with a risk for thrombosis or stroke (albeit poorly defined) to enter the thrombogenic state of pregnancy untreated? Our retrospective case analysis identified that more than 80% of thrombotic episodes in women with APS were associated with pregnancy or oral contraceptives.[76] Although controversial, we consider treatment with heparin and low-dose aspirin warranted based on maternal thrombotic risk alone. We continue to treat patients with APS through the first month postpartum to prevent postpartum thrombosis.

Many questions remain in the treatment of pregnancies in women with APS. To expedite answers, the Fetal Loss Subcommittee of the Kingston Antiphospholipid Study Group organized a Registry to record prospectively pregnancy treatments (if any) and outcomes in women with APS. Any interested individuals or centers may participate in the Registry. It is hoped that the patients submitted to the Registry will form the basis of a successful funding proposal in the future. Interested individuals may inquire by writing *The KAPS Fetal Loss Registry, Room 2B200 Medical Center, 50 North Medical Drive, Salt Lake City, Utah 84132.*

Subclinical Autoimmunity

The idea that a subclinical autoimmune condition may in some way cause pregnancy loss is derived primarily from the observation that a seemingly larger than expected proportion of patients with RPL have detectable levels of autoantibodies. If anything, the recognition of APS has stimulated further exploration of autoantibodies among RPL patients. The literature in this area, however, is marked by differences in autoantibody measurements, types of assays, and a variety of conclusions. Most of the published reports have focused on antinuclear antibodies (ANA). The study of Clauvel and colleagues,[87] which includes no controls and involves only 14 highly selected patients, can be dismissed. Edelman and associates[88] found ANA in 6 of 130 (5%) women with RPL, compared with only 1 of 50 controls. The titers of all positive samples were less than or equal to 1:200. One additional patient was positive for anti-DNA (native) antibodies. After a small series suggested that certain autoantibodies might be more prevalent in RPL patients,[89] Cowchock and colleagues investigated 61 women with unexplained RPL and 21 women with recognizable RPL and 3 of 21 (14%) women with explained RPL, a difference that was not statistically significant. Twelve patients had positive titers at or beyond 1:500 dilution (10 in the unexplained group and 2 in the explained group). Of either group, only three women with unexplained

RPL had anti-DNA (native) antibodies (the difference between groups was not statistically significant). Maier and Parke[91] found that 20% of 20 women with unexplained RPL and 14% of 14 women with explained RPL had positive ANA tests, all at titers less than or equal to 1:256. None of 24 controls had positive tests, but there was no statistical difference between any of the groups. One ANA-positive patient also had anti-DNA (native) antibodies.

In a much larger study, Harger and coworkers[92] found that a similar proportion (16%) of women with RPL, normal nonpregnant controls, and pregnant controls had a positive ANA. There was a significantly higher proportion of women with RPL who had ANA at greater than or equal to 1:80 compared with controls. The next pregnancy outcomes of the RPL patients with positive ANA at greater than or equal to 1:80, however, did not differ significantly from the outcomes of ANA-negative RPL patients (live births, 52% versus 67%). In the three studies in which it was addressed, 17%,[90] 71%,[88] and 100%[91] of the RPL patients with positive ANA also had aPL. Taken together, the currently available data do not support performing ANA or anti-DNA determinations in patients with RPL. Moreover, no reasonable recommendation is currently available regarding the management of RPL patients with positive tests.

Other autoantibodies or autoimmune aberrations have been implicated in otherwise unexplained RPL. At least one investigation suggests that anti-Ro antibody is associated with miscarriage, but substantial data exist to the contrary.[93] A veritable myriad of autoantibodies detected by one screening "profile" were associated with pregnancy loss.[94] The study had several major flaws, however;[95] one was that every patient underwent 33 separate autoantibody assays (11 antigens, 3 isotypes). It is well known that a relatively large proportion of apparently normal women tested for multiple autoantibodies are positive in at least one test.[96] Because of these problems, clinicians should not order autoantibody profiles in the evaluation of RPL.

A possible role for subclinical thyroid disease, or for antithyroid autoantibodies, in some cases of RPL has been suggested. The prospective investigation of Edelman and colleagues[88] found antithyroglobulin autoantibodies in 7 of 130 (5%) women with RPL and antimicrosomal autoantibodies in 10 of 130 (8%). Only three controls had either of these autoantibodies detected. The serendipitous findings of a prospective study are also quite interesting. The authors screened 552 women for antithyroid autoantibodies at their first prenatal visit.[97] Twenty percent of the patients were positive for either antithyroglobulin or antimicrosomal antibodies. Pregnancy loss occurred in a significantly higher proportion of those with the antibodies (17% versus 8.4%). These studies require confirmation before clinicians should consider the tests to be useful markers of a subset of patients with RPL. Moreover, further investigation is needed to assess which therapies are efficacious.

Summary

Currently available data suggest the proportion of patients with RPL who have LA or significant levels of aCL and who meet the criteria for APS is small. If a patient with APS decides to attempt another pregnancy, she may benefit from treatment with subcutaneous heparin and low-dose aspirin. Autoimmune conditions implied by the presence of autoantibodies other than aPL need to be independently confirmed as causes of RPL before testing for such conditions can be recommended.

INFECTIONS

Whether an infectious agent may cause or is a common cause of RPL remains controversial. For an infectious agent to cause multiple pregnancy losses, it seems reasonable to expect the following criteria:

1. Organisms must be present for at least one to several years. In other words, the infection must be chronic.
2. The colonization or infection cannot make the patient so ill as to impair ovulation or sexual function.
3. The organism must infect the gestational tissues (decidua, trophoblast, or fetus). A less likely alternative is for the organism to have systemic effects that directly affect the uterus or gestational tissues.

Because no infectious agent meets all three criteria, none has been proved to cause RPL. Nonetheless, case reports and circumstantial evidence suggest that several infectious agents might be responsible for RPL.

Treponema pallidum and *Borrelia burgdorferi*

T. pallidum, which causes syphilis, has been unequivocally identified in first-trimester abortuses.[98] Syphilis is an unlikely cause of RPL, however, because it is such an uncommon infection. Lyme disease, caused by the treponeme *B. burgdorferi,* is now recognized as a common cause of adult arthritis in some areas of the United States. Similar to syphilis, the infection is chronic if left untreated. Although the spirochete has been found in fetal tissue from a fetal death at 12 weeks' gestation,[99] the relationship of Lyme disease to RPL is unknown.

Chlamydia trachomatis

C. trachomatis infections of the female genital tract are among the most common sexually transmitted bacterial infections in the United States. Because this organism may cause a chronic genital tract infection, investigators have hypothesized that it may be an infectious cause of RPL. One serologic study supported this hypothesis.[100] Nevertheless, microbiologic studies suggest that *C. trachomatis* is not a cause of late first-trimester or early second-trimester pregnancy loss. In 361 patients cultured before 16 weeks' gestation, no significant difference was found in positive endocervical cultures between controls and miscarriage patients.[101] Another study of 18 women with positive endocervical cultures for *Chlamydia* observed no spontaneous miscarriages, but the mean age of enrollment was 14 to 15 weeks' gestation.[102] Currently no conclusive evidence exists that *Chlamydia* is a cause of early pregnancy loss or RPL.

Listeria monocytogenes

The gram-positive, rod-shaped bacterium *L. monocytogenes* is a well-recognized cause of isolated pregnancy loss in humans. The organism appears to have a propensity for the placenta and fetus, causing septicemia, pneumonia, and meningitis in the infant. The most characteristic clinical picture is low-grade chorioamnionitis resulting in premature labor in the latter half of pregnancy. Among non–farm worker adults, the disease tends to occur in epidemics, probably spread through improperly pasteurized dairy products. The organism may be carried in the endocervix or vagina[103] and possibly spread by venereal transmission.[107] Some believe that pregnant women are particularly susceptible to infection with listeriosis.[105]

Case reports implicate *Listeria* as a cause of sporadic first-trimester and second-trimester pregnancy loss;[106] one study strongly suggests that *Listeria* may play a role in RPL. The investigators isolated *Listeria* from the cervix of 25 of 34 women with RPL and none of 87 controls.[107] Four subsequent studies, however, found no association between *Listeria* and miscarriage.[108–111] At present, the preponderance of evidence weighs against *Listeria* playing a role in anything but an exceptional case of RPL.

Mycoplasmas

Two mycoplasmas, *Mycoplasma hominis* and *Ureaplasma urealyticum,* are commonly detected in the genitourinary tract of sexually active adults. Although the vagina or endocervix is the usual site of colonization, upper tract colonization and infection have been abundantly demonstrated.

Mycoplasmas were first linked to pregnancy loss in a few case reports published in the late 1960s.[112, 113] A subsequent study found that nearly one third of 104 midtrimester miscarriages were culture-positive for mycoplasmas.[114, 115]

Stray-Pedersen and colleagues[116] first drew an association between mycoplasmas and RPL; 28% of women with RPL had colonization of the endometrium with *U. urealyticum,* whereas only 7% of controls were colonized ($P < 0.01$). The rate of endocervical colonization was high in both RPL patients and controls with no difference between the two groups. This suggests that although a substantial proportion of all patients may have endocervical colonization, some women presenting with RPL may be susceptible to intrauterine colonization. Another study, however, showing a high frequency of endocervical colonization cast a doubt on a causative role for mycoplasmas in RPL; these investigators found that more than a quarter of the culture-positive women had a genetic or anatomic explanation for their pregnancy losses.[43] Munday and associates[117] found a similar frequency of positive endocervical mycoplasma cultures in women with spontaneous miscarriage (67%), threatened miscarriage (75%), and normal pregnancies (67%).

Several investigators have studied the effect of antibiotic treatment on the subsequent pregnancy outcome in women with positive mycoplasma cultures. Quinn and colleagues[118] treated culture-positive patients before conception or before conception and during pregnancy. Among retrospectively studied "controls," the pregnancy loss rate was 96% (22 of 24). For those treated before conception with doxycycline, the pregnancy loss rate was 49% (18 of 37); for those treated with doxycycline both before conception and during pregnancy with erythromycin, it was only 17% (2 of 12). The data of Harger and associates[43] are not as encouraging. In their study, all culture-positive patients and their husbands were treated with doxycycline. Of 19 successfully treated women who had a subsequent pregnancy, 13 (68%) had a live birth. Six of 7 (86%) women, however, who were treatment failures (persistent positive cultures) also had live births, as did 10 of 14 (71%) women who received no treatment. Although more has been written about mycoplasmas than any other infectious agent, no conclusive evidence exists that this organism is a cause of RPL.

Toxoplasma gondii

The protozoan parasite *T. gondii* most commonly infects humans through ingestion of raw or undercooked infected meat or by inadvertent ingestion of fecal material containing the *Toxoplasma* oocytes. Infection rates vary considerably among different populations. Primary infection results in a parasitemia that is usually asymptomatic. The parasite, which may initially lodge in certain tissues, appears to be well contained thereafter by the immune system.

Maternal primary infection with *T. gondii* can result in infection of the midtrimester or third-trimester fetus and is a well-recognized cause of fetal death.[119] One report shows that *T. gondii* infection of the first-trimester fetus may occur in apparently immunocompetent seropositive women.[120] Despite a few suggestive cases, the data linking toxoplasmosis to RPL are scant. Kimball and coworkers[121] found a statistically higher frequency of *Toxoplasma* antibodies among RPL patients (31%) compared with women with sporadic spontaneous miscarriages. Nevertheless, two other investigations failed to confirm this finding,[122, 123] suggesting that serologic testing for toxoplasmosis is not useful in the evaluation of RPL.

The most intriguing data regarding a possible connection between *Toxoplasma* and RPL comes from the work of Stray-Pedersen and Lorentzen–Stry.[123] They found immunohistologic evidence of *T. gondii* tachyzoites in the endometrium of 6 of 41 (15%) women with habitual miscarriage compared with only 1 of 59 (2%) patients with other obstetric or gynecologic problems. In no case, however, could the organism be grown from the endometrium, and five of seven women with *Toxoplasma*-positive endometria were serologically negative. As a practical point, immunohistologic staining of endometrial biopsy specimens for *T. gondii* tachyzoites is not clinically available, and the weight of evidence indicates that *Toxoplasma* serology is not helpful and may be misleading.

Viral Agents

Several known viruses have been linked to sporadic cases of first-trimester pregnancy loss or fetal death owing to primary maternal infection. These include rubella, herpes simplex virus (HSV), cytomegalovirus (CMV), measles virus, and coxsackievirus. Of these viruses, HSV and CMV establish a chronic, latent infection that conceivably could cause RPL.

Even though no data are available to suggest CMV as a cause of RPL, two studies implicate HSV. One, a retrospective analysis, found evidence of HSV infection in a significantly greater proportion of women with previous miscarriage than in those without previous miscarriage.[124] In the second study, the authors found a statistically insignificant trend toward positive immunohistochemical staining for HSV in endometrial or chorionic villus material taken from women with RPL.[125] The authors also found that luteal phase endometria were more likely to stain positive for HSV than follicular phase endometria, suggesting that HSV activation might be hormonally driven. This interesting hypothesis and other aspects of a possible link between viral infections and RPL deserve further investigation. On the whole, there is currently little to suggest that chronic viral infection results in RPL. Regarding CMV and HSV, serologic evaluation of patients is of little value because a relatively high proportion of adult women (with or without RPL) have antibodies to CMV and HSV.

Summary and Conclusions

Of the organisms covered in this chapter, *U. urealyticum* is perhaps the one most strongly implicated as an infectious cause of RPL, even though the association remains controversial. In the evaluation of a woman with RPL, it seems reasonable to culture the endometrium for this mycoplasma, which can be done at the time of endometrial biopsy for luteal phase evaluation. Because endocervical cultures are likely to be positive in a large proportion of patients (with or without RPL), these cultures are not particularly helpful. Couples in whom the woman has a positive endometrial culture should be treated with doxycycline. Indeed, orally administered tetracycline medications are relatively benign, with few, if any, serious adverse effects. Because of this, and the cost of mycoplasma cultures, many physicians empirically treat all couples with RPL with a 10- to 14-day course of doxycycline.

IDIOPATHIC CATEGORY

Unfortunately, the previously discussed detection methods reveal no recognized cause of miscarriage in the majority of RPL patients. Epidemiologic studies have not been enlightening because they have focused primarily on the relationship of environmental toxins and drugs to all spontaneous miscarriages rather than to recurrent miscarriage.[126] The incidence of spontaneous miscarriage is reportedly higher in patients with endometriosis and subsequently lower after conventional endometriosis treatment.[127] Although some RPL patients seem to have a concomitant infertility problem, no convincing relationship to endometriosis has been established. The presence of anti-P antibody has been rather convincingly shown to be an uncommon cause of spontaneous miscarriage. When this antibody is present, treatment with plasmapheresis is reportedly successful.[128]

Potential psychological factors related to early pregnancy loss are the most difficult of all to evaluate objectively. Certainly the mechanism of action for this cause would be difficult to explain. No definite evidence links specific events (e.g., intercourse, physical activity, or emotionally stressful events) to RPL. After observing the pregnancies in women who have a variety of psychiatric disorders and emotional states, we conclude that psychological factors are more often the result, not the cause, of this frustrating experience.

Because the majority of recurrent miscarriage patients have none of the demonstrable causes previously discussed, it has been proposed that alloimmune factors may be responsible. Despite a variety of hypotheses, the mechanisms that prevent a pregnant woman from rejecting her semiallogenic conceptus are incompletely understood. The immune system is a complex, integrated system with two fundamental components: (1) humoral immunity mediated by antibodies that are produced by B lymphocyte–derived plasma cells and (2) cellular immunity mediated by activated T lymphocytes. It is now thought that the principal manner by which these cells communicate is through the elaboration of soluble regulatory and chemotactic factors, collectively called cytokines.

Immunologic responses are regulated by genes of the major histocompatibility complex (MHC), located on chromosome 6. MHC class I antigens (HLA A, B, C) and MHC class II antigens (HLA DR, DP, DQ) determine immunologic compatibility of tissues. Class I MHC antigens are important recognition structures in rejection responses mediated by cytotoxic T lymphocytes. Class II MHC antigens present antigens to helper T lymphocytes and help initiate immune responses. The older traditional concept of *help and suppression,* however, probably does not adequately describe the complex nature of immune recognition.

In random matings, the conceptus is immunologically distinct from the mother (i.e., histoincompatible), and one might intuitively suppose that this would lead to rejection of the conceptus by the mother. Current theory, however, suggests that the histoincompatible conceptus paradoxically evokes an immunotolerant or immunotrophic[129] response from the mother that is necessary for successful implantation and growth. Following the same line of reasoning, it has been hypothesized that histocompatibility between mother and conceptus results in a defective maternal immune response leading to spontaneous miscarriage. The large majority of RPL couples, however, are histoincompatible, making the fetus histoincompatible with the mother. Moreover, recurrent miscarriage is not a common problem in genetically histocompatible inbred animals.

Reproductive immunologists propose several hypotheses to explain the immunotolerance of the mother to the conceptus. These are broadly classified in terms of local events at the maternal-fetal interface or peripheral factors measured in the maternal circulation.

Local Suppressive Factors

The presence of eicosanoids, cytokines, and soluble factors that modulate and possibly suppress immune responses in the late luteal phase (secretory) endometrium and decidua of normal pregnancies is absent in both animals and humans with RPL.[130, 131] These factors are hormonally dependent and are important for the immunoregulation of implantation and growth of the conceptus. Throughout the menstrual cycle and pregnancy, macrophages are present in the endometrium. A few B lymphocytes are present, but T lymphocytes, which are rare in proliferative endometrium, increase until the midsecretory phase and then decline.[132] T lymphocytes are also present in first-trimester decidua but lack the receptor for interleukin-2 (Il-2), a marker of T cell activation.[133] A heterologous group of larger granular lymphocytes in the endometrium and decidua are neither T cells nor B cells, but in vitro they express natural killer (NK), natural suppressor, and antibody-dependent and antibody-independent and allogeneic cytotoxicity. NK cells differ from T cells in that they are not "antigen driven"; they form a part of the innate system for nonspecific immune surveillance that requires no priming.[134] Although it has been suggested that decidual cells may suppress immune responses by releasing prostaglandins,[134] the actual level of prostaglandins in maternal endometrium and their cellular origin remain to be defined.

Cytokines appear to be the language of the trophoblast/decidua system: Some products of activated lymphocytes and macrophages are probably immunosuppressive, some may be immunotropic, and some may cause miscarriage when expressed. Supernatants from decidual cell suspensions contain factors capable of blocking the action of Il-2. This activity at the maternal-fetal interface is believed to direct an immunosuppressive response, thereby safeguarding the conceptus from immune attack.[135] The lack of class I MHC antigens on syncytiotrophoblast, together with the atypical nature of HLA antigen expression on cytotrophoblast and the complete absence of class II MHC determinants on either trophoblast layer, precludes trophoblast involvement, either as a classic immunogen for maternal sensitization or as a target for MHC-directed cytotoxic T cells. Certain products of immune cells, however, have toxic or deregulating effects on fetal tissues if present during specific intervals of development. For example, class I MHC antigen expression may be induced by gamma interferon (γ-INF). Theoretically secretion of γ-INF by lymphocytes in the endometrium of some women could induce class I MHC antigen expression, providing a mechanism for cytotoxic lymphocyte attack that culminates in miscarriage.[136] Granulocyte-macrophage colony-stimulating factor, which is present in decidual cell supernatants, enhances trophoblast growth and prevents spontaneous fetal resorption,[137] whereas injections of tumor necrosis factor dramatically increase the percent of fetal resorption in animal models.[138] The interrelationship of molecular changes in the preimplantation endometrium and decidua is a rapidly developing area that has not been thoroughly studied in humans. Currently there are no practical clinical tests for these factors.

Circulating Blocking Factors

Although circulating blocking antibodies and other pregnancy-maintaining factors have been widely accepted as necessary for normal pregnancy, they have never been well characterized biochemically or immunologically. Blocking factors are usually identified by in vitro tests, such as the mixed lymphocyte reaction (MLR). The clinician, however, should be aware of several pitfalls with these assays. A wide variability in the proliferative response has been found among different patients and between the same couples tested at different times. Also, no uniform method exists for reporting the results. Our data indicate that the presence of blocking factors depends on the equation used for calculation of MLR data.[139]

A number of studies have reported the presence of blocking antibodies in women with successful pregnancies and their absence in women with RPL.[140, 141] Investigators found that sera from women with RPL inhibit the development of in vitro mouse preimplantation embryos and that a lymphocyte-derived, progesterone-induced blocking factor has an antiabortive effect.[142] Other investigators, however, have cast doubt on this concept because (1) blocking antibodies frequently do not appear until late in the first or second trimester of the first pregnancy, (2) agammaglobulinemic women have normal pregnancies, and (3) animals rendered incapable of producing immunoglobulins or mounting a humoral immune response also have successful pregnancies.[143] Because only a small percentage of pregnant women make antibodies directed against paternal HLA, it is doubtful that the production of antipaternal cytotoxic antibodies is a useful marker in the management of RPL. Finally, patients with RPL reportedly have a factor in their peripheral blood that inhibits in vitro development of preimplantation mouse embryos.[144] Whether this embryotoxic factor disappears in a subsequent successful pregnancy or is clinically useful is presently unknown.

Tests advocated to detect immunologic abnormalities in couples with recurrent miscarriages are expensive. Moreover, there is no consensus on which tests are clinically important and how they should be used to determine which patients may benefit from immunologic treatment. Perhaps nothing has generated more controversy and confusion over the past few years for physicians and their recurrent miscarriage patients.

Immunotherapy

Pretransplant blood transfusions in allograft recipients have been used to decrease the chance of immunologic rejection. Long-term survival of kidney grafts is reportedly increased with either donor-specific or third-party blood; the buffy coat appears to be responsible for this beneficial effect. In animal models, it has also been shown that the rate of fetal resorptions or abortions is decreased by prior immunization with spleen cells from a paternally related strain. This background information has led to similar clinical therapeutic approaches to improve the maternal immune response and to prevent rejection of the fetus in recurrent miscarriers.

A variety of immunization regimens have been used for treating RPL patients for whom all nonimmunologic causes have been ruled out (Table 19–9),[145–156] but only three prospective, randomized trials have been done (Table 19–10).[157–159] Immunization with paternal lymphocytes has shown successful pregnancy rates of 50% to 83%; random donor leukocyte injections have produced successful pregnancy rates from 71% to 95% with similar results using high-dose intravenous immunoglobulin.

Although potential maternal and fetal risks are associated with immunization using any type of cells or blood products, few complications have been reported in hundreds of treated mothers or their offspring observed for more than 5 years. Likewise, the prevalence of fetal or neonatal problems has not been higher than one would expect compared with the general population of untreated recurrent miscarriage patients matched for age.

Immunotherapy for potential alloimmune causes of RPL is

TABLE 19–9. Results of Immunotherapy in Recurrent Miscarriage Patients

Investigator (Reference)	Cell Source	Route	Patients	Live Births
Beer (146)	Paternal	ID	121	100 (83%)
Mowbray (150)	Paternal	ID, SC, IV	244	181 (74%)
Takakuwa (155)	Paternal	ID	42	33 (78%)
Smith (154)	Paternal	ID, SC, IV	58	29 (50%)
Carp (147)	Paternal	ID, SC, IV	81	61 (75%)
Alexander (145)	Paternal	ID, SC, IV	30	24 (80%)
Reznikoff (153)	Paternal	ID, SC, IV	35	30 (80%)
McIntyre (149)	Third party	IV	23	20 (87%)
Unander (156)	Third party	IV	105	100 (95%)
Beer (146)	Third party	ID	21	15 (71%)
Johnson (148)	Trophoblast	IV	21	16 (76%)
Peters (152)	Immunoglobulin	IV	4	3 (75%)
Mueller-Eckhardt (151)	Immunoglobulin	IV	38	27 (71%)
Totals			843	639 (76%)

ID, Intradermal; SC, subcutaneous; IV, intravenous.

TABLE 19–11. Suggested Routine Evaluation for Recurrent Miscarriage*

History
Determine pattern and trimester of pregnancy losses and whether a live fetus was present; unusual exposure to environmental toxins, drugs, infections; previous gynecologic disorders or surgery, including dilatation and curettage; and previous diagnostic tests and treatments

Physical
Habitus; abnormalities on pelvic examination, including abnormal discharge; findings suggestive of diethylstilbestrol exposure; or uterine anomalies

Tests
1. Hysterosalpingogram
2. Luteal phase endometrial biopsy
3. Parental chromosome analysis
4. Screening test for lupus anticoagulant (aPTT) and anticardiolipin
5. Other laboratory tests only if suggested by history and physical evaluation
6. Immunologic tests are an option and last resort if everything is negative and immunotherapy is planned before attempting another pregnancy

*Ultrasound examinations at 6 weeks' gestation in next pregnancy and chromosome analysis of products of conception from any subsequent spontaneous miscarriage.

still controversial, and cautious interpretation of the results is warranted at this time. The major questions that remain are: (1) What is the actual success rate with and without immunotherapy? (2) Exactly which patients should be offered immunotherapy? (3) If effective, what is the optimum source of white cells and what is the best regimen? (4) Are there any unanticipated long-term risks?

SUMMARY

What pertinent information can the clinician glean from this chapter to use in the future management of RPL patients? Our recommendations for an efficient, cost-effective diagnostic workup in patients with RPL are summarized in Table 19–11. In well-selected cases, treatment of maternal factors is effective and rewarding. Although nothing remarkable may be found during an initial evaluation, even this information can be used in a positive way to reassure and counsel the couple about their favorable chances of eventually achieving a successful pregnancy. Further attempts at pregnancy without treatment may be justified, depending on the situation and the wishes of the couple. If further immunologic evaluation and experimental immunotherapy is necessary, it is perhaps best to refer these patients to research centers.

Finally, a sympathetic attitude by the physician is impor-

TABLE 19–10. Published Prospective, Randomized Trials of Immunotherapy in Recurrent Miscarriage Patients

Investigator (Reference)	Cell Source	Route	Patients	Live Births
Mowbray (159)	Paternal	ID, SC, IV	22	17 (77%)
	Maternal	ID, SC, IV	27	10 (37%)
Ho (158)	Paternal	ID	20	23 (65%)
	Third party	ID	6	5 (83%)
	Maternal	ID	28	14 (50%)
Cauchi (157)	Paternal	ID, SC, IV	21	13 (62%)
	Saline	ID, SC, IV	25	19 (76%)

ID, Intradermal; SC, subcutaneous; IV, intravenous.

tant. Establishment of trust and rapport permits tactful and thorough discussions with a patient and her husband. This is of critical importance because physicians often fail to appreciate the severity of grief reactions experienced by RPL patients. Education and understanding help prevent multiple expensive and unproductive tests as well as "doctor hopping" in a desperate attempt to find a physician with a magic solution. Importantly, high live birth rates do occur in RPL patients who receive emotional support and who visit their physicians frequently.[159]

REFERENCES

1. Branch DW, Scott JR. Pregnancy loss terminology (letter). Am J Obstet Gynecol 1990; 163:245–246.
2. Poland BJ, Miller JR, Jones DC, et al. Reproductive counselling in patients who have had a spontaneous abortion. Am J Obstet Gynecol 1977; 127:685–697.
3. Roman E. Fetal loss rates and their relation to pregnancy order. J Epidemiol Commun Health 1984; 38:29–43.
4. Warburton D, Clarke Fraser F. Spontaneous abortion risks in man: data from reproductive histories collected in a medical genetics unit. Hum Genet 1964; 16:1–19.
5. Simpson JL. Fetal wastage. In: Gabbe SG, Niebyl JR, Simpson JL, editors. Obstetrics. Normal and Problem Pregnancies. New York: Churchill Livingston, 1991:783.
6. Kajii T, Ferrier A, Nikawa N, et al. Anatomic and chromosomal anomalies in 639 spontaneous abortions. Hum Genet 1980; 55:87–93.
7. Davison EV, Burn J. Genetic causes of early pregnancy loss. In: Huisjes HJ, Lind T, editors. Early Pregnancy Failure. Edinburgh: Churchill Livingston, 1990:55.
8. Szulman AE, Surti U. The clinicopathologic profile of the partial hydatidiform mole. Obstet Gynecol 1981; 59:597.
9. Jacobs PA, Szulman AE, Funkhouser J, et al. Human triploidy: relationship between parental origin of the additional haploid complement and development of partial hydatidiform mole. Ann Hum Genet 1982; 46:223–232.
10. Hassold T, Chin D, Yamane J. Parental origin of autosomal trisomies. Ann Hum Genet 1984; 48:1–24.
11. Meulenbroek GH, Geraedts JT. Parental origin of chromosome abnormalities in spontaneous abortions. Hum Genet 1982; 62:129–133.
12. Sperling K. Frequency and origin of chromosome abnormalities in man. In: Obe G, editor. Mutations in Man. Berlin: Springer-Verlag, 1984:128–149.
13. Alberman E. Maternal age and spontaneous abortion. In: Bennett MJ,

Edmonds DK, editors. Spontaneous and Recurrent Abortion. Oxford: Blackwell Scientific Publications, 1987:746–764.

14. Chandley AC. The origin of chromosomal aberrations in man and their potential for survival and reproduction in adult human populations. Ann Genet 1981; 24:5–11.

15. Simpson JL, Golbus MS, Martin AO, Sarto GE. Genetics in Obstetrics and Gynecology. New York: Grune & Stratton, 1982:126–147.

16. Hassold T. A cytogenetic study of repeated spontaneous abortions. Am J Hum Genet 1980; 32:723–734.

17. Warburton D, Kline J, Stein Z, et al. Does the karyotype of a spontaneous abortion predict the karyotype of a subsequent abortion? Evidence from 273 women with two karyotyped spontaneous abortions. Am J Hum Genet 1987; 41:465–482.

18. Campana M, Serra A, Neri G. Role of chromosome aberrations in recurrent abortion: a study of 269 balanced translocations. Am J Med Genet 1986; 24:341–356.

19. Simpson JL, Elias S, Meyers CM, et al. Translocations are infrequent among couples having repeated spontaneous abortions but no other abnormal pregnancies. Fertil Steril 1989; 51:811–832.

20. Boue A, Gallano P. A collaborative study of the segregation of inherited chromosome structural rearrangements in 1356 prenatal diagnoses. Prenat Diag 1984; 4:45–60.

21. Mikkelson M. Cytogenetic findings in first trimester chorionic villi biopsies: a collaborative study. In: Fraccaro C, Simoni G, Brambati B, editors. First Trimester Fetal Diagnosis. Berlin: Springer-Verlag, 1985:109–120.

22. Thompson JS, Thompson MW: Genetics in Medicine. Philadelphia: WB Saunders, 1986:113–114.

23. Klein J, Vincek V, Kasahara M, Figueroa F. Is there a t complex in man? In: Beard RW, Sharp F, editors. Early Pregnancy Loss. London: Springer-Verlag, 1988:269–273.

24. Gill TJ, MacPherson TA, Ho HN, et al. Immunological and genetic factors affecting implantation and development in the rat and in the human. In: Gill TJ, Wegmann TG, Nisbet-Brown E, editors. Immunoregulation and Fetal Survival. New York: Oxford University Press, 1987:137–155.

25. Maxson WS. Hormonal causes of recurrent abortion. Clin Obstet Gynecol 1986; 29:941–952.

26. Rock JA, Zacur HA. The clinical management of repeated early pregnancy wastage. Fertil Steril 1983; 39:123–143.

27. Lee CS. Luteal phase defects. Obstet Gynecol 1987; 42:267–274.

28. McNeely MS, Soules MR. The diagnosis of luteal phase deficiency: a critical review. Fertil Steril 1988; 50:1–15.

29. Csapo AI, Puikkinen M. Indispensibility of the human corpus luteum in the maintenance of early pregnancy: luteectomy evidence. Obstet Gynecol Surv 1978; 33:69–82.

30. Maclin VM, Radwanska E, Binor Z, Dmowski WP. Progesterone: estradiol ratios at implantation in ongoing pregnancies, abortions, and nonconception cycles resulting from ovulation induction. Fertil Steril 1990; 54:238–244.

31. Regan L, Owen EJ, Jacobs HS. Hypersecretion of luteinising hormone, infertility, and miscarriage. Lancet 1990; 336:1141–1144.

32. Noyes RW, Hertig AT, Rock J. Dating the endometrial biopsy. Fertil Steril 1950; 1:3–24.

33. Tho PT, Byrd JR, McDonough PG. Etiologies and subsequent reproductive performance of 100 couples with recurrent abortion. Fertil Steril 1979; 32:389–395.

34. Daya S, Ward S, Burrows E. Progesterone profiles in luteal phase defect cycles and outcome of progesterone treatment in patients with recurrent spontaneous abortion. Am J Obstet Gynecol 1988; 158:225–232.

35. Wentz AC, Herbert CM, Maxson WS, Garner CH. Outcome of progesterone treatment of luteal phase inadequacy. Fertil Steril 1984; 41:856–862.

36. Check JH, Chase JS, Nowroozi K, et al. Progesterone therapy to decrease first-trimester spontaneous abortions in previous aborters. Int J Fertil 1987; 32:192–199.

37. Daya S. Efficacy of progesterone support for pregnancy in women with recurrent miscarriage. A meta-analysis of controlled trials. Br J Obstet Gynaecol 1989; 96:275–280.

38. Goldstein P, Berrier J, Rosen S, et al. A meta-analysis of randomized control trials of progesterone agents in pregnancy. Br J Obstet Gynaecol 1989; 96:265–274.

39. Patton P, Novy MJ. Reproductive potential of the anomalous uterus. Semin Reprod Endocrinol 1988; 6:217–233.

40. Branch DW. Operations for cervical incompetence. Clin Obstet Gynecol 1986; 29:240–254.

41. Gast MJ, Martin CM. Pregnancy in a woman with a uterine septum. J Reprod Med 1992; 37:85–88.

42. Portuondo JA, Camara MM, Echanojauregui AD, et al. Müllerian abnormalities in fertile women and recurrent aborters. J Reprod Med 1986; 31:616–637.

43. Harger JH, Archer DF, Marchese SG, et al. Etiology of recurrent pregnancy loss and outcome of subsequent pregnancies. Obstet Gynecol 1983; 62:574–581.

44. Thompson JP, Smith RA, Welch JS. Reproductive ability after metroplasty. Obstet Gynecol 1966; 28:363–373.

45. Scott JR. Habitual abortion—recommendations for a reasonable approach to an enigmatic problem. In: Soules MR, editor. Controversies in Obstetrics and Gynecology. New York: Elsevier, 1989:95–106.

46. Kaufman RH, Adam E, Binder GL, et al. Upper genital tract and pregnancy outcome in offspring exposed in diethylstilbesterol. Am J Obstet Gynecol 1980; 137:299–311.

47. Malini S, Valdes C, Malinaki LR. Sonographic diagnosis and classification of anomalies of the female genital tract. J Ultrasound Med 1984; 3:397–404.

48. Doyle MB. Magnetic resonance imaging in müllerian fusion defects. J Reprod Med 1992; 37:33–38.

49. Fayez JA. Comparison between abdominal and hysteroscopic metroplasty. Obstet Gynecol 1986; 68:399–432.

50. Harris EN. Syndrome of the black swan. Br J Rheumatol 1986; 26:324–343.

51. Alarcon-Segovia D, Deleze M, Oria C, et al. Antiphospholipid antibodies and the antiphospholipid syndrome in systemic lupus erythematosus. A prospective study of 500 consecutive cases. Medicine 1989; 68:353–365.

52. Hughes GRV. The Prosser White oration: connective tissue disease and the skin 1983. Clin Exp Dermatol 1984; 9:535–544.

53. Chartash EK, Lans DM, Paget SA, et al. Aortic insufficiency and mitral regurgitation in patients with systemic lupus erythematosus and the antiphospholipid syndrome. Am J Med 1989; 86:407–419.

54. Harris EN. The second international anti-cardiolipin standardization workshop/The Kingston anti-phospholipid antibody study (KAPS) group. Am J Clin Pathol 1990; 4:476–489.

55. Chamley LW, Pattison NS, McKay EJ. Separation of lupus anticoagulant from anticardiolipin antibodies by ion-exchange and gel filtration chromatography. Haemostasis 1991; 21:25–32.

56. Exner T, Sahan N, Trudinger B. Separation of anticardiolipin antibodies from lupus anticoagulant on a phospholipid-coated polystyrene column. Biochem Biophys Res Commun 1988; 155:1001–1007.

57. Beaumont JL. Syndrome hemorrhagique acquis du a un anticoagulant circulant. Sangre 1954; 25:1–16.

58. Laurell AB, Nilsson IM. Hypergamma-globulinemia, circulating anticoagulant, and biologic false positive Wassermann reaction: a study of two cases. J Lab Clin Med 1957; 49:694–703.

59. Nilsson IM, Astedt B, Hedner U, et al. Intrauterine death and circulating anticoagulant, "antithromboplastin." Acta Med Scand 1975; 197:153–172.

60. Kochenour NK, Branch DW, Hershgold E, et al. The lupus anticoagulant—a recently discovered and treatable cause of recurrent abortion and fetal death (abstr.). Proceedings of the 31st Annual Meeting of the Society of Gynecologic Investigation, San Francisco, 1984:11.

61. Branch DW, Scott JR. Clinical implication of anti-phospholipid antibodies: the Utah experience. In: Harris EN, Exner T, Hughes GRV, Asherson RA, editors. Phospholipid-Binding Antibodies. Boca Raton, FL: CRC Press, 1991:335–341.

62. Harris EN, Spinnato JA. Should anticardiolipin tests be performed in otherwise healthy pregnant women? Am J Obstet Gynecol 1991; 165:1272–1277.

63. Branch DW, Hales K, Rote NS, et al. Incidence of antiphospholipid antibodies in pregnancy (abstr.). Am J Reprod Immunol 1987; 14:1.

64. Lockwood CJ, Romero R, Feinburg RF, et al. The prevalence and biologic significance of lupus anticoagulant and anticardiolipin antibodies in a general obstetric population. Am J Obstet Gynecol 1989; 161:369–383.

65. Pattison NS, Chamley LW, McKay EJ. Prevalence of antiphospholipid antibodies in a normal pregnant population (abstr.). Clin Exp Rheumatol 1988; 6:210.

66. Barbui T, Cortelazzo S, Galli M, et al. Antiphospholipid antibodies in early repeated abortions: a case-controlled study. Fertil Steril 1988; 50:589–603.

67. Out HJ, Bruinse HW, Christiaens GCML, et al. Prevalence of antiphospholipid antibodies in patients with fetal loss. Ann Rheum Dis 1991; 50:553–564.

68. Parke AL, Wilson D, Maier D. The prevalence of antiphospholipid antibodies in women with recurrent spontaneous abortion, women with successful pregnancies, and women who have never been pregnant. Arthritis Rheum 1991; 34:1231–1246.

69. Parazzini F, Acaia B, Faden D, et al. Antiphospholipid antibodies and recurrent abortion. Obstet Gynecol 1991; 77:854–858.

70. Petri M, Golbus M, Anderson R, et al. Antinuclear antibody, lupus anticoagulant, and anticardiolipin antibody in women with idiopathic habitual abortion. A controlled, prospective study of 44 women. Arthritis Rheum 1987; 30:601–623.

71. Creagh MD, Malia RG, Cooper SM, et al. Screening for lupus anticoagulant and anticardiolipin antibodies in women with fetal loss. J Clin Pathol 1991; 44:45–47.

72. Haddow JE, Rote NS, Dostal-Johnson D, et al. Lack of an association between late fetal death and antiphospholipid antibody measurements in the second trimester. Am J Obstet Gynecol 1991; 165:1308–1313.

73. Infante-Rivard C, David M, Gauthier R, Rivard G-E. Lupus anticoagulants, anticardiolipin antibodies, and fetal loss: a case-controlled study. N Engl J Med 1991; 325:1063–1078.

74. Branch DW, Scott JR, Kochenour NK, et al. Obstetric complications associated with lupus anticoagulant. N Engl J Med 1985; 313:1322–1326.

75. Lubbe WF, Palmer SJ, Butler WS, et al. Fetal survival after prednisone suppression of maternal lupus anticoagulant. Lancet 1983; 1: 1361–1363.

76. Branch DW, Silver RM, Dudley DJ, Scott JR. Antiphospholipid syndrome: outcome of treated pregnancies: an update of the Utah experience (abstr.). Am J Obstet Gynecol 1992; 166:279.

77. Cowchock FS, Reece EA, Balaban D, et al. Repeated fetal losses associated with antiphospholipid antibodies: a collaborative randomized trial comparing prednisone to low-dose heparin treatment. Am J Obstet Gynecol 1992; 166:1318–1323.

78. Gatenby PA, Cameron K, Shearman RP. Pregnancy loss with phospholipid antibodies: improved outcome with aspirin containing treatment. Aust NZ Obstet Gynecol 1989; 29:294–342.

79. Lockshin MD, Druzin ML, Qamar T. Prednisone does not prevent recurrent pregnancy fetal death in women with antiphospholipid antibody. Am J Obstet Gynecol 1989; 160:439–443.

80. Lubbe WF, Liggins GC. Role of lupus anticoagulant and autoimmunity in recurrent pregnancy loss. Semin Reprod Endocrinol 1988; 6:181–190.

81. Ordi J, Barquinero J, Vilardelli, et al. Fetal loss treatment in patients with antiphospholipid antibodies. Ann Rheum Dis 1989; 48:798–802.

82. Reece EA, Gabrielli S, Cullen MT, et al. Recurrent adverse pregnancy outcome and antiphospholipid antibodies. Am J Obstet Gynecol 1990; 163:162.

83. Rosove MH, Tabsh K, Wasserstrum N, et al. Heparin therapy for pregnant women with lupus anticoagulant or anticardiolipin antibodies. Obstet Gynecol 1990; 75:630–634.

84. Beaufils M, Uzan S, Donsimoni R, et al. Prevention of pre-eclampsia by early antiplatelet therapy. Lancet 1985; 1:840–852.

85. Wallenburg HCS, Dekker GA, Makovitz JW, et al. Low-dose aspirin prevents pregnancy-induced hypertension and pre-eclampsia in angiotensin-sensitive primigravidae. Lancet 1986; 1:1–15.

86. Trudinger BH, Stewart GJ, Cook CM, et al. Monitoring lupus anticoagulant-positive pregnancies with umbilical artery flow velocity waveforms. Obstet Gynecol 1988; 72:215–234.

87. Clauvel JP, Tchobroutsky C, Danon F, et al. Spontaneous recurrent fetal wastage and autoimmune abnormalities: a study of 14 cases. Clin Immunol Immunopathol 1986; 39:523–542.

88. Edelman PH, Rouquette AM, Verdy E, et al. Autoimmunity, fetal losses, lupus anticoagulant: beginning of systemic lupus erythematosus or new autoimmune entity with gynaeco-obstetrical expression? Hum Reprod 1986; 1:295–297.

89. Cowchock FS, DeHoratius RJ, Wapner RJ, Jackson LG. Subclinical autoimmune disease and unexplained abortion. Am J Obstet Gynecol 1984; 152:367–371.

90. Cowchock FS, Smith JB, Gocial B. Antibodies to phospholipids and nuclear antigens in patients with repeated abortions. Am J Obstet Gynecol 1986; 155:1002–1015.

91. Maier DB, Parke A. Subclinical autoimmunity in recurrent aborters. Fertil Steril 1989; 51:280–293.

92. Harger JH, Rabin BS, Marchese SG. The prognostic value of antinuclear antibodies in women with recurrent pregnancy losses: a prospective controlled study. Obstet Gynecol 1989; 73:419–428.

93. Lockshin MD, Harpel PC, Druzin ML, et al. Lupus pregnancy: II. Unusual pattern of hypocomplementemia and thrombocytopenia in the pregnant patient. Arthritis Rheum 1985; 28:58–72.

94. Gleicher N, El-Roeiy A, Confino E, Friberg J. Reproductive failure because of autoantibodies: unexplained infertility and pregnancy wastage. Am J Obstet Gynecol 1989; 160:1376–1380.

95. Branch DW. Critique of Gleicher N, El-Roeiy A, Confino E, Friberg J: Reproductive failure because of autoantibodies: unexplained infertility and pregnancy wastage. Am J Obstet Gynecol 1989; 160:1381–1382.

96. Patton PE, Coulam CB, Bergstralh E. The prevalence of autoantibodies in pregnant and nonpregnant women. Am J Obstet Gynecol 1987; 157:1345–1350.

97. Stagnaro-Green A, Roman SH, Cobin RH, et al. Detection of at-risk pregnancy by means of highly sensitive assays for thyroid antibodies. JAMA 1990; 264:1422–1425.

98. Harter CA, Benirschke K. Fetal syphilis in the first trimester. Am J Obstet Gynecol 1976; 124:705–720.

99. MacDonald AB, Benach JL, Burgdorfer W. Gestational Lyme disease. Rheum Dis Clin North Am 1989; 15:657–670.

100. Quinn PA, Petric M, Barkin M, et al. Prevalence of antibody to *Chlamydia trachomatis* in spontaneous abortion and infertility. Am J Obstet Gynecol 1987; 156:291–296.

101. Harrison HR, Alexander ER, Weinstein L, et al. Cervical *Chlamydia trachomatis* and mycoplasmal infections in pregnancy. JAMA 1983; 250:1721–1737.

102. Martin DH, Koutsky L, Eschenbach DA, et al. Prematurity and perinatal mortality in pregnancies complicated by maternal *Chlamydia trachomatis* infections. JAMA 1982; 247:1585–1590.

103. Gray ML. Genital listeriosis as a cause of repeated abortion. Lancet 1960; 2:315–325.

104. Toaff R, Krochik N, Rabinovitz M. Genital listeriosis in the male. Lancet 1962; 2:482–493.

105. Charles D, Larsen B. Infectious agents as a cause of spontaneous abortion. In: Bennett MJ, Edmonds DK, editors. Spontaneous and Recurrent Abortion. Oxford: Blackwell Scientific Publications, 1987:149–167.

106. Pezeshkian R, Fernando N, Carne CA, Simanowitz MD. Listeriosis in mother and fetus during the first trimester of pregnancy. Case report. Br J Obstet Gynaecol 1984; 91:85–102.

107. Rappaport F, Rabinovitz M, Toaff R, Krochik N. Genital listeriosis as a cause of repeated abortion. Lancet 1960; 2:1273–1284.

108. Lawler FE, Wood WS, King S, et al. *Listeria monocytogenes* as a cause of fetal loss. Am J Obstet Gynecol 1964; 89:915–923.

109. MacNaughton MC. *Listeria monocytogenes* in abortion. Lancet 1962; 2:484.

110. Rabau E, David A. *Listeria monocytogenes* in abortion. Lancet 1963; 1:228.

111. Ruffolo EH, Wilson RB, Weed LA. *Listeria monocytogenes* as a cause of pregnancy wastage. Obstet Gynecol 1962; 19:533–536.

112. Knudsin RB, Driscoll SG. Mycoplasmas and human reproductive failure. Surg Gynecol Obstet 1970; 131:89–92.

113. Knudsin RB, Driscoll SG. Strain of *Mycoplasma* associated with human reproductive failure. Science 1967; 157:1573–1593.

114. Harwick HJ, Uppa JP, Purcell RH, et al. *Mycoplasma hominis* septicemia associated with abortion. Am J Obstet Gynecol 1967; 99:725–727.

115. Sompolinsky D, Solomon F, Elkina L, et al. Infections with mycoplasma and bacteria in induced midtrimester abortion and fetal loss. Am J Obstet Gynecol 1975; 121:610–623.

116. Stray-Pedersen B, Eng J, Reikvam TM. Uterine T-mycoplasma colonization in reproductive failure. Am J Obstet Gynecol 1978; 130:307–332.

117. Munday PE, Porter R, Falder PF, et al. Spontaneous abortion—an infectious aetiology? Br J Obstet Gynaecol 1984; 91:1177–1180.

118. Quinn PA, Shwechuk AB, Shuber J, et al. Efficacy of antibiotic therapy in preventing spontaneous pregnancy loss among couples colonized with genital mycoplasmas. Am J Obstet Gynecol 1983; 145:239–251.

119. Foulon W, Naessens A, Mahler T, et al. Prenatal diagnosis of congenital toxoplasmosis. Obstet Gynecol 1990; 76:769–789.

120. Fortier B, Aissi E, Ajana F, et al. Spontaneous abortion and reinfection by *Toxoplasma gondii*. Lancet 1991; 338:444–459.

121. Kimball AC, Kean BH, Fuchs F. The role of toxoplasmosis in abortion. Am J Obstet Gynecol 1971; 111:219–231.

122. Southern PM. Habitual abortion and toxoplasmosis. Is there a relationship? Obstet Gynecol 1972; 39:45–63.

123. Stray-Pedersen B, Lorentzen-Stry A. Uterine Toxoplasma infections and repeated abortions. Am J Obstet Gynecol 1977; 128:716–721.

124. Bujko M, Sulovic M, Zivanovic V, et al. Herpes simplex virus infection

in women with previous spontaneous abortion. J Perinat Med 1988; 16:193–196.

125. Robb JA, Benirschke K, Barmeyer R. Intrauterine latent herpes simplex virus infection. I. Spontaneous abortion. Hum Pathol 1986; 17:1196–1203.

126. Pernoll ML. Abortion induced by chemicals encountered in the environment. Clin Obstet Gynecol 1986; 29:953–958.

127. Wheeler JM, Johnston BM, Malinak LR. The relationship of endometriosis to spontaneous abortion. Fertil Steril 1983; 39:656–670.

128. Rock JA, Shirey RS, Braine HG, et al. Plasmapheresis for the treatment of repeated early pregnancy wastage associated with anti-P. Obstet Gynecol 1985; 66(3 Suppl):57S–60S.

129. Wegman TG. Maternal T cells promote placental growth and prevent spontaneous abortion. Immunol Lett 1988; 17:297–302.

130. Clark DA, Chaput A, Tutton D. Active suppression of host-vs-graft reaction in pregnant mice: VII. Spontaneous abortion of allogeneic CBA/J × DBA/2 fetuses in the uterus of CBA/J mice correlates with deficient non-T suppressor cell activity. J Immunol 1986; 136:1668–1675.

131. Toder V, Strassburger D, Irlin Y, et al. Nonspecific immunopotentiators and pregnancy loss: complete Freund adjuvant reverses high fetal resorption rate in CBA × DBA12 mouse combination. Am J Reprod Immunol 1990; 24:63–66.

132. Daya S, Clark DA, Devlin MC, et al. Preliminary characterization of two types of suppressor cells in the human uterus. Fertil Steril 1985; 44:778–785.

133. Hill JA, Anderson DH. Immunological mechanisms of female infertility. Bailliere's Clin Immunol Allergy 1988; 2:551–574.

134. Redman CWG, Ferry BL, Jackson MC, et al. Immune cell populations in the human early pregnancy decidua. In: Wegman TG, Gill TJ, Nisbet-Brown E, editor. Molecular and Cellular Immunobiology of the Maternal Fetal Interface. New York: Oxford University Press, 1991:110–128.

135. Daya S, Rosenthal KL, Clark DA. Immunosuppressor factor(s) produced by decidua-associated suppressor cells: A proposed mechanism for fetal allograft survival. Am J Obstet Gynecol 1987; 56:344–350.

136. Feinman MA, Kliman HJ, Main EK. HLA antigen expression and induction by interferon in cultured human trophoblasts. Am J Obstet Gynecol 1987; 157:1429–1434.

137. Chaouat G, Menu E, Clark DA, et al. Control of fetal survival in CBA × DBA/2 mice by lymphokine therapy. J Reprod Fertil 1990; 89:447–458.

138. Berkowitz RS, Hill JA, Kurtz CB, et al. Effects of products of activated leukocytes (lymphokines and monokines) on the growth of malignant trophoblast cells in vitro. Am J Obstet Gynecol 1988; 158:199–203.

139. Park MI, Edwin SS, Scott JR, Branch DW. Interpretation of blocking activity in maternal serum depends on the equation used for calculation of mixed lymphocyte culture results. Clin Exp Immunol 1990; 82:363–368.

140. Rocklin RE, Kitzmiller JL, Carpenter CG, et al. Maternal-fetal relation: absence of an immunologic blocking factor from the serum of women with chronic abortions. N Engl J Med 1976; 295:1209–1213.

141. Stimson WH, Strachman AF, Shepherd A. Studies on the maternal immune response to placental antigens: absence of a blocking factor from the blood of abortion-prone women. Br J Obstet Gynaecol 1979; 86:41–46.

142. Szekeres-Bartho J, Chaouat G. Lymphocyte-derived progesterone-in-duced blocking factor corrects resorption in a murine abortion system. Am J Reprod Immunol 1990; 23:26–28.

143. Scott JR, Rote NS, Branch DW. Immunologic aspects of spontaneous abortion and fetal death. Obstet Gynecol 1987; 70:645–656.

144. Abir R, Zusman I, Ben Hur H, et al. The effects of serum from women with miscarriages on the in vitro development of mouse pre-implantation embryos. Acta Obstet Gynecol Scand 1990; 69:27–33.

145. Alexander SA, Latinne D, Debruyere M, et al. Belgian experience with repeat immunization in recurrent spontaneous abortions. In : Beard RW, Sharp W, editors. Early Pregnancy Loss. London: Springer-Verlag, 1988:355–365.

146. Beer AE. Pregnancy outcome in couples with recurrent abortions following immunologic evaluation and therapy. In: Beard RW, Sharp F, editors. Early Pregnancy Loss. London: Springer-Verlag, 1988:337–349.

147. Carp HJA, Toder V, Gazit E, et al. Immunization by paternal leukocytes for prevention of primary habitual abortion: results of a matched controlled trial. Gynecol Obstet Invest 1990; 29:16–21.

148. Johnson PM, Chia KV, Griffith HB, et al. Trophoblast membrane infusion for unexplained recurrent miscarriage. Br J Obstet Gynaecol 1988; 95:342–347.

149. McIntyre JA, Faulk WP, Nichols-Johnson VR, et al. Immunologic testing and immunotherapy in recurrent spontaneous abortion. Obstet Gynecol 1986; 67:169–174.

150. Mowbray JF, Underwood JL, Michel M, et al. Immunization with paternal lymphocytes in women with recurrent miscarriage. Lancet 1987; 2:679–680.

151. Mueller-Echardt G, Heine O, Polten B. IVIG to prevent recurrent spontaneous abortion. Lancet 1991; 337:728–730.

152. Peters AJ, Coulam CB. Pregnancy outcome after the use of intravenous immunoglobulin for the treatment of recurrent spontaneous abortion (abstr.). Fertil Steril Program Suppl 1990; 821.

153. Reznikoff-Etievant MF, Durieux I, Huchet J, et al. Human MHC antigens and paternal leucocyte injection in recurrent spontaneous abortions. In: Beard RW, Sharp F, editors. Early Pregnancy Loss. London: Springer-Verlag, 1988:375–384.

154. Smith JB, Cowchock S. Immunologic studies in recurrent spontaneous abortion: effects of immunization of women with paternal mononuclear cells on lymphocytotoxic and mixed lymphocyte reaction blocking antibodies and correlation with sharing of HLA and pregnancy outcome. J Reprod Immunol 1988; 14:99–113.

155. Takakuwa K, Goto S, Hasegawa I, et al. Result of immunotherapy on patients with unexplained recurrent abortion: a beneficial treatment for patients with negative blocking antibodies. Am J Reprod Immunol 1990; 23:37–41.

156. Unander AM, Linholm A. Transfusions of leukocyte-rich erythrocyte concentrates: a successful treatment in selected cases of habitual abortion. Am J Obstet Gynecol 1986; 154:516–520.

157. Cauchi MN, Lim D, Young DE, et al. Immunotherapy for recurrent spontaneous abortions. Am J Reprod Immunol 1991; 25:16–17.

158. Ho HG, Gill TH, Hsieh HH, et al. Immunotherapy for recurrent spontaneous abortions. Am J Reprod Immunol 1991; 25:10–15.

159. Mowbray JF, Gibbings C, Liddel H, et al. Controlled trial of treatment of recurrent spontaneous abortion by immunization with paternal cells. Lancet 1985; 2:941–943.

160. Stray-Pederson B, Stray-Pederson S. Etiologic factors and subsequent reproductive performance in 195 couples with a prior history of habitual abortion. Am J Obstet Gynecol 1984; 148:140–146.

CHAPTER 20

Unexplained Infertility*

JOHN A. COLLINS

When the diagnostic test results of an infertility evaluation are normal for both partners, the delay in conception cannot be explained. Delayed conception in apparently normal couples with infertility can occur for a variety of reasons. First, some couples are truly normal, but their conception has been randomly delayed, because successful human conception occurs in only one out of five or six ovulatory cycles with coital exposure. Other apparently normal infertile couples are truly subfertile, either because of advancing age in the female partner or because of the presence of latent, undetectable defects in the process leading to conception. Finally, the unexplained infertility category includes couples with true sterility, in whom the latent defect is unremediable. The existence of such defects provides evidence of the need for research in fertilization and implantation in the human.

The clinical management of unexplained infertility calls on a range of clinical problem-solving skills and often requires the application of advanced reproductive technology. There is a dilemma, however, in that treatment-independent pregnancy occurs frequently in this category of infertile couples and therefore it is as important to understand the natural course of unexplained infertility as it is to know the effect of treatment. Attaining a desirable outcome is the challenge of unexplained infertility.

The discussion that follows is based on clinical evidence, and where possible, test results and outcomes are correlated with the outcome of interest in the clinical management of infertility: a normal live birth.

DEFINITION AND DIAGNOSTIC PROTOCOLS

Definition

There is some disagreement about the definition of unexplained infertility. Based on the normal distribution of fe-

cundity, 10% to 14% of normal couples will not have conceived after 1 year of regular exposure.[38] The unsuccessful group includes those who are sterile, as well as those who are subfertile. When the diagnostic assessment of infertility reveals no abnormality, the appropriate diagnosis is unexplained infertility. Thus, it is evident that the definition of unexplained infertility rests on the definition of a complete diagnostic assessment of infertility. There is general agreement about the standard investigations (laboratory assessment of ovulation, evaluation of tubal patency, and semen analysis).[61] The debate centers on whether the results of additional testing correlate with fertility. Even the agreed-on standard investigation, however, is not an in-depth evaluation. For example, no assessment of ovulation available confirms the completion of a normal ovulatory process. Lacking that ideal, mid-luteal progesterone assessment appears to be the most cost-effective compromise. Tubal patency but not tubal function can be evaluated by hysterosalpingography; laparoscopy may exclude the presence of endometriosis or adhesions, but it does not further elucidate tubal function. The semen analysis enumerates normal spermatozoa but does not evaluate their fertilizing capacity. Normal is defined as 20 $\times$ 10^6 spermatozoa per milliliter, with 50% forward motility and 50% normal morphology.[62]

Whether additional investigations contribute to effective diagnosis is controversial. The controversy arises in part because some clinicians regard abnormal test results by themselves as evidence for a cause of the infertility, whereas others insist that the results must be reliable in identifying conditions that can be shown to impair fertility. For example, delays in histologic maturation of the endometrium do exist, and an endometrial cause of infertility would be plausible. In question is whether the delayed endometrial maturation correlates with fertility. That evidence is required to conclude that an abnormal test result from an endometrial biopsy represents an endometrial cause of infertility. The search for such a correlation between fertility and luteal phase defect defined by histologic or hormonal evaluation has not been productive.[20, 60] For similar reasons, it has been concluded that the postcoital test "lacks validity as a test for infertility," and this test is not consistently included in the conventional diagnostic assessment protocol for infertility.[22] Computerized measurements of sperm movement characteristics have so far failed to produce a result that is superior to semen analysis

*Portions of the data collection and analysis presented were funded by the National Health Research and Development Program, National Department of Health and Welfare, Ottawa, Canada (Project No. 6606-2628-44), and by Contract No. 91-R-515 from the Royal Commission on New Reproductive Technology, Ottawa, Canada. The views expressed are those of the author and not necessarily those of the National Department of Health and Welfare or the Royal Commission.

in the prediction of fertility. The penetration of zona-free hamster eggs by human spermatozoa yields an assay with only marginal ability to discriminate between fertile and infertile men.[39, 24] With respect to antisperm antibody, no clear correlations have been demonstrated between fertility and the presence of antibody to sperm in the serum of either male or female partners.[8] In vitro fertilization (IVF) as a diagnostic evaluation offers useful information, but it is not a practical diagnostic test. Furthermore, even among partnerships where there has been a failure of fertilization, the failed fertilization is an inconclusive finding, because successful fertilization frequently occurs in subsequent attempts.

The diagnosis of unexplained infertility is one of exclusion. If a cause of infertility can be identified, then by definition unexplained infertility cannot exist. There is no consensus, however, about which diagnostic tests are needed to rule out a cause of infertility. Such clinical disagreement is normal, given the different views of evidence and the variety of clinical experience. The debate about postcoital testing is a good example of the issues. This debate is not about whether the existence of cervical infertility is a possibility; it concerns whether the postcoital test is an accurate diagnostic test for the detection of any contribution of cervical function to fertility. The uncertainty about postcoital and other diagnostic tests underscores the need for basic and clinical research to improve the diagnostic evaluation of infertility.

Thus, the definition of unexplained infertility can be based on normal findings in a diagnostic assessment that includes a laboratory assessment of ovulation, evaluation of tubal patency, and semen analysis. This definition may not be unanimously accepted, but it is based on published evidence summarizing studies that correlate test results with fertility, which is the criterion standard.

Diagnostic Protocols

For those who practice evidence-based medicine, the value of a given diagnostic test depends on whether the test results correlate with the outcome. The outcome of primary interest for tests of fertility is live birth, and the value of these diagnostic tests lies in their ability to predict this outcome. Nearly all of the available data on infertility outcomes deal with pregnancy rather than live birth, but both expressions of the outcome have a similar relationship to test results. In this pragmatic way, the commonly used diagnostic tests for infertility can be sorted into the following three categories:

1. Test results have an established correlation with pregnancy: semen analysis, tubal patency testing by hysterosalpingogram or laparoscopy, and mid-luteal plasma progesterone. In each instance, an unequivocal abnormal test result (azoospermia, bilateral occlusion, or anovulation) implies unarguably impaired fertility without therapy.

2. Test results are inconsistently correlated with pregnancy: zona-free hamster penetration test, postcoital test, cervical mucus penetration test, hysteroscopy, and antisperm antibody assays. For these tests, abnormal results frequently are associated with subsequent fertility without therapy.

3. Test results do not appear to be correlated with pregnancy: endometrial dating, varicocele assessment, *Chlamydia* testing, falloposcopy, and salpingostomy. For these tests, data

exist that confirm the lack of correlation with pregnancy, or such followup studies do not exist.

Among 20 studies reporting on the outcome of unexplained infertility, virtually all required semen analysis, a laboratory assessment of ovulation, and tubal patency testing by laparoscopy or hysterosalpingogram. Postcoital testing also was required in most studies, but sperm antibody tests were a prerequisite for the diagnosis in only 1 of 20 studies.[52]

PREVALENCE OF UNEXPLAINED INFERTILITY

A true estimate of the prevalence of unexplained infertility in the population is impossible. It is possible, however, to estimate the unexplained proportion of infertile couples included in various studies. Twenty-one studies from 1950 to 1991 included 14,141 couples, of whom 2,425 (17.2%) had unexplained infertility (Fig. 20–1).[2, 6, 10, 12, 16, 18, 23, 25, 30, 32, 33, 35, 44–46, 49, 51, 54, 57, 58, 61] The proportion with unexplained infertility in the individual studies ranged from 0 to 26%. The variability in the reported percentages may be attributed to the characteristics of the patient group in each reporting infertility clinic, but it may also arise from the definition of unexplained infertility applied by the authors of each report. For example, if for one author the presence of an abnormal postcoital test would constitute a diagnosis of cervical infertility, the proportion with unexplained infertility in that study would be lower.

Different diagnostic protocols, however, do not entirely explain the variability in the proportion of couples with unexplained infertility. In a recent study from 11 Canadian infertility clinics, all of which used a uniform protocol, the proportion with unexplained infertility ranged from 8% to 37% (in all 562 of 2198 couples [26%]).[58] These differences in the likelihood of unexplained infertility were evaluated by means of logistic regression. This analysis took into account the clinical and demographic characteristics that were associated with a diagnosis of unexplained infertility compared with any other infertility diagnosis (Table 20–1). Age of the female partner was the only significant predictor that the diagnosis would be unexplained infertility rather than another specific infertility diagnosis. The duration of infertility, the male partner's age, the pregnancy history in the partnership, and coital frequency were not associated. Various estimates of socioeconomic status (occupation and family in-

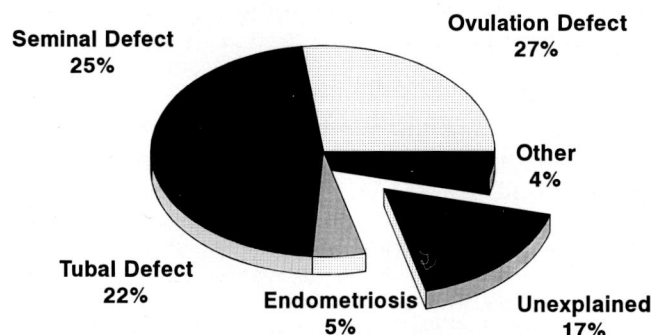

FIGURE 20–1. Primary clinical diagnoses among 14,141 cases in 21 published reports.[2, 6, 10, 12, 16, 18, 23, 25, 30, 32, 33, 35, 44–46, 49, 51, 54, 57, 58, 61]

TABLE 20–1. Predictors of Unexplained Infertility		
Variables	**Adjusted Odds Ratio (95% confidence interval)**	**P Value***
Female partner aged >30 years	1.56 (1.31, 1.92)	0.0001
Secondary infertility		0.41
Duration of infertility		0.25
Male partner's age		0.98
Coital frequency		0.33
Male professional		0.25
Female professional		0.98

*P value to enter or remove the term (logistic regression model). Data from Vutyavanich T, Collins JA. An overview of the Canadian Infertility Therapy Evaluation Study. J Soc Obstet Gynecol Can 1991;13:29–34.

come) also were not predictors of unexplained infertility. In univariate analysis, there was a small excess of professional women in the unexplained category, but this was due entirely to the correlation between professional occupations and older age. For a couple with a female infertile partner older than 30 years of age, the likelihood of being in the unexplained category was 1.56 (95% confidence interval [CI] 1.31, 1.92). Women who have no reason for their infertility other than age would usually present among the couples with unexplained infertility; therefore, the excess of older women in this category logically follows.

In summary, about one in five infertile couples have unexplained infertility, but the proportion is variable for reasons that cannot be accurately defined. When the likelihood of such a diagnosis is evaluated among individual couples, however, female age is the most important of the known factors. Thus, when published studies are compared, differences in female age contribute in a major way to differences in the proportion of reported couples with unexplained infertility.

POSSIBLE REASONS FOR UNEXPLAINED INFERTILITY

It is not known whether the decrease in fecundity with advancing female age is attributable to impaired follicular development, fertilization, or implantation. It is possible that the effect of age impacts on a broad range of prerequisites to conception. Setting aside the contribution from female age, unexplained infertility may arise from chance delays in conception, or it may be the result of undetectable defects in reproduction.

On theoretical grounds, it seems reasonable to consider that couples with normal but lower than average fecundity would form a large proportion of those with unexplained infertility. The logic goes as follows. First, any infertility diagnostic test would be likely to be normal among such couples, unless falsely abnormal results occurred. Second, couples in the lower range of normal fertility form a higher proportion of the population than subfertile and sterile couples. Third, such truly normal couples should have a better prognosis than those with evidence of infertility pathology such as tubal disease.

On this last point, the hypothesis that unexplained infertility represents delayed conceptions among couples with normal but below average fecundity can be tested. If chance delays in conception lead to a high proportion of the unexplained infertility, this favorable diagnosis should be associated with a shorter duration of infertility when compared with other infertility diagnostic groups. In contrast, however, the duration of infertility is distributed similarly among groups with unexplained infertility and other infertility diagnoses.[11] Therefore, the category of unexplained infertility probably includes a substantial proportion of couples who have defects in one or more of the processes of gamete preparation, fertilization, and implantation. These defects, although severe in some instances, are undetectable with currently available diagnostic tests.

Given the present highly developed state of reproductive technology, it may be surprising that the diagnostic assessment of infertility is so insensitive. With respect to the male partner, however, no combination of diagnostic tests can provide a complete profile of sperm fertilizing ability. Semen analysis estimates the number of normal motile spermatozoa, but normal, motile spermatozoa are not necessarily capable of fertilization. Measures of the ability to penetrate cervical mucus are being developed, but the predictive value of this assessment with respect to fertility has not been established.[22] No clinical tests are available to evaluate capacitation or the ability of sperm to negotiate the uterotubal junction. Various tests have been developed to evaluate the acrosomal reaction and the ability of sperm to bind to and penetrate through zona pellucida, but none of these is both reliable and practical. The interaction between the sperm membrane and the oocyte plasma membrane can be assessed only in part by means of the zona-free hamster oocyte test, and even the IVF of oocytes is an imperfect as well as expensive test of sperm fertilizing capacity.

Similar limitations affect the diagnostic assessment of the female partner, so there is the potential for the existence of undetectable defects in follicular development, ovulation, fertilization, and the prerequisites for recognition and maintenance of early pregnancy. Diagnostic tests for ovulation are unable to confirm that the ovulatory process is complete. The occurrence of ovulation can be assumed only when there is evidence of progesterone secretion during the luteal phase. Even the disappearance of one or more follicles on sonographic evaluation does not ensure that an ovum has been released. With respect to tubal function, tests of tubal patency do not assess the characteristics of bidirectional tubal motility that may be required for the transport of capacitated sperm to the site of fertilization and the subsequent movement of the fertilized embryo toward the uterus. The additional visual information from salpingostomy and falloposcopy has yet to be evaluated as an assessment of tubal function. Measures of luteal adequacy that might predict implantation success are evolving, but no current evaluation of luteal function reveals how numerous peptide and other factors contribute to the vascular, biochemical, and immunologic preparation of the endometrium for the successful implantation of a developing embryo. Briefly, the male and female prerequisites for successful conception are numerous, and many remain inaccessible even after the most comprehensive diagnostic assessment.

There are, then, several possible reasons for unexplained infertility. First, a minority of couples with unexplained infertility are truly normal, with normal but below average fecundity. Second, a higher proportion of couples have im-

Authors

Barnea et al, 1985..
Collins, 1989..
Daly, 1989..
Fisch et al, 1977..
Hull et al, 1985..

Iffland et al, 1989..
Kliger, 1984..
Lenton et al, 1977..
Rousseau et al, 1983..
Sorensen, 1980..

Templeton, 1982..
Trimbos-Kemper, 1984..
Van Dijk et al, 1979..
Welner et al, 1988..
Wright et al, 1979..

0   10   20   30   40

Mean Female Partner's Age (Years)

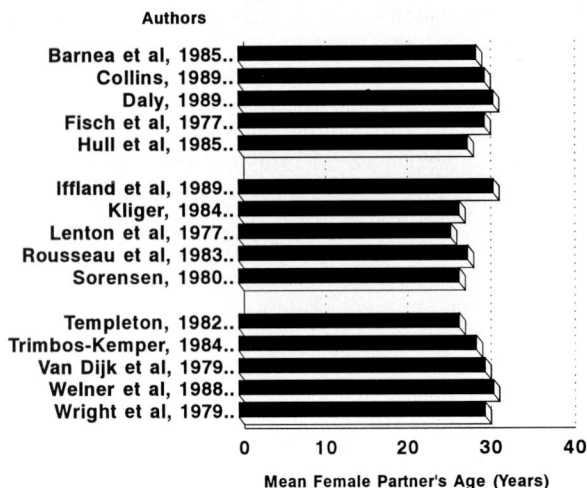

FIGURE 20–2. Mean female partner's age in published reports on unexplained infertility.

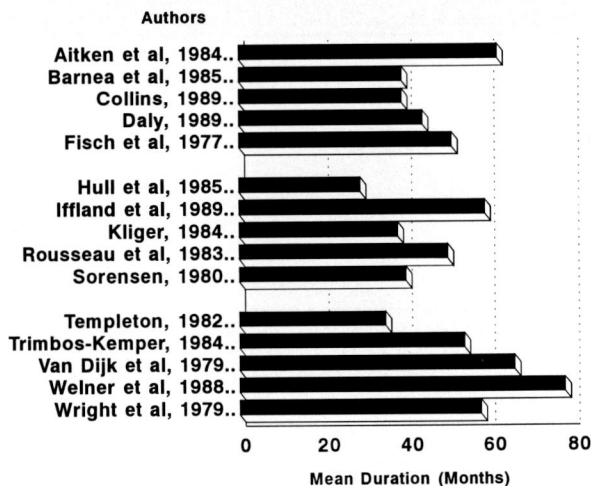

Authors

Aitken et al, 1984..
Barnea et al, 1985..
Collins, 1989..
Daly, 1989..
Fisch et al, 1977..

Hull et al, 1985..
Iffland et al, 1989..
Kliger, 1984..
Rousseau et al, 1983..
Sorensen, 1980..

Templeton, 1982..
Trimbos-Kemper, 1984..
Van Dijk et al, 1979..
Welner et al, 1988..
Wright et al, 1979..

0   20   40   60   80

Mean Duration (Months)

FIGURE 20–3. Mean duration of infertility in published reports on unexplained infertility.

paired fecundity related to female age beyond 30 years. Third, most couples with unexplained infertility may have a variety of undetectable disorders in reproductive processes. Given that some couples with unexplained infertility remain sterile, some of the undetectable biologic defects must be extremely severe indeed.

CLINICAL CHARACTERISTICS OF REPORTED GROUPS

As discussed in the section on prevalence, the age of the female partner is significantly older among groups with unexplained infertility, but other prognostic characteristics for infertility are distributed similarly in this diagnostic category and in groups with a specific infertility diagnosis. In the group of followup studies that have been assembled for the next section on the long-term untreated prognosis, the mean female age ranged from 26 to 31 years, and the weighted aggregate was 29 years (Fig. 20–2). The mean duration of infertility ranged from 20 to 78 months, and the weighted aggregate was 40 months (Fig. 20–3). In some of the studies assembled for this review, the basis for selection was primary infertility.[17, 31, 63] In the remainder of the studies, the proportion with primary infertility ranged from 39% to 90%, and the weighted mean proportion was 66% (Fig. 20–4). Thus, about one third of reported couples with unexplained infertility have secondary infertility. If a couple has previously been able to conceive, then at some time all of the necessary prerequisites for conception were functional. Unexplained infertility in such a couple is especially enigmatic. In the Canadian data, secondary infertility was defined as infertility occurring after the prior occurrence of a pregnancy in the same partnership, and 25% of the couples were in this category.[7] With respect to socioeconomic status, couples with unexplained infertility do not differ from those with specific causes of infertility.[50]

Correlation with Pregnancy

The duration of infertility was a significant prognostic factor in numerous studies of unexplained infertility.[7, 30, 35, 37, 47, 49]

The relationship between duration of infertility and pregnancy rate is shown in Figure 20–5. The pregnancy rate appears to be approximately 2% lower per additional month, or one fourth lower for each additional year of infertility.[7]

Age of the female partner also is an important contributor to the prognosis with unexplained infertility. In one study, pregnancy rates were reduced by one third when the female partner was 35 years of age or older.[30] In another study, the independent influence of the female partner's age was significant only in the couples where the duration of infertility exceeded 3 years.[11] Among such couples, the mean age of the female partner at registration was 31 years, and the cumulative pregnancy rate after 24 months was 28%. The effect of older age reduced the probability of conception by a factor of 0.9, or about one tenth of the expected pregnancy rate for every additional year of female partner's age beyond 31 years. No study has revealed an independent association between the age of the male partners and the pregnancy rate among couples with unexplained infertility.

Secondary infertility also is associated with a better prog-

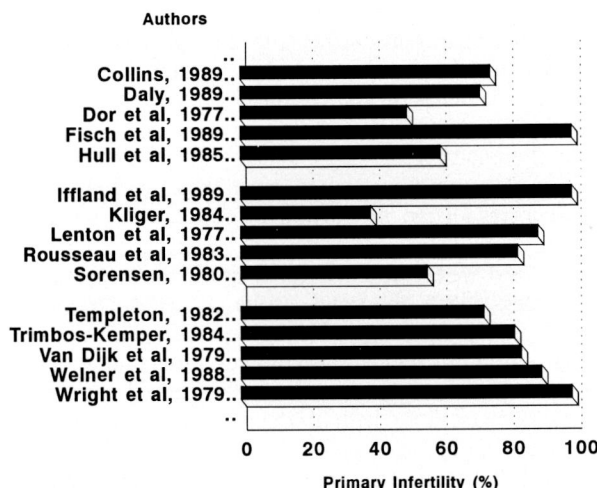

Authors

Collins, 1989..
Daly, 1989..
Dor et al, 1977..
Fisch et al, 1989..
Hull et al, 1985..

Iffland et al, 1989..
Kliger, 1984..
Lenton et al, 1977..
Rousseau et al, 1983..
Sorensen, 1980..

Templeton, 1982..
Trimbos-Kemper, 1984..
Van Dijk et al, 1979..
Welner et al, 1988..
Wright et al, 1979..

0   20   40   60   80   100

Primary Infertility (%)

FIGURE 20–4. Proportion of couples with primary infertility in published reports on unexplained infertility.

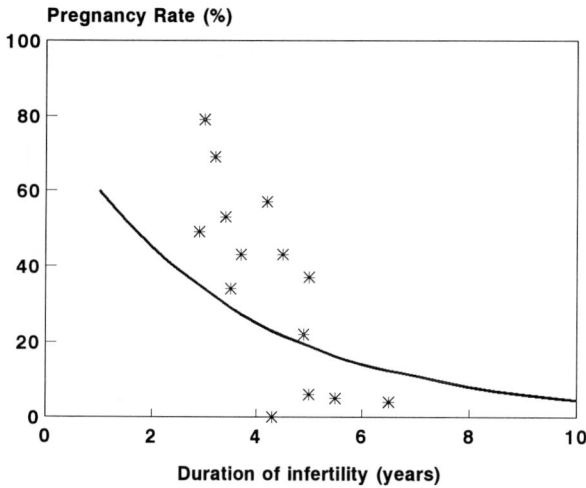

FIGURE 20–5. Duration of infertility and pregnancy rate in published reports on unexplained infertility. Mean duration of infertility and pregnancy rate, citations as in Figure 20–3; *, regression curve, Collins, 1989.[7]

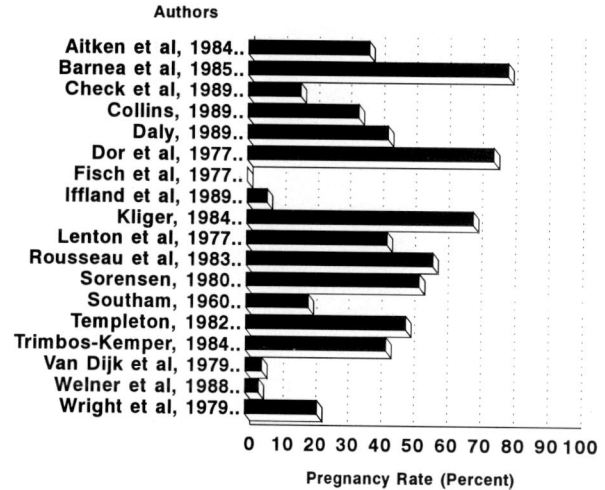

FIGURE 20–6. Pregnancy rate among cases reported in published reports on unexplained infertility.

nosis.[37, 53] When secondary infertility was defined as a previous pregnancy in the present relationship, the pregnancy rate was nearly double the rate with primary infertility.[7]

Higher socioeconomic status has been significantly associated with better fertility in an analysis of all diagnostic groups.[58] This trend also was present among couples with unexplained infertility, but in the smaller group the association with economic status was not significant.

NATURAL COURSE OF UNEXPLAINED INFERTILITY

In the course of the clinical management of infertility, the physician who has made a diagnosis first makes a forecast about the natural course of the diagnosed condition and then estimates the effect of treatment on the predicted outcome. When the diagnosis is unexplained infertility, the long-term prognosis may be quite good, but studies have not formulated the clinical findings into a prediction that could help in making treatment decisions. Much of the information about the untreated prognosis is based on the short-term experience of control subjects taking part in clinical trials.[17, 19] After reviewing published reports, this section on the long-term prognosis for the untreated couple with unexplained infertility focuses first on definitions, then it evaluates those factors that may contribute to the prognosis, and finally, a prediction score is developed that can be used in practice to estimate the prognosis for the individual couple.

Published Reports

Eighteen trials or case series provide information about the simple pregnancy rate among untreated couples with unexplained infertility (Fig. 20–6). The lowest pregnancy rate occurred in a study of 4 months' duration, and the highest in a study of 16 months' duration, so that the duration of followup is an obvious factor that may influence the published pregnancy rate. Other factors, however, include the

mean duration of infertility, the mean age of female partners, and the percentage of patients with primary infertility in each study group. When multiple regression analysis was performed on the data from these studies, the mean duration of infertility was found to account for 73% of the variability in the reported pregnancy rates. The number of months of followup contributed a further 13% of the variability.[52]

Two further studies reported cumulative pregnancy rates. Infertile couples under observation are frequently lost to followup, or they may adopt, and a few couples resolve the infertility issue and withdraw from treatment. Such losses to followup during observation are preferably analyzed by means of life table analysis, yielding cumulative pregnancy rates. In one study the cumulative pregnancy rate was 72% after 24 months, and the mean duration of infertility was 29 months.[30] In another study, 340 couples with a mean duration of infertility of 39 months were followed for as long as 42 months (mean of 22 months); the simple pregnancy rate was 34%, and the cumulative pregnancy rate at 36 months after registration was 46%.[7]

Definitions of Outcome and Untreated Status

The outcome of interest to couples is live birth rather than conception. Pregnancy outcomes among 381 untreated cou-

TABLE 20–2. Pregnancy Outcomes Among 381 Untreated Couples with Unexplained Infertility

Outcome	No. of Couples	Percentage of 123	Percentage of 381
Pregnancy	123		32
Live birth	84	68	22
Abortion	21	17	6
Premature	6	5	2
Perinatal loss	6	5	2
Ectopic	6	5	2

Data from Vutyavanich T, Collins JA. An overview of the Canadian Infertility Therapy Evaluation Study. J Soc Obstet Gynecol Can 1991;13:29–34.

TABLE 20–3. Other Outcomes Among 381 Infertile Couples with Unexplained Infertility

Outcome	No. of Couples	Percentage of 381 Couples
Continued followup	127	33
Lost to followup	94	25
Resolved	29	8
Adopted	8	2

Of 562 couples with unexplained infertility, 181 (32%) received treatment. Data from Vutyavanich T, Collins JA. An overview of the Canadian Infertility Therapy Evaluation Study. J Soc Obstet Gynecol Can 1991;13:29–34.

ples with unexplained infertility are shown in Table 20–2. Other outcomes among these couples included loss to followup, resolution, and adoption (Table 20–3). For the purposes of the development of a prediction score for the long-term prognosis, it seems appropriate to make use of live birth rather than pregnancy, given the relatively high proportion of pregnancy losses.

Untreated status is more difficult to define in nonrandomized studies. Whenever a group of couples has been assembled for observation, decisions about treatment depend on individual clinical circumstances and patient choice. Some couples will have had treatment before their enrollment in the study; others require some investigations before treatment, and still others will have no treatment. Thus, untreated status could be defined in four ways, according to whether either partner received treatment before registration or after registration in a given observational study. Definitions used here were the following:

A—All couples are included, and observations including events such as live birth among couples treated after registration are excluded. The months of observation prior to treatment are included in the life table.

B—As in definition A, but couples who are treated prior to registration are excluded.

C—Excludes couples who receive treatment after registra-

TABLE 20–4. Predictors of the Untreated Probability of Pregnancy Among 562 Couples with Unexplained Infertility

Clinical Characteristics at the Time of Registration	Probability of Pregnancy (95% confidence interval)	P Value
Duration of infertility (yr)	0.74 (0.64, 0.84)	0.009
Secondary infertility	1.7 (1.1, 2.7)	0.006
Female partner's age (yr)	0.91 (0.84, 0.97)	0.015
Male partner's income more than $34,000*	1.7 (1.1, 2.5)	0.01
Coitus twice per week or more	1.6 (1.0, 2.3)	0.072
Male partner <40 years of age	1.0 (0.5, 2.0)	0.98
(Duration of infertility <3 years)†	1.7 (1.1, 2.7)	0.0004
(Female partner's age <30 years)	1.6 (1.1, 2.4)	0.006

*1986 Canadian dollars.

†The duration and female age variables were converted to two groups (above and below average) and evaluated in a separate analysis including pregnancy history, income, coital history, and male age. In each proportional hazards analysis, laparoscopy was a time-dependent variable, and observations were censored at the start of treatment for 181 treated couples. Data from Vutyavanich T, Collins JA. An overview of the Canadian Infertility Therapy Evaluation Study. J Soc Obstet Gynecol Can 1991;13:29–34.

TABLE 20–5. Estimated Area Under the ROC Curve by Definition of Untreated Status

Definition	Area Under the Curve (95% confidence interval)*	
	Training Set	Validation Set
All patients: Definition A	0.56 (0.03)	0.55 (0.03)
Untreated only: Definition C	0.56 (0.04)	0.56 (0.04)

*Predictor score estimated from proportional hazards model (Table 20–4). In Definition A, treated patients are considered not pregnant and censored at the beginning of treatment.

ROC, receiver-operating characteristics.

tion, but this definition includes couples who received treatment before registration.

D—Untreated couples, as in definition C, but couples who were treated before registration also are excluded here, so that under definition D there is no prior history of treatment, and no treatment under observation.

The four different definitions of untreated status were compared to evaluate the effect of selection according to previous treatment and treatment after registration (Fig. 20–7). The lowest cumulative pregnancy rate is associated with the least restrictive definition (Definition A). The exclusion of couples who have received treatment either before or after registration yields untreated cohorts with a superior prognosis, and this superior prognosis may arise from selection factors. Thus, the most conservative and the least problematic estimate of the likelihood of live birth follows from the definition that includes all couples in the denominator and excludes the pregnancies of all treated couples from the numerator.

Prognostic Factors

The potential prognostic factors were entered into proportional hazards analysis to develop a prediction score. To avoid the loss of cases because of missing occupation data, male partner's income was estimated from occupation or postal code, and the upper quartile (>$34,000 in 1986 Canadian dollars) was taken to represent higher social class. The analysis included all couples but excluded any conception among the 181 couples who had treatment (Definition A above). The significant clinical predictors of live birth were duration of infertility, pregnancy history, female partner's age, and male income. In a related analysis, each of the continuous predictor variables was dichotomized to provide an odds ratio (OR), or relative likelihood of pregnancy. Duration of infertility less than 3 years, secondary infertility, female age younger than 30 years, and the upper quartile of male income all were associated with a 60% to 70% better expectation of live birth (Table 20–4).

Evaluating the Prediction Score

To evaluate the prediction score, the proportional hazards analysis was repeated in a randomly selected training sample consisting of one half of the 562 cases. The score that was

Cumulative Live Birth Rate

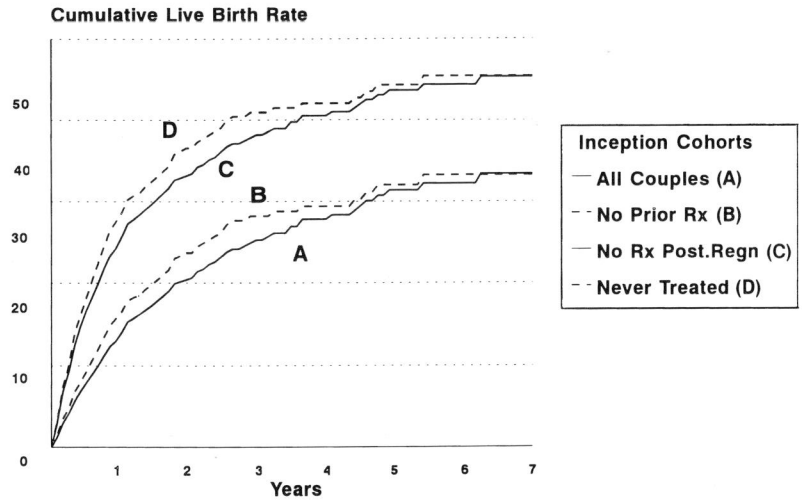

FIGURE 20–7. Cumulative live birth rates for untreated, unexplained infertility. Inception cohorts (A through D) are defined in the text.

derived from the coefficients of this analysis was applied to the remaining cases (the validation sample). Reproducibility of the prediction score was estimated by evaluating the score against the observed outcome in the training and validation groups. The resulting data yield a receiver-operating characteristics curve (ROC), which evaluates the accuracy of the prediction (Fig. 20–8). The prediction score yields an area under the curve equal to 0.56 (95% CI 0.53, 0.59) in the training sample (Table 20–5). Confidence limits for areas under the curves indicate that there is no significant difference in the performance of the score in the training or validation sample. Also, making use of a selected inception cohort (Definition C) did not improve the accuracy of the prediction. A score of 0.50 denotes a prediction with no more value than guessing, whereas a score of 1.0 reflects a perfect prediction score. The similar scores in both training and validation samples indicate that the prediction of the outcome of unexplained infertility is reproducible; also, it is significantly superior to 0.50, but falls far short of ideal. When future research gives rise to new diagnostic tests, the value of such tests can be tested by similar means. If a prediction score that includes the new test results significantly increases the area under the curve, the test results add important information to the prediction score available from clinical data alone.

Using the Prediction Score in Practice

The demands of clinical practice require the best possible estimate of the prognosis without treatment to facilitate treatment decisions. As a starting point, the cumulative rate of conceptions leading to live birth, shown in Figure 20–6 for Definition A, can be estimated with 95% CI at various projected times (Table 20–6). The baseline estimate for 6 months is 13.6% (95% CI 10.5, 16.8). This is the prognosis for the average couple, but this estimate can be tailored according to the characteristics of the couple, using adjustment factors derived from the proportional hazards analysis. For example, a couple with primary infertility of 2 years' duration, a female partner aged 32 years, and an average income has a 6-month expectation of conception leading to live birth equivalent to 23% (13.6 × 1.7). The adjustment factor for duration less than 3 years has been applied, but the adjustment factors for secondary infertility, female age and income do not apply. Although only a few infertile couples prefer to continue under observation without treatment, clearly those with one or more good prognostic factors would have sound reasons to do so.

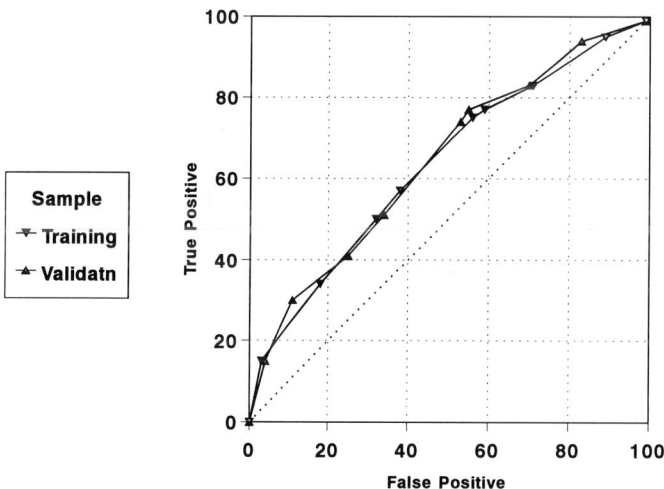

FIGURE 20–8. Receiver-operating characteristics (ROC) curve: accuracy of the prediction score at tenth percentile cut points in the training sample (n = 278) and the validation (Validatn) sample (n = 284).

TABLE 20–6. Untreated Prognosis for an Individual Couple with Unexplained Infertility

Baseline Estimate	Cumulative Rate of Conceptions Leading to Live Birth (95% confidence interval)
6 months	13.6 (10.5, 16.8)
12 months	22.1 (18.0, 26.1)
24 months	29.3 (24.4, 34.2)
Adjustment Factors	
Duration <3 years	1.7
Secondary infertility	1.7
Female <30 years	1.6
Highest income quartile	1.7

EFFECTIVENESS OF TREATMENT

Medical practice is a thoughtful process. Making decisions about treatment is more satisfying when each therapy has a specific biologic rationale, known effectiveness, and minimal hazards. For unexplained infertility, this orderly sequence is incomplete. In the absence of a known defect, there can be no biologic rationale for therapy. Also, knowledge of the effectiveness of therapy is deficient because there are few randomized studies. In any condition such as infertility when spontaneous cure is possible, the effect of treatment can be judged only by comparison with the effect of no treatment. Among such comparative studies, the randomized clinical trial is the most powerful design because it minimizes bias. Cohort studies are in a second class of quality, because treatment is chosen rather than being allocated by chance. Because few comparative studies have been published, there is an unavoidable tendency to compare treated subjects reported in one study and untreated subjects reported elsewhere. Numerous factors affect the observed pregnancy rates in such studies, and for that reason, treatment effects should be developed within the context of a single study. For these reasons, a key factor in the interpretation of clinical studies on the effectiveness of treatment is the quality of study design.

Although there are numerous studies on treatment for unexplained infertility, those that are comparative were frequently assembled as historical cohort (or retrospective) studies. Thus, some subjective judgment on the inclusion of cases could detract from the integrity and impartiality of the resulting statistics. Also important are the baseline differences in prognostic factors that are likely to exist among groups assembled in this way. A further bias arises from the comparison of groups followed for different periods. This bias is of particular interest in the field of infertility because we tend to think of the average pregnancy rate among groups, or the average fecundability. In practice, however, when a group of infertile couples is assembled, fecundability is higher during the early months of observation. This stands to reason, because couples who are more likely to get pregnant conceive early in the observation period. Unless new couples are added, the remainder are less fertile. Thus, there is a "period effect" because the likelihood of pregnancy is altered during followup. This period effect manifests as a steep rise in the cumulative pregnancy rate curve in the first 6 months, and a flattening of the curve after a year or more.[9] As a result, a group of patients followed during three cycles of procedures would not be comparable with a similar group followed for a longer period.[9] The period effect is most evident when the outcome is expressed as approximate fecundability, and the contrast can be seen readily in a comparison of untreated groups. The cumulative pregnancy rate for an untreated cohort of couples with unexplained infertility is shown in Figure 20–9. This group of 381 patients was defined as group C in Figure 20–7, which showed live birth rates. The average pregnancy rate per month (approximate fecundability) was 4.1% after 6 months but only 1.9% after 24 months of followup; Figure 20–9 shows graphically this difference in the slopes of the respective lines. Because of this source of bias, as well as the more obvious biases referred to earlier, evidence from studies that do not include random allocation is inadequate to assess the effects of treatment for fertility.

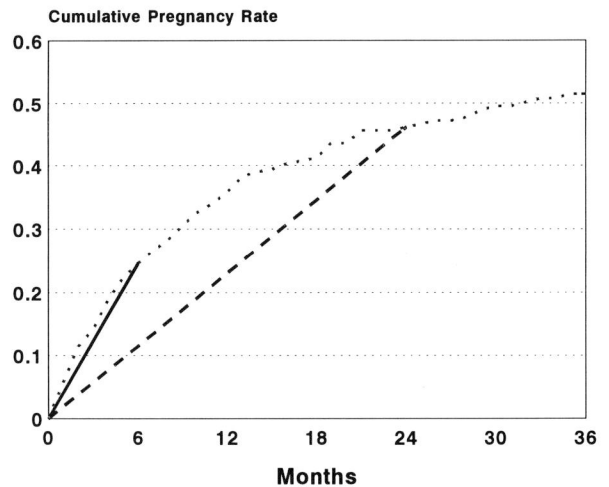

FIGURE 20–9. Cumulative pregnancy rate in 381 untreated couples with unexplained infertility (...). Average fecundability after 6 months (—); 24 months (- - -).

In the treatment sections that follow, the individual studies are described, and for each study the OR representing the likelihood of conception is given with its 95% CI. The OR approximates the relative risk as an expression of the relative value of treatment, and ORs are often used in meta-analysis, a technique for combining published data. Meta-analysis is a useful way to summarize data on the effectiveness of the various empiric treatments for unexplained infertility. In studies of events such as these infertility reports, the meta-analysis consists of combining the individual study ORs into a common odds ratio (COR), (also called the *summary OR* or the *typical OR*). The COR evaluates whether the treatment may be considered proven (the lower 95% confidence limit exceeds unity). If the OR is higher than one but the CI includes unity, the treatment would be considered promising, but as yet unproved. A χ^2 test of association is reported for the COR together with a P value for the significance of the association between the treatment and the occurrence of conception. The COR is more meaningful if the results of the individual studies tend toward the same result, that is, the ORs are not dissimilar, or heterogeneous. The test for homogeneity is the Breslow-Day statistic; if the associated P value is greater than 0.05, there is no significant heterogeneity.[4] The presence of significant heterogeneity would suggest that some factor other than treatment was contributing to the variability in the observed treatment effects. CORs, confidence limits, tests of association, and tests for homogeneity all help summarize the published data on the value of individual treatments.

Bromocriptine

Three studies with relatively small sample sizes have evaluated bromocriptine compared with placebo treatment. The observed pregnancy rates in these randomized trials were not measurably different in the treated group. The COR is 1.1 (95% CI 0-5-26) and the χ^2 test of association is not significant (Fig. 20–10). The test of homogeneity unambiguously indicates that these studies are not dissimilar. Bromocriptine

Authors

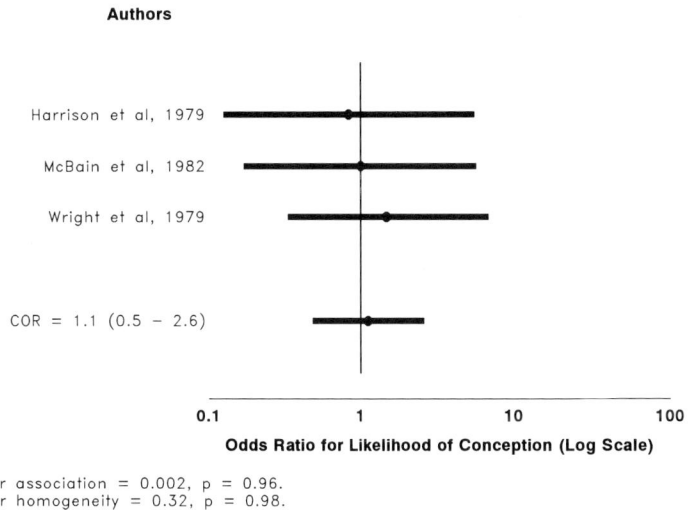

FIGURE 20–10. Bromocriptine treatment for normoprolactinemic unexplained infertility. Odds ratio and 95% confidence
intervals for individual studies are as follows: Harrison et al,
1979[27]: 0.8 (0.1–5.5); McBain and Pepperell, 1982[42]: 1.0 (0.2–
5.7); Wright et al, 1979[63]: 1.5 (0.3.–6.8). COR, common odds
ratio.

Test for association = 0.002, p = 0.96.
Test for homogeneity = 0.32, p = 0.98.

is, for practical purposes, not a useful empiric therapy for
unexplained infertility.[27, 42, 63]

Danazol

Two studies have evaluated danazol for the treatment of
unexplained infertility.[31, 56] Those studies were small, but
there was not a significant improvement in the pregnancy
rate. The expense of danazol and its prolonged contraceptive
effect indicate that this drug would be a poor choice as an
empiric therapy for unexplained infertility.

Intrauterine Insemination

Two studies have evaluated intrauterine insemination (IUI)
as a treatment for unexplained infertility.[34, 40] In the first of
these, patients were randomly allocated to a balanced set of
treatments arranged by cycle. In half of the cycles there was
cointervention with clomiphene, but the pregnancy rate in
cycles with IUI was not significantly superior to cycles with
timed intercourse. In the second study, patients were allo-

cated to a first cycle of IUI or a single episode of timed
intercourse, and in subsequent cycles the treatments were
alternated. Among 73 couples with unexplained infertility,
there were six pregnancies in 145 IUI cycles and three pregnancies in 123 cycles of timed intercourse, a difference that
was not significant. The combined results indicate that IUI
has promise but remains unproven, and further study is
needed (Fig. 20–11).

Although the evidence is inconclusive, IUI alone seems to
have no proven benefit among couples with unexplained
infertility. However, the treatment does appear to be reasonably safe, and it does not alter the frequency of antisperm
antibody detected by immunobead testing.[21, 29]

Clomiphene

The rationale of empiric treatment such as clomiphene
rests on the possibility that augmenting fertility in this way
may compensate for relative subfertility in one or the other
partner. In clomiphene cycles, the augmentation may consist
of a simple increase in the recruitment and maturation of

Authors

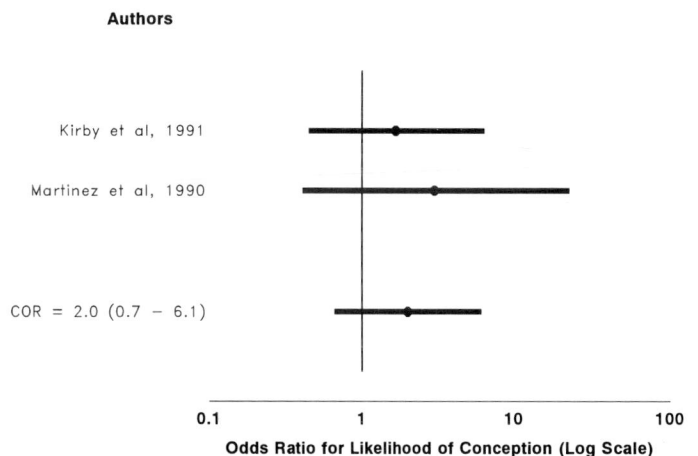

FIGURE 20–11. Intrauterine insemination for unexplained infertility. Odds ratios and 95% confidence limits for the individual
studies are as follows: Kirby et al, 1991[34]: 1.7 (0.5–6.4); Martinez
et al, 1991[40]: 3.0 (0.4–22.5). COR, common odds ratio.

Test for association = 0.91, p = 0.34.
Test for homogeneity = 0.24, p = 0.62.

follicles or in modification of unidentified or undetectable defects in the ovulatory process.

This empiric use of clomiphene has been evaluated in four comparative trials, one of which included IUI with clomiphene therapy, compared with natural cycles and timed intercourse.[15] One study assessed clomiphene with or without human chorionic gonadotropin (hCG) in the luteal phase.[17] Another study evaluated clomiphene with or without hCG for the induction of ovulation[26]; only one study evaluated clomiphene alone.[19] Despite this heterogeneity in the interventions, the results were similar in all four trials. The combined data suggest that clomiphene use for 4 to 6 months may improve fertility by as much as two times (Fig. 20–12). The 95% CI for this result does not include unity, confirming the χ^2 estimate that this typical OR represents a significant treatment effect. When the results of different studies are combined in this way, some measure is needed of the variability from study to study. The Breslow-Day statistical test for homogeneity in the clomiphene studies yielded a P value of 0.94, indicating unambiguously that the inter-study comparisons are not significantly dissimilar.[4] Thus, despite the different inclusion criteria (including patients with treated endometriosis in the case of Deaton and associates in 1990) and the different treatment protocols (clomiphene alone, or with hCG, or with IUI), the treatment effect appears mainly to be associated with the presence or absence of clomiphene.

The better fecundity with clomiphene does not appear to be related to the size of the lead follicle, the number of dominant follicles checked by ultrasound, or the highest dosage.[15] In one randomized trial, the greatest relative increase in conception rates occurred when clomiphene was given to women who had been infertile for more than 3 years.[19]

Clomiphene has been widely used for more than two decades, and its side effects are reasonably predictable. As an empiric therapy for couples with unexplained infertility, this relatively simple therapy may be clinically justified. Use of clomiphene may not be effective where the duration of infertility is less than 36 months, and it is not yet known whether there is value in continuing clomiphene administration after 6 months.

Human Menopausal Gonadotropins With or Without Intrauterine Insemination

Superovulation with human menopausal gonadotropins (hMGs) might improve pregnancy rates among patients with unexplained infertility simply by exposing a larger number of oocytes to the chance of fertilization. It is often used in conjunction with IUI, because the latter can be optimally timed in this way. It is assumed that a combination of superovulation with IUI thus might further improve fertility.

At least five studies have evaluated whether hMG with or without IUI is an effective treatment for unexplained infertility. In 1989, Daly compared hMG and IUI with no treatment in a group of 67 couples with unexplained infertility, all of whom were shown by ultrasonographic monitoring to be free of abnormal follicular dynamics.[14] Welner and associates compared the effects of hMG alone in a group of 39 women (mean duration of infertility 83 months) with a group of 48 women (mean duration of infertility 78 months) who did not receive such therapy.[59] Serhal and coworkers compared hMG and IUI with IUI alone in a group of 30 couples, 15 of whom were allocated to each treatment group.[48] Crosignani and colleagues, in a large multicenter, randomized trial, evaluated several treatments, including hMG alone and hMG with IUI.[13] A further randomized trial included diagnostic and treatment stratification with crossover from cycle to cycle, and the results of this study did not directly address whether hMG with IUI is an effective treatment for unexplained infertility.[41]

ORs derived from the results of these studies suggest that hMG with IUI treatment may be superior to the control treatments, (no treatment, IUI alone, and hMG alone) (Fig. 20–13). The confidence limits for the COR and the P value are indicative of a highly significant result. The treatment effects were not heterogeneous among the studies despite the use of different control groups.

Whether this treatment effect is associated with hMG and IUI or is due to bias cannot be ensured from the available studies. First, for example, treatment allocation was random in only one study. Also, the data are selected. In Daly's study, for example, the primary concern was hMG treatment of problems in follicular dynamics; the hMG/IUI and untreated cohorts were included as comparison groups. The European trial compared gamete intrafallopian transfer (GIFT), IVF, and intraperitoneal insemination or IUI after hMG with hMG alone. The global comparison was only marginally significant ($P = 0.052$). These design issues may, however, be less important than the period effect referred to in Figure 20–9. The data for Figure 20–13 shown in Table 20–7 indicate that for three of the comparisons, there were more months or cycles of observation in the control group. Thus, control group fecundability is likely to be lower simply because of longer followup. The period effect helps explain why similar results are seen, despite the use of different controls. Additionally, although it may seem that time to conception is reduced by hMG/IUI treatment, this effect is mainly due to differences in the length of followup. Thus, from the best evidence available, it would be prudent to conclude that hMG and IUI is a promising therapy but that the efficacy of

	Treatment Groups		**Control Groups**		
Authors	*Number Pregnant*	*Number of Cycles*	*Number Pregnant*	*Number of Cycles*	**Control**
Daly, 1989[14]	6	55	20	571*	No treatment
Serhal et al, 1989[48]	6	19	1	30	IUI
Crosignani et al, 1991[13]	36	158	9	78	hMG
Serhal et al, 1989[48]	6	19	3	49	hMG

TABLE 20–7. hMG and IUI Treatment for Unexplained Infertility

*Estimated from fecundability.
hMG, human menopausal gonadotropin; IUI, intrauterine insemination.

Authors

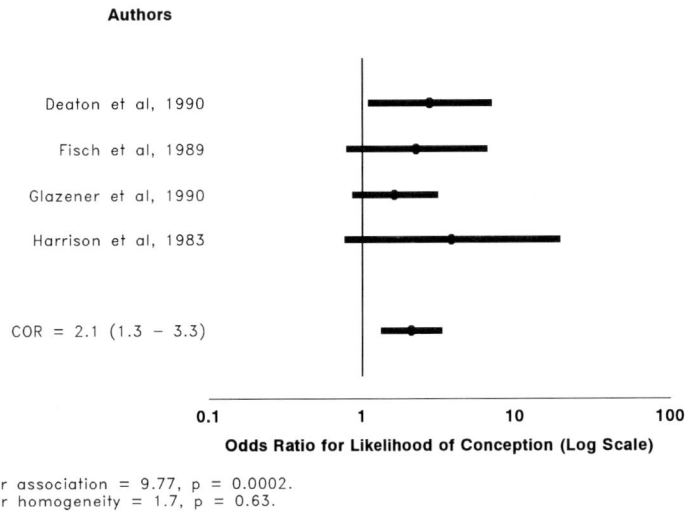

Deaton et al, 1990

Fisch et al, 1989

Glazener et al, 1990

Harrison et al, 1983

COR = 2.1 (1.3 − 3.3)

0.1   1   10   100

Odds Ratio for Likelihood of Conception (Log Scale)

Test for association = 9.77, p = 0.0002.
Test for homogeneity = 1.7, p = 0.63.

FIGURE 20–12. Clomiphene treatment for unexplained infertility. COR: commons odds ratio. Odds ratios and 95% confidence intervals for the individual studies are as follows: Deaton et al, 1990[15]: 2.8 (1.1–7.0); Fisch et al, 1989[17]: 2.3 (0.8–6.6); Glazener et al, 1990[19]: 1.6 (0.9–3.1); Harrison and O'Moore, 1983[26]: 3.85 (0.77–19.3).

this treatment is untested by satisfactory studies. Also uncertain is whether hMG and IUI have independent effects or act solely in partnership.

In Vitro Fertilization and Its Variants

A wide variety of reproductive technology is available as a last resort in the treatment of almost all infertile patients, including those with unexplained infertility. The prognosis with unexplained infertility compared with other infertility diagnoses does not appear to be impaired.[28, 64] IVF and GIFT procedures have been compared in two studies, and there was no significant preference for either treatment.[13, 36] Among 1042 IVF and GIFT cycles in 1989 for female unexplained infertility, there were 184 (17.7%) clinical pregnancies, of which 58 were in IVF and 126 were GIFT cycles.[28] The combined results of IVF and GIFT yielded 149 deliveries (14.3% per cycle). No studies are available that have evaluated IVF or GIFT with respect to an untreated or placebo group in a randomized design. One cohort study compared conception rates during 99 cycles of GIFT and 894 months of observation among 76 couples with unexplained infertil-

ity.[43] The average fecundability was 14% with GIFT and 2% with observation (Fig. 20–14, *square markers*). There was an average of 1.7 cycles of GIFT compared with 12.2 months of observation. A similar result can be seen among untreated couples if they are divided into groups followed for different lengths of time (see Fig. 20–14, *diamond markers*). Among the untreated couples whose followup was shown previously in Figures 20–7 and 20–9, fecundability in the group that was followed for 3 months or less was 22% compared with 2% in the group with longer followup.[9] This is another example of the unexpected bias that can occur in nonexperimental studies, and this bias underlines the need for randomized, comparative studies. Given a sufficiently large sample, such a comparison could be conducted within one or two cycles, so that the untreated group would not be disadvantaged and the study design would be ethically acceptable. The European trial referred to earlier compared the results of IVF treatment and GIFT treatment with hMG alone. The results of each treatment were not significantly different in the first cycle, but in the combined results of two cycles, pregnancy rates with GIFT (28%) and IVF (25%) were higher than the pregnancy rates with hMG alone (15.2%). It is likely that IVF and GIFT are effective therapies; certainly the world

Authors

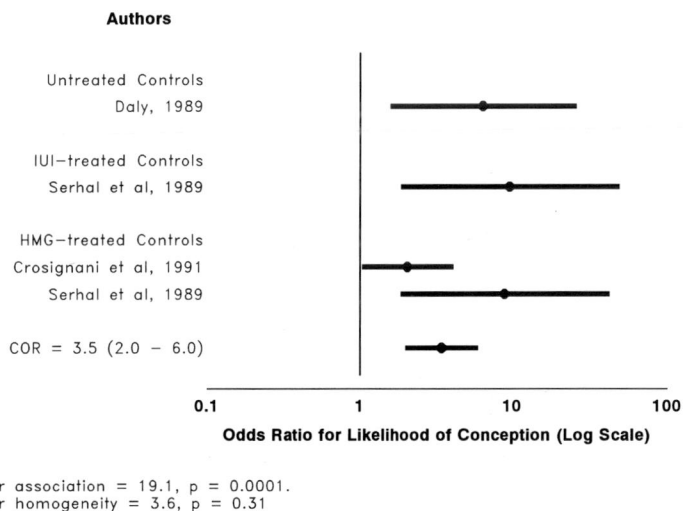

Untreated Controls
Daly, 1989

IUI–treated Controls
Serhal et al, 1989

HMG–treated Controls
Crosignani et al, 1991
Serhal et al, 1989

COR = 3.5 (2.0 − 6.0)

0.1   1   10   100

Odds Ratio for Likelihood of Conception (Log Scale)

Test for association = 19.1, p = 0.0001.
Test for homogeneity = 3.6, p = 0.31

FIGURE 20–13. Superovulation with intrauterine insemination (IUI) treatment for unexplained infertility. Odds ratios and 95% confidence intervals for the individual studies are as follows: Daly, 1989[14]: 6.4 (1.6–25.6); Serhal et al, 1989 (IUI-treated controls)[48]: 9.6 (1.9–48.7); Crosignani et al, 1991[13]: 2.1 (1.0–4.1); Serhal et al, 1989 (HMG-treated controls)[48]: 8.9 (1.9–41.9). COR, common odds ratio; HMG, human menopausal gonadotropin.

Conceptions Resulting in Live Births

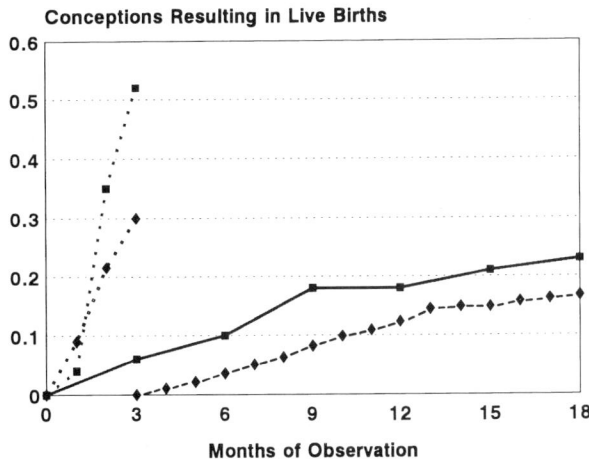

Months of Observation

Data selected according to length of follow-up.

FIGURE 20–14. Cycles of gamete intrafallopian transfer (GIFT) (...) and untreated observations (–) reported for 76 couples with unexplained infertility from Newcastle, UK (solid square markers).[43] Untreated couples with followup ≤3 months (...) and >3 months (- - -) selected by length of followup (diamond markers).[9]

is not waiting for evidence of that effectiveness. Nevertheless, it is not too late for well-designed studies that might provide a better estimate of the true treatment effect.

The factors affecting treatment decisions among couples with unexplained infertility include issues other than the efficacy of therapy. On the issue of efficacy, however, only clomiphene therapy has been demonstrated, by means of acceptable clinical evidence in the form of repeated randomized trials, to be an effective treatment with proven superiority over no therapy. On the basis of the best available evidence, hMG or IUI, or both, are promising treatments, but the benefit is unproven. No studies exist to demonstrate a benefit for IVF methodology.

MANAGEMENT OF UNEXPLAINED INFERTILITY

Unexplained infertility is an especially frustrating form of infertility, given the enigma of the underlying factors and the uncertainty about the efficacy of treatment. The benefits of treatment are linked with hazards, so that each decision should be tailored to the needs of the individual couple. Given the range and intensity of feelings that may be associated with infertility, and the differences in risk-taking behavior that must exist within each couple, the optimal role of the physician is one of providing information and advice. The final decision should rest with the couple.

Applying the Treatment Factor to the Prognostic Model

As indicated earlier, in the course of clinical problem solving, the physician who has arrived at a diagnosis next makes a forecast about the natural course of the diagnosed disorder and then estimates the effect of treatment. This estimate of the benefits expected from therapy should be presented to

patients with information about the cost of treatment and the expected hazards. Presenting a balanced view about treatment provides patients with more realistic information and is essential for continued communication.

Although prognostic models such as the prediction score in the section on the natural course of infertility are limited in comparison with the reality of clinical and biologic variability, the information can serve to help estimate the role of treatment. For example, in a typical couple (average income, aged in their 30s, prolonged primary infertility) who remain untreated for the next 6 months, the likelihood of pregnancy leading to live birth is 13.6% (95% CI 10.5, 16.8), or approximately 2% per month (see Table 20–6). In the example of this typical couple, no adjustment factors would apply, so the next step is to estimate the effect of therapy on this baseline prognosis. Table 20–8 shows the relative effect of treatment on fertility among couples with unexplained infertility, as derived from studies cited in the earlier section. In the case of clomiphene treatment, the COR was 2.1. Thus, for the given couple, a trial of clomiphene might be expected to double the fecundability from approximately 2% to 4% per month.

Offering treatment in which the 6-month prognosis is only moderately increased (from 14% to approximately 28%) is for some physicians a troublesome prospect. Using objective evidence as the basis of decision making offers advantages, however. First, the objective provision of data allows the couple to at least consider what may have been on their minds: the possibility of not choosing any treatment at this time. Second, offering evidence in this way maintains physician credibility. Because it is likely that most patients with prolonged infertility will fail to conceive during any single treatment regimen, the physician who has provided objective data will remain a credible source of counseling when the same couple is considering a further treatment decision.

The lack of a proven rationale for therapy, and the lack of proven effectiveness for many of the treatments, suggests that patients' wishes should count heavily in the choice. The couple may benefit from participating in the development of a plan for the management of their infertility, a plan that may include a sequential approach to treatment. In such a plan, the simplest and possibly most effective treatment would form the initial program of management. For couples with a short duration of infertility, the best initial choice may be continued observation. For couples with a duration of infertility less than 3 years, unless there are other considerations, the benefits of any active intervention are unproven. The first therapy will usually be clomiphene, but after that the choices become problematic. Whether or not hMG and IUI are effec-

TABLE 20–8. Relative Effect of Treatment on Fertility Among Couples with Unexplained Infertility	
Treatment	**Treatment Effect Relative to Controls (95% confidence interval)**
Clomiphene	2.1 (1.3, 3.4)*
IUI	2.0 (0.7, 6.1)†
hMG ± IUI	2.3 (1.4, 3.7)‡

*Typical odds ratio (see Fig. 20–11).
†Typical odds ratio (see Fig. 20–12).
‡Typical odds ratio (see Fig. 20–13).
hMG, human menopausal gonadotropin; IUI, intrauterine insemination.

tive, the cost is lower than the cost of IVF or GIFT. If hMG and IUI therapy is chosen, the average reported duration of hMG and IUI therapy is two or three cycles. IVF or GIFT usually is the final treatment either because the expense is so much higher, or because there are long waiting lists in countries where national insurance includes IVF therapy.

Providing information, counseling, and education for couples with unexplained infertility is a demanding part of the role of an infertility clinical service. Some couples often feel despair when they hear an honest prognosis, and others are despondent after the completion of a therapy without success. Thus, infertile couples need access to knowledgeable counseling by social workers, psychologists, or interested psychiatrists. Counseling has more value if the professional involved has a knowledge of the clinical and biologic basis of infertility, and this is especially true in the case of unexplained infertility.

Summary

About one in five infertile couples have unexplained infertility, often because of undetectable disorders among the prerequisites for conception. Some of these disorders are age related; the likelihood of this diagnosis is 56% greater if the female partner is older than 30 years of age. Two thirds of reported cases have primary infertility, and the mean duration of infertility ranges from 20 to 78 months. In the typical untreated couple, the cumulative rate of conceptions leading to live birth is 22% (95% CI 18%, 26%) in 12 months. If the duration of infertility were less that 3 years, the predicted rate would be 1.7 times higher, or 37%. Treatment is indicated after 3 or more years' duration of infertility. Clomiphene treatment for 4 to 6 months has been demonstrated in repeated trials to improve fertility by two times or more. Other treatments such as hMG and IUI alone or in combination remain unproven; hMG with IUI is a promising treatment, but the side effects of hMG are noteworthy. The effectiveness of IVF and related methods also is unproven, although after several years of unexplained infertility, even such costly treatment is warranted in many instances.

Acknowledgments

The Investigators of the Canadian Infertility Therapy Evaluation Study Group were as follows: William Wrixon, M.D., Halifax, Nova Scotia; Rodolphe Maheux, M.D., and Nacia Faure, M.D., Laval, Quebec; Togas Tulandi, M.D., and D. Robert A. McInnes, M.D., Montreal, Quebec; John F. Jarrell, M.D., Hamilton, Ontario; R. Hugh Gorwill, M.D., and Robert L. Reid, M.D., Kingston, Ontario; David C. Cumming, M.D., and Josef Z. Scott, M.D., Edmonton, Alberta; Timothy C. Rowe, M.D., and Peter F. McComb, M.B., Vancouver, British Columbia; Patrick J. Taylor, M.B., H. Anthony Pattinson, M.B., and Arthur Leader, M.D., Calgary, Alberta; John McCoshen, Ph.D., and Ronald A. Livingston, M.B., Winnipeg, Manitoba; John E. H. Spence, M.D., and Peter Garner, M.B., Ottawa, Ontario; Charles W. Simpson, M.D., and David R. Popkin, M.D., Saskatoon, Saskatchewan; Serge Belisle, M.D., and Youssef Ain-Melk, M.D., Sherbrooke, Quebec; Stanley E. Brown, M.D., and Earl R. Plunkett, M.D., London, Ontario, Canada.

REFERENCES

1. Aitken RJJ, Best FSM, Warner P, Templeton A. A prospective study of the relationship between semen quality and fertility in cases of unexplained infertility. J Androl 1984;5:297–303.

2. Anderson AJB. Ugeskrift fur Laeger. Infertilitet 1968;130:633–635.

3. Barnea ER, Holford TR, McInnes DRA. Long-term prognosis of infertile couples with normal basic investigations: a life-table analysis. Obstet Gynecol 1985;66:24–26.

4. Breslow NE, Day NE. Combination of results from a series of 2 × 2 tables: control of confounding. In: Davis W, editor. Statistical Methods in Cancer Research: Volume 1. The Analysis of Case-Control Studies. Cedex, France: IARC Scientific Publications, 1980:136–157.

5. Check JH, Chase JS, Nowroozi K, et al. Empirical therapy of the male with clomiphene in couples with unexplained infertility. Int J Fertil 1989;34:120–122.

6. Cocev D. Results of studies and treatment of sterility in families in Blagogengrade district during a period of five years. Akush Ginekol (Sofia) 1972;11:133–135.

7. Collins JA. Natural course of unexplained infertility. In: Proceedings of the Serono Symposium on Unexplained Infertility: Basic and Clinical Aspects, 1989. Rome: Serono Aries Publishers, 1989:71–85.

8. Collins JA, Crosignani PG. Unexplained infertility: a review of diagnosis, prognosis, treatment efficacy and management. Int J Gynecol Obstet 1992;39:267–275.

9. Collins JA, Enkin M. Is GIFT (gamete intrafallopian transfer) the best treatment for unexplained infertility? [letter; comment] Br J Obstet Gynaecol 1992;99:169–170.

10. Collins JA, Rand CA, Wilson EH, et al. The better prognosis in secondary infertility is associated with a higher proportion of ovulation disorders. Fertil Steril 1986;45:611–616.

11. Collins JA, Rowe TC. Age of the female partner is a prognostic factor in prolonged unexplained infertility: a multicentre study. Fertil Steril 1989;52:15–20.

12. Cox LW. Infertility: a comprehensive programme. Br J Obstet Gynaecol 1975;82:2–6.

13. Crosignani PG, Walters DE, Soliani A. The ESHRE multicentre trial on the treatment of unexplained infertility: a preliminary report. Hum Reprod 1991;6:953–958.

14. Daly DC. Treatment validation of ultrasound-defined abnormal follicular dynamics as a cause of infertility. Fertil Steril 1989;51:51–57.

15. Deaton JL, Gibson M, Blackmer KM, et al. A randomized, controlled trial of clomiphene citrate and intrauterine insemination in couples with unexplained infertility or surgically corrected endometriosis. Fertil Steril 1990;54:1083–1088.

16. Dor J, Homburg R, Rabau E. An evaluation of etiologic factors and therapy in 665 infertile couples. Fertil Steril 1977;28:718–722.

17. Fisch P, Casper RF, Brown SE, et al. Unexplained infertility: evaluation of treatment with clomiphene citrate and human chorionic gonadotropin. Fertil Steril 1989;51:828–833.

18. Frank R. A clinical study of 240 infertile couples. Am J Obstet Gynecol 1950;60:645–654.

19. Glazener CMA, Coulson C, Lambert PA, et al. Clomiphene treatment for women with unexplained infertility: placebo-controlled study of hormonal responses and conception rates. Gynecol Endocrinol 1990;4:75–83.

20. Glazener CMA, Kelly NJ, Hull MGR. Luteal deficiency not a persistent cause of infertility. Hum Reprod 1988;3:213–217.

21. Goldberg JM, Haering PL, Friedman CI, et al. Antisperm antibodies in women undergoing intrauterine insemination. Am J Obstet Gynecol 1990;163:65–68.

22. Griffith CS, Grimes DA. The validity of the postcoital test. Am J Obstet Gynecol 1990;162:616–620.

23. Gunaratne M. The epidemiology of infertility: A selected clinic study. Ceylon Med J 1979;24:36.

24. Gwatkin RBL, Collins JA, Jarrell JF, et al. The value of semen analysis and sperm function assays in predicting pregnancy among infertile couples. Fertil Steril 1990;53:693–699.

25. Harrison RF, O'Moore RR, O'Moore A. Stress and fertility: some modalities of investigation and treatment in couples with unexplained infertility. Int J Fertil 1986;31:153–159.

26. Harrison RF, O'Moore RR. The use of clomiphene citrate with and without human chorionic gonadotropin. Ir Med J 1983;76:273–274.

27. Harrison RF, O'Moore RR, McSweeney J. Idiopathic infertility: a trial of bromocriptine versus placebo. Ir Med J 1979;72:479–482.

28. Hartz SC. Medical Research International, Society of Assisted Reproductive Technology. The American Fertility Society. In vitro fertilization–embryo transfer (IVF-ET) in the United States: 1989 results from the IVF-ET registry. Fertil Steril 1991;55:14–23.

29. Horvath PM, Beck M, Bohrer MK, et al. A prospective study on the lack of development of antisperm antibodies in women undergoing intrauterine insemination. Am J Obstet Gynecol 1989;160:631–637.

30. Hull MGR, Glazener CMA, Kelly NH, et al. Population study of causes, treatment and outcome of infertility. Br Med J 1985;291:1693–1697.

31. Iffland CA, Shaw RW, Beynon JL. Is danazol a useful treatment in unexplained primary infertility? Eur J Obstet Gynecol Reprod Biol 1989;32:115–121.

32. Insler V, Potashnik G, Glassner M. Some epidemiological aspects of fertility evaluation. In: Insler V, Bettendorf G, Geissler KH, editor. Advances in Diagnosis and Treatment of Infertility. New York: Elsevier North Holland 1981:165–177.

33. Johansson CJ. Clinical studies on sterile couples with special reference to the diagnosis, etiology, and prognosis of infertility. Acta Obstet Gynecol Scand 1957;36(Suppl 5):161–168.

34. Kirby CA, Flaherty SP, Godfrey BM, et al. A prospective trial of intrauterine insemination of motile spermatozoa versus timed intercourse. Fertil Steril 1991;56:102–107.

35. Kliger BE. Evaluation, therapy, and outcome in 493 infertile couples. Fertil Steril 1984;41:40–46.

36. Leeton J. Rogers P, Caro C, et al. A controlled study between the use of gamete intrafallopian transfer (GIFT) and in vitro fertilization and embryo transfer in the management of idiopathic and male infertility. Fertil Steril 1987;48:605–607.

37. Lenton EA, Weston GA, Cooke ID. Long-term follow-up of the apparently normal couple with a complaint of infertility. Fertil Steril 1977;28:913–919.

38. Leridon H, Spira A. Problems in measuring the effectiveness of infertility therapy. Fertil Steril 1984;41:580–586.

39. Mao C, Grimes DA. The sperm penetration assay: can it discriminate between fertile and infertile men? Am J Obstet Gynecol 1988;159:279–286.

40. Martinez AR, Bernardus RE, Voorhorst FJ, et al. Intrauterine insemination does and clomiphene citrate does not improve fecundity in couples with infertility due to male or idiopathic factors: a prospective, randomized, controlled study. Fertil Steril 1990;53:847–853.

41. Martinez AR, Bernardus ER, Voorhorst FJ, et al. Pregnancy rates after timed intercourse or intrauterine insemination after human menopausal gonadotropin stimulation of normal ovulatory cycles: a controlled study. Fertil Steril 1991;55:258–265.

42. McBain JC, Pepperell RJ. Use of bromocriptine in unexplained infertility. Clin Reprod Fertil 1982;1:145–150.

43. Murdoch AP, Harris M, Mahroo M, et al. Is GIFT (gamete intrafallopian transfer) the best treatment for unexplained infertility? Br J Obstet Gynaecol 1991;98:643–647.

44. Newton J, Craig S, Joyce D. The changing pattern of a comprehensive infertility clinic. J Biosoc Sci 1974;6:477–482.

45. Ratnam SS, Chew PC, Tsakok M. Experience of a comprehensive infertility clinic in the Department of Obstetrics and Gynaecology, University of Singapore. Singapore Med J 1976;17(3):157–159.

46. Raymont A, Arronet GH, Arrata WSM. Review of 500 cases of infertility. Int J Fertil 1969;14:141–153.

47. Rousseau S, Lord J, Lepage Y, Van Campenhout J. The expectancy of pregnancy of "normal" infertile couples. Fertil Steril 1983;40:768–772.

48. Serhal PF, Katz M, Little V, Woronowski H. Unexplained infertility—the value of pergonal superovulation combined with intrauterine insemination. Fertil Steril 1988;49:602–606.

49. Sorensen SS. Infertility factors: their relative importance and share in an unselected material of infertility patients. Acta Obstet Gynecol Scand 1980;59:513–520.

50. Southam AL. What to do with the "normal" infertile couple? Fertil Steril 1960;11:543–549.

51. Southam AL, Buxton CL. Factors influencing reproductive potential. Fertil Steril 1957;8:25–35.

52. Taylor PJ, Collins JA. Unexplained infertility. New York: Oxford Medical Publications, 1992.

53. Templeton AA, Penney GC. The incidence, characteristics, and prognosis of patients whose infertility is unexplained. Fertil Steril 1982;37:175–182.

54. Thomas AK, Forrest MS. Infertility: a review of 291 infertile couples over eight years. Fertil Steril 1980;34:106–111.

55. Trimbos-Kemper GC, Trimbos J, van Hall E. Pregnancy rates after laparoscopy for infertility. Eur J Obstet Gynecol Reprod Biol 1984;18:127–132.

56. van Dijk JG, Frolich M, Brand EC, van Hall EV. The "treatment" of unexplained infertility with danazol. Fertil Steril 1979;31:481–485.

57. Verkauf BS. The incidence and outcome of single-factor, multifactorial, and unexplained infertility. Am J Obstet Gynecol 1983;147:175–181.

58. Vutyavanich T, Collins JA. An overview of the Canadian Infertility Therapy Evaluation Study. J Soc Obstet Gynecol Can 1991;13:29–34.

59. Welner S, DeCherney AH, Polan ML. Human menopausal gonadotropins: a justifiable therapy in ovulatory women with long-standing idiopathic infertility. Am J Obstet Gynecol 1988;158:111–117.

60. Wentz AC, Kossoy LR, Parker RA. The impact of luteal phase inadequacy in an infertile population. Am J Obstet Gynecol 1990;162:937–945.

61. West CP, Templeton AA, Lees MM. The diagnostic classification and prognosis of 400 infertile couples. Infertility 1982;5:127–144.

62. World Health Organization. WHO laboratory manual for the examination of human semen and semen–cervical mucus interaction. Cambridge: Cambridge University Press, 1987:1–26.

63. Wright CS, Steele SJ, Jacobs HS. Value of bromocriptine in unexplained primary infertility: a double-blind controlled trial. Br Med J 1979;1:1037–1039.

64. Yovich JL, Matson PL. Early pregnancy wastage after gamete manipulation. Br J Obstet Gynaecol 1988;95:1120–1127.

Surgical Management of the Infertile Female

WILLIAM R. KEYE, JR.

CHAPTER 21

Principles of Surgical Management of the Infertile Female

G. DAVID ADAMSON

Many important advances have occurred in the past 20 years in the surgical management of the infertile female. These began with the advent of diagnostic laparoscopy and, soon after, the introduction of minor operative laparoscopic procedures such as tubal ligation. Operative laparoscopy did not progress much further during the interval when microsurgery at laparotomy became popular during the late 1970s and early 1980s. Diagnostic hysteroscopy was only infrequently performed. However, the last decade has seen the emergence of operative laparoscopy and hysteroscopy as important surgical techniques, with lasers stimulating a great deal of the progress. More recently, the focus has returned to discussion of the appropriateness of endoscopic techniques, with an emphasis on surgical principles, outcome assessment, and the roles of surgery and in vitro fertilization (IVF). This chapter outlines contemporary principles of the surgical management of the infertile female (Table 21–1).

PREOPERATIVE SURGICAL PRINCIPLES

Patient Selection

FACTORS AFFECTING SURGICAL DECISION MAKING

The surgeon's role in presenting surgical options is to evaluate patients thoroughly and determine their values and aims. Patients need to be educated about their investigations, treatments, probabilities of success, and ability to absorb the financial, time, physical, and emotional costs of surgery. Especially, they need to be educated about their surgical and nonsurgical options. Patients' decisions regarding treatment choices should be respected and validated unless the decisions are medically unsound. Patients should be referred for other consultations if either they or the surgeon are not comfortable with the management decision.

Patient selection for surgical procedures is a complex proc-

TABLE 21–1. Surgical Principles in Infertility Surgery

Knowledge of disease and treatment modalities
Experienced surgeon
Adequate facilities, personnel, and equipment
Appropriate patient selection
Informed consent
Proper patient position
Careful pelvic evaluation
Maximum exposure
Use of magnification
Minimum tissue trauma
Excellent hemostasis
Removal of all diseased tissue
Avoidance of foreign body material
Confirmation of tissue pathology

ess. The eventual probability of a good surgical outcome is highly dependent on preoperative decisions regarding the surgical options. These decisions are frequently made when the patient is experiencing a great deal of stress and psychological vulnerability. The surgeon must be aware of issues involved in the meaningful presentation of surgical options to each patient (Table 21–2).

The quality of scientific information regarding reproductive surgery has improved dramatically in the past 20 years.

TABLE 21–2. Factors Affecting Surgical Decision Making

1. There is often limited or incomplete data from prospective randomized surgical trials.
2. The surgeon who is counseling the patient may be unaware of all the data that are available.
3. Patients make decisions in different ways.
4. Physicians frame options based on their unique experiences and biases.
5. Patients may have irrational fears or concerns.
6. Religious, moral, and ethical issues can complicate the surgeon's and patient's decisions.
7. Patients may have strong personal preferences for certain treatments.

Nevertheless, we still have only limited data on which to base decisions. Well-designed and controlled clinical trials are difficult to do and not often performed.[1–3] Although it is unreasonable to expect all surgeons to be experts in experimental design, it is necessary to have an appreciation of the limitations of current surgical knowledge. Factors affecting pregnancy rates among infertile couples include characteristics of the infertile group, such as age, duration of infertility, and previous pregnancy history, as well as the expected spontaneous cure rate.[4, 5]

Surgeons need to keep abreast of developments by reading the literature and attending continuing medical education meetings. If they do not, they may provide the patient with inaccurate or outdated information. They need to appreciate that people make decisions in different ways, some intuitively, some based on experience, and others with a straightforward analysis of the facts. Numerous basic misconceptions about decision making can easily lead the surgeon and patient to choose inappropriate management involving surgery.[6] Contemporary decision making involves a shared responsibility between surgeons and patients. Surgeons bring knowledge and expertise to the decision while patients bring their aims and values. Surgeons should encourage their patients to employ cost-benefit analysis techniques in their decision making. Despite such objective approaches, some patients will make irrational decisions because many people have a tendency to maximize short-term gains and avoid risks or costs in the near future as opposed to taking a longer-term approach to a problem. For example, a patient may opt for a 20% chance of pregnancy with in vitro fertilization rather than a 60% chance with laparoscopic adhesiolysis because of her desire to get pregnant as quickly as possible and avoid surgery. Other patients may have unrealistic feelings about low probability events and have fear or anxiety that greatly exceeds the actual risks or pain of the procedure.[7] Distinguishing between a reasonable and unreasonable concern is often difficult. Patients may have values or beliefs that are unique to them, and surgeons may "frame" options more or less favorably, depending on their biases. It is imperative that surgeons be aware of these issues in decision making when selecting patients for surgery. Usually, the best approach is to present the available choices in alternative ways to allow patients to evaluate the different options from different perspectives.

Finally, surgical decision making is becoming increasingly complex because of ethical issues regarding treatment.[8] The first question which must be asked is, "What are the indications for surgical intervention?" In couples in whom the prognosis is good without any intervention at all, the surgeon must be careful not to use unnecessary treatment.[4, 9] Patient preferences can also create ethical dilemmas. General guidelines for dealing with patient preferences have been recommended by Brett and McCullough.[10] Surgeons are under no obligation to render useless health care, regardless of its safety, just because a patient requests it. A general consensus exists that surgeons have the right not to participate in nonemergency care, although exceptions sometimes occur. Brett and McCullough also recommended that "decisions in individual cases should not ultimately be made on the basis of economic considerations unless the society has developed formal guidelines for the use of the medical resource in question."[10] At this time, American society has not developed formal guidelines that ration health care on an economic basis. Until such guidelines are formulated, surgical care for individual patients should not be rationed based on arbitrary financial considerations. Patients should be offered second opinions whenever significant issues involving surgical decision making are difficult to resolve. It is important to establish the religious, moral, and ethical values of the couple and surgeon early in any decision-making process. Should there be significant variance or nonacceptance of all views, then alternative sources of health care should be identified for the benefit of all involved. Ethical dilemmas exist when options for care conflict with the patient's autonomy, quality of life, or social justice. The most important principle is to avoid harm when making surgical decisions.

EVALUATION OF PELVIC STATUS

Surgeons must perform a comprehensive history and physical examination. A pelvic examination includes vulvar examination followed by speculum examination of the vagina and the cervix. A bimanual examination involves careful assessment of uterine and adnexal size, shape, position, mobility, and consistency. Rectovaginal examination is also mandatory prior to surgery. The finding of uterine enlargement raises the possibility of myomas, adenomyosis, or, rarely, sarcoma. Abnormal contour may reflect uterine developmental abnormalities. Adnexal enlargement may be associated with self-limiting functional cysts, benign neoplasms, or malignancy. Hydrosalpinges must also be considered. Decreased mobility may be a result of adhesions resulting from pelvic inflammatory disease, endometriosis, or malignancy. Rectovaginal nodularity or thickening may be a sign of endometriosis. Such findings help the surgeon decide on subsequent preoperative tests or medical treatment and may influence the timing, nature, and approach to surgery.

Preoperative laboratory tests frequently include hysterosalpingogram and ultrasonography, and, much less often, magnetic resonance imaging (MRI) and computed tomography (CT) scanning. Selective tubal cannulation or balloon tuboplasty under radiographic control is increasingly used in preoperative assessment and, sometimes, treatment. Diagnostic laparoscopy, hysteroscopy, and salpingoscopy may also provide valuable prelaparotomy information but are more frequently performed as both diagnostic and therapeutic procedures at the same time.

EVALUATION OF OTHER FACTORS

Nonsurgical infertility factors affecting outcome must also be considered in evaluating the desirability of a surgical procedure. These include duration of infertility, sperm quality, ovulation status, and prior pregnancy history.[4, 11, 12] A most important factor affecting egg quality is the patient's age.[13] Cycle day 3 serum follicle-stimulating hormone (FSH) levels can also be helpful in assessing ovarian function, irrespective of age. Because many women have subtle reduction in ovarian function in their 30s, it is recommended that a cycle day 2, 3, or 4 FSH level be obtained on all women 35 years of age or over before surgery and also on all women with ovulation dysfunction. Surgeons need to familiarize themselves with normal ranges in their laboratories. An FSH level less than 15 mIU/mL is generally within normal limits; 15 to 25 mIU/mL indicates some reduction in ovarian function and a reduced prognosis; 25 to 40 mIU/mL a perimenopausal state, and higher than 40 mIU/mL a menopausal state. In most situations, it is inappropriate to operate on patients with an FSH level greater than 20 mIU/mL because their prognosis will be severely compromised. Data show that fertility is reduced moderately by age alone until the mid to late 30s when there is approximately a 25% reduction in fertility by age 37, 45% by age 40, 70% by age 43, and 90% by age 45.[14] Clinical spontaneous abortion rates also increase dramatically from approximately 10% at age less than 30, to 18% age 35 to 39, and 34% age 40 to 44.[15] The risk of obstetric complications and abnormal fetuses also increases with age.[16]

Consultations with gastroenterologists, urologists, or other specialists as indicated should be scheduled to help ensure that the operation produces the maximum benefits. Alternatives to treatment, or treatment in combination with surgery, such as the use of gonadotropin-releasing hormone (GnRH) agonists, should be considered and implemented as indicated.

DETERMINATION OF PROGNOSIS

Surgeons need to determine the prognosis based on realistic surgical outcomes in their hands. Literature success rates for various procedures often represent the best outcomes by experienced surgeons (Table 21–3).[11, 17–20] It is not to be expected that less experienced surgeons who perform a procedure less frequently, or who have less skill, will obtain the same results as published experts. It is each surgeon's responsibility to know their own success rate and to tell the patient what it is. These results may be altered for a given patient because of unique features of her disease or the surgeon's experience. The role of second-look laparoscopy in reducing postoperative adhesions needs to be considered as an adjunct to the initial surgery. Although no studies have yet proved a subsequent increased pregnancy rate, many surgeons believe that second-look laparoscopy is beneficial.[21–23] Second-look laparoscopy should be discussed with all patients. It is indicated more often following laparotomy, when the risk of de novo adhesion formation is higher. It is reasonable to recommend second-look laparoscopy when there is more than mild adhesive disease, moderate or greater endometriosis, or ovarian disease that has been treated at the primary surgery.

TABLE 21–3. Postoperative Pregnancy Rates by Procedure[11, 17–20]

Procedure	Pregnancy Rate (%)
Salpingolysis/ovariolysis	25–69
Fimbrioplasty	27–70
Salpingostomy (tubal reconstruction)	21–39
Salpingostomy (ectopic pregnancy)	38–80
Tubal anastomosis	52–82
Tubal anastomosis (uterotubal obstruction)	37–69
Tubal cannulation (uterotubal obstruction)	27–37
Repeat tuboplasties	6–20
Fulguration of endometrial implants	40–82
Recurrent endometriosis	40–47
Myomectomy	16–82
Intrauterine adhesiolysis	40–70

These patients are at highest risk for reduced fecundity because of adhesion formation. Patients who do not have adnexal disease, or who have extensive, severe disease, or who have had multiple procedures for adhesiolysis, are not likely to benefit much from second-look laparoscopy, and it is generally not indicated. Second-look laparoscopy is also generally not indicated for patients who will soon be undergoing IVF.

CONTRAINDICATIONS TO SURGERY

Contraindications to infertility surgery must be specifically considered prior to operation. Relative contraindications include advanced maternal age (see earlier) and end-stage tubal, uterine, or pelvic disease. Poor sperm quality is also a relative contraindication unless therapeutic donor insemination is an acceptable option. Absolute contraindications are active salpingitis, ovarian failure, and any medical condition making major surgery or pregnancy a significant health risk. These conditions include acquired immunodeficiency syndrome or human immunodeficiency virus–positive patients, and those with significant psychiatric or social problems that preclude parenting.

OPTIONS AND COST-BENEFIT ANALYSIS

After thoroughly understanding all the preoperative information, the patient can use a modified form of cost-benefit analysis to decide which options to pursue, including surgery. The expected benefit from any option or choice is equal to the product of the choice's outcome's utility multiplied by the probability of the outcome occurring. Value can be considered the intrinsic or objective worth of anything. It is often difficult to assign value because any given person will be influenced by personal, subjective criteria. A more useful term is *utility,* which is the subjective measure of value; the utility of any outcome is unique for each patient and example. How much value a given individual couple places on having their own biologic child, an adopted child, or a donor gamete child, for example, is the utility of each of those outcomes. The actual utility of an outcome is also difficult to measure and requires extensive discussion between the patient and her partner. The probability of surgical success is largely determined by the surgeon's information base and surgical skills. It is most useful to give the couple a percentage chance of success over a 1, 2, or 3-year interval based on estimated life table pregnancy rates, giving due consideration to each couples' unique circumstances. These can be difficult to obtain, although there are sources in the literature.[4, 9, 11] It is also frequently useful to give the couple a range of success. In addition, success should be presented in terms of live births for the patient. The loss rate from spontaneous abortions and ectopic pregnancies must be factored into the "success" rate. Given an ordered set of choices from the patient and a realistic estimate of the probability of success from the physician, the overall expected benefit from any given option can be determined.

Once the expected benefit is determined and the options prioritized, the costs associated with pursuing the option need to be considered. The costs include financial expenditure, the amount of time required to pursue the option, physical health risks, and emotional costs. These costs can also be considered as negative utilities. Once the benefits and costs all have been evaluated, it is obvious that the choosing of any option will imply that the expected benefit of that option is greater than the expected cost of the investigation and treatment. For an option to be chosen, then:

$$\text{Utility} \times \text{Probability of occurrence} > \text{Financial cost} + \text{Time cost} + \text{Physical cost} + \text{Emotional cost}$$

This process can be made somewhat more scientific, although also more complex, by using formal decision analysis, which is a scientific method of choosing between trade-offs.[24] A decision tree model can be established to evaluate different options. Each option can be evaluated by assigning to it a negative or positive utility, for example a number between −1 to +1, and a probability of it occurring. The product of utility multiplied by probability calculates an expected benefit for that option. The sum of the expected benefit for all of the possible outcomes yields a total expected benefit for that option. Each option can then be evaluated against the others. Figure 21–1 shows how this method might be used.[24]

The decision tree just discussed could represent the choice between tubal surgery to repair a single remaining tube after a prior salpingectomy for an ectopic pregnancy (option A) with the probability of intrauterine pregnancy (outcome 1 =

0.50) or subsequent ectopic pregnancy (outcome 2 = 0.20) versus pursuing IVF (option B) with the possibility of single (outcome 1 = 0.20) or multiple births (outcome 2 = 0.05) versus another ectopic pregnancy (outcome 3 = 0.04), with theoretical patient utilities assigned to each outcome. For this particular patient and clinical situation, option A, surgery, has a higher expected benefit of 0.45 compared with option B, IVF, of 0.15.

The structure of decision trees can be classified into just a few patterns. Therefore, a large number of surgical decisions can be described by a small number of decision trees. These decision trees can be simplified or expanded depending on the clinical situation.[24] At least the two best options should be included and options not clearly inferior to the best two should also be included. Probabilities should be derived from the literature and personal data. Probabilities can be modified if the characteristics of the patient do not match those in the data base for baseline probabilities.

Experienced Surgeon

Surgical treatment of infertility requires a surgeon who is familiar with the pathophysiology of infertility and possible

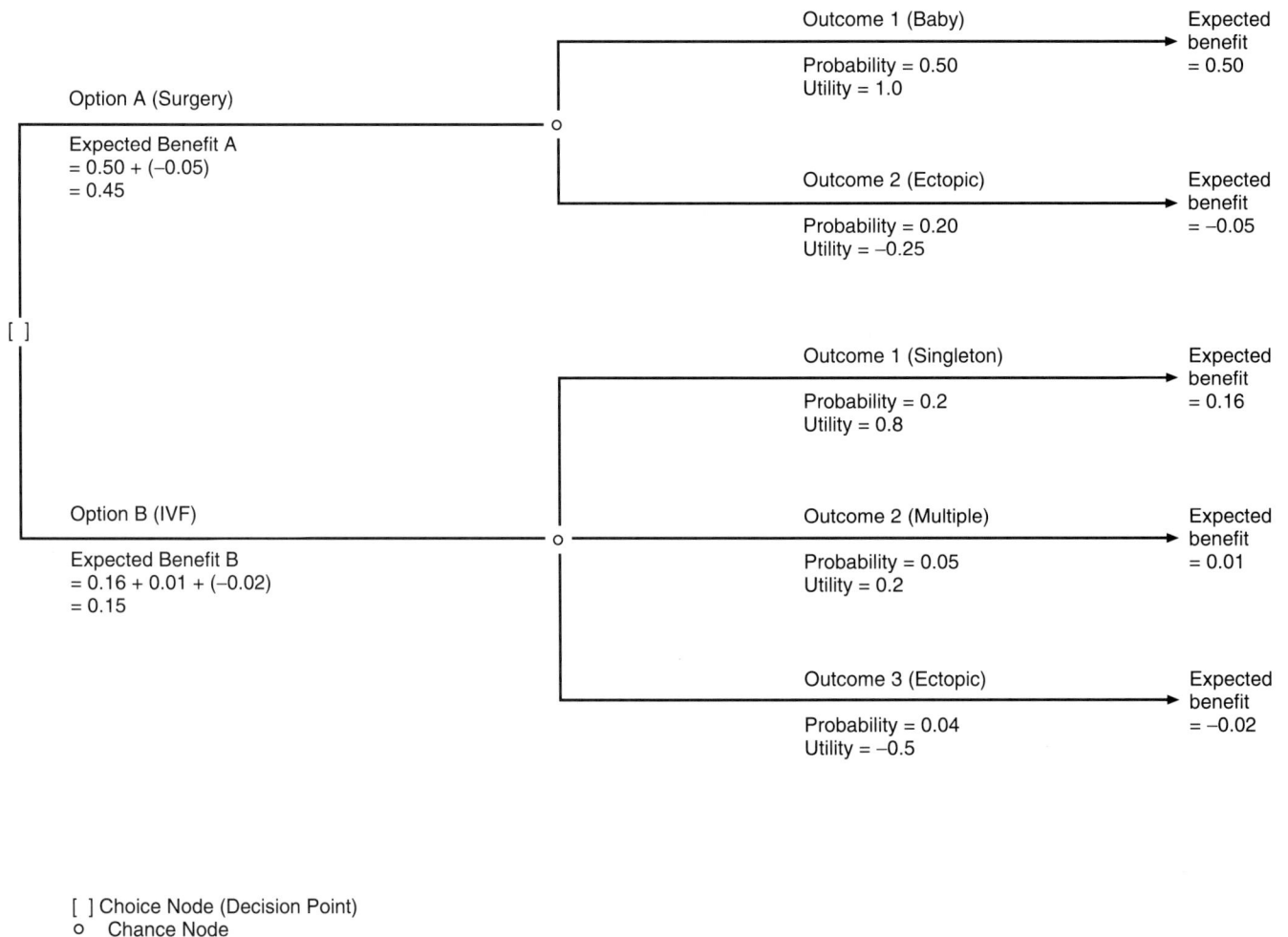

Option A (Surgery)
Expected Benefit A
= 0.50 + (−0.05)
= 0.45

Outcome 1 (Baby)
Probability = 0.50
Utility = 1.0
Expected benefit = 0.50

Outcome 2 (Ectopic)
Probability = 0.20
Utility = −0.25
Expected benefit = −0.05

Option B (IVF)
Expected Benefit B
= 0.16 + 0.01 + (−0.02)
= 0.15

Outcome 1 (Singleton)
Probability = 0.2
Utility = 0.8
Expected benefit = 0.16

Outcome 2 (Multiple)
Probability = 0.05
Utility = 0.2
Expected benefit = 0.01

Outcome 3 (Ectopic)
Probability = 0.04
Utility = −0.5
Expected benefit = −0.02

[ ] Choice Node (Decision Point)
o   Chance Node

FIGURE 21–1. Decision analysis. Example of surgery vs. in vitro fertilization (IVF). (Modified from Clarke JR. Decision making in surgical practice. World J Surg 1989; 13:245–251.)

therapeutic options, including no treatment, medical treatment, IVF, laparotomy, or laparoscopic surgery. Initially, surgeons acquire their skills in residency programs and then gradually increase their skills through experience. To acquire new surgical skills rapidly, the surgeon needs didactic and hands-on experience through courses, preceptorships, and assisting in the operating room. Each surgeon must then acquire surgical experience treating less severe problems before advancing to more complex procedures. Surgeons need to have a comprehensive understanding of normal and diseased pelvic anatomy, different surgical techniques, and the principles and application of mechanical, electrosurgical, and laser energy. Surgeons need to develop hand-eye coordination working from a video monitor with different instruments for operative laparoscopy or hysteroscopy, and operating microscopes for microsurgical procedures. Most important, each surgeon needs to develop an appreciation of the limitations of infertility surgery in his or her hands. This is obtained by ongoing careful evaluation of personal results and use of sound surgical judgment.

Adequate Facilities, Personnel, and Equipment

The technology available for reproductive surgery has increased dramatically in the past few years. Several principles regarding the surgical setting for infertility treatment can be stated. The facility needs to have an adequate-sized operating room for the equipment and adequate time for performance of the operation. Backup support, such as the ability to perform a laparotomy in the case of planned endoscopic procedures, provide blood transfusion, evaluate a frozen section, or transfer the patient to an acute care hospital from an ambulatory care facility, are mandatory.

Trained and motivated personnel, preferably who have worked together with the surgeon, are important for more complex cases. Also, more difficult cases can almost always be performed faster, better, and more safely with an assistant surgeon (preferably one who is also an experienced laparoscopist, hysteroscopist, or microsurgeon) who has worked with the surgeon.

Necessary equipment for operative laparoscopy includes an operative laparoscope with good optics, a high-resolution video camera and monitors, and an appropriate selection of instruments and energy sources. For hysteroscopy, appropriate carbon dioxide (CO_2) gas insufflators or fluid-distending media, as well as diagnostic and operative instruments are needed. A resectoscope and a laser may also be useful in some situations. For laparotomy, powered operative microscope and appropriate microsurgical instruments are needed for reanastomosis and fimbrioplasty. For many laparotomies, surgical loupes with 3 to 6× magnification may be as helpful as the operating microscope. All equipment needs to be checked before use, and critical equipment must be available from secondary sources in case of failure.

Informed Consent

Preoperatively, the patient needs to be thoroughly informed of the nature of the surgery, its indications, alternative approaches to management, potential complications and risks, and its potential benefits. Extensive education, including discussions, written material, and possibly videotapes, can be helpful. Emotional support needs to be provided and determination made if the patient's physical health is acceptable for surgery.

At the preoperative visit surgeons have the responsibility to review their protocol for surgery, perform a history and physical examination, and provide patients with general information about surgery and specific information about their own operation. Whenever possible, such information should be provided in a written form for the patient to review before and after the preoperative visit. At this visit the patient can also be prescribed the appropriate analgesics, bowel preparation medications, antibiotics, antiemetics, and tranquilizers or sleeping pills on a short-term basis if appropriate. The need for an empty bowel, bladder, and stomach at the time of surgery should be reemphasized. The patient's history should be evaluated for factors that may alter the surgical approach. These could include previous laparotomy with complications, abdominal adhesions, previous bowel disease and peritonitis, colostomy, obesity, pelvic kidney, or risk of malignancy. This could involve a decision to alter the type of incision, perform a laparotomy, a hysteroscopy, dilation and curettage, salpingoscopy, hysterosalpingography, or open laparoscopy. A few gynecologists prefer routine use of open laparoscopy because of theoretically increased safety of the procedure. However, open laparoscopy does increase the time required to enter the abdominal cavity and can hinder mobility of the laparoscopic sheath. Other surgeons use open laparoscopy in selected patients with suspected intra-abdominal adhesions. However, there are no data that justify its routine use or demonstrate reduced morbidity in patients with intra-abdominal adhesions.

Indications for In Vitro Fertilization

IVF is the appropriate approach for patients with severe pelvic disease, in particular those with extensive, dense adhesions; severe intraluminal fimbrial agglutination; large hydrosalpinges; fibrotic tubes with thick walls; sterilization involving residual tubal length shorter than 3 to 4 cm or removal of a significant portion of the distal tube; women having had two ectopic pregnancies; women with failed reconstructive pelvic surgery, especially those not amenable to laparoscopic surgery; and those with bilateral, bipolar disease.

IVF should also be strongly considered for women in the 35- to 38-year age range and as the treatment of choice for women 38 to 39 years of age unless a surgical approach has a high chance of success. Women 40 years of age and older have a much poorer prognosis regardless of treatment. A special circumstance in which surgery in older women is often successful involves reversal of tubal sterilization in women with proven fertility, normal ovulation, and a partner with normal sperm.[25]

Couples who have male factor infertility, ovulation dysfunction, significant cervical factor, prolonged duration of infertility, or multiple factors causing infertility are generally better candidates for IVF than reconstructive pelvic surgery.

IVF offers the advantages of sperm processing, microoperative techniques, and gamete donation in selected couples.

IVF is the primary assisted reproductive technology treatment for patients with tubal disease. Carefully selected patients with minimal intraluminal damage may be candidates for gamete intrafallopian transfer (GIFT). At this time there is no documented benefit to performing zygote intrafallopian transfer rather than GIFT, or for transcervical GIFT.

Patients should not undergo IVF if they have significant concerns of a religious, moral, or ethical nature regarding the procedure. Patients also should not undergo IVF if they have medical risks that may be severely compounded by multiple pregnancy and if they are reluctant to agree to pregnancy reduction. Financial considerations may also make reconstructive surgery a more favorable option than IVF.

When considering reconstructive surgery and IVF one must recognize that only about three to five IVF cycles can be performed per year and therefore the fecundity per cycle needs to be compared with the monthly fecundity over 12 cycles that may occur following reconstructive surgery. Therefore, an improved fecundity associated with each cycle of IVF may be insufficient to overcome the larger number of cycles providing an opportunity for conception following tubal surgery.

It is clear that IVF has a major role to play in the surgical patient and also that surgery has a potentially major role to play in the IVF patient. Both modalities are complementary in offering patients optimal chances for pregnancy. It is the surgeon's responsibility to identify comprehensively the couple's situation and factors affecting prognosis for tubal surgery and IVF. Given this information, the surgeon can provide the couple with the appropriate information to help them decide which treatment modality may initially be the most appropriate. Frequently, one treatment modality may be followed by the other should the initial one not be successful. In this way the highest pregnancy rates can be achieved at the least cost for the patient. Increasing sophistication both in reconstructive pelvic surgery and the assisted reproductive technologies should ensure even higher success rates for both of these modalities in the future.

INTRAOPERATIVE PRINCIPLES OF INFERTILITY SURGERY

Anesthesia

Appropriate anesthesia is an important part of infertility surgery, especially operative laparoscopy. A well-trained anesthesiologist who is motivated to provide balanced general endotracheal anesthesia is required. Frequently, a nasogastric tube is indicated to deflate the stomach to avoid injury to the stomach during passage of the Veress needle or trocars. Some surgeons and anesthesiologists believe a nasogastric tube is mandatory. Careful monitoring of electrocardiogram, oximeter, and end-tidal volume can significantly improve safety for the patient. In selected patients, diagnostic hysteroscopy can be performed in an office setting with a mild tranquilizer and paracervical block.

Patient Position

At laparotomy the patient needs to be positioned supine so that the operative microscope and other equipment can be placed appropriately.

At laparoscopy the patient is placed in a modified lithotomy position, with her arm at her side on the side at which the surgeon stands. The other arm may be extended if carefully supported or placed at her side so that operating from either side can be performed if necessary. Trendelenburg position will help move the bowel out of the pelvis after the Veress needle and pneumoperitoneum have been established or at laparotomy once the cavity is entered. The legs need to be well supported, and if supported under the knee, mobilized approximately every 2 hours to help prevent compression injury to the nerves.

At hysteroscopy the legs need to be in a modified lithotomy position so that the surgeon can operate without hindrance.

Selection of Surgical Approach

Operative endoscopy has become the preferred operative treatment for most infertility surgery. The noted exceptions are tubal reanastomosis and myomectomy involving multiple, large, or intramural myomas. Compared with laparotomy, the laparoscopic modality provides significant additional benefits to patients, physicians, and society. The advantages of operative laparoscopy and laser technology are both general in nature as well as unique for specific conditions. However, operative endoscopy also has some limitations not associated with laparotomy (Table 21–4).

VISUALIZATION

Contemporary laparoscopes, light sources, and video equipment afford an excellent view of the pelvis for both the surgeon, operative assistants, and other operating room personnel.[26] The magnification provided by the laparoscope's 6 to 8× magnification when in close proximity to lesions may be particularly important for diagnosis of the multiple morphologic presentations of endometriosis; for operating on the bowel, ureter, or vessels; or for salpingolysis, ovariolysis, fimbrioplasty, and salpingostomy.[27, 28] Although magnification is not as great as that provided by the operating microscope, this is probably only a limiting factor in performing tubal reanastomosis and possibly fimbrioplasty. The laparoscope's angle of view of the pelvis affords superior visualization in the cul-de-sac, under the ovaries, and in the upper abdomen

---

TABLE 21–4. Characteristics of Laparoscopic Surgery

Advantages
 Improved visualization
 Simultaneous diagnosis and treatment
 Less tissue trauma
 Reduced de novo adhesion formation
 Lower complication rates
 Shorter, easier recovery
 Reduced social costs because recovery is faster
Disadvantages
 Two-dimensional view
 Resolution of television monitor less than direct vision
 Decreased tactile sense
 Coordination of movement with assistant surgeon more difficult
 Complications associated with instrument insertion and
  pneumoperitoneum
 Unipolar electrosurgery complications unique to laparoscopy

relative to laparotomy. A high level of operative precision can be attained because of this improved visualization. This precision can be enhanced by palpation with instruments to ascertain tissue consistency.

Nevertheless, operative laparoscopy has some unique disadvantages and complications not associated with laparotomy. The laparoscopic view is two dimensional rather than three dimensional as at laparotomy. Also, the resolution of the video monitor is not as good as direct vision at laparotomy. The surgeon must control the surgical field almost entirely through the two-dimensional video monitor, a more difficult process than operating at laparotomy. Coordination of intraoperative movements with the assistant surgeon is also more difficult. Fatigue can occur more easily because of the need to view the monitor in one place at all times.

SIMULTANEOUS DIAGNOSIS AND TREATMENT

Diagnostic laparoscopy provides a relatively safe and simple method of diagnosing most anatomic gynecologic disease states. The choice of therapy can also be determined at the time of diagnostic laparoscopy. When appropriate, operative laparoscopy enables treatment to be initiated and possibly completed at the same time. Medical and surgical treatment modalities sometimes have the same results, but surgical treatment completed at the time of diagnosis has a distinct advantage over medical therapy because of decreased time, cost, and side effects.[11] The patient can also be spared a second operation (laparotomy) if operative laparoscopy can be performed at the time of diagnosis.[29] However, it is more important to give the patient the best operation possible in the particular surgeon's hands rather than to compromise by performing a poor operation at laparoscopy.

TISSUE TRAUMA

Operative laparoscopy offers several advantages to laparotomy with respect to surgical tissue trauma. The abdominal cavity is not open to the drying air of the operating room, preserving tissue integrity. This is especially true when copious irrigation is performed throughout the procedure. The tissue is also not cooled by room air at laparoscopy, further reducing tissue trauma. However, at laparoscopy tissue can be cooled by CO_2 gas at room temperature if constant irrigation is not carried out. Tissue is not exposed to foreign bodies such as talc from gloves. Most important, under ideal circumstances, tissue is not grasped, squeezed, or abraded by handling and packing off the bowel as occurs at laparotomy. This maintains serosal integrity and reduces the risk of de novo adhesion formation. These advantages are especially pronounced when treating disease that is difficult to visualize at laparotomy, such as under the ovaries and deep in the cul-de-sac. However, although palpation of structures can be performed with instruments, tactile sense is less than that obtained digitally at laparotomy.

ADHESION FORMATION

It is possible that operative laparoscopy produces superior results to laparotomy with respect to the reformation of adhesions removed at the initial surgery, but this has not yet been conclusively demonstrated.[23] However, studies strongly suggest that de novo adhesion formation is less frequent following operative laparoscopy compared with laparotomy.[1, 21, 23, 30] The reduced de novo adhesion formation may be due to reduced tissue trauma or a reduction in oozing from small vessels immediately after surgical injury owing to the increased intra-abdominal pressure created by the pneumoperitoneum. Earlier ambulation and absence of packing off the bowel may also result in less ileus and subsequent mechanical disruption of early-forming adhesions by bowel peristalsis.

COMPLICATION RATES

Complication rates for operative laparoscopy are low. One American study reported a 1.8% intraoperative and 0.9% postoperative complication rate, with only one patient in 821 requiring laparotomy.[31] Another American study had similar low complication rates.[32] A French study of 1429 laparoscopies reported three laparotomies and an overall morbidity of 1.2%.[33] A large German study of 249,467 laparoscopies had a serious complication rate of 1.97% and a laparotomy rate of 1.66%. Death occurred in approximately 1 in 35,000 cases.[34] It is believed that these rates are comparable to or better than those at laparotomy.[31] However, no well-controlled studies have directly compared laparoscopy and laparotomy complication rates. The most serious common laparoscopic injuries are injuries to the internal organs, especially bowel, hemorrhage, and anesthetic complications. The earlier postoperative ambulation following operative laparoscopy should reduce the rate of pneumonia and thrombophlebitis.[35] Laparoscopic surgery may be safer than laparotomy for the surgeon because of a lower risk of percutaneous injury from scalpels or other sharp instruments.[36]

Although the rate of complications associated with operative laparoscopy may be lower than that of laparotomy, certain complications are unique to laparoscopy.[37] Anesthesia complications such as respiratory embarrassment because of increased intra-abdominal CO_2 gas pressure and deep Trendelenburg position can occur. Subcutaneous emphysema, pneumothorax, and pneumomediastinum are more common. Cervical laceration and uterine perforation may occur with placement of manipulating instruments. Inadvertent Verres needle placement and CO_2 embolism can result in cardiovascular collapse, as can laceration of a major blood vessel. Injury to organs from blind placement of instruments occurs more often than at laparotomy. This risk may be reduced by careful placement of Veress needles and laparoscopic trocars. In addition, secondary instruments should be inserted under direct vision. Unipolar electrosurgical injury poses a greater risk at laparoscopy than at laparotomy. These injuries may also be less recognizable at laparoscopy than at laparotomy. Hemorrhage may be more difficult to control because of reduced ability to apply pressure. In addition, some operations, such as myomectomy, may take longer at laparoscopy. It is important for all surgeons to be aware of these differences between laparotomy and laparoscopy.

Surgical Approach to Adnexal Masses

Laparoscopic treatment of adnexal masses has been controversial because of concern that diagnosis of an ovarian cancer may be missed, that contamination of the pelvis with an ovarian cancer may result in reduced survival, and that unnecessary laparoscopic surgery may be performed in a cancer patient who needs laparotomy. This issue was highlighted by a questionnaire review that collected 42 cases of ovarian masses treated laparoscopically that were eventually determined to be malignant.[38] Capsule rupture and delay of treatment raised concern about the appropriateness of the laparoscopic approach to adnexal masses. Although delay of treatment can be avoided, capsule rupture inevitably occurs in at least some patients who have an ovarian malignancy treated laparoscopically. Whether or not such rupture affects prognosis is actively debated.[39, 40] A set of guidelines for laparoscopic surgery in the management of ovarian cysts has recently been presented by a group of gynecologic oncologists, reproductive endocrinologists, and ultrasonographers.[41] These have been summarized in Table 21–5.

Patient history is an important factor in determining approach. The menopausal patient should have bilateral oophorectomy for adnexal mass, without spillage of any cystic contents. Laparotomy should be performed immediately if this is not possible. A patient with family history of ovarian cancer should be strongly considered for laparotomy. Younger patients with a short duration of symptoms and minimal probability of malignancy should be considered for laparoscopy. Pelvic findings are also important. Large (>5 cm), firm, and fixed masses are much more likely to be malignant and also much more likely to present difficult surgical technique problems. Such cases are almost always better managed at laparotomy. However, large masses that are believed to be endometriomas can likely be treated effectively at laparoscopy.[42]

Preoperative testing can also help determine the best approach. Nonmalignant lesions tend to be smaller than 5 cm in diameter, unilocular, unilateral, completely cystic, have a smooth border, and not be associated with peritoneal fluid. Findings other than these increase the chance of malignancy

and the desirability of performing a laparotomy. Tumor markers such as CA 125, alpha-fetoprotein and human chorionic gonadotropin generally lack sufficient sensitivity and specificity to independently identify the best approach but may be helpful in conjunction with other tests and may help to follow the course of the disease postoperatively. Additional studies that some consider may be helpful include MRI or CT scan, carcinoembryonic antigen, needle aspiration for cytology, and ovarian cystoscopy and biopsy.

The patient should be informed that the risk of an ovarian neoplasm being malignant increases with age from 8% at less than 20 years, to 35% at ages 40 through 49, with the risk of low malignant potential neoplasms being 0% and 6%, respectively.[43] Each patient needs to be made aware of the controversies surrounding laparoscopic management of adnexal masses and participate in the decision regarding surgical approach.

However, most adnexal masses are not malignant. Therefore, many experienced laparoscopists believe that by following careful guidelines, the risk of unwittingly treating an adnexal malignancy at laparoscopy can be reduced to one in several hundreds of patients.

Peritoneal washings should be obtained on entering the abdominal cavity. These should be evaluated and immediate laparotomy performed if suspicious or malignant cells are found. Careful exploration of the entire abdominopelvic cavity for evidence of malignant lesions should be performed. Biopsies of suspicious lesions should be obtained for frozen section. The ovary should be evaluated carefully for excrescences or other suspicious findings and biopsies obtained if indicated for frozen section. Oncology consultation should be considered. Removal of the adnexal lesion should be performed without rupturing the cyst and avoiding leakage into the pelvic cavity by the use of bags or other laparoscopy technologies.

Because the actual extent of harm to the patient should a malignancy be opened is controversial, many laparoscopists believe that adnexal masses can reasonably be approached laparoscopically. Should an adnexal mass be found to be malignant, contemporary management would dictate immediate laparotomy for staging and treatment. It is possible that adnexal malignancies may be treated laparoscopically in the future.[44] Although some surgeons are concerned by the possible spillage of endometriotic or dermoid cyst contents at laparoscopy, there are no data to prove that such spillage causes a worsened prognosis. With the increasing availability of sophisticated technology, such as plastic bags, even small amounts of spillage now often can be prevented at laparoscopy most the time.

Diagnosis and Preparation for Therapeutic Intervention

Careful, systematic initial evaluation of the pelvic and abdominal cavity at laparoscopy or laparotomy, or uterine cavity at hysteroscopy, is mandatory prior to undertaking therapeutic intervention. The type and degree of disease then can be determined and optimal approach decided. All organs and structures must be carefully evaluated. Potential additional needed equipment for the operation can be requested from the circulating staff who will be able to anticipate the sur-

---

TABLE 21–5. Guidelines for Laparoscopic Surgery in the Management of Ovarian Cysts

History
 Patient age
 Menopausal status
 Duration of symptoms
 Differential diagnosis
 Cancer (personal and family)
Physical Examination
 Size
 Consistency
 Fixation
Ultrasonography
 Size, unilocular or multilocular, unilateral or bilateral, cystic or solid,
  smooth or irregular border, peritoneal fluid present or absent
Tumor Markers
 CA 125, alpha-fetoprotein, human chorionic gonadotropin
Informed Consent
Intraoperative
 Peritoneal washings
 Exploration of all peritoneal surfaces and biopsy as indicated
 Exploration of ovarian mass for external excrescences or other suspicious
  findings
 Frozen section
Laparotomy
 Immediate for suspicious or confirmed malignant masses
 Avoidance of cyst rupture

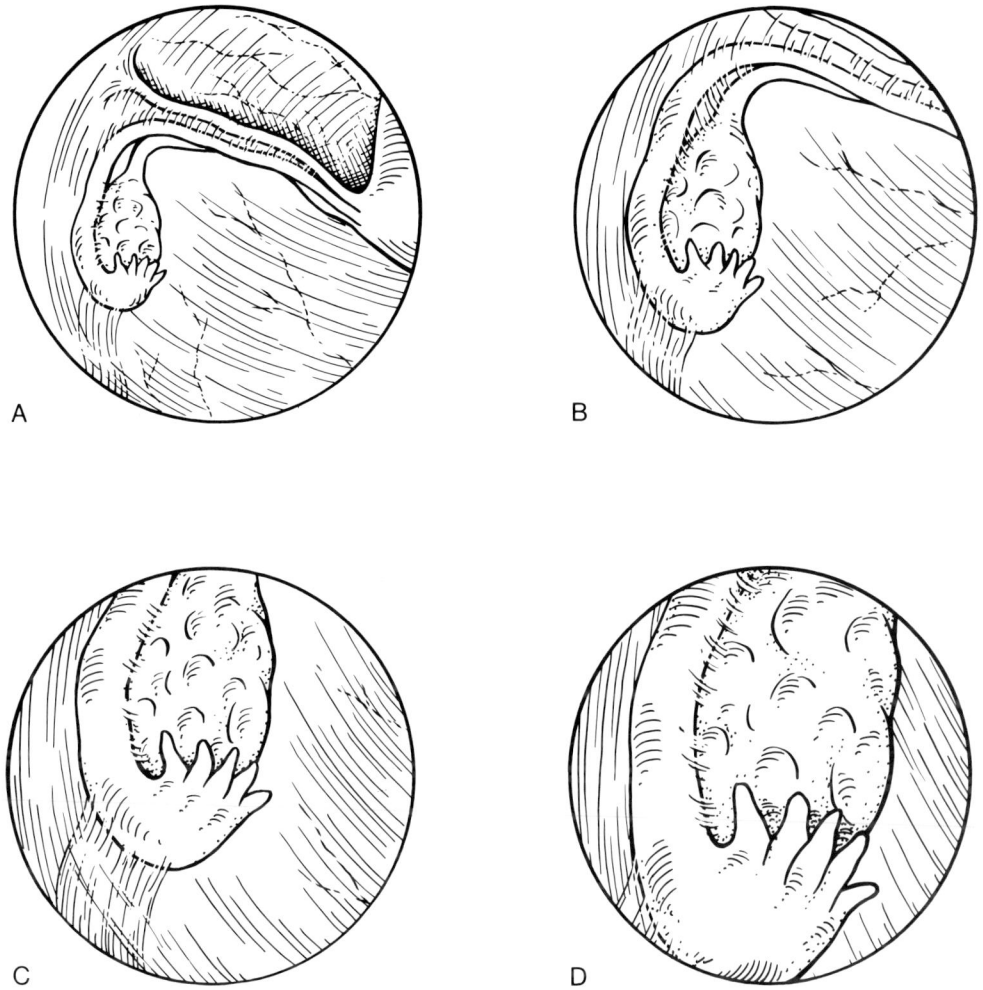

FIGURE 21–2. Magnification and demagnification with the laparoscope. *A,* Half size (demagnified), at approximately 5 cm from the structure. *B,* Actual size, at approximately 4 cm from the structure. *C,* Magnified ×2, at approximately 3 cm from the structure. *D,* Magnified ×4, at approximately 2 cm from the structure.

geon's requirements. Additional incisions or enlargement of the existing incision then can be performed if needed. Having adequate exposure is critical to the success of infertility surgery. For most infertility laparotomies, a Pfannenstiel incision is adequate. For microsurgical procedures, a generous incision is usually necessary to allow easy and gentle manipulation of the pelvic organs into the microscope's surgical field of view. A midline incision may be required for large myomas. At laparoscopy at least two, and often three, lower abdominal incisions may be needed. Usually, 5-mm ports are sufficient, but for knot tying, morcellation, and removal of larger pieces of tissue, 10- to 12-mm ports are more satisfactory. A 20-mm port is available for removal of large masses of tissue. At hysteroscopy, operative intervention is facilitated by the use of dilators to obtain easy access of larger instruments such as resectoscopes. Use of a laminaria preoperatively can minimize the risk of cervical laceration or injury in selected cases.

Visualization of Surgical Field

At operative laparoscopy, visualization of the pelvis under direct vision without the camera at the beginning and end of surgery facilitates diagnosis of subtle disease such as various types of endometriotic lesions and confirms their removal.

The laparoscope magnifies tissue so that when the laparoscope is about 1 cm from tissue, the magnification is approximately six times, at 2 cm four times, at 3 cm two times, and at 4 cm no magnification. At distances greater than 4 cm, demagnification occurs and structures appear smaller through the laparoscope (Fig. 21–2). Hysteroscopes provide similar magnification and demagnification. At laparotomy, magnifying loupes up to approximately 6× magnification are available and operating microscopes to approximately 30×. As magnification increases, visualization is improved in the observed area, but it is important to recognize that overall perspective of the surgical field is decreased.

The most important surgical principle is control of the surgical field. Control of the surgical field involves an awareness of the anatomy of the entire surgical field, knowledge of the characteristics and location of tissue being operated on, and a perspective on the relative location of the tissue being operated on to contiguous structures, especially those being avoided such as ureter, bowel, and vessels. Control also involves the ability to deliver the energy being used in a precise and knowledgeable manner. Maximum control should be maintained at all times. At operative laparoscopy and hysteroscopy, the surgeon is working without binocular vision and also with a camera that is placed at a distance from the surgical field. In addition, instruments are being used rather than hands to grasp. Depending on surgical procedures being performed, small movements of the hand may result in larger movement of the instrument. Therefore, the apparent control of the surgical field is less than one has at laparotomy, although the actual degree of control can be maximized significantly with surgical experience.

All surgical techniques should attempt to maximize exposure, minimize trauma, and produce the desired result in the minimum amount of time. Hemostasis must be carefully maintained at all times. It is important to place the appropriate instruments through the appropriate abdominal incisions to optimize surgical technique. This often requires moving instruments from site to site throughout the operation. Irrigation and aspiration can significantly assist in good visualization and in the maintenance of a clean surgical field. For procedures with a relatively high risk of complications, it is necessary to evaluate whether the benefit of the procedure outweighs the risk. For some surgeons this may occur relatively frequently. Alternative methods of treatment should be carried out in such situations.

Selection of Energy Source

LASER ENERGY

The last 10 years have witnessed the widespread application of lasers in the treatment of gynecologic disease. Lasers have also been an important factor spurring the dramatic developments in laparoscopic surgery. Some important advantages of lasers are (1) the ability to select from a variety of wavelengths that produce different tissue effects; (2) the ability to control precisely the laser energy and thereby the tissue effect; (3) the "no-touch" surgical capability of the laser; and (4) the availability of different delivery systems (Table 21–6). Lasers also have some important disadvantages (see Table 21–6).

The CO_2 laser was the first laser to be used extensively in gynecology and remains the most commonly used. Other lasers have also gained recognition for their utility. Some of these lasers and their properties are listed in Table 21–7.

The different tissue-absorption characteristics of different lasers occur because of both the different wavelengths of the photons (which are the laser energy) and the characteristics of the tissue with which the photons interact. With the CO_2 laser, absorption of photons by the tissue water results in instantaneous heating and conversion of tissue water to water vapor. The resulting rapid tissue expansion results in an explosion of the tissue; this process is called *vaporization*. The CO_2 laser generally has a depth of penetration of less than 1 mm and produces a discrete and reproducible lesion. The CO_2 laser, because of these properties, is highly specific but

a poor coagulating instrument. The laparoscopic CO_2 laser beam can work at any distance from tissue with a fairly constant tissue effect. This enables the surgeon to work close when magnification is needed or further away when not necessary. When the CO_2 laser beam is delivered directly through the operating channel of the laparoscope, the surgeon's second hand is not needed to deliver energy to the pelvis and can be used for manipulation of other instruments. Tissue does not have to be touched or moved to be operated on, reducing tissue trauma and facilitating dissection in anatomically difficult areas.

The neodymium:YAG (Nd:YAG) laser has a wavelength associated with absorption by tissue proteins and significant forward scattering of the photons in the laser beam at the time the tissue is struck. This results in a markedly increased thermal effect of the Nd:YAG laser beam deep in the tissue compared with the surface on which the laser beam strikes. This can be dangerous if the deeper tissue heats up and explodes, an effect called the "popcorn" effect and one to be avoided. Newer delivery systems and sculpted fibers avoid this problem. The Nd:YAG laser can also be used with a touch or no-touch technique. Nevertheless, the Nd:YAG laser, although having little precision, is an excellent coagulator, and therefore has some useful applications. The argon and KTP-532 lasers are absorbed by hemoglobin molecules, and heat is distributed much more widely in the tissue than with the CO_2 laser but less than the Nd:YAG laser. Therefore, the argon and KTP-532 lasers cut better than Nd:YAG and less than CO_2 lasers and have better coagulation properties than the CO_2 laser and less than the Nd:YAG.

Tissue effects vary significantly depending on the power density of the laser beam. Power density is directly related to the power in watts from the laser and inversely related to the square of the diameter of the laser beam. Therefore, small spot sizes generally result in significantly greater penetration and destruction of tissue over a smaller area than a large spot size, which produces a much shallower, but also wider lesion. These variations in effect can also be altered by the use of sapphire laser tips with Nd:YAG lasers, sculptured fibers with Nd:YAG, KTP-532, or argon lasers, rigid waveguides, and contact versus noncontact Nd:YAG, KTP-532, and argon laser surgery. Knowledge of the different physical properties and clinical relevance of these differences is essential prior to using lasers.[45]

A principle that always needs to be considered when using a laser is that thermal injury is time related and independent of power density. This means that the degree of thermal injury to the tissue increases with the duration of time that the laser beam dwells on any given portion of the tissue. Carbon char can be created, especially by the CO_2 laser. Carbonization occurs after vaporization where there is burning at the base of the lesion leaving it black with carbon char. The long-term effect of these carbon particles is probably innocuous but unknown. These particles should be washed away with the irrigation fluid and aspirated out of the pelvis.

Training and credentialing of personnel to use lasers can be time consuming and expensive. This is true not only for the physician who must invest a significant amount of time and money to become well trained but also for the nursing and hospital staff who must become familiar with the equipment. However, investment in this aspect of a laser program is imperative if high-quality service is to be provided.

TABLE 21–6. Characteristics of Laser Surgery

Advantages
  Unique characteristics of different lasers
  Precision of laser energy
  "No touch" technique
  Multiple delivery systems
Disadvantages
  Unique characteristics of different lasers
  Cost of equipment
  Need for specialized training for surgeon and operating room personnel

TABLE 21–7. Characteristics of Surgical Lasers

	Laser Medium			
Characteristics	CO_2	Argon	KTP532	Nd:YAG
Type	Gas	Gas	Crystal	Crystal
Wavelength	10.6 μ	0.488 + 0.514 μ	0.532 μ	1.06 μ
Absorbed by	Water	Hemoglobin/melanin	Hemoglobin/melanin	Tissue protein
Penetration	1 mm	2–3 mm	2–3 mm	5–7 mm
Delivery	Mirror system	Fiberoptic	Fiberoptic	Fiberoptic
Coagulation	Low	Fair	Fair	High
Cutting	High	Low	Low	Fair

ELECTROSURGICAL ENERGY

Electrosurgical principles are poorly understood by many gynecologists. Nevertheless, an understanding of electrosurgery is critically important if this energy source is to be used effectively and safely in reproductive surgery. Concepts of current, voltage, and resistance, which are related through Ohm's Law (current = voltage divided by resistance) are imperative. Power is the energy produced or consumed over time and is equal to current multiplied by volts.

Direct current involves the flow of electrons in only one direction. With alternating current, the direction of flow is constantly being reversed. The number of times the current changes direction per second is called the *frequency*. The concept of capacitance, or storage of charge, is also important to understand. Most important in the understanding of electrosurgery is the difference between unipolar and bipolar surgery. With unipolar surgery a small electrode that is used by the surgeon is the active electrode, and a large "ground" electrode is placed at a remote site to carry the electron flow out of the body. Very-high-power density current is concentrated at the small surface area of the active electrode resulting in tissue effects, whereas the current at the larger ground electrode is dispersed over a wider area so that the low-power density does not affect the tissue. With unipolar electrosurgery, the flow of electrons from the active or surgically controlled electrode to the ground electrode follows the path of least resistance and cannot be controlled by the surgeon. With bipolar electrosurgery, the flow of electrons occurs between one electrode of the surgical instrument to the second electrode of the instrument and therefore results in a much more controllable and localized thermal injury to the tissue.

It is also important to understand the difference between cutting current and coagulation current. With cutting current, the tissue is heated so rapidly the cells are vaporized. This type of energy is produced by a sine wave or nonmodulated current. Superficial coagulation or hemostasis is best obtained by producing sparks to coagulate or char tissue without cutting the tissue. This is called *fulguration*. This requires a much higher voltage than cutting current. The voltage is high enough to produce sparks but low enough that the tissue is not vaporized. Intermittent short bursts of high voltage produces this result and are called *coagulation, or modulated current*. Desiccation occurs when electrical current is passed through the tissue, causing heating and drying of the tissue when water leaves in a vaporous state from the tissue. This results in coagulation of deeper tissues and is best obtained with a high-frequency, low-voltage current in contact with the tissue. A special situation with unipolar electrosurgery exists at laparoscopy, where the use of mal-functioning instruments or those with both conductive and nonconductive materials in the instruments passing through the abdominal wall, can result in unrecognized current flow to organs out of the surgical field and subsequent organ injury. Newer equipment is available to prevent this problem. All surgeons must have an understanding of basic electrosurgical principles to use this energy source effectively and safely.[46]

MECHANICAL ENERGY

The use of scissors to dissect is obviously the oldest and most widely used energy source. Advantages include their easy availability, familiarity, "feel" for the tissue, and cost. Disadvantages include the fact that nondisposable scissors frequently are too dull to work well, are associated with more bleeding because of lack of thermal effect, and often require more tissue manipulation. Disposable instruments that usually cut well are expensive.

CHOICE OF ENERGY SOURCE

The choice of energy source is primarily dependent on the surgeon. The CO_2 laser has the advantage of being extremely precise and causing limited thermal injury away from the site of impact. Superpulse lasers provide more energy over a shorter period than continuous wave lasers and therefore produce less thermal injury. The newer ultrapulse laser also provides very high power, which allows even faster dissection than with superpulse lasers and the ability to vary the amount of power and the amount of coagulating effect. This laser is therefore desirable for precise work around the bowel, ureter, and other critical structures. Some surgeons prefer the Nd:YAG, argon, or KTP-532 lasers because of the ability to use fibers and their coagulating effect. This coagulating effect would seem to be much less desirable when performing more precise dissection. The use of sculptured tips can improve their precision. Many surgeons prefer electrosurgery because of their familiarity with it, its easy availability, and low cost. A major difficulty with unipolar electrosurgery is the risk of injury to other organs from unrecognized electrical energy burns. Some surgeons prefer scissors dissection. Several innovative instruments for stapling, suturing, and bowel anastomosis currently are only available as disposable instruments. Their cost is sometimes justified by benefits provided to the patient through their use.

Operating Room Safety

Operating room safety is important. Numerous regulatory bodies exist at the federal, state, and local levels to help ensure operating room safety.[47] National standards and regulations have been developed by the American National Standards Institute (ANSI), which is a nongovernmental organization of experts who determine appropriate standards in various fields. The published standards are referred to and identified as ANSI Z136.1 (ANSI, Inc., 1430 Broadway, New York, NY 10018). Another agency is the Center for Devices and Radiological Health, which is the regulatory arm of the Food and Drug Administration, which is chartered by Congress to standardize the manufacture of laser units. A third federal agency is the Occupational Safety and Health Administration. This regulatory agency is responsible for ensuring worker safety. In addition to federal regulations, states also have agencies whose responsibility is to ensure operating room safety. Local ordinances and hospital policy may also add further regulations to the operating room. It is important that surgeons be aware of and abide by these safety standards.

Principles of safety can be reduced to several issues easily remembered by surgeons. Surgeons and operating room personnel need to be familiar with the operating principles and actual operation of equipment they use. They need to know the purpose and meaning of dials and switches necessary to operate equipment. They need to know the appropriate clinical use of the equipment. Equipment should be placed so as to minimize the possibility of confusion between instruments and foot pedals, such as those providing electrosurgical or laser energy. Equipment should be located so as to minimize interference with tasks performed by all operating room personnel, including surgeons, assistants, anesthesiologists, scrub nurses, and circulators. Electrical, suction, and other lines should be placed so as to minimize interference with the operative field and with the movement of operating room personnel. Any malfunctioning equipment should not be used, and backup equipment for essential instruments should be available. Personnel should exercise care when moving about the operating room. Appropriate precautions to prevent electrical, fire, or laser injury should be followed rigorously. The surgeon must give especial attention to the safety of the patient, who is asleep and more vulnerable to injury.

Potential hazards to surgical personnel include direct injury from the laser or electrosurgical instruments. Equipment can also be physically hazardous because of its physical size and high-voltage electronics. Inhalation of particulate matter in the laser plume can cause tracheobronchial irritation, pneumonitis, and possible transmission of viral particles, tumor cells, or deoxyribonucleic acid fragments, which can cause infection or have mutagenic properties. Precautions to prevent inhalation should be taken.

Special Techniques—Reduction of Adhesion Formation

Numerous factors contribute to adhesion formation.[48] These include tissue trauma, which can be reduced by gentle tissue handling and avoidance of exposure to air drying by constant irrigation and shorter operating times. Infection can also cause adhesion formation, but its risk can be reduced by the use of prophylactic antibiotics. Ischemia is a major cause of adhesions but can be reduced by not placing the tissue on tension with sutures. Deperitonealized surfaces regenerate a new serosal layer if other pelvic structures do not contact the fibrin mesh on the deperitonealized surface.

Methods used to minimize postoperative adhesion formation include the use of dextran, heparin, steroids, fibrinolytic agents, nonsteroidal anti-inflammatory agents, and progesterone. All these methods are of unproven efficacy. The placement of large volumes of fluid in the pelvis has also been popularized more recently and may be of some benefit in producing a fluid bath, but again prospective randomized studies have not yet confirmed the efficacy of this treatment. Interceed TC7 (Ethicon, Inc., Somerville, NJ) and Gore-Tex (WL Gore and Associates, Inc., Flagstaff, AZ) are newer modalities for adhesion prevention that show some promise but require further evaluation.

Hemorrhage can facilitate adhesion formation when the fibrin clot provides a matrix for invasion by fibroblasts. Use of magnification and bipolar electrosurgery can reduce oozing, as can avoidance of aspirin and nonsteroidal anti-inflammatory drugs for several weeks before surgery. Techniques for hemostasis include the injection of a dilute solution of vasopressin into the base of a myoma for myomectomy. It is also important to control bleeding quickly at laparoscopy and hysteroscopy because bleeding that would ordinarily be insignificant at laparotomy can quickly obscure the surgeon's view, resulting potentially in the need for laparotomy or transfusion. Hemostasis can also be improved by coagulating or isolating a vessel before cutting it. Hemostasis may be facilitated by use of the CO_2 laser as well as fiber lasers. The microbipolar and large bipolar forceps should also be available at all times. The maintenance of hemostasis increases the surgeon's ability to perform the surgery without using clips, staples, sutures, or Roeder loops, which are foreign bodies that can increase adhesion formation. Foreign bodies such as suture should be used as little as possible because these have been shown to be associated with adhesion formation.[49] It is possible that the multiple end-organ effects caused by the hypoestrogenism associated with GnRH agonist use may result in an improved pelvic milieu and fewer postoperative adhesions (Table 21–8).

ADJUVANT USE OF GnRH AGONISTS TO IMPROVE RESULTS OF REPRODUCTIVE SURGERY

It is possible, although not proved, that the use of GnRH agonists may improve results of infertility surgery.[50] The potential benefits include a reduction in size and endocrinologic activity of endometriotic lesions and possible reduction of adhesions. Metastatic endometriosis is treated. In addition, reduced vascularity in the pelvis may result in less blood loss, less tissue trauma, shorter operating time, and less inflammatory response. Reduced inflammation in the pelvis may result in decreased immunologic response from antibodies, macrophages, or antiendometrial antibodies, or other substances such as interleukins and growth hormones.[51] However, no properly designed studies have been performed that conclusively show that GnRH agonist use preoperatively or postoperatively improves pregnancy rates.[52]

Reduction of adenomyosis by GnRH agonist treatment may result in less operative bleeding and may promote proximal tubal patency if adenomyosis, endometriosis, or other hormonally related conditions have caused an obstruction. Pretreatment with GnRH agonists reduces the vascularity of

TABLE 21–8. Potential Benefits of Preoperative GnRH Agonists on Adhesion Formation Following Operative Endoscopy

Causes of Adhesion Formation	Potential Benefits of GnRH Agonists
Tissue trauma	Smaller incisions
	Fewer incisions
	Decreased tissue dissection
	Decreased bleeding in tissue
	Hysterectomy less likely with myomectomy
	Laparoscopic/hysteroscopic approach more likely
	Avoidance of uterine cavity at laparotomy for myomectomy
	Shorter operating time with smaller myomas
Infection	Endoscopic or vaginal approach more likely
	Decreased tissue dissection
	Shorter operating time with smaller myomas
Ischemia	Decreased sutures with smaller myomas
	Decreased need for coagulation
	Decreased tissue dissection
	Decreased operative blood loss
	Availability of autologous donation
Denuded surface apposition	Decreased tissue dissection
	Better visualization, decreased tissue manipulation
	Fewer incisions
	Smaller incisions
	Hysteroscopic approach
Foreign body	Decreased need for sutures
	Laparoscopic/hysteroscopic approach
	Decreased operative blood loss
Hemorrhage	Decreased dissection
	Decreased bleeding
	Reduced operating time
	Better visualization
	Laparoscopic/hysteroscopic approach

GnRH, gonadotropin-releasing hormone.

the cornual region, which may facilitate tubal reanastomosis and potentially improve patency rates. The usual duration of treatment preoperatively or postoperatively is 2 to 6 months.

GnRH agonist use can prevent the development of ovarian cysts and may be of some benefit in highly selected patients prior to ovarian surgery. In addition, agonists have been shown to reduce both uterine and myoma size by an average of approximately 50% after 3 to 4 months of treatment. However, variation in response is marked between patients and myomas. Regrowth of myomas and return to pretreatment uterine size also occurs within several months following discontinuation of agonist use. However, the agonist may be of benefit preoperatively.[50, 53, 54] Reduction in myoma volume has several potential benefits. The feasibility of myomectomy rather than hysterectomy is increased, as is the possibility of a laparoscopy approach rather than a laparotomy. Reduced uterine volume also means that fewer and smaller incisions may be required, thus facilitating operative technique, decreasing operative time, and reducing blood loss and the risk of postoperative infection. Less tissue trauma occurs, more normal tissue is preserved, and risk of adhesions may be decreased. The smaller uterine and myoma size also results in less risk of injury to other critical organs and allows easier ovarian assessment. It may also allow a Pfannenstiel rather than a vertical midline incision to be performed. Further, a vaginal hysterectomy may be possible, resulting in less febrile morbidity, fewer transfusions, and decreased recovery time.

The reduction in blood flow to the pelvic organs may have several advantages.[55] The mean volume of blood lost at myomectomy and hysterectomy is reduced, as is the risk of blood transfusion.[56] The major potential complication of GnRH agonist treatment is profuse hemorrhage occurring 5 to 10 weeks after therapy is initiated.[57, 58] This occurs mainly with large submucosal myomas that have degenerated, allowing vessels within the myoma to bleed. Treatment requires immediate transfusion and myomectomy or hysterectomy.

The smaller uterine and myoma size resulting from preoperative GnRH agonists may allow the physician to pursue a hysteroscopic approach to submucous or intrauterine myomas. The use of a dilute solution of vasopressin injection (Pitressin is commonly prepared in concentrations ranging from 5 U in 100 mL to 20 U in 20 mL of normal saline) may result in less blood loss with myomectomy. Some surgeons are concerned about the use of any vasopressin because of the potential for cardiovascular side effects.

GnRH agonists have also been used prior to endometrial ablation because their use results in decreasing uterine blood loss or even amenorrhea prior to surgery.[59] This improves the patient's hematologic status and may provide a much clearer surgical field and less intraoperative bleeding.[60] Many clinicians feel that such preoperative treatment allows for a shorter operating time and improved outcome. GnRH agonists may also facilitate falloposcopy through reduction in endometrial and tubal mucosa thickness.[61] The use of GnRH agonists prior to surgery may reduce patient symptomatology, including pain and bleeding, allowing the patient time to undergo adequate preoperative evaluation and to facilitate scheduling of the procedure based on medical and patient needs.

The actual benefits of GnRH agonists in reproductive surgery are largely speculative. As noted, there are many potential uses for GnRH agonists, but prospective, randomized trials are needed to determine their efficacy compared with other treatment modalities and no treatment. The most common current use is to reduce myoma size before treatment by laparotomy, laparoscopy, or hysteroscopy.

No data are available to justify the routine use of postoperative hydrotubation to improve postsurgical patency and pregnancy rates.[62] It is also not proved that second-look laparoscopic adhesiolysis improves pregnancy rates.[63] Second-look procedures are generally not beneficial if performed by laparotomy but have been shown to reduce adhesions by approximately half when performed laparoscopically.[22, 64, 65] The timing of the second-look laparoscopy may be important, with earlier second-look laparoscopy patients having less dense and vascularized adhesions.[66] Early second-look laparoscopy should occur between approximately 10 days to 12 weeks after the initial surgery.

POSTOPERATIVE PRINCIPLES

Good postoperative care requires that the patient have realistic expectations. In cases in which extensive laparoscopic surgery has been performed, the patient may well not be prepared to go home within the usual 2 to 3 hours after the operation. She needs to understand that all patients recover differently and that extensive surgical treatment within the pelvis, even though through smaller incisions, is still associated with a more difficult recovery than a strictly diagnostic laparoscopy. The surgical center should follow up with patients after they have been sent home, as should the surgeon's office, to determine whether any problems were encountered in the early postoperative period. Patients should be seen or called by the physician within 1 or 2 days postoperatively so that the results of the operation can be discussed and the patient's welfare evaluated.

Superficial sutures should be removed by 2 to 4 days after laparoscopy so that skin scarring does not occur. Deep fascial sutures in laparoscopic puncture sites and laparotomy incisions should, of course, be left in situ. The patient should be instructed to maintain a light diet for several days and drink fluids as much as possible. Early ambulation is important, as is sufficient rest and avoidance of strenuous exercise for 2 weeks following hysteroscopy and laparoscopy. Coitus should be avoided for at least 2 weeks after laparoscopy or hysteroscopy and until all vaginal bleeding has stopped.

Following laparotomy, the patient will usually be hospitalized for 1 to 3 days. Tubal reanastomosis patients may sometimes be discharged within 24 hours to be followed 1 or 2 days later in the office. Patients with more extensive dissection and longer operations require somewhat longer hospital stays. Generally, patients should have nothing by mouth the day of surgery, and may have clear fluids on postoperative day 1. Full fluids can generally be tolerated towards the end of postoperative day 1. A mechanical soft diet can be initiated when the patient is passing flatus, usually later on postoperative day 1 or early on postoperative day 2. A glycerin suppository on the afternoon of postoperative day 1 often encourages bowel function, as does early ambulation. The patient can then gradually increase to a full diet.

Careful monitoring of intravenous fluids, electrolytes, and intake and output is mandatory while the patient is on intravenous fluids. These can be discontinued once the patient is drinking sufficiently without vomiting, usually about 24 hours following surgery.

On postoperative day 1, ambulation should be encouraged, and the Foley bladder catheter should be removed. Deep respirations using a Voldyne or other mechanical device helps reduce atelectasis and the risk of pneumonia. Intermittent leg and foot exercises help reduce the risk of thrombophlebitis. A hemogram, electrolytes, and chemistry panel should be obtained on postoperative day 1 to rule out bleeding, electrolyte imbalance, or organ dysfunction.

For pain, patients often require intramuscular narcotics, nonnarcotics, or intravenous analgesics controlled by the patient. Oral analgesics are sufficient for some patients. Most patients should be able to discontinue parenteral medication within 12 to 36 hours of surgery and all pain medications within a week of surgery.

Patients should be monitored postoperatively for vital signs, increasing pain, bleeding, or other signs of deterioration. The most important symptoms and signs to observe are those pertaining to cardiovascular stability, respiratory status, bowel function, operative site bleeding, wound infection, genitourinary infection or ureteral obstruction, and thrombophlebitis. Known medical problems must be carefully monitored and consultation sought as appropriate.

At discharge, the patient should have written and oral instructions regarding diet, exercise, rest, work, and sexual activity. These will, of course, depend on the individual patient. In general, however, patients should be on a regular diet within 5 days, get frequent walking of gradually increasing duration, not lift any weight heavier than 10 lb, and not participate in any formal exercise programs other than walking. The patient should be seen in the office about 1 week following surgery. The wound can be checked, pelvis evaluated, and general health status determined. The patient can usually be cleared medically to drive an automobile at 1 week. She should return 6 weeks postoperatively for a final checkup when recovery should almost be complete. A pelvic examination should be performed. The patient can usually return to work, activities of daily living, exercise, and sexual intercourse at that time.

Oral analgesics should be sufficient for pain relief once the patient is home. Complaints of pain not resolved by oral analgesics are sufficient to mandate an office visit. The patient should be seen by the physician for temperature elevations greater than 100.5°F occurring later than 2 days postoperatively. Urinary symptoms that arouse suspicion of complication include frequency, dysuria, hematuria, anuria, or flank pain. Bowel symptoms of diarrhea, constipation, blood in the stool, abdominal distention, increasing abdominal pain, nausea, and vomiting mandate a careful history and physical examination. Patients with reddened or tender wounds or calf tenderness should be seen, as well as those with cardiorespiratory symptoms. In addition, any altered or deteriorating health condition should alert the surgeon to the possibility of a postoperative complication and the need for immediate followup and consultation if necessary.

Management plans should be based on the surgical results, prognosis, and patient's desires. Other infertility factors such as ovulation, male, and cervical factor should be treated as clinically indicated. Hysterosalpingogram may be performed 3 to 12 months postoperatively for diagnostic and possibly therapeutic purposes in selected patients. A repeat laparoscopy should be performed 9 to 24 months postoperatively if the patient has not conceived and if the overall clinical situation and prognosis justifies a repeat operation. If the patient had a limited prognosis following the initial surgery or has additional important fertility problems, IVF, adoption, or childfree living should be seriously considered as alternative approaches.

CONCLUSION

The past decade has seen major developments that have provided many advantages to patients, physicians, and society. Many of these developments have depended on an exponential growth of technology. Earlier, these included the widespread use of microsurgery and microsurgical techniques. This was followed by the use of the CO_2, Nd:YAG, argon, and KTP-532 lasers. More recently, endoscopy and associated instrumentation have developed dramatically, allowing much more sophisticated operations to be performed without laparotomy.

Currently, tubal cannulation and balloon tuboplasty under hysteroscopic, radiographic, or ultrasonographic control are being evaluated for their ability to treat proximal tubal occlusion and gain access to the fallopian tube for placement of gametes. Falloposcopy for diagnosis and treatment is improving our management of the fallopian tube.

The optimal applications of many of these technologies are yet to be determined. Well-designed and performed studies are necessary.[67] However, these technologies appear to be just beyond their infancy; their many obvious advantages to patients and society should ensure their continued growth.

The trend toward conservative surgery and retaining reproductive organs will make reproductive (nonextirpative) surgery even more important. Cost containment will result in more conservative surgical approaches, as well as medical treatment of conditions currently treated surgically, such as ectopic pregnancy. Advances in imaging technologies will result in more accurate preoperative diagnosis and selective treatment of disease.

We will likely continue to see dramatic breakthroughs in endoscopic equipment, surgical techniques, and laser technology in the future. These will include smaller flexible and directable instruments and cameras, three-dimensional video systems, the use of virtual reality, linkage by computer of diagnostic and treatment modalities, miniaturized robotics, and development of telepresence. Almost all intra-abdominal surgery, including cancer surgery, may be performed endoscopically by experienced laparoscopists working in teams. Smaller lasers, such as the diode laser and more powerful lasers, such as the free-electron laser, will become available. Laser technology will deliver almost any type of laser energy in a highly controllable fashion to the surgical site. Use of lasers for photodynamic therapy will be common. Training, credentialing, and reimbursement of endoscopic and laser surgeons will become more sophisticated, standardized, and regulated. These developments will make it imperative that all gynecologists continue to learn about reproductive surgery to optimize care of their patients.

Despite the exponential growth in these technologic advances for treating female infertility, the basic principles of surgical management remain unchanged. These principles are proper patient selection, careful preoperative preparation, intraoperative minimization of tissue trauma through meticulous surgical technique, and thoughtful postoperative integration of the surgical result into a comprehensive management approach. It is evident that surgery is not an exact science but rather "a complex series of mental, moral, and physical acts which for working purposes is called surgical judgment."[68] All the principles involved in the surgical management of the infertile female can be effectively implemented if we constantly strive to improve our surgical judgment.

REFERENCES

1. Gant NF. Infertility and endometriosis: comparison of pregnancy outcomes with laparotomy versus laparoscopy techniques. Am J Obstet Gynecol 1992;166(4):1072–1081.
2. Grimes DA. Frontiers of operative laparoscopy: a review and critique of the evidence. Am J Obstet Gynecol 1992;166(4): 1062–1071.
3. Olive DL. Analysis of clinical fertility trials: a methodologic review. Fertil Steril 1986;45(2):157–171.
4. Collins JA, Wrixon W, Janes CB, Wilson EH. Treatment-independent pregnancy among infertile couples. N Engl J Med 1983;309(20):1201–1206.
5. Leridon H, Spira A. Problems in measuring the effectiveness of infertility treatment. Fertil Steril 1984;41(4):580–586.
6. Kahneman D, Slovic T, Tversky A. Judgement Under Uncertainty: Heuristics and Biases. Cambridge: Cambridge University Press, 1982.
7. Brock DW, Wartman SA. When competent patients make irrational choices. N Engl J Med 1990;322(22):1595–1599.
8. Ethical dilemmas of infertility. Contemp OB/GYN 1987; March;170–192.
9. Barnea ER, Holford TR, McInnes DRA. Long-term prognosis of infertile couples with normal basic investigations: a life table analysis. Obstet Gynecol 1985;66(1):24–26.
10. Brett AS, McCullough LB. When patients request specific interventions: defining the limits of the physician's obligation. N Engl J Med 1986;315(21):1347–1351.
11. Adamson GD, Hurd SJ, Pasta DJ, et al. Laparoscopic endometriosis treatment: is it better? Fertil Steril 1993;59(1):35–44.
12. Evans S, Schiff I. Pre- and post-operative assessment of the tubal surgery patient. In: DeCherney AH, Polan ML, editors. Reproductive Surgery. Chicago: Year Book Medical, 1987:48–63.
13. Sauer MV, Paulson RJ, Lobo RA. Reversing the natural decline in human fertility: an extended clinical trial of oocyte donation to women of advanced reproductive age. JAMA 1992;268(10):1275–1279.
14. Menken J, Trussel J, Larsen U. Age and infertility. Science 1986;233(4771):1389–1394.
15. Gindoff PR, Jewelewicz R. Reproductive potential in the older woman. Fertil Steril 1986;46(6):989–1001.
16. Barad DH. Epidemiology of infertility. Infertil Reprod Med Clin North Am 1991;2(2):255–266.
17. Silverberg KM, Hill GA. Reproductive surgery versus assisted reproductive technologies: selecting the correct alternative. J Gynecol Surg 1991;7:67.
18. Thurmond AS, Rosch J. Nonsurgical fallopian tube recanalization for treatment of infertility. Radiology 1990;174(2):371–374.
19. Wallach EE. Myomectomy: a guide to indications and technique. Contemp OB/GYN 1988;74–88.
20. Witt BR. Pelvic factors and fertility. Infertil Reprod Med Clin North Am 1991;2(2):371–390.
21. Diamond MP, Daniell JF, Feste J, et al. Adhesion reformation and de novo adhesion formation after reproductive pelvic surgery. Fertil Steril 1987;47(5):864–866.
22. Jansen RPS. Early laparoscopy after pelvic operations to prevent adhesions: safety and efficacy. Fertil Steril 1988;49(1):26–31.
23. Operative Laparoscopy Study Group. Post-operative adhesion development following operative laparoscopy: evaluation at early second-look procedures. Fertil Steril 1991;55(4):700–704.
24. Clarke JR. Decision making in surgical practice. World J Surg 1989;13(3):245–251.
25. Trimbos-Kemper TCM. Reversal of sterilization in women over 40 years of age: a multi-center survey in the Netherlands. Fertil Steril 1990;53(3):575–577.
26. Nezhat C, Crowgey SR, Nezhat F. Videolaseroscopy for the treatment of endometriosis associated with infertility. Fertil Steril 1989;51(2):237–240.
27. Adamson GD. Diagnosis and clinical presentation of endometriosis. Am J Obstet Gynecol 1990;162(2):568–569.
28. Redwine DB. Age-related evolution in colour appearance of endometriosis. Fertil Steril 1987;48(6):1062–1063.
29. Bruhat MA, Mage C, Chapron C, et al. Present-day endoscopic surgery in gynecology. Eur J Ob Gyn Reprod Biol 1991;41(1):4–13.
30. Nezhat CR, Nezhat FR, Metzger DA, Luciano AA. Adhesion reformation after reproductive surgery by videolaseroscopy. Fertil Steril 1990;53(6):1008–1011.
31. Carbon Dioxide Laser Laparoscopy Study Group. Initial report of the carbon dioxide laser laparoscopy study group: complications. J Gynecol Surg 1989;5:269–272.
32. Peterson HB, Hulka JF, Phillips JM. American Association of Gynecologic Laparoscopists' 1988 membership survey on operative laparoscopy. J Reprod Med 1990;35(6):587–589.
33. Von Theobald P, Marie G, Herlicoviez M, et al. Morbidite et mortalite de la coelioscopie: etude retrospective d'une serie de 1,429 cas. Rev fr Gynecol Obstet 1990;85(11):611–614.
34. Riedel HH, Lehmann-Willenbrock E, Mecke H, Semm K. The frequency distribution of various pelviscopic (laparoscopic) operations, including complication rates—statistics of the Federal Republic of Germany in the years 1983–1985. Zent bl Gynakoll 1989;111(2):78–91.
35. Method MW, Keith CG. Economic impact of gynecologic endoscopy. In: Sanfilippo JS, Levine RL, editors. Operative Gynecologic Endoscopy. New York: Springer-Verlag, 1989:299–307.
36. Tokars JI, Bell DM, Culver DH, et al. Percutaneous injuries during surgical procedures. JAMA 1992;267(21):2899–2904.
37. Murphy AA. Operative laparoscopy. Fertil Steril 1987;47(1):1–18.
38. Maiman M, Seltzer V, Boyce J. Laparoscopic excision of ovarian neo-

plasm subsequently found to be malignant. Obstet Gynecol 1991;77(4):563–565.

39. Dembo AJ, Davy M, Stenwig AE, et al. Prognostic factors in patients with stage I epithelial ovarian cancer. Obstet Gynecol 1990;75(2):263–273.

40. Webb MJ, Decker DG, Mussey E, Williams TJ. Factors influencing survival in stage I ovarian cancer. Am J Obstet Gynecol 1973;116(2):222–228.

41. Seltzer VL, Maiman M, Boyce A, et al. Laparoscopic surgery in the management of ovarian cysts. Female Patient 1992;17:16.

42. Adamson GD, Subak LL, Pasta DJ, et al. Comparison of CO_2 laser laparoscopy with laparotomy for management of endometriomata. Fertil Steril 1992;57(5):965–973.

43. Koonings PP, Campbell K, Mishell DR Jr, et al. Relative frequency of primary ovarian neoplasms: a 10-year review. Obstet Gynecol 1989;74(6):921–926.

44. Reich H, McGlynn F, Wilkie W. Laparoscopic management of stage I ovarian cancer: a case report. J Reprod Med 1990;35(6):601–605.

45. Keye WR. Laser Surgery in Gynecology and Obstetrics. Chicago: Year Book Medical, 1989.

46. Duffy S, Reid PC, Smith JH, et al. In vitro studies of uterine electrosurgery. Obstet Gynecol 1991;78(2):213–220.

47. Lotze EC, Grunert GM. The use of lasers in infertility surgery. Clin Obstet Gynecol 1989;32(3):576–585.

48. Drollette CM, Badawy SZA. Pathophysiology of pelvic adhesions: modern trends in preventing infertility. J Reprod Med 1992;37(2):107–121.

49. Nezhat C, Nezhat F, Silfen SL, et al. Laparoscopic myomectomy. Int J Fertil 1991;36:275–280.

50. Adamson GD. Use of GnRH agonists to improve results of operative laparoscopy and hysteroscopy. Infertil Reprod Med Clin North Am 1993;4(1):65–81.

51. Homm RJ, Garza DE, Mathur S. Immunological aspects of surgically induced experimental endometriosis: variation in response to therapy. Fertil Steril 1989;52(1):132–139.

52. Silverberg KM. Combination therapy for endometriosis. Infertil Reprod Med Clin North Am 1992;3(3):683–695.

53. Andreyko JL, Blumenfeld Z, Marshall LA, et al. Use of an agonistic analog of gonadotropin-releasing hormone (nafarelin) to treat leiomyomas: assessment by magnetic resonance imaging. Am J Obstet Gynecol 1988;158(4):903–910.

54. Friedman AJ, Barbieri RL, Benacerraf BR, Schiff I. Treatment of leiomyomata with intranasal or subcutaneous leuprolide, a gonadotropin-releasing hormone agonist. Fertil Steril 1987;48(4):560–564.

55. Zawin M, McCarthy S, Scoutt L, et al. Monitoring therapy with a gonadotropin-releasing hormone analog: utility of MR imaging. Radiology 1990;175(2):503–506.

56. Friedman AJ, Rein MS, Harrison-Atlas D, et al. A randomized, placebo-controlled double-blind study evaluating leuprolide acetate depot treatment before myomectomy. Fertil Steril 1989;52(5):728–733.

57. Friedman AJ. Vaginal hemorrhage associated with degenerating submucous leiomyomata during leuprolide acetate treatment. Fertil Steril 1989;52(1):152–154.

58. Thorp JM Jr, Katz VL. Submucous myomas treated with gonadotropin-releasing hormone agonists and resulting in vaginal hemorrhage: a case report. J Reprod Med 1991;36(8):625–626.

59. Brooks PG, Serden SP. Preparation of the endometrium for ablation with a single dose of leuprolide acetate depot. J Reprod Med 1991;36:477–478.

60. Feste J. Use of GnRH agonists in endoscopic and reproductive surgery. In: Barbieri RL, Friedman AJ, editors. Gonadotropin-Releasing Hormone Analog. New York: Elsevier, 1991:103–119.

61. Kerin J, Daykhovsky L, Grundfest W, Surrey E. Falloposcopy: a microendoscopic transvaginal technique for diagnosing and treating endotubal disease incorporating guide wire cannulation and direct balloon tuboplasty. J Reprod Med 1990;35(6):606–612.

62. Rock JA, Siegler AM, Meisel MB, et al. The efficacy of postoperative hydrotubation: a randomized prospective multicenter clinical trial. Fertil Steril 1984;42(3):373–376.

63. Gomel V, Taylor PJ. Surgical endoscopy. In: Gomel V, Taylor PJ, Yutzpe AA, et al, editors. Laparoscopy and Hysteroscopy in Gynecologic Practice. Chicago: Year Book Medical, 1986:140.

64. Kistner RW. Management of endometriosis in the infertile patient. Fertil Steril 1975;26(12):1151–1166.

65. Lauritsen JG, Pagel JD, Vangsted P, et al. Results of repeated tuboplasties. Fertil Steril 1982;37(1):68–72.

66. DeCherney AH, Mezer HC. Timing of post-operative laparoscopic evaluation of tubal surgery patients. Fertil Steril 1983;39:402–403.

67. McDonough PG. The need for technology assessment in the reproductive sciences. Am J Obstet Gynecol 1992;166(4):1082–1086.

68. Laufman H. Surgical judgment. In: Davis L, editor. Christopher's Textbook of Surgery, 9th edition. Philadelphia: WB Saunders, 1968:1459.

CHAPTER 22

Operative Instrumentation for Infertility Surgery

JOSEPH FESTE

In the last two decades, many advances have been made in the types of instrumentation used for infertility surgery. For instance, newer, more advanced laparoscopic instruments have been developed over the last 10 years that have allowed many operations that formerly would have been performed via laparotomy to be performed by laparoscopy. This shift has benefited patients by reducing discomfort and convalescence. This chapter discusses various types of instruments used for infertility surgery and is subdivided into categories of tools used for laparoscopy, hysteroscopy, and laparotomy procedures. Special mention is also made of lasers, electrosurgical equipment, and photographic documentation. Occasionally references to original prototype equipment are offered only to illustrate improvements. Of course, many of these instruments are produced by several companies. It is not my intention to promote any particular manufacturer but to discuss those instruments that I believe to be most useful and advanced.

LAPAROSCOPY

Until recently, laparoscopy was performed primarily to make a diagnosis, to treat minor cases of endometriosis, or to ligate fallopian tubes. Now operative laparoscopy has become the wave of the present and future with respect to many gynecologic procedures. Basic and advanced tools used for laparoscopy are discussed.

Laparoscopes

There are basically two types of laparoscopes available for use in gynecologic surgery. The first is used primarily for diagnostic purposes, and the second is used for more invasive operative procedures. The diagnostic laparoscope was the first one to be developed and is used simply to view the contents of the peritoneal cavity. The most commonly used diagnostic laparoscope is 10.5 mm in diameter, is 31 cm in length, and has a 7.2-mm optical channel. Laparoscopes range in size, however, from 1.8 to 10.5 mm in diameter. The larger the optical channel, the larger the field of visualization (Fig. 22–1). Diagnostic laparoscopes not only have larger optical channels, but also bring in more light through the fiberoptic bundles than do operative laparoscopes of the same diameter. By and large, most diagnostic laparoscopes are comparable in structure and efficiency. Laparoscopes with smaller diameters are available; however, photographic documentation for patient records or publication is of better quality when the larger diameter laparoscopes are used. A new optical catheter system with an external diameter of 1.8 mm is available for office laparoscopy (Fig. 22–2). This rigid laparoscope can be used under local anesthesia in an office setting for diagnostic purposes only. I have found it particularly helpful to use this instrument to decide which patients should be admitted for a second-look laparoscopy after an extensive laparoscopic or laparotomy procedure.

Two major types of operative laparoscopes are readily available: (1) The first has an eyepiece that is offset but parallel to the telescope and is called the *two right angle laparoscope* (Fig. 22–3). It allows the surgeon to look in the same direction as that of a diagnostic laparoscope. Earlier operative laparoscopes had large operative channels (up to

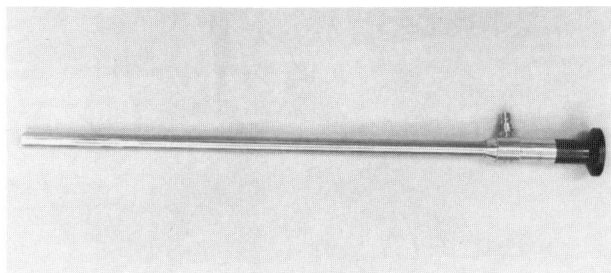

FIGURE 22–1. Diagnostic (10.5-mm) laparoscope. (Courtesy of Olympus Corporation, Lake Success, NY.)

281

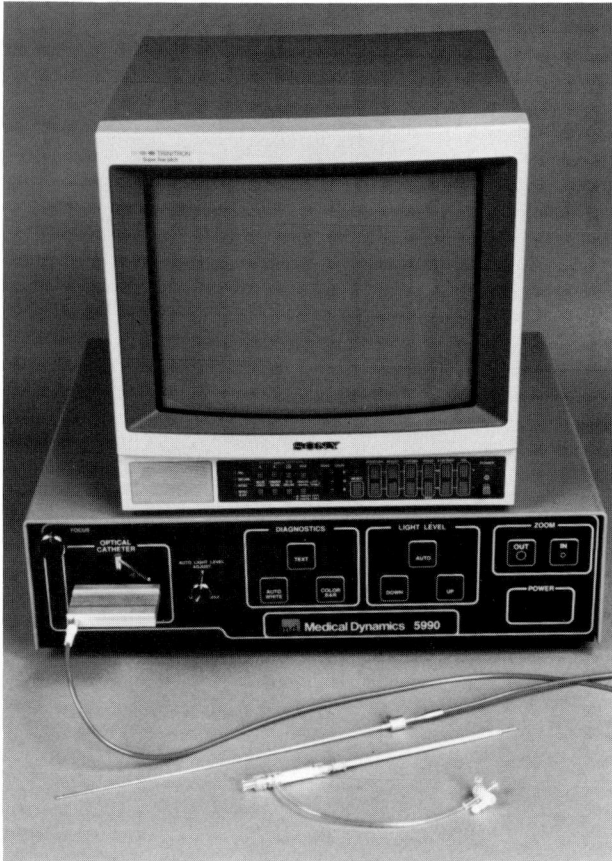

FIGURE 22–2. Optical catheter system with 1.8-mm rigid endoscope. (Courtesy of Medical Dynamics, Englewood, CO.)

7.3 mm in diameter), whereas newer laparoscopes have 5.5 to 6 mm channels that accommodate most accessory instruments as well as a CO_2 laser beam or fiberoptic laser introduced through an accessory sheath. (2) The second laparoscope has a 45-degree angulated eyepiece and is commonly used when operating off a video monitor. Often surgeons who have back problems prefer this type of eyepiece because the angulation minimizes the need to bend over the patient to look into it (Fig. 22–4).

Cannulas and Trocars

Introduction of a laparoscope or accessory instrument into the abdominal cavity requires use of a cannula and trocar.

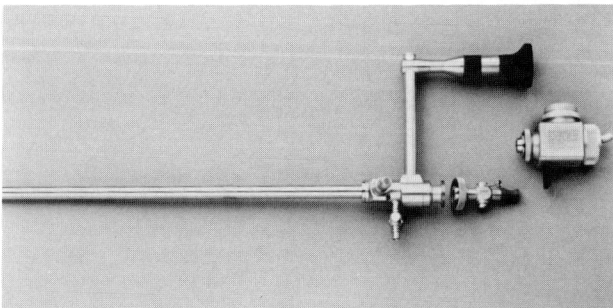

FIGURE 22–3. Operative right-angle laparoscope. (Courtesy of R. Wolf Medical Instruments Corp., Vernon Hills, IL.)

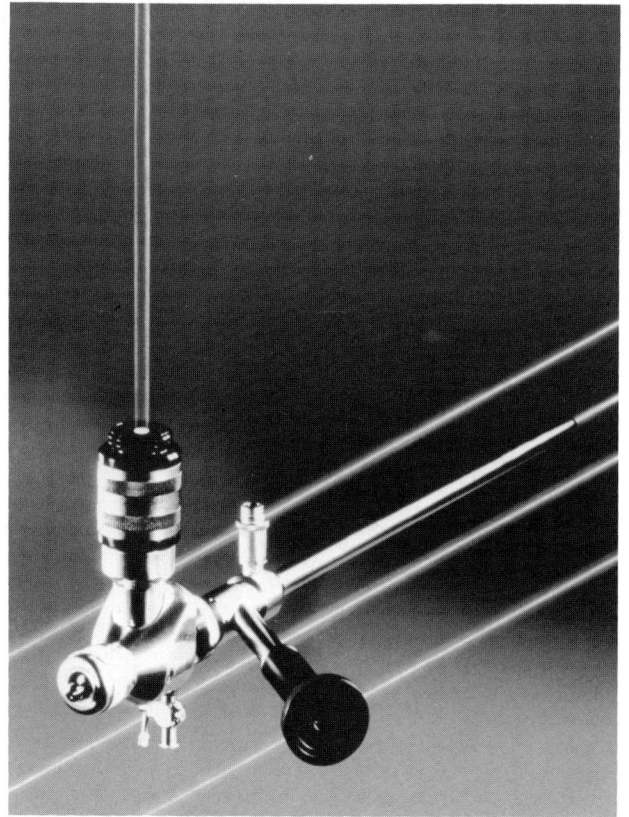

FIGURE 22–4. Forty-five–degree angulated eyepiece for an operative laparoscope. (Courtesy of Olympus Corporation, Lake Success, NY.)

Reusable metal cannulas and trocars have been available ever since the first laparoscope was developed. Trocars are made with either pyramidal or conical tips, and there has been a great deal of discussion in the industry about which shape is safer to use. In theory, the conical tip should prevent more tearing of the tissue as it enters the abdomen. There have been no studies reported, however, to determine the efficacy of the conical over the pyramidal shaped trocars. There are several disadvantages, however, to use of these metal instruments. If the trocar becomes bent or dulled, it is difficult to insert through the abdominal wall; it may lead to unnecessary tearing or injury to intra-abdominal organs if the instrument is thrust too quickly or deeply through the skin layers. A bent cannula may also prevent the laparoscope from passing through it.

Reusable instruments require proper cleaning and have interchanging parts that may become lost or misplaced. The increased incidence of acquired immunodeficiency syndrome (AIDS) and the persistent problem of exposure to hepatitis add to the significance of these disadvantages.

Many of these problems may be eliminated with the use of disposable products. The cannulas are well designed, and trocars are extremely sharp. The presence of a safety shield is intended to prevent the trocar from injuring vital structures after entering the peritoneum (Fig. 22–5A and B). Each disposable trocar has a Luer-Lok connector, which accommodates gas tubing from an insufflator. This is particularly important when more than one insufflator is used to provide more than 6 L/minute of carbon dioxide flow. A good deal of concern has been stated regarding the cost of the disposable trocars as well as other disposable instruments. Much of this

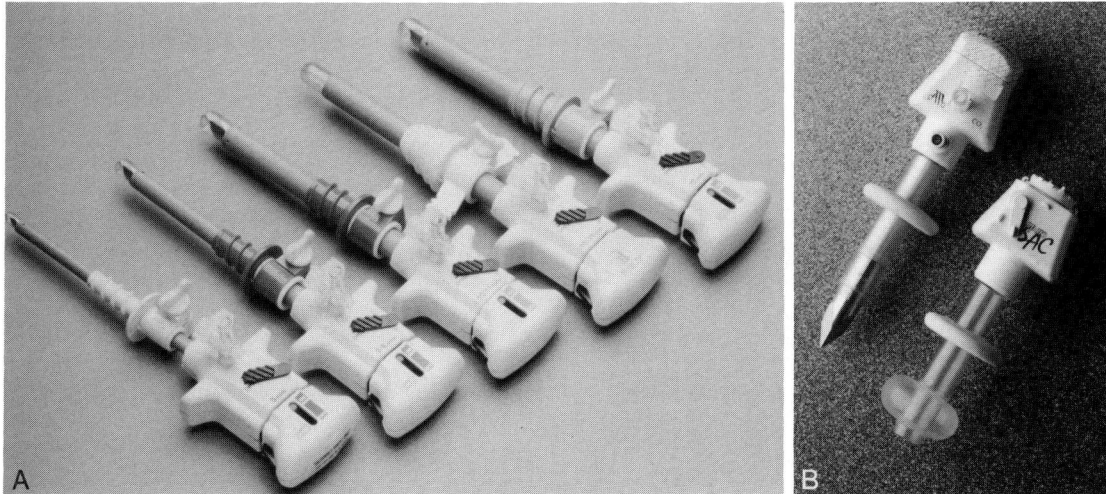

FIGURE 22–5. *A,* Ethicon disposable trocars with safety shield. Sizes are 5 mm, 7/8 mm, 10/11 mm, and 12 mm. The second trocar from the right is used in open laparoscopy cases. (*A* courtesy of Ethicon, Inc., Cincinnati, OH.) *B,* Marlow disposable trocar with pyramidal tip and balloon insufflation device that secures the cannula in place. (*B* courtesy of Marlow Surgical Technologies, Inc., Willoughby, OH.)

apparent cost is due to cost shifting by hospitals to make up for deficiencies in other areas. Many of these instruments can save a good deal of operating time, which, in itself, can be as high as $25 to $35 per minute in some hospitals. In addition, there is concern about the environmental impact of disposable surgical equipment. Manufacturers of these disposables are aware of and evaluating these concerns. Yet one must consider both the proper selection of patients and surgical skills in determining when a surgeon should use disposables.

Insufflators for Laparoscopy

The first insufflators available for laparoscopy were designed to provide a flow rate of 1 L/minute. This flow rate was feasible only when the diameter of the tubing or accessory port on the laparoscope was no smaller than the point of exit on the insufflator machine. With the increase in advanced operative laser laparoscopic procedures, the need to clear out large volumes of laser plume has necessitated the use of much higher gas flow rates. As a result, many of the insufflators now provide flow rates of up to 12 L/minute made possible by special adaptations of the machine, which

provides continuous flow from the supply tank (Fig. 22–6). Before the high flow is instigated, the operating surgeon must make certain that the cannula is in the peritoneal cavity to avoid unnecessary subcutaneous emphysema. Equally important is prevention of excessive distention of the peritoneal cavity, which can lead to a decrease in venous return or, in some cases, a pneumothorax.[1-3]

To prevent overdistention of the peritoneal cavity, several manufacturers have produced an insufflator that circulates carbon dioxide gas through a filter to remove laser or cautery plume as well as liquids. Theoretically this keeps the volume of gas constant with an intra-abdominal pressure of no more than 15 mm Hg. Inadvertent loss of gas, however, in or around the cannula sleeves requires the periodic addition of more carbon dioxide to the abdominal cavity to maintain an adequate pneumoperitoneum (Fig. 22–7).

Light Sources and Cables

There are basically three types of light source available: a single 150-watt lightbulb, a high-powered mercury vapor, and a xenon bulb. The latter two are frequently used for

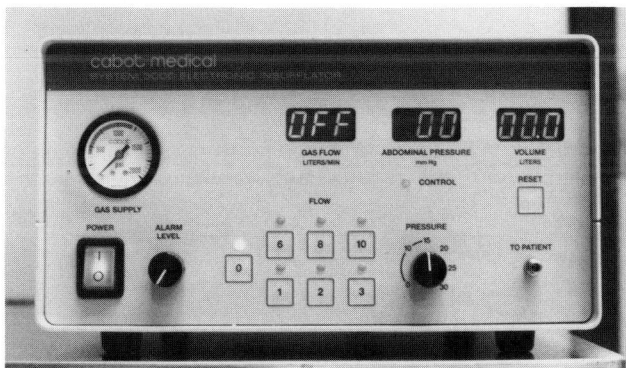

FIGURE 22–6. High-flow insufflator that warns of excessive pressures and automatically vents off excess carbon dioxide gas. (Courtesy of Cabot Medical, Langhorne, PA.)

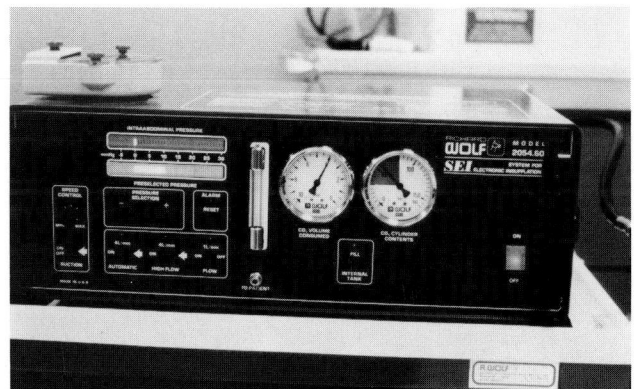

FIGURE 22–7. High-flow insufflator that recirculates carbon dioxide gas and filters out plume. (Courtesy of R. Wolf Medical Instruments Corp., Vernon Hills, IL.)

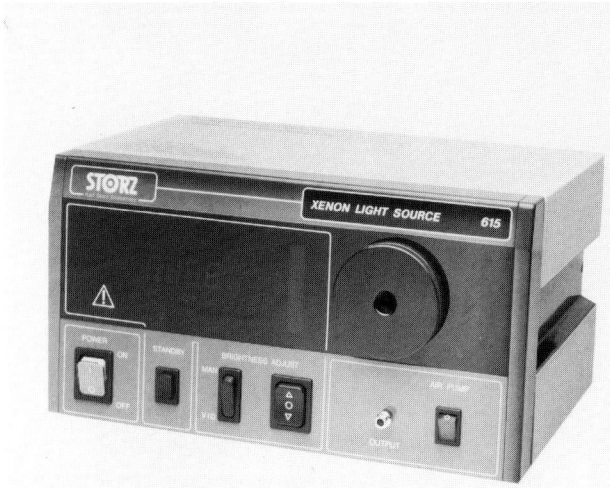

FIGURE 22–8. Xenon high-intensity light source. (Courtesy of Karl Storz Endoscopy, Culver City, CA.)

video photography (Fig. 22–8). Some of the light sources have a combination of a 150-watt bulb and a flash unit adapted for photography. Whatever the light source, care must be taken with these because heat generated by these units can burn a hole in a drape or burn a patient if the end of the attached cable is not monitored carefully.

Special cables that contain fiberoptic bundles have been developed that transmit light from the source to the endoscope. (Fig. 22–9). The amount of available light is directly proportional to the diameter of the cable and the efficiency of the attachment at each end of the cable. Light is lost at either end, but this loss is minimized by using condensing lenses at the attachment to the endoscope to concentrate the light over the endoscope connecting post.

Because of the tendency of the fibers to break in the

fiberoptic cables, usually from improper handling, several manufacturers have developed liquid cables to overcome this problem. In addition, the amount of light lost at the junction of the cable to the endoscope is minimal when compared with the fiberoptic systems. These cables, however, are not as flexible as the fiberoptic ones and tend to be unwieldy while operating. These cables can be filled with either alcohol or water. They may last longer than fiberoptic cables but cannot be sterilized at high temperatures.

One of the unfortunate problems associated with all light cables is that none of them fit all endoscopes. Consequently, special adapters are necessary to allow attachment of these cables to various endoscopes. Although there may be some loss of light intensity through these adapters, this loss is minimal and not noticeable unless one is using a video or taking 35-mm photographs.

Ancillary Instrumentation

A wide range of ancillary instruments is available for use during endoscopic procedures. These instruments are made to fit either through a second, third, or fourth puncture cannula or through the operative channel of the laparoscope. Personal preference dictates which instrument to put through which cannula or laparoscope. Most ancillary instruments vary from 3 to 7 mm in diameter; however, a few 7 to 18 mm diameter instruments are also available. Following is a discussion of these instruments.

DEVICES FOR HYDRODISSECTION (AQUADISSECTION)

To evacuate large volumes of fluids and gas during prolonged endoscopic cases, several manufacturers have developed irrigation/suction devices. These machines allow for high pressure irrigation that is needed to lavage blood and debris attached to the pelvic viscera or peritoneum (Fig. 22–10). The aspirator component removes fluids, blood clots, gas, and plume efficiently. The cannula end may be used as a

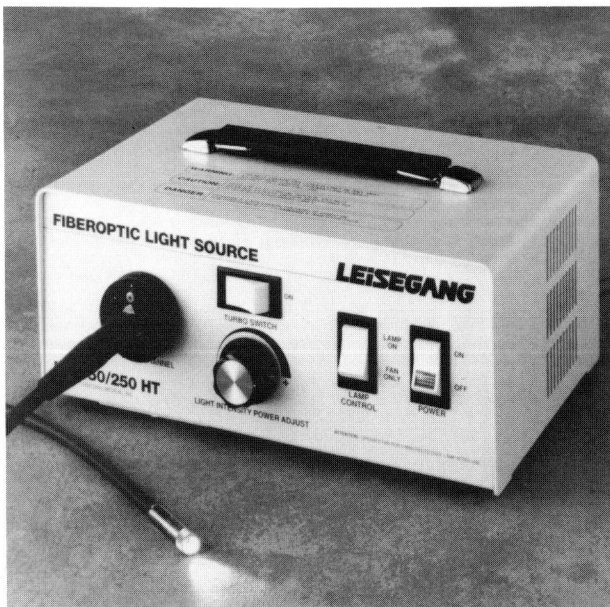

FIGURE 22–9. Leisegang fiberoptic light source and cable. (Courtesy of Leisegang Medical, Inc., Boca Raton, FL.)

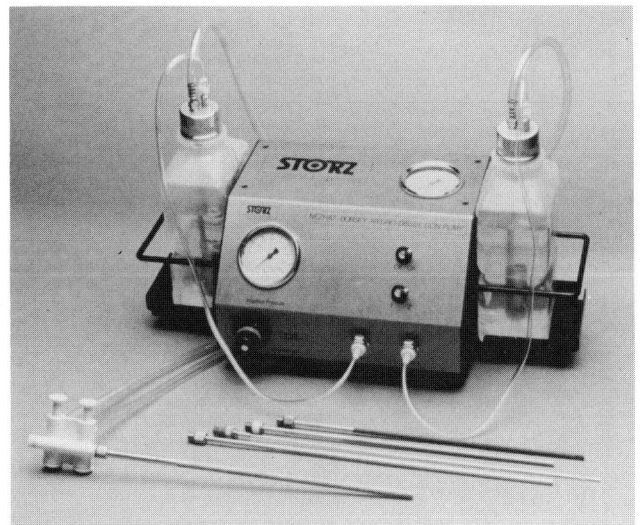

FIGURE 22–10. Suction-irrigation pump with cannula device. (Courtesy of Karl Storz Endoscopy, Culver City, CA.)

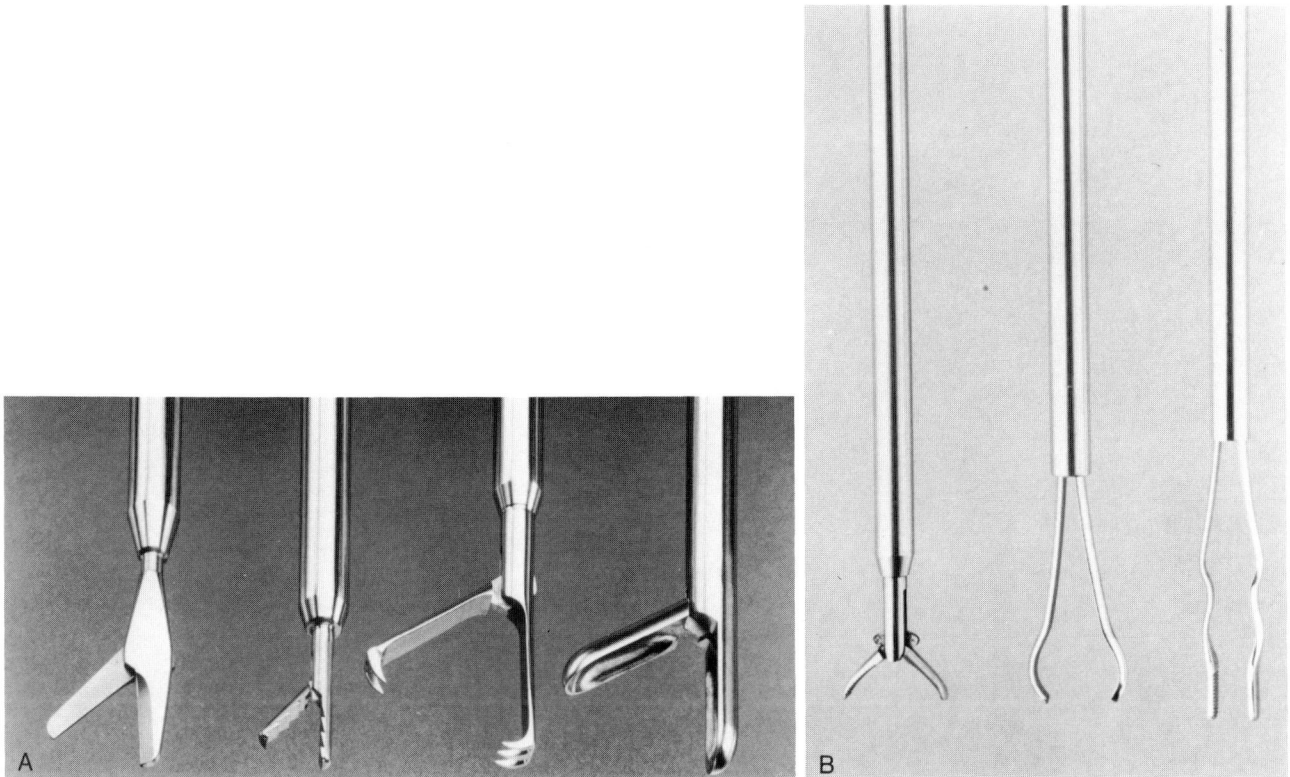

FIGURE 22–11. *A,* A variety of accessory instruments for laparoscopic use. Scissors (far left) and three different types of graspers are shown. *B,* Three other types of tissue graspers for laparoscopic use.

blunt probe for tissue dissection or manipulation of pelvic viscera. All of these cannulas are fitted with a valve that prevents inadvertent loss of peritoneal gas.

The continual evacuation of fluids and gas requires use of a high-flow insufflator to maintain an adequate pneumoperitoneum. Most of these devices have at least a liter-sized container for delivering fluid and one of the same size for collecting fluid. A circulating nurse must watch the levels in each of these containers to keep the system flowing efficiently. Alternatively, there are several disposable units that work off of the hospital wall suction system and deliver the fluids from an intravenous bag with a special mechanism to pressurize the flow of fluid.

GRASPING FORCEPS, SCISSORS, PROBES, AND BIOPSY FORCEPS

There are a multitude of forceps, and scissors available for laparoscopic use. Figure 22–11*A* and *B* shows a variety of these instruments. There is wide variation in the shape, size, and configuration of each type of instrument. Most of these instruments have unipolar coagulation capabilities, and most are 5 mm in diameter. A few instruments are made longer than 27 cm so they can be used through the operative channel of a laparoscope. Microscissors are helpful in dissecting ureters from lateral pelvic walls. Several new instruments are available for use through an ancillary cannula that allow grasping or stabilization of the ovary. A long aspirating needle is available for evacuation of benign cysts. Also, biopsy forceps of several sizes may be used for biopsy of the ovary or peritoneal surface. Laser instruments, which may also be

used for cutting or biopsy purposes, are discussed later in this chapter.

SUTURES, STAPLE DEVICES, CLIPS AND ENDOSUTURES

Endoscopic suturing has become more popular in recent years as new instrumentation (i.e., sutures, needle holders) has allowed these procedures to be performed more efficiently. One special suture, the "Endoloop," (Ethicon) (Fig. 22–12) has been used frequently for laparoscopic removal of fallopian tubes or entire adnexae. When ligating large pedicles, it is often preferable to use up to three loops to ensure complete vascular occlusion. Of course, bipolar cautery may be used as an alternative in most of these instances.

Staple devices are now in use that contain six rows of vascular, titanium staples introduced through an 11 to 12 mm ancillary cannula. On firing the instrument, the staples

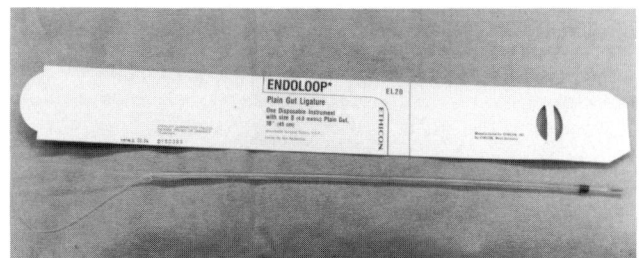

FIGURE 22–12. Ethicon special suture ligature device used for removal of organs such as the fallopian tubes, ovaries, and appendix. (Courtesy of Ethicon, Inc., Cincinnati, OH.)

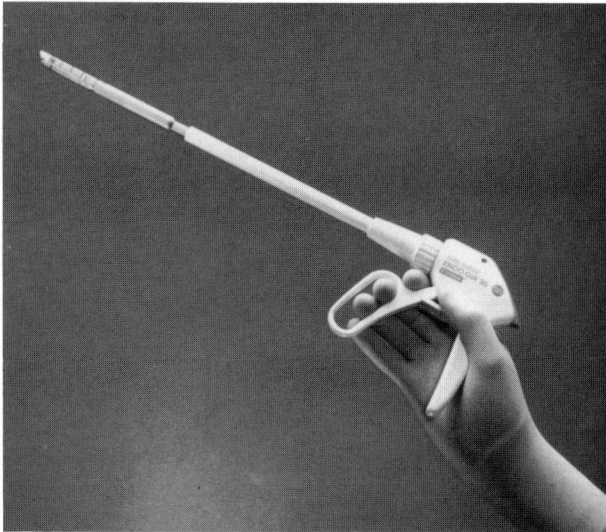

FIGURE 22–13. Endo GIA stapler device. (Courtesy of United States Surgical Corporation, Norwalk, CT.)

FIGURE 22–15. *A,* "Knot pusher" to deliver an extracorporeal knot through a 5-mm trocar. *B,* Close-up of "knot pusher" end. (*A* and *B* courtesy of R. Wolf Medical Instruments Corp., Vernon Hills, IL.)

are set, and the pedicle is cut automatically through the middle of the six rows (Fig. 22–13). These disposable devices make possible the performance of a salpingo-oophorectomy, a salpingectomy, appendectomy, or laparoscopic-assisted vaginal hysterectomy while minimizing the use of suture or cautery.

Several companies make single-clip or multiple-clip applicators used through a 10 to 11 mm cannula (Fig. 22–14). These clips are useful for the isolation of individual bleeding points, where a suture by laparoscopy would be time-consuming and difficult to place. The staples are used more often to "tack up" tissue or for hernia repairs.

An experienced laparoscopist may apply endoscopic sutures with either a curved or a straight needle using an intracorporeal or extracorporeal technique for knot-tying. The extracorporeal knot is pushed down a 5.5-mm ancillary cannula with an instrument called a "knot pusher" (Fig. 22–15A and B). A square knot is tied and passed down the cannula to secure a bleeding point or to bring two pieces of tissue together.

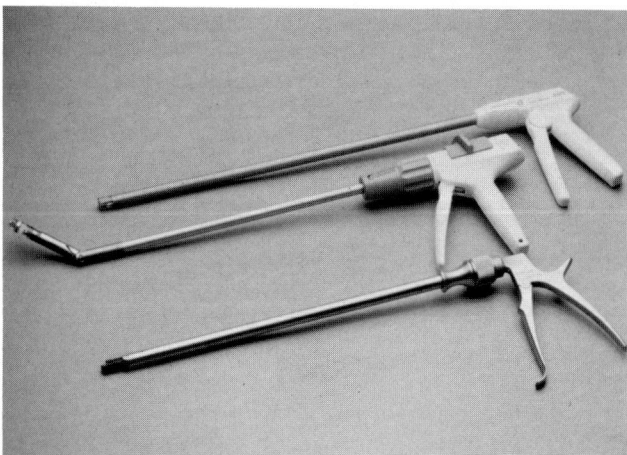

ELECTROSURGICAL EQUIPMENT

For years, the use of electrosurgical units via endoscopy was met with disapproval.[4] Visceral injuries caused by the early unipolar units led to significant concern about using this modality during endoscopy. New electrosurgical generators, however, are low-voltage, high-frequency, solid-state units with insulated circuitry. These units offer both unipolar and bipolar capabilities (Fig. 22–16). Whenever a unipolar accessory is used, the patient must be grounded with a proper pad. Most companies make disposable grounding pads that have a conductive jelly as well as a sensor plate that gives a warning if the patient is not properly grounded. All units have the ability to blend the cutting and coagulation currents, which alters its operative performance. As opposed to unipolar cautery, in which the current travels from an ingoing electrode to the patient and then to the grounding pad, the bipolar units use two paddles between which the electric current flows. Thus, the bipolar unit current flows in

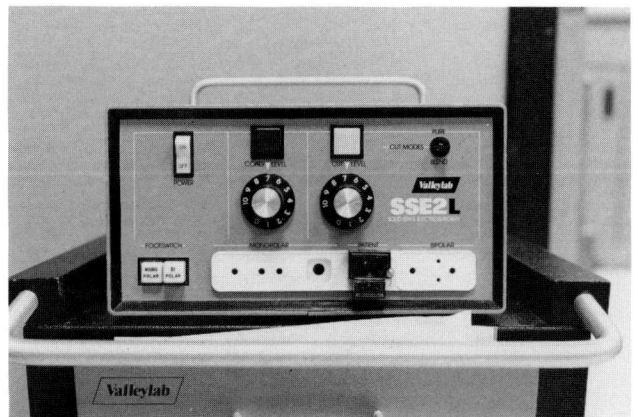

FIGURE 22–14. Several types of single-clip applicators and disposable staple devices. (Courtesy of Ethicon, Inc., Cincinnati, OH.)

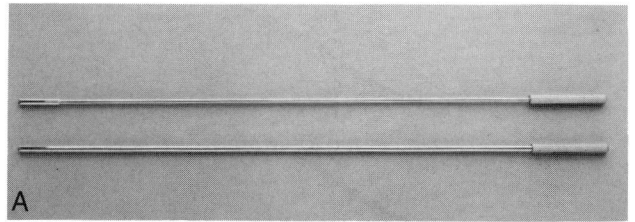

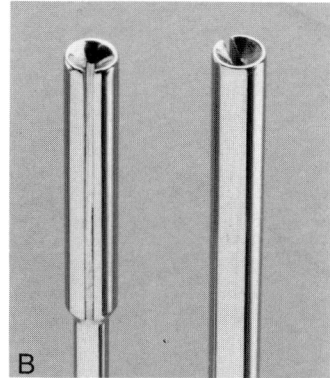

FIGURE 22–16. Electrosurgical generator. (Courtesy of Valleylab, Boulder, CO.)

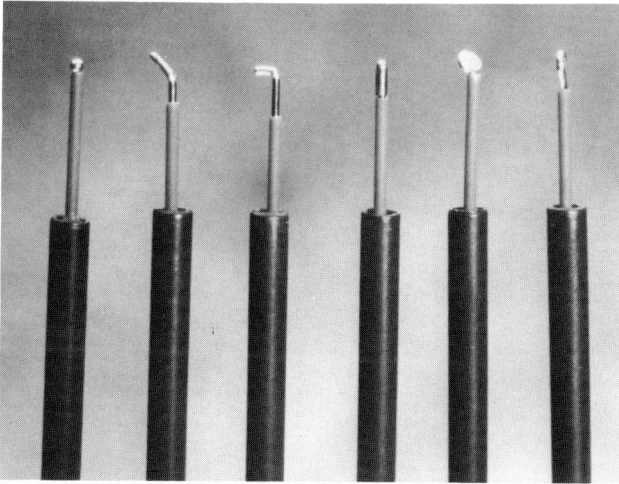

FIGURE 22–17. A variety of accessory tip probe configurations. (Courtesy of Valleylab, Boulder, CO.)

one electrode to the tissue to be coagulated and then out the other electrode. With the bipolar system, no grounding pad is necessary.

Many of the unipolar electrodes may be rounded, hooked, conical, or blade shaped (Fig. 22–17). Even though the likelihood of a "spark gap" is highly unlikely, one must be extremely careful when using the unipolar cautery at laparoscopy. A bipolar electrode coupled to an aspirator is useful for providing hemostasis during laparoscopic procedures.

An electrosurgical device, the Argon Beam Coagulator, has been developed for use during laparotomy cases as well as endoscopic procedures (Fig. 22–18). This unit provides both a hand piece for laparotomy cases and accessory instrument for laparoscopic use. The device delivers a monopolar current through a stream of argon gas that is polarized by the current into millions of smaller, superficial sparks (Fig. 22–19). Thus, coagulation is superficial with a depth of tissue destruction of no more than 1 to 2 mm. In addition, the argon gas dries the field of any fluids in front of the beam to allow better coagulation of the vessels. If used properly, this instrument is able to coagulate vessels as large as 5 to 6 mm in diameter effectively. Yet because coagulation can be controlled at a superficial level, this device may carefully be used effectively to ablate tissues or lesions that lie over vital structures without harm to the latter. There are, however, no studies comparing the safety and efficacy of this device with standard unipolar coagulation devices.

CARBON DIOXIDE LASER INSTRUMENTATION

For more than 15 years, lasers have played an important role in surgery.[5] Figure 22–20 demonstrates frequent laser wavelengths used in surgery. By far the most commonly used laser over the last decade has been the carbon dioxide laser (CO_2 laser). It emits a wavelength of 10,600 nm, which is absorbed by water. In addition, its effect is not influenced by tissue color.

Most available CO_2 laser systems deliver power as low a few milliwatts up to 100 watts of energy (Fig. 22–21). An articulating arm allows laser energy to be delivered via a free hand piece, laparoscope, or micromanipulator. These units require delicate handling because even a small bump to the

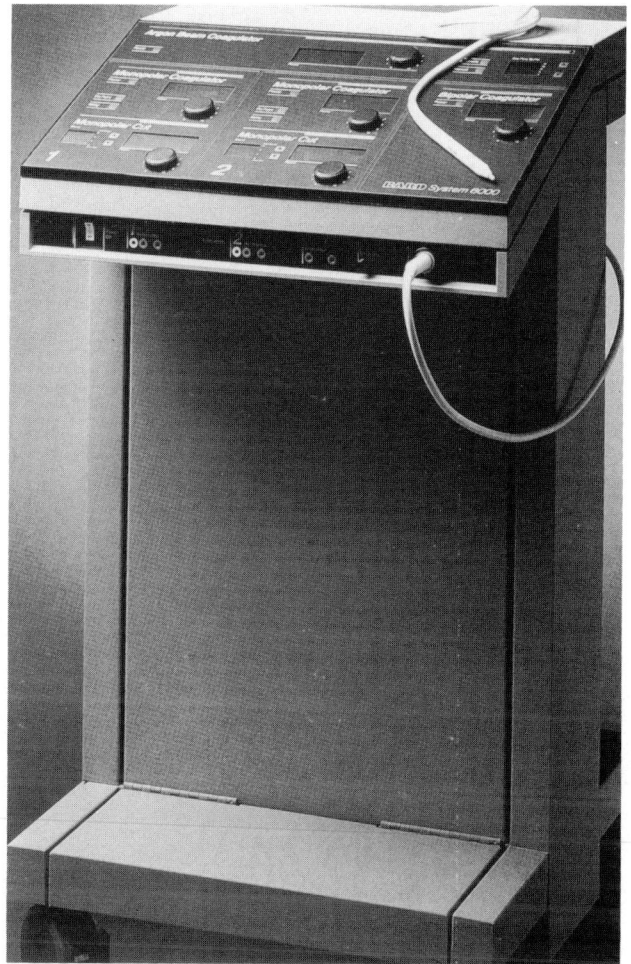

FIGURE 22–18. Argon beam coagulator. (Courtesy of Bircher, Irvine, CA.)

articulating arm can knock the mirrors out of alignment requiring repair before the next usage. Newer, improved models have better fixation of the mirrors, and this problem now occurs less frequently. Most of the units are equipped

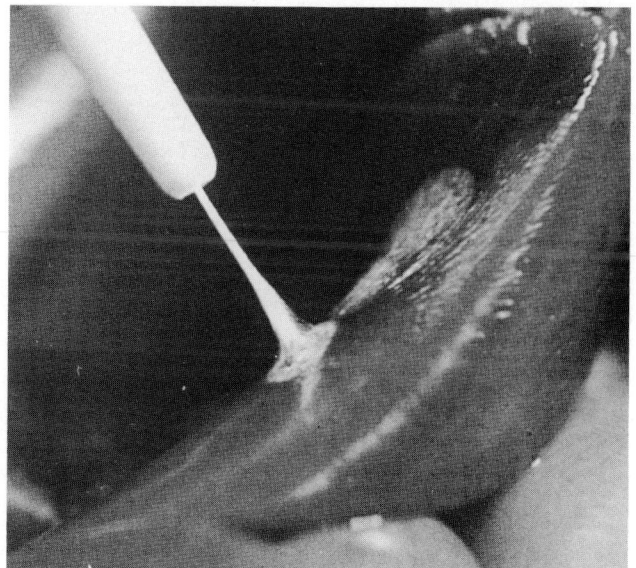

FIGURE 22–19. Argon beam coagulator delivers a monopolar current through a stream of argon gas. (Courtesy of Bircher, Irvine, CA.)

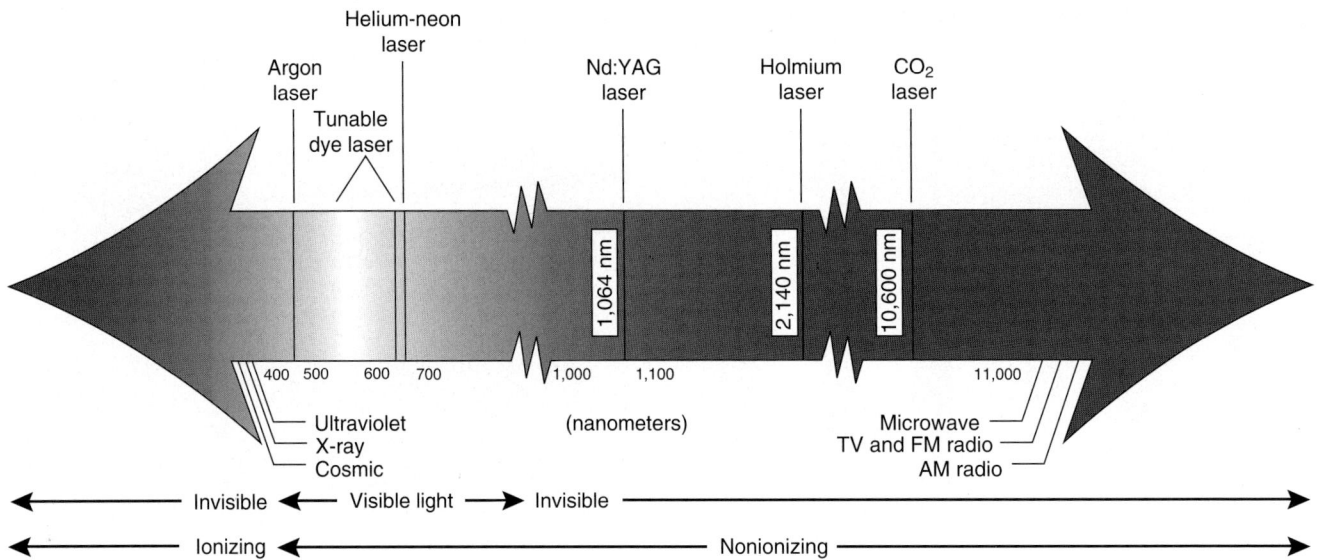

FIGURE 22–20. Electromagnetic radiation spectrum.

with superpulse or ultrapulse features that allow the surgeon to operate with less thermal effect on the tissues than occurs with the standard continuous mode (Fig. 22–22). Because of the large amount of power generated by these units, the inexperienced surgeon needs to use extreme caution during

procedures. Table 22–1 illustrates advantages of CO_2 laser systems.

The CO_2 laser laparoscope is currently distributed in the United States by many companies. Both single and double puncture laser laparoscopic systems are available. Operative laser laparoscopes currently available have either a 10.7 or 12.7 mm outer diameter with a 5 or 6 mm operating channel. The operating channel can be used either for the delivery of standard 5-mm accessory instruments such as forceps or, with an adapter, for the delivery of a CO_2 laser beam. If the CO_2 laser is used through the laparoscope, the surgeon simply attaches the articulated arm, which has a special focusing lens, to the operating laparoscope.

Should there be a misalignment of the beam down the operative channel, a small joystick and mirror allows the surgeon to focus and align the beam as it passes through the operating channel of the scope and impacts on the tissue. The surgeon then attaches the CO_2 insufflation tubing to the

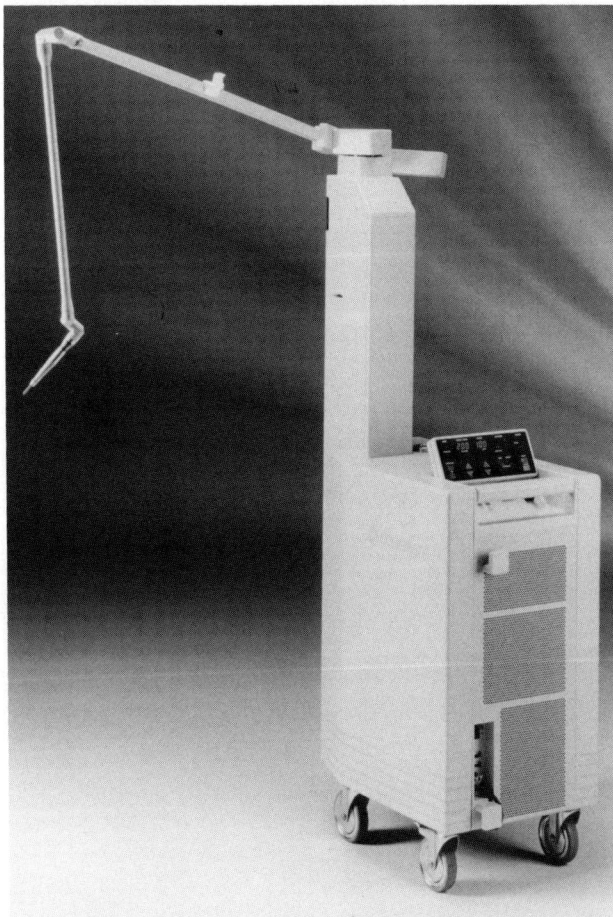

FIGURE 22–21. Carbon dioxide laser delivery system. (Courtesy of Coherent, Palo Alto, CA.)

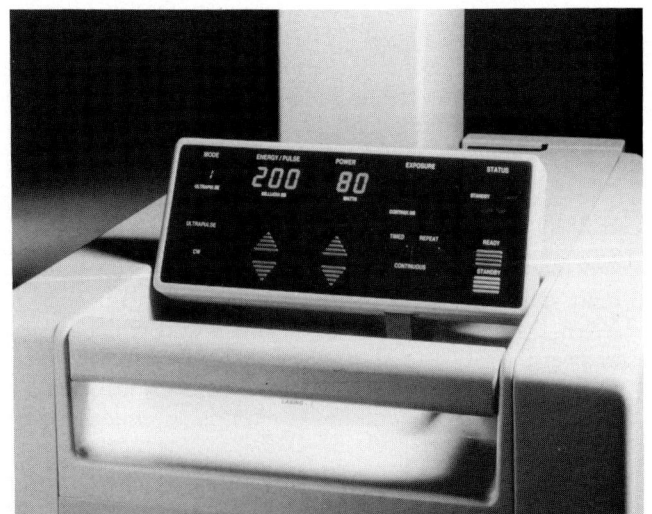

FIGURE 22–22. Carbon dioxide laser delivery system with continuous and ultrapulse modes within the same unit. (Courtesy of Coherent, Palo Alto, CA.)

TABLE 22–1. Advantages of the Carbon Dioxide Laser

The beam can be precisely controlled to incise or destroy tissue.
The area of destruction is sharply limited, and the zone of tissue devitalization is narrow
The depth of destruction is better visualized than with other laser wavelengths
Hemostasis is adequate, which improves visualization and reduces trauma
Application to regions of difficult access is good
Spot sizes of 0.2–2 mm in diameter are available depending on the laser focusing and delivery device

operating channel just distal to the mirror to deliver carbon dioxide down the beam channel. This prevents fogging of the mirror and lens and also displaces smoke from the channel. This is extremely important because excess smoke reduces the power of the beam as it emerges from the laser channel.

The alignment of the CO_2 laser and helium/neon (HeNe) beam is tested by directing and firing the beam at a moist tongue blade. The laparoscope is then reintroduced into the abdomen, and the orange-red HeNe aiming beam is sighted before firing. A second puncture site for suction/irrigation may be used to manipulate and irrigate pelvic structures as well as to vent off laser plume. The operator should keep the suction probe close to the impact site of the laser beam and immediately suction off the smoke to maintain adequate visualization of the tissues. If smoke accumulates despite this maneuver, high-flow insufflators and smoke evacuation systems (Fig. 22–23) can be used to maintain a clean environment.

For those surgeons who prefer to operate with a second puncture CO_2 laser probe, a double-ring device measuring 8 mm in external diameter can be used. The probe attaches to the same zinc selinide focusing lens or lens and mirror that is used with the operating laparoscope. The carbon dioxide insufflation tubing is attached to the probe so the gas flows down the channel in a manner similar to the flow down the operating scope. The laser plume is drawn out the outer ring channel of the probe. This second puncture probe is also available with a backstop, which minimizes the risk of inadvertent injury to intraperitoneal structures by the laser beam.

The focusing lens is a 300 to 315 mm lens that provides for the laser beam a focal point 2 cm from the end of either the operating scope or the second puncture probe (Fig. 22–

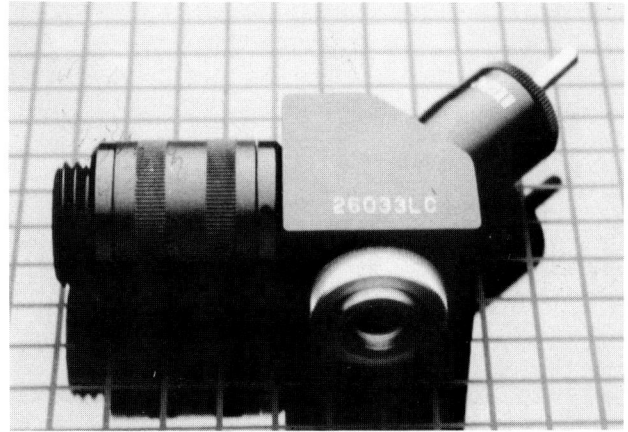

FIGURE 22–24. Focusing lens that focuses for the laser beam 2 cm from the end of the operating laparoscope or laser probe. (Courtesy of Edward Weck and Company, Research Triangle Park, NC.)

24). This long focal length produces a spot diameter of approximately 0.5 mm. Unfortunately, with this system, it is difficult to defocus the laser by pulling the scope away from the tissue. This limits the range of power densities. In addition, the long focal length of the second puncture system results in an instrument that is longer than necessary for comfortable use with multiple techniques.

Lens and mirror attachments with focal lengths of 250 and 300 mm have been developed. These laser laparoscopes give the system greater flexibility. For example, use of the 250-mm lens with a shorter second puncture probe (230 mm) results in an instrument that is much less cumbersome and allows higher power densities and a smaller diameter of the focused beam. Conversely, the 250-mm lens, when aimed and fired through the longer operating channel of the laser scope, results in a significantly defocused beam and less power density. Carbon dioxide fibers and wave guides are also available, which can eliminate the need for focusing systems. The fibers, unfortunately, have a large spot size that limits their use. The mere fact that the carbon dioxide energy comes out of the end of the wave guide makes this device more safe because the surgeon can see where the laser beam is emitted, thereby decreasing the chances of bowel inadvertently coming in front of the laser beam as one operates.

ARGON LASER INSTRUMENTATION

In an attempt to overcome some of the limitations of the CO_2 laser, the argon laser has been used at laparoscopy, hysteroscopy, and microsurgical procedures. The argon laser, with wavelengths of 488 and 514.5 nm, is selectively absorbed by pigmented tissues rich in hemoglobin and hemosiderin (Fig. 22–25). Thus, endometrial implants absorb the energy of the argon laser much more effectively than surrounding tissues that are not so richly pigmented. In addition, the argon laser can be delivered through a flexible quartz fiber, which can, in turn, be passed through the operating channel of a standard operative laparoscope.

Although the original argon laser system generated only 5 watts of energy, a present model can generate and deliver between 15 and 20 watts. Thus, the power density delivered at the tip of the 600-μ diameter quartz fiber makes it possible

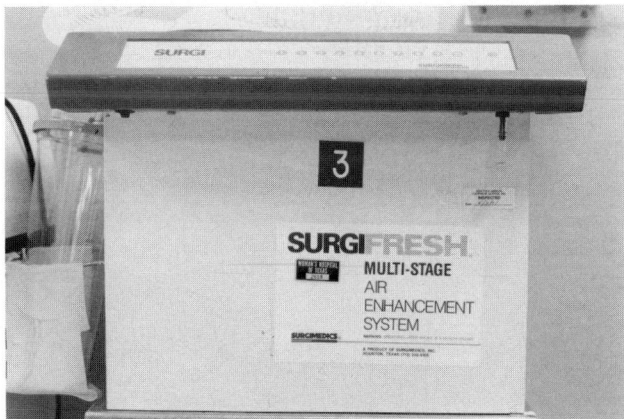

FIGURE 22–23. Smoke evacuation system (Courtesy of SurgiMedics, Inc., Houston, TX.)

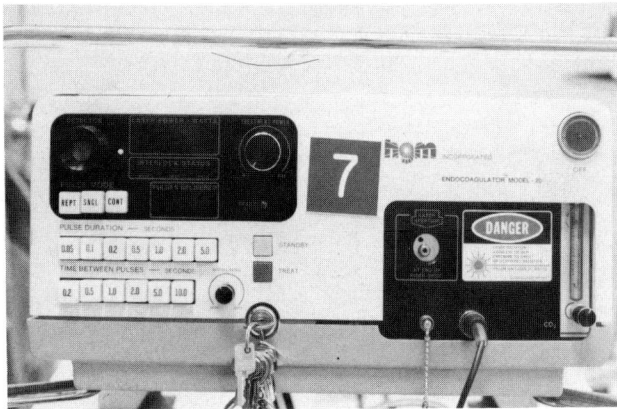

FIGURE 22–25. Argon laser delivery system. (Courtesy of HGM, Inc., Salt Lake City, UT.)

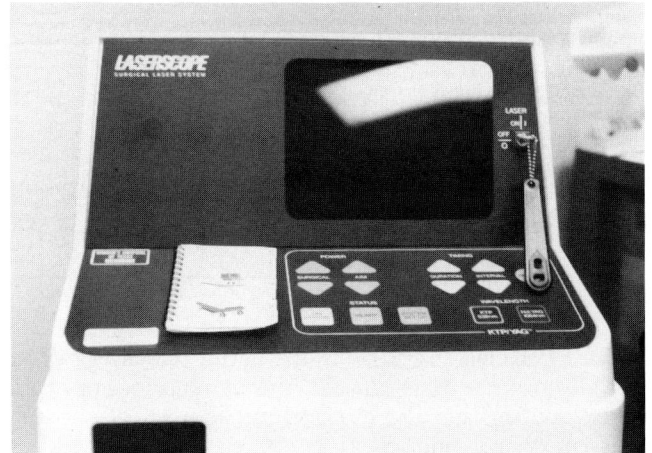

FIGURE 22–26. KTP laser delivery system. (Courtesy of Laserscope, San Jose, CA.)

to vaporize as well as coagulate tissue. The surgeon must wear colored goggles or glasses to prevent inadvertent retinal damage. The advantages and disadvantages of the argon laser are listed in Table 22–2.

KTP (DOUBLED FREQUENCY Nd:YAG LASER) INSTRUMENTATION

The KTP (potassium-titanyl-phosphate) laser produces a visible light of 532 nm wavelength and can be delivered by a 300 or 600 μ, flexible quartz fiber (Fig. 22–26). This fiber can pass through the operating channel of a hysteroscope or laparoscope and can be used with an operating microscope for microsurgery.

The KTP-532 laser beam is generated by doubling the frequency of a neodymium-yttrium-aluminum-garnet (Nd:YAG) laser and passing the beam through a KTP crystal, in which the wavelength is halved from 1064 to 532 nm. The resulting 532-nm beam is easy to see because of its lime-green color. It has a tissue depth of penetration ranging from 0.3 mm to more than 2 mm, depending on the power density. It is selectively absorbed by reddish pigments and, as a result, is effective for coagulation of blood vessels and ablation of endometriosis in the pelvis. Some newer laser units have wavelength capacity with both KTP and Nd:YAG lasers available in the same machine (Fig. 22–27).

Clinically the KTP/532 laser and argon laser are identical endoscopically for hysteroscopy and laparoscopy. Hysteroscopic procedures performed include intrauterine incision of septa, vaporization of submucous fibroids, excision of benign intrauterine polyps, and vaporization of intrauterine adhesions. The procedures can be performed with minimal bleeding. It is often recommended to perform a laparoscopy at the

time of advanced operative hysteroscopic procedures to monitor for potential uterine perforation. The risk of penetration, however, with the argon or KTP laser fiber is minimized by keeping the fiber tip off of the endometrium.

This laser is not used for endometrial ablation because the depth of penetration is not sufficient to destroy the basalis layer of the endometrium. With respect to uterine septa, bleeding that was previously encountered with other forms of hysteroscopic removal rarely occurs with the KTP/532 or argon laser owing to the coagulating effects of the beam. As

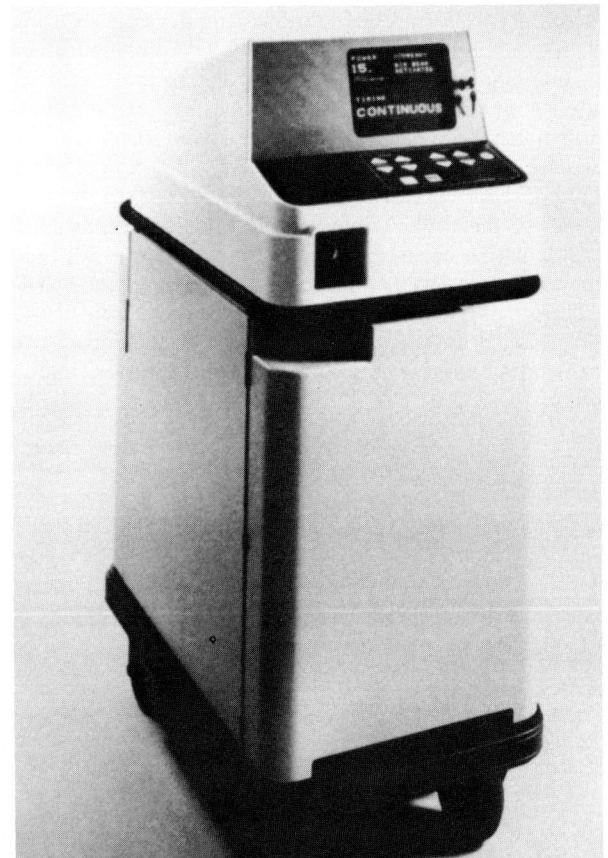

FIGURE 22–27. Dual-wavelength capability unit: both KTP-532 and neodymium:YAG lasers. (Courtesy of Laserscope, San Jose, CA.)

TABLE 22–2. Advantages and Disadvantages of Argon and KTP/532 Laser Laparoscopy	
Advantages	**Disadvantages**
Both vaporization and coagulation possible	Eye filter needed
Minimal lateral scatter	Possible breakage of fibers
Shallow depth of penetration	Cost of laser (relative to CO_2)
Energy passes through water	Somewhat deeper coagulation than the CO_2 laser

for the treatment of intrauterine adhesions, laser ablation is effective and precise and is therefore one other alternative to the use of scissors and electrosurgical loops.

The KTP/532 and argon lasers have been used extensively during laparoscopic procedures to aid in the surgical treatment of pelvic endometriosis, pelvic adhesions, ectopic pregnancies, subserosal uterine fibroids, and hydrosalpinx. The fiber itself can be placed close to the tissue for coagulation or can directly touch the tissue for dissecting purposes. The advantages and disadvantages of the KTP are similar to those of the argon laser because both are "green" lasers and have similar wavelengths.

Nd:YAG LASER

The Nd:YAG laser is a solid-state laser that emits in the near-visible infrared portion of the electromagnetic spectrum at 1064 nm wavelength (Fig. 22–28). Most of the units today are air cooled rather than water cooled and require 110 volts rather than the 208 single-phase electrical requirements of the first laser units. These systems can create short pulses with peak powers exceeding 100 watts or deliver continuous outputs ranging between 50 and 100 watts. As with the argon and KTP lasers, this wavelength is delivered through fiberoptic quartz fibers. One particular unit has a special sapphire tip that enhances the precision of the YAG laser and limits the depth of coagulation (Fig. 22–29). By and large, the YAG

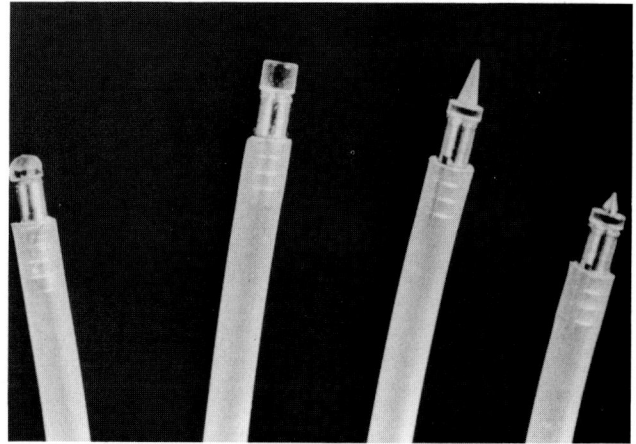

FIGURE 22–29. Variety of sapphire tips for the YAG laser.

laser is a coagulating laser with rather deep tissue penetration. The sapphire tips have allowed more control of this wavelength so it can be used more safely at laparoscopy. Because the laser energy passes through water, the YAG laser is ideal to be used at hysteroscopy for ablation to the endometrium, incision of uterine septa, or excision of endometrial polyps or submucous fibroids. The disadvantages of the YAG laser are similar to the KTP and argon with few exceptions. Greater care must be taken when using YAG energy because the danger of a uterine perforation is much greater owing to its deeper and wider thermal damage capability.

LAPAROTOMY

Although in the 1970s and 1980s laparotomy was the most common surgical procedure used in the treatment of infertile patients, in the last 10 years, there has been a definite trend toward what has been called *minimally invasive surgery* or advanced operative laparoscopy. There will always be situations, however, in which a laparotomy incision is necessary. In this chapter, the most updated instrumentation for infertility surgery by laparotomy is discussed. Over the last several years, there have actually been few new instruments developed for microsurgery.

Operating Microscope and Magnifying Loupes

Even though magnification is not required for all infertility surgery, there are many procedures in which its use is necessary or even mandatory. It is therefore necessary for the infertility surgeon to have a working knowledge of the operating microscope, its function, and capabilities.

Zeiss of West Germany in 1951 introduced the first commercially available microscope for the otorhinolaryngologist. From that time on, there have been a number of manufacturers developing microscopes for the industry. Not only have the microscopes been developed for magnification, but also various types of operating loupes with magnifying power ranging from 1.8× to 8× with field of view from 100 to 20 mm have been marketed (Fig. 22–30). The newest operating microscopes can provide magnification from 2× to 40×.

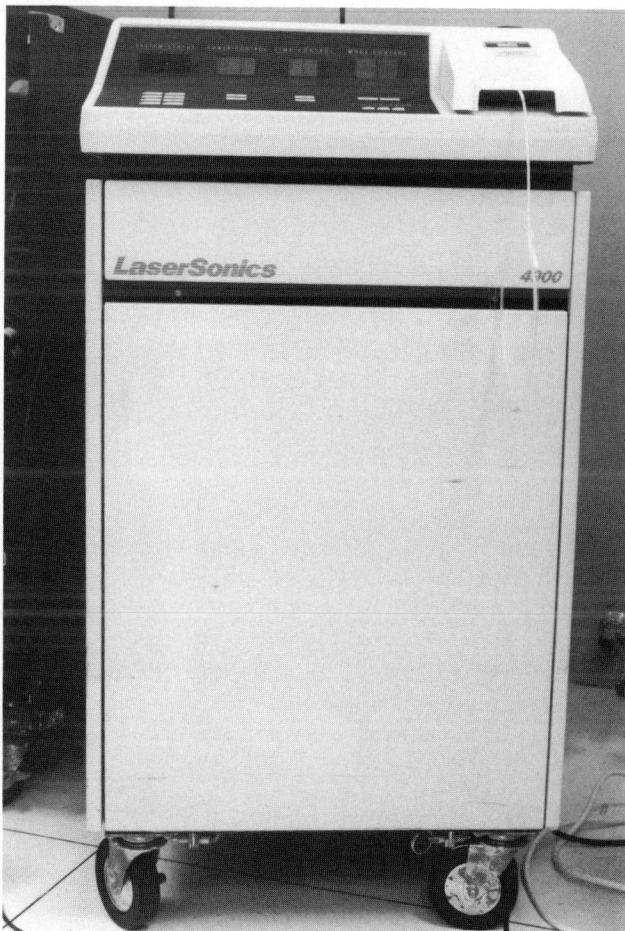

FIGURE 22–28. YAG laser delivery system. (Courtesy of LaserSonics, Milpitas, CA.)

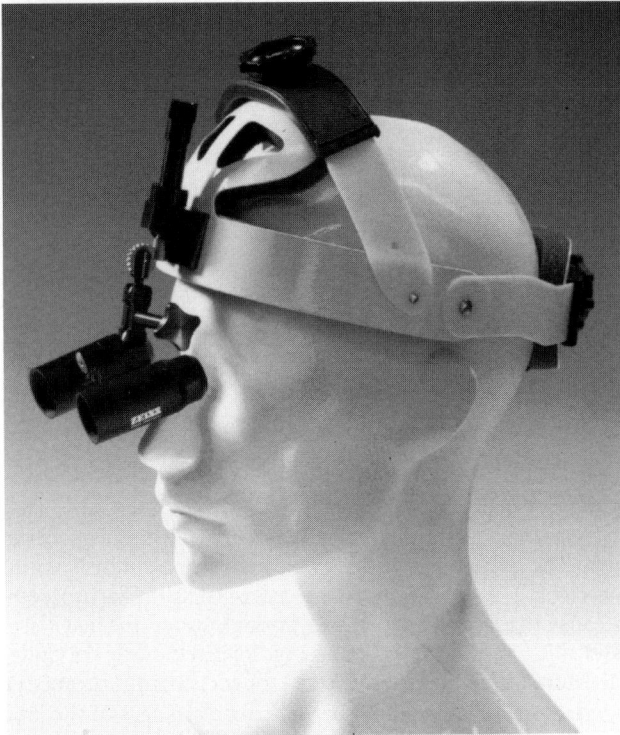

FIGURE 22–30. Zeiss operating loupes. (Courtesy of Zeiss Optical, Inc., Thornwood, NY.)

however, are extremely knowledgeable and eager to give on-site demonstrations of these applications.

Electrosurgical and Laser Equipment

The more important laser and electrosurgical units are described in the section on laparoscopy. Electrosurgical and laser delivery systems for microsurgery at laparotomy are different and must be described separately.

The electrosurgical units must all have three separate output transformers: a general surgical, micromonopolar, and microbipolar. Some of the newer units also have an argon beam coagulator, which has proved to be an excellent modality for hemostasis. The delivery system for the microsurgical unit is important. It should be lightweight, with easy fingertip control for cutting and coagulation of proper length, and should be able to accommodate electrodes for both conventional surgery and microsurgery. Every unit must be properly grounded when using the monopolar coagulation or cutting. A 100-μ monopolar, insulated microelectrode is preferred for most dissections. A well-designed, hand-controlled microbipolar forcep is an important and necessary instrument for microsurgery. Even though foot-controlled models are avail-

Any higher magnification is not practical for our specialty. There are operating loupes that have magnification over 4×, but they are cumbersome and difficult to operate with. Many surgeons experience a lot of neck discomfort owing to limited head movement or dizziness if there is too much head movement. If magnification of more than 4× is necessary, an operating microscope should be used.

Present-day microscopes are stereomicroscopes with Galilean optics (Fig. 22–31). These optics originated from the old Galilean telescopes used to observe distant objects. To convert this telescope into a microscope, a large positive lens was placed in front of the focal plane. This lens determines the focal length of the microscope and represents the working distance. Modification of the working distance is affected by changing the objective lens and is altered by using telescopes of different power or a zoom system. Of course, working distances vary with each surgical procedure. For example, the range of an ideal working distance for the gynecologist is between 250 and 300 mm. In an obese patient, one may need a 350-mm lens. In contrast, the ophthalmologist uses a working distance of 150 to 200 mm, whereas the otolaryngologist uses 320 to 400 mm. An important accessory for the operating microscope is the beam splitter. Insertion of a beam splitter between the magnification changer and the binocular tube permits separation of the light beam without changing any of the optical parameters. The beam splitter allows the surgeon to view the operating field directly while the image is projected onto a video screen. This benefits all assistants in the operating room and permits documentation using still photography, television, or cinematography. Space does not permit a detailed discussion of the mechanisms for obtaining documentation. The representatives of each manufacturer,

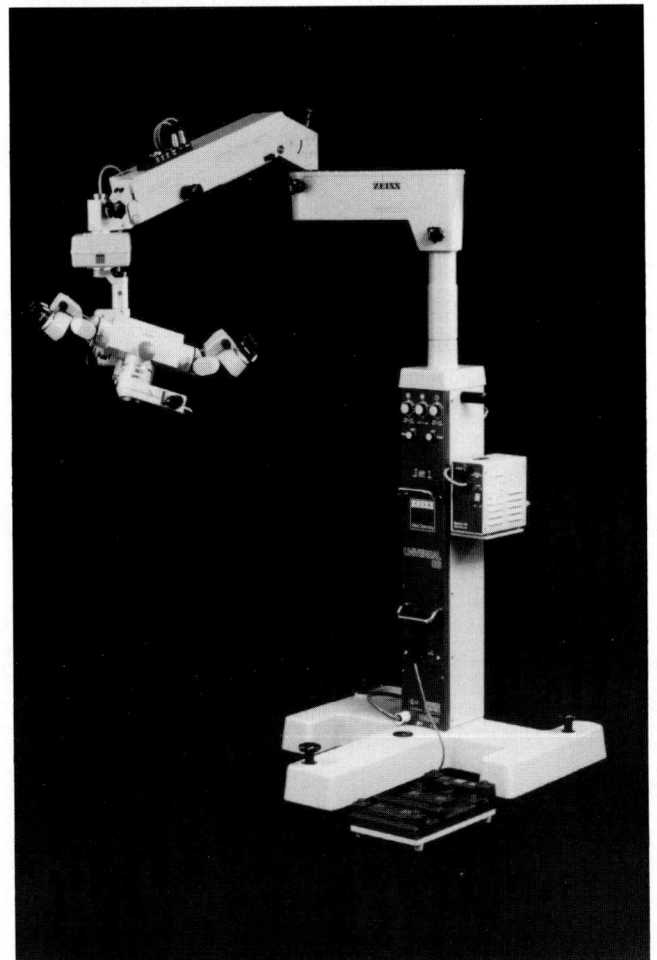

FIGURE 22–31. Zeiss operating microscope. (Courtesy of Zeiss Optical, Inc., Thornwood, NY.)

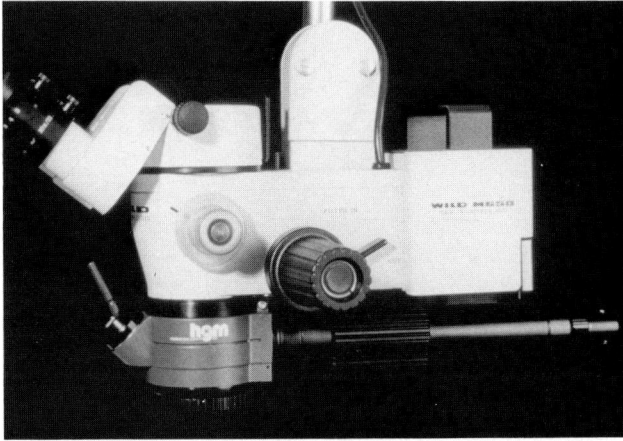

FIGURE 22–32. Micromanipulator used with the microscissors and argon laser during microsurgery. (Courtesy of HGM, Inc., Salt Lake City, UT.)

able, the hand-controlled instruments are preferable. It is a good idea to minimize the number of foot pedals used during a surgical procedure to avoid a situation in which the wrong one is pressed.

Laser energy can be an extremely beneficial tool for microsurgery. The laser beam is directed toward the operative field by attaching a micromanipulator, or joystick, below the objective of the operating microscope (Fig. 22–32). To set the laser beam properly, the microscope is first focused on the tissue at maximum magnification. At this point, both the laser beam and the optical focus are the same. If the magnification is then decreased, the laser beam is always in focus. The reason for the need to have the beam in focus with the objective lens is based on the fact that a defocused beam creates a significant decrease in the power density of the laser, which, in turn, increases the coagulation and decreases its cutting ability. If one is using a fiberoptic laser, the micromanipulator also has a filter specific for that wavelength superimposed between the objective and the eyepiece to prevent laser damage to the retina of the eye. If a filter is present, one must wear protective glasses while looking through the eyepiece of the microscope.

Instruments and Sutures

A vast array of sizes and shapes of instruments for microsurgery exists. Only a few select instruments, however, are needed for most cases. In general, the instrument must fit properly in the hand and usually is grasped in the same way as a pencil. The working end of the instrument, certainly its most important part, should be somewhat blunt for delicate handling of the tissues. Instruments that are too sharp on the end increase the likelihood of tissue trauma and thus increase the chances of adhesion formation.

Microforceps are available with teeth or without teeth (Fig. 22–33). Forceps without teeth should have thin, rounded tips to allow for easy tying of suture, and an ideal length for these forceps is about 14 cm. There are several types of needle holders; the two most common and useful have a spring-loaded ratchet to secure the needle. Another important feature of a needle holder is the jaw configuration. The curved jaw shape is preferable to the conventional flat jaw

because this permits better control and fitting of the needle within the needle holder (Fig. 22–34).

There are a variety of scissors used in microsurgery, but only two configurations are really necessary. The microdissecting scissors have slightly rounded tips and thin, curved blades (Fig. 22–35). These scissors are used primarily for microdissection and cutting microsuture. Iris scissors are straight, sturdier, and used primarily to cut across tissue segments or dense adhesions. Neither of these scissors should be used to cut standard nonmicrosurgical suture because of eventual damage to the scissor blades.

Another essential microsurgical instrument is an irrigator. Commonly, a 20-ml syringe with a blunt needle tip is used. There are other devices, however, that can provide constant flow of irrigating fluid from an intravenous bag that prevents the need to change syringes constantly.

Manipulating probes are also important in microsurgery. Different types are used with electrosurgical energy or laser energy. For electrosurgery, Teflon-coated metal rods allow atraumatic manipulation of tissue and at the same time do not conduct the electricity from the microelectrode (Fig. 22–36). For laser surgery, however, the Teflon would be vaporized to a toxic gas, so a titanium rod that has been ebonized must be used to prevent scatter of the laser beam. The titanium rod absorbs and dissipates the heat of the laser, preventing damage to tissue beyond the target of the laser beam.

The proper selection of sutures for microsurgical procedures is fairly standard. The most common sutures are polyethylene, nylon, or polyglycolic acid. In animal studies, polyglycolic acid sutures appear to provoke the least tissue reaction when evaluated after 80 days, even though the other two sutures have minimal effect.[6] The most common suture size is 7–0 to 11–0 for fallopian tube anastomosis. The smaller suture would obviously be used in the intramural portion of the tube. Needle selection is another difficult problem because so many sizes and shapes are available. Probably the most frequently used is the tapered 3/8 circle, 130-μ,

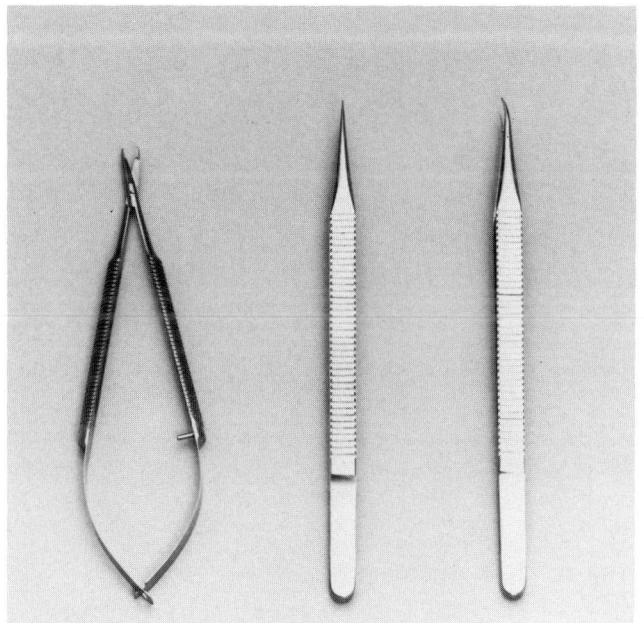

FIGURE 22–33. Microforceps. (Courtesy of Cohen Micro Instruments.)

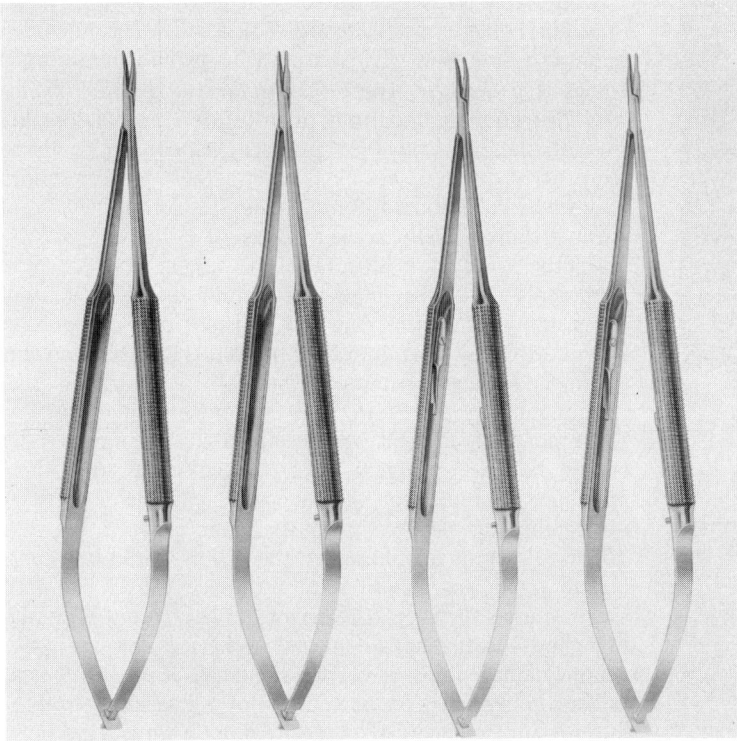

FIGURE 22–34. Microneedle holders with varying jaw configurations. (Courtesy of Elmed, Addison, IL.)

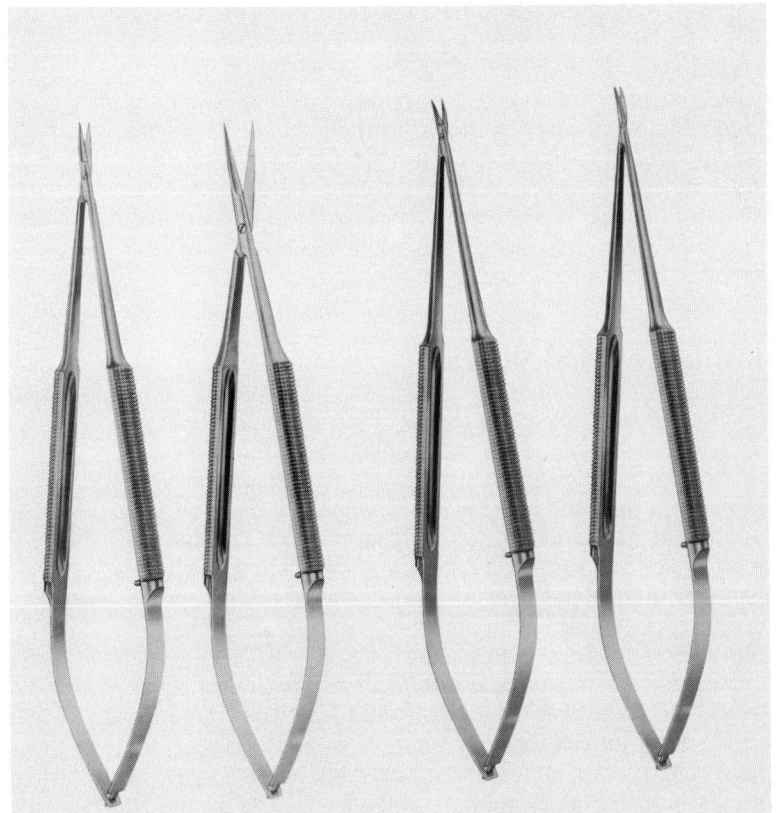

FIGURE 22–35. Microscissors for dissection. (Courtesy of Elmed, Addison, IL.)

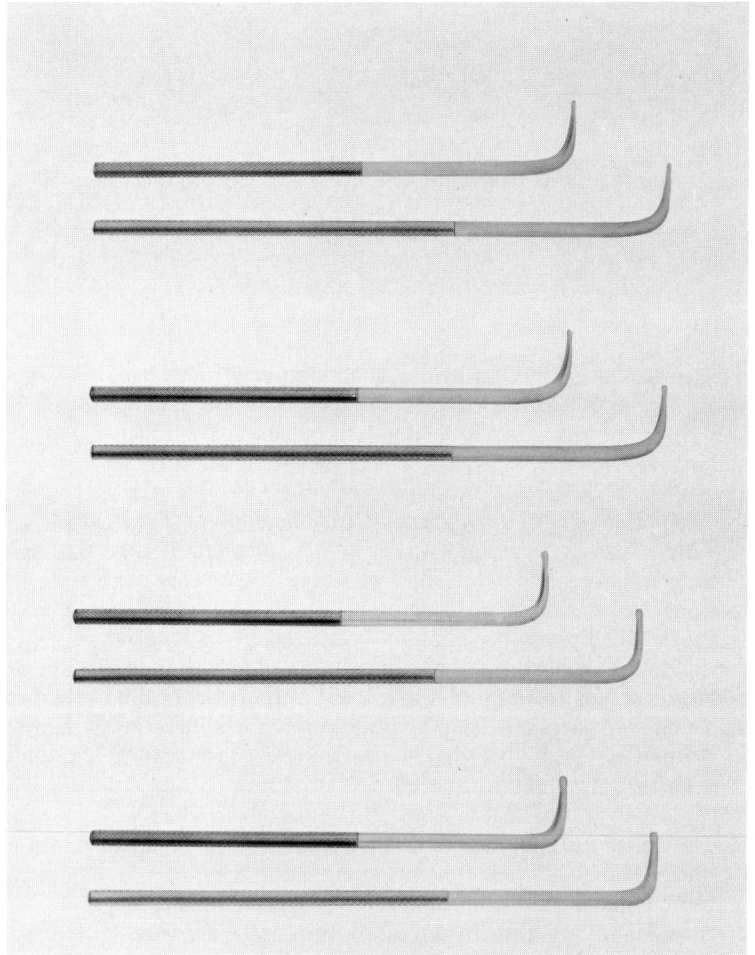

FIGURE 22–36. Teflon-coated metal rods for backstops when performing electrosurgical dissections. (Courtesy of Elmed, Addison, IL.)

3.7-mm needle. A taper cut needle is preferred to allow easier tissue penetration.

Hysteroscopy

Over the last decade, interest in hysteroscopy has greatly increased. Advances in surgical technique and instrumentation have provided the gynecologist with methods for treating conditions such as septate uterus and submucous fibroids that were previously untreatable or were treated only through major intra-abdominal incision.[7, 8]

There are essentially two types of hysteroscopes for operative hysteroscopy, rigid and flexible. The rigid hysteroscope was the first one developed for operative hysteroscopy. It consists of a telescope containing fiberoptic bundles for image and light transmission. The outer sheath contains three or four side channels for the introduction of instruments or distention media. The four-channel instrument is the most popular because of its wide versatility (Fig. 22–37). It has an 8-mm outer diameter, whereas the three channel instrument has a 6 to 7 mm outer diameter. The deflection angles vary from 0 degrees up to 70 degrees. For working in the cornu of the uterus, a moderate degree of deflection is helpful (at least 25 degrees) to give better visualization of this area. This is particularly important when canalizing the proximal fallopian tube with Novy catheters or similar catheters. Several ancillary instruments are used through the operative channels of the hysteroscope. The most practical are the scissors, biopsy forceps, graspers, and blunt dissectors. Some rigid hysteroscopes have an instrument called an *albaran,* which is used to direct an instrument within the endometrial cavity (Fig. 22–38). This is particularly valuable when a fiberoptic laser is used within the uterine cavity either to ablate the endometrium or to incise polyps, submucous fibroids, or intrauterine adhesions.

The resectoscope is an electrosurgical device adapted for use within the endometrial cavity (Fig. 22–39). This instrument has telescopes similar to other hysteroscopes, but the

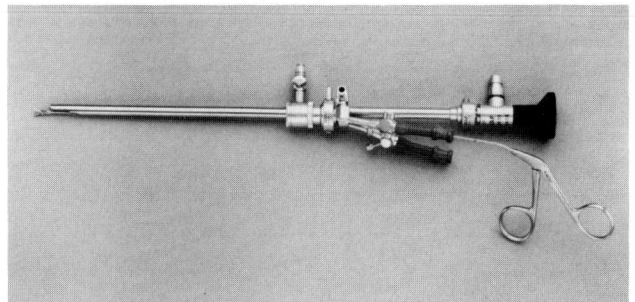

FIGURE 22–37. Four-channel hysteroscope with hysteroscopic scissors introduced through an accessory operative channel. (Courtesy of R. Wolf Medical Instruments Corp., Vernon Hills, IL.)

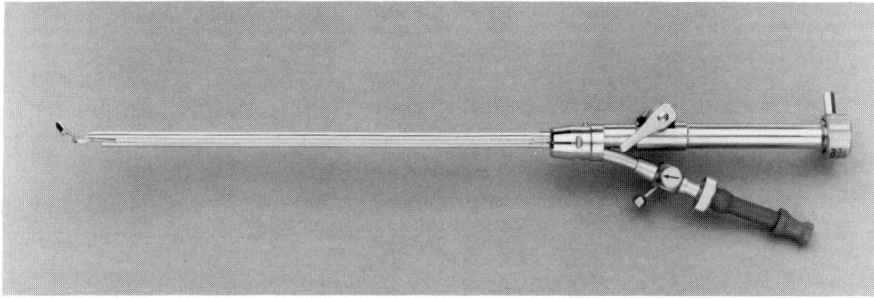

FIGURE 22–38. Albarran device used to direct an instrument or filter within the endometrial cavity. (Courtesy of R. Wolf Medical Instruments Corp., Vernon Hills, IL.)

outer sheath is adapted to hold a small loop or a roller ball or bar. The loop is particularly useful for excising submucous fibroids or polyps or even for endometrial ablation. The roller ball or bar is used specifically for endometrial ablation (Fig. 22–40). Most hysteroscopists now prefer the roller bar over the YAG laser or resectoscope ablation of the endometrium. The YAG laser is sometimes preferred for ablation of the cornu area because an acute angle occasionally prevents the roller bar from reaching this area.

The flexible hysteroscope has not been available as long as the rigid model. Flexible scopes are now available with outer diameters as small as 4 mm for diagnostic purposes or 5 mm for operative purposes. The 1-mm operative channel can accommodate a laser fiber that can be used to incise a septum or to excise polyps, submucous fibroids, or intrauterine adhesions. This operative channel may also be used with the YAG laser to ablate the endometrium. For the purpose of evaluating the proximal fallopian tube, there is even a scope of 1 to 3 mm in diameter. With respect to distention media for diagnostic and operative hysteroscopy, the first agent introduced by Rubin[9] was carbon dioxide. This gas normally provides excellent visibility; however, troublesome bubbles and debris at times can obscure the view. It is important that the rate of flow not exceed 80 to 100 cc per minute; therefore, the use of a laparoscopic insufflator is strictly prohibited. Cases of death from carbon dioxide embolus have been re-

ported in the past.[10] Dextran 70 was introduced by Edstrom and Fernstrom in 1970 as an alternate distention medium. This medium is optically clear, electrolyte free, nonconductive, biodegradable, and immiscible with blood. These attributes make it a desirable distention medium except for one problem. Dextran is extremely thick and sometimes difficult to push through the in-flow channel. It can obstruct the operative channels if allowed to dry or accumulate. Therefore, the instruments must be cleaned thoroughly after each use. Cases of anaphylactic shock have been reported with the use of dextran 70, although the incidence is low (approximately 1 per 10,000 cases). Respiratory failure and coagulopathies have also been reported.[11]

Other fluid media, such as 5% or 10% dextrose in water or regular saline, have a low viscosity. The use of saline is prohibited, however, if electrosurgical instruments are used. In these instances, one must use 1.5% glycine, sorbitol, or other similar nonconductive fluids. The advantages of the low-viscosity fluids include lower cost, ready availability, reduced pain, and less risk of extravasation. A more thorough discussion of hysteroscopy appears in Chapter 26.

DOCUMENTATION: VIDEO, STILL PHOTOGRAPHY, CINEMATOGRAPHY

For many years, still photography has been the predominant mode of documentation for endoscopic and microsurgical procedures. This has now largely been replaced by video monitoring and documentation and computerized digital freeze-frame photography.

Documentation with 35-mm still photography has long been used for teaching purposes as well as patient education

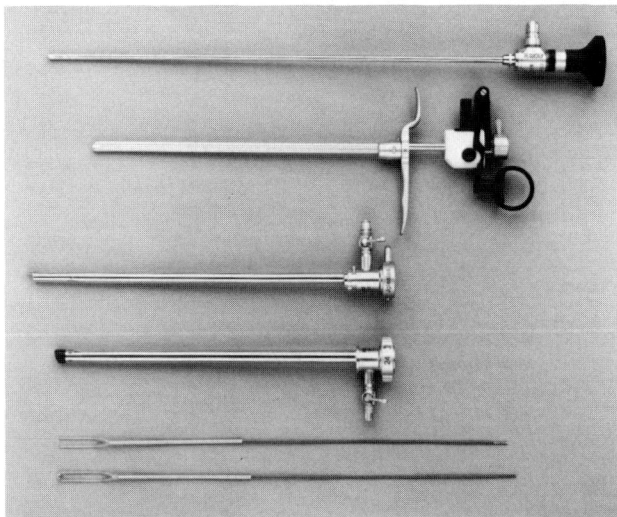

FIGURE 22–39. Hysteroscopic resectoscope for removal of submucous fibroids or incision of septate uterus. From top to bottom: telescope, loop holder, inner and outer sheath, loop, and rollerball. (Courtesy of R. Wolf Medical Instruments Corp., Vernon Hills, IL.)

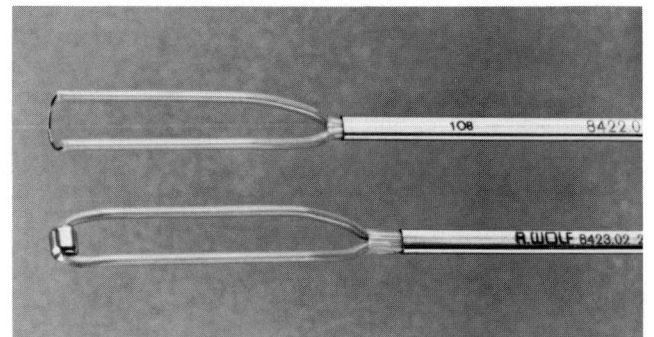

FIGURE 22–40. Wire loop (*top*) or rollerbar (*bottom*) for use with the resectoscope. (Courtesy of R. Wolf Medical Instruments Corp., Vernon Hills, IL.)

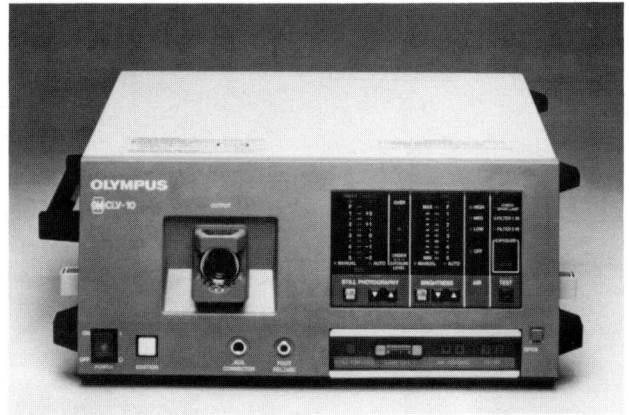

FIGURE 22–41. Endoscopic light source with available flash unit. (Courtesy of Olympus Corporation, Lake Success, NY.)

and charting. Almost any single reflex camera (SLR) can be adapted for use during laparoscopy, hysteroscopy, or laparotomy. The most frequently used camera is the Olympus OM 1 with special endoscopic adapter. When the camera is attached to the endoscope, the surgeon can scan the field through the viewfinder of the camera. In most instances, the ground-glass focusing screen must be replaced with a clear glass screen. Most endoscopic cameras are equipped with this device. The most popular lens is the 90-mm lens, which classically produces a circular picture that occupies about 75% of the viewing frame. A focal length of 120 mm takes up almost 100% of the frame.

As far as the proper selection of film, the slower the film, the less grainy the picture. I have used successfully a 64 ASA film with an Olympus flash and have pushed the film to 100 ASA in the developing process. Most endoscopic photography requires more than the ordinary 150-watt lightbulb to obtain good pictures. The best pictures and slides are obtained either with a halogen or xenon bulb and a high-quality flash unit (Fig. 22–41).

With respect to documentation for endoscopic surgery, the large, cumbersome tube cameras have been replaced with modern digital chip cameras weighing a little more than 2 oz (Fig. 22–42A and B). One-chip and three-chip cameras are now available, each having features significantly improved over the earlier model. These high-resolution monitors and cameras now produce video footage that is much clearer and

truer to color than older models. Yet until the lines of resolution in both the cameras and monitors approach the quality of resolution of our own eyes, operating entirely off a video monitor is not the same as using direct vision. One option the surgeon has is to use a *beam splitter,* which is essentially a camera that allows projection of an image onto the video screen, so the surgical assistant and operating room personnel can view the procedure while the surgeon is looking directly through the camera and viewing the field during the operation.

The availability of video documentation has become an important asset in the education process. The ability to observe actual surgical procedures without having to be in the operating room has improved the quality of physician and patient education. The use of videos for patient or referring physician review has been beneficial in planning surgery or evaluating one's treatment without actually having been present. These videotapes can be reviewed by credentialing committees for approval of a candidate's operative privileges.

Another valuable addition to the video system is the instant Polaroid printer (Fig. 22–43). From the camera output, these printers can produce exact images that are seen on the screen. Either full-frame images or prints that contain four or nine images per page can be generated. Although the quality of the prints are not reproducible for publication, they are extremely valuable for chart documentation and for demonstrating to patients and their families any anatomic pathology.

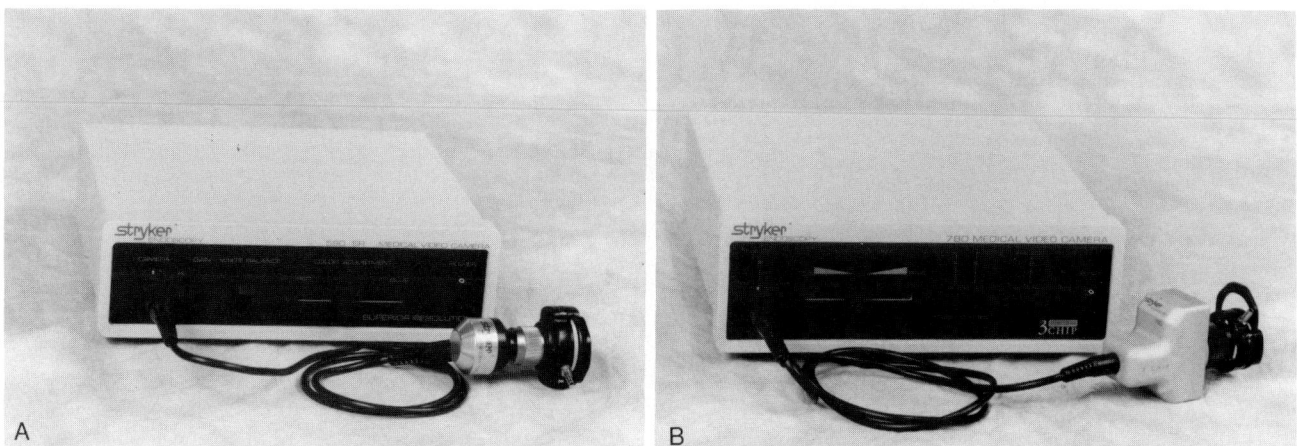

FIGURE 22–42. *A,* Single-chip camera *B,* Three-chip camera. (*A* and *B* courtesy of Stryker Endoscopy, Kalamazoo, MI.)

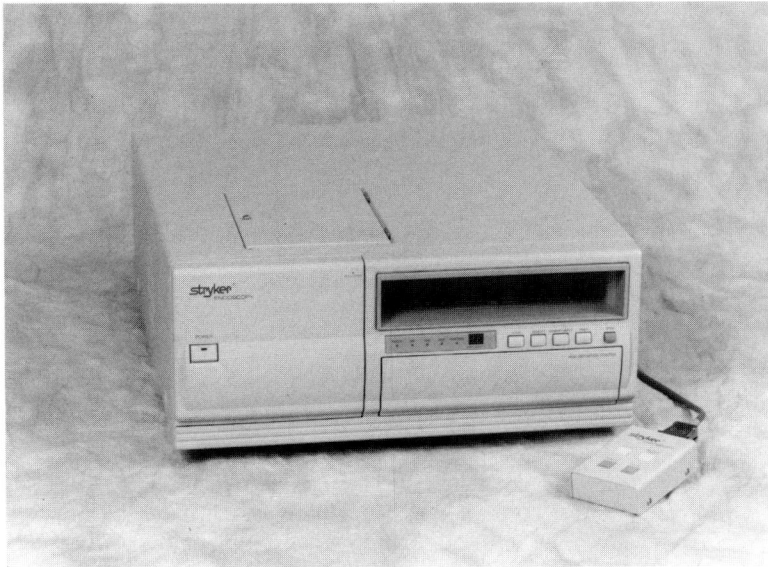

FIGURE 22–43. High-resolution Polaroid printer. (Courtesy of Stryker Endoscopy, Kalamazoo, MI.)

The printer also keeps photographs in memory for further printouts at the end of the procedure.

For more efficient record keeping, a character generator is available for all of the video systems (Fig. 22–44). This allows the surgeon to put the patient's demographics and any other information on the videotape. This particular feature is useful for documentation of surgery both for credentialing committees and for medicolegal encounters.

The most recent development in video systems is the digital camera unit (DCU), which is a computer-based capture device that connects to the video system through the existing video output (NTSC or S-VHS) (Fig. 22–45). The DCU captures images directly from the video camera. There is no need to interrupt the procedure to attach or detach any equipment to take photos. Photography is accomplished by pressing a foot pedal, and there are no exposure or focusing settings. The system is camera dependent for photographic quality. The computer processor contains the image capture hardware and software, which captures 24-bit color images. These images may contain more than 16 million colors and more than 1000 TV lines of resolution, compared with 256 colors and 200 TV lines of resolution for the common instant printer.

The image to be photographed is projected onto the computer monitor much as the image is projected onto the video monitor. The outboard disk drive is used to store the images on a large-capacity removable disk. Approximately 100 images per disk may be stored. The DCU is controlled by a simple computer trackball, which controls the on/off function as well as disk ejection and replacement. No keyboard or computer commands are used in this system, thus simplifying its use. To capture and save the image in less than 5 seconds, specialized software is required that is unique to the DCU.

Operation of the DCU is simple. Its monitor projects the same video image that is on the video monitor. Photographs

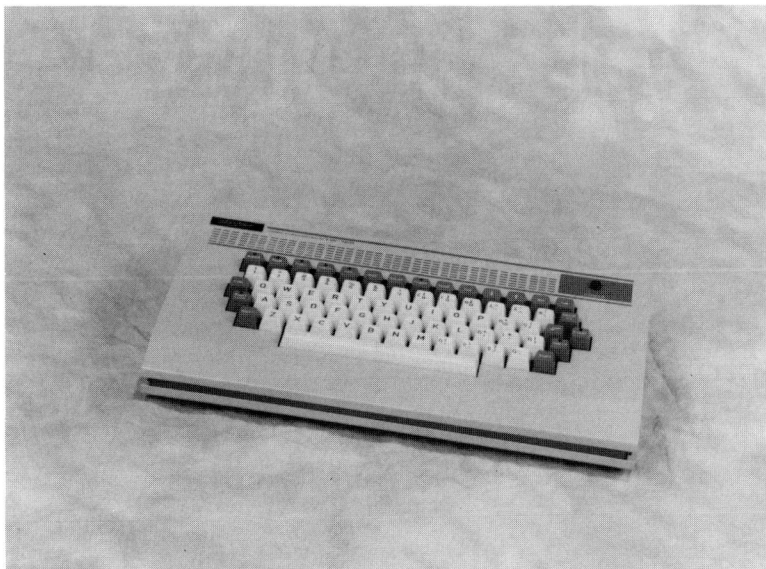

FIGURE 22–44. Character generator. (Courtesy of Stryker Endoscopy, Kalamazoo, MI.)

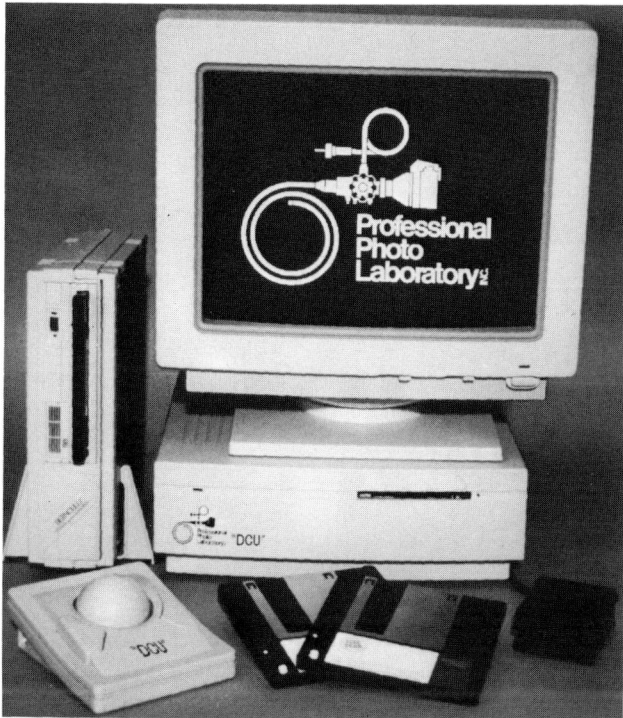

FIGURE 22–45. Digital camera unit. (Courtesy of Professional Photo Laboratory, Inc., Marina Del Ray, CA.)

are taken by pressing a footswitch briefly while the image on the DCU monitor is frozen for 5 seconds. During this time, the operator checks the frozen image for sharpness, and if the image is not of good quality, another photograph may be taken. When the procedure is over, the disk is removed and sent for processing.

SUMMARY

Undoubtedly progress in the field of gynecologic surgery has been greater in the last decade than at any time in the past. Evidence is in the increased proportion of outpatient surgeries that has revolutionized the surgical care of the infertile woman. In some instances, the available technology has outstripped clinical applications. Every day new instrumentation is being developed to further our skills in both endoscopic and microsurgical techniques. There is no question that the future of our profession is limited only by our creativity.

REFERENCES

1. Gussain NH. Bilateral pneumothorax associated with laparoscopy. A case report of a rare hazard and review of literature. Anesthesia 1973; 28:79–81.
2. Fitzgerald TB, Johnstone MW. Diaphragmatic defects and laparoscopy. BMJ 1970; 2:604.
3. Steptoe NC. Laparoscopy in Gynecology. Edinburgh: ES Livingston, 1967:30–34.
4. Levy BS, Soderstrom RM, Dail DH. Bowel injuries during laparoscopy: gross anatomy and histology. J Reprod Med 1985; 30:168–179.
5. Keye WR Jr. Laser Surgery in Gynecology and Obstetrics. Chicago Year Book Medical Publishers, 1990.
6. Sanz LE. Sutures. A primer in structure and function. Contemp Obstet Gynecol 1990; 35:99–106.
7. Valle RF, Scianna JJ. Current status of hysteroscopy in gynecologic practice. Fertil Steril 1979; 32:619.
8. Valle RF. Technique of panoramic hysteroscopy. In: Baggish MS, Barbot J, Valle RF, editors. Diagnostic and Operative Hysteroscopy. A Text and Atlas. Chicago: Year Book Medical Publishers, 1989:79–101.
9. Rubin IC. Uterotubal Insufflation. St. Louis: CV Mosby, 1947.
10. Corson SC, Hoffman JJ, Jakowski J, Chapman CA. Cardiopulmonary effects of direct venous CO_2 inflation in ewes. A model for CO_2 hysteroscopy. J Reprod Med 1988; 33:440–444.
11. McLucas B. Hyskon complication in hysteroscopic surgery. Obstet Gynecol 1991; 46:196–200.

CHAPTER 23

Imaging of the Reproductive Tract in Infertile Women: Hysterosalpingography, Ultrasonography, and Magnetic Resonance Imaging

MICHAEL R. SOULES and LAURENCE A. MACK

When an infertile couple presents to a physician, the initial emphasis should be on an accurate diagnosis of the condition(s) that is inhibiting their ability to conceive. Various tests are undertaken, as described earlier in this book. One of these basic tests, which is a cornerstone of an infertility evaluation, is hysterosalpingography. Ultrasonography is an imaging technique that has not reached the status of being a standard infertility test, yet it has assumed a major role in both the diagnosis and the treatment of infertility. Magnetic resonance imaging (MRI) has a much more limited role in the diagnosis of infertility and should be appropriately viewed as an ancillary modality to be reserved for special situations. This chapter addresses each of these imaging modalities as they pertain to female infertility. Imaging of the male reproductive tract has a much more limited role as part of an infertility evaluation and is not addressed in this chapter.

HYSTEROSALPINGOGRAPHY

After a history and physical examination, an infertility evaluation consists of a series of diagnostic tests. These tests are performed in a logical sequence that proceeds from the less complex to more invasive and expensive procedures. Unless specific information points toward uterotubal disease, a hysterosalpingogram (HSG) should be performed (Fig. 23–1)

after completion of an ovulation assessment, semen analysis, and postcoital test. If information is obtained that indicates an increased likelihood of uterotubal disease, it would be appropriate to obtain a HSG earlier in the evaluation. Examples of such information would be (1) history of salpingitis (pelvic inflammatory disease), (2) a positive Chlamydia culture or IgG titer ($\geq$1:32),[1] (3) status post postpartum dilatation and curettage (risk of Asherman's syndrome), (4) history of appendicitis with rupture, (5) a previous ectopic pregnancy, (6) prior pelvic surgery, (7) exposure to diethylstilbestrol (DES), (8) repetitive pregnancy loss, (9) a previous HSG that was abnormal, or (10) menorrhagia or metrorrhagia.[2]

A common misconception is that a laparoscopy suffices for a HSG. This is a fallacy that can lead to significant errors of omission in an infertility evaluation. Certain disease states are most amenable to diagnosis with HSG (e.g., Asherman's syndrome) or are capable only of diagnosis by HSG (e.g., salpingitis isthmica nodosa). Information concerning the intrauterine contour, intrauterine pathology, and location of tubal obstruction is available only with the use of HSG as opposed to laparoscopy. A laparoscopy allows the visualization of external uterine anatomy as well as external tubal anatomy (e.g., adhesions) and tubal ovarian relationships. Therefore, the two procedures, HSG and laparoscopy, are *complementary*.[3] The HSG is less expensive and less invasive than laparoscopy and generally should be *performed before the operative procedure*. If intrauterine pathology is identified at the time of

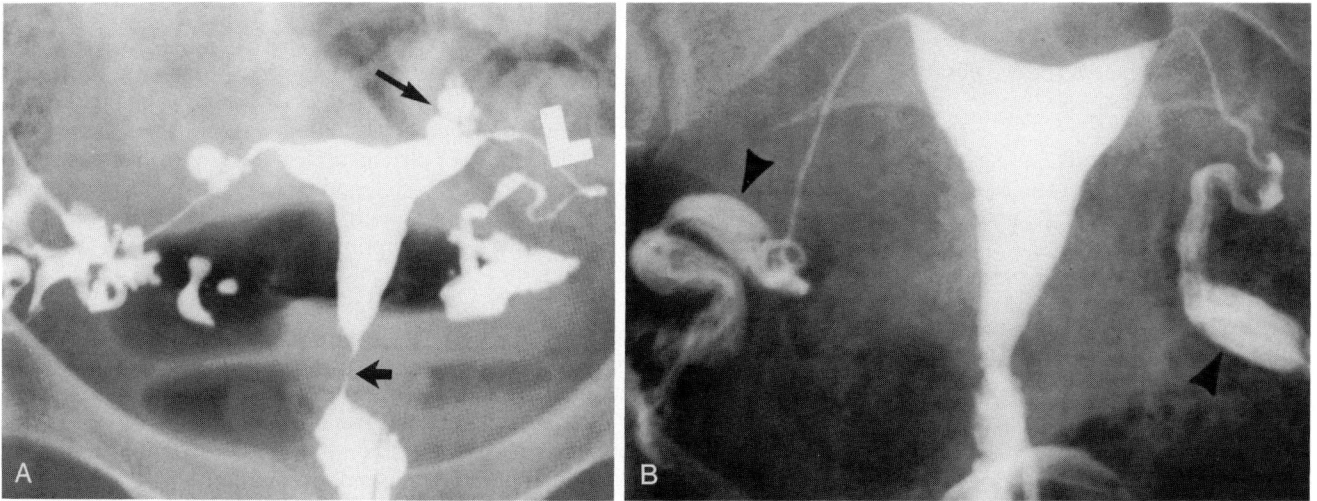

FIGURE 23–1. Normal hysterosalpingograms. *A,* Normal hysterosalpingogram performed with oil-soluble contrast medium. The oil-based medium is noted for being thicker, and the image appears more dense and opaque on the radiograph. This particular radiograph illustrates a narrow isthmus (*shorter arrow*) between the cervix and the main body of the uterus. Beads of oil can be seen where the medium spilled on the left side of the pelvis (*longer arrow*). *B,* This figure illustrates a normal radiograph using water-soluble contrast medium that yields an image that is less opaque. When water-soluble medium is used, the rugations (*arrowheads*) in the ampullar portion of the tube can be visualized and are used as a sign of normalcy of the tube. Oil- and water-soluble media have different properties, as discussed in the text. It is legitimate to use either medium for the performance of a hysterosalpingogram.

HSG, this can be verified and perhaps treated by a hysteroscopy performed at the time of laparoscopy. If tubal pathology is found with an HSG, this fact can be verified (and in some cases can be treated) with a laparoscopy.

A HSG is a test of uterine-tubal anatomy and *not function.* The physiologic capability of the uterus and tubes is not revealed with a HSG. There may be tests that demonstrate uterine-tubal physiology available in the future, such as the transport of radioactive albumin through the reproductive tracts as described elsewhere,[4] but no such tests are clinically relevant yet. Pregnancy alone is currently the only functional determinant of uterine-tubal physiology.

The use of hysterosalpingography should not be limited to the diagnosis of infertility. There are clear and relevant indications to perform a HSG in fertile women or women who have not attempted conception. Some examples of such indications are (1) persistent abnormal uterine bleeding to exclude polyps, (2) uterine myomas on pelvic examination to determine whether there is distortion of the cavity (submucous fibroids), (3) repetitive pregnancy loss to exclude a uterine anomaly. Furthermore, hysterosalpingography is not exclusively a diagnostic technique but has therapeutic aspects as well. Not only is there an increase in the pregnancy rate after a HSG, but also tubal catheterization techniques have been developed to be used in conjunction with HSG (selective salpingography).

History

It was not long after the advent of roentgenology (1895) that physicians were experimenting with the instillation of radiopaque media into every conceivable orifice. In 1910, Rindfleisch[5] was the first to attempt uterine radiography when he injected a bismuth solution into the uterine cavity. From his description of the results of the first HSG, we can assume his patient probably had a uterine anomaly. An American physician, William Cary[6] published an article in 1914 extolling the use of a radiopaque medium called collargol for the investigation of sterility. This medium was soon abandoned (it caused marked peritoneal irritation). In 1920, Rubin described a technique for nonoperative determination of tubal patency by insufflating oxygen into the uterine cavity. Tubal patency was determined by the sound of the gas entering the peritoneal cavity or the presence of the gaseous medium under the diaphragm. This test was to be performed for a number of years (using carbon dioxide and not oxygen) and was known as Rubin's test. The use of this procedure has now been virtually eliminated in favor of HSG. HSG became an accepted procedure after an efficacious and apparently safe contrast medium was developed in France in 1921. This medium was a chemical combination of 40% iodine in poppy seed oil known as Lipiodol. It was used for bronchograms, central nervous system (CNS) ventriculograms, and arteriograms. In 1925, Heuser[7] first described the use of Lipiodol for HSGs. HSG has been a common and useful procedure ever since this discovery of an effective medium.

Indications and Contraindications

The primary indications for performing a HSG are infertility, abnormal uterine bleeding, and repetitive pregnancy loss. The following outline lists the major anatomic or pathologic entities that are commonly found. Most of these potential findings are discussed and illustrated later in this section.

A. Uterine pathology.
   1. Leiomyomata uteri (submucous).
   2. Endometrial polyps.
   3. Intrauterine synechiae (adhesions).
B. Congenital uterine anomalies.
   1. Unicornuate uterus.
   2. Bicornuate uterus.

3. Septate uterus.
4. Uterus didelphys.
5. T-shaped uterus (DES exposure).
6. Uterine hypoplasia.
C. Oviduct anatomy.
   1. Proximal obstruction (e.g., fibrosis, debris).
   2. Distal tubal obstruction (e.g., hydrosalpinx).
   3. Tuberculosis.
   4. Peritubal adhesions.
D. Evaluation of recurrent pregnancy loss.
   1. Congenital uterine anomalies.
   2. Intrauterine synechiae.
   3. Incompetent cervical os.
E. Miscellaneous.
   1. Uterine or tubal fistulas.
F. Postoperative uses.
   1. Status post salpingoplasty.
   2. Status post metroplasty.
   3. Status post cesarean section—scar evaluation.
   4. Status post uterine perforation.
   5. Status post tubal ligation.

The contraindications to hysterosalpingography are infection (e.g., cervicitis, endometritis, or salpingitis), bleeding, and pregnancy. A HSG is capable of causing endometritis or salpingitis (pelvic inflammatory disease). This risk is compounded when active infection is present. Therefore, if there is a known infection at the time of procedure, the HSG is contraindicated until the infectious problem is resolved. Although it is unnecessary to do specific tests to rule out pelvic infection in every infertile woman before a HSG, it is advisable to maintain a high level of awareness toward this possibility. There are several ways to check for pelvic infection before a HSG: (1) Inquire regarding a history of prior pelvic infection, (2) do a pelvic examination checking for tenderness, (3) order a complete blood count and sedimentation rate, and (4) obtain a *Chlamydia* titer. (The first two items should be part of the performance of every HSG; the latter two items are optional if there is a suspicion of pelvic infection.)

Active uterine bleeding is a contraindication to HSG for three reasons: (1) There is an increased potential for intravasation of media, (2) the blood and clots obscure uterine pathology (sometimes clots appear to be intrauterine masses), and (3) the potential for retrograde menstruation and induction of endometriosis exists. Pregnancy is an obvious contraindication to HSG both in the short-term in regards to disruption of the pregnancy and in the long-term in regards to radiation exposure. Yet early in the history of hysterosalpingography, this procedure was performed specifically for the diagnosis of early pregnancy.[7, 8] These early investigations reported no untoward effects on the pregnancy after a HSG. Also pertaining to pregnancy has been concern regarding the outcome of pregnancies that occur in the same menstrual cycle as the x-ray procedure. A report in 1976 noted only 4 spontaneous abortions in 47 pregnancies conceived immediately after a HSG.[9] There were no congenital anomalies.[9] It would not be unreasonable to recommend the use of barrier contraception or abstinence during the menstrual cycle in which a HSG is to be performed; however, this is not a general recommendation in current practice.

Technique

There are two issues pertaining to the timing of a HSG. The first aspect of timing of a HSG concerns the phase of the menstrual cycle. A HSG should be performed in the late follicular phase of the menstrual cycle after the menstrual flow has been completed and before ovulation. By so timing a HSG, complications with the menstrual flow are obviously avoided as well as disruption of an early pregnancy. Although a HSG performed in the luteal phase of the cycle usually still reveals important information regarding uterine-tubal anatomy, it has a potential for disrupting or harming an embryo or early pregnancy. Furthermore, late in a cycle, the thicker endometrium can lead to false-positive diagnoses, such as intrauterine filling defects and proximal tubal obstruction (a ball-valve effect). The second aspect of timing pertains to the allowance of a 3- to 6-month waiting period after a HSG before the performance of further tests. This postprocedure waiting period is to allow a window of opportunity for conception to occur in selected patients. The patients for whom this recommendation applies are those couples with unexplained infertility (all tests up to and including the HSG are normal) and the female partner is less than 35 years of age. If the waiting period passes without conceiving, a laparoscopy is usually the next appropriate step.

It is important that the infertility practitioner be present at, and preferably perform, the HSG procedure. Presence at the procedure ensures knowledge of (1) any technical difficulties and (2) information available from the fluoroscopic phase of the procedure. In some HSG procedures, the fluoroscopic findings (e.g., ease of tubal spill, shift of an intrauterine bubble [alias a filling defect]) are more informative than the permanent radiographs.

It is pertinent to review the following step-by-step performance of an HSG (Fig. 23–2):

1. Perform a bimanual examination to rule out an unexpected pregnancy or adnexal mass.
2. Insert speculum and thoroughly cleanse the cervix with an antiseptic (i.e., iodine) solution.
3. Warm the medium to body temperature to help reduce tubal spasm.
4. Fill the introducer with medium to eliminate any bubbles.
5. Use an acorn-tip cannula on the introducer, and place the tip just inside the external cervical os while applying countertraction with a tenaculum. The tip should not be longer than 1 to 2 cm so as to not bypass the cervical anatomy. *Note:* A local anesthetic can be injected at 12 o'clock on the cervix with a 21- to 25-gauge spinal needle to help alleviate pain in association with placement of a tenaculum. The use of an intracavitary balloon device to introduce the medium is not recommended because it obscures the cervical and lower uterine anatomy.
6. Remove the speculum because it may obscure the findings.
7. Make certain that there is a right or left marker in place on the field.
8. After obtaining a scout radiograph, apply gentle traction on the cervix to bring the uterus into a horizontal position relative to the x-ray tube.

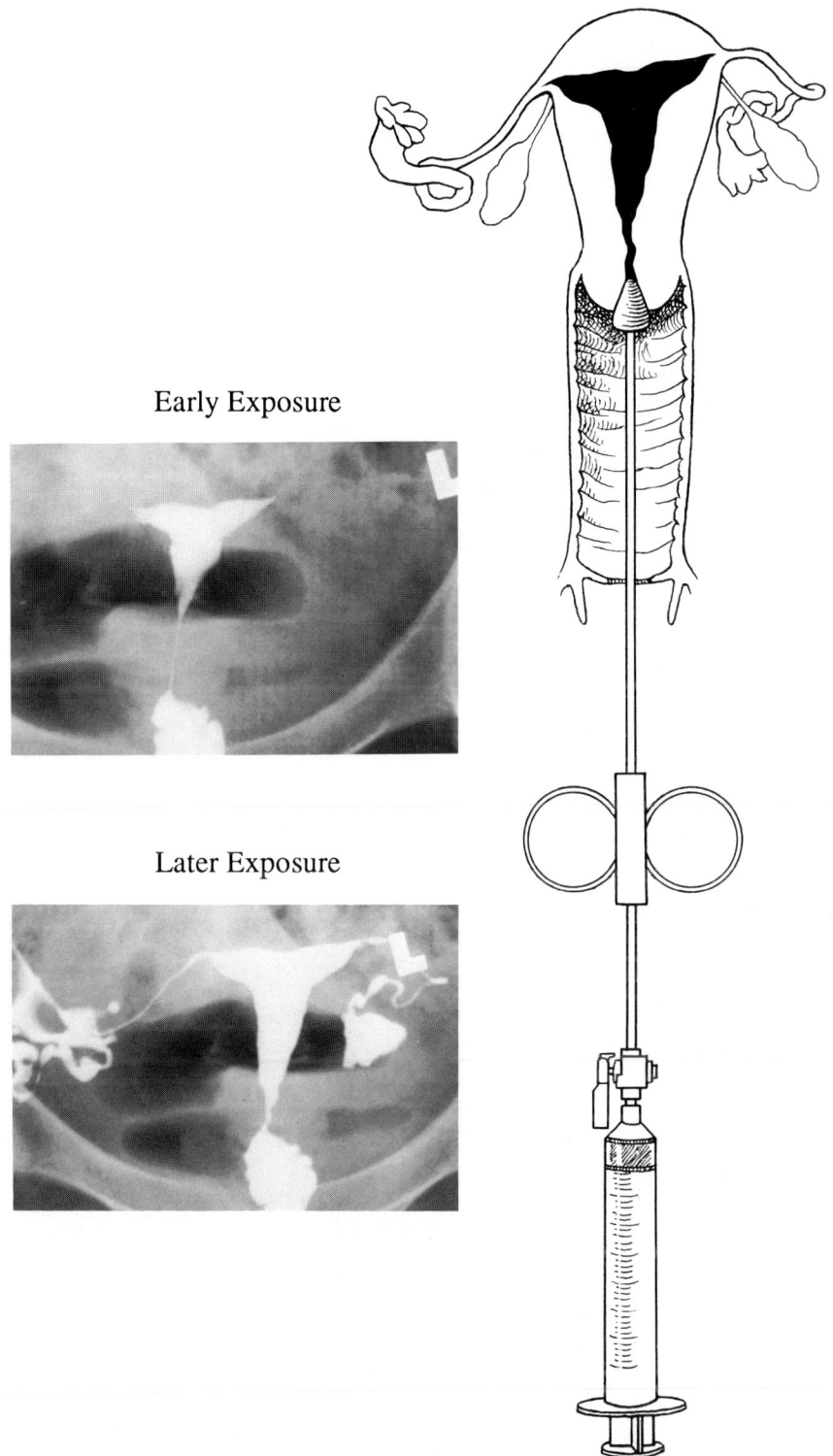

Early Exposure

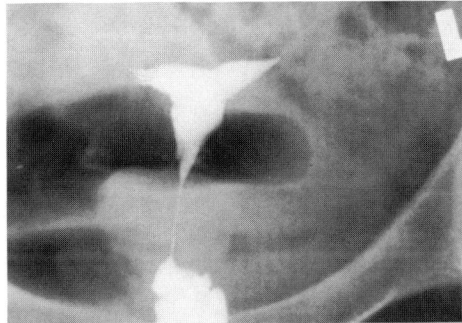

Later Exposure

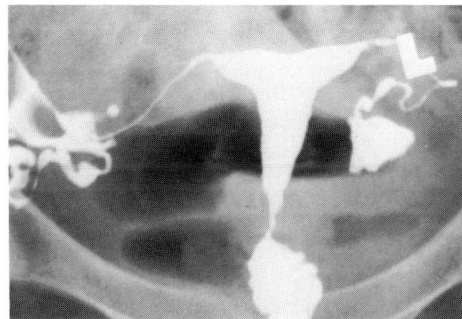

FIGURE 23–2. Performing a hysterosalpingogram. This drawing illustrates a simple and effective technique for performing a hysterosalpingogram. Either oil- or water-soluble contrast medium is placed in a syringe that, in turn, is attached to a rigid cannula with an acorn tip. The acorn tip has been trimmed rather short so that it seals the cervix but does not bypass the cervix. In this setup, it is necessary to place a tenaculum on the cervix. Inward pressure on the cannula and outward traction on the tenaculum will provide a sufficient seal. The medium should be injected slowly, with pertinent radiographic exposures made as the study progresses. Early and later exposures are illustrated.

9. Inject the medium in a slow, steady fashion while watching its progress by fluoroscopy. Usually only 5 to 10 mL of medium is sufficient for the entire procedure.

10. Obtain an early radiograph of the uterine cavity when it first fills with medium because further medium can sometimes obscure intracavitary pathology.

11. Continue medium injection and intermittent fluoroscopy, and expose one to three radiographs as the tubes fill and spill.

12. Turn the patient toward her right or left side, if necessary, to delineate the uterus and tubes better.

13. Inject only as much medium as necessary to confirm tubal spillage; excessive medium into the peritoneal cavity only obscures the relevant anatomy.

After completion of the procedure, it may be necessary to order a delayed radiograph. If oil-soluble contrast medium (OSCM) was used, it is necessary to obtain a 24-hour delayed

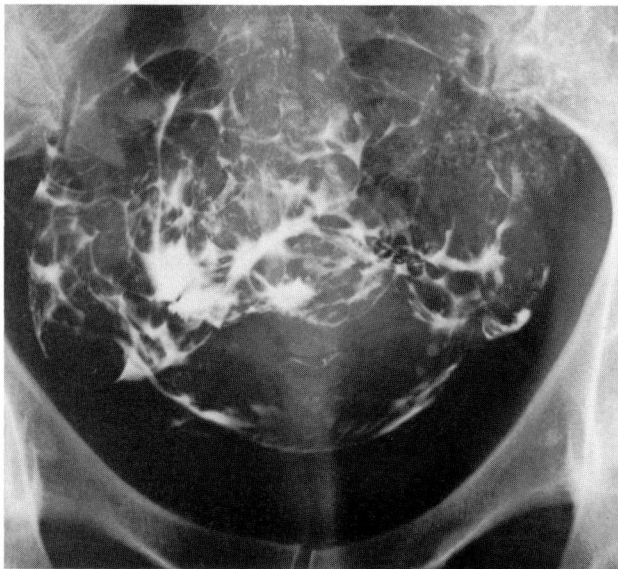

FIGURE 23-3. Delayed radiograph. This delayed radiograph is an exposure made 24 hours after a hysterosalpingographic procedure using oil-soluble contrast medium (OSCM). A delayed radiograph is usually necessary when OSCM is used. In a normal study, the medium will be diffusely dispersed throughout the pelvis after 24 hours, as noted here. Retention of medium in a tube or loculation of medium in one aspect of the pelvis would be abnormal.

film to check for medium dispersion (primarily to confirm tubal obstruction and rule out pelvic adhesions) (Fig. 23–3). A delay interval as short as 1 hour has been recommended for OSCM, but, although the information about tubal status was equal, there was less accuracy in terms of adhesions with the shorter interval.[10] A delayed radiograph is necessary with the use of water-soluble contrast medium (WSCM) only to confirm distal tubal obstruction—a 10-minute delay interval is appropriate with WSCM. Some extra procedures that have been found to be helpful in certain patients undergoing a HSG are injection of air, use of an internal calibration device, and a simple protocol to follow when confronted with proximal tubal obstruction. The injection of room air through the

cannula can be used to create an air-contrast interface in the uterine cavity to delineate pathology better (Fig. 23–4) and also can be used to confirm tubal patency (air bubbles are seen to percolate through the tube) on fluoroscopy. An internal calibration device is occasionally helpful to determine the uterine size, cervical width, and so forth. This can be easily accomplished by measuring the actual distance of the threads on the end of the cannula. Then a set of calipers can be used on the ensuing radiographs to make reasonably accurate anatomic measurements. When confronted with proximal tubal obstruction, it may indicate true intramural tubal blockage, or it may only be tubal spasm. If confronted with proximal tubal obstruction, the first step is to continue to apply steady pressure with the syringe and simply wait 3 to 5 minutes. Often the medium progresses past this apparent obstruction (spasm) with the allowance of more time. If simply waiting is unsuccessful, the administration of a smooth muscle relaxant medication is reasonable but unproven. Several "studies" give anecdotal information that most women with proximal obstruction respond to such medications.[11, 12] An example would be the parenteral administration of 2 mg of glucagon. It is not known whether waiting longer or a placebo medication would yield similar results.

Media

PROPERTIES AND HANDLING CHARACTERISTICS

There are many different radiopaque media that have been used over the years for hysterosalpingography. These media fall into two general categories dependent on whether they have an oil or water base (OSCM and WSCM). The pros and cons of each type of media were thoroughly discussed in a specific review article on this subject published in 1982.[13] The various media tend to have different handling properties, which primarily depend on their relative viscosities. *Handling properties* refers to the ease with which the medium is transferred from a syringe through a cannula into the uterus and out through the fallopian tubes. A medium with good han-

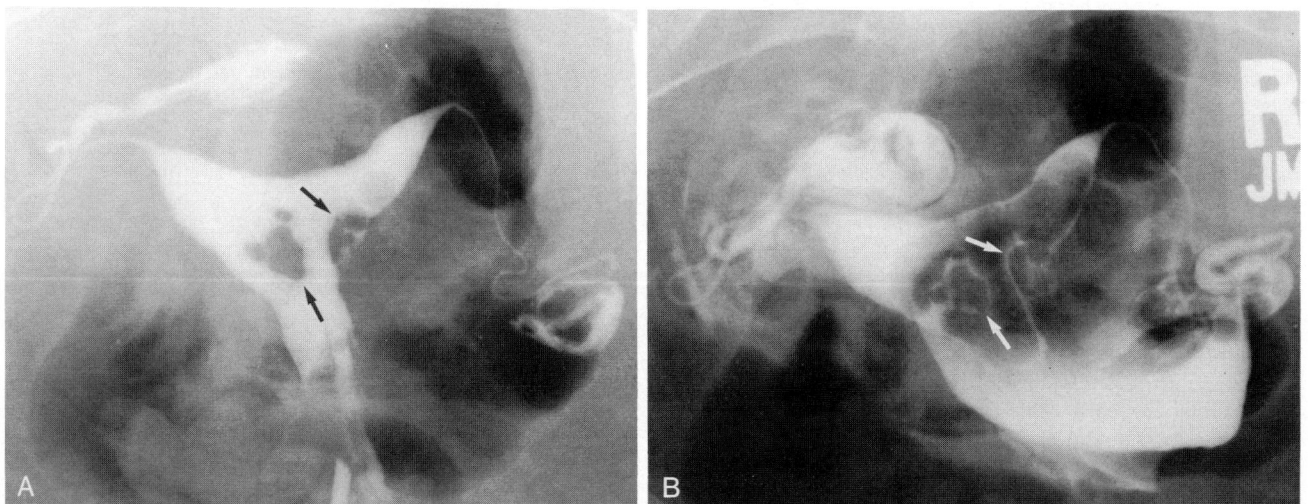

FIGURE 23-4. Use of air contrast. *A,* This radiograph illustrates what appears to be two filling defects in the middle of the uterine cavity (*black arrows*). *B,* A few moments later, room air was introduced behind the contrast medium. The introduction of air into the uterine cavity outlines the two areas in question and confirms them to be filling defects (*white arrows*). This patient has Asherman's syndrome.

dling properties flows easily throughout the entire system, with few air bubbles. The currently available media, whether oil or water based, are the products of an evolutionary process and tend to have similar handling properties that are quite acceptable.

There appears to be general agreement in the literature that OSCM provide a more clear radiographic image. Radiographs from HSGs with OSCM have a distinctive appearance that is both sharper and more contrasting than WSCM images (see Fig. 23–1A and B). The denser image associated with oil media is generally a positive trait except perhaps in relation to the definition of the ampullary portion of the fallopian tube. Longitudinal rugations are visible on a radiograph of the normal tube ampulla when this structure is outlined with WSCM (see Fig. 23–1B) but not with OSCM (see Fig. 23–1A). The finding of ampullary rugations is suggestive of a normal tubal mucosa. One study reported higher pregnancy rates in those infertile women with tubal disease who retained ampullary rugations, as opposed to those women in whom no ampullar rugations could be demonstrated.[14]

Water-soluble HSG media are rapidly absorbed, whereas the oil media are slowly absorbed. These relative absorption rates represent one of the most pronounced clinical differences between these classes of media. WSCM dissipates and is absorbed within minutes after passing through the tubes and into the peritoneal cavity after a normal examination. When the fallopian tubes are obstructed, an aqueous medium persists longer in the distal tubes but rarely for more than an hour. The OSCM have been known to persist for months to years, especially when there is tubal obstruction. Residual Ethiodol has been reported to persist in the pelvis for 1 to 4 months after HSG.[15] The most recent literature on radiopaque media for HSG has focused on the application of newer WSCM for this procedure. These new media are either of low osmolality (assumed to cause less pain from peritoneal irritation) or contain iodine in a nonionic form (less likely to result in an allergic reaction to iodine).[16, 17] The handling properties of these new media are essentially the same as the older WSCM. Although the newer media do have some attractive features, these limited benefits must be weighed against a marked increase in cost compared with older WSCM, such as Sinografin, Renografin-60, or Conray-60.

THERAPEUTIC EFFECT

HSG has often been claimed to have a therapeutic as well as a diagnostic function in infertile women. The early published claims of a therapeutic effect of HSG tended to recount the same story: an apparent increase in the spontaneous pregnancy rate after HSG in an otherwise normal infertility evaluation. The next generation of publications on this subject attempted to compare pregnancy rates after HSGs with water-based and lipid-based media.[18, 19] The primary methodologic deficiency in these studies was lack of randomization. Apparently various practitioners involved in this study preferred a certain medium and used that medium on all of their patients. Therefore, the spontaneous pregnancy rates after HSG in these studies may reflect the differences in pregnancy rates between patients of various practitioners but not the difference between HSG media.

More recently, there have been three well-designed studies (prospective, randomized) that have compared the spontaneous pregnancy rate in infertility patients after a HSG with either WSCM or OSCM. In 1983, it was reported there was a significant increase in the pregnancy rate in couples with unexplained infertility when a HSG was performed with an OSCM (Ethiodol) compared with a WSCM (Sinografin).[20] When this study examined the pregnancy rate in all types of infertility (n = 121), there were no media-related differences in the subsequent pregnancy rate. A similar study (n = 106) was published in 1986 that compared HSG with an OSCM (Ethiodol) and with a WSCM (Renografin-60).[21] No differences in the postprocedure pregnancy rate were found even in the subgroup with unexplained infertility. In 1991, Rasmussen and colleagues[22] published a randomized, prospective trial in which they compared the post-HSG pregnancy rates in women in whom the procedures were performed with three different WSCM (Omnipaque, n = 101; Hexabrix, n = 102; Urografin, n = 97) and an OSCM (Ethiodol, n = 98). No differences were noted among the groups in demographic patterns, infertility diagnosis, or diagnosis made at the time of HSG. After a 1-year follow-up, significantly (P < 0.01) more patients became pregnant after HSG with the OSCM compared with all three WSCM.[22] A rabbit study demonstrated a significant decrease in tubal transport of surrogate ova in animals exposed to Sinografin compared with Ethiodol.[23] This finding would favor the data that pregnancy rates after HSG are superior with an OSCM. From all these accumulated data, it seems clear that there is more of a therapeutic effect in terms of pregnancy after a HSG with OSCM compared with WSCM. Most of these pregnancies occur in the 4 to 6 months following the procedure (justifying a waiting period after a HSG in selected patients). The mechanism whereby a HSG promotes pregnancy remains speculative (e.g., dislodging mucous plugs that block the lumen, inhibition of peritoneal macrophages). At this time, it is recommended that OSCM be used for routine HSG.

Complications

As is true for most medical procedures, there are a number of potential risks associated with hysterosalpingography. It is the duty of the practitioner who orders or performs a HSG to make certain that the benefits outweigh the risks for each individual who undergoes this procedure. Some of the risks associated with a HSG are directly related to the medium selected, and other risks are independent of the medium used. Certain rare complications, such as uterine perforation with the instillation apparatus and postexamination hemorrhage, do occur.

IODINE ALLERGY

Both the lipid-based and water-based media use iodine as their contrast agent. Therefore, the potential for hypersensitivity reactions to iodine is present with any of the HSG media. An allergic reaction to iodine is so rare that it has never been reported in the medical literature in association with a HSG. The newer nonionic media (Table 23–1) are thought to have a lower incidence of iodine allergy, but they do not entirely eliminate the possibility. The risk-to-benefit ratio needs to be weighed before performing a HSG in a

TABLE 23–1. Radiopaque Media for Hysterosalpingography

Generic Name	Trade Name	Iodine (mg/mL)	Osmolality (mOsm/kg)	Type
Ethiodized poppy seed oil	Ethiodol	475	—	Oil
Diatrizoate meglumine and iodipamide meglumine	Sinografin	380	—	H₂O Ionic
Diatrizoate meglumine 52%	Renografin-60	292	1420	H₂O Ionic
Diatrizoate meglumine 66%	Renografin-76	370	1940	H₂O Ionic
Iothalamate meglumine 60%	Conray-60	282	1400	H₂O Ionic
Ioxaglate	Hexabrix	320	600	H₂O Ionic
Iopamidol	Isovue 370	370	796	H₂O Nonionic
Ioxitol	Ioxilan	350	280	H₂O Nonionic
Diatrizoate sodium	Hypaque	300	1515	H₂O Ionic
Iohexol	Omnipaque	300	672	H₂O Nonionic

woman who claims to have an iodine allergy. The reaction would probably consist of urticaria or a rash, or both, and would be more likely after uterine intravasation of medium.

PELVIC INFECTION

One of the major complications of HSG is exacerbation of salpingitis/pelvic peritonitis (pelvic inflammatory disease). This complication is independent of either class of media—OSCM or WSCM. In some patients, a severe pelvic peritonitis with serious sequelae, such as abscess formation and tubal obstruction, can occur after HSG. Six of the 11 reported deaths attributed to HSG were the result of peritonitis (all occurred before the modern antibiotic era).[24, 25] The patients at increased risk for this complication are those with a prior history of salpingitis or tubal disease present at the time of the x-ray examination. The pathogenesis is probably a physical disruption of a delicate balance between a smoldering tubal infection and host defense mechanisms. These infections can also occur secondary to ascending bacteria associated with the HSG procedure. Several reports on HSG have tabulated infectious complication rates; these are summarized in Table 23–2.

The authors generally reported the more severe cases, which required hospitalization. The incidence and severity of pelvic peritonitis do not appear to be influenced by the type of radiographic medium. The article by Stumpf and March[31] (see Table 23–2) found no protective effect with a prophylactic oral antibiotic. Their study, however, primarily examined the use of ampicillin, which does not provide antibiotic coverage for *Chlamydia trachomatis* and anaerobic organisms.[31] A later study followed a similar protocol but used doxycycline, which provides superior coverage for pelvic pathogens.[32] This study found that doxycycline prevented salpingitis after a HSG even when it was not initiated until after the procedure (in women with demonstrated tubal disease). It would be naive to believe, however, that all salpingitis can be prevented with the use of an oral antibiotic before or after an HSG. It appears that a low but significant infectious complication rate after HSG is inevitable. Proper antiseptic preparation of the cervix and endocervix before injection of the contrast medium helps keep the incidence of salpingitis low. In those women at risk for peritonitis after this procedure (patients with a history of salpingitis, known tubal/adhesive disease, or a positive *Chlamydia* titer), the risk-to-benefit ratio needs to be consulted. An assessment of the white blood cell (WBC) count and the erythrocyte sedimentation rate (ESR) can be helpful to determine whether there is any active infection. In women at risk for salpingitis in whom it is elected to proceed with a HSG, the prophylactic (preprocedure initiation) use of

TABLE 23–2. Peritonitis After Hysterosalpingography

Year	Investigator	No. Hysterosalpingograms	Medium	Reported Incidence of Peritonitis (%)
1945	Bang[25]	900	Lipiodol and other oil based	1.7
1950	Marshak et al[26]	2500	Lipiodol	0.3
1956	Norris[27]	961	Lipiodol	0.6
1959	Whitelaw & Miller[28]	157	Sinografin	1.3
1960	Measday[29]	623	Oil and water based	1.1
1960	Palmer[15]	258	Ethiodol	1.2
1969	Geary et al[30]	500	Lipiodol	0.4
1980	Stumpf & March[31]	448	Sinografin	3.1
1983	Pittaway et al[32]	278	Conray or Sinografin	1.4

oral doxycycline is recommended. In women not known to be at risk, in whom distal tubal disease (hydrosalpinx) is found at HSG, the use of doxycycline beginning immediately after the procedure and continued for 5 days is recommended. All women undergoing a HSG should be warned about the risk of salpingitis and apprised of the common symptoms. (Symptoms usually begin within 24 to 48 hours.) The practitioner who orders or performs a HSG should have a 24-hour emergency system in place for the rare patient who develops salpingitis.

PAIN

Discomfort or pain is commonly experienced by women undergoing HSG. There is usually a certain amount of discomfort associated with application of the tenaculum and the introduction of the cannula. Much more variable is the prevalence and severity of pain associated with the procedure itself. This is often directly related to the skill and experience of the physician(s) performing the examination. In addition to this physician factor, there appears to be a medium-dependent pain factor. It has been stated that OSCM cause less peritoneal irritation than WSCM.[15, 26] A prospective study that surveyed the pain associated with HSG when water-soluble medium (Salpix) and oil-soluble medium (Ethiodol) were randomized found a significant increase in pain with the WSCM.[33] A study published in 1949 comparing the absorption characteristics of various water-soluble and lipid-soluble media indicated that the pain associated with peritoneal spill varied little among the different media.[34] Most of the WSCM referenced in these studies are no longer used. The pain associated with peritoneal irritation is postulated to be secondary to the high osmolality of the WSCM (see Table 23–1). Although some newer WSCM are of lower osmolality and should cause less peritoneal irritation, this was not found when Hexabrix was compared with Renografin-60.[16] The pain with WSCM seems to vary somewhat in intensity among the different WSCM, is transient, and rarely requires analgesia before or after the examination. Although increased pain from peritoneal spill of WSCM appears to be a real phenomenon, it should not be a major factor in the selection of a radiopaque medium. If a practitioner wishes to use a WSCM, I would recommend Sinografin, Renografin-60, or Conray-60 as proven media that cause minimal pain and are less expensive than the newer water-soluble media.

INFLAMMATION; GRANULOMA FORMATION

The persistence of oil-soluble medium in the pelvis for months to years after HSG has already been noted. Such persistence of OSCM has the potential to induce a foreign body reaction (granuloma formation) in the uterine and tubal tissue. In the early literature on HSG, there were a number of reports (but no incidence figures) on granuloma formation in association with both OSCM and WSCM that are no longer available. Reports on HSG with currently available oil-soluble and water-soluble media seem to ignore the potential side effect of granuloma formation. In a 1980 report on Ethiodol, the authors mention that they have never seen any cases with granuloma formation, but they do not mention how frequently they looked.[35] Therefore, no study to date has established the prevalence of granuloma formation after HSG with oil-based or water-based media.

A rabbit study in which Ethiodol was documented to persist in induced hydrosalpinges for up to 8 weeks noted no granuloma formation nor inflammation within the tube.[23] There are other reports, however, in animal models (guinea pig, rabbit) that have noted inflammation of reproductive organs and peritoneal surfaces up to 30 days after exposure.[36–38] When all the evidence is weighed together, it appears there can be a transient inflammatory reaction involving the uterus, oviducts, and surrounding tissues after exposure to a radiopaque medium.

Altogether OSCM appears to have a greater potential than WSCM to induce granuloma formation. The real question is how frequently HSG media lead to granuloma formation in partially obstructed or completely obstructed but operable fallopian tubes and how significant granuloma formation is when it occurs. Implicit in this entire discussion is the belief that granuloma formation is detrimental to a woman's fertility potential. All media pass quickly through normal oviducts; thus there is only slight potential for granuloma formation. Surveying all the evidence, granuloma formation and inflammation are still considered to be undesirable and should be avoided if possible. Therefore, it is recommended that WSCM be used for a HSG when a patient is at high risk for or known to have distal tubal obstruction.

EMBOLI

The most dramatic side effect of HSG is venous or lymphatic intravasation of the medium. Lymphatic intravasation results in a reticular pattern of small vessels in the broad ligament (Figs. 23–5 and 23–6). When venous intravasation occurs in a patient, the medium quickly passes through the uterine or ovarian veins to the lungs (see Figs. 23–5 and 23–6). Such emboli can occur with oil-soluble or water-soluble media, but in the latter, the medium is quickly dissipated, and no embolic symptoms or side effects have ever been reported except when carboxymethylcellulose was transiently

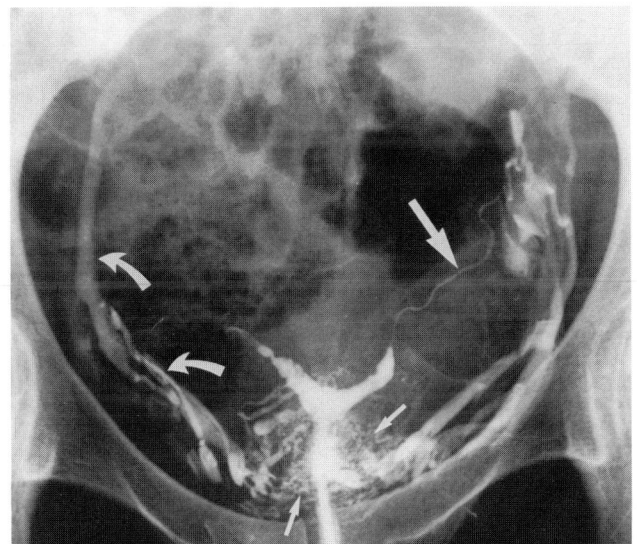

FIGURE 23–5. Intravasation of medium. This radiograph illustrates lymphatic (*small arrows*) and venous intravasation of water-soluble medium during the performance of a hysterosalpingogram. The uterus is small and has an arcuate tendency. Only the left tube is visualized (*large arrow*). The uterine and internal iliac veins (*curved arrows*) are seen on both sides of the pelvis.

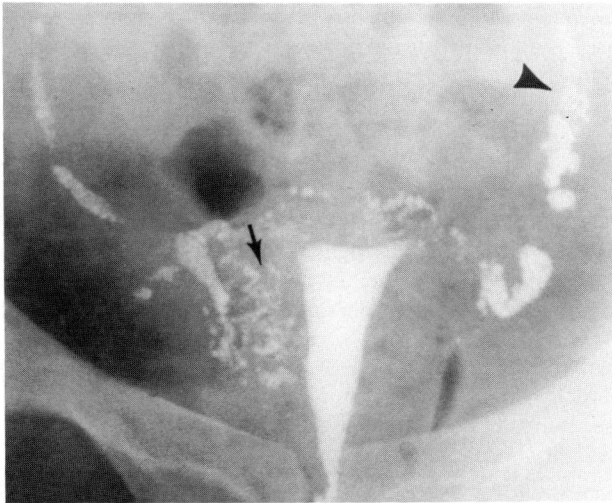

FIGURE 23–6. Intravasation of medium. This radiograph illustrates lymphatic (*small arrow*) and venous (*arrowhead*) intravasation of oil-based contrast medium. The fallopian tubes are not seen. Note that the medium forms small beads when it comes into contact with blood.

enced after an oil embolus include chest pain, cough, dyspnea, light-headedness, confusion, headache, and, rarely, cardiorespiratory failure and death. Likewise, a number of physical signs and laboratory findings have been reported after oil emboli: hematuria, hemoptysis, hemolysis, fever, leukocytosis, pneumonia, lipuria, and medium in peripheral vessels, most notably in vessels of the brain. It is therefore apparent that the OSCM can be dispersed widely throughout the body. The presence of symptoms and their nature generally depend on the volume of medium that enters the circulation. There have been five deaths attributed to emboli after HSG (four with oil-based media).[24, 40]

Although intravasation occurs with the use of Ethiodol (the dominant OSCM in use today), there have been no recent reports of any serious embolus-related side effects. The nearly universal use of fluoroscopy at the time of HSG in recent times has allowed the examiner to detect immediately any intravasation and promptly stop the flow of contrast medium. Although the intravasation of OSCM remains a potential serious complication of HSG, it has rarely been experienced as a significant clinical problem in recent years.

used as a thickening agent. There has been serious concern ever since the advent of HSG that emboli with OSCM may be detrimental to the patient (see Fig. 23–6). This concern has not been without merit.

Intravasation with OSCM has been reported to vary between 0% and 6.3% (Table 23–3). There is nearly complete agreement in the literature on this subject that certain predisposing conditions are usually present when intravasation occurs: (1) tubal disease or obstruction, (2) recent uterine operation (e.g., dilatation and curettage); (3) uterine malformation; (4) misplacement of the HSG cannula; and (5) excessive injection pressure or quantity of media. There have been more than 200 reported cases in the medical literature of OSCM intravasation during HSG. The early reports between 1920 and 1940 are lengthy accounts that generally recount a series of minor postembolic signs and symptoms noted during a hospitalized observation period followed by complete recovery.[41, 42] The reports in the period between 1950 and 1980 generally state the incidence of oil emboli in their experience and have not hospitalized the patients nor followed the patients as closely as in the early reports.[27, 35] In these latter reports, it has generally been concluded that most oil emboli are innocuous and should not be regarded as a major complication of the HSG.

It has been estimated that only about 20% of the patients with episodes of intravasation of OSCM experience any symptoms.[40] The reported sequelae that have been experi-

RADIATION

The radiation dose to female tissues and especially to the ovaries imposes the risk of future complications with every HSG. The main danger is in regard to induced mutations in the genetic material of ova, with the effects exhibited in future generations. Although this risk is real with any pelvic radiation, the magnitude of the risk is uncertain and apparently quite small. It would be difficult to study this situation, and no investigation has ever been attempted to quantify the long-term effects of pelvic irradiation in general or HSG in particular. The general tenet has been to minimize the radiation exposure with all diagnostic radiographic procedures. The total radiation dose from a HSG procedure depends on a number of variables: (1) the size and shape of the patient, (2) the position of the ovaries at the time of the examination, (3) the x-ray machine used with its specific radiation output characteristics, (4) the distance between the ovaries and the machine, (5) the duration of fluoroscopy, (6) the amount of image magnification, and (7) the number of permanent radiographic exposures during the procedure.

The ovarian radiation exposure has been estimated for a HSG. Studies using a thermoluminescent dosimeter in the posterior fornix have estimated the average ovarian radiation dose to be 500 to 1000 mRad (range 100 to 2000 mRad).[42, 43] These average doses were corroborated using a dosimeter in a water phantom with radiation exposures designed to mimic

Year	Investigator	No. Hysterosalpingograms	Medium	Reported Incidence of Intravasation (%)
1950	Marshak et al[26]	300	Lipiodol	0.0
1952	Palmer[39]	295	Lipiodol-F	4.3
1954	Zachariae[40]	505	Iodized oils	2.0
1956	Norris[27]	961	Lipiodol	6.3
1960	Palmer[15]	258	Ethiodol	3.9
1980	Bateman et al[35]	533	Ethiodol	2.4

TABLE 23–3. Intravasation with Oil-Soluble Medium

a HSG.[45] Exposure was determined to be somewhat higher with selective salpingography and fallopian tube recanalization (200 to 2750 mRad).[46] To put these doses into perspective, the average radiation dose with an excretory urogram and barium enema is about 1000 and 6000 mRad. Once again, the practitioner who orders or performs a HSG needs to consider the risk-to-benefit ratio, in this instance in terms of the radiation exposure. The main factors that determine the radiation dose for any given HSG study (aside from the equipment used) include the anatomy of the patient and the experience of the radiographer. With more experience, a given radiographer requires less fluoroscopy time and fewer radiographs. The radiation dose with HSG does not depend on the contrast medium. Although the use of OSCM usually requires a delayed radiograph at 24 hours, this particular radiograph is not necessarily an additional exposure. The total number of radiographs as well as the fluoroscopy time required for HSG should be quite comparable among oil-based and water-based media.

Uterine/Tubal Pathology

This section focuses on specific abnormalities that can affect the female reproductive organs. Specifically, these are abnormalities that can be effectively diagnosed by hysterosalpingography.

UTERINE PATHOLOGY

The anatomy of the cervical canal can be examined with a HSG (Fig. 23–7). A normal cervical canal is 1 to 2 cm long with a convoluted border at HSG, which represents the cervical glands. A cervical canal that is more than 1 cm wide is suspicious for an incompetent cervix. A normal nulliparous uterus is 3 to 5 cm from the external cervical os to the fundal-cavitary border. The fundal measurement from the tubal-uterine junctions is 3 to 4 cm. A hypoplastic uterus may sometimes be found in the course of performing a HSG

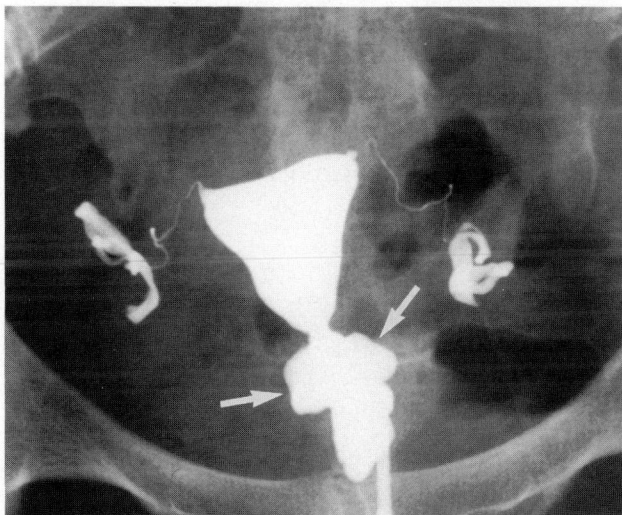

FIGURE 23–7. Cervical pathology. This radiograph is normal except for the appearance of the cervix. The upper region of the cervical canal has lateral extensions in both directions (*arrows*). This woman had a prior low transverse cesarean section, and this ballooning of the cervix is presumably secondary to that procedure.

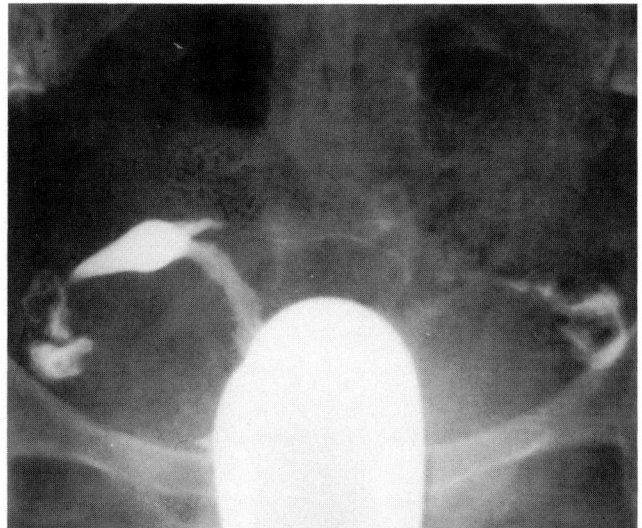

FIGURE 23–8. Hypoplastic uterus. This radiograph illustrates an underdeveloped uterus. Although a speculum should not be left in place during the performance of a hysterosalpingogram, its presence in this radiograph illustrates the relative small size of the uterus. Small uterine size can be congenital or secondary to lack of stimulation from quiescent ovaries.

(Fig. 23–8). A hypoplastic uterus is one that appears small on the permanent radiograph and is confirmed to be so when actual measurements are taken. Most of the time when this condition is found, the woman has not been exposed to normal ovarian function (e.g., primary gonadal failure). Rarely a woman with normal ovarian function can have a hypoplastic uterus. During pregnancy, a hypoplastic uterus usually undergoes normal growth and development.

Within the uterine cavity, there can be abnormal growths of tissue that would appear as filling defects on a HSG. When confronted with shadows within the endometrial cavity on a radiograph, it is important to ascertain whether they are present on every film. An initial scout radiograph should be performed before each HSG study to locate any background shadows that overlie the uterus. If intracavitary defects are seen at fluoroscopy, it is helpful to have the patient turn about 30 degrees to the right or left to see if the shadows move. Intrauterine polyps present as single or multiple discrete round filling defects (Fig. 23–9). Air bubbles can masquerade as discrete round filling defects but are seen to move freely about the cavity, especially with lateral positioning. Fibroids (leiomyomata uteri) arise from the myometrium, vary widely in size, and can be located next to the endometrium (submucous). When fibroids protrude into the endometrial cavity, they usually present a picture of a semilunar filling defect(s) (Fig. 23–10A) or large filling defects within the cavity (Fig. 23–10B).

The endometrial cavity can be partially or completely obliterated by scar tissue. The condition of intrauterine synechiae is also known as Asherman's syndrome (Fig. 23–11A and B). This syndrome presents as secondary amenorrhea or hypomenorrhea and is usually secondary to instrumentation (e.g., dilatation and curettage) of the uterine cavity in the postpartum interval.

OVIDUCT ANATOMY AND PATHOLOGY

The delineation of tubal anatomy and patency is a critical facet of hysterosalpingography. It is important to recall that

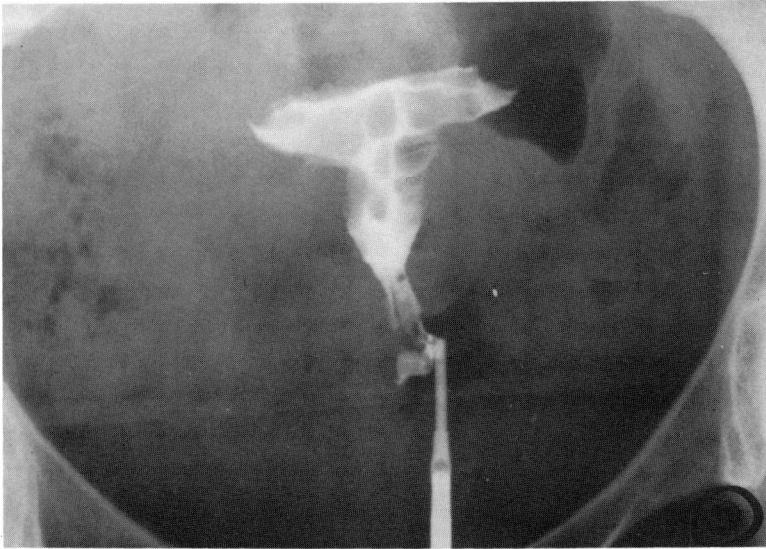

FIGURE 23–9. Uterine polyps. This radiograph illustrates a uterus with a number of round, symmetrical filling defects. The number, shape, and position of these defects led to a presumptive diagnosis of uterine polyps, which was confirmed at hysteroscopy.

the tube is anatomically and functionally divided into four segments: intramural (interstitial), isthmus, ampulla, and fimbria. The initial segment of tube visualized at HSG is the intramural portion. Figure 23–12 illustrates the location of the intramural-isthmic junction. This junction is more lateral relative to the uterine cavity than most initial observers expect, which is a function of the magnification used in the procedure.

Proximal tubal obstruction is present when radiopaque medium fails to traverse the intramural or isthmic portion of either tube (Fig. 23–13). (The issue of tubal spasm was addressed in the technique section; selective salpingography is addressed at the end of this chapter.) The obstruction can be functional (spasm), partial (mucous plug), or complete. When proximal obstruction is complete, the pathology has

been found to be fibrosis, salpingitis isthmica nodosa (SIN), endometriosis, or chronic tubal inflammation.[47] Complete obstruction was found always to involve the intramural tubal segment and extend a variable distance into the isthmic segment. Salpingitis isthmica nodosa can also be present in conjunction with tubal patency (Fig. 23–14).

Midtubal obstruction refers to blockage in the isthmic-ampullary tubal segments. Obstruction at this site rarely, if ever, occurs spontaneously. It is usually encountered when checking whether a post–tubal ligation patient has a fistula or investigating proximal tubal length before a planned tubal ligation reversal (Fig. 23–15).

Distal tubal obstruction is a common sequela to salpingitis (dependent on the number of infectious episodes and their severity). The inflamed ends of the fallopian tubes, in an

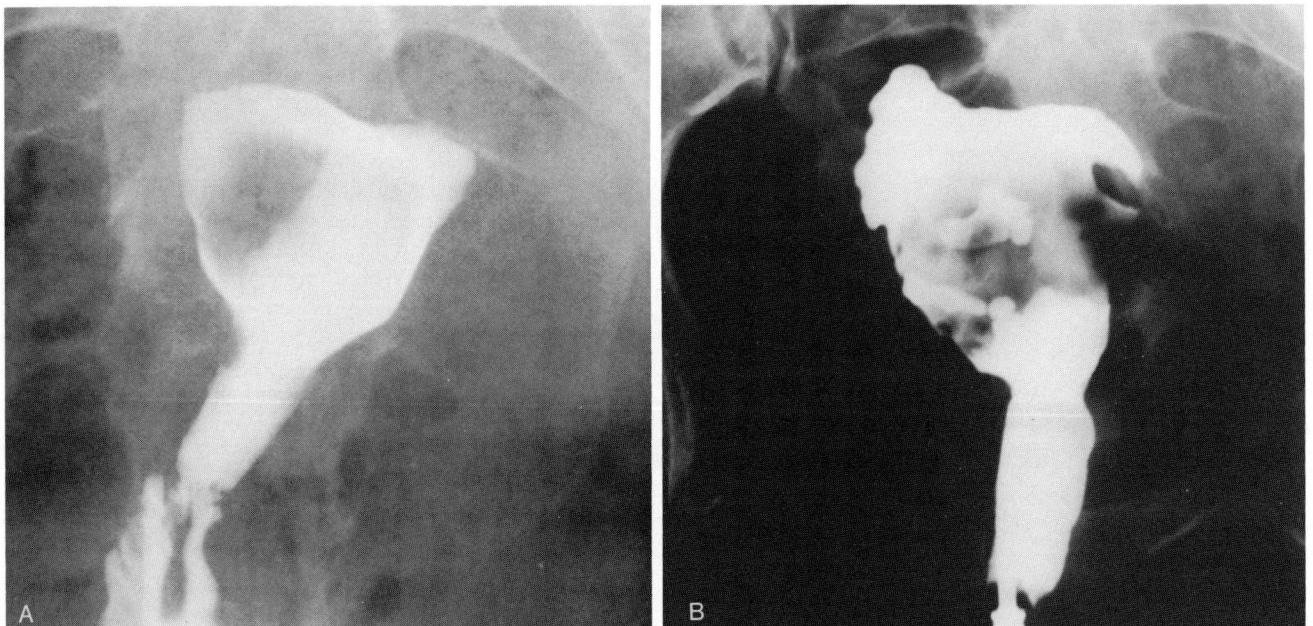

FIGURE 23–10. Leiomyomata uteri. *A,* This radiograph illustrates a single submucous fibroid that was protruding into the uterine cavity. *B,* This radiograph illustrates a uterus in which multiple myomas are impinging on the cavity. Note that these myomas do not give the appearance of complete filling defects but, instead, displace medium in the cavity and, therefore, cause the image in that area to be less opaque.

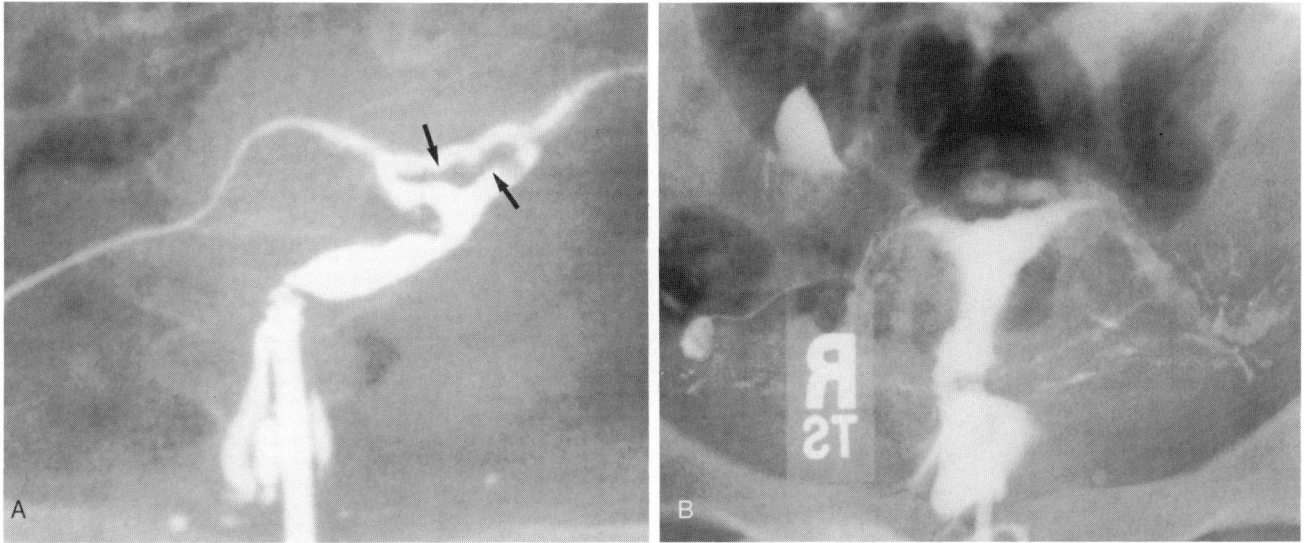

FIGURE 23–11. Asherman's syndrome. *A,* This radiograph illustrates a central filling defect within the uterine cavity *(arrows)*. This patient had a postpartum dilation and curettage for endometritis. She was experiencing menstrual abnormalities but not total amenorrhea. *B,* A repeat radiograph in the same patient 3 months after performance of an operative hysteroscopy. The synechiae have been resected, and the uterine cavity appears normal.

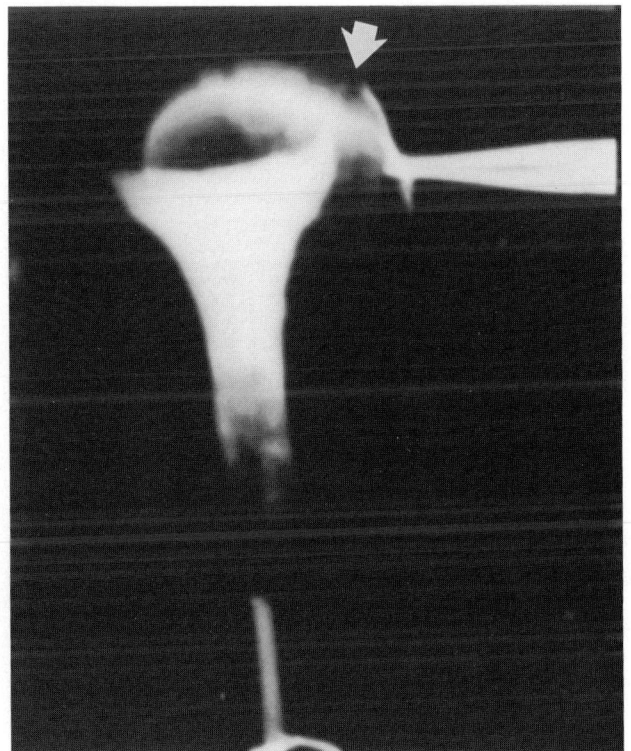

FIGURE 23–12. Intramural tubal segment. This radiograph was performed with water-soluble medium using a hysterectomy specimen. A surgical clamp was placed where the isthmic segment of the tube met the outer surface of the uterus. Injection of medium through the cervix illustrates the length of the intramural segment of the tube *(arrow)* relative to the uterine cavity.

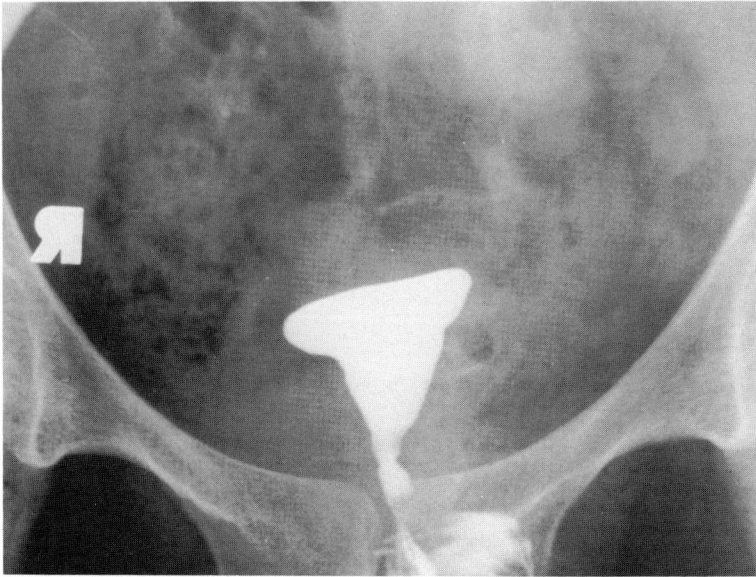

FIGURE 23–13. Proximal tubal obstruction. This radiograph illustrates the uterine cavity, but there is no fill of the intramural segments of the fallopian tubes. When this image persists throughout a hysterosalpingogram study, it leads to confusion as to the patient's proper diagnosis—tubal spasm (a transient functional condition) or complete obstruction of the intramural segments of the tubes.

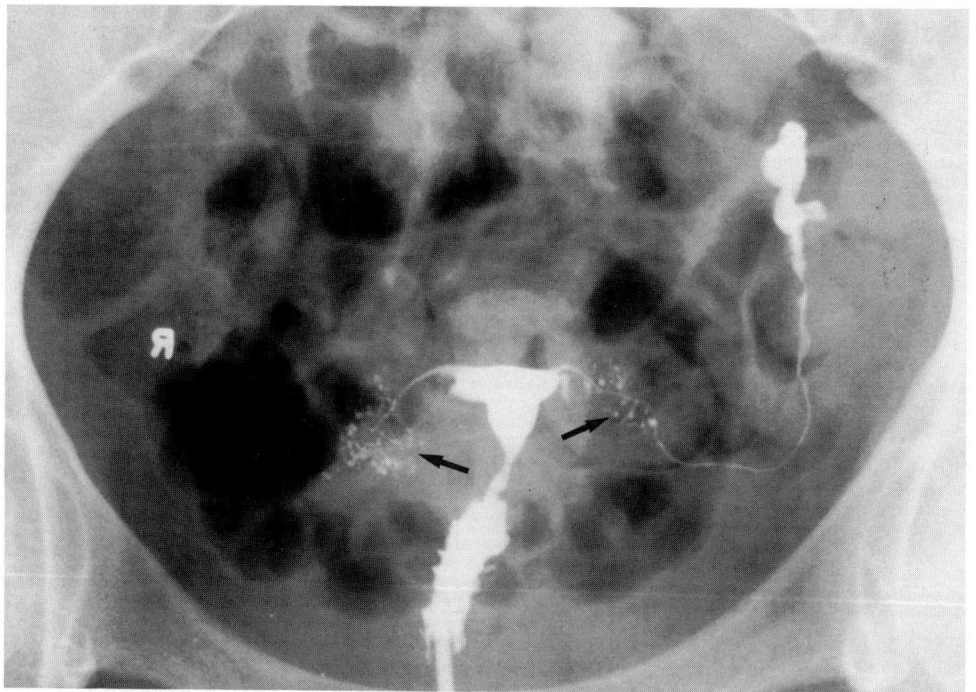

FIGURE 23–14. Salpingitis isthmica nodosum. This radiograph illustrates bilateral diffusion of medium into small pockets (*arrows*) adjacent to the isthmic portion of the fallopian tubes. This condition is known as *salpingitis isthmica nodosum* and indicates the patient has had salpingitis.

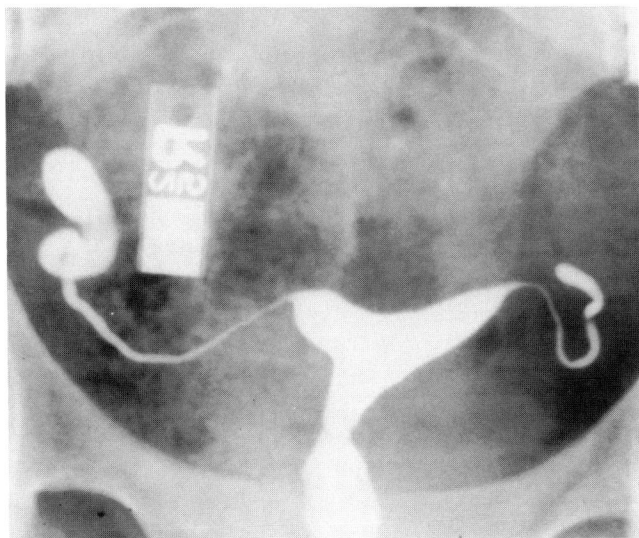

FIGURE 23–15. Midsegment tubal obstruction. This radiograph illustrates bilateral tubal obstruction in the vicinity of the ampullary isthmic junction. More ampulla is seen in the right compared with the left tube. An obstruction in this location rarely, if ever, occurs secondary to intrinsic tubal pathology. In this case, the obstruction was due to a prior tubal ligation.

attempt to wall off spread of the infection, retract and scar. This sequence of events often leads to permanent obstruction. After the infection has subsided (with or without the use of antibiotics), the pus-filled abscess cavity gradually reverts to a space filled with serous fluid—a hydrosalpinx. The presence of hydrosalpinges at hysterosalpingography is not always as easy to demonstrate as one might expect (Figs. 23–16 and 23–17).

Pelvic adhesions can be a major cause of infertility. Severe pelvic adhesions can be present along with bilateral tubal patency. Pelvic adhesions can be detected with a HSG when it is noted that the medium does not disperse normally throughout the pelvis after spillage. Sometimes the medium loculates within what is thought to be a pocket among adhesions. When OSCM is used, a delayed (24-hour) radiograph is the best method to detect adhesions (Fig. 23–18). A practitioner, however, can never be certain that a particular patient does not have pelvic adhesions based on a HSG alone. It is estimated that a HSG performed properly by experienced practitioners detects pelvic adhesions in approximately 50% of cases in which they are present.

UTERINE ANOMALIES

The vagina, cervix, uterus, and oviducts are formed embryologically from the paired müllerian ducts. The müllerian ducts undergo elongation, fusion, canalization, and septal resorption between 8 and 20 weeks from a pregnant woman's last menses. This process can deviate from normal at every step (i.e., failure to fuse, lack of septal resorption) and result in various uterine (müllerian) anomalies.[48] When a uterine anomaly is present, there is always a change in the internal (cavitary) uterine anatomy and often, but not always, a change in the external uterine anatomy. An example of an anomaly encompassing both internal and external changes would be a bicornuate uterus in which two separate uterine horns would be apparent both at HSG and when the external surface of the uterus was examined (i.e., laparoscopy). An example of a uterine anomaly with internal but not external changes would be a septate uterus. Generally a HSG is the best and therefore the preferred method for the initial investigation of a uterine anomaly. Sometimes a HSG is performed to find out whether a woman has a uterine anomaly (i.e., evaluation of recurrent spontaneous abortion), and other times a HSG is used to define a known anomaly (i.e., a uterus didelphys with two cervices present on pelvic examination).

A unicornuate uterus consists of a single uterine horn and fallopian tube (Fig. 23–19). The contralateral horn and tube are absent. There is often (in about 50% of cases) a significant renal anomaly on the contralateral side. A bicornuate uterus has a single cervix but two uterine horns (Fig. 23–20). A normal pregnancy can occur in either uterine horn; however, spontaneous abortions are considered to be causally related to this anomaly in some women. Some women can have a

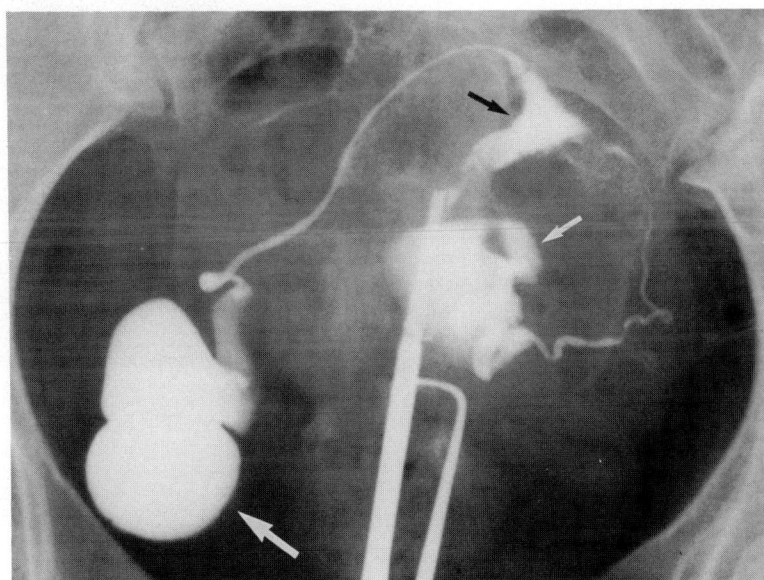

FIGURE 23–16. Bilateral hydrosalpinges. This radiograph illustrates bilateral distal tubal obstruction (hydrosalpinges). In this radiograph, the uterus is indicated by a *black arrow*, one tube is in the foreground *(large white arrow)*, and the other is in the background *(small white arrow)*. A hydrosalpinx is distinguished by dilation of the ampullar portion of the tube as well as a rounded, blunt end at the site of obstruction.

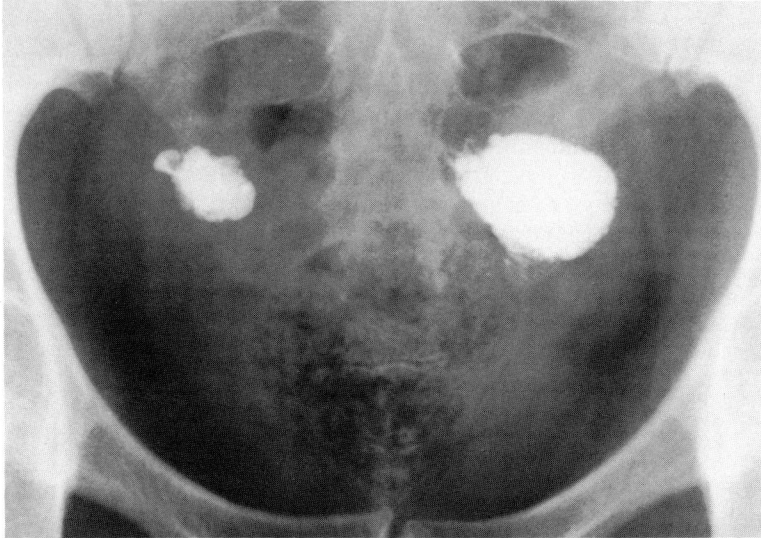

FIGURE 23–17. Bilateral hydrosalpinges—delayed exposure. This radiograph illustrates bilateral retention of oil-based contrast medium in the distal end of obstructed fallopian tubes. This exposure was made approximately 1 week after the initial hysterosalpingographic study. Normal tubes will not retain oil-based medium more than several hours.

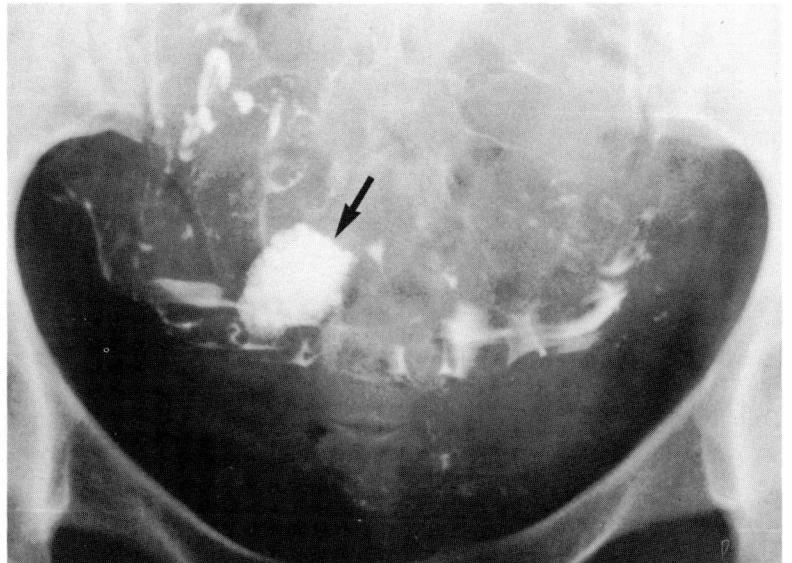

FIGURE 23–18. Pelvic adhesions. This is a 24-hour delayed radiograph after a hysterosalpingographic study using oil-based medium. There is unilateral retention of medium in a confined area *(arrow)* that is highly suspicious for pelvic adhesions.

Selective Salpingography/Retrograde Salpingoplasty

It has been estimated that proximal tubal obstruction is encountered in 10% to 20% of HSGs (Fig. 23–24A).[49] (In some clinics, the incidence is less—5% to 10%.) This finding may represent only a functional condition (i.e., tubal spasm), a reversible obstruction (i.e., luminal plug), or complete blockage (i.e., fibrosis). In the past, the standard approach to proximal tubal obstruction was confirmation of this condition by injecting a saline/dye mixture into the uterus at laparoscopy followed by a laparotomy with a cornual-isthmic tubal anastomosis. In 1987, the first report appeared describing a technique of transcervical retrograde catheterization of selected fallopian tubes.[51] The technique consists of confirming proximal obstruction with a standard HSG followed by passing a relatively large catheter (i.e., 9 French) through the cervix into the uterine cavity. Under fluoroscopic guidance and using appropriate guidewires, a medium-size (i.e., 5 French) catheter is "wedged" into the proximal tubal ostia followed by injection of a standard WSCM. If the particular tube remains occluded, an attempt is made to thread the guidewire through the ostia and into the isthmus of the tube.

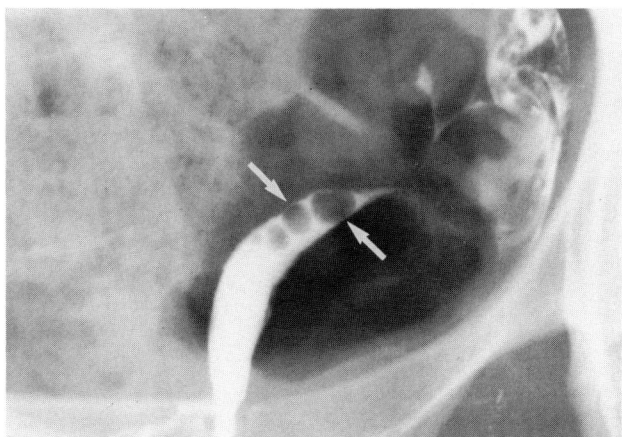

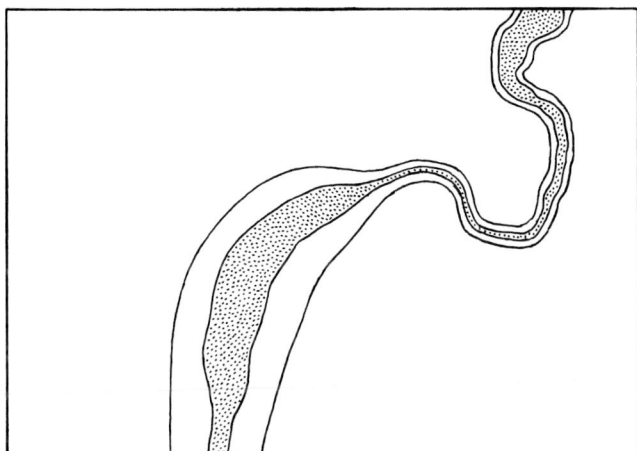

FIGURE 23–19. Unicornuate uterus. This radiograph and accompanying drawing illustrate a uterus with a single horn and single fallopian tube. The round filling defects (*arrows*) in the radiograph are merely transient air bubbles.

bicornuate uterus with one of the horns being rudimentary and not communicating with the primary uterine cavity. The HSG in this latter situation would appear the same as in a woman with a unicornuate uterus. A septate uterus (Fig. 23–21) cannot be distinguished from a bicornuate uterus with only a HSG. Although a bicornuate uterus generally demonstrates a wider separation of the two cavities on a HSG, this is not always the case. The septate anomaly is much more common than the bicornuate anomaly and can also be a cause of pregnancy wastage in a significant minority (25%) of affected patients. The didelphys uterine anomaly occurs when there is a fusion defect leading to the presence of two separate cervices and two uterine cavities (Fig. 23–22). There is often a communication between the two cavities at the level of the cervix. Functionally, each uterine cavity is separate, and the potential pregnancy complications are the same as with a unicornuate uterus (i.e., premature labor, malpresentation, postpartum hemorrhage). The DES uterine anomaly is not spontaneous but iatrogenic. The internal shape of the uterine cavity is altered when a female fetus is exposed in utero to exogenous estrogen.[49] The uterine cavity after DES exposure has a T shape and an irregular "shaggy" border (Fig. 23–23). The DES-induced uterine anomaly makes a woman more prone toward spontaneous abortion and premature labor.

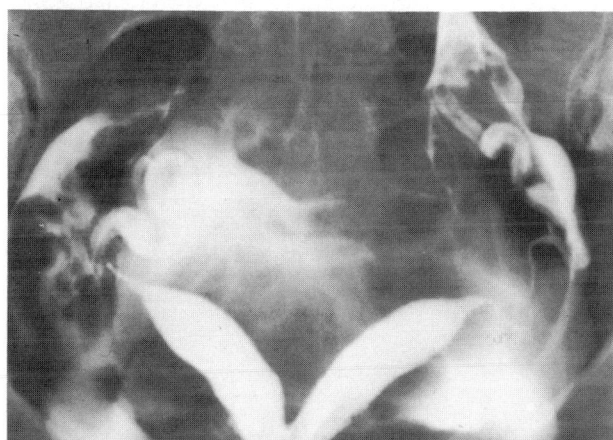

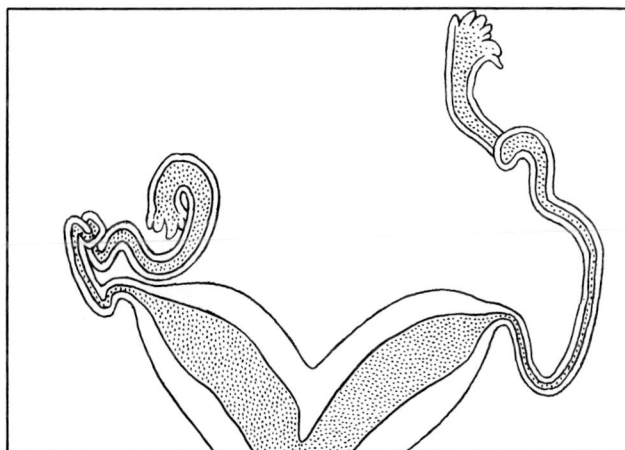

FIGURE 23–20. Bicornuate uterus. This radiograph and accompanying drawing illustrate two separate uterine horns with their respective fallopian tubes. There is spill of medium into the peritoneal cavity as well. As illustrated in the drawing, a bicornuate uterus has an external uterine contour consisting of two horns.

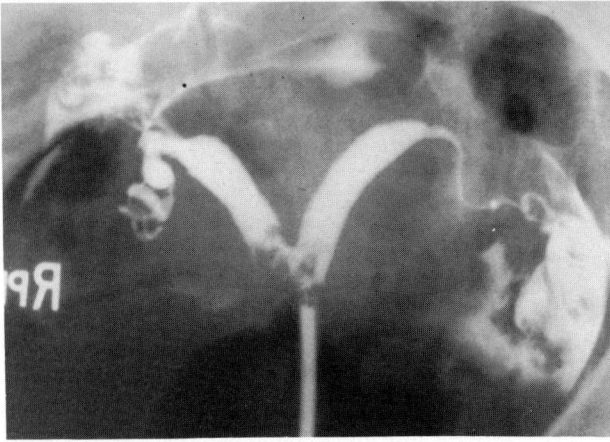

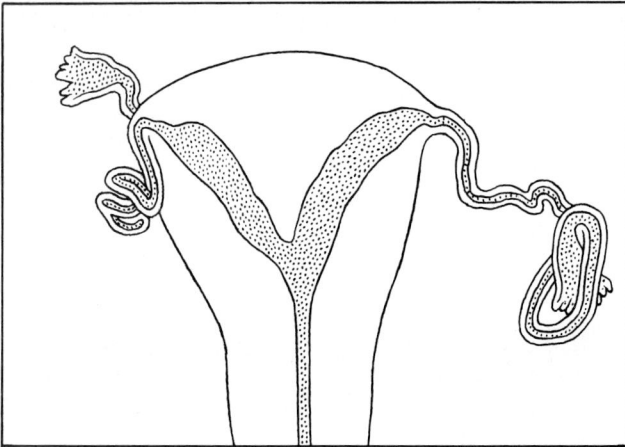

FIGURE 23–21. Septate uterus. This radiograph and accompanying drawing illustrate a uterus that appears to have two separate horns. However, as illustrated in the drawing, a septate uterus has a normal external uterine contour.

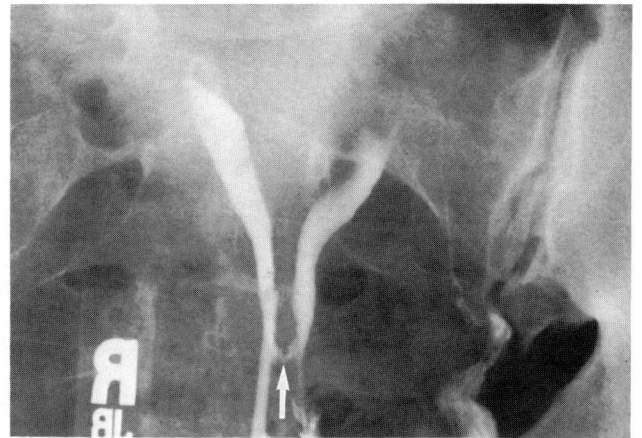

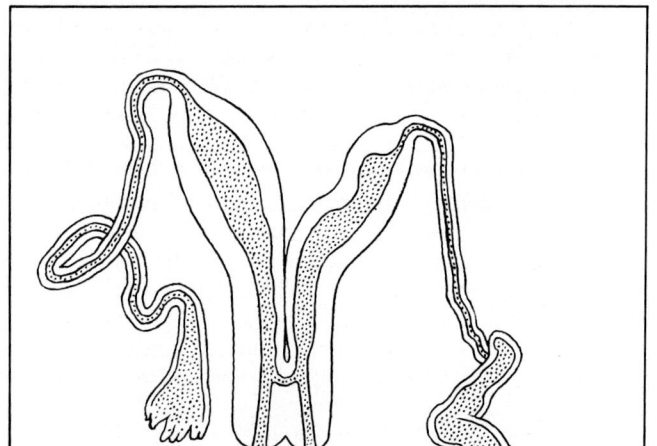

FIGURE 23–22. Uterine didelphys. A uterine didelphys has two cervical openings and two separate uterine horns with associated fallopian tubes. This radiograph and accompanying drawing illustrate two separate uteri, side by side, except for a small interconnecting fistula (*arrow*) at the level of the cervix.

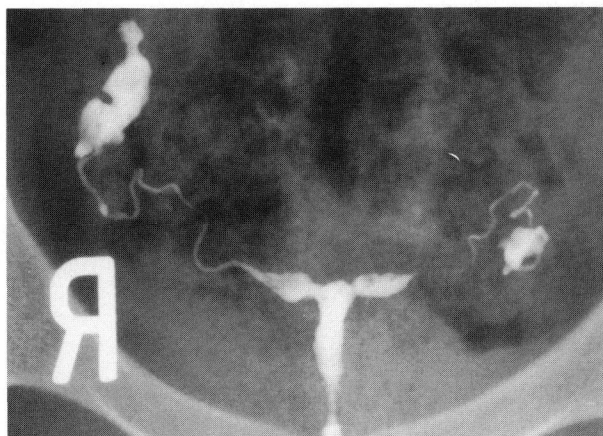

FIGURE 23-23. Diethylstilbestrol uterus. This radiograph demonstrates a small T-shaped uterus with an irregular endometrial border that has the classic appearance associated with estrogen exposure in utero during the first and second trimesters of pregnancy.

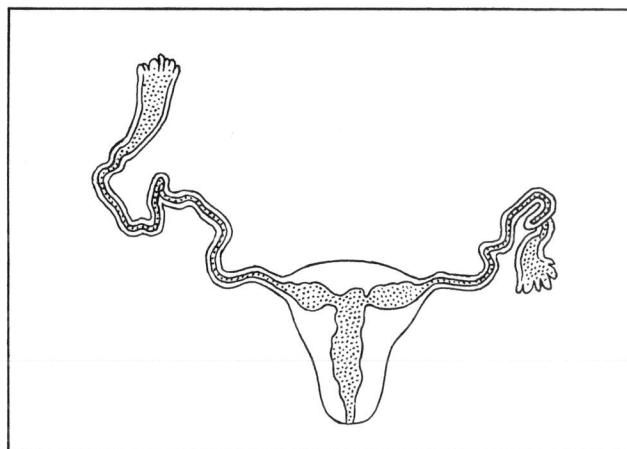

If the guidewire successfully traverses the proximal tube, a 3 French catheter is advanced over the guidewire (Fig. 23–24B) through which WSCM is injected and distal tubal anatomy is demonstrated (Fig. 23–24C).[52] Even after successful recanalization, the distal tube may demonstrate obstruction or dilatation, or there may be pelvic adhesions. It is recommended that the procedure be performed under antibiotic coverage. A common regimen is doxycycline, 100 mg twice a day for 5 days, with the initial dose given 12 hours preceding the procedure. A series of reports have appeared that describe the experience and results with this technique (Table 23–4).[52-57] Approximately 85% of proximally obstructed oviducts are successfully recanalized with an estimated 30% reocclusion rate. About 30% to 40% of women in whom at

TABLE 23-4. Success Rates of Selective Salpingography and Fallopian Tube Recanalization*

Indication/ Reference Source	No. Patients	Recanalization	Early Pregnancy Rate† (%) Early Pregnancy (Average Months of Follow-up)	Ectopic Pregnancy	Reocclusion (estimated)
Primarily for Diagnosis					
Thurmond & Rösch[52]	100	86	39(8)	6	30
Kumpe et al[53]	22	88	23(8)	9	30
Winfield et al[54]	20	NA	15	5	NA
Amendola et al[55]	12	89	17	0	NA
Primarily for Treatment					
Thurmond & Rösch[52]	20	95	48(9)	0	25
			58(12)	0	
Confino et al[56]	77	92	34(12)	4	32

*Note: Diagnostic indications included unilateral or bilateral obstruction, presence of distal disease, and other factors not controlled. Indications for treatment included bilateral obstruction and absence of significant distal disease or pelvic adhesions by laparoscopy. The technique used by all researchers, with the exception of Confino et al, was a vacuum cup hysterosalpingography device with nonballoon fallopian tube catheters. Confino et al[56] used a balloon hysterosalpingography device with balloon fallopian tube catheters. NA, Not available.

†Viable intrauterine pregnancy as seen at ultrasound study.

Adapted from Confino E, Tur-Kaspa I, DeCherney A, et al. Transcervical balloon tuboplasty. JAMA 1990; 264:2079–2082. Copyright 1990, American Medical Association.

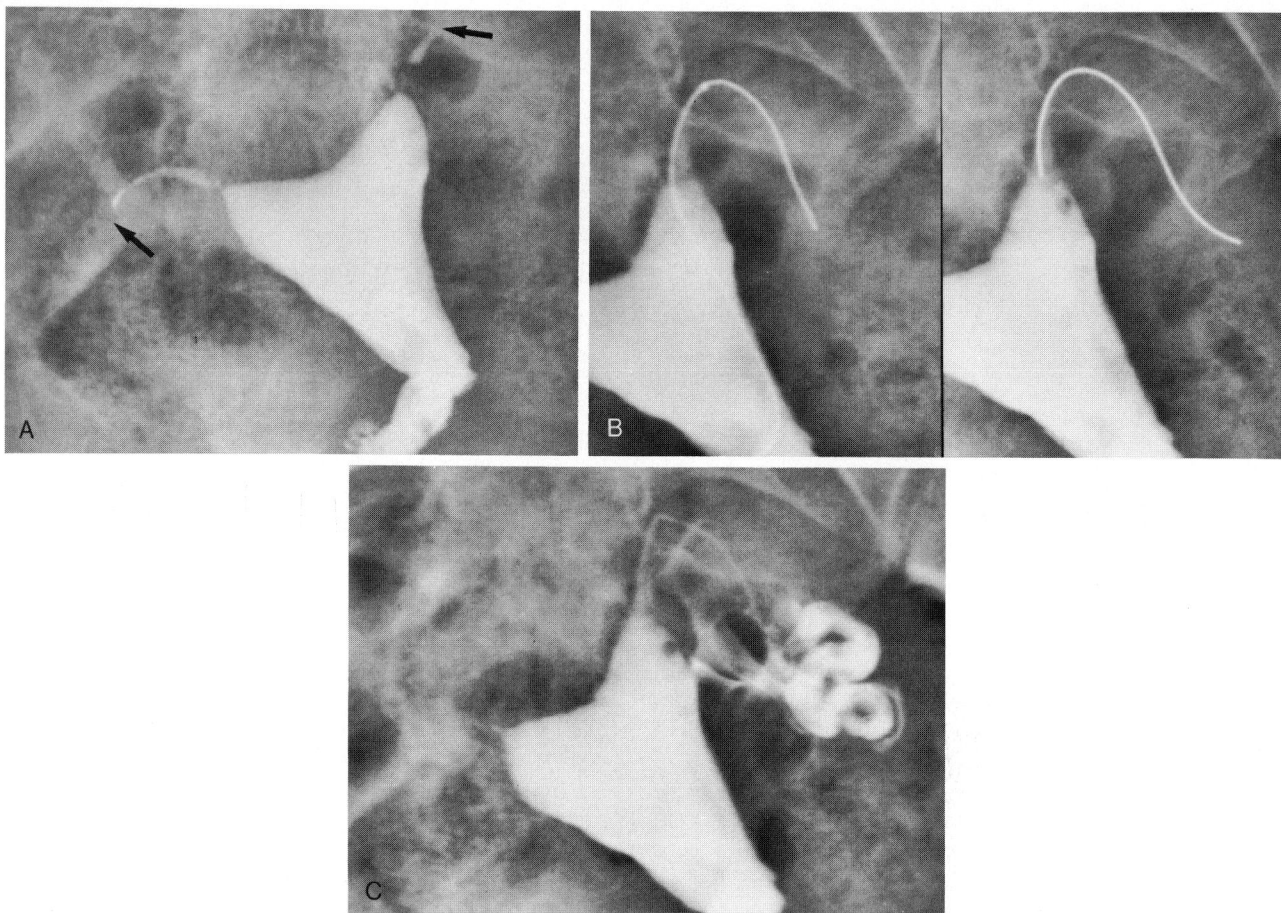

FIGURE 23–24. Selective salpingography. *A,* This radiograph illustrates a uterine cavity (with an arcuate tendency) and the intramural tubal segments. There is proximal tubal obstruction at approximately the intramural-isthmic junction bilaterally *(arrows). B,* The radiologist has proceeded to introduce a 3 Fr catheter over a flexible guide wire. The guide wire and catheter have traversed the obstruction, and the tip of the catheter is now in the isthmic portion of the left tube. *C,* The guide wire and catheter have been removed, and the medium is now able to traverse the full length of the left tube and spillage is noted. The radiologist will now attempt to cannulate and open up the contralateral right tube.

least one tube was successfully recanalized conceive within 6 to 12 months. About 5% to 10% of these pregnancies are ectopic (tubal).[57]

It is difficult to separate the diagnostic from the therapeutic aspects of selective salpingography. The placement of the guidewire and a small catheter through the tubal lumen probably dislodges debris and breaks up fine adhesions in many cases. The underlying disease can only be surmised and not actually determined when selective salpingography demonstrates proximal tubal patency. When proximal obstruction persists and selective salpingography was unsuccessful, it has been reported that 93% of resected tubal segments are diseased (fibrosis, chronic salpingitis, and SIN).[58] Procedures similar to selective salpingography using a coaxial balloon catheter have been reported.[56] The patency and pregnancy rates are quite similar between the two procedures. Enough experience has been gained with these retrograde techniques (selective salpingography, transcervical balloon tuboplasty) to make the following recommendation: When persistent bilateral proximal tubal obstruction is encountered in an infertile woman, a retrograde catheterization procedure should be attempted before resorting to tubal surgery or in vitro fertilization. If patency (recanalization) is demonstrated,

at least a 6-month interval should be allowed as a window of opportunity for pregnancy to occur.

ULTRASONOGRAPHY, COMPUTED TOMOGRAPHY, AND MAGNETIC RESONANCE IMAGING

The last 15 years have been marked by rapid development and dissemination of imaging modalities. Ultrasonography (US), computed tomography (CT) and MRI have been made widely available during this period. Advances in sonographic technology have rapidly been followed by new applications, many of which have had tremendous impact on the evaluation and treatment of infertility. Although CT has had limited application to the evaluation of this group of patients, it may be helpful in the evaluation of pre-existing conditions that contribute to the process. MRI applications are still in a phase of development as new techniques and technology are being introduced. Its use in the evaluation of developmental anomalies as well as uterine and adnexal pathology has been widely reported. Topics to be discussed include evaluation of pre-existing conditions, monitoring of ovulation, evaluation of the endometrium, and evaluation of early pregnancy.

Equipment

ULTRASONOGRAPHY

There has been rapid evolution of US equipment over the past 15 years. Gray scale resolution has improved with the introduction of electronically focused transducers. The development of endovaginal transducers has revolutionized pelvic imaging. Images produced by these transducers, by allowing the use of relatively high-frequency transducers (5 to 7 mHz), by avoiding the scattering effects of subcutaneous fat, and by placing the transducer closer to the areas of interest, are substantially better than comparable transabdominal scans. Use of endovaginal probes obviates the need for a full urinary bladder, which has led to a higher level of patient acceptance. Transabdominal imaging retains a role in providing orienting images in examination of large masses and in visualization of cephalically displaced structures.

Duplex Doppler (DD) and color Doppler imaging (CDI) are the most recent technologic advances for use in both transabdominal and endovaginal scanning. DD permits determination of the presence, the direction, and the velocity of flow in a given vessel. Information concerning resistance in the vascular bed can be derived from this information through the use of various parameters, such as the resistive and pulsatility indices. CDI uses color to indicate direction and mean velocity of blood flow. The high sensitivity of current devices allows visualization of vessels that are poorly visualized on standard gray-scale images. This technique facilitates the placement of Doppler sample volumes as well as providing a qualitative estimate of vascularity.

MAGNETIC RESONANCE IMAGING

Since its introduction a decade ago, MRI has also been widely applied to evaluation of the female pelvis. This technique uses strong, homogeneous magnetic fields in conjunction with radiofrequency pulses to interrogate the molecular environment of atoms with unpaired protons. Nearly all work to date has concentrated on hydrogen atoms. T2-weighted images are obtained by using long pulse repetition and echo times. Such images reflect the incoherent exchange of energy among neighboring spins and molecular environment of the hydrogen atoms.[59] T2-weighted images are important in evaluation of the female pelvis because these images are best at defining internal organ anatomy and most disease processes.[60] T1-weighted images are produced by pulse sequences with short pulse repetition and echo times. Such images are primarily influenced by the adjacent molecular lattice of hydrogen atoms and measure the loss of longitudinal magnetization after a radiofrequency pulse. T1-weighted images are helpful in increasing diagnostic accuracy, especially in evaluation of fat-containing or blood-containing lesions. Images may be enhanced by the use of surface coils, which provide stronger local magnetic gradients and improved signal-to-noise ratios. Advances in pulse-sequence software, such as fast-spin-echo and gradient-recalled techniques, have resulted in improvements in image quality. Use of paramagnetic contrast material, such as gadolinium-DTPA, provides additional information about vascularity of structures.

COMPUTED TOMOGRAPHY

CT uses conventional x-rays to create axial images of the body. Since its introduction 20 years ago, numerous changes in the technique have occurred. Availability of high-output x-ray tubes and more efficient radiation detectors has improved resolution and decreased scanning times. Most recently, introduction of helical scanning with continuous gantry rotation combined with continuous table motion has increased scan speed. For pelvic scanning, use of oral and rectal contrast material is imperative to distinguish bowel from other structures. Intravenous contrast material may also be helpful in detecting vessels, urinary tract structures, and mass lesions.

Technique

Transabdominal US requires a full urinary bladder for adequate visualization of pelvic structures. The full bladder pushes the intestines cephalad and provides a relatively reproducible location for mobile pelvic structures. This technique provides orienting images, which may be helpful in defining the complex relationships between pelvic structures. Specific areas of interest can be identified for further examination with endovaginal transducers. Disadvantages include patient discomfort associated with the maintenance of a full bladder and the possibility that large masses may be pushed out of the pelvis and obscured by overlying bowel gas. Variability of bladder filling may make comparison between studies difficult, and the bladder may deform structures, causing diagnostic confusion.

Endovaginal scanning is accomplished using transducers specially designed for this application, although use of standard abdominal probes has been reported. Transducers are covered with latex sheaths. Acoustic contact is established within the sheath using standard acoustic gel and between transducer and pelvic structures using sterile lubricant. In specific applications, in which bactericidal components of lubricant are undesirable, saline or transport media may be substituted. Between patients, current recommendations mandate that the transducers be cleansed with one of several antiseptic solutions, such as glutaraldehyde (Cidex).

MRI requires little patient preparation. Because the technique requires that the patient be placed within the bore of the magnet, claustrophobia and obesity are limiting factors. Between 1% and 5% of patients do not tolerate the procedure for these reasons. Glucagon may be used to decrease bowel motion and resultant image artifact. Although various bowel contrast materials have been investigated, no single agent has proved useful in all applications, and their use is investigational. Gadolinium-DTPA is receiving increased application in pelvic MRI. This agent, which markedly reduced the T1 of blood, can be used in similar fashion to intravenous contrast material in CT.

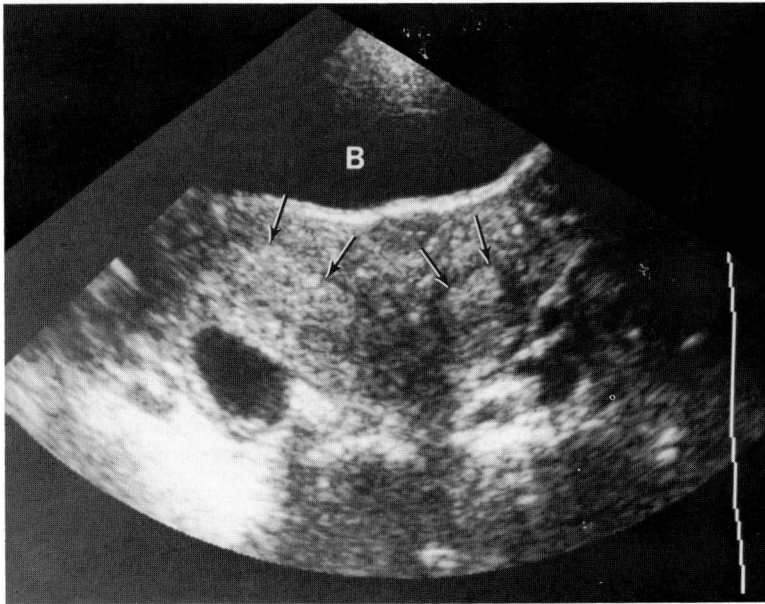

FIGURE 23–25. Bicornuate uterus. The transverse sonogram through a full urinary bladder demonstrates the character appearance of bicornuate uterus. Note the increased intercornual distance and characteristic lobulated appearance. *Arrows* indicate uterine cavities. B, bladder.

Evaluation of Clinical Conditions

UTERINE ANOMALIES

One percent to 5% of women may have müllerian anomalies, but only 20% of these patients are infertile.[61, 62] US and MRI, used in conjunction with HSG, are helpful in precisely defining these anomalies. HSG is best at defining the shape of the uterine cavity. When used alone, however, HSG had an accuracy of only 55% in distinguishing between septate and bicornuate uterus.[63] When combined with US, the diagnostic accuracy improved to 90%.

US and MRI contribute by better defining the outer contour of the uterus and the extent and composition of the septum. Bicornuate uterus has a characteristic lobulated appearance of outer contour, increased intercornual distance, and outward fundal concavity (Fig. 23–25).[61] On occasion, this sonographic appearance may be mimicked by the presence of myomas. In this circumstance, MRI signal intensities distinguish between this possibility and bicornuate uterus. MRI signal may also be helpful in determining the composition of the septum. When composed entirely of myometrium, the septum demonstrates characteristic medium intensity signal on T1-weighed images and high signal on T2-weighted

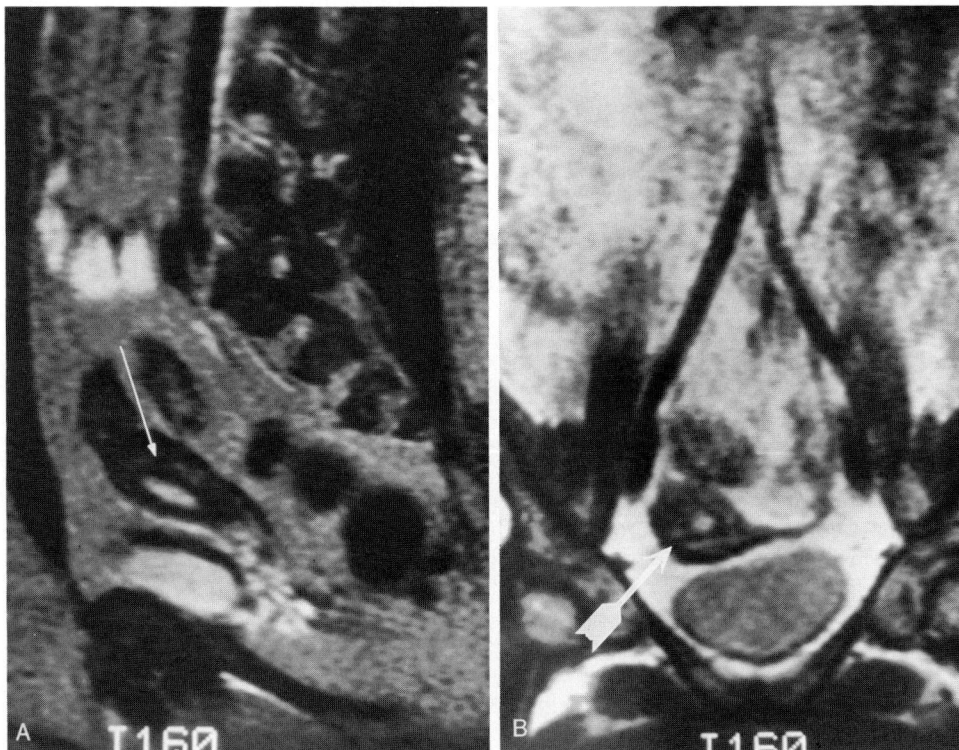

FIGURE 23–26. Unicornuate uterus. *A,* Sagittal T2-weighted body coil magnetic resonance imaging (MRI) shows a single horn of a unicornuate uterus *(arrow)*. *B,* Coronal spin density-weighted MRI shows a small unicornuate uterus *(arrow)*. (*A* and *B* courtesy of Dr. Mark Schiebler.)

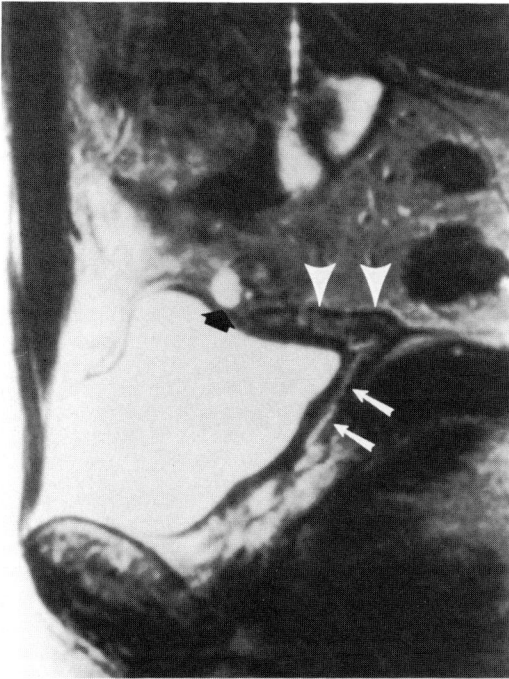

FIGURE 23–27. Hypoplastic uterus and vagina in a patient with infertility. Sagittal T2-weighted images show a small vaginal canal (*arrows*) leading to an extremely small hypoplastic uterus (*arrowheads*). A small ovarian cyst is also noted (*black arrow*). (Courtesy of Dr. Mark Schiebler.)

images. If the inferior portion of the septum is of fibrous origin, low signal on both T1- and T2-weighted images may be expected. In patients with septate uterus, the outer contour is normal with normal intercornual distance. The septum in such patients is characteristically fibrous and demonstrates low signal intensities on T1- and T2-weighted images. Other congenital anomalies, including unilateral agenesis/hypoplasia, unicornuate uterus, and obstruction of duplicated tracts, may also be identified through a combination of these imaging modalities (Figs. 23–26 and 23–27). When such uterine anomalies are identified, further examination to detect renal anomalies is essential.[65]

UTERINE LEIOMYOMAS

Uterine leiomyomas are common uterine neoplasms that may be associated with infertility or early pregnancy loss. US has been used extensively to identify these lesions. The most common sonographic appearance is that of a well-marginated hypoechoic or heterogeneous uterine mass (Fig. 23–28).[66] The echo architecture, however, depends on the relative amounts of fibrous tissue and smooth muscle present as well as the degree of degeneration. This results in considerable variation in sonographic appearance. Pitfalls in the diagnosis of uterine myomas have been studied. Baltarowich and associates[67] reported on 44 patients with atypical sonographic appearance of myomas in whom the lesions were interpreted as adnexal masses in 19 cases, as bicornuate uteri in 4 cases, and as pregnancy-related conditions in 13 cases. Endovaginal scans are helpful in patients with small mural, submucous, or cervical myomas.[68] The smaller field of view and decreased soft tissue penetration from high-frequency transducers, however, limit utility in patients with large, echodense, or

pedunculated lesions. US may be used to monitor myoma size after treatment. Sauer and colleagues[69] found sonography best in monitoring the size of myomas in patients with lesions greater than 6 cm in diameter.

MRI has also been used to evaluate size and position of leiomyomas. These lesions usually have medium intensity signal on T1-weighted images and homogeneous low intensity signal on T2-weighted images (Fig. 23–29). This low signal on T2-weighted images distinguishes myomas from most other types of uterine pathology. Myomas with degeneration, however, may exhibit increased signal on such pulse sequences and make MRI findings less specific. Zawin and associates[70] reported a high degree of accuracy in diagnosis, especially in patients with large uteri. In addition, MRI may be helpful in distinguishing myomas from other pelvic masses when US is not able to define the origin of such pathology precisely.[71]

ENDOMETRIOSIS

Endometriosis has varied appearance on US. By transabdominal technique, lesions are hypoechoic in 80% of cases.[72] Internal septations, loculations, and variable wall thickness are common sonographic findings (Fig. 23–30). Using endovaginal transducers, low-level internal echoes are commonly observed.[73] This characteristic sonographic finding is thought to reflect the presence of degraded blood products found within the endometrioma. The findings unfortunately are not specific and tubo-ovarian abscess, ovarian teratoma, hemorrhagic ovarian cyst, and mucinous cystadenoma may mimic the common sonographic findings in endometrioma. In addition, small implants of endometriosis are not visible by US. For these two reasons, US plays a limited role in this disease process. In a series of 37 patients studied by transabdominal US and laparoscopy, US had a sensitivity of only 11% in detecting endometriosis.[74]

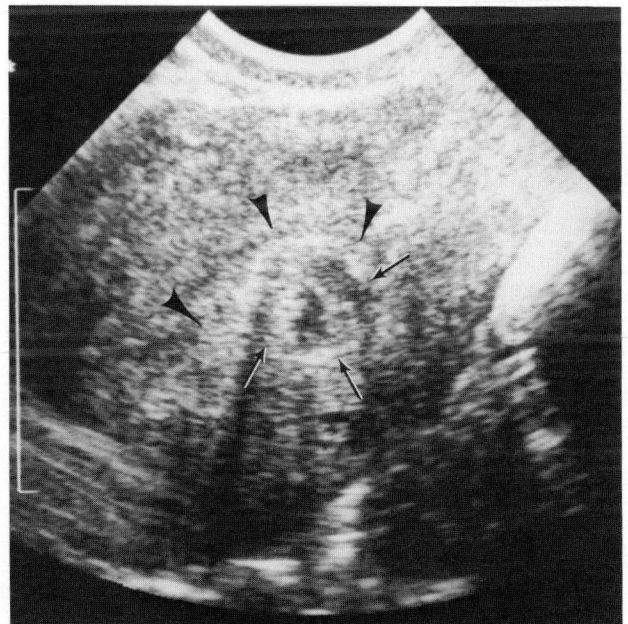

FIGURE 23–28. Uterine leiomyoma. Endovaginal scan demonstrates a small submucosal leiomyoma (*arrows*) deforming the endometrial cavity (*arrowheads*).

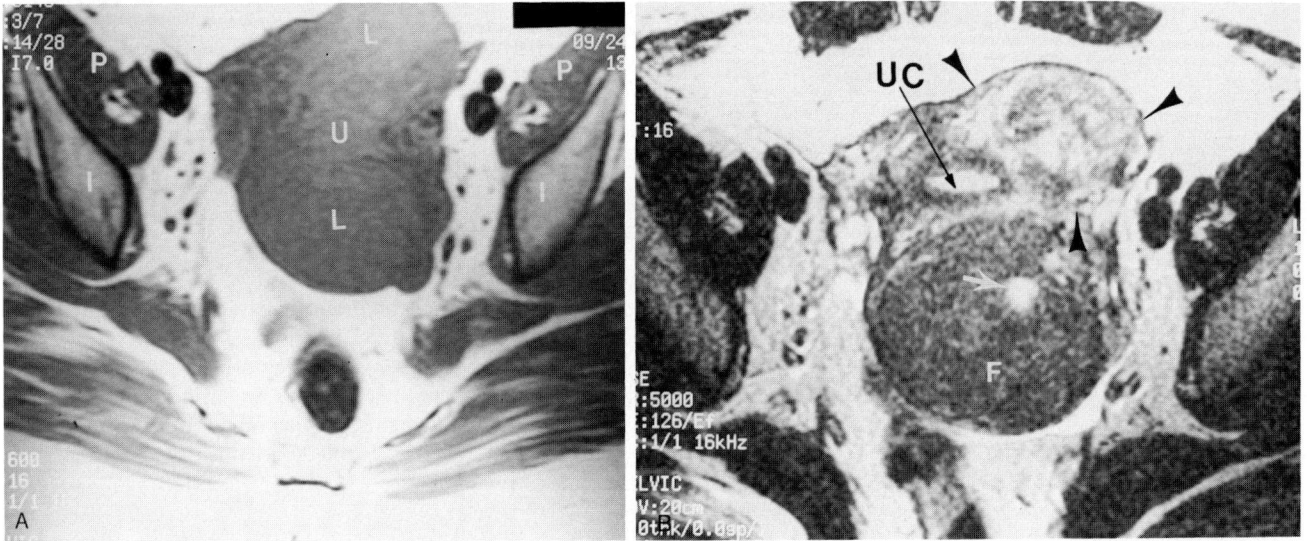

FIGURE 23–29. Magnetic resonance imaging of leiomyomas. *A,* Axial T1-weighted image demonstrates markedly irregular uterine margins. The deforming masses are of medium-level signal. Internal uterine architecture is not well seen. P, psoas; I, iliac bone; L, leimyoma; U, uterus. *B,* Axial fast spin echo T2-weighted images in the same patient show that the larger posterior leiomyoma (F) demonstrates predominantly low-level signal intensity with small areas of increased signal activity caused by focal degeneration *(white arrow).* The more anterior leiomyoma *(arrowheads)* demonstrates heterogeneous, predominantly high-level signal intensity compatible with a degenerating leiomyoma. UC, uterine cavity. (*A* and *B* courtesy of Dr. Mark Schiebler.)

A spectrum of findings has also been reported in the examination of endometriosis by MRI. Large endometriomas can be reliably identified. Togashi and associates[75] reported that hyperintense signal on T1-weighted images combined with hypointense signal on T2-weighted scans and focal hyperintense areas ("shading") was most diagnostic of endometrioma. Their sensitivity in diagnosing endometrial cysts from other adnexal masses was 90%, specificity was 98%, and accuracy was 96%. Other authors have found MRI to be less reliable, with sensitivity of only 64%.[76] The problem stems from variable signal patterns from hemorrhage of different ages. In addition, hemorrhage from other causes, including hemorrhagic cyst, pelvic inflammatory disease, ovarian carcinoma, teratoma, and cystadenoma, may have similar appearances. Small endometrial implants are not readily visualized

by MRI.[77] For this reason, the primary role of both US and MRI is monitoring of therapy once the diagnosis has been established laparoscopically.

MALE GENITALIA

Scrotal US is important in the evaluation of the infertile couple. Nashan and coworkers[78] found abnormalities in 40% or 658 male patients referred from an infertility clinic. The most common abnormality seen was varicocele, which was diagnosed in 21% of their patients. Of these, 24% were not suspected clinically. More recently, Petros and colleagues[79] described the use of CDI in the evaluation of patients with oligospermia (Fig. 23–31; see color section in the center of the book). Their results were similar, with detection of varicoceles in 29% of patients with normal clinical examinations. Other abnormalities that may be detected include cysts of the epididymis, testicular microlithiasis, and primary testicular tumors.[80]

OVARIAN FOLLICLES

US plays an important role in monitoring the development of ovarian follicles. Initial reports used transabdominal US to visualize the ovaries through a filled urinary bladder.[81, 82] US is used to assess the number and size of developing follicles. This information, most often in the form of follicle diameter, is used together with serum estradiol levels to infer the maturity of the follicles. Ovaries are identified on transabdominal scans by their characteristic relationship to the iliac vessels and sonographic appearance. In the absence of factors that might modify their location, such as surgery or pelvic inflammatory disease, the ovaries can be identified along the pelvic sidewall between the internal and external iliac vessels. In the presence of pre-existent disease, their location may vary with anterior, lateral, or posterior locations possible. Ovaries may also be identified by their characteristic sono-

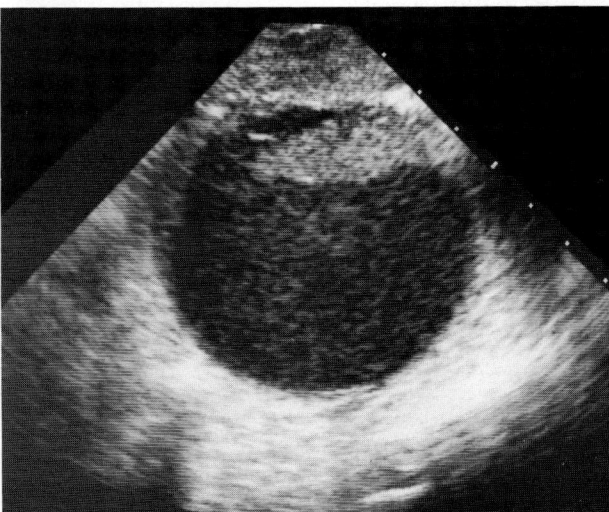

FIGURE 23–30. Endometrioma. Endovaginal scan demonstrates characteristic sonographic findings of a hypoechoic mass with homogeneous low-level echoes.

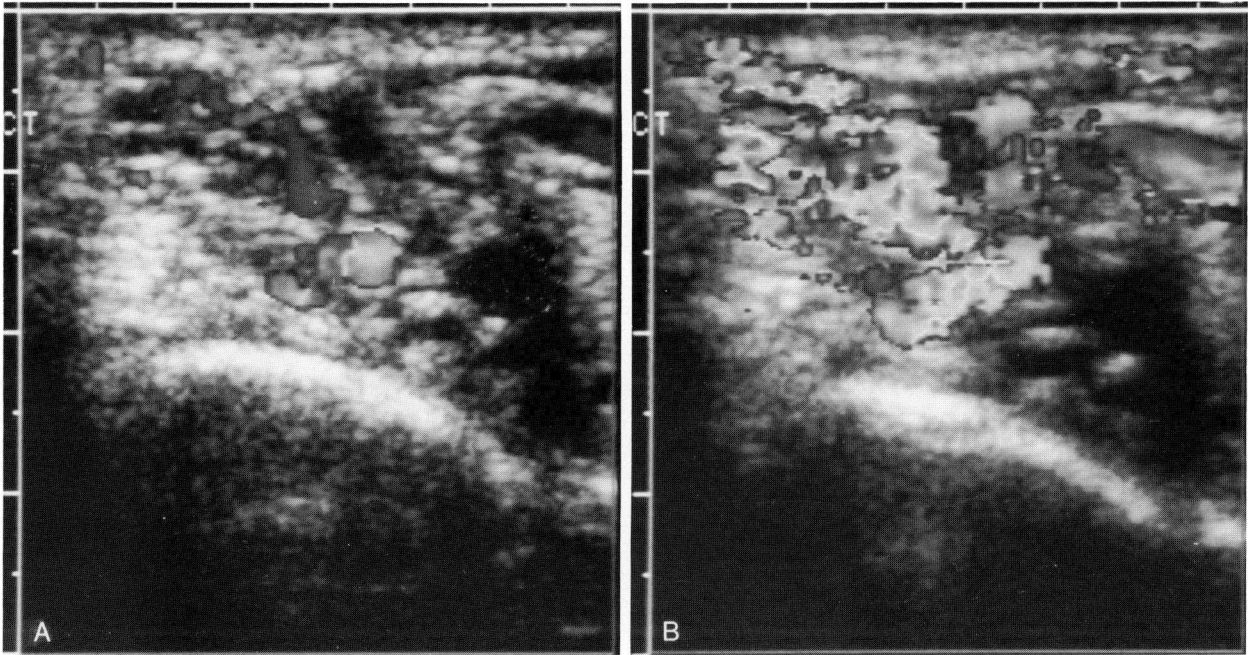

FIGURE 23–31. Varicocele. Color Doppler imaging with patient erect demonstrates changing appearances before (A) and following (B) Valsalva maneuver.

graphic appearance. The outer cortical layer contains multiple follicles arranged in a circular array. These small cystic structures are easily visualized and serve as identifying landmarks. An inner medullary zone may also be visualized as a zone of increased echogenicity. Visualization in two orthogonal planes is important to prevent errors in localization. Although serpiginous broad ligament vessels may mimic ovarian appearances, their vascular nature is apparent on orthogonal imaging. Color flow and Doppler imaging may also help in difficult cases.

More recent studies have used endovaginal transducers to study ovarian follicle size.[83] These transducers have the advantage of increased resolution. Such examinations, however, are more technically difficult because of the absence of orienting landmarks, which aid in transabdominal scans, and because the empty urinary bladder increases the variability of ovarian position on endovaginal examinations.

Several sources of error in the examination of ovarian follicles have been identified. Using transabdominal technique, Prins and Vogelzang[84] suggested that interobserver variability and variability in bladder filling were the most important factors contributing to variation in measurement. Because of significant interobserver variability, the number of individuals evaluating a single patient should be limited when transabdominal scans are used. Higgins and associates[85] have suggested that this variability is reduced with endovaginal scans. Other reports have confirmed that endovaginal technique produces more reproducible results, which are more closely correlated with findings at laparoscopy and follicle aspiration (Fig. 23–32).[86]

Characteristic sonographic findings have been described that were thought to be helpful in predicting ovulation. A hypoechoic rim surrounding the follicle has been reported as predictive of ovulation. This finding was reported to be secondary by early separation of the granulosa cell layer from the theca cell layer and increased vascularity and edema of the thecal tissue following the luteinizing hormone surge.[87]

The appearance of a small echogenic mound of tissue projecting into the follicle, representing the cumulus oophorus, has also been described.[88] More recent studies with endovaginal technique have contradicted these reports. Zandt-Stastny and coworkers[89] found no sonographic evidence of imminent ovulation in 22 menstrual cycles. These authors have suggested that slice thickness and side-lobe artifacts may have accounted for previous findings when transabdominal technique was used.

US has been used to evaluate blood flow to the ovary. The dual blood supply of this structure from both branches of uterine and ovarian arteries increases variability of such as-

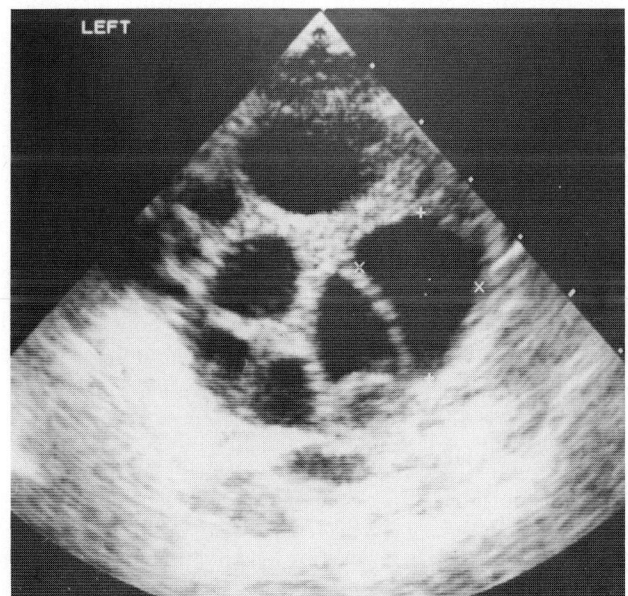

FIGURE 23–32. Ovarian follicles. Endovaginal scan in a patient undergoing in vitro fertilization demonstrates multiple follicles. Two orthogonal measurements of an individual follicle are indicated by cursor locations.

sessment. Patterns of change in vascular resistance, however, have been described. The overall trend is for vascular resistance to be high early in the follicular phase, decrease progressively in the late follicular and early luteal phases, and then rise late in the luteal period.[90] The pulsatility index is significantly higher in the nondominant ovary when compared with the dominant ovary.[91]

ENDOMETRIUM

Characteristic changes of the endometrium during the menstrual cycle have been evaluated by US and MRI. The normal uterus is characterized by visualization of three layers on T2-weighted magnetic resonance images or ultrasound studies. The outer myometrium is intermediate in signal intensity or echogenicity. It surrounds a low signal intensity and low echogenicity junctional zone, which is thought to represent the inner third of myometrium.[92] The inner layer representing endometrium is echogenic on US and high intensity on T2-weighted MRI.

The proliferative phase is characterized by increasing thickness of the endometrium. Early in this phase, the echogenicity is similar to adjacent structures. As ovulation approaches, however, the endometrium becomes more echoic. Increased reflectivity from distended and tortuous glands has been suggested as a cause for this finding.[93] During the secretory phase, the endometrium increases more slowly in thickness to reach its maximum thickness and echogenicity.[94] US had a sensitivity of 100% and a specificity of 62% for detecting normal endometrial development in a series of 18 women with ovarian failure.[95]

Similar endometrial growth patterns have been observed on serial MRI scans.[96] Endometrial thickness demonstrated a phase of more rapid growth from day 8 to day 16 and slower rates of growth from day 4 to 8 and day 16 to 24. MRI provides better demonstration of the so-called junctional zone between endometrium and outer myometrium. This area of low signal on T2-weighted images surrounds the higher signal of the endometrium. Although the junctional zone may be visualized as a hypoechoic rim on sonograms, the margins of this region are less well defined on US. Reports have demonstrated that this area contains compact smooth muscle with less extracellular matrix and increased nuclear area when compared with the myometrium proper.[97, 98] Myometrial thickness demonstrates linear increase in thickness during the follicular phase with slower rates of increase during the luteal phase.[99]

Divergence from normal US patterns have been observed during ovulation induction with various agents. Fleischer and associates[100] and Randall and Templeton[101] both described decrease in endometrial thickness during clomiphene citrate cycles. Rogers and colleagues[102] reported more prominent endometrial echogenicity and increased thickness after gonadotropin-releasing hormone agonist plus human menopausal gonadotropin (hMG) compared with a clomiphene citrate/hMG regimen in assisted reproductive technology patients.

The role of US in evaluating endometrial readiness for implantation has also been studied. Considerable variability exists in published reports. Although some investigators have found correlation between endometrial thickness and conception, others have failed to observe this correlation.[103–105]

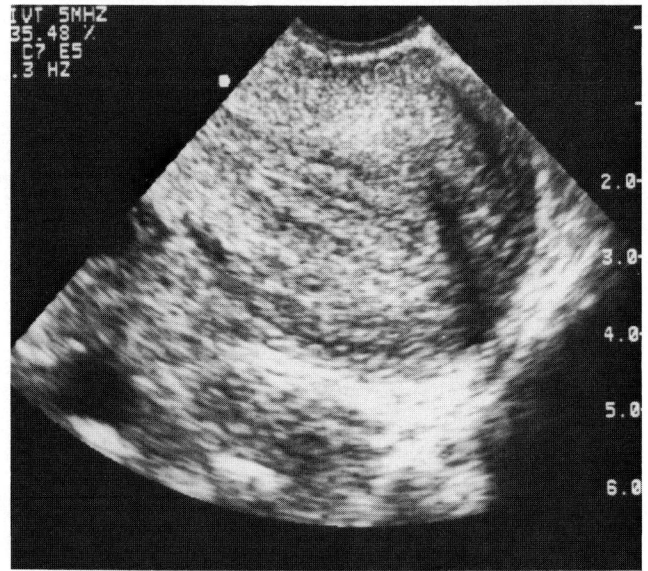

FIGURE 23–33. Ultrasonogram of the endometrium. Endovaginal sagittal uterine image demonstrates the characteristic three-layered appearance that has been associated with increased success of in vitro fertilization.

Correlation has also been noted with the sonographic appearance of the endometrium. Higher rates of conception have been reported in patients who developed a multilayered appearance than those in whom the endometrium remained homogeneously echogenic (Fig. 23–33).[106, 107] This correlation is greater than when simple measurement of endometrial thickness is used. Although differences in criteria make comparison between various series difficult, the rates of conception with favorable endometrial appearances are 23% to 33% compared with 0 to 3% with less favorable appearances.

Most recently, evaluation of the uterus by DD and CDI has been described. CDI is especially important because it allows rapid identification of small vessels for subsequent Doppler interrogation. These studies have demonstrated characteristic changes in uterine blood flow during the menstrual cycle. Decrease in uterine vascular impedance with increasing uterine perfusion accompanies the rise in estrogen and progesterone.[108] Uterine wave form analysis also demonstrates characteristic changes with decreasing uterine vascular resistance starting on the day before ovulation.[109] de Ziegler and colleagues[110] demonstrated that this effect is closely related to serum E_2 levels. Progesterone did not have a significant effect on the estrogen-mediated vasodilation in their group of patients. Failure of the uterus to demonstrate increased perfusion in the midsecretory phase has been suggested as a cause for infertility in patients undergoing in vitro fertilization.[111]

EARLY PREGNANCY (UTERINE AND ECTOPIC)

US plays a central role in the evaluation of early pregnancy and of its complications. US must answer two central questions in patients with biochemical evidence of pregnancy. The first question that must be resolved at the time of initial evaluation is the location of the pregnancy. The second question that may be more difficult to resolve and may require more than one sonogram is whether the pregnancy, if intrauterine, is normal or abnormal.

Human chorionic gonadotropin (hCG) values play a crucial role in these evaluations. Sonographic expectations based on biochemical values are especially important in addressing both issues just described. Scans interpreted in the absence of quantitative hCG values may provide limited information. It is important to distinguish between a threshold of a sonographic finding, the first level at which a given finding might be visualized, and the discriminatory level of this finding, the value at which all patients would be expected to exhibit a given ultrasound observation. Only discriminatory values are helpful in the assessment of ectopic pregnancy.

The earliest sonographic finding of intrauterine pregnancy is the visualization of a gestational sac. This appears as a fluid collection surrounded by echogenic trophoblastic tissue (Fig. 23–34). Implantation within the endometrium gives rise to the characteristic eccentric location. The gestational sac can consistently be recognized by 5 weeks' menstrual age when the mean sac diameter is 5 mm.[112] The hCG discriminatory value for visualization of a gestational sac varies with technique. The hCG threshold using transabdominal scans is 3600 to 6500 mU (First International Reference Preparation).[113, 114] Using endovaginal scans, this discriminatory value is 1000 to 2000 units (1st IRP).[115, 116] Care must be taken so intrauterine fluid or decidual reaction is not confused with a true gestational sac.

Failure to visualize an intrauterine gestation with an hCG titer above the discriminatory level should strongly raise the suspicion of ectopic pregnancy. Uterine findings in ectopic pregnancy are nonspecific. The lack of gestational sac may be accompanied by a variable degree of endometrial prominence. An endometrial thickness of greater than 10 mm predicts ectopic pregnancy with a sensitivity of 50%, a specificity of 84%, and a negative predictive value of 84%.[117] The presence of intrauterine fluid is a potential source of error. The presence of fluid collections within the uterus may cause difficulty because such pseudosacs may resemble an intrauterine gestation. Pseudogestational sac may be differentiated

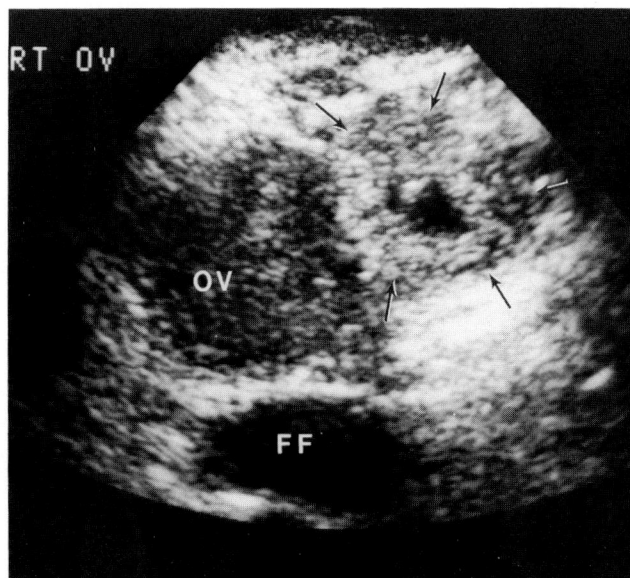

FIGURE 23–35. Ectopic pregnancy. Endovaginal scans demonstrate a hyperechoic adnexal ring (arrows) adjacent to the right ovary (OV). FF, free intraperitoneal fluid.

from intrauterine pregnancy by its central location and the lack of fetal pole or yolk sac.[118] Doppler may also be helpful in making this differentiation. Dillon and associates[119] have demonstrated that characteristic low-resistance trophoblastic flow is absent in pseudogestational sac, but present in the vast majority of intrauterine gestations.

Adnexal appearances are important in the sonographic diagnosis of ectopic pregnancy. The most specific sonographic finding is the visualization of an embryo within the ectopic pregnancy. Only a minority (15% to 28%) of patients, however, demonstrate this finding, limiting its utility.[115, 120] The most common finding is the visualization of a hyperechoic adnexal ring separate from the ovary (Fig. 23–35). The increased marginal echogenicity of these extrauterine gestational sacs reflects the presence of chorionic villi. Embryos, yolk sacs, or other recognizable internal structures are frequently absent. These structures are visualized 46% to 71% of the time with transvaginal sonography.[115, 121] CDI may be helpful with visualization of characteristic trophoblastic vascularity surrounding the hyperechoic ring (Fig. 23–36). Pulsed Doppler sampling of vessels within this ring of vascularity demonstrates the low resistance characteristic of trophoblastic flow. Use of Doppler technique has been reported to increase sensitivity from 77% to 87%.[122, 123] This flow pattern may be absent in ectopics with low hCG values, in early ectopics, and in ectopic demises. False-positive results have been reported in patients with pelvic inflammatory disease, corpus luteum, and uterine fibroids. These causes for false-positive CDI findings may be excluded by the absence of a positive hCG, intraovarian origin, location and clinical history, respectively.

The presence of echogenic intraperitoneal free fluid is an important secondary finding in patients with ectopic pregnancy (Fig. 23–37). Although the presence of any fluid within the peritoneum is more common in this group of patients, Nyberg and others[124] have demonstrated that the visualization of echogenic free fluid had a specificity of 98% and a positive predictive value of 92% regardless of other

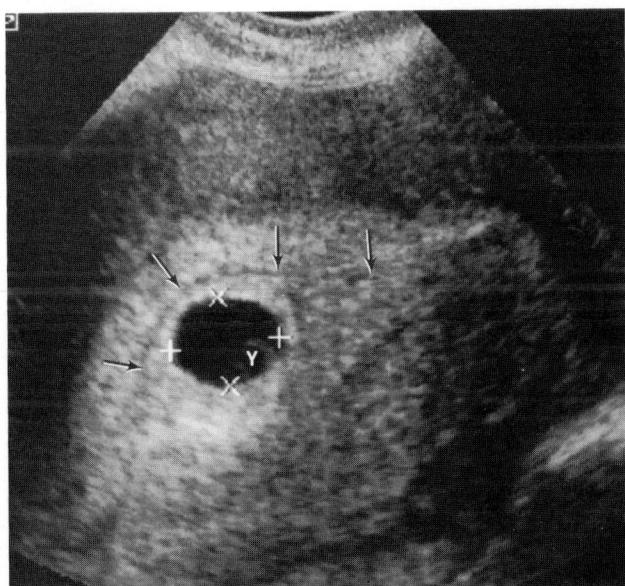

FIGURE 23–34. Early gestation. Endovaginal scan demonstrates a small gestational sac (cursors) that is eccentrically implanted. Arrows show the endometrial canal. Y, yolk sac.

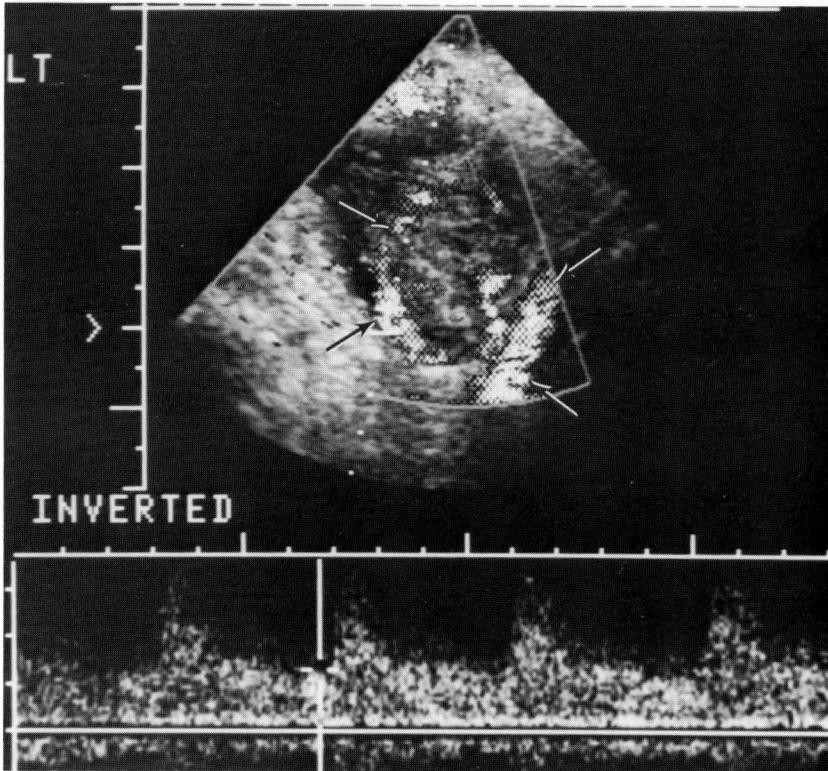

FIGURE 23–36. Ectopic pregnancy. A black-and-white photo of color Doppler and duplex image (arrows) of ectopic pregnancy demonstrates the characteristic ring of vascularity. Doppler waveforms demonstrate the characteristic low-resistance pattern.

sonographic findings. In addition, the visualization of echogenic free fluid was the only finding in 15% of cases in this report. False-positive cases have been noted in patients with hemorrhagic corpus luteum cysts.

The determination of whether an intrauterine pregnancy is normal or abnormal may be less decisive and require more than one sonogram. Several sonographic findings have been associated with poor pregnancy outcome. Bradycardia with cardiac rates of less than 85 beats/minute is associated with poor prognosis.[125] Disparity of mean gestational sac diameter with crown-rump length is also associated with poor outcome. Bromley and colleagues[126] demonstrated poor outcome if the gestational sac minus the crown-rump length is less than 4 mm. Failure to achieve a number of sonographic

milestones has been associated with poor prognosis. Levi and associates[127] noted that pregnancies that failed to demonstrate a yolk sac when the mean sac diameter was greater than 8 mm were abnormal. More recently, Kurtz and coworkers[128] have published a prospective series that suggests that detection of the yolk sac is not an early predictor of pregnancy outcome. Yolk sacs with diameters of greater than 6 mm have also been associated with poor outcome.[129] Yolk sacs that are calcified or too echogenic have also been associated with a similarly poor outcome.[130] The failure to visualize an embryo when the mean sac diameter exceeds 18 mm is considered to be diagnostic of a nonviable pregnancy.[127] Similarly, Levi and associates[131] have demonstrated that cardiac motion should be visualized in a viable pregnancy when the crown-

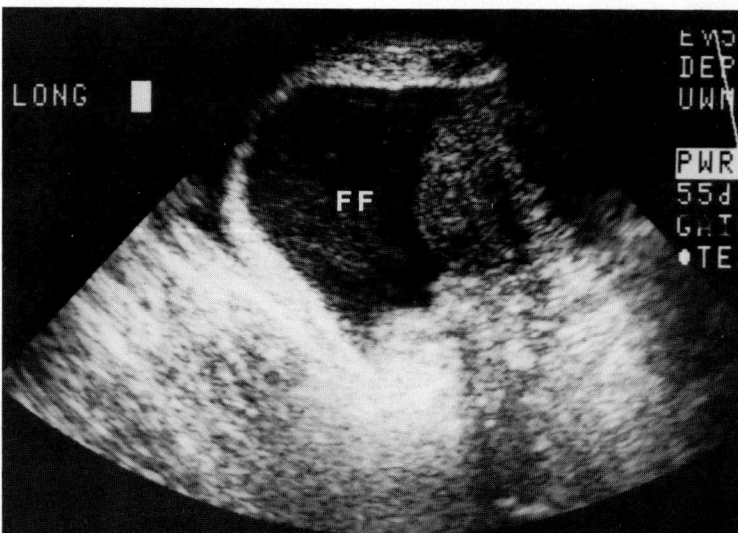

FIGURE 23–37. Echogenic intraperitoneal fluid. Scans in this patient with surgically confirmed ectopic pregnancy demonstrate the characteristic appearances of echogenic-free fluid with low-level echoes. FF, free intraperitoneal fluid.

rump length is greater than 5 mm. Other indicators of poor outcome include less than expected levels of hCG for a given gestational sac size and gestational sac growth of less than 6 mm per week.[132, 133]

REFERENCES

1. Moore DE, Foy HM, Daling JR, et al. Increased frequency of serum antibodies to chlamydia trachomatis in infertility due to distal tubal disease. Lancet 1982; 3:574–577.
2. Mueller BA, Daling JR, Moore DE, et al. Appendectomy and the risk of tubal infertility. N Engl J Med 1986; 315:1506.
3. Snowden EU, Jarrett JC II, Dawood MY. Comparison of diagnostic accuracy of laparoscopy, hysteroscopy, and hysterosalpingography in evaluation of female infertility. Fertil Steril 1984; 41:709.
4. Stone SC, McCalley M, Braunstein P, Egbert R. Radionuclide evaluation of tubal function. Fertil Steril 1985; 43:757.
5. Rindfleisch W. Darstellung des cavum uteri. Berl Klin Wochenschr No (Apr) 1910; 17:780.
6. Cary WH. Note on determination of patency of fallopian tubes by the use of collargol and x-ray shadow. Am J Obstet Dis Woman Child 1914; 69:462.
7. Heuser C. Lipiodol in the diagnosis of pregnancy. Lancet 1925; 2:1111.
8. Miller HA, Martinez DB. Iodinized oil in the diagnosis of pregnancy. Radiology 1928; 11:191.
9. Goldenberg RL, White R, Magendantz HG. Pregnancy during the hysterogram cycle. Fertil Steril 1976; 27:1274–1276.
10. Reshef E, Daniel WW, Foster JC, et al. Comparison between 1-hour and 24-hour follow-up radiographs in hysterosalpingography using oil based contrast media. Fertil Steril 1989; 52:753–755.
11. Alper MM, Garner PR, Spence JEH. Hyoscine butylbromide to relieve utero-tubal obstruction at hysterosalpingography. Br J Radiol 1985; 58:915–916.
12. Gerlock AJ, Hooser CW. Oviduct response to glucagon during hysterosalpingography. Radiology 1976; 119:727–728.
13. Soules MR, Spadoni LR. Oil versus aqueous media for hysterosalpingography: a continuing debate based on many opinions and few facts. Fertil Steril 1982; 38:1–11.
14. Young PE, Egan JE, Barlow JJ, Mulligan WJ. Reconstructive surgery for infertility at the Boston Hospital for Women. Am J Obstet Gynecol 1970; 108:1093.
15. Palmer A. Ethiodol hysterosalpingography for the treatment of infertility. Fertil Steril 1960; 11:311.
16. Winfield AC, Maxson WS, Harding DR, et al. Hexabrix as a contrast agent for hysterosalpingography. Radiology 1984; 152:232–233.
17. Davies AC, Keightley A, Borthwick-Clarke A, Walters HL. The use of a low-osmolality contrast medium in hysterosalpingography: comparison with a conventional contrast medium. Clin Radiol 1985; 36:533–536.
18. Mackey RA, Glass RH, Olson LE, Vaidya R. Pregnancy following hysterosalpingography with oil- and water-soluble dye. Fertil Steril 1971; 22:504.
19. DeCherney AH, Kort H, Barney JB, DeVore GR. Increased pregnancy rate with oil-soluble hysterosalpingography dye. Fertil Steril 1980; 33:407.
20. Schwabe MG, Shapiro SS, Haning RV. Hysterosalpingography with oil contrast medium enhances fertility in patients with infertility of unknown etiology. Fertil Steril 1983; 40:604–606.
21. Alper MM, Garner PR, Spence JEH, Quarrington AM. Pregnancy rates after hysterosalpingography with oil- and water-soluble contrast media. Obstet Gynecol 1986; 68:6–9.
22. Rasmussen F, Lindequist S, Larsen C, Justesen P. Therapeutic effect of hysterosalpingography: oil- versus water-soluble contrast media—a randomized perspective study. Radiology 1991; 179:75–77.
23. Patton DL, Soules MR, Engel CC, Halbert SA. Induced hydrosalpinges in rabbits: comparison of hysterosalpingographic media and development of an animal model. Fertil Steril 1984; 42:466–473.
24. Siegler AM. Dangers of hysterosalpingography. Obstet Gynecol Surv 1967; 22:284.
25. Bang J. Complications of hysterosalpingography. Acta Obstet Gynecol Scand 1950; 29:383.
26. Marshak RH, Poole CS, Goldberger MA. Hysterography and hysterosalpingography. Surg Gynecol Obstet 1950; 91:182.
27. Norris S. The hysterogram in the study of sterility. Can Med Assoc J 1956; 75:1016.
28. Whitelaw MJ, Miller EB. New water soluble medium (Sinografin) for hysterosalpingography. Fertil Steril 1959; 10:227.
29. Measday B. An analysis of the complications of hysterosalpingography. J Obstet Gynaecol Br Commonw 1960; 67:663.
30. Geary WL, Holland JB, Weed JC. Uterosalpingography. Am J Obstet Gynecol 1969; 104:687.
31. Stumpf PG, March CM. Febrile morbidity following hysterosalpingography. Feril Steril 1980; 33:487.
32. Pittaway DE, Winfield AC, Maxson W, et al. Prevention of acute pelvic inflammatory disease after hysterosalpingography: efficacy of doxycycline prophylaxis. Am J Obstet Gynecol 1983; 147:623–633.
33. Moore DE. Pain associated with hysterosalpingography: ethiodol versus salpix media. Fertil Steril 1982; 38:629–631.
34. Brown WE, Jennings AF, Bradbury JT. The absorption of radio-opaque substances used in hysterosalpingography. Am J Obstet Gynecol 1949; 58:1041.
35. Bateman BG, Nunley WC, Kitchin JD. Intravasation during hysterosalpingography using oil-base contrast media. Fertil Steril 1980; 34:439.
36. Eisenberg AD, Winfield AC, Page DL, et al. Peritoneal reaction resulting from iodinated contrast material: comparative study. Radiology 1989; 172:149–151.
37. Moore DE, Segard JH, Winfield AC, et al. Effects of contrast agents on the fallopian tube in a rabbit model. Radiology 1990; 176:721–724.
38. Thurmond AS, Hedgpeth PL, Scanlan RM. Selective injection of contrast media: inflammatory effects on rabbit fallopian tubes. Radiology 1991; 180:97–99.
39. Palmer A. Lipiodol "F" for use in hysterosalpingography. Fertil Steril 1952; 3:210.
40. Zachariae F. Venous and lymphatic intravasation in hysterosalpingography. Acta Obstet Gynecol Scand 1954; 34:131.
41. Meaker SR. Accidental injection of iodized oil into uterine veins. Am J Obstet Gynecol 1934; 28:568.
42. Roblee MA, Moore J. Lipiodol pulmonary emboli following hysterosalpingography. South Med J 1945; 38:89.
43. Shirley RL. Ovarian radiation dosage during hysterosalpingogram. Fertil Steril 1971; 22:83–85.
44. Sheikh HH, Yussman MA. Radiation exposure of ovaries during hysterosalpingography. Am J Obstet Gynecol 1976; 124:307–310.
45. Seppänen S, Lehtinen E, Holli H. Radiation dose in hysterosalpingography: modern 100 mm fluorography vs. full-scale radiography. Radiology 1978; 127:377–380.
46. Hedgpeth PL, Thurmond AS, Fry R, et al. Radiographic fallopian tube recanalization: absorbed ovarian radiation dose. Radiology 1991; 180:121–122.
47. Fortier KJ, Haney AF. The pathologic spectrum of uterotubal junction obstruction. Obstet Gynecol 1985; 65:93–98.
48. Soules MR, Pagon RA, Burns MW, Matsumoto AM. Normal and abnormal sexual development, ambiguous genitalia, and mullerian and wolffian duct anomalies. In: Carr BR, Blackwell RE, editors. Textbook of Reproductive Medicine. Norwalk, CT: Appleton & Lange, 1993:67–88.
49. Haney AF, Hammond CB, Soules MR, Creasman WT. DES induced upper genital tract abnormalities. Fertil Steril 1979; 31:142.
50. Thurmond AS, Novy M, Rösch J. Terbutaline in diagnosis of interstitial fallopian tube obstruction. Invest Radiol 1988; 23:209–210.
51. Thurmond AS, Novy M, Uchida BT, Rösch J. Fallopian tube obstruction: selective salpingography and recanalization. Radiology 1987; 163:511–514.
52. Thurmond AS, Rösch J. Nonsurgical fallopian tube recanalization for treatment of infertility. Radiology 1990; 174:371–374.
53. Kumpe DA, Zwerdlinger SC, Rothbarth LJ, et al. Proximal fallopian tube occlusion: diagnosis and treatment with transcervical fallopian tube catheterization. Radiology 1990; 177:183–187.
54. Winfield AC, Moore D, Segars J, et al. Selective fallopian tube canalization [abstr]. AJR Am J Roentgenol 1990; 154:195.
55. Amendola MA, Banner MP, Pollack HM, Sondheimer S. Preliminary experience with fluoroscopic transcervical fallopian tube recanalization [abstr]. AJR Am J Roentgenol 1990; 154:196.
56. Confino E, Tur-Kaspa I, DeCherney A, et al. Results of transcervical balloon tuboplasty. JAMA 1990; 264:2079–2082.
57. Thurmond AS. Selective salpingography and fallopian tube recanalization. AJR Am J Roentgenol 1991; 156:33–38.
58. Letterie GS, Sakas EL. Histology of proximal tubal obstruction in cases of unsuccessful tubal canalization. Fertil Steril 1991; 56:831.
59. Edelman RR, Kleefield J, Wentz KU, Atkinson DJ. Basic principles of magnetic resonance imaging. In: Edelman RR, Hesslink JR, editors.

Clinical Magnetic Resonance Imaging. Philadelphia: WB Saunders, 1990:3–38.

60. McCarthy S. Magnetic resonance imaging in the evaluation of infertile women. Magn Reson Q 1990; 4:239–249.

61. Carrington BM, Hricak H, Nuruddin RN, et al. Mullerian duct anomalies: MR imaging evaluation. Radiology 1990; 176:715–720.

62. Hill LM. Infertility and reproductive assistance. In: Nyberg DA, Hill LM, Bohn-Velez M, Mendelson EB, editors. Transvaginal Ultrasound. St. Louis: Mosby-Year Book, 1992.

63. Reuter KL, Daly DC, Cohen SM. Septate versus bicornuate uteri: errors in imaging diagnosis. Radiology 1989; 172:749–752.

64. Johnson J, Hillman BJ. Uterine duplication, unilateral imperforate vagina and normal kidneys. AJR Am J Roentgenol 1986; 147:1197–1198.

65. Wiseman DA, Taylor PJ. Infertility. In: Rumack C, Wilson S, Charboneau W, editors. Diagnostic Ultrasound. St. Louis: Mosby-Year Book, 1991:983–1008.

66. Karasock S, Lev-Toaff AS, Toaff ME. Imaging of uterine leiomyomas. AJR Am J Roentgenol 1992; 158:799–805.

67. Baltarowich OH, Kurtz AB, Pennell RG, et al. Pitfalls in the sonographic diagnosis of uterine fibroids. AJR Am J Roentgenol 1988; 151:725–728.

68. Fedele L, Bianchi S, Dorta M, et al. Transvaginal ultrasonography versus hysteroscopy in the diagnosis of uterine submucous myomas. Obstet Gynecol 1991; 77:745–748.

69. Sauer MV, Agnew C, Worthen N, et al. Reliability of ultrasound in predicting uterine leiomyoma volume. J Reprod Med 1988; 33:612–614.

70. Zawin M, McCarthy S, Scoutt LM, Comite F. High-field MRI and US evaluation of the pelvis in women with leiomyomas. Magn Reson Imaging 1990; 8:371–376.

71. Weinreb JC, Barkoff ND, Demopoulos R. The value of MR imaging in distinguishing leiomyomas from other solid pelvic masses when sonography is indeterminate. AJR Am J Roentgenol 1990; 154:295–299.

72. Athey PA, Diment DD. The spectrum of sonographic findings in endometriomas. J Ultrasound Med 1989; 8:487–491.

73. Kupfer MC, Schwimmer SR, Lebovic J. Transvaginal sonographic apperance of endometriomata: spectrum of findings. J Ultrasound Med 1992; 11:129–133.

74. Friedman H, Vogelzang RL, Mendelson EB, et al. Endometriosis detection by US with laparoscopic correlation. Radiology 1985; 157:217–220.

75. Togashi K, Nishimura K, Kimura I, et al. Endometrial cysts: diagnosis with MR imaging. Radiology 1991; 180:73–78.

76. Arrive L, Hricak H, Martin MC. Pelvic endometriosis: MR imaging. Radiology 1989; 171:687–692.

77. Zawan M, McCarthy S, Scoutt L, Comite F. Endometriosis: appearance and detection at MR imaging. Radiology 1989; 171:693–696.

78. Nashan D, Behre HM, Grunert JH, Nieschlag E. Diagnostic value of scrotal sonography in infertile men: report on 658 cases. Andrologia 1990; 22:387–395.

79. Petros JA, Andriole GL, Middleton WD, Picus DA. Correlation of testicular color Doppler ultrasonography, physical examination and venography in the detection of left varicoceles in men with infertility. J Urol 1991; 145:785–788.

80. Doherty FJ. Ultrasound of the nonacute scrotum. Semin US CT MRI 1991; 12:131–156.

81. O'Herlihy C, de Crespigny LJ, Lopata A, et al. Preovulatory follicular size: a comparison of ultrasound and laparoscopic methods. Fertil Steril 1980; 34:24–26.

82. Fleischer AC, Darnell J, Rodier J, et al. Sonographic monitoring of ovarian follicular development. J Clin Ultrasound 1981; 9:275–280.

83. Schwimmer SR, Lebovic J. Transvaginal pelvic ultrasonography: accuracy in follicle and cyst size determination. J Ultrasound Med 1985; 4:61–63.

84. Prins GS, Vogelzang RI. Inherent sources of ultrasound variability in relation to follicular measurements. J IVF Embryo Transfer 1984; 1:221–225.

85. Higgins RV, van Nagell JR Jr, Woods CH, et al. Interobserver variation in ovarian measurements using transvaginal sonography. Gynecol Oncol 1990; 39:69–71.

86. Yee B, Barnes RB, Vargyas JM, Marrs RP. Correlation of transabdominal and transvaginal ultrasound measurements of follicle size and number with laparoscopic findings for in vitro fertilization. Fertil Steril 1987; 47:828–832.

87. Ritchie WGM. Sonographic evaluation of normal and induced ovulation. Radiology 1986; 161:1–10.

88. Hackeloer BJ, Fleming R, Robinson HP, et al. Correlation of ultrasonic and endocrinologic assessment of human follicular development. Am J Obstet Gynecol 1979; 135:122–128.

89. Zandt-Stastny D, Thorsen MK, Middleton WD, et al. Inability of sonography to detect imminent ovulation. AJR Am J Roentgenol 1989; 152:91–95.

90. Taylor KJW. Pulsed Doppler ultrasound of the pelvis and the first trimester of pregnancy. In: Taylor KJW, Burns PN, Wells PNT, editors. Clinical Applications of Doppler Ultrasound. New York: Raven Press, 1988:246–262.

91. Scholtes MCW, Wladimiroff JW, van Rijen HJM, Hop WCJ. Uterine and ovarian flow velocity waveforms in the normal menstrual cycle: a transvaginal Doppler study. Fertil Steril 1989; 52:981–984.

92. Scoutt LM, Flynn SD, Luthringer DJ, et al. Junctional zone of the uterus: correlation of MR imaging and histologic examination of hysterectomy specimens. Radiology 1991; 179:403–407.

93. Winfield AC, Fleischer AC, Moore DE. Diagnostic imaging of fertility disorders. Curr Probl Diagn Radiol 1990; 19:1–18.

94. Fleischer AC, Kalemeris GC, Entman SS. Sonographic depiction of the endometrium during normal cycles. Ultrasound Med Biol 1986; 12:271–277.

95. Grunfeld L, Walker B, Bergh PA, et al. High-resolution endovaginal ultrasonography of the endometrium: a noninvasive test for endometrial adequacy. Obstet Gynecol 1991; 78:200–204.

96. Janus CL, Wiczyk HP, Laufer N. Magnetic resonance imaging of the menstrual cycle. Magn Reson Imag 1988; 6:669–674.

97. Scoutt LM, Flynn SD, Luthringer DJ, et al. Junctional zone of the uterus: correlation of MR imaging and histologic examination of hysterectomy specimens. Radiology 1991; 179:403–407.

98. Brown HK, Stoll BS, Nicosia SV, et al. Uterine junctional zone: correlation between histologic findings and MR imaging. Radiology 1991; 171:409–413.

99. Haynor DR, Mack LA, Soules MR, et al. Changing appearance of the normal uterus during the menstrual cycle: MR studies. Radiology 1986; 161:459–462.

100. Fleischer AC, Herbert CM, Hill GA, et al. Transvaginal sonography of the endometrium during induced cycles. J Ultrasound Med 1991; 10:93–95.

101. Randall JM, Templeton A. Transvaginal sonographic assessment of follicular and endometrial growth in spontaneous and clomiphene citrate cycles. Fertil Steril 1991; 56:208–212.

102. Rogers PAW, Polson D, Murphy CR, et al. Correlation of endometrial histology, morphometry, and ultrasound appearance after different stimulation protocols for in vitro fertilization. Fertil Steril 1991; 55:583–587.

103. Fleisher AC, Herbert CM, Sacks GA, et al. Sonography of the endometrium during conception and nonconception cycles of in-vitro fertilization and embryo transfer. Fertil Steril 1986; 46:442–447.

104. Glissant A, deMouson J, Fryman R. Ultrasound study of endometrium during in vitro fertilization cycles. Fertil Steril 1985; 44:786–790.

105. Gonen Y, Casper RF, Jacobson W, Blankier J. Endometrial thickness and growth during ovarian stimulation: a possible predictor of implantation in in vitro fertilization. Fertil Steril 1989; 52:446–449.

106. Sher G, Herbert C, Maassarani G, Jacobs MH. Assessment of the later proliferative phase endometrium by ultrasonography in patients undergoing in-vitro fertilization and embryo transfer (IVF:ET). Hum Reprod 1991; 6:232–237.

107. Welker BG, Gembruch U, Diedrich K, et al. Transvaginal sonography of the endometrium during ovum pickup in stimulated cycles for in vitro fertilization. J Ultrasound Med 1989; 8:549–553.

108. Schiller VL, Grant EG. Dopper ultrasonography of the pelvis. Radiol Clin North Am 1992; 40:735–742.

109. Kurjak A, Kupesic-Urek S, Schulman H, Zalud I. Transvaginal color flow Doppler in the assessment of ovarian and uterine blood flow in infertile women. Fertil Steril 1991; 56:870–873.

110. de Ziegler D, Bessis R, Frydman R. Vascular resistance of uterine arteries: physiological effects of estradiol and progesterone. Fertil Steril 1991; 56:775–779.

111. Goswamy RK, Williams G, Steptoe PC. Decreased uterine perfusion—a cause of infertility. Hum Reprod 1988; 3:955–959.

112. Fossum GT, Davajan V, Kletzky OA. Early detection of pregnancy with transvaginal US. Fertil Steril 1988; 49:788–791.

113. Kadar N, DeVore G, Romero R. Discriminatory hCG zone; its use in

the sonographic evaluation for ectopic pregnancy. Obstet Gynecol 1981; 58:156–161.

114. Nyberg DA, Filly RA, Mahony BS, et al. Early gestation: correlation of hCG levels and sonographic identification. AJR Am J Roentgenol 1985; 144:951–954.

115. Nyberg DA, Mack LA, Laing FC, Jeffrey RB. Early pregnancy complications; endovaginal sonographic fijndings correlated with hCG levels. Radiology 1988; 167:619–622.

116. Cacciatore B, Titinen A, Stenman U-H, Ylostalo P. Normal early pregnancy: serum hCG levels and vaginal ultrasonography findings. Br J Obstet Gynaecol 1990;97:899–903.

117. Stabile I, Cambell S, Grudzinskas JG. Can ultrasound reliably diagnose ectopic pregnancy? Br J Obstet Gynaecol 1988; 95:1247–1252.

118. Nyberg DA, Laing FC, Filly RA, et al. Ultrasonographic differentiation of the gestational sac of early intrauterine pregnancy from the pseudo-gestational sac of ectopic pregnancy. Radiology 1983; 146:755–759.

119. Dillon EH, Feyock AL, Taylor KJW. Pseudogestational sacs: Doppler US differentiation from normal or abnormal intrauterine pregnancies. Radiology 1990; 176:359–364.

120. Thorsen MK, Lawson TL, Aiman EJ, et al. Diagnosis of ectopic pregnancy: endovaginal vs. transabdominal sonography. AJR Am J Roentgenol 1990; 155:307–310.

121. Rempen A. Vaginal sonography in ectopic pregnancy: a prospective evaluation. J Ultrasound Med 1988; 7:381–387.

122. Emerson DS, Cartier MS, Alltieri LA, et al. Diagnostic efficacy of endovaginal color Doppler flow imaging in an ectopic pregnancy screening program. Radiology 1992; 183:413.

123. Pellerito JA, Taylor KJW, Quedens-Case C, et al. Ectopic pregnancy: evaluation with endovaginal color flow imaging. Radiology 1992; 183:407.

124. Nyberg DA, Hughes M, Mack LA, Wang K. Extrauterine findings of ectopic pregnancy at transvaginal US: importance of echogenic fluid. Radiology 1991; 178:823–826.

125. Laboda LA, Estroff JA, Benacerraf BR. First trimester bradycardia: a sign of impending fetal loss. J Ultrasound Med 1989; 8:320–321.

126. Bromley B, Harlow BL, Harlow BL, et al. Small sac size in the first trimester: a predictor of poor fetal outcome. Radiology 1991; 178:375–377.

127. Levi CS, Lyons EA, Lindsay DJ. Early diagnosis of nonviable pregnancy with endovaginal US. Radiology 1988; 167:383–385.

128. Kurtz AB, Needlemen L, Pennell RG, et al. Can detection of the yolk sac in the first trimester be used to predict the outcome of pregnancy? A prospective sonographic study. AJR Am J Roentgenol 1992; 158:843–847.

129. Lindsay DJ, Lovett IS, Lyons EA, et al. Yolk sac diameter and shape at endovaginal US: predictors of pregnancy outcome in the first trimester. Radiology 1992; 183:115–118.

130. Harris RD, Vincent LM, Askin FB. Yolk sac calcification: a sonographic finding associated with intrauterine demise in the first trimester. Radiology 1988; 166:109–110.

131. Levi CS, Lyons EA, Zheng XH, et al. Endovaginal US: demonstration of cardiac activity in embryos of less than 5.0 mm in crown-rump length. Radiology 1990; 176:71–74.

132. Nyberg DA, Mack LA, Laing FC, Patten RM. Distinguishing normal from abnormal gestational sac growth in early pregnancy. J Ultrasound Med 1987; 6:23–27.

133. Nyberg DA, Filly RA, Duarte-Filho DL, et al. Abnormal pregnancy: early diagnosis by ultrasound and serum chorionic gonadotropin levels. Radiology 1986; 158:393–396.

CHAPTER 24

Diagnostic Laparoscopy in Infertility

VICTOR GOMEL and PATRICK J. TAYLOR

The investigation of the infertile couple cannot be considered to be complete until a diagnostic laparoscopy has been performed.[1] The value of this procedure is greatest when it is carried out at the appropriate time in the overall scheme of investigation of the couple and when meticulous attention is paid to the technical details. The surgeon must always be aware of the potential complications that may arise.

No investigation should ever be ordered unless the physician has clearly established the goals of the test and the actions to be taken dependent on the findings. All of these issues are addressed in this chapter.

TIMING

Laparoscopy is an invasive procedure and should be one of the later investigations. The details of the evaluation of the infertile couple are described elsewhere. For the purpose of this discussion, it is sufficient to remark that after completion of the initial investigations, it is possible to assign couples to one of the three broad categories that follow:

1. The apparently ovulatory woman and the man in whom a cause for infertility has been determined.
2. The anovulatory woman.
3. The apparently ovulatory woman and normozoospermic man.

The Apparently Ovulatory Woman and the Man in Whom a Cause for Infertility Has Been Determined

In most cases, investigation of the tubal or peritoneal factors should be deferred for four to six cycles, during which treatment for the male factor is instituted. If pregnancy does not occur, the status of the pelvis of the female partner should be evaluated. This evaluation should precede treatment of the male factor if there are clinical grounds to suspect the presence of tubal or peritoneal disease or if the woman is of advanced reproductive years. Significant clinical findings include history of pelvic infection, intrauterine device use, endometriosis, previous tubal and ovarian surgery, and abnormal findings at the time of pelvic examination.[2] It must be noted that in approximately 60% of patients with hydrosalpinges, neither a prior history of pelvic pain or pelvic infection is elicited nor abnormal pelvic findings are detected during the physical examination.[3]

The Anovulatory Woman

The cause for anovulation can usually be determined by intelligent use of hormonal assays. Consistently elevated follicle-stimulating hormone (FSH) levels may be indicative of gonadal dysgenesis, premature ovarian failure, or resistant ovary syndrome. If indicated, differentiation may be made by laparoscopic visualization and ovarian biopsy. In the last condition, primordial follicles are identified in the specimen. Such is not the case with either gonadal dysgenesis or premature ovarian failure. If it is clear that exogenous gonadotropin administration is required, it is sensible to perform laparoscopy before instituting this therapy.

If simpler methods (clomiphene, clomiphene and human chorionic gonadotropin, or gonadotropin-releasing hormone) are to be used, their ease of administration and relatively low cost allow deferral of laparoscopy until after four to six ovulatory cycles have occurred, without pregnancy. In the woman of advanced reproductive years or in whom there is a strongly suggestive history of lesions of the lower genital tract, laparoscopy should precede induction of ovulation.

The Apparently Ovulatory Woman and the Normozoospermic Man

Tubal obstruction occurs in 12% to 33% of infertile couples.[4–6] In an ovulatory woman with a normozoospermic man, tubal and peritoneal factors should be sought.

Two methods of evaluation, the hysterosalpingogram (HSG) and laparoscopy, play complementary roles. Hysterosalpingography should be the initial investigation. Advantages of initial HSG include (1) identification of cornual occlusion or cornual lesions, even in the presence of tubal patency; (2) immediate identification of distal tubal occlusion and assessment of the intratubal architecture; (3) given that most pathologically damaged tubes are now repaired laparoscopically, prior knowledge that damage exists, which permits the surgeon to schedule operative room time effectively; and (4) identification of intrauterine lesions or congenital uterine malformations. In such cases, hysteroscopy should complement laparoscopy.

If the HSG is abnormal, the laparoscopic determination of the exact nature of the abnormality and, when possible, correction should be undertaken immediately. If the HSG is normal, except in the woman of advanced reproductive years, laparoscopy should be deferred for 6 months. During this time, some women conceive. In those who do not, laparoscopy may detect unsuspected periadnexal adhesions or endometriosis. These lesions are detected in approximately 10% of patients.[1]

TECHNIQUE

Any discussion of laparoscopy must pay due attention to the method by which the procedure is performed and the steps to be taken to assess the reproductive organs. Because operative laparoscopy is described in Chapter 21, this discussion deals with diagnosis only. In many instances, however, it is to the patient's advantage to treat immediately any lesions encountered at the time of the diagnostic laparoscopy. If the surgeon has not been trained in operative laparoscopy, the wisdom of embarking on laparoscopy in infertile patients, for purely diagnostic purposes, must be questioned.

It is only by meticulous attention to detail, thorough familiarity with the instruments, and extensive knowledge of the intrapelvic structures, and increasing experience that laparoscopy can be performed safely, accurately and to the maximum benefit of the patient.[7]

Instruments

The instruments required for the performance of diagnostic laparoscopy are simple and few in number, but because it may be necessary to move immediately to operative laparoscopy, the complete operative set must always be at instant readiness. The basic diagnostic set must contain the following:

1. A cold light source and transmission cables.
2. An insufflator and tubing.

Although 150-watt light sources and constant flow rate insufflators are perfectly suitable for diagnostic purposes, most surgeons use a more powerful light source that is video compatible and an insufflator with automatic rapid flow capability in case it becomes necessary to perform immediate reparative surgery.

3. Video equipment. Although video equipment is not necessary for diagnosis, its use greatly facilitates operative laparoscopy.

4. A Veress needle.
5. A principal trocar and cannula. These should be of a diameter that can accommodate the telescope. The trocar may have a pyramidal or conical tip. The cannula may be equipped with a flap or trumpet valve.
6. A telescope. Those of 5 mm diameter are suitable for diagnostic purposes only. The distal lens may provide direct (180 degrees) or Foroblique (30 degrees) angles of observation.
7. Ancillary trocars/cannulas.
8. A calibrated blunt probe. A thorough survey can be performed only if bowel is displaced and the intrapelvic organs can be manipulated. Instruments introduced through a second portal rather than through an operative laparoscope separate the visual from the manipulative axes. This separation is essential if the pelvic organs are to be assessed completely.
9. A suction cannula. It may be necessary to aspirate fluid from the pelvis to enable visualization of underlying structures. This cannula may also be used as a probe.
10. A uterine cannula with which the uterus can be mobilized and through which a chromopertubation solution can be injected.
11. A standard minor gynecologic tray equipped with the usual specula, tenaculums, and sterile drapes.

It is the responsibility of the surgeon to ensure that all of the equipment is in perfect working order before the patient enters the operating room.

Anesthesia—Positioning of the Patient and Placement of the Uterine Cannula

The use of general anesthesia is preferable. Because of the risks of hypercarbia associated with laparoscopy, patients should be intubated and ventilated.

Anesthesia is induced with the patient in the supine position. Although the anesthesiologist may wish to use an arm board during the induction, once the patient is asleep, the arm should be placed by her side. This increases the working space for the surgeon and decreases the risk of brachial plexus injury. Care must be taken to ensure that the patient's hands are not at risk from moving parts of the operating table.

The patient is placed in the dorsal lithotomy position (Fig. 24–1). Low lithotomy stirrups or Lloyd-Davis stirrups are used. The buttocks should protrude 1 to 2 inches from the distal end of the table to facilitate manipulation with the uterine cannula. Once properly positioned, the abdomen, perineum, and vagina are cleansed with antiseptic solution, and the patient is draped. Preoperative shaving of the pubic hair is not recommended.

The surgeon, who is double gloved, performs a bimanual examination of the pelvis to assess the nature of the reproductive organs and the fullness of the bladder. Patients should void immediately preoperatively, thus avoiding the need for catheterization. If the bladder is full, however, it should be drained.

A speculum is placed, a tenaculum is fixed to the anterior lip of the cervix, and the uterine cannula is inserted and locked to the tenaculum. The speculum is removed. The

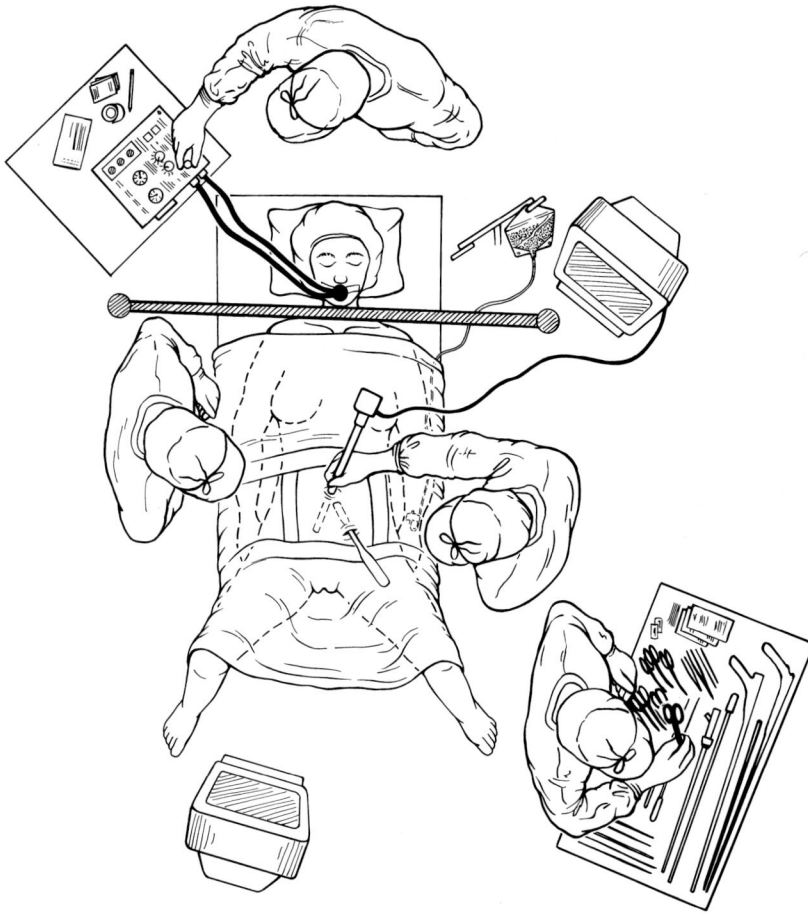

FIGURE 24–1. Positioning of the patient for laparoscopy.

surgeon removes the outer pair of gloves before beginning the laparoscopy.

A diagnostic laparoscopy is carried out in the following, systematic, step-by-step fashion:

- Induction of the pneumoperitoneum.
- Introduction of the primary trocar and cannula.
- Introduction of the telescope.
- Introduction of ancillary trocar and cannula and instruments.
- The survey.
- Removal of the instruments and closure of the incisions.
- Documentation.

Pneumoperitoneum

"It is this step above all that is critical in the avoidance of major complications and in ensuring proper visualization and room to perform any necessary intraperitoneal manipulations."[7] This statement was made in 1986, reflecting the then-standard method of laparoscopy. Since then, direct insertion of the primary trocar and cannula, with subsequent induction of pneumoperitoneum, has been advocated.[8] This latter approach may reduce operating time by a minute or two, but it is more hazardous in patients with a scarred abdomen or in those who are extremely thin or in whom an abdominal mass is present. We therefore continue to induce pneumoperitoneum using a Veress needle in all patients.

The abdomen is inspected for the presence of scars. Palpation and percussion delineate the presence and limits of any tumors or distention of the gastrointestinal tract. If any of these are noted, a different site of placement of the Veress needle may have to be chosen. If it is obvious that the stomach is distended, a nasogastric tube should be passed and the organ deflated.

The Veress needle is usually introduced intraumbilically. The thumb and forefinger of the nondominant hand are placed on either side of the umbilical margin and used to exert traction in a caudal direction. A natural fold is exposed in the umbilicus, and incision is made in this fold of sufficient size to permit introduction of the principal trocar and cannula (Fig. 24–2).

The Veress needle is grasped between the thumb and forefinger of the dominant hand, in such a way that movement of the internal blunt cannula is not impeded. The hypogastric parietes are grasped by the nondominant hand and elevated. The Veress needle is inserted in the incision at an angle of 45 degrees and advanced toward the hollow of the pelvis (Fig. 24–3). With experience, the surgeon will come to recognize the sensation as each layer of the abdominal wall is penetrated, culminating in the rapid advance of the blunt cannula as the peritoneal cavity is entered. An audible click is heard as the hub of the internal cannula strikes the proximal part of the external sharp sheath.

A syringe test is performed to confirm that the tip of the needle is correctly placed (Figs. 24–4 and 24–5). The Veress

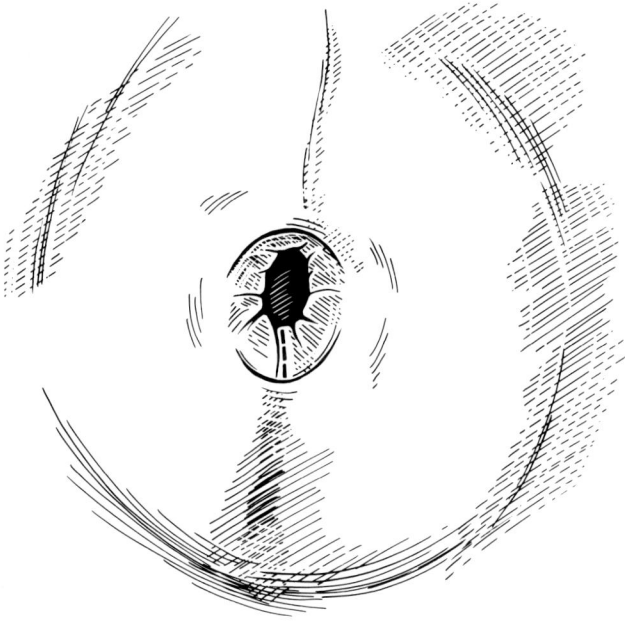

FIGURE 24–2. A vertical infraumbilical incision.

needle is connected to a 20-mL syringe that contains 10 mL of normal saline. The plunger is gently withdrawn. No gas or blood should enter the saline. Five milliliters are injected. Correct placement of the needle tip is indicated if traction on the plunger fails to recover the saline. If blood-stained or feces-stained fluid returns, the Veress needle has entered a vessel or bowel. Once the surgeon is satisfied that the insufflation needle is correctly positioned, the gas line is connected. Gas flow should be set at 1 L/minute (Fig. 24–6). The pressure should not rise by more than 5 mm Hg over the baseline pressure of the system. If the insufflation pressure is high and such simple maneuvers as grasping the abdominal wall and shaking it gently (this may dislodge omentum from the needle tip) or increasing the angle of the needle (thus preventing it from impinging on the anterior abdominal wall) fail to correct the pressure, the needle should be removed.

If the gas pressures are satisfactory, percussion over the liver reveals loss of dullness within 1 minute when the flow rate is 1 L/minute. If dullness does not disappear, the tip of the needle is either in the preperitoneal space or in a viscus, and the needle should be withdrawn.

Assuming that the gas is flowing into the peritoneal cavity, flow should continue, either at a rate of 1 L/minute or, if the insufflator is equipped with a rapid flow system, the rate may now be increased to 3 L/minute. The optimal volume of gas to be insufflated depends on the depth of anesthesia, the size of the patient, and the diameter of the primary trocar to be used.

If the abdomen is scarred, if there are intra-abdominal masses or distended loops of bowel, or if the original insufflation attempt has produced preperitoneal emphysema, it may be necessary to use an alternative site through which to introduce the Veress needle. Alternative sites include the area located midway between the pubic symphysis and the umbilicus, immediately supraumbilically in the midline, the lateral border of the rectus at either the left or right McBurney's point, or at the lateral border of the rectus 2 fingerbreadths below the left costal margin.

If the Veress needle is introduced in the lower abdomen, it should be angled toward the center of the hollow of the sacrum. If introduced in the midline above the umbilicus, an angle of approach should be undertaken similar to the traditional intraumbilical approach. If introduced beneath the left costal margin, the needle must be directed so as not to place the intrathoracic structures at risk.

Pneumoperitoneum may also be effected transvaginally by introducing the Veress needle (or preferably a modified one with a metallic stop near its tip) into the pouch of Douglas. The vaginal approach should be undertaken only in a patient who has a uterus, in whom there is no reason to suspect that the cul-de-sac is obliterated, and in whom bimanual pelvic examination reveals no evidence of thickening or masses within the cul-de-sac.[7]

Introduction of the Primary Trocar and Cannula

The primary trocar and cannula are held in the dominant hand, with the thumb fixing the trocar firmly against the upper limit of the cannula (Fig. 24–7). The ulnar border of the other hand is placed on the abdominal wall, the hand encircling the instrument to act as a backstop should sudden

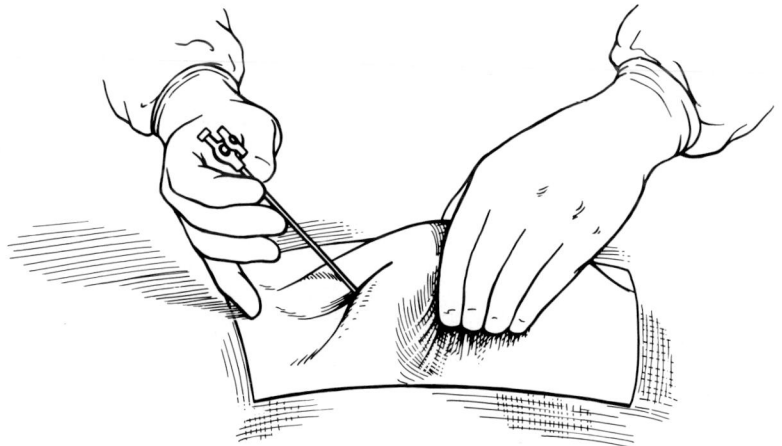

FIGURE 24–3. Insertion of the Veress needle.

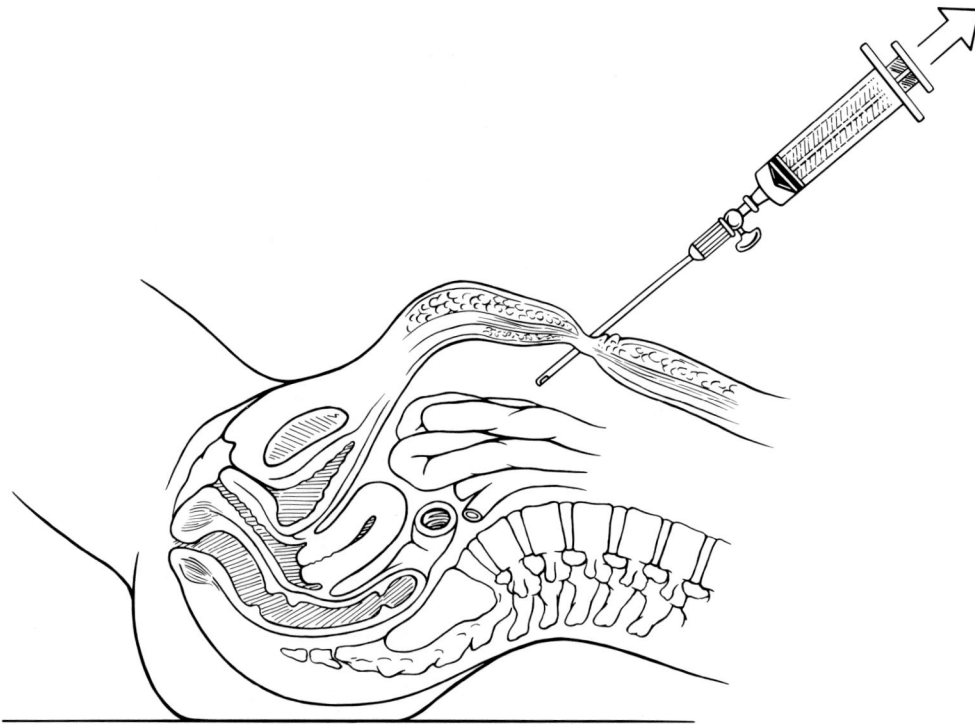

FIGURE 24–4. Aspiration through the Veress needle.

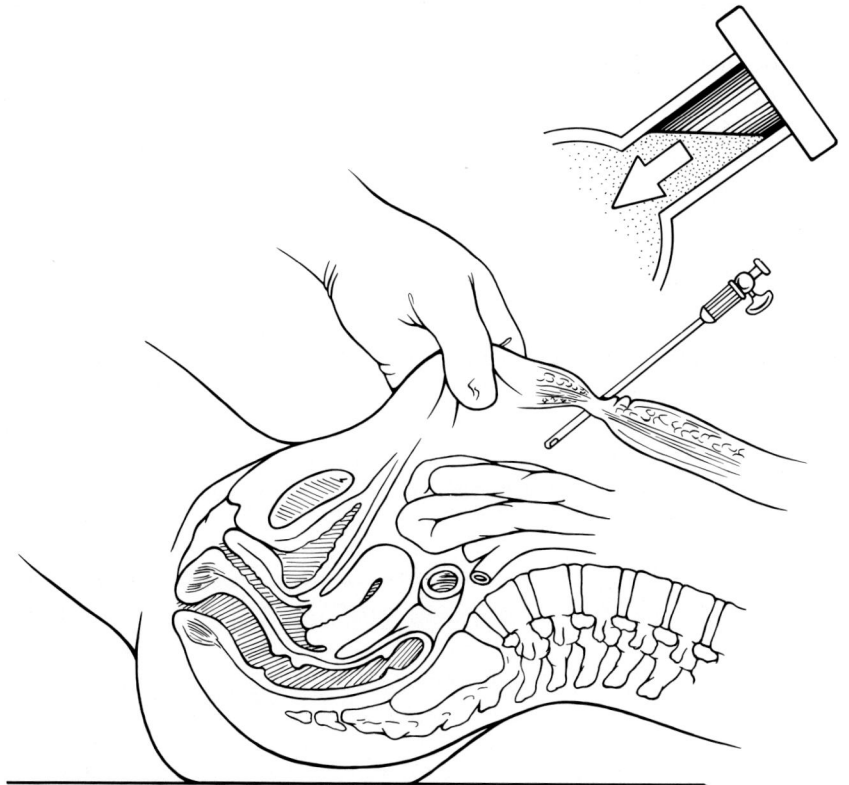

FIGURE 24–5. Establishing the intraperitoneal position of the Veress needle by the "hanging drop" test.

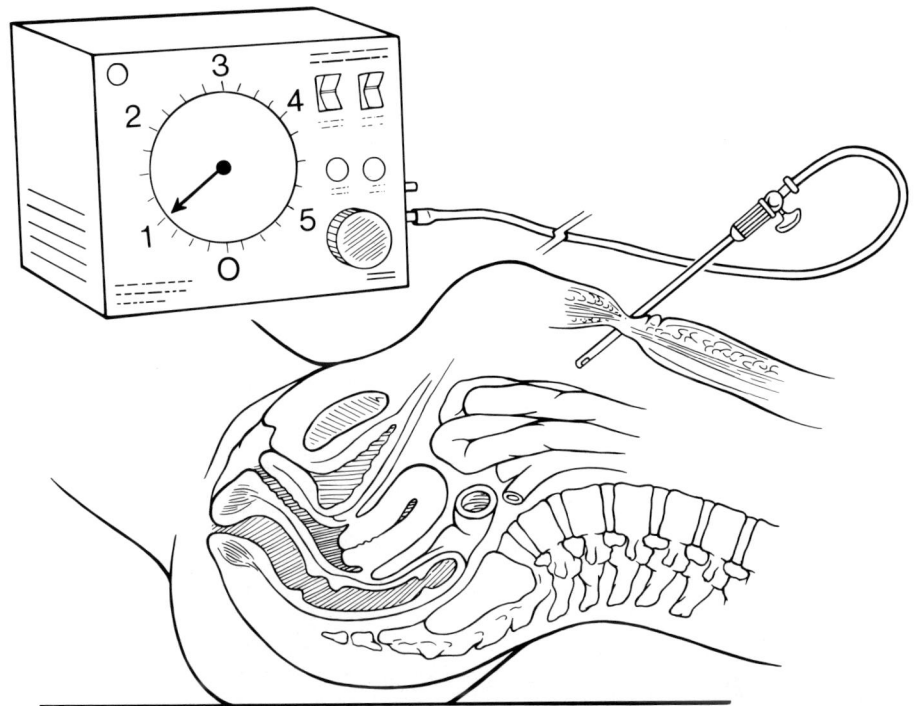

FIGURE 24–6. Insufflation of CO_2 at 1 L/min.

penetration of the parietes occur. The trocar and cannula are initially introduced through the previously made incision for a distance of about 2 cm in the subcutaneous tissue. The uterus is acutely anteverted by using the previously placed uterine cannula, thus creating a space in the pouch of Douglas. The principal trocar and cannula are shifted to a 45-degree angle, which aims them at this space. The direction of insertion must always be in the midline to avoid trauma to the structures, particularly the major vessels of the lateral pelvic walls.

The trocar and cannula are advanced. Some cannulas are hollow with a small hole in the distal end and another, larger hole in the proximal end. Gas can be heard to escape from the proximal aperture once the tip has entered the peritoneal cavity. At this point, the trocar is grasped firmly and the cannula advanced so it enters the peritoneal cavity while containing the sharp tip of the cannula within its sleeve. The trocar is then removed.

Introduction of the Telescope

The telescope is connected to the light source. The telescope is introduced into the cannula, and viewing begins as the telescope traverses the sheath. If the telescope is thrust violently through the sheath, any organ that has been impaled inadvertently is dislodged, and the trauma may not be recognized. As soon as the peritoneal cavity is entered, the bowel and other organs along the track of insertion are immediately inspected to assure the surgeon that no trauma has

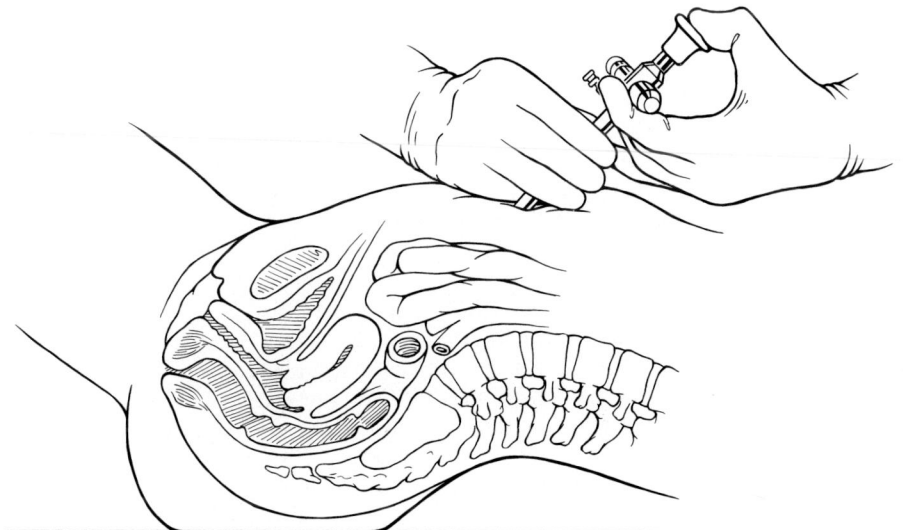

FIGURE 24–7. Insertion of the trocar.

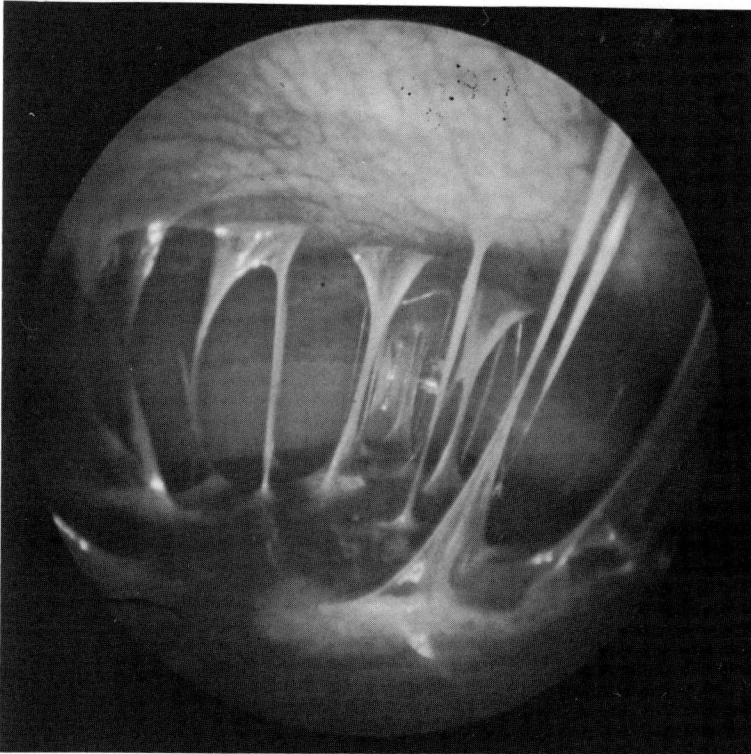

FIGURE 24–8. Laparoscopic view of perihepatic adhesions. (Courtesy of William R. Keye, Jr., M.D.)

resulted from insertion of the sharp instruments. The telescope is next turned through 180 degrees so the upper abdomen may be inspected. Often, perihepatic scarring is the only evidence that acute pelvic inflammatory disease has occurred (Fig. 24–8). The table at this point is still in the horizontal position. If upper abdominal visualization is difficult, it may be necessary to tilt the table to raise the head.

Introduction of Ancillary Trocars and Cannulas

Preparations are made for insertion of the ancillary instruments. A thorough pelvic assessment cannot be performed unless, at a minimum, a calibrated probe is inserted. The appropriate-sized secondary trocar and cannula may be inserted in the midline or laterally within the area of safety bounded by the obliterated umbilical arteries. It is most usual to introduce the probe in the midline 2 fingerbreadths above the symphysis (Fig. 24–9). Once the site has been selected, the operating room lights are dimmed and the abdominal wall is transilluminated with the laparoscope to delineate the presence of any large blood vessels. When the surgeon is satisfied that the area is avascular, it should be indented with the index finger and viewed from inside the abdomen. The point of indentation is readily recognized, and the surgeon can be assured that no vital structures lie beneath it. An incision of sufficient size to accommodate a secondary trocar and cannula is made, and the instruments are inserted under direct visual control. It is often helpful once again to antevert the uterus so a clear space exists within the pouch of Douglas. If it proves difficult to insert the second trocar and cannula without placing bowel at risk, the angle of attack can be directed toward the tip of the laparoscope, which is with-

drawn to within the primary cannula. Further insertion of the secondary trocar and cannula then occurs into the safety of the metal sheath. Once the secondary trocar and cannula are in place, the trocar is withdrawn and the blunt probe inserted.

Although the steps of insertion of the Veress needle and primary and secondary trocars, cannulas, the laparoscope, and probe are standard in the average patient, special precautions should be taken in the obese and the extremely thin.

The obese patient must be positioned in such a way that flexion of the thighs does not result in folding of the abdominal pannus. It may be advantageous to insert the Veress

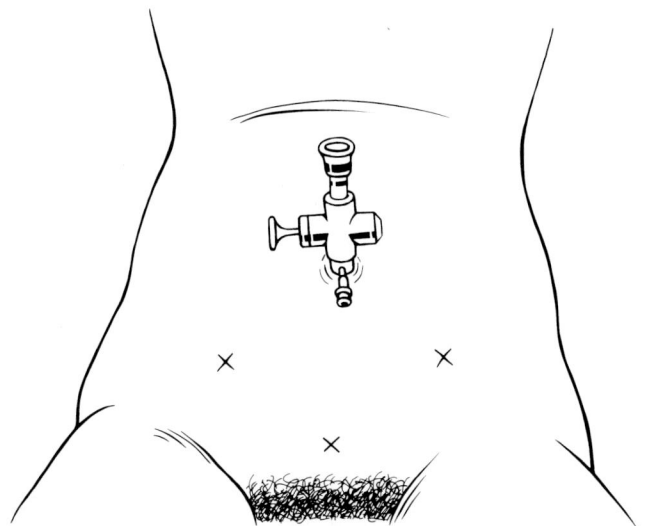

FIGURE 24–9. Sites for insertion of trocars.

needle before placing the thighs in the stirrups. A longer Veress needle may be required. In these patients, insertion of the Veress needle and primary trocar and cannula intraumbilically ensures that they pass through the thinnest part of the abdominal wall. It is in such women that, if no contraindications exist, transvaginal insufflation through the posterior fornix should be considered.

Paradoxically the extremely thin patient is at greater risk. The distance between the anterior abdominal wall and the abdominal aorta is short. It is possible to incise this vessel with the scalpel used to make the initial intraumbilical incision. Great care, therefore, must be taken. The force required to introduce the Veress needle is less, so it should be grasped close to its tip and the abdominal wall completely elevated by the nondominant hand. Insertion should be at a shallower angle, almost parallel to the abdominal wall.

Survey

It is critical that the survey be performed meticulously and in a systematic fashion. The inspection of the upper abdominal organs has already been described. Once the probe has been inserted, the telescope is once again reversed and the liver, gallbladder, transverse descending and ascending colon, and small bowel are inspected (Fig. 24–10). The patient is placed in a deep Trendelenburg position. The caecum and appendix are assessed. It may be necessary to use the blunt probe to manipulate the caecum so the appendix can be visualized (Fig. 24–11). The uterine cannula can be used to manipulate the uterus, using the fundus to push the redundant loops of bowel from the pelvis. Any remaining bowel should be displaced with the blunt probe so the cul-de-sac adnexa and uterus are clearly visible.

A general panoramic inspection is first performed with the laparoscope at some distance from the pelvic organs (Fig. 24–12). This allows an immediate impression to be formed. It may be necessary to move the uterus both from side to side and in the anteroposterior directions with the uterine cannula. The telescope is then advanced and, beginning with the uterus, the entire pelvis is scrutinized in a systematic fashion. The uterine cannula is used to place the uterus in retroversion, and its anterior surface and uterovesical pouch are inspected. The uterus is then anteverted, and fundus and posterior surface are assessed (Fig. 24–13; see color section in the center of the book). The telescope next enters the pouch of Douglas. Any fluid is noted, and, if excessive, the probe is replaced with an aspirating cannula and the fluid removed. If this step is not taken, areas of endometriosis beneath the fluid may be missed (Fig. 24–14; see color section in the center of the book). Once the floor of the cul-de-sac has been thoroughly inspected, each uterosacral ligament in turn is examined from its posterior to its anterior insertions.

Starting on one side, the adnexa is thoroughly scrutinized (Figs. 24–15 through 24–19; for Figs. 24–15, 24–18, and 24–19, see color section in the center of the book). The anterior surface of the ovary is inspected, and then the gonad is elevated with the probe so its posterior surface and the ovarian fossa can be inspected, as can the entire extent of the posterior leaf of the broad ligament. The tube is inspected systematically. The fimbriae are visualized and manipulated gently with the probe and viewed en face. Examination continues throughout the length of the oviduct from the distal to the proximal segment. Particular attention is paid to any evidence of fusiform swelling of the uterotubal junction, which may be due to salpingitis isthmica nodosa or endometriosis. The other ovary and tube are similarly assessed. Tubal inspection is followed by chromopertubation. If there is no evidence of distal tubal occlusion, dilute methylene blue

Text continued on page 342

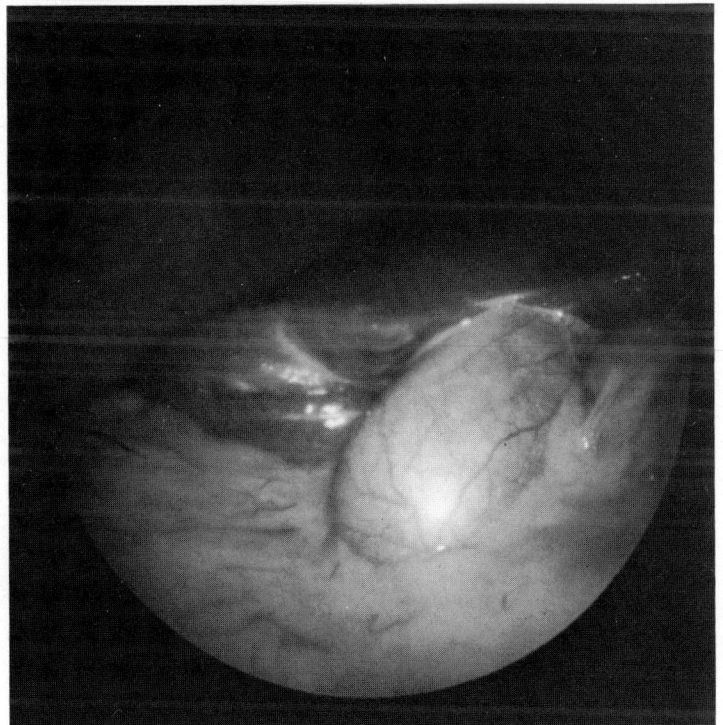

FIGURE 24–10. Laparoscopic view of grossly normal liver and gallbladder. (Courtesy of William R. Keye, Jr., M.D.)

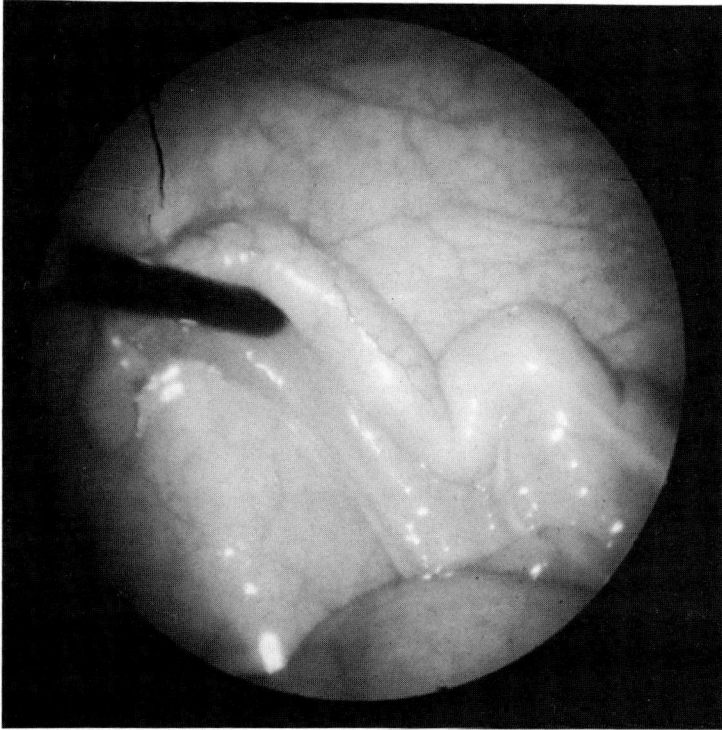

FIGURE 24–11. Laparoscopic view of the appendix. (Courtesy of William R. Keye, Jr., M.D.)

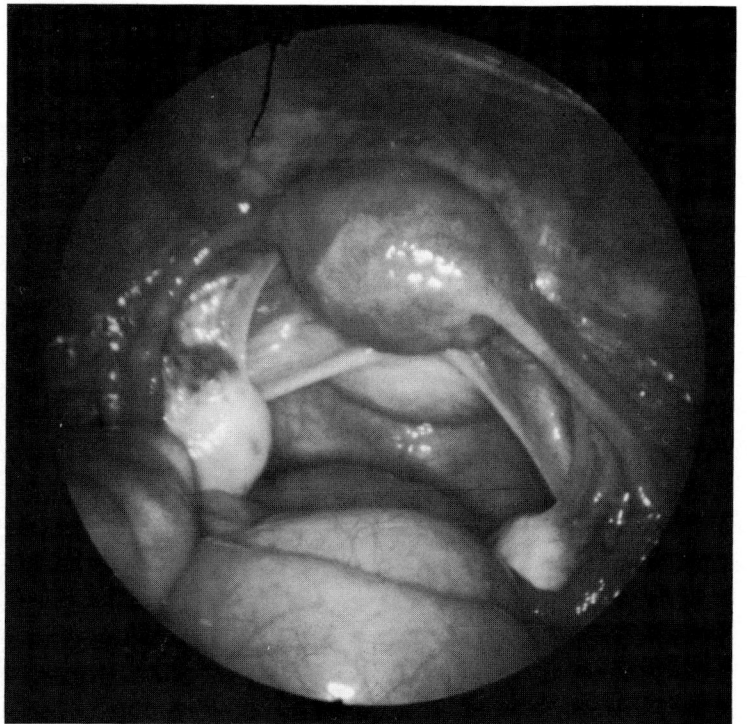

FIGURE 24–12. Panoramic view of the pelvis. (Courtesy of William R. Keye, Jr., M.D.)

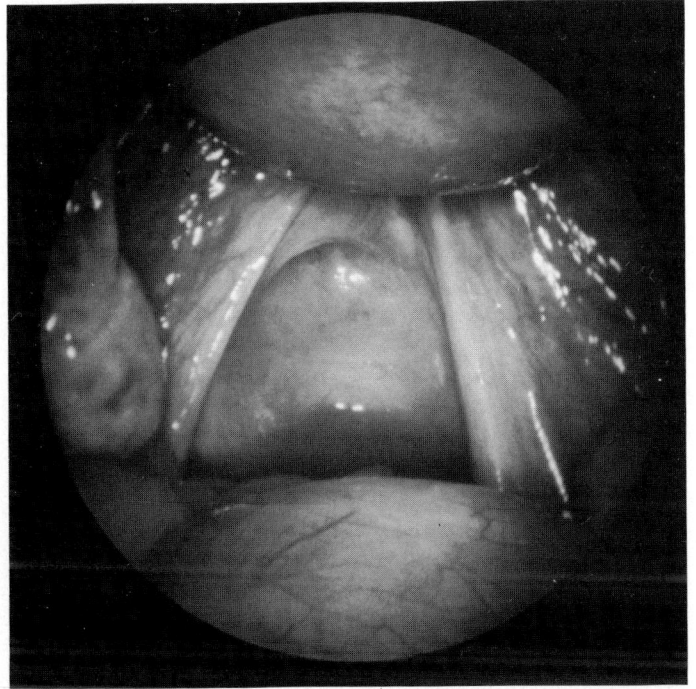

FIGURE 24–13. View of the normal cul-de-sac and uterosacral ligaments. (Courtesy of William R. Keye, Jr., M.D.)

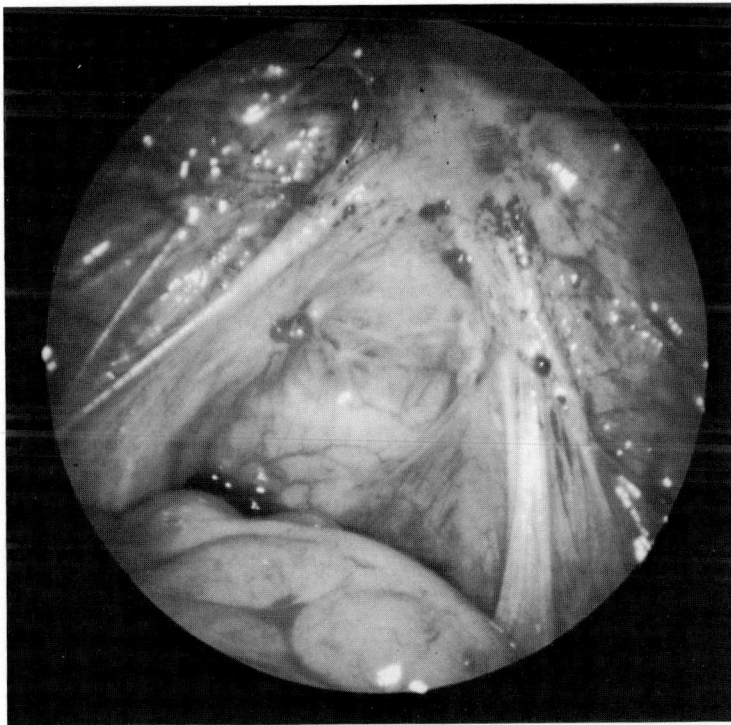

FIGURE 24–14. Laparoscopic view of the cul-de-sac in a woman with endometriosis. (Courtesy of William R. Keye, Jr., M.D.)

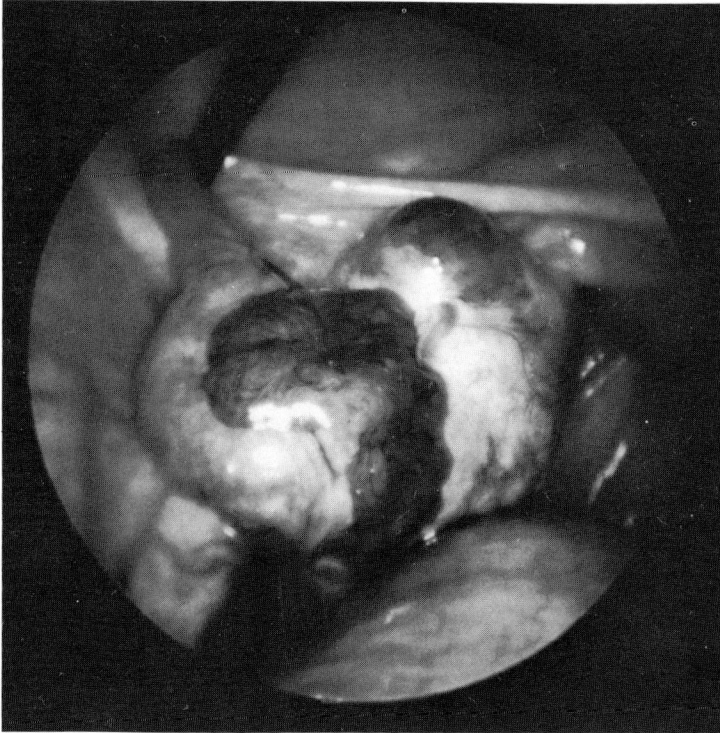

FIGURE 24–15. Normal adnexa. (Note the corpus luteum on the ovary and the spill of methylene blue from the fimbriated end of the fallopian tube.) (Courtesy of William R. Keye, Jr., M.D.)

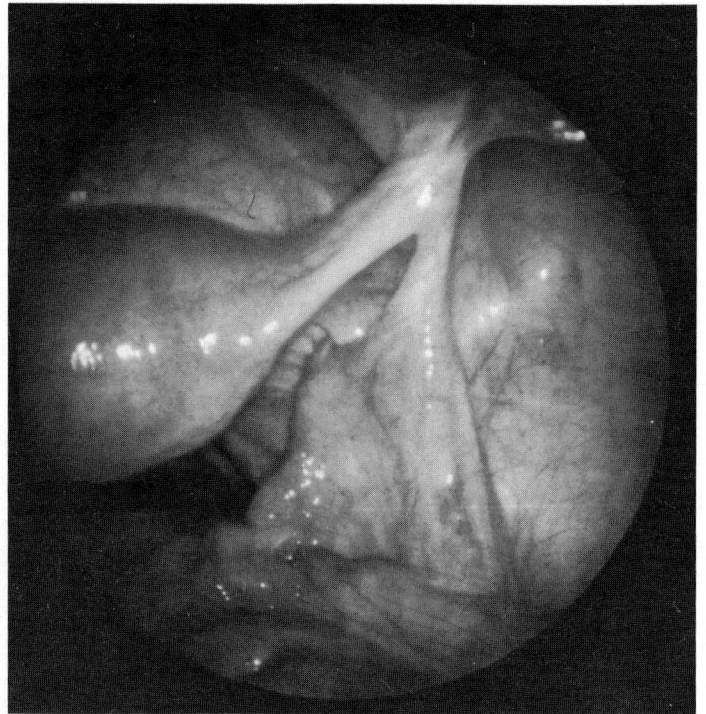

FIGURE 24–16. Scarring of the round ligament and the fallopian tube to the anterior abdominal wall resulting from a previous anterior suspension of the uterus. (Courtesy of William R. Keye, Jr., M.D.)

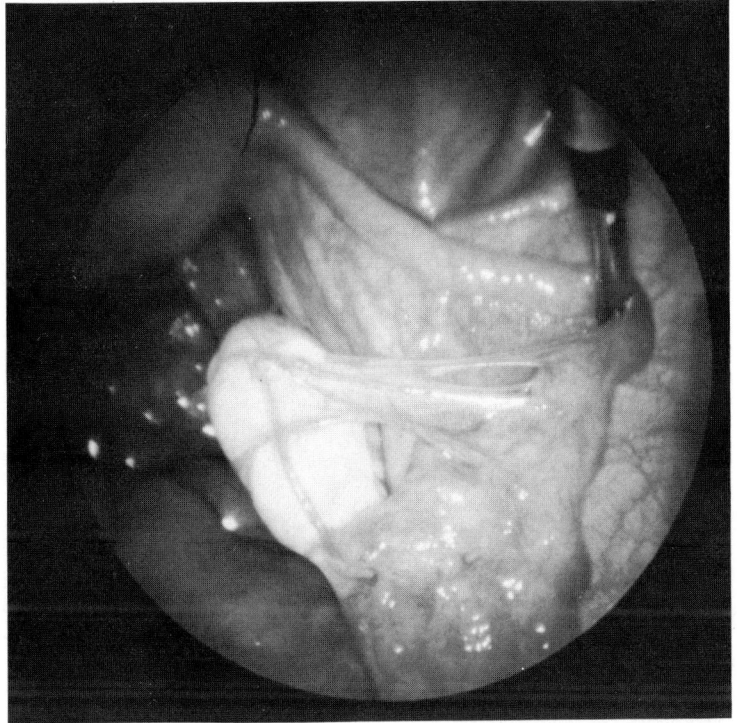

FIGURE 24–17. Laparoscopic view of tubo-ovarian adhesions. (Courtesy of William R. Keye, Jr., M.D.)

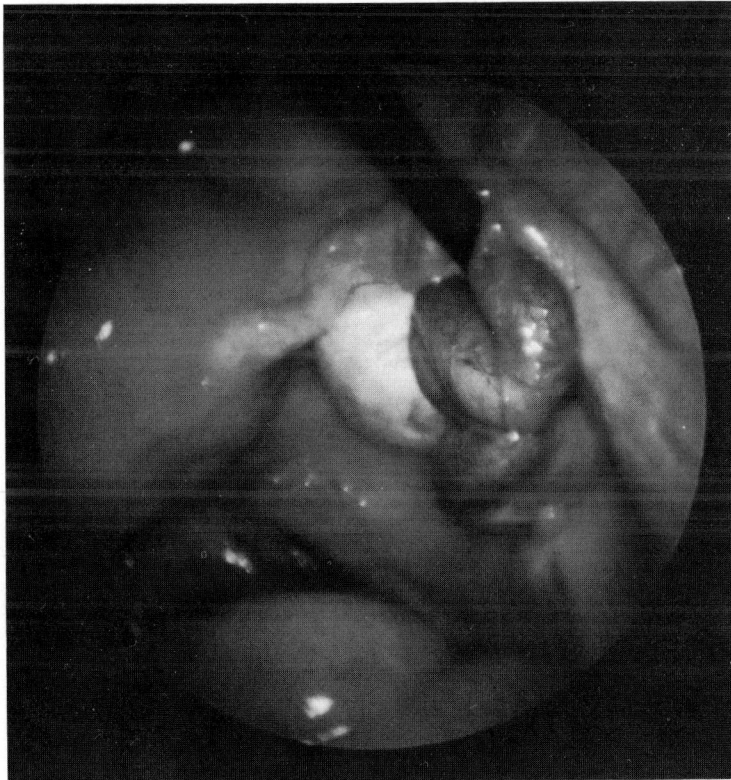

FIGURE 24–18. Laparoscopic view of an adnexa with a hydrosalpinx. (Courtesy of William R. Keye, Jr., M.D.)

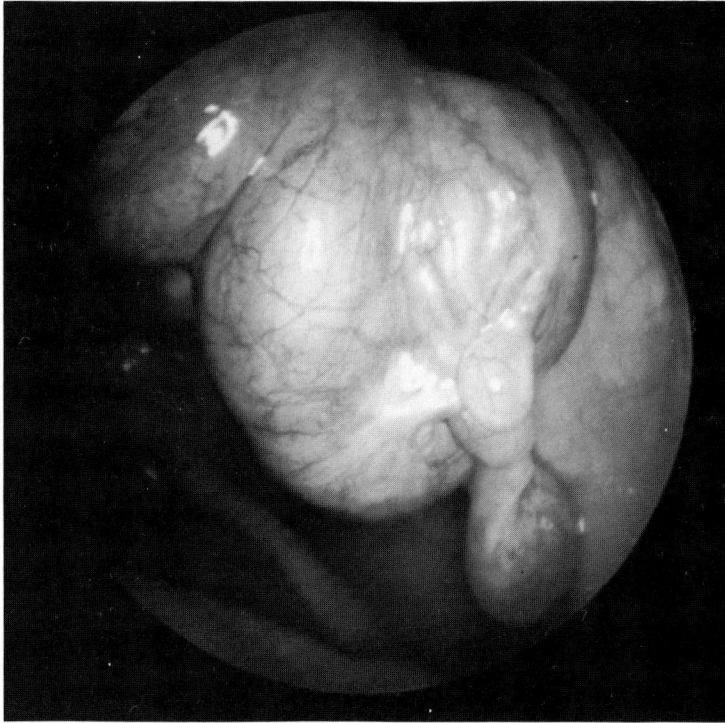

FIGURE 24–19. Close-up view of the distal end of a hydrosalpinx. (Courtesy of William R. Keye, Jr., M.D.)

dye or indigo carmine may be injected through the uterine cannula. If there is evidence of hydrosalpinx formation and it is proposed to perform salpingoscopy, saline is used so it will distend the tube but not stain the mucosa. The passage of the dye solution is followed through the uterotubal junction along the isthmus and ampulla. The fimbriae are once again inspected. The procedure is then repeated on the other tube. If there is concern that fine perifimbrial adhesions exist, it may be necessary to flood the pelvis with saline and inspect the fimbriae under water with the lens in close approximation. This technique is valuable for displaying such fine adhesion. This systematic approach ensures that the entire pelvis has been visualized thoroughly.

Removal of the Instruments and Closure of the Incisions

Once the surgeon is satisfied that the entire pelvis has been scrutinized thoroughly, a final survey is performed of the entire pelvis and abdomen to ensure that no unsuspected trauma or bleeding has occurred. The ancillary instruments and their cannulas are removed. The laparoscope is used to inspect the internal side of puncture sites to ensure that no bleeding is occurring. The telescope is removed. The patient is kept in the Trendelenburg position, and the valve of the principal cannula is opened so the gas can be expelled. Every endeavor should be made to ensure that all the gas is removed to reduce the incidence of postoperative shoulder pain. The abdominal wall is compressed with the nondominant hand, and the cannula is removed with the valve in the open position. This pressure prevents introduction of the room air. Keeping the valve open prevents the creation of negative pressure and perhaps sucking bowel or omentum into this puncture site.

Once the instruments have been removed, the incisions may be closed with subcuticular sutures or Steri-strips.

Documentation

Even if an absolutely meticulous pelvic survey has been performed, little value accrues if detailed records of the findings are not kept, particularly if the patient requires referral to a colleague or simply moves to another physician's care. Immediately on completion of the procedure, a detailed operative report should be dictated. Many surgeons still find that a simple sketch of the findings is immensely helpful. If video equipment is available, a short videotape of the findings can be made. This videotape then becomes part of the patient's permanent record and can, if necessary, be relayed to a colleague.

Complications of Diagnostic Laparoscopy in the Infertile Patient

Complications arising in the performance of laparoscopy range from the relatively common failure to complete the procedure to the fortunately extremely rare death. Complications include those associated with (1) the pneumoperitoneum, (2) trocar insertion, (3) other events, and (4) anesthesia.

Failure to complete the procedure may be due to an inability to establish a proper pneumoperitoneum or to the discovery of extensive intraperitoneal adhesions that are not amenable to laparoscopic dissection. Induction of the pneumoperitoneum may lead to extraperitoneal insufflation, mediastinal emphysema, pneumothorax, and pneumo-omentum. The Veress needle may enter a hollow viscus, the liver, or the spleen. Penetration of a blood vessel may lead to bleeding or gas embolism.

Injuries caused by the large trocar and cannula are generally the most serious. Bleeding can occur in the abdominal wall. Major blood vessels, including the aorta, vena cava, iliac arteries, and veins, can be torn. A hollow or solid viscus can be entered. Most such injuries require immediate repair either by laparoscopic means or by the performance of a laparotomy. Similarly, damage can occur from carelessly placed second and third portals. If a blood vessel or viscus is damaged, it is wise to consult the appropriate surgical specialist to assist in repairing the damage.

Other less serious events may occur and include cervical bleeding from the tenaculum site, uterine perforation, shoulder pain caused by the irritant effects of carbon dioxide on the diaphragm, reactivation of quiescent pelvic inflammatory disease, and the development of incisional hernias. In addition, the brachial plexus and the nerves of the leg are at risk of pressure damage.

The risks of general anesthesia are those for any anesthetic, but, in addition, patients undergoing laparoscopy are particularly vulnerable to the development of cardiac arrhythmias occasioned by both splinting of the diaphragm because of the head-down position and the increased intra-abdominal pressure and the absorption of carbon dioxide.

It is difficult to give precise figures for the incidence of the various complications because most reports depend on mail surveys. Data derived from these surveys must be regarded as soft, relying as they do on the recall of the respondents and the recognized reluctance of surgeons who have high personal complication rates to reply to such surveys. Suffice it to say that proper training, skill of the surgeon, correct selection of patients, and meticulous attention to the details of technique are the key factors in the safe performance of any surgical procedure.

Contraindications to Diagnostic Laparoscopy in the Infertile Patient

The contraindications to diagnostic laparoscopy in the general population, which include severe cardiorespiratory disease, acute generalized peritonitis, severe ileus, intestinal obstruction, or abdominal and diaphragmatic hernia, are rarely encountered in the infertile young woman. Contraindications in the infertile patient may be more related to the patient's infertility. If, for example, the findings at the time of laparoscopy would not alter the outcome for the patient, it is probably inappropriate to submit her to the surgery and the associated risks. If, for example, a woman in her late 40s wishes to pursue in vitro fertilization using donor oocytes to overcome her infertility, the laparoscopic findings will not influence the likelihood of success or failure of that particular procedure.

GOALS OF DIAGNOSTIC LAPAROSCOPY IN THE INFERTILE PATIENT AND ACTIONS TO BE TAKEN DEPENDENT ON THE FINDINGS

Laparoscopy should not be undertaken simply as a fishing expedition. In the majority of cases of infertility, the goals of the procedure can be stated as follows: (1) to establish beyond any doubt that the reproductive organs are entirely normal and as the final investigation required to establish a firm diagnosis of unexplained infertility; (2) to identify, stage, and permit development of a rational therapeutic plan for patients with endometriosis; (3) to identify and stage the sequelae of chronic pelvic inflammatory processes, particularly of the tubes and ovaries, so a decision can be made as to whether the lesions are best treated by laparoscopy, microsurgery, or in vitro fertilization.

Unexplained Infertility

All necessary investigations should be performed before making a diagnosis of unexplained infertility, a diagnosis that, by definition, is one of exclusion. The final step should always be a diagnostic laparoscopy. In some circumstances, in prior discussion with the patient, she and her partner have expressly stated (often owing to her age and the prolonged nature of their infertility) that because no simple cause has been found, the only option they would exercise would be in vitro fertilization. In these cases, the laparoscopic findings, although of interest, will not affect the outcome of their management. For statistical purposes, a diagnosis of unexplained infertility cannot be made unless a laparoscopy has been performed.

Endometriosis

Endometriosis is an enigma. Its pathophysiology is poorly understood as is its relationship to infertility. Nevertheless, every endeavor should be made to identify and stage the disease process. The classification currently used is the American Fertility Society revised classification, which is presently being revised once again. In staging the disease, it is essential to remember the pleomorphic nature of the implants.

Three types of lesions may be recognized: peritoneal implants, adhesions, and intraovarian cysts. A wide variety of peritoneal lesions can be identified. It would appear that clear and flame-colored ones represent early and active stages of the disease (Fig. 24–20; see color section in the center of the book). The classic black powder burns with or without the whitish scarred areas are the late stages (Fig. 24–21; see color section in the center of the book). The adhesions associated with endometriosis may be fleshy or dense and affect any part of the pelvis (Fig. 24–22; see color section in the center of the book). Ovarian cysts are filled with chocolate-colored material and are usually readily apparent (Fig. 24–23; see color section in the center of the book). A definite diagnosis of endometriosis can be made only by evaluation of biopsy specimens, and every endeavor should be made to obtain such specimens laparoscopically. The biopsy technique is beyond the scope of this chapter and is discussed elsewhere.

Unless a systematic and thorough evaluation is performed, the diagnosis of endometriosis frequently is missed. Often, the lesions exist behind the ovaries, and the fact that the ovaries are adherent to the pelvic sidewall is not identified unless a probe is used in an attempt to mobilize them and, if necessary, separate them from the ovarian fossa. If the ovary is enlarged or appears to contain an endometrioma and is intimately adherent, undue force should not be used because the

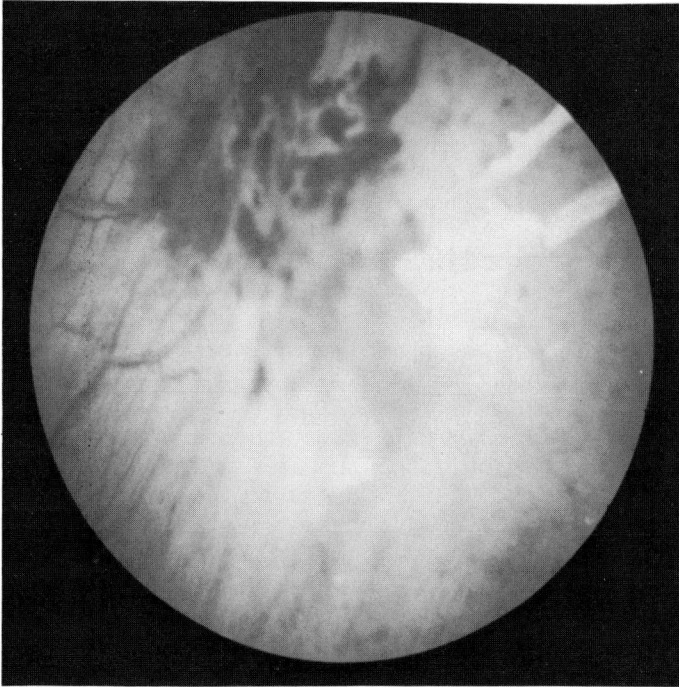

FIGURE 24–20. Laparoscopic view of a flame-like lesion of endometriosis. (Courtesy of William R. Keye, Jr., M.D.)

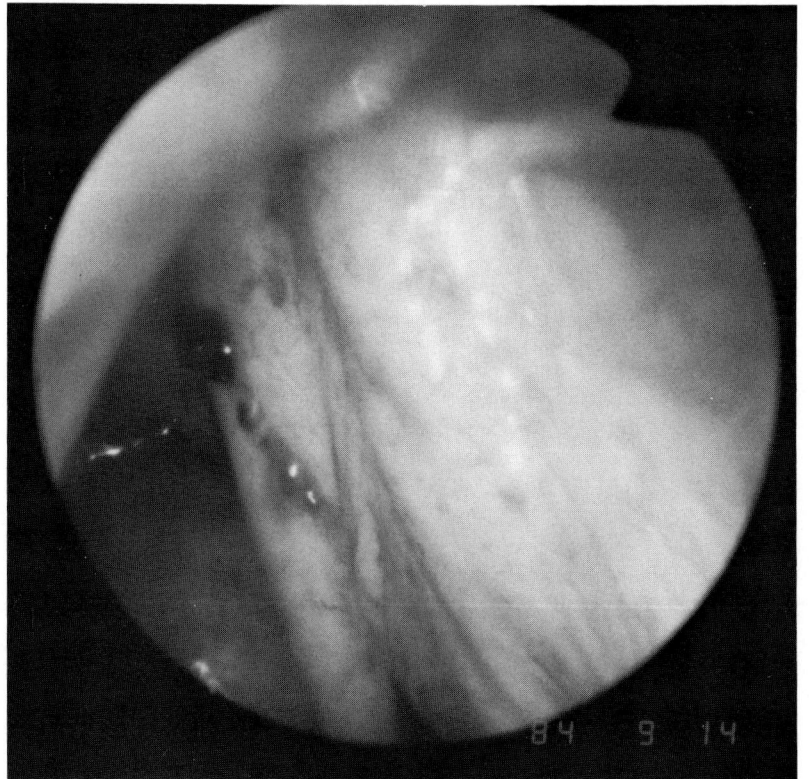

FIGURE 24–21. Laparoscopic view of a darkly pigmented lesion of endometriosis. (Courtesy of William R. Keye, Jr., M.D.)

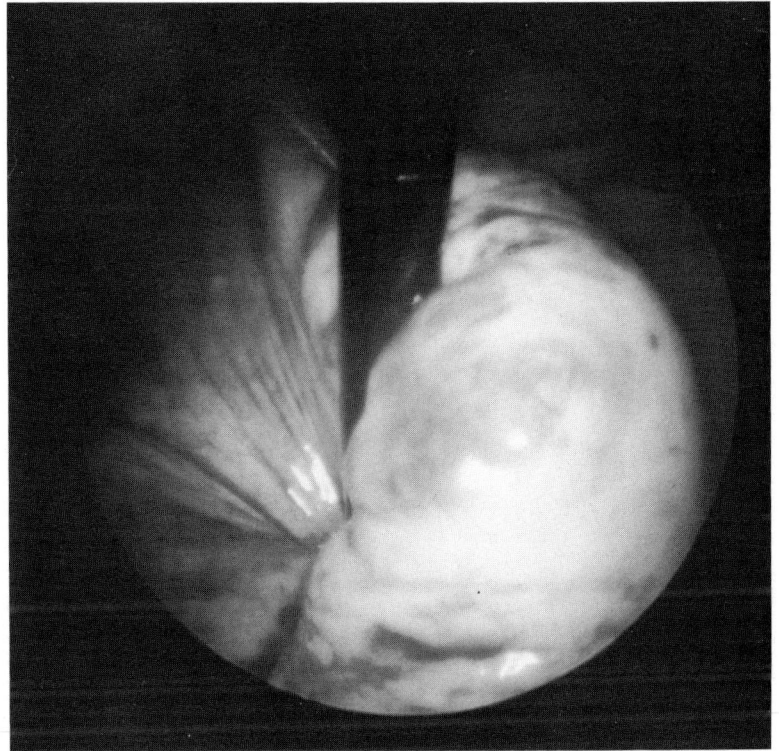

FIGURE 24–22. Laparoscopic view of a retro-ovarian adhesion secondary to endometriosis. (Courtesy of William R. Keye, Jr., M.D.)

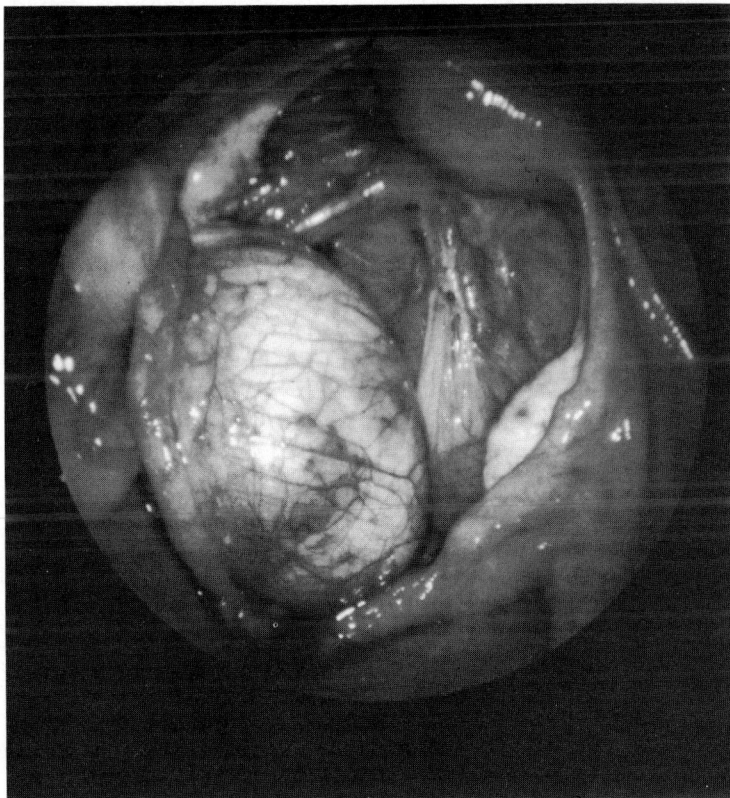

FIGURE 24–23. Laparoscopic view of the pelvis and left ovarian endometrioma. (Courtesy of William R. Keye, Jr., M.D.)

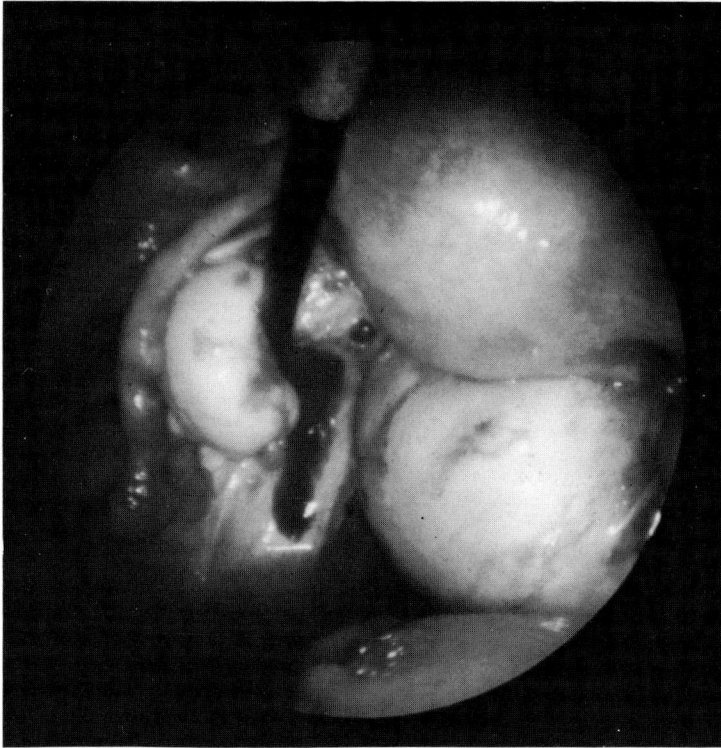

FIGURE 24–24. Rupture of endometrioma with spill of chocolate-colored material. (Courtesy of William R. Keye, Jr., M.D.)

cyst may rupture, spilling its contents into the pelvis (Fig. 24–24; see color section in the center of the book). Traumatic manipulation may also cause bleeding. If the ovaries are enlarged and adherent to each other behind the uterus, the so-called kissing ovaries, the diagnosis of endometriosis is almost certain (Fig. 24–25).

If adhesions are identified, in the absence of any obvious ovarian cysts or endometriotic implants, biopsy specimens should be taken from the adhesions. Often, glands and stroma typical of the condition are identified. The entire peritoneum should be scrutinized closely with the lens in approximation because the magnification may allow identification of suspicious areas that should undergo biopsy.

Management of the patient with endometriosis depends on the severity of the disease and the patient's symptoms. To date there is no convincing evidence to suggest that ablation of implants in stages 1 and 2 disease offers any advantages over no treatment when the outcome of interest is pregnancy. Nevertheless, most surgeons ablate such lesions during the diagnostic laparoscopy. In patients with more severe endometriosis, it may be possible immediately to perform laparoscopic reparative surgery. In other instances, it may be necessary simply to record the findings and undertake preoperative medical therapy to suppress the lesions before finally embarking on definitive laparoscopic surgery or microsurgery for the particular purpose of extirpating the disease.

Sequelae of Chronic Pelvic Inflammatory Processes

The likelihood exists that changes secondary to pelvic inflammation have been determined in most instances by the history and the preliminary HSG. If the HSG findings suggest

that laparoscopic reparative surgery would be feasible, the operating room should be booked for sufficient time. Immediate laparoscopic repair can follow if, on inspection, the condition appears amenable to such an approach. Even if the HSG is normal, periadnexal adhesive disease may be encountered. This condition may also be treated laparoscopically.

Thus, the goals of the diagnostic laparoscopy in postinflammatory patients are to stage and assess the degree of tubal and periadnexal damage and to identify those patients who should undergo laparoscopic correction, those best treated by microsurgery, and those for whom in vitro fertilization would be the optimum choice.

The goals for any infertile couple should be the birth of a live baby or the ability to feel that they have exhausted all reasonable attempts to achieve a pregnancy. For the woman with tubal damage, there are only two realistic options: reparative surgery or in vitro fertilization, techniques that should be regarded as complementary rather than antagonistic. The decision as to which route to take is influenced by both technical and nontechnical considerations.

Nontechnical considerations include age, cost, and wishes of the couple. Age of the female partner exerts a demonstrably detrimental effect on conception and successful outcome, which becomes most marked after the fortieth birthday. In the reproductively inclined older woman, although reparative surgery may be technically feasible, it may be more appropriate to offer her in vitro fertilization, saving surgery for a last-ditch attempt should the assisted reproductive approach fail. The younger woman may well be advised to consider surgery, reserving in vitro fertilization as a "court of last appeal" if the surgery is unsuccessful. The cost and financial means of the couple cannot be underestimated. The final decision always rests with the couple and is influenced by their perception of the facts and their own value system. It is the physician's role ·

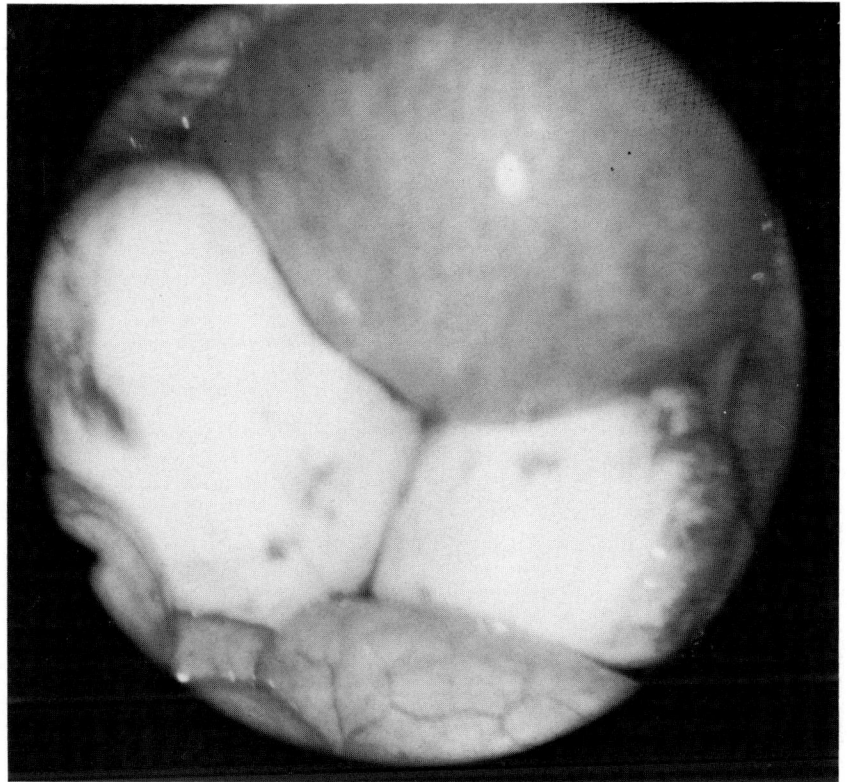

FIGURE 24–25. Kissing ovaries of endometriosis. (Courtesy of William R. Keye, Jr., M.D.)

at all times to respect the patient's final decision, although this does not mean that the physician's own value system is not worthy of respect. The physician must also provide accurate information with regard to probable outcome of any suggested form of treatment.[9]

From the purely technical point of view, diagnostic laparoscopy allows the physician to perform the assessment, which allows an accurate medical prognosis to be made. For some patients, in vitro fertilization is the only reasonable option. These situations arise if the tubes are inoperable, that is to say, absent or severely damaged. Tubal disease may be coincident with another important infertility factor. For example, if the female partner is anovulatory or there is a significant male factor and six cycles of appropriate treatment have been completed unsuccessfully and the HSG now reveals bilateral hydrosalpinges, it is probably more appropriate to proceed directly to in vitro fertilization and spare the patient a diagnostic laparoscopy.

In all other situations, the decision-making process requires comparison of the take-home baby rate and the cumulative pregnancy rates after multiple cycles of in vitro fertilization with the probable outcome following tubal reconstructive surgery.[9]

If the only lesion detected is periadnexal adhesive disease, laparoscopic salpingo-ovariolysis can be performed at the time of the diagnostic laparoscopy. The subsequent live birth rate is approximately 50% to 60%; ectopic pregnancies occur in about 5% of patients who have undergone this procedure. If, in addition, it is necessary to perform fimbrioplasty, the birth rate falls to between 40% and 48%.[3, 10–14] If the tubes are occluded distally, the live birth rate following microsurgical salpingostomy and salpingo-ovariolysis varies between 19% and 35%.[3, 15] Laparoscopic salpingostomy in appropriately selected cases may yield similar results.[14, 16–19]

The factors that affect the outcome of salpingostomy include distal ampullary diameter, tubal wall thickness, extent of adhesions, type of adhesions, and the nature of the tubal endothelium. All but the last of these factors can be assessed directly by laparoscopy. The nature of the tubal endothelium can be inferred by evaluation of the hysterosalpingogram or by direct observation. The distended ampulla may be visualized at the time of laparoscopy using a hysteroscope inserted through the distal end of the tube, after placement of a small incision.

A scoring system for distal tubal occlusion permits estimation of the likely surgical outcome.[20] In unfavorable cases, in vitro fertilization would be the treatment of choice. In those deemed favorable, live birth rates between 50% and 70% have been achieved by microsurgical salpingostomy.[21, 22] For these patients, the decision must be made at the time of diagnostic laparoscopy whether or not to proceed to immediate laparoscopic salpingostomy or to undertake reconstructive microsurgery. The decision as to which approach to recommend must be based on local outcome experience when the two procedures are compared. It is becoming apparent, however, that in most instances, if the tubes cannot be repaired laparoscopically because of the severity of disease, it is unlikely that microsurgery will be successful.

Pathologic proximal tubal occlusion presents a more challenging problem. Data would suggest that in some circumstances, transcervical fallopian tube cannulation will be of value both in elucidating false-positive HSG results and in perhaps overcoming occlusion associated with the presence of spasm, a mucous plug, or tubal synechiae.[23]

In the face of apparent proximal occlusion, however, diagnostic laparoscopy should be performed to assess the remainder of the tube and pelvic architecture. In a number of cases, chromopertubation demonstrates proximal patency. If, in addition, the tube appears otherwise healthy, no further treatment is required. If there is distal occlusion with the demonstration of proximal patency, a salpingostomy may be indicated. If proximal occlusion is confirmed and the rest of the tube appears normal, exclusive of periadnexal adhesions, concurrent tubal cannulation may be undertaken. If cannulation fails or if there is clear evidence of proximal tubal disease, microsurgical correction yields a live birth rate between 37% and 58% and ectopic pregnancy between 5% and 7%.[3, 24–26]

In the face of apparent proximal and distal occlusion, cannulation may be attempted if the cornu appears externally normal and the tube otherwise amenable to salpingostomy. If cannulation proves to be successful, a salpingostomy may be undertaken. If cannulation fails or if there is clear evidence of proximal tubal disease (i.e., salpingitis isthmica nodosa), cannulation is unnecessary, and in vitro fertilization would be the only recommended option.

CONCLUSIONS

In the investigation of the infertile couple, diagnostic laparoscopy represents one of the major advances that have been made in the last 30 years. It is an invasive procedure and should be carried out late in the investigative workup. Hysterosalpingography and laparoscopy are complementary and not competitive investigations.

In the infertile woman, the goals of the diagnostic laparoscopy are to determine that no pelvic disease exists, so a final diagnosis of unexplained infertility can be made, or to detect, stage, and direct management for endometriosis and tubal and ovarian inflammatory disease.

A well-performed diagnostic laparoscopy is of inestimable value. A poorly performed diagnostic laparoscopy is of little service to the patient or physician.

REFERENCES

1. Taylor PJ, Collins JA. Unexplained Infertility. New York: Oxford University Press, 1992:88.
2. Cummings DC, Taylor PJ. Historical predictability of abnormal laparoscopic findings in the infertile woman. J Reprod Med 1979; 23:295–298.
3. Gomel V. Microsurgery in Female Infertility. Boston: Little, Brown, 1983:2.
4. Collins JA, Wrixon W, Janes LB, Wilson EH. Treatment-independent pregnancy among infertile couples. N Engl J Med 1983; 309:1201–1206.
5. Hull MGR, Glazener CMA, Kelly NJ, et al: Population study of causes, treatment, and outcome of infertility. Br Med J 1985; 291:1693–1697.
6. Kliger BE. Evaluation, therapy, and outcome in 493 infertile couples. Fertil Steril 1984; 41:40–46.
7. Gomel V, Taylor PJ, Yuzpe AA, Rioux JE. Laparoscopy and Hysteroscopy in Gynecologic Practice. Chicago: Year Book Medical Publishers, 1986.
8. Jarret JC II. Laparoscopy: direct trocar insertion without pneumoperitoneum. Obstet Gynecol 1990; 75:725–727.
9. Gomel V, Taylor PJ. In vitro fertilization versus reconstructive tubal surgery. Assist Reprod Genet 1992; 9:306–309.
10. Gomel V. Laparoscopic tubal surgery in infertility. Obstet Gynecol 1975; 46:47–48.
11. Gomel V. Salpingo-ovariolysis by laparoscopy in infertility. Fertil Steril 1983; 340:607–610.
12. Bruhat MA, Mage G, Hanhes H, et al. Laparoscopy procedures to promote fertility: ovariolysis and salpingolysis results of 93 selected cases. Acta Eur Fertil 1983; 14:476–479.
13. Fayez JA. An assessment of the role of operative laparoscopy in tuboplasty. Fertil Steril 1983; 39:476–479.
14. Dubuisson JB, Borquet deJoliniere J, Aubriot FX, et al. Terminal tuboplasties by laparoscopy: 65 consecutive cases. Fertil Steril 1990; 54:401–403.
15. Gomel V. Salpingostomy by microsurgery. Fertil Steril 1978; 29:380–387.
16. Gomel V. Salpingostomy by laparoscopy. J Reprod Med 1975; 18:265–268.
17. Daniell JF, Herbert CM. Laparoscopic salpingostomy utilizing the CO_2 laser. Fertil Steril 1984; 41:558–563.
18. Bruhat MA, Dubuisson JB, Pouly JL, et al. La Coeliochirurgie in Encycl Med Chir Techn Chirurg Urol-Gynecol. Vol 6. Paris: Editions Techniques, 1989:38.
19. McComb P, Paleoulogou A. The intussusception salpingostomy technique for the therapy of distal oviductal occlusion at laparoscopy. Obstet Gynecol 1991; 78:443–447.
20. Gomel V. Distal tubal occlusion. Fertil Steril 1988; 49:946–948.
21. Gomel V, Erenus M. Prognostic value of the American Fertility Society's (AFS) classification for distal tubal occlusion. Presented at the 46th Annual Meeting of the AFS (1990), Washington, DC, Abstracts. S106.
22. Boer-Meisel M, Egbert R, te Velde ER, et al. Predicting the pregnancy outcome in patients treated for hydrosalpinx: a prospective study. Fertil Steril 1986; 45:23–29.
23. Kerrin JF, Surrey ES, Williams DB, et al. Falloposcopic observations of endotubal isthmic plugs as a cause of reversible obstruction and their histological characterization. J Laparoendoscop Surg 1991; 1:103–110.
24. Gomel V. Tubal reanastomosis by microsurgery. Fertil Steril 1977; 28:59–65.
25. Donnez J, Casanas-Roux F. Prognostic factors influencing the pregnancy rate after microsurgical cornual anastomosis. Fertil Steril 1986; 46:1089–1092.
26. McComb P, Gomel V. Cornual occlusion and its microsurgical reconstruction. Clin Obstet Gynecol 1980; 23:1229–1241.

CHAPTER 25

Diagnostic Hysteroscopy

RAFAEL F. VALLE

There is no better examination of an organ than that performed visually. This type of exploration, however, is feasible only during surgery or at autopsy. Modern endoscopes have provided a new dimension of visual exploration of organs in vivo without the need for major invasive surgery.

The uterus is a versatile organ that plays a significant role in reproduction. Although uterine pathology affecting fertility may not exceed 10% of couples with infertility, successful reproduction can sometimes be significantly affected. Therefore, uterine evaluation is important in patients with pathology of the uterus.

Although the uterus has been evaluated externally with the aid of laparoscopy, its inner recesses and cavity finally became accessible to visualization with the introduction of hysteroscopy. Safe and appropriate media to distend the uterine cavity permitted this potential space to be converted to an actual cavity that can be viewed panoramically. Although crude early attempts to perform hysteroscopy demonstrated the usefulness of this approach, problems with instrumentation, adequate illumination, and appropriate uterine distention interfered with the clinical application of hysteroscopy. By the early 1970s, the uterine cavity could be illuminated properly by the transmission of intense light via fiberoptics and proper instrumentation that could be safely and easily used transcervically.

Many methods to explore the uterine cavity have been available to gynecologists, among them uterine sounding and tactile appraisal, exploration with forceps or curettes, and radiography using radiopaque materials to outline any filling defects in the uterine cavity. All these methods had significant drawbacks, however, that limited their value as diagnostic tools for the evaluation of the uterine cavity. The recent addition of ultrasonography has provided valuable information about the uterus, particularly during pregnancy, but even this valuable method does not afford the clarity and precision of direct visualization.

Although the interest in modern hysteroscopy arose specifically to achieve transcervical tubal sterilization using methods such as electrocoagulation, sclerosing substances, and mechanical plugs, this new method of intrauterine investigation offers great potential in the diagnosis and treatment of intrauterine pathology and direct access to the fallopian tubes.[1-3]

INSTRUMENTATION AND DISTENDING MEDIA

As with any other endoscopic procedure, hysteroscopy requires the appropriate instrumentation, including the hysteroscope, the light source for illumination, and the distending medium to obtain a panoramic view of the uterine cavity.

Hysteroscopes

The modern hysteroscopes are of two kinds. The first type is the *diagnostic hysteroscope*, which usually is no larger than 4 mm in outside diameter (OD), with a diagnostic sheath providing a single channel for insufflation of carbon dioxide (CO_2) gas and lacking an operative channel. The telescope has a Foroblique view of 30 degrees and, in general, is the same telescope used with operative sheaths of 7 mm OD or larger. Smaller-caliber telescopes are available; however, they provide less light intensity, and photography may be impaired.

Although most rigid endoscopes are similar, a special hysteroscope designed by J. Hamou* permits standard $1 \times$ magnification and $20 \times$ magnification for the panoramic view. An additional ocular transforms the endoscope into a contact hysteroscope with magnifications of $60 \times$ and $150 \times$, which can evaluate cells at their nucleoplasmatic level. This instrument, the colpomicrohysteroscope, can be used for cervical and endocervical evaluations as an adjuvant to colposcopy, cytology, and histology in the evaluation of cervical and endocervical lesions (Figs. 25–1 to 25–3).

Flexible and steerable hysteroscopes are also available for diagnosis with a 3.3 mm OD; these permit better exploration of the uterotubal cones and tubal apertures (Fig. 25–4).

The second type is the *operative hysteroscope*. This endoscope, using a telescope of 4 mm OD, requires a larger sheath of 7 mm OD or wider to permit introduction of instruments through an operating channel.

Flexible operative hysteroscopes of 4.9 mm OD are also

---

*Karl Storz Endoscopy-America, Inc., Culver City, CA 90232-3578.

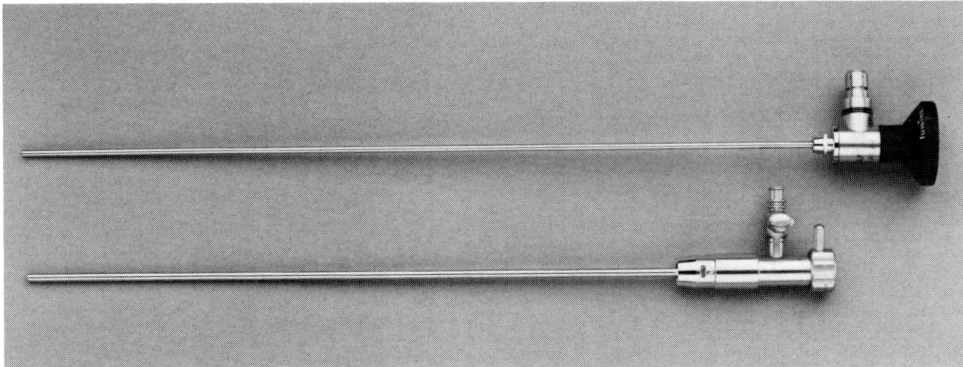

FIGURE 25–1. Unassembled diagnostic hysteroscope. Telescope, 2.8 mm OD (*top*), and diagnostic sheath, 3.3 mm OD (*bottom*). (Courtesy of R. Wolf Medical Instruments Corporation, Vernon Hills, IL.)

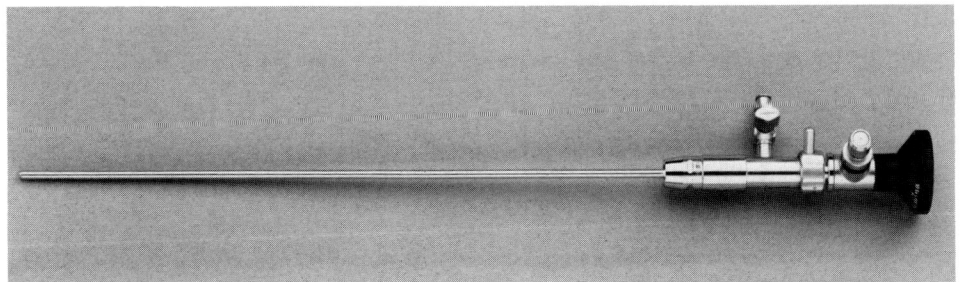

FIGURE 25–2. Assembled diagnostic hysteroscope. (Courtesy of R. Wolf Medical Instruments Corporation, Vernon Hills, IL.)

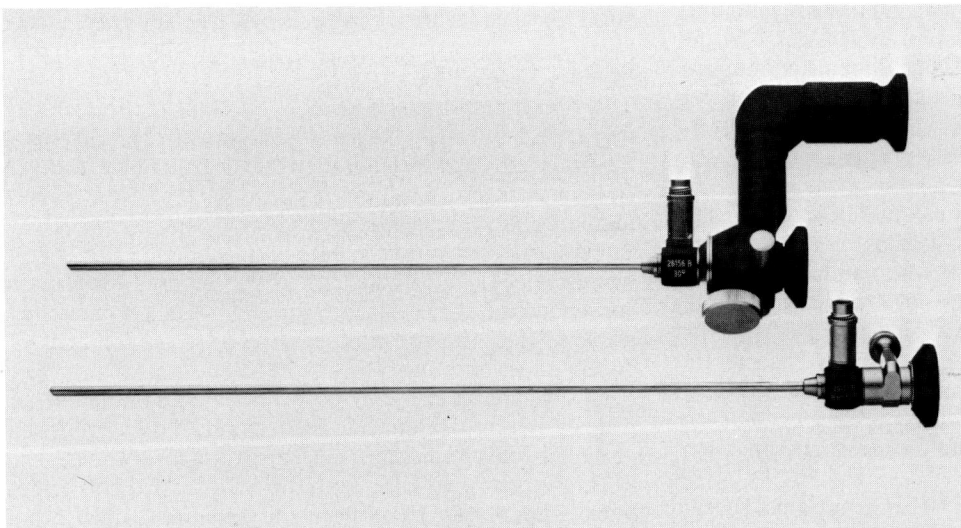

FIGURE 25–3. Focusing hysteroscope (*top*). Microcolpohysteroscope (*bottom*) with double ocular for varying magnification. (Courtesy of Karl Storz Endoscopy-America, Inc., Culver City, CA.)

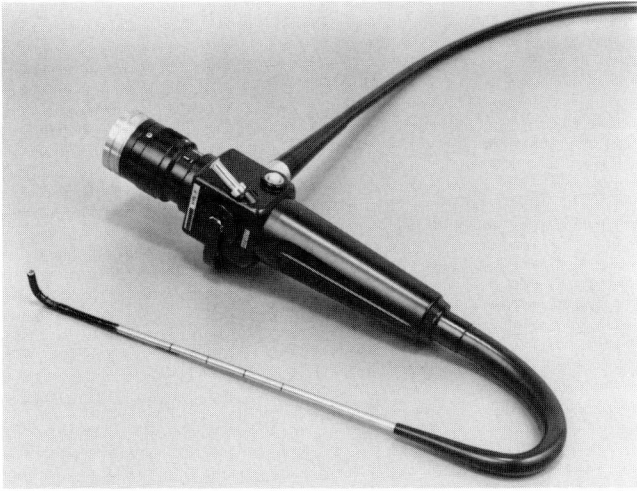

FIGURE 25–4. Diagnostic flexible hysteroscope, 3.3 mm OD. (Courtesy of Fujinon, Inc., Wayne, NJ.)

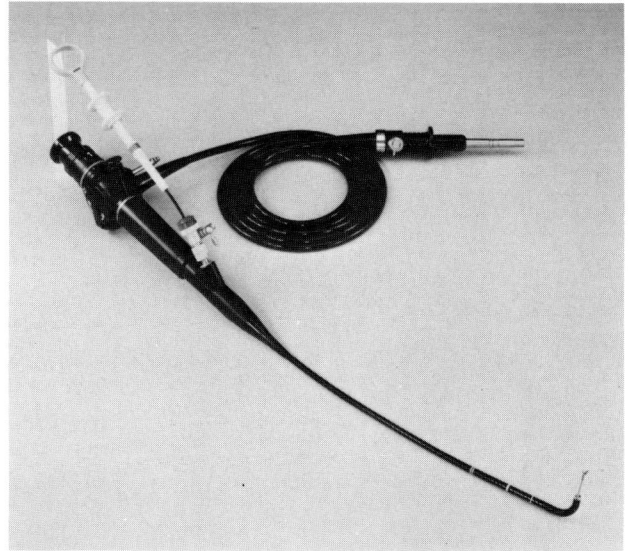

FIGURE 25–5. Operative flexible hysteroscope, 4.9 mm OD, with biopsy forceps in place. (Courtesy of Olympus Corporation, Lake Success, NY.)

available, providing a 2.5-mm inner diameter (ID) for the introduction of flexible instruments or catheters. Although their use is increasing, perhaps their greatest usefulness is in tubal cannulations and delivery of fiberoptic lasers (Fig. 25–5).

Ancillary instrumentation includes rigid, semirigid, and flexible grasping forceps, biopsy forceps, scissors, and catheters (Figs. 25–6 to 25–13).

The *resectoscope* has been adapted for gynecologic purposes and specifically designed for continuous flow of low-viscosity fluids provided by two concentric sheaths that do not communicate. Their OD varies and is available in 5, 8, and 9 mm OD. They are specifically used to remove lesions such as submucosal leiomyomas and polyps using a loop electrode. The roller-ball or roller-bar electrode is used for endometrial ablation. These two electrodes are interchangeable and, because they are activated by monopolar electrical current, the fluids required to distend the uterine cavity during these procedures should not contain electrolytes (Figs. 25–14 to 25–17).

Significant improvements and technologic advances in the manufacturing of video cameras with high resolution, light weight, and maneuverability have made videohysteroscopy an almost routine method for endoscopic evaluation and for use particularly during operative procedures. High-resolution images projected on the video screen with magnification and clarity permit the operator to work with comfort and share every step of the procedure with assistants, anesthesiologists, and all personnel involved in the operating suite, improving the team awareness and serving as a valuable teaching tool (Figs. 25–18 and 25–19).

Media Used to Distend the Uterine Cavity

In general there are two types of distending media: liquid media and CO_2 gas.

Text continued on page 356

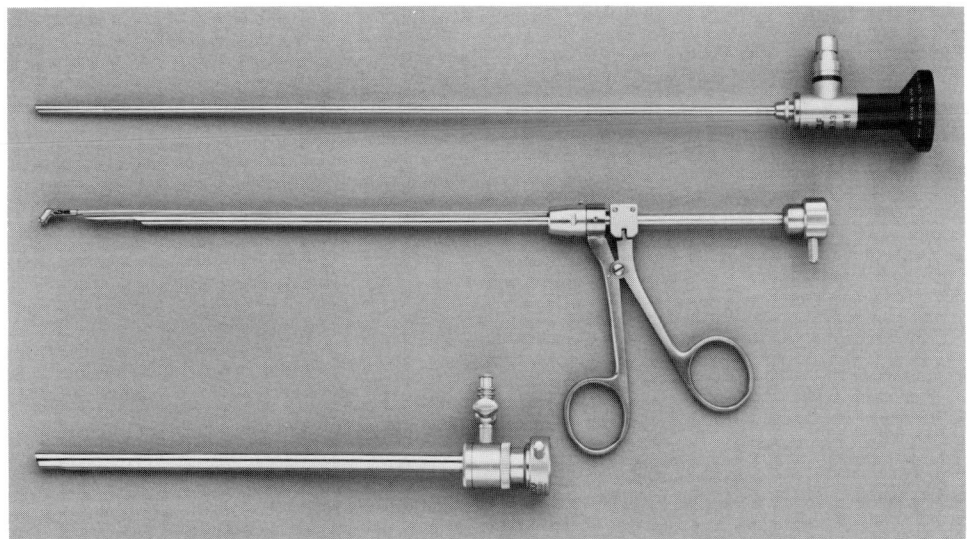

FIGURE 25–6. Unassembled operative hysteroscope. Telescope, 4 mm OD (*top*); fixed optic biopsy forceps (*middle*); and operative sheath, 7 mm OD assembled (*bottom*). (Courtesy of R. Wolf Medical Instruments Corporation, Vernon Hills, IL.)

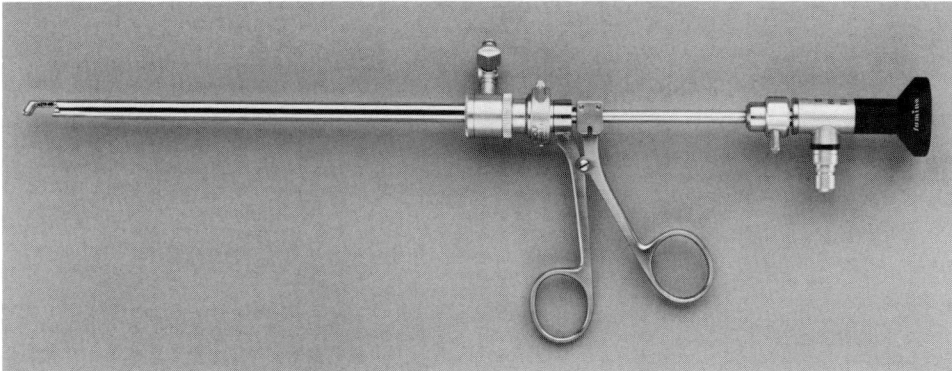

FIGURE 25–7. Assembled operative hysteroscope with fixed optic biopsy forceps. (Courtesy of R. Wolf Medical Instruments Corporation, Vernon Hills, IL.)

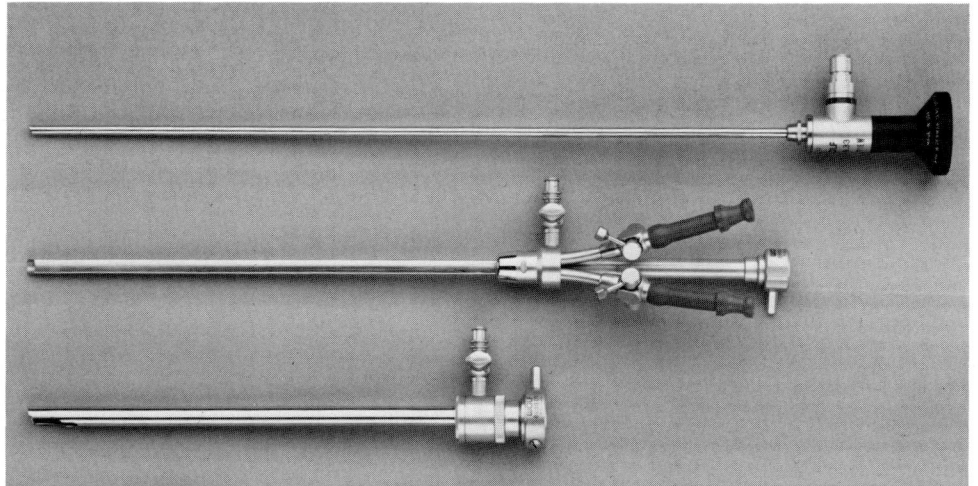

FIGURE 25–8. Unassembled double-channel operative hysteroscope. (Courtesy of R. Wolf Medical Instruments Corporation, Vernon Hills, IL.)

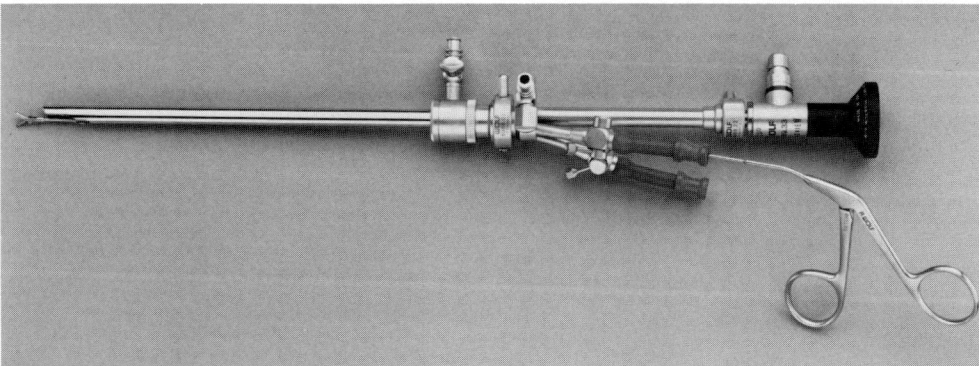

FIGURE 25–9. Assembled double-channel operative hysteroscope with semirigid biopsy forceps in place. (Courtesy of R. Wolf Medical Instruments Corporation, Vernon Hills, IL.)

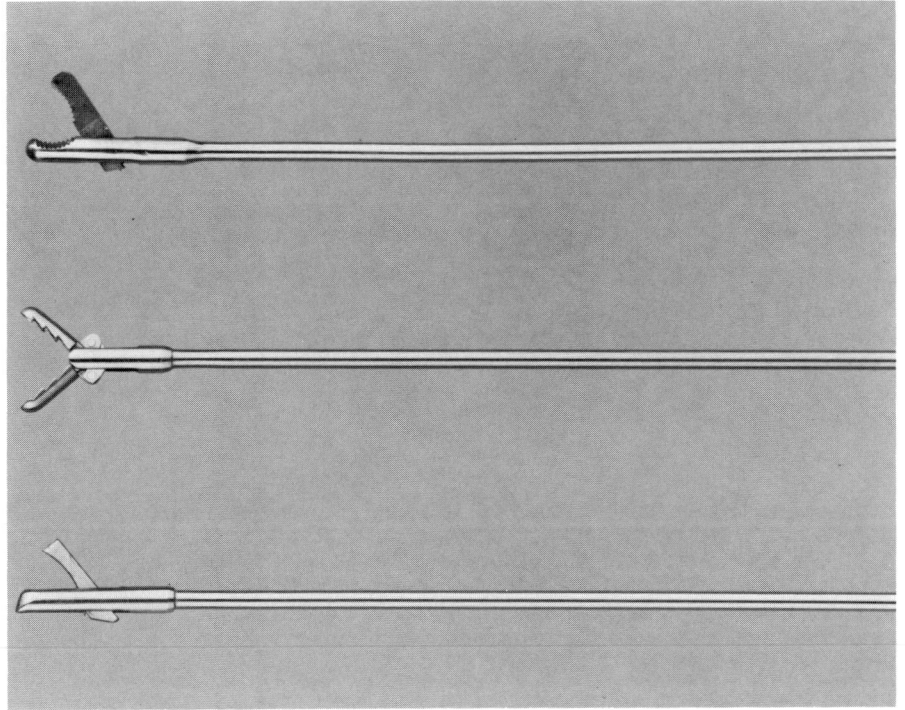

FIGURE 25–10. Semirigid hysteroscopic operative instruments. *Top* to *bottom*, Serrated scissors, grasping forceps, biopsy forceps. (Courtesy of Linvatec [Weck Endoscopy], Raleigh, NC.)

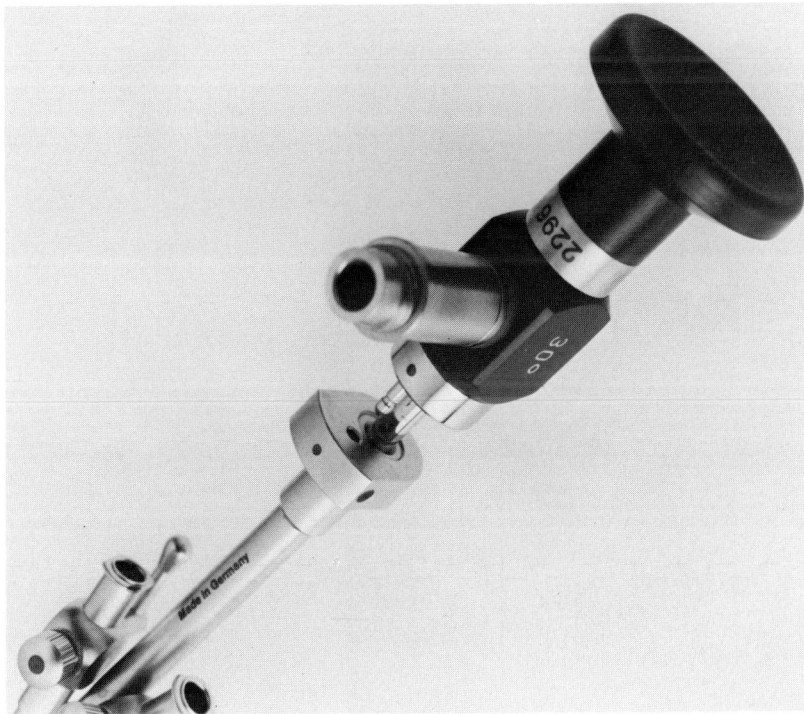

FIGURE 25–11. Close-up view of proximal end of Weck-Baggish hysteroscope with snap-locking mechanism. An operative sheath with double channel is shown. (Courtesy of Linvatec [Weck Endoscopy], Raleigh, NC.)

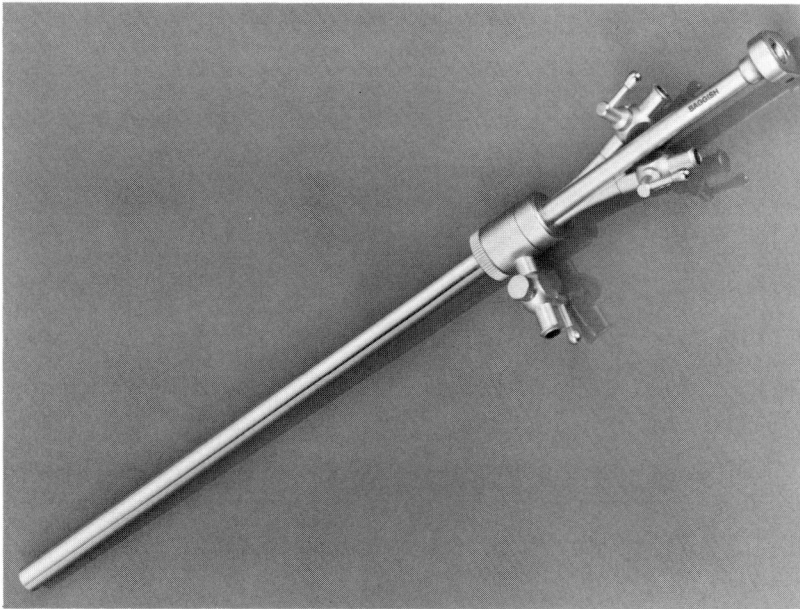

FIGURE 25–12. Double-channel built-in operative sheath (Weck-Baggish hysteroscope). (Courtesy of Linvatec [Weck Endoscopy], Raleigh, NC.)

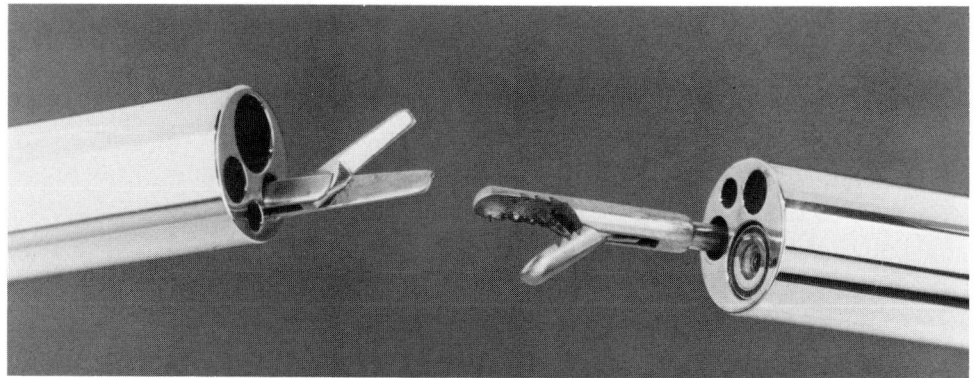

FIGURE 25–13. Close-up view of the distal end of double-channel hysteroscopes with biopsy forceps (*right*) and scissors (*left*) in place. (Courtesy of Linvatec [Weck Endoscopy], Raleigh, NC.)

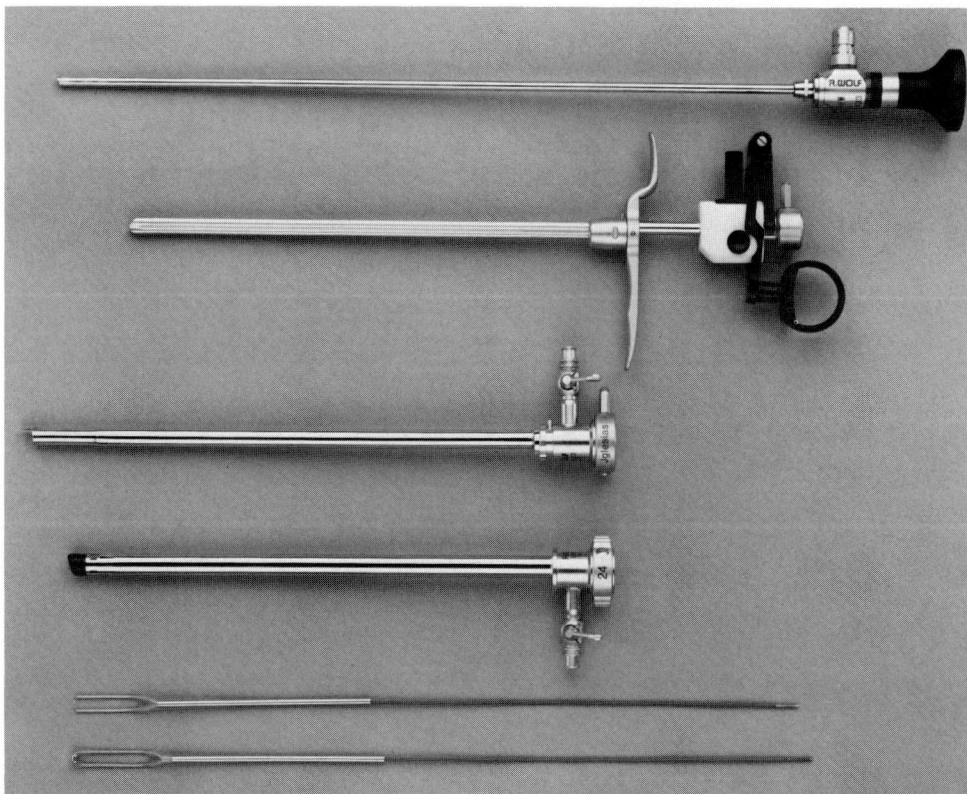

FIGURE 25–14. Unassembled gynecologic resectoscope 24 Fr OD. *Top* to *bottom*, Telescope, supporting bridge, inner cannula (inflow), outer cannula (outflow), electrodes. (Courtesy of R. Wolf Medical Instruments Corporation, Vernon Hills, IL.)

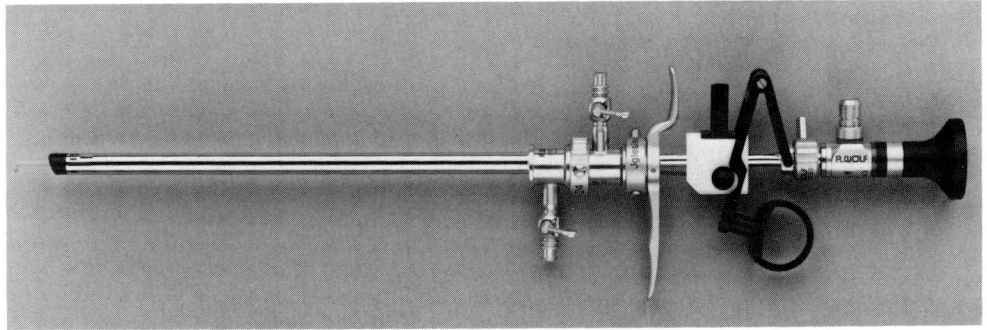

FIGURE 25–15. Assembled gynecologic resectoscope with cutting-loop electrode in place. (Courtesy of R. Wolf Medical Instruments Corporation, Vernon Hills, IL.)

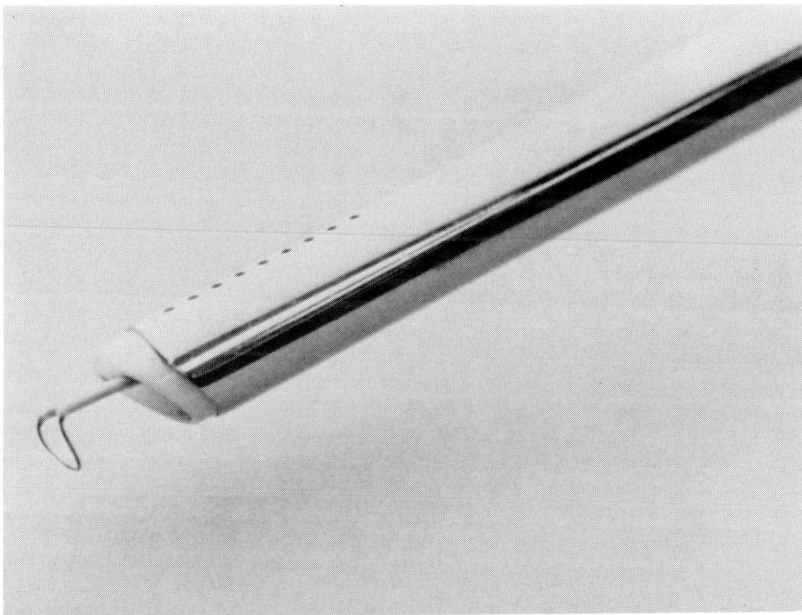

FIGURE 25–16. Distal end of resectoscope with cutting loop in place. (Courtesy of Karl Storz Endoscopy-America, Inc., Culver City, CA.)

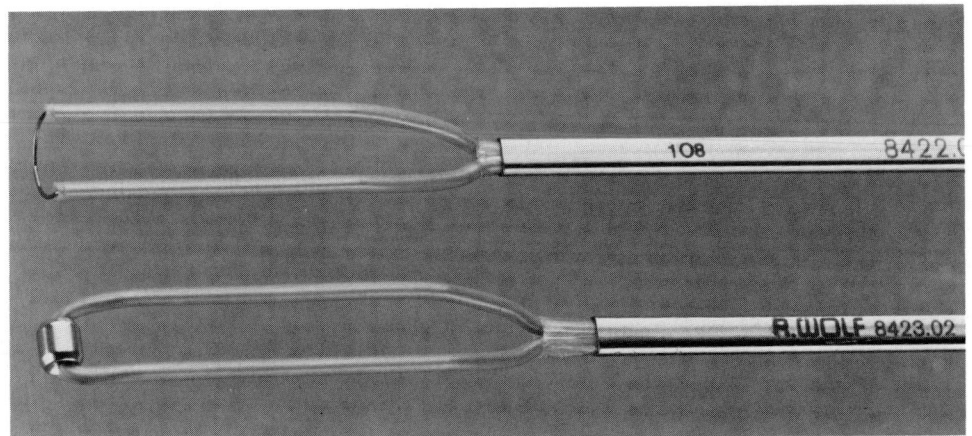

FIGURE 25–17. Electrodes for use with resectoscope. A cutting loop (*top*), and roller bar (*bottom*) are shown. (Courtesy of R. Wolf Medical Instruments Corporation, Vernon Hills, IL.)

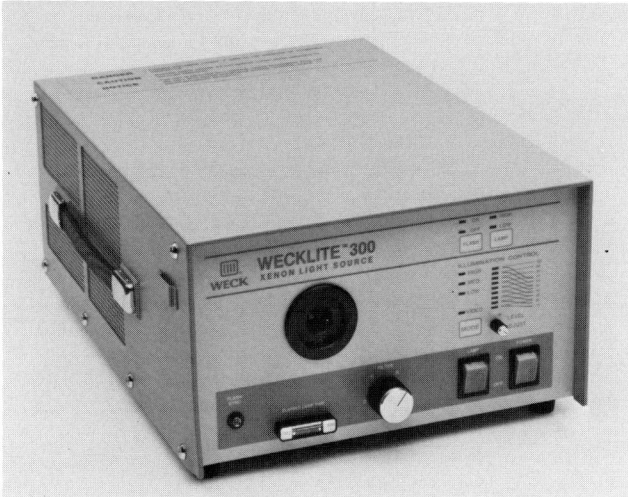

FIGURE 25–18. Xenon light source (Wecklite 300). (Courtesy of Linvatec [Weck Endoscopy], Raleigh, NC.)

LIQUID MEDIA

The liquid media used to distend the uterine cavity are of low or high viscosity. Low-viscosity media may or may not contain electrolytes. The choice of which low-viscosity fluid is used depends on the type of energy used during the performance of any operative procedure through the hysteroscope. Because lasers do not use a flow of electrons, the medium chosen may contain electrolytes. Examples of media containing electrolytes include normal saline, dextrose 5% in half normal saline or in saline, and Ringer's lactate solution. When electrocoagulation is used, fluids devoid of electrolytes should be selected. Examples of nonelectrolyte fluids include glycine 1.5%, sorbitol 3% to 5%, or a mixture of sorbitol, mannitol, and 5% dextrose in water.

When low-viscosity fluids are used, the rate of flow and the quantity used are important. Therefore, the amount of fluid infused and the amount recovered should be carefully monitored to avoid excessive absorption of the media and possible pulmonary edema.

High-viscosity fluids, such as dextrans (particularly 32% dextran 70 in 10% dextrose [Hyskon]), provide clarity of vision. They do not mix well with blood, so that when a small amount of bleeding occurs, visualization is still good. However, these substances are polysaccharides and may therefore produce allergic reactions. In addition, in the event of intravasation they may, because of their hyperosmotic properties, draw fluids into the vascular system, causing pulmonary edema.

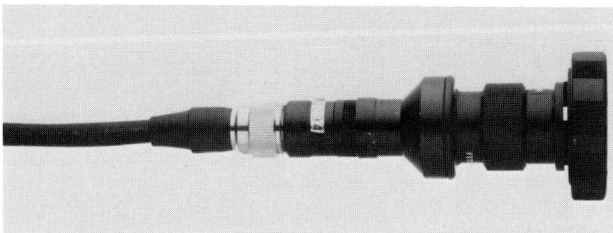

FIGURE 25–19. Video camera for endoscopic use. (Courtesy of Karl Storz Endoscopy-America, Inc., Culver City, CA.)

When low-viscosity fluids are used, it is important to calculate the amount of fluid absorbed by the patient and be aware of the potential for fluid overload if excessive quantities are absorbed. Similar precautions are important with high-viscosity fluids such as 32% dextran 70, particularly during operative procedures.

CO_2 GAS

Because of the small space the diagnostic sheaths provide for instillation of the distending medium, the best medium for distention of the uterine cavity during diagnostic hysteroscopy is CO_2. Also, small endoscopes do not require previous cervical dilation; therefore, less debris, blood clots, or trauma to the endocervical canal may occur, permitting a nontraumatic insertion under direct vision. To deliver the CO_2 gas into the uterine cavity, a special insufflator designed for hysteroscopy is required. This insufflator controls the flow rate (at 40 to 60 mL/min) and the intrauterine pressure (not to exceed 150 mm Hg) (Figs. 25–20 to 25–22).

TECHNIQUES OF PANORAMIC HYSTEROSCOPY

Two types of techniques are used for panoramic hysteroscopy: diagnostic and operative.

Diagnostic hysteroscopy with endoscopes less than 4 mm OD is useful for office hysteroscopy and can be performed with or without local anesthesia in the office. A small volume (4 mL) of a local anesthetic, such as chloroprocaine hydrochloride (Nesacaine 1%) is infiltrated superficially at the base of the uterosacral ligaments, and a small dot (0.5 mL) is injected superficially in the anterior cervical lip. The anterior lip of the cervix is then grasped with a tenaculum. The hysteroscope is attached to its gas source, and a light-transmitting cord is attached to the hysteroscope. The hysteroscope is then introduced into the ectocervix and gently guided into the endocervical canal, following the small microcavity performed by the gas (Fig. 25–23). If visualization is impaired, the endoscope should be withdrawn gently until

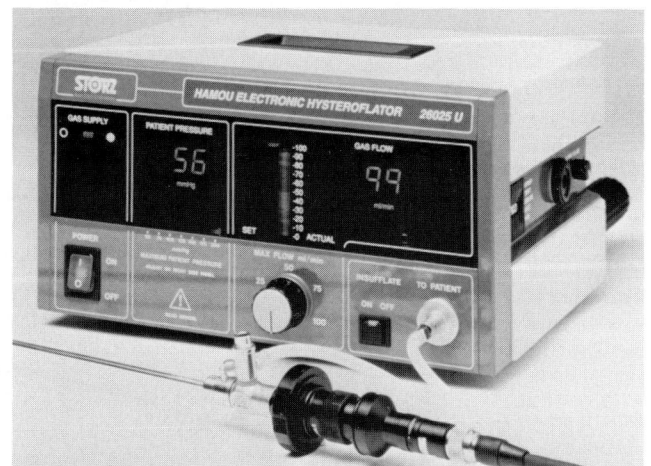

FIGURE 25–20. Electronic hysterosuflator with digital display of CO_2 gas flow and pressure. (Courtesy of Karl Storz Endoscopy-America, Inc., Culver City, CA.)

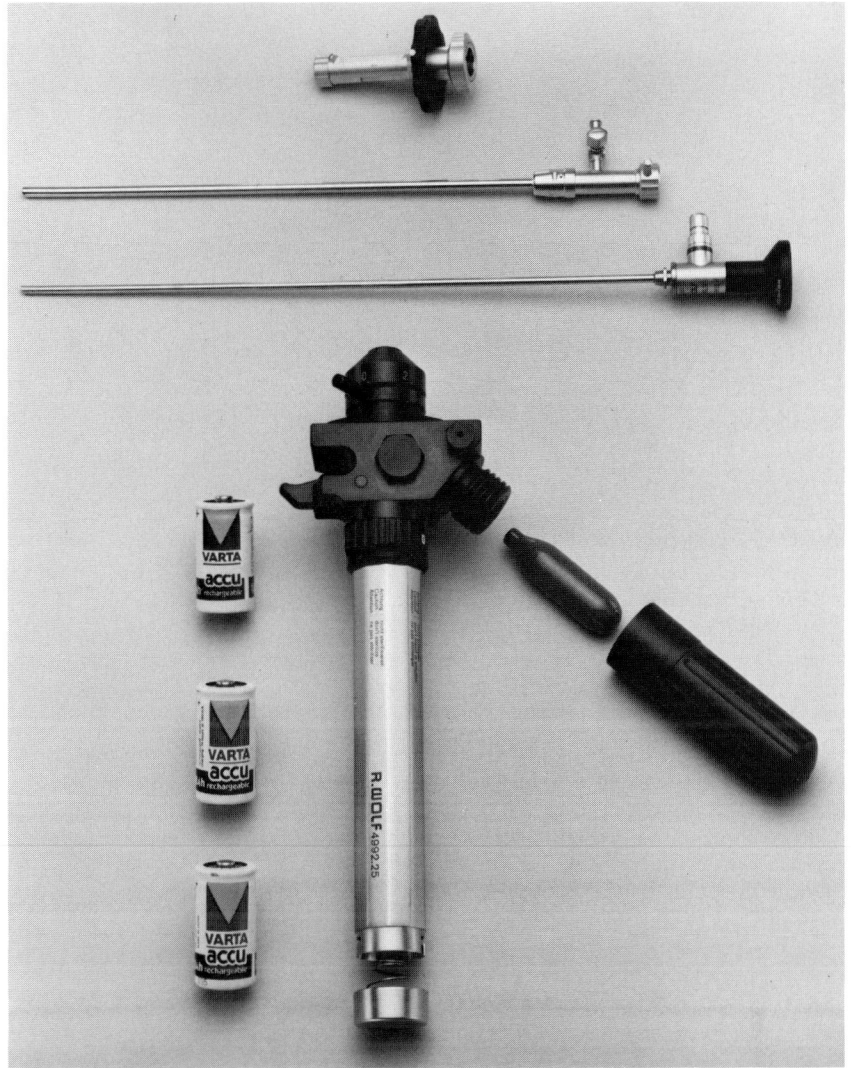

FIGURE 25–21. Unassembled all-in-one hysteroscope. *Top,* Hysteroscopic sheath and telescope. *Bottom,* Batteries, handle, and CO_2 gas cartridge. (Courtesy of R. Wolf Medical Instruments Corporation, Vernon Hills, IL.)

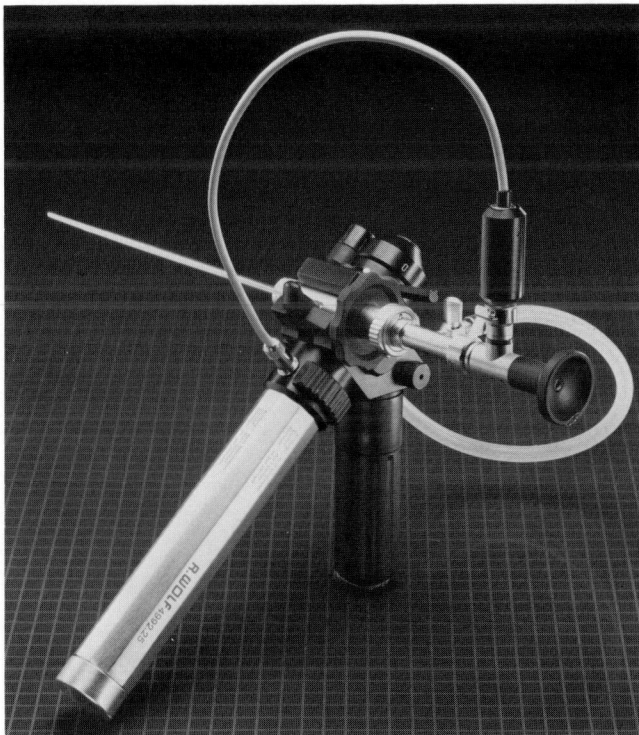

FIGURE 25–22. Assembled all-in-one hysteroscope. (Courtesy of R. Wolf Medical Instruments Corporation, Vernon Hills, IL.)

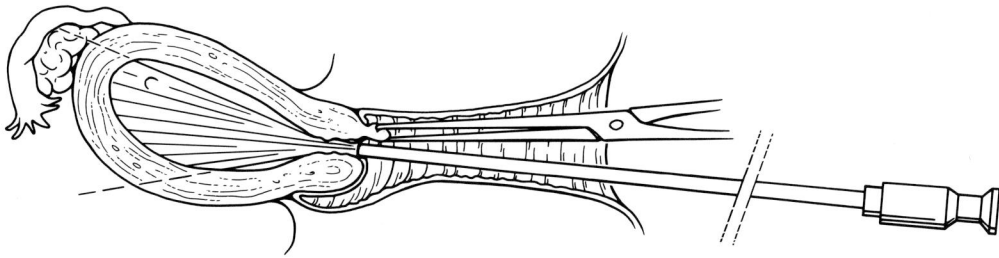

FIGURE 25–23. Initial insertion of hysteroscope in endocervical canal.

the microcavity is created again. The hysteroscope should then be advanced to the internal cervical os, where the evaluation and systematic exploration of the uterine cavity begins. Once the examination is completed, the endoscope is withdrawn under direct vision, and the uterine cavity and endocervical canal are checked once more as the endoscope is withdrawn.

The distal end of most hysteroscopes is beveled and corresponds to the Foroblique vision (30-degree angle). This angle must be taken into consideration, particularly at the introduction of an endoscope through the endocervical canal. The orientation of most hysteroscopes provides deflected vision away from the corresponding transmitting light cable connection. Therefore, when the cord is down, the hysteroscope is directed in a slightly upward direction. When the light-transmitting cord is up, the direction of view is somewhat down. With the resectoscope, this direction of view is generally reversed, with the light-transmitting cable up (Figs. 25–24 and 25–25).

Operative hysteroscopy is the second type of panoramic technique. Because most operative hysteroscopes have operating sheaths of 7 mm OD or larger, cervical dilation is necessary in most patients. The endocervical canal is dilated to the size of the sheath; sometimes an obturator is necessary to insert the operative sheath and avoid abrasion of the endocervical canal. The obturator is removed and replaced with the operating bridge and telescope. The exploration begins at the internal os in a manner similar to that performed in the diagnostic evaluation. The instrument is withdrawn under direct vision and then the endocervical canal is explored while the instrument is being withdrawn (Fig. 25–26).

In most instances when operative hysteroscopy is performed, liquid media are used, particularly those of low viscosity. It is therefore important to wash the uterine cavity by inserting a polyethylene catheter of 2.6 mm OD through the operating channel. This washing procedure permits removal of debris, blood clots, and mucus usually produced after cervical dilation. When the fluid returning through the catheter is clear, visualization may begin. Selective suctioning of clots or debris can also be done under direct vision. This maneuver may be rendered obsolete by the new continuous-flow hysteroscopes now being introduced.

Use of the resectoscope requires steps similar to those of the operative technique, but suctioning is not necessary, because the continuous flow provided by the resectoscope helps cleanse the uterine cavity before the electrodes are activated.

INDICATIONS FOR HYSTEROSCOPY

Determining indications and applications for a new technique is difficult. A potential application could be defined without proven benefit in accepted clinical studies. How

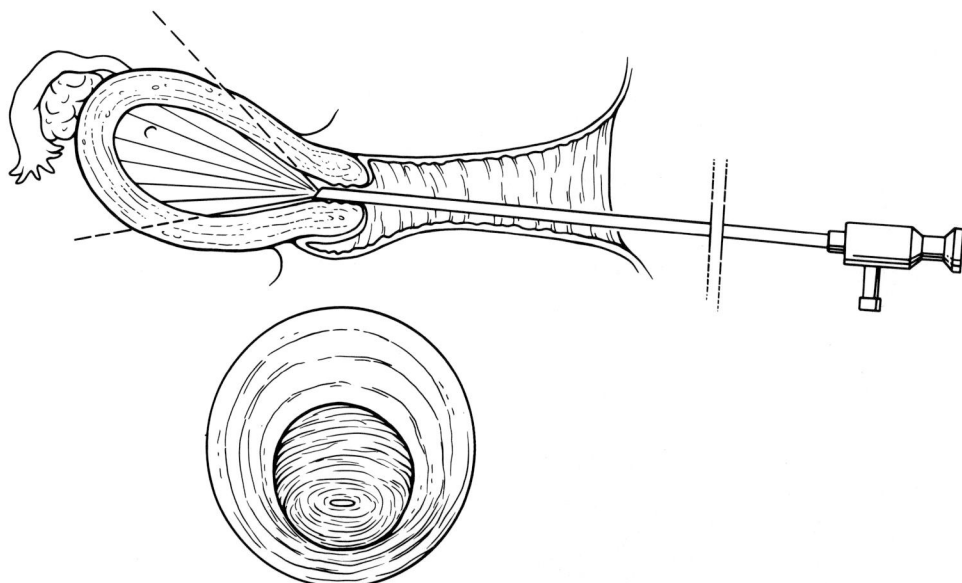

FIGURE 25–24. Schematic representation of initial insertion of hysteroscope. Note upward diversion of view by Foroblique lens.

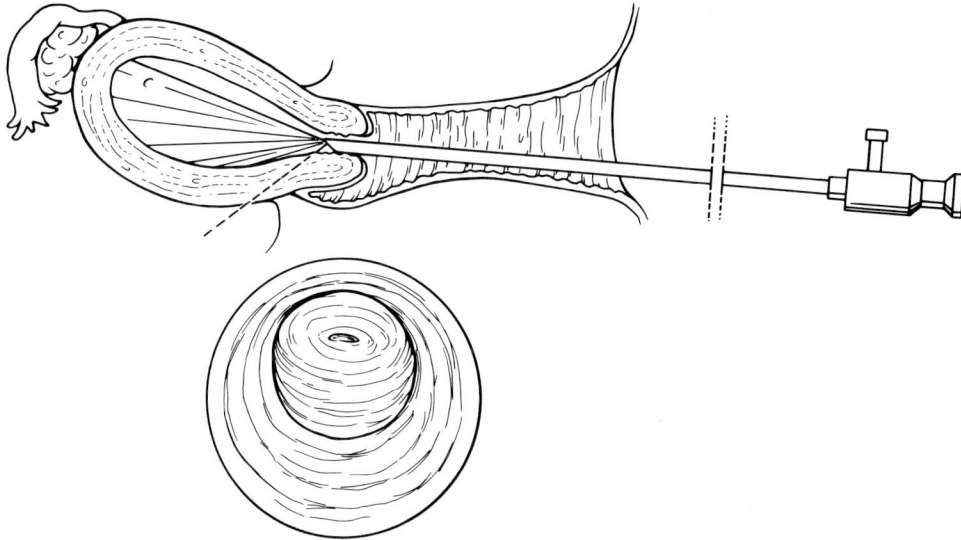

FIGURE 25–25. Hysteroscope with Foroblique view downward.

many patients or trials are required to support a proven clinical study is not clear. Specific clinical indications for hysteroscopy are now being established to define better the usefulness of hysteroscopy in clinical practice. An indication is defined in this section as any application of hysteroscopy that has been shown by at least one investigator to be of value in the diagnosis or treatment, or both, of patients with gynecologic problems.

Although attempts have been made to obtain biopsies and cannulate the fallopian tubes transcervically since the late 1920s,[4] the diagnostic capabilities of the technique were used more frequently in the early years of hysteroscopy than any intrauterine surgery. The principal indication for hysteroscopy was abnormal uterine bleeding. Pathologic lesions such as polyps, submucous leiomyomas, focal areas of hyperplasia of the endometrium, and carcinoma were identified. The ability to determine the location, extension, and topography of these lesions prompted early attempts at intrauterine surgery, such as those initiated by Norment in the 1950s.[5–8]

Current Indications for Hysteroscopy

Technologic refinements in instrumentation and experience have made hysteroscopy simpler and safer than ever before. In addition, recent experience has confirmed some indications and added new applications. The current indications for hysteroscopy are outlined in Table 25–1.

ABNORMAL UTERINE BLEEDING

Abnormal uterine bleeding in the premenopausal and postmenopausal woman continues to be the leading indication for hysteroscopy. Hysteroscopy permits visual evaluation of the uterine cavity, increases the accuracy in diagnosing suspected intrauterine pathology, and offers the opportunity to obtain targeted biopsies of abnormal or suspicious endometrial lesions. Despite the fact that dilation and curettage has been the most frequently performed gynecologic surgical procedure for diagnosis and treatment of abnormal uterine bleeding, focal lesions of the endometrium or lesions located at the uterotubal cones may be missed by the curette. Furthermore, even relatively large pathologic lesions in the endometrial cavity, such as submucous leiomyomas and endometrial polyps, may be missed by the blind curettage (Tables 25–2 and 25–3).

To use curettage selectively in patients with recurrent or persistent abnormal uterine bleeding, the visualization provided by hysteroscopy aids in selecting patients who may require selective curettage and helps in determining the site to which the curette is to be guided. Although biopsy of the endometrium by suction curettage, using the mechanical aspirators such as the Vabra* aspirator or the Vakutage,† increases the accuracy and adequacy of tissue samples, it still

---

*Berkeley Medevices, Inc., Berkeley, CA.
†Warner-Chilcott, Morris Plains, NJ.

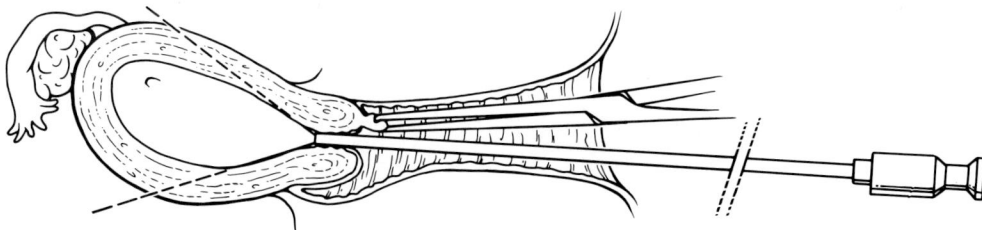

FIGURE 25–26. Hysteroscope withdrawn to explore the endocervical canal.

TABLE 25-1. Indications for Hysteroscopy

Evaluate unexplained abnormal uterine bleeding in premenopausal
or postmenopausal patient

Diagnose and transcervically remove submucous leiomyoma/polyp

Locate, retrieve "lost" intrauterine device, other foreign body

Evaluate infertile patient with abnormal hysterosalpingogram

Diagnose, surgically treat intrauterine adhesions

Diagnose, surgically treat uterine septum

Explore endocervical canal, uterine cavity in repeated spontaneous
abortions

Evaluate failed first-trimester elective abortion

Ablate endometrium of patient with intractable menorrhagia

Cannulate fallopian tubes

TABLE 25-3. Adequacy of Dilation and Curettage (D & C) (Polyps)

Study	No. Patients	Diagnosed (%)	Missed (%)
Bibbo M, et al, 1982 (Vakutage/ D & C or hysterectomy)	840	83	17
Burnett JE, 1964 (D & C /hysterectomy)	1298 specimens (121 [9.3%] had polyps)	53	47
Grimes DA, 1982 (Vabra review)	111	80–83	17–20
Valle RF, 1981 (hysteroscopy/ D & C)	553 (179 had polyps)	100/10	0/90

remains inadequate for the diagnosis of endometrial polyps, submucous leiomyomas, and focal pathologic lesions of the endometrium.

The endometrial biopsy is an excellent method of assessing the overall endometrial response to ovulation, diagnosing lesions that occupy a large portion of the endometrium (Table 25–4). When hysteroscopy has been used as an adjuvant in the evaluation of patients with abnormal uterine bleeding, a significant rate of detection of abnormal findings has been achieved, ranging from 40% to 85% in published studies.[9, 10] Although hysteroscopy increases diagnostic precision in patients with intrauterine lesions, its use does not exclude other methods of evaluation. Rather, it complements them and improves their accuracy of diagnosis and therapy. Because hysteroscopic visualization of the endometrium alone may not provide an accurate diagnosis, a biopsy of the suspicious lesion should be obtained for further pathologic study (Figs. 25–27 to 25–32).

INFERTILITY

Hysterosalpingography (HSG) is a useful method for evaluation of the uterine cavity; nonetheless, its sensitivity and specificity have been challenged, because transient distortion of the uterine cavity by blood, mucus, debris, and air bubbles may produce false-positive results. Errors in technique, the choice of a radiocontrast agent, and interpretation of findings may also contribute to the failure of the HSG to diagnose intrauterine lesions. The ability to observe the inside of the uterus directly may confirm that an abnormal shadow seen on the hysterogram is the result of an intrauterine lesion. It also facilitates a direct biopsy of the lesion under visual con-

trol. The confirmation of abnormal hysterographic findings by subsequent hysteroscopy varies from 43% to 66% in different studies that compare these two techniques.[9, 11]

The abnormal hysterogram is the main indication for hysteroscopy in the infertile patient. The false shadow may be rectified, and biopsies of suspicious lesions can be obtained and the lesions removed transcervically under hysteroscopic control. Polyps, submucous leiomyomas, uterine septa, and intrauterine adhesions may be diagnosed and treated.[11]

Hysteroscopy and HSG nonetheless are not exclusive of each other but are complementary. The hysterosalpingogram, usually performed as part of the infertility evaluation, is one of the routine screening methods for evaluating the uterine cavity and fallopian tubes because of its ease of performance, simplicity, low cost, and valuable information obtained. Only those patients with abnormal hysterosalpingograms become candidates for hysteroscopy, in the absence of other symptomatology requiring intrauterine visualization. The low yield of diagnostic hysteroscopy in infertile women with a normal HSG does not justify routine hysteroscopy in infertile patients. The hysterosalpingogram offers additional information not amenable to hysteroscopic diagnosis, such as intratubal defects, diverticuli, tubal epithelial ruggae, and tubal patency. Used in combination, these two techniques make possible a complete systematic evaluation of the uterine cavity providing a precise diagnosis and selective transcervical treatment (Table 25–5).[12–14]

SUBMUCOUS LEIOMYOMAS

Hysteroscopy is the best method to confirm submucous leiomyomas and endometrial polyps, because these lesions distort the symmetry of the uterine cavity and are easily visualized on panoramic view. Although large endometrial polyps, particularly those that are pedunculated, are easily removed under hysteroscopic guidance, the removal of sub-

TABLE 25-2. Adequacy of Dilation and Curettage (D & C)

Study	No. Patients	Adequate Curettage	Incomplete Curettage
Englund S, et al, 1957 (D & C /hysteroscopy)	124	44 (35%)	80 (65%)
Gribb JJ, 1960 (D & C /hysteroscopy)	58	9 (15.4%)	49 (84.6%)
Stock RJ, Kanbour A, 1975 (D & C /hysterectomy)	50	<½ of cavity in 30 (60%)	<⅔ of cavity in 42 (84%)
Word B, et al, 1958 (D & C /hysterectomy)	512	10% of lesions missed by curettage	

TABLE 25-4. Endometrial Sampling: Adequacy of Specimens

Procedure	Percentage
Dilation and curettage (two studies >300 cases each)	77–94
Vabra aspiration (four studies >300 cases each)	95–99

From Grimes DA. Diagnostic dilation and curettage: a reappraisal. Am J Obstet Gynecol 1982; 142:1.

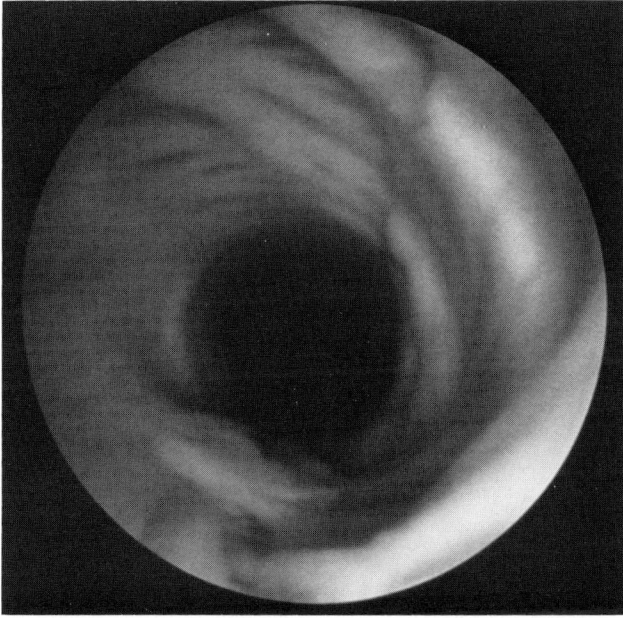

FIGURE 25–27. Hysteroscopic view of the endocervical canal.

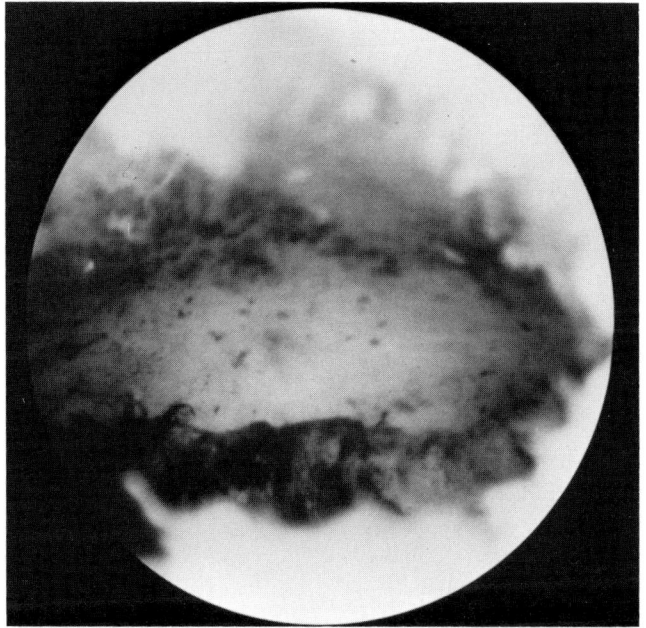

FIGURE 25–29. Intrauterine visualization during secretory phase.

mucous leiomyomas is more difficult and requires a great deal more skill. Pedunculated submucous leiomyomas can be removed intact after direct transection of the pedicle or by morcellation using the resectoscope (Figs. 25–33 to 25–36). Myomas with thick pedicles are removed by shaving the lesion progressively from its adhering pedicle to the uterine wall. Sessile myomas can be partially removed and shaved down to the level of the endometrium. Following this treatment the treated area undergoes secondary epithelialization. In the absence of additional leiomyomas, complete hysteroscopic myomectomy for pedunculated submucous leiomyomas has provided a cure for anemia, dysmenorrhea, and

abnormal uterine bleeding in practically all patients treated. Partially shaved sessile submucous leiomyomas need a close followup because of persistent symptoms in more than 30% of patients.[15–19]

INTRAUTERINE ADHESIONS

Hysteroscopy is the standard surgical method of treatment for intrauterine adhesions, permitting selective division of these adhesions without damage to the surrounding endometrium and offering an excellent tool to establish the symmetry and normal architecture of the uterine cavity. Following treatment, more than 90% of the patients have resumed normal menstruation, and 75% to 80% have achieved preg-

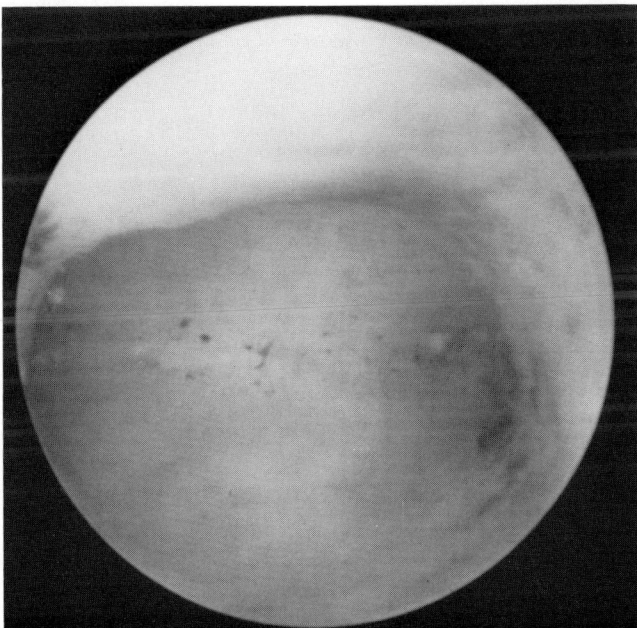

FIGURE 25–28. Visualization of the endometrial cavity in early proliferative phase.

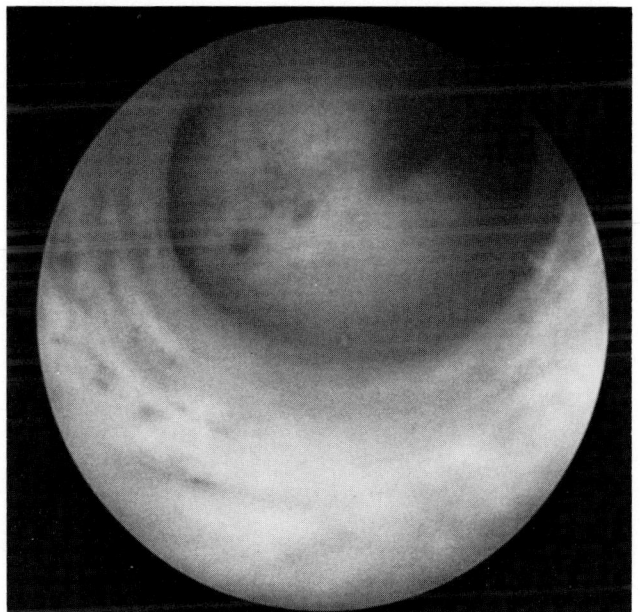

FIGURE 25–30. Atrophic endometrium in postmenopausal patient.

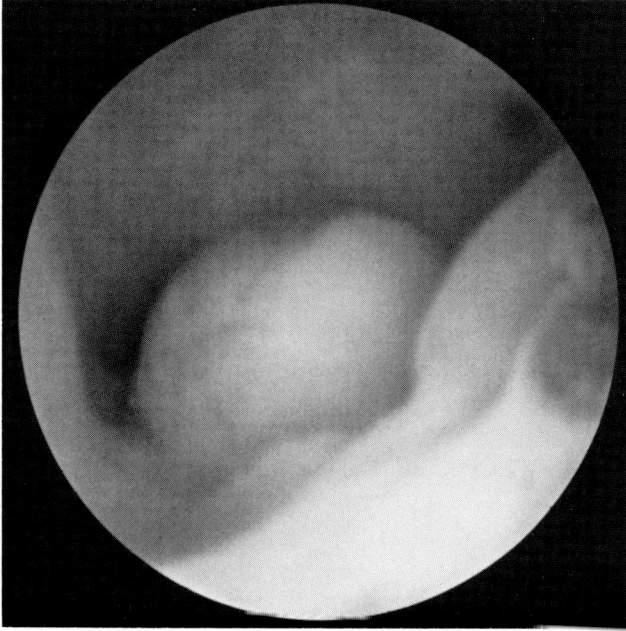

FIGURE 25–31. Sessile endometrial polyp in right cornual area.

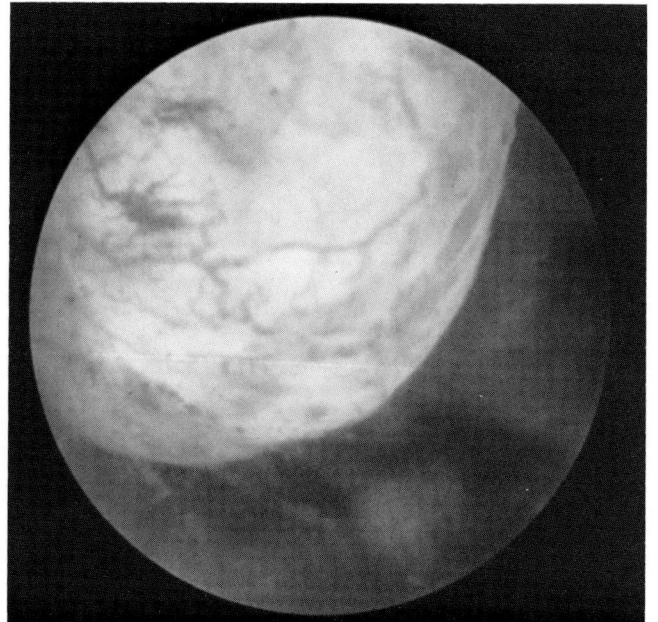

FIGURE 25–32. Submucous leiomyoma with typical peripheral vascularization.

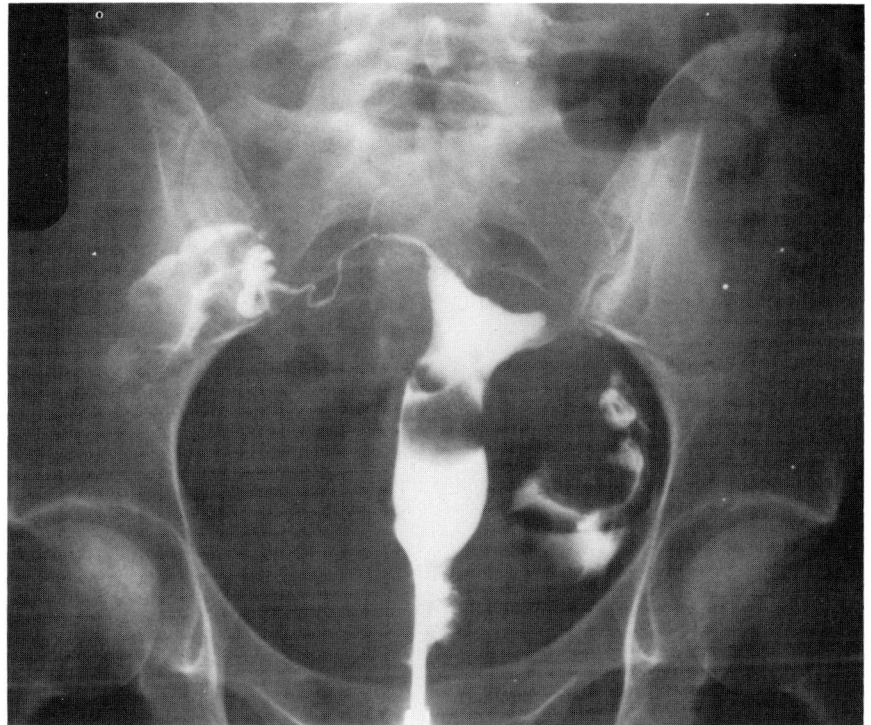

FIGURE 25-33. Hysterosalpingogram showing large filling defects in the lower portion of the uterine cavity.

nancy; of those, 50% to 60% have delivered an infant at term.[20-22] Nonetheless, the reproductive outcome is closely related to the type of adhesions treated as well as to the extent of uterine cavity involvement; therefore, it is useful when evaluating and treating these patients to classify the adhesive disease according to these criteria. Although extensive, thick adhesions have been difficult to treat, even with hysteroscopy, the visual approach to these adhesions has improved treatment and decreased the risk of uterine damage and creation of new adhesions. Hysteroscopy helps delineate the extent of uterine cavity occlusion and the type of adhesions present, providing an accurate appraisal of the severity of this condition and offering a useful prognostic index for the outcome of therapy.

Three stages of intrauterine adhesions may be defined:

- *Mild adhesions*: filmy adhesions (endometrial) that produce partial or complete uterine cavity occlusion
- *Moderate adhesions*: fibromuscular adhesions, characteristically thick, covered with endometrium that may bleed on division; these adhesions partially or totally occlude the uterine cavity

TABLE 25-5. Comparison of Hysteroscopy and Hysterosalpingography	
Hysteroscopy	**Hysterosalpingography**
Direct visualization of uterine cavity	Indirect visualization (contrast medium's shadow)
Diagnosis and specification of intrauterine lesions	Recognition and presumptive diagnosis
Possibility of targeted biopsies and surgical therapy	No possibility
Precise localization of abnormalities (polyps, myomas, malformations, adhesions, carcinoma and precursors)	Localization of abnormalities is less precise
Direct access to tubal lumen (biochemical or biophysical studies, selective chromopertubation)	No direct access (indirect study, possible spasm)
No evaluation of fallopian tubes possible	Evaluation of tubal lumen, patency, epithelial folds and abnormalities
Requires special instrumentation and experience, more expensive	Simple instrumentation, easy to perform, less expensive

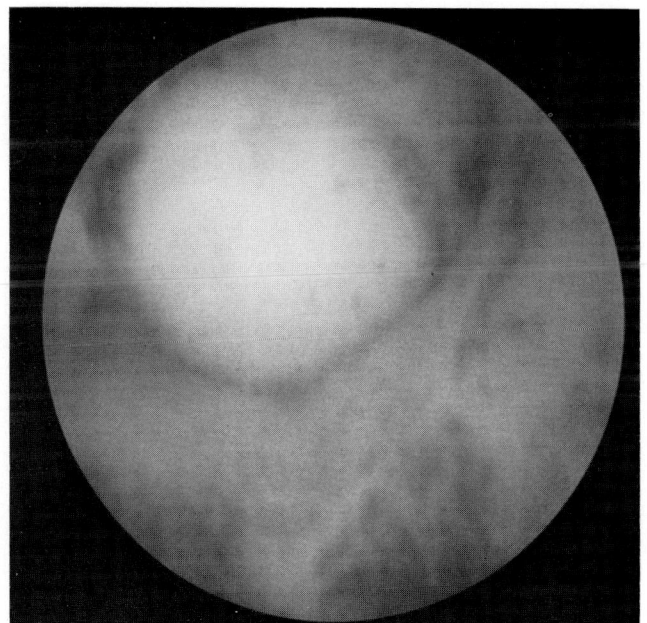

FIGURE 25-34. Submucous leiomyoma at hysteroscopy.

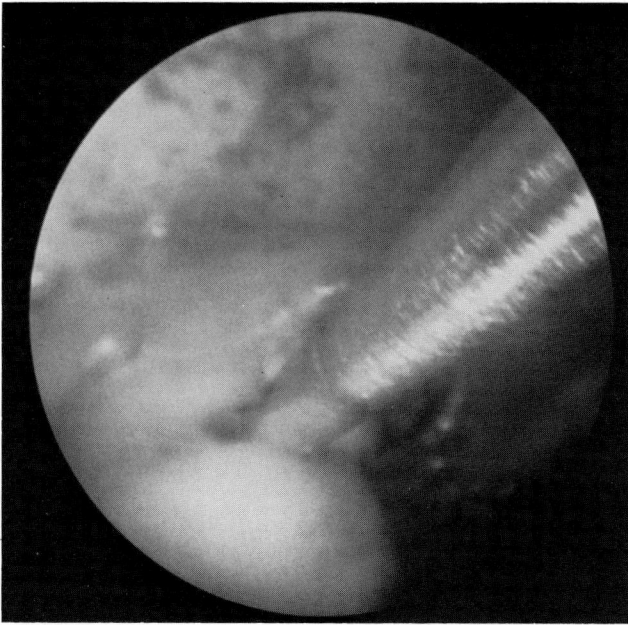

FIGURE 25–35. Hysteroscopic resection of a myoma (scissors shown).

■ *Severe adhesions*: composed of connective tissue only, lacking any endometrial lining, and unlikely to bleed on division. These adhesions may also partially or totally occlude the uterine cavity

This classification is based on the degree of intrauterine involvement shown by HSG and the extent and type of intrauterine adhesions found at hysteroscopy.[22] Because of the difficulty in treating severe adhesions composed of connective tissue, particularly when occlusion of the uterine cavity is extensive, increased awareness of the entity of intrauterine adhesions following postpartum and postabortal curettage or trauma to the uterine cavity may enhance early diagnosis by evaluating with a hysterosalpingogram those patients who

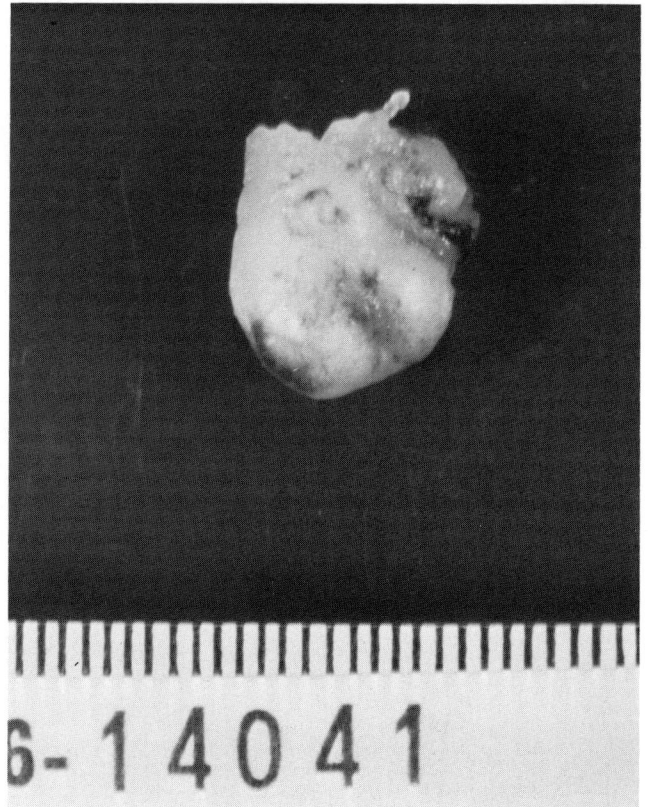

FIGURE 25–36. Myoma after removal.

develop menstrual abnormalities following trauma to the endometrium in the postpartum or postabortal period; best results are achieved when adhesions are mild and filmy. The modern management of intrauterine adhesions should include hysteroscopy because it is the most accurate method of diagnosis and treatment (Figs. 25–37 to 25–43).

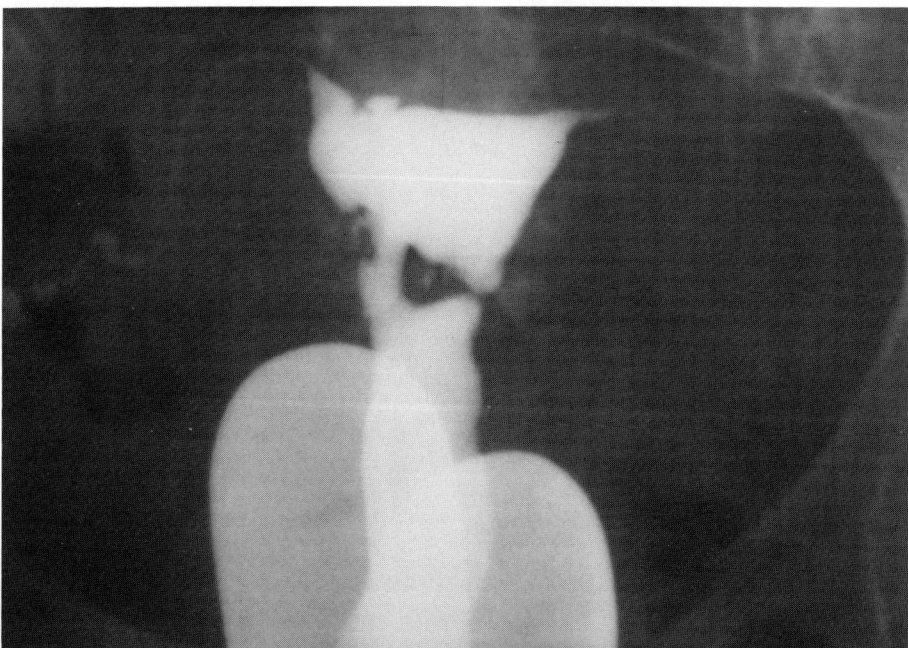

FIGURE 25–37. Hysterosalpingogram showing filling defects in the uterine cavity compatible with adhesions.

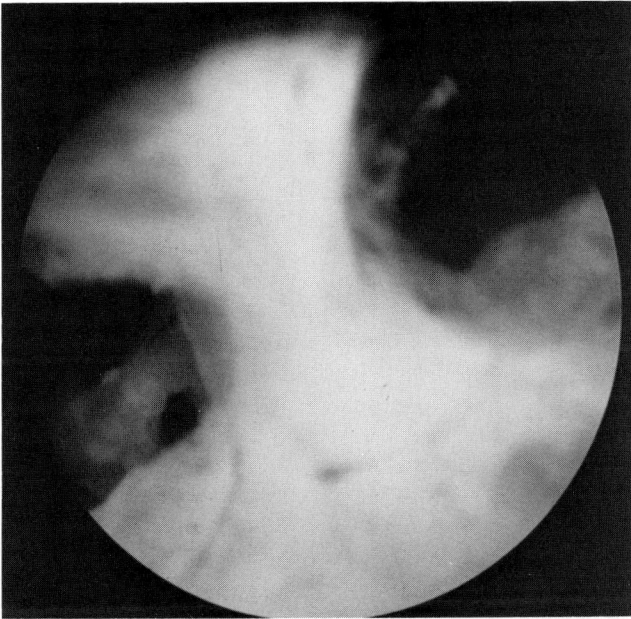

FIGURE 25–38. At hysteroscopy, an hourglass adhesion unifying uterine walls.

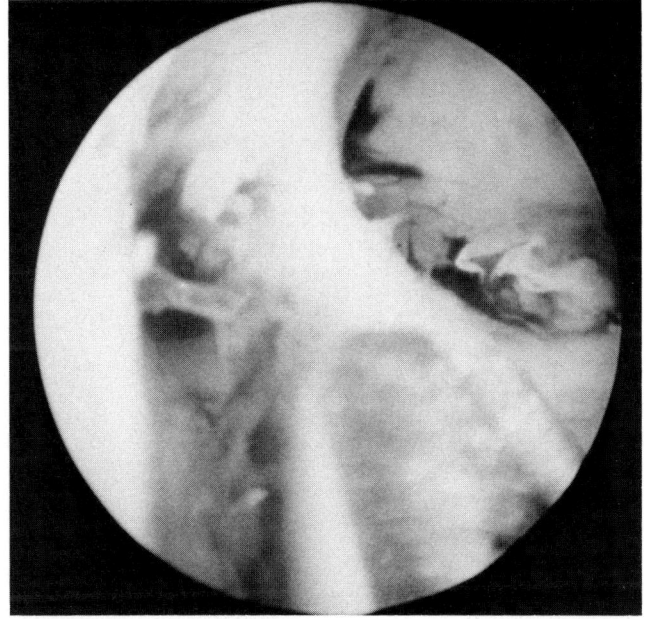

FIGURE 25–40. Right-sided marginal adhesion, with hysteroscopic scissors approaching the adhesion for division.

UTERINE ANOMALIES: SEPTUM

The septate uterus is the most common uterine malformation associated with reproductive wastage. The classic clinical picture is that of repeated early mid-trimester pregnancy wastage, with signs of labor and bleeding. This condition has classically been treated by abdominal metroplasty, with excision of the septum through a wedge uterine excision (Jones) or incision of the septum without excision to prevent reduction of size of the uterine cavity (Tompkins).[23, 24] Both operations require a laparotomy and division of the uterine corpus.

To avoid laparotomy and uterine bisection, which can predispose to pelvic adhesions and secondary infertility, the septate uterus has been treated with hysteroscopy using transcervical division of the septum (Figs. 25–44 to 25–46). Experience is increasing; the results compare well with those achieved by abdominal metroplasty but promise to surpass them.

Hysteroscopic metroplasty has become the treatment of choice for the symptomatic septate uterus because of its relative simplicity, low morbidity, excellent success, and avoidance of laparotomy and uterine bisection. Furthermore, a woman treated by this procedure does not require a cesarean section, because the myometrium has not been incised. In

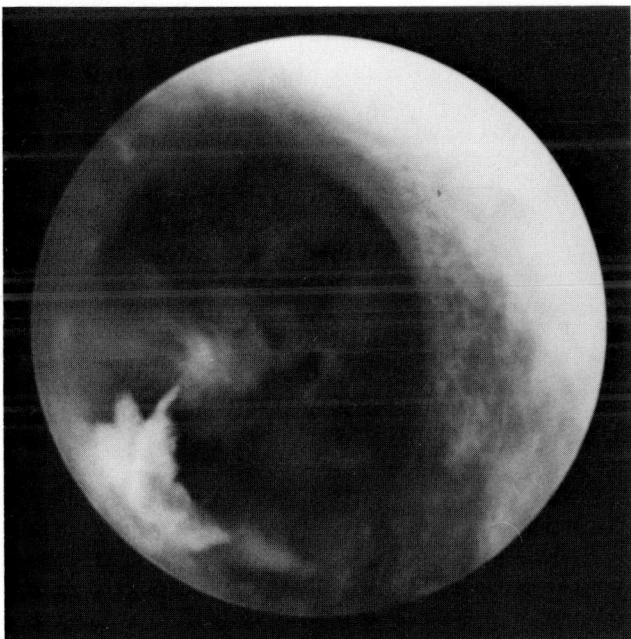

FIGURE 25–39. Following hysteroscopic treatment of adhesions, the uterine cavity's symmetry is reestablished.

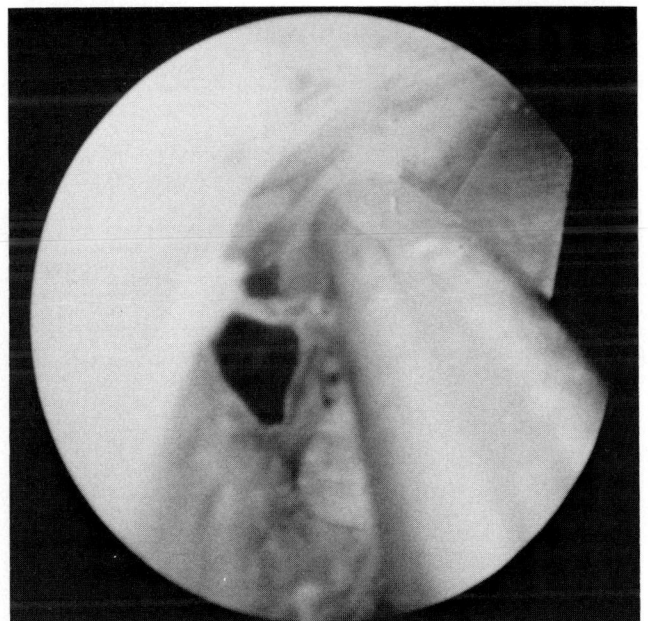

FIGURE 25–41. Hysteroscopic division of adhesion (scissors).

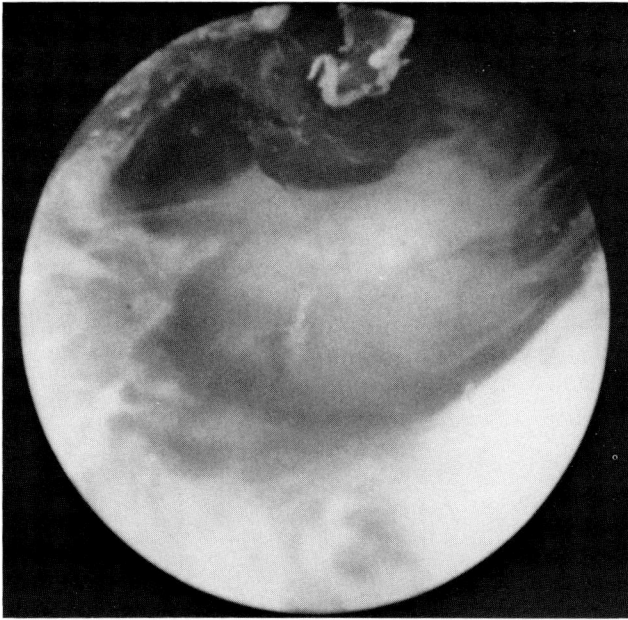

FIGURE 25–42. Normal uterine cavity's symmetry reestablished after hysteroscopic treatment.

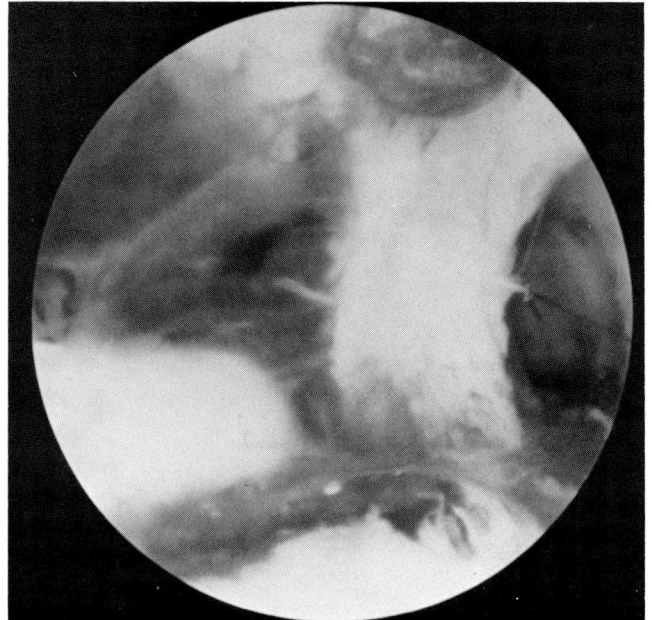

FIGURE 25–43. Extensive uterine cavity occlusion with thick connective tissue adhesions.

addition, the woman can attempt pregnancy after only a month following the surgery and after the completion of adjuvant hormonal therapy (estrogens-progesterone). The reproductive outcome of these patients has been excellent, when treatment has been provided. Because of recurrent pregnancy wastage following treatment, most women achieve pregnancy, and of those who do, about 90% deliver a viable infant.[25–28] In patients with pregnancy wastage, the fertility potential is preserved and the viable pregnancy rate approaches 90%.

OTHER CLINICAL APPLICATIONS

Hysteroscopy is also of value in exploring the cervical canal in patients with repeated pregnancy losses; the internal cervical os can be seen and anatomic defects can be diagnosed. A dynamic appraisal of the endocervical canal is possible during the hysteroscopic examination, because many of these patients demonstrate a loss of the anatomic relationship between the corpus and the cervix, losing the sphincter-like

action of the internal cervical os. Also, uterine anomalies can be observed directly.

When an early first-trimester pregnancy termination fails, and the pathologic and histologic examination of the contents evacuated does not demonstrate chorionic villi, an ectopic pregnancy should be suspected, particularly if the pregnancy test is persistently positive. When laparoscopy fails to find tubal pathology or lesions of the ovary or peritoneum consistent with an ectopic pregnancy, hysteroscopy may be of value. Occasionally, hysteroscopy may detect an anomalous uterus, such as a septate or bicornuate uterus with an early pregnancy in a horn or other site not curetted. This visual evaluation can guide a suction curettage for the transcervical termination of the missed pregnancy.[29]

The clinical use of intrauterine devices (IUDs) for fertility control has greatly decreased, but many women still use these devices, and occasionally the filaments are lost and not seen at the external cervical os. Unnecessary radiation may occur when radiographs are used for diagnostic purposes. On many occasions, unnecessary and potentially traumatic manipula-

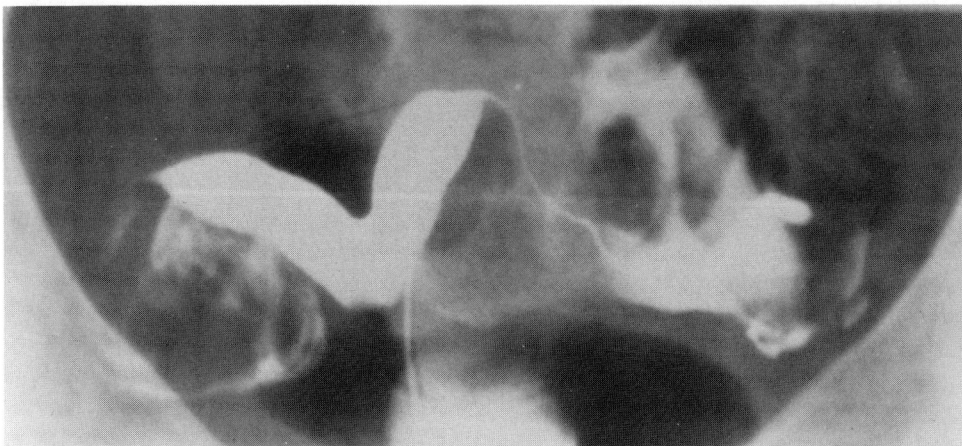

FIGURE 25–44. Hysterosalpingogram showing a divided uterine cavity, suggesting a uterine septum.

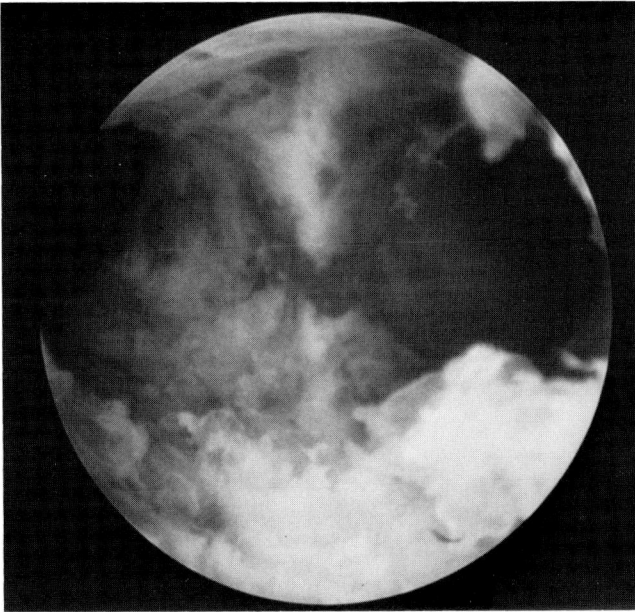

FIGURE 25–45. Hysteroscopic view of a uterine septum.

tions are performed that are troublesome and uncomfortable for the patient. Furthermore, these manipulations may fail to remove the device. With direct visualization of the endometrial cavity, the IUD can be easily located, its possible embedment ruled out, and the device removed transcervically without unnecessary damage or injury to surrounding endometrium. Therefore, hysteroscopy remains the best alternative in the evaluation and treatment of these patients.[30, 31]

Although blind tubal cannulations of the fallopian tubes were attempted by Smith[32] and Gardner[33] well over 100 years ago, and partial tubal cannulations were performed hysteroscopically in the 1920s,[4] it was not until the late 1960s[34] and early 1970s[35] that true hysteroscopic tubal cannulations were safely performed.

The introduction of tubal cannulation for sterilization purposes by Quinones-Guerrero and associates[35, 36] in 1972 paved the way to more refined techniques of tubal cannulations now in use, particularly with the introduction of softer and thinner catheters better suited to be guided under hysteroscopy into the tubal openings. These new catheters, which are the approximate size of 3-Fr, can be guided over a flexible guide wire less than 0.5 mm in diameter.[37]

Tubal cornual occlusions demonstrated by HSG are assessed by laparoscopy to rule out spurious occlusions due to a spasm. When the obstruction is confirmed on laparoscopy, hysteroscopy is performed, and an attempt is made to cannulate the tubes. When cannulation is unsuccessful, true occlusion secondary to fibrosis is likely and microsurgery will be necessary for the reestablishment of patency. However, many patients have tubes obstructed with mucous plugs or amorphous material that is easily dislodged by cannulation. Thus, hysteroscopy not only confirms the diagnosis of true tubal obstruction but often provides by direct cannulation of the tube the reestablishment of patency, thus sparing these patients a laparotomy and microsurgery.

Hysteroscopic tubal cannulation, therefore, offers an excellent diagnostic method and appropriate therapeutic alternative for patients with nonfibrotic tubal obstructions. Because laparoscopy is performed concomitantly, additional laparoscopic therapeutic procedures may be performed, because some patients may also demonstrate periovarian and peritubal adhesions that can be treated concomitantly with hysteroscopic tubal cannulation (Fig. 25–47).

Future Indications for Hysteroscopy

There are several potential applications of hysteroscopy under investigation, but not enough data are available to confirm their clinical usefulness. These applications are listed in Table 25–6.

The topographic changes of the endometrium during the

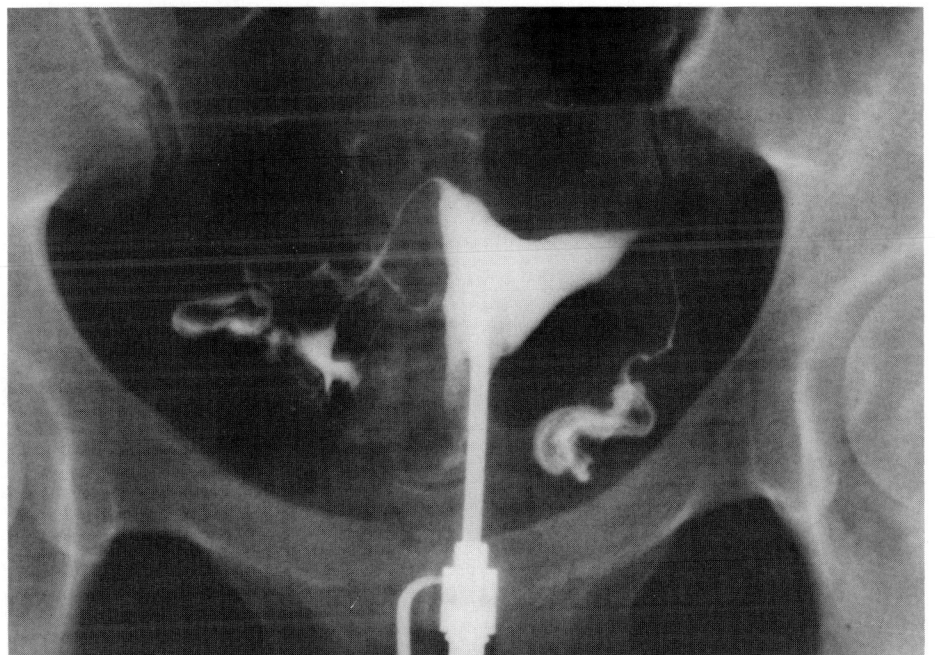

FIGURE 25–46. Hysterosalpingogram showing a normal uterine cavity after hysteroscopic division of a uterine septum.

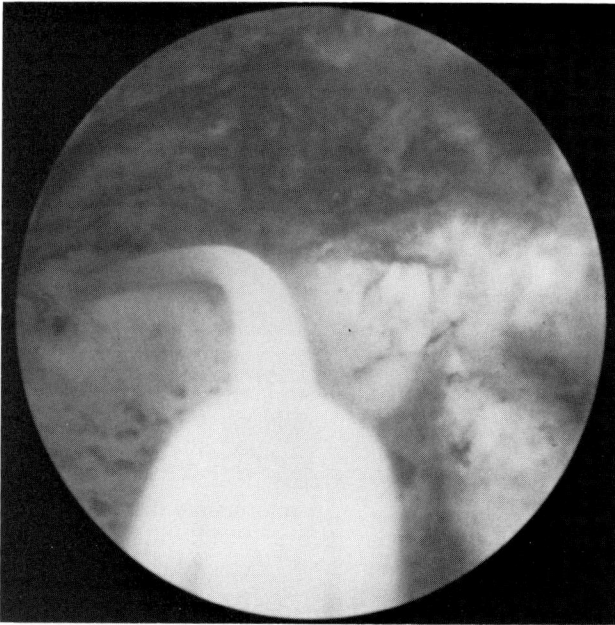

FIGURE 25–47. Hysteroscopic tubal cannulation for tubal obstruction. A soft 3 Fr catheter is inserted in the tubal lumen.

TABLE 25–6. Hysteroscopic Indications Under Investigation
Study of endometrial surface changes in various phases of menstrual cycle
Study of intratubal milieu, biochemistry of tubal secretions, tubal motility with open-ended catheters
Delivery of flexible mini-endoscopes at the uterotubal junctions for intratubal observations
Tubal occlusion by electrocoagulation, cryocoagulation, instillation of chemical substances, or placement of mechanical plugs
Application to new reproductive technologies (intratubal insemination, gamete and zygote intrafallopian transfer)
Study of endometrium to assess adequate maturity prior to in vitro fertilization–embryo transfer
Chorionic villus sampling under hysteroscopy
Embryoscopy-fetoscopy

proliferative and secretory phases of the menstrual cycle are being studied using the magnification provided by the hysteroscope. This is making it possible to describe the topographic changes of the endometrium during the normal menstrual cycle. For example, the changing pattern of superficial endometrial vascularization can be methodically examined during the menstrual cycle and correlated to the endometrial maturation.[38] Eventually, these topographic changes may be correlated with receptivity of the endometrium to the early embryo for implantation and investigation extended to women who have problems with a failure of implantation of embryo transfers.[39]

As experience in the evaluation of patients with known carcinoma of the endometrium increases, the importance of observing the extension of the carcinoma into the endocervical canal is beginning to be accepted. However, this examination will remain the responsibility of gynecologic oncologists, who can better interpret the findings and plan the appropriate therapy.

Smaller hysteroscopes with better-built operative channels have been introduced, and cannulation of the fallopian tubes is now feasible for obtaining studies of tubal secretions and evaluating ascending spermatozoa. This approach has also permitted the insertion of gametes or zygotes into the fallopian tubes via the hysteroscope. Tubal insemination is being evaluated by this approach.

The hysteroscope remains an attractive tool to eventually achieve tubal sterilization in an office setting, despite the present lack of a practical technique that is safe, effective, and reversible; nonetheless, once these technologic problems are solved, hysteroscopy may become the best technique used on an ambulatory basis to obtain tubal occlusion.[40]

Although transcervical visualization of the first 4 to 5 mL of the proximal fallopian tube can now be accomplished, the availability of a slender, flexible endoscope with sufficient resolution and clarity could provide accurate visualization of the entire intratubal lumen.[41]

Direct endoscopic chorionic villi sampling is being investigated and may provide better samples of vascularized villi, permitting accurate diagnosis in a safer and more accurate way than is provided under sonographic guidance.[42, 43] The microhysteroscope, with its detailed evaluation of the endocervical canal, may enhance our ability to diagnose early abnormal endocervical abnormalities, and the magnification provided by the instrument may facilitate the tailoring of the size of cervical conizations.[44] Used as a colpomicroscope, this new instrument may help in the evaluation of the cervical transformation zone as a screening method for early detection of carcinoma precursors of the cervix.[45, 46]

The most common indications for hysteroscopy are the evaluation of abnormal, persistent, or recurrent uterine bleeding; the evaluation of an abnormal hysterogram; the surgical treatment of intrauterine adhesions; the division of uterine septa; the removal of submucous leiomyomas; and the location and removal of misplaced intrauterine devices.

Although experience in hysteroscopy builds confidence and skill in the interpretation of pathologic lesions, skill in hysteroscopy is necessary before relying on visualization alone. Because hysteroscopic visualization of the endometrium may not provide accurate diagnosis, particularly when pathologic lesions are seen, hysteroscopically directed biopsies of these suspicious lesions should be obtained for histopathologic confirmation. Operative hysteroscopy requires additional experience and dexterity and a fundamental knowledge and expertise in diagnostic hysteroscopy. Therefore, the indications for operative hysteroscopy should be tailored to the endoscopist's experience. Hysteroscopy, therefore, may be used whenever intrauterine visualization enhances and refines diagnosis and increases the accuracy and precision of therapy.

CONTRAINDICATIONS FOR HYSTEROSCOPY

Absolute Contraindications

Absolute contraindications are pelvic inflammatory disease (PID) and profuse uterine bleeding (Table 25–7).

Pelvic Inflammatory Disease. The potential of spreading infection either systematically by hematogenous or lymphatic routes, or through the peritoneal cavity, makes PID an abso-

TABLE 25–7. Absolute Contraindications for Hysteroscopy

Pelvic inflammatory disease (vaginal, cervical, uterine, or tubal infection)
Profuse and excessive uterine bleeding

lute contraindication. Infection must be ruled out in those patients presenting with symptoms or history of recent pelvic infection by appropriate cervical cultures before hysteroscopy is undertaken, to prevent exacerbation of existing infection, and meticulous attention to technique exercised to avoid introduction of new bacteria to the endometrial cavity.

Profuse Uterine Bleeding. Regardless of the distending medium used, hysteroscopy cannot be performed satisfactorily when bleeding is excessive. If bleeding is not excessive, proper evacuation and washing of the endometrial cavity prior to uterine distention may allow an adequate uterine visualization.

Relative Contraindications

Relative contraindications to hysteroscopy, as discussed in the following sections, imply a special modification of the technique and careful attention to the nature and aims of this approach (Table 25–8).

Pregnancy. Hysteroscopy is contraindicated during pregnancy because the possibility of infection or interruption of a wanted pregnancy outweighs the value of intrauterine observation. Under special circumstances, such as removal of misplaced IUDs in early pregnancy or investigational studies of the early embryo, visualization could be performed in selected patients with a modified technique, converting the hysteroscopic examination to an amnioscopic one. Pregnancy should be ruled out, and hysteroscopy should not be attempted if the patient is pregnant and wishes to continue with an undisturbed pregnancy. The importance of the information to be obtained should be balanced against the possible adverse sequelae (interruption of the pregnancy or infection). Also, with small-caliber endoscopes, hysteroscopy is possible in early pregnancy when chorionic villus sampling or embryoscopy through a chorionic window is attempted. These latter procedures are still experimental.

Cervical Malignancy. Because of the possibility of spreading disease with cervical manipulation, patients with known carcinoma of the cervix should be excluded. Under meticulous and controlled protocols, the endocervical canal could be evaluated with a small-caliber endoscope to assess the extent of an adenocarcinoma of the cervix. Nonetheless, these

TABLE 25–8. Relative Contraindications for Hysteroscopy

Pregnancy
Carcinoma of the cervix
Menstruation
Known adenocarcinoma of the endometrium
Severe cervical stenosis
Recent uterine perforation
Slight to moderate uterine bleeding
Operator's inexperience

observations should be done in conjunction with gynecologic oncologists to establish the proper therapy.

Menstruation. Hysteroscopy should not be performed at this time of the menstrual cycle. The potential risks of infection during menstruation are increased with the possibility of pushing necrotic debris and menstrual blood through the fallopian tubes into the peritoneal cavity during hysteroscopy; furthermore, visualization is hindered by blood and debris, despite uterine washes and flushings. Hysteroscopy should be performed following menstruation.

Adenocarcinoma of the Endometrium. When the endoscopist is inexperienced in the evaluation and treatment of this condition, a known carcinoma of the endometrium of a patient is a relative contraindication for hysteroscopy. It may be indicated, however, when done in collaboration with a gynecologic oncologist, who can evaluate the extent of the corporeal adenocarcinoma and map its extension to the cervical canal.

Cervical Stenosis. When this condition cannot be overcome by the usual methods of dilation of the endocervical canal, it becomes a contraindication to hysteroscopy; if the endoscope, even of a smaller caliber, cannot be passed under direct vision, the procedure cannot be performed safely.

Recent Uterine Perforation. The inability to distend the uterine cavity impedes the panoramic view and may predispose to a new perforation or reopening of a recent perforation. Nonetheless, a perforation with a small sound or a small-caliber endoscope may not preclude uterine distention if appropriate precautions are taken. When a perforation has occurred, it is advisable to wait 3 months before any intrauterine manipulation is attempted.

Operator's Inexperience. Performance of hysteroscopy without supervision by clinicians never trained in the technique may convert a simple technique into a potential source of complications. Of all the contraindications, the one of greatest concern is cervical infection. Fortunately, active infections following a hysteroscopic examination have been rare. Nonetheless, a strict adherence to technique, proper indications, and avoidance of contraindications provides the best basis for a safe examination that is free of sequelae. The combination of a proper indication, absence of contraindications, meticulous technique, and an experienced surgeon will pave the way for a procedure performed without serious complications.

COMPLICATIONS OF HYSTEROSCOPY

Like any other surgical technique, hysteroscopy has potential complications. Some are related to the procedure itself, such as laceration of the cervix while applying the tenaculum to the uterine cervix and uterine perforation. Because these potential complications are due to poor attention to details or faults in the technique, they are usually preventable. The hysteroscope should be advanced gently, delicately, and always under direct vision.

The appropriate selection, evaluation, and preparation of patients for hysteroscopy help prevent infection. To avoid contamination of the cervical canal and uterine cavity during the procedure, sterile techniques should be maintained, and the procedure should be performed under meticulous protocols. Complications also may occur secondary to the distending medium used; when CO_2 gas exceeds the flow rate of 100 mL/min, hypercarbia, arrhythmias, acidosis, and even gas emboli may occur. These problems can be avoided by using only machines specifically designed for hysteroscopy, which electronically calibrate the appropriate flow rate of 40 to 60 mL/min and do not permit intrauterine pressures of more than 100 to 150 mm Hg.[47]

When using 32% dextran 70 for operative procedures, it is important to measure the amount of instilled and the amount recovered, not permitting more than 300 mL of this substance to be absorbed by the patient. Intravasation of dextran under pressure may produce noncardiogenic pulmonary edema, perhaps owing to a toxic effect of dextran at the capillary levels of the lungs and the release of tissue thromboplastin within the alveolar tissue. Furthermore, the hyperosmotic properties of these dextrans pull fluid intravascularly and may trigger pulmonary edema. Because of the effects dextran has on coagulation factors, a coagulopathy, similar to disseminated intravascular coagulation, with decrease in platelets and prolonged partial thromboplastin time and low fibrinogen, may ensue. This condition should be recognized and immediately treated accordingly with diuretics and respiratory supportive measures and, if coagulopathy ensues, with appropriate therapy.[48, 49]

When low-viscosity fluids are used to distend the uterine cavity during operative hysteroscopy, the most frequent complication may be due to fluid overload and electrolyte imbalance, particularly if no electrolytes are used in the distending solution. Therefore, the volume of fluids administered as well as the volume recovered should be meticulously measured. The differential, which indicates the approximate amount of fluid absorbed by the patient, should be determined and should not exceed 1 L.

Diagnostic hysteroscopy carries practically no morbidity, but operative hysteroscopy, owing to the complex surgical nature of the procedures and the time required to complete the operations, may predispose the patient to complications.

Other complications specifically related to the operation may occur. For example, perforation of the uterus may occur during the removal of submucous leiomyomas or the division of intrauterine adhesions or a uterine septum. Complications may also be related to the energy used during operative procedures. For example, the resectoscopic electrode may cause coagulation beyond the intended depth, thus producing necrosis of the uterine wall and bowel injury.[50] This applies as well to fiberoptic lasers, such as the neodymium: YAG, KTP-532, and argon types.

To decrease the chances of damage to the uterus or other surrounding organs during operative hysteroscopy, when the operations require extensive manipulations and dissections, laparoscopy should be used to monitor these operations. This is particularly important during division of uterine septa or severe and extensive intrauterine adhesions, during tubal cannulations for tubal obstructions, and during resection of sessile leiomyomas with the resectoscope.

It is important for beginning hysteroscopists to continually strive to increase their skills in using the hysteroscope for diagnosis and therapy. After mastering diagnostic hysteroscopy and minor surgical procedures, the physician can advance to more difficult operations that require more experience and dexterity. This approach ensures the effective and relatively simple use of hysteroscopy in a clinical setting.

SUMMARY

Intrauterine visualization has been facilitated by several technologic advancements that have permitted the easy and atraumatic use of the hysteroscope. In addition, improved visualization has been made possible by improved lens systems and fiberoptics for light transmission. The uterine cavity can be distended safely with a variety of media, permitting an excellent panoramic view and extensive intrauterine operations.

Small-caliber endoscopes that can be introduced atraumatically to explore the endocervical canal and uterine cavity without previous cervical dilation permit safe, simple, and effective hysteroscopy in an office setting. Office hysteroscopy has become increasingly popular by decreasing morbidity, expense, and inconvenience to patients.

The indications for operative hysteroscopy have expanded dramatically in the past decade. Thus, procedures such as the division of uterine septa, the treatment of intrauterine adhesions, the removal of submucous leiomyomas, and the treatment of tubal cornual obstructions that have previously required a laparotomy can be performed effectively with less morbidity through the hysteroscope.

Indications for hysteroscopy are well defined, particularly for the evaluation of patients with abnormal uterine bleeding, evaluation of the abnormal hysterogram, treatment of intrauterine adhesions, resection of uterine septa, removal of submucous leiomyomas, tubal cannulation, and endometrial ablation. New indications are under investigation, including the evaluation of the endometrium during the menstrual cycle and transcervical salpingoscopy.

Knowledge of the technique of diagnostic and operative hysteroscopy, its proper indications, and absolute and relative contraindications, as well as awareness of its possible complications, will serve as the background for the utilization of hysteroscopy in a safe and effective manner, with maximum benefits to patients.

Hysteroscopy is the best method of intrauterine evaluation and an excellent aid in diagnosis and treatment of intrauterine pathology.

REFERENCES

1. Porto R, Gaujoux J. Une Nouvelle Methode d' hysteroscopie. J Gynecol Obstet Biol Reprod 1972;1:691.
2. Quinones-Guerrero R, Aznar-Ramos R, Alvarado-Duran A. Tubal electrocauterization under hysteroscopic control. Contraception 1973;7:195.
3. Sciarra JJ, Butler JC, Speidel JJ, editors. Hysteroscopic Sterilization. New York: Intercontinental Medical Book, 1974.
4. von Mikulicz-Radecki F, Freund A. Ein neues Hysteroskop und seine proktische Anwendung in der Gynaekologie. Z Geburtshilfe Gynaekol 1927;92:13.
5. Ahumada JC, Gandolfo-Herrera R. Histeroscopia. Rev Med Lat Am 1935;21:265.
6. Norment WB. Hysteroscope in diagnosis of pathological conditions of uterine canal. JAMA 1952;148:917.
7. Norment WB. The hysteroscope. Am J Obstet Gynecol 1956;71:426.
8. Norment WB, Sikes CH, Berry FX, Bird J. Hysteroscopy. Surg Clin North Am 1957;37:1377.
9. Valle RF, Sciarra JJ. Current status of hysteroscopy in gynecologic practice. Fertil Steril 1979;32:619.
10. Valle RF. Hysteroscopic evaluation of patients with abnormal uterine bleeding. Surg Gynecol Obstet 1981;153:521.
11. Valle RF. Hysteroscopy in the evaluation of female infertility. Am J Obstet Gynecol 1980;137:425.

12. Valle RF. Hysteroscopy in the evaluation of infertility. In: Winfield AC, Wentz AC, editors. Diagnostic Imaging in Infertility. Baltimore: Williams & Wilkins, 1992:117–150.

13. Fayez JA, Mutie G, Schneider PJ. The diagnostic value of hysterosalpingography and hysteroscopy in infertility investigation. Am J Obstet Gynecol 1987;156:558.

14. Snowden EU, Jarret JC, Dawood MY. Comparison of diagnostic accuracy of laparoscopy, hysteroscopy, and hysterosalpingography in evaluation of female infertility. Fertil Steril 1984;41:709.

15. Sciarra JJ, Valle RF. Hysteroscopy: a clinical experience with 320 patients. Am J Obstet Gynecol 197;127:340.

16. Valle RF. Hysteroscopic removal of submucous leiomyomas. J Gynecol Surg 1990;6:89.

17. Neuwirth RS. Hysteroscopic management of symptomatic submucous fibroids. Obstet Gynecol 1983;62:509.

18. Loffer FD. Removal of large symptomatic intrauterine growths by the hysteroscopic resectoscope. Obstet Gynecol 1990;76:836.

19. Corson SL, Brooks PG. Resectoscopic myomectomy. Fertil Steril 1991;55:1041.

20. March GM, Israel R. Gestational outcome following hysteroscopic lysis of adhesions. Fertil Steril 1981;36:455.

21. Sanfilippo JS, Fitzgerald MR, Badawy SZA, et al. Asherman's syndrome: a comparison of therapeutic methods. J Reprod Med 1982;27:328.

22. Valle RF, Sciarra JJ. Intrauterine adhesions: hysteroscopic diagnosis, classification, treatment, and reproductive outcome. Am J Obstet Gynecol 1988;158:1459.

23. Jones HW, Jones GES. Double uterus as an etiological factor in repeated abortion: indication for surgical repair. Am J Obstet Gynecol 1953;65:325.

24. Tompkins P. Comments on the bicornuate uterus and twinning. Surg Clin North Am 1962;42:1049.

25. Valle RF, Sciarra JJ. Hysteroscopic treatment of the septate uterus. Obstet Gynecol 1986;67:253.

26. DeCherney AH, Russell JB, Graebe RA, Polan ML. Resectoscopic management of Müllerian fusion defects. Fertil Steril 1986;45:726.

27. March CM, Israel R. Hysteroscopic management of recurrent abortion caused by septate uterus. Am J Obstet Gynecol 1987;156:834.

28. Daly DC, Maier D, Soto-Albors C. Hysteroscopic metroplasty: six years' experience. Obstet Gynecol 1989;73:201.

29. Valle RF, Sabbagha RS. Management of first-trimester pregnancy termination failures. Obstet Gynecol 1980;55:625.

30. Siegler AM, Kemmann EK. Location and removal of misplaced or embedded intrauterine devices by hysteroscopy. J Reprod Med 1976;16:139.

31. Valle RF, Sciarra JJ, Freeman DW. Hysteroscopic removal of intrauterine devices with missing filaments. Obstet Gynecol 1977;49:55.

32. Siegler AM, Valle RF, Lindemann HJ, Mencaglia L. Tubal cannulation. In: Therapeutic Hysteroscopy: Indications and Techniques. St. Louis: CV Mosby, 1990:164.

33. Gardner AK. The Causes and Curative Treatment of Sterility with a Preliminary Statement of the Physiology of Generation. New York: DeWitt and Davenport, 1856.

34. Menken FC. Endoscopic observations of endocrine processes and hormonal changes. In: Ruiz-Albretch F, Ramirez-Sanchez J, Willowitzer H, editors. Simposio sobre Esteroides Sexuales. Museo Nocional, Bogota, Colombia, June 24–26, 1968. Berlin: Saladruck, 1969:276.

35. Quinones-Guerrero R, Alvarado-Duran A, Aznar-Ramos R. Tubal catheterization: applications of a new technique. Am J Obstet Gynecol 1972;114:674.

36. Alvarado A, Quinones-Guerrero R, Aznar R. Tubal instillation of quinacrine under hysteroscopic control. In: Sciarra JJ, Butler JC, Speidel JJ, editors. Hysteroscopic Sterilization. New York: Intercontinental Medical Book, 1974:85.

37. Novy MJ, Thurmond AS, Patton P, et al. Diagnosis of cornual obstruction by transcervical fallopian tube cannulation. Fertil Steril 1988;50:434.

38. van Herendael B, Stevens M, Flakiewicz-Kula A, Hansch C. Dating of the endometrium by microhysteroscopy. Gynecol Obstet Invest 1987;24:114.

39. Bordt J, Belkien L, Vancaillie T, et al. Ergebnisse diagnostischer hysteroskopien in einem IVF/ET-Programm. Geburts u Frauenheilk 1984;44:813.

40. Valle RF. Hysteroscopic sterilization. In: Baggish MS, Barbot J, Valle RF, editors. Diagnostic and Operative Hysteroscopy: A Text and Atlas. Chicago: Year Book Medical, 1989:195–203.

41. Kerin J, Dayhovsky L, Segalowitz J, et al. Falloposcopy: a microendoscopic technique for visual exploration of the human fallopian tube from the uterotubal ostium to the fimbria using a transvaginal approach. Fertil Steril 1990;54:390.

42. Mencaglia L, Ricci G, Perino A, et al. Hysteroscopic chorionic villi sampling: a new approach. Acta Eur Fertil 1986;17:491.

43. Ghilardini G, Gualerzi C, Fachi F, et al. Chorionoscopy and chorionic villi sampling. Acta Eur Fertil 1986;17:495.

44. West JH, Charnock MF. The influence of microcolpo-hysteroscopy on cone biopsy practice. J Obstet Gynaecol 1989;9:323.

45. Hamou J, Salat-Baroux J, Coupez F, DeBrux J. Microhysteroscopy: a new approach to the diagnosis of cervical intraepithelial neoplasia. Obstet Gynecol 1984;63:567.

46. Valle RF. Future growth and development of hysteroscopy. Obstet Gynecol Clin North Am 1988;15:111–126.

47. Gallinat A. The effect of carbon dioxide during hysteroscopy. In: Van der Pas H, Van Herendael B, van Lith D, Keith L, editors. Hysteroscopy. Boston: MTP Press, 1982:19–27.

48. Zbella EA, Moise J, Carson SA. Noncardiogenic pulmonary edema secondary to intrauterine instillation of 32% dextran 70. Fertil Steril 1985;43:479.

49. Mangar D, Gerson JI, Constantine RM, Leuzi V. Pulmonary edema and coagulopathy due to Hyskon (32% dextran-70) administration. Anesth Analg 1989;68:686.

50. Peterson HB, Hulka JF, Phillips JM. American Association of Gynecologic Laparoscopists' 1988 Membership Survey on Operative Hysteroscopy. J Reprod Med 1990;35:590.

CHAPTER 26

Tubal Microendoscopy: Salpingoscopy and Falloposcopy

JOHN F. KERIN,
ANTHONY C. PEARLSTONE,
and ERIC S. SURREY

The last decade has witnessed the transformation of tubal microendoscopy from theory to reality. The key role of the human fallopian tube in reproduction as well as its involvement with several prevalent disease processes underscores the potential applications of such technology. Two distinct approaches have been used to image endotubal anatomy. *Salpingoscopy* refers to procedures using transfimbrial access for performing tubal endoscopy. This technique requires an incision (either via laparoscopy or laparotomy) to enter the peritoneal cavity, followed by the introduction of an endoscope via the distal tubal opening. To date, this approach has not been successful at imaging the intramural segment of the fallopian tube. In contrast, *falloposcopy* is a nonincisional, transvaginal technique for tubal microendoscopy that accesses the oviduct via the uterotubal ostium. Such an approach is capable of imaging the interior anatomy of the entire fallopian tube. This chapter reviews the current status of each of these procedures as well as highlights advances in this field.

SALPINGOSCOPY

Instrumentation and Distention Media

Reports of successful salpingoscopy were first published in the early 1980s.[1-3] Since that time, a number of investigators have used a variety of flexible and rigid endoscopes of small diameter to perform this procedure (Table 26–1).[4-16] The optical systems currently used in rigid endoscopes provide clear images with a panoramic field of view. Flexible endoscopes, however, are thought to be less traumatic to the endosalpinx.[4] In addition, the only salpingoscope that has, to date, been reported to access and image the isthmic portion of the tube effectively has used flexible, fiberoptic technol-

ogy.[11] Thus, although both types of instrumentation have potential utility, the flexible systems seem to offer the greatest promise. Several rigid and flexible endoscopes are currently marketed specifically for distal tubal imaging procedures (salpingoscopes). A number of other endoscopes, however, might serve this purpose equally well (see Table 26–1).

Independent of the salpingoscope used, distention of the tubal lumen is necessary to image the endosalpinx effectively. Although carbon dioxide gas has been used successfully,[1, 5] a liquid medium (lactated Ringer's[3] or a saline solution[8]) is thought to be preferable. Carbon dioxide has been reported to flatten the ampullary folds, which prevents an adequate examination.[4] Furthermore, its drying effect is also a potential concern.

Technique

Rigid and flexible salpingoscopy have been performed both at laparotomy[7] and at laparoscopy.[4, 12] At laparotomy, the salpingoscope is introduced into the distal tubal ostium by manually stabilizing and aligning the oviduct.[7] At laparoscopy, the salpingoscope is introduced into the peritoneal cavity either via the operative channel of an appropriately equipped laparoscope[8] or through an auxiliary port. The fallopian tube is then aligned and stabilized with an atraumatic forceps along its antimesenteric border.[7] Under laparoscopic monitoring, the salpingoscope is introduced into the distal ostium of the tube. Aside from this step, the procedure is identical at laparotomy and laparoscopy. After introduction of the endoscope into the ostium, irrigation using a balanced salt solution is initiated to provide tubal distention. The salpingoscope is then gently advanced toward the cornua until resistance is sensed. This usually occurs at the ampulloisthmic junction, unless a more distal stenosis or obstruction is identified. One group has reported successfully accessing the isthmic portion of the tube using a flexible, fiberoptic endoscope.[11] When the salpingoscope has been advanced to the most proximal point that gentle technique allows, imaging is then performed by withdrawing the endoscope while maintaining irrigation. Imaging proceeds systematically in a retrograde fashion through the ampulla and out the distal tube. These maneuvers optimize visualization. The salpingoscope is usually attached to a camera system that allows the study to be observed on a video screen and simultaneously recorded.

Certain cases require antecedent adhesiolysis to mobilize the oviduct and allow access to the distal tubal ostium. In addition, hydrosalpinges are entered by making a small incision at the site of occlusion.[6]

Normal Anatomy

Salpingoscopic descriptions of the distal fallopian tube in presumably normal women have been reported.[3, 6] The infundibulum is characterized by several large, radially arranged folds. The normal ampulla demonstrates three to six major folds, with several minor folds interspersed between them. The major and minor folds are approximately 4 and 1 mm in height.[6] Secondary folds, with a delicate vascular pattern, arise from the major folds (Fig. 26–1). The ampulloisthmic junction has several folds, regularly distributed, that diverge from the isthmus toward the ampulla.[3] To date, no systematic salpingoscopic descriptions of the isthmic or intramural tubal segments have been published.

Pathology

A variety of endotubal abnormalities have been observed during salpingoscopy. Pathologic entities include fimbrial agglutination,[7] intraluminal synechiae (both bridge and cobweb types),[3] stenoses,[4] and prominent vascular patterns suggestive of inflammation (Fig. 26–2; see color section in the center of the book).[6] Other findings, including flattening, increased separation, or loss of the major folds[6] as well as mucosal atrophy,[4] have been noted in association with hydrosalpinges. A classification of disease severity for hydrosalpinges, based on the extent and character of mucosal abnormality, has been described.[8] One difficulty, however, in integrating the results of salpingoscopic investigations to date has been the lack of

a general, standardized classification system for pathologic (and normal) findings. Such a system has been prospectively validated in falloposcopic studies[17] and is reviewed in detail later in this chapter. This system has also been adapted for use in salpingoscopic examinations.[11]

Indications

GENERAL CONSIDERATIONS

Currently there are no generally accepted indications for salpingoscopy. Mounting data, however, support its utility in the evaluation of hydrosalpinges. The following discussion reviews the available data on hydrosalpinges as well as on other conditions in which this technology has potential clinical application.

HYDROSALPINGES

The importance of the endotubal mucosa as a prognostic variable in the outcome of surgical treatment for hydrosalpinges is recognized.[18] In the past, this has been assessed indirectly by a preoperative hysterosalpingogram (HSG).[19] Several studies have compared the results of HSG with concomitant salpingoscopy.[3, 4, 8] These investigations demonstrated a false-negative (normal muscosa by HSG with abnormal salpingoscopy) rate for HSG of 45% (range 42% to 48%). They also found a false-positive rate (abnormal muscosa by HSG with normal salpingoscopy) of 30% (range 21% to 40%) for HSG.

Salpingoscopic examination has been reported to be predictive of luminal patency after microsurgical tuboplasty. In one series, postoperative reocclusion occurred in 12 of 17 women with bilateral salpingoscopic abnormalities, compared with patency in 12 of 14 patients with at least one endoscopically normal tube.[14]

The prognostic value of salpingoscopy for tuboplasty outcome has also been assessed using pregnancy as an end point. In the largest series to date, Henry-Suchet and colleagues[13] determined the predictive value of salpingoscopy in 136 women who underwent simultaneous tuboplasty. When the 80 women with normal salpingoscopic findings were compared with 56 women with abnormal ampullary mucosae, statistically significant differences were found in the rate of total pregnancies (50% versus 19%), intrauterine pregnancies (46% versus 9%), and ongoing pregnancies (43% versus 0%). The length of followup ranged from 1 to 3 years. Four percent of women with normal mucosa (8% of conceptions) had ectopic pregnancies, compared with 10% of women (55% of conceptions) with abnormal salpingoscopic examinations. Several other studies have reported consistent findings.[10, 12, 14] It is noteworthy that Henry-Suchet and colleagues observed normal uterine pregnancies only in women with at least one salpingoscopically normal tube, independent of the HSG findings. On the basis of these observations, these authors concluded that salpingoscopy is superior to HSG for predicting the chances for pregnancy after tuboplasty.

SUSPECTED TUBAL DISEASE

Pelvic abnormalities, including adhesions and fimbrial agglutination, have been associated with abnormal salpingos-

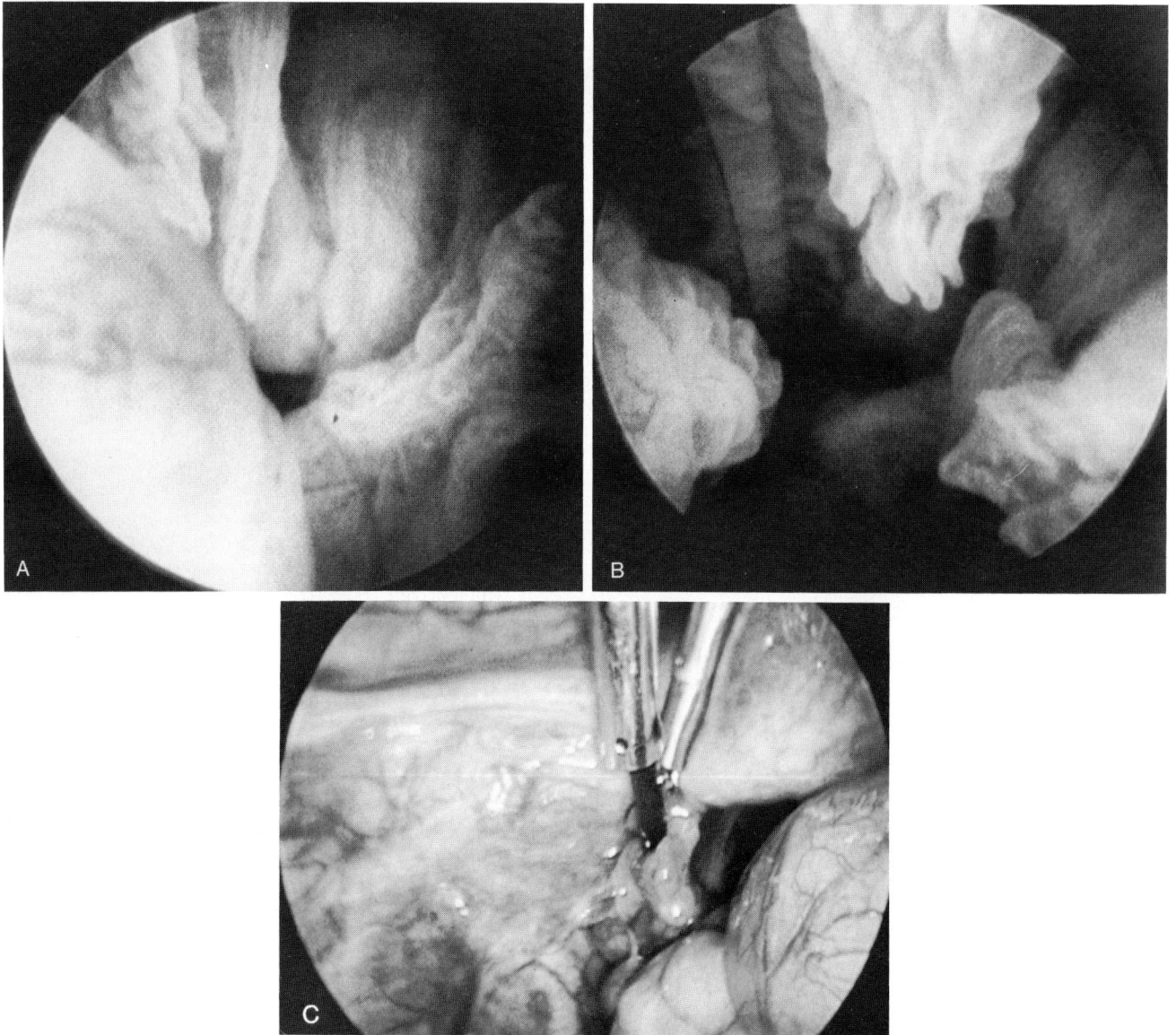

FIGURE 26–1. Salpingoscopic views of normal distal tubal anatomy. A, The infundibulum is characterized by several large, radially oriented folds. B, The normal ampullary mucosa is characterized by three to six major folds, with secondary folds arising from them and several minor folds between them. C, Laparoscopic view of a salpingoscope in the distal fallopian tube. (A and B from Brosens I, Boeckx W, Delattin P, et al. Salpingoscopy: a new preoperative diagnostic tool in tubal infertility. Br J Obstet Gynaecol 1987; 94:768–773. Reprinted by permission of Blackwell Scientific Publications Ltd.)

copic findings in 57% to 75% of cases.[7, 16] Conversely, relying solely on the pelvic findings in lieu of an endoscopic study would result in a 25% to 43% false-positive rate. Thus, salpingoscopy seems to offer a modality for correctly classifying such patients.

ENDOMETRIOSIS

Shapiro and associates[7] reported that four of six patients with mild endometriosis (by the revised American Fertility Society classification system) had intratubal abnormalities in at least one fallopian tube. Nezhat and associates[9] then undertook a prospective salpingoscopic study involving 100 women with minimal-to-moderate endometriosis and 20 normal controls. Neither group had any evidence of intratubal pathology, and only five women in the endometriosis

group had perifimbrial adhesions. Thus, at present, the evidence suggests that the presence of lesser stages of pelvic endometriosis per se should not be considered an indication for salpingoscopy.

UNEXPLAINED INFERTILITY

In infertile women with normal pelvic findings at laparoscopy, salpingoscopic abnormalities have been reported in 27% to 37% of tubes.[4, 16] In one series, Cornier[4] performed salpingoscopy in 54 patients with unexplained infertility (mean duration of 4 years). In 40 tubes (37%), periostial, ampullary, or fimbrial adhesions were detected by salpingoscopy, despite normal laparoscopic examinations. In 17 instances, these adhesions were bluntly lysed, with 11 of 17 women (65%) becoming pregnant in an average of 3 to 4

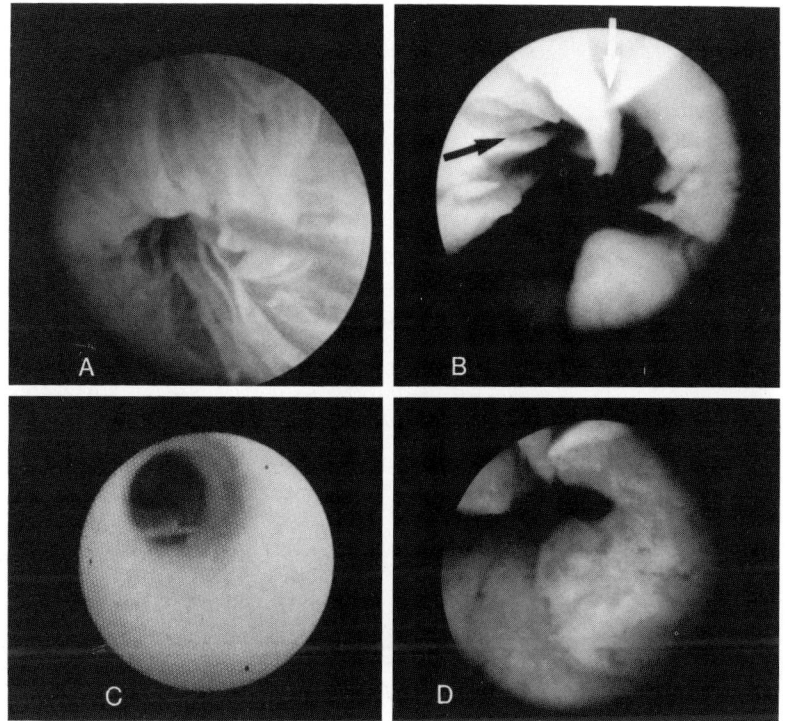

FIGURE 26–2. Salpingoscopic view of a normal ampulla (*A* and *B*). Primary and secondary folds are indicated by the *white* and *black arrows*, respectively. An intraluminal isthmic adhesion is demonstrated with a view obtained via a flexible salpingoscope (*C*). The ampullary lumen in a patient with a severe hydrosalpinx (*D*) is devoid of primary and secondary folds, with abnormal vessel formation. (*A* through *D* from Herschlag A, Seifer DB, Carcangiu ML, et al. Salpingoscopy: light microscopic and electron microscopic correlations. Reprinted with permission from The American College of Obstetricians and Gynecologists [Obstetrics and Gynecology, 1991, 77, 399–405].)

months. This uncontrolled study, although interesting, awaits confirmation. These data do suggest that further investigation on the utility of salpingoscopy in the evaluation of unexplained infertility is warranted.

ECTOPIC PREGNANCY

Cornier[4] also described four cases of early suspected ectopic gestation that could not be localized by laparoscopy alone. Salpingoscopy identified the implantation site in two of these women. The role of salpingoscopy in the diagnosis or management of ectopic gestation remains to be determined.

ASSISTED REPRODUCTIVE TECHNOLOGIES

In addition to a possible role in assessing the relative efficacy of reconstructive surgery versus in vitro fertilization in the management of tubal infertility, it has been suggested that salpingoscopy may be of value in patients scheduled for assisted reproductive technologies (ART) procedures who still have apparently functional tubes.[8] Specifically, such information might be used to assess the suitability of patients for tubal transfer procedures. To date, there are no prospective data on this issue.

Contraindications

No specific contraindications have been set forth in the literature to date. Certainly contraindications to laparotomy or laparoscopy would be relevant. Further, active pelvic infection should be considered as a contraindication.

Failure Rate and Complications

Failure to achieve access to one or both fallopian tubes has been reported in anywhere from 0 to 16% of cases.[6–9] This is most often secondary to extensive pelvic adhesions. The most commonly reported complication has been a small amount of usually self-limited bleeding from the tubal site of forceps stabilization. The frequency of this occurrence has not been quantified. One tubal abscess[4] associated with salpingoscopy has been described in the more than 500 cases (more than 800 tubes) reported in the literature to date.[1–16] No cases of perforation or other intraoperative or postoperative complications attributable to this procedure have been described.

Limitations

Although the overall correlation between salpingoscopy and simultaneous histopathology has been found to be good (correlation coefficient 0.71), this relationship is reported to vary depending on the severity of the tubal disease.[11] Specifically, in a small series, Hershlag and coworkers[11] reported that salpingoscopy correctly identified normal, mildly diseased, and severely diseased oviducts but underdiagnosed two of seven cases with moderate histologic abnormalities. This indicates that salpingoscopy may underdiagnose subtle but significant tubal lesions. An incisional requirement and the inability to image the intramural segment have already been noted as limitations of this procedure.

Future

Current data indicate that salpingoscopy is a relatively safe procedure with several potential applications. Additional, prospective studies using a standardized classification system are required to delineate its role in clinical practice.

FALLOPOSCOPY

History

A description and an illustration of the passage of a wire probe through the intramural segment of the human oviduct using a transvaginal approach were presented by Gardner[20] in 1856. In 1962, Sweeney[21] studied the course the intramural oviduct took through each lateral uterine horn to the uterotubal junction in 100 posthysterectomy uterine specimens. He noted that the course of the tube through the uterine wall was variable in both caliber and direction. The intramural oviduct was tortuous in 69% of cases, and he concluded that it was not feasible to pass probes from the uterine cavity to the oviduct lumen. Mohri and colleagues[22] attempted to pass a flexible fiberoptic endoscope transcervically in 1970. A number of technical problems were encountered in this study, including difficulties in tubal cannulation and poor image quality as well as evidence of procedure-related intratubal trauma (bleeding). With these discouraging results, no further work on this topic was reported for more than a decade. In 1987, Brand and coworkers[23] attempted ex vivo transcervical tubal microendoscopy on 14 specimens, succeeding in only six cases (43%). Contemporaneously De Cherney[24] cautioned overenthusiastic investigators about the complex, narrow, and tortuous nature of the intramural oviduct, noting that harm might result from persevering with retrograde cannulation procedures. In 1990, Kerin and associates,[25, 26] however, were the first to report successful nonincisional, transvaginal tubal microendoscopy of the entire oviductal length, which they named *falloposcopy*. This achievement resulted from the integration of innovations in optics, bioengineering, and surgical technique.

Instrumentation and Media

Falloposcopy was first described as a coaxial procedure using a hysteroscope to visualize the uterotubal ostium, accessory instruments to cannulate the tubal lumen (including steerable guide wires and soft Teflon catheters), and a small endoscope (falloposcope) for tubal imaging. In addition, other instrumentation has also been used in falloposcopically monitored tuboplasty procedures. This section briefly describes this technology. It should be noted that an alternative approach for tubal access and falloposcope delivery, known as the linear-everting catheter (LEC), has been developed and is currently undergoing testing.[27] This promising technology is reviewed at the end of this chapter.

HYSTEROSCOPE-FALLOPOSCOPE SYSTEM

Modifications of angioscopic instrumentation[28, 29] were undertaken to develop a series of effective falloposcopes (Olympus PF-5X, Olympus Corp., Lake Success, New York; Intramed Laboratories, San Diego, California; Medical Dynamics Inc., Englewood, Colorado; Advanced Interventional Systems, Costa Mesa, California; Imagyn Medical, Inc., San Clemente, California). These flexible falloposcopes measure 1.5 m in length and 0.5 mm in outside diameter (OD) and have atraumatic leading ends to minimize the risk of damage or perforation. Flexible operating hysteroscopes are used to guide the falloposcope into the uterotubal ostium under direct vision (Intramed Laboratories, Olympus Corp., and Imagyn Medical, Inc.). This instrumentation is illustrated in Figure 26–3. The falloposcopic images are of sufficient definition to assess the status of the epithelial lining as well as to identify intraluminal stenoses, dilatation, polyps, and obstructions.

ACCESSORY EQUIPMENT INCLUDING GUIDE WIRES, CANNULAS, IRRIGATION SYSTEMS, WIRE GUIDE DILATORS, AND BALLOON CATHETERS

The accessory equipment used in these procedures is directed into the uterotubal ostium via the operating channel of the flexible hysteroscope under video monitoring. Flexible guide wires (Cook OB/GYN, Spencer, Indiana; Glidewire, Medi-tech, Watertown, Massachusetts; Target Therapeutics, San Jose, California), 0.3 to 0.8 mm in OD, and over-the-wire, soft Teflon catheters (Cook OB/GYN and Target Therapeutics) of up to 1.3 mm OD are used to gain tubal access. An irrigation system using gravity or pump fed (Angiopump, Olympus) lactated Ringer's solution is used for both uterine and tubal distention. Balloon catheters (Advanced Cardiovascular Systems, Temecula, California, and Target Therapeutics) with shaft diameters of 1 mm and inflated balloon diameters ranging from 2 to 5 mm over lengths of 2 cm can be used for tuboplasty procedures. Steerable wire dilators can also be used to break down intraluminal adhesions and dilate tubal stenoses, including the "Stubbie" (Target Therapeutics; OD 0.5 mm, taper length 7 cm, and overall length 175 cm), fixed core straight safety wire guides, and a slightly more flexible Teflon-coated straight Newton wire guide (Cook OB/GYN; OD 0.97 mm, overall length 125 cm).

Technique

DIAGNOSTIC FALLOPOSCOPY

After the induction of general anesthesia, the uterine cavity is gently sounded and the flexible hysteroscope inserted without prior cervical dilation. Uterine distention with lactated Ringer's solution permits end-on viewing of the tubal ostia. A guide wire enclosed in a Teflon catheter and preloaded into the hysteroscope operating channel is directed to the ostium under video monitoring. The guide wire is then advanced into the tubal ostium for a distance of 12 to 15 cm. If resistance is experienced, the guide wire is not advanced further. The Teflon catheter is then passed over the wire for a similar distance or until resistance is detected. Force is never used. The wire is then withdrawn.

The falloposcope is then introduced (via a Tuohy-Borst type **Y** adapter) into the Teflon catheter under video monitoring until it exits from the distal end of the catheter, either beyond the fimbria and into the peritoneal cavity or at some point within the tubal lumen. Lactated Ringer's solution is fed into the other arm of the **Y** adapter, to flow between the falloposcope and the lumen of the Teflon catheter. This irri-

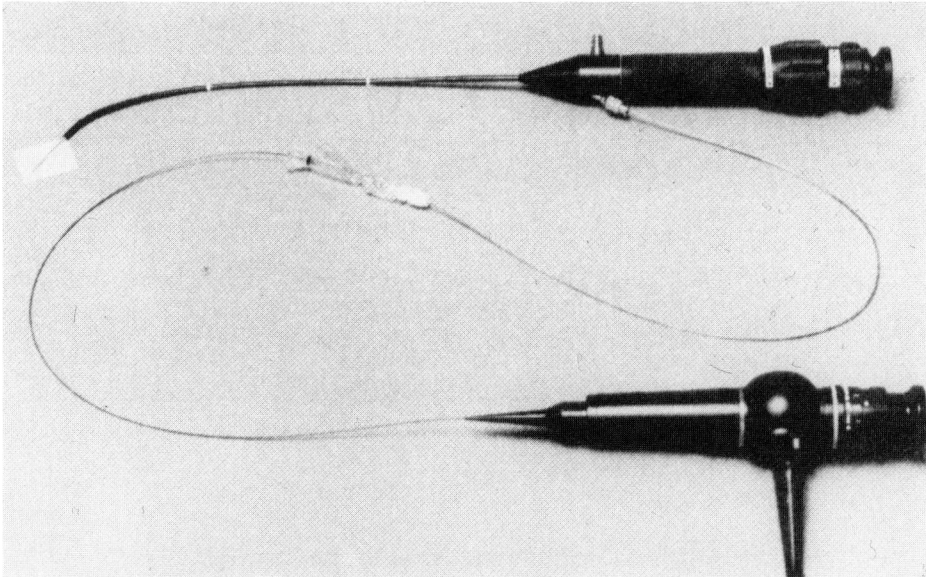

FIGURE 26–3. A falloposcope (Olympus PF-5X; Lake Success, NY) with an OD of 0.5 mm ("baby scope," *bottom instrument*), shown passing through a **Y**-adapter Teflon cannula assembly. The falloposcope in its Teflon sheath assembly is seen passing through the operating channel of a steerable miniature hysteroscope ("mother scope," *top instrument*), which has a working optical fiber OD of 3.3 mm (Intramed Laboratories, San Diego, CA). The leading end of the falloposcope (on a white background) can be seen extending 2 cm beyond the operating-channel opening of the hysteroscope. Focusing and steerability of the hysteroscope are manually operated below the eye piece. The 10-cm markings can be seen on the 30-cm hysteroscope working optical fiber. (From Kerin J, Daykhovsky L, Segalowitz J, Surrey E, Anderson R, Stein A, et al. Falloposcopy: a microendoscopic technique for visual exploration of the human fallopian tube from the uterotubal ostium to the fimbria using a transvaginal approach. Fertil Steril 1990;54:390–400. Reproduced with permission of the publisher, The American Fertility Society.)

gation facilitates movement of the falloposcope within the catheter and displaces the tubal epithelium off the falloposcope lens to permit visualization of the epithelial surface anatomy. This coaxial cannulation technique maintains a 0.3-mm space between the falloposcope (OD 0.5 mm) and the internal diameter of the Teflon sheath (0.8 mm) and allows for a flow rate of about 10 to 15 mL/minute.

Falloposcopic imaging of the endotubal surface anatomy involves slowly drawing the falloposcope-cannula system back from the fimbria toward the uterine cavity. It is important that the distal tip of the falloposcope and its end-on viewing lens be flush with the end of the protective Teflon sheath. In that way, irrigation fluid can gently lift the tubal endothelium off the lens, permitting a lens-fluid-endothelium interface to optimize image quality. If the lens directly contacts the epithelium, a "white-out" occurs. That is likely to happen if there is (1) inadequate irrigation; (2) contact with a lumenal stenosis, adhesion, or blockage; (3) protrusion of the falloposcope 1 mm or more beyond its Teflon sheath; or (4) an attempt to advance the falloposcope in an antegrade fashion from the uterotubal ostium toward the fimbria. Thus, white-outs are minimized with good irrigation, proper lens-to-sheath positioning, and retrograde falloposcopy. The technique of tubal endoscopy differs from that used in small blood vessel endoscopy because a patent vessel is naturally distended by the circulating blood, whereas the normal tubal lumen is largely a potential space occupied by mucous secretions and its secondary, branching epithelial extensions.

Dual video monitoring is used simultaneously for both continuous hysteroscopic and falloposcopic recordings. The advancing falloposcope tip can be seen laparoscopically as a bright light transilluminating through the tubal wall. Women undergoing hysteroscopy-falloposcopy are given perioperative antibiotic prophylaxis.

OPERATIVE FALLOPOSCOPY

Because falloposcopic-assisted tuboplasty is a new technique, it is recommended that it be performed under laparoscopic control until the risks of such procedures are fully established. Furthermore, laparoscopic manipulation of the tube often aids negotiation through intraluminal adhesions or strictures, provides access for surgical repair of external tubal disease, and allows visual assessment of tubal patency after a tuboplasty.

A guide wire is passed gently through the tubal ostium under hysteroscopic control and advanced until resistance is sensed. This distance from the ostium is noted and the site visualized laparoscopically. An over-the-wire Teflon catheter is then advanced to the point of resistance, and the guide wire is removed and replaced by a falloposcope. The area of resistance is evaluated falloposcopically. Intratubal pathology (Table 26–2), extrinsic tubal disease, or even marked tortuosity of an otherwise normal tube may be responsible for the resistance.[30]

Once the site, nature, and extent of the endotubal lesion has been characterized falloposcopically, specific management is then undertaken. When pathology is encountered that does not yield to the guide wire or aquadissection techniques, a Stubbie wire (Target Therapeutics) or a fixed core safety wire guide (Cook OB/GYN) can be used. Under laparoscopic observation, such wire dilators can be carefully advanced against the site of obstruction. If the obstruction is due to thin adhesions or a mild-to-moderate stenosis, it usu-

TABLE 26–2. Falloposcopic Description and Frequency Distribution of Endotubal Lesions per Tube Following 112 Falloposcopic Examinations

Type of Lesion	Intramural	Isthmic	Ampullary	Fimbrial	Incidence
Falloposcopically normal	52	52	52	52	52/112 (46%)
Obstructive debris	1	6	0	0	7/112 (6%)
Thin, nonobstructive adhesions	4	9	6	10	29/112 (26%)
Thick, nonobstructive adhesions	3	7	5	4	19/112 (17%)
Stenosis	3	7	6	2	18/112 (16%)
Fibrotic obstruction	4	9	7	6	26/112 (23%)
Polyps	2	4	1	0	7/112 (6%)
Hydrosalpinx	0	0	7	0	7/112 (6%)
Salpingitis isthmica nodosum	1	5	0	0	6/112 (5%)
Number of lesions/segment	18	47	32	22	
% of total lesions (N = 119)	15	39	27	19	

From Kerin JF, Williams DB, San Roman GA, et al. Falloposcopic classification and treatment of fallopian tube lumen disease. Fertil Steril 1992; 57:731. Reprinted with permission of the publisher, The American Fertility Society.

ally bypasses them and proceeds along the tubal lumen. If the obstruction is too resistant, the wire may take the path of least resistance and perforate the tube proximal to the obstruction. An alternative method is to use an appropriate sized balloon catheter with a fixed or coaxial wire system. It is introduced into the site of obstruction, and the balloon is then dilated at the lesion site for 50 to 60 seconds. The overlying tube blanches from stretching of the tubal wall. On deflating the balloon, the tube's pink color returns rapidly, and the catheter is withdrawn (if the stenosis is considered dilated), or the balloon is advanced another 0.5 to 1 cm and inflated again. At the completion of the tuboplasty procedure, falloposcopic re-evaluation of the stricture, adhesion, or obstruction is performed to assess the results. After removal of the falloposcope, chromotubation via the intratubal Teflon catheter can be performed to test for patency under laparoscopic visualization. Alternatively, aquadissection under moderate pressure can be used in an attempt to dislodge lumenal debris and blood clot or to lyse any remaining filmy intraluminal adhesions. Representative images from falloposcopic procedures are presented in Figures 26–4 through 26–7. (For Figs. 26–5 through 26–7, see color section in the center of the book.)

Normal Anatomy

UTEROTUBAL OSTIUM

In the relaxed state, the healthy ostial opening is sharp in outline, circular or ovoid in shape, and easily seen provided that the falloposcopy is done between day 6 and 10 of the proliferative phase of the menstrual cycle (see Fig. 26–4). Falloposcopy performed during the late proliferative and luteal phase is sometimes associated with difficulty visualizing the ostium owing to epithelial overgrowth. The thicker endometrium tends to make the ostial opening slightly smaller, and sometimes the polypoid secretory endometrium is carried into the intramural tube, making cannulation more difficult. The upper uterine cavity (uterotubal gutter) funnels toward the tubal ostium, which is situated at the bottom of a shallow, saucer-shaped indentation and measures 1 to 1.5 mm in diameter. Owing to fluid distention of the intramural tube, four to six longitudinal folds of its epithelium can be seen (see Fig. 26–5). As the tube contracts, the fourfold to sixfold puckering of the ostium appears to be continuous with these longitudinal intramural folds (see Fig. 26–4). No anatomic valve mechanism can be identified.

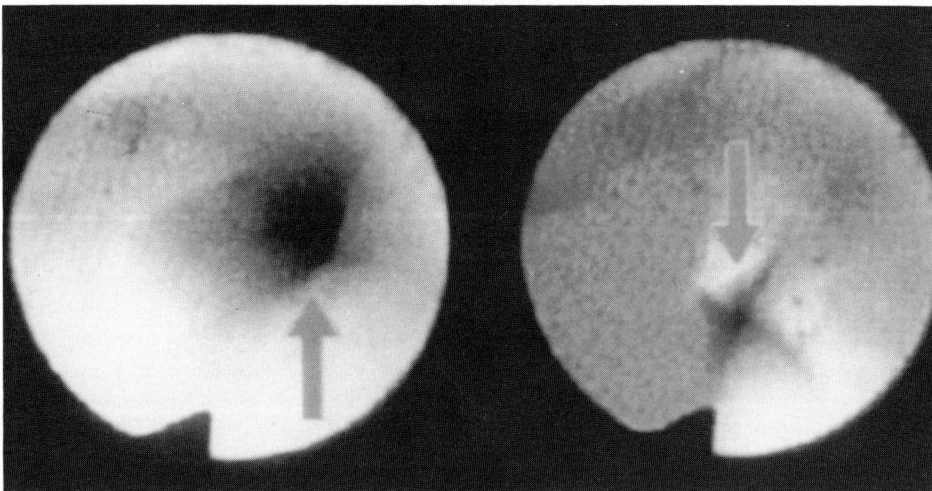

FIGURE 26–4. *Left,* Hysteroscopic view of the uterotubal ostium (*arrow*) in the relaxed state; ostium diameter is 1.3 mm. *Right,* Same ostium (*arrow*) 2 s later contracting; note the typical four-segment puckering of the contracted ostium. (From Kerin J, Daykhovsky L, Segalowitz J, Surrey E, Anderson R, Stein A, et al. Falloposcopy: a microendoscopic technique for visual exploration of the human fallopian tube from the uterotubal ostium to the fimbria using a transvaginal approach. Fertil Steril 1990;54:390–400. Reproduced with permission of the publisher, The American Fertility Society.)

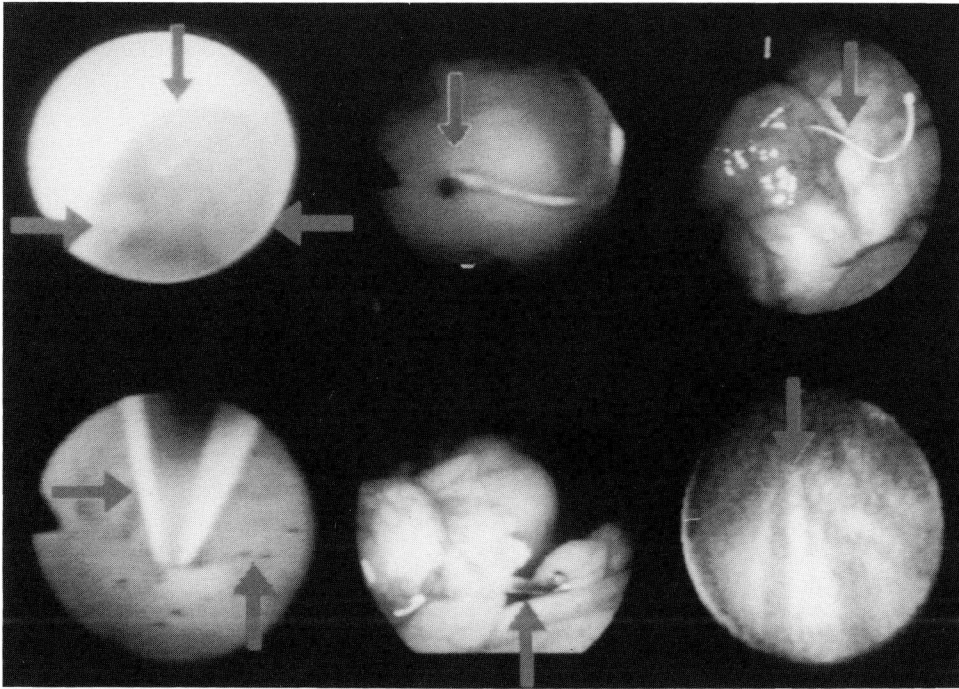

FIGURE 26–5. *Upper left,* End-on view via a miniature flexible hysteroscope into the uterotubal ostium (*arrows*) of the delicate longitudinal folds of the intramural epithelium. *Upper middle,* Flexible guide wire entering ostium (*arrow*). *Upper right,* Same platinum-tipped guide wire (*arrow*) exiting the fimbria. *Lower left,* Falloposcope enclosed in its Teflon catheter entering the ostium (*arrows*). The openings of individual proliferative endometrial glands can be seen. *Lower middle,* Close-up laparoscopic view of the same transparent Teflon cannula enclosing the falloposcope, exiting the fimbria (*arrow*). *Lower right,* Normal individual epithelial secondary branching villi containing central vascular cores, at the level of the mid-ampulla in the same tube (*arrow*). (From Kerin JF, Williams DB, San Roman GA, Pearlstone AC, Grundfest WS, Surrey ES. Falloposcopic classification and treatment of fallopian tube lumen disease. Fertil Steril 1992;57:731–741. Reproduced with permission of the publisher, The American Fertility Society.)

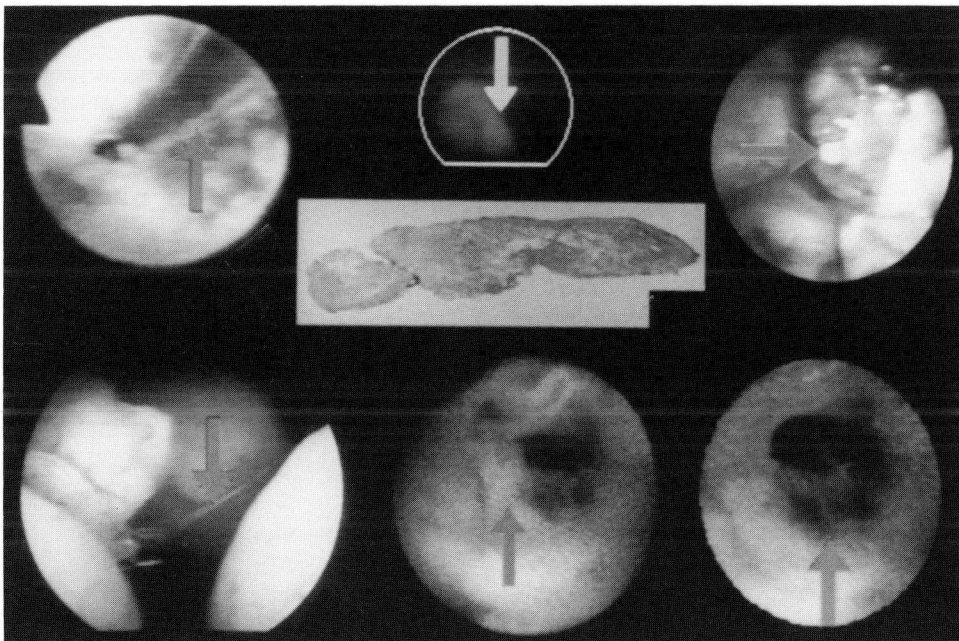

FIGURE 26–6. *Upper left,* Selective tubal cannulation (*arrow*) and aquadissection using Indigo carmine–colored lactated Ringer's solution as a contrast medium. *Upper middle (top),* The proximal white end (*arrow*) of a tubal plug occupying the isthmic lumen as contrasted against the Indigo carmine solution. *Upper middle (bottom),* A low-power microscopic view (×40) of the same entire isthmic plug measuring 3 × 0.7 × 0.7 mm, which is an intact cast consistent with an origin from the isthmic lumen. It is composed of a mixture of endothelial cells and amorphous debris.[33] *Upper right,* Mobilization of the same plug seen in the previous view (*arrow*), followed by the appearance of Indigo carmine fluid, indicating the achievement of patency. *Lower left,* A fine, clear elastic fimbrio-ovarian mucus connection (*arrow*) extending from the tip of the falloposcope and attached to the ovarian surface overlying a preovular follicle.[31] *Lower middle,* Stringy, nonobstructive adhesions (*arrow*) in a pale devascularized fibrotic and atrophic epithelium. *Lower right,* Weblike fenestrated nonobstructive isthmic adhesions (*arrow*). (From Kerin JF, Williams DB, San Roman GA, Pearlstone AC, Grundfest WS, Surrey ES. Falloposcopic classification and treatment of fallopian tube lumen disease. Fertil Steril 1992;57:731–741. Reproduced with permission of the publisher, The American Fertility Society.)

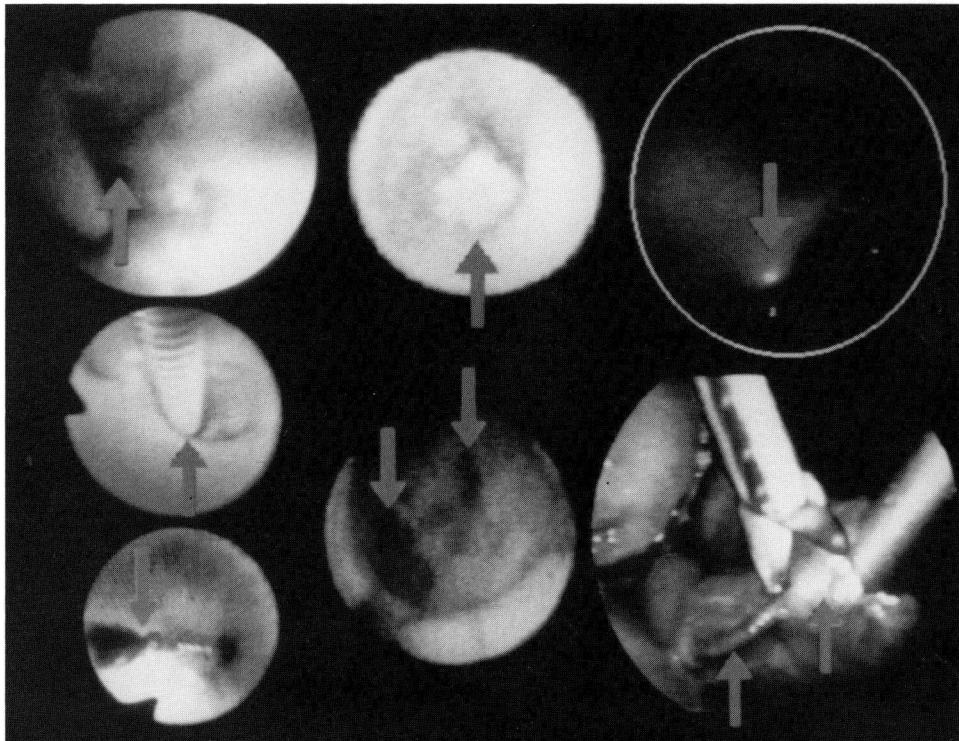

FIGURE 26–7. *Upper left,* A 0.3-mm flexible guide wire (*arrow*) both entering and exiting the ostium owing to a block just distal to the uterotubal junction in the medial isthmus. *Upper middle,* Identification of the lesion (*arrow*) with the falloposcope in the medial isthmus, which is blocked by polypoid extensions of fibrotic tissue arising from a devascularized epithelium. *Upper right,* A simultaneous laparoscopic view of the falloposcopic light transilluminating the tube wall just proximal to the isthmic block (*arrow*). The laparoscope light has been dimmed to highlight the falloposcope light and the site of the block. *Lower left (top),* A ribbed flexible wire dilator entering the same ostium (OD = 0.6 mm) (*arrow*), which successfully bypassed the block and exited the fimbria, following which free tubal patency was demonstrated. *Lower left (bottom),* The leading wire of a balloon catheter entering the ostium (*arrow*) followed by the deflated balloon (OD = 1 mm). *Lower middle,* Falloposcopic view of lysed isthmic luminal adhesions following successful direct balloon tuboplasty. The red areas (*arrows*) are patches of blood at the site of the divided adhesions. Posttuboplasty patency was demonstrated. The inner crescent-shaped lining of the Teflon catheter can be seen (ID = 0.8 mm). *Lower right,* A guide wire has been passed to the fimbrial level. The wire is flexed into a U owing to perifimbrial adhesions (*arrow*). The wire is deliberately used to expose the delicate interfimbrial adhesions to facilitate accurate laparoscopic scissor division of these adhesions. The rest of the tubal lumen was falloposcopically normal. The external tube was also normal. (From Kerin JF, Williams DB, San Roman GA, Pearlstone AC, Grundfest WS, Surrey ES. Falloposcopic classification and treatment of fallopian tube lumen disease. Fertil Steril 1992;57:731–741. Reprinted with permission of the publisher, The American Fertility Society.)

INTRAMURAL OVIDUCT

The normal intramural oviduct ranges from 1.5 to 2.5 cm in length and takes a straight to slightly curved course to the uterotubal junction. The lumen reaches its narrowest point at the uterotubal junction and ranges from 0.8 to 1.4 mm in diameter. The intramural oviduct is pale pink in color and contains four to six flattened epithelial folds, which are continuous with the puckering of the ostium during ostial contractions.[26] HSG studies frequently demonstrate the presence of a small, ampulla-like dilation or bulge in the proximal intramural lumen. The base of this bulge is formed medially by the ostium "membrane" and is frequently seen on HSG as a small triangle, which has its base facing the uterus and apex into the isthmic lumen. If a guide wire or cannula system is not facing the long axis of the intramural oviduct in a coaxial alignment, the wire may be deflected off the intramural bulge, bunch up, bend excessively, or turn around and re-enter the uterus via the ostium. The less flexible cannulas and endoscopes tend to get stuck in the intramural bulge as it narrows about 1 to 1.5 cm distal to the ostium "membrane" (Fig. 26–8).

ISTHMIC OVIDUCT

The isthmic lumen is the narrowest extrauterine tubal segment and extends from the uterotubal junction to the ampulloisthmic junction. The ampulloisthmic junction is difficult to define exactly, but on falloposcopic examination it is characterized by a short segment of about 0.5 cm, which displays a more abrupt change in lumen diameter and a change to ampullary-type epithelium.[26] The isthmic lumen measures about 2 to 3 cm in length and 1 to 2 mm in diameter. Its epithelium is pink in color and lined by four to six longitudinal folds. Occasional rhythmic contractions of the intramural and isthmic segments can be observed and appear to be more frequent in the late follicular phase, when estrogen levels are maximally elevated.[26] The isthmic oviduct commonly takes a 40- to 60-degree bend as it exits beyond the uterotubal junction and starts its variable, straight-to-serpiginous course anterior to the ovary. If care is not taken, perforation at the uterotubal junction or in the first 2 cm of the curved isthmic oviduct is likely, despite the fact that the muscular layers of the isthmus are the thickest and most clearly defined of the major oviductal segments.

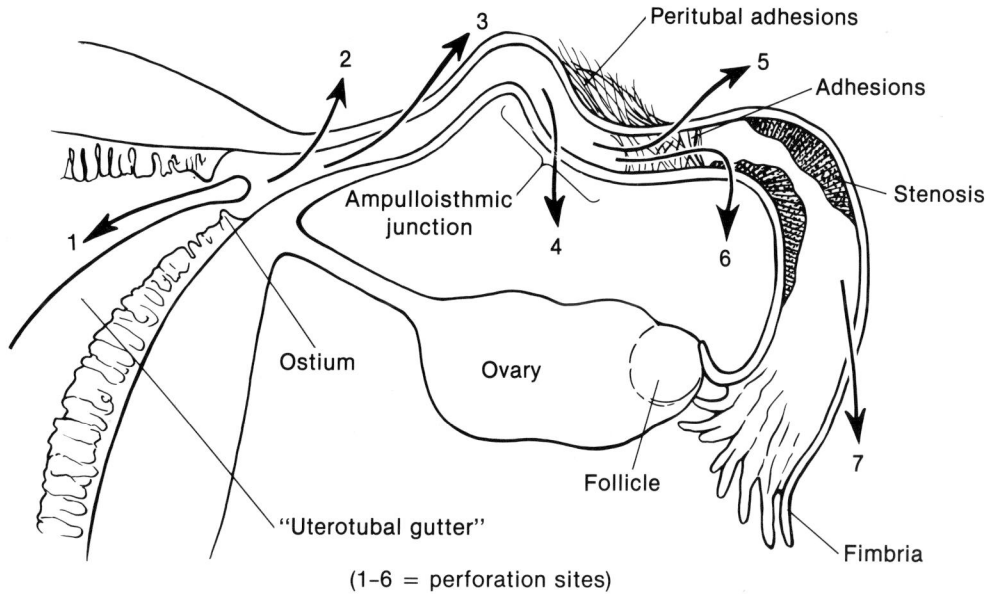

FIGURE 26–8. Diagrammatic representation of the "uterotubal gutter," ostium, and segments of the oviduct. (Nos. 1 through 7 are perforation sites.) The vulnerable sites and predisposing factors for perforation are illustrated. (From Kerin JF, Pearlstone AC, Surrey ES. Cannulation of the fallopian tube and falloposcopy: difficulties and complications. In: Corfman RS, Diamond MP, DeCherney AH, editors. Complications of Laparoscopy and Hysteroscopy. Oxford, Blackwell Scientific, 1993.)

AMPULLARY OVIDUCT

Beyond the ampulloisthmic junction, there is a rapid increase in lumen diameter from 1.5 to 4 mm over the first 1 to 2 cm of the ampullary oviduct, which further increases to a diameter of 8 to 10 mm just proximal to the fimbria. It is the longest but most variable in length of all the oviductal segments, ranging from 5 to 10 cm. The epithelium changes from pale pink to a rich red color owing to the well-vascularized secondary epithelial folds that occupy the lumen.[26] The ampullary oviduct is cavernous and thin-walled and prone to perforation if natural or acquired sharp bends are present along its course.

FIMBRIA AND TRANSVAGINAL PERITONEOSCOPY

The fimbria are characterized by extensions of the rich vascular endothelium as they float freely in and out of view against the dark background of fluid in the peritoneal cavity. Limited outlines of ovary, small bowel, mesentery, and omentum can be observed as the falloposcope extends beyond the fimbria. During the periovular period, fine mucous strands connecting the fimbria to the preovular follicle have been observed[31] and may play a role in oocyte capture by the fimbria (see Fig. 26–6).

Pathology

CHARACTERIZATION OF SITE AND TYPE OF ENDOTUBAL DISEASE

A variety of endotubal lesions have been described at falloposcopy. In one study, 55 women between the ages of 26 and 44 years who had known or suspected tubal disease underwent a hysteroscopy-falloposcopy procedure.[32] A total

of 84 tubes were available for falloposcopy, and 75 tubes were successfully imaged. The type, frequency, and location of the endotubal lesions were tabulated.

A total of 69 lesions were characterized falloposcopically in 43 diseased tubes, accounting for an average of 1.6 lesions per tube. The remaining 32 tubes were considered to be falloposcopically normal (42%). The most common lesions were thin-to-thick intraluminal, nonobstructive adhesions (27 of 69, 39%) followed by stenosis (13 of 69, 19%), obstruction (11 of 69, 16%), and polyps (7 of 69, 10%). The most common site of an endotubal lesion was within the isthmus (31 of 69, 45%), followed by the intramural segment (20 of 69, 29%) and the ampullary-fimbrial segment (18 of 69, 26%). An expanded series reported similar findings (see Table 26–2).[17]

FALLOPOSCOPIC CLASSIFICATION OF ENDOTUBAL LESIONS

A falloposcopic classification and scoring system for defining the location, nature, and extent of tubal lumen disease has been developed to standardize the evaluation of these endoscopic findings.[17] A series of parameters, including degree of patency, abnormal epithelial changes, abnormal vascular patterns, degree of adhesion formation, amount of dilatation, and abnormal intraluminal contents, are ascribed a score of 1 (normal), 2 (mild-to-moderate disease), and 3 (severe disease) for each of the four segments of the left and right tube. A total minimum score of 20 for each tube reflects normality, a score between 20 and 30 reflects mild-to-moderate endotubal disease, and a score greater than 30 reflects severe endotubal disease (Fig. 26–9). A standardized form containing the classification system is divided into three sections. The top section covers the history; the middle section contains the scoring chart; and the lower section contains a diagram of the tubes, uterus, and ovaries; treatment sum-

FALLOPOSCOPIC CLASSIFICATION AND LOCALIZATION OF TUBAL LUMEN DISEASE

Patient's Name _____ Date _____ Phone # _____
Age _____ G _____ P _____ Sp Ab _____ VTP _____ Ectopic _____ Infertile: Yes _____ No _____
Other Significant History (i.e. surgery, Infection, etc.) _____

HSG _____ Sonography _____ Photography _____ Laparoscopy _____ Laparoatomy _____
Cycle Details _____
Semen Details _____

SITE of DISEASE	RIGHT TUBE				LEFT TUBE			
	INTRAMURAL	ISTHMIC	AMPULLARY	FIMBRIAL	INTRAMURAL	ISTHMIC	AMPULLARY	FIMBRIAL
PATENCY Patency __ __ __ 1 Stenosis __ __ __ 2 Obstruction __ __ __ 3								
EPITHELIUM Normal __ __ __ 1 Pale, Atropic __ __ __ 2 Flat, featureless __ __ __ 3								
VASCULARITY Normal __ __ __ 1 Intermediate __ __ __ 2 Poor psllor __ __ __ 3								
ADHESIONS None __ __ __ 1 Thin, weblike __ __ __ 2 Thick __ __ __ 3								
DILITATION None __ __ __ 1 Minimal __ __ __ 2 Hydrosalpinx __ __ __ 3								
* OTHER __ __ __ 2-3								
CUMULATIVE SCORE								

TOTAL SCORE   RIGHT TUBE = _____ (NORMAL = 20)   LEFT TUBE = _____ (NORMAL = 20)

A cumulative score for each tube of: 20 = Normal Tubal Lumen; > 20 but < 30 = Moderate Endotubal Disease; > 30 = Severe Endotubal Disease.
* Mucus Plugs or Tubal Debri, Endotubal Polyps, Endometriosis, Salpingitis Isthmica Nodosa, Inflammatory, Infective, Neoplastic conditions and absent tubal segments are each assigned a score of 2 to 3 depending on the significance of the lesion.

Treatment (Specify R & L Tube Surgical Procedures).

Nothing _____
Aquadissection _____
Guidewire Cannulation _____
Wire Dilitation _____
Direct Balloon Tuboplasty _____
Other _____

Prognosis for Conception:

_____ Excellent (> 75%)
_____ Good (50-75%)
_____ Fair (25-50%)
_____ Poor (< 25%)

Recommended Followup Treatment: _____
_____
_____
Surgeons _____
_____

RIGHT   LEFT

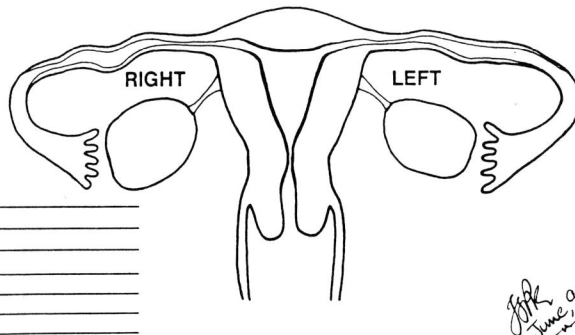

FIGURE 26–9. Falloposcopic classification and scoring system for the quantification and localization of fallopian tube lumen disease. (From Kerin JF, Williams DB, San Roman GA, Pearlstone AC, Grundfest WS, Surrey ES. Falloposcopic classification and treatment of fallopian tube lumen disease. Fertil Steril 1992;57:731–741. Reprinted with permission of the publisher, The American Fertility Society.)

mary; pregnancy prognosis; and a recommendation for future treatment. This system is also used to guide management during tuboplasty procedures. If the tube is falloposcopically normal throughout its intramural, isthmic, ampullary, and fimbrial segments (normal score = 20 points), no further procedures are performed. If the tube contains intraluminal debris, endotubal plugs,[33] or filmy adhesions, simple tubal cannulation and aquadissection procedures are performed (see Fig. 26–6).[25] If thickened intraluminal adhesions, polypoid structures, or obstructions are detected, the passage of flexible dilatation wires with OD up to 0.8 mm (Cook OB/GYN, Target Therapeutics) are used in an attempt to treat these lesions.[32] When there are thick intraluminal adhesions or fibrotic obstructions, small balloon catheters with OD of 1.0 mm in the deflated state and up to 2.5 mm in the inflated state can be used[25, 32] (Fig. 26–10).

VALIDATION OF CLASSIFICATION SYSTEM

In one series, 75 women with a provisional diagnosis of endotubal disease (including obstruction, stenosis, and fail-

ure of peritoneal spill) following hysterosalpingographic or laparoscopic investigation were subjected to falloposcopy.[17] A total of 112 tubes were available for adequate falloposcopic evaluation. The endotubal lumens were falloposcopically normal in 52 tubes (46%) and contained mild-to-moderate disease in 33 (29%), and severe to fibrotic obstructive disease in 27 (25%). Within a year of the procedure, pregnancies occurred in 6 of 28 (21%) women with at least one falloposcopically normal tube, in 2 of 22 (9%) in whom there was mild-to-moderate disease, and in 0 of 16 (0%) in whom there was severe endotubal disease.

Indications

The initial experience with falloposcopy has been quite favorable.[34] This technique, however, has been performed within one center and awaits validation from separate studies. Falloposcopy is currently being evaluated in a multicenter study under the supervision of an approved Food and Drug Administration (FDA) protocol. At present, the procedure is

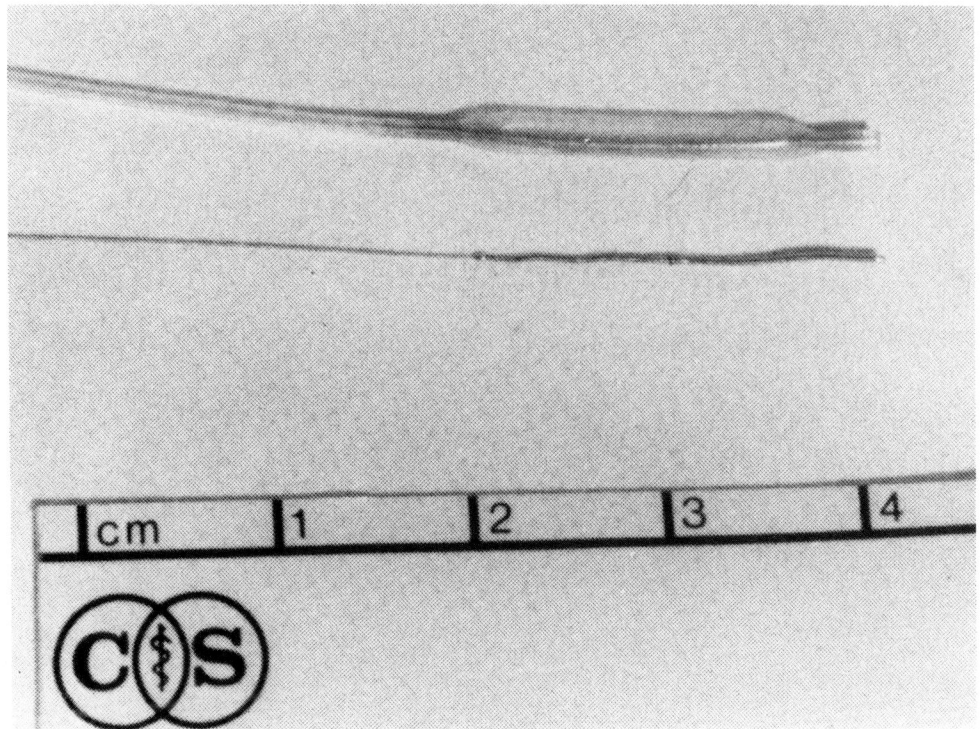

FIGURE 26–10. *Upper,* Close-up of soft balloon cannula with a 1-mm OD and collapsed balloon. The balloon distends to a 2-mm OD over a length of 2 cm. *Lower,* Guide wire with a small ball valve located 1 cm proximal to the floppy tip. This ball valve locks into place to seal the distal end of the balloon for inflation (Stealth catheter system). (From Kerin J, Daykhovsky L, Grundfest W, Surrey E. Falloposcopy: a microendoscopic transvaginal technique for diagnosing and treating endotubal disease incorporating guide wire cannulation and direct balloon tuboplasty. J Reprod Med 1990;35:606–612.)

confined to research protocols monitored by hospital Institutional Review Board (IRB) committees. Based on our experience to date, the following represent potential indications for this procedure:

1. Failure to demonstrate tubal patency by conventional investigations (HSG and chromohydrotubation under laparoscopic monitoring). This is particularly relevant when there is failure to demonstrate patency of the proximal tubal lumen.

2. Demonstration of tubal stenosis. Falloposcopic assessment of the type, extent, and severity of a lesion can be obtained and a tuboplasty performed, if indicated. An analysis of the effects of various tuboplasty techniques in relation to the nature of the lesion treated has been reported.[30] The combined technique of aquadissection and guide wire cannulation disrupted thin, nonobstructive adhesions in 9 of the 15 procedures attempted (60%). The techniques of flexible wire dilatation and direct balloon tuboplasty disrupted thick, nonobstructive adhesions in 4 of 12 procedures (33%) and significantly dilated tubal stenoses in 5 of 13 procedures (39%). When the tubal lumen was totally obstructed by a fibrotic process (11 cases), however, attempts to bypass the obstruction on six occasions with direct balloon tuboplasty failed in all cases.

3. Recurrent tubal ectopic pregnancies in which the affected tube is patent. The status of the lumen can be assessed to define the degree of tubal damage and determine if there is a lesion (such as nonobstructive intraluminal lesion) that may predispose to its recurrence.

4. Unexplained infertility in which conventional tests for tubal patency have not revealed an endotubal lesion. Falloposcopy may isolate areas of epithelial damage or other intraluminal pathology, which may compromise tubal function and predispose to ongoing infertility.

5. The presence of extensive peritubal disease, which may be associated with endotubal disease.

6. Display of perifimbrial adhesions by falloposcopic distention from within the tube, to facilitate accurate laparoscopic adhesiolysis.

7. Falloposcopic guidance and verification of cannula placement for transvaginal tubal transfer of gametes and embryos.

8. Assist in the diagnosis and management of ectopic gestations.

Contraindications

Contraindications to falloposcopy include inability to tolerate general or regional anesthesia, active genital infection, intrauterine pregnancy, and active uterine bleeding sufficient to preclude endoscopic visualization. The need for anesthesia may be obviated in the near future through the use of nonhysteroscopic techniques for falloposcope delivery.[35, 36]

Failure Rate and Complications

The technical failure rate for coaxial falloposcopy (defined as a failure to advance the falloposcope in the absence of luminal obstruction) is 7% (9 of 121 procedures). Up to 6% of tubes are fibrotically obstructed at the uterotubal ostium to a degree precluding falloposcopy.[32] In more than 120 procedures, no known complications (including bleeding, perforation, infection, or other adverse sequelae) have been attributed to diagnostic falloposcopy. After 60 endotuboplasties, there have been six perforations (four partial, two complete) yielding a perforation rate of 10% in these cases. It should be noted that such perforations have been associated

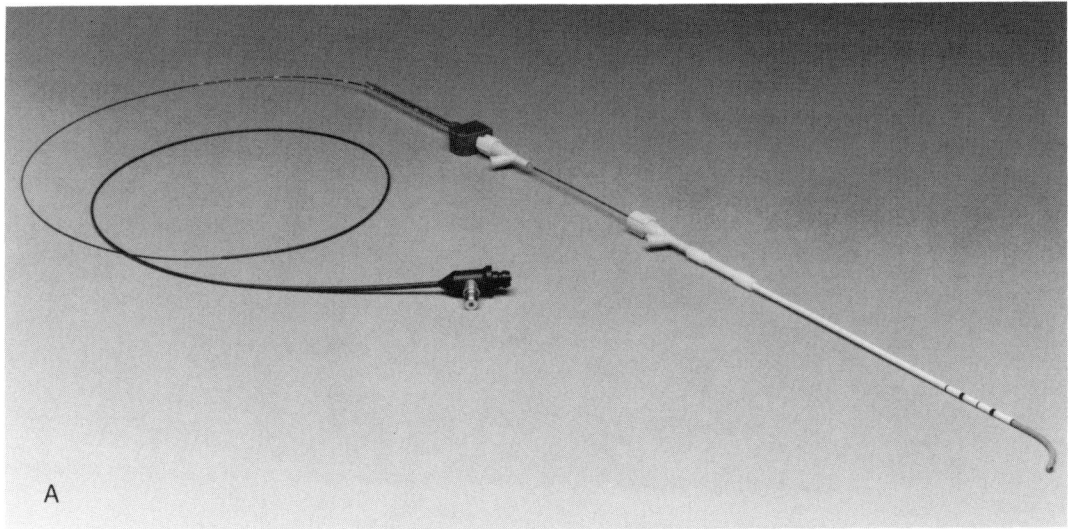

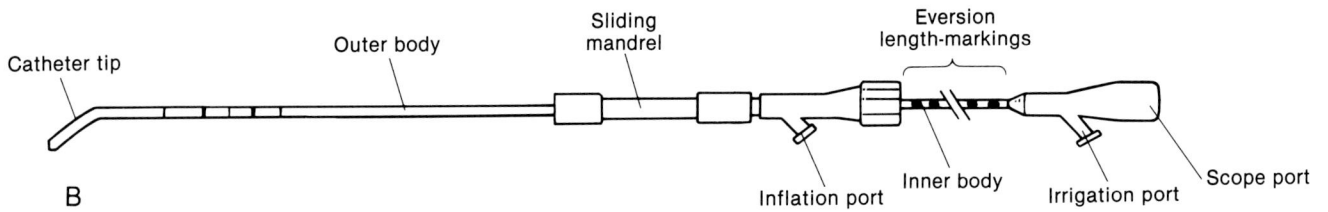

FIGURE 26–11. Linear-everting catheter system. *A*, Actual photograph. *B*, Labeled diagram. (*A* and *B* from Pearlstone AC, Surrey ES, Kerin JF. The linear-everting catheter: a non-hysteroscopic, transvaginal technique for access and microendoscopy of the fallopian tube. Fertil Steril 1992;58:854–857. Reprinted with permission of the publisher, The American Fertility Society.)

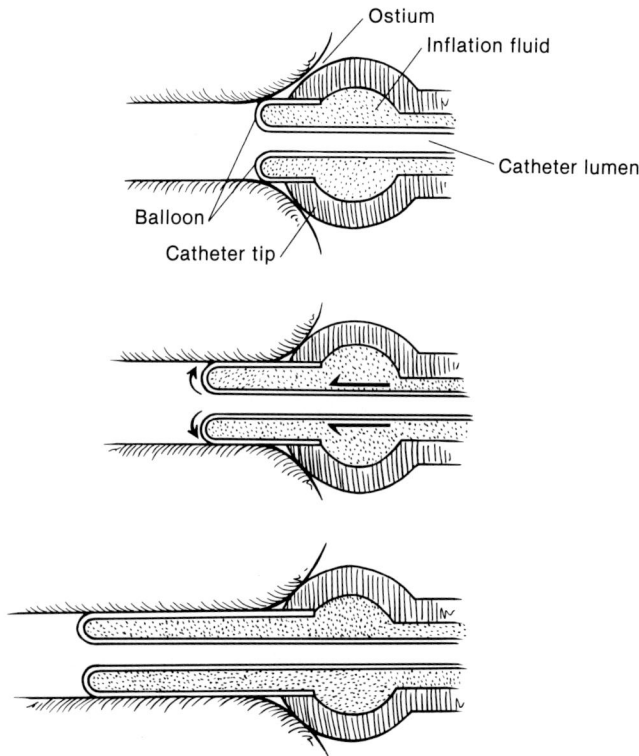

FIGURE 26–12. Mechanism of eversion with the linear-everting catheter system. (From Pearlstone AC, Surrey ES, Kerin JF. The linear-everting catheter: a non-hysteroscopic, transvaginal technique for access and microendoscopy of the fallopian tube. Fertil Steril 1992;58:854–857. Reprinted with permission of the publisher, The American Fertility Society.)

only with cases involving attempts to treat severe, fibrotic endotubal disease. As mentioned, tuboplasty has not been successful in these cases. These perforations were monitored laparoscopically and did not result in any adverse sequelae.

Recent Developments

Modifications of falloposcopy continue to evolve at a rapid rate. One of the most promising innovations has been the development of the linear everting catheter system.[27] This technology offers an alternative to the coaxial approach for falloposcopic guided transvaginal oviductal cannulation. The linear everting catheter consists of inner and outer catheter bodies joined circumferentially at their distal tips by a flexible, distensible membrane or balloon (Fig. 26–11). When the membrane is pressurized, advancing the inner body results in balloon eversion. The membrane slowly unrolls from the catheter tip, in a manner similar to a carpet being unrolled onto a floor. The catheter is introduced through a nondilated cervix and does not require hysteroscopic guidance.

Using a falloposcope delivered through the linear everting catheter central lumen, the uterotubal ostium is visualized, and the pressurized balloon is then everted through the ostium and along the tube (Fig. 26–12). Eversion is performed in gradual increments, with attention paid to maintaining the falloposcope within the balloon's protective cover. When the desired degree of eversion is achieved, systematic imaging of the endosalpinx is performed in a retrograde manner.[27] The linear everting catheter system offers a number of advantages relative to currently available alternatives. The everting balloon mechanism serves to minimize endotubal shear forces while facilitating delivery of the falloposcope. The flexible balloon system is also able to conform to variations in tubal anatomy, which can be advantageous during procedures in tortuous or stenotic tubes. Finally, the ability to deliver the linear everting catheter transcervically without the need for dilation or concomitant hysteroscopy may obviate the need for anesthesia.[35] Such properties make this system a potentially attractive method for falloposcopic guided tubal transfer procedures. The initial experience with the linear everting catheter system has been promising.[27, 37, 38]

CONCLUSION

Tubal microendoscopy is at an early but rapidly evolving stage of development. Both salpingoscopy and falloposcopy have revealed evidence of intratubal pathology that previously had been inaccessible to other in vivo diagnostic modalities. Using innovative delivery systems, falloposcopy seems to exemplify the potential applications of minimally invasive endoscopic technology. Prospective, multicenter studies are necessary to define appropriate clinical indications for these microendoscopic procedures.

REFERENCES

1. Hamou J. Microhysteroscopy: a new procedure and its original applications in gynecology. J Reprod Med 1981;26:375–382.
2. Scarselli G, Mencaglia L, Tantini C, et al. Intraoperative microsalpingoscopy of the ampullar fallopian tube. Acta Eur Fertil 1982;13:35–38.
3. Henry-Suchet J, Tesquiter L, Pez JP, Loffredo V. Prognostic value of tuboscopy vs. hysterosalpingography before tuboplasty. J Reprod Med 1984;29:609–612.
4. Cornier E. Ampullosalpingoscopy. In: Siegler AM, editor. The Fallopian Tube: Basic Studies and Clinical Contributions. New York: Futura, 1986:383–390.
5. Mencaglia L, Hamou J, Perino A, Cosmi E. Transcervical and retrograde salpingoscopy: evaluation of the fallopian tube in infertile women. In: Siegler AM, editor. The Fallopian Tube: Basic Studies and Clinical Contributions. New York: Futura, 1986:377–381.
6. Brosens I, Boeckx W, Delattin P, et al. Salpingoscopy: a new pre-operative diagnostic tool in tubal infertility. Br J Obstet Gynaecol 1987;94:768–773.
7. Shapiro BS, Diamond MP, DeCherney AH. Salpingoscopy: an adjunctive technique for evaluation of the fallopian tube. Fertil Steril 1988;49:1076–1079.
8. Puttemans P, Brosens I, Delattin P, et al. Salpingoscopy versus hysterosalpingography in hydrosalpinges. Hum Reprod 1987;2:535–540.
9. Nezhat F, Winer WK, Nezhat C. Fimbrioscopy and salpingoscopy in patients with minimal to moderate pelvic endometriosis. Obstet Gynecol 1990;75:15–17.
10. Nezhat C, Winer WK, Cooper JD, et al. Endoscopic infertility surgery. J Reprod Med 1989;34:127–134.
11. Hershlag A, Seifer DB, Carcangiu ML, et al. Salpingoscopy: light microscopic and electron microscopic correlations. Obstet Gynecol 1991;77:399–405.
12. De Bruyne F, Puttemans P, Boeckx W, Brosens I. The clinical value of salpingoscopy in tubal infertility. Fertil Steril 1989;51: 339–340.
13. Henry-Suchet J, Loffredo V, Tesquier L, Pez JP. Endoscopy of the tube (tuboscopy): its prognostic value for tuboplasties. Acta Eur Fertil 1985;16:139–145.
14. Cornier E, Feintuch MJ, Bouccara L. La fibrotuboscopie ampullaire. J Gynecol Obstet Biol Reprod 1984;1:49–53.
15. Cornier E. L'ampullosalpingoscopie per-coelioscopique. J Gynecol Obstet Biol Reprod 1985;14:459–466.
16. Marana R, Muscatello P, Muzii L, et al. Perlaparoscopic salpingoscopy in the evaluation of the tubal factor in infertile women. Int J Fertil 1990;35:211–214.
17. Kerin JF, Williams DB, San Roman GA, et al. Falloposcopic classification and treatment of fallopian tube lumen disease. Fertil Steril 1992;57:731–741.
18. Boer-Meisel ME, te Velde ER, Habbema JDF, Kardaun JWPF. Predicting the pregnancy outcome in patients treated for hydrosalpinx: a prospective study. Fertil Steril 1986;45:23–29.
19. Schlaff WD, Hassiakos DK, Damewood MD, Rock JA. Neosalpingostomy for distal tubal obstruction: prognostic factors and impact of surgical technique. Fertil Steril 1990;54:984–990.
20. Gardner AK: The Causes and Curative Treatment of Sterility with a Preliminary Statement of the Physiology of Generation. New York: DeWitt & Davenport, 1856.
21. Sweeney WJ: The interstitial portion of the uterine tube: its gross anatomy, course, and length. Obstet Gynecol 1962;19:3–8.
22. Mohri T, Mohri C, Yamadori F. Tubaloscope. Endoscopy 1970;4:226–230.
23. Brand E, Daykhovsky L, Grundfest W. Salpingoscopy: a method for direct examination of the fallopian tube. Surg Endosc 1987;1:221–223.
24. DeCherney AH: Anything you can do I can do better . . . or differently! Fertil Steril 1987;48:374–376.
25. Kerin J, Daykhovsky L, Grundfest W, Surrey E: Falloposcopy: a microendoscopic transvaginal technique for diagnosing and treating endotubal disease incorporating guide wire cannulation and direct balloon tuboplasty. J Reprod Med 1990;35:606–612.
26. Kerin J, Daykhovsky L, Segalowitz J, et al. Falloposcopy: a microendoscopic technique for visual exploration of the human fallopian tube from the uterotubal ostium to the fimbria using a transvaginal approach. Fertil Steril 1990;54:390–400.
27. Pearlstone AC, Surrey ES, Kerin JF. The linear everting catheter: a nonhysteroscopic, transvaginal technique for access and microendoscopy of the fallopian tube. Fertil Steril 1992;58:854–857.
28. Grundfest WS, Litvack F, Sherman T, et al. Delineation of peripheral and coronary detail by intraoperative angioscopy. Ann Surg 1985;202:394–400.
29. Grundfest W, Litvack F, Sherman T, et al. The current status of angioplasty and laser angioscopy. J Vasc Surg 1987;5:667–673.
30. Kerin J, Pearlstone AC, Surrey ES. Cannulation of the fallopian tube and falloposcopy: difficulties and complications. In: Corfman R, Diamond MP, DeCherney A (eds). Complications of Laparoscopy and Hysteroscopy. Boston: Blackwell Scientific, 1992:223–235.

31. Kerin JF, Williams DB, Serden SP, et al. Falloposcopic identification of a fimbrio-ovarian mucus connection as a possible mechanism for tubal oocyte capture. J Laparoendosc Surg 1991;1:97–101.
32. Kerin JF, Surrey E, Daykhovsky L, Grundfest WS. Development and application of a falloposcope for transvaginal endoscopy of the fallopian tube. J Laparoendosc Surg 1990;1:47–56.
33. Kerin JF, Surrey ES, Williams DB, et al. Falloposcopic observations of endotubal isthmic plugs as a cause of reversible obstruction and their histological characterization. J Laparoendosc Surg 1991;1:103–110.
34. Kerin JF, Pearlstone AC, Surrey ES. Cannulation of the fallopian tube and falloposcopy: difficulties and complications. In: Corfman RS, Diamond MP, DeCherney AH, editors. Complications of Laparoscopy and Hysteroscopy. Oxford: Blackwell Scientific, 1993:223–235.
35. Bauer O, Diedrich K, Bacich S, et al. Transcervical access and intraluminal imaging of the fallopian tube in the non-anesthetized patient: preliminary results using a new fallopian tube access technology. Hum Reprod 1992;7:7–11.
36. Kerin JF. Non-hysteroscopic falloposcopy: a proposed method for visual guidance and verification of tubal cannula placement for endotuboplasty, gamete and embryo transfer procedures. Fertil Steril 1992;57:1133–1135.
37. Confino E, Surrey E, Pearlstone A, et al. Linear everting catheter for transcervical falloposcopy: preliminary results of a multicenter trial [Abstract]. Presented at the 48th Annual Meeting of the American Fertility Society, New Orleans, LA, October 31–November 5, 1992.
38. Kerin J, Scudamore I, Surrey E, et al. Collaborative evaluation of falloposcopy using a non-hysteroscopic linear eversion catheter delivery system [Abstract]. Presented at the 48th Annual Meeting of the American Fertility Society, New Orleans, LA, October 31–November 5, 1992.

CHAPTER 27

Developmental Anomalies of the Reproductive Tract

JOHN A. ROCK and
SANFORD M. MARKHAM

Embryonic development of the female reproductive tract represents a complicated, yet dependable process that begins in the 4th week of gestation and is completed sometime after the 16th week. During this time the fallopian tubes, the uterus, and the vagina develop to their final state in a predictable manner that is repetitive and generally efficient. When the process malfunctions, however, the developmental defects of the reproductive tract that result can significantly impact involved women in a variety of ways, from amenorrhea to increased pregnancy wastage.

This chapter begins with a brief review of the embryology of the reproductive tract and the general incidence of developmental defects followed by a simple classification of uterovaginal anomalies. Techniques currently used in the evaluation and management of reproductive tract anomalies are then discussed in detail, including treatment alternatives and pregnancy outcomes.

EMBRYOLOGY

After maturing for 4 to 5 days in the fallopian tube, the zygote reaches the uterus on approximately the 6th day after ovulation and implants on the uterine cavity wall. The resulting embryonic disk gives rise shortly to the formation of a primitive streak. This germ layer takes a linear shape, with epithelium of the superior end developing into ectoderm and the inferior end simultaneously developing into endoderm. A third primitive germ layer, the mesoderm, is formed between the endoderm and the ectoderm around the 16th day. From the mesoderm, nephrogenic cords develop approximately 3 weeks after fertilization and give rise to the development of the mesonephric tubules and ducts in the 4th week and to the mesonephros early in the 5th week. The paramesonephric ducts develop lateral to the mesonephric ducts as a result of an evagination of the coelomic epithelium late in the 5th or early in the 6th week following fertilization (Fig. 27–1).

The paramesonephric ducts (müllerian ducts) give rise to the fallopian tubes, the uterus, the cervix, and the upper two thirds of the vagina. By the end of the 7th week of pregnancy, the müllerian ducts fuse in the caudal region to form a single structure consisting of the uterus, the cervix, and the upper vagina. The tip of this structure abuts on the developing posterior wall of the urogenital sinus immediately between the two orifices of the mesonephric ducts (wolffian ducts) (Fig. 27–2).[1]

It is believed that the point where the tip of the müllerian duct abuts on the posterior wall of the urogenital sinus is of critical importance,[2] because this point is the site of the future vaginal orifice. The urogenital sinus, also of mesodermal origin, proliferates and forms a column of squamous epithelium known as the *vaginal plate,* which displaces the tip of the müllerian duct cephalad from the wall of the urogenital sinus.[2]

By the end of the first trimester, a mesenchymal thickening occurs around a portion of the caudal end of the fused müllerian ducts and gives rise to the endocervix.[1] This thickening includes portions of the wolffian ducts and is important because in all other areas of the developing reproductive tract, the wolffian ducts are external to the wall of the müllerian duct.[2] This is significant when remnants of the wolffian ducts persist into adult life (Fig. 27–3).

Only in the vaginal portion of the fused müllerian ducts does the columnar epithelium convert into squamous epithelium.[1] In cases of persistent complete transverse vaginal septum, the upper portions of the vagina, if present, do not undergo this conversion and remain lined by mucin-secreting epithelium.[2]

By the 18th to 20th week after conception, smooth muscle appears in the wall of the reproductive canal, and by the 24th week, the muscle portion of the uterine wall is well developed.[1] Cervical glands appear by the 15th week, whereas early endometrial glands are not noted until the 19th week after conception.

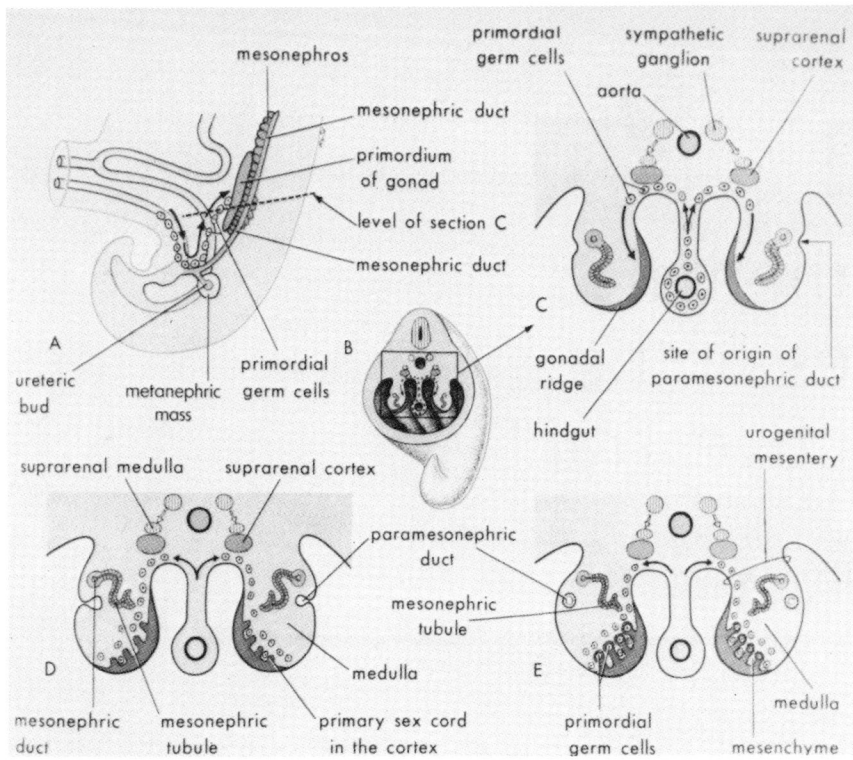

FIGURE 27–1. *A,* Sketch of a 5-week embryo, illustrating the migration of primordial germ cells from the yolk sac. *B,* Three-dimensional sketch of the caudal region of a 5-week embryo, showing the location and extent of the gonadal ridges on the medial aspect of the urogenital ridges. *C,* Transverse section showing the primordium of the suprarenal glands (adrenal glands), the gonadal ridges, and the migration of primordial germ cells into the developing gonads. *D,* Transverse section through a 6-week embryo showing the primary sex cords and the developing paramesonephric ducts. *E,* Similar section at later stage showing the indifferent gonads and the mesonephric and paramesonephric ducts. (From Moore KL. The Developing Human: Clinically Oriented Embryology. 4th edition. Philadelphia: WB Saunders, 1988.)

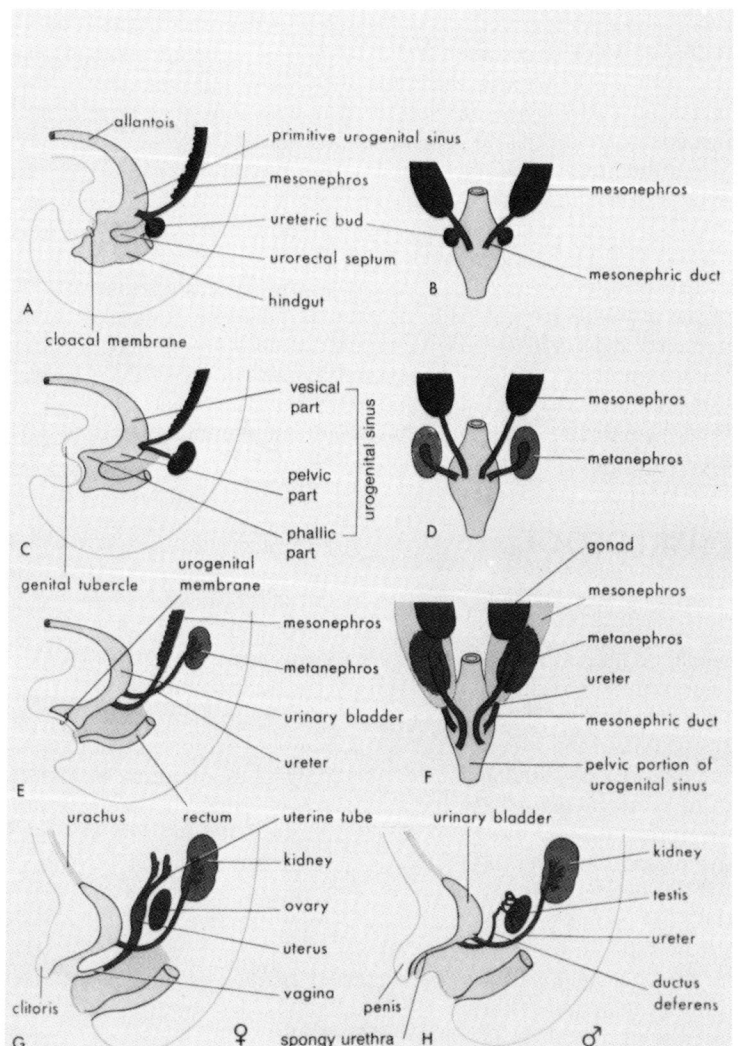

FIGURE 27–2. Diagrams showing (1) division of the cloaca into the urogenital sinus and rectum, (2) absorption of the mesonephric ducts, (3) development of the urinary bladder, urethra, and urachus, and (4) changes in the location of the ureters. *A,* Lateral view of the caudal half of a 5-week embryo. *B, D,* and *F,* Dorsal views. *C, E, G,* and *H,* Lateral views. The stages shown in *G* and *H* are reached by the 12th week. (From Moore KL. The Developing Human: Clinically Oriented Embryology. 4th edition. Philadelphia: WB Saunders, 1988.)

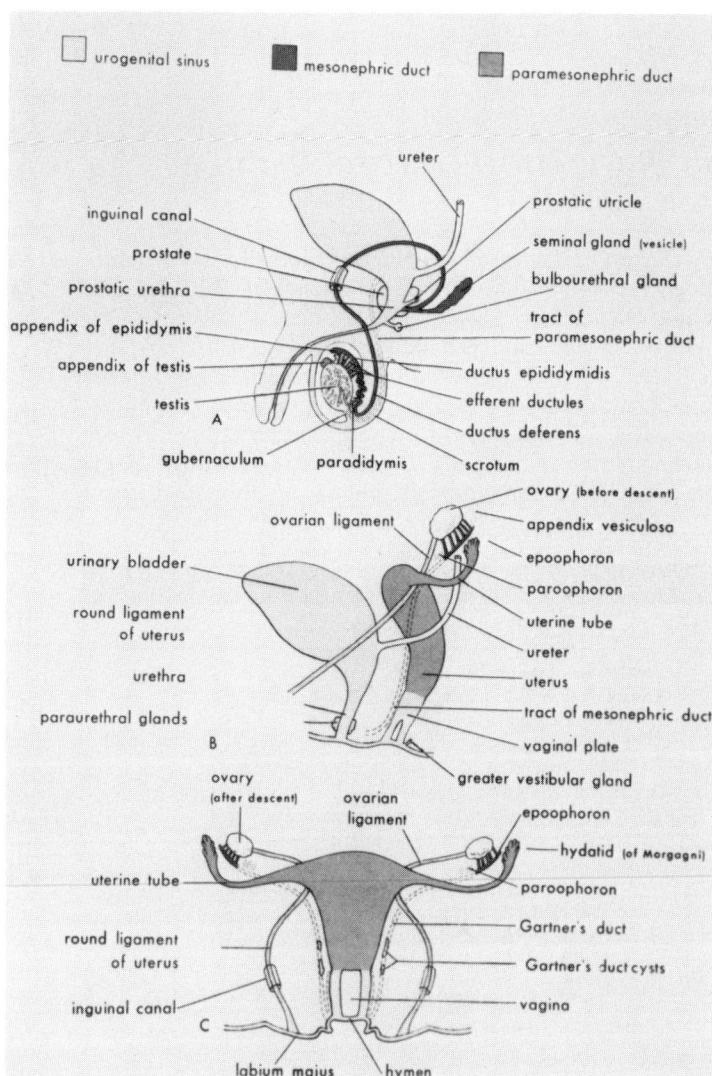

FIGURE 27–3. Schematic drawings illustrating development of the male and female reproductive systems from the genital ducts and the urogenital sinus. Vestigial structures are also shown. *A,* Reproductive system in a newborn male. *B,* Female reproductive system in a 12-week fetus. *C,* Reproductive system in a newborn female. (From Moore KL. The Developing Human: Clinically Oriented Embryology. 4th edition. Philadelphia: WB Saunders, 1988.)

It has been suggested that development of the müllerian ducts occurs in three stages. The first stage takes place at the beginning of the 10th week and consists of fusion of the medial aspects of the more caudal portions of the müllerian ducts starting in the middle and progressing simultaneously in both directions, resulting in the formation of a median septum. Between the 10th and 13th weeks, the second stage consists of a rapid cell proliferation, with the filling in of the triangular space between the two uterine cornua forming a thick upper median septum. Between the 13th and the 20th week, the third stage consists of degeneration of the upper uterine septum, starting with the lower uterine region and proceeding cranially to the top of the fundus.[3]

Although the most significant anomalies of the gonads are associated with failure of the germ cells to develop in the urogenital ridge,[2] defects in the development of the genital ducts and external genitalia are associated with the presence or absence of circulating hormones in utero,[4] with the lack of appropriate fusion of the müllerian ducts, or with a lack of degeneration of the uterine septum or of the vaginal plate. The resulting malformations and their management are the focus of this chapter.

INCIDENCE

The incidence of müllerian anomalies resulting from inappropriate fusion or lack of degeneration of the uterine septum or vaginal plate is uncertain. It is quite likely that most of these defects go unnoticed and undiagnosed, particularly in women who are uninterested in pregnancy, or in those whose defect did not result in an adverse pregnancy outcome. One review of müllerian duct anomalies suggested a frequency of 0.1% to 0.5%.[5] In another review of 167 women having laparoscopic sterilization, 1.2% were found to have a bicornuate uterus.[6] Of interest in this same review was the finding that müllerian anomalies were significantly higher in women having oligomenorrheic periods exceeding 1 year.[6] In still another review, müllerian duct anomalies were found in 1% to 5% of women.[7] This diversity in incidence suggests that the existing data may be focusing on different populations of women and that the actual occurrence rate may never be determined. The incidence of these anomalies is, however, frequent enough to warrant their consideration in all women, particularly those presenting with symptoms such as pregnancy wastage, abnormal uterine bleeding, amenorrhea, and intractable dysmenorrhea, or in those who are found on examination to have pelvic anatomic defects or renal anomalies.

CLASSIFICATION OF UTEROVAGINAL ANOMALIES

The most common developmental anomalies of the reproductive tract are the uterovaginal anomalies. Although this group encompasses a wide variety of defects, a recent classification system developed by Rock and Keenan (Table 27–1)[8] allows a simple division of anomalies into four classes based on disorders of vertical or lateral fusion of the müllerian ducts. The disorders of lateral fusion are further broken down into asymmetrical disorders with obstruction of the uterus or vagina, or both, and symmetrical disorders without

---

TABLE 27–1. Uterovaginal Anomalies

Class	Definition
I	Dysgenesis of the müllerian ducts
II	Disorders of vertical fusion of the müllerian ducts
	A. Transverse vaginal septum
	1. Obstructed
	2. Unobstructed
	B. Cervical agenesis or dysgenesis
III	Disorders of lateral fusion of the müllerian ducts
	A. Asymmetrical—obstructed disorder of the uterus or the vagina usually associated with ipsilateral renal agenesis
	1. Unicornuate uterus with a noncommunicating rudimentary anlagen or horn
	2. Unilateral obstruction of a cavity of a double uterus
	3. Unilateral vaginal obstruction associated with a double uterus
	B. Symmetrical—unobstructed
	1. Didelphic uterus
	a. Complete longitudinal vaginal septum
	b. Partial longitudinal vaginal septum
	c. No longitudinal vaginal septum
	2. Bicornuate uterus
	a. Complete
	(1) Complete longitudinal vaginal septum
	(2) Partial longitudinal vaginal septum
	(3) No longitudinal vaginal septum
	b. Partial
	(1) Complete longitudinal vaginal septum
	(2) Partial longitudinal vaginal septum
	(3) No longitudinal vaginal septum
	3. Septate uterus
	a. Complete
	(1) Complete longitudinal vaginal septum
	(2) Partial longitudinal vaginal septum
	(3) No longitudinal vaginal septum
	b. Partial
	(1) Complete longitudinal vaginal septum
	(2) Partial longitudinal vaginal septum
	(3) No longitudinal vaginal septum
	4. Arcuate uterus
	5. T-shaped uterine cavity (DES drug related)
	6. Unicornuate uterus
	a. With a rudimentary horn
	(1) With communicating endometrial cavity
	(2) Without endometrial cavity
	b. Without rudimentary horn
IV	Unusual configurations of vertical and lateral fusion defects

DES, diethylstilbestrol.
Adapted from Thompson JD, Rock JA. Te Linde's Operative Gynecology. Philadelphia: JB Lippincott, 1992.

---

obstruction. Anomalies of the external genitalia are less common and are not included in this classification because their occurrence is generally associated with inappropriate hormone stimulation in the early developmental period, and the defects produced are varied and not subject to a meaningful classification system.

SYMPTOMS, DIAGNOSIS, AND MANAGEMENT OF ANOMALIES

Anomalies of the reproductive tract may occur at any point along the route of the developing paramesonephric tract (müllerian ducts) from the fimbriated end of the fallopian tube to the lower third of the vagina. Anomalies of the lower third of the vagina and of the external female genitalia generally occur as the result of inappropriate intrauterine androgen stimulation between the 6th and 30th week of gestation, whereas anomalies of the remainder of the reproductive tract occur as a result of a defect in lateral or vertical fusion of the müllerian ducts between the 8th and 17th weeks of gestation. The most common defects occur in the area of the uterus and the upper vagina and represent anomalies that can be surgically corrected in a high proportion of cases. For this reason, the bulk of this chapter addresses anomalies of dysgenesis and of lateral or vertical fusions, focusing on current diagnosis and management.

Class I: Dysgenesis of the Müllerian Ducts

Congenital absence of the entire müllerian duct system is an uncommon event. Agenesis or dysgenesis of the lower portions of the müllerian ducts, however, is not an infrequent occurrence. Dysgenesis of the uterus with agenesis of the upper two thirds of the vagina (Mayer-Rokitansky-Küster-Hauser syndrome) is reported to occur in 1 in 4000 to 5000 females[9] and represents a common cause of primary amenorrhea second only to gonadal dysgenesis. As many as 40% of patients with this syndrome have defects in the urinary tract system,[8] and 12% or more have skeletal anomalies.[10] The kidney defects include congenital unilateral absence of a kidney, a pelvic kidney, malrotation of the kidney, or a partial double collecting system on one side. Skeletal anomalies most commonly involve the lumbar spine but may also include fusion of the cervical vertebrae.

The etiology of the Meyer-Rokitansky-Küster-Hauser syndrome is unknown. A genetic association has been suggested.[11, 12] One report identified five sisters with this syndrome.[13] The karyotype of patients with Meyer-Rokitansky-Küster-Hauser syndrome, however, is characteristically 46XX.[8] Proof of a genetic etiology is lacking, and this syndrome is now believed to be due to an error in the growth and development of the caudal portions of the paramesonephric tract.

Patients with uterovaginal dysgenesis or agenesis are generally not diagnosed until puberty. This defect should be suspected, however, in all children who are found to have a blind or absent vagina. In these patients the external female genitalia appear quite normal, as do other secondary sexual characteristics. Because of this, the diagnosis is usually suspected after puberty when patients fail to develop menses and an absent vagina or shortened blind vaginal pouch is found. Although these patients are usually asymptomatic of cyclic abdominal pain due to an absence of the uterus, some patients may have a rudimentary uterine anlage that has sufficient endometrium allowing for a periodic sluff resulting in cyclic low abdominal cramps and pain.[8] Excision of the uterine anlage is usually required to control the symptoms in these patients.

Prior to puberty the differentiation of patients with an imperforate hymen or transverse vaginal septum from those with müllerian dysgenesis or agenesis is most difficult. On physical examination, the vagina may be totally absent, or there may be a shallow vaginal pouch as long as 3 cm. The diagnosis of müllerian dysgenesis or agenesis is based on documentation of the presence or absence of the uterus and the vagina. In the past a definitive diagnosis has required a diagnostic laparoscopy.[14] More recently, it is believed that sonography, an examination under anesthesia,[8] or magnetic resonance imaging (MRI)[15, 16] can provide an accurate diagnosis, reducing the need for laparoscopy.

Once the diagnosis is made, management, if desired, is directed primarily to the creation of a functional vaginal vault. These patients have normal ovarian function and therefore do not need hormone replacement therapy. Natural pregnancy is impossible. However, ovulation induction with oocyte retrieval for in vitro fertilization using a surrogate for embryo transfer is a possibility.[17]

The creation of a functional vaginal vault in patients with uterovaginal agenesis or dysgenesis may be accomplished by one of two routes: dilation or surgery. Two separate dilation procedures, the Frank technique[18] and the Ingram technique,[19] have proved to be of benefit. The Frank technique involves the active creation of a vaginal vault. This is accomplished by applying pressure to the center of the hymenal region with progressively larger Lucite vaginal dilators (Fig. 27–4) two or three times per day for 30 minutes each session until a vault of approximately 7 to 10 cm in length and 2.5 cm in diameter is produced.[20] Once the vault has reached this size, a dilator is kept in the vagina at night until the patient is sexually active.

The Ingram technique is a passive dilation technique in which the patient is instructed to sit on a racing-type bicycle seat positioned on a stool 24 in. above the floor. A series of graduated Lucite dilators of progressive lengths and diameters are positioned at the introital dimple and held in place by a light girdle or support. Passive pressure is applied by the patient gently sitting on the stool for 15 to 30 minutes at a session for a total of approximately 2 hours per day. As the new vault is developed, increasing-sized dilators are used until a final size of 7 to 10 cm in length and 2.5 cm in diameter has been achieved.

Because functional success rates for these procedures approach 95%,[8] it is suggested that a dilation procedure be used as initial management in all patients with vaginal agenesis, with surgical procedures reserved for unsuccessful outcomes.

In the past, a number of surgical procedures have been devised to create a vaginal vault in female patients with vaginal agenesis. The most popular has been the technique of McIndoe[21] modified by Counsellor and Flor.[22] The modified McIndoe procedure for the surgical creation of a functional vaginal vault may be used both in patients presenting

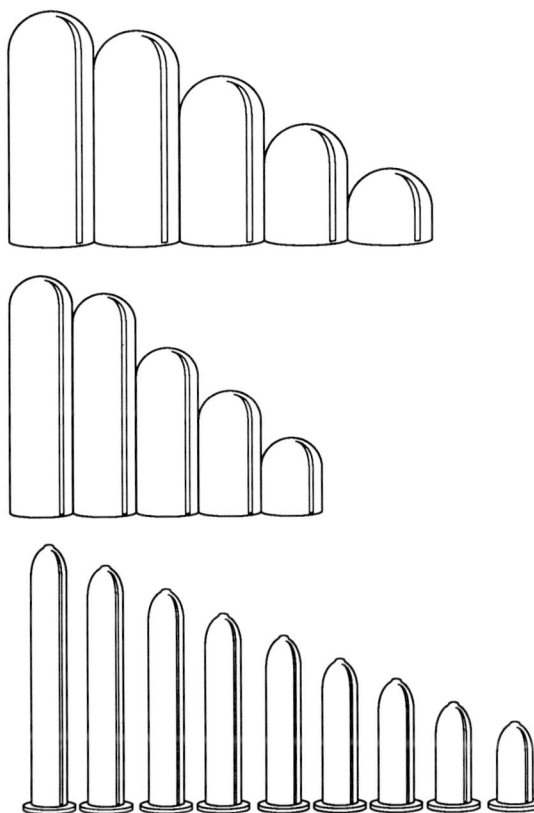

FIGURE 27–4. Ingram passive dilator set.

with vaginal agenesis with no prior surgery and in those who have experienced a failed surgical procedure. This procedure is accomplished under general anesthesia with the patient in the dorsal lithotomy position. Prior to surgery the patient should undergo a standard bowel preparation, and at the time of surgery she should be placed on prophylactic antibiotics. The success of the McIndoe procedure is directly related to obtaining a satisfactory split-thickness skin graft. This graft is obtained most easily by use of the Padgett electrodermatome. It is recommended that the graft be taken from either buttock using, where possible, skin within the patient's swim suit line to avoid a visible scar (Fig. 27–5A and B). This is accomplished by placing the patient in the Sims' position. Using the Padgett electrodermatome, a graft of 0.017 to 0.018 in. can be obtained with a width measuring approximately 10 cm and a length twice the new vaginal vault depth.[8] This length is necessary to completely cover a vaginal mold. This foam rubber mold is cut to resemble a large vaginal vault (Fig. 27–6A and B) and is covered with two plain condoms to compress the rubber mold to the desired vaginal size (Fig. 27–6C and D). The split-thickness graft is folded over the mold and then sewn onto the mold with the skin surface inward using interrupted vertical mattress sutures of 5-0 nonreactive material (Fig. 27–6E and F). The vaginal mold with the skin graft should be kept moist with normal saline while the neovaginal vault is being developed.

With the patient returned to the dorsal lithotomy position, a transverse incision is made at the site of the vaginal dimple, and a neovaginal space is created by digital pressure on both sides of the medial raphe. The dissection is extended laterally

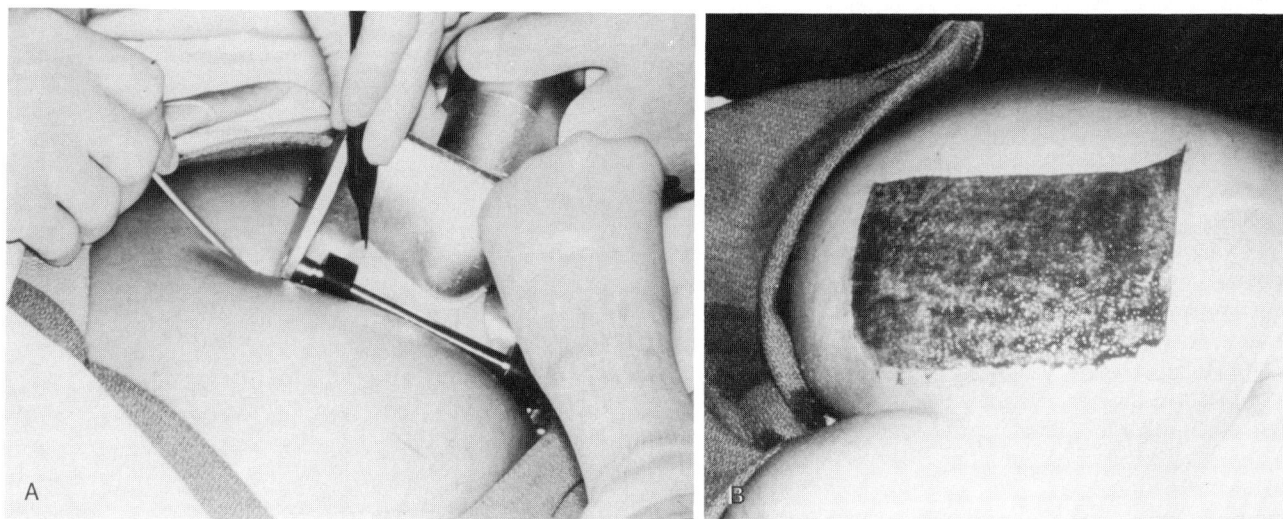

FIGURE 27–5. *A,* A split-thickness graft is taken from the buttock with a Padgett electrodermatome. The graft is 0.45-mm thick, 10-cm wide, and 15- to 18-cm long, twice the planned vaginal depth. Either buttock may be used. *B,* The donor site is low enough to be covered by most swim suits. (*A* and *B,* Photographs by Lester V. Bergman courtesy LTI Medica® and the Upjohn Company. Copyright 1987 by Learning Technology Incorporated.)

first and then toward the midline. The digital dissection is ultimately carried out to the level of the peritoneum, taking care not to expose too large an area of peritoneum so as not to develop an enterocele during the postoperative period. The medial raphe is then dissected free, and the neovaginal space is completed.

The previously cut split-thickness graft sewn onto the vaginal mold is inserted into the neovaginal space, and the edges of the graft are sutured to the cut edges on the vaginal epithelium (Fig. 27–6G and H and Fig. 27–7). The mold and the graft are held in position by placing several large braided sutures through the labia majora to prevent expulsion of the form. A suprapubic catheter is recommended for bladder draining postoperatively.

Postoperatively, the patient should be placed on a low-residue diet and kept on bedrest for 7 days. The antibiotics should be continued until the original vaginal mold is removed the first time. The labial sutures are removed 4 days after surgery, and 7 days after the surgery, the patient is returned to the operating room where the mold is removed along with the suprapubic catheter and the neovagina carefully irrigated with normal saline. The original condom-covered mold is then cleansed and reinserted into the neovaginal vault. A second vaginal mold, similar to the first, is made at this time and given to the patient for later use at home. After 24 hours, the patient is instructed in the technique of vaginal mold removal and reinsertion and is started on daily removal of the mold followed by a low-pressure, clear, warm water douche followed by reinsertion of the mold. This is accomplished for 6 weeks, after which the soft mold is replaced by a Silastic form (see Fig. 27–11H) that is used at night until the patient is sexually active.

Also of importance in the success of this procedure are the preoperative planning and discussions with the patient and her family. Time must be taken to thoroughly review the procedure and the commitment that the patient must be prepared to make during both the early and late postoperative periods if maximal results are to be achieved in creating a neovagina and in keeping the neovagina functional. It is

also suggested that the patient, along with other members of her immediate family, undergo psychological counseling to reinforce the dedicated motivation that is necessary and to ensure with reasonable certainty that the patient will follow through with necessary postoperative instructions.

In addition to the modified McIndoe procedure using a split-thickness graft, other techniques for a neovaginal creation have been described but have some disadvantages over the McIndoe procedure, including a more extensive surgical procedure, prolonged operating time, more visible graft site scarring, or more complications. These techniques include (1) vaginal replacement using an isolated colocecal segment[23]; (2) neovaginal construction using a rectus abdominous musculocutaneous flap[24]; (3) vaginal reconstruction using an axial subcutaneous pedicle flap from the inferior abdominal wall[25]; and (4) use of an amnion graft in the creation of a neovagina.[26]

Müllerian dysgenesis or agenesis with resulting absent vagina and absent or hypoplastic uterus is a defect that precludes both normal sexual relations and natural pregnancy. Although the surgical creation of a functioning uterus is not yet possible, the development or surgical creation of a functional vagina is quite possible and should be considered in all appropriate patients. The Frank or the Ingram procedure for the development of a functioning vaginal vault should meet with good success, particularly in patients without previous attempts at surgical neovaginal creation. In those patients who have been unsuccessful with dilation attempts or those who are unwilling or unable to use these procedures, the use of a split-thickness skin graft with surgical neovaginal creation offers a high success rate when performed by trained specialists.[8]

Class II: Disorders of Vertical Fusion of the Müllerian Ducts

Vertical fusion disorders of the müllerian ducts include transverse vaginal septa and cervical agenesis or dysgenesis.

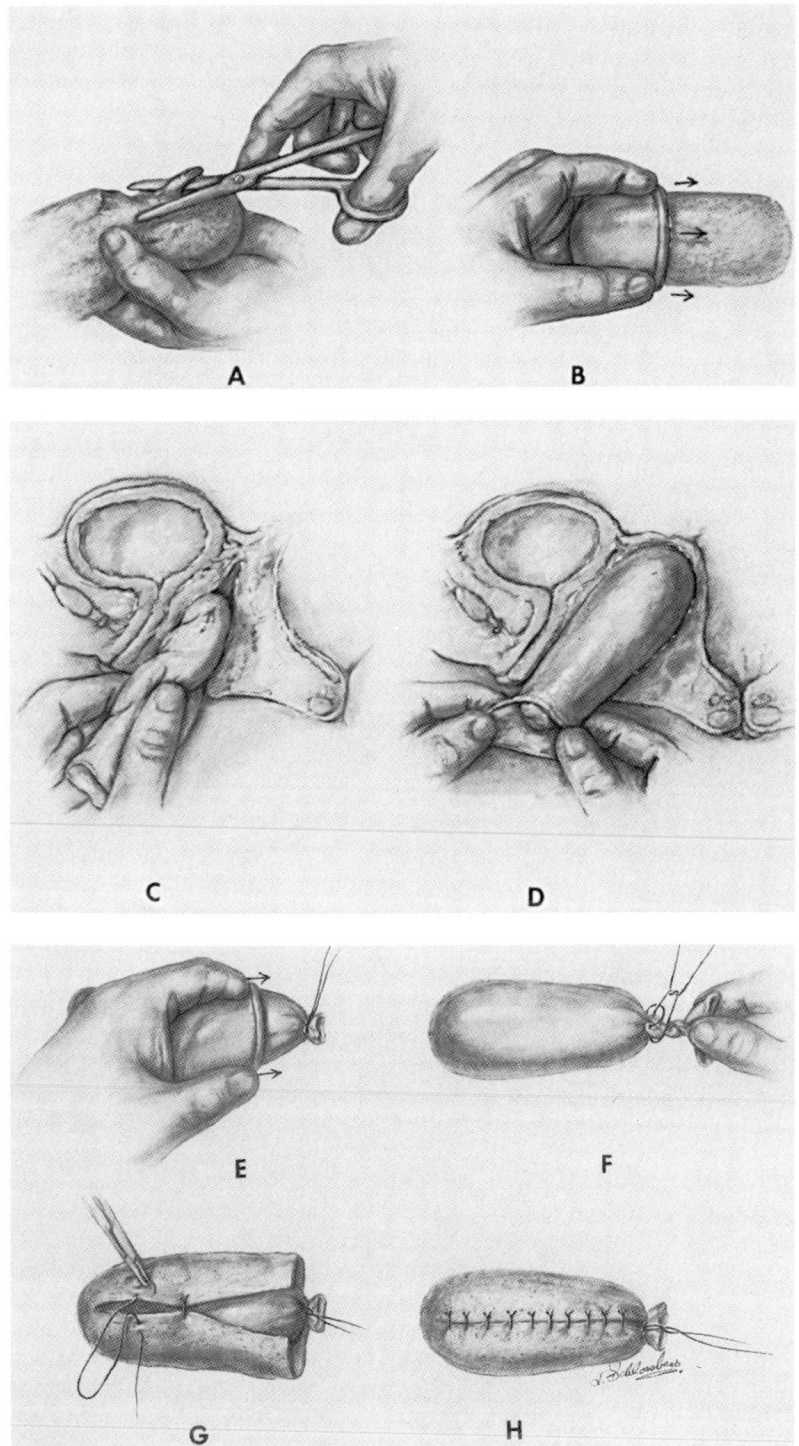

FIGURE 27–6. Counsellor-Flor modification of the Mc-Indoe technique. *A,* A form is cut from a foam rubber block. *B,* A condom is placed over the form. *C,* The form is compressed and placed into the vagina. *D,* Air is allowed to expand the foam rubber, which accommodates the neovaginal space. The condom is closed and the form is removed. *E,* A second condom is placed over the form and *F,* tied securely. *G,* The graft is then sewn over the form with interrupted No. 5-0 nonreactive sutures. *H,* The undersurfaces of the sutured edges of the graft are exteriorized. The vaginal form is ready for insertion into the neovagina. (*A* to *H* From Thompson JD, Rock JA, editors. Te Linde's Operative Gynecology. 7th edition. Philadelphia: JB Lippincott, 1992:617.)

Transverse vaginal septa are generally correctable through reconstructive surgical procedures. Cervical agenesis or dysgenesis has been managed surgically[27]; however, the results have been somewhat disappointing. Combined cervical agenesis with a transverse vaginal septum or with a partial agenesis of the upper vagina has been reported.[28, 29] Like isolated cervical agenesis, combined cervical and vaginal defects are not easily correctable by surgical procedures, and in patients for whom reconstructive attempts have been made, significant complications have been encountered.

TRANSVERSE VAGINAL SEPTA

Transverse vaginal septa are a relatively uncommon reproductive tract anomaly, with data suggesting an occurrence rate of 1 in 30,000.[30] It is likely, however, that the true incidence is somewhat less than these data suggest. These septa may be divided into two groups: (1) those resulting in an obstructed vagina (complete or imperforate) and (2) those that do not obstruct the vaginal canal (incomplete or perforate). These septa result from one of several developmental

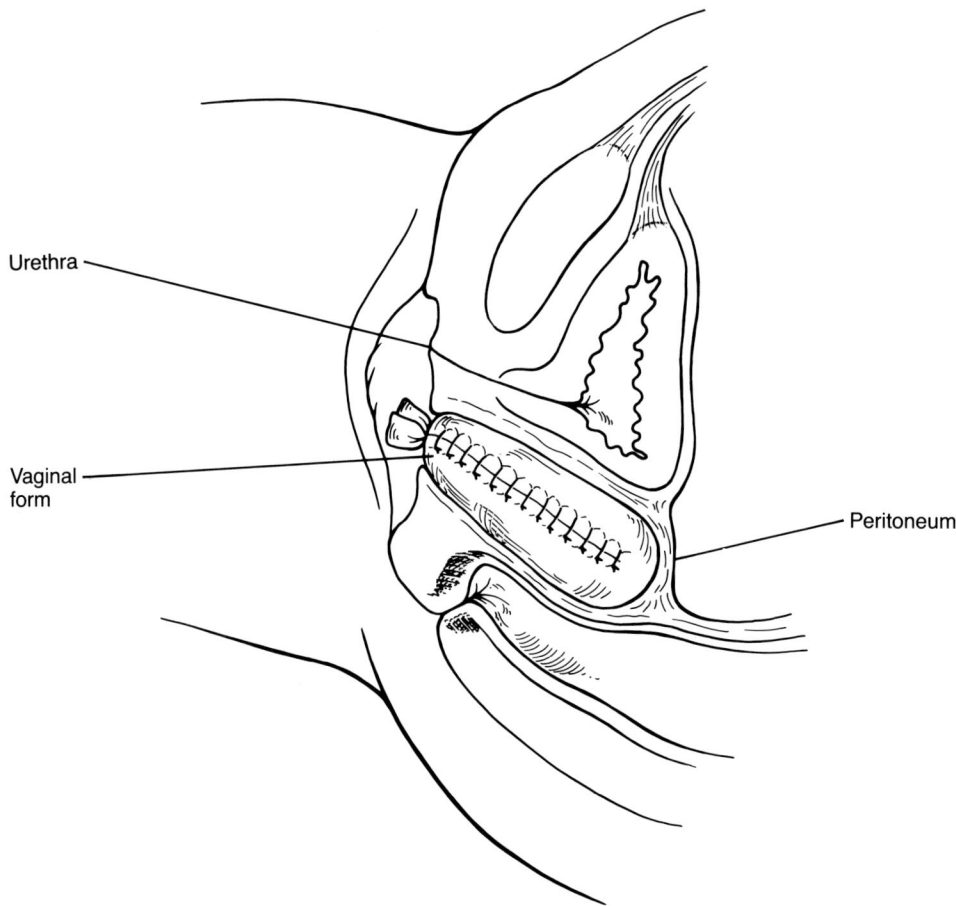

FIGURE 27–7. The vaginal form has been inserted into the neovaginal space, and the edges of the graft have been sutured to the cut edges of the vaginal epithelium. (From Rock JA, Jones HW Jr. Construction of a neovagina for the patient with a flat perineum. Am J Obstet Gynecol 1989; 160:849.)

defects, including a failure of complete canalization of the primordial vaginal plate or a lack of union of the urogenital sinus with the caudal extension of the paramesonephric ducts.[8] Some evidence suggests that one type of complete vaginal septum may be the result of expression of an uncommon autosomal recessive gene.[31]

These septa most frequently occur in one of three areas of the vaginal canal: (1) the upper vagina or high transverse septa; (2) the middle vaginal septa; and (3) the lower vaginal septa (Fig. 27–8). The most common location of these defects is in the upper vagina at the junction of the middle and the upper third of the canal. Septa occurring in this area may be quite wide and are occasionally associated with an underdeveloped vagina caudal to the septa. These cases are examples of the more extreme forms of transverse vaginal septa.

The diagnosis of a complete vaginal septum is most commonly made at the time of puberty. With the onset of menstruation, cyclic pelvic pain is initially experienced; however, after a period, hematocolpos or hematometra frequently develops (Fig. 27–9), giving rise to increasing pelvic pressure and pain. A diagnosis before puberty is difficult except when the obstructed outflow tract results in hydromucocolpos. These defects are often mistaken for an intact hymen.

Although incomplete septa may go unnoticed, they are most frequently diagnosed during pregnancy or during a routine gynecologic examination.[32] These patients have cyclic menses, with the amount of flow being somewhat dependent on the size of the opening in the septum. Presenting symptoms may vary from light but prolonged menses combined with intermenstrual spotting to relatively normal menstrual cycles.

The diagnosis of a transverse vaginal septum begins with suspicion of its presence. It should be suspected in any patient found to have an abnormal vagina or in whom a pelvic mass is palpated, as well as in postpubertal patients who have cyclic pain or pelvic pressure. In contrast with vaginal agenesis, a vaginal vault can usually be visualized, with a reduced length dependent on the location of the septum. Rectal examination allows identification of the uterus and the cervix, and in most instances, of a thickening between the cervix and the visualized vault apex. When hematocolpos or hematometra is present, the resulting distortion may be significant and make identification of the cervix or uterus by palpation extremely difficult. Hematocolpos is more frequent in transverse septa of the lower or middle vagina because of the greater distensibility of the vaginal wall (see Fig. 27–9). In high septa, little vaginal vault remains, and as a result hematometra is more frequent. In patients with hematocolpos, bulging of the vaginal outlet is uncommon; however, if bulging and discoloration occur, a diagnosis of intact hymen should be suspected.

The incidence of associated urologic defects is considerably less with transverse vaginal septa than with agenesis of the müllerian ducts. However, the distended vagina secondary to hematocolpos may compress and displace the bladder anteriorly and the ureters laterally, with resulting hydroureter and

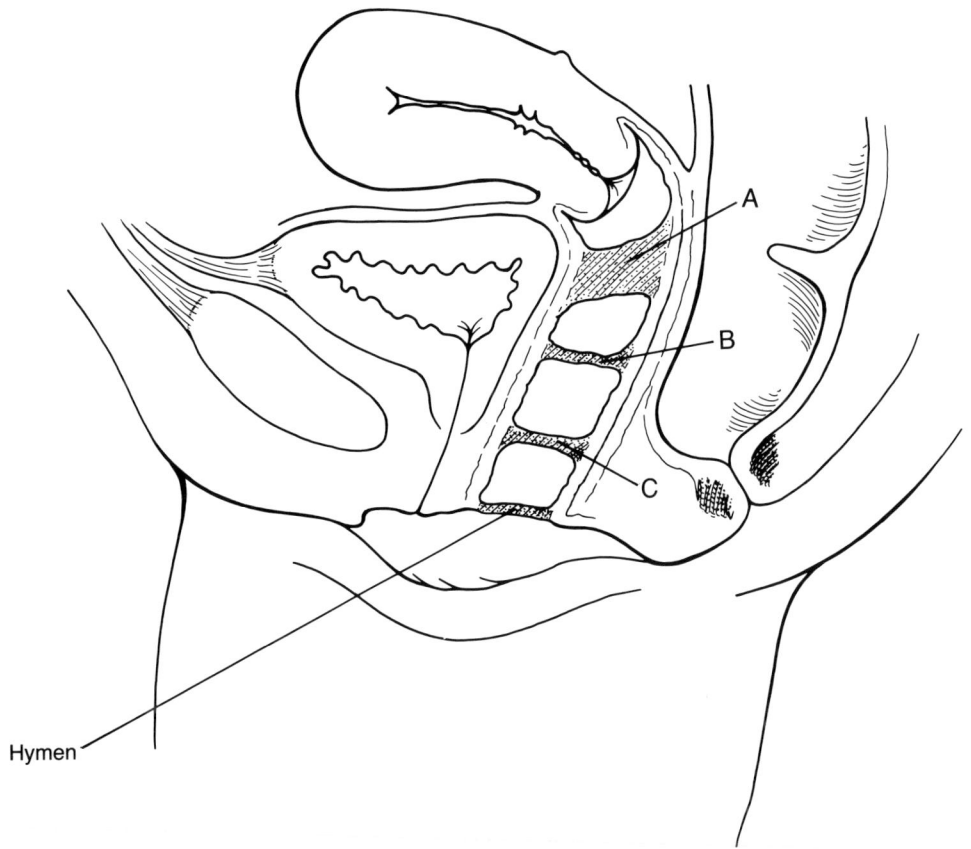

FIGURE 27–8. Transverse vaginal septa of the (*A*) upper vagina or high vaginal septum; (*B*) middle vaginal septum; (*C*) lower vaginal septum. (From Rock JA, Zacur HA, Dlugi AM, et al. Pregnancy success following surgical correction of imperforated hymen and complete transverse vaginal septum. Reprinted with permission from The American College of Obstetricians and Gynecologists [Obstetrics and Gynecology, 1982; 59:450].)

Hymen

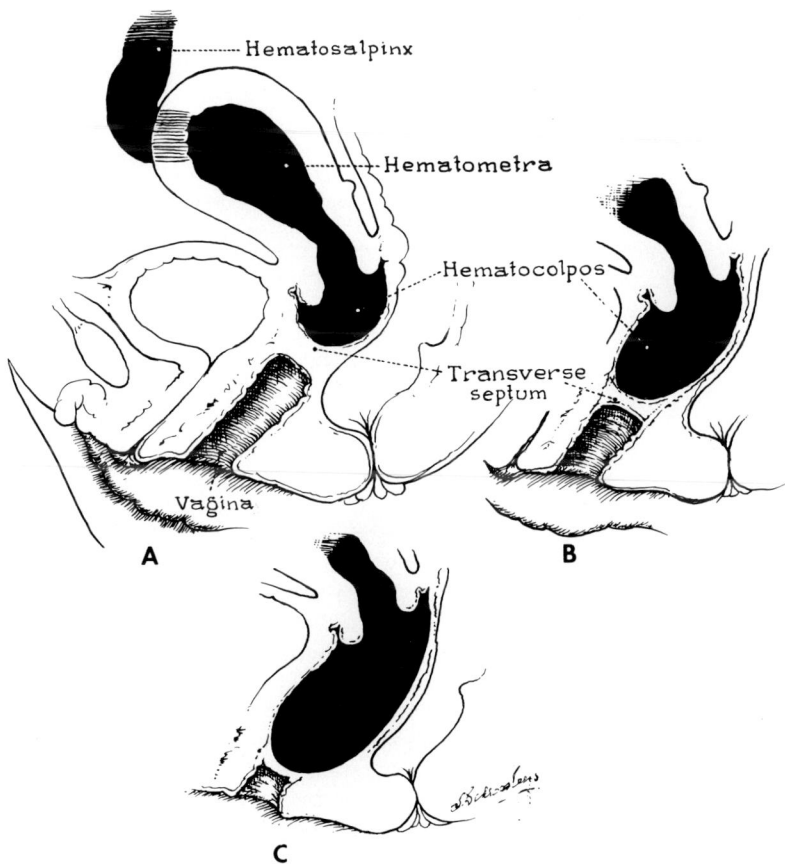

Hematosalpinx

Hematometra

Hematocolpos

Transverse septum

Vagina

A

B

C

FIGURE 27–9. Positions of a septum responsible for complete vaginal obstruction. *A,* High; *B,* Mid; and *C,* Low transverse vaginal septum. Note the position of the hematocolpos. Lower vaginal septa allow more blood to accumulate in the upper vagina. The vaginal mass shown in *C* may be more readily appreciated on rectovaginal examination. (*A* to *C* from Thompson JD, Rock JA, editors. Te Linde's Operative Gynecology. 7th edition. Philadelphia: JB Lippincott, 1992:621.)

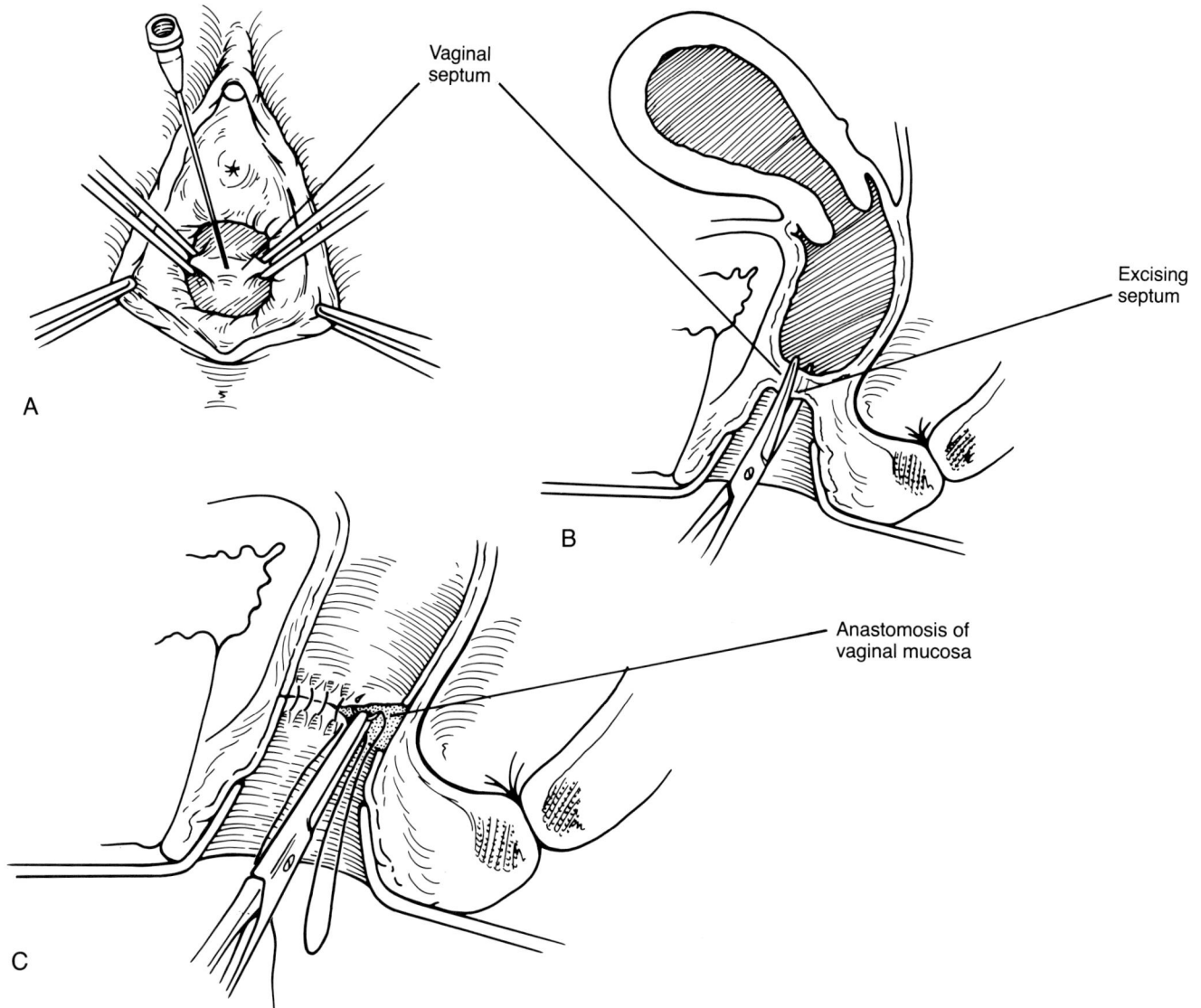

FIGURE 27–10. Excision of a transverse vaginal septum. *A,* A needle is passed through the septum to assess its length and to identify a blood-filled space above it. *B,* A transverse incision is made over the center of the septum or in the area of the greatest bulge, and the septum is excised. *C,* The vaginal mucosa is anastomosed between the upper and lower vagina using an interrupted delayed-absorbable suture. (Reprinted with permission from Seminars in Reproductive Endocrinology, volume 4, issue 1, page 23, 1986, Thieme Medical Publishers, Inc.)

hydronephrosis. Additionally, the rectum and the sigmoid colon may be compressed posteriorly, leading to constipation and intestinal obstruction.

The diagnosis of transverse vaginal septa is not improved by standard radiographic assessment except when a needle can be inserted through the septum and contrast media injected into the upper vaginal space. MRI, however, offers new hope in recognizing vaginal septa both through the identification of the septum location and of menstrual blood in the upper vagina and in the uterus, which appears like contrast media.[33]

Management of these vertical fusion defects consists of excision of the transverse septum. The most effective operation is done from a vaginal approach. Because of distortion, however, occasionally an exploratory laparotomy is necessary, at which time a sound may be passed through the uterine fundus and the cervix to tent the vaginal septum, allowing better identification and safer resection. When the septum is

identified in relation to the bladder and rectum (Fig. 27–10A), a needle may be passed through the septum to assess the length of the defect and identify the space above the septum that generally contains old blood. In septa of the lower and middle vagina, a transverse incision is made over the center of the septum or in the area of the greatest bulge. The septum is then excised using scissors or a sharp scalpel (Fig. 27–10B), and the vaginal mucosa anastomosed between the upper and lower vagina using an interrupted delayed-absorbable suture (Fig. 27–10C). During the dissection of the septum, a previously placed urethral catheter can serve as an anterior guide, and a double-gloved finger in the rectum properly identifies the rectum and serves as a posterior guide, preventing injury. Lateral margins of the septum should be excised widely to prevent postoperative stricture formation. As described in the McIndoe procedure, a soft foam rubber vaginal mold may be cut to a size somewhat larger than the repaired vaginal vault and covered and compressed by a

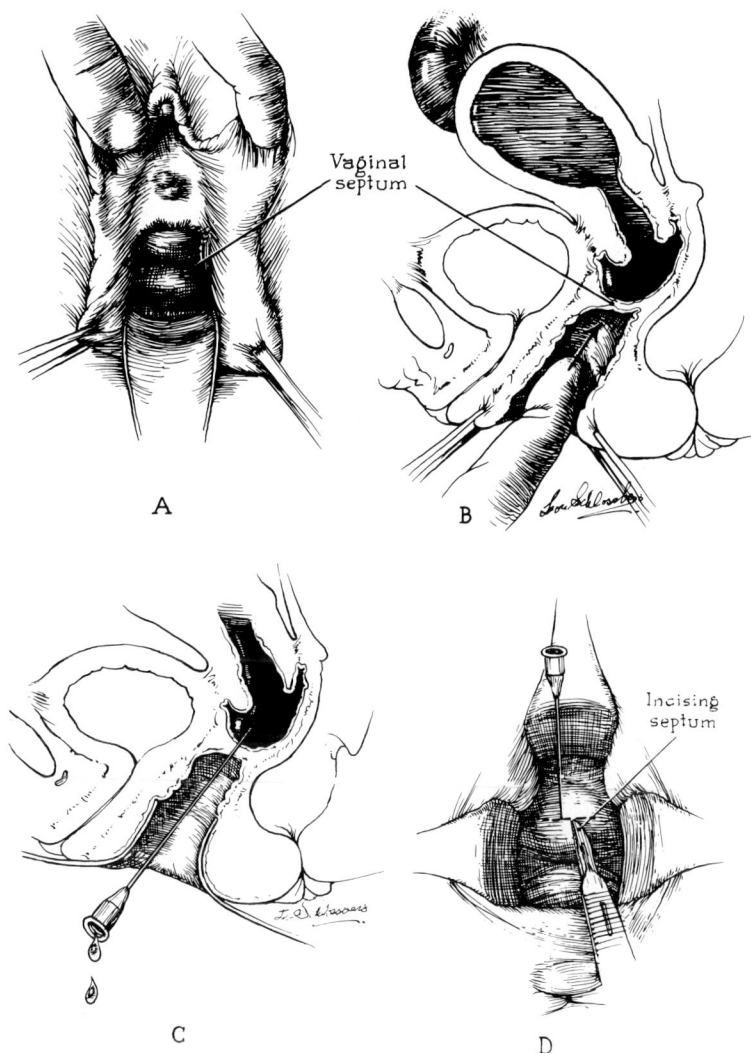

FIGURE 27–11. High transverse vaginal septum. *A,* The neovaginal space is dissected, revealing a high obstructing vaginal membrane. *B,* This may be palpated with the middle finger. *C,* A needle is then placed into the mass. *D,* The incision is made over the needle with a sharp knife.

Illustration continued on following page

sterile plain condom. This form is placed in the vagina for 7 to 10 days and then removed to evaluate the healing process. After this time, the form should be replaced for a 4- to 6-week period with daily removal and cleansing by the patient and with periodic examination to determine complete healing. Sexual activity is permitted after this point. However, if this approach is impractical, vaginal dilation may be necessary to prevent constriction. In such instances a Silastic vaginal form may be used at night until sexual activity is established or until the constrictive phase of the healing process is completed.

Prior to surgical correction of a transverse vaginal septum, the lower vaginal vault and the lower surface of the septum are covered by squamous epithelium, whereas the upper vaginal vault and the upper surface of the septum are covered by glandular epithelium. After surgical excision of the septum, the upper vaginal epithelium is transformed into squamous epithelium over time.

High transverse or upper vaginal septa are generally more difficult to repair and require the same dedication of the patient as required for McIndoe procedures. The increased width of the high transverse septum results in a significant atretic portion of vagina, which makes anastomosis of the upper and lower vaginal epithelium impossible after septal excision. In these instances, it is frequently necessary to create a space between the rectum and the bladder to accurately identify the defect. Once the septum has been fully identified, excision is accomplished in much the same manner as lower septa (Fig. 27–11*A* to *G*).

Because the vaginal epithelium cannot usually be anastomosed in high transverse vaginal septa, some type of extended use of a vaginal form is necessary to prevent stenosis and obstruction of the surgical site. An indwelling Lucite form (Fig. 27–11*H*) consisting of a bulbous upper end and an open central channel for menstruation is recommended. The form can be held in place by a retaining harness or girdle and, in most instances, should be left in place for 4 to 6 months to allow for complete epithelization of the surgical site. During this time, periodic examinations should be accomplished to assess the completeness of healing. After removal of the form sexual activity is permitted; however, daily vaginal dilation should be accomplished by the patient for an additional 2 to 4 months. An alternative is the use of a split-thickness graft or a **Z**-plasty or flap procedure; however, in either case, a vaginal form must be used for 4 to 6 months to prevent vaginal constriction. Recent data from Hurst and Rock[33a] suggest that preoperative dilation of a high transverse vaginal septum facilitates repair of the septum. In their arti-

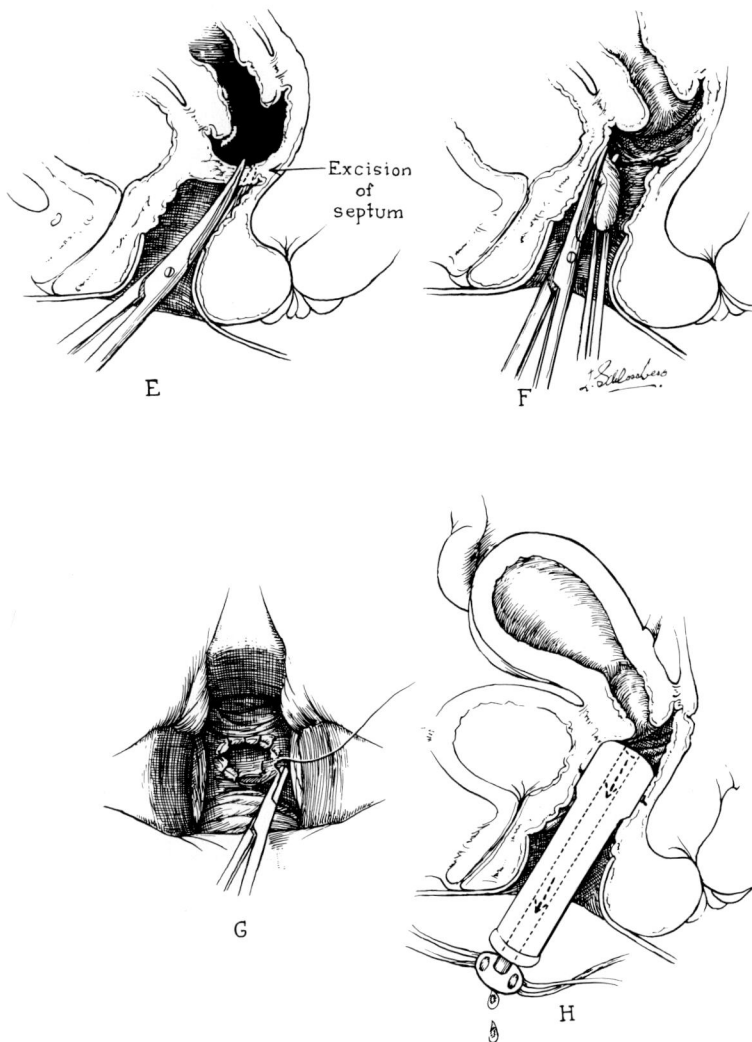

FIGURE 27–11 *Continued E* and *F,* The high transverse vaginal septum is usually thick, and considerable bleeding may occur when excised with Mayo scissors. *G,* After the septum is removed, the wall of the septum is oversewn with interrupted sutures of No. 2-0 chromic catgut. Because the distance between the septum and the upper vagina is too great to allow anastomosis, an acrylic resin (Lucite) form is placed in the vagina such that epithelialization may occur over the form while vaginal patency is maintained. *H,* The form is in place and fitted with a plastic retainer. Rubber strips may be placed through the retainer and attached to a waist belt to allow constant upper pressure so that the form is retained in the upper vagina. Modification of this method includes a small adapter to allow drainage through the acrylic resin (Lucite) form, preventing the accumulation of old blood and mucus in the upper vagina. (*A* to *H* from Thompson JD, Rock JA, editors. Te Linde's Operative Gynecology. 7th edition. Philadelphia: JB Lippincott, 1992:624–625.)

cle, the authors describe an alternative approach to management of a patient with a transverse vaginal septum that includes (1) ultrasound-directed needle aspiration combined with broad-spectrum antibiotic prophylaxis to decompress the hematocolpos and to relieve the acute pain; (2) continuous endometrial suppression to prevent recurrence of the hematocolpos; and (3) vaginal dilation prior to resection of the septum to lengthen the lower vagina. Hurst and Rock believe that such an approach simplifies the septal excision and improves the results.

CERVICAL AGENESIS OR DYSGENESIS

Agenesis, or atresia, of the uterine cervix is an infrequent müllerian anomaly with fewer than 50 cases reported in the medical literature by 1989.[29, 34] This anomaly may occur in several configurations: (1) total absence of the cervix (Fig. 27–12); (2) a cervix containing only stromal tissue with no cervical canal (Fig. 27–13); or (3) a cervix without canalization but with small linear inclusions of endocervical-like tissue (Fig. 27–14).[35] Additionally, this anomaly frequently occurs in association with absence of a portion or all of the vagina.[36] Similar to vaginal septa, cervical agenesis most often is not diagnosed until puberty when cyclic low abdominal

pain without menses causes the patient to seek a gynecologic evaluation.

The diagnosis of cervical agenesis is extremely challenging. Cervical agenesis is frequently mistaken for vaginal atresia or

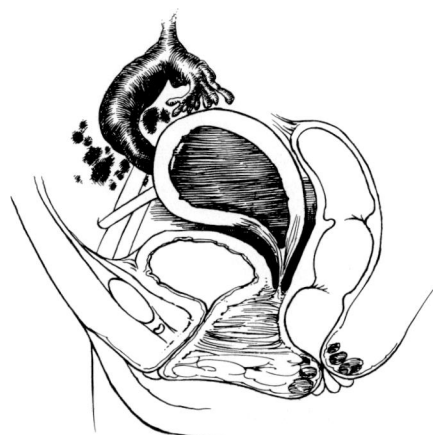

FIGURE 27–12. Congenital absence or dysgenesis of the cervix: cervical agenesis. (From Thompson JD, Rock JA, editors. Te Linde's Operative Gynecology. 7th edition. Philadelphia: JB Lippincott, 1992:625.)

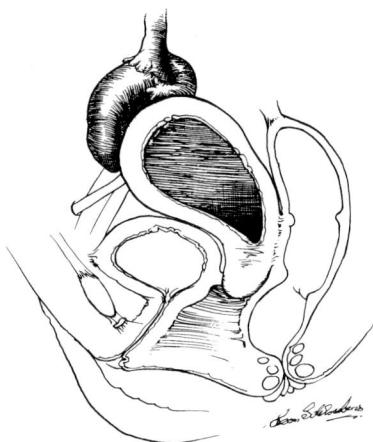

FIGURE 27–13. Congenital absence or dysgenesis of the cervix: a bulbous cervical stroma without an endocervical canal. (From Thompson JD, Rock JA, editors. Te Linde's Operative Gynecology. 7th edition. Philadelphia: JB Lippincott, 1992:627.)

for a transverse vaginal septum because of the common occurrence of an upper vaginal pouch.[35] Standard radiographic assessment or rectovaginal examination is not definitive in making a diagnosis. Ultrasonography may be helpful[37] in the evaluation of this defect. An increasing number of reports suggest, however, that MRI offers the best support in achieving a preoperative diagnosis.[38]

Management of cervical atresia is difficult, particularly when a functioning uterine corpus is present along with both an absent cervix and an absent or partially absent vagina. In these instances it has been extremely hard to maintain an open passage through the vagina and the cervix through which menstruation could occur. Until recently, preservation of the reproductive organs in these patients resulted in numerous complications, including endometriosis, scarring and adhesions, infection, and abdominal and pelvic pain.[35] In the last 9 years several reports have suggested techniques for achieving an open cervicovaginal outflow tract. One report[28] described the construction of a neovagina and a neocervical canal by a series of stents covered with split-thickness skin grafts. Another report[39] described the combination of a McIndoe vaginoplasty with a split-thickness neocervical canal skin graft that resulted later in a 38-week pregnancy delivered by cesarean section. In another report[34] a polyethylene tube and a stainless-steel stem pessary were used to stent a newly created vaginal canal during the process of healing. These cases represent the exception. In most cases repeated dilations have been necessary and, ultimately, the problems of recurrent stenosis, infection, and in many instances, endometriosis, lead to the eventual removal of the uterus.

Of interest is a case in which histologic sections of an atretic cervix revealed endocervical glands within the normal lamina propria and with muscle bundles running deep in the cervix, arranged in a linear fashion, and extending as a complete uninterrupted bridge around the closed end of the cervix.[29] Not all patients with cervical agenesis have this continuous muscle bridge. In some, the muscle bundles do not bridge across the closed end of the cervix but instead come to a junction at a central position normally occupied by the cervical canal. Patients without the muscle bridge may represent those cases that, with creation of a neocervical

canal, would not result in the stenosis and postoperative obstruction that is frequently seen. Perhaps in the future, MRI of patients with cervical agenesis will be able to identify these two types and therefore aid in the decision to carry out reconstructive surgery. However, with successful canalization of the cervix, endocervical glands do not develop and, therefore, natural conception would be impeded.

In addition to the one pregnancy noted earlier, other pregnancies have occurred in patients with cervical agenesis using assisted reproductive technologies.[40]

Currently, the recommended management of cervical agenesis in most patients remains a hysterectomy. For these patients, the surgeon should be prepared to accomplish a vaginoplasty such as the McIndoe procedure at the same time to provide a functional vagina. This is most important in patients who have vaginal dissection at the time of hysterectomy because postoperative vaginal scarring makes future vaginoplasty difficult and with less acceptable outcome.

Class III: Disorders of Lateral Fusion of the Müllerian Ducts

In contrast with vertical fusion disorders of the müllerian ducts, which involve primarily the vagina and cervix, lateral fusion disorders involve the uterine fundus and cervix, and, infrequently, the vagina. These anatomic defects are the result of a complete or partial failure of medial fusion of the two müllerian ducts giving rise to a complete or partial duplication of the uterus, the cervix, and the vagina. A partial failure can result in a single vagina with two cervices and uteri, a single vagina and cervix and two uterine corpora, or a failure of absorption of the uterine septum between the two fused müllerian ducts. These disorders may be divided into (1) asymmetrical defects, which usually result in obstruction, and (2) symmetrical defects, which usually are nonobstructed. The symmetrical defects are further subdivided into six groups: (1) didelphic uterus, (2) bicornuate uterus, (3) septate uterus, (4) arcuate uterus, (5) T-shaped (diethylstilbestrol [DES] drug related) uterine cavity, and (6) unicornuate uterus.

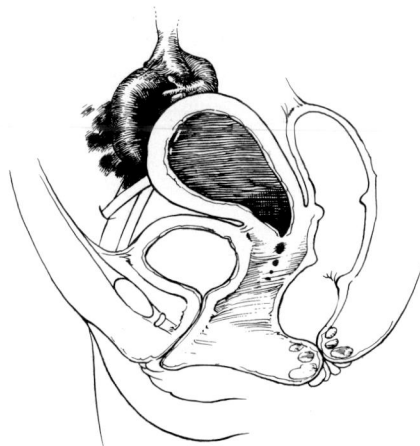

FIGURE 27–14. Congenital absence or dysgenesis: a malformed cervix with islands of endocervical glands present. (From Thompson JD, Rock JA, editors. Te Linde's Operative Gynecology. 7th edition. Philadelphia: JB Lippincott, 1992:627.)

Because a large number of these anomalies go unnoticed, the incidence of these defects is uncertain. A review of the medical literature suggests a conflicting incidence rate. One report suggests an incidence of lateral fusion defects from 0.1% to 0.3% based on pelvic examination at the time of delivery, and an incidence rate of from 1.1% to 3.5% based on hysterosalpingogram (HSG) reviews.[41]

The likely time of diagnosis of lateral fusion disorders depends on the type of defect that exists. Defects leading to an obstruction of the uterus, the cervix, or the vagina, like vertical fusion defects, commonly are diagnosed after puberty because of obstructed menstruation with resulting cramping and abdominal pain. These disorders are usually associated with ipsilateral renal agenesis or other urologic defects. Unobstructed disorders may be diagnosed at a variety of times secondary to mechanical problems such as difficulty with tampon insertion or with coitus due to a vaginal septum. These defects may also be discovered during an evaluation for dysmenorrhea or menorrhagia or during a routine gynecologic examination. Most lateral fusion disorders, however, are diagnosed by HSG during an evaluation for pregnancy wastage or for infertility.[35]

In spite of the success of identification of lateral fusion defects by HSG, the specific disorder frequently cannot be determined by this procedure. That is to say, septate uteri cannot easily be differentiated from arcuate or bicornuate uteri (Fig. 27–15A to C). In the past, the true diagnosis was made through use of several procedures including a pelvic examination, an HSG, or laparoscopy or hysteroscopy. More recently, pelvic ultrasonography and MRI have proved helpful in identifying the actual type of lateral fusion defect and therefore aiding significantly in preoperative planning. Ultra-

sonography has been shown to have the same sensitivity as and a somewhat greater specificity than HSG in the demonstration of uterine abnormalities.[42] Other studies confirm the capability of ultrasonography in screening for[43] and diagnosing[44] uterine malformations.

In spite of the past use of HSG and the more recent advances in ultrasonography, both procedures have some drawbacks. HSG is an invasive procedure, and the radiation exposure, although small, is of concern to some physicians. Ultrasonography is a noninvasive procedure but lacks some aspects of resolution that would be helpful in differentiating a fibrous septum from a uterine wall with both fibrous and muscle tissue.

MRI is an extremely effective means of diagnosing müllerian duct anomalies. MRI eliminates the invasiveness of HSG and shows greater resolution of tissue densities than does ultrasonography, therefore imparting the ability to characterize septal tissue.[45] This ability of MRI to provide exceptional soft-tissue contrast results in a relatively clear definition of zonal anatomy of the uterus[46] and, therefore, the ability to differentiate bicornuate uteri from septate and arcuate uteri as well as the capability to image and diagnose didelphic uterus and unicornuate uteri. The ability to preoperatively differentiate between the septate and arcuate uterus and the bicornuate uterus is of considerable importance because the surgical correction of the septate uterus is now accomplished primarily by operative hysteroscopy, whereas reconstructive surgery of a bicornuate uterus is accomplished through abdominal surgery. Such a differentiation is possible with a reported 100% sensitivity by MRI.[47]

MRI procedures are expensive and are not available in all locations. As a result, HSG still remains the most commonly

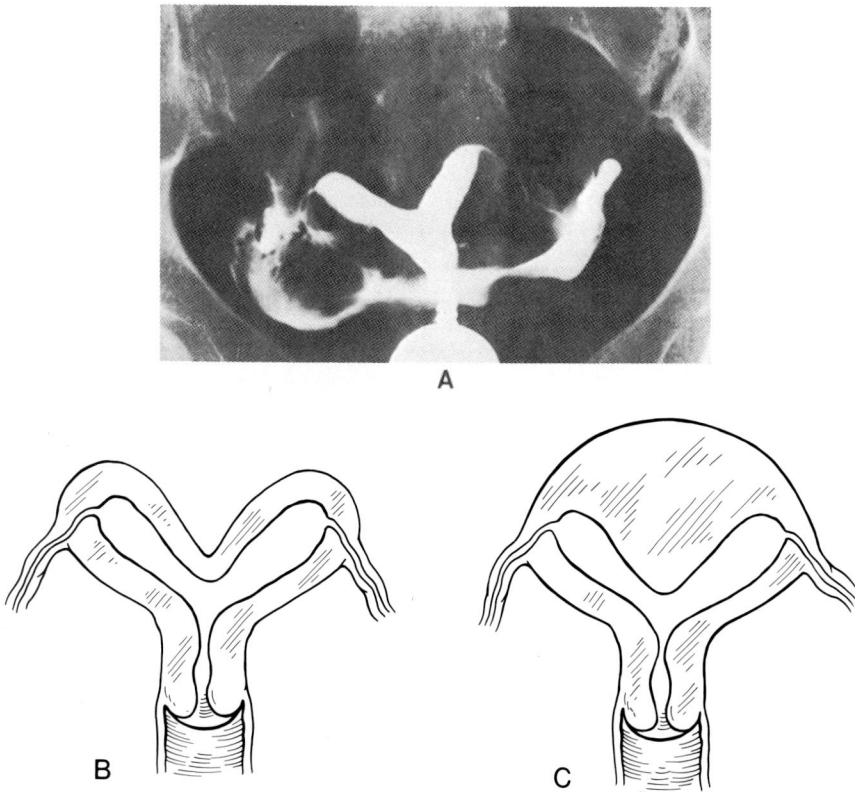

FIGURE 27–15. *A,* Hysterogram of a double uterus. A bicornuate *(B)* and a septate uterus *(C)* are types of double uteri. Visualization of the fundus is required to determine the type of uterus. *(B and C* adapted from Thompson JD, Rock JA, editors. Te Linde's Operative Gynecology. 7th edition. Philadelphia: JB Lippincott, 1992:630.)

used diagnostic modality in determining müllerian duct defects. However, HSG techniques alone are inadequate to distinguish between a septate and a bicornuate uterus. Some recent data suggest that if the angle of divergence of two straight uterine cavities as seen on HSG is 75 degrees or less, the defect is most likely a septate uterus, and additional studies may be unnecessary. If the cavities seen on HSG are not straight, but instead curved, or if the angle of divergence of the cavities is wider than 75 degrees but less than 105 degrees, a diagnosis by HSG cannot be substantiated, and a luteal phase ultrasonography evaluation taking advantage of the thickened endometrium contrasted with the myometrium and intervening space is necessary to rule out a bicornuate uterus.[48] No matter what modality is used, it is important to have an accurate understanding of the müllerian defect before surgical correction is attempted. From a practical point of view, an HSG, combined with an ultrasonographic evaluation, would be expected to provide necessary information for preoperative planning in most instances. Septum versus uterine wall differentiation, however, may require MRI assessment.

ASYMMETRICAL DISORDERS OF LATERAL FUSION

Asymmetrical disorders of lateral fusion of the müllerian ducts are the result of normal development of one duct and abnormal development of the contralateral duct owing either to a failure of development or to incomplete development. The underdeveloped or poorly developed duct may have the defect present at any point along the duct or throughout the entire route of the duct. Additionally, the actual defect may involve the musculature, endometrium, ligamentous attachments, cervix, or fallopian tube individually or in combination. On the opposite side, a relatively normal unicornuate uterus is found. The underdeveloped horn may or may not communicate with the normal side. If the underdeveloped side has an endometrium, cyclic abdominal pain will occur at menarche secondary to the obstructed outflow tract. In these patients, the diagnosis may be clouded by the fact that the normal horn cycles in an appropriate fashion with periodic vaginal menstrual discharge. As in all patients with an obstructed outflow tract and a patent fallopian tube, increased retrograde menstruation results in a high incidence of pelvic endometriosis. For this reason, early diagnosis and surgical intervention are important.

Unicornuate Uterus with Noncommunicating Rudimentary Anlagen or Horn. Surgical management of a unicornuate uterus with a noncommunicating rudimentary anlage or horn is based on the presence or absence of functioning endometrium in the noncommunicating abnormal horn. If functioning endometrium is not present, excision of the rudimentary horn is not indicated unless other reasons for reconstructive surgery are present. If functioning endometrium is present, a simple excision of the horn along with its fallopian tube is recommended. A functioning endometrium may be suspected on the basis of cyclic symptoms of abdominal pain and diagnosed with an ultrasonographic scan showing a fluctuating endometrial thickness in association with the pain or a laparoscopic visualization of retrograde menstruation or a dilated, obstructed fallopian tube. Prior to surgical excision of a rudimentary uterine horn, an assessment of the urinary tract is necessary because of the

associated incidence of ipsilateral renal agenesis and the possibility of ureteral distortion when the kidney is present.

Unilateral Obstruction of a Cavity in a Double Uterus. A less common asymmetrical disorder is a unilateral obstruction of a cavity of a double uterus secondary to failure of cervical development or canalization or hypoplasia of the lower uterine segment or cervix. In these patients the presenting complaint is significant dysmenorrhea beginning with menarche. Pelvic examination usually identifies a palpable mass secondary to a dilated uterine horn with trapped menstrual discharge (Fig. 27–16A and B). Surgical management of this defect involves an incision into the anterior wall of the dilated horn with evacuation of menstrual discharge, excision of the septum between the two cavities, and anastomosis of the two cavity walls using interrupted myometrial sutures of medium-sized (2-0) nonreactive material reinforcing a continuous locking stitch in the muscularis adjacent to the uterine cavity. The procedure is completed with an outer layer of interrupted nonreactive suture uniting the outer muscularis and the serosa. As with other asymmetrical müllerian defects, a preoperative urinary tract assessment should be accomplished.

Unilateral Vaginal Obstruction Associated with a Double Uterus. A third group of asymmetrical obstructive disorders is the combination of a double uterus associated with a unilateral partial or complete vaginal obstruction. These defects are divided into three groups: (1) complete unilateral vaginal obstruction without uterine cavity communication between the double uteri; (2) incomplete unilateral vaginal obstruction without uterine communication; and (3) complete unilateral vaginal obstruction with lateral communication between the double uterine cavities (Fig. 27–17A to C). The presenting complaints in each of these groups include abdominal pain and dysmenorrhea. In groups 1 and 3, a perivaginal mass can usually be palpated. In these same two groups, menses are regular, and the pelvic pain is cyclic. In group 2, intermenstrual bleeding with foul-smelling mucopurulent discharge is common.

The diagnosis is suspected with a careful pelvic examination revealing an upper vaginal defect. The diagnosis may be supported with an ultrasonographic scan defining the two uterine cavities or by an MRI scan revealing a double uterus and an obstructed upper vagina with trapped menstrual blood. Surgical management of all three groups of unilateral vaginal obstruction involves careful excision of the vaginal septum. Abdominal exploration is generally unnecessary unless other defects are apparent. There is no need to repair small communications between uterine cavities at the same time.

A unilateral vaginal septum often may be quite thick. For this reason, an incision should first be made into the obstructed upper vaginal space, and once the cavity is defined, the septal excision should be completed, taking caution to firmly grasp the entire septal wall to prevent retraction and slippage during suturing.

SYMMETRICAL DISORDERS OF LATERAL FUSION

Symmetrical disorders of lateral fusion may be divided into six separate groups depending on the degree and location of the defect. These groups include (1) didelphic uterus, (2) bicornuate uterus, (3) septate uterus, (4) arcuate uterus (5)

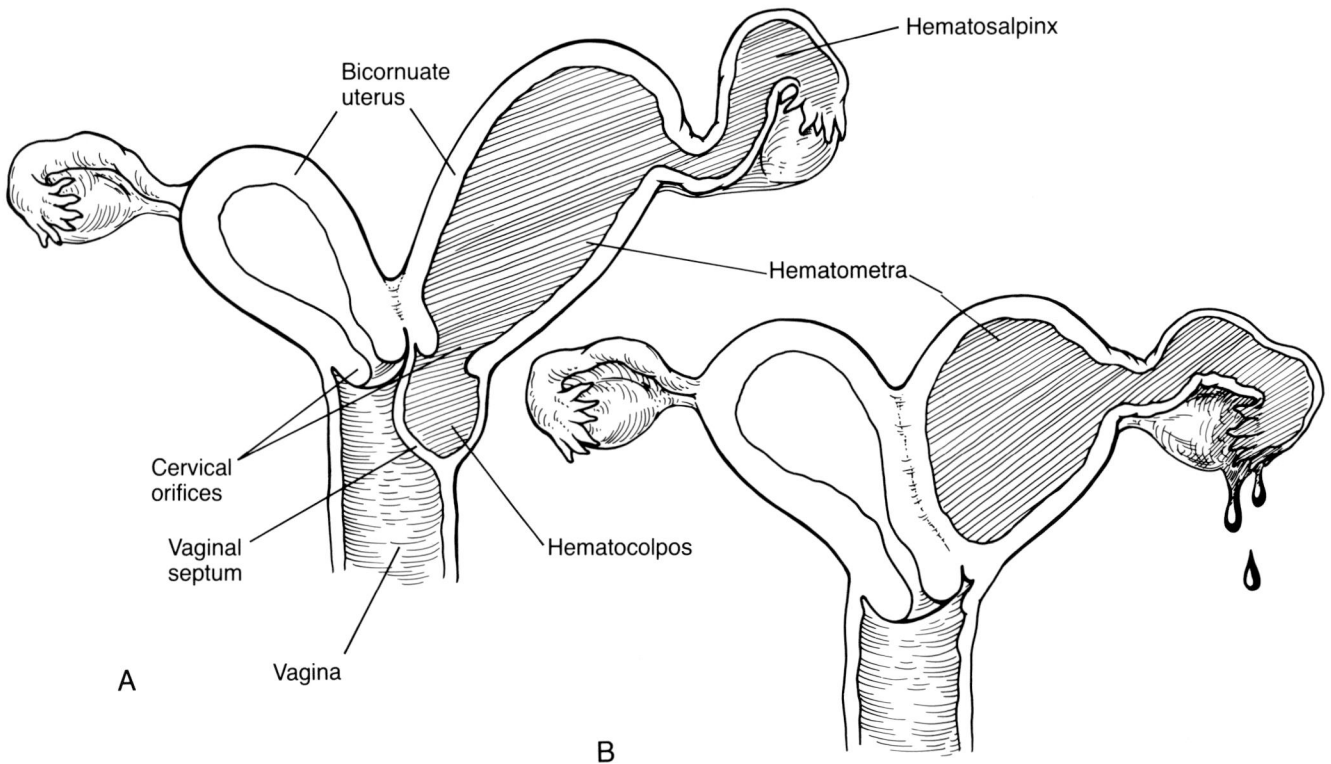

FIGURE 27–16. *A,* Double uterus with unilateral, complete vaginal obstruction and ispilateral renal agenesis. *B,* A double uterus with a noncommunicating horn and hematometra. (*A* and *B* adapted from Thompson JD, Rock JA, editors. Te Linde's Operative Gynecology. 7th edition. Philadelphia: JB Lippincott, 1992.)

T-shaped uterine cavity (DES drug related), and (6) unicornuate uterus (Fig. 27–18). Aside from the fifth group, which is not depicted in the figure, these disorders all reflect a defect in fusion of the müllerian ducts, a defect in the development of a single müllerian duct, or a defect in the reabsorption of the septum between the developing müllerian ducts. Some of these defects are correctable surgically, whereas others are either excised or best left untouched. The surgical management of some of these disorders has undergone significant changes in the last decade owing to the advancement of operative hysteroscopic techniques. A prerequisite for successful use of these newer techniques is an accurate diagnosis of the müllerian defect.

Didelphic Uterus. Surgical management of a didelphic uterus is dependent on the nature of the presenting complaints. Because both uterine horns have normal outflow tracts, cyclic pain and dysmenorrhea are not more frequent than in normal uteri. This defect is usually associated with a partial or complete longitudinal vaginal septum. These septa may be associated with dyspareunia because of the reduction in size of either vaginal canal. Surgical management in these cases would be limited to simple excision of the longitudinal vaginal septum. Such an excision, although generally uncomplicated, may become quite difficult owing to an unusual thickness or vascularity of the septum. Excision in these instances should be carried out with a Foley catheter in the urethra and bladder to delineate these structures from the anterior excision area and a double-gloved finger in the rectum to delineate this structure from the posterior excision area. Anastomosis of the two mucosal surfaces should be accomplished once the septum has been completely excised.

Conversely, because most patients with a didelphic uterus have a longitudinal vaginal septum, the finding of such a septum during a routine examination should result in suspicion of a didelphic uterus.

In patients with a didelphic uterus without obstruction, surgical reconstruction of the uterus and cervix is usually not indicated. In these disorders, successful pregnancy rates are among the highest of the uterine anomalies[49]; however, not all data support this conclusion.[50] A unification procedure is therefore not indicated in most cases of didelphic uterus and, when accomplished, is technically difficult with disappointing results, particularly if the cervix is involved in the unification procedure.

Bicornuate Uterus. A bicornuate uterus may occur in several forms: (1) those with a complete wall and septum extending inferiorly to the cervix and (2) those with only a partial wall and septum. Both of these forms may exist with a complete longitudinal vaginal septum, with a partial longitudinal vaginal septum, or with no vaginal septum. Surgical reconstruction of a bicornuate uterus is accomplished through one of several unification metroplasty techniques, the purpose of which is to increase the volume of the uterine cavity and to remove an intervening wall and septum that may interfere with pregnancy outcome. Patients with a bicornuate uterus usually do not have difficulty in becoming pregnant. They do, however, experience an increased incidence of pregnancy wastage. When pregnancies progress into the third trimester or to term, additional difficulties in delivery may occur because of malpresentation.[8] The cause of reproductive failure earlier in pregnancy remains unclear. It has been suggested that reduced intrauterine space interferes

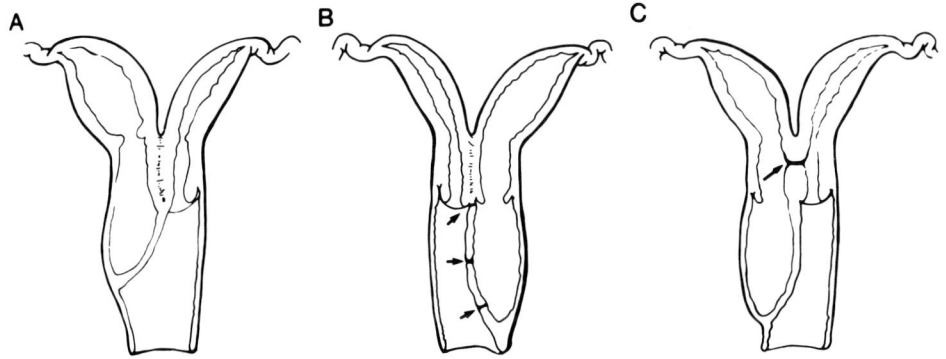

FIGURE 27–17. Double uterus, complete or incomplete vaginal obstruction, and ipsilateral renal agenesis. *A,* Complete vaginal obstruction. *B,* Incomplete vaginal obstruction. *C,* Complete vaginal obstruction with a lateral communicating double uterus. (*A* to *C* from Rock JA, Jones HW Jr. The double uterus associated with an obstructed hemivagina and ipsilateral renal agenesis. Am J Obstet Gynecol 1980; 138:340.)

with placental or fetal growth,[52] and in the case of uterine septum, reduced vascular supply results in an unfavorable implantation site.[51] If this is true, it is likely that the vascular bed is similarly less than optimal in a bicornuate uterus.

Abdominal unification procedures for surgical reconstruction of a bicornuate or septate uterus include (1) the Strassmann metroplasty; (2) the modified Jones metroplasty; and (3) the Tompkins metroplasty (Fig. 27–19). These procedures are accomplished through a transverse abdominal incision. Because each technique involves a significant uterine incision, hemostasis becomes quite important and requires special attention. Hemostasis may be adequately achieved by the use of tourniquets or vasoconstrictive agents such as vasopressin. For the most effective results, tourniquets should be placed around the junction of the lower uterine segment passing laterally through a broad ligament avascular space just outside the uterine vessels. Because of a significant blood supply to the uterus from the ovarian vessels, it is also

necessary to place tourniquets around both infundibulopelvic ligaments using a similar hole in an avascular space below the ligament. When vasopressin is used, 20 U is diluted with 20 mL of normal saline and injected into the anterior and posterior walls of the uterine corpora.

All three abdominal uterine metroplasty procedures have resulted in successful reconstruction of müllerian duct lateral fusion defects. The Strassmann metroplasty procedure is the most commonly used technique for unification of a bicornuate uterus and should be considered to be the procedure of choice in these defects. The Strassmann technique may also be used in the unification of a didelphic uterus, although this is not a frequently accomplished procedure because of less

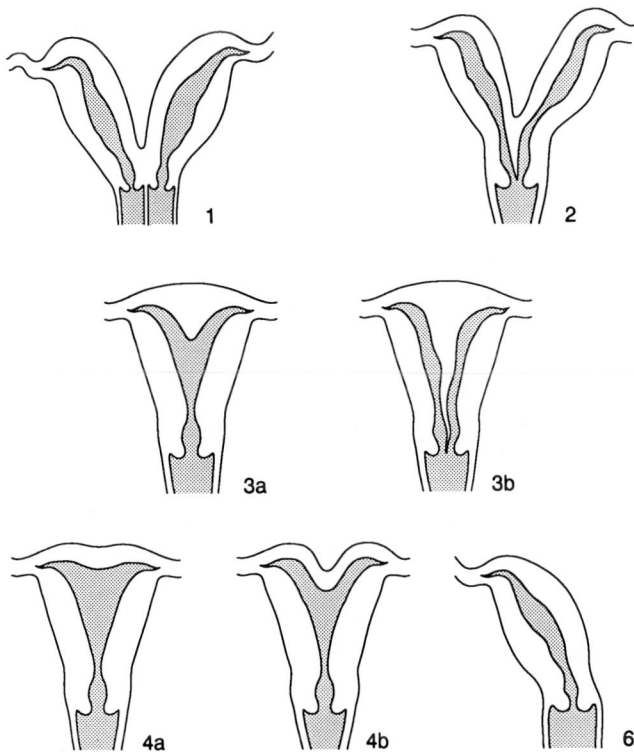

FIGURE 27–18. Diagram of the various forms of double uteri. See text for explanation.

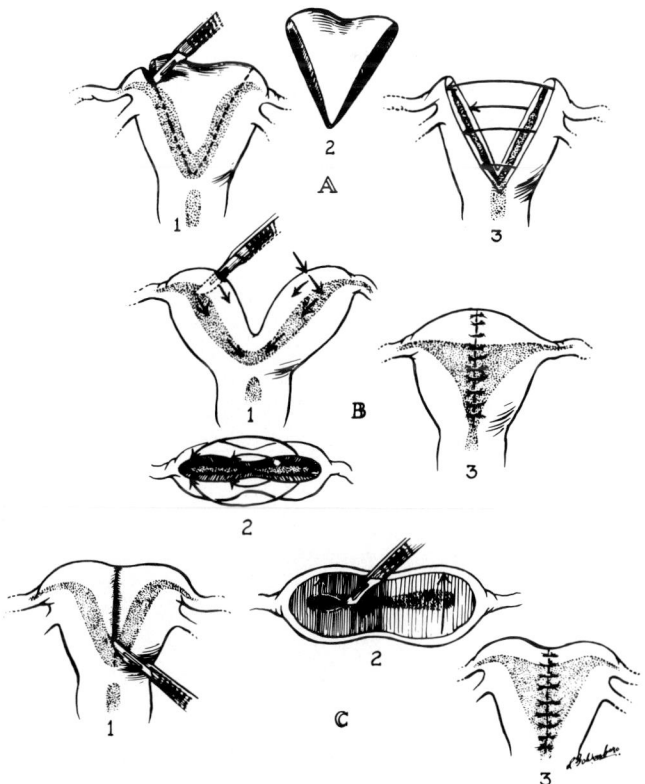

FIGURE 27–19. *A,* Diagram of a method of repairing a small septate uterus by excision of a wedge. *B,* Diagram of the Strassmann technique of repair. This technique is applicable to a bicornuate uterus but not as applicable to a septate uterus. *C,* Repair of a septate uterus by the Tompkins technique. (*A* to *C* from Jones HW Jr, Rock JA. Reparative and Constructive Surgery of the Female Generative Tract. ©1983, the Williams & Wilkins Co., Baltimore.)

than desirable results. Before a Strassmann metroplasty is started, careful inspection of the pelvis should be accomplished after the abdominal cavity is opened because, not infrequently, a broad peritoneal band will be identified running from the bladder wall posteriorly to the anterior wall of the rectum and sigmoid colon and passing between the two lateral uterine corpora of the bicornuate uterus (Fig. 27–20). This band should be excised to allow visualization and space for the metroplasty. Once this is accomplished and hemostatic procedures instituted, the metroplasty should proceed without complication. The two uterine corpora are incised on their median surfaces in a longitudinal axis deep enough to expose the uterine cavity. The incision is carried inferiorly to a point below the junction of the two uterine corpora and, if necessary, to the cervix so that when the two sides are joined, a single uterine cavity and endocervical canal remain. If the cervix is duplicated, it is suggested that they not be joined because the resulting complications, including incompetent cervix, do not justify the additional procedure. Equally important is the care that must be taken with the superior end of the incision in order not to come too close to or damage the tubal ostium or the interstitial segment of the fallopian tube.

Closure of the uterus in all abdominal metroplasty procedures should be carried out in three layers of interrupted suture, with the first layer directed so that the knots are tied within the uterine cavity. It is suggested that this first inner layer encompass both endometrium and the inner myometrium. The second layer should approximate the middle myometrium, and the third layer, the outer myometrium. No. 2-0 nonreactive suture on a tapered atraumatic needle has proven to be most effective. Finally, the serosal edges should be approximated with a No. 3-0 or 4-0 nonreactive suture using a stitch exposing the least amount of suture and knots. Application of adhesion retardants such as oxidized regenerated cellulose (Interceed) or a surgical membrane (Gore-Tex) may be beneficial. The most effective adhesion retardant, however, has proved to be careful surgical technique resulting in a smooth symmetrical closure with serosal borders in close approximation and minimal exposed suture material.

The modified Jones metroplasty, although better suited for septate uteri, may be used in the reconstruction of partial bicornuate uteri and is accomplished in much the same manner as the Strassmann technique. In these cases, an incision is made into the uterine cavity starting on the anterior surface of each uterine corpora and directed inferiorly and medially toward the junction of the two corpora. A similar incision is made posteriorly removing a **V**-shaped wedge of tissue representing the medial wall of the bicornuate uterus. Care must be taken to avoid the tubal ostium or the interstitial portion of the fallopian tube during both the initial incision and the closure. Closure of the uterine walls should use the same suture technique as in the Strassmann metroplasty.

The Tompkins metroplasty is also more suited for surgical reconstruction of a septate uterus but may be useful in the repair of some types of partial bicornuate uteri that present with a normal-appearing fundal surface, no visible separation of the uterine corpora, and a thin intervening wall. This technique is accomplished by making a single midline incision in the septal wall between the two uterine cavities and carrying the incision interiorly until the endometrial cavity is reached. The central septal wall is then incised in a lateral fashion from a point 1 cm medial to the tubal ostium to a similar point on the opposite fundal surface. This incision is extended interiorly until the uterine cavity is entered. No septum is excised, and the uterine wall is closed in the same manner as in the Strassman procedure. In both types of bicornuate uterus, a metroplasty procedure should be accompanied by the excision of a partial or complete vaginal septum.

Septate Uterus. The septate uterus may also occur in several forms: (1) those with a complete septum extending

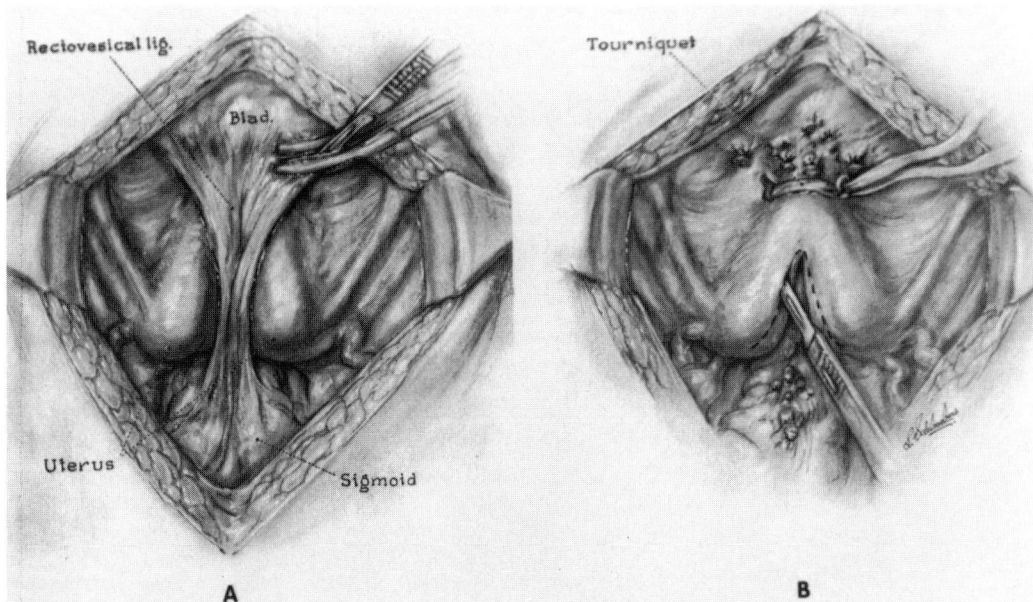

FIGURE 27–20. Strassmann metroplasy with modifications. *A,* If a rectovesical ligament is found, it should be removed. *B,* An incision is made on the medial side of each hemicorpus and carried deep enough to enter the uterine cavity. The edges of the myometrium will evert to face the opposite side. (From Thompson JD, Rock JA, editors. Te Linde's Operative Gynecology. 7th edition. Philadelphia: JB Lippincott, 1992.)

inferiorly to the cervix and (2) those with a partial or incomplete longitudinal vaginal septum. Similar to the bicornuate uterus, both these forms may also exist with a complete longitudinal vaginal septum, with a partial longitudinal vaginal septum, or with no vaginal septum.

It is important to differentiate accurately between a septate uterus and a bicornuate uterus for several reasons. First, reproductive failure is reported to be higher in septate uteri,[8] making surgical intervention of greater importance. Second, transcervical metroplasty has now become the surgical procedure of choice in the management of septate uterus. Transcervical metroplasty for bicornuate uteri, on the other hand, is considered to be unsafe and ineffective.

In the past, surgical management of the septate uterus was accomplished through use of the modified Jones metroplasty or the Tompkins metroplasty. The Strassmann metroplasty is not applicable to septate uterus repair. More recently, hysteroscopic incision or resectoscopic resection of the septum of a septate uterus has proved to be not only more effective but to result in fewer complications than a metroplasty by the abdominal approach.[53-56] For this reason abdominal metroplasty of a septate uterus is now only rarely accomplished, and generally only in patients with an extremely wide septum.

The technique for transcervical repair of a partial uterine septum involves either the use of a hysteroscopic incision of the septum using operating scissors or a resectoscopic excision of the septum using an electric current (Fig. 27–21A). The resectoscopic excision is believed to be less time consuming and simpler to accomplish and is currently the procedure of choice. Patients selected for transcervical procedures should be suppressed with either a gonadotropin-releasing hormone agonist or with danazol for 2 to 3 months prior to their surgery to reduce the endometrial thickness to a minimum. The procedure should be performed simultaneously with a laparoscopy to reduce the risk of uterine perforation. The uterine septum is then incised or excised until tubal ostium can be visualized and there is no intervening septal tissue. Antibiotic coverage should be started before the procedure and continued for 5 days to reduce the risk of an ascending infection. Unusual postoperative bleeding may be managed by inserting a large Foley catheter into the uterine cavity for 4 to 6 hours.

A complete uterine septum separating two uterine cavities with two cervices may also be excised by transcervical resectoscopic means. In these cases, a No. 8 Foley catheter is placed through one cervix, and a marking dye such as indigo carmine is injected into the cavity. The resectoscope is passed through the opposite cervix, and the cavity is distended with dextran 70 (Hyskon). The septal excision is begun in a lateral plane directed toward the other lower uterine cavity until the Foley bulb is visualized and the second cavity entered (Fig. 27–21B). The septum is then excised in a superior direction until both tubal ostia are visualized without an intervening septum.[57] When the septum is found to be unusually wide, a modified Jones or Tompkins abdominal metroplasty may be indicated.

The differentiation of a partial septate uterus from an arcuate uterus is based on the finding of an arcuate configuration of the uterine fundus on ultrasonographic examination or at laparoscopy and the identification of an abbreviated septum in the fundal cavity. Septa of any size associated with repeated pregnancy wastage and in the absence of other identifiable causes of abortion should be considered for surgical correction.

At the time of a transcervical or an abdominal metroplasty

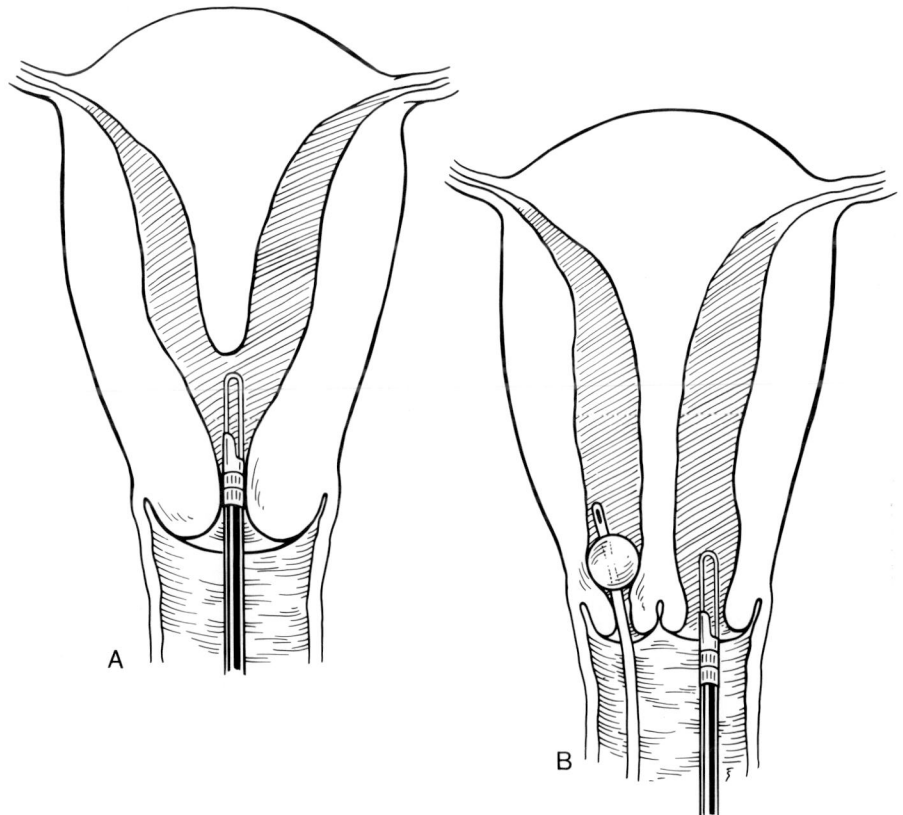

FIGURE 27–21. Resectoscopic metroplasty. *A,* A septate uterus with a single cervix. The septum may be incised with the straight loupe of the resectoscope. *B,* A Foley catheter is placed in one cavity of a complete septate uterus (American Fertility Society class VA uterus). The resectoscope is inserted in the opposite cavity, and the septum incised until the Foley catheter is visualized. The septum is then incised. The septum may be easily incised with the resectoscope until the internal ossa are visible. (*A* and *B* from Thompson JD, Rock JA, editors. Te Linde's Operative Gynecology. 7th edition. Philadelphia: JB Lippincott, 1992.)

for surgical correction of a septate uterus, an existing partial or complete vaginal septum should be excised in the same manner as previously described.

In selecting patients for surgical correction of a septate uterus, other causes of pregnancy wastage should be ruled out prior to surgical intervention. Additionally, because of the fact that some patients with a septate uterus will carry a pregnancy to viability, surgical correction should be limited to those patients who have experienced two or more spontaneous abortions. In patients older than 38 years of age, this requirement may be relaxed. In patients who have elected to undergo assisted reproductive technologies, to manage one or more causes of infertility, surgical correction of the septum should be considered before in vitro fertilization.

Arcuate Uterus. Differentiation of an arcuate uterus from a partial septate or a partial bicornuate uterus is sometimes difficult. The term *arcuate* refers to the double curvature of the uterine fundus found in some patients and represents a minimal distortion from normal uterine architecture. Defects found by HSG or visualized during hysteroscopy are minimal and appear as a residual flat septum protruding into the cavity. No convincing data currently identify an arcuate uterus as a cause of pregnancy wastage or of other gynecologic symptoms; therefore, this defect does not usually require surgical correction.

T-Shaped Uterine Cavity (DES Drug Related). Between the late 1940s and 1970, DES was widely used in the United States to prevent spontaneous abortion, prematurity, intrauterine fetal death, and toxemia.[58] It has been estimated that between 2 million and 3 million women received DES during this period, exposing from 1 million to 1.5 million female progeny to the drug in utero.[59] It is also estimated that from 50% to 75% of those exposed females developed anatomic abnormalities in the developing müllerian ducts leading to infertility, pregnancy wastage, and ectopic pregnancy.[60] One review of 267 DES-exposed females demonstrating uterine abnormalities on HSG reported the following structural defects: (1) T-shaped uterus with a small cavity (31%); (2) T-shaped uterus (19%); (3) small uterine cavity (13%); (4) T-shaped uterus with constriction (13%); (5) multiple constriction rings (4%); and (6) other anomalies (8%).[61] Additionally, 44% of these 267 females had structural changes of the cervix consisting of an anterior cervical ridge, a cervical collar, a hypoplastic cervix, or a pseudopolyp. In another study of 16 women who were exposed to DES in utero, a high incidence of a unique tubal morphologic feature consisting of a foreshortened, convoluted tube with a "withered" fimbria and a pinpoint os was noted.[62]

The diagnosis of these uterine defects is best appreciated through the use of HSG; however, pelvic ultrasonography with water contrast (normal saline) injected in the uterine cavity may be used in patients who are sensitive to iodine radiographic dyes.

Management of uterine cavity deformities secondary to DES exposure rests only with diagnosis and counseling of patients as to the increased risk factor in pregnancy outcome (see section on management outcome). No surgical techniques currently available have a proven benefit in enlarging the uterine cavity or in altering the uterine cavitary deformities. Unlike all other müllerian duct congenital deformities, however, the incidence of DES-exposed T-shaped uterine cavity defects would be expected to markedly decrease as the

DES-exposed female population passes through its childbearing years. It remains to be seen whether female offspring of the DES-exposed offspring will also sustain some structural defects.

Unicornuate Uterus. A unicornuate uterus may result from a variety of müllerian duct developmental defects, including a complete absence of development of one duct to an underdeveloped, unfused duct. The resulting defects include a single uterine horn structure with or without a rudimentary horn. It is essential to determine the presence of a rudimentary horn because some rudimentary horns may have small functioning cavities that may or may not communicate with the unicornuate major cavity. In the case of a small functioning cavity in a rudimentary horn, surgical excision is indicated to prevent the increased risk of pelvic endometriosis, occurring as a result of the noncommunicating horn, and a pregnancy implantation in either a communicating or a noncommunicating horn.

A unicornuate uterus without rudimentary horn has been evaluated and reviewed in combination with didelphic uteri.[63] Most patients with an isolated unicornuate uterus are asymptomatic. However, some data suggest an increased abortion rate and an increased incidence of premature labor.[14] No surgical treatment for this defect has been universally proved to be effective or accepted. Some data have suggested a reduction in premature labor in unicornuate uteri through the use of cervical cerclage[64]; however, the wisdom or benefit of this approach is controversial. It has been a general observation that pregnant patients with an isolated unicornuate uterus experience improved obstetric outcomes in successive pregnancies.

Class IV: Unusual Configurations of Vertical and Lateral Fusion Defects

Anomalies of the müllerian duct system occur not infrequently with a variety of other developmental problems, the most common of which include urinary tract defects. Unilateral agenesis of a kidney and ureter is a common association.[8] Anomalies of the external genitalia and vagina have also been associated with bladder exstrophy.[65]

Less frequent associations have occurred with a wide range of genetic defects, including the hand-foot-uterus syndrome, an autosomal dominant syndrome presenting with extremity defects and lack of fusion of the müllerian ducts[66]; the McKusick-Kaufman syndrome, an autosomal recessive syndrome with multisystem involvement, including müllerian duct defects[67]; and a localized chromosomal mosaicism etiology of congenital defects of the external genitalia.[68]

In such patients, surgical management may be used to correct the vaginal, cervical, or uterine malformations in a manner described earlier in this chapter, provided the surgical management is appropriate to the overall management plan of the patient with other somatic defects.

OUTCOME OF MANAGEMENT

Outcome of management of uterovaginal anomalies may be measured in several ways. Disorders of vertical fusion of the müllerian ducts are usually assessed by the functional capability of the neovagina, whereas disorders of lateral fusion of the müllerian ducts are usually assessed by pregnancy outcome. In both instances, an additional assessment would be in the improvement of symptoms of abdominal and pelvic pain. Finally, changes in the incidence of pelvic endometriosis must be considered, although this outcome change cannot be accurately assessed or proved.

Management of dysgenesis of the müllerian ducts rests with the creation of a functional neovaginal vault by means of nonsurgical techniques described earlier. Although success rates vary in different reports, the active dilation technique of Frank is reported to be successful in slightly fewer than 50% of cases, whereas the passive technique of Ingram may be expected to result in success in 70% of cases.[35]

Surgical creation of a neovagina originally resulted in some serious complications, including severe constriction, infection, and granulation tissue formation. The more recent modified McIndoe procedure has proved to be extremely successful, even when used with dilation or surgical failures. One report of 94 patients recorded an 83% success rate (100% take of the skin graft), with 14% achieving a somewhat less than full graft take but later epithelization and a functional neovagina and only 3% with a graft failure.[35]

Malignancies have been reported in the neovagina and seem to be related to the type of transplant or graft tissue. In one reported series, two adenocarcinomas and seven squamous cell carcinomas were described.[69] Condylomata acuminata formation has also been reported.[70] Other complications of vaginal atresia or neovaginal construction, although rare, include (1) rectovaginal fistula[71]; (2) vaginal prolapse[72]; (3) pelvic pain associated with a functioning uterine anlagen[72]; and (4) the development of endometriosis in patients with a functioning rudimentary horn and retrograde menstruation.[74]

Although natural pregnancy is not possible with dysgenesis of the müllerian ducts, successful stimulation and retrieval of oocytes in patients with Mayer-Rokitansky-Küster-Hauser syndrome has been reported[75] and offers hope in these patients if surrogacy is not objectionable.

Management of disorders of vertical fusion of the müllerian ducts rests with excision of the vaginal septum or removal of the uterus in patients with a cervical deformity, with the possibility of neocanalization of the cervix in a few selected cases. Excision of complete transverse vaginal septa is generally more difficult if the septum is high or unusually thick. In these instances, there is a higher incidence of vaginal stricture and granuloma formation. In wide septa, skin grafting is occasionally necessary. As a result of these problems, outcome results vary widely. One report on outcomes of surgical management of transverse vaginal septa found a 100% success rate in developing a patent vagina with successful coital function in a series of 26 patients.[35] Of these patients, 7 of 19 successfully achieved pregnancy. Other reports have described pregnancy following repair of vaginal atresia as an isolated defect.[76] Successful pregnancies have been reported in patients with repair of a congenital partial cervical atresia.[39, 77] Additionally, assisted reproductive technologies using zygote intrafallopian transfer have resulted in a successful pregnancy in a patient with cervical atresia.[40]

Disorders of lateral fusion of the müllerian ducts are by far the most common of the uterovaginal anomalies. Management of these disorders is directed toward the elimination of abdominal and pelvic pain, a reduction in the incidence of

pelvic endometriosis, or an improvement in pregnancy outcome. To support the impression that endometriosis is more prevalent in patients with müllerian anomalies, one study reviewed the case histories of 64 women with müllerian defects who had undergone intra-abdominal surgery.[78] In this study, 10 of 13 of these women with a functioning endometrium and patent fallopian tubes but obstructed outflow tracts were found to have pelvic endometriosis, whereas only 16 of 43 of these women without obstruction had endometriosis (77% versus 37%; $P < .01$). The same study additionally found 8 of 9 women with hematocolpos or hematometra had endometriosis, whereas only 18 of 47 patients with functioning endometrium but no hematocolpos or hematometra had the disease (89% versus 38%; $P < .01$). Other reports[79, 80] support these findings and, therefore, surgical correction of all müllerian defects with functioning endometrium and obstructed outflow tracts would seem justified. The reduction or elimination of abdominal or pelvic pain also resulting from an obstructed outflow tract is commonly observed following reparative surgeries of lateral fusion defects.[35]

Obstetric consequences of uterovaginal anomalies include an increased incidence of (1) mid-trimester abortion, (2) premature labor, (3) malpresentation, and (4) retained placenta.[82] In a study of 186 pregnancies in 150 women with müllerian duct anomalies (didelphic 25, bicornuate 59, septate 45, arcuate 9, unicornuate 12), breech presentation and transverse lie occurred in 61% and 11% of the patients, respectively.[82] In the same study, preterm delivery occurred in 25% of the pregnancies, and 83% of the deliveries were by cesarean section.

In another study, 96 women with recurrent abortion were evaluated by HSG, and more than two thirds were found to have defects compatible with müllerian anomalies.[83] This same study compared these results with 96 other women who had undergone HSG before artificial insemination and who later had a full-term normal delivery. In this latter group, approximately 20% were found to have some type of müllerian defect. These data suggest a relationship between recurrent first-trimester abortion and müllerian defects and should be included in the list of obstetric consequences of uterovaginal anomalies. Current data suggest, however, that these patients do not have difficulty in conceiving.[81]

In an 8-year study of 42 women with 101 pregnancies, all with uncorrected uterine anomalies (didelphic 10, bicornuate 61, septate 25, unicornuate 5), 60% of the pregnancies in the didelphic and unicornuate groups reached term, whereas 39% of the bicornuate group and 48% of the septate group reached term.[84] These results are supported by other data suggesting that uncorrected septate uteri have a poorer reproductive prognosis.[85] In the group of 42 women just discussed,[84] high-risk obstetric care was given in an attempt to provide a more favorable outcome, but less than optimal results were observed. As a result, the authors concluded that traditional indications for metroplasty should continue to be used. This impression, however, is not totally accepted by others.[86]

Surgical reconstruction or correction of uterine anomalies in the presence of repeatedly poor obstetric outcomes without other detectable factors is an appropriate procedure. Although the greatest benefit is believed to occur with the surgical correction of the bicornuate or septate uterus, some obstetric benefit has been reported in patients with didelphic uterus.[87, 88] In these studies, however, it is unclear whether the actual defect was a didelphic uterus or possibly a complete bicornuate uterus. Because an uncorrected didelphic uterus has been observed to have improved obstetric outcome with successive pregnancies, it is recommended that surgical intervention of a true didelphic uterus be reserved for the rare patient with proven recurrent abortion in the absence of all other causes that may reflect on an adverse outcome.

The benefits of metroplasty for a bicornuate or septate uterus in the presence of poor obstetric outcome have been well publicized. One study reviewed previous studies on the reproductive performance of women with uterine anomalies before and after metroplasty.[89] This work reviewed 764 pregnancies in women with bicornuate or septate uterus with the following results before and after metroplasty: term births 7% (before)/74% (after); premature births 8%/9%; abortions 84%/17%; and living children 9%/77%. These authors additionally added 19 women with bicornuate or septate uteri in which a 98% abortion rate occurred before metroplasty and an 86% live infant rate after metroplasty. In these patients, a Strassmann technique was performed in cases of bicornuate uteri and a Tompkins technique in cases of subseptate anomalies.

More recently, hysteroscopic treatment of uterine septum has produced the same success rates with markedly reduced morbidity and cost.[90, 91] In one study, 35 patients with uterine septum were followed over a 4-year period, and in those with only a septal defect as a cause for poor obstetric outcome, 100% experienced spontaneous abortion before hysteroscopic metroplasty, whereas following the procedure, a 68% live infant rate was observed.[90] These data support the view that surgical intervention is an indicated procedure in cases of septate uteri when poor pregnancy outcome has been documented and other factors ruled out.

Some data suggest that women with congenital uterine anomalies also have a higher incidence of cervical incompetence.[88, 92, 93] In one study, 29 cases of cervical incompetence were found among 98 women with congenital uterine anomalies, with the highest incidence rate of cervical incompetence occurring in the bicornuate group (38%).[93] In this group, an improvement in obstetric performance was observed after cerclage, increasing the term delivery rate from 26% to 63%. Cervical structural defects not infrequently occur with uterovaginal deformities. A positive obstetric history combined with physical findings indicative of cervical incompetence supports the need for a preconceptual cervical cerclage procedure to promote a more favorable obstetric outcome in women with müllerian duct defects.

Reproductive performance in patients with a T-shaped uterine cavity (DES exposure) is also reduced. A study of 69 women with DES-related cervicovaginal anomalies revealed 62 pregnancies in which 36 pregnancy failures occurred (58%).[94] Of these failures, first- and second-trimester abortions accounted for 83%. In this same group, uterine anomalies were found in all 25 patients undergoing HSG. In another study of reproductive performance in 106 patients exposed in utero to DES, a corrected fetal wastage of 37% was noted, with a premature delivery rate of 6%.[95] Fetal wastage is believed to be due to a combination of anatomic defects that include both a small, deformed cavity and to an increased incidence of cervical incompetence. An earlier report on DES-exposed offspring suggested a higher-than-expected incidence of incompetent cervix and suggested that these women need frequent speculum examinations during pregnancy, with the performance of a cerclage at the first sign of cervical incompetence.[96] The same author recommended an HSG on all DES-exposed women and a prophylactic cerclage if evidence of an incompetent endocervical canal or dilated internal os is found. In our experience, an HSG using a cervical injection technique showing a cervical canal width of 1 cm or wider is highly suggestive of an incompetent cervix. The positive and negative predictive value of such a finding is yet to be substantiated; therefore, a prophylactic cerclage in DES-exposed women cannot be supported.

Reproductive performance in women with a unicornuate uterus is reduced to a degree similar to that found with didelphic uterus.[97, 98] In a series of 19 women with unicornuate uteri, 13 had a total of 29 pregnancies in which 58.6% resulted in abortion, 10.3% in premature labor, and 27.6% in term births.[97] One pregnancy occurred in a rudimentary uterine horn that ruptured. In another study of 18 women with a unicornuate uterus followed for 1 to 6 years, 12 had a total of 38 pregnancies, with 21 ending in spontaneous abortion, 3 in premature labor, and 14 in term births.[98] In this review, 4 women had a cavitary noncommunicating horn, 12 a noncavitary rudimentary horn, and 2 no rudimentary horn.

Outcomes of patients presenting with unusual configurations of vertical and lateral fusion defects are similar to those with vertical and lateral defects and are dependent on the type and extent of concurrent abnormalies. In many of these patients, a functional vagina and pregnancy are not an issue. Of greatest importance in patients with multiple genetic and congenital defects is the diagnosis of an obstructed outflow tract in the presence of a functioning endometrial cavity. In these patients surgical intervention to correct the obstruction would be supportive to the overall management plan.

SUMMARY

Embryonic development of the reproductive tract is generally a predictable and efficient process. Defects in müllerian duct development do occasionally occur, however, with a reported incidence of approximately 1% in all women. These defects are conveniently divided into four classes, including agenesis or dysgenesis of the müllerian ducts, disorders of vertical fusion of the müllerian ducts, disorders of lateral fusion of the müllerian ducts, and unusual configurations of vertical and lateral fusion defects. Disorders of vertical fusion include transverse vaginal septum and cervical agenesis or dysgenesis. Disorders of lateral fusion are separated into asymmetrical and symmetrical defects, the latter including didelphic uterus, bicornuate uterus, septate uterus, arcuate uterus, T-shaped defects of the uterine cavity (DES exposure), and unicornuate uterus.

Agenesis or dysgenesis of the müllerian ducts may be discovered by observing an abnormal vagina during an early pelvic examination but is usually suspected in a phenotypic and genotypic female with secondary sexual characteristics with primary amenorrhea.

Disorders of vertical fusion and asymmetrical disorders of lateral fusion of the müllerian ducts usually result in obstructed outflow tracts and are therefore suspected when cyclic or acyclic abdominal or pelvic pain occurs without visible menstruation at the appropriate time for menarche in an otherwise normal female.

Symmetrical disorders of lateral fusion of the müllerian ducts may not be suspected until the patient presents with a history of poor obstetric outcome or infertility.

The diagnosis of these developmental problems of the female reproductive tract is made by careful abdominal and pelvic examination supported with an HSG and with pelvic sonography or MRI. Occasionally, laparotomy and hysteroscopy are required to appreciate the full extent of the defects.

Management of these defects is directed toward (1) the desire for a functional vagina; (2) the management of abdominal and pelvic pain secondary to an obstructed outflow tract; (3) the reduction in the incidence of resulting pelvic endometriosis; or (4) the improvement of obstetric outcome.

The creation of a neovagina in patients with agenesis of the müllerian ducts may be accomplished by mechanical or surgical means. Mechanical techniques should be attempted first, and if unsuccessful, surgical procedures such as the modified McIndoe technique should be accomplished. Both of these techniques are effective in the development of a functional vagina in an appropriately motivated patient.

Management of both vaginal septa and asymmetrical disorders of lateral fusion of the müllerian ducts requires careful dissection and excision of the septum or the noncommunicating rudimentary anlagen. Management of symmetrical disorders of lateral fusion (unobstructed) is dependent on their effect on reproduction. If the patient is able to conceive and carry the pregnancy close to term, surgical intervention is unwarranted. These defects, however, are reported to increase the incidence of first- and second-trimester abortion, premature labor, malpresentation, and retained placenta. Generally, didelphic uterus is not effectively unified through surgical reconstruction without a significant surgical risk and an unacceptable complication rate. Unicornuate uteri and T-shaped uterine cavity defects (DES exposure) are not amenable to surgical correction.

Bicornuate uteri and septate uteri, on the other hand, are effectively managed by surgical reconstruction. A variety of abdominal metroplasty techniques are useful in correcting a bicornuate uterus. These include the modified Jones and the Strassmann techniques. Septate uteri may be corrected abdominally by use of the Tompkins technique; however, septate uteri currently are better managed by means of a transcervical hysteroscopic resection unless the septum is extremely wide.

Unilateral renal agenesis frequently occurs with müllerian duct abnormalities and should be assessed as a part of the workup for reproductive tract anomalies. Additionally, the possibility of cervical incompetence must be considered in all patients with müllerian duct abnormalities.

Although müllerian duct anomalies are less frequent than other reproductive tract pathologic disorders, a suspicion of their presence is the first step in the diagnosis, and their consideration must be included as a part of the differential diagnosis in any patient presenting with an abnormal vagina, primary amenorrhea, unexplained abdominal or pelvic pain, or a history of poor pregnancy outcome.

REFERENCES

1. O'Rahilly R. The embryology and anatomy of the uterus. In: Norris H, Hertig A, editors. The Uterus. Baltimore: Williams & Wilkins, 1973:17–39.
2. Parmley T. Embryology of the female genital tract. In: Kurman RJ, editor. Blaustein's Pathology of the Female Genital Tract. New York: Springer-Verlag, 1987:1–14.
3. Musset R. Necessity for a global classification of uterine malformations. Gynecol Obstet 1967;66:145–166.
4. Jost A. Embryonic sexual differentiation. In: Jones HW Jr, Scott WW, editors. Hermaphroditism, Genital Anomalies, and Related Endocrine Disorders. 2nd edition. Baltimore: Williams & Wilkins, 1971:16–64.
5. Stein AL, March CM. Pregnancy outcome in women with müllerian duct anomalies. J Reprod Med 1990;35(4):411–414.
6. Sorensen SS. Estimated prevalence of müllerian anomalies. Acta Obstet Gynecol Scand 1988;67:441–445.
7. Carrington BM, Hricak H, Nuruddin RN, et al. Müllerian duct anomalies: MR imaging evaluation. Radiology 1990;176:715–720.
8. Rock JA, Keenan DL. Surgical correction of uterovaginal anomalies. In: Sciarra JJ, editor. Gynecology and Obstetrics. Volume 1. New York: Harper & Row, 1992:1–20.
9. Rock JA, Azziz R. Genital anomalies in childhood. Clin Obstet Gynecol 1987;30(3):682–696.
10. Speroff L, Glass RH, Kase NG. Amenorrhea. In: Speroff L, Glass RH, Kase NG, editors. Clinical Gynecological Endocrinology and Infertility. Baltimore: Williams & Wilkins, 1989:165–211.
11. Lischke JH, Curtis CH, Lamb F, et al. Discordance of vaginal agenesis in monozygotic twins. Obstet Gynecol 1973;41:920–924.
12. Verp MS, Simpson JL, Elias S, et al. Heritable aspects of uterine anomalies: I. Three familial aggregates with müllerian fusion anomalies. Fertil Steril 1983;40:80–85.
13. Jones HW JR, Merut S. Familial occurrence of congenital absence of the vagina. Am J Obstet Gynecol 1972;114:1100–1101.
14. Buttram VC, Reiter RC. Uterine anomalies. In: Buttram VC, Reiter RC, editors. Surgical Treatment of the Infertile Female. Baltimore: Williams & Wilkins, 1985:149–199.
15. Fedele L, Dorta M, Brioschi D, et al. Magnetic resonance imaging in Mayer-Rokitansky-Kuster-Hauser syndrome. Obstet Gynecol 1990;76:593–596.
16. Carrington BM, Hricak H, Nuruddin RN, et al. Müllerian duct anomalies: MR imaging evaluation. Radiology 1990;176:715–720.
17. Yovich JL, Hoffman TD. IVF surrogacy and absent uterus syndromes. Lancet 1988;2(8608):331–332.
18. Frank RT. The formation of an artificial vagina without operation. Am J Obstet Gynecol 1938;35(6):1053–1055.
19. Ingram JM. The bicycle seat stool in the treatment of vaginal agenesis and stenosis: a preliminary report. Am J Obstet Gynecol 1981;140:867–873.
20. Rock JA, Reeves LA, Retto H, et al. Success following vaginal creation for müllerian agenesis. Fertil Steril 1983;39(6):809–813.
21. McIndoe A. Treatment of congenital absence and obliterative conditions of the vagina. Br J Plast Surg 1950;2(4):254–267.
22. Counsellor VS, Flor FS. Congenital absence of the vagina. Surg Clin North Am 1957;37(5):1107–1117.
23. Turner-Warwick R, Kirby RS. The construction and reconstruction of the vagina with the colocecum. Surg Gynecol Obstet 1990;170(2):132–136.
24. Lilford RJ, Johnson N, Batchelor A. A new operation for vaginal agenesis: construction of a neo-vagina from a rectus abdominus musculocutaneous flap. Br J Obstet Gynecol 1990;170(2):132–136.
25. Chen ZJ, Chen MY, Chen C, et al. Vaginal reconstruction with an axial subcutaneous pedicle flap from the inferior abdominal wall: a new method. Plast Reconstr Surg 1989;83(6):1005–1012.
26. Soong YK, Lai IM. Amnion graft in treatment of congenital absence of the vagina: report of three cases. Taiwan I Hsueh Hui Tsa Chih 1987;86(11):1232–1235.
27. Jacob JH, Griffin WT. Surgical reconstruction of the congenitally atretic cervix: two cases. Obstet Gynecol Surv 1989;44(7):556–569.
28. Cukier J, Batzofin JH, Connors JS, et al. Genital tract reconstruction in a patient with congenital absence of a vagina and hypoplasia of the cervix. Obstet Gynecol 1986;68:32S–36S.
29. Markham SM, Huggins GR, Parmley TH, et al. Cervical agenesis combined with vaginal agenesis diagnosed by magnetic resonance imaging. Fertil Steril 1987;48(1):143–145.

30. Lodi A. Vaginal malformations in the Mangiagalli University Hospital from 1906–1950. Am J Obstet Gynecol 1951;73:1246.
31. McKusick VA, Weilbaecher RG, Gragg GW. Recessive inheritance of a congenital malformation syndrome. JAMA 1968;204(2):113–118.
32. Sueldo CE, Rotman CA, Cooperman NR, et al. Transverse vaginal septum: a report of four cases. J Reprod Med 1985;30(2):127–131.
33. Hricak H, Chang YC, Thurnher S. Vagina: evaluation with MR imaging: I. Normal anatomy and congenital anomalies. Radiology 1988; 169(1):169–174.
33a. Hurst BS, Rock JA. Preoperative dilatation to facilitate repair of the high transverse vaginal septum. Fertil Steril 1992;57:1351–1353.
34. Jacob JH, Griffin WT. Surgical reconstruction of the congenitally atretic cervix: two cases. Obstet Gynecol Surv 1989;44(7):556–569.
35. Rock JA. Surgery for anomalies of the müllerian ducts. In: Thompson JD, Rock JA, editors. Te Linde's Operative Gynecology. 7th edition. Philadelphia: JB Lippincott, 1992:603–646.
36. Jeffcoate TNA. Advancement of the upper vagina in the treatment of hematocolpos and hematometra caused by vaginal aplasia: pregnancy following the construction of an artificial vagina. J Obstet Gynaecol Br Common 1969;76:961–968.
37. Sherer DM, Beyth Y. Ultrasonographic diagnosis and assisted surgical management of hematotrachelos and hematometra due to uterine cervical atresia with associated vaginal agenesis. J Ultrasound Med 1989;8(6):321–323.
38. McCarthy S. Magnetic resonance imaging in the evaluation of the infertile couple. Magn Reson Q 1990;6(4):239–249.
39. Hampton HL, Meeks GR, Bates GW, et al. Pregnancy after successful vaginoplasty and cervical stenting for partial atresia of the cervix. Obstet Gynecol 1990;76(5):900–901.
40. Thijssen RFA, Hollanders JMG, Willemsen WNP, et al. Successful pregnancy after ZIFT in a patient with congenital cervical atresia. Obstet Gynecol 1990;76(5 Pt 2):902–904.
41. Buttram VC Jr, Reiter RC. Uterine anomalies. In: Buttram VC Jr, Reiter RC, editors. Surgical Treatment of the Infertile Female. Baltimore: Williams & Wilkins, 1985:149–199.
42. Randolph JR Jr, Ying YK, Maier DB, et al. Comparison of real-time ultrasonography, hysterosalpingography, and laparoscopy/hysteroscopy in the evaluation of uterine abnormalities and tubal patency. Fertil Steril 1986;46(5):828–832.
43. Nicolini U, Bellotti M, Bonazzi B, et al. Can ultrasound be used to screen uterine malformations? Fertil Steril 1987;47(1):89–93.
44. Nasri MN, Setchell ME, Chard T. Transvaginal ultrasound for diagnosis of uterine malformations. Br J Obstet Gynecol 1990;97:1043–1045.
45. Carrington BM, Hricak H, Nuruddin RN, et al. Müllerian duct anomalies: MR imaging evaluation. Radiology 1990;176:715–720.
46. Mintz MC, Grumbach K. Imaging of congenital uterine anomalies. Semin Ultrasound CT MR 1988;9(2):167–174.
47. Fedele L, Dorta M, Brioschi D, et al. Magnetic resonance evaluation of double uteri. Obstet Gynecol 1989;74:844–847.
48. Reuter KL, Daly DC, Cohen SM. Septate versus bicornuate uteri: errors in imaging diagnosis. Radiology 1989;172:749–752.
49. Musich JR, Behrman SJ. Obstetric outcome before and after metroplasty in women with uterine anomalies. Obstet Gynecol 1978;52:63–66.
50. Jones WS. Obstetric significance of female genital anomalies. Obstet Gynecol 1957;10:113–127.
51. El-Mahgoub SE. Unification of a septate uterus: El-Mahgoub's operation. Int J Gynecol Obstet 1978;15(5):400–404.
52. Mizuno K, Koike J, Ando K. Significance of Jones-Jones operation on double uterus: vascularity and dating of endometrium in uterine septum. Jpn J Fertil Steril 1978:23:9.
53. Chervenak FA, Neuwirth RS. Hysteroscopic resection of the uterine septum. Am J Obstet Gynecol 1981;141:351–353.
54. Daly DC, Walters CA, Sopto-Albors CE, et al. Hysteroscopic metroplasty: surgical technique and obstetrical outcome. Fertil Steril 1983;39:623–628.
55. DeCherney AH, Russell JB, Graebe RA, et al. Resectoscopic management of müllerian fusion defects. Fertil Steril 1986;45(5):726–728.
56. Hassiakos DJ, Zourlas PA. Transcervical division of uterine septum. Obstet Gynecol Surv 1990;45(3):165–173.
57. Rock JA, Murphy AA, Cooper WA, Jr, et al. Resectoscopic techniques for the lysis of a class V complete uterine septum. Fertil Steril 1987;48(3):495–496.
58. Smith OW. Diethylstilbesterol in the prevention and treatment of complications of pregnancy. Am J Obstet Gynecol 1948;56(5):821–834.
59. Stillman RJ. In utero exposure to diethylstilbesterol: adverse effects on the reproductive tract and reproductive performance in male and female offspring. Am J Obstet Gynecol 1982;142(7):905–921.
60. Richmond JB. Physician's advisory: Health effects of the pregnancy use of diethylstilbesterol. DES Task Force, Summary Report. Washington, DC: Department of Health, Education, and Welfare, October 4, 1978.
61. Kaufman RH, Adam E, Binder GL, et al. Upper genital tract changes and pregnancy outcome in offspring exposed in utero to diethylstilbesterol. Am J Obstet Gynecol 1980;137(3):299–308.
62. DeCherney AH, Cholst I, Naftolin F. Structure and function of the fallopian tubes following exposure to diethylstilbesterol (DES) during gestation. Fertil Steril 1981;36(6):d741–d745.
63. Buttram VC. Müllerian anomalies and their management. Fertil Steril 1983;40(2):159–163.
64. Heinonen PK, Saarikoski S, Pystynen P. Reproductive performance of women with uterine anomalies: an evaluation of 182 cases. Acta Obstet Gynecol Scand 1982;61:157–162.
65. Jones HW Jr. An anomaly of the external genitalia in female patients with exstrophy of the bladder. Am J Obstet Gynecol 1973;117:748–756.
66. Longmuir GA, Conley RN, Nicholson DL, et al. The hand-foot-uterus: a case study. J Manipulative Physio Ther 1986;9(3):213–217.
67. Vince JD, Martin NJ. McKusick-Kaufman syndrome: report of an instructive family. Am J Med Genet 1989;32(2):174–177.
68. Seely JR, Seely BL, Bley R, Jr, et al. Localized chromosomal mosaicism as a cause of dysmorphic development. Am J Hum Genet 1984;36(4):899–903.
69. Baltzer J, Zander J. Primary squamous cell carcinoma of the neovagina. Gynecol Oncol 1989;35(1):99–103.
70. Buscema J, Rosenshein NB, Shah K. Condylomata acuminata formation arising in a neovagina. Obstet Gynecol 1987;69(3 Pt 2):528–530.
71. Buss JG, Lee RA. McIndoe procedure for vaginal agenesis: results and complications. Mayo Clin Proc 1989;64(7):758–761.
72. Peters WA III, Uhlir JK. Prolapse of a neovagina created by self-dilatation. Obstet Gynecol 1990;76 (5 Pt 2):904–906.
73. Murphy AA, Krall A, Rock JA. Bilateral functioning anlagen with the Rokitansky-Mayer-Kuster-Hauser syndrome. Int J Fertil 1987; 32(4):316–319.
74. Acien P, Lloret M, Chehab H. Endometriosis in a patient with Rokitansky-Kuster-Hauser syndrome. Gynecol Obstet Invest 1988;25(1):70–72.
75. Egarter C, Huber J. Successful stimulation and retrieval of oocytes in a patient with Mayer-Rokitansky-Kuster syndrome. Lancet 1988; 1(8597):1283.
76. Bergman KS, Schwaitzberg SD, Harris BH. Pregnancy following repair of vaginal atresia. J Pediatr Surg 1988;23(11):1063–1064.
77. Fraser IS. Successful pregnancy in a patient with congenital partial cervical atresia. Obstet Gynecol 1989;74(3 Pt 2):443–445.
78. Olive DL, Henderson DY. Endometriosis and müllerian anomalies. Obstet Gynecol 1987;69(3 Pt 1):412–415.
79. Acien P. Endometriosis and genital anomalies: some histologic aspects of external endometriosis. Gynecol Obstet Invest 1986;22(2):102–107.
80. Tang LC, Ngan HY, Tang MH. Rudimentary uterine horn with adenomyosis and pelvic endometriosis in a 23-year-old girl. J Adolesc Health Care 1986;7(4):265–267.
81. Rock JA, Schlaff WD. The obstetric consequences of uterovaginal anomalies. Fertil Steril 1985;43(5):681–692.
82. Stein AL, March CM. Pregnancy outcome in women with müllerian duct anomalies. J Reprod Med 1990;35(4):411–414.
83. Portuondo JA, Camara MM, Echanojauregui AD, et al. Müllerian abnormalities in fertile women and recurrent aborters. J Reprod Med 1986;31(7):616–619.
84. Ludmir J, Samuels P, Brooks S, et al. Pregnancy outcome of patients with uncorrected uterine anomalies managed in a high-risk obstetric setting. Obstet Gynecol 1990;75(6):906–910.
85. Fedele L, Dorta M, Brioschi D, et al. Pregnancies in septate uteri: outcome in relation to site of uterine implantation as determined by sonography. AJR 1989;152:781–784.
86. Treffers PE. Pregnancy outcome of patients with uncorrected uterine anomalies managed in a high-risk obstetrics setting [Letter]. Obstet Gynecol 1990;76(6):1147–1148.
87. Fedele L, Zamberletti D, D'Alberton A, et al. Gestational aspects of uterus didelphys. J Reprod Med 1988;33(4):353–355.
88. Maneschi M, Maneschi F, Pariato M, et al. Reproductive performance in women with uterus didelphys. Acta Eur Fertil 1989;20(3):121–124.
89. Spirtos NJ, Evans TN, Magyar DM, et al. The reproductive performance of women before and after metroplasty. Int J Fertil 1987;32(1):46–49.
90. Guarino S, Incandela S, Maneschi M, et al. Hysteroscopic treatment of uterine septum. Acta Eur Fertil 1989;20(5):321–325.
91. Daly DC, Maier D, Soto-Albors C. Hysteroscopic metroplasty: six years' experience. Obstet Gynecol 1989;73(2):201–205.

92. Surico N, Tavassoli K, Mora MS, et al. Cervical cerclage as a pregnancy treatment in the presence of a malformed uterus. Panminerva Med 1987;29(1):53–56.
93. Golan A, Langer R, Wexler S, et al. Cervical cerclage—its role in the pregnant anomalous uterus. Int J Fertil 1990;35(3):164–170.
94. Berger MJ, Goldstein DP. Impaired reproductive performance in DES-exposed women. Obstet Gynecol 1980;55(1):25–27.
95. Veridiano NP, Delke I, Rogers J, et al. Reproductive performance of DES-exposed female progeny. Obstet Gynecol 1981;58(1):58–61.
96. Goldstein DP. Incompetent cervix in offspring exposed to diethylstilbesterol in utero. Obstet Gynecol 1978;52(1 Suppl):73S–75S.
97. Fedele L, Zamberletti D, Vercellini P, et al. Reproductive performance of women with unicornuate uterus. Fertil Steril 1987;47(3):416–419.
98. Maneschi M, Maneschi F, Fuca G. Reproductive impairment of women with unicornuate uterus. Acta Eur Fertil 1988;19(5):273–275.

CHAPTER 28

Management of Uterine Myomata

GERSON WEISS

Uterine myomata are the most common tumors of the female reproductive tract. These tumors go by many names, including fibroids, leiomyomata uteri, fibroma, or fibromyoma. The term *fibroid* has been firmly established in the literature for many years and is used interchangeably with myomata in this chapter. These tumors are generally firm and well circumscribed. They are made up of smooth muscle in an interdigitating pattern separated by fibrous connective tissue. Uterine myomata are predominately tumors of the reproductive years. These tumors appear to be hormonally responsive, being stimulated by estrogens and androgens and resolving after menopause or after ovariectomy. Women have roughly a 40% chance of developing a detectable myoma during their reproductive years.[1] Fibroids are more common in black women.

The high occurrence rate of fibroids makes these tumors familiar to practicing obstetrician-gynecologists. Myomata therapy is a major indication for operative gynecologic procedures. Roughly 60% of all pelvic laparotomies are performed for myomata.[2]

BIOLOGY OF UTERINE MYOMATA

Uterine fibroids are thought to be monoclonal in origin. This conclusion is arrived at both by glucose-6-phosphate dehydrogenase isoenzyme patterns and cytogenetic patterns.[3, 4] Clonal chromosomal rearrangements occur in roughly half of the tumors observed. Alterations occur in chromosomes 1, 2, 6, 7, 12, 14, 22, and X. The most frequent gene rearrangements are reciprocal translocations or insertions observed in region 12q14–15. Specific chromosomal abnormalities do not correlate with specific histologic tumor types.[59] A variety of substances have been implicated in the growth of uterine myomata. These substances include the insulin-like growth factors I and II,[5] epidermal growth factor,[6] growth hormone,[7] estrogens, and androgens. Fibroids are metabolically active. They are rich in aromatase, capable of converting androgens into estrogens.[8] They are also rich in 17β-hydroxysteroid dehydrogenase, the enzyme that converts estradiol-17β to estrone.[9] Fibroids are also rich in 5α-reductase, the hormone that converts testosterone into 5α-dihydrotestosterone. This enzyme is present within fibroids in higher concentration than in other uterine components.[10]

The smooth muscle cells of uterine myomata produce prostaglandin $F_2\alpha$, E_2, and prostacyclin. Prostacyclin is produced in the largest concentration.[11] Because these agents are active in altering uterine vascular tone as well as uterine contractility, the presence of fibroids with their associated prostaglandin and prostacyclin receptors may be responsible for uterine dysfunctional activity.

Fibroids have been shown to contain elevated levels of prolactin. Fibroids have been demonstrated to synthesize prolactin in vitro.[12] Fibroid prolactin is identical to pituitary and decidual prolactin. In most cases, it appears not to be secreted. A case of symptomatic circulating hyperprolactinemia, however, has been reported in which the prolactin arose from a uterine myoma. This prolactin was not responsive to bromocriptine. Within 3 days of myomectomy, however, prolactin levels returned to normal.[13]

Occasionally fibroids have been shown to produce erythropoietin. In some cases, this has resulted in polycythemia.[14] Certainly patients with fibroids and elevated hematocrit should be evaluated for the presence of ectopic erythropoietin.

LOCATION OF UTERINE MYOMATA

Fibroids are generally classified according to their position in the uterus (Fig. 28–1). The most common are intramural myomata, situated within the muscle wall. Submucous myomata are under the endometrium. They displace the endometrium above them. Occasionally these tumors can become pedunculated. Subserous fibroids are located beneath the uterine serosa. They may be either sessile and produce asymmetric uterine irregularity or pedunculated and attached to the uterus by a pedicle. These tumors may occasionally be intraligamentous, growing from the uterus into the broad ligament. In this position, they are most likely to affect the ureters. Occasionally uterine myomata may be adherent to other structures in the pelvis and simultaneously lose their

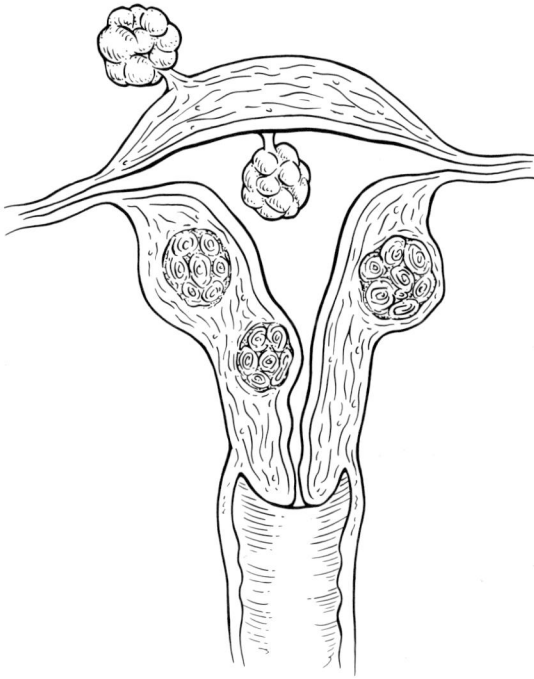

FIGURE 28–1. Localization of fibroids in relation to the uterus.

uterine blood supply and their attachment to the uterus. These tumors are called parasitic.

DIAGNOSIS OF UTERINE MYOMATA

The majority of fibroids are asymptomatic. The diagnosis of myomata is usually entertained on feeling an enlarged uterus of irregular contour or firm masses producing uterine irregularity or distortion. From a practical point of view, this is usually a sufficient diagnostic maneuver to establish the diagnosis. If the mass is shaped like a fibroid, feels like a fibroid, is part of the uterus, and can be differentiated from adnexa, there is an overwhelming likelihood that the mass is, in fact, a fibroid. It is important, however, to keep in mind that many other masses may become attached to the uterus and may be difficult to differentiate from uterine myomata by pelvic examination. Obviously an ovarian fibroma would be almost impossible to differentiate from a pedunculated uterine myoma. Many inflammatory masses or solid ovarian tumors can be confused with uterine myomata. Even inflammatory adnexa adherent to the uterus can at times be difficult to differentiate from a uterine myoma, especially a myoma that has incurred a vascular accident. Even inflammatory bowel disease adherent to the uterus has been confused with myomata. Differentiation from ovarian tumors is essential. A particular problem is the differentiation by physical examination alone of ovarian endometriomata from uterine fibroids. Ovarian endometriomata may be indurated and are frequently adherent to the posterior uterus. This differentiation becomes extremely difficult when the pelvic mass is greater than the size of a 12- to 14-week pregnancy and thus totally fills the pelvis. Thus, differentiation of masses from adnexa might be impossible by physical examination. Because of this caveat, a diagnosis of "pelvic mass" should be

made until a more definitive diagnosis of uterine myoma could be confirmed.

Our diagnostic acuity has improved with the advent of modern imaging technology. Transabdominal and transvaginal ultrasonography has been useful in defining uterine myomata. Transvaginal ultrasonography is particularly useful in the presence of a small uterus. Larger uteri or masses are best observed via transabdominal ultrasonography. The pattern generated by uterine myoma depends on its components, the relative amounts of muscle and connective tissue. The degree of degeneration or calcification also clearly alters the ultrasonographic pattern. Myomas typically result in sonographic patterns that demonstrate irregularity of the uterine contour. This is the most common ultrasonographic finding.[15] Uterine enlargement is also common. Irregularity of the contour may be general or focal. Calcifications are suggested by hyperechoic foci with acoustic shadowing (Fig. 28–2). Hypoechoic areas can be seen with cystic degeneration (Fig. 28–3). Ultrasonography cannot, however, distinguish uterine myomata from adenomyosis if they are present concurrently. Fibroids have been mistaken for uterine anomalies. Differentiation from ovarian tumors is also essential (Figs. 28–4 and 28–5).[16] Sonographic differentiation of ovaries from fibroids has allowed conservative management of even large fibroids, which could previously not have been differentiated from the ovary based on physical examination alone. Practically, sonographic definition of fibroids is usually adequate. This is a readily available test that is relatively inexpensive.

There are situations in which sonographic identification of fibroids is difficult. These situations include observations of patients who are markedly obese or are pregnant. When the fibroids are pedunculated or small, when adenomyosis and fibroids should be differentiated, or when they are multiple and large, differentiation may be difficult by sonography. In these cases, magnetic resonance imaging (MRI) can be a useful alternative.[17, 18] Use of MRI is expensive, and the

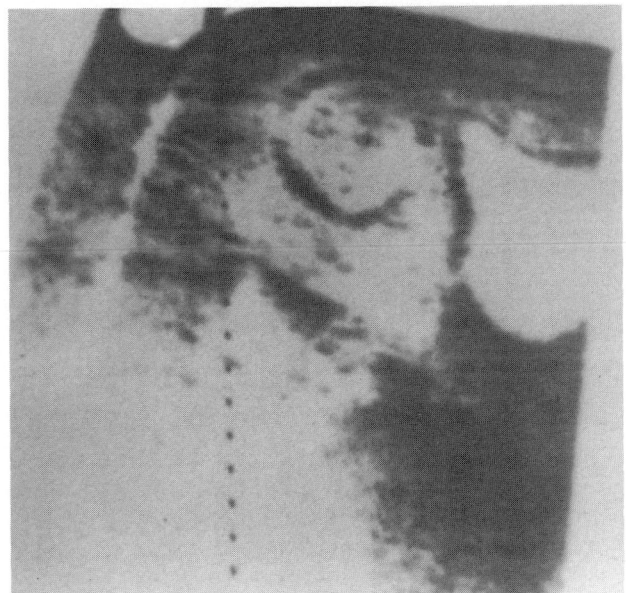

FIGURE 28–2. Longitudinal scan with an extensively calcified myoma resembling a fetal head. (From Snyder JR, Goldstein SR, Weinreb JC. Imaging of fibroids: modern diagnostic techniques. Clin Consult Obstet Gynecol 1990; 2:13–19.)

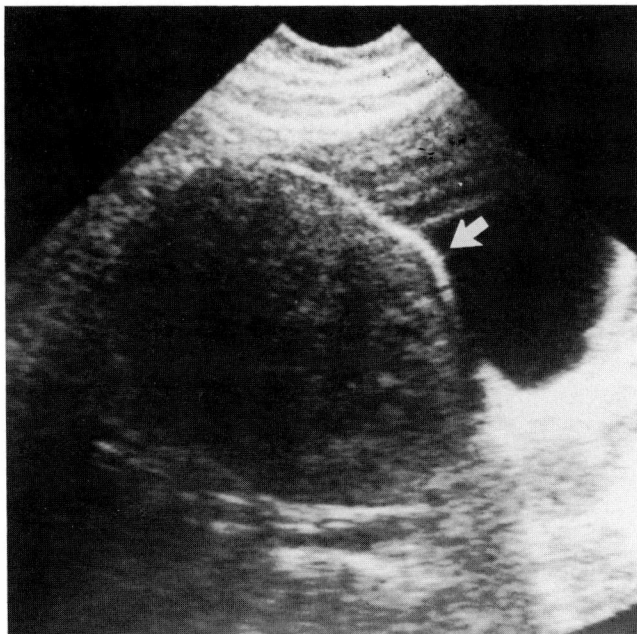

FIGURE 28–3. Longitudinal scan showing an enlarged fibroid uterus with a hypoechoic texture. *Arrow* indicates anterior wall contour irregularity. (From Snyder JR, Goldstein SR, Weinreb JC. Imaging of fibroids: modern diagnostic techniques. Clin Consult Obstet Gynecol 1990; 2:13–19.)

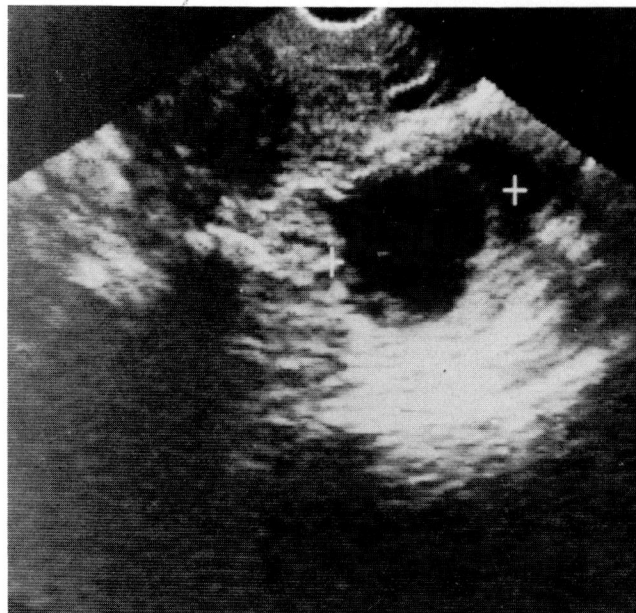

FIGURE 28–5. Endovaginal scan of patient in Figure 28–4. Posterior mass (*cursors*) is in reality a septated cystic mass (mucinous cystadenoma). (From Snyder JR, Goldstein SR, Weinreb JC. Imaging of fibroids: modern diagnostic techniques. Clin Consult Obstet Gynecol 1990; 2:13–19.)

equipment is not universally available. MRI, however, does not use ionizing radiation and has no known biologic risk. MRI is more sensitive in soft tissue than ultrasonography or computed tomography. MRI has additional advantage over computed tomography because computed tomography uses ionizing radiation. An acoustic window such as a full bladder is not required for MRI evaluation. On MRI, myoma are well-

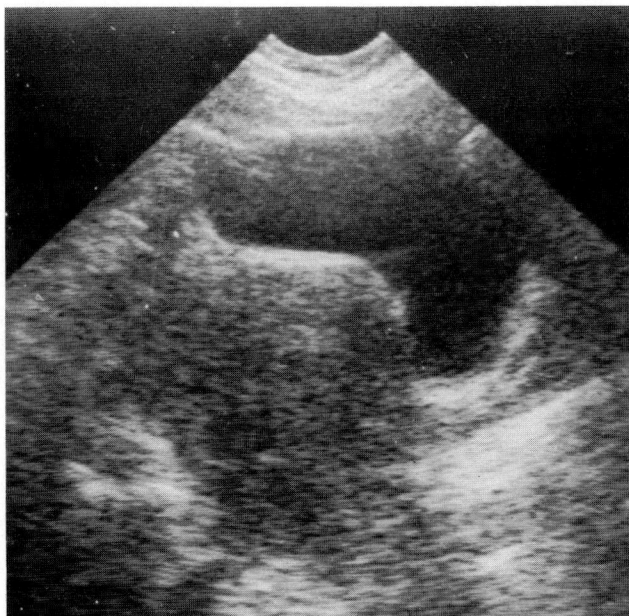

FIGURE 28–4. Longitudinal scan presumably showing a 10-week-size fibroid uterus. (From Snyder JR, Goldstein SR, Weinreb JC. Imaging of fibroids: modern diagnostic techniques. Clin Consult Obstet Gynecol 1990; 2:13–19.)

defined dark masses differentiated from normal myometrium. Occasionally they may be hyperintense owing to the degenerative or hemorrhagic changes within the tumors. It is important to recognize that no imaging technique can differentiate between benign tumors and sarcomatous degeneration. MRI can detect lesions as small as 3 mm, and they can clearly be localized. This may be important in localizing submucous lesions. These lesions have been associated with miscarriage or hypermenorrhea. One report describes many cases in which sonographically interpreted adnexal masses were shown to be uterine myoma using MRI.[19] MRI can serve as an alternative to ultrasonography as a method of evaluation of uterine fibroids. This may be useful when the ultrasound study is inconclusive. Figure 28–6 shows varying patterns of uterine myomata using MRI. Figure 28–7 demonstrates the ease of differentiation of uterine myomata from endometrium and normal myometrium using pelvic MRI.

SYMPTOMS OF MYOMATA

Abnormal Bleeding

Prolonged menses and increased menstrual flow (menorrhagia) are the most common abnormal bleeding patterns associated with the presence of uterine myomata.[20] Any abnormal bleeding pattern, however, can coexist with the presence of these tumors. The first clinical objective is to differentiate the presence of the myoma as the cause of bleeding from any other pathologic or endocrine condition that causes abnormal bleeding. Both endometrial tissue sampling and imaging technology may be important in making this differentiation. It would certainly also be important to determine the patient's hormonal status. Hypothyroid patients may also have prolonged menses. Abnormal bleeding is common in

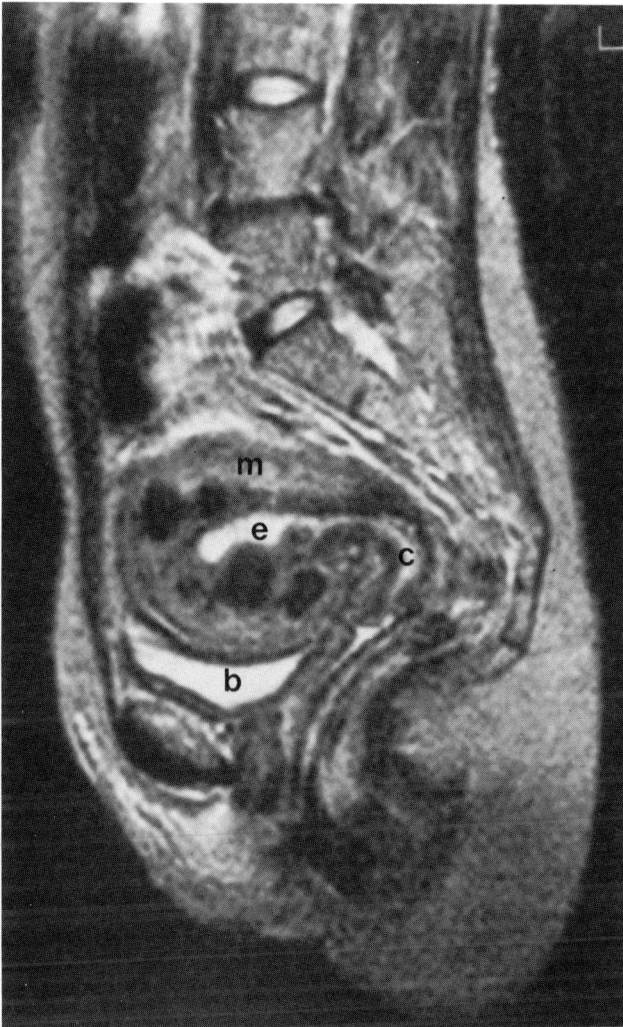

FIGURE 28–6. Sagittal magnetic resonance imaging (MRI) of the pelvis. Numerous well-circumscribed, low-density masses measuring up to 2 cm are uterine myomas. MRI provides a detailed road map of fibroids and their relation to the endometrium (e), cervix (c), myometrium (m), and bladder (b). (From Snyder JR, Goldstein SR, Weinreb JC. Imaging of fibroids: modern diagnostic techniques. Clin Consult Obstet Gynecol 1990; 2:13–19.)

hyperprolactinemic patients. Abnormal bleeding from myomata may mimic bleeding secondary to endometrial hyperplasia or adenocarcinoma as well as bleeding from coagulopathies.

The cause of the fibroid-associated bleeding is not always clear. Certainly multiple tumors may significantly increase the endometrial surface area, thus increasing the bleeding surface. Fibroids may mechanically interfere with surface blood supply. The tumors may also interfere with the ability of myometrial fibers to constrict the endometrial arteries and thus increase blood flow. Surface ulceration of submucous fibroids can also be a cause of bleeding.

Discomfort

A large myomatous uterus can produce a heavy feeling or general discomfort in the pelvis. There can be pressure on the bladder producing urinary frequency. Constipation owing

to rectal pressure is another symptom of fibroids. This is especially true with either a large fibroid uterus or a retroflexed fibroid uterus. Pressure on the ureter, especially at the pelvic brim where the ureter cannot be displaced laterally, can produce hydronephrosis. It may be necessary to diagnose this condition by an intravenous pyelogram.

Some large uterine fibroids may cause chronic pelvic pain. Recent onset of dysmenorrhea in women in their later reproductive years may be a symptom of fibroids. Pedunculated submucosal fibroids may produce severe cramping pains, especially with menses. Accidents, such as hemorrhage or infarction of a fibroid, can produce acute severe pain. A pedunculated subserosal fibroid that twists on its pedicle may infarct and cause a focal pelvic peritonitis with severe pain, tenderness over the mass, fever, and leukocytosis.

DEGENERATIVE COMPLICATIONS OF UTERINE MYOMATA

Alteration in the blood supply to uterine myomata, which can occur with changes in a woman's hormonal status, can produce a variety of degenerative changes. The most common degenerative change is hyalinization. This results in a homogeneous pattern in the fibroids and replacement of smooth muscle cells with hyalinized connective tissue. Calcification of uterine myomata can occur. This is, however, more common in postmenopausal women. The calcifications can be diffuse, localized, or present only on the surface of the tumors. Cystic degeneration, local areas of softening, or

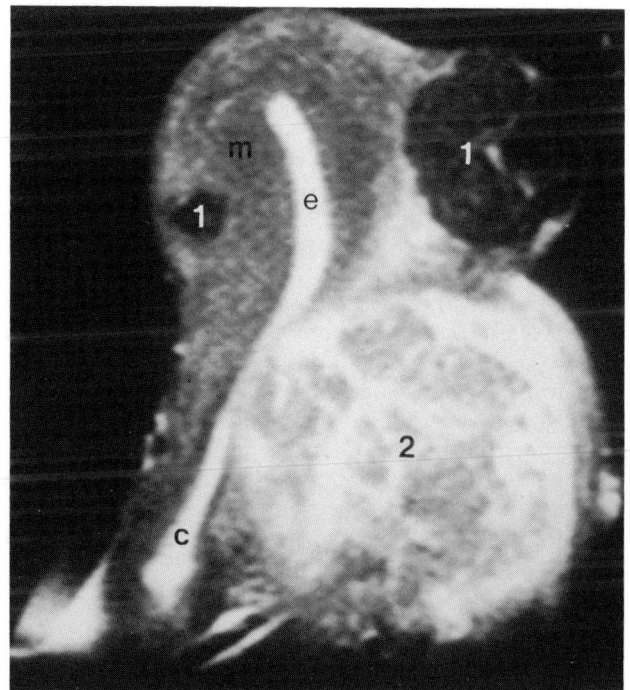

FIGURE 28–7. Magnetic resonance imaging of uterus and cervix specimen. There are two subserosal, nondegenerated, low-signal intensity fibroids (1), which measure 3 mm and 1.8 cm. A larger inhomogeneous high-signal intensity mass (2) represents a degenerated submucosal fibroid. Endometrium (e) cervix (c), are myometrium (m) are identified. (From Snyder JR, Goldstein SR, Weinreb JC. Imaging of fibroids: modern diagnostic techniques. Clin Consult Obstet Gynecol 1990; 2:13–19.)

liquefaction of fibroids can also occur. Fatty degeneration is also observed in fibroids.

Red or carneous degeneration in fibroids is due to aseptic necrosis associated with hemorrhage into the tumor. This process produces pain and tenderness. Necrosis of a fibroid can occur from acute compromise of the tumor's blood supply, as can occur if there is torsion of a pedunculated fibroid.[21] This occurrence is associated with the acute onset of generally severe abdominal pain, tenderness over the mass, and other signs and symptoms of focal peritonitis.

Sarcomatous degeneration of the uterine myomata is a rare event, with approximately a 0.1 to 0.2% occurrence. This event is so uncommon that its possibility should not influence the clinical management of a patient with uterine myomata.

Uterine myomata occasionally become infected. On rare occasions, the infection may even produce abscesses within the tumor (pyomyoma).[22] Submucosal fibroids are most likely to become infected because these tumors are so close to an exposed endometrial surface. One possible route of infection is trauma to the surface of the myoma at the time of an endoscopic procedure or uterine curettage. Infected uterine myomata may be difficult to treat because of a decreased blood flow to the center of the tumor. Removal of the abscessed tumors is usually required.

MYOMATA AND INFERTILITY

Because uterine myomata increase in frequency in advancing reproductive years and because there is a current tendency for women to delay childbirth into these years, the occurrence of fibroids in patients desiring pregnancy is likely to increase. The presence of fibroids has been associated with infertility. Most studies that make this association are not tightly controlled for age, position of the fibroids, size, and other factors affecting fertility. In the absence of clear data defining the conditions under which uterine myomata cause infertility, a reasonable and rational approach can be undertaken. This approach requires an understanding that initial decision making may be shown to be inaccurate by later developed data. Intuitively, it would be reasonable to state that several superficial, subserosal, small leiomyomata on the uterine fundus are unlikely to be related or causal to infertility. It would be easier to make a case for an association if a woman has no other infertility factors and has an irregular fibroid uterus with fibroid masses the size of an 18 week pregnancy markedly distorting and stretching the intramural portion of the fallopian tube and distorting the uterine cavity. Likewise, recurrent pregnancy loss in a patient with multiple submucosal uterine myomata would suggest a causal relationship.

A variety of theories have been proposed to explain the relationship of infertility to fibroids. It has been proposed that ovarian compression by large fibroids could result in an infertile state.[23] Other investigators have associated fibroids with anovulation.[24] These theories have not withstood the test of time. Others have proposed that uterine function is severely altered by prostaglandin-induced uterine contractions. It has been proposed that this alteration adversely affects sperm migration into the tubes.[25] Clearly if fibroids produce bilateral cornual obstruction, this could be a defini-

tive structural cause of infertility. In most situations, this is not the case. It is likely that fibroids distort the endometrium and interfere with endometrial blood flow in a manner that inhibits appropriate nidation and implantation. Although there are no clear data to this point, it seems reasonable that a pregnancy could implant better on a well-vascularized endometrium over a normal myometrium as opposed to a stretched, possibly atrophic endometrium covering a relatively avascular myoma. There is clear evidence of reduced blood flow in leiomyomata themselves compared with blood flow in uteri of nonaffected women.[26, 27] It is thus reasonable to suggest that this decrease in blood flow produces an environment that is either less receptive for the initial implantation or less receptive to continued fetal growth. Decreased endometrial blood flow could result in either infertility or recurrent pregnancy loss.

Accepting the theory that myoma-associated infertility is most likely to be the product of an altered local environment, one would then be able to select most effectively patients who are infertile and have fibroids for individualized therapy. Uterine myomata that interfere neither with tubal structure nor the endometrium and its underlying myometrial architecture are unlikely to result in infertility and are best left alone. Removal of fibroids is not always a benign procedure. Postoperatively, many patients may develop adhesive disease, which may further complicate infertility management and may interfere with tubal function. Thus localization of fibroids becomes imperative. One common technique is the use of a hysterosalpingogram. This would allow definition of the contour of the endometrial cavity. It would also allow detection of significant filling defects, which would represent the presence of fibroids (Fig. 28–8). A caveat here is that although the contour of the uterus and presence of filling defects can be noted, the size of these lesions cannot be determined from a hysterosalpingogram because the relative

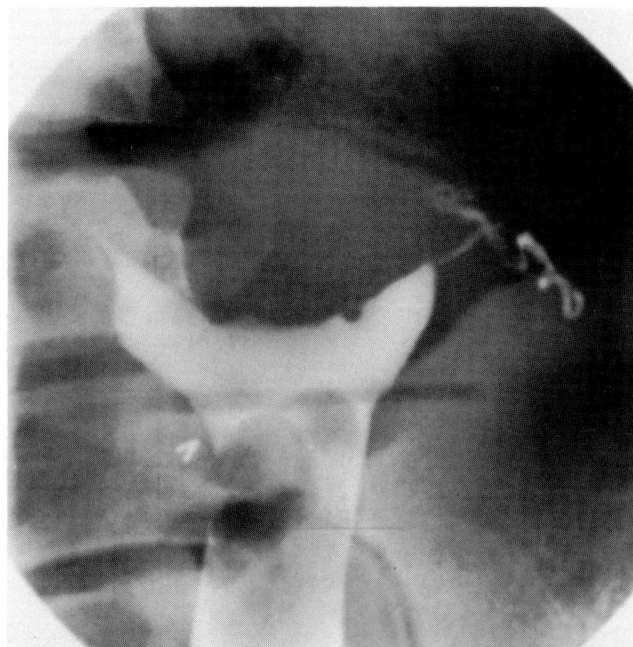

FIGURE 28–8. Hysterosalpingogram of a patient with a large fibroid uterus. Note distortion of the endometrial cavity, the large fundal filling defect, and the defect caused by a large intracavitary myoma.

position of the lesion from the x-ray plate may vary and thus will alter the size of the image on that plate. As previously shown, clear determination of fibroid position can be noted by MRI.

The presence of significant submucous fibroids can clearly be determined by hysteroscopy. As seen later, a hysteroscopic approach for therapy can also be undertaken. Hysteroscopy is rarely needed for diagnosis because less invasive technology, such as hysterosalpingography or other imaging techniques, can usually provide equivalent answers.

Laparoscopy may be necessary to determine the concurrent presence of other infertility factors. This technique is rarely needed to diagnose fibroids because they can usually be determined to be present by a combination of physical examination and the imaging technology previously mentioned. These factors notwithstanding, it is not uncommon for the fibroids first to be recognized at the time of a laparoscopic evaluation of tubal or peritoneal factors causing infertility. In many cases, determining the presence of uterine myomata at the time of laparoscopy is insufficient to determine if these fibroids are likely to be the cause of infertility. This relationship can best be determined by observation of the positions of the myomata with respect to the endometrial cavity.

INDICATIONS FOR THERAPY OF UTERINE MYOMATA IN INFERTILE PATIENTS

It is obvious that if indications exist for therapy of fibroids irrelevant to the presence of infertility, these conditions would also apply to infertile patients (Table 28–1). Thus, an infertile patient who is in pain owing to hemorrhage or ischemia in a fibroid must be treated. The indication here is relief of pain rather than infertility. Certainly the therapy should be designed in a way to optimize future fertility. Likewise, an infertile patient who has chronic anemia and menorrhagia secondary to fibroids should be treated for this condition. In this case, it is likely that the fibroids are distorting the endometrium, and so therapy would treat not only the abnormal bleeding and anemia, but also might improve chances of pregnancy.

Before undertaking treatment of uterine myomata to improve fertility, two conditions must be met. The first is that a complete evaluation of other causes of infertility must be undertaken. This would bring the presence of fibroids and the fibroids' relationship to infertility into clearer perspective. Uterine myomata producing tubal distortion may be a reason to remove fibroids in patients with no other causes of infer-

tility. This would hardly be an appropriate procedure, however, in a patient with concomitant hydrosalpinges because her infertility would be treated by in vitro fertilization, which does not require normal tubal anatomy. When faced with a patient with small superficial fibroids and anovulation, the appropriate clinical response would be first to correct the anovulation and only consider dealing with the fibroids if pregnancy still does not occur and there are no other fertility factors. Even then there should be some indication that whatever fibroids are present are in such position as to produce uterine dysfunction.

The other condition that must be met, as previously alluded to, is that if the uterine myomata present are to be related to infertility, this would mean that the tumors would have to be of either significant size or in specific position to affect reproductive function. By way of example, submucous myomata are likely to be causal of infertility. Small subserosal myomata are not likely to be related to infertility. An 8-cm fibroid that totally replaces the posterior wall of the uterus is more likely to be a direct fertility factor than a 2-cm intramural myoma. Before removing a fibroid and incurring the risk of fertility-compromising pelvic adhesions, it should be clear that the fibroid has the potential to affect fertility adversely (see Table 28–1).

MEDICAL THERAPY OF UTERINE MYOMATA

The advent of gonadotropin-releasing hormone (GnRH) agonist therapy has allowed for the first time effective medical therapy for uterine myomata, which can result in their actual shrinkage. Myomata are usually estrogen dependent. Withdrawal of estrogen results in tumor shrinkage. GnRH agonists, after an initial 1- to 3-week period of pituitary desensitization, can result in a state of profound hypoestrogenism. This hypoestrogenic state continues for as long as therapy is maintained. It is, however, rapidly reversed on cessation of therapy.[28]

The principles of GnRH agonist therapy are independent of the specific agent used. The agonist must be given in doses adequate to suppress endogenous estrogen levels to below 45 pg/mL. The average shrinkage of myomata is more than 50%. The range for individual tumors varies from no change to more than 90%. Maximum tumor shrinkage usually occurs by 8 to 12 weeks of therapy (Table 28–2). Regrowth of the myomata rapidly occurs when therapy is discontinued, according to most, but not all, clinical studies. Although medical therapy is highly effective, long-term use is obviated by side effects of therapy. These hypoestrogenic side effects include unpleasant hot flashes and bone demineralization. Therapy obviously induces an anovulatory state, preventing pregnancy for the duration of therapy (Fig. 28–9). If concomitant ovulation induction is desirable while the patient is on GnRH agonist therapy, human menopausal gonadotropins can be used as replacement therapy.[60] The transient nature of GnRH agonist therapy precludes this method as definitive treatment of fibroids. In selected cases, there may be advantages to medical therapy as adjunctive treatment. Advantages to this treatment include:

1. Allowance of definitive therapy to be delayed until ad-

TABLE 28–1. Indications for Myomectomy in Infertile Patients

Conditions irrelevant to infertility
  Fibroid-related pain
  Fibroid-related menorrhagia and/or anemia
  Other fibroid-related noxious symptoms
Conditions relevant to infertility
  Significant distortion of endometrial cavity
  Occlusion of tubal orifices
  Size resulting in significant uterine distortion

TABLE 28–2. Medical Management of Fibroids*

Authors†	N	Agonist	% Shrink‡	Time to Max (wk)§	Nonsurgical Pregnancy* (%)
Filicori, 1983[29]	1	D-Trp-6 8 μg/kg SQ/day	77	12	—
Healy, 1984[30]	1	6 μg q 45 min SQ infusion buserelin (200 μg/day)	85	16	—
Maheux, 1984[31]	3	Buserelin 200 μg tid × 7 days, then 500 μg SQ/day	84	24	—
Maheux, 1985[32]	10	Buserelin as in 1984	0–80	24	0/4
Healy, 1986[33]	5	Buserelin 20 μg SQ/day	55	8–12	0/2
Coddington, 1986[34]	6	Histrelin 4 μg/kg/SQ/day	35–65	8	—
Kessel, 1988[35]	14	D-Trp-6 or histrelin 20–50 μg SQ/day	34–40	12	2/5‖
Friedman, 1987[36]	14	7 = LA 500 μg SQ/day	45	12	—
		7 = LA 1600 μg IN/day	Ineffective	12	—
Friedman, 1988[37]	16	8 = LA 500 μg SQ/day¶	51	12	—
		8 = LA + Provera 20 mg qd	15	24	—
Friedman, 1989[38]	38	3.75 mg LA depot/month	40	12	—
Lumsden, 1987[39]	13	3.6 mg goserelin depot/month	40	12**	—
Andreyko, 1988[40]	11	Nafarelin 800 μg IN daily	57	12	—
Maheux, 1987[41]	9	Buserelin 400 μg IN tid	71	12	—
Perl, 1987[42]	10	D-Trp-6 100 μg SQ/day	45	9	—
Friedman, 1991[43]	63	3.75 mg LA depot/month	45	24	—
Nakamura, 1991[47]	25	Buserelin 300 μg IN tid	35	16	—

*Summary of pertinent clinical parameters in GnRH agonist–treated leiomyomatous women.

†Superscript numbers refer to references from Santoro article.

‡% Shrink, maximum percent shrinkage of uterus, when given, or myomas.

§Time to Max, time to maximum shrinkage of uterus, when given or myomas.

‖Submucosal myomas, one obstructing tube.

¶Slight and significant increase in Ca^{++} and PO_4 in serum. Slight and significant increase in alkaline phosphatase. No change in single photon absorptiometry of wrist in 24 weeks.

**Thirty-three percent decrease in blood lost at hysterectomy.

SQ, subcutaneous; IN, intranasal; LA, leuprolide acetate.

From Santoro NF. Medical management of uterine leiomyomata. Clin Consult Obstet Gynecol 1990; 2:29.

equate iron reserves are replenished and there is preoperative normalization of hematocrit. It would also be possible to use this time to store autologous blood for intraoperative transfusion.

2. Several authors have stated that there is a reduction of intraoperative blood loss by the preoperative use of GnRH agonists.[39–41]

3. It is possible that the surgical approach to the tumor may be simplified. A large submucous fibroid, which before GnRH agonist treatment may have required laparotomy for removal, can potentially be approached by an endoscope transcervically after tumor shrinkage.

Because tumor response is variable, not all patients are helped by the preoperative use of GnRH agonists. GnRH agonists have the disadvantage of requiring at least 2 to 3 months of expensive therapy before maximum response is achieved. In many cases, it may not be worth the expense to wait for whatever benefit is derived. Some surgeons have thought that, on occasion, the overlying myometrium is adherent to the myomata after GnRH agonist therapy, making development of the tissue planes more difficult.

There is an ever-increasing panoply of GnRH agonists available. The principle of therapy is that the agent must be simple to use, require minimal attention by the patient, and achieve adequate blood levels. Long-acting agents would seem to be more appropriate than agents requiring single or multiple patient-initiated administrations daily. In the near future, GnRH antagonists will become available for clinical usage. These agents will not have the initial increase in estro-

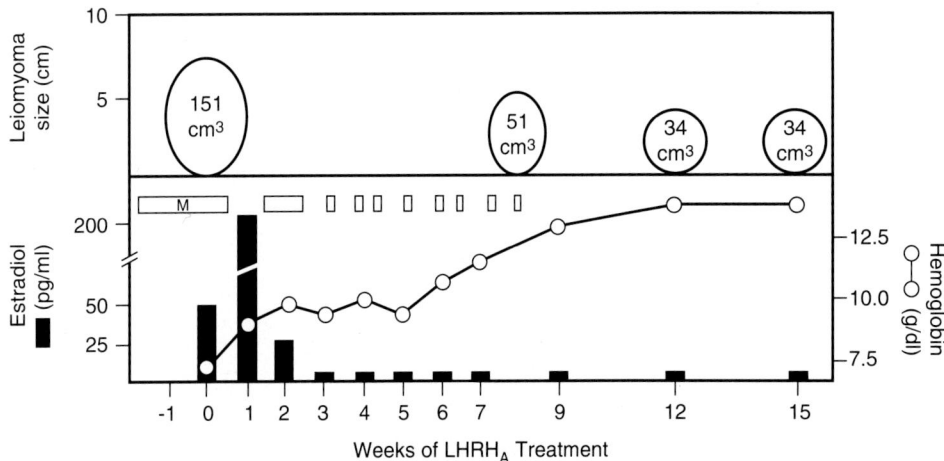

FIGURE 28–9. Behavior of large submucosal myoma during treatment with a gonadotropin-releasing hormone agonist (D-Trp-6 LHRH$_A$ [D-Ttp-6 GnRH]). Note 77% size reduction in 12 weeks' attainment of amenorrhea by 8 weeks, suppression of estradiol levels in 3 weeks, and normalization of hemoglobin levels. (From Filicori M, Hall DA, Loughlin JS, et al. A conservative approach to the management of uterine leiomyomata: pituitary desensitization by a luteinizing hormone-releasing hormone analogue. Am J Obstet Gynecol 1983; 147:726–727.)

gen seen with GnRH agonists. There will be no need to wait 1 to 3 weeks for desensitization. Thus, these agents will be more appropriate for the medical therapy of uterine myomata. GnRH therapy of fibroids is not devoid of complications. Severe hemorrhage was encountered in women in whom GnRH therapy caused necrosis of submucous myomata.[44]

The concern of some surgeons is that the myoma will resolve under medical therapy to a point where they would not be found during exploration. This fear has not been realized practically, probably because the agonists are not able to shrink significant myoma totally.

ENDOSCOPIC MANAGEMENT OF UTERINE MYOMATA IN INFERTILE PATIENTS

Laparoscopic Approach

It is not unusual for myomata to be observed during a diagnostic laparoscopy in an infertile patient. The technology is clearly available to ablate small surface or subserosa myomata or to remove pedunculated fibroids through the laparoscope. This can be done by a variety of techniques, which include laser surgery or electrocoagulation. Several principles clearly apply. The first is that one should remove fibroids only if there is either a clear indication for therapy, such as pain or abnormal bleeding, or if the fibroids are clearly likely to be cause infertility. It is unlikely that fibroids that are amenable to a laparoscopic approach would meet these criteria. Fibroids that can be removed laparoscopically would not impinge on the endometrial cavity and are likely to be fairly small. Thus it is not reasonable to anticipate that fertility would be improved by ablation of fibroids that can be laparoscopically removed. Another basic principle in surgery is to do no harm. A more sophisticated statement of that principle is that there should be a favorable risk-to-benefit ratio in any therapy. Because it is unlikely that fibroids removable through the laparoscope would be causes of infertility, there would be minimal benefit to the patient in their removal. That these small fibroids may in later years become large fibroids harmful to the patient has yet to be clearly established because most fibroids do not produce problems requiring therapy. Ablation or removal of these lesions, however, may be attended by postoperative scarring and adhesion formation, which may involve the adnexa and decrease the patient's chance of conception. Thus, a basic rule of thumb might be that if the myoma can be removed laparoscopically, it is unlikely to be a cause of infertility, and there would be little indication for its removal.

Hysteroscopic Approach

There are major advantages to a hysteroscopic approach for the management of infertility-related fibroids. The procedure can be done on an outpatient basis. After a hysteroscopic approach, the patient may be allowed a vaginal delivery. There are several common indications for hysteroscopic myomectomy. Submucosal tumors may produce menorrhagia

or abnormal uterine bleeding, mandating removal. Pedunculated submucosal myomata may behave as if they were foreign bodies in the endometrial cavity. There is significant pain attendant to the uterus' attempt to reject or deliver these masses through the cervix. Thus, removal is required to relieve pain. Submucosal fibroids are most likely to be associated with infertility by interfering with normal implantation. These tumors have also been related to recurrent early pregnancy loss, probably because of improper nidation and growth of the placental base.[45]

PREOPERATIVE EVALUATION

If patients have abnormal bleeding, curettage or endometrial biopsy should be performed to rule out endometrial cancer. As previously mentioned, imaging techniques may be helpful in confirming the presence of the fibroid tumor, location, exact size, and position. Generally, a hysteroscopic approach can be used if the uterine cavity does not exceed 10 cm in length. For a hysteroscopic procedure, tumor masses should not be greater than 3 cm in diameter, with at least half of the mass protruding into the cavity. GnRH agonists can be used to shrink the size of uterine myomata, making the hysteroscopic approach more practical. GnRH agonist therapy has the additional advantage of thinning the endometrium, thus making surgery easier.

PROCEDURE

Many surgeons like to perform a laparoscopy simultaneously in patients having any operative hysteroscopic resection. This has the advantage of communication from the laparoscopic observer, who can frequently anticipate, by surface blanching and the presence of light transilluminating the uterus, that the hysteroscope may be dangerously close to uterine perforation. A warning may thus avoid this complication. Before hysteroscopic resection is undertaken, it is imperative that the landmarks such as tubal ostia are clearly identified. A variety of electrosurgical resectoscopic instruments can be used; cutting current is used, and the instruments are drawn forward toward the surgeon. Usually tissue fragments float away, but on occasion they have to be removed with forceps. Pedunculated tumors can be grasped and may then be avulsed or twisted off. Inspection of the base is then necessary to determine if anything further need be done to deal with local bleeding.[46]

POSTOPERATIVE MANAGEMENT

Occasionally balloon tamponade using a Silastic rubber balloon is needed to deal with postoperative bleeding. The patient then has to be observed in the hospital and the balloon removed after 6 to 12 hours of tamponade. Most surgeons treat all postoperative patients with at least 2 weeks of exogenous estrogen therapy to stimulate endometrial development and potentially to prevent intrauterine adhesion formation. A relatively high dose of estrogen is needed to obtain rapid endometrial thickening. A reasonable protocol is to start therapy at the time of surgery using premarin, 1.25 mg twice daily, for 6 weeks. Provera, 10 mg, should be added during the last 2 weeks of treatment to decidualize the endometrium and allow for synchronous endometrial shedding at hormonal withdrawal. Many surgeons use antibiotic therapy as well, especially if tamponade is required. The success of hysteroscopic myomectomy and transabdominal myomectomy is equivalent. Complications of the procedure include hemorrhage and uterine perforation. Occasionally a laparotomy may be necessary to repair damage or stop bleeding. Additional potential complications include damage to other intra-abdominal structures, fluid overload from the distention medium, or allergic reactions to the distention medium used during hysteroscopy.

Surgical Therapy

In general gynecologic parlance, surgical therapy for uterine myomata includes either myomectomy or hysterectomy. Obviously in the context of infertility, myomectomy is the only option. The indications as previously discussed include all conditions related to uterine myomata that would require therapy unrelated to infertility, such as persistent abnormal bleeding and complications of large pelvic masses, including hydronephrosis and pain. Additional infertility-related indications include uterine distortion, which interferes with normal reproductive function. The obvious advantage of myomectomy over hysterectomy is that it allows retention of the uterus for further reproductive function. If it is clear that reproductive function is not desired and there is an indication for surgery for fibroids, hysterectomy would be the more appropriate procedure. Retention of the uterus after myomectomy, although allowing for subsequent pregnancy, has the disadvantages of allowing regrowth of undetected fibroids that may require additional therapy and recurrence of potentially noxious symptoms, such as pain or abnormal bleeding. Generally, myomectomies are attendant to greater blood loss and more operative morbidity than hysterectomies. Performance of a myomectomy allows continuation of menstrual function, which may be viewed by individual women as either a disadvantage or an advantage. Clearly, in many women, retention of the uterus may have significant psychological advantage. It has been stated that loss of the uterus may result in feelings of defeminization, a symbolic castration, or permanent loss of all reproductive function. In an era in which egg donation can allow pregnancy beyond the usual age of fertility, these issues should clearly be discussed and explored with patients having uterine myoma requiring therapy.

Myomectomies are clearly contraindicated in the presence of age advanced enough to preclude a reasonable chance of a successful pregnancy, that is, 43 years old; the clear possibility of sarcoma or other uterine malignancy; bleeding diathesis; or pregnancy.

Preoperative evaluation should include hemoglobin evaluation and a pregnancy test. Autologous blood donation should certainly be considered because it is not unusual to require blood transfusion during extensive myomectomy procedures. Preoperative imaging procedures minimize the risk that the pelvic mass is other than a fibroid.

It has generally been cautioned that whenever a patient undergoes an extensive myomectomy procedure, an unanticipated hysterectomy may have to be performed. Although this is highly unlikely in most operative procedures, a clear discussion of this risk should occur at the time that an informed consent is obtained. Potential reasons for hysterectomy include technical problems during attempts to stop bleeding that result in devitalization of the uterus; severe adenomyosis, which precludes the formation of clear tissue planes; or the occurrence of previously unrecognized malignancies, such as an ovarian malignancy diagnosis based on a frozen section examination. Hemorrhage itself would rarely be an indication for hysterectomy because it can be stopped surgically. Obviously adequate blood for replacement must be available. If abnormal bleeding had been present before surgery, endometrial sampling should have occurred to rule out a concurrent endometrial malignancy.

Most surgeons schedule myomectomies at any time of convenience, a practice to which I ascribe. Some, however, prefer to perform this procedure in the proliferative phase, a time of relatively decreased uterine swelling and pelvic edema.

The choice of the abdominal incision is the surgeon's option. It is important that there be adequate exposure to deal with deep or posterior fibroids. As a rule of thumb, one would need greater exposure for an extensive myomectomy than for a hysterectomy.

Hemostasis can most efficiently be obtained by expeditious surgical technique. Some surgeons believe that delivering the entire uterine mass through the abdominal incision may place vessels on stretch and decrease bleeding. After a bladder flap is lowered, a soft Penrose drain passed through the avascular spaces of the broad ligament bilaterally and compressed in the midline compresses the uterine vessels and may decrease blood loss (Fig. 28–10). To prevent ischemic necrosis, the tourniquet should be loosened at 10-minute intervals.[48] Atraumatic clamps applied to the infundibulopelvic ligaments may also decrease blood loss. Some surgeons elect to use local infiltration with a dilute solution of Pitressin (Parke-Davis, Morris Plains, New Jersey).[49] This is an aqueous solution of synthetic vasopressin (8-arginine vasopressin) essentially free of oxytocin. A 1-mL ampule contains 20 pressor units. This may be diluted in 30 mL of normal saline and infiltrated along the site of the uterine incisions. This technique decreases blood loss. Because vasopressin is a potential hypertensive agent and alters urine output, it is important to consult with and inform the anesthesiologist before it is used. A vertical midline uterine incision is usually adequate to remove most fibroids without excessive blood loss.

The choice of cutting instruments for myomectomy is also the surgeon's option. Choices include electrocautery, laser, or sharp knife. There is no clear advantage of one instrument over the other. There may be decreased blood loss from tiny superficial vessels using either electrocautery or laser, but these methods of cutting may cause greater local tissue damage. Especially when operating near the tubal insertions, there may be some advantage to the greater precision offered by a sharp scalpel.

The principles of a successful myomectomy for infertility include use of as few incisions as possible with care to avoid the intramural portions of the fallopian tubes.[50] The direction of dissection for significant fibroids is from a lateral to a medial direction and from an inferior to a superior direction. This decreases blood loss and avoids damage to lateral blood vessels. Before the procedure is started, a moment should be taken to inspect the uterus carefully and determine where the tubal insertions are and where the uterine vessels are. It is also important to determine the relative positions of fi-

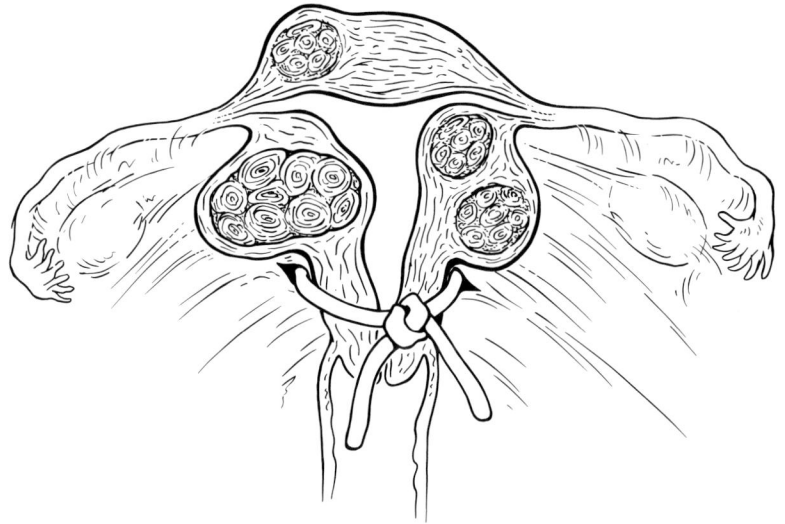

FIGURE 28–10. Compression of uterine vessels by a Penrose drain passed through the avascular space in the broad ligament after the bladder is advanced.

broids and the ureters. By determining where the tubal insertions are, one can thereby determine best where the endometrial cavity is. It is necessary to keep in mind where the cavity is so one can then differentiate anterior from posterior fibroids. Certainly a large posterior intramural fibroid is best removed from a posterior uterine incision. If its position relative to the endometrial cavity is not known, the surgeon may inadvertently take an anterior approach and remove the myoma after incising both sides of the endometrium. This would certainly be a traumatic approach with a much more protracted repair.

When the myoma is identified, an incision is made down to the myoma. Fairly large myomata can be removed through relatively small incisions. The myoma is surrounded by a condensation of fibroconnective tissue, the so-called capsule. It is important to incise through the capsule to the surface of the myoma before attempting to remove the myoma (Fig. 28–11). An incision that does not go through the capsule would then result in dissection, which tears through normal myometrium and causes myometrial damage and increases hemorrhage. It is thus more appropriate to cut into the myoma or up to it to identify it rather than fail to bring the incision down far enough and cause uterine damage.

Once the myoma is identified, it is usually dissected free from its bed. The myoma is first grasped with a tenaculum or towel clip and placed on traction (Fig. 28–12). It is then released from its bed by digital dissection, dissection with a

blunt object such as the handle of the scalpel or cautery (Fig. 28–13). This process is helped by pressure from behind the fibroid mass or lateral to it, expressing the tumor out through the incision. The tumor is then totally removed by either blunt dissection or twisting while the tenaculum is held under tension. Significant bleeding points in the wall of the uterus can be grasped with atraumatic clamps. A single feeder artery supplying the tumor can often be identified, clamped, and ligated.[51] In most cases, the mass can be removed without bothering to clamp the most dependent portions of the capsule. This area is usually not a vascular base but simply the last part of the capsule to be separated from the myoma. It can be dissected free with blunt dissection in a way similar to removal of the rest of the tumor.

It is preferable to remove adjacent myomata through a single uterine incision. The position of the endometrium should be ascertained for deep myomata. If they are not pedunculated, but impinge on or slightly protrude into the endometrial cavity, the myoma can usually be dissected free from endometrium without incising the endometrium. When down this deeply into the myometrium, it is appropriate to palpate the endometrial cavity to detect pedunculated submucous fibroids, which can then be removed after incision of the endometrium. The endometrium need not be incised if there are no pedunculated fibroids. Some surgeons prefer to stain the endometrium by instilling relatively concentrated methylene blue dye transcervically via a cannula or pediatric

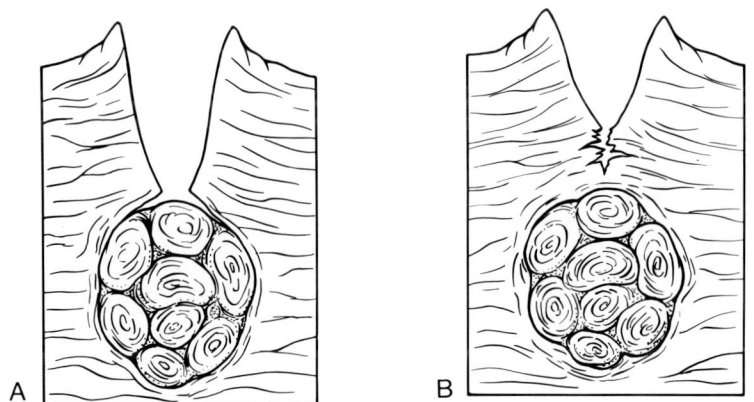

FIGURE 28–11. Incision up to (A) or into the myoma provides the proper dissection plane. An incision that does not reach the fibroid (B) will result in tearing of uterine tissue without dislodging the fibroid.

A   B

After fibroid removal, redundant hypertrophic uterine tissue may be present. This tissue should not be removed because it involutes after closure of the uterus.

Uterine incisions are best repaired by absorbable suture; 0 or 2–0 suture for larger incisions or deeper layers is appropriate. Superficial closure can be effected by 3–0 or 4–0 suture. It is important to eliminate and close all deep dead space. It is also important to build up the myometrium directly over the endometrium supporting this area. Continuous sutures are usually adequate. It is important to remember that locking sutures devitalize tissue. A slight hemorrhagic ooze is not unusual after myomectomy. It is appropriate, however, to leave the uterus as dry as possible and with minimal surface trauma in the hope that this will avoid adhesion formation. Adhesion formation can also be minimized by covering raw areas on the surface of the uterus. Imbricating sutures are useful in this regard. Effective hemostasis and good surgical technique are probably the best procedures for decreasing adhesion formation. Many physicians have their favorite medications, solutions, or wetting agents for the prevention of adhesions. None are universally accepted, and none have withstood the test of time. It would, however, make sense to use physiologic solutions to irrigate the pelvis to avoid surface tissue damage and edema caused by solutions of nonphysiologic tonicity or nonphysiologic ion concentration. Removal of clots at the end of the procedure is also worthwhile. Uterine suspension has been recommended to correct retroversion and prevent adhesions, but there are no available data that this procedure is helpful in decreasing future symptoms or improving fertility.

Postoperative care includes the principles of rapid ambulation. There should be close attention to immediate postoperative hematocrit as well as the hematocrit on the first 2 postoperative days because there is a tendency to drop hematocrit levels significantly in the postoperative period. A transient temperature elevation occurs, not unusually, 2 to 3 days after extensive myomectomy. Some surgeons use prophylactic antibiotics preoperatively and extending into the first postoperative day in an attempt to prevent infection.

Occasionally surgeons encounter adenomyomatosis when

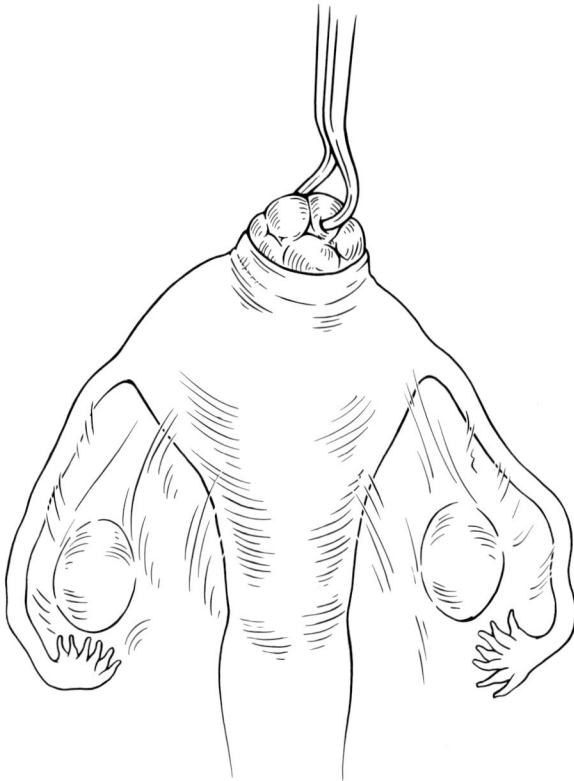

FIGURE 28–12. Incision over a superficial sessile fibroid will allow adequate uterine tissue for closure.

Foley catheter. This stain can serve as an aid to identification of the endometrium.

Sessile subserosal myomata can frequently be removed by circumferentially inscribing their surface, dissecting the tumor free, and then closing the remaining condensed myometrium without disturbing the body of the uterus. Pedunculated fibroids can be removed safely by clamping and ligation of the base.

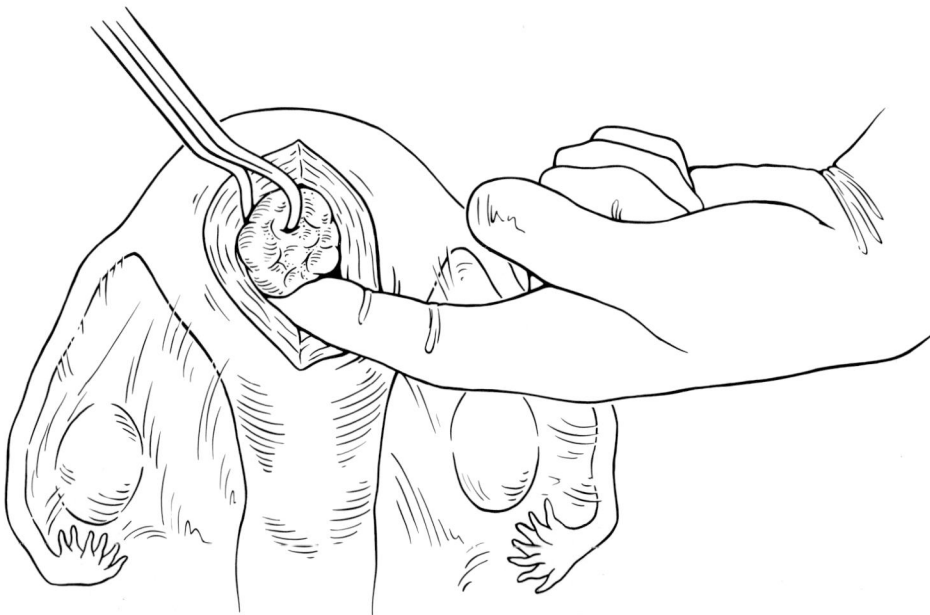

FIGURE 28–13. Removal of the myoma is effected by digital dissection, traction, and twisting of the tumor.

performing an operation for fibroids. These tumor-like nodules of adenomyosis and associated uterine scarring and induration do not have clear tissue planes and are difficult to dissect specifically from the uterus. If the uterus is to be maintained in such cases, cytoreductive surgery to eliminate the more severe areas may be necessary. Although clear tissue planes may not be present, it is usually possible to eliminate the central endometriotic core of these lesions.

Although there is much discussion as to whether a cesarean section is indicated if the endometrial cavity had been entered during the course of a myomectomy, there are little hard data to speak to this issue. It appears reasonable that this decision should be a judgment call of the surgeon. A small incision in the endometrial cavity may not require a cesarean section. Multiple incisions into the uterus with significant compromise to the uterine integrity whether or not the cavity is entered may require subsequent cesarean section. This is a decision best made by the operating surgeon at the time of myomectomy. This information should be clearly imparted to the patient in the postoperative period and included in the operative note. In any event, the occurrence of a myomectomy should alert the patient's obstetrician to the potential risk of uterine rupture.[52] Although there are few well-controlled studies on the results of myomectomy, reviews summarizing many studies have suggested an average postoperative pregnancy rate of 40%.[51] Most reports suggest that myomata-associated infertility is significantly improved postsurgically. One report, however, suggests that myomectomy in infertile women with no other infertility factors may actually decrease fertility.[53] It is important to recognize that one significant postoperative risk of myomectomy is adhesion formation, which may interfere with tubo-ovarian function.

UTERINE MYOMATA DURING PREGNANCY

As previously mentioned in this chapter, submucous myoma may be a cause of recurrent early pregnancy loss. This loss can be reduced by removal of myomata impinging and interfering with the endometrial cavity. Women whose pregnancies become established in the presence of fibroids are subject to specific risks. Antepartum bleeding can occur owing to the presence of fibroids. Pain from a vascular accident in the tumor is best managed expectantly. There appears to be an increased incidence of preterm labor in the presence of fibroids.[54] The obstetrician should be alert to these problems. Significantly sized lower segment myomata may produce obstruction of labor. Dystocia may also occur from interference with the efficiency of uterine contractions. The net effect of these problems is an increased incidence of cesarean section in women with myomata in pregnancy.[55]

Rare fetal complications have been reported in the presence of fibroids. Mechanical compression of the fetus has been implicated in cases of limb reduction anomalies, localized malformations,[56] and congenital torticollis.[57]

Although it is clear that there are specific risks associated with fibroids in pregnancy, most pregnancy outcomes are quite favorable. Women with fibroids should not be discouraged from undergoing pregnancy.

REFERENCES

1. Robboy SJ, Mehta K, Norris HJ. Malignant potential and pathology of leiomyomatosis tumors of the uterus. Clin Consult Obstet Gynecol 1990;2:2–9.
2. Merrill JA, Creasman WT. Benign lesions of the uterine corpus. In: Scott JR, DiSaia PJ, Hammond CB, Spellacy WN, editors. Danforth's Obstetrics and Gynecology. 6th edition. Philadelphia: JB Lippincott, 1990:1027.
3. Townsend DE, Sparkes RS, Baluda MC, McClelland G. Unicellular histogenesis of uterine leiomyomas as determined by electrophoresis of glucose-6-phosphate dehydrogenase. Am J Obstet Gynecol 1970;107:1168–1173.
4. Rien MS, Friedman AJ, Barbieri RL, et al. Cytogenetic abnormalities in uterine leiomyomata. Obstet Gynecol 1991;77:923–926.
5. Chandrasekhar Y, Heiner J, Osuamkpe C, Nagamani M. Insulin-like growth factor I and II binding in human myometrium and leiomyomas. Am J Obstet Gynecol 1992;166:64–69.
6. Fayed YM, Tsibris JCM, Langenberg PQ. Human uterine leiomyoma cells: binding and growth responses to epidermal growth factor, platelet-derived growth factor, and insulin. Lab Invest 1989;60:30–37.
7. Spellacy WM, LeMaire WJ, Buhl WC. Plasma growth hormone and estradiol levels in women with uterine myomas. Obstet Gynecol 1972;40:829.
8. Folkerd EJ, Newton CJ, Davidson K, et al. Aromatase activity in uterine leiomyomata. J Steroid Biochem 1984;20:1195–1200.
9. Pollow K, Sinnecker G, Boquoi E, Pollow B. In vitro conversion of estradiol-17-beta into estrone in normal human myometrium and leiomyoma. J Clin Chem Clin Biochem 1978;16:493–502.
10. Reddy VV, Rose LI. 4-3-Ketosteroid 5α-oxidoreductase in human uterine leiomyoma. Am J Obstet Gynecol 1979;135:415–418.
11. Bamford DS, Jogee M, Williams KL. Prostacyclin formation by the pregnant human myometrium. Br J Obstet Gynaecol 1980;87:215–218.
12. Daly DC, Walters CA, Prior JC, et al. Prolactin production from proliferative phase leiomyoma. Am J Obstet Gynecol 1984;148:1059–1063.
13. Kenigsberg D, Chapitis J, Zuna R, Riddick D. Hyperprolactinemia arising from a uterine tumor [abstr]. Soc Gynecol Invest 1987;34:157.
14. Weiss DB, Aldor A, Aboulafia Y. Erythrocytosis due to erythropoietin-producing uterine fibromyoma. Am J Obstet Gynecol 1975;122:358–360.
15. Gross BH, Silver TM, Jaffe MH. Sonographic features of uterine leiomyomas: an analysis of 41 proven cases. J Ultrasound Med 1983;2:401–406.
16. Killackey MA, Neuwirth RS. Evaluation and management of the pelvic mass: a review of 540 cases. Obstet Gynecol 1988;71:319–322.
17. Togashi K, Ozasa H, Konish I, et al. Enlarged uterus: differentiation between adenomyosis and leiomyoma with MR imaging. Radiology 1989;171:531–534.
18. Dudiak DM, Turner DA, Patel SK, et al. Uterine leiomyomas in the infertile patient: preoperative localization with MR imaging versus ultrasound and hysterosalpingography. Radiology 1988;167:627–630.
19. Baltarowich OH, Kurtz AB, Pennell RG, et al. Pitfalls in the sonographic diagnosis of uterine fibroids. AJR Am J Roentgenol 1988;151:725–728.
20. Merrill JA, Creasman WT. Benign lesions of the uterine corpus. In: Scott JR, DiSaia PJ, Hammond CB, Spellacy WN, editors. Danforth's Obstetrics and Gynecology. 6th edition. Philadelphia: JB Lippincott, 1990:1033.
21. Merrill JA, Creasman WT. Benign lesions of the uterine corpus. In: Scott JR, DiSaia PJ, Hammond CB, Spellacy WN, editors. Danforth's Obstetrics and Gynecology. 6th edition. Philadelphia: JB Lippincott, 1990:1030.
22. Weiss G, Shenker L, Gorstein F. Suppurating myoma with spontaneous drainage through the abdominal wall. NY State J Med 1976;76:572–573.
23. Rubin A, Ford JA. Uterine fibromyomata in urban blacks. S Afr Med J 1974;48:2060–2062.
24. Miller NF, Ludovici PP. On origin and development of uterine fibroids. Am J Obstet Gynecol 1955;70:720–740.
25. Countinho EM, Maia HS. The contractile response of the human uterus, fallopian tubes, and ovary to prostaglandins in vivo. Fertil Steril 1971;22:539–543.
26. Farrer-Brown G, Beilby JOW, Tarbit MH. Venous changes in the endometrium of myomatous uteri. Obstet Gynecol 1971;38:743–751.
27. Forssman L. Distribution of blood flow in myomatous uteri as measured by locally injected 133 Xenon. Acta Obstet Gynecol Scand 1976;55:101–104.

28. Santoro NF. Medical management of uterine leiomyomata. Clin Consult Obstet Gynecol 1990;2:29–34.

29. Filicori M, Hall DA, Loughlin JS, et al. A conservative approach to the management of uterine leiomyomata: pituitary desensitization by a luteinizing hormone-releasing hormone analogue. Am J Obstet Gynecol 1983;147:726–727.

30. Healy DL, Fraser HM, Lawson SL. Shrinkage of a uterine fibroid after subcutaneous infusion of a LHRH agonist. Br Med J 1984;289:1267–1268.

31. Maheux R, Guilloteau C, Lemay A, et al. Regression of leiomyomata uteri following hypoestrogenism induced by repetitive luteinizing hormone-releasing hormone agonist treatment: preliminary report. Fertil Steril 1984;42:644–646.

32. Maheux R, Guilloteau C, Lemay A, et al. Luteinizing hormone-releasing hormone agonist and uterine leiomyomata: a pilot study. Am J Obstet Gynecol 1985;152:1034–1038.

33. Healy DL, Lawson SR, Abbott M, et al. Toward removing uterine fibroids without surgery: subcutaneous infusion of a luteinizing hormone-releasing hormone agonist commencing in the luteal phase. J Clin Endocrinol Metab 1986;63:619–625.

34. Coddington CC, Collins RL, Shawker HT, et al. Long-acting gonadotropin hormone-releasing hormone analog used to treat uteri. Fertil Steril 1986;45:624–629.

35. Kessel B, Liu J, Mortola J, et al. Treatment of uterine fibroids with agonist analogs of gonadotropin-releasing hormone. Fertil Steril 1988;49:538–541.

36. Friedman AJ, Barbieri RL, Benacerraf BR, Schiff I. Treatment of leiomyomata with intranasal or subcutaneous leuprolide, a gonadotropin-releasing hormone agonist. Fertil Steril 1987;48:560–564.

37. Friedman AJ, Barbieri RL, Doubilet PM, et al. A randomized, double-blind trial of a gonadotropin-releasing hormone agonist (leuprolide) with or without medroxyprogesterone acetate in the treatment of leiomyomata uteri. Fertil Steril 1988;49:404–409.

38. Friedman AJ, Atlas DH, Barbieri RL, et al. A randomized, placebo-controlled, double-blind study evaluating the efficacy of leuprolide acetate depot in the treatment of uterine leiomyomata. Fertil Steril 1989;51:251–256.

39. Lumsden MA, West CP, Baird DT. Goserelin therapy before surgery for uterine fibroids. Lancet 1987;1:36–37.

40. Andreyko JL, Blumenfeld Z, Marshall LA, et al. Use of an agonistic analog of gonadotropin-releasing hormone (nafarelin) to treat leiomyomas: assessment of magnetic resonance imaging. Am J Obstet Gynecol 1988;158:903–910.

41. Maheux R, Lemay A, Merat P. Use of intranasal luteinizing hormone-releasing hormone agonist in uterine leiomyomas. Fertil Steril 1987;47:229–233.

42. Perl V, Marquez J, Schally AV, et al. Treatment of leiomyomata uterine with D-Trp-6-luteinizing hormone-releasing hormone. Fertil Steril 1987;48:383–389.

43. Friedman AJ, Hoffman DI, Comite F, et al. Treatment of leiomyomata uteri with leuprolide acetate depot: a double-blind, placebo-controlled, multicenter study. Obstet Gynecol 1991;77:720–725.

44. Friedman AJ. Vaginal hemorrhage associated with degenerating submucous leiomyomata during leuprolide acetate treatment. Fertil Steril 1989;52:152–154.

45. Neuwirth RS, Richart RM. Hysteroscopic resection of submucous leiomyoma. Contemp Obstet Gynecol 1985;25:103–123.

46. Neuwirth RS. Operative hysteroscopy. In: Baggish M, Barbot J, Valle R, editors. Diagnostic and Operative Hysteroscopy: A Text and Atlas. Chicago: Year Book Medical Publishers, 1989;179–185.

47. Nakamura Y, Yoshirmura Y, Yamada H, et al. Treatment of uterine leiomyomata with a luteinizing hormone-releasing hormone agonist: the possibility of nonsurgical management in selected perimenopausal women. Fertil Steril 1991;55:900–905.

48. Rubin IC. Uterine fibromyomas and sterility. Clin Obstet Gynecol 1958;1:501–518.

49. Kistner RW: Malignant neoplasms. In: Kistner RW, editor. Gynecology: Principles and Practice. 3rd edition. Year Book Medical Publishers, Chicago:1979:255.

50. Lock FR. Multiple myomectomy. Am J Obstet Gynecol 1969;104:642–650.

51. Buttram VC, Reiter RC. Uterine leiomyomata: etiology, symptomatology and management. Fertil Steril 1981;36;433–445.

52. Roopnarinesingh S, Ramsewak S: Rupture of the uterus in patients with previous myomectomy. J Obstet Gynecol 1985;6:32–36.

53. Berkeley AS, DeCherney AH, Polan ML: Abdominal myomectomy and subsequent fertility. Surg Gynecol Obstet 1983;156:319–322.

54. Davis JL, Ray-Maziemder S, Hobel CJ, et al. Uterine leiomyomas in pregnancy: A prospective study. Obstet Gynecol 1990;75:41–44.

55. Bardeguez AD. Uterine leiomyomas in pregnancy. Clin Consult Obstet Gynecol 1990;2:53–57.

56. Graham JM, Miller ME, Stephan MJ, Smith DW. Limb reduction anomalies and early in utero limb compression. Pediatrics 1980;96:1052–1056.

57. Romero R, Chervenak FA, DeVore G, et al. Fetal head deformation and congenital torticollis associated with uterine tumor. Am J Obstet Gynecol 1981;141:839–840.

58. Snyder JR, Goldstein SR, Weinreb JC. Imaging of fibroids: Modern diagnostic techniques. Clin Consult Obstet Gynecol 1990;2:13–19.

59. Meloni AM, Surti U, Contento AM, et al. Uterine leiomyomas: cytogenetic and histologic profile. Obstet Gynecol 1992;80:209–217.

60. Gagliardi CL, Emmi AM, Weiss G, Schmidt, CL. Gonadotropin-releasing hormone agonist improves the efficiency of controlled ovarian hyperstimulation/intrauterine insemination. Fertil Steril 1991;55:939–944.

CHAPTER 29

Lesions Affecting the Uterine Cavity

CRAIG A. WINKEL

The uterus functions in a variety of complex roles in human reproduction: as a conduit for the transport of sperm to the fallopian tubes, as a unique environment for the implantation of the embryo, as a source of energy and nutrients for the developing fetus, as an incubator for the growing fetus, and as the force that expels the fetus during parturition. Apart from parturition, dysfunction of the uterus in general, and the endometrium specifically, may lead to failure of conception or early pregnancy wastage. Unfortunately, today, our ability to detect abnormalities of the uterus and endometrium that might result in failure of reproduction is limited primarily to those tests that identify structural rather than functional abnormalities. As a result of these deficiencies, the precise magnitude of the role that the uterus and endometrium play in infertility is difficult to determine. It has been estimated, however, that among carefully evaluated couples, abnormalities of the uterus per se may account for between 5% and 10% of the cases of infertility. These difficulties notwithstanding, it is important for the clinician to have a thorough understanding of the techniques for evaluation of the uterus and endometrium to allow for complete investigation of possible causes of reproductive failure in the infertile couple.

EMBRYOLOGY OF THE UTERUS AND ENDOMETRIUM

It seems appropriate to begin a discussion of infertility and the endometrium with the embryologic development of the uterus. In all vertebrates in classes below the marsupials, the müllerian ducts remain separate and open directly into the permanent cloaca. In the mammals that develop placentae, there are various degrees of fusion of the müllerian ducts near their caudal ends. In the primates, the union of the two müllerian ducts results in the development of a single uterus and vagina.

The müllerian ducts in the human embryo become apparent at about the 37th day of gestational age. The müllerian ducts in the early embryo tend to follow the general course of the mesonephric ducts (Fig. 29–1). At their cranial ends, the müllerian ducts maintain a position lateral to that of the mesonephric ducts. The müllerian ducts run parallel to the mesonephric ducts until near the caudal end of these ducts, at which point the müllerian ducts cross over the mesonephric ducts and come to lie medially. In the human embryo, at about 2 months of gestational age, the caudal ends of the two müllerian ducts reach to a point just caudal to the urogenital sinus and extend as far as the müllerian tubercle, a midline projection that is formed by the entrance of the mesonephric ducts into the posterior wall of the cloaca. It is not until about the 20th week that the müllerian ducts actually communicate with the urogenital sinus.[1]

Well before the 20th week of gestational age, the caudal ends of the müllerian ducts, which are compressed together between the lateral mesonephric ducts in the genital cord, fuse to form a single structure with a single canal (Fig. 29–2). At this time, the paired cranial ends of the müllerian ducts develop ostia, and the flared ends become the fimbria of the fallopian tubes. The more caudal part of the müllerian ducts that originates from the fused portion differentiates into the uterus and the vagina.[2]

Because the müllerian ducts develop within the urogenital folds, their course is one that contains two bends that correspond to the bends in the urogenital folds. As a result, the

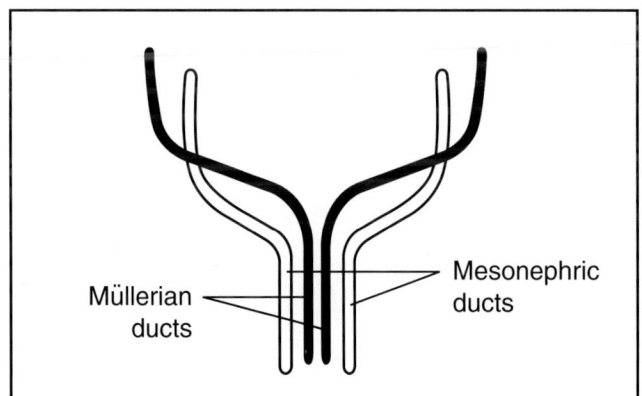

FIGURE 29–1. The müllerian ducts follow the general course of the mesonephric ducts in the early embryo.

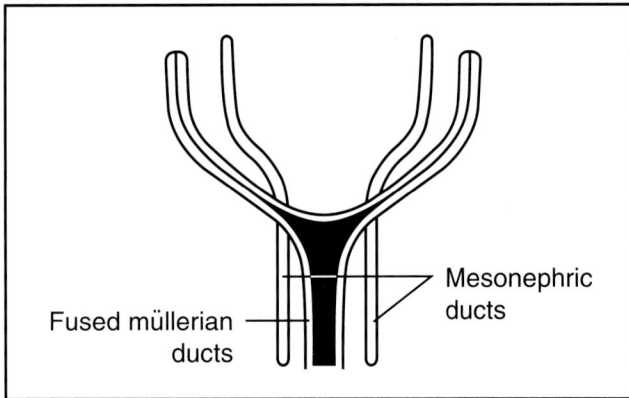

FIGURE 29–2. By the 20th week of gestational age, the caudal portions of the müllerian ducts fuse to form the developing uterus while the cranial portions remain unfused. This configuration persists in the normal human female.

müllerian ducts may be divided into three segments relative to these two bends. The cranial portion of the müllerian ducts runs a longitudinal course that we recognize as that of the fallopian tube in the woman. The middle portion of the müllerian ducts takes a somewhat transverse course that becomes the uterine fundus and corpus, whereas the most caudal segment again runs longitudinally and eventually develops into the uterine cervix and vagina (Fig. 29–3A). The latter segment, fused with its sister, constitutes the uterovaginal primordium.

As development of the embryo proceeds, the cranial wall of the middle or transverse limbs of the müllerian ducts commences to bulge upward, thus changing the concave surface of the intervening tissue into a convex surface. This results in the unfused portions of the müllerian ducts being added to the uterus as its fundus and corpus (Fig. 29–3B). The cervix and vagina then develop from the fused primordium.

The eventual muscular walls of the female genital tract commence their development as a covering, well-defined

layer of dense mesenchymal tissue. It has been demonstrated that the endometrial lining of the uterine canal becomes defined at about the seventh month of fetal life. At about the same time, endometrial glands develop and evaginate toward the myometrium.[3] These glands remain quiescent, small and rather atypical, however, until puberty. A distinction between the lining of the uterus and that of the vagina is not possible before the fourth month of fetal life. In contrast to the rest of the female genital tract, at that time the canal of the vagina becomes lined with stratified epithelium. Shortly thereafter, a plug of columnar cells obliterates the vaginal canal for a period of time, until the vaginal canal reappears at about 5 months of age.

Failure of these events to occur in the order and at the times described can result in permanent uterine as well as vaginal anomalies. These anomalous conditions are relatively easy to understand if one keeps in mind the normal course of events that has been summarized. Complete duplication of the uterus and the vagina, as is observed normally in the monotremes and the lower marsupials, is the result of total failure of the paired müllerian ducts to fuse (Fig. 29–4A). Duplication of the uterus but not the vagina, as is seen in most rodents, is caused by an arrest in fusion of the portion of the müllerian ducts just cranial to the vagina (Fig. 29–4B). The development of a bipartite (or septate) uterus, as is observed in carnivores and ruminants, is the result of fusion of the uterine portion of the müllerian ducts only at their caudal ends, with the cranial, uterine portion more or less separated by a median partition (Fig. 29–4C). A bicornuate uterus, as is observed in sheep, develops owing to imperfect fusion and absorption of the fundal segments of the müllerian ducts that leave paired pouches at the upper ends of the uterus (Fig. 29–4D). Congenital absence of one or both müllerian ducts, the result of either failure to form or some embryonic accident, may result in complete absence of the vagina, uterus, and tubes or the development of a unicornuate uterus or a unicornuate remnant (Fig. 29–4E). Finally, failure of the uterus to grow beyond that formed as a fetus may result in the presence of an infantile uterus in the woman.[4]

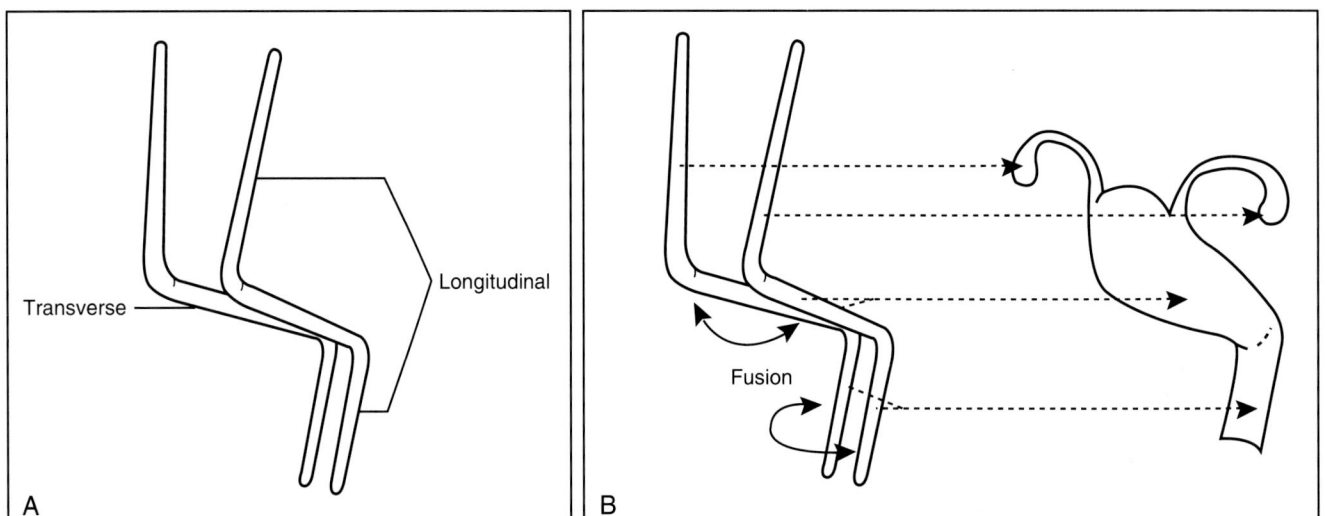

FIGURE 29–3. The three-dimensional relationship of the müllerian ducts during embryologic life. A, The longitudinal and transverse portions of the müllerian ducts. B, The corresponding derivation of the uterus and fallopian tubes.

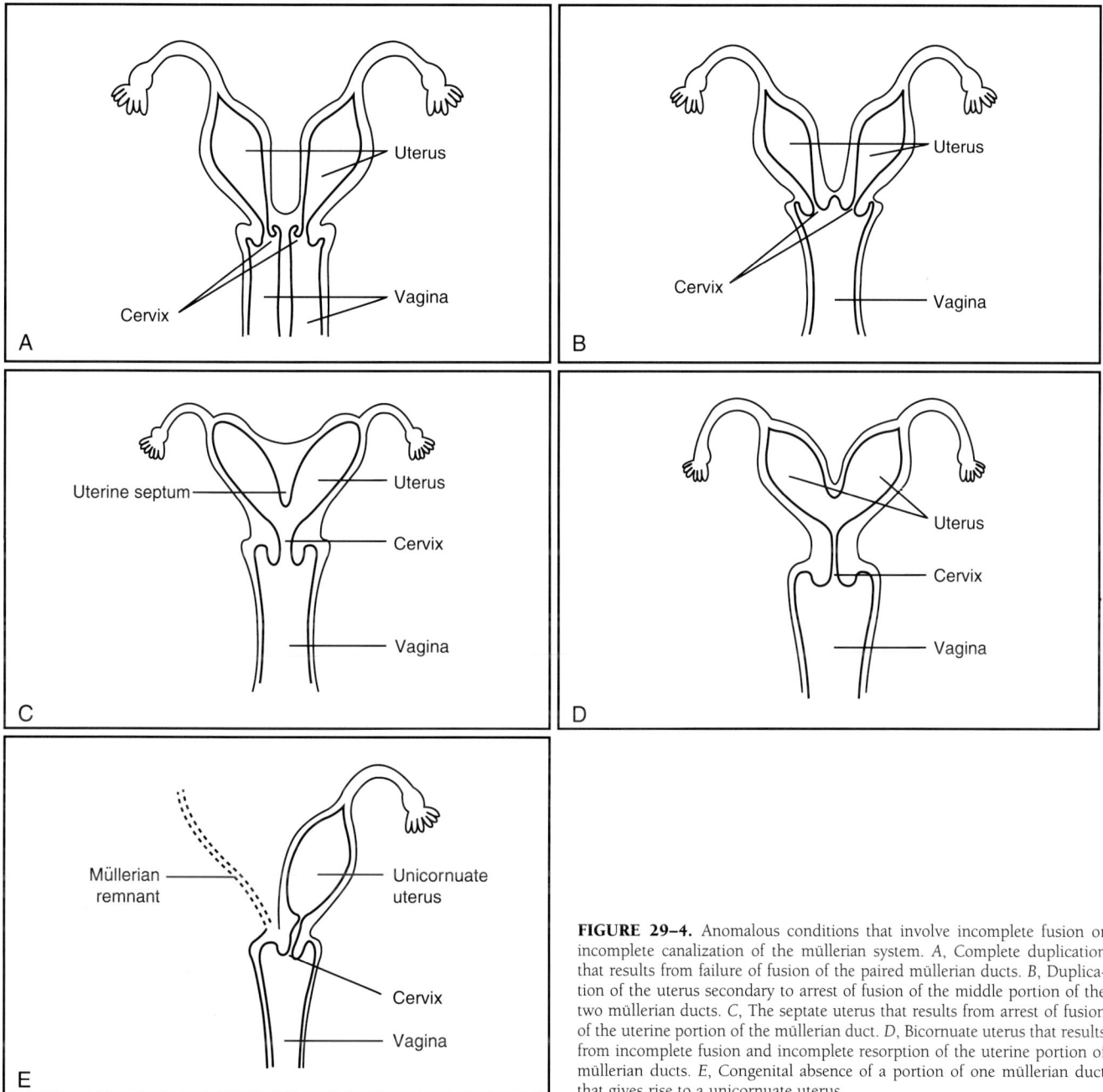

FIGURE 29–4. Anomalous conditions that involve incomplete fusion or incomplete canalization of the müllerian system. *A*, Complete duplication that results from failure of fusion of the paired müllerian ducts. *B*, Duplication of the uterus secondary to arrest of fusion of the middle portion of the two müllerian ducts. *C*, The septate uterus that results from arrest of fusion of the uterine portion of the müllerian duct. *D*, Bicornuate uterus that results from incomplete fusion and incomplete resorption of the uterine portion of müllerian ducts. *E*, Congenital absence of a portion of one müllerian duct that gives rise to a unicornuate uterus.

ENDOMETRIAL RESPONSE TO OVARIAN HORMONES

The factors that regulate the cyclic synthesis and secretion of steroid hormones by the ovaries are discussed elsewhere in this book. A review, however, of the effects of the various sex steroid hormones of ovarian origin on the endometrium is crucial to development of an understanding of potential ways in which endometrial abnormalities might lead to infertility or early pregnancy wastage.

The endometrium is a relatively unique tissue in the human because few tissues—the mucosa of the gut, the squamous epithelium of the skin, and the vagina, and the endometrium of the ovulatory woman—undergo significant replication as a part of their normal function. It has been observed that the endometrium is shed and regenerated not less than 400 times during the reproductive life of an ovulatory woman. More impressively, it has been calculated that the 5 g of endometrium normally attained at the midsecretory phase of the menstrual cycle (day 20) would grow to nearly 1800 pounds if the rate of growth at that stage of the cycle continued without interruption for 365 days.[5]

The endometrium makes up the lining of the uterine cavity. On gross inspection, the endometrium is a thin, pink, membranous layer of tissue that on magnification is seen to have a large number of minute openings. These openings are actually the ostia of the endometrial glands that are responsible for the secretion of material thought to be important in the nutrition of the early embryo. Because of the functional changes in response to ovarian steroid hormones, the thickness of the endometrium during the menstrual cycle may vary between 0.5 and 5.0 mm.

The endometrium comprises surface epithelium that consists of a single layer of high columnar, ciliated cells; glands; and interglandular mesenchymal stroma in which are located the endometrial blood vessels. The ciliated cells tend to be grouped in discrete patches. Interestingly, the ciliated cells demonstrate no secretory activity, whereas the nonciliated cells appear to produce the secretions attributed to the endometrium. The function of the ciliated cells remains to be elucidated completely, but it has been demonstrated that the ciliated cells located from the fallopian tube to the internal os of the cervix develop a ciliary current that is directed toward the cervix and may be important in the movement of the fertilized ovum into the endometrial cavity.

The uterine glands are actually tubular-shaped invaginations of the endometrial epithelia that extend through the entire depth of the endometrium to the myometrium and even occasionally interdigitate for a short distance between the myometrial cells. The glands thus are not true glands in the histologic sense. They are lined by a single layer of columnar epithelium similar to the rest of the epithelial surface of the endometrium. This single layer of cells is separated from the underlying endometrial stroma by a well-defined basement membrane. The endometrial glands secrete a slightly alkaline fluid that moistens the uterine cavity.

The endometrium undergoes specific changes in structure and presumably function under the direct control of the hormones secreted during the ovarian cycle. During the follicular phase of the ovarian cycle, the principal ovarian hormone, estradiol-17β, stimulates proliferation of the endometrium. Commencing as a thin layer, perhaps no more than 2 mm in thickness, the effect of estrogen is to stimulate mitosis in both endometrial glandular epithelial cells and in the stroma. This mitotic activity continues until 2 to 3 days after ovulation has occurred. In the superficial portion of the endometrium, the stromal cells are packed loosely because repair following menstruation is progressing. In the deeper layers, the stromal cells are relatively dense. The glands tend to be strictly tubular and rather widely spaced.

As the proliferative effects of estrogen continue and as the stimulation increases as a result of progressive elevations in circulating levels of estradiol, the endometrium becomes thicker. The glandular and stromal elements proliferate simultaneously. The glands become taller and pseudostratified as the time of ovulation approaches. Nonetheless, the glands remain widely spaced in the superficial layers of the endometrium but become tortuous and rather crowded in the deeper layers. Histologic "dating" (assigning the day of an idealized 28-day menstrual cycle to which the endometrium corresponds based on histologic criteria) of the endometrium during the proliferative phase of the menstrual cycle is difficult, if not impossible, because of the great variation among women. Although the luteal phase of the ovarian cycle, which corresponds to the secretory phase of the endometrial cycle, is of remarkably constant duration, the follicular phase of the ovarian cycle may be associated with extreme variability in length from cycle to cycle.

At the time that ovulation occurs, there is the onset of synthesis and secretion of progesterone by the ovary. The changes in endometrial morphology in response to stimulation by progesterone are so predictable that it becomes pos-

sible for the pathologist to "date" the endometrium with significant accuracy. Under the influence of progesterone, there is a loss of fluid from the endometrium, and thus endometrial thickness may decrease slightly. At the same time, during the secretory phase of the endometrial cycle, the three layers of the endometrium become easily identified: the basalis layer adjacent to the myometrium, the compacta layer that lies immediately beneath the epithelial surface, and the spongiosa that lies between the compacta and the basalis layers. The basalis layer undergoes relatively few histologic changes despite the wide fluctuations in ovarian steroid production. The glands become tortuous in the spongiosa but maintain their straight configuration in the compacta. The lumen of the glands becomes filled with secretions during the late secretory phase.

Late in the secretory phase of the endometrial cycle, the endometrium becomes highly vascular. This appears to be an ideal situation for the implantation of an embryo. During this phase of the cycle, the stromal cells immediately surrounding each blood vessel undergo hypertrophy that results in the appearance reminiscent of the decidua of pregnancy. At about the sixth to seventh day postovulation, at a time when implantation would be expected to occur, the endometrium attains its greatest thickness, about 5 to 6 mm. At the same time, there is a remarkable proliferation of changes in the morphology of the blood vessels within the endometrial stroma. The vessels become tortuous, and in the compacta zone, arterioles develop that branch into fine capillaries. Because this proliferation of vessels occurs more rapidly than the increasing thickness of the entire endometrium, the vessels approach closer and closer to the surface of the endometrium. This disparity in growth of vessels and stroma is mimicked in disparity of growth of the endometrial stroma and glands, and, as a result, the glands become highly coiled and closely packed. It appears that the stimulatory effect of estrogen on both glandular and stromal elements is inhibited partially by the action of progesterone. In this way, the stroma slows its rate of growth, whereas the glands do not.

During the 2 or 3 days that precede the onset of menstruation, there are dramatic changes in the endometrium. Initially and in concert with the decline in secretion of progesterone by the corpus luteum that has failed to be rescued by human chorionic gonadotropin of trophoblastic origin, there is an influx of polymorphonuclear cells and macrophages. In addition, there is a rapid increase in the coiling of the endometrial vessels. This is believed to result in increased resistance to flow, and as a consequence blood flow to the endometrium is diminished. The result is relative vascular stasis. Shortly thereafter, predictable and significant periods of vasoconstriction occur. This leads to hypoxia and presumably damage to the vessel walls. The intermittent nature of the vasoconstriction allows for repeated escape of blood into the tissue. Ultimately there is necrosis and liquefaction of the superficial one to two thirds of the endometrium that results in the commencement of menstruation. Thereafter, with the onset again of ovarian synthesis and secretion of estrogen, the cycle begins again in the endometrium.

DIAGNOSTIC EVALUATION OF THE UTERUS

As mentioned previously, diagnostic evaluation of the uterus and the endometrium for the purpose of detection of disorders that might contribute to infertility or early pregnancy wastage is limited primarily to tests for the presence of structural rather than functional abnormalities. Although there are a number of tests of organic pathology, such as endometrial biopsy, hysterosalpingography, hysteroscopy, laparoscopy, ultrasonography, endometrial culture, and endometrial steroid hormone receptor analysis, that are available and used routinely today, there are relatively few tests of endometrial function: production of endometrial proteins, alterations in immunohistochemistry of the endometrium, characterization of endometrial enzymes, and sonographic detection of changes in endometrial thickness and sonolucency. Because a number of these tests and techniques are the subject of whole chapters in this book, the following discussion is limited primarily to the role of each of these as a diagnostic tool for the evaluation of the infertile woman.

ENDOMETRIAL BIOPSY

Although we have innumerable reports in the medical literature that concern the normal patterns of synthesis and secretion of sex steroid hormones by the ovaries, the associated plasma concentrations of each of these hormones that can be expected to be observed on a given day of the ovarian cycle, the response of the endometrium to these fluctuations in hormone levels remains critical to the success of the reproductive process. Regardless of whether the plasma hormone concentrations fall into the range of values that might be expected, the endometrial response determines whether embryo growth, implantation, placentation, and fetal development proceed.

Dating of the Endometrium

As discussed previously, it has been demonstrated that endometrial histology follows a remarkably consistent pattern of morphologic change in response to the changes in circulating sex steroid hormone concentrations. Bernirschke[6] has summarized the major histologic changes that occur in the endometrium throughout the menstrual cycle. It is apparent that the histologic changes that can be observed during the proliferative phase of the endometrial cycle are too variable to allow for precise assignment of a "date" related to the day of an idealized 28-day menstrual cycle mainly because of the fact that variation in cycle length almost always arises from variation in the length of the follicular phase of the ovarian cycle. At the same time, it has been demonstrated repeatedly that the length of the duration of function of the corpus luteum is surprisingly consistent from cycle to cycle in the human.[7] For these reasons, "dating" of the endometrium tends to be limited to the secretory phase of the endometrial cycle.

Examination of endometrial histology may provide a great deal of information related to reproductive function. In a sense, the endometrium may serve as an internal bioassay of the individual woman's ovarian function. Moreover, endometrial histology may provide information that relates to the quality of the hormonal preparation of the endometrium and its role in implantation as well as the presence of endometrial abnormalities, such as hyperplasia and endometritis.

Even before Noyes and colleagues[7] described the criteria already alluded to for the dating of the endometrium, investigators encountered women in whom the histology of the endometrium appeared to lag in its maturation behind the actual date of the endometrial cycle. The first published report regarding what has come to be known as luteal phase defect was recorded in 1949, when Jones[8] suggested that this finding might be associated with infertility. Since then, literally hundreds of publications have appeared in which the authors have supported or refuted this as a diagnosis and a cause of infertility. The subject of luteal phase defect is covered elsewhere in this book, and so comments are limited to the role that the endometrial function may play in this defect as a cause of either infertility or early pregnancy wastage. Despite the near universal availability of sophisticated techniques for assessment of the concentrations of circulating sex steroid hormones,[9–11] measurement of numbers of endometrial steroid hormone receptors,[12–14] and other biochemical activities, biopsy of the endometrium retains its place as the most widely used method for assessment of endometrial functional capacity.[15–20]

Technique for Sampling the Endometrium

The technique for taking an endometrial biopsy requires some description because sampling of the endometrium is one of the primary means by which the clinician can test the endometrium for functional normality. Originally the technique of endometrial biopsy for detection of luteal phase defect involved the use of the rigid Novak curette,[8] and the diagnosis of luteal phase deficiency was made when the day of dating of the endometrium lagged by more than 2 days behind the cycle date, as calculated retrospectively based on the day of onset of the next menses.[15, 16] At this time, however, there is lack of consensus in the literature whether an endometrial biopsy is out of phase when "dating" is suggestive of 2 days' lag or more than 2 days' lag. Today there are a variety of instruments that can be used for the performance of the endometrial biopsy: flexible suction cannula, the Gynocheck endometrial sampler,[21, 22] and the endometrial Pipelle curette, to name a few. In general, the devices that may be used can be divided into two types. The first type is used to aspirate tissue from the endometrial lining during abrasion or scraping of the curette against the wall of the uterine cavity. These instruments provide tissue specimens suitable for histologic examination and assessment of day of cycle. The second type of device is used to obtain a collection of endometrial cells for cytologic screening by insertion of a plastic or metal brush or a sponge into the endometrial cavity and literally wiping the wall of the cavity with the device. These devices provide cytologic specimens on which histologic assessment of day of cycle is nearly impossible.

Although there are few studies of the reliability of the various instruments when used for endometrial biopsy, it is possible that the instrument used might artifactually alter the results. Honore and associates[23] reported a reduced incidence of finding "out of phase" endometrium when the endometrial Pipelle was used to perform endometrial biopsy compared with the Novak curette despite no difference in adequacy of the tissue sample. It has been suggested that the narrower lumen of the Pipelle as well as its less rigid nature causes less trauma to the tissue and thus adds no artifact to the histologic specimen.

As compared with the 4-mm Novak curette, the endometrial Pipelle seems to be well tolerated by patients, perhaps because of its smaller (3.1 mm) external diameter. The latter instrument is associated with an acceptable specimen as frequently or more often than is the use of the Novak curette. The technique used with the Pipelle is relatively simple (Fig. 29–5A). The vagina and cervix should be cleansed with an aseptic solution such as iodine. The Pipelle is inserted into the uterine cavity through the cervix. Occasionally it is necessary to anesthetize the cervix by local injection of an anesthetic agent and to grasp the anterior lip of the cervix with a tenaculum to stabilize the cervix or to straighten the endocervical canal (Fig. 29–5B). The inner plunger of the Pipelle is then pulled back with a twisting motion, while the outer cannula is rotated and withdrawn from the endometrial cavity. This combined action creates suction at the lateral opening in the tip of the Pipelle, thereby drawing tissue into the cannula. As the cannula is withdrawn, the tissue is sheared off, and a specimen is retained within the cannula. With the use of this technique, an acceptable specimen can be obtained most of the time and with good patient tolerance.[24]

Endometrial Assessment

IMMUNOHISTOCHEMICAL EVALUATION

As discussed, one of the uses of an endometrial specimen in the evaluation of the infertile woman or the woman who suffers repeated pregnancy loss is histologic dating of the endometrium. There are, in addition, several other studies that can be performed on the endometrium in an attempt to define the cause of the reproductive dysfunction. The characterization of several proteins synthesized by the endometrial cells[25-29] as well as demonstration of their regulation by circulating hormone levels allows for the evaluation of endometrial function by immunohistochemical techniques.

The protein, α_2-PEG (pregnancy-associated endometrial α_2-globulin), is associated mainly with the glandular epithelium. Another endometrial protein, the 24K protein, is a secretory product of the luminal epithelium of the endometrium. Immunohistochemical assessment of the endometrium for the presence of these two proteins may allow for characterization of the functional response of the endometrium to the hormonal environment. α_2-PEG appears in significant amounts precisely 5 to 6 days after ovulation,[30] about the time that blastocyst implantation occurs. Thereafter the glandular content of this protein increases remarkably until the onset of menses. In the same specimens of endometrium, the 24K protein was found to appear in the glandular epithelium on only days 2 and 3 postovulation, thereafter disappearing from the endometrial glands. This protein then began to appear in the luminal epithelium at about the first or second day after the expected day of implantation.[30] It has been suggested that the sequential appearance of these two proteins in the endometrium around the time of embryo implantation might serve as a physiologic marker of this event.

The appearance of the 24K protein in the decidua of pregnancy as well as the appearance of this protein in endometrium at the time noted is supportive of the theory that this protein is regulated synergistically by both estrogen and progesterone. Although the specific functions of this protein are not known completely, it has been suggested that it may play a role in the attachment of the blastocyst to the uterine wall.[26, 28] The secretion of α_2-PEG does not appear to be linked directly to estrogen or progesterone because the appearance of α_2-PEG in the endometrium commences well after the start of the luteal phase and the secretory changes thereby induced. Instead, it seems that prolonged stimulation by progesterone as well as perhaps other endocrine requirements for decidualization may regulate the secretion of α_2-PEG.[29] Interestingly, the N-terminal amino acid sequence of α_2-PEG has been determined and there is considerable homology with the amino acid sequence of the β-lactoglobulin group.[27] This finding is suggestive that α_2-PEG may play a role in the transfer of retinol to the trophoblast during the process of implantation.[25]

An issue that remains to be clarified regarding immunohistochemical assessment of the presence of these two endometrial proteins is the clinical usefulness of such evaluation. In addition to histologic evaluation of an endometrial biopsy specimen, it would seem that immunohistochemical evaluation might detect information of a specific biochemical nature that simple histology might not. By way of example, in one

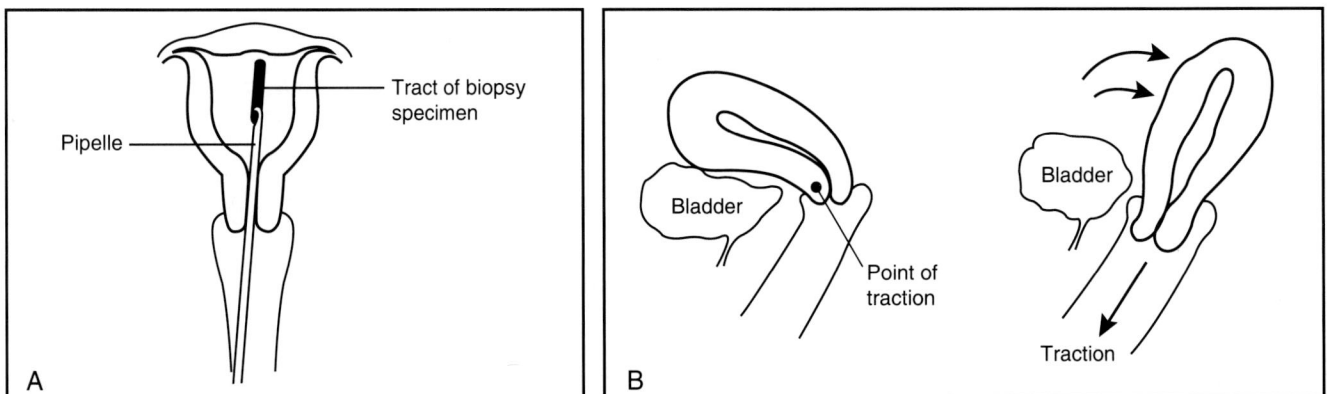

FIGURE 29–5. A, The endometrial pipelle is withdrawn from the fundus while applying suction, thereby aspirating a thin specimen of endometrium from the uterine cavity. B, Angulation between the uterus and the vagina may make sounding of the uterus difficult. By grasping the anterior lip of the cervix at the point of traction (A) and applying traction along the line of the vagina (B), the uterus rotates on its axis, thereby bringing the uterine cavity and vaginal canal into alignment.

study, no "out-of-phase" endometrial biopsy specimens were found to be immunohistochemically normal, whereas about a third of "in-phase" biopsy specimens were determined to have immunohistochemical abnormality.[30] Thus, atypical biochemistry of the endometrium was not reflected morphologically in all cases. Such findings might have obvious clinical impact. During treatment with clomiphene citrate for ovulation induction, histologic evaluation of the endometrium may be suggestive of normal morphology, but biochemical deviation from normalcy may be found immunohistochemically.[31] Similarly, the hypersecretion associated with progesterone supplementation during the luteal phase of the ovarian cycle may not be depicted histologically but is obvious when performing immunohistochemical staining for the presence of α_2-PEG and the 24K protein.[32]

Further studies of the endometrium of infertile women are suggestive that additional markers of endometrial deficiency, despite morphologic normality, do exist. The normal secretory differentiation of the endometrium is associated with the development on the endometrial cell surfaces of a peptide-associated sialo-oligosaccharide of the sulfated lactosaminoglycan family[33, 34] to which a monoclonal antibody (D9B1) has been raised.[35, 36] The cell surface epitopes to which this antibody binds are produced and secreted by endometrial gland cells mainly between the third and seventh days after the onset of the luteinizing hormone surge.[37] In women with a luteal phase defect, there appears to be a strong correlation between infertility and reduced production of the D9B1 epitope.[35] Unfortunately, to date, a specific function for the glycoprotein that carries the D9B1 epitope is unknown. Its temporal distribution, however, in the endometria of women with normal fertility is known to coincide with the timing of embryo implantation.[37]

UTERINE SECRETIONS

To establish a pregnancy, it is clear that viable embryos need an endometrium that is prepared adequately to achieve attachment and then implantation. It is important also to remember that the human embryo survives unattached in uterine luminal fluid for 3 days within the endometrial cavity before the processes of implantation begin. Significant advances in our understanding of ovarian function have been gained from hormonal monitoring of women who undergo in vitro fertilization. Nonetheless, implantation rates remain relatively low. Indeed, it has been estimated that 65% to 90% of apparently normal embryos fail to implant after embryo transfer.[38, 39] It is possible, and even likely, that the preparation of the endometrium that results from exposure to the hormonal milieu created during the follicular and then the early luteal phase of the ovarian cycle is representative of only a part in the whole scheme of events necessary for successful implantation. Along this line of thinking, it seems reasonable to hypothesize that the secretions of the endometrial epithelium in which the embryo must develop during its residence in the uterine cavity and before its implantation into the wall of the endometrium play a significant role in the success of achieving an ongoing pregnancy. From the study of animal models, it has been demonstrated that implantation succeeds only when the protein milieu of the intracavitary fluid is favorable,[40, 41] a finding that correlates also with appropriate morphologic transformation of the endo-

metrium. From these studies as well as others,[42–46] it has been shown that histologically normally transformed endometrium must offer an adequate luminal secretory milieu to the blastocyst around the time of implantation to ensure a stage of receptivity in the blastocyst that in turn facilitates implantation. A complete understanding of the mechanism(s) by which receptivity of the embryo is developed and acts to promote implantation remains to be elucidated. Identification of some of the proteins that are believed to be components of the "receptive" uterine luminal milieu, however, has been accomplished. Two of these luminal proteins, identical electrophoretically, chromatographically, immunologically, and by various biologic tests to the pregnancy-specific, placental proteins PP12 and PP14, have been identified.[47–54]

Because there has been some success in identifying these two proteins, not only in uterine luminal fluid, but also in peripheral plasma, there have been attempts at the development of blood tests to evaluate and predict the period of receptivity to embryo implantation. Although the presence of these proteins can be established in blood, correlation with successful implantation remains to be established. This may be because other sources of synthesis of the same or similar proteins may exist. In addition, just as peripheral concentrations of gonadotropin-releasing hormone (GnRH) are likely not reflective of hypothalamic-hypophyseal portal blood concentrations of GnRH, it is unlikely that peripheral plasma levels are reflective of the substantial synthesis and secretion into the lumen of endometrial proteins.

Nonetheless, several facts appear supportive of the concept that alterations in the milieu created by the endometrium in response to ovarian stimulation might play a role in early pregnancy wastage and infertility. Although it is unlikely that a single protein will ever serve as a marker of receptivity of the endometrium to the peri-implantation blastocyst, it does appear that various patterns of proteins present in endometrial secretions might correlate with the functional state of the endometrium. Certain protein patterns, for example, have been demonstrated to provide reliable information for implantation in the rabbit.[55–57] Among women treated with clomiphene citrate, a variety of individual responses with regard to patterns of proteins present in endometrial secretions was noted:[58]

1. A physiologically normal pattern associated with receptivity.

2. A quiescent pattern associated with no endometrial response to stimulation and thus no receptivity.

3. A pseudoproliferative pattern suggestive of partial endometrial response only and thus no receptivity.

4. A pattern suggestive of abortive secretion as though there was an interruption in normal secretions and thus no receptivity.

From these sorts of studies, it must be concluded that alterations in endometrial function, aside from deviations that might be demonstrable based purely on morphologic screening, do exist. What remains is to determine the best means by which to test the functional capacity of the endometrium.

BIOCHEMICAL EVALUATION

It is believed generally that the response of the endometrium, morphologically as well as functionally from the starting point of synthesis of endometrial proteins and then release of those proteins into the uterine lumen, is controlled by the steroid hormone milieu that is created simultaneously during the development and maturation of the ovum and embryo by the ovary. We have discussed already the morphologic changes that occur within the endometrium as well as the changes in function of the endometrium that occur to enable implantation of the embryo. It seems appropriate at this time to consider also the biochemical events that must occur within the endometrial cells to enable the endometrium to respond appropriately to the changing hormonal milieu.

During the follicular phase of the ovarian cycle, the major steroid secretory product from the ovary is estradiol-17β, a potent estrogen. The response of endometrial cells to estrogen is mediated by estrogen receptors that have been found to be present within the nuclei of both endometrial stromal and epithelial cells.[59-65] During the luteal phase of the ovarian cycle, the ovary produces prodigious amounts of progesterone in concert with rather modest amounts of estradiol-17β. During the secretory phase of the endometrial cycle, embryo endometrial interaction takes place. Among the biochemical events that allow for this interaction to progress successfully is the interplay of progesterone with the progesterone receptor also located within the nuclei of endometrial stromal and epithelial cells.[59-66]

The regulation of endometrial estrogen receptor formation is rather poorly understood, but suffice it to say that estradiol-17β is believed to stimulate the formation of the nuclear estrogen receptor.[64] The regulation of the formation of the progesterone receptor within the endometrium has been studied in considerable depth because it has been suggested that deficiency in the ability of the endometrium to respond to the effect of progesterone secreted by the corpus luteum of the ovary results in either early pregnancy loss or failure of implantation.[67-69] The progesterone receptor is regulated positively by the action of estradiol-17β.[61, 70] Thus, during the early secretory phase of the endometrial cycle, progesterone receptor concentration is greatest,[71] presumably because of the heretofore unopposed action of estrogen during the follicular phase of the ovarian cycle. Although an inherently large variation among individuals in endometrial progesterone receptor content can be demonstrated, there appears to be a progressive decrease in the number of progesterone receptors from the day following ovulation until about day 6 of the secretory phase (about the time of implantation).[63, 65, 67, 68, 71] Because one of the actions of progesterone within the endometrium is to stimulate the activity of the enzyme estradiol-17β dehydrogenase,[72] it is thought that the action of progesterone to increase the synthesis of this enzyme results in increased metabolism of estradiol-17β to weak estrogens and thus reduced estrogenic stimulation of the formation of additional progesterone receptors. Although it is clear that these events occur in normal endometrium, there appears to be no conclusive evidence that alterations in either activity of the enzyme estradiol-17β dehydrogenase or the content of endometrial progesterone receptor is altered significantly in women thought to have a luteal phase defect. Indeed, the authors of some studies have demonstrated apparent reductions in secretory phase progesterone receptor numbers in women with luteal phase defect,[68] whereas other authors have not.[71, 72]

An interesting finding associated with the study of estrogen and progesterone receptor content of endometrium and women with infertility has been the apparent finding of reduced estrogen receptors in the endometrium of such women during the follicular phase of the endometrial cycle.[73] This finding, along with the findings of reduced progesterone receptor content of the endometrium during the follicular phase among such women,[72] is supportive of the hypothesis of DiZerega and Hodgen,[74] who suggested that luteal phase dysfunction was actually a sequela to poor folliculogenesis.

In addition to these biochemical events that transpire in the endometrium, it is clear that the endometrium has the ability to produce prolactin.[75] Based on studies of endometrial cells in culture, Ying and colleagues[76] found correlation between normality of endometrial function in vivo and prolactin production in vitro. For example, it has been demonstrated that the decidualized endometrium of women with evidence of luteal phase dysfunction has reduced capacity for the formation of prolactin in vitro.[76] The significance of this finding remains to be determined, as does the significance of the actions of prolactin within the endometrial cavity. It may be that the factors that play a role in normal endometrial function just happen to stimulate the production of prolactin by this tissue. Thus, the production of prolactin may serve as a marker of endometrial function.

Although one or more causes can now be identified for many cases of subfertility, especially based on endometrial abnormalities, there remain many situations in which specific abnormalities cannot be identified. For this reason, investigators have continued to look for ways in which to assess the endometrium that might provide a clue to the cause of infertility among these women. As a result, a host of issues have been addressed. Although no definitive answers have been supplied, it seems appropriate in the context of this discussion to mention these investigations.

Another area of endometrial function that has been addressed is that of endometrial binding of oxytocin. Oxytocin, which is produced and secreted by the posterior pituitary gland, has been shown to bind to high-affinity binding sites in both the mammary glands[77] and the myometrium.[78] It has been demonstrated that oxytocin is produced also by the corpus luteum,[79] binds to specific binding sites within the endometrium,[80] and thus may play a role in the normal function of the endometrium. Because oxytocin has been shown to stimulate the production of the luteolytic prostaglandin, $PGF_2\alpha$,[81] and because intermittent surges of oxytocin from the regressing corpus luteum of sheep has been demonstrated to be associated with intermittent surges of secretion of $PGF_2\alpha$ from the endometrium in that species,[82] it seems reasonable to suggest that oxytocin may play a role in the alterations in endometrial function associated with luteolysis in the human. Baker and colleagues[83] have studied this subject and found that subfertile women had lower midcycle and higher midluteal phase endometrial concentrations of oxytocin binding sites than did normal women. In these women, treatment with clomiphene appeared to be associated with elevations in oxytocin binding during the midcycle of these subfertile women. The potential explanation for this change offered by these authors was based on the findings in other studies that estrogen stimulates the formation of oxytocin binding sites.[84] Although these findings are interesting and suggestive potentially of a marker other than progesterone receptors for the action of estrogen in the endometrium, clinical significance of such data is purely speculative.

With respect to endometrial function and infertility, there are several reports in the medical literature suggestive of associations between other diseases and abnormal endometrium. It has been suggested that women with endometriosis are predisposed to ovarian dysfunction that may present as though the primary abnormality involves the endometrium. For example, there is an apparent association between luteal phase endocrine alterations described with this disease[85–89] and altered histologic changes in endometrium that may be interpreted as a luteal phase defect. Furthermore, it has been demonstrated that women with endometriosis have apparently lower rates of embryo implantation than women with infertility based on tubal disease.[90] It has been demonstrated that women with minimal and mild endometriosis suffer alterations in endometrial morphology that cannot be explained based on aberrations in endocrine function. Fedele and colleagues[91] found that women with endometriosis demonstrated abnormalities in endometrium during the proliferative phase of the cycle that were characterized by decreased ratios of ciliated-to-nonciliated endometrial cells. In addition, there is also an associated decrease in cellular height in the endometrium of these women.[91] Because various authors[92–94] have reported immunoglobulin (Ig)G, IgA antiendometrial antibodies, and C3 and C4 complement deposits in endometrial tissue of patients with endometriosis, a relationship between the change in ciliated cells and endometriosis might be explained based on some associated immunologic abnormality. Furthermore, elevated circulating levels of antiendometrial autoantibodies have been found in women with endometriosis.[95, 96] Taken together, these findings, along with the apparent cellular changes, are suggestive of a possible autoimmune reaction at the endometrium that is triggered by the presence in abnormal sites of endometrial implants. Further studies are warranted to clarify this possibility.

Also, there is an association between β-thalassemia and infertility. Although most patients with this abnormality suffer from failure of pubertal development and hypogonadotropism,[97, 98] the possibility exists that these patients may also have some endometrial abnormality. It has been demonstrated that the gonadal failure is due in large part to iron deposition within the hypothalamus, pituitary gland, and ovaries. In addition, defective maturation of the hypothalamus has been suggested as a possible cause of the defective gonadal function in these individuals.[99] A limited number of pregnancies have been reported among women with β-thalassemia who are transfusion dependent,[100–104] most the result of treatment with an iron chelating agent such as desferrioxamine. It has been demonstrated that women with β-thalassemia also have large deposits of iron within the endometrium.[105] Typically these deposits are found in the apical part of the endometrial cells above the nuclei. These iron deposits may contribute to the infertility observed among women with this disease by interfering with embryo implantation, especially because treatment with iron chelating agents that results in pregnancy is associated with a dramatic decrease in endometrial deposits of iron. Thus, in the patient with β-thalassemia in whom pregnancy is desired, treatment should be directed not only at ovulation induction, but also at evaluation of the endometrium for hemosiderosis and the use of iron chelating agents to reduce these iron deposits.

EVALUATION OF THE ENDOMETRIAL CAVITY

Hysterosalpingography

Hysterosalpingography has been a mainstay in the diagnostic evaluation of the infertile woman. Many clinicians believe that the primary indication for the performance of a hysterosalpingogram (HSG) is the assessment of tubal patency. The HSG, however, may be of considerable value in the evaluation of the endometrial cavity and may lead to the identification of intracavitary pathology, such as leiomyomata, polyps, and synechiae, as well as the "forgotten" or "lost" intrauterine contraceptive device (IUD).

The ideal contrast material for visualization of the endometrial cavity and the fallopian tubes has been discussed by many authors. Both aqueous and oil-based contrast agents have their advocates. Although most clinicians agree regarding the diagnostic efficacy of the HSG, several have suggested that the HSG when performed using an oil-based contrast medium may serve a therapeutic role as well,[106–111] resulting in a 35% spontaneous pregnancy rate within 3 months of the procedure. Alper and associates[112] and deBoer and colleagues[113] found some therapeutic value to the HSG but could detect no significant difference in therapeusis when either aqueous or oil-soluble contrast material was used. There may be some difference, however, between the aqueous and oil-soluble media if the sharpness of the radiographic picture is considered. Although some authors have found equal sharpness with either medium for visualization of the fallopian tubes, the oil-based medium appears to provide a more distinct image for visualization of the endometrial cavity.[113] This may be due to the higher iodine concentration and the separation of the oily contrast phase and the watery mucous phase within the uterus. An aqueous contrast medium is likely to penetrate the excretory ducts of the endometrial glands and to blend with the uterine secretions, giving rise to an unclear image. Furthermore, the lower iodine concentration of the aqueous medium creates a less dense image of the uterine cavity. The same physiochemical properties enable the oil-based contrast medium to yield a more detailed image of the uterine mucosa,[111, 112] as evidenced by more frequent visualization of tubal mucosal folds. Water-soluble contrast agents, however, seem to provide better definition of tubal mucosal folds.

Although either aqueous or oil-soluble contrast media may be used in the performance of the HSG, a word of caution should be mentioned for those who choose to use the oil-soluble material. The oil-based contrast media may persist in the peritoneal cavity for months to years and if present in occluded fallopian tubes may even lead to the generation of a granuloma and foreign body reaction.[106, 108, 111, 112, 114] Moreover, a well-known complication of HSG is venous or lymphatic intravasation of contrast material. If an oil-based material is used and intravasation occurs, oil embolization can result. This may result rarely in serious cardiovascular problems.[111, 112] The aqueous contrast materials are resorbed completely within 15 minutes, and intravasation has little effect.

NORMAL HYSTEROSALPINGOGRAM

The uterus is a pyriform organ that measures about 7 by 4 by 3 cm. The wall of the uterus, which consists of both myometrium and endometrium, is 1.5 to 2.0 cm in thickness and totally encloses the endometrial cavity, which is only a potential space. The cavity of a uterus of normal size is distended fully by the instillation of 2 to 3 mL of contrast material, which results in the characteristic appearance at hysterosalpingography.

The uterine cavity on HSG consists of two rather discrete areas that have quite different appearances. The superior portion, the endometrial cavity itself, extends from the internal os of the cervix inferiorly to the dome-shaped fundus superiorly. The endometrial cavity accounts for about 50% of the uterus in the woman but somewhat less than 50% in the prepubertal child. The appearance of the endometrial surface as depicted by the contrast medium may vary somewhat during the menstrual cycle. Although generally rather smooth and regular, during the postovulatory phase of the cycle, the secretory endometrium may display a fuzzy, slightly irregular contour.

The inferior portion of the uterine cavity as it appears on HSG consists of the endocervical canal and is defined as the span between the internal cervical os above to the external os below. The mucosal surface of this area is notably irregular, often with an exaggerated pattern of in-pouchings and out-pouchings. The endocervical canal frequently cannot be visualized if a Foley catheter or balloon device is used in the performance of HSG. Although some importance of the internal cervical os has been suggested, on HSG this is only the area that separates the endometrial cavity from the endocervical canal rather than a specific structure per se.

The appearance of the endometrial cavity at the time of HSG may vary depending on the axis in which the uterus lies relative to the x-ray film. For example, if the cavity lies at nearly a right angle to the x-ray film, the cavity tends to have a linear shape. With traction on the cervix during the procedure, the uterus is deflexed, thereby bringing the endometrial canal to lie nearly parallel to the x-ray film and thus provide an image similar to what one would expect to see.

UTERINE DEFECTS

The detection of abnormalities of the endometrial cavity may be important because such abnormalities may be associated with failure of embryo implantation or pregnancy loss. The most common disorders of the endometrial cavity can be noted at the time of HSG and are perceived generally as filling defects because they displace the contrast material within the uterine cavity.

The most common filling defects tend to be benign neoplasms, most often endometrial polyps and leiomyomata. Endometrial polyps appear on HSG as smooth, well-defined, sessile or pedunculated filling defects that may be various sizes but most commonly are of less than 1 cm in diameter (Fig. 29–6). Most of the time, endometrial polyps are solitary, but it is not impossible to find a woman with multiple polyps on HSG.

Leiomyomata may be associated with a variety of appearances on HSG depending on the size, number, and location of the tumors. Submucosal tumors may give an appearance on HSG similar to that depicted by a sessile endometrial polyp. The intramural tumors usually distort the endometrial cavity without encroaching on the endometrial lining. These tumors yield a picture in contrast to that seen with endome-

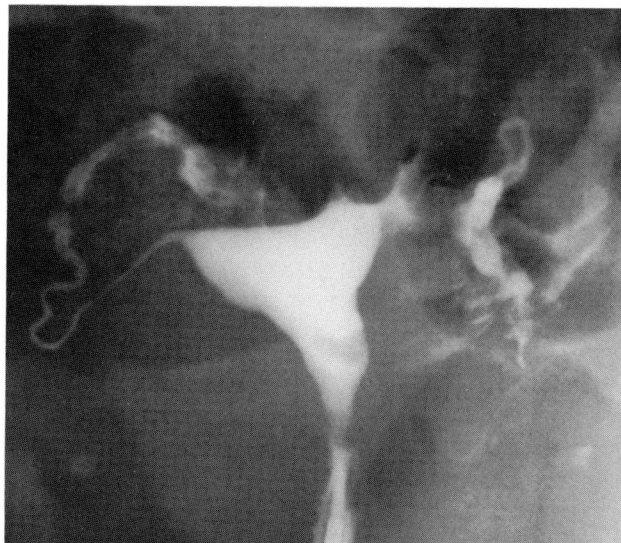

FIGURE 29–6. A small endometrial polyp is observed as a partial filling defect in the lower uterine segment.

trial polyps (Fig. 29–7). With multiple intramural myomas, the endometrial cavity not only may be distorted in configuration, but also may be increased in size. It is not unusual to find the woman with an 18 week–sized uterus and a cavity that requires 30 mL or more of contrast material to fill.

The finding of a malignant tumor at the time of HSG is not impossible but is rather rare in the patient population that is investigated for infertility. As might be anticipated, a malignant tumor is associated usually with an irregular appearance and frequently a rather large filling defect within the endometrial cavity. Hysterosalpingography, however, is not the best means of diagnosis in the event of an endometrial or uterine malignancy, and accessory procedures, such as sonography, computed tomography, and magnetic resonance imaging (MRI), are of value in such a situation.

The HSG should be scheduled routinely between the 5th and the 10th day of the ovarian cycle. By not performing the HSG before the fifth day of the cycle, the risk of intravasation

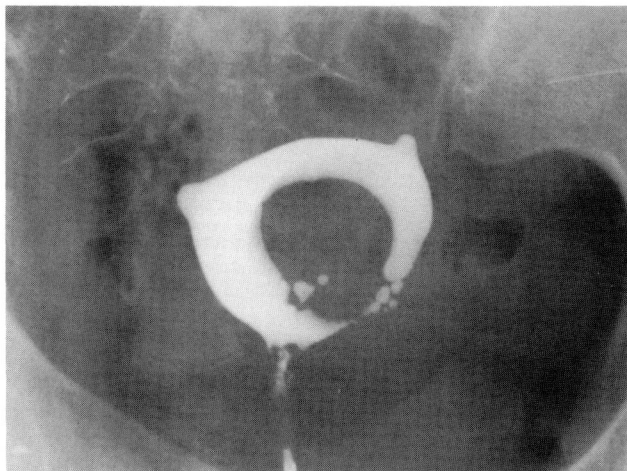

FIGURE 29–7. Hysterosalpingogram in which a large intracavitary leiomyoma presents as a filling defect in the uterine cavity.

of contrast material, which is more likely to occur during or immediately following menstruation when venous channels are most likely to be opened, can be diminished. Likewise, by performing the HSG no later than the 10th day of the ovarian cycle, inadvertent radiation of an intrauterine pregnancy can be avoided. Occasionally, and it is hoped rarely, HSG is performed in the presence of an early pregnancy. The appearance is similar to that observed with an endometrial polyp. For this reason, it is probably prudent, if such a defect were detected, to perform a pregnancy test before undertaking any surgical procedure. The greater question that arises, however, is how to manage the woman who is pregnant and has undergone hysterosalpingography. Although considerable debate still exists concerning the issue of termination of the pregnancy, it has been suggested that radiation exposure of less than 10 rad to the embryo or fetus during the first 6 weeks of gestation results in little risk of developmental abnormality.[115]

Foreign bodies, such as retained products of conception and "lost" or "forgotten" IUDs, may occasionally be demonstrated at the time of HSG. The picture observed with retained products of conception may be mistaken for that of a malignant neoplasm, that is to say, an irregular, not infrequently large intracavitary mass. The history of recent pregnancy, spontaneous abortion, or pregnancy termination as well as symptoms of irregular uterine bleeding may be of value in making the correct diagnosis. The "forgotten" IUD is frequently a surprise at the time of HSG. Although it may sound like an uncommon cause of infertility, numerous reports in the literature attest to the occurrence of this as a cause of infertility.[116–118] Although HSG can be of value in localizing an IUD, precise location is generally accomplished more effectively by ultrasonography.

Artifacts of the procedure, on occasion, may be associated with images that are confusing or may be suggestive of intrauterine filling defects. Air bubbles, blood clots, or even displaced globules of cervical mucus may give the appearance of a filling defect. In most cases, however, such filling defects have little relationship to truly pathologic conditions. For the most part, artifacts yield images of round, linear, or ovoid densities. In addition, such densities are frequently found to be mobile during the procedure. For this reason, the performance of hysterosalpingography under fluoroscopic control is recommended highly.[119] It should also be noted that after removal of an intrauterine device, residual molding of the uterus may result in apparent filling defects at the time of HSG.[120, 121]

ASHERMAN'S SYNDROME

An important finding at the time of HSG is the presence of intrauterine filling defects associated with intrauterine adhesions or synechiae. Amenorrhea traumatica (atretica) or posttraumatic intrauterine pathology has been recognized since the end of the 19th century and is associated typically with clinical manifestations of amenorrhea or hypomenorrhea, infertility, and early pregnancy loss. The cause, clinical manifestations, and radiologic picture on HSG make this an important consideration in the woman with infertility.

In 1894, Fritsch[122] published the first report on a patient who developed amenorrhea following curettage performed a few weeks postpartum. Thereafter, reports appeared in 1927[123] and in 1946[124] that enumerated approximately 44 additional cases associated with similar symptoms. It was not until Asherma,[126] in 1948, published his report that the clinical significance of this problem became obvious. Thence, in 1956, Netter and colleagues[127] coined the eponym *Asherman's syndrome* to describe this condition.

Although the principle cause of Asherman's syndrome or intrauterine adhesions is believed to be trauma to the endometrium, it must be remembered that some cases of secondary amenorrhea with severe intrauterine adhesions (IUA) may arise secondary to infection, especially with tuberculosis[128] or even spontaneously after pregnancy. Although it has been suggested that infection always precedes the formation of IUA,[129] in most cases, infection cannot be demonstrated. In addition, the postpartum state is not an obligate precursor for the development of this disease because IUA have been described following curettage after miscarriage.[130, 131] Moreover, the presence of congenital anomalies is believed to be associated with a predisposition to the formation of these adhesions.[132] Regardless of this debate, it is clear that trauma to the uterus may lead to the formation of IUA regardless of the actual state of the uterus at the time. The obstetric antecedents of IUA have been described by Lancet and Kessler[133] and include previous delivery, spontaneous and induced abortions, or combinations of these events.

The actual mechanism by which the formation of the intrauterine adhesions occurs remains to be determined. Asherman believed that the juxtaposition of the denuded walls of myometrium after the complete removal of the endometrial lining was sufficient to allow the development of fibrous bands between the two walls.[127] Indeed, it was his supposition that too vigorous and aggressive curettage might initiate the problem, but it is well known that adhesions might be observed after simple manual exploration of the uterus[130] or even after gentle suction curettage.[134] It has also been suggested that constitutional factors in a given individual might influence the formation of adhesions.[130] Along these lines, it was suggested that vascular changes near the endometrium that result in fibrosis of this tissue might predispose to the formation of adhesions.[135] There are experimental data obtained in the study of the rat that are supportive of this concept.[136]

As mentioned already, infection does not invariably play a role in the cause of Asherman's syndrome. Endometrial tuberculosis may result frequently in the formation of IUA. It has been suggested that uterine tuberculosis accounts for about 1% of patients with Asherman's syndrome.[133] Obviously tuberculous disease may be associated with the development of IUA more often in those countries in which the prevalence of tuberculosis is high.

The consequences of Asherman's syndrome may be quite varied. Some patients may note amenorrhea or hypomenorrhea, whereas others may experience periodic discomfort—likely the result of development of hematometra if the adhesions block the egress of menstrual fluid from the cervix. Under these circumstances, hematosalpinx and even pelvic endometriosis may develop. At the same time, the disease may be associated with absolutely no symptoms other than infertility. Indeed, women with Asherman's syndrome who experience pelvic pain, dysmenorrhea, or local symptoms are relatively rare. It is estimated that about 6% to 80% of patients experience alteration in menstrual function with this disease.[130, 133] This wide range is suggestive that the degree of alteration in menstrual function is likely related to the severity of adhesions. The most important consequences of Asherman's syndrome, however, are infertility and altered reproductive function. This may present as primary or secondary infertility, repeated spontaneous abortion, missed abortion, or preterm labor.[130, 133, 136–138]

Although pathologic study of the adhesions is seldom undertaken because of technical difficulties, some findings have been described. The adhesions usually connect the uterine walls anterior-posteriorly, but transverse bands also may be seen. In addition, shelf-like protrusions from one uterine wall have been described.[134, 139, 140] Following examination of the adhesions after curettage, three types of adhesions have been described:[136] endometrial (65%), fibrous (25%), and muscular (10%). Thus, the cellular makeup of the adhesions may be endometrial, fibroblast, or myometrial.[141] Often the adhesions are relatively avascular, but exaggerated vascularity and even adenomatous formation have been described.[142]

The diagnosis of IUA is quite simple by HSG. Although intrauterine adhesions are included as filling defects within the uterine cavity, they do not represent true filling defects: Rather the adhesion or synechiae causes focal or regional obliteration of part of the endometrial cavity as the opposing walls of the uterus adhere to each other. The typical defect is characterized as irregular and angular and often has faceted margins (Fig. 29–8). On HSG, the defects may vary significantly in size, shape, and number. The adhesions may nearly completely obliterate the cavity or may present as "fuzzy" margins at the edges of the endometrial cavity. Although frequently obvious even to the inexperienced, it is possible for the adhesions to produce subtle changes that are missed at initial observation. If the adhesions are quite extensive, intravasation of contrast material may occur frequently.

The treatment for Asherman's syndrome has changed dramatically over the last few years. Initial methods for division of the adhesions included primarily blind, sharp curettage.[126, 134] Hysteroscopically directed lysis of adhesions with diathermy or scissors[140] and hysteroscopically directed

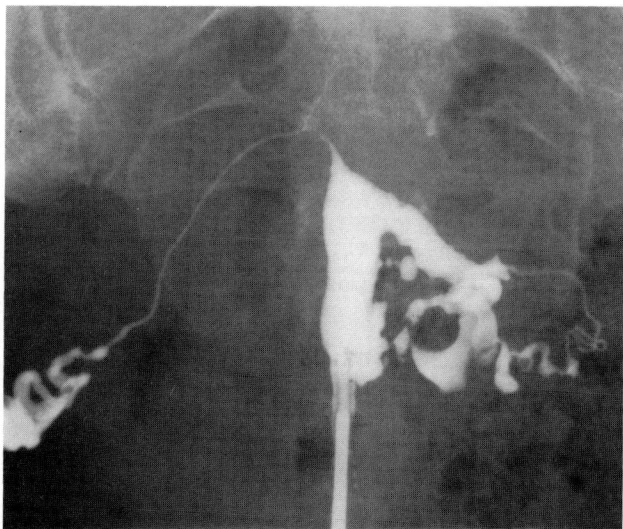

FIGURE 29–8. Hysterosalpingogram demonstrating large irregular filling defect consistent with intrauterine synechia observed classically with Asherman's syndrome.

curettage[143] have been suggested also. Finally, it has been demonstrated that distention of the uterine cavity with a Foley catheter balloon without hormonal therapy may alleviate the problem.[134] The hysteroscopic use of laser energy of different wavelengths has been found to be a highly effective means of removing the intrauterine adhesions.[144–146] The results of studies of comparison of each of the techniques for lysis of uterine synechiae—sharp curettage, electrocautery, or laser—have yet to be reported. Thus, the efficacy of each of the various procedures with regard to recurrence of IUA, pregnancy rate, and pregnancy outcome remains somewhat controversial and highly subjective. The techniques for hysteroscopy and hysteroscopic lysis of adhesions are discussed elsewhere in this book. After lysis of adhesions, it is a good idea to treat the patient with estrogen for a minimum of 1 month after surgery to stimulate growth and regeneration of the endometrium. It has been recommended also that an IUD or Foley catheter be inserted to keep the opposing uterine wall separated. This author has not found the latter to be necessary in most situations.

Ultrasonography

Since the introduction of sonographic technology in medicine, new approaches for the morphologic characterization of different organs as well as new invasive techniques have been developed. The principle uses in the past for ultrasonography in gynecology have been aimed primarily at detection of pelvic or adnexal masses and serial monitoring of the ovarian follicle during folliculogenesis. Repeated sonographic determinations, however, have been demonstrated to have some usefulness in detection of endometrial changes during the menstrual cycle.[147–150] Several investigators have attempted to characterize the hormonally induced changes in endometrial morphology by ultrasonographic techniques. Serial changes in the endometrium can be detected through stimulated ovarian cycles using transvaginal sonographic equipment.[151] Along these lines, it can be demonstrated that two aspects of the endometrium appear to change as the endometrium matures during the ovarian cycle: thickness and reflectivity.[152] Reflectivity of the endometrium can be graded based on the gray-scale appearance of endometrial texture compared with that of the myometrial wall.[151, 152] The grades of endometrium relative to the proliferative and secretory changes have been described as follows:

- *Grade D*: Almost anechogenic endometrium in the presence of a prominent midline echo. This pattern is usually observed during the early proliferative phase (Fig. 29–9A).
- *Grade C*: Solid area of reduced reflectivity that appears darker than the surrounding myometrium. This pattern is detected usually during the midproliferative phase (Fig. 29–9B).
- *Grade B*: The endometrial reflectivity is similar to that of the surrounding myometrium and is indistinguishable on gray-scale. This pattern is seen usually during the later proliferative phase close to the time of the estrogen peak (Fig. 29–9C).
- *Grade A*: The endometrium is brighter than the myometrium. This pattern is associated with impending ovulation (Fig. 29–9D).

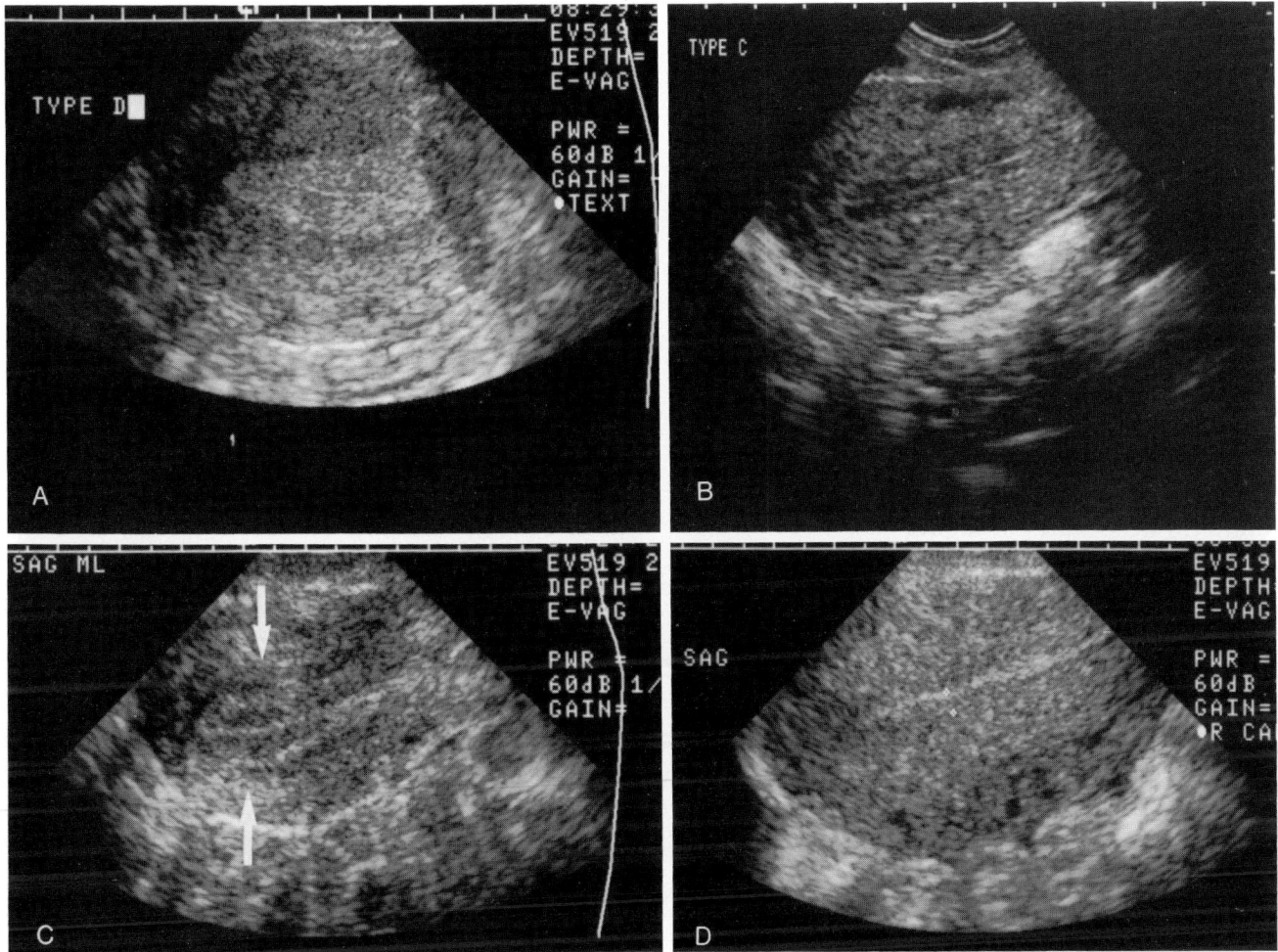

FIGURE 29–9. Sonographic grading of the endometrium relative to proliferative and secretory changes. *A*, Grade D endometrium. *B*, Grade C endometrium. *C*, Grade B endometrium. *D*, Grade A endometrium.

The thickness of the endometrium that is determined sonographically is actually the combined thickness of two layers of opposing endometrium. The endometrium increases in thickness during the follicular phase of the ovarian cycle in concert with exposure to increasing concentrations of estrogen. An endometrial thickness of less than 5 mm is observed usually in the early follicular to midfollicular phase of the cycle. At the time of ovulation, one expects to see a grade A pattern of reflectivity associated with endometrium 10 to 14 mm in thickness. After ovulation has occurred and progesterone is produced, the "triple line" appearance that is representative of the follicular phase of the cycle disappears, and the hyperechogenic endometrium of 13 mm thickness or more is seen in conjunction with the secretory changes that occur morphologically in the endometrium (see Fig. 29–9A to D).

Although there is some correlation between the changes in the endometrium that are detected sonographically and the levels of estrogen and progesterone in plasma, this relationship is not perfect.[153, 154] Attempts at identifying endometrial abnormalities based on sonographic findings have met with limited success to date. Whether such determinations will prove to be clinically useful in the future remains to be determined. Nonetheless, there does appear to be some prognostic value in sonographic measurement of changes within the endometrium. It has been demonstrated, for example, that the maximal thickness of the endometrium achieved during a clomiphene-induced ovulatory cycle is less at the time of ovulation than that which is observed during a spontaneous ovulatory cycle.[155] Furthermore, it has been demonstrated that with conception the endometrium continues to thicken throughout the luteal phase of the cycle,[155] an occurrence that is not observed during nonconception, normal secretory phases. The changes in endometrial thickness that are observed during the proliferative phase of the cycle are comparable in both stimulated and unstimulated cycles in most other studies.[156]

The use of Doppler flow studies to evaluate uterine perfusion have met with some success in the detection of apparent abnormalities among some women. Doppler ultrasound studies of the ascending branch of the uterine artery were performed in a group of women who were participating in in vitro fertilization. A small but significant decrease in perfusion of the uterus after embryo transfer was detected in women who failed to conceive.[157] The clinical significance of this finding is difficult to determine. It remains unclear whether the reduced perfusion is the result of alterations in hormonal response or the primary factor in the failure to conceive. Nonetheless, it is intriguing to hypothesize that some women with infertility may have a primary defect in uterine blood flow as a cause for their subfertility.

Finally, new combined techniques that use ultrasonographic equipment and the principles of hysterosalpingography have been reported.[158] The feasibility and clinical efficacy of such procedures remain to be elucidated. A nonechogenic contrast medium for ultrasonography, however, is used. The contrast medium may be insufflated transcervically in a manner similar to that used for HSG. The flow of multiple fractions of the contrast medium through the fallopian tubes has been found to correlate well with normal and abnormal anatomy of the fallopian tubes, and a diagnosis of tubal patency with this technique has been found to be confirmed 100% of the time. The usefulness of this technique for evaluation of the uterine cavity per se has not been addressed.

Magnetic Resonance Imaging

The advent of MRI has improved diagnostic accuracy in the workup of women with a variety of causes of infertility. The role of MRI in evaluation of the endometrium, however, remains to be determined. On the surface, attention to detail in MRI technique can yield precise data regarding female pelvic anatomy generally and the uterus specifically. For gynecologic imaging, T2-weighted images are essential because internal organ anatomy and most pathologic states are demonstrated most effectively with long repetition time/echo time technique. The alternate T1-weighted scan may add diagnostic specificity once anatomy is determined and provide information regarding fatty or hemorrhagic lesions. The characteristic architecture of the body of the uterus, the cervix, and the vagina is defined clearly on T2-weighted scans (Fig. 29–10).[158] Within the corpus of the uterus, it is possible to identify the entire thickness of the endometrium (actually the combined thicknesses of opposing endometrial walls) as the relatively high signal central stripe. The surrounding low signal band is representative of the inner portion of the myometrium.[159] The junctional zone between the endometrium and the myometrium is seen as a low T1, T2, water content area.[160] The myometrium that surrounds the junctional zone can be quite variable in its signal intensity but is almost always intermediate in comparison with the endometrium and the junctional zone.

The relative size or thickness of the tissue layers within the uterus depends primarily on the hormonal status of the woman at the time the MRI is performed.[161–164] During the follicular phase of the ovarian cycle, the average dimension of the endometrial "stripe" is usually found to be about 5 mm, whereas during the luteal phase of the ovarian cycle, the secretory changes result in an endometrial "stripe" approximating 10 mm.[161] The junctional zone itself does not really undergo any significant changes in dimension throughout the cycle despite the relatively dramatic changes in circulating levels of hormones. Because normal anatomy is well depicted on MRI, developmental or congenital anomalies are relatively easy to identify.[165] Such anomalies as partial or complete uterine duplication, the presence of a rudimentary uterine horn, and müllerian agenesis are easy to define by MRI. Specific discussion of congenital uterine anomalies and their diagnosis and treatment is covered elsewhere in this book.

With the exception of situations in which uterine leiomyomata (Fig. 29–11), large endometrial tumors, adenomyomas, or hematometra exist, the usefulness of MRI for diagnosis of endometrial abnormalities that might affect fertility has not been tested. It is unclear whether MRI will add more information to that contributed by sonography.

INFLAMMATORY CONDITIONS

Inflammatory conditions of the endometrium may involve a variety of infective agents that can lead initially to acute

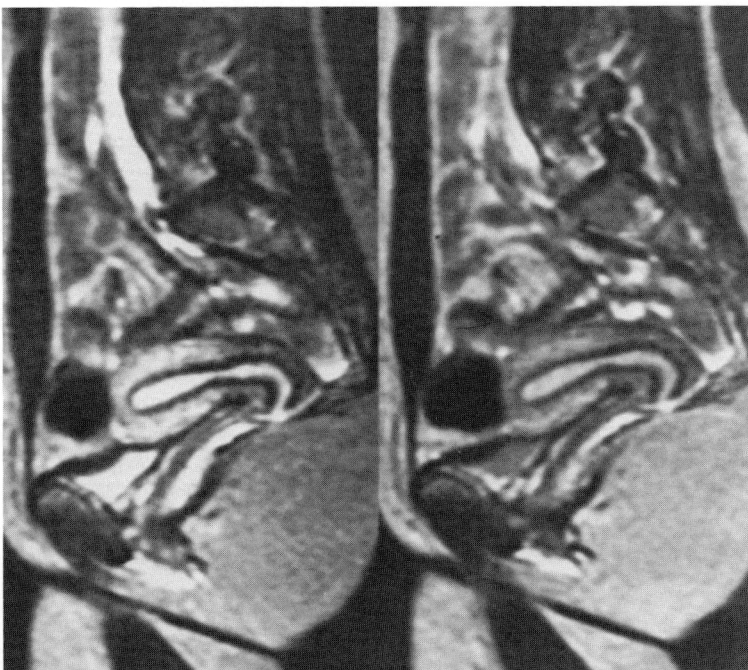

FIGURE 29–10. T2-weighted image of the normal uterus.

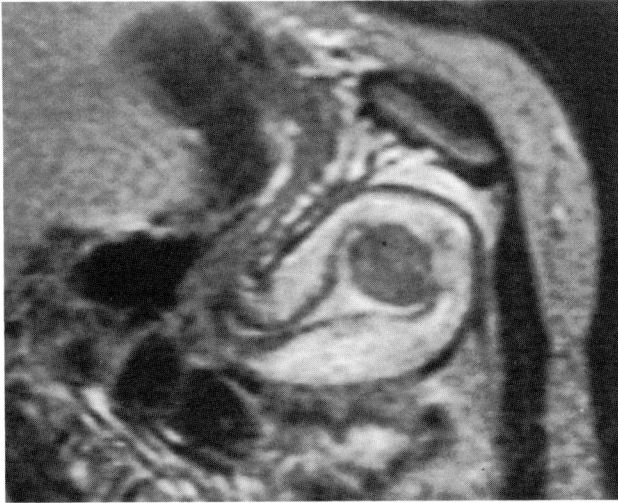

FIGURE 29–11. T2-weighted image of the uterus with submucosal myoma.

conditions but ultimately to chronic endometritis and pelvic inflammatory disease that result in temporary or permanent sterility. Among these endometrial infective agents are bacteria, mycoplasma, viruses, and various parasites.[166] Despite the fact that such infections do occur, the results of a number of studies are suggestive that the endometrial cavity and the endometrium itself normally are sterile.[167–169] Indeed, most authors agree that colonization of the endocervical canal by any number of these offending agents is the most likely source of endometrial infection.[167–170] A number of authors have attempted to study the incidence of colonization of the endometrium by bacteria as well as other organisms, and their different results may well be the result of differences in techniques used—most often the method of approach to the endometrial cavity. Ansbacher and colleagues[167] and Sparks and associates[169] used a transfundal approach to culture the endometrium at the time of removal of the uterus during the performance of abdominal hysterectomy. These authors declared the endometrial cavity to be sterile. Grossman and associates,[171] using a similar technique, found a variety of organisms in about a fourth of the hysterectomy specimens examined. Most importantly, various results have been described depending on the population of women examined. In one study of infertile women from Nigeria, nearly 40% of the subjects were found to have a variety of organisms within the endometrial cavity.[172]

Acute endometritis is associated usually with an ascending infection of the reproductive tract and is almost always accompanied by signs and symptoms of acute pelvic inflammatory disease. A number of factors may predispose to endometrial infection in addition to sexual activity. Dilatation of the cervix has been suggested to remove normal physiologic barriers to ascending infection.[173] Instrumental dilatation may carry into the uterus contaminants from the vagina, endocervix, or endocervical canal. Furthermore, the removal of mucus from the cervix during the process of dilatation may favor the establishment of endometrial infection. Additional predisposing conditions include retention of products of conception or blood within the uterus during the postpartum state that act as effective culture media for the establishment of

infection. Finally, trauma to the cervix that may be incurred during biopsy, cauterization, or conization may interfere with normal cervical secretions and thus lower natural resistance to invading organisms.

Under normal circumstances, cervical mucus contains IgA of cervical origin that acts as a natural barrier to ascending organisms.[172] In addition, the endometrium produces a number of substances, including IgA, that have local antibacterial activity.[168, 174] The protective functions of these substances can be disturbed by instrumentation of the endometrium during the insertion of an IUD, by conditions that depress immunity, by overwhelming infection, or simply by damage to the endometrium.[174]

Chronic endometritis is an inflammation of the endometrium that is characterized by the presence of plasma cells within the stroma of the endometrial tissue. Other inflammatory cells are usually present and include lymphocytes, histocytes, giant cells, and fibroblasts. Although acute endometritis may cause severe symptoms, chronic endometritis may be associated with infertility and pregnancy wastage. The mechanisms by which reproductive failure occurs with endometrial infection remain open to speculation, but the general consensus is that the inflammatory process itself may interfere with blastocyst implantation and subsequent growth. The condition of chronic endometritis frequently is associated with no signs other than infertility. For this reason, the clinician must be suspicious if no cause for infertility can be identified. Under most circumstances, culture of the endometrium that is removed by biopsy as well as histologic evaluation of the biopsy specimen provides confirmation of the diagnosis and identifies the offending organism. The best time to undertake these studies is the follicular phase of the ovarian cycle.

A variety of infectious agents have been implicated in the pathogenesis of chronic endometritis. Tuberculous endometritis is detected rarely in the United States but may be found in up to 10% to 15% of infertile women in developing countries. Unfortunately, genital tuberculosis is associated with a dismal outcome regarding future fertility, and therapy is aimed primarily at eradication of the disease rather than at restoration of childbearing potential. The diagnosis of tuberculous endometritis may be made based on histologic examination of an endometrial specimen and the finding of granulomatous changes as well as the finding of typical acid-fast bacilli on culture and staining.

Perhaps the most subtle cause of endometritis is infection with *Chlamydia trachomatis*. Although infertility of tubal origin is a well-recognized consequence of acute pelvic inflammatory disease, most women with tubal disease do not have evidence of acute salpingitis.[176–178] This and the finding of a high prevalence of antibodies to *C. trachomatis* in women with infertility has led to the conclusion that tubal infection with this organism is a likely cause of tubal dysfunction, infertility, and ectopic pregnancy.[179–181] Despite treatment with an appropriate antibiotic, usually tetracycline, a number of patients demonstrate residual or recurrent disease. It is now recognized that up to 20% of women at risk for chlamydial infection can be demonstrated to have *C. trachomatis* colonizing the endometrium, despite no clinical evidence of endometritis.[182, 183] At the present time, no clear evidence is available to implicate endometrial infection with *C. trachomatis* as the primary cause of infertility in these women.

Instead, it is more likely that the presence of *C. trachomatis* within the endometrial cavity should be taken as evidence of the likelihood of tubal infection also and that the latter is the cause of reproductive failure.

SUMMARY

As stated at the beginning of this discussion, the endometrium plays a significant role in the physiology of reproduction. The events that lead to ovulation occur simultaneously with the changes in the endometrium in preparation for the arrival of the conceptus. Although the endometrial canal serves as a conduit for the transport of sperm to the fallopian tube, little is known regarding the impact of endometrial morphology and biochemistry on this activity. With arrival of the conceptus within the endometrial canal, the endometrium begins to play a significant role in the events surrounding embryo nourishment, implantation, placentation, and subsequent growth of the fetus. A great deal remains to be elucidated regarding each of these functions of the endometrium. Today science is only beginning to scratch the surface of what we need to know about the endometrium to evaluate and treat the infertile woman. Even though our understanding has advanced tremendously in the past few years, we still have a long way to go.

REFERENCES

1. Koff AK. Development of the vagina in the human fetus. Carnegie Contrib Embryo 1933; 24:59–90.
2. Felix W. The development of the urogenital organs. In: Manual of Human Embryology. Philadelphia: JB Lippincott, 1912:916.
3. Baumgartner EA, Nelson MT, Dock W. Development of the uterine glands in man. Am J Anat 1920; 27:203–219.
4. Arey LB. Developmental Anatomy: A Textbook and Laboratory Manual of Embryology. Philadelphia: WB Saunders, 1940:239–278.
5. Pritchard JA, MacDonald A, Gant NF. Williams Obstetrics. 17th edition. Norwalk, CT: Appleton-Century-Crofts, 1985; 65–77.
6. Bernirschke K. The endometrium. In: Yen SSC, Jaffe RB, editors. Reproductive Endocrinology: Physiology, Pathophysiology and Clinical Management. Philadelphia: WB Saunders, 1978:241–260.
7. Noyes RW, Hertig AT, Rock J. Dating the endometrium. Fertil Steril 1950; 1:3–25.
8. Jones GES. Some newer aspects of the management of infertility. JAMA 1949; 141:1123–1129.
9. Abraham GE, Maroulis GB, Marshall JR. Evaluation of corpus luteum function using measurement of plasma progesterone. Obstet Gynecol 1977; 44:522–525.
10. Cumming DC, Honore LH, Scott JZ, Williams KP. The late luteal phase: comparison of simultaneous endometrial biopsy and serum progesterone levels. Fertil Steril 1985; 43:715–719.
11. Chryssikopoulos A, Gregoriou O, Vitoratos N, Liapis A. The diagnosis of luteal phase defect using different diagnostic criteria. Gynecol Endocrinol 1990; 4:193–204.
12. McRae MA, Blasco L, Lyttle CR. Serum hormones and their receptors in women with normal and inadequate corpus luteum function. Fertil Steril 1984; 42:58–63.
13. Jacobs MH, Balasch J, Gonzalez-Merlo JM, et al. Endometrial cytosolic and nuclear progesterone receptors in the luteal phase defect. J Clin Endocrinol Metab 1987; 64:472–475.
14. Levy C, Robel P, Gautay JP, et al. Estradiol and progesterone receptors in human endometrium: normal and abnormal menstrual cycles and early pregnancy. Am J Obstet Gynecol 1980; 136:646–651.
15. Wentz AC. Endometrial biopsy in the evaluation of infertility. Fertil Steril 1980; 33:121–124.
16. Rosenfeld DL, Chudow S, Bronson RA. Diagnosis of luteal phase inadequacy. Obstet Gynecol 1980; 56:193–196.
17. Balasch J, Vanrell JA, Creus M, et al. The endometrial biopsy for diagnosis of luteal phase deficiency. Fertil Steril 1985; 44:699–701.
18. Davidson BJ, Thrasher TV, Seraj IM. An analysis of endometrial biopsies performed for infertility. Fertil Steril 1987; 48:770–774.
19. Annos T, Thomson IE, Taymor ML. Luteal phase deficiency and infertility: difficulty encountered in diagnosis and treatment. Obstet Gynecol 1980; 55:705–710.
20. Jones GES. Luteal phase defects. In: Behrman J, Kistner R, editors. Progress in Infertility. Boston: Little, Brown, 1975:299–324.
21. Smith RNJ. Use of Gynocheck endometrial tissue sampler in infertility. Br J Obstet Gynaecol 1990; 97:454–455.
22. Meekins JW, Haddad NG: Use of the Gynocheck endometrial tissue sampler in infertility. Br J Obstet Gynaecol 1991; 98:115.
23. Honore LH, Cumming DC, Fahmy N. Significant difference in the frequency of out-of-phase endometrial biopsies depending on the use of the novak curette or the flexible polypropylene endometrial biopsy cannula ("Pipelle"). Gynecol Obstet Invest 1988; 26:338–340.
24. Henig I, Chan P, Tredway DR. Evaluation of the pipelle curette for endometrial biopsy. J Reprod Med 1989; 34:786–789.
25. McGuire WL, Dressler LG, Sledge GW, et al. An estrogen-regulated protein in normal and malignant endometrium. J Steroid Biochem 1986; 24:155–159.
26. Bell SC. Secretory endometrial/decidual proteins and their function in early pregnancy. J Reprod Fertil 1988; 36(suppl):109–125.
27. Ciocca DR, Asch R, Adams DJ, McGuire WL. Evidence for modulation of a 24K protein in human endometrium during the menstrual cycle. J Clin Endocrinol Metab 1983; 57:496–499.
28. Julkunen M, Seppala M, Janne OA. Complete amino acid sequence of human placental protein 14: a progesterone-regulated uterine protein homologous to β-lactoglobulins. Proc Natl Acad Sci 1988; 85:8845–8849.
29. Waites GT, Wood PL, Walker RA, Bell SC. Immunohistological localization of human endometrial secretory protein, pregnancy-associated endometrial alpha$_2$-globulin (alpha$_2$-PEG), during the menstrual cycle. J Reprod Fertil 1988; 82:665–672.
30. Manners CV. Endometrial assessment in a group of infertile women on stimulated cycles for IVF: immunohistochemical findings. Hum Reprod 1990; 5:128–132.
31. Birkinfeld A, Beier HM, Schenker JG. Review: the effect of clomiphene citrate on early embryonic development, endometrium and implantation. Hum Reprod 1986; 1:387–395.
32. Dallenbach-Hellweg G. The endometrium in natural and artificial luteal cycles. Hum Reprod 1988; 3:165–168.
33. Aplin JD, Hoadley ME, Seif MW. Hormonally regulated secretion of keratin sulphate by endometrial epithelium. Biochem Soc Trans 1989; 17:136–137.
34. Hoadley ME, Alpin JD, Seif MW. Menstrual cycle-dependent expression of keratin sulphate in human endometrium. Biochem J 1990; 266:757–763.
35. Seif M, Aplin JD, Buckley CH. Luteal phase defect: the possibility of immunohistochemical changes. Fertil Steril 1986; 51:273–279.
36. Graham RA, Seif MW, Alpin JD, et al. An endometrial factor in unexplained infertility Br Med J 1990;300:1428–1431.
37. Smith RA, Seif MW, Rogers AW, et al. The endometrial cycle: the expression of a secretory component correlated with luteinizing hormone peak. Hum Reprod 1989; 4:236–242.
38. Rogers PA, Milne BJ, Trounson AO. A model to show human uterine receptivity and embryo viability following ovarian stimulation for in-vitro fertilization. J In Vitro Fertil Embryo Transfer 1986; 3:93–98.
39. Macnamee MC, Edwards RG, Howles CM. The influence of stimulation regimens and luteal phase support on the outcome of IVF. Hum Reprod 1988; 3:43–52.
40. Beier HM. Die hormonelle Steuerung der Uterussekretion und fruhen Embryonalentwicklung des Kaninchens. Habilitationsschrift, Medizinische Fakultat der Christian-Albrechts-Universitat Kiel 1973:1–216.
41. Beier HM. Oviductal and uterine fluids. J Reprod Fertil 1974; 37:221–237.
42. Beier HM. Physiology of uteroglobin. In: Spilman CH, Wilks JW, editors. Novel Aspects of Reproductive Physiology. Vol 8. New York: SP Medical and Scientific Books, 1978:219–248.
43. Beier HM. Uteroglobin and other endometrial proteins: biochemistry and biological significance in beginning pregnancy. In: Beier HM, Karlson P, editors. Proteins and Steroids in Early Pregnancy. New York: Springer Verlag, 1982:38–71.
44. Beier HM, Mootz U. Significance of maternal uterine proteins in the establishment of pregnancy. In: Whelan J, editor. Maternal Recognition of Pregnancy. Ciba Foundation Series 64, Excerpta Medica, 1979:111–140.

45. Beier HM, Karlson P. Proteins and Steroids in Early Pregnancy. New York: Springer Verlag, 1982:346.

46. Beier HM, Mootz U, Hegele-Hartung C. Studies on the establishment of mammalian pregnancy: synchronization of the maternal and the embryonic systems. In: Holstein AF, Voigt KD, Grablin D, editors. Reproductive Biology and Medicine. Colloquium of the DFG held at Steinhorst Castle. Berlin: Diesbach Verlag, 1989:210–223.

47. Bohn H, Kraus W. Isolierung und charakterisierung eines neuen plazentaspezifischen proteins (PP12). Arch Gynecol 1980; 229:279–281.

48. Joshi SG, Ebert KM, Schwartz DP. Detection and synthesis of a progesterone-dependent protein in the human endometrium. J Steroid Biochem 1980; 19:751–757.

49. Sutcliffe RG, Joshi SG, Paterson WF, Bank JF. Serological identity between human alpha uterine protein and human progestogen-dependent endometrial protein. J Reprod Fertil 1982; 65:207–209.

50. Rutanen E-M, Bohn H, Seppala M. Radioimmunoassay of placental protein 12: levels in amniotic fluid, cord blood and serum of healthy adults, pregnant women and patients with trophoblastic disease. Am J Obstet Gynecol 1982; 144:460–463.

51. Bell SC, Hales MW, Patel S, et al. Protein synthesis and secretion by the human endometrium and decidua during early pregnancy. Br J Obstet Gynaecol 1985; 92:793–803.

52. Bell SC. Secretory endometrial and decidual proteins: studies and clinical significance of a maternally derived group of pregnancy-associated serum proteins. Hum Reprod 1986; 1:129–143.

53. Julkunen M. Human decidua synthesizes placental protein 14 (PP14) in vitro. Acta Endocrinol 1986; 112:271–277.

54. Koistinen R, Kalkinen N, Huhtala M-L, et al. Placental protein 12 is a decidual protein that binds somatomedin and has an identical N-terminal amino acid sequence with somatomedin-binding protein from human amniotic fluid. Endocrinology 1986; 118:1375–1378.

55. Beier HM. Hormone and hormonantagonisten in der implantationforschung. In: Schirren C, editor. Endokrinologie und Immunologie der Implantation bie Tier und Mensch. Fortschr Fertilitatsforsch Bd 13. Berlin: Grosse Verlag, 1986:2–15.

56. Beier HM, Elger W, Hegel-Hartung C. Effects of antiprogestins on the endometrium during the luteal phase after postovulatory treatment. In: Naftolin F, DeCherney A, editors. The Control of Follicle Development, Ovulation and Luteal Function: Lessons from In Vitro Fertilization. New York: Raven Press, 1987:331–343.

57. Hegele-Hartung C, Beier HM. Distribution of uteroglobin in the rabbit endometrium after treatment with an anti-progestin (ZK 98.734): an immunocytochemical study. Hum Reprod 1986; 1:497–505.

58. Beier-Hellwig K, Sterzik K, Bonn B, Beier HM. Contribution to the physiology and pathology of endometrial receptivity: the determination of protein patterns in human uterine secretions. Hum Reprod 1989; 4:115–120.

59. Bayard F, Damilano S, Robel P, Beaulieu EE. Cytoplasmic and nuclear estradiol and progesterone receptors in human endometrium. J Clin Endocrinol Metab 1978; 46:635–648.

60. Levy C, Eychenne B, Robel P. Assay of nuclear estradiol receptor by exchange on a glass fiber filter. Biochem Biophys Acta 1980; 630:301–305.

61. Levy C, Robel P, Gautay JP, et al. Estradiol and progesterone receptors in human endometrium: normal and abnormal menstrual cycles and early pregnancy. Am J Obstet Gynecol 1980; 136:646–651.

62. Beaulieu EE, Atger M, Best-Belpomme M, et al. Steroid hormone receptors. Vit Horm 1975; 33:649–736.

63. Kreitman-Gimbl B, Bayard B, Nixon WE, Hodgen GD. Patterns of estrogen and progesterone receptors in monkey endometrium during the normal menstrual cycle. Steroids 1980; 35:471–479.

64. Kreitzmann-Gimbal B, Goodman AL, Bayard F, Hodgen GD. Characterization of estrogen and progesterone receptors in monkey endometrium: methodology and effects of estradiol and/or progesterone on endometrium in castrated monkeys. Steroid 1979; 34:749–770.

65. Tsibris JCM, Cazenave CR, Cantor B, et al. Distribution of cytoplasmic estrogen and progesterone receptors in human endometrium. Am J Obstet Gynecol 1978; 132:449–454.

66. Haukkamaa M, Luukkainen TY. The cytoplasmic receptor of human endometrium during the menstrual cycle. J Steroid Biochem 1974; 5:447–452.

67. Saracoglu OF, Aksel S, Yeoman RR, Wiebe RH. Endometrial estradiol and progesterone receptors in patients with luteal phase defects and endometriosis. Fertil Steril 1985; 43:851–855.

68. Laatikainen T, Anderson B, Karkkainen J, Wahlstrom T. Progestin receptor levels in endometrium with delayed or incomplete secretory changes. Obstet Gynecol 1983; 65:592–595.

69. Keller DW, Wiest WG, Askin FB, et al. Pseudocorpus luteum insufficiency: a local defect of progesterone action on endometrial stroma. J Clin Endocrinol Metab 1979; 48:127–132.

70. Milgrom E, Thi L, Baulieu EE. Mechanisms regulating the concentration and the conformation of progesterone receptor(s) in the uterus. J Biol Chem 1973; 248:6366–6374.

71. Gravanis A, Zorn J-R, Tanguy G, et al. The "dysharmonic luteal phase" syndrome: endometrial progesterone receptor and estradiol dehydrogenase. Fertil Steril 1984; 42:730–736.

72. Jacobs MH, Balasch J, Gonzales-Merlo JM, et al. Endometrial cytosolic and nuclear progesterone receptors in the luteal phase defect. J Clin Endocrinol Metab 1987; 64:472–475.

73. Abbassi R, Kreitzmann-Gimbal B, Rifka SM, Falk RJ. Total estradiol and progesterone receptor concentration in patients with luteal phase defects [abstr]. American College of Obstetricians and Gynecologists Annual Meeting, 1986:14.

74. DiZerega GS, Hodgen GD. Luteal phase dysfunction in infertility: a sequel to aberrant folliculogenesis. Fertil Steril 1981; 35:489–499.

75. Nakajima ST, Brumstead JR, Riddick DH, Gibson M. Absence of progestational activity of oral spironolactone. Fertil Steril 1989; 52:155–158.

76. Ying YK, Maier DB, Randolph JF, et al. Stimulation of uterine prolactin secretion by human chorionic gonadotropin and progesterone in the cynomolgus monkey. Fertil Steril 1988; 50:976–979.

77. Soloff MS, Rees HD, Sar M, Stump WE. Autoradiographic localization of radioactivity from [^{3}H]-oxytocin in the rat mammary gland and oviducts. Endocrinology 1975; 96:1475–1477.

78. Soloff MS, Schwartz TL, Steinberg AH. Oxytocin receptors in human uterus. J Clin Endocrinol Metab 1974; 38:1952–1056.

79. Flint APF, Sheldrick EL. Ovarian secretion of oxytocin in sheep. J Physiol 1982; 330:61–62.

80. Roberts JS, McCracken JA, Gavagan JE, Soloff MS. Oxytocin stimulated release of prostaglandin F_2 from ovine endometrium in vitro. Endocrinology 1976; 99:1107–1114.

81. Sharma SC, Fitzpatrick RJ. Effect of oestradiol 17 and oxytocin treatment on PGF_2 release in the anoestrous ewe. Prostaglandins 1974; 6:97–105.

82. Fairclough RJ, Moore LG, McGowan LT, et al. Temporal relationship between plasma concentrations of 13, 14-dihydro-15-keto-prostaglandin F and neurophysin I/II around luteolysis in sheep. Prostaglandins 1980; 20:199–208.

83. Baker PN, Peat ML, Symonds EM, Maynard PV. Endometrial oxytocin binding sites in normal women and subfertile patients. Postgrad Med J 1990; 66:195–199.

84. Sheldrick EL, Flint APF. Endocrine control of uterine oxytocin receptors in the ewe. J Endocrinol 1985; 106:249–258.

85. Dmowski WP, Cohen HR, Wilheilm JL. Endometriosis and ovulatory failure: does it occur? In: Greenblatt RB, editor. Recent Advances in Endometriosis. Princeton, NJ: Excerpta Medica, 1976:129.

86. Brosens IA, Koninkx PR, Corveleyn PA. A study of plasma progesterone, oestradiol-17-beta, prolactin and of the luteal appearance of the ovaries in patients with endometriosis and infertility. Br J Obstet Gynaecol 1978; 85:246–250.

87. Cheeseman KL, Cheeseman SD, Chatterton RT, Cohen MR. Alterations in progesterone metabolism and luteal function in infertile women with endometriosis. Fertil Steril 1983; 40:590–595.

88. Tummon IS, Maclin VM, Radwanska E, et al. Occult ovulatory dysfunction in women with minimal endometriosis or unexplained infertility. Fertil Steril 1988; 50:716–720.

89. Doody MC, Gibbons WE, Buttram VC Jr. Linear regression analysis of ultrasound follicular growth series: evidence for an abnormality of follicular growth in endometriosis. Fertil Steril 1988; 49:47–51.

90. Yovich JL, Matson PL, Richardson PA, Hilliard C. Hormonal profile and embryo quality in women with severe endometriosis treated by in vitro fertilization and embryo transfer. Fertil Steril 1988; 50:308–313.

91. Fedele L, Marchini M, Bianchi S, et al. Structural and ultrastructural defects in preovulatory endometrium of normo-ovulating infertile women with minimal and mild endometriosis. Fertil Steril 1990; 53:989–993.

92. Weed JC, Arquenburg PC. Endometriosis: can it produce an autoimmune response resulting in infertility? Clin Obstet Gynecol 1980; 23:885–893.

93. Saiffudin A, Buckley CH, Fox H. Immunoglobulin content of the endometrium in patients with endometriosis. Int J Gynaecol Pathol 1983; 2:255–263.

94. Bartosik D, Damjanov I, Viscarello RR, Riley JA. Immunoproteins in

the endometrium: clinical correlates of the presence of complements fractions C3 and C4. Am J Obstet Gynecol 1987; 156:11–15.

95. Mathur S, Perss MR, Williamson HO, et al. Autoimmunity to endometrium and ovary in endometriosis. Clin Exp Immunol 1982; 50:259–266.

96. Wild RA, Shivers CA. Antiendometrial antibodies in patients with endometriosis. Am J Reprod Immunol Microbiol 1985; 8:84–86.

97. Canale VC, Steinherz P, New M, Erlandoson M. Endocrine function in thalassaemia major. Ann NY Acad Sci 1974; 232:333–345.

98. Landau H, Spitz IM, Cividalli G, Rachmilewiz EA. Gonadotropin, thyrotropin and prolactin reserve in beta-thalassaemia. Clin Endocrinol (Oxf) 1978; 9:163–173.

99. Modell B. Total management of thalassaemia major. Arch Dis Child 1977; 52:489–500.

100. Walker EH, Wetton MJ, Beaven GH. Successful pregnancy in a patient with thalassaemia major. J Obstet Gynaecol Br Commonw 1969; 76:549–553.

101. Perkins RP. Inherited disorders of hemoglobin synthesis and pregnancy. Am J Obstet Gynecol 1971; 118:120–151.

102. Necheles T. Obstetric complications associated with hemoglobinopathies. Clin Haematol 1973; 2:497–514.

103. Thomas RM, Skalicka AE. Successful pregnancy in transfusion dependent thalassaemia. Arch Dis Child 1980; 55:572–574.

104. Meadows KA. A successful pregnancy outcome in transfusion dependent thalassaemia major. Aust NZ J Obstet Gynaecol 1984; 24:43–44.

105. Birkenfeld A, Goldfarb AW, Rachmilewitz EA, et al. Endometrial glandular haemosiderosis in homozygous beta-thalassaemia. Eur J Obstet Gynaecol Reprod Biol 1989; 31:173–178.

106. Cooper RA, Jabamoni R, Pieters CT. Fertility rates after hysterosalpingogram with Sinografine. Am J Radiol 1983; 141:105–106.

107. DeCherney AH, Kort H, Barney JB, DeVore GR. Increased pregnancy rate with oil soluble hysterosalpingography dye. Fertil Steril 1980; 33:407–410.

108. Mackey RA, Glass RH, Olson LE, Vaidye R. Pregnancy following hysterosalpingography with oil and water soluble dye. Fertil Steril 1971; 22:504–507.

109. Schutte HE. Comparative study: Endografin (Diatrizoate), Vasurix-polyvidone (acetrizoate), Dimer X (Iocarnate) and Hexabrix (Ioxaglate) in hysterosalpingography. Diag Imaging 1982; 51:227–283.

110. Schwabe MG, Shapiro SS, Haning RV. Hysterosalpingogram with oil contrast medium enhances fertility in patients with infertility of unknown etiology. Fertil Steril 1983; 40:604–606.

111. Soules MR, Spadoni LR. Oil versus aqueous media for hysterosalpingography, a continuing debate based on many opinions and a few facts. Fertil Steril 1982; 38:1–11.

112. Alper MM, Garner PR, Spence JEH, Quarrington AM. Pregnancy rates after hysterosalpingography with oil- and water-soluble contrast media. Obstet Gynecol 1986; 66:6–9.

113. deBoer AD, Vemer HM, Willemsen WNP, Sanders FBM. Oil or aqueous contrast media for hysterosalpingography: a prospective, randomized, clinical study. Eur J Obstet Gynaecol Reprod Biol 1988; 28:65–68.

114. Eisenberg AD, Winfield AC, Page DL, et al. Peritoneal reaction resulting from iodinated contrast material: a comparative study. Radiology 1989; 172:149–151.

115. Winfield AC, Wentz AC. Diagnostic Imaging in Infertility. Baltimore: Williams & Wilkins, 1987.

116. Leeton J, Buttery B. The "forgotten" intrauterine device: an unusual cause of infertility. Aust NZ J Obstet Gynaecol 1988; 28:150–151.

117. Ron-El R, Weintraub Z, Langer R, et al. The importance of ultrasonography in infertile women with "forgotten" intrauterine devices. Am J Obstet Gynecol 1989; 161:211–212.

118. Rowe T, McComb P. Unknown intrauterine devices and infertility. Fertil Steril 1987; 47:1038–1039.

119. Winfield AC, Fleischer AC, Moore DE. Diagnostic imaging of fertility disorders. In: Keats TE, Bragg DG, Evens RG, et al, editors. Current Problems in Diagnostic Radiology. Chicago: Yearbook Medical Publishers, 1990:5–38.

120. Adel SK, Ghoneim MA, Sobrero AJ. Hysterography study of long-term effects of intrauterine contraceptive devices. Fertil Steril 1971; 22:651–662.

121. Viglione CA, Cuttino JT Jr, Clark RL. Molding of the uterus following intrauterine contraceptive device removal: documentation by hysterosalpingography. Urol Radiol 1987; 9:188–190.

122. Fritsch H. Ein Fall von volligen Schwund de Gebarmutterhohle nach Auskratzung. Zentralbl Gynaekol 1984; 18:1337.

123. Bass B. Ueber die Verwachsungen in der Cervix uteri nach Curettagen. Zentralbl Gynakol 1927; 51:223.

124. Stamer S. Partial and total atresia of the uterus after excochleation. Acta Obstet Gynaecol Scand 1946; 26:263.

125. Topkins PT. Traumatic intrauterine synechiae: the Asherman syndrome. Am J Obstet Gynecol 1962; 83:1599–1608.

126. Asherman JG. Amenorrhea traumatica (atretica) J Obstet Gynaecol Br Emp 1948; 55:23–30.

127. Netter A, Musset R, Lambert R, Salomon Y. Traumatic uterine synechiae. Am J Obstet Gynecol 1956; 71:368–375.

128. Solal R, Bouchara J, Legros M. Les synechies uterines tuberculeuses. Presse Med 1960; 68:2126–2129.

129. Rabau E, David A. Intrauterine adhesions: etiology, prevention and treatment. Obstet Gynecol 1963; 22:626.

130. Schenker JG, Margalioth EJ. Intrauterine adhesions: an updated appraisal. Fertil Steril 1982; 37:593–610.

131. Polishuk Z, Graff G, Halevy S. The outcome of pregnancies after induced abortion. Harefuah 1966; 69:229–234.

132. Stillman RJ, Asarkof N. Association between mullerian duct malformations and Asherman's syndrome in infertile women. Obstet Gynecol 1985; 65:673–677.

133. Lancet M, Kessler I. A review of Asherman's syndrome, and results of modern treatment. Int J Fertil 1988; 33:14–24.

134. Klein SM, Garcia C-R. Asherman's syndrome: a critique and current view. Fertil Steril 1973; 24:722–735.

135. Polishuk Z, Siew FP, Gordon R, Lebenshart P. Vascular changes in traumatic amenorrhea and hypomenorrhea. Int J Fertil 1977; 22:189–192.

136. Foix RQ, Bruno RQ, Davison T, Lema B. The pathology of postcurettage intrauterine adhesions. Am J Obstet Gynecol 1966; 96:1027.

137. Toaff R, Ballas S. Traumatic hypomenorrhea-amenorrhea (Asherman's syndrome). Fertil Steril 1978; 30:379–387.

138. Toaff R. Quelques observations sur les adherences uterines posttraumatiques. Rev Franc Gynecol Obstet 1966; 61:550.

139. Sugimoto O. Diagnostic and therapeutic hysteroscopy for traumatic intrauterine adhesions. Am J Obstet Gynecol 1978; 131:539–547.

140. Lancet M, Mass N. Concomitant hysteroscopy and hysterography in Asherman's syndrome. Int J Fertil 1981; 26:267–272.

141. Truc JB, Paniel BJ, Chantraine J. Traitment des synechies. J Obstet Gynecol Biol Reprod 1986; 15:470–475.

142. Glezerman M, Levin S, Bernstein D. Asherman's syndrome—a self limiting disease? Int J Obstet Gynecol 1978; 15:522.

143. Sanfilippo JS, Fitzgerald MR, Badawy SA, et al. Asherman's syndrome: a comparison of therapeutic methods. J Reprod Med 1982; 27:328–330.

144. March CM, Israel R, March AD. Hysteroscopic management of intrauterine adhesions. Am J Obstet Gynecol 1978; 130:653–657.

145. Newton JR, MacKenzie WE, Emens MJ, Jordan JA. Division of uterine adhesions (Asherman's syndrome) with the nd-YAG laser. Br J Obstet Gynaecol 1989; 96:102–104.

146. Tadir Y, Raif J, Dagan J. Hysteroscope for CO_2 laser application. Laser Surg Med 1984;4:153–156.

147. Duffield SE, Picker RH. Ultrasonic evaluation of the uterus in the normal menstrual cycle. Med Ultra 1981; 5:70.

148. Fleischer AC, Kalemeris GC, Entman SS. Sonographic depictions of the endometrium during normal cycles. Ultrasound Med Biol 1986; 12:271–277.

149. Pupols AZ, Wilson SR. Ultrasonographic interpretation of physiological changes in the female pelvis. J Can Assoc Radiol 1984; 35:34–39.

150. Sakamoto C, Yoshimitsu K, Nakamura G, et al. Sonographic study of the endometrial response to ovarian hormones in patients receiving ovarian stimulation. Int J Gynaecol Obstet 1988; 27:407–414.

151. Smith B, Porter R, Ahuja K, Craft I. Ultrasonic assessment of endometrial changes in stimulated cycles in an in vitro fertilization and embryo transfer program. J In Vitro Fertil Embryo Transfer 1984; 1:233–238.

152. Drugan A, Blumenfeld Z, Erlik Y. The use of transvaginal sonography in infertility. In: Timor-Tritsch IE, Rottem S, editors. Transvaginal Sonography. New York: Elsevier, 1988:45.

153. Hall DA, Hann LE, Ferrucci JT, et al. Sonographic morphology of the normal menstrual cycle. Radiology 1979; 133:185–188.

154. Sakamoto C, Nakano H. The echogenic endometrium and alterations during the menstrual cycle. Int J Gynaecol Obstet 1982; 220:255–259.

155. Imoedemhe DAG, Shaw RW, Kirkland A, Chan R. Ultrasound measurement of endometrial thickness on different ovarian stimulation regimens during in vitro fertilization. Hum Reprod 1987; 2:545–547.

156. Itskovitz J, Boldes R, Levron J, Thaler I. Transvaginal ultrasonography in the diagnosis and treatment of infertility. J Clin Ultrasound 1990; 18:248–256.

157. Goswamy RK, Williams G, Steptoe PC. Decreased uterine perfusion—a cause of infertility. Hum Reprod 1988; 3:955–959.

158. Hricak H, Alpers C, Crooks LE, Sheldon PE. Magnetic resonance imaging of the female pelvis: initial experience. AJR Am J Roentgenol 1983; 141:1119–1128.

159. Lee JKT, Gersell DJ, Balfe DM, et al. The uterus: in vitro MR-anatomic correlation of normal and abnormal specimens. Radiology 1985; 157:175–179.

160. McCarthy S, Scott G, Majumdar S, et al. Uterine junctional zone: MR study of water content and relaxation properties. Radiology 1989; 171:241–243.

161. McCarthy S, Tauber C, Gore J. Female pelvic anatomy: MR assessment of variations during the menstrual cycle and with use of oral contraceptives. Radiology 1986; 160:119–123.

162. Zawin M, McCarthy S, Scoutt L, et al. Monitoring therapy with a gonadotropin releasing hormone analog: utility of MR imaging. Radiology 1990; 175:503–506.

163. Haynor DR, Mack LA, Soules MR, et al. Changing appearance of the normal uterus during the menstrual cycle: MR studies. Radiology 1986; 161:459–462.

164. Demas BE, Hricak J, Jaffe RB. Uterine MR imaging: the effects of hormonal stimulation. Radiology 1986; 159:123–126.

165. McCarthy S. Magnetic resonance imaging in the evaluation of infertile women. Magn Reson Q 1990; 6:239–249.

166. Hunt JE, Wallach EE. Uterine factors in infertility: an overview. Clin Obstet Gynecol 1974; 17:44–64.

167. Ansbacher R, Boyson WA, Morris JA. Sterility of the uterine cavity. Am J Obstet Gynecol 1967; 99:394–396.

168. Moyer DL, Mishell DR, Bell J. Reactions of human endometrial histology with the bacterial environment of the uterus following short-term insertion of IUD. Am J Obstet Gynecol 1970; 106:799–809.

169. Sparks RA, Purrier BGA, Watt PJ, Elstein M. The bacteriology of the cervix and the uterus. Br J Obstet Gynaecol 1977; 84:701–704.

170. Gorbach SL, Menda KB, Thadepalli H, Keith L. Anaerobic microflora of the cervix of healthy women. Am J Obstet Gynecol 1973; 117:1053–1055.

171. Grossman JH, Adams RL, Hierholzer WJ, Androile VT. Endometrial and vaginal cuff bacteria recovered at elective hysterectomy during a trial of antibiotic prophylaxis. Am J Obstet Gynecol 1978; 130:312–316.

172. Emembolu JO. Endometrial flora of infertile women in Zaria, Northern Nigeria. Int J Gynaecol Obstet 1989; 30:155–159.

173. Wallach EE. Uterine factors in infertility. Keio J Med 1987; 36:223–227.

174. Mishell DR, Bell JH, Good RG, Moyer DL. The intrauterine device. A bacteriologic study of the endometrial cavity. Am J Obstet Gynecol 1966; 96:119–126.

175. Mardh PA, Ripa T, Svensson L, Westrom L. Chlamydia trachomatis infection in patients with acute salpingitis. N Engl J Med 1977; 296:1377–1379.

176. Gump DW, Gibson M, Ashikaga T. Evidence of prior pelvic inflammatory disease and its relationship to Chlamydia trachomatis antibody and intrauterine contraceptive device use in infertile women. Am J Obstet Gynecol 1983; 146:153–159.

177. Jones RB, Ardery BR, Hui SL, Cleary RE. Correlation between serum antichlamydia antibodies and tubal factor as a cause of infertility. Fertil Steril 1982; 38:553–558.

178. Moore DE, Foy HM, Daling JR, et al. Increasing frequency of serum antibodies to Chlamydia trachomatis in infertility due to distal tubal disease. Lancet 1982; 2:574–577.

179. Hartford SL, Silva PD, diZerega GS, Yonekura ML. Serologic evidence of prior chlamydial infection in patients with tubal ectopic pregnancy and contralateral tubal disease. Fertil Steril 1987; 47:118–121.

180. Kane JL, Woodland RM, Forsey T, et al. Evidence of chlamydial infection in infertile women with and without fallopian tube obstruction. Fertil Steril 1984; 42:843–848.

181. Anestad G, Lunde O, Moen M, Dalaker K. Infertility and chlamydial infection. Fertil Steril 1987; 48:787–790.

182. Jones RB, Mammel JB, Shepard MK, Fisher RR. Recovery of Chlamydia trachomatis from endometrium of women at risk for chlamydial infection. Am J Obstet Gynecol 1986; 155:35–39.

183. Shepard MK, Jones RB. Recovery of Chlamydia trachomatis from endometrial and fallopian tube biopsies in women with infertility of tubal origin. Fertil Steril 1989; 52:232–238.

CHAPTER 30

The Fallopian Tube: Pathophysiology

PETER F. McCOMB and
BETTINA G. FLEIGE-ZAHRADKA

This chapter reviews the normal function of the oviduct and then, in the light of this, diseases of the oviduct. The fallopian tube is one part of the apparatus that preserves the basic aquatic nature of reproduction in higher forms of life. To put this another way, life began in the sea. With evolution to become higher mammals, we have wrapped the fertilization process within the oviduct, while maintaining the essential fluid basis. An awareness of this original function allows some insight as to why the oviduct is constructed the way it is and also as to how it functions.

NORMAL ANATOMY

The fallopian tube is a tubular structure of approximately 9 to 11 cm in length; there is wide interindividual variation. It is the site of ovum retrieval, ovum and sperm transport,

sperm capacitation, fertilization, and, later, embryo transport (Figs. 30–1 [see color section in the center of the book] and 30–2).[1] The tubal environment also provides vital nutrient support for the dividing embryo. These mechanisms occur in various anatomic sections of the normal tube.

Cyclic changes in anatomic (ciliation, epithelial height), endocrinologic, and mechanical patterns[2–5] have been postulated or proved.[6] Although studies have elucidated certain aspects of tubo-ovarian interaction, not all have been verified in the human.[6–9]

The oviduct is made up of the fimbria, the infundibulum, the ampulla, the isthmus, and the intramural (interstitial) tube.

The *fimbria*, the most distal portion of the oviduct, is relatively free and motile. The only attachment to the ovary is via the fimbria ovarica, one of about 25 fimbrial folds. Even this attachment is inconstant.

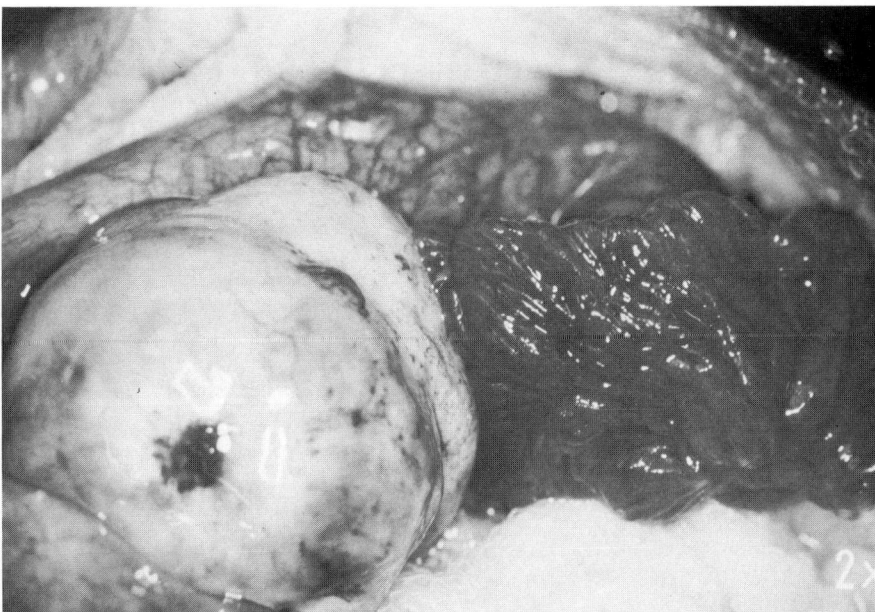

FIGURE 30–1. The fallopian tube.

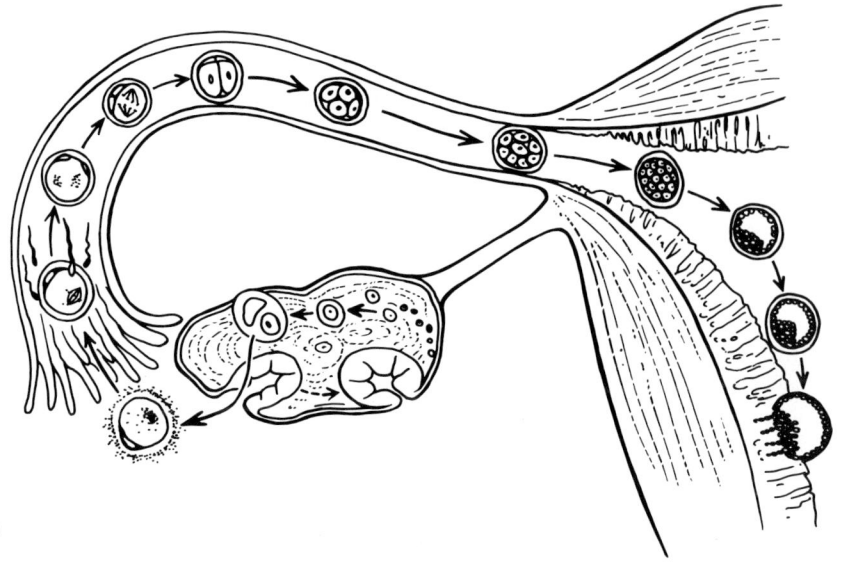

FIGURE 30–2. Schematic representation of the function of the fallopian tube.

The fimbriae attach to the *infundibulum,* a trumpet-shaped portion of the fallopian tube 1 cm long. Like the fimbriae it is thin walled and densely ciliated (60% to 80%)[3, 10] and has a complex pattern of mucosal folds. Ovum retrieval and initial transport are effected by the close spatial relationship of the fimbriae to the site of ovulation.[11]

The *ampulla* comprises approximately two thirds of the total tubal length. Its luminal diameter decreases from 1 cm at the ampulloinfundibular junction to 1 to 2 mm at the ampulloisthmic junction. The seromuscular layer is thin and comprises an incomplete internal longitudinal, a middle circular, and an external longitudinal layer. The mucosal folds within the ampulla are complex. The lumen is packed with these folds. Approximately 40% to 50% of ampullary cells are ciliated.[3] The inner longitudinal spiral myosalpingeal layer found in the ampulla is lost at the ampulloisthmic junction.

The *isthmus* represents approximately one third of tubal length (3 to 3.5 cm), and the lumen is considerably narrower than the ampulla (0.5 to 1 mm). The muscular layers are well developed. Isthmic ciliation is less profuse (25% to 30%)[3] compared with the ampulla. There are four primary mucosal folds (Fig. 30–3).

The *intramural* or *interstitial segment* of the tube is short (10 mm) and narrow with a straight, arched, or convoluted course through the endometrium.[12] It has been described as a uterotubal junction or erroneously as a sphincter, although no anatomic correlation to a sphincter has been documented.

At the site of junction of the endometrial funnel with the intramural portion of the tube, an abrupt change from endometrial to tubal mucosa occurs. Complete ciliation is not immediately evident in all cases.[12] A well-developed inner longitudinal muscle layer surrounded by a circular layer is present. The uterine cornu can be incised tangentially at the level of the junction of the intramural tube and endometrial cavity without loss of integrity of the uterus.[13]

The *vascular supply* to the oviduct is derived from the uterine and ovarian arteries. There is a capillary bed within the lateral mesosalpinx and oviduct where the two supplies meet, culminating in a rich vascularity.[7] This vascular bed

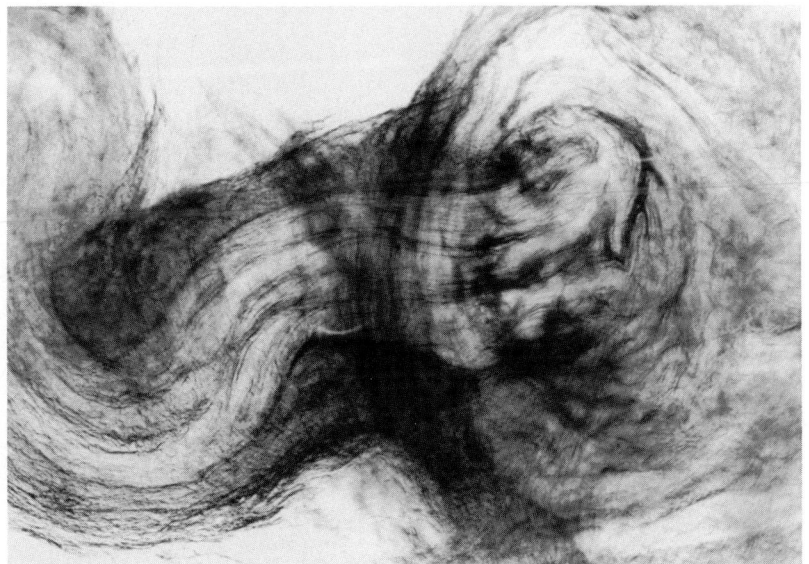

FIGURE 30–3. Uterotubal junction prepared by the Orsini tissue clearing technique.

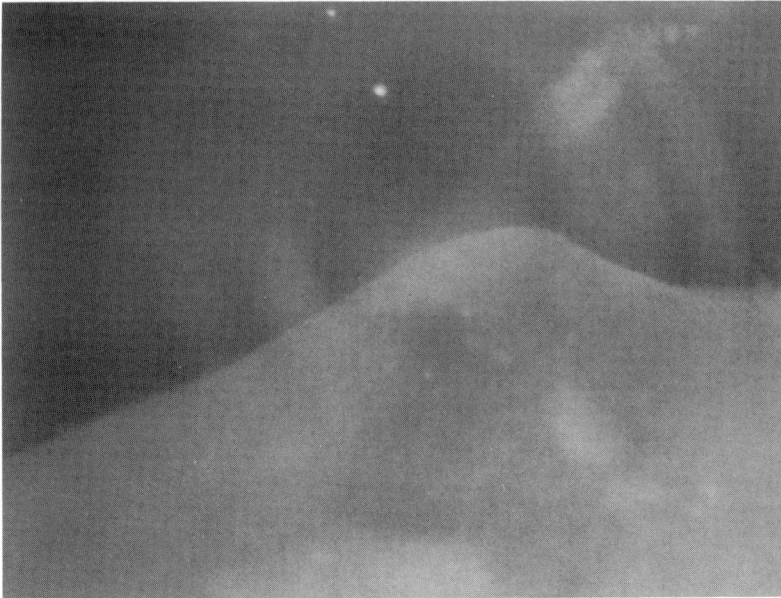

FIGURE 30–4. Magnified photography. The preovulatory follicle "in vivo." Time elapsed for Figures 30–4 to 30–7 is 15 minutes.

responds to vasoconstrictor solutions (often used, for example, for removal of an ectopic pregnancy).

The uterine artery ascends to supply the cornu and to then course laterally beneath the isthmus to dissipate in the lateral mesosalpinx. At tubal surgery the most prominent and easily injured vessels are those underlying the isthmus.

The function of the *autonomic nerve supply* to the oviduct is uncertain. It is notable that oviductal transplantation procedures with attendant denervation of the tube have yielded successful pregnancies.[14–16]

NORMAL PHYSIOLOGY

A "working model" of the fallopian tube may be described as follows. Much of the detail has been inferred from animal studies, especially the rabbit.

At about the time of ovulation (Figs. 30–4 to 30–6), the fimbria is close to the ipsilateral ovary, with some access to the opposite ovary. Bowel invests the adnexa so that there is only a potential space within the pelvis. Peritoneal fluid lubricates the single cell mesothelial layer of the ovary, serosal surfaces, and peritoneum. Motion is conferred to the pelvis by body movement, bowel peristalsis, and some contraction of the ovarian and tubal mesenteries. With ovulation the sticky cumulus oophorus unfolds from the follicular cavity (Fig. 30–7) and adheres to the follicular stigma assisted by blood clot formation and fibrin deposition. As the fimbria brushes the ovary (Figs. 30–8 and 30–9 [for Fig. 30–9, see color section in the center of the book]), the granulosa cells of the cumulus oophorus are exposed to the fluid currents generated by the rapidly beating cilia that surface the anemone-like folds of the fimbria (Figs. 30–10 to 30–14). These currents draw the cloud of granulosa cells toward the ostium

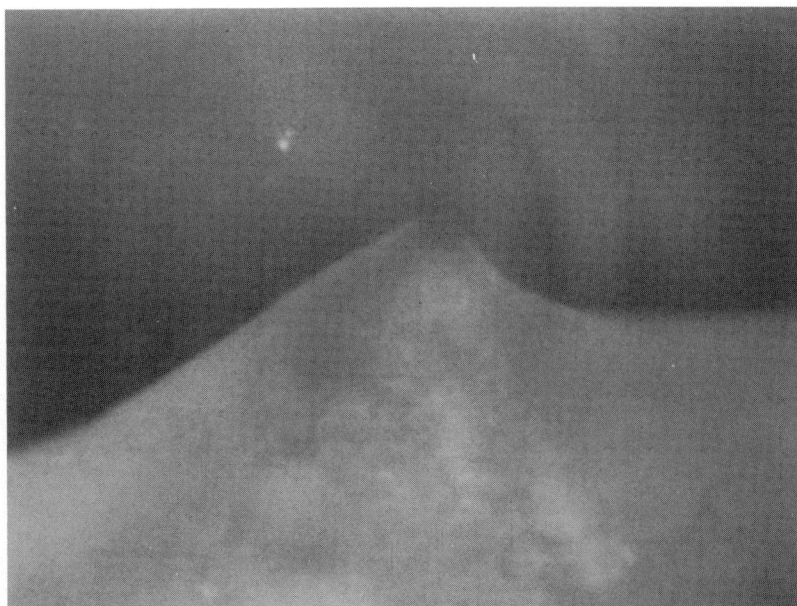

FIGURE 30–5. Magnified photography. The follicle has formed a stigma. This is the clear (but unruptured) apex of the follicle.

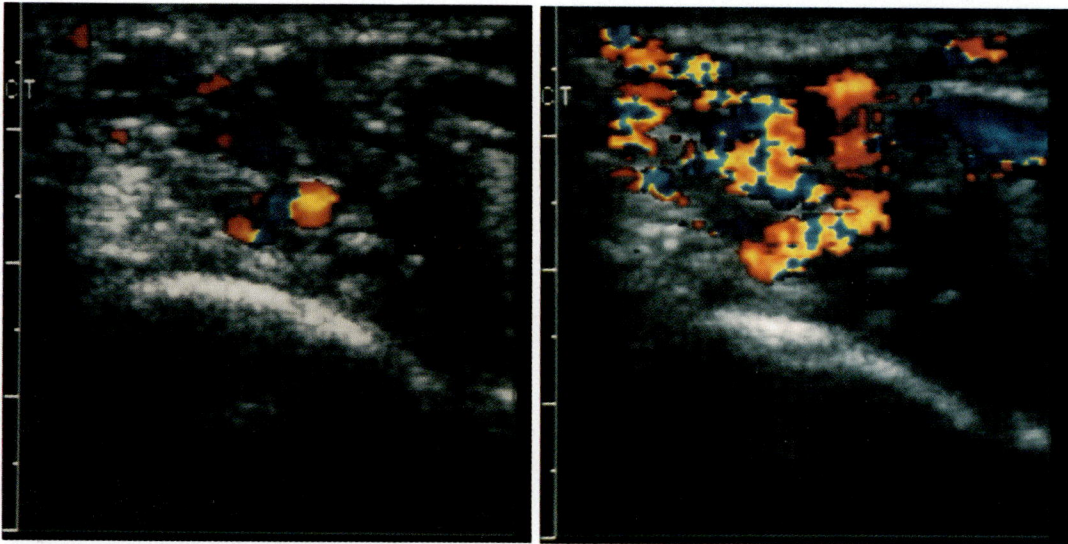

FIGURE 23–31. Varicocele. Color Doppler imaging with patient erect demonstrates changing appearances before (A) and following (B) Valsalva maneuver.

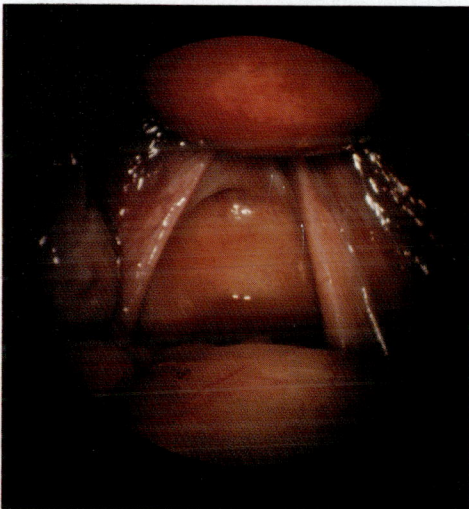

FIGURE 24–13. View of the normal cul-de-sac and uterosacral ligaments. (Courtesy of William R. Keye, Jr., M.D.)

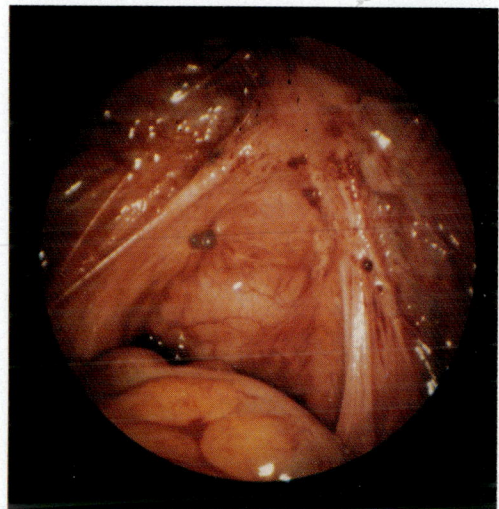

FIGURE 24–14. Laparoscopic view of the cul-de-sac in a woman with endometriosis. (Courtesy of William R. Keye, Jr., M.D.)

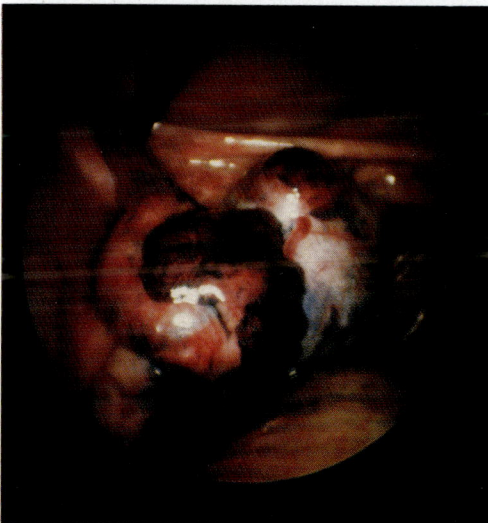

FIGURE 24–15. Normal adnexa. (Note the corpus luteum on the ovary and the spill of methylene blue from the fimbriated end of the fallopian tube.) (Courtesy of William R. Keye, Jr., M.D.)

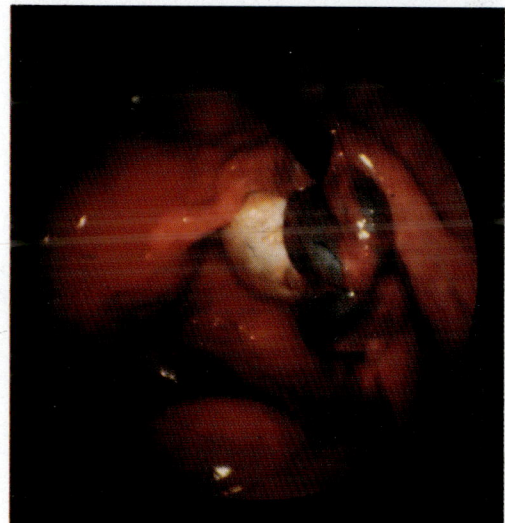

FIGURE 24–18. Laparoscopic view of an adnexa with a hydrosalpinx. (Courtesy of William R. Keye, Jr., M.D.)

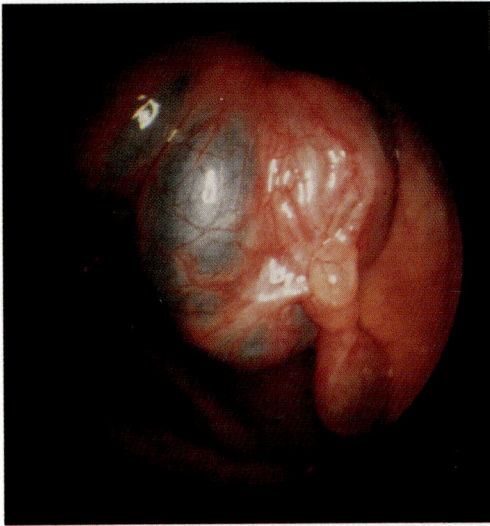

FIGURE 24–19. Close-up view of the distal end of a hydrosalpinx. (Courtesy of William R. Keye, Jr., M.D.)

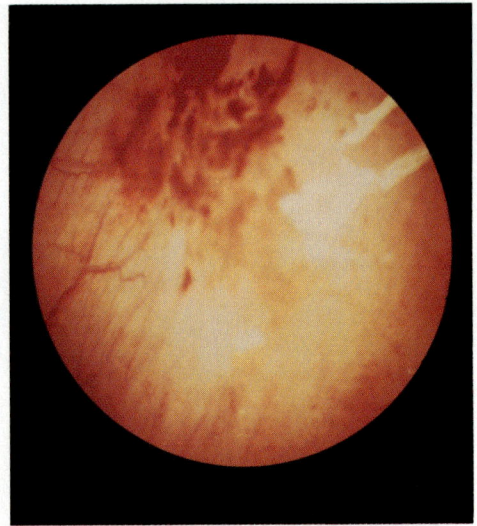

FIGURE 24–20. Laparoscopic view of a flame-like lesion of endometriosis. (Courtesy of William R. Keye, Jr., M.D.)

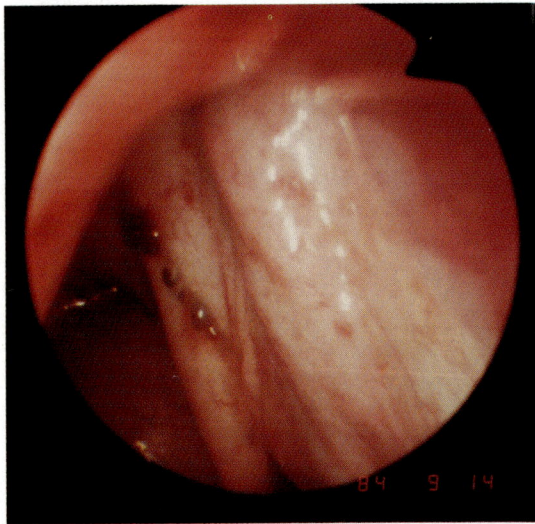

FIGURE 24–21. Laparoscopic view of a darkly pigmented lesion of endometriosis. (Courtesy of William R. Keye, Jr., M.D.)

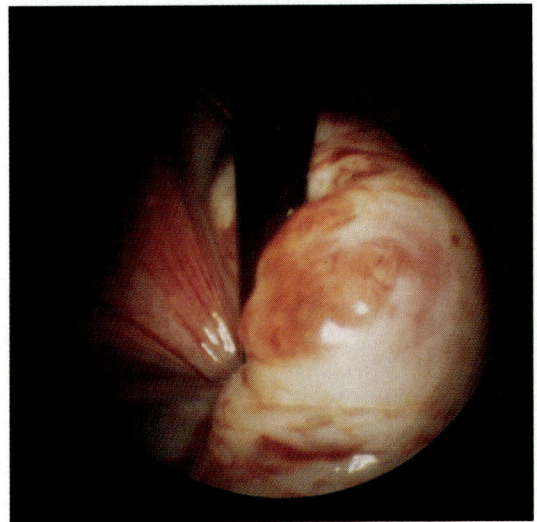

FIGURE 24–22. Laparoscopic view of a retro-ovarian adhesion secondary to endometriosis. (Courtesy of William R. Keye, Jr., M.D.)

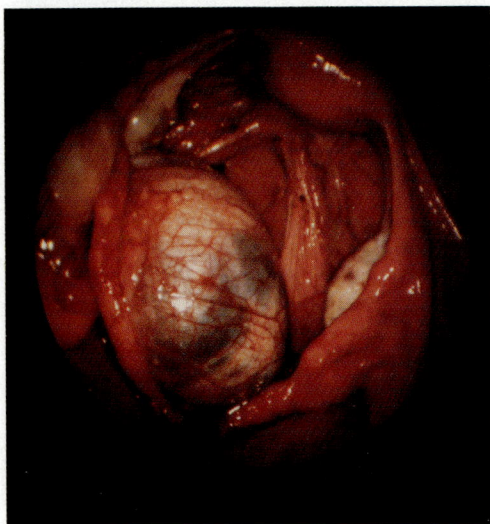

FIGURE 24–23. Laparoscopic view of the pelvis and left ovarian endometrioma. (Courtesy of William R. Keye, Jr., M.D.)

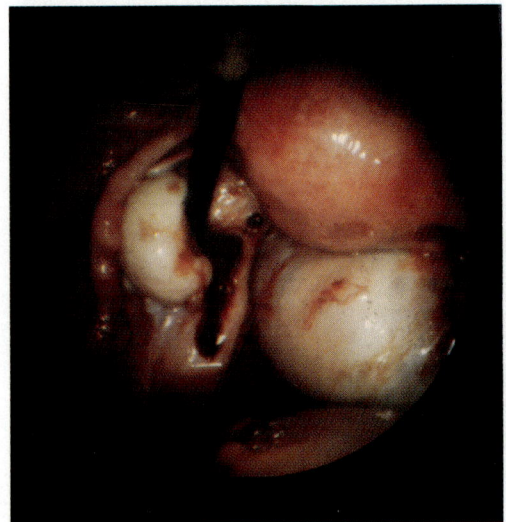

FIGURE 24–24. Rupture of endometrioma with spill of chocolate-colored material. (Courtesy of William R. Keye, Jr., M.D.)

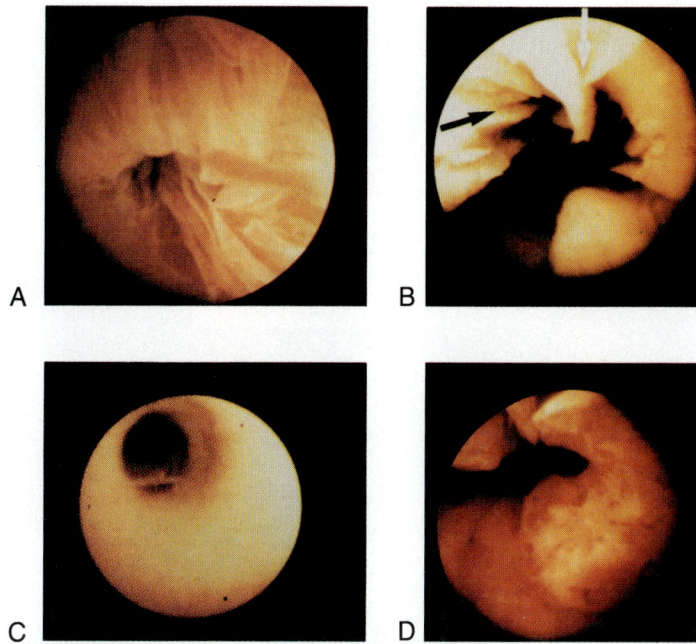

FIGURE 26–2. Salpingoscopic view of a normal ampulla (*A* and *B*). Primary and secondary folds are indicated by the *white* and *black arrows*, respectively. An intraluminal isthmic adhesion is demonstrated with a view obtained via a flexible salpingoscope (*C*). The ampullary lumen in a patient with a severe hydrosalpinx (*D*) is devoid of primary and secondary folds, with abnormal vessel formation. (*A* through *D* from Herschlag A, Seifer DB, Carcangiu ML, et al. Salpingoscopy: light microscopic and electron microscopic correlations. Reprinted with permission from The American College of Obstetricians and Gynecologists [Obstetrics and Gynecology, 1991, 77, 399–405].)

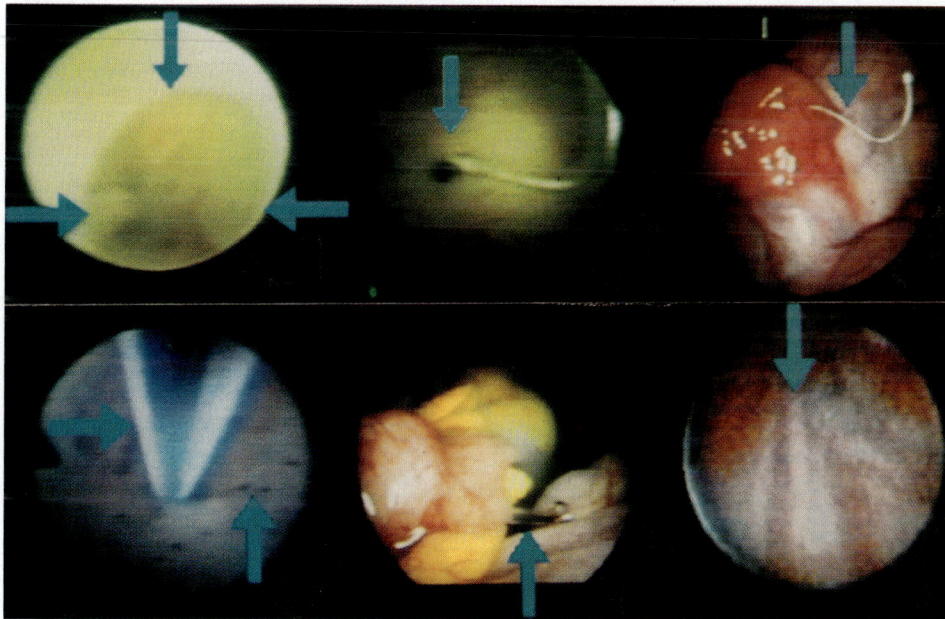

FIGURE 26–5. *Upper left,* End-on view via a miniature flexible hysteroscope into the uterotubal ostium (*arrows*) of the delicate longitudinal folds of the intramural epithelium. *Upper middle,* Flexible guide wire entering ostium (*arrow*). *Upper right,* Same platinum-tipped guide wire (*arrow*) exiting the fimbria. *Lower left,* Falloposcope enclosed in its Teflon catheter entering the ostium (*arrows*). The openings of individual proliferative endometrial glands can be seen. *Lower middle,* Close-up laparoscopic view of the same transparent Teflon cannula enclosing the falloposcope, exiting the fimbria (*arrow*). *Lower right,* Normal individual epithelial secondary branching villi containing central vascular cores, at the level of the mid-ampulla in the same tube (*arrow*). (From Kerin JF, Williams DB, San Roman GA, Pearlstone AC, Grundfest WS, Surrey ES. Falloposcopic classification and treatment of fallopian tube lumen disease. Fertil Steril 1992;57:731–741. Reproduced with permission of the publisher, The American Fertility Society.)

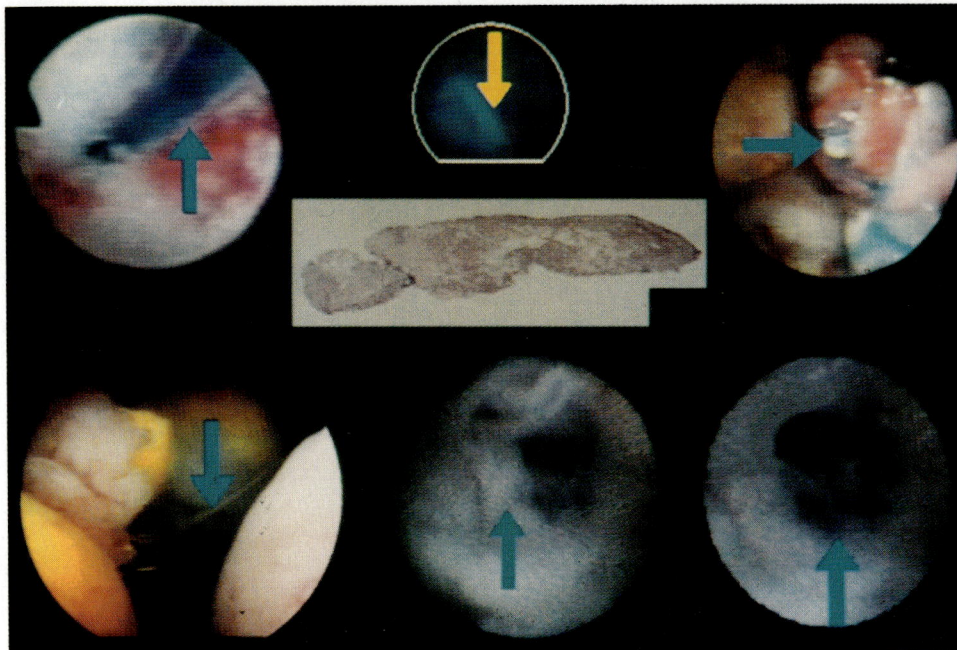

FIGURE 26–6. *Upper left*, Selective tubal cannulation (*arrow*) and aquadissection using Indigo carmine–colored lactated Ringer's solution as a contrast medium. *Upper middle (top)*, The proximal white end (*arrow*) of a tubal plug occupying the isthmic lumen as contrasted against the Indigo carmine solution. *Upper middle (bottom)*, A low-power microscopic view (×40) of the same entire isthmic plug measuring 3 × 0.7 × 0.7 mm, which is an intact cast consistent with an origin from the isthmic lumen. It is composed of a mixture of endothelial cells and amorphous debris.[33] *Upper right*, Mobilization of the same plug seen in the previous view (*arrow*), followed by the appearance of Indigo carmine fluid, indicating the achievement of patency. *Lower left*, A fine, clear elastic fimbrio-ovarian mucus connection (*arrow*) extending from the tip of the falloposcope and attached to the ovarian surface overlying a preovular follicle.[31] *Lower middle*, Stringy, nonobstructive adhesions (*arrow*) in a pale devascularized fibrotic and atrophic epithelium. *Lower right*, Weblike fenestrated nonobstructive isthmic adhesions (*arrow*). (From Kerin JF, Williams DB, San Roman GA, Pearlstone AC, Grundfest WS, Surrey ES. Falloposcopic classification and treatment of fallopian tube lumen disease. Fertil Steril 1992;57:731–741. Reproduced with permission of the publisher, The American Fertility Society.)

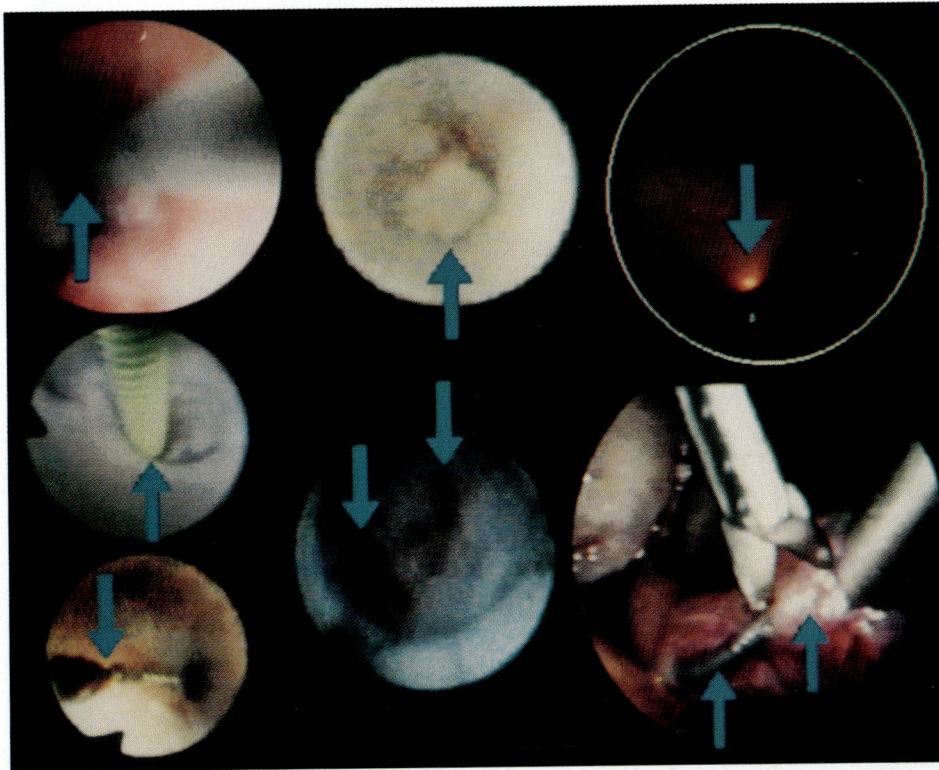

FIGURE 26–7. *Upper left*, A 0.3-mm flexible guide wire (*arrow*) both entering and exiting the ostium owing to a block just distal to the uterotubal junction in the medial isthmus. *Upper middle*, Identification of the lesion (*arrow*) with the falloposcope in the medial isthmus, which is blocked by polypoid extensions of fibrotic tissue arising from a devascularized epithelium. *Upper right*, A simultaneous laparoscopic view of the falloposcopic light transilluminating the tube wall just proximal to the isthmic block (*arrow*). The laparoscope light has been dimmed to highlight the falloposcope light and the site of the block. *Lower left (top)*, A ribbed flexible wire dilator entering the same ostium (OD = 0.6 mm) (*arrow*), which successfully bypassed the block and exited the fimbria, following which free tubal patency was demonstrated. *Lower left (bottom)*, The leading wire of a balloon catheter entering the ostium (*arrow*) followed by the deflated balloon (OD = 1 mm). *Lower middle*, Falloposcopic view of lysed isthmic luminal adhesions following successful direct balloon tuboplasty. The red areas (*arrows*) are patches of blood at the site of the divided adhesions. Posttuboplasty patency was demonstrated. The inner crescent-shaped lining of the Teflon catheter can be seen (ID = 0.8 mm). *Lower right*, A guide wire has been passed to the fimbrial level. The wire is flexed into a U owing to perifimbrial adhesions (*arrow*). The wire is deliberately used to expose the delicate interfimbrial adhesions to facilitate accurate laparoscopic scissor division of these adhesions. The rest of the tubal lumen was falloposcopically normal. The external tube was also normal. (From Kerin JF, Williams DB, San Roman GA, Pearlstone AC, Grundfest WS, Surrey ES. Falloposcopic classification and treatment of fallopian tube lumen disease. Fertil Steril 1992;57:731–741. Reprinted with permission of the publisher, The American Fertility Society.)

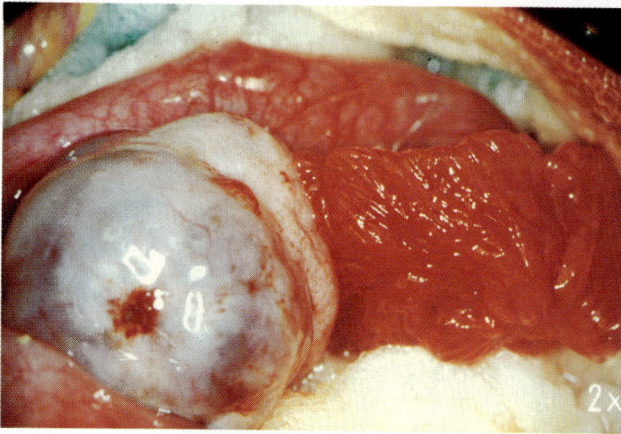

FIGURE 30–1. The fallopian tube.

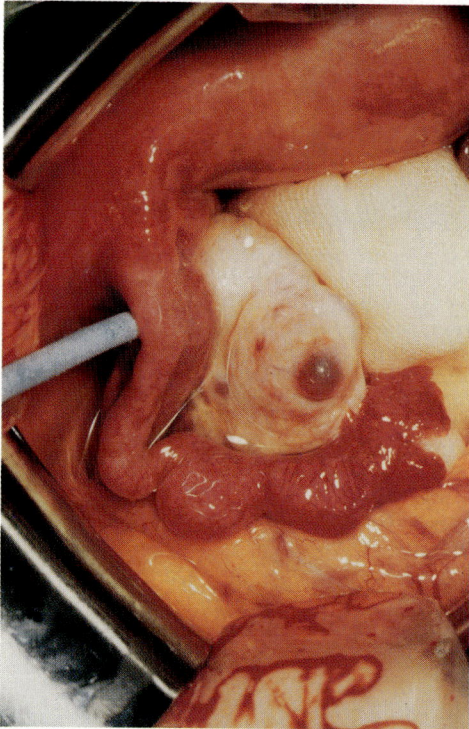

FIGURE 30–28. Microsurgical laparotomy. Unilateral rudimentary uterine horn formation mimics unilateral proximal tubal occlusion.

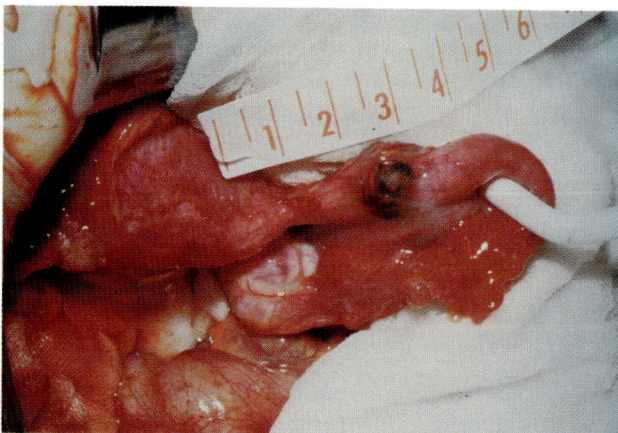

FIGURE 30–54. Microsurgical laparotomy. Tubal endometriosis is evident. A nodule of endometriosis occludes the midtube.

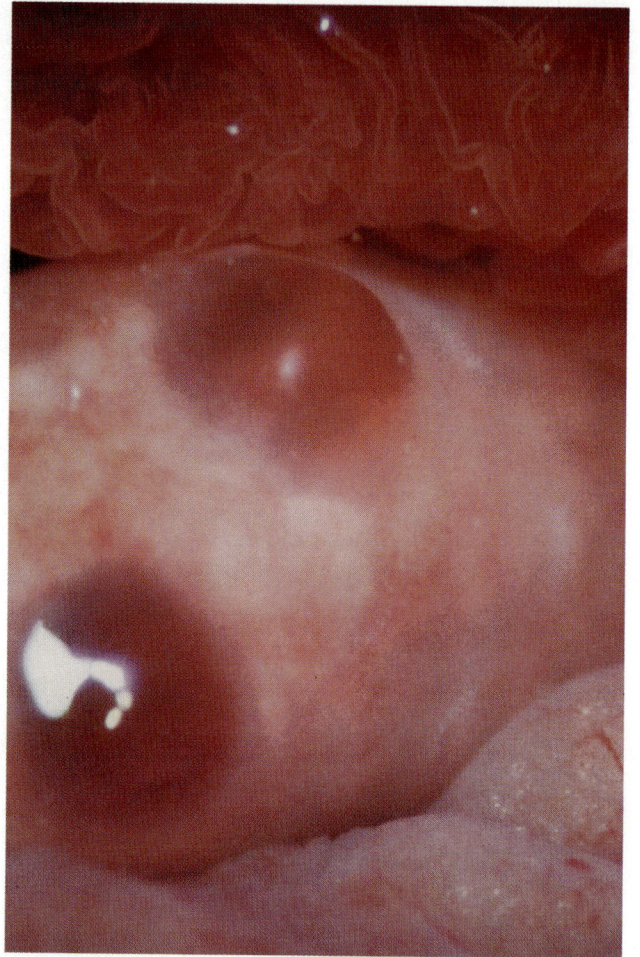

FIGURE 30–9. Relationship of fimbria to ovary in the preovulatory state. The fimbria sweeps across the ovarian surface.

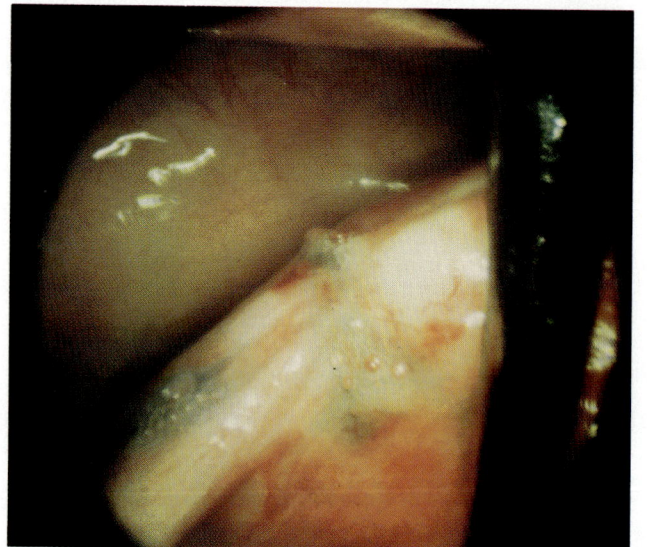

FIGURE 30–49. Laparoscopy. A view of the proximal oviduct is shown. Normal supple myosalpinx has been replaced by salpingitis isthmica nodosa. Note the mucosal diverticula that have penetrated the myosalpinx to reach the tubal serosa.

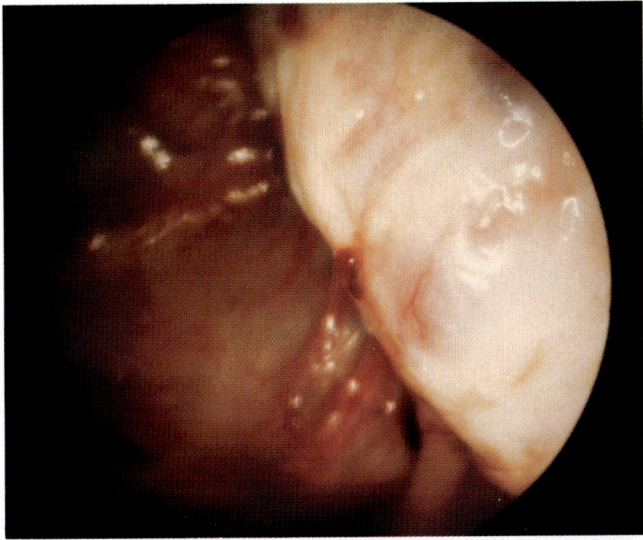

A

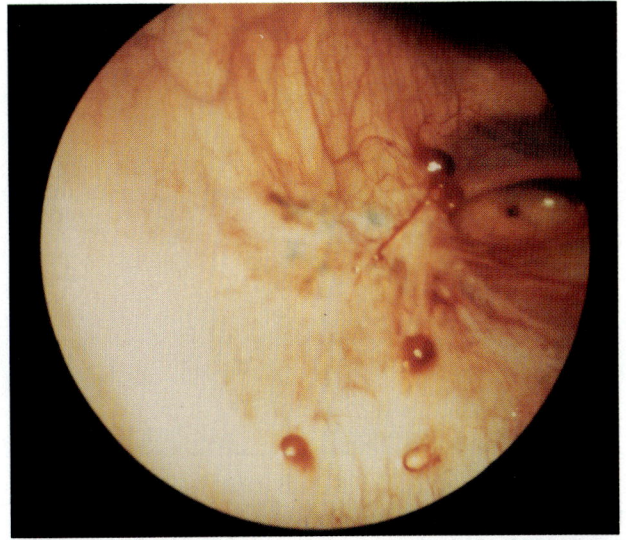

B

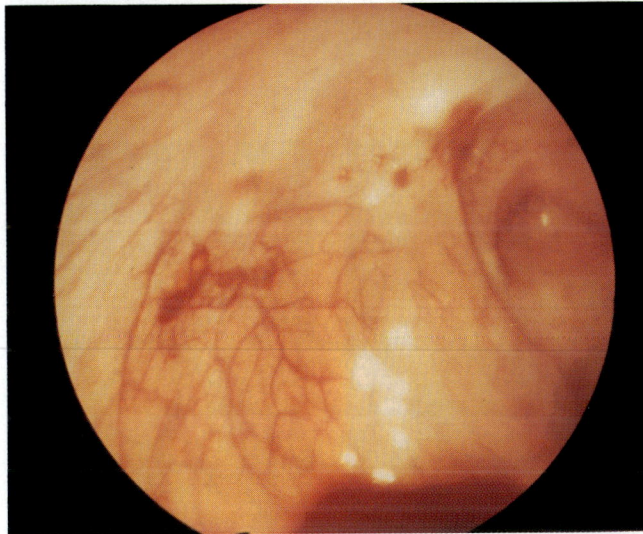

C

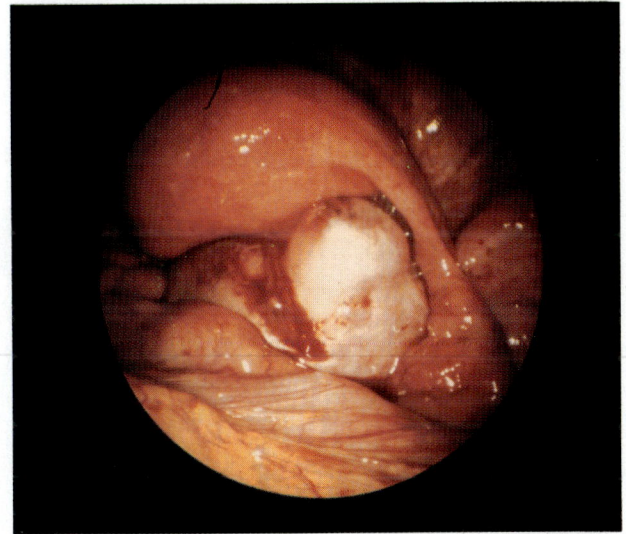

D

FIGURE 33–3. Examples of the gross appearance of endometriotic lesions. *A*, Adhesion from the ovarian fossa to an implant on the surface of the ovary. *B*, Superficial pigmented lesions. *C*, Peritoneal pocket and superficial pigmented lesions. *D*, Endometrioma of the ovary. (Courtesy of William R. Keye, Jr., M.D.)

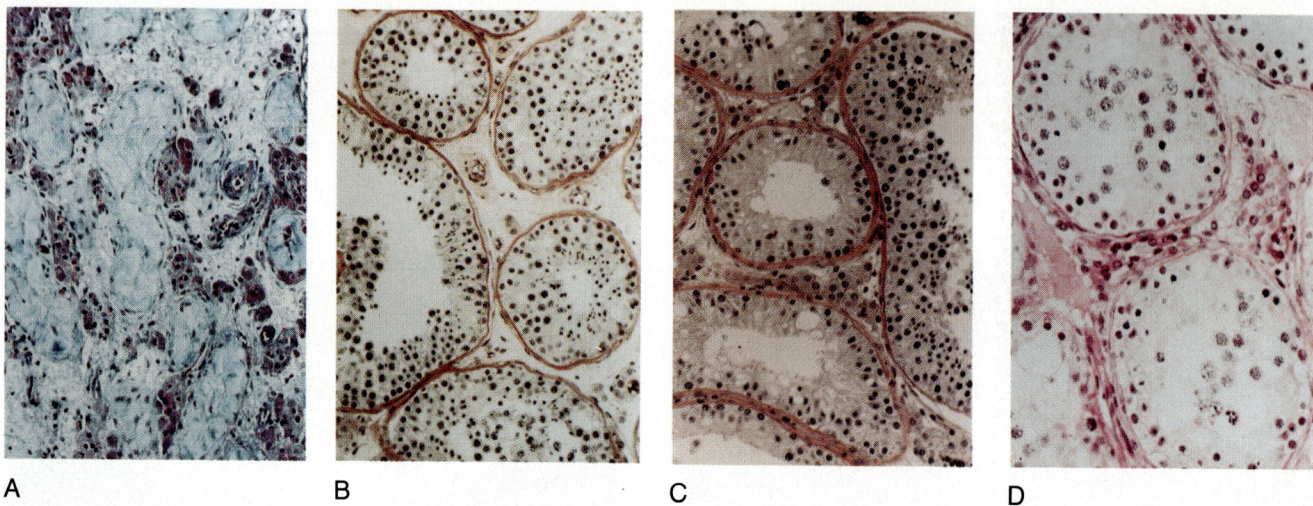

FIGURE 37–3. Testis biopsies from (*A*) a man with testicular damage from mumps orchitis. Note the severe germ cell loss and seminiferous tubule sclerosis with clumped Leydig cells in the interstitium; (*B*) an infertile man with idiopathic oligozoospermia, demonstrating a hypospermatogenesis pattern; (*C*) another infertile man with idiopathic oligozoospermia, demonstrating more severe hypospermatogenesis than that found in the previous man; and (*D*) an infertile male with idiopathic azoospermia, demonstrating a maturation arrest pattern with very few spermatids present. (Reprinted from Paulsen CA. In: Santen RJ, Swerdloff RS, editors. Male Reproductive Dysfunction: Diagnosis and Management of Hypogonadism, Infertility, and Impotence. New York: Marcel Dekker, 1986, p. 202 by courtesy of Marcel Dekker, Inc.)

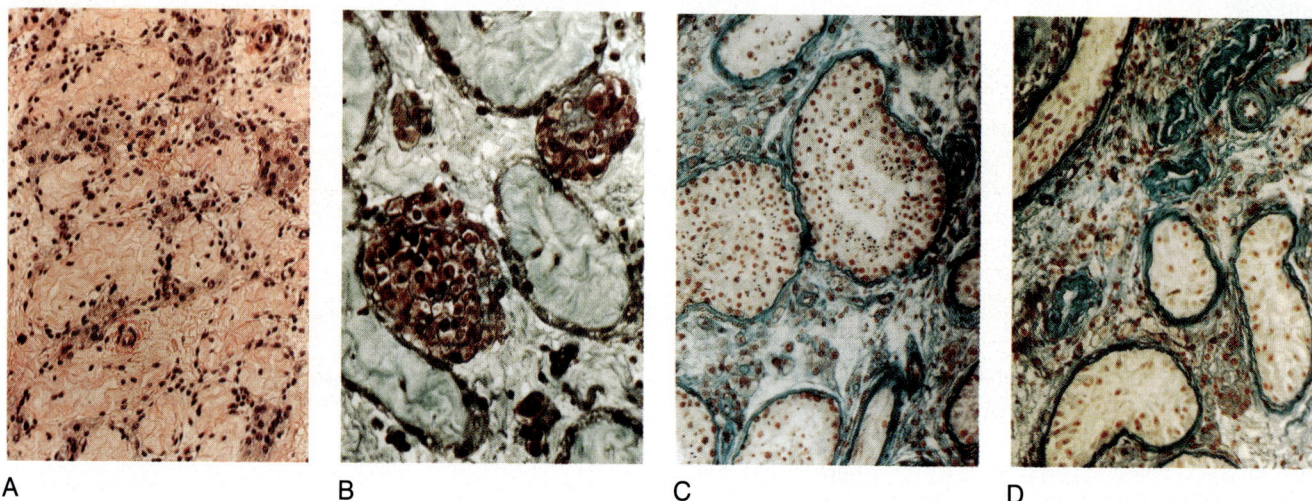

FIGURE 37–4. Testis biopsies from men with Klinefelter's syndrome, demonstrating (*A*) total sclerosis of seminiferous tubules and Leydig cells that are dispersed throughout the interstitium; (*B*) reticular fibers surrounding hyalinized seminiferous tubules and Leydig cells that are present in adenomatous clumps; (*C*) a variable pattern of germ cell damage with some seminiferous tubules showing active spermatogenesis; and (*D*) a variable pattern of germ cell loss with a mixture of hyalinized seminiferous tubules and tubules containing only Sertoli cells. (Reprinted from Paulsen CA. In: Santen RJ, Swerdloff RS, editors. Male Reproductive Dysfunction: Diagnosis and Management of Hypogonadism, Infertility, and Impotence. New York: Marcel Dekker, 1986, p. 201 by courtesy of Marcel Dekker, Inc.)

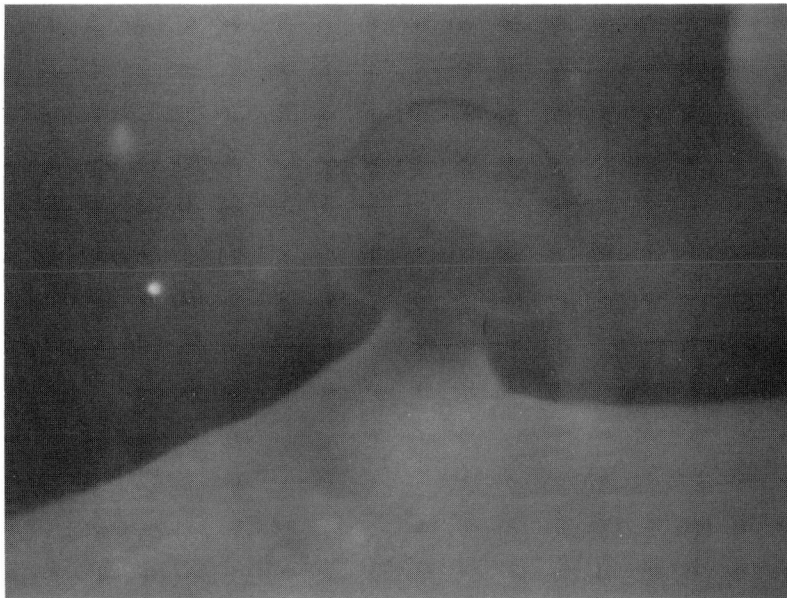

FIGURE 30–6. Magnified photography. The follicle has ruptured. Follicular fluid is released before expulsion of the cumulus.

FIGURE 30–7. Magnified photography. The cumulus "unfolds," bearing the oocyte. Bleeding from the capillaries at the stigma helps attach the cumulus oophorus to the surface of the ovary. Note the visible white spot within the cumulus; this is the oocyte.

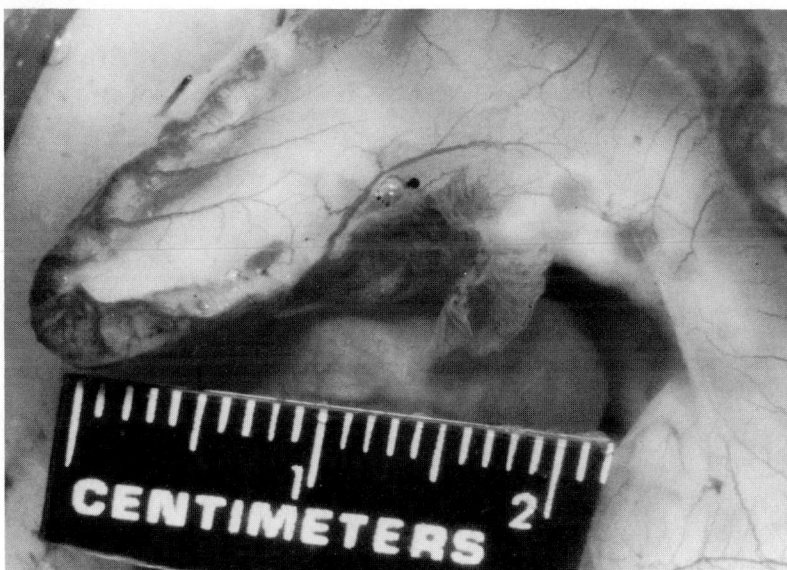

FIGURE 30–8. Exposed "in vivo" intact adnexum of the rabbit. The fimbria caresses the ovary.

447

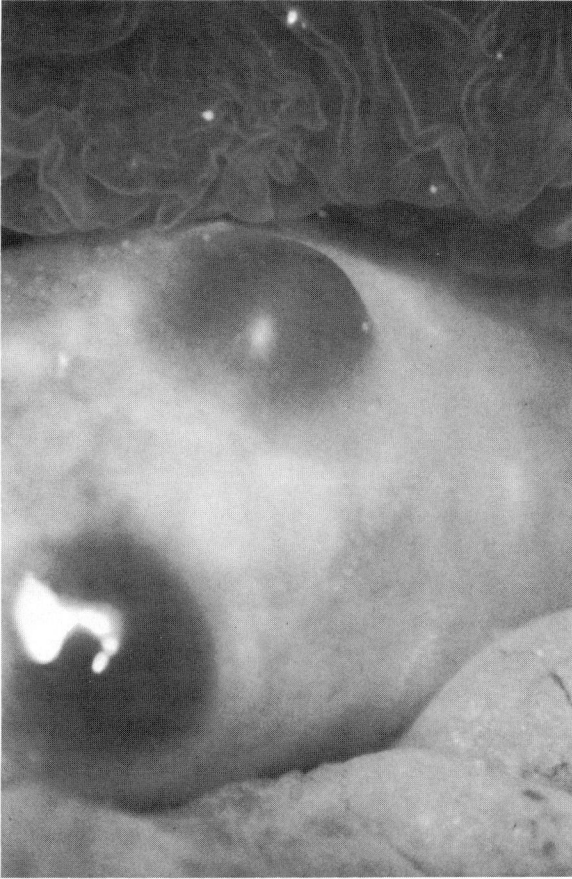

FIGURE 30–9. Relationship of fimbria to ovary in the preovulatory state. The fimbria sweeps across the ovarian surface.

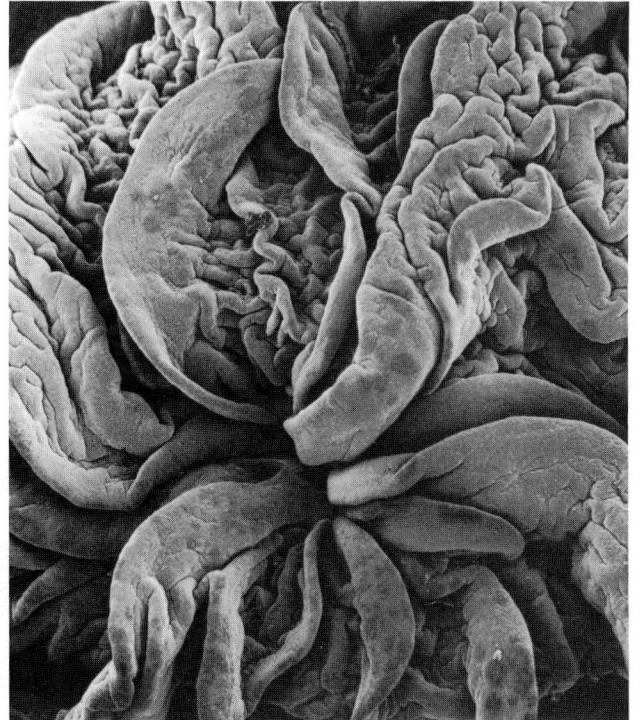

FIGURE 30–10. Scanning electron microscopy. The intact fimbria (rabbit) is shown. The complex mucosal folds transport the cumulus oophorus by the generation of fluid currents. (Original magnification ×8.5)

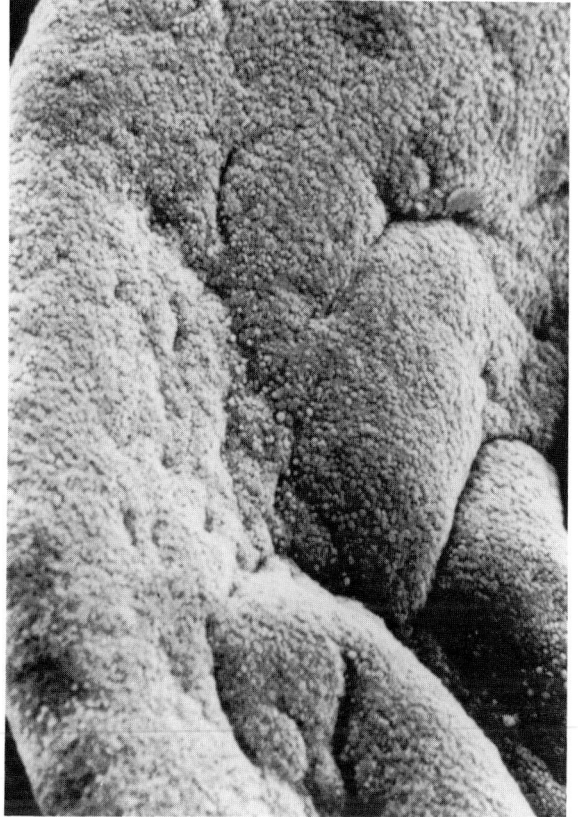

FIGURE 30–11. Scanning electron microscopy. Higher magnification discloses lush populations of ciliated cells intermingled with secretory cells. (Original magnification ×800)

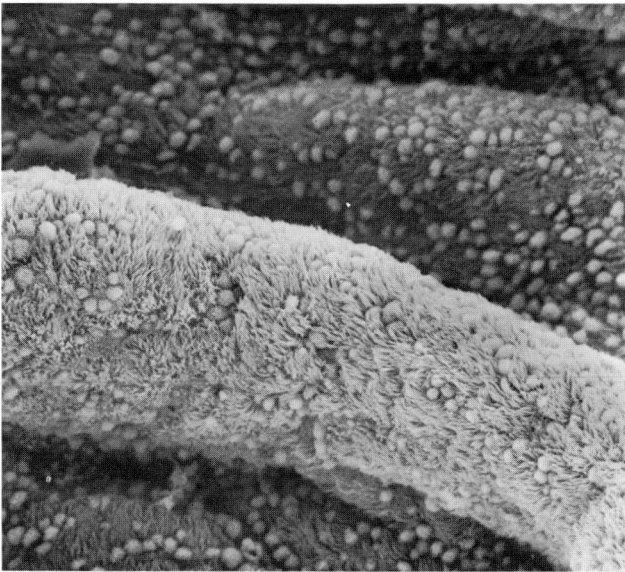

FIGURE 30–12. Scanning electron microscopy. Further magnification of the ampullary mucosa shows the density of ciliated cells. (Original magnification ×1200)

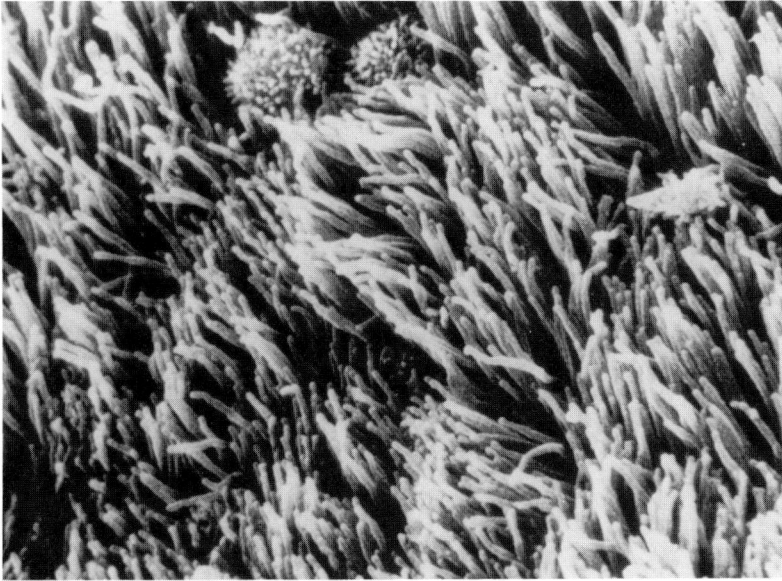

FIGURE 30–13. Scanning electron microscopy. High magnification details the ciliated cells. (Original magnification ×2800)

of the fallopian tube. As the cumulus is surrounded by more ciliary surface area, it is more tenaciously held. The ovum is carried within the cumulus toward the infundibulum (Fig. 30–15), where the granulosa cells become completely contained within the ampulla. This process may take minutes to hours. The transport rate across the fimbrial mucosa is about 0.1 mm/s.[17]

Once in the ampulla, the cumulus complex has reached a stable environment conducive to fertilization. The complex tertiary mucosal folds are displaced laterally as the cumulus travels through (Fig. 30–16). Ciliary-induced fluid currents (Fig. 30–17) are the major transport mechanism to carry the cumulus to the ampulloisthmic junction,[17] that is, fully two thirds of the distance from fimbria to uterus. The time elapsed is minutes from the fimbria and hours from first follicular release. The cumulus complex lodges at the ampul-

loisthmic junction due predominantly to the volume of the cloud of granulosa cells, the diminutive diameter of the isthmic lumen (1 mm) and the reduced numbers of cilia within the isthmus. It is considered that fertilization most often occurs within the ampulla and particularly at the ampulloisthmic junction.

Once ejaculation of sperm has occurred, spermatozoa are deposited in the vagina as a coagulum. At about the time detumescence of the elastic vaginal tissues has restored a degree of occlusion to the vagina, liquefaction of the seminal coagulum releases the spermatozoa. The periovulatory mucus is cascading from the cervical os. The spinnbarkeit of the mucus causes the previously entangled mucopolysaccharide molecules to align longitudinally; this allows the sperm to form phalanges as they self-propel by axonemal flagellation into the clear, copious mucus of the cervical canal. This mucus thereafter acts as a reservoir for the sperm. Through

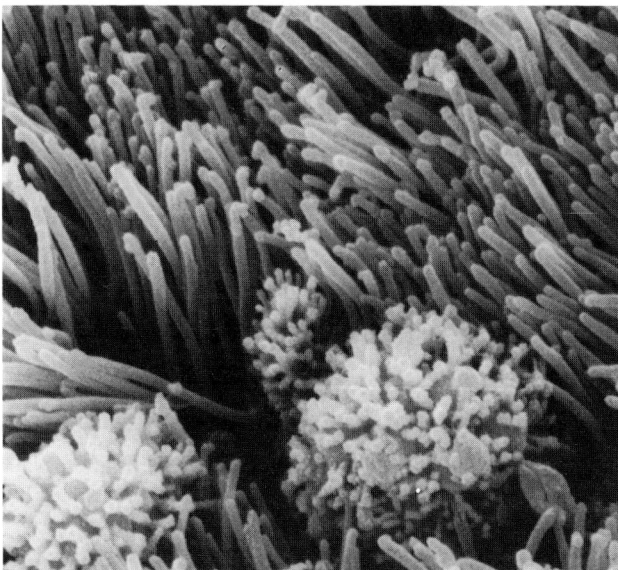

FIGURE 30–14. Scanning electron microscopy. Very high magnification shows detail of the cilia. Note the adjacent secretory cells. (Original magnification ×3400)

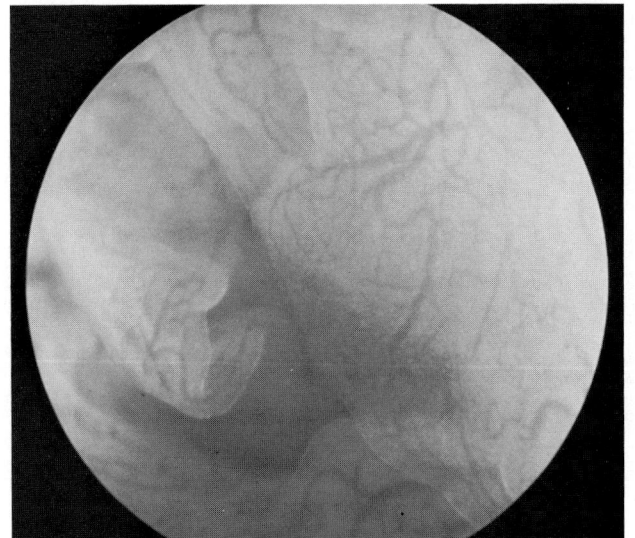

FIGURE 30–15. Salpingoscopy. Telescopic magnification of the infundibulum and lateral ampulla shows the mucosal folds and vascular pattern of the normal fallopian tube.

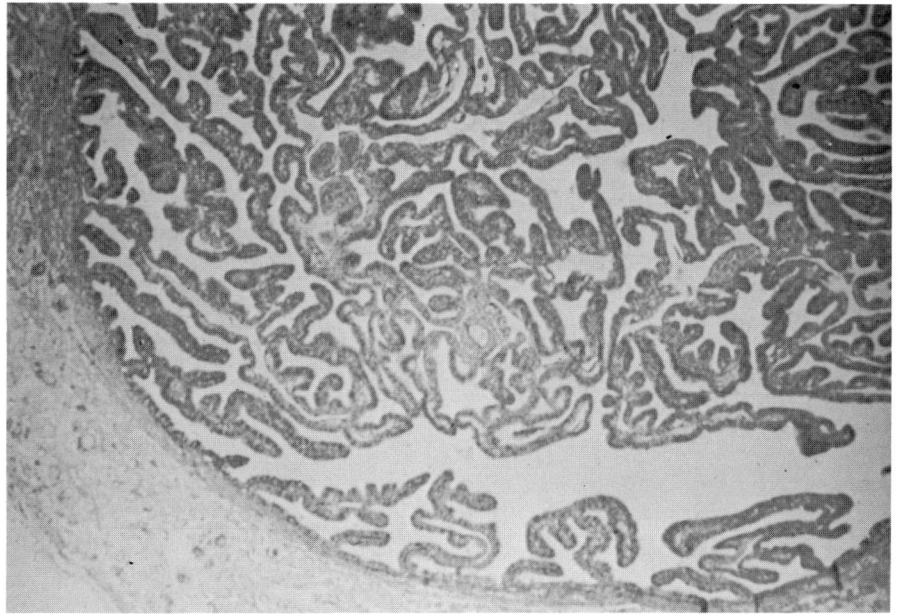

FIGURE 30–16. Histologic section of the ampulla. The profusion of mucosal folds is demonstrated in this section.

the uterine cavity, the intramural oviduct, and the isthmus, the spermatozoa appear to move by a combination of self-propulsion and retrograde myometrial and myosalpingeal contraction. Selection of the quickest and most robust sperm cell takes place. Sperm transport is thought to be a result of a combination of mechanisms including its innate motility, cilial propulsion, fluid flow, and tubal contractility.[18] The number of sperm successfully reaching the fallopian tube is much smaller than that in the ejaculate, a fact partially explained through selection via motility mechanisms. Others postulate that the uterotubal junction functions as a barrier.

Following capacitation of mature spermatozoa in the female oviduct, sperm acquire a hyperactivated motility, which allows them to reach and penetrate the zona pellucida. Capacitation appears to require a minimum oviductal stay of several hours. The acrosome reaction—which is triggered by binding to the zona pellucida and which is necessary for penetration of the zona pellucida—occurs only in capacitated spermatozoa. Once the spermatozoa reach the cumulus mass within the ampulla, fertilization may occur. The granulosa cells that surround the oocyte do not interfere with the ability of sperm to fertilize the oocyte. The rapid ciliary transport from fimbria delivers the cumulus oocyte complex to the constant nurturing milieu of the proximal ampulla.

After some 24 hours within the proximal ampulla, the cumulus cells dissipate to facilitate entry of the fertilized ovum/embryo into the isthmus. There is no consensus as to how embryo transport through the human isthmus to the uterine cavity occurs. The embryo stays within the isthmus for 2 days. Direct observation of the transilluminated rabbit isthmus documents brisk to-and-fro motion of the embryo due to myosalpingeal contraction (Fig. 30–18). This is ac-

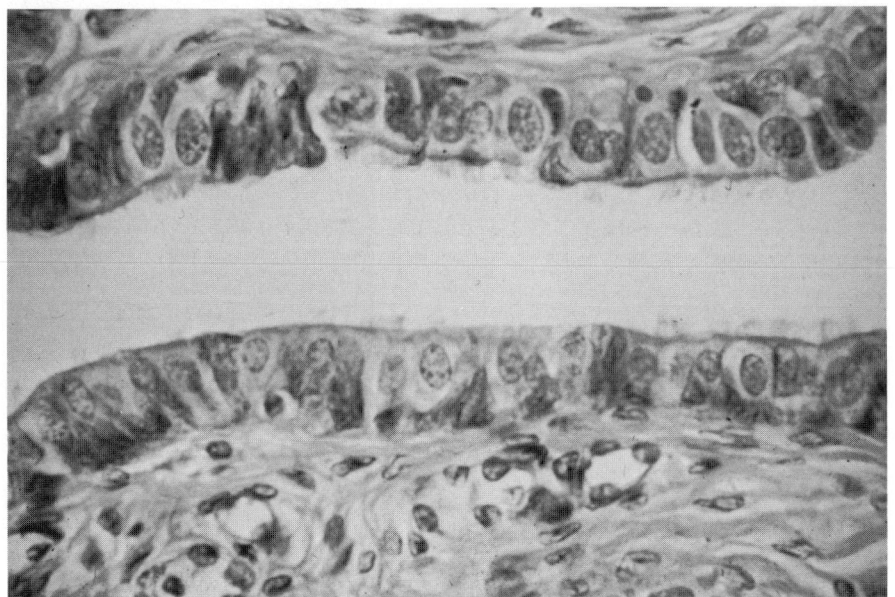

FIGURE 30–17. Histologic section of ampullary mucosal fold. The ciliated cells generate fluid currents to transport the cumulus.

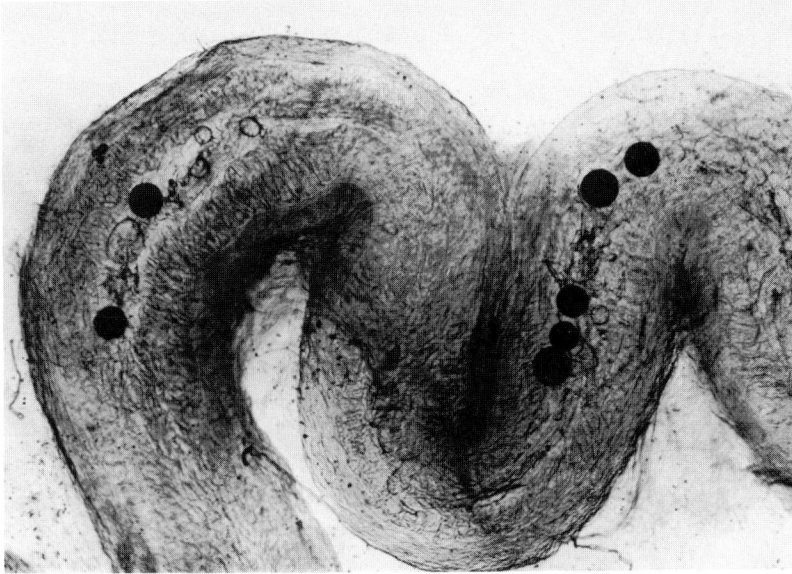

FIGURE 30–18. Oviductal isthmus prepared by the Orsini tissue clearing technique. Surrogate ova as well as the zona pellucidae of ova are seen to be evenly distributed through the isthmic segment.

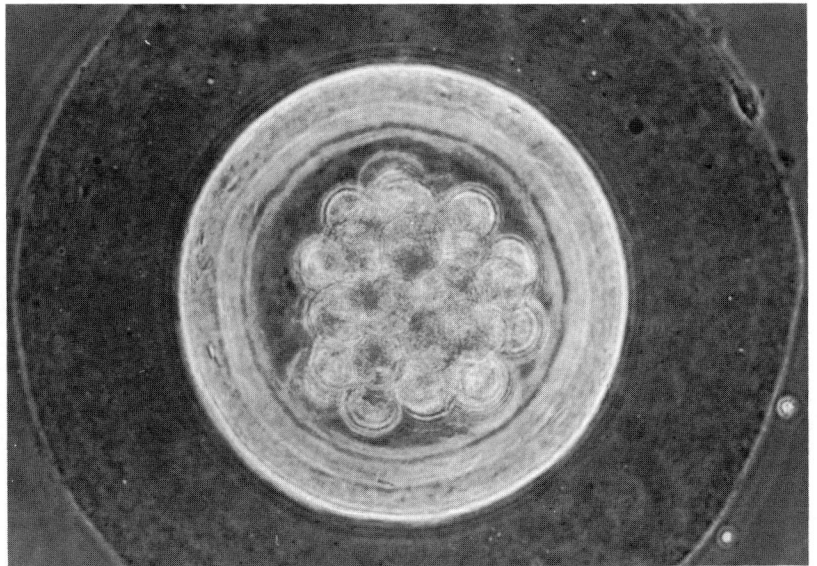

FIGURE 30–19. Morula stage. The diameter is approximately 100 μ.

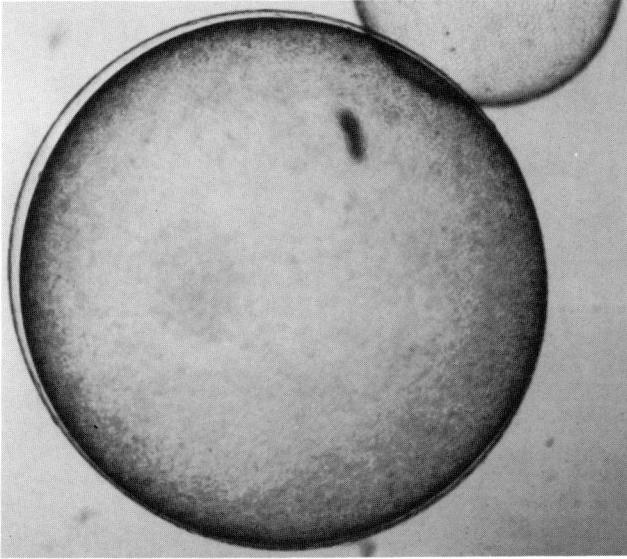

FIGURE 30–20. Expanded blastocyst stage. The diameter is approximately 3 mm.

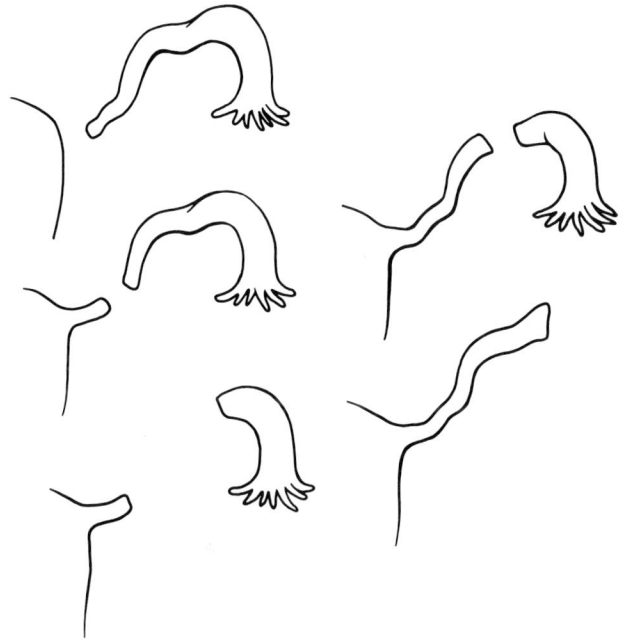

FIGURE 30–21. The different forms of "segmental deletion" associated with sterilization.

companied by gradual descent of the morula (Fig. 30–19) to the uterine cavity,[18] where at 4 days after ovulation the embryo hatches from the zona pellucida to become an expanded blastocyst (Fig. 30–20). Still another 3 days elapse before implantation. There is evidence, once more in the rabbit, that a function of the isthmic myosalpinx (see Fig. 30–3) adjacent to the uterus is to thrust the embryo from the isthmus into the uterine cavity. Fertility in women is little reduced even when a substantial loss of isthmic length has occurred (compared with the ampulla), suggesting that if this mechanism occurs in the human, only a short isthmic segment may be needed to perform this function.[19] Before considering the disease states of the oviduct, it is appropriate to review the effects of deletion of tubal segments and deletion of transport function.[19, 20]

EFFECTS ON TUBAL PHYSIOLOGY DUE TO DELETION OF STRUCTURE OR FUNCTION

Structural Deletion

The most frequent structural deletion is that caused by sterilization of women (Fig. 30–21). We can determine the role of each tubal segment, especially with respect to any essential function that it may perform. With a sterilization procedure, the remaining tubal segments are healthy with normal muscular, ciliary, and nutritive functions. One must also consider the effect of the anastomosis on the tubal function (Figs. 30–22 and 30–23).

At the outset, one may observe that the process of fertilization is literally essential to the survival of the species. This is reflected in backup mechanisms that may be required if failure or loss of a primary oviductal function occurs.

The *fimbria* has proved to be dispensable.[21–23] This became evident with the failure rate associated with the fimbriectomy sterilization procedure. In cases of failed sterilization by fimbriectomy, a tongue of fimbrial tissue (usually in the region

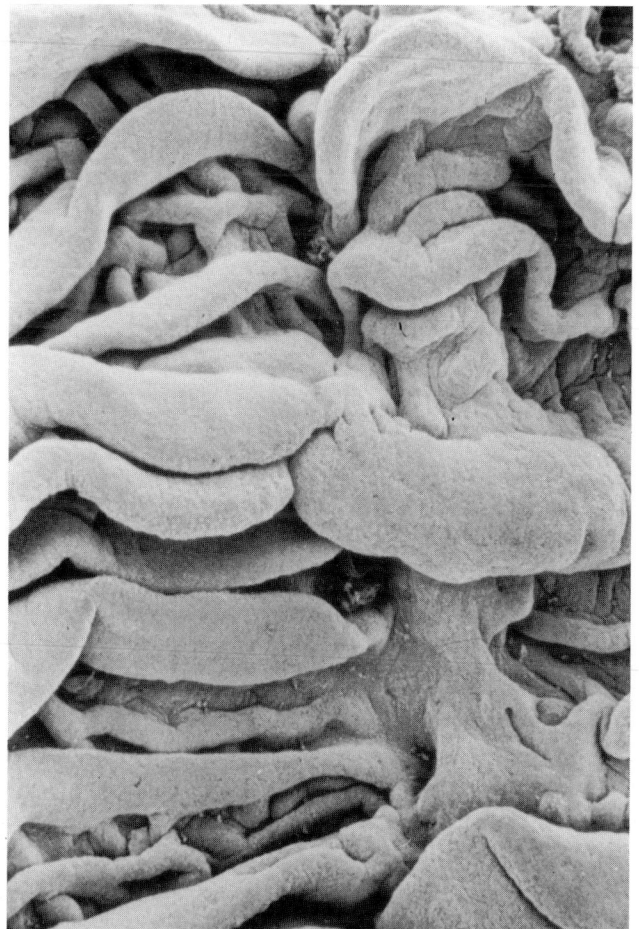

FIGURE 30–22. Scanning electron microscopy. The slit-open ampulla demonstrates the mucosal pattern after end-to-end microsurgical anastomosis. (Original magnification ×32)

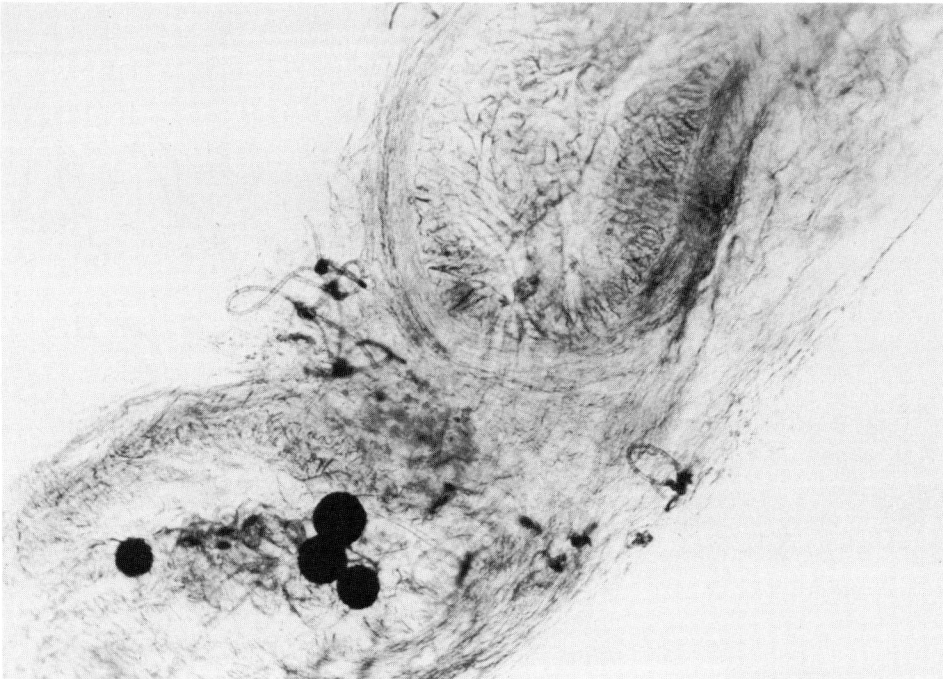

FIGURE 30–23. Oviductal isthmus prepared by the Orsini tissue clearing technique. A microsurgical anastomosis in the isthmus segregates the surrogate ova.

of the fimbria ovarica) protrudes from a crack in the tubal wall. The function of the fimbria is dependent primarily on the ciliary mucosa and the surface area of the mucosa[23] that is available. The ampulla also is richly endowed with ciliated cells. For example, at the surgical reversal of a fimbriectomy, the ampullary mucosa can be fashioned to create a neofimbria (Figs. 30–24 and 30–25), albeit with decreased surface area, that can function.

The *ampulla* appears to be essential for successful pregnancy. When sterilization reversal is attempted in the absence of the ampulla, for example by anastomosing fimbria directly to isthmus, intrauterine pregnancy is rare. The essential function of the ampulla may be as a nutritive site for fertilization (as a containment location for the cumulus oophorus). At least 50% of the ampulla should be present if one is to anticipate successful pregnancies after either ampullary anastomoses or fimbriectomy reversals.

The *isthmus* and the *intramural oviduct* seem to be the most functionally redundant parts of the human oviduct.[24] Ampullomyometrial anastomosis can lead to successful intrauterine pregnancy. Loss of isthmic length does decrease fertility, but not as much as does loss of ampullary length.

Functional Deletion

There are two forms of functional deletion: ciliary, and muscular.

Muscular deletion is seen with a failed sterilization. Usually, the sterilization has been attempted by electrical coagulation of the tubal segment. At reoperation the surgeon is often able to identify only mucosal tissue between the interrupted tubal segments. Histologic section of this intervening tissue demonstrates typically a tunnel of oviductal mucosa linking the tubal parts. The muscularis has been successfully transected at the time of the sterilization and has contracted and re-

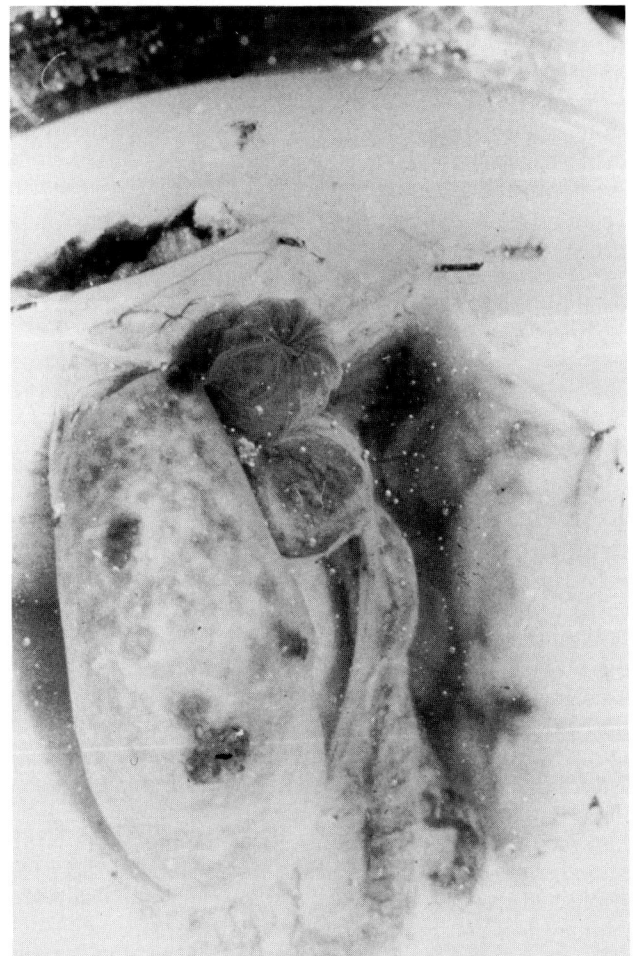

FIGURE 30–24. Exposed "in vivo" surgically modified adnexum of the rabbit. The "neofimbria" with lush everted ampullary mucosa nestles close to the ovary.

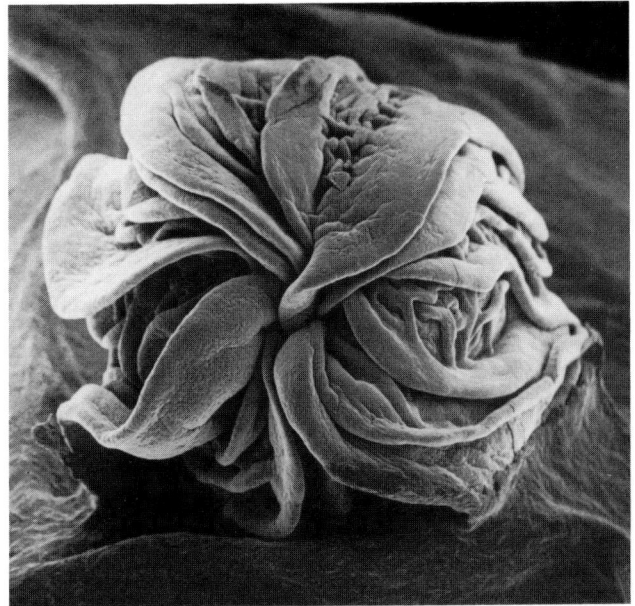

FIGURE 30–25. Scanning electron microscopy. This is the same neofimbria as in Figure 30–24. Note the preservation of the mucosal folds. (Original magnification ×15)

tracted. This points to the ability of the ciliary mucosa alone to facilitate transport of the spermatozoa toward the ovary and the embryo toward the uterus. Conversely, it can be concluded that the myosalpinx is not essential for oviductal transport of either the gametes or the embryo.

Ciliary deletion has been induced in the rabbit by reversing a segment of ampulla and thereby reversing the direction of ciliary beat. Infertility was induced in virtually all animals despite the preservation of normal myosalpingeal contractility.[17]

In women, ciliary deletion is typified by the "immotile cilia" syndrome. Only a small number of those women described as having Kartagener's syndrome (situs inversus, bronchiectasis) or "ciliary dyskinesia" will have absolutely immotile cilia.[25] Various intraciliary ultrastructural defects

(Fig. 30–26) may be related to varied forms and degrees of ciliary dyskinesis. These defects may involve the mechano-chemical coupling between the adenosine triphosphatase–containing outer dynein arms of the A fiber with the B fiber and other skeletal derangements (Fig. 30–27). In women who have ciliary immotility documented by phase-contrast microscopy, there is associated infertility.[26] This points to the essential nature of ciliary transport through the oviduct.

PATHOPHYSIOLOGY

Most tubal lesions interfere with fertility by distortion of normal anatomy. Interference through alteration of normal function is less well understood.

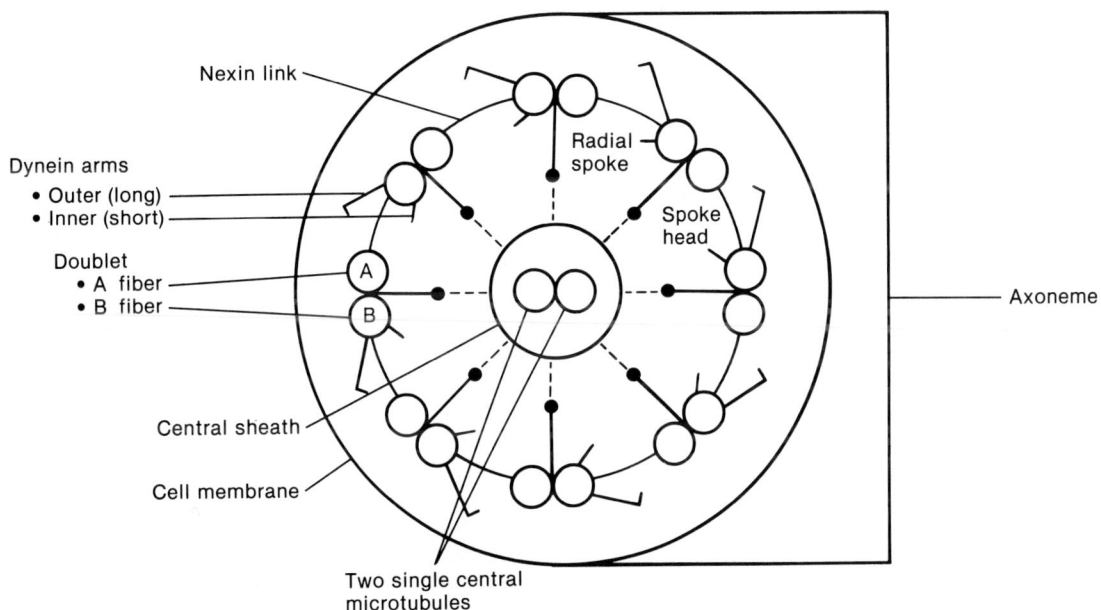

FIGURE 30–26. This schematic representation of a cilium illustrates the ultrastructure. The adenosine triphosphatase containing outer dynein arms, radial spokes, central sheath, and the doublets all may be deficient, with differing functional consequences.

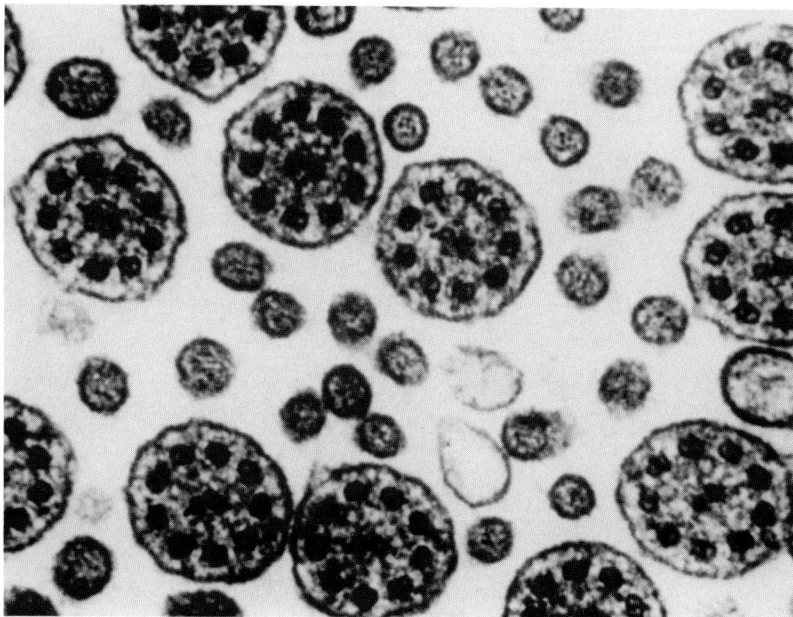

FIGURE 30–27. Transmission electron microscopy. Cilia in cross section from a woman with immotile cilia. Multiple ultrastructural anomalies were present, including absence of the outer dynein arms.

It is important to differentiate between those oviductal lesions that are due to disease as opposed to those that are iatrogenically caused.

Lesions in Otherwise Normal Tubes

The segmental deletion due to *sterilization* leaves tubal tissue that is intrinsically normal.

One exception to this is the endometriosis that may damage the proximal segment of oviduct after a sterilization.[27, 28] It is postulated that the menstrual fluid that would ordinarily traverse the oviduct to reach the peritoneal cavity instead becomes loculated in the proximal tubal stump. The endometrial tissue so entrapped initiates endometrial gland formation within the isthmic myosalpinx. The subsequent reactive fibrosis further damages the proximal stump to render it useless for reconstruction. Development of these poststerilization lesions does appear to accord with the time elapsed since the sterilization.[29]

Congenital Tubal Abnormalities

Congenital tubal abnormalities range from 1 in 500 to 700 deliveries and are classified as complete absence, segmental absence and duplication, accessory ostia, and multiple lumina.[30]

Complete absence of the oviduct may occur with or without absence of the ipsilateral ovary. Autoamputation may explain some of these occurrences.[31]

Coelomic invagination has been postulated as the causative mechanism for accessory ostia and multiple lumina. An association with infertility and ectopic pregnancy has been suggested.[32, 33] Segmental absence is uncommon. Distal segmental absence of the oviduct has been noted with absence of the ipsilateral ovary.[34] Isthmic and infundibular segmental deletions are also reported but are rare.

We have seen an unusual case of elongated fallopian tubes. In this woman the ovaries were located at the pelvic brim, superior to the normal location.

The presence of a rudimentary uterine horn may be misdiagnosed as an occluded proximal tube (Fig. 30–28; see color section in the center of the book).

Iatrogenic tubal resection at inguinal hernia repair is another instance in which the tube will be otherwise normal.[35]

Segmental oviductal resection for ectopic tubal pregnancy may have been performed in apparently normal tubal tissues. However, the pelvic inflammatory disease (PID) and salpingitis isthmica nodosa (SIN) that are so often associated with tubal pregnancy make this less likely.

Iatrogenic Tubal Lesions

Tubal lesions can be classified as proximal, midtubal, and distal. These lesions are almost always either of the fimbria (distal) or the intramural oviduct (proximal). Less often, there will be combined proximal and distal lesions (Fig. 30–29), and least often a midtubal lesion will be encountered.

The most common and best described lesion is *distal tubal occlusion,* with consequent distention of the oviductal ampulla, that is, a hydrosalpinx. Hydrosalpinx formation is often associated with intraperitoneal stigmata of previous PID. It is usually associated with intrinsic tubal damage and peritubal scarring (Figs. 30–30 and 30–31).

Midtubal occlusion is the least common site for tubal obstructive disease[20] and may be combined with either distal or proximal obstruction. It can be associated with endometriosis, previous ectopic pregnancy, or infections such as tuberculosis.

Proximal tubal obstruction has been receiving increasing interest and research. It occurs less often than distal obstruction, and its etiology and treatment are considerably more controversial. SIN, inflammatory disease, obliterative fibrosis, endometriosis, polyps, and previous ectopic pregnancy are among the most commonly implicated lesions.

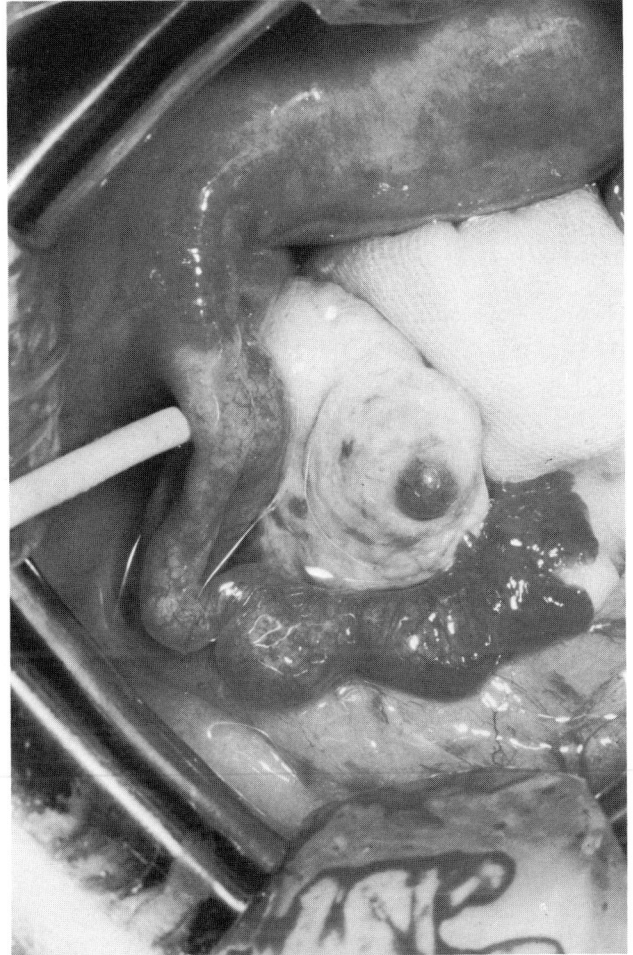

FIGURE 30–28. Microsurgical laparotomy. Unilateral rudimentary uterine horn formation mimics unilateral proximal tubal occlusion.

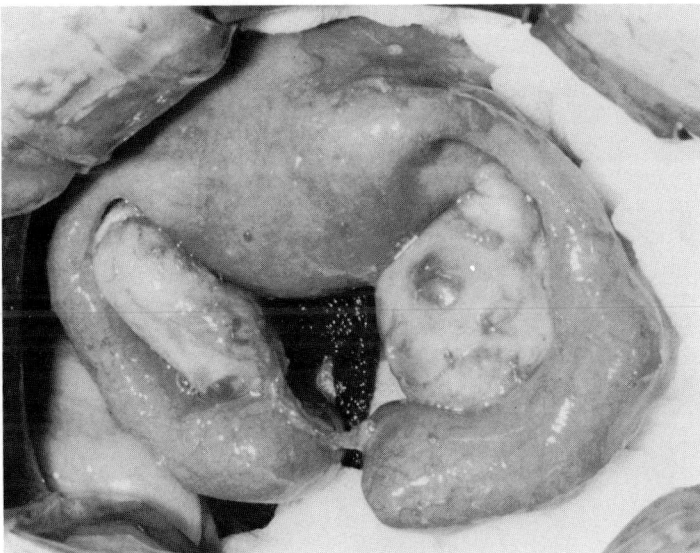

FIGURE 30–29. Microsurgical laparotomy. Bipolar disease is evident. There is cornual disease as well as hydrosalpinx. The prognosis for fertility is poor.

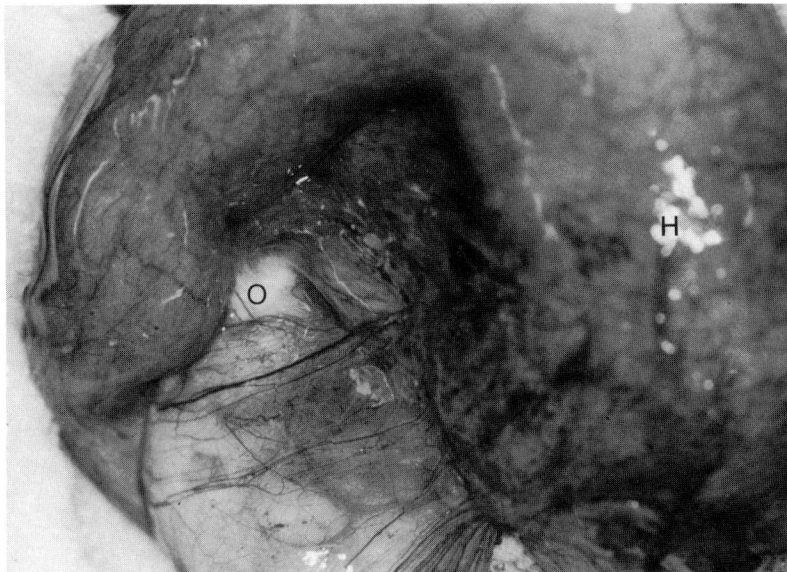

FIGURE 30–30. Distal tubal disease. The triad of peritubal scarring, tubal occlusion, and ciliary damage is present. O, ovary; H, hydrosalpinx.

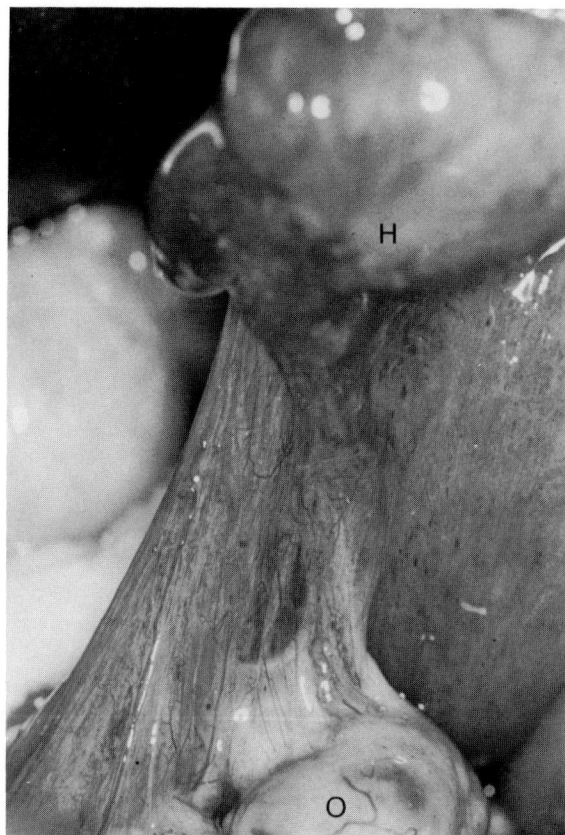

FIGURE 30–31. Distal tubal disease. The scarring between the tube and the ovary is demonstrated. O, ovary; H, hydrosalpinx.

EVOLUTION OF DAMAGE

Tuboperitoneal factors are recognized as the cause of infertility in approximately 50% of women. *Inflammatory diseases* and their sequelae probably constitute the most frequent and best described lesions. They can be classified into acute, chronic, and granulomatous inflammatory processes.

PID and its sequelae appear to be on the rise in industrialized countries. The majority represent sexually transmitted disease, although postoperative, postinstrumentation, puerperal or secondary (associated with appendicitis, diverticulitis, or *Mycobacterium tuberculosis*) infections do occur.

Only about 40% of women with tuboperitoneal infertility and evidence of previous intraperitoneal inflammation have a history of PID. Pathologic changes such as deciliation, flattened mucosal folds, and degeneration of secretory cells are observed in patients with both overt and silent PID.[37]

The classic concept is that of an ascending, mono-organism (*Neisseria gonorrhoeae*) infection. Evidence has accumulated that most cases of PID represent a multiorganism infection commonly involving *Chlamydia trachomatis* and anaerobic organisms. Significant regional differences in the prevalence of pathogens appear to exist. A hematogenous (i.e., tuberculosis) or lymphatic (streptococci, staphylococci, and coliform bacilli) spread is postulated for certain organisms, but the more common pathway of bacterial infection appears to involve an ascent of pathogens from the endocervix via the endometrium to the endosalpinx. In particular, gonococci tend to invade and spread along mucosal surfaces.

Endometriosis is the next most ubiquitous disease that can distort and destroy the pelvic structures. The scarring that results from endometriosis is typically dense and refractory to dissection.

Pathophysiology

DISTAL TUBAL DISEASE

The degree of damage to the pelvis may range from a few filmy peritubal adhesions with tubal patency to a "frozen pelvis" and an occluded distal oviduct (Figs. 30–32 to 30–35).

The anatomic distortion may be categorized as peritubal, occlusive-tubal, and ciliary.

The *peritubal adhesions* are best considered as to their potential for repair

1. If the fallopian tube is freely mobile with space (Figs. 30–36 and 30–37) between the tube, ovary, and pelvic sidewall, and the adhesions are easily transected (Fig. 30–38), the prospects for restoration of tubal function are reasonable.

2. If the adhesive process has fused the tube to the ovary (Fig. 30–39)—usually with increased density of adhesions—the probability of successful correction is diminished.

3. If the ovary oviduct, or both, have fused additionally to the pelvic sidewall, often with loss of ovarian volume, the prospects for effective repair are guarded.

Occlusive-tubal damage may be represented by fimbria encased completely or in part by adhesions, fimbrial phimosis, or total tubal occlusion: the hydrosalpinx. Each is attended by a different extent of mucosal damage. Intratubal adhesions may further reduce potential transport function (Fig. 30–40).

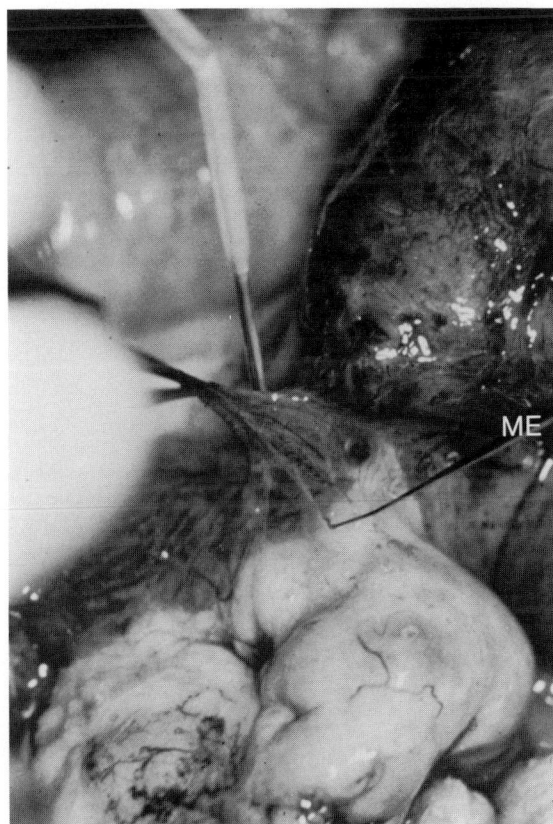

FIGURE 30–32. Distal tubal disease. The scarring is resected with the microelectrode (ME) from the ovarian surface.

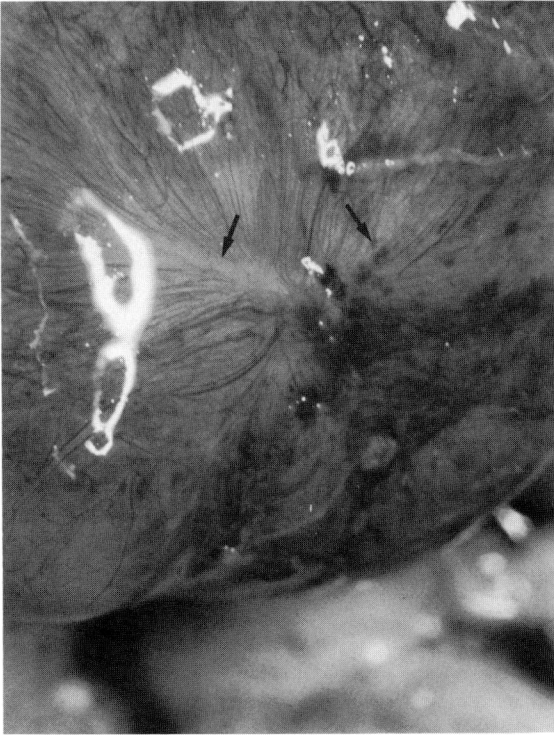

FIGURE 30–33. Distal tubal disease. Hydrosalpinx is evident. Lines of fusion of the fimbrial lappets are shown by *arrows*.

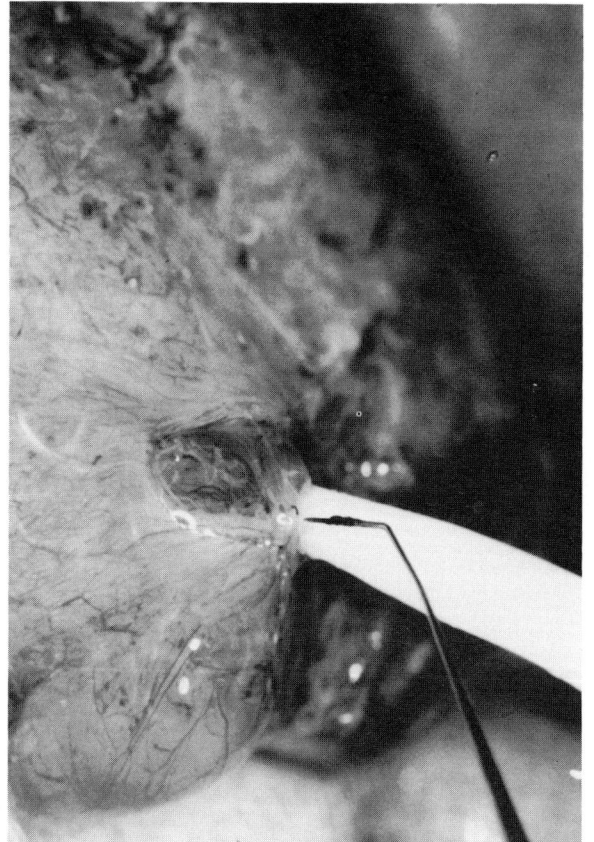

FIGURE 30–34. Distal tubal disease. Hydrosalpinx is evident. The lines of fusion are incised to restore patency.

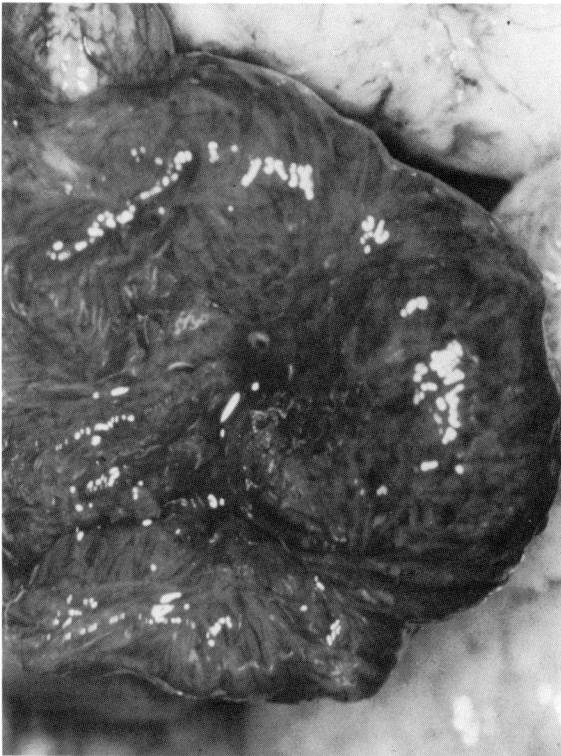

FIGURE 30–35. Distal tubal disease. Hydrosalpinx is evident. The tubal mucosa has been everted. The quality appears to be reasonable.

The *ciliated cells* are also ablated by inflammation to a varied extent.[37, 38] A direct ciliostatic effect of *Mycoplasma hominis* has been reported.[39]

In terms of tubal function, the physical quality of the oviduct is the best predictor. Recently, prospective scoring systems have been proposed for prediction of fertility based on tubal wall thickness, the extent and character of adhesions, and the percentage of ciliated cells in the fimbrial mucosa.[40, 41]

Of these, the most important physical attribute is the ciliated mucosa, because this confers motion on the cumulus.

Surgery is capable of restoring patency in more than 75% of hydrosalpinges.[42] However, the subsequent intrauterine pregnancy rate ranges from only 10% to 35%. This discrepancy between patency and function further emphasizes the crucial nature of ciliary transport.[43, 44] Distal tubal disease induces poor retrieval and ampullary containment of the cumulus oophorus. Scarring, limited tubo-ovarian mobility, reduced ovarian surface, and compromised ovulatory function may compound the abnormal transport.

Delay in retrieving or transporting the cumulus complex may result in blastocyst formation within the oviduct and an ectopic implantation.[5]

MIDTUBAL DISEASE

A recent review of the etiology of midtubal lesions determined their frequency as follows: tuberculosis, chronic (arrested) ectopic pregnancy, obliterative salpingitis, endometriosis, mature cystic teratoma (associated with ectopic pregnancy),[45] and intratubal (endosalpingeal) adhesions. Of all these predisposing conditions, successful pregnancy ensues most often after tubotubal anastomosis for excision of a chronic ectopic pregnancy. The defect in tubal function is contingent on the extent of tubal damage. Where the insult is great, as in the chronic granulomatous inflammation of tuberculosis, the oviduct is affected from endosalpinx through myosalpinx to serosa. Consequently, pregnancy rates are poor. Where occlusion is the only insult, anastomosis of the relatively healthy segments of tube is more likely to yield successful pregnancies.

Tuberculosis. Tuberculosis as tuberculous salpingitis has been estimated to account for 1% of infertility in the United States as compared with 10% in India.[46]

The damage associated with tubal tuberculosis is diffuse. Although the initial oviductal infection is mucosal, thereafter the muscularis and serosa are involved. Tuberculosis has a proclivity to infect tubal mucosal epithelium (as it does the endometrium) by hematogenous spread.

At first the disease is a microscopic infection secondary to a primary focus (usually respiratory). It then may progress to become nodular, albeit with preservation of fimbria, or ad-

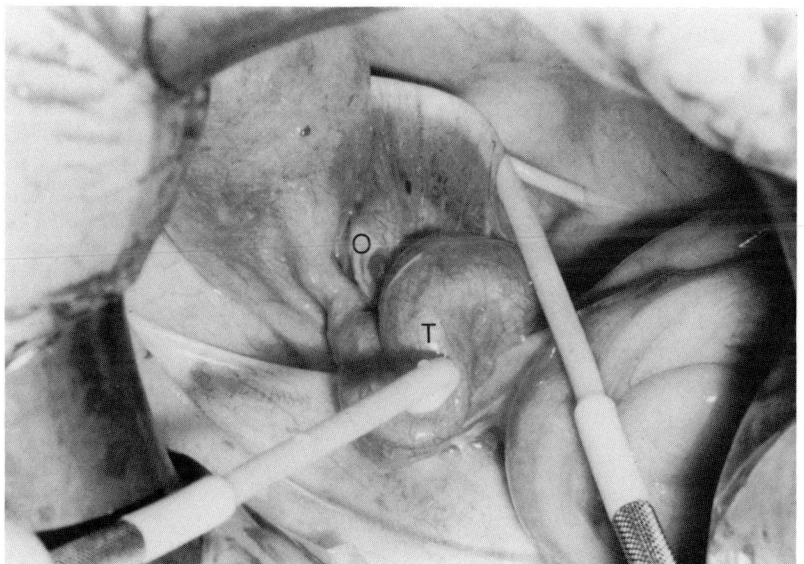

FIGURE 30–36. Microsurgical laparotomy. Distal tubal disease is evident. Filmy adhesions are demonstrated between the tube and the ovary. O, ovary; T, tube.

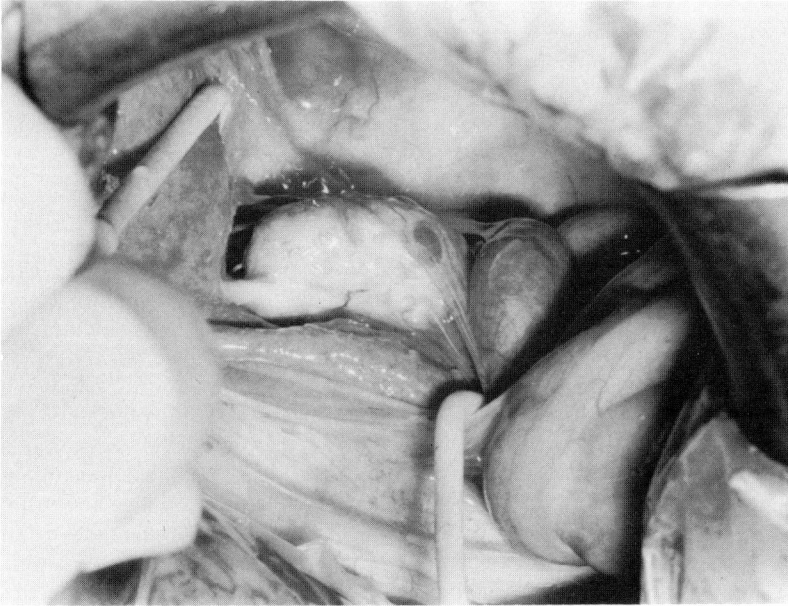

FIGURE 30–37. Microsurgical laparotomy. Distal tubal disease is evident. Filmy adhesions are shown between the ovary and the uterus.

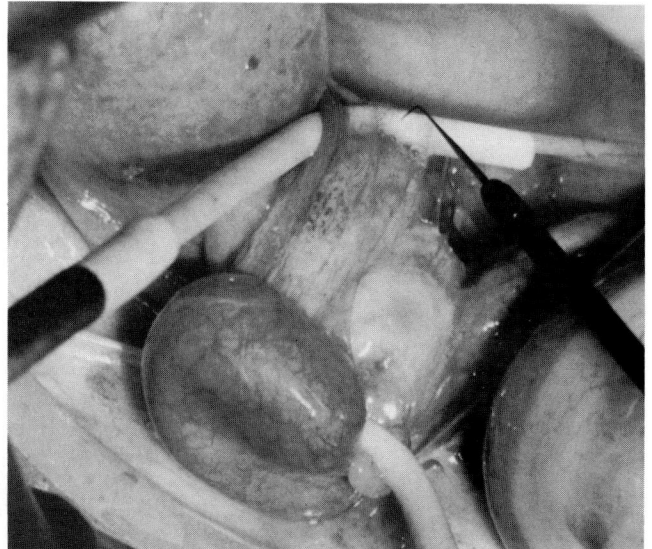

FIGURE 30–38. Microsurgical laparotomy. Distal tubal disease is evident. Transection of the adhesions is done to disclose the hydrosalpinx.

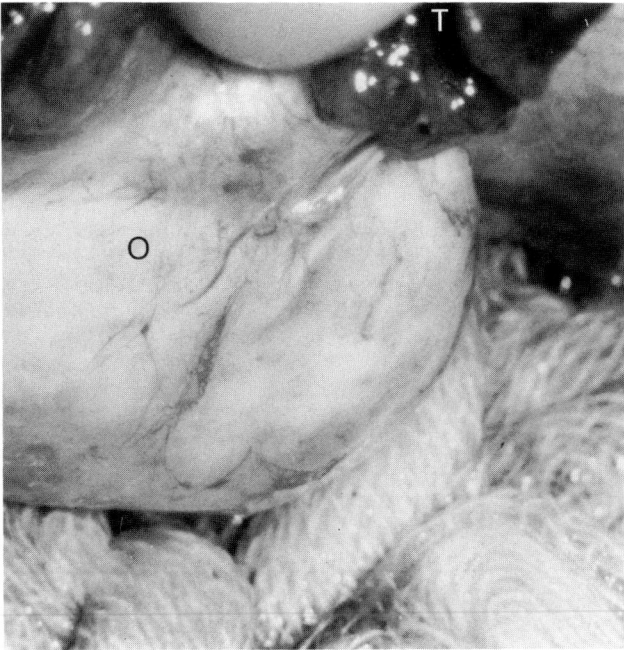

FIGURE 30-39. Microsurgical laparotomy. Fusion of the tube to the ovary is evident. T, tube; O, ovary.

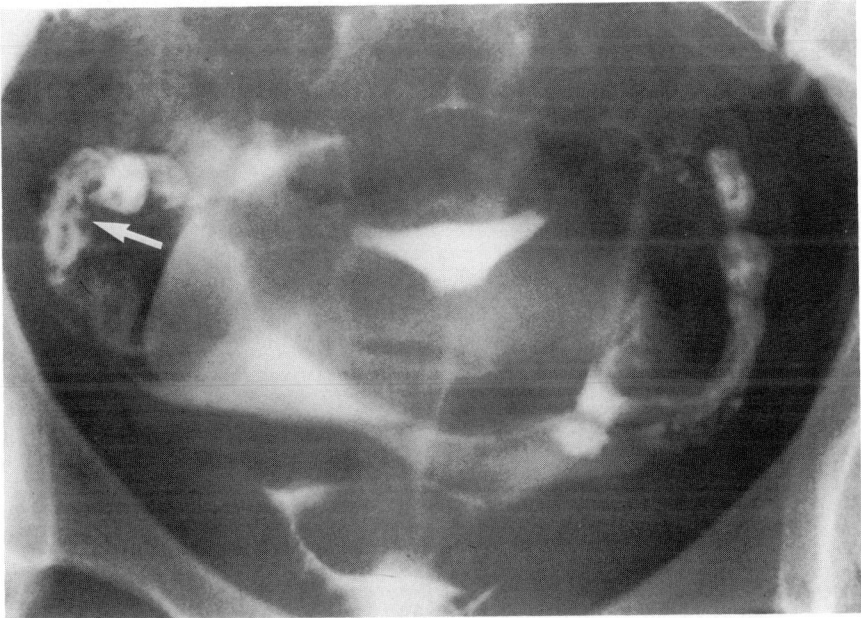

FIGURE 30-40. Hysterosalpingogram. Intratubal adhesions (*arrow*) are evident. Note the "leopard skin" appearance of the ampullary mucosa.

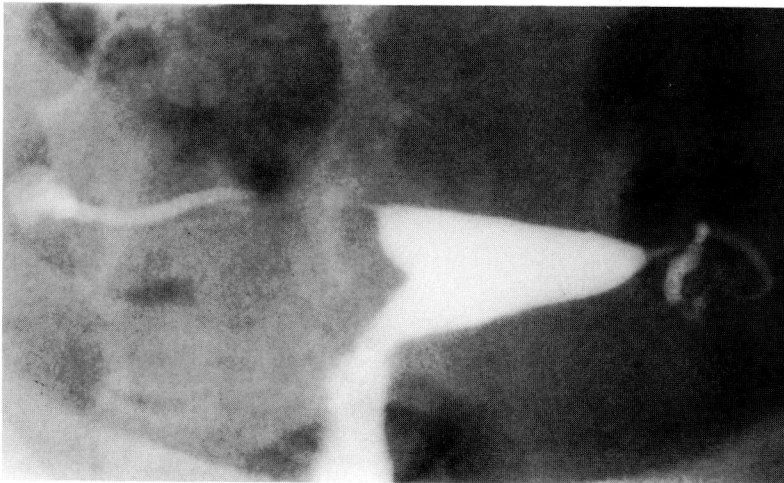

FIGURE 30–41. Hysterosalpingogram. Tuberculosis is evident. Note the "stove pipe" appearance of the proximal tube that culminates in proximal ampullary occlusion.

hesive with distortion of the adnexa. In the exudative form of tuberculous salpingitis, caseated granulomata can coalesce to simulate a pyosalpinx.

The consequence of this infection is to obstruct the tube (most often at the proximal ampulla) and to further interfere with ovum retrieval and transport by the adhesion formation. The rigidity of the oviduct reflects the transmural damage. The extensive tubal damage caused by this disease is such that tubal repair cannot yield functional fallopian tubes. Furthermore, reactivation of the infection may follow an attempt at surgical repair.[7]

These histologic hallmarks are manifested radiographically and especially at hysterosalpingography (HSG) by the following[47]:

1. A rigid isthmus culminating in a midampullary occlusion
2. A beaded appearance of the lumen with dilation alternating with stenosis
3. A "rosette" or "Maltese Cross" image of the distal oviduct (Fig. 30–41)
4. Intratubal adhesions with or without diverticula
5. Associated features such as calcified pelvic lymph nodes and intrauterine synechiae

Other Causes. Tuberculous salpingitis is only one manifestation of granulomatous salpingitis. A number of organisms and disease processes may provoke similar responses: *M. tuberculosis, Actinomyces, Enterobius vermicularis, Schistosoma (haematobium* and *mansoni),* sarcoidosis and inflammatory bowel disease may produce granulomatous lesions in the female genital tract. Foreign body material such as mineral oil and talc have been implicated as well.[48]

PROXIMAL TUBAL DISEASE

Proximal Tubal Obstruction. In a series of 500 HSG studies, the incidence of proximal tubal obstruction (Fig. 30–42) was found to be about 33% of all cases with tubal occlusion.[36] In one series, obliterative fibrosis was the most common finding with 38% and chronic tubal inflammation the next most commonly identified lesion with 21%.[49] Less common causes of proximal obstruction include tubal endo-

metriosis (this includes endometrial colonization), chronic ectopic pregnancy, and congenital disease. Tubal polyps rarely lead to complete obstruction.

One study reported that 11 of 18 cases of purported proximal tubal obstruction failed to have histologic evidence of occlusion. Amorphous tubal casts or plugs were found in 6, no pathology in 3, and some pathology but no obstruction in 8 patients.[50] This finding highlights the need to investigate extensively with repeated evaluations of tubal patency before surgery is undertaken to minimize the false positive findings.

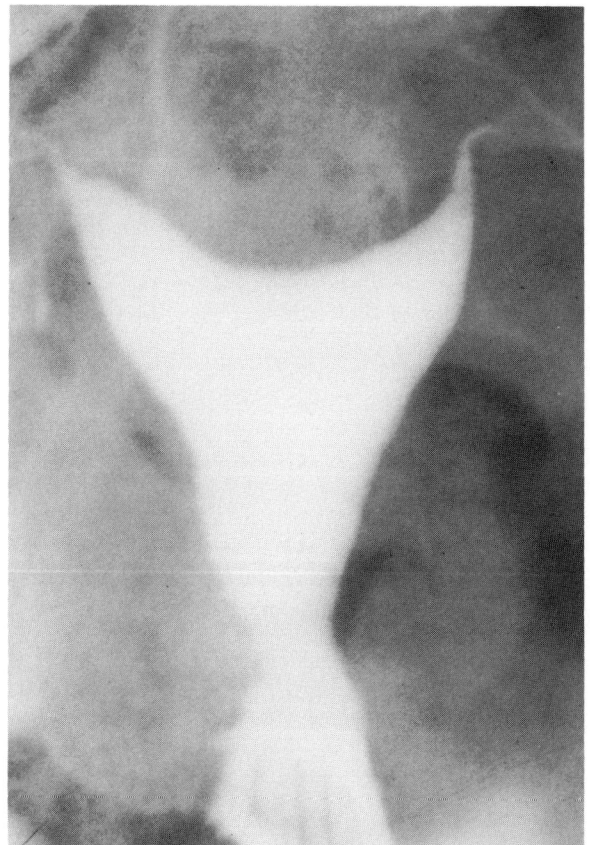

FIGURE 30–42. Hysterosalpingogram. Proximal tubal obstruction at the level of the midintramural tube is shown.

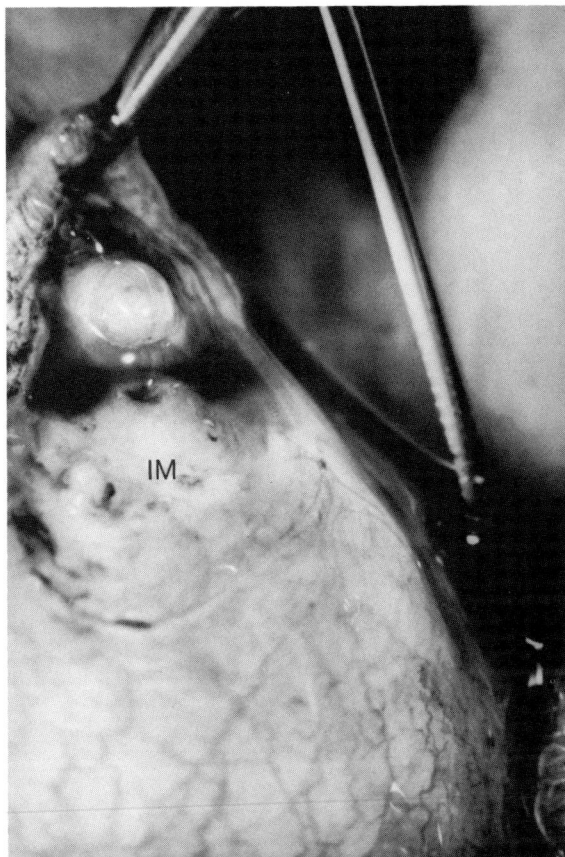

FIGURE 30–43. Uterine cornu. The intramural oviduct (IM) is identified as it traverses the myometrium.

Ancillary measures such as selective HSG or tubal cannulation can assist.

Tubocornual obstruction usually affects the intramural tube (Figs. 30–43 and 30–44) and the contiguous isthmus. More extensive disease tends to encroach laterally into the isthmus.

A recent study examined pregnancy rates following unilateral tubocornual anastomosis (TCA) and contralateral salpingostomy and found a 80% pregnancy rate.[51] This is more consistent with rates found following pure TCAs than after salpingostomies. Taking into consideration the poor success after repair of bipolar disease (disease located at both ends of the oviduct), it is postulated that proximal tubal occlusion represents one extreme of a disease spectrum. An ascending infective process is thought to first involve the tubocornual junction. This may lead to obstruction at the tubocornual junction and thereby impede further ascent of the infectious agent. When the inflammation does not cause obstruction, the infection may spread transmucosally to involve the distal tube to culminate in distal occlusion. Bipolar damage reflects progression of the proximal disease in the presence of distal occlusion and therefore represents involvement of the entire length of the oviduct. This explains the poor success of tubal reconstruction in this situation.[52, 53]

Tubal Polyps. Tubal polyps have been described in association with tubal infertility, although their exact correlation with infertility is still unclear. Polyps have been identified in as many as 10% of HSGs performed for the investigation of infertility[54] and 11% of hysterectomy specimens.[55] They usu-

ally occur in the intramural segment and less often in the isthmus. Microscopically, tubal polyps are composed of endometrial-type mucosa (Figs. 30–45 and 30–46) with a broad-based attachment ranging from 2 to 3 mm to 1 cm.[56] Obstruction of the tubal lumen is possible but rare. Associated pelvic endometriosis has been found in some 41% of patients.[56]

A higher incidence of infertility has been found in a group of patients with tubocornual polyps, but pregnancy rates do not differ[57] when comparing these patients to unaffected patients with unexplained infertility. Despite this, microsurgical removal of tubal polyps in patients with otherwise unexplained infertility has been advocated.[58, 59] However, the studies suffer from small sample sizes and lack of control groups. Therefore, no firm treatment recommendations can be made at present.

Obliterative Fibrosis. In this form of occlusion the tubal lumen is completely obliterated by densely collagenous connective tissue. No other preceding or predisposing condition can be identified. The tubal epithelium is completely destroyed.[49] Obliterative fibrosis has been viewed as a nonspecific response of the tubal epithelium to a variety of stimuli, including inflammation or infection.[49] On inspection or palpation, the tube may appear completely normal.

Salpingitis Isthmica Nodosa. SIN was first described by Chiari[60] in 1887 as epithelial inclusions within the tubal wall (Fig. 30–47). In its more advanced stage, the fibrosis induced by SIN may occlude the tube. It is considerably less common

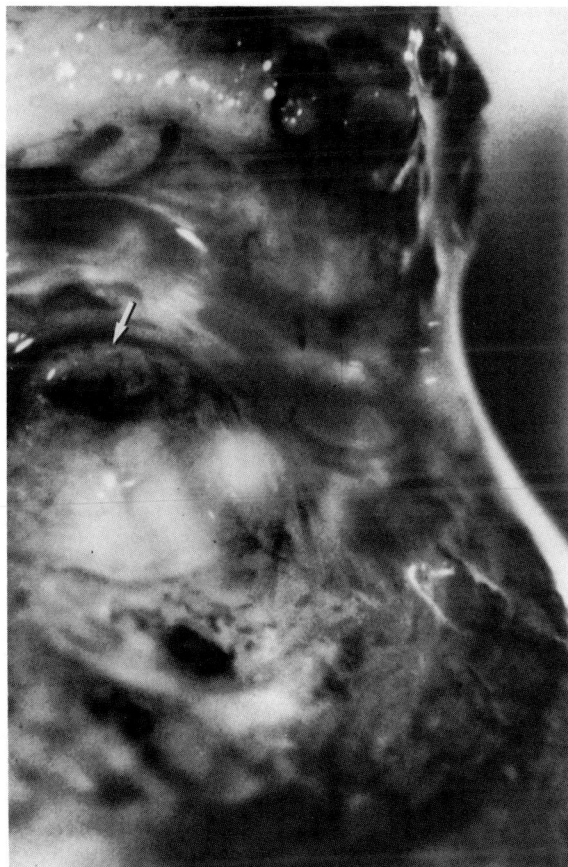

FIGURE 30–44. Uterine cornu. Proximal tubal occlusion often spares the intramural tube. The *arrow* points to the normal vascular pattern.

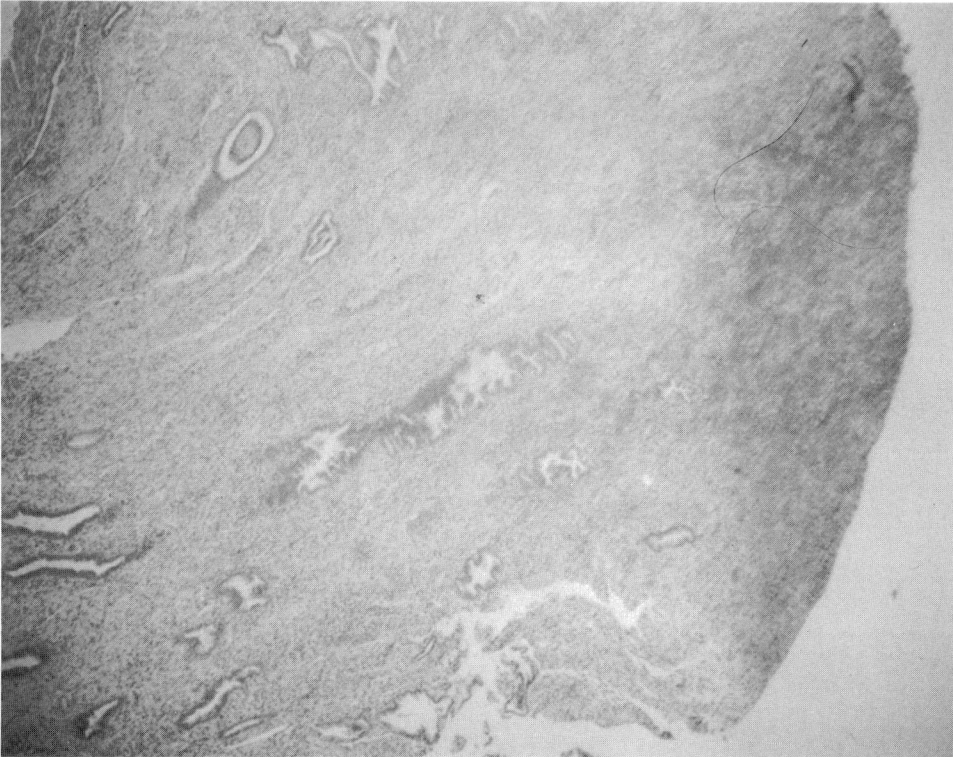

FIGURE 30–45. Histologic section. A cornual polyp is evident. The polyp is derived from endometrium.

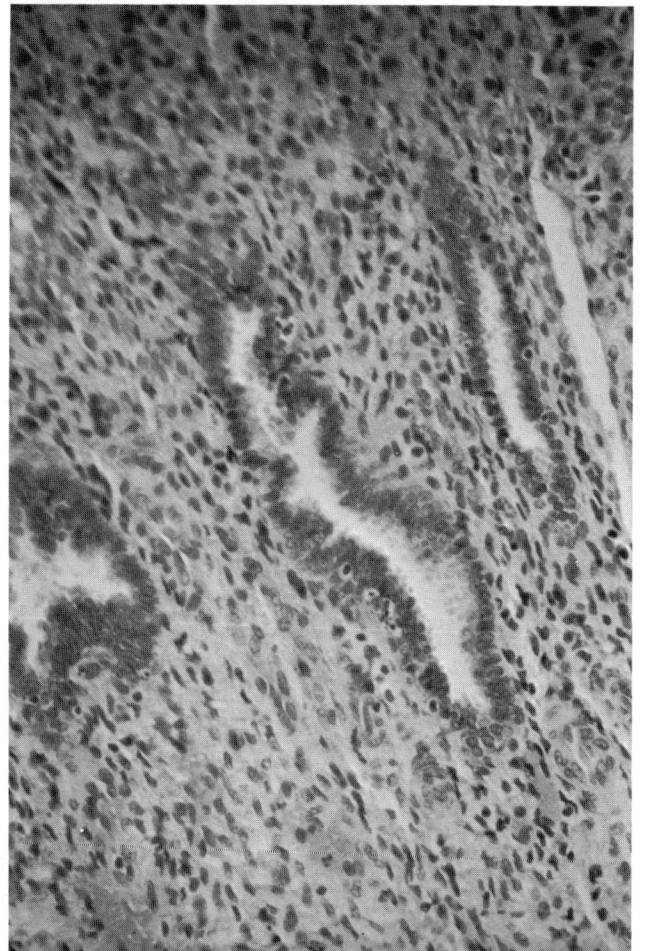

FIGURE 30–46. Histologic section. A cornual polyp showing secretory changes within the endometrial tissue is evident.

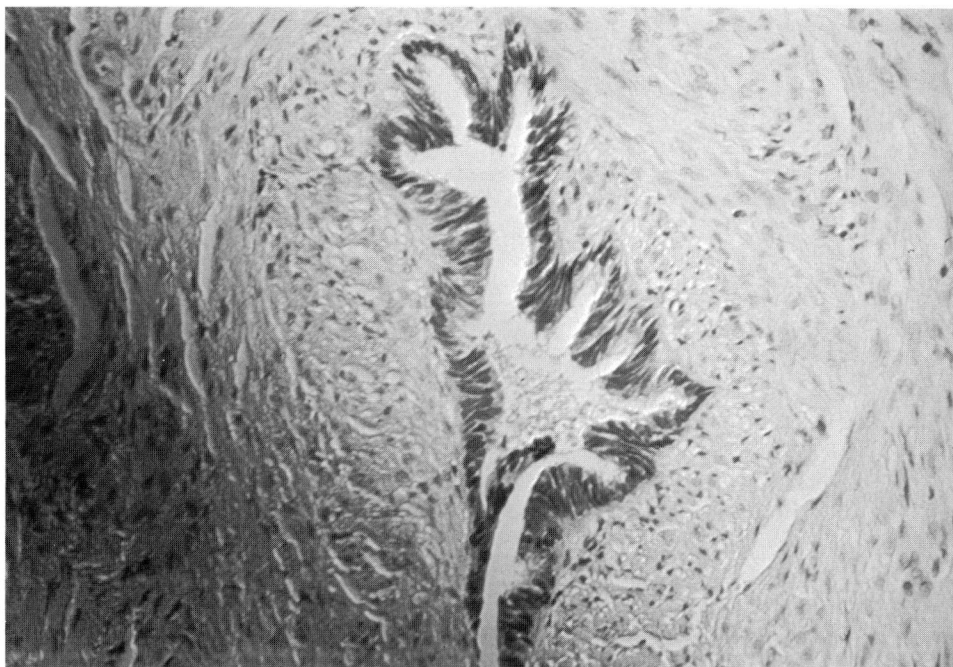

FIGURE 30–47. Histologic section of cornual tissue containing salpingitis isthmica nodosa. Tubal epithelium lines a diverticulum.

than distal tubal disease but is thought to be responsible for as much as 5% of female infertility. At elective sterilization, less than 1% of tubes show evidence of SIN.[61] SIN is identified as the causative histologic abnormality in 23% to 60%[48, 62–64] of cases of proximal tubal occlusion. Of 37 cases of women with isthmic ectopic pregnancy and no other predisposing factors, 46% were found to have SIN in the involved tube.[65] Others have found SIN in 57% of fallopian tubes in a series of 100 ectopic pregnancies.[66] Despite this prevalence, only recently has SIN been acknowledged and thus sought as a potential cause of ectopic pregnancy. Both clinician and pathologist must operate with a high index of suspicion to identify SIN. The documentation of SIN within a woman's fallopian tubes has implications for future management and followup for both infertility and ectopic pregnancy.

Age Distribution. SIN is a disease of woman in the reproductive age group with an age range of 26 to 30 years.[66, 67] It has rarely been described in premenarchal or postmenopausal women. A higher incidence has been noted in the black population in North America and in Jamaicans in retrospective, uncontrolled series.[66, 68]

Site. In one study that established the radiologic appearance of SIN, SIN was identified in 45 patients (in 70 tubes) from 1194 HSG studies.[67] Of these lesions, 35.7% were bilateral, 50% located only in the proximal tube, 28% only in the midtubal region, and 3% only in the distal tube. In 7% the entire tube and in 11% both proximal and midportion were involved. Other authors have reported as many as 85% bilaterality and more than 65% isthmic involvement.[69] A histologic review of 100 ectopic pregnancies found the lesions of SIN located predominantly in the isthmus (63%) rather than the ampulla (37%).[66]

Histology. Histologically, SIN is characterized by nodular hyperplasia and hypertrophy of the muscularis surrounding pseudogland-like structures that are lined by tubal epithelium. The lining epithelium consists of columnar to cuboidal cells with occasional ciliated cells. An attempt to grade the

severity of SIN has proposed that the depth of glandular invasion into the myosalpinx be taken into consideration. No clinical correlation with outcome is available.[66] In a large number of cases, endometrial-like stromal cells may be seen clustered around the diverticula. In contrast, if tubal epithelium is not present, and if both endometrial stroma and endometrial glands are seen, a diagnosis of endometriosis must be made, as distinct from SIN. There is no documented correlation of SIN with endometriosis clinically.

Few have been able to identify histologically the direct connection from the tubal lumen to the pseudogland that is seen at HSG and thereby show direct extension of tubal epithelium from the oviductal lumen to the diverticular pouch.[66] In one case of ectopic pregnancy, implantation was observed within an SIN diverticulum. This prompted the assumption that the mechanical arrest of ovum transport may lead to nidation within a pseudogland.

Apart from isthmic and ampullary pregnancies, SIN has also been reported as the underlying cause in a case of interstitial pregnancy.[70]

Many authors have found histologic evidence of chronic inflammation manifested as lymphocytic infiltration coexisting with SIN as well as evidence of previous infection elsewhere in the pelvis.[64] Others have not been able to demonstrate a difference in the presence of chronic salpingitis in tubes that contain an ectopic pregnancy as well as SIN compared with tubes that contain an ectopic without SIN.[66]

Various synonyms have been used for SIN, including tubal diverticulosis, adenomyosalpingitis, epitheliomyosis, adenosalpingitis, adenomyohyperplasia, and adenomyosis. Some have used the term *endosalpingiosis* interchangeably[69] with SIN, although these are considered two distinct entities by most. Others have described SIN and adenomyosis-like features within the tubal wall following tubal electrocautery.[71] This is in contrast with the usual histologic diagnosis of endometriosis after tubal sterilization. These postcauterization lesions lack the feature of (reactive) muscular hypertrophy and have been coined *endosalpingoblastosis* as opposed to

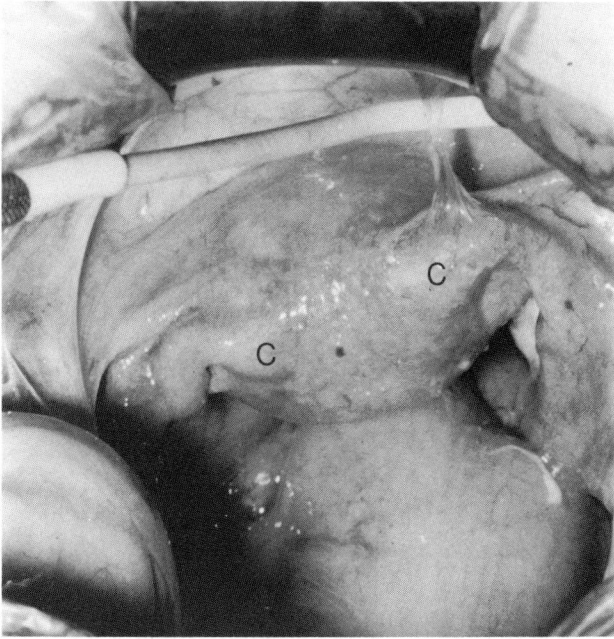

FIGURE 30–48. Microsurgical laparotomy. Salpingitis isthmica nodosa is evident. The adhesion to the cornu (C) signifies the presence of SIN. The cornua are bulbous and firm.

endosalpingiosis. Because both uterine and tubal features may be found in the same specimen, their origin is postulated to be from pluripotent coelomic stem cells.[71] We suggest that the terminology remain as *SIN*.

Diagnosis. The mainstays of diagnosis are the distinctive radiologic and laparoscopic appearances. SIN is radiologically characterized by single or multiple diverticula or tracts in close proximity to the tube. The incidence reported varies from 3.9% to 8.7%[72] of HSGs, likely because of differences in the populations studied or because of differing indications for the HSGs. The differential diagnosis includes contrast extravasation (this disappears on late films), tubal endometriosis, and tuberculosis (these are usually associated with other radiologic features).

At laparoscopy one characteristically notes a nodular, fusiform enlargement with thickening and induration of the isthmus (Fig. 30–48). With injection of a contrast medium, characteristic diverticula may become visible (Fig. 30–49; see color section in the center of the book). The serosa is usually smooth and intact. In one study a hysteroscopic finding of endosalpingeal hyperplasia of the tubal ostium correlated with SIN on histology in six cases.[73]

Etiology. Divergent theories as to the etiology of SIN have been advanced: congenital, inflammatory, hormonal, and mechanical.

SIN has rarely been reported in prepubertal females, although a case report of this occurrence in a diethylstilbestrol (DES)-exposed adolescent does exist.[74] Infertility and ectopic

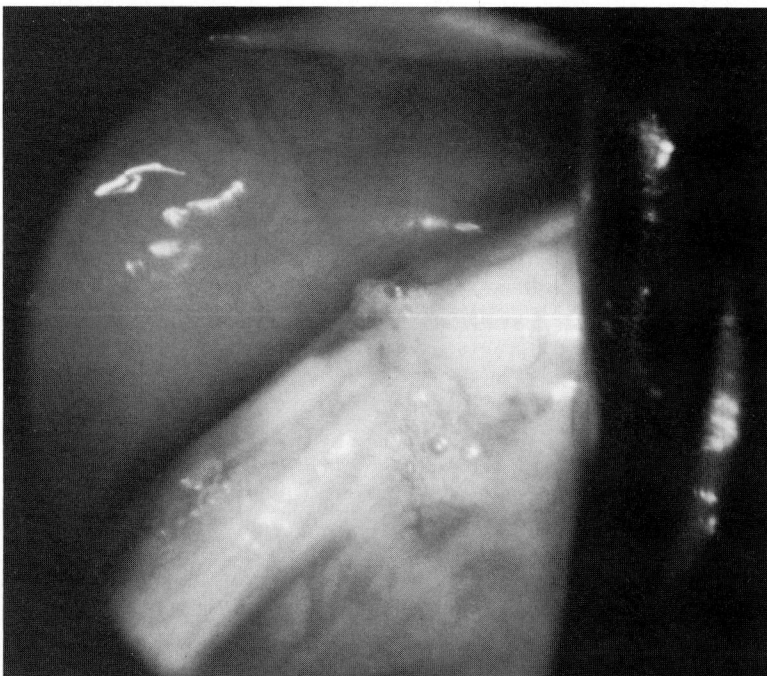

FIGURE 30–49. Laparoscopy. A view of the proximal oviduct is shown. Normal supple myosalpinx has been replaced by salpingitis isthmica nodosa. Note the mucosal diverticula that have penetrated the myosalpinx to reach the tubal serosa.

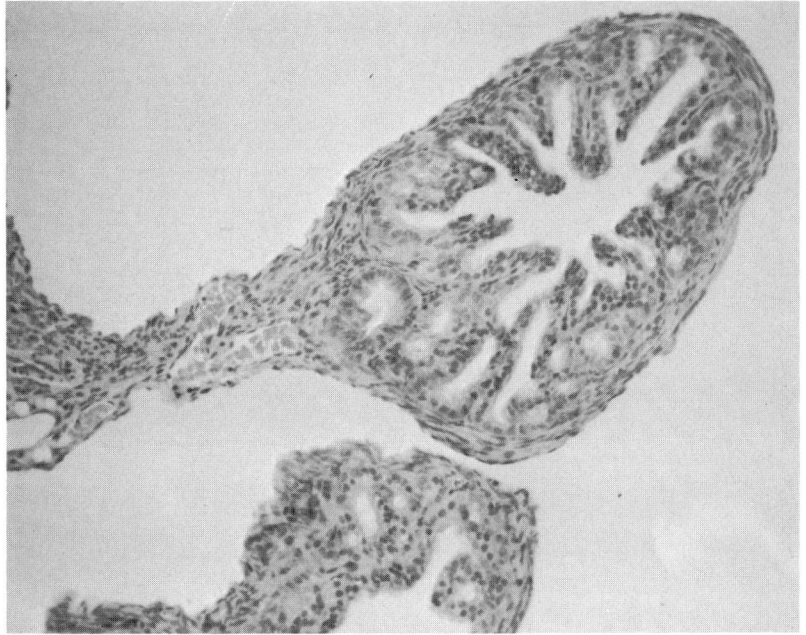

FIGURE 30–50. Histologic section. A mouse oviduct is shown. Diverticular formation has been induced by administration of diethylstilbestrol to the neonatal mouse.

pregnancies are common sequelae in DES-exposed women, but SIN has not frequently been described in association with DES exposure. Neonatal mice injected with DES manifested SIN-like tubal lesions (Fig. 30–50). Continuing hormonal stimulation produces a steady progression of the tubal lesion as well as ovarian cyst formation. This is indirect evidence of a possible hormonal mechanism in the genesis of SIN in women. The absence of muscular hypertrophy in the animal model could implicate a cofactor, possibly inflammation in humans.[75] Others support this theory with the observation that the SIN disease process is similar to adenomyosis. That is, a hormonally sensitive müllerian tissue derivative responds to unknown stimuli by slow proliferation.[76]

Others postulate that chronic tubal spasm of the thick isthmic muscle results in pulsion diverticula akin to diverticulosis coli.[61]

The cause of SIN is thus still unclear, although it is likely to be an acquired condition. An inflammatory-infectious etiology is favored by most investigators. The evidence supporting this view is circumstantial based predominantly on historical, histologic, serologic, and radiologic evidence of associated inflammation or infection.[49, 64, 66, 76]

In retrospective series an association has been found between SIN and primary infertility and ectopic pregnancy. This causal linkage[61, 65] has prompted some to advocate TCA whenever SIN is detected despite patency in the diseased tubes. The decision to advise a TCA in these circumstances is based on the severity of the SIN lesion, the length of time of preceding infertility, and other intercurrent factors such as history of ectopic pregnancy.

SIN appears to be a progressive disease, with an initial increase in size of lesions (Fig. 30–51) eventually leading to complete obliteration of the tubal lumen (Fig. 30–52) despite lack of evidence of a continuing stimulus.[77] This observation suggests that a recent HSG should be available for evaluation before reconstructive surgery is undertaken. It is also recom-

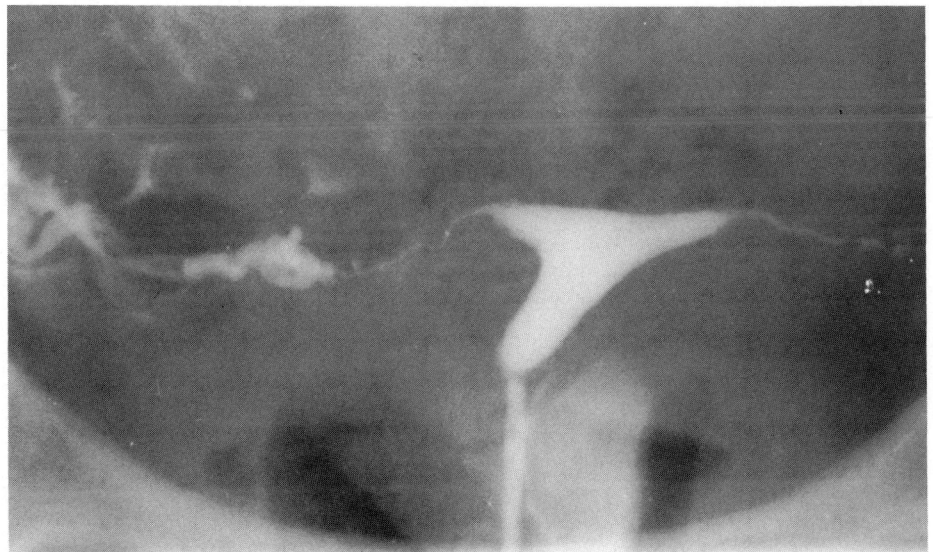

FIGURE 30–51. Hysterosalpingogram. Salpingitis isthmica nodosa is evident. This is seen as diverticula extending from the isthmus.

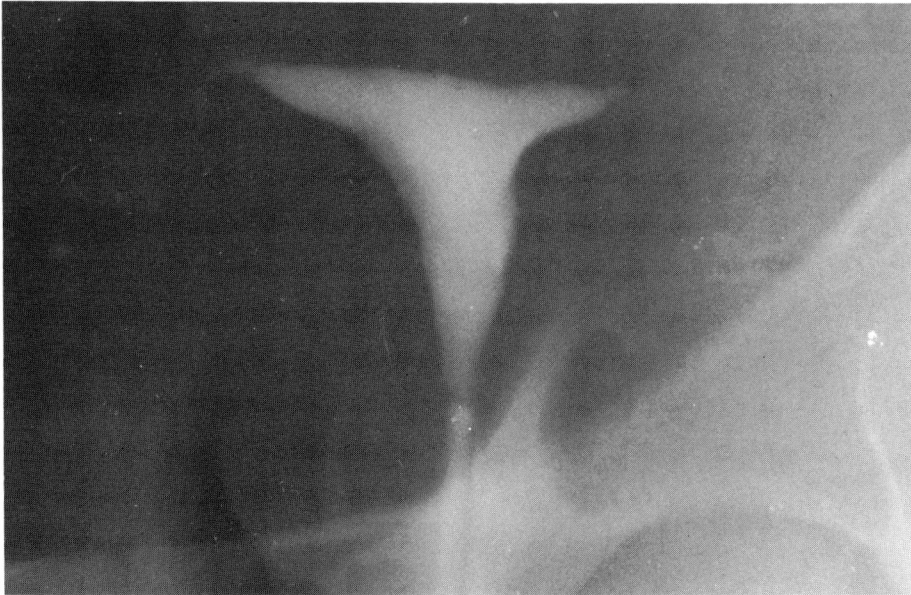

FIGURE 30–52. Hysterosalpingogram. Salpingitis isthmica nodosa (SIN) is evident. This is the same woman as in Figure 30–51 6 years later. The SIN has progressed to frank occlusion.

mended that an HSG be performed after an ectopic pregnancy to investigate for SIN.

Clinical Implications. Recent studies employing microsurgical TCA have shown good success rates with 57.7% pregnancies and 15% ectopic pregnancies in all cases of tubocornual obstruction.[13] This high rate of success is upheld even when SIN is identified as the underlying disease process.[6, 13] These results were again confirmed in a recent article examining pregnancy rates in unilateral TCA and contralateral salpingostomy.[52] Other authors have reported lower overall success (44% intrauterine pregnancies) and a worse outcome for cases of "endosalpingiosis" (likely SIN) with only 26% pregnancies. In these series the best outcomes with TCA have been found with preserved intramural portion of tube and in the absence of tubal inclusions and endometriosis.[62, 69]

SIN is a distinct disease of the proximal tube that has only recently been associated with a high incidence of infertility and ectopic pregnancy. The progressive nature of SIN poses unique diagnostic and therapeutic challenges to both pathologist and clinician. Of all the current pathophysiologic conditions of the oviduct, this disease most warrants research.

Endosalpingiosis. Endosalpingiosis was initially described by Sampson in 1930.[78] It has been defined as tubal type epithelium in an ectopic location, that is, involving peritoneal surfaces. These lesions usually appear as small, clear cysts, microscopically lined by fallopian tube–type epithelium. As with SIN, it has been found in association with ectopic pregnancy and has been described following salpingectomy.[78] These endosalpingeal outpouchings are distinguished from SIN by the absence of characteristic myosalpingeal hypertrophy. Such lesions have been noted in tubes following tubal ligation (Fig. 30–53).

Endometriosis. Endometriosis that is intrinsic to the oviduct is a relatively uncommon finding with an incidence of 7%[62] to 14%[49, 64, 69] in patients operated on for isthmic tubal occlusion (Fig. 30–54; see color section in the center of the book) and infertility. Unlike SIN, there are no synonyms for endometriosis that involves the oviduct. Other foci of endometriosis are often identified elsewhere in the pelvis (reported prevalence of 30%[64] to 100%).[49] Fertility outcome after TCA for proximal tubal endometriosis has been reported as relatively poor, with a 0 to 12% pregnancy rate as compared with 41% to 44% overall for TCA in two series.[62, 69] In these series endometriosis was histologically identified only in conjunction with a radiologic finding of numerous diverticular lesions. A high recurrence rate is postulated for tubal

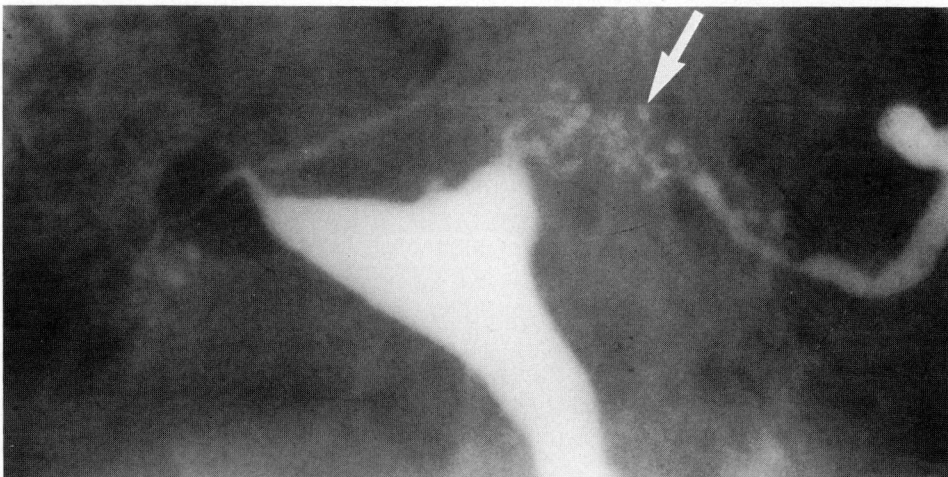

FIGURE 30–53. Hysterosalpingogram. Endometriosis (*arrow*) of the proximal oviduct secondary to tubal sterilization is evident.

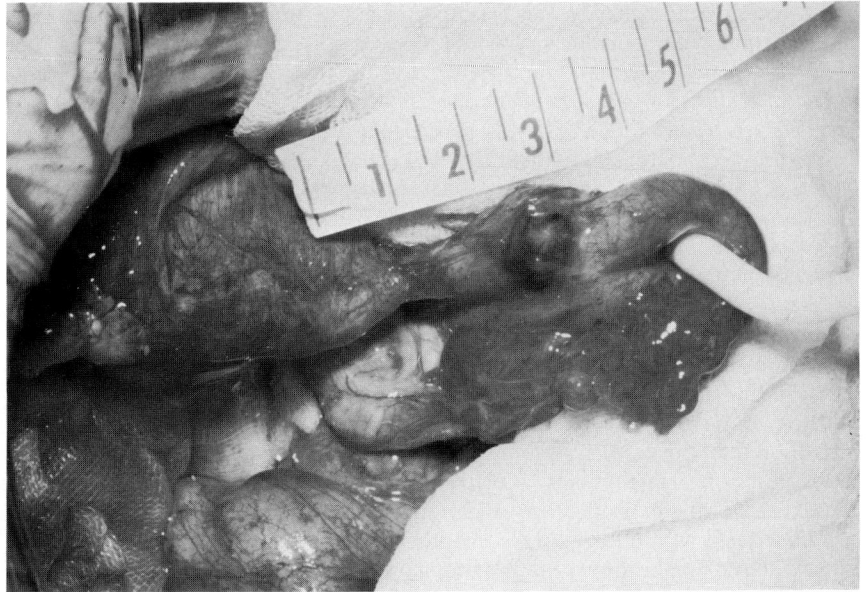

FIGURE 30–54. Microsurgical laparotomy. Tubal endometriosis is evident. A nodule of endometriosis occludes the midtube.

endometriosis with a reocclusion rate of 63% at 1 year. It is suggested that in known cases of tubal endometriosis, the excision of a generous portion of isthmic tube might be advisable in an attempt to decrease recurrence rates.[18] This and other studies have linked pregnancy rates to the length of preserved tube.[79] Another series of TCA reported pregnancies in two of four patients with endometriosis.[13]

Endometriosis that affects the pelvis generally may involve the oviducts extrinsically by scarring. This scars the ovary to the pelvic sidewall and ampulla to ovary initially; it then may proceed to cul-de-sac obliteration and fusion of bowel, ovary, uterus, and oviducts. Curiously, the fimbriae tend to be spared and frequently remain patent (Fig. 30–55).

ECTOPIC PREGNANCY

The ectopic implantation of a pregnancy is a gross perturbation of normal transport into and through the fallopian tube.[5]

Whereas 95% of ectopic pregnancies pertain to the oviduct, the other 5% may implant elsewhere in the peritoneal cavity, the omentum, and the ovary.[80]

The incidence of ectopic pregnancy has increased significantly over the last two decades. This has been attributed predominantly to the concurrent prevalence of PID, manifested as chronic salpingitis and follicular salpingitis.[81, 82]

SIN has become increasingly implicated as a predisposing condition over the last decade. Yet the etiologic relationship of SIN to PID has not been elucidated. In those gestation-bearing oviducts fully 45% to 57% contain SIN[66, 83] compared with 5% in control oviducts. Previous ectopic pregnancy, prior reconstructive pelvic surgery, in utero DES exposure, use of an intrauterine device (although this may relate to salpingitis), and history of infertilty are additional factors. All these entities relate to tubal damage. Those women subfertile with ciliary dyskinesia do not have a proclivity to tubal pregnancy, although impaired tubal transport is the postulated reason for their fertility lack. This points to the effect of the disease on the oviduct as the most important factor predis-

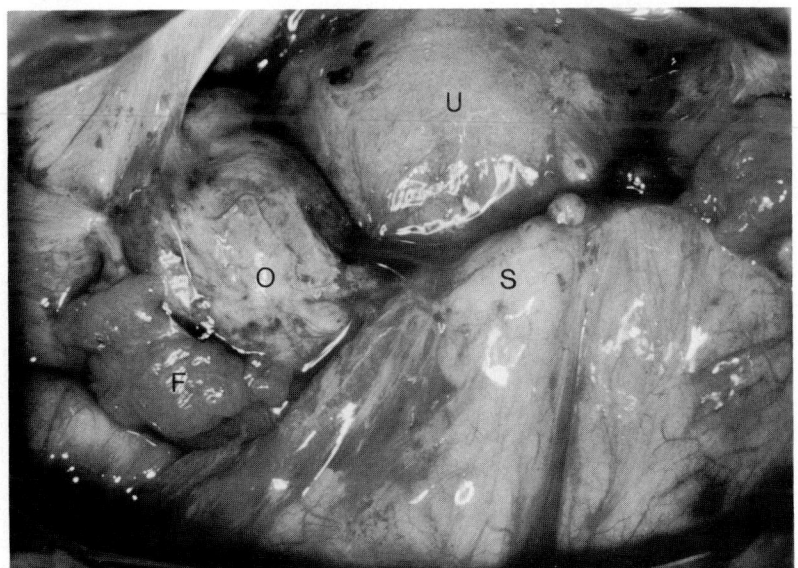

FIGURE 30–55. Endometriosis. Fusion of the pelvic organs has occurred. The fimbriae are spared. U, uterus; O, ovary; S, sigmoid colon; F, fimbria.

posing to ectopic pregnancy. This is supported by the finding of deciliation within oviducts containing an ectopic gestation.[84]

The *ampulla* is the most frequent site of an ectopic tubal pregnancy (75% to 80%).[80] This is perhaps surprising, because the site of SIN is most often isthmic (63.2% isthmic, 36.8% ampullary).[66] It may be postulated that the morula/blastocyst within the nonaffected segment of isthmus is undergoing to-and-fro excursions conferred by myosalpingeal contractility. The hypertrophic and fibrotic SIN "splints" the proximal isthmus and is a functional barrier to the passage of the embryo.[61, 85] Accordingly, the blastocyst is more likely to be exposed to the distal isthmus and proximal ampulla at the time that implantation is to take place. The nutritive ampullary mucosa may be more receptive to implantation than the adjacent isthmic epithelium. Another factor predisposing to ampullary implantation may be the increased size of the expanded blastocyst: this would be better accommodated within the ampulla than the isthmus. Hence, SIN of the proximal isthmus and intramural tube may predispose to ampullary ectopic pregnancy.

The *isthmus* is the next most likely site for an ectopic pregnancy. The occurrence of an isthmic ectopic pregnancy is considered evidence of underlying isthmic disease.

The ectopic trophoblast may penetrate the myosalpinx to become extraluminal in some instances.

These observations are pertinent to the surgical management. With an ampullary ectopic pregnancy, one may conserve the ampulla by linear salpingotomy because it is likely to be normal. An isthmic ectopic pregnancy is often treated by segmental resection, although subsequent intrauterine pregnancy may occur after linear salpingotomy of the isthmic segment. The extraluminal site of a proportion of ectopic pregnancies mandates that the site of implantation be evaluated at surgery, and, in particular, that follow-up human chorionic gonadotropin levels are determined to exclude persistence of trophoblastic tissue.

The consequences of the linear salpingotomy on gamete transport have been evaluated: near normal[86] ampullary structure and ciliary transport is preserved.

Cornual (interstitial) ectopic pregnancies are uncommon and frequently associated with underlying disease. For this reason, if the ectopic pregnancy is removed with conservation of the cornu, investigation to exclude SIN and related conditions is warranted.

Arrested (Chronic) Ectopic Pregnancy

Arrested ectopic pregnancies are found within the cornu, the isthmus, and the ampulla. The causation is the same as for acute tubal pregnancies. The differential diagnosis includes endometriosis, adenomatoid tumor, leiomyoma, tuberculosis, and SIN. The transected chronic ectopic is often yellow, fatty, and friable. Ghost villi may be seen by light microscopy; otherwise, direct immunostaining for human chorionic gonadotropin may confirm the diagnosis.

CONCLUSION

The pathophysiology of the fallopian tube is a changing subject. Societal mores influence directly the form and prevalence of oviductal disease, infertility, and ectopic pregnancy.

Such change is reflected in one tubal lesion in particular, SIN.

An understanding of the function of the oviduct allows fertility to be assessed when there is oviductal disease and to be predicted after therapy of diseases of the fallopian tube.

REFERENCES

1. Gomel V, McComb P. Microsurgery in reproductive physiology. In: Gomel V, editor. Microsurgery in Female Infertility. Boston: Little, Brown, 1983:29–50.
2. Bonilla-Musoles F, Ferrer-Barriendos J, Pelliger A. Cyclical changes in the epithelium of the fallopian tube. Clin Exp Obstet Gynecol 1983;10:79–86.
3. Donnez J, Casanas-Roux F, Caprasse J, et al. Cyclic changes in ciliation, cell height, and mitotic activity in human tubal epithelium during reproductive life. Fertil Steril 1985;43:554–559.
4. Helm G, Owman C, Sjoeberg NO, Walles B. Motor activity of the human fallopian tube in vitro in relation to plasma concentration of oestradiol and progesterone, and the influence of noradrenaline. J Reprod Fertil 1982;64:233–242.
5. Jansen RPS. Endocrine response in the fallopian tube. Endo Rev 1984;5:525–551.
6. McComb PF, Moon Y. Prostaglandin E and F concentration in the fimbria of the rabbit fallopian tube increases at the time of ovulation. Acta Eur Fertil 1985;16:423–426.
7. Gomel V, McComb P. Microsurgery in gynecology. In: Silber SJ, editor. Microsurgery, Baltimore: Williams & Wilkins, 1979:143–184.
8. McComb P, Bourdage RJ, Halbert SA. Suppressed ovulatory function and oviductal microsurgery in the rabbit. Fertil Steril 1981;35:481–482.
9. McComb P, Delbeke L. Decreasing the number of ovulations in the rabbit with surgical division of the blood vessels between the fallopian tube and ovary. J Reprod Med 1984;29:827–829.
10. Critoph FN, Dennis KJ. Ciliary activity in the human oviduct. Br J Obstet Gynaecol 1977;84:216–218.
11. Gaddum-Rosse P, Blandau RJ. In vitro studies on ciliary activity within the oviduct of the rabbit and pig. Am J Anat 1973;136:91–104.
12. Merchant RN, Prabhu SR, Chougale A. Uterotubal junction: morphology and clinical aspects. Int J Fertil 1983;28:199–205.
13. McComb P. Microsurgical tubocornual anastomosis for occlusive cornual disease: reproducible results without the need for tubouterine implantation. Fertil Steril 1986;46:571–574.
14. McComb P, Filmar S, Pabuccu R. Successful transplantation of a free fimbrial graft to the peritoneum. J Reprod Med 1989;34:55–58.
15. McComb PF. Free autologous graft of fimbria to ampulla with subsequent oviductal function. J Reprod Med 1992;37:223–226.
16. Winston RML, McClure-Browne JC. Pregnancy following autograft transplantation of fallopian tube and ovary in the rabbit. Lancet 1974;2:494–495.
17. McComb P, Gomel V. The effect of segmental ampullary reversal on the subsequent fertility of the rabbit. Fertil Steril 1979;31:83–85.
18. Harper MJK. Gamete and zygote transport. In: Knobil E, Neill J, editors. The Physiology of Reproduction. New York: Raven Press, 1988:103–134.
19. McComb P, Gomel V. The influence of fallopian tube length on fertility in the rabbit. Fertil Steril 1979;31:3–6.
20. McComb P, Halbert SA. Reproduction in rabbits after excision of the oviductal isthmus, ampullary-isthmic junction and utero-isthmic junction. Fertil Steril 1981;35:640–677.
21. Halbert SA, McComb P, Patton DL. Function and structure of the rabbit oviduct following fimbriectomy: I. Distal ampullary salpingostomy. Fertil Steril 1981;35:349–354.
22. Halbert SA, McComb P, Patton DL. Function and structure of the rabbit oviduct following fimbriectomy: II. Proximal ampullary salpingostomy. Fertil Steril 1981;35:355–358.
23. Coppo M, McComb P, Halbert S. The functional potential of the fimbria in the rabbit. J Reprod Med 1984;29:731–735.
24. Halbert SA, McComb PF, Bourdage RJ. The structural and functional impact of microsurgical anastomosis on the rabbit oviductal isthmus. Fertil Steril 1981;36:653–658.
25. Lurie M, Tur-Kaspa I, Weill S, et al. Ciliary ultrastructure of respiratory and fallopian tube epithelium in a sterile woman with Kartagener's syndrome. Chest 1989;95:578–581.
26. McComb P, Verdugo P, Langley L. The oviductal cilia and Kartagener's syndrome. Fertil Steril 1986;46:412–416.

27. Donnez J, Casanas-Roux F, Ferin J, Thomas K. Tubal polyps, epithelial inclusions, and endometriosis after tubal sterilization. Fertil Steril 1984;41:564–568.

28. Rock JA, Parmley TH, King TM, et al. Endometriosis and the development of tuboperitoneal fistulas after tubal ligation. Fertil Steril 1981;35:16–20.

29. Vasquez G, Winston RML, Boeckx W, Brosens I. Tubal lesions subsequent to sterilization and their relation to fertility after attempts at reversal. Am J Obstet Gynecol 1980;138:86–92.

30. Paterson PJ, Chan CLK. Congenital absence of fallopian tube segments. Aust NZ J Obstet Gynaecol 1985;25:130–131.

31. Bates GW, Abide JK. Bilateral autoamputation of the fallopian tubes. Fertil Steril 1982;38:253–254.

32. Beyth Y, Kopolovic J. Accessory tubes: a possible contributing factor in infertility. Fertil Steril 1982;38:382–383.

33. Yablonski M, Sarge T, Wild RA. Subtle variations in tubal anatomy in infertile women. Fertil Steril 1990;54:455–458.

34. Wanermann J, Wulwick R, Brenner S. Segmental absence of the fallopian tube. Fertil Steril 1986;46:525–527.

35. Urman CB, McComb P. Midtubal obstruction after inguinal hernia repair. J Reprod Med 1991;36:175–176.

36. Donnez J, Casanas-Roux F, Nisolle-Pochet M, et al. Surgical management of tubal obstruction at the uterotubal junction. Acta Eur Fertil 1987;18:5–9.

37. Patton DL, Moore DE, Spadoni LR, et al. A comparison of the fallopian tube's response to overt and silent salpingitis. Obstet Gynecol 1989;73:622–630.

38. Vasquez G, Winston RML, Boeckx W, et al. The epithelium of human hydrosalpinges: a light optical and scanning microscopic study. Br J Obstet Gynecol 1983;90:764–770.

39. Baldetorp B, Mardh P-A, Weström L. Studies on ciliated epithelia of the human genital tract. STD 1983;11(Suppl):363–365.

40. Boer-Meisel ME, te Velde ER, Habbema JDF, Kardaun JWPF. Predicting the pregnancy outcome in patients treated for hydrosalpinx: a prospective study. Fertil Steril 1986;45:23–29.

41. Donnez J, Casanas-Roux F. Prognostic factors of fimbrial microsurgery. Fertil Steril 1986;46:200–204.

42. McComb PF, Paleologou A. The intussusception technique for the therapy of distal oviductal occlusion at laparoscopy. Obstet Gynecol 1991;78:443–447.

43. Bateman BG, Nunley WC, Kitchin JD III. Surgical management of distal tubal obstruction—are we making progress? Fertil Steril 1987;48:523–542.

44. Donnez J, Casanas-Roux F, Ferin J, Thomas K. Fimbrial ciliated cell percentage and epithelial height during and after salpingitis. Eur J Obstet Gynecol Reprod Biol 1984;17:293–299.

45. Kutteh WH, Albert T. Mature cystic teratoma of the fallopian tube associated with an ectopic pregnancy. Obstet Gynecol 1991;78:984–986.

46. Schaefer G. Tuberculosis of the female genital tract. Clin Obstet Gynecol 1970;13:965–998.

47. McComb P, Gomel V, Rowe T. Investigation of tuboperitoneal causes of female infertility. In: Insler V, Lunenfeld B, editors. Infertility. London: Churchill Livingstone, 1986:213–240.

48. Campbell JS, Nigam S, Hurtig A, et al. Mineral oil granulomas of the uterus and parametrium and granulomatous salpingitis with Schaumann bodies and oxalate deposits. Fertil Steril 1964;15:278–287.

49. Fortier J, Haney AF. The pathologic spectrum of uterotubal junction obstruction. Obstet Gynecol 1985;65:93–98.

50. Sulak PJ, Letterie GS, Coddington CC, et al. Histology of proximal tubal obstruction. Fertil Steril 1987;48:437–440.

51. McComb PF, Lee NH, Stephenson MD. Reproductive outcome after unilateral tubocornual anastomosis and contralateral salpingostomy by microsurgery. Fertil Steril 1991;55:1011–1013.

52. McComb PF, Lee NH, Stephenson MD. Reproductive outcome after microsurgery for proximal and distal occlusions in the same fallopian tube. Fertil Steril 1991;56:134–135.

53. Patton PE, Williams TJ, Coulam CB. Results of microsurgical reconstruction in patients with combined proximal and distal tubal occlusion: double obstruction. Fertil Steril 1987;48:1–4.

54. Reasbeck J, Wynn-Williams G, Gillett W. Tubal intramural polyps: incidence and radiographic demonstration. Aust Radiol 1988;32:117–121.

55. Lisa JR, Gioia J, Rubin IC. Observations of the interstitial portion of the fallopian tube. Surg Gynecol Obstet 1954;99:159–169.

56. Gordts S, Boeckx W, Vasquez G, Brosens I. Microsurgical resection of intramural polyps. Fertil Steril 1983;40:258–259.

57. Glazener CMA, Loveden LM, Richardson SJ, et al. Tubo-cornual polyps: their relevance in subfertility. Hum Reprod 1987;2:59–62.

58. McLaughlin DS. Successful pregnancy outcome following removal of bilateral cornual polyps by microsurgical linear salpingotomy with the aid of the CO_2 laser. Fertil Steril 1984;42:939–941.

59. Stangel JJ, Chervenak FA, Mouradian-Davidian M. Microsurgical resection of bilateral fallopian tube polyps. Fertil Steril 1981;35:580–582.

60. Chiari H. Zur pathologischen Anatomie des Eileitercatarrhs. Z Heilkunde 1887;8:457–473.

61. Honore LH. Salpingitis isthmica nodosa in female infertility and ectopic pregnancy. Fertil Steril 1978;29:164–168.

62. Donnez J, Casanas-Roux F. Histology: a prognostic factor in proximal tubal occlusion. Eur J Obstet Gynecol Reprod Biol 1988;29:33–38.

63. Jansen RPS. Tubal resection and anastomosis: II. Isthmic salpingitis. Aust NZ J Obstet Gynaecol 1986;26:300–304.

64. Punnonen R, Soederstroem KO, Alanen A. Isthmic tubal occlusion: etiology and histology. Acta Eur Fertil 1984;15:39–42.

65. Homm RJ, Holtz G, Garvin AJ. Isthmic ectopic pregnancy and salpingitis isthmica nodosa. Fertil Steril 1987;48:756–760.

66. Majmudar B, Henderson PH, Semple E. Salpingitis isthmica nodosa: a high-risk factor for tubal pregnancy. Obstet Gynecol 1983;62:73–78.

67. Creasy JF, Clark RL, Cuttino JT, Groff TR. Salpingitis isthmica nodosa: radiologic and clinical correlates. Radiology 1985;154:597–600.

68. Persaud V. Etiology of tubal ectopic pregnancy: radiologic and pathologic studies. Obstet Gynecol 1970;36:257–263.

69. Donnez J, Casanas-Roux F. Prognostic factors influencing the pregnancy rate after microsurgical cornual anastomosis. Fertil Steril 1986;46:1089–1092.

70. Petersen LK, Clausen I. Repeated contralateral ectopic pregnancy. Int J Gynecol Obstet 1989;29:185–187.

71. McCausland A. Endosalpingiosis ("endosalpingoblastosis") following laparoscopic tubal coagulation as an etiologic factor of ectopic pregnancy. Am J Obstet Gynecol 1982;143:12–22.

72. Karasick S, Karasick D, Schilling J. Salpingitis isthmica nodosa in female infertility. J Can Assoc Radiol 1985;36:118–121.

73. Vancaillie T, Schmidt EH. The uterotubal junction. J Reprod Med 1988;33:624–629.

74. Shen CC, Bausal M, Purrazzella R, et al. Benign glandular inclusions in lymph nodes, endosalpingiosis, and salpingitis isthmica nodosa in a young girl with clear cell adenocarcinoma of the cervix. Am J Surg Pathol 1983;7:293–300.

75. Newbold RR, Bullock BC, McLachlan JA. Diverticulosis and salpingitis isthmica nodosa (SIN) of the fallopian tube. Am J Pathol 1984;117:333–335.

76. Benjamin CL, Beaver DC. Pathogenesis of salpingitis isthmica nodosa. Am J Clin Pathol 1951;21:212–222.

77. McComb PF, Rowe TC. Salpingitis isthmica nodosa: evidence it is a progressive disease. Fertil Steril 1989;51:542–525.

78. Sampson JA. Postsalpingectomy endometriosis (endosalpingiosis). Am J Obstet Gynecol 1930;20:443–480.

79. Gomel V. Results of reconstructive infertility surgery. In: Gomel V, editor. Microsurgery in Female Infertility. Boston: Little, Brown, 1983:236.

80. Breen JL. A 21-year survey of 654 ectopic pregnancies. Am J Obstet Gynecol 1970;106:1004–1019.

81. Stock RJ. Histopathology of fallopian tubes with recurrent tubal pregnancy. Obstet Gynecol 1990;75:9–14.

82. Weström L, Bengtsson LPH, Mardh P-A. Incidence, trends, and risks of ectopic pregnancy in a population of women. Br Med J 1970;282:15–18.

83. Green LK, Kott ML. Histopathologic finding in ectopic tubal pregnancy. Int J Gynecol Pathol 1989;8:255–262.

84. Vasquez G, Winston RML, Brosens I. Tubal mucosa and ectopic pregnancy. Br J Obstet Gynaecol 1983;90:468–474.

85. Wrork DH, Broders AC. Adenomyosis of the fallopian tube. Am J Obstet Gynecol 1942;44:412–432.

86. McComb PF. Linear ampullary salpingotomy heals better by secondary versus primary closure. Acta Eur Fertil 1985;16:401–404.

CHAPTER 31

Treatment of Disorders of the Fallopian Tube

MICHAEL P. DIAMOND and
ALAN B. COPPERMAN

An early surgical attempt to correct infertility secondary to tubal damage was made in 1909 by Estes,[1] who directly implanted an ovary into the endometrial cavity. He reported a 15% pregnancy rate but no term pregnancies. Attempts have since been made to replace the damaged fallopian tube with plastic prostheses,[2] vermiform appendices,[3] and homotransplanted and allotransplanted fallopian tubes. Today, however, in vitro fertilization and other reproductive technologies have success rates far beyond that expected from experimental procedures, and only certain procedures involving reconstructive tubal surgery remain efficacious.

The operating microscope was first used in 1921, employed at that time to drain middle ear infections. It was not until the 1970s, however, that its potential benefits were first explored by the gynecologist. Optimal microsurgery requires an experienced surgeon who has had advanced training because the first attempt at microsurgical reconstruction yields better results than subsequent attempts at revision.[4] The term *microsurgery* refers not simply to magnification, but to meticulous hemostasis, minimized tissue handling, prevention of tissue desiccation, avoidance of contamination by foreign bodies such as talc, and use of fine suture material with minimal reactivity.[5]

Importantly, although the principles of gynecologic microsurgery were described for the performance of infertility procedures at laparotomy, their application should not be limited to this specialized situation. Rather, these principles should be applied to the extent possible in all surgical procedures regardless of whether infertility is an issue and regardless of whether the procedure is performed by laparotomy or laparoscopy. Additionally, several corollaries to the principles of gynecologic microsurgery should be recognized. Not only is it important to minimize tissue handling, but also when tissue handling must be performed, it should be done as atraumatically as possible. In this way, tissue injury can be minimized. Also, it is important not only to attain hemostasis, but also to do so in a manner that leaves as little devitalized tissue as possible. Thus large avascular pedicles should not be created, and areas of coagulation should be minimized so as not to leave large areas of eschar. The use of magnifica-

tion, either with a microscope or loupes, is often helpful for precise identification of bleeding sites and for tubal anastomosis. Although it is generally considered that magnification improves the clinical outcome of many infertility procedures, well-designed studies demonstrating such improvement have not been performed. Lastly, one of the principles of gynecologic microsurgery that has been taught for many years may not be correct. Precise reapproximation of tissue planes, rather than reducing adhesions, may actually predispose to the postoperative development of adhesions. This may be due to increased tissue handling at these sites, the sutures or clips used for approximation, or tissue ischemia induced by closure.

An analysis of tubal function and dysfunction must be preceded by an understanding of normal tubal anatomy and physiology. The fallopian tube is a complex organ composed of sequential, varied anatomic components organized to allow conception and the timely transfer of the blastocyst to the endometrial cavity (Fig. 31–1). At ovulation, ovarian ligament and fimbrial activity facilitate ovum pickup from the ruptured graafian follicle. The ovum is then transferred to the ampullary section of the oviduct for fertilization, and most likely aided by ampullary secretions[6] for maturation of the spermatozoa and subsequent fertilization followed by division of the zygote. The oviduct itself undergoes cyclic changes, including changes in cell height, ciliation, and secretory activity during the menstrual cycle. The isthmus and the cornua maintain a tonic state, thereby preventing premature delivery of the zygote into the endometrial cavity. Under hormonal stimulation and on establishment of an adequate endometrium, the isthmus and cornua expel the blastocyst into the endometrial cavity for implantation.

Before undergoing tubal surgery, the presenting couple must be studied to search for other causes of infertility. The basic evaluation includes analysis of seminal fluid and tests for ovulation and tubal patency. Some recommend that fertility surgery be performed during the proliferative phase of the menstrual cycle to decrease the likelihood of infection (occurring during menstruation secondary to shedding) and to work in a less vascular operative field. Demonstration of

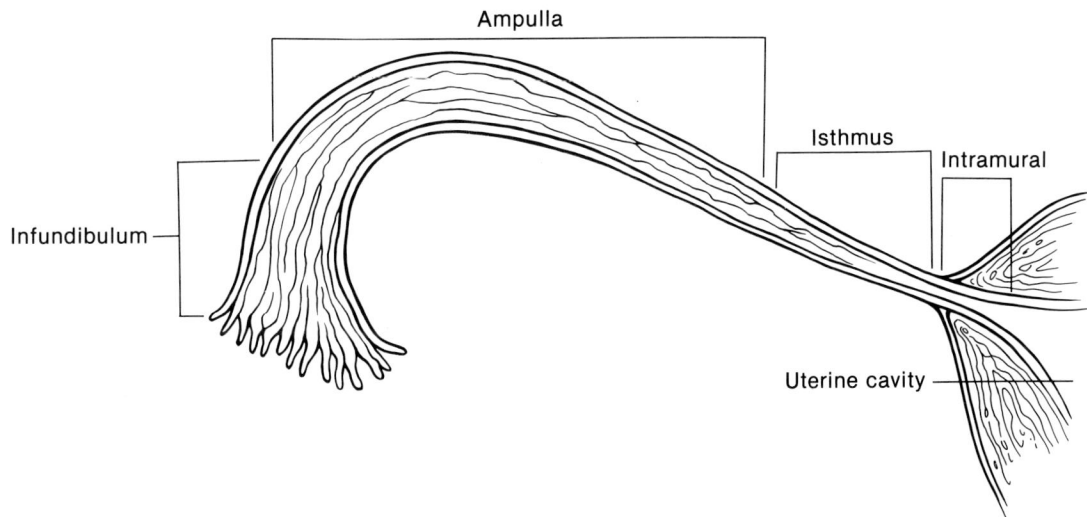

FIGURE 31–1. Anatomy of the fallopian tube.

improved outcome in the preovulatory phase of the cycle, however, is lacking. Similarly, the theoretical advantage of operating in the luteal phase owing to the potential adhesion-preventing abilities of a high progesterone environment has not been demonstrated.

A variety of microsurgical procedures are performed on fallopian tubes and adjacent pelvic structures. Common indications for microsurgery include microsurgical lysis of adhesions (salpingolysis and ovariolysis), fimbrioplasty, salpingostomy, tubal anastomosis and reanastomosis, tubal-cornual anastomosis, endometriosis, myomectomy, ovarian cystectomy, and management of ectopic pregnancy.

In a comparative paper, Fayez and Suliman[7] compared microsurgical with macrosurgical technique. They compared 128 macrosurgical tuboplasties performed between 1971 and 1977 with 73 subsequent comparable operations using microsurgical technique (at least $10\times$ magnification, microsurgical instruments, irrigation rather than sponging, and microcauterization rather than suture ligature). They found that microscopic techniques improved results in all categories evaluated and recommended that microscopic technique be exercised in all tuboplasty procedures. Other analyses have concurred,[8] showing up to a twofold improvement in success rate for both distal and proximal tubal disease treated by microsurgical techniques.

Oelsner and colleagues'[9] study on rabbits further demonstrated the necessity of adequate training and experience for successful microsurgery. Although only 30% of the first group of 20 rabbits to undergo fallopian tube reanastomosis conceived, there was a 100% pregnancy rate in the fifth and final group of 20 animals.

Although often the optimal procedure, relative and absolute contraindications to tubal microsurgery exist. These include tuberculosis of the oviducts, a "frozen pelvis" (in which there are extensive adhesions involving most if not all pelvic organs), the high-risk surgical patient, the patient with contraindications to pregnancy, an inexperienced surgeon, and a patient with a documented recent episode of salpingitis or pelvic peritonitis. An additional consideration is that much of tubal surgery may now be performed endoscopically. Although endoscopic surgery allows for good magnification

and takes advantage of rapid recovery time, smaller scars, and reduced cost, the question that remains to be assessed is the relative efficacy of procedures performed at laparotomy and laparoscopy.

The advances made in tubal reconstructive surgery have not been without drawbacks. The association between ectopic pregnancy and history of prior tubal surgery is well documented. A history of tubal surgery places the patient in a higher risk group for ectopic pregnancy; 3% to 20% of these patients encounter an ectopic pregnancy after the corrective surgery.[10] When the risk of ectopic pregnancy is unacceptably high or when the patient is reluctant to be exposed to a high risk of ectopic pregnancy, in vitro fertilization–embryo transfer (IVF-ET) could be offered as an alternative. In view of the fact that patency rates after tubal surgery are higher than pregnancy rates, it has been suggested that postoperative fallopian tubes most likely experience some loss of function despite the achievement of anatomic patency.

With the improvement of IVF-ET rates, there has been a reanalysis of the efficacy of distal tuboplasty. In a retrospective study,[11] 64 patients who had undergone distal tuboplasty (fimbrioplasty, salpingostomy, and neosalpingostomy) experienced a cumulative postoperative pregnancy rate of 42% and ectopic rate of 17%. These authors concluded that because of the economic burden and technical difficulties associated with IVF, distal tuboplasty remains an appropriate operation. Additional studies[12, 13] have shown even better success rates. Alternatively, technologic advances have enabled one center[14] to achieve a live or ongoing pregnancy rate of 42.7% after three cycles at IVF-ET and 85.3% after six cycles in one group of patients. This success establishes IVF-ET as an effective alternative to surgery for tubal obstruction in some cases. Supporting the authors' position was a comparative analysis of the two modalities[15] from Norway revealing a total cost of $17,000 per live birth following tubal surgery (based on $4000 per operation, multiple operations, and lost work time) and $12,000 after IVF treatment (at their estimated price in Norway of only approximately $1500 per treatment cycle). Furthermore, life-table analyses in that series demonstrated a highly significant increased rate of deliveries after a complete IVF treatment (72.3% per patient) compared with tubal surgery (23.7%, $P<0.001$). These authors also noted a narrowing of indications for tubal surgery and a nearly 50% reduction in the number of tubal operations performed in their hospital. Clearly prospective studies assessing relative efficacy of tubal surgery and assisted reproductive technologies are needed. At the present time, recommendations for tubal surgery or IVF-ET need to be individualized; we believe that the surgical approach is still often appropriate.

FIMBRIOLYSIS

In tubes appropriate for fimbriolysis, the fimbrial surface is essentially healthy, but some fimbria have become attached and phimotic, probably as a result of previous inflammatory exudate. The individual fimbriae are gently "teased" or dissected apart. Both ovariolysis and fimbriolysis are amenable to laparoscopy, and much routine lysis of adhesions can even be performed at diagnostic laparoscopic procedures. The adhesions are often the result of extragenital disease, such as appendicitis, and the endosalpinx is usually spared to a much greater extent than with ascending pelvic infections. The relatively high pregnancy rate of 52% and low ectopic rate of 3.5% following microsurgical lysis of adhesions in a combined series[16] seem to be a result of retained functional tubal integrity.

FIMBRIOPLASTY

In cases of more severe tubal disease, a fimbrioplasty is required. Fimbrioplasty refers to a surgical procedure performed for repair of a partial occlusion of the fimbriated end of the oviduct. In contrast, neosalpingostomy refers to the repair of the totally occluded distal tube. Extensive fimbrial agglutination is the result of pelvic inflammatory disease in the majority of cases and therefore commonly involves the endosalpinx. Fimbrioplasty procedures are performed when there are remnants of fimbriae that appear to be attached to one another. The procedure may include lysis of adhesions within the fimbria, tubal dilatation, incision of a peritoneal ring, or incision of the tubal wall to recover fimbria (Fig. 31–2). The purpose of this procedure is to open the obstructed fallopian tube and salvage enough function of the fimbriae to allow successful entrapment and transport of the oocyte.

Traditional deagglutination and dilatation have given way to finer microsurgical technique. The most commonly encountered condition requiring microsurgical fimbrioplasty appears as a ring of scar tissue that has compressed a tuft of fimbria. The mild form may represent the condition referred to as tubal phimosis. In the severe form, the tube appears similar to a hydrosalpinx until a small opening is located.

After the lysis of any peritubal adhesions that may be present, indigo carmine is injected through a cervical cannula. Attention is turned to the distal end of the tube, often slightly distended by the dye. The scarred serosal layer of the tube is then gently lifted and transected. Under magnification, the avascular line of scar formation can be seen and incised, allowing the often normal fimbria to "pop out." Adhesions between the fimbriae can then be divided sharply,

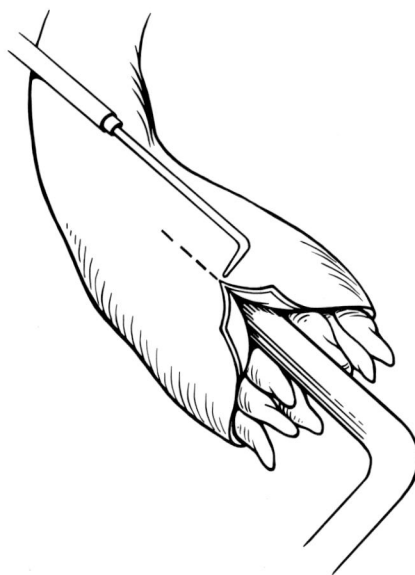

FIGURE 31–2. Incision of the distal fallopian tube to expose fimbria.

with cautery, or via laser (Fig. 31–3). Once the serosa is opened, it can be sutured back to the fallopian tube to free the fimbriae and keep the fallopian tubes patent (Fig. 31–4). Postoperative hydrotubation, once routine and thought to be vital to the success of the operation, has been shown to be ineffective. Good prognostic factors for successful fimbrioplasty include a thin as opposed to a thick tubal wall, a small as opposed to a large degree of ampullary dilatation, and a high fimbrial ciliated cell percentage.[17] One series[18] of microsurgical fimbrioplasty resulted in pregnancy in 68% of 40 patients, of which 25 were intrauterine and 2 were ectopic.

At the present time, fimbrioplasty remains the primary mode of therapy for incomplete distal tubal occlusion, with IVF-ET reserved for those patients failing to attain pregnancy during a predetermined period of treatment postfimbrioplasty. This length of time varies, depending on the severity

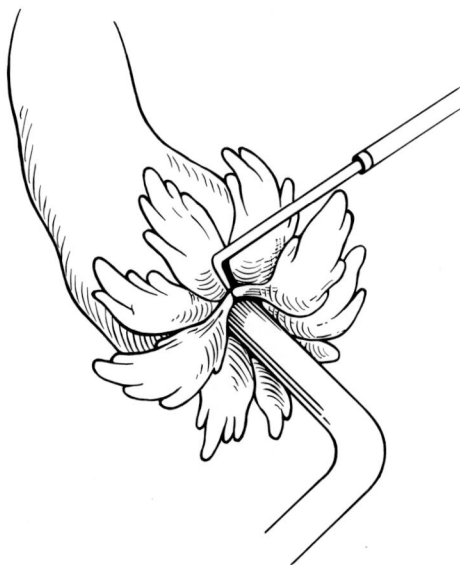

FIGURE 31–3. Division of an adhesion within the fimbria.

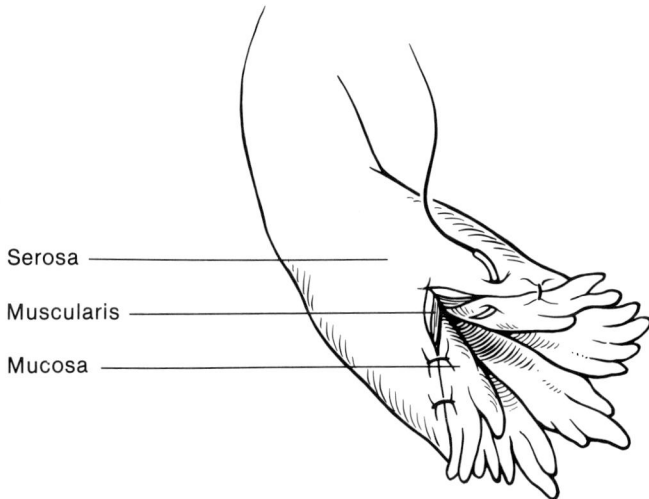

FIGURE 31-4. Placement of tiny sutures to maintain distal patency.

TABLE 31-1. Rock Classification of the Extent of Tubal Disease with Distal Tubal Obstruction

Extent of Disease	Findings
Mild	Absent or small hydrosalpinx ≤15 mm diameter
	Inverted fimbria easily recognized when patency achieved
	No significant peritubal or periovarian adhesions
	Preoperative hysterogram reveals a rugal pattern
Moderate	Hydrosalpinx 15–30 mm diameter
	Fragments of fimbria not readily identified
	Periovarian and/or peritubal adhesions without fixation, minimal cul-de-sac adhesions
	Absence of rugal pattern on preoperative hysterogram
Severe	Large hydrosalpinx ≥30 mm diameter
	No fimbria
	Dense pelvic or adnexal adhesions with fixation of the ovary and tube to the broad ligament pelvic sidewall, omentum, or bowel
	Obliteration of the cul-de-sac
	Frozen pelvis (adhesion formation so dense that the limits of organs are difficult to define)

Reprinted with permission from The American College of Obstetricians and Gynecologists (Obstetrics and Gynecology, 1978, 52:597).

of tubal disease, associated infertility factors, patient age, and financial constraints.[19]

NEOSALPINGOSTOMY

This procedure is designed to reopen the distal end of an occluded oviduct that has no recognizable fimbria externally whatsoever, in an attempt to create a new tubal ostium. Distal tubal occlusion, as discussed previously, is most commonly a sequela of pelvic inflammatory disease and is often complicated by endosalpinx involvement. Hydrosalpinges may be opened by cutting the surrounding white scarred peritoneal bands with microsurgical thermoelectric needles, a scalpel, pointed scissors, or laser. Small balloons, hypodermic needles, glass medicine droppers, plastic dilators, and glass catheters may each be inserted into the tubal lumen to serve as guides to increase the length and width of the incision, based on the individual preference of the surgeon. If necessary, cuffs are made, and the new opening is secured with fine (e.g., 5–0 or smaller) sutures (Fig. 31–5). In the past, these ostia were protected postoperatively by hoods, caps, or stents; such practice is no longer performed.

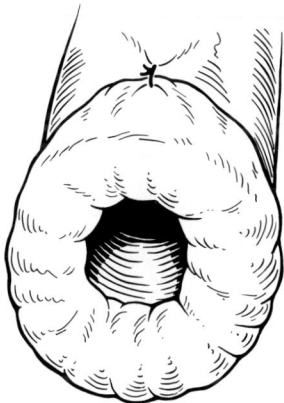

FIGURE 31-5. Appearance of the distal fallopian tube after a neosalpingostomy.

The tubal patency rate after neosalpingostomy is approximately 90% to 95%, whereas actual term pregnancy rates range only from 20% to 25%.[20] This discrepancy may be the result of intraluminal tubal pathology. In some series,[21] subsequent conceptions were more likely to occur more than 1 year after surgery. This phenomenon may be the result of slow mucosal healing from hydrosalpinx-induced damage. Other studies,[22] however, have demonstrated a higher pregnancy rate in the first postoperative year. Further, salpingostomy patients who do not conceive during the first year after surgery had continued evidence of deciliation.[23]

Prognostic factors for successful neosalpingostomy were reviewed in one series of 95 women.[24] Pregnancy rate was inversely related to the extent of tubal distortion (dilation, rugal integrity, and status of the fimbria) and degree of adnexal adhesions. Using the Rock classification system for distal tubal obstruction (Table 31–1), patients with mild disease had an 80% pregnancy rate, with moderate disease a 31% rate, and with severe disease a 16% rate. A second series[25] reported a patency rate of 96% but an overall live birth rate of only 13%. These authors recommended that patients with severe adhesions and poor tubal status be primarily directed to IVF-ET programs rather than to microsurgery. In a multicenter study,[26] use of the carbon dioxide (CO_2) laser for neosalpingostomy did not change the term pregnancy rate. Thus at the current time, there does not appear to be any significant advantage to the use of any single modality.

TUBAL IMPLANTATION

Ascending inflammation is postulated as the mechanism of initiation of most proximal occlusive tubal disease.[27] Previous tubal sterilization and endometriosis account for much of the rest. In one series of histologic evaluation of uterotubal junction obstruction, the most frequent lesion encountered was obliterative fibrosis (38.1%), followed by salpingitis isthmica nodosa (SIN) (23.8%), intramucosal endometriosis (14.3%), and chronic tubal inflammation (21.4%).

The management of proximal tubal obstruction presents a challenge to the reproductive surgeon. The traditional approach to therapy has been tubouterine implantation (Fig. 31–6). When the initial insult is severe, however, there is often distal sparing, with even the intramural portion patent. Often only a small segment of the tube, however, is severely damaged, and adjacent sections, including the intramural segment, appear to be normal. Consequently, the preferred procedure is often the isthmic uterine anastomosis: anastomosis of the tubal isthmus to the intramural portion of the fallopian tube (Fig. 31–7). In one series,[29] 54% of patients undergoing this technique subsequently had intrauterine pregnancies, and in another series,[30] a 58% pregnancy rate ensued. The two surgical options in patients undergoing correction of cornual occlusion were compared.[31] The patency rate in the implantation group was 70% and the pregnancy rate was 39%, whereas in the anastomosis group, the patency rate was 94% and the pregnancy rate was 69%. The author concluded that, when feasible, tubouterine anastomosis should be the procedure of choice for the repair of cornual occlusion[32] regardless of cause. An alternate technique includes reimplantation of the distal segment at a point between the origin of the ovarian ligaments on the posterior aspect of the uterus. This technique, however, is associated with a high rate of dehiscence and is no longer recommended.

Because approximately two thirds of fallopian tubes resected for proximal tubal obstruction based on preoperative hysterosalpingogram reveal the absence of luminal occlusion, the distinction between true pathologic occlusion and either spasm or plugging is crucial in determining therapy. Hysteroscopic or fluoroscopic cannulation of the fallopian tube may be a safe diagnostic and even therapeutic procedure in some of these cases.[33] Consequently, for most patients with pathologic proximal tubal obstruction, a trial tubal recannulation procedure is often attempted before progressing to performance of a tubal anastomosis. In addition, direct lavage[34] or even placement of a narrow catheter, such as a ureteral stent,[35] may be beneficial in restoring tubal patency.

A comparison of results in the world literature for microsurgery in cases of isolated proximal tubal occlusion secondary to surgical sterilization, previous infection, or endometriosis and results reported for IVF-ET suggests that microsurgical tubocornual anastomosis may remain the procedure of choice for proximal tubal occlusion.[36] Balloon tuboplasty, however, may eventually play an increasing role in the treatment of this disease and as previously stated may often be attempted before progressing to anastomosis. In one series[37] patients with combined proximal and distal tubal occlusion had a postoperative conception rate at 2.5 years of 12%, with no live births in 31 patients. This poor surgical

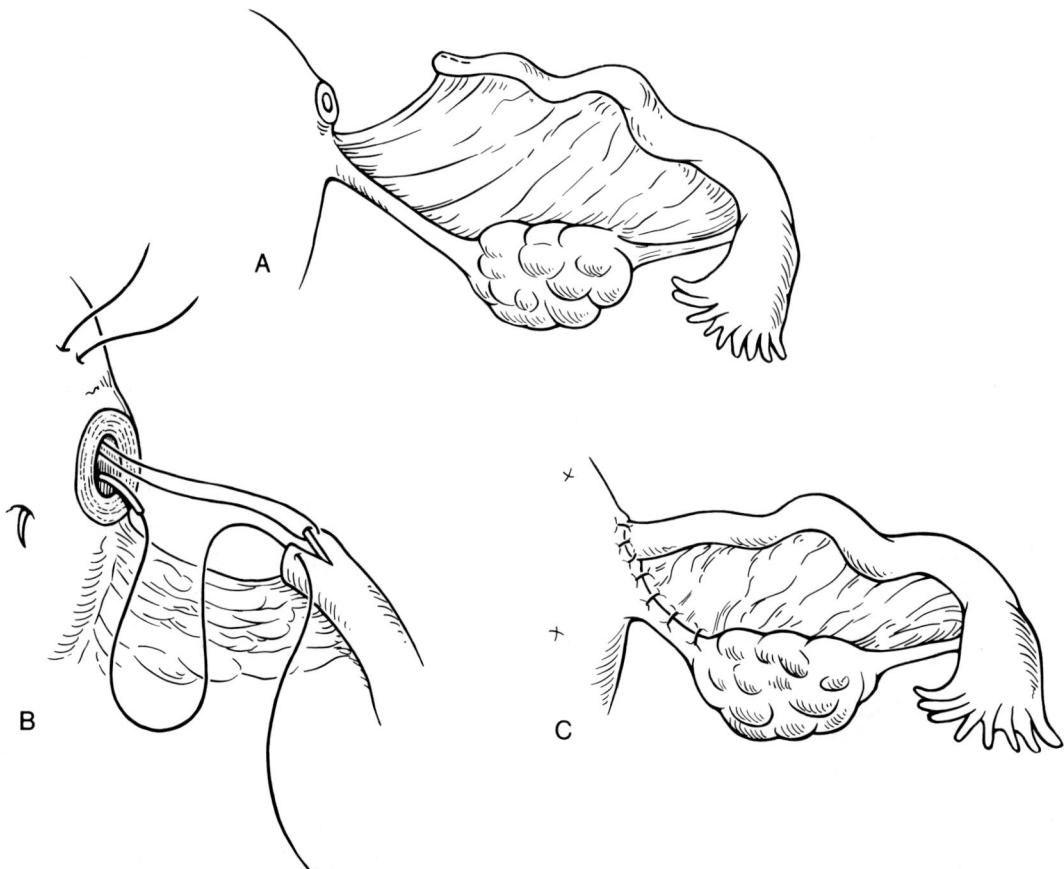

FIGURE 31–6. Tubouterine implantation. *A*, Preparation of the fallopian tube with excision of the occluded segment. (The site of a proposed slit in the antimesenteric wall is denoted by a *dotted line*). *B*, The initial placement of sutures through the fallopian tubes and uterus. *C*, The final appearance after all sutures have been tied.

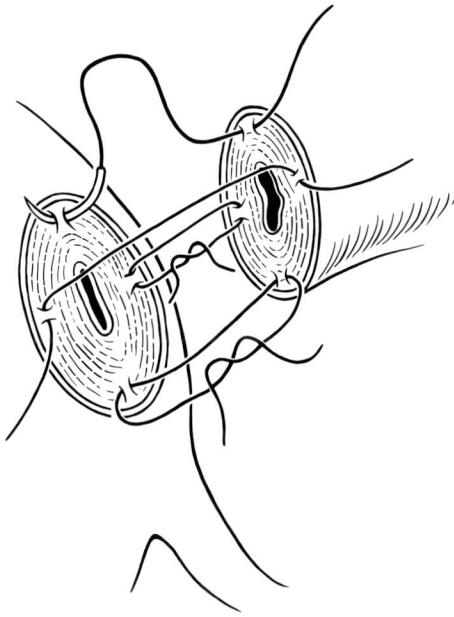

FIGURE 31–7. The placement of sutures for an isthmointerstitial anastomosis.

outcome suggests that IVF-ET should be strongly considered as an alternative in these patients; however, surgical treatment of bipolar tubal disease remains an option and has yielded an overall approximate birth rate of 20%.[5] Other factors found to influence the pregnancy rate included maximized tubal length, preserved intramural portion, absence of chronic inflammation, absence of tubal inclusions, and absence of tubal endometriosis.[38] Deep resection of the intramural tube and cases with technical difficulty also show a reduced pregnancy rate.[39]

TUBAL ANASTOMOSIS

The resection and anastomosis of the fallopian tube is indicated in those cases of infertility in which midtubal obstruction has been diagnosed by hysterosalpingogram and confirmed by laparoscopy. The tubal blockage can be a result of pelvic inflammatory disease, prior tubal sterilization (to be discussed separately), or even a segmental resection performed as a treatment of an ectopic pregnancy. First, the proximal scarred end of the distal segment of the fallopian tube is transected. A probe is inserted through the fimbriae and passed through the open fallopian tube. The distal end of the proximal segment of tube is then transected. Patency of this stump should be documented by the spillage of indigo carmine injected through a cervical cannula. The reanastomosis can be done over 2–0 nylon suture or over a splint. Reanastomosis is performed using fine monofilament nylon or polyglycolic acid sutures. (Our choice is often 8–0, although others use 6–0 to 10–0 suture). The first layer unites the tubal muscularis, often excluding the endosalpinx. Although the suture is theoretically attempted to be placed so as not to include the endosalpinx, if it is included, the stitch is not removed. Approximately four or five of these sutures are placed circumferentially until the tube is completely closed. The second layer reapproximates the tubal serosa and

the outer portion of the muscle of the fallopian tube. Spillage of injected dye should now be demonstrated through the fimbriated end. In the past, reanastomosis procedures were performed using a splint, which was then left in place for several weeks until mucosal healing was completed. These have fallen out of favor because animal studies revealed inflammation and fibrosis at the anastomosis site and a lower pregnancy rate.[40] Subsequent human studies[41] have supported these findings.

Because each portion of the fallopian tube plays a role in ovum pickup, transfer, or fertilization, fertility may be impaired by the absence of even one segment. It seems that an intact ampullary segment is more critical for achieving pregnancy than is an intact isthmus. The chances for pregnancy with a total tubal length of less than 3 to 4 cm are decreased, and tubal reanastomosis should not be recommended when the reconstructed tube is not expected to be at least 4 cm.[42]

REVERSAL OF PREVIOUS STERILIZATION

It is estimated that 1% to 2% of women seek a reversal of a previous sterilization. Presently using microsurgical technique, high pregnancy rates following reversals are common. Creative surgical approaches have been taken in the past to reverse sterilization procedures, in response to the varied anatomic remnants encountered. One approach, described by Haney,[43] was to combine segments of both oviducts to provide a single reconstructed fallopian tube. Numerous attempts have been made to find a nonsuture technique for fallopian tube anastomosis. One possibility, cyanoacrylate, led to severe scar formation.[44] Another attempt has involved the CO_2 laser, which has been used to "weld" the two ends together. An experimental model for anastomoses using "fibrin glue," a biologic tissue-adhesive allogenic fibrinogen, has proved efficacious in the animal model.[45] Lastly, Hurteau and associates[46] evaluated a mechanical stapling device and also had reasonable success in the animal model.

A 1985 compilation of several large series of macrosurgical reversals of sterilization[48] documented a cumulative pregnancy rate of 67.7%, with 54.5% live births, 8.6% abortions, and 4.4% tubal pregnancies. More recently, however, with the implementation of microsurgical technique, better results have been achieved. Hulka and Halme[49] reported the outcomes of 79 reversal-of-sterilization procedures. The group reported an overall 91% tubal patency rate and in selected cases of isthmic-to-isthmic anastomoses a live-birth pregnancy rate of 83%.

Among women desiring reversal of previous tubal ligations, the method of tubal occlusion is a major prognostic factor in subsequent pregnancy outcome. The best results are obtained with Hulka clips or Fallope rings; the worst outcome is obtained after unipolar cautery. Intermediate pregnancy rates are achieved after segmental resection or bipolar cautery.

Silber and Cohen[50] prospectively analyzed the prognostic significance of tubal length in sterilization reversal and concluded that subsequent intrauterine pregnancy was directly related to tubal length. This held as long as there was at least 1 cm of ampulla. Rock and colleagues[51] confirmed a relationship between tubal length and outcome, finding that pregnancy was least likely to occur in women with shortened oviducts of less than 4 cm. In a different study,[52] a logistic regression analysis of 215 patients, localization of the anastomosis, the number of anastomosed tubes, and the presence of other infertility factors were selected as the most important prognostic factors. A separate analysis of 113 women undergoing reversal of sterilization agreed,[53] concluding that factors affecting pregnancy rate include length of tube, type of sterilization performed, anastomotic site, and availability of both tubes for reconstruction. Age, parity, and interval from sterilization to reversal surgery did not affect the pregnancy rate. Of note, 50% of intrauterine pregnancies were conceived within 6 months of reversal surgery.

An analysis performed by Seiler[54] showed sterilization performed by coagulation to be reversible less often than noncoagulation procedures. This difference was attributed to the extensive tubal destruction that followed coagulation. He found a longer time interval to conception following reversal and a higher ectopic pregnancy rate but no statistical difference in the actual pregnancy rate.

A multicenter survey of sterilization reversal in 78 women over the age of 40[55] reported an intrauterine pregnancy rate of 45% and an ectopic pregnancy rate of 4%. The authors of the study concluded that microscopic reversal of sterilization in women between ages 40 and 45 years is an acceptable infertility treatment.

The efficacy of the CO_2 laser as an adjunct to conventional microsurgical techniques was studied in patients undergoing reversals of elective tubal sterilizations. Although the laser has been suggested to have technical advantages (precision, hemostasis, improved preservation of normal tissues), there was no advantage in 1-year conception rate (43.7% in the nonlaser group and 42.9% in the laser group).[56]

Sterilization by fimbriectomy had once been thought to be irreversible. This was based on the recognition of the highly specialized and unique role of ovum pickup performed by intact fimbriae. Failures of Kroener fimbriectomy[57] were thought primarily to be the result of tuboperitoneal fistulas.[58, 59] It has been shown in both animal[60] and human models,[61] however, that reversal is possible. After fimbriectomy and ampullary cuff salpingostomy in rabbits, scanning electron microscopy of the "neofimbria" demonstrates populations of ciliated and secretory cells similar to those of intact fimbria.[62] The technique for reversal involves the creation of a new ostium by transverse salpingostomy and a cuff-eversion technique and has been described to yield a success rate of approximately 40%.[61] Successful reversal is associated with protrusion of the endosalpinx to form a neofimbria. The probability of success of this procedure when a portion of the ampulla remains makes this procedure a viable alternative to IVF.

TUBAL TRANSPLANTATION

Actual fallopian tube transplantation has been performed to bypass unsalvageable or absent fallopian tubes. Both homologous[47] and autologous grafting have been performed on many animal species. A few women have undergone vascularized fallopian tube transplants, obtained from women undergoing total abdominal hysterectomies. The recipient operations lasted more than 4 hours in each case, and although vascular patency was achieved, immunologic rejection universally occurred.

BALLOON TUBOPLASTY

A phenomenon in tubal surgery has been the introduction of tuboscopy or falloposcopy and tubal recanalization. Salpingoscopy has been promoted as a means of determining the extent of internal tubal disease.[63] Laparoscopic employment of a rigid salpingoscope can allow evaluation of the ampullary mucosa and the extent of intratubal adhesions, neither of which are accurately assessed by hysterosalpingography.[64] The transvaginal approach provides an alternate (and perhaps less invasive) way to obtain this information.[65] Information regarding damage of the tubal mucosa is potentially valuable to patients who might consider IVF-ET as an alternative. Additionally, salpingoscopy may help the reproductive surgeon better select patients for a gamete intrafallopian transfer procedure and may provide a better estimation of the risk of ectopic pregnancy than laparoscopic external appraisal can provide. Although severe endotubal disease can be accurately diagnosed using the salpingoscope, moderate histopathologic changes may be missed salpingoscopically.[66]

Transcervical tubal cannulation procedures, essentially an adaptation of established balloon angioplasty techniques, may facilitate the recanalization of proximally occluded oviducts. In a multicenter study,[67] 77 women with confirmed bilateral proximal tubal occlusion underwent the procedure. A minimum of unilateral recanalization was accomplished in 92% of patients. Of the patients whose tubes were canalized and whose tubes showed no distal obstruction, 34% had confirmed clinical pregnancies, whereas only one was diagnosed with an ectopic pregnancy. Similar results have been achieved by transcervical tubal cannulation techniques, which do not involve the use of balloon catheters. Transcervical tubal catheterization thus appears to represent a useful technique to treat selected cases of tubal interstitial obstruction. Long-term sequelae of cornual catheterization on tubal histology and function, however, remain to be established.

Transcervical tubal cannulation procedures and tuboplasty may also prove helpful in the management of an often refractory problem to the reproductive surgeon, SIN. SIN seems to be an acquired form of tubal diverticulosis and has been implicated as the culprit in cases of female infertility and ectopic pregnancies.[68] Although there has been a report[65] of successful guidewire cannulation and direct balloon tuboplasty in a case of isthmic stricture secondary to SIN, however, the nature of this disorder may make it less amenable to this form of therapy. In his series of patients with SIN and tubal patency, McComb[69, 70] concurred, recommending resection of the diseased portion of tube and anastomosis. Homm and colleagues[71] added that resection and anastomosis may optimize fertility and reduce the recurrence rate for ectopic pregnancy.

PREVENTION OF POSTOPERATIVE ADHESIONS

Postoperative adhesions frequently complicate pelvic surgery, being documented after 75% to 84% of various pelvic procedures.[72, 73] Along with use of optimal microsurgical technique as described previously, surgical adjuvants have been used in an attempt to decrease adhesion occurrence. Usage of these adjuvants is widespread among reproductive surgeons.[74] Classes of surgical adjuvants include fibrinolytic agents, anticoagulants, anti-inflammatory agents, antibiotics, and barriers.[75] Antibiotics are usually recommended in microsurgical procedures because of the potential detrimental effects of an infection; however, there are no studies that clearly demonstrate efficacy. In theory, anti-inflammatory agents, such as dexamethasone and promethazine (Phenergan), should be helpful, but again efficacy has not been shown in human clinical trials (although they are believed by many to make patients feel better). Although 32% dextran-70 (Hyskon) has been evaluated extensively, its efficacy in human clinical trials is mixed. Although efficacy was shown in two human clinical trials, in two others no benefit was demonstrated. It is most likely to be beneficial in reducing adhesions in the posterior cul-de-sac, which is the most dependent part of the pelvis. Currently the only product approved for the reduction of postoperative adhesion development is Intercede TC-7. This product, which is composed of oxidized regenerated cellulose, has been shown in human clinical trials to reduce adhesion reformation after adhesiolysis significantly. No adjuvant, however, represents a panacea for prevention of postoperative adhesions. The most important factor in reducing postoperative adhesions is the use of microsurgical principles and therefore the minimization of tissue injury at the time of surgery. Adjuvants are not a means of compensating for poor surgical technique.

SUMMARY

It is clear that there have been great advances made in microsurgery and specifically in tubal surgery over the past 20 years. Careful analysis of all new data must be performed to determine whether surgical intervention is more efficacious than IVF-ET. Despite the advances in assisted reproductive technologies, reconstructive tubal surgery retains an important role in the treatment of the infertile patient.

REFERENCES

1. Greentree LB. The Estes operation: one possible alternative to a "test tube" baby. Fertil Steril 1979; 32:130–132.
2. Wood C, Leeton J, Taylor R. A preliminary design and trial of an artificial human tube. Fertil Steril 1971; 22:446–449.
3. O'Neil JJ. The use of the vermiform appendix as a fallopian tube. Am J Obstet Gynecol 1966; 95:219–222.
4. Thie JL, Williams TJ, Coulam CB. Repeat tuboplasty compared with primary microsurgery for postinflammatory tubal disease. Fertil Steril 1986; 45:784–787.
5. Diamond MP. Surgical aspects of infertility. In: Sciarra J, editor. Gynecology and Obstetrics. Philadelphia: Harper & Row, 1988: 1–2.
6. Verhage HG, Fazleabas AT, Donnelly K. The in vitro synthesis of estrogen-dependent proteins by the baboon (Papia anubis) oviduct. Endocrinology 1988; 122:1639–1645.
7. Fayez JA, Suliman OS. Infertility surgery of the oviduct: comparison between macrosurgery and microsurgery. Fertil Steril 1982; 37:73–78.
8. Williams TJ. Surgical procedures for inflammatory tubal disease. Obstet Gynecol Clin North Am 1987; 14:1037–1048.
9. Oelsner G, Boeckx W, Verhoeven H, et al. The effect of training in microsurgery. Am J Obstet Gynecol 1985; 152:1054–1058.
10. Lavy G, Diamond MP, DeCherney AH. Ectopic pregnancy: its relationship to tubal reconstructive surgery. Fertil Steril 1987; 47:543–556.
11. Williams KM, Griffin WI. Distal tuboplasty: is it appropriate? South Med J 1988; 81:872–877.
12. Russell JB, DeCherney AH, Laufer N, et al. Neosalpingostomy; comparison of 24- and 72-month follow-up time shows increased pregnancy rate. Fertil Steril 1986; 45:296–298.
13. DeCherney AH, Kase N. A comparison of treatment for bilateral fimbrial occlusion. Fertil Steril 1981; 35:162–166.
14. Hassiakos DK, Muasher SJ, Veeck LL, Jones HS Jr. In vitro fertilization: effective alternative to surgery for distal tubal occlusion. VA Med Q 1981; 118:26–30.
15. Holst N, Maltau JM, Forsdahl F, Hansen LJ. Handling of tubal infertility after introduction of in vitro fertilization: changes and consequences. Fertil Steril 1991; 55:140–143.
16. Lavy G, Diamond MP, DeCherney AH. Ectopic pregnancy: its relationship to tubal reconstructive surgery. Fertil Steril 1987; 47:543–556.
17. Donnez J, Casanas-Roux F. Prognostic factors of fimbrial microsurgery. Fertil Steril 1986; 46:200–204.
18. Patton Grant W Jr. Pregnancy outcome following microsurgical fimbrioplasty. Fertil Steril 1982; 37:150–155.
19. Diamond MP, Cunningham T, Linsky CB, et al. Interceed TC7 as an adjuvant for adhesion reduction: animal studies. In: DiZerega GS, Malinak LR, Diamond MP, Linsky CB. Treatment of Post Surgical Adhesions. New York, Wiley-Liss, 1990:131–144.
20. Daniell JF, Diamond MP, McLaughlin DS, et al. Clinical results of terminal salpingostomy using the CO_2 laser: report of the intra-abdominal laser study group. Fertil Steril 1986; 45:175–178.
21. Gomel V. Salpingostomy by microsurgery. Fertil Steril 1978; 29:380–387.
22. Godo G, Koloszar S, Sas M. Up to date surgical management of tubal infertility due to inflammations of the pelvis. Acta Chir Hung 1988; 29:197–204.
23. Donnez J, Casanas-Roux F. Prognostic factors of fimbrial microsurgery. Fertil Steril 1986; 46:200–204.
24. Schlaff WD, Hassiakos DK, Damewood MD, Rock JA. Neosalpingostomy for distal tubal obstruction: prognostic factors and impact of surgical technique. Fertil Steril 1990; 54:984–990.
25. Laatikainen TJ, Tenhunen AK, Venesmaa PK, Apter DL. Factors influencing the success of microsurgery for distal tubal occlusion. Arch Gynecol Obstet 1988; 243:101–106.
26. Daniell JF, Diamond MP, McLaughlin DS, et al. Clinical results of terminal salpingostomy with the use of the CO_2 laser: report of the Intraabdominal Laser Study Group. Fertil Steril 1986; 45:175–178.
27. McComb PF, Lee NH, Stephenson MD. Reproductive outcome after unilateral tubocornual anastomosis and contralateral salpingostomy by microsurgery. Fertil Steril 1991; 55:1011–1013.
28. Fortier KJ, Haney AF. The pathologic spectrum of uterotubal junction obstruction. Obstet Gynecol 1985; 65:93–98.
29. Gomel V. Tubal reanastomosis by microsurgery. Fertil Steril 1977; 28:59–66.
30. McComb P. Microsurgical tubocornual anastomosis for occlusive cornual disease: reproducible results without the need for tubouterine implantation. Fertil Steril 1986; 46:571–577.
31. Fayez JA. Comparison between tubouterine implantation and tubouterine anastomosis for repair of cornual occlusion. Microsurgery 1987; 8:78–82.
32. Sulak PJ, Letterie GS, Coddington CC, et al. Histology of proximal tubal occlusion. Fertil Steril 1987; 48:437–440.
33. Deaton JL, Gibson M, Riddick DH, Brumsted JR. Diagnosis and treatment of cornual obstruction using a flexible tip guidewire. Fertil Steril 1990; 43:232–236.
34. Sulak PJ, Letterie GS, Hayslip CC, et al. Hysteroscopic cannulation and lavage in the treatment of proximal tubal occlusion. Fertil Steril 1987; 48:493–494.
35. Daniell JF, Miller W. Hysteroscopic correction of cornual occlusion with resultant term pregnancy. Fertil Steril 1987; 48:490–492.
36. Marana R, Quagliarello J. Proximal tubal occlusion: microsurgery versus IVF—a review. Int J Fertil 1988; 33:338–340.
37. Patton PE, Williams TJ, Coulam CB. Results of microsurgical reconstruction in patients with combined proximal and distal tubal occlusion: double obstruction. Fertil Steril 1987; 48:670–674.
38. Donnez J, Casanas-Roux F, Nisolle-Pochet M, et al. Surgical management of tubal obstruction at the uterotubal junction. Acta Eur Fertil 1987; 18:5–9.
39. Gillett WR, Herbison GP. Tubocornual anastomosis: surgical considerations and coexistent infertility factors in determining the prognosis. Fertil Steril 1989; 51:241–246.
40. Winston RML: Reversal of female sterilization. Int Plann Parent Fed Med Bull 1978; 12:1.

41. Meldrum DR. Microsurgical tubal reanastomosis—the role of splints. Obstet Gynecol 1981; 57:613–619.

42. Hershalg A, Diamond MP, DeCherney AH. Tubal physiology: an appraisal. J Gynecol Surg 1989; 5:3–25.

43. Haney AF. Utilization of contralateral fallopian tube segments in tubal reanastomosis. Fertil Steril 1982; 37:701–703.

44. Smith D. The use of tissue adhesive for oviduct anastomosis. In: Philips JM, editor. Microsurgery in Gynecology. St. Louis: Christian Board of Publications, 1977.

45. Scheidel PH, Wallwiener DR, Wiedemann RA, Hepp HK. Experimental anastomosis of the rabbit fallopian tube using fibrin glue. Fertil Steril 1982; 38(4):461–474.

46. Hurteau GD, Bradley G. Evaluation of the stapled anastomosis in experimental salpingoplasty. Fertil Steril 1966; 17:323–331.

47. DeCherney AH, Naftolin F. Homotransplantation of the human fallopian tube: report of a successful case and description of a technique. Fertil Steril 1980; 34:14–16.

48. Siegler AM, Hulka J, Peretz A. Reversibility of female sterilization. Fertil Steril 1985; 43:499–510.

49. Hulka JF, Halme J. Sterilization reversal: results of 101 attempts. Am J Obstet Gynecol 1988; 159:767–774.

50. Silber SJ, Cohen R. Microsurgical reversal of female sterilization: the role of tubal length. Fertil Steril 1980; 33:598–601.

51. Rock JA, Guzick DS, Katz E, et al. Tubal anastomosis: pregnancy success following reversal of Falope ring or monopolar cautery sterilization. Fertil Steril 1987; 48:13–17.

52. te Velde FR, Roer ME, Looman CW, Habbema JD. Factors influencing success or failure after reversal of sterilization: a multivariate approach. Fertil Steril 1990; 54:270–277.

53. Spivak MM, Librach CL, Rosenthal DM. Microsurgical reversal of sterilization: a six year study. Am J Obstet Gynecol 1986; 154:355–361.

54. Seiler JC. Factors influencing the outcome of microsurgical tubal ligation reversals. Am J Obstet Gynecol 1983; 146:292–298.

55. Trimbos-Kemper TC. Reversal of sterilization in women over 40 years of age: a multicenter survey in the Netherlands. Fertil Steril 1990; 53:575–577.

56. McLaughlin DS, Bonaventura LM, Jarrett JC 2d. Tubal reanastomosis: a comparison between microsurgical and microlaser techniques. Microsurgery 1987; 8:83–88.

57. Kroener WF Jr. Surgical sterilization by fimbriectomy. Am J Obstet Gynecol 1969; 104:247–254.

58. Metz KG. Failures following fimbriectomy. Fertil Steril 1977; 28:66–71.

59. Metz KG. Failures following fimbriectomy: a further report. Fertil Steril 1978; 30:269–273.

60. Perez LE, Flores JJ, Bajpai VK, et al. Fertility following fimbriectomy and tubo-ovarian microsurgery in the rabbit. Fertil Steril 1981; 35:573–579.

61. Novy MJ. Reversal of Kroener fimbriectomy sterilization. Am J Obstet Gynecol 1980; 137:198–206.

62. Halbert SA, McComb PF, Patton DL. Function and structure of the rabbit oviduct following fimbriectomy. I. Distal ampullary salpingostomy. Fertil Steril 1981; 35:349–354.

63. Shapiro BS, Diamond MP, DeCherney AH. Salpingoscopy: an adjunctive technique for evaluation of the fallopian tube. Fertil Steril 1988; 49:1076–1079.

64. DeBruyne F, Puttemans P, Boeckx W, Brosens I. The clinical value of salpingoscopy in tubal infertility. Fertil Steril 1989; 51:339–340.

65. Kerin J, Daykhovsky L, Segalowitz J, et al. Falloposcopy: a microendoscopic technique for visual exploration of the human fallopian tube from the uterotubal ostium to the fimbria using a transvaginal approach. Fertil Steril 1990; 54:390–400.

66. Hershlag A, Seifer DB, Carcangiu ML, et al. Salpingoscopy: light microscopic and electron microscopic correlations. Obstet Gynecol 1991; 77:399–405.

67. Confino E, Tur-Kaspa I, DeCherney AH, et al. Transcervical balloon tuboplasty. A multicenter study. JAMA 1990; 264:2079–2082.

68. Honore LH. Salpingitis isthmica nodosa in female infertility and ectopic tubal pregnancy. Fertil Steril 1978; 29:164–168.

69. McComb P. Microsurgical tubocornual anastomosis for occlusive cornual disease: reproducible results without the need for tubouterine implantation. Fertil Steril 1986; 46:571–577.

70. McComb P. The determinants of successful surgery for proximal tubal disease. Fertil Steril 1986; 46:1002–1004.

71. Homm RJ, Holtz G, Garvin AJ. Isthmic ectopic pregnancy and salpingitis isthmica nodosa. Fertil Steril 1987; 48:756–760.

72. Diamond MP, Daniell JF, Feste J, et al. Pelvic adhesions at early second look laparoscopy following carbon dioxide laser surgery procedures. Infertility 1984; 7:39–44.

73. DeCherney AH, Mezer HC. The nature of posttuboplasty pelvic adhesions as determined by early and late laparoscopy. Fertil Steril 1984; 41:643–649.

74. Holtz G. Current use of ancillary modalities for adhesion prevention. Fertil Steril 1985; 44:174–176.

75. Diamond MP, DeCherney AH. Pathogenesis of adhesion formation/reformation: application to reproductive pelvic surgery. Microsurgery 1987; 8:103–107.

CHAPTER 32

Management of the Ectopic Pregnancy

LISA BARRIE SCHWARTZ and
ALAN H. DeCHERNEY

Ectopic pregnancy has become an "epidemic,"[23] more than tripling in incidence between 1965 and 1985.[2–4] This trend parallels the increased prevalence of sexually transmitted diseases and pelvic inflammatory disease, more widespread use of intrauterine devices, higher rates of tubal ligations, and greater availability of reconstructive tubal surgery for infertility. Although ectopic pregnancies have been reported anywhere outside of the uterus (such as in the ovary, cervix, and abdomen), this chapter is limited to a discussion of tubal ectopic pregnancy.

A tubal pregnancy has more than one possible fate. Not only may it progress to tubal rupture and intraperitoneal hemorrhage, it can also resorb spontaneously or terminate as a tubal abortion with spontaneous expulsion of the products of conception via the fimbriated end. Therefore, our ability to detect tubal pregnancies so early has led to the diagnosis of previously undiagnosable cases destined for spontaneous resolution. In this regard, Mashiach and Oelsner[5] diagnosed 13 tubal pregnancies laparoscopically without instituting treatment. Only 3 of the 13 women required a subsequent laparotomy because of pain or tubal rupture with hemorrhage, and the other 10 had an uneventful followup with spontaneous resolution of symptoms. However, even in the cases that are destined for eventual spontaneous resolution, intervention is still strongly recommended to minimize morbidity, such as distorted pelvic anatomy and adhesions[6] from possible chronic ectopic pregnancies.

However, earlier detection often means diagnosis prior to rupture, tissue destruction, and blood loss. The ability to diagnose and intervene earlier is due to three diagnostic modalities: laparoscopy, transvaginal ultrasonography, and β-human chorionic gonadotropin (hCG) levels. This past decade has brought the greatest advances in the diagnosis and management of ectopic pregnancy since 1883, when Lawson Tait described treatment when he performed the first successful salpingectomy for ectopic pregnancy,[7] although accurate diagnosis remained elusive at that time. These advances have already benefited the patient population. Recent statistics show that despite the increased frequency of ectopic pregnancies, the case fatality rate has declined from 3.5 to 0.4 deaths per 1000 ectopic pregnancies from 1970 to 1985.[8]

DIAGNOSIS

Clinical suspicion of an ectopic pregnancy in a patient with an acute abdomen or orthostatic symptoms, or both, for whom emergent surgery is indicated requires a rapid, sensitive urine pregnancy test and culdocentesis. (A "positive culdocentesis" refers to the aspiration of more than 5 mL of freely flowing nonclotting blood from the pouch of Douglas, whereas a "negative culdocentesis" is indicated by the presence of clear fluid and a "nondiagnostic culdocentesis" reflects the inability to obtain enough fluid.) When bloody fluid is aspirated, hematocrit levels higher than 15% in the fluid are generally associated with ectopic pregnancies. A positive pregnancy test combined with a positive culdocentesis almost always is associated with an ectopic pregnancy. In one series, a positive culdocentesis in a patient with a positive pregnancy test corresponded with an ectopic pregnancy in 99.2% of cases.[9] In this study, 82 of 106 (77.3%) unruptured ectopics and 50 of 57 (88%) ruptured ectopics had a positive culdocentesis.[9] Other possible causes of a positive culdocentesis include hemorrhagic corpus luteal cyst, tubal reflux, other sources of intra-abdominal hemorrhage, or prior attempts at culdocentesis.

The approach to the evaluation of a clinically stable patient suspected of having an ectopic pregnancy is a completely modern problem because in the past it was not possible to identify such patients. The characteristic triad of pain, vaginal bleeding, and a history of amenorrhea raises suspicion. The evaluation begins with a rapid and sensitive serum pregnancy test. A positive result requires followup with a β-hCG level and pelvic ultrasonography. It has been shown that the sac of a normal intrauterine pregnancy is visualized on transabdominal ultrasonography when the β-hCG level is higher than

6000 to 6500 mIU/mL (International Reference Preparation [IRP]).[10]*

Romero and associates established that the absence of an intrauterine sac on transabdominal ultrasonogram in conjunction with β-hCG levels higher than 6500 mIU/mL signified an ectopic pregnancy in 87% of cases.[10, 11] This criteria has a 100% sensitivity, 96% specificity, and a negative predictive value of 100%. Vaginal ultrasonography, in combination with the improved methods to quantify β-hCG, has lowered this discriminatory zone to approximately 1400[12] to 2000 mIU/mL (IRP). (The exact value depends on the experience of the examiner and quality of the ultrasonogram image.) The ability to detect the intrauterine gestational sac when the β-hCG level is near 2000 mIU/mL is due to the increased resolution and image quality obtainable with the closer proximity of the transvaginal ultrasound transducer to the pelvic structures, enabling the detection of an intrauterine pregnancy about 1 week earlier than with the classic transabdominal scanner.

The use of serum progesterone levels in combination with β-hCG levels has been suggested to further aid in distinguishing an abnormal gestation from a normal intrauterine pregnancy. A progesterone level lower than 15 ng/mL was consistently associated with either an ectopic gestation or nonviable intrauterine pregnancy in two studies of 99 patients.[13, 14] Conversely, a progesterone value higher than 15 ng/mL excluded the diagnosis of ectopic pregnancy in all cases.[13, 15, 16] More recent studies suggested that progesterone levels may be helpful in terms of a range rather than a cutoff of a specific value. Also more recently, serum estradiol levels were evaluated as an aid in diagnosing ectopic pregnancies.[17] Mean estradiol levels were significantly lower in 100 ectopic pregnancies in comparison with control subjects who had either normal intrauterine pregnancies or threatened abortions. The authors reported an estradiol level cutoff of 650 pg/mL: all the ectopic pregnancies had values lower than this, and all but one of the control subjects had values higher than this level, for a reported 100% sensitivity and 99% specificity in diagnosing an intrauterine pregnancy.[17] The authors recommended the evaluation of serum estradiol levels in conjunction with progesterone values to improve the ability to distinguish ectopic from intrauterine pregnancies.[17] However, further investigation of the clinical usefulness of such hormonal levels is necessary before widespread clinical application is initiated.

The absence of a sac on ultrasound examination when the level of β-hCG is lower than the discriminatory level (<6000 mIU/mL for abdominal ultrasound and <1400 mIU/mL for vaginal ultrasound) is nondiagnostic, and management from that point depends on the clinical situation. For the stable patient, serial quantitative β-hCG levels and ultrasound examination should be followed until the diagnosis becomes clarified. Because β-hCG blood levels are known to double every 2 to 3 days,[18, 19] an abnormal increase is suggestive of a nonviable pregnancy, and the next step is to distinguish between an abnormal intrauterine gestation (such as a missed abortion and blighted ovum) and an extrauterine gestation.

An absent double decidual intrauterine sac on ultrasound examination ("double sac sign") has been defined as a pseudodecidual sac representing a decidual cast and has been associated with an intrauterine pregnancy in only 4 of 68 women.[20] The finding of a complex adnexal mass on transabdominal ultrasound examination associated with or without cul-de-sac fluid in patients with β-hCG levels lower than 6000 mIU/mL has been shown, in a prospective study by Romero and colleagues,[21] to aid in the diagnosis of ectopic pregnancy. Falling β-hCG levels may be indicative of a miscarriage in process but may also occur when there is spontaneous resolution or abortion of a tubal pregnancy. β-hCG levels are monitored until the level exceeds either 2000 or 6500 mIU/mL, following which either transvaginal or transabdominal ultrasound, respectively, is performed to search for an intrauterine fetal sac. If present, the tentative diagnosis of a normal intrauterine pregnancy is made and serial ultrasound examination is performed until a fetal pole with heart motion is identified. If no fetal sac is seen, the presumed diagnosis is an ectopic pregnancy, and laparoscopy should be performed to evaluate the pelvis for a more definitive diagnosis. Laparoscopy is also recommended for patients with subnormal increases in serial quantitative β-hCG levels.

The laparoscope was described in 1964[22] as a diagnostic aid providing easy visualization of the pelvis and, therefore, of ectopic pregnancies. Since then, the laparoscope has become the standard means of evaluating the hemodynamically stable patient with the presumptive diagnosis of an ectopic pregnancy. The accuracy of diagnosing ectopic pregnancies in successful laparoscopies has been reported to be 98.5%.[23] However, proper timing of laparoscopy is essential. If laparoscopy is performed too early, the ectopic can initially be missed and the patient may then have to undergo a second laparoscopy when the ectopic has enlarged enough to be visualized through the laparoscope. In fact, studies have reported that early ectopics are missed at laparoscopy in 3% to 4% of cases.[23, 24] Figure 32–1 outlines this current management protocol for early diagnosis (and subsequent treatment) of ectopic gestations.

With advanced technology and more sophisticated instrumentation, the laparoscope was found to be a powerful therapeutic tool, in addition to its already well-known diagnostic capabilities. Thus, over the past 15 years, the diagnosis, management, and treatment of ectopic gestations has been dramatically revolutionized. The evolution has been that of emergent radical intra-abdominal surgical treatment of acute rupture and life-threatening hemorrhage to early conservative surgical or medical management of an asymptomatic patient with emphasis on preserving fertility and minimizing morbidity.

TREATMENT

Laparotomy: Salpingectomy

The historical approach to the management of ectopic pregnancies was based on making the diagnosis at the time of a laparotomy performed on a hemodynamically unstable patient experiencing acute tubal rupture. In contrast with the present, there was less time for consideration of the patient's desire for future fertility, and the circumstances were not ideal when the consent was obtained in an emergency situation. The standard methods used in the 1950s, now considered more radical, involved immediate laparotomy with re-

---

*There are two distinct hCG standards provided by the World Health Organization: the IRP yields a value that is approximately double the hCG value calculated by the second International Standard.

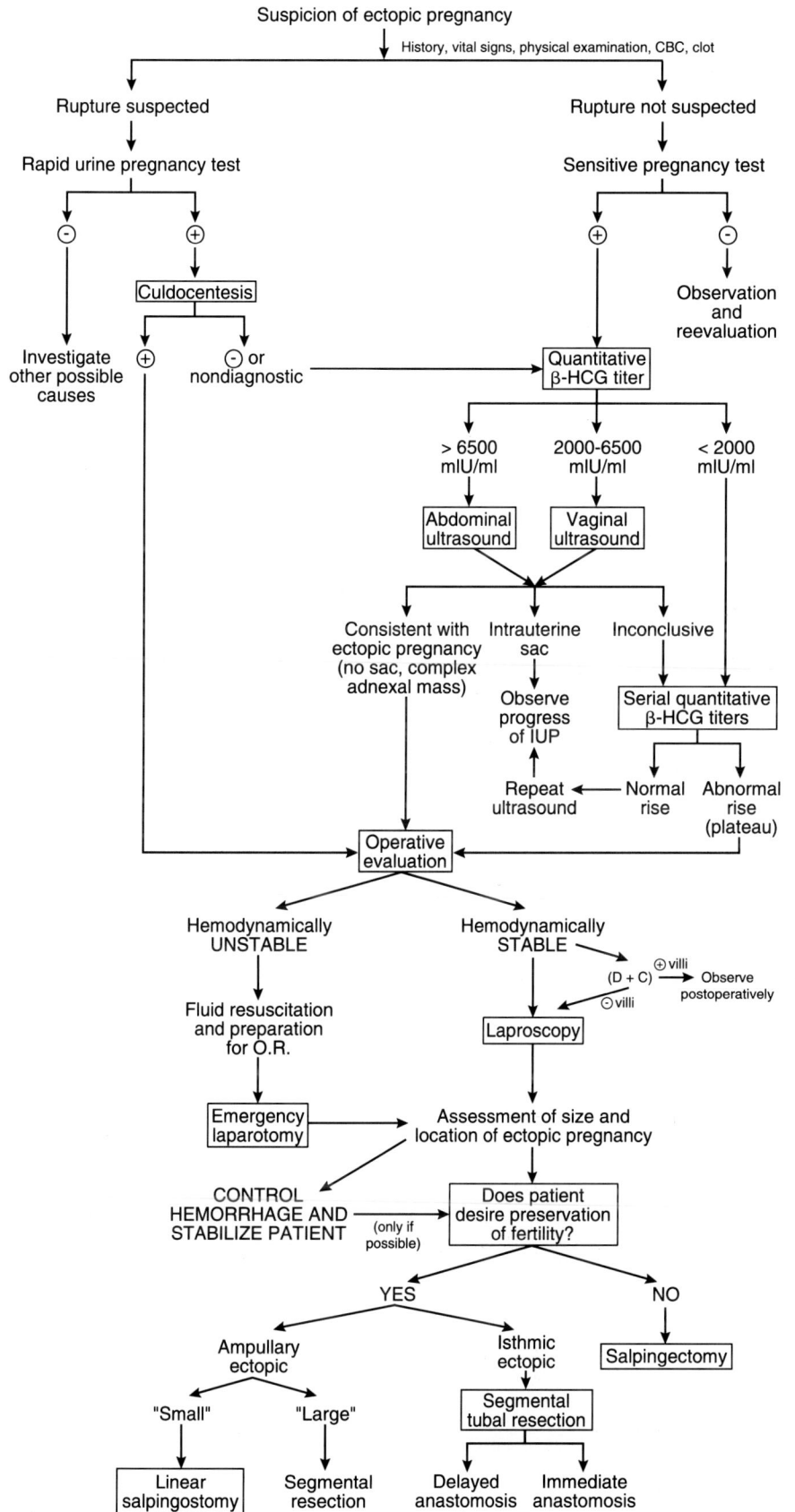

FIGURE 32–1. Alternatives in diagnosis and management of ectopic pregnancy. CBC, complete blood count; IUP, intrauterine pregnancy; β-HCG, β-human chorionic gonadotropin; D + C, dilation and curettage; O.R., operating room.

section of the involved tube and adjoining ovary.[25] The rapidity and ease of salpingectomy were used to treat the frequent presentation of massive hemorrhage and shock or extensive tubal destruction. Ipsilateral oophorectomy, also known as *paradoxical oophorectomy*, was often advocated to ensure that ovulation would subsequently occur on the same side as the remaining tube.[26] However, the potential for transmigration of the oocyte to the contralateral fallopian tube in at least 15% of pregnancies,[27] the subsequent finding of equivalent conception rates following salpingectomy with and without ipsilateral oophorectomy,[28, 29] the possibility that the remaining ovary would subsequently become diseased, and the more recent availability of in vitro fertilization–embryo transfer (IVF-ET) all have led to the recommendation that "elective" oophorectomy at the time of salpingectomy for ectopic pregnancy be abandoned.

The technique of salpingectomy at laparotomy involves identifying the tube and then successively grasping the mesosalpinx with Kelly clamps beginning at the fimbriated end of the tube (Fig. 32–2). The individual pedicles are ligated with fine, nonreactive absorbable sutures. This procedure is continued along the base of the tube until the cornua is reached. In the past, cornual resection (removal of a small wedge of tissue at the base of the tube) had been advocated at the time of salpingectomy to prevent future implantation in the stump.[30] However, subsequent studies have shown that cornual resection not only failed to prevent interstitial pregnancies but was associated with more blood loss at the time of surgery and possible uterine rupture during subsequent pregnancies.[31–33] Therefore, it is no longer recommended unless the pregnancy is in the interstitial portion of the fallopian tube.

Although necessary for the treatment of patients with ectopic pregnancies associated with either irreparable tubal damage or hemodynamic instability or for those patients who no longer desire fertility (i.e., failed tubal ligation), salpingectomy is not ideal for other patients with otherwise healthy-appearing tubes desiring future reproductive capability. However, salpingectomy is an alternate option for the patient who does not want to take the chance of persistent gestational tissue that can result after a less aggressive approach.

Laparotomy: Salpingostomy

Since Stromme's initial report of conservative surgery for ectopic pregnancy in 1953,[34] salpingostomy at laparotomy evolved and replaced salpingectomy as the standard treatment for unruptured ampullary ectopic pregnancies. Again, this more conservative approach has become more common because of our ability to make the diagnosis before rupture of the fallopian tube. As noted earlier, this procedure has become the standard approach for young, stable patients with minimally diseased tubes desiring future fertility.

A series of prospective studies have demonstrated salpingostomy to be as effective as salpingectomy for treatment of ectopic pregnancy and as successful with regard to future fertility without increasing the rate of subsequent tubal pregnancy as had originally been anticipated.[18, 25, 35–37] Numerous reports have demonstrated subsequent intrauterine pregnancy rates of 40% to 60% and repeat ectopic rates of 10% to 15% (Table 32–1).[18, 25, 36, 38, 39] Timonen and Nieminen[25] reported a 49% intrauterine pregnancy rate and an 11.5% repeat ectopic rate following salpingectomy compared with a 53% pregnancy rate and a 15.7% repeat ectopic rate after salpingostomy. DeCherney and Kase[18] reported a 42% intrauterine pregnancy rate and a 12% repeat ectopic rate following more radical surgery (i.e., salpingectomy or sal-

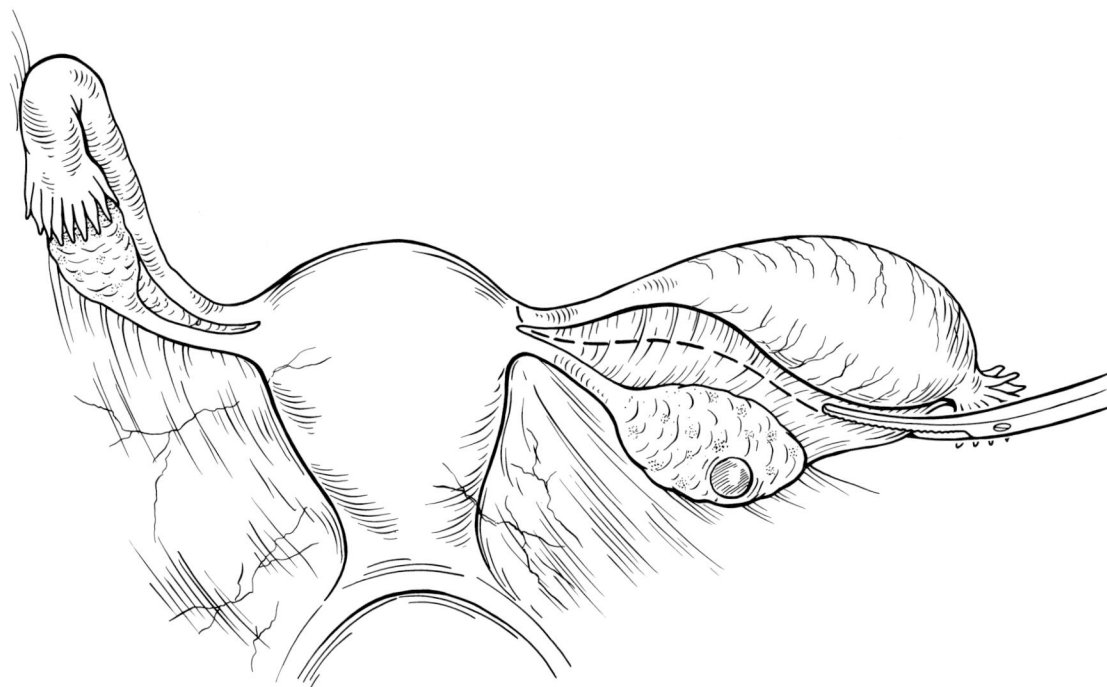

FIGURE 32–2. Salpingectomy performed at laparotomy for a right tubal pregnancy. Kelly clamps are used to clamp the mesosalpinx, which is incised and then sutured.

TABLE 32–1. Summary of Results of Surgery for Ectopic Pregnancy

Authors	Mode of Surgery	Type of Surgery	No. of Patients	Patent Tubes (%)	Repeat Ectopic Pregnancies (%)	Intrauterine Pregnancies (%)	Live Births (%)
Timonen and Nieminen (1967)[25]	Laparotomy	Salpingectomy (and other radical surgery)	827	—	11.5	49.3	30.4
	Laparotomy	Salpingostomy (and other conservative surgery)	240	—	15.7	53	27.2
Stromme (1973)[38]	Laparotomy	Salpingotomy (and other conservative surgery)	45	—	15	71	—
Bukovsky et al (1979)[39]	Laparotomy	Salpingotomy	23	100	4	70	55
DeCherney and Kase (1979)[18]	Laparotomy	Salpingectomy (and other radical surgery)	50	—	12	42	—
	Laparotomy	Salpingostomy	48	88.9	11.6	39.6	(overall 40)
Bruhat et al (1980)[40]	Laparoscopy	Salpingotomy	25	52	12	72	72
DeCherney et al (1981)[41]	Laparoscopy	Salpingotomy	16	100	0	50	—
Langer et al (1982)[36]	Laparotomy	Salpingostomy (fimbrial expression in 13 cases)	54	—	12	80	71
Cartwright et al (1986)[42]	Laparoscopy	Salpingostomy (and other conservative surgery)	23	75	12.5	50	—
Pouly et al (1986)[43]	Laparoscopy	Salpingostomy	118	77.8	22	64.4	—
DeCherney and Diamond (1987)[44]	Laparoscopy	Salpingostomy	79	—	16	62	—
Vermesh et al (1989)[45]	Laparotomy	Salpingostomy	19	89	16	42	—
	Laparotomy	Salpingostomy	20	80	6	50	—

pingo-oophorectomy) as compared with a 39.6% intrauterine pregnancy rate and a repeat ectopic rate of 11.6% after more conservative techniques (i.e., linear salpingostomy) in a group of 50 patients treated for ectopic pregnancies. Bukovsky and associates,[39] Langer and colleagues,[36] and Stromme[38] all noted a 70% to 71% intrauterine pregnancy rate following salpingostomy with similar ectopic rates of 12% in the last two studies. Many of these small descriptive studies are difficult to interpret because they are complicated by other factors, such as including fimbrial expression in the conservatively treated groups and cornual resections, salpingo-oophorectomies, and even hysterectomies in the radically treated groups.

To determine if those patients who subsequently conceived had fertilization of the oocyte in the tube that had been operated on, several investigators have reviewed pregnancy rates in patients who had salpingostomies performed on a sole remaining fallopian tube.[35, 37, 43, 46] One study demonstrated normal tubal function and subsequent fertility following linear salpingostomy for unruptured ectopic pregnancies in 15 patients with a single remaining fallopian tube.[35] This group had a 53% term pregnancy rate and 20% repeat ectopic rate, which was based on a 100% followup for at least 1 year. In a similar group of 13 patients, Valle and Lifchez[37] reported an 85% term pregnancy rate without any recurrent ectopics after 664 months of followup. In Pouly and associates' series of 321 ectopic pregnancies, 11 of 24 (45.8%) women attempting conception following salpingostomy (laparoscopic) for removal of an ectopic pregnancy from the sole remaining fallopian tube established an intrauterine pregnancy, and 7 patients (29.2%) had a second ectopic.[43] Oelsner and coworkers[46] reported the results of conservative microsurgery for 22 women with an ectopic in their single tube. Of 21 patients who desired pregnancy, 76% subsequently conceived, with 47.6% intrauterine and 42.8% repeat ectopic

pregnancy rates.[46] Thus, these pregnancy rates are similar to those of the radically and conservatively treated groups reviewed earlier, which suggests that normal tubal function can be restored following conservative treatment of ectopic pregnancy.

Salpingostomy with delayed secondary closure of the tubal incision has been shown to be as effective as salpingostomy with one- or two-layer suture closure of the tubal incision (salpingotomy). Animal and human studies have illustrated acceptable tubal repair, limited adhesion formation, and similar pregnancy rates[40, 41, 47, 48] with both methods. Salpingostomy has become the preferred method over salpingotomy, partly owing to surgical expediency.

The surgical technique of salpingostomy at laparotomy involves creating a linear incision along the antimesenteric border over the area of maximal tubal bulge using microelectrocautery or a laser (Fig. 32–3A).[49] The ectopic gestation and clot are evacuated through the linear incision (Fig. 32–3B and C). Hemostasis along the edges is then obtained with cautery, laser, or fine, nonreactive absorbable sutures. If bleeding is uncontrollable despite these measures, salpingectomy should be performed. The tenets of microsurgery should be applied, including minimal tissue handling, use of fine, nonreactive sutures and atraumatic instruments, meticulous hemostasis, and copious irrigation. Intraoperative adjuvants, such as Hyskon and Interceed, can be used at the end of the procedure to reduce postoperative adhesion formation.

Laparotomy: Segmental Resection

The experience with linear salpingostomy primarily applies to treatment of unruptured ampullary ectopic gestations. Unlike ampullary pregnancies that are extratubal growing be-

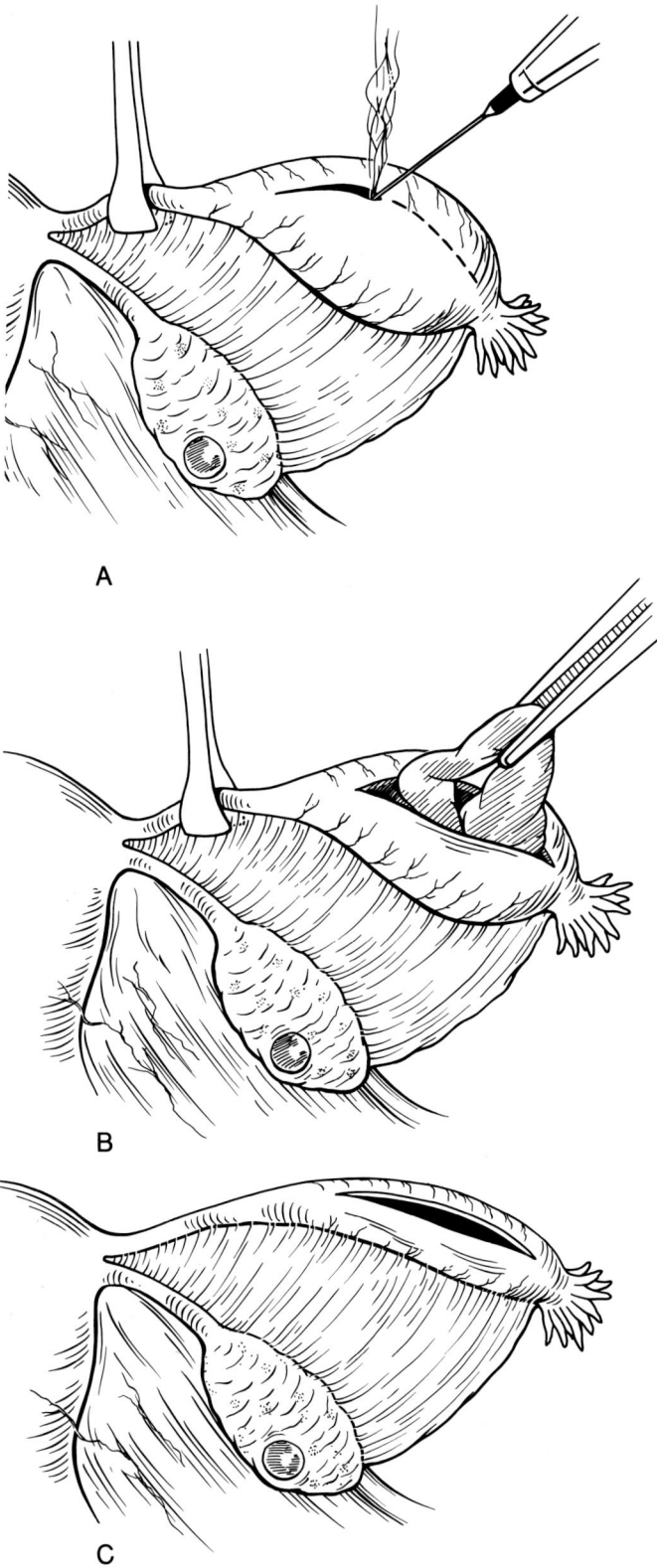

FIGURE 32–3. Salpingostomy performed at laparotomy for a right tubal pregnancy. *A*, After securing the fallopian tube with a Babcock clamp, an incision is made in the antimesenteric border of the tube over the ectopic pregnancy. *B*, The pregnancy is then removed with a forceps. *C*, The incision is left open to heal.

tween the serosa and tubal lumen, isthmic pregnancies more frequently grow within the lumen of the tube, destroying the surrounding luminal epithelium.[50] For this reason, segmental resection of the affected portion of the fallopian tube has been the recommended treatment approach for isthmic ectopic pregnancies (Fig. 32–4*A* and *B*).[51, 52] Following such surgery, both immediate and delayed tubal anastomosis can

be performed. However, deferral of the anastomosis has been advocated so that it can be done electively without the interference of tubal edema and intraperitoneal blood clots.[18] One series[53] compared unruptured isthmic ectopics treated with segmental resection (i.e., partial salpingectomy of the involved segment of the tube) with delayed microsurgical anastomosis to linear salpingostomy and reported higher patency

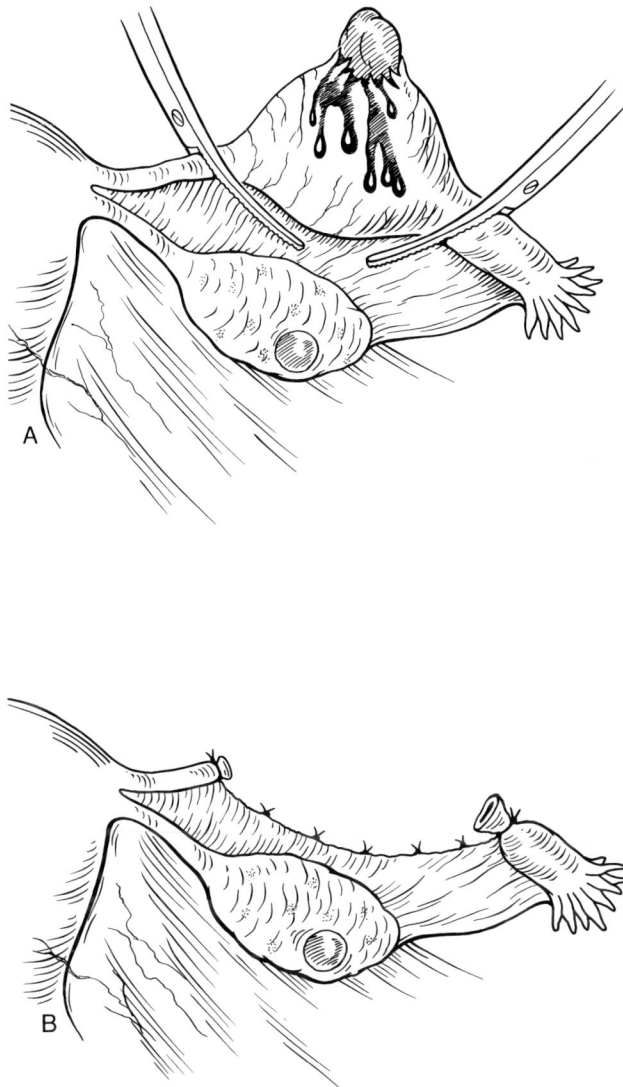

FIGURE 32–4. Segmental resection of the right fallopian tube performed at laparotomy. *A,* Kelly clamps are placed across the fallopian tube and the mesosalpinx. *B,* The tube and mesosalpinx are sutured.

and pregnancy rates in the former group. Four of the six patients who were managed by segmented resection and delayed microsurgical anastomosis subsequently conceived, whereas none of the four patients managed by linear salpingostomy subsequently conceived. On the other hand, Pouly and associates[43] treated 22 patients with isthmic ectopic pregnancies by laparoscopic salpingostomy and had a 54.5% subsequent intrauterine pregnancy rate. Isthmic ectopic pregnancy remains a relative contraindication to laparoscopic salpingostomy.

Ectopic pregnancies in the infundibular portion of the tube between the fimbria and the ampulla are rare; they have been treated in the past by "milking" or "squeezing" the pregnancy out through the distal end of the tube. Because of delayed hemorrhage and lower success rates reported following such a procedure, linear salpingostomy has replaced "fimbrial expression" as the currently recommended surgical technique for this condition (Fig. 32–4).[54] In contrast, tubal abortions, in which the ectopic is already partially or completely extruded from the fimbriated end, should be treated by removing any remaining products of conception.[54] Table 32–2

summarizes the recommended surgical approaches to conservative management of ectopic pregnancy based on its location.

OPERATIVE LAPAROSCOPY

Successful laparoscopic removal of a small, unruptured ampullary tubal ectopic pregnancy was first achieved by Shapiro and Adler in 1973.[55] Since then, the laparoscopic approach to the treatment of unruptured tubal pregnancy has become common and in most communities is now the standard of care. A comparison of salpingostomy at laparotomy versus salpingostomy at laparoscopy revealed significantly shorter hospital stay, convalescence, and operating time in the latter group.[56] Other investigators have studied conservative laparoscopic surgery in terms not only of morbidity but also of prognosis for future tubal patencies and pregnancy rates (see Table 32–1).[40, 41, 45, 57] Bruhat and colleagues[40] successfully treated 57 of 60 patients with laparoscopic salpingostomy or tubal aspiration, following which 18 of 25 (72%) women desiring pregnancy had normal pregnancies and 3 (12%) had another ectopic. Another group[41] reported laparoscopic salpingostomy treatment of 18 stable patients with unruptured ampullary ectopic pregnancies smaller than 3 cm in diameter, following which 50% of those patients trying to conceive were successful without any repeat ectopic gestations. These authors reported the advantages of these laparoscopic treatments of ectopic pregnancies to include decreased operative time (average 45 minutes), shortened hospitalization (average 1.5 days), and smoother hospital course compared with laparotomy. Cartwright and coworkers[42] reported on 27 patients managed laparoscopically with salpingostomy for small unruptured ectopics. Six of eight patients subsequently tested had tubal patency, and five of eight patients attempting conception became pregnant, one of which had a repeat tubal pregnancy in the operated tube. Pouly and associates[43] reported conservative laparoscopic salpingostomy treatment of 321 ectopics, and of 118 patients desiring subsequent pregnancy, the intrauterine pregnancy rate was 64.4% and the ectopic rate was 22%. Another series[44] reported a 62% intrauterine pregnancy rate and 16% repeat

TABLE 32–2. Summary of Currently Recommended Surgical Approaches to Conservative Management of Ectopic Pregnancy*	
Location	**Recommended Surgical Management**
Cornual	Cornual resection at laparotomy
Interstitial	Resect pregnancy with tubal preservation followed by delayed microsurgical anastomosis at laparotomy
Isthmic	Laparoscopic partial salpingectomy of the involved segment followed by delayed microsurgical anastomosis‡
Ampullary	Laparoscopic linear salpingostomy†, ‡
Infundibular	Laparoscopic linear salpingostomy†, ‡
Fimbria	Laparoscopic linear salpingostomy or enucleation†, ‡
Tubal abortion	Laparoscopically remove any remaining products of conception through the distal end†, ‡
Ovarian	Laparoscopic excision with preservation of adnexa‡, §

*Based on its location for the patient who desires future fertility.
†Proceed to partial salpingectomy if hemostasis cannot be accomplished.
‡Proceed to laparotomy if technically difficult at laparoscopy.
§Proceed to oophorectomy if technically difficult.

ectopic rate after laparoscopic linear salpingostomy for small, unruptured ampullary ectopic pregnancies. Unfortunately, these reports are based on descriptive studies without a control group and only short-term followup. In addition, some of these studies combined salpingostomy, salpingotomy, tubal aspiration, and partial salpingectomy in their analysis of conservative laparoscopic management. Furthermore, incomplete followup of the patients was common. In contrast with the studies cited earlier, Vermesh and colleagues[45] performed a prospective, randomized clinical trial comparing the treatment of 60 patients with unruptured ectopics by linear salpingostomy via laparoscopy versus laparotomy. Ipsilateral tubal patency was demonstrated in 16 of 20 (80%) patients undergoing laparoscopic salpingostomy and 17 of 19 (89%) patients undergoing salpingostomy by laparotomy. The subsequent pregnancy rates were 56% (10 of 18, 9 of which were intrauterine pregnancies and 1 was an ectopic pregnancy) in patients who underwent laparoscopic salpingostomy and 58% (11 of 19, 8 of which were intrauterine pregnancies and 3 were ectopics) in those treated with salpingostomy at laparotomy. Although they found statistically similar outcomes with regard to tubal patency, pregnancy rates, and persistent trophoblast disease (1 patient from each group), laparoscopic salpingostomy was associated with significant reduction in patient morbidity, hospitalization, and cost.

Hemodynamic instability and cornual ectopic location remain absolute contraindications to the laparoscopic approach. More relative contraindications have included hemoperitoneum, tubal rupture, excessive tubal diameter, isthmic location, severe pelvic adhesive disease, and concurrent severe medical illnesses. Both Vermesh and associates[45] and Pouly and colleagues[43] have increased the recommended upper limit of the tubal diameter approachable by laparoscopic methods from 3 to 4 to 6 cm (Tables 32–3 and 32–4).

The technique of laparoscopic salpingostomy is similar to that performed at laparotomy. Use of diluted vasopressin solution (20 U of vasopressin in 20 mL of physiologic saline) injected into the antimesenteric border of the fallopian tube overlying the ectopic bulge before performing linear salpingostomy diminishes incisional bleeding. A 22-gauge spinal needle can be introduced directly into the peritoneal cavity through the abdominal wall and directed into the antimesenteric bulge. A linear salpingostomy incision can be made using electrocautery, laser (carbon dioxide, potassium-titanyl-phosphate, argon, neodymium-YAG), or laparoscopic scissors once the tube has been stabilized. This usually requires multiple abdominal puncture sites, including at least two or three suprapubic and one umbilical. The length of the tubal incision should be about two thirds the length of the ectopic bulge. Extrusion of the products of conception sometimes occurs spontaneously but usually requires assistance, which can be accomplished using atraumatic or spoon forceps. Irrigating inside the tube through the salpingostomy incision has

been advocated to aid in creating a plane of separation between the trophoblast and the implantation site. Removal of large tissue fragments can be accomplished by using either the larger trochar sleeve or the operating channel of the laparoscope, or by morcellation. In this regard, the recent availability of disposable laparoscopic instruments, especially those instruments for retrieving tissue, such as a bag that is pulled through the trochar, is useful. Careful attention to the tissue as it enters the trochar is important to prevent the products of conception from dropping unnoticed back into the pelvis, where it may reimplant. Irrigation of the salpingostomy and implantation sites aids in identifying and treating remaining trophoblastic tissue or residual bleeding.

Finally, with the advent of even more sophisticated laparoscopic instruments, sutures, operating techniques, and video equipment, the reality of performing more invasive procedures, previously requiring laparotomy, through the laparoscope has been reached. In this way, salpingectomies can be performed through a laparoscopic approach. The location, diameter, and integrity of the ectopic as well as the patient's desire for future fertility dictate the specific operation performed. For cases of failed salpingostomy, tubal rupture with persistent bleeding, isthmic location of the ectopic pregnancy, or a severely damaged tube, a partial or complete salpingectomy through the laparoscope is now commonly performed instead of a laparotomy.[58, 59] Two or three Endoloop sutures (0 chromic catgut) may be placed proximal to the ectopic bulge before the tube is sharply transected (Fig. 32–5A and B). Alternatively, electrocautery and laparoscopic scissors may be used in a sequential fashion to coagulate and then cut the tubal segments and mesosalpinx proximal and distal to the ectopic. To accomplish a complete salpingectomy, the mesosalpinx is sequentially coagulated and then cut before the proximal portion of the tube is coagulated and cut free from the cornua (Fig. 32–6). The tubal segment can be removed from the abdomen in the same way already described for the large products of conception in association with salpingostomy. For patients who preoperatively request sterilization, the uninvolved tube can also be removed using these same techniques, or a portion of this tube can be cauterized as is usually performed in laparoscopic tubal sterilization.

Electrocautery can be used for coagulative destruction of the ectopic gestation. Such a technique may be useful for the patient with an isthmic ectopic who does not desire future fertility. The disadvantage of this method is the inability to confirm the diagnosis histologically, and for this reason electrocauterization of the ectopic gestation is not the preferred technique.

TABLE 32–4. Contraindications for Laparoscopic Treatment of Ectopic Pregnancy

Absolute Contraindications
- Hemodynamic instability
- Cornual ectopic pregnancy

Relative Contraindications
- Hemoperitoneum
- Tubal rupture
- Excessive tubal diameter
- Isthmic location
- Severe pelvic adhesive disease
- Concurrent severe medical illness

TABLE 32–3. Indications for Laparotomy for Ectopic Pregnancy

- Hemodynamic instability
- Cornual ectopic pregnancy
- Severe pelvic adhesive disease
- Tubal diameter greater than 6 cm

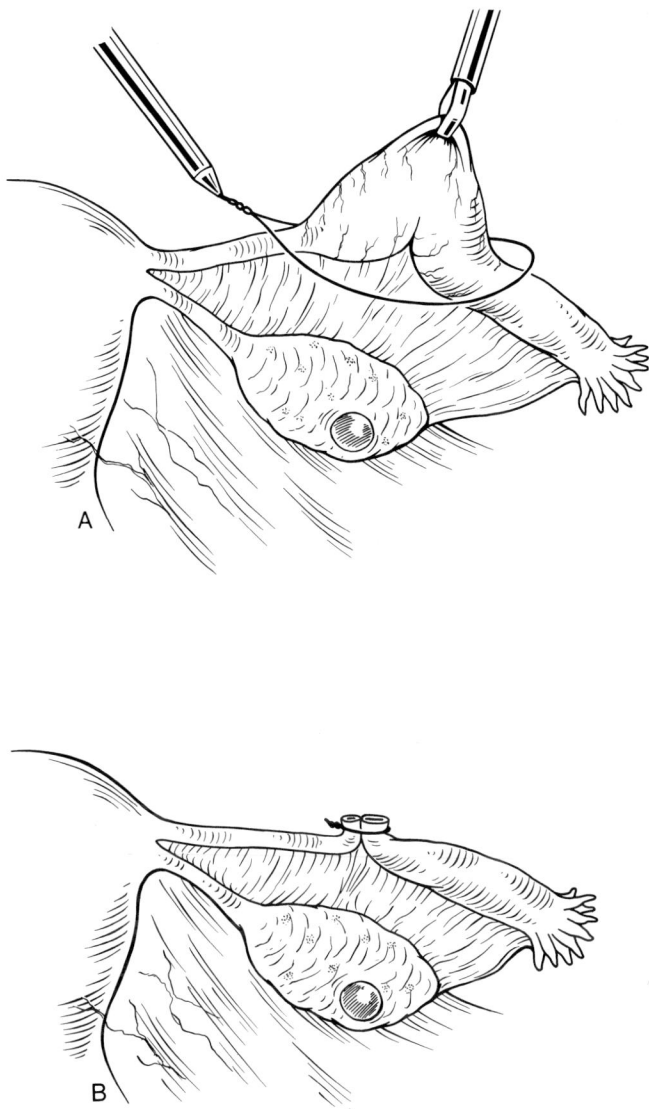

FIGURE 32–5. A segmental resection of a tubal pregnancy performed at laparoscopy. *A*, The tube is elevated and a pre-tied suture is looped around the ectopic. *B*, The segment of the fallopian tube containing the pregnancy is excised and removed, leaving the two stumps secured by the suture.

NONOPERATIVE MEDICAL APPROACH

The evolution of the management of ectopic gestations has continued to progress rapidly, and we are now at the point that nonsurgical treatment is an option in well-selected cases. Although an acutely ruptured symptomatic ectopic pregnancy remains a surgical emergency, recent studies support the efficacy of medical management of properly selected cases such as small, unruptured ampullary ectopics. Theoretical benefits of a medical approach include decreased tissue trauma and peritoneal adhesion formation.

The most experience stems from the use of methotrexate, a cytotoxic drug that has been widely used to treat gestational trophoblastic disease. This drug inhibits dihydrofolate reductase, an enzyme that converts dihydrofolic acid to tetrahydrofolic acid and thus interferes with the synthesis of deoxyribonucleic acid. Because of its rapid growth, the trophoblast is extremely sensitive to this agent. A series of recent reports confirmed the efficacy of the application of methotrexate in

various dosages and routes of administration for both primary treatment of small, unruptured ectopics and followup use for persistent trophoblastic tissue.[60–72] Other agents such as systemic RU-486[60] and local injection of prostaglandins or potassium chloride have also been investigated.[60, 63]

Early reports described the use of methotrexate on an inpatient basis.[61, 64, 66] In 1986, Ory and associates[61] treated six patients with laparoscopically confirmed, nonruptured ampullary ectopics (<4 cm in diameter with <100 mL of blood in the peritoneal cavity) with four doses of intravenous methotrexate (1 mg/kg) alternating every other day with 0.1 mg/kg leucovorin (also four doses in total). Five of the six subjects experienced resolution of the ectopic pregnancy, with the sixth patient eventually requiring a salpingectomy. However, morbidity from the methotrexate included mild stomatitis, gastritis, and transiently elevated transaminase levels. Rodi and coworkers,[64] using a similar dosing regimen, inclusion criteria, and monitoring, reported on seven women. All patients responded after a full course, with a median time to resolution (undetectable levels of β-hCG) of 31 days (range 5 to 50 days). Followup hysterosalpingogram in four of five patients demonstrated patency, and the fifth patient had an intrauterine pregnancy prior to the scheduled hysterosalpingogram.

A trial by Stovall and colleagues[67] in 1989 evaluated a less complicated approach to the use of methotrexate treatment of ectopics. These investigators described outpatient chemotherapy of unruptured ectopic pregnancy in 37 of 116 laparoscopically documented ectopics using "individualized" dosing regimens. Titrating the doses of methotrexate to the rate of decrease in β-hCG levels reduced the total amount administered, side effects, and cost. All the patients in their study had an unruptured ectopic smaller than 3 cm in diameter diagnosed at laparoscopy. Methotrexate (1 mg/kg) was administered intramuscularly, alternating with intramuscular citrovorum (0.1 mg/kg) on a daily basis, beginning just after laparoscopy. This regimen was continued until there was a

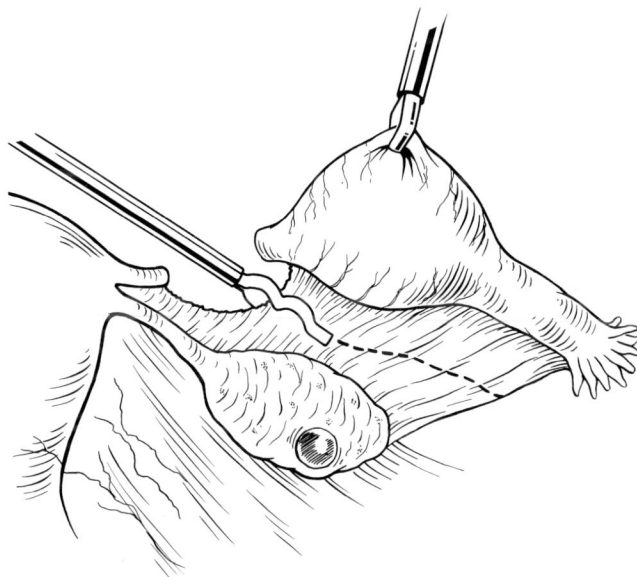

FIGURE 32–6. A salpingectomy performed at laparoscopy for a right tubal pregnancy. After elevating the tube with a forceps, a Kloeppinger forceps is used to coagulate the tube and adjacent mesosalpinx. The tube is excised by cutting along the line of coagulation.

15% or greater decrease in two consecutive daily β-hCG titers or until the blood progesterone level was lower than 1 ng/mL. No more than four doses of methotrexate were given without a drug-free interval of at least 1 week. Most patients required two doses. Complete blood counts and aspartate aminotransferase were monitored. Only one patient required a second course of methotrexate, which was given for plateauing levels. However, two patients experienced tubal rupture and required laparotomy, one of whom had fetal cardiac activity within the fallopian tube on ultrasonographic examination.[67] This, combined with the experience of Sauer and colleagues,[66] who described two ruptures in their series both with ultrasound-detected fetal heartbeats, led to the recommendation that the presence of fetal cardiac activity is an absolute contraindication to systemic chemotherapeutic treatment of ectopic pregnancies.

In a subsequent series of 57 patients, Stovall and colleagues[68] reported a descriptive study of reproductive performance following treatment of ectopics by their methotrexate protocol outlined earlier. The mean time to return of menses was 26.0 (range 0 to 157) days. Nineteen of 23 patients (82.6%) demonstrated patency of the affected fallopian tube on hysterosalpingogram. Eleven of 14 patients (78.6%) desiring a pregnancy were successful, one of whom had an extrauterine gestation. In a subsequent report of 100 similar cases,[70] only four patients failed treatment, and only five patients had mild side effects after the fourth dose. Followup hysterosalpingograms of 58 patients revealed an 84.5% ipsilateral tubal patency. Final reproductive outcome included 31 intrauterine and 4 recurrent ectopic pregnancies. Because of the small number of cases, it is difficult to compare tubal patency and intrauterine and recurrent ectopic pregnancy rates following surgical versus medical treatment in any sort of a meaningful way. However, most researchers report subsequent tubal patency after systemic methotrexate to be 53% to 100%, with an average of 71%,[63] which compares well with the incidence of patency for various surgical methods (see Table 32–1).[73]

The methotrexate protocols described so far have required laparoscopic diagnosis, which by nature taints the benefit of nonsurgical treatment. Stovall and associates[69] recently reported an algorithm for the nonlaparoscopic diagnosis and treatment of ectopic pregnancy that was 100% accurate in their randomized trial (Fig. 32–7), and applied it successfully in 50 other patients reported in a more recent publication.[70] They later combined this nonsurgical diagnostic technique with an outpatient single-dose methotrexate regimen[71] to describe a minimally invasive diagnostic and treatment approach to the care of the hemodynamically stable patient with an unruptured ectopic pregnancy less than 3.5 cm in diameter. Previously, medical protocols have required multiple methotrexate doses. Stovall's group recently reported on a single 50 mg/m² intramuscular methotrexate dose without citrovorum rescue for treatment of unruptured ectopic pregnancy less than 3.5 cm in greatest diameter in 30 patients.[71] The β-hCG levels continued to rise for at least 3 days in all patients after treatment, with the levels starting to decline by day 7. Their plan was that any patient whose β-hCG level did not decline by 15% between days 4 and 7 would receive another 50 mg/m² intramuscular methotrexate dose 1 week after the first dose. Patients with declining β-hCG levels by day 7 were followed weekly until their β-hCG level was lower than 15 IU/L. They recommended a second course of

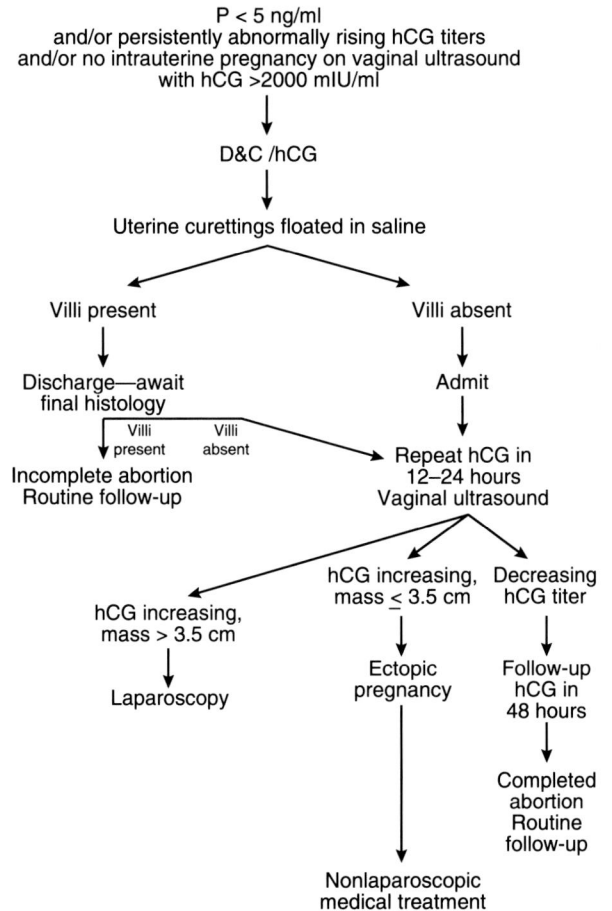

FIGURE 32–7. The Stovall algorithm for the nonsurgical diagnosis of ectopic pregnancy. hCG, human chorionic gonadotropin; D&C, dilation and curettage.

methotrexate for a plateau or increase in levels. No patient required a second dose or experienced any side effects. Twenty-nine patients were successfully treated, and only one patient (whose ectopic had cardiac activity) required surgery for tubal rupture.[71] In terms of followup, in a more recent study[74] the same group reported that the mass of an ectopic pregnancy may remain after the β-hCG determination is negative in an adequately treated patient, and an increase in mass size alone did not appear to predict tubal rupture.

Others have described local methotrexate injection into the ectopic site at the time of laparoscopy[16, 62] to reduce side effects. Pansky and associates[62] described the treatment of 27 hemodynamically stable patients with small unruptured ampullary ectopic pregnancies with an injection of 12.5 mg of methotrexate (diluted in 2 mL of physiologic solution) into the ectopic site at laparoscopy. Twenty-four of the patients underwent an unremarkable course and required no further intervention. Three patients required a laparotomy for rising titers. In another similar series,[16] nine outpatients were treated with a 15-mg methotrexate injection into the gestational mass at the time of laparoscopy. Eight had complete resolution over the next 10 to 33 days, and one required a laparotomy for plateauing β-hCG levels. There were no complications, and two patients subsequently conceived. Still others have reported success with local injection, at the time of laparoscopy, of other agents such as prostaglandin F₂α,[1, 75, 76] hyperosmolar glucose solution,[77] and potassium chloride.[63] Although potassium chloride lacks the side effects of methotrexate, its main disadvantage is that it acts mainly by causing asystole of the fetal heart, leading to fetal death, but has no direct effect on the growth of trophoblastic tissue, which may continue. Successful local injection of these drugs at the time of transabdominal[78] and transvaginal[79, 80] ultrasonography has also been reported. Ultrasound-guided injection of prostaglandin E_2 has been a less successful approach than methotrexate.[81, 82] Currently, the systemic use of methotrexate is the preferred route for administration with regard to the modern medical treatment of ectopic pregnancies. The local injection of particular compounds or solutions for this purpose is still investigative.

PERSISTENT ECTOPIC PREGNANCY

Methotrexate therapy has also been suggested for noninvasive treatment of patients with persistent ectopic pregnancies,[65, 83, 84] a well-recognized complication of salpingostomy, and the result of the continued growth of trophoblastic tissue after incomplete removal of the ectopic pregnancy. The clinical manifestations of a persistent ectopic can be that of acute symptoms of pain or hypotension, or a persistent or rising β-hCG level following conservative surgery. Although the incidence is unclear at the present time, Pouly and colleagues[43] reported that 15 of 321 (4.8%) patients treated for an ectopic with conservative laparoscopic surgery had subsequent persistent disease. Consistently, the incidence has been reported to vary between 0% and 10% in a series of studies.[18, 43, 45, 85, 86] Formerly, the treatment of choice was repeat surgery to complete the removal of the trophoblastic tissue, frequently requiring salpingectomy. This is obviously less than optimal for a young, healthy patient population in whom preservation of fertility is strongly desired. More recently, Rose and coworkers[65] described three such patients successfully treated with methotrexate and citrovorum factor rescue, thus avoiding the need for reoperation. They administered methotrexate as an intravenous bolus of 100 mg/m² over 1 hour followed by 200 mg/m² as a 12-hour infusion. Citrovorum factor, 10 mg/m² every 12 hours for four doses, was given parenterally on an outpatient basis 24 hours after the methotrexate was initiated.

Although the goal of less invasive surgical therapy is important, the prevention and early diagnosis of this condition are even more imperative. One group[57] noted that early surgical therapy (<2 cm, <42 days of amenorrhea) increased the subsequent risk for occurrence of persistent trophoblastic disease. They postulated that this was due to incomplete evacuation of the products of conception caused by ill-defined cleavage planes between the trophoblast and implantation site in the absence of intratubal hemorrhage and clot. In another review of eight cases of persistent tubal pregnancy,[87] four of the five tubes examined histopathologically showed the implantation sites with associated chorionic villi to be medial (toward the uterus) to the previous surgical incision sites. This was also noted in two other cases in which the entire tube had been removed after attempted conservative surgical procedures failed because of uncontrolled bleeding. The recommendation was made for irrigation or exploration of the tube medial to the apparent site of implantation at the time of initial uncontrolled bleeding.[87] To control bleeding and enhance complete removal of the ectopic pregnancy,

others have suggested placement of a mesosalpingeal ligature[88] or vasopressin injection into the mesosalpinx[43] at the time of conservative surgery to reduce vascular supply and therefore initiate a more complete and rapid involution of the implantation site. In yet another report,[86] preoperative and postoperative hCG levels predicted and detected patients at risk of developing persistent trophoblast disease. In this study, 7 of 98 patients, who underwent conservative surgery for ectopic pregnancies by laparoscopy or laparotomy, had biochemical and histologic evidence of persistent trophoblastic activity. A second operation was needed in 7 of 31 patients with preoperative hCG levels higher than 3000 IU/L, whereas only one such intervention was necessary in the remaining patients with preoperative hCG levels lower than 3000 IU/L. Eight of the 22 patients with hCG levels higher than 1000 IU/L on the second day and 7 of 11 patients with hCG levels higher than 1000 IU/L on the seventh day after surgery needed a second surgical procedure, whereas 86 of 87 patients with hCG levels lower than 1000 IU/L on the seventh day after surgery had an uneventful course.[86] For early documentation of persistent disease, it is recommended to routinely follow serial quantitative β-hCG levels after conservative treatment until they become negative over time.[83] Vermesh and coworkers[89] showed that by postoperative day 12, the diagnosis of persistent ectopic pregnancy is suspected if β-hCG levels did not fall below 10% of their initial value. Consideration of biweekly β-hCG levels after laparoscopic salpingostomy may be most appropriate, especially for patients with less than 6 weeks of amenorrhea who had small ectopic pregnancies (<2 cm). Management of persistent ectopic pregnancies depends on the symptomatology of the individual patient as well as the medical-surgical history, the trend of the serial β-hCG levels, and, finally, the individual surgeon's experience.

AVAILABILITY OF IN VITRO FERTILIZATION

With the advent of the assisted reproductive technology (ART), IVF, and ET, with its associated continuously improving pregnancy rates, the furor over conserving as much tube as possible following surgical removal of ectopic pregnancies may begin to dampen. The ability to achieve an intrauterine pregnancy via IVF-ET while bypassing an absent or defective fallopian tube may lessen the concern regarding tubal integrity following ectopic pregnancy surgery. In fact, in patients planning for or actually participating in IVF, laparoscopic salpingectomy for an ectopic pregnancy may even be preferable to salpingostomy by perhaps reducing the risk of developing another ectopic during future IVF.

REPRODUCTIVE POTENTIAL FOLLOWING AN ECTOPIC PREGNANCY

The reproductive potential of patients with previous tubal pregnancies varies depending on prior tubal integrity, ectopic location, treatment approach, condition of the contralateral tube, and other infertility factors. The fertility rates following radical and more conservative surgery have already been reviewed in the preceding sections (see Table 32–1). In summary, pregnancy results seem to remain in the same range regardless of approach (i.e., laparoscopy versus laparotomy, salpingostomy versus salpingectomy). Use of microsurgical techniques and surgical adjuvants both have been applied in an effort to improve future fertility and decrease the occurrence of repeat ectopic pregnancies. Postoperatively, it has been recommended that patients should be evaluated with a hysterosalpingogram at 4 to 6 months and laparoscopy at 1 year if pregnancy has not occurred.[54]

Reproductive potential following two tubal pregnancies has also been described. In one series,[90] 23 patients with two previous ectopic pregnancies were followed over the subsequent 5 years, and of 13 of the women attempting to conceive, 4 had an intrauterine pregnancy, and 1 had a repeat ectopic pregnancy. Tulandi and associates[91] followed 24 women with two previous ectopic pregnancies (all initially had a salpingectomy, followed by a salpingostomy in their remaining tube at laparotomy) and found that 50% of the patients who tried to conceive had an intrauterine pregnancy; the incidence of a third ectopic pregnancy was 27.8%. Halatt[31] showed that 4 of 7 patients (57.1%) who conceived after two tubal pregnancies had a third ectopic pregnancy. Conversely, Valle and Lifchez[37] reported that all nine patients who had two previous ectopic pregnancies and desired future fertility subsequently had term intrauterine pregnancies.

While attempting to optimize successful future reproductive potential, it must not be forgotten that Rh-negative women can become sensitized during an ectopic pregnancy with an Rh-positive fetus, creating an increased risk of fetal hydrops in a future pregnancy. Thus, Rh-negative women should receive RhoGAM.[92] This is especially important in young patients, many of whom desire future fertility.

CONCLUSION

During the past decade, the incidence of ectopic pregnancy has dramatically increased, although morbidity and mortality rates have significantly declined. Earlier detection before acute tubal rupture and massive intraperitoneal hemorrhage requiring emergent laparotomy is a key effector of these trends. The advent of newer diagnostic modalities such as laparoscopy, transabdominal-transvaginal ultrasonography, and rapid, sensitive quantitative β-hCG determinations have led to the occurrence of earlier diagnosis of an asymptomatic patient. The subsequent diagnosis of smaller unruptured ectopics paved the way toward implementation of more conservative surgical approaches. The remarkable journey from the classic salpingo-oophorectomy approach at laparotomy to linear salpingostomy with tubal preservation at laparoscopy seems to be superseded only by more recent advances employing medical treatments such as methotrexate and options of future fertility with ART. The net result has been to decrease patient morbidity and medical expenses, seemingly without compromising pregnancy rates.

All these factors have remarkably converted the clinical presentation of an ectopic pregnancy from an acute, life-threatening disease to a more benign condition, enabling physicians to "tailor make" treatment approaches to appropriately fulfill the wishes of their patients, especially those interested in future reproductive capability.

REFERENCES

1. Doyle MB, DeCherney AH, Diamond MP. Epidemiology and etiology of ectopic pregnancy. Obstet Gynecol Clin North Am 1991; 18(1):1–17.

2. Centers for Disease Control. Current trends: ectopic pregnancies—United States, 1979–1980. MMWR 1984; 33:201.

3. Centers for Disease Control. Ectopic pregnancy: United States, 1981–1983. MMWR 1986; 35:289.

4. Stock RJ. The changing spectrum of ectopic pregnancy. Obstet Gynecol 1988; 71:885.

5. Mashiach S, Oelsner G. Nonoperative management of ectopic pregnancy: a preliminary report. J Reprod Med 1982; 27:127.

6. Cole T, Corlett RC Jr. Chronic ectopic pregnancy. Obstet Gynecol 1982; 59:63.

7. Tait RL. Five cases of extrauterine pregnancy operated upon at the time of pregnancy. Br Med J 1884; 1:1250.

8. Lawson HW, Atrash HK, Saftlas AF, et al. Ectopic pregnancy surveillance, United States, 1970–1985. MMWR 1988; 37:9.

9. Romero R, Copel JA, Kadar N, et al. Value of culdocentesis in the diagnosis of ectopic pregnancy. Obstet Gynecol 1985; 65:519.

10. Kadar N, DeVore G, Romero R. Discriminatory hCG zone: its use in the sonographic evaluation for ectopic pregnancy. Obstet Gynecol 1981; 58 (2):156–161.

11. Romero R, Kadar N, Jeaty P, et al. The value of the discriminatory hCG zone in the diagnosis of ectopic pregnancy. Obstet Gynecol 1985; 66:357.

12. Fossum GT, Davanajan V, Kletzky OA. Early detection of pregnancy with transvaginal ultrasound. Fertil Steril 1988; 49:788.

13. Matthew CP, Coulson PB, Wild RA. Serum progesterone levels as an aid in the diagnosis of ectopic pregnancy. Obstet Gynecol 1986; 68:390.

14. Yeko TR, Gorrill MJ, Hughes LH, et al. Timely diagnosis of early ectopic pregnancy using a single blood progesterone measurement. Fertil Steril 1987; 48:1048.

15. Buck RH, Joubert SM, Norman RJ. Serum progesterone in the diagnosis of ectopic pregnancy: a valuable diagnostic test? Fertil Steril 1988; 50:752–755.

16. Wolf GC, Witt BR. Outpatient laparoscopic management of ectopic pregnancy with a local methotrexate injection. J Reprod Med 1991; 36:489–492.

17. Guillaume J, Benjamin F, Sicuranza BJ. Serum estradiol as an aid in the diagnosis of ectopic pregnancy. Obstet Gynecol 1990; 76:1126–1129.

18. DeCherney AH, Kase N. The conservative surgical management of unruptured ectopic pregnancy. Obstet Gynecol 1979; 54:451.

19. Kadar N, Caldwell B, Romero R. A method of screening for ectopic pregnancy and its indications. Obstet Gynecol 1980; 58:162.

20. Nyberg DA, Laing FC, Filly RA, et al. Ultrasonographic differentiation of the gestational sac of early intrauterine pregnancy from the pseudogestational sac of ectopic pregnancy. Radiology 1983; 146:755.

21. Romero R, Kadar N, Castro D, et al. The value of adnexal sonographic findings in the diagnosis of ectopic pregnancy. Am J Obstet Gynecol 1988; 158:52.

22. Frangenheim H, Turanli I. Die Vorteile der Kuldoskopie und der Laparoskopie beider Diagnose der Extrauteringraviditat. Feburtshilfe Frauenheikd 1964; 24:4744.

23. Samuelson S, Sjovall A. Laparoscopy in suspected ectopic pregnancy. Acta Obstet Gynecol Scand 1972; 51:31.

24. Gonzalez FA, Wayman M. Ectopic pregnancy: diagnosis. Gynecol Obstet 1981; 3:181.

25. Timonen S, Nieminen U. Tubal pregnancy: choice of operative method of treatment. Acta Obstet Gynecol Scand 1967; 46:327.

26. Jeffcoate TNA. Salpingectomy or salpingo-oophorectomy. Br J Obstet Gynaecol 1955; 135:74.

27. Bronson RA. Tubal pregnancy and infertility. Fertil Steril 1977; 28:221–228.

28. Bender S. Fertility after tubal pregnancy. J Obstet Gynecol Br Emp 1956; 63:400.

29. Schenker JG, Eyal F, Polishuk WK. Fertility after tubal pregnancy. Surg Gynecol Obstet 1972; 135:74.

30. Fulsher RW. Tubal pregnancy following homolateral salpingectomy. Am J Obstet Gynecol 1959; 78:355.

31. Halatt JG. Repeat ectopic pregnancy: a study of 123 consecutive cases. Am J Obstet Gynecol 1975; 122:520.

32. Kalchman GG, Meltzer RM. Interstitial pregnancy following homolateral salpingectomy. Am J Obstet Gynecol 1966; 96:1139.

33. Novy MJ. Surgical alternatives for ectopic: is conservative treatment best? Contemp Obstet Gynecol 1983; 20:91.

34. Stromme WB. Salpingotomy for tubal pregnancy. Obstet Gynecol 1953; 1:472.

35. DeCherney AH, Maheux R, Naftolin F. Salpingostomy for ectopic pregnancy in the sole patient oviduct: reproductive outcome. Fertil Steril 1989; 37:619.

36. Langer R, Bukovsky I, Herman A, et al. Conservative surgery for tubal pregnancy. Fertil Steril 1982; 38:427.

37. Valle JA, Lifchez AS. Reproductive outcome following conservative surgery for tubal pregnancy in women with a single fallopian tube. Fertil Steril 1983; 39:316–320.

38. Stromme WB. Conservative surgery for ectopic pregnancy: a twenty-year review. Obstet Gynecol 1973; 41:215–223.

39. Bukovsky I, Langer R, Herman A, et al. Conservative surgery for tubal pregnancy. Obstet Gynecol 1979; 53:709–711.

40. Bruhat MA, Manhes H, Mage G, Pouly JL. Treatment of ectopic pregnancy by means of laparoscopy. Fertil Steril 1980; 33:411.

41. DeCherney AH, Romero R, Naftolin F. Surgical management of unruptured ectopic pregnancy. Fertil Steril 1981; 35:21.

42. Cartwright PS, Herbert CM III, Maxson WS. Operative laparoscopy for the management of tubal pregnancy. J Reprod Med 1986; 31:589–591.

43. Pouly JL, Mahnes H, Mage G, et al. Conservative laparoscopic treatment of 321 ectopic pregnancies. Fertil Steril 1986; 46:1093.

44. DeCherney AH, Diamond MP. Laparoscopic salpingostomy for ectopic pregnancy. Obstet Gynecol 1987; 70:948.

45. Vermesh M, Silva PD, Rosen GF, et al. Management of unruptured ectopic gestation by linear salpingostomy: a prospective randomized clinical trial of laparoscopy versus laparotomy. Obstet Gynecol 1989; 73:400.

46. Oelsner G, Rabinovitch O, Morad K, et al. Reproductive outcome after microsurgical treatment of tubal pregnancy in women with a single fallopian tube. J Reprod Med 1986; 3:483–486.

47. Nelson LM, Margara RA, Winston RM, et al. Primary and secondary closure of ampullary salpingotomy compared in the rabbit. Fertil Steril 1986; 45:292.

48. Tulandi T, Guralnick M. Treatment of tubal ectopic pregnancy by salpingotomy with or without tubal suturing and salpingectomy. Fertil Steril 1991; 55:53–55.

49. DeCherney AH, Maheux R. Modern management of tubal pregnancy. Curr Probl Obstet Gynecol 1983; 6:1.

50. Budowick M, Johnson TR Jr, Genadry R, et al. The histopathology of the developing tubal ectopic pregnancy. Fertil Steril 1980; 34:169.

51. DeCherney AH, Naftolin F, Graebe R. Isthmic ectopic pregnancy: segmental resection and anastomosis to conserve fertility. Fertil Steril 1984; 41:458.

52. Senterman M, Jibodh R, Tulandi T. Histopathologic study of ampullary and isthmic tubal ectopic pregnancy. Am J Obstet Gynecol 1988; 159:399.

53. DeCherney AH, Boyers SP. Isthmic ectopic pregnancy: segmental resection as a treatment of choice. Fertil Steril 1985; 44:301.

54. DeCherney AH, Meyer WR. Ectopic pregnancy. In: Sciarra JJ, Droegemueller W, editors. Gynecology and Obstetrics. Philadelphia: JB Lippincott, 1991:1–20.

55. Shapiro HI, Alder DH. Excision of an ectopic pregnancy through the laparoscope. Am J Obstet Gynecol 1973; 117:290.

56. Brumsted J, Kessler C, Gison C, et al. A comparison of laparoscopy and laparotomy for the treatment of ectopic pregnancy. Obstet Gynecol 1988; 71:889.

57. Seifer DB, Gutmann JN, Doyle MB, et al. Persistent ectopic pregnancy following laparoscopic linear salpingostomy. Obstet Gynecol 1990; 76:1121–1125.

58. Dubuisson JB, Aubriot FX, Cardone V. Laparoscopic salpingectomy for tubal pregnancy. Fertil Steril 1987; 47:225.

59. Taracani JC. Endoscopic salpingectomy. J Reprod Med 1981; 26:541.

60. Kenigsberg D, Porte J, Hull M. Medical treatment of residual ectopic pregnancy: RU 486 and methotrexate. Fertil Steril 1987; 47:702–703.

61. Ory SJ, Villanueve AL, Sand PK, et al. Conservative treatment of ectopic pregnancy with methotrexate. Am J Obstet Gynecol 1986; 154:1299–1306.

62. Pansky M, Bukovsky I, Golan A, et al. Local methotrexate injection: a nonsurgical treatment of ectopic pregnancy. Am J Obstet Gynecol 1989; 161:393–396.

63. Pansky M, Golan A, Bukovsky I, et al. Nonsurgical management of tubal pregnancy: necessity in view of the changing clinical appearance. Am J Obstet Gynecol 1991; 164:888–895.

64. Rodi IA, Sauer MV, Gorrill MJ. The medical treatment of unruptured ectopic pregnancy with methotrexate and citrovorum rescue: preliminary experience. Fertil Steril 1986; 46:811–813.

65. Rose PG, Cohen SM. Methotrexate therapy for persistent ectopic pregnancy after conservative laparoscopy management. Obstet Gynecol 1990; 76:947–949.

66. Sauer MV, Gorrill MJ, Rodi IA, et al. Nonsurgical management of unruptured ectopic pregnancy: an extended clinical trial. Fertil Steril 1987; 48:752.

67. Stovall TG, Ling FW, Buster JE. Outpatient chemotherapy of unruptured ectopic pregnancy. Fertil Steril 1989; 51:435–438.

68. Stovall TG, Ling FW, Buster JE. Reproductive performance after methotrexate treatment of ectopic pregnancy. Am J Obstet Gynecol 1990; 162:1620–1624.

69. Stovall TG, Ling FW, Carson SA, et al. Nonsurgical diagnosis and treatment of tubal pregnancy. Fertil Steril 1990; 54:537–538.

70. Stovall TG, Ling FW, Gray LA, et al. Methotrexate treatment of unruptured ectopic pregnancy: a report of 100 cases. Obstet Gynecol 1991; 77:749–753.

71. Stovall TG, Ling FW, Gray LA. Single-dose methotrexate for treatment of ectopic pregnancy. Obstet Gynecol 1991; 77:754–757.

72. Tanaka T, Hayashi H, Kutsuzawa T, et al. Treatment of interstitial ectopic pregnancy with methotrexate: report of a successful case. Fertil Steril 1982; 37:851–852.

73. Mitchell DE, McEwain HF, McCarthy JA, et al. Hysterosalpingographic evaluation of tubal patency after ectopic pregnancy. Am J Obstet Gynecol 1987; 157:618–621.

74. Brown DL, Felker RE, Stovall TG, et al. Serial endovaginal sonograph of ectopic pregnancies treated with methotrexate. Obstet Gynecol 1991; 77:406–409.

75. Linblom B, Kallfelt B, Hahlin M, Hamberger L. Local prostaglandin $F_2\alpha$ injection for termination of ectopic pregnancy. Lancet 1987; 4:776.

76. Vejtorpm, Vejerslew L, Ruge S. Local prostaglandin treatment of ectopic pregnancy. Hum Reprod 1989; 4:464.

77. Lang P, Weiss P, Mayer H. Local application of hyperosmolar glucose solution in tubal pregnancy. Lancet 1989; 1:922.

78. Robertson DE, Moye MAH, Hansen JN, et al. Reduction of ectopic pregnancy by injection under ultrasound control. Lancet 1987; 2:974–975.

79. Timor-Tritsch I, Baxi I, Peisner DB. Transvaginal salpingocentesis: a new technique for treating ectopic pregnancy. Am J Obstet Gynecol 1989; 160:459–461.

80. Tulandi T, Bret P, Atri M, et al. Treatment of ectopic pregnancy by transvaginal intratubal methotrexate administration. Obstet Gynecol 1991; 77:627–630.

81. Ribic Paucelj M, Novak-Antolic Z, Urhovec I. Treatment of ectopic pregnancy with prostaglandin E_2. Clin Exp Obstet Gynecol 1989; 16:106–109.

82. Feichtinger W, Kemeter P. Conservative treatment of ectopic pregnancy by transvaginal aspiration under sonographic control and injection of methotrexate. Lancet 1987; 1:381–382.

83. Rivlin ME. Persistent ectopic pregnancy: complication of conservative surgery? Int J Fertil 1985; 30:10–14.

84. Seifer DB, Diamond MP, DeCherney AH. Persistent ectopic pregnancy. Obstet Gynecol Clin North Am 1991; 18:153–159.

85. Dimarchi JM, Kososa TS, Kobara TY, et al. Persistent ectopic pregnancy. Obstet Gynecol 1987; 70:555–558.

86. Lundorff P, Hahlin M, Sjöblom P, et al. Persistent trophoblast after conservative treatment of tubal pregnancy: prediction and detection. Obstet Gynecol 1991; 77:129–133.

87. Stock RJ. Persistent tubal pregnancy. Obstet Gynecol 1991; 77:267–270.

88. Kelly RW, Martin SA, Strickler RC. Delayed hemorrhage in conservative surgery for ectopic pregnancy. Am J Obstet Gynecol 1979; 133:225–226.

89. Vermesh M, Silva PD, Sauer MV, et al. Persistent tubal ectopic gestation: patterns of circulating β-human chorionic gonnadotropin and progesterone, and management options. Fertil Steril 1988; 50:584.

90. DeCherney AH, Silidker JS, Mezer HC, et al. Reproductive outcome following two ectopic pregnancies. Fertil Steril 1985; 43:82.

91. Tulandi T. Reproductive performance of women after two tubal ectopic pregnancies. Fertil Steril 1988; 50:164.

92. Grimes DA. Rh immunoglobin utilization after ectopic pregnancy. Am J Obstet Gynecol 1981; 140:246.

CHAPTER 33

Endometriosis: Pathophysiology and Presentation

JOUKO HALME and VICKEN SAHAKIAN

Endometriosis is the presence of endometrial tissue, glandular and stromal, outside the uterine cavity. Although endometriosis is one of the most common and fascinating gynecologic disorders, its pathogenesis and pathophysiology still remain an enigma. This chapter presents the current concepts and the available newest information dealing with the pathophysiology and the presentation of this intriguing disorder.

EPIDEMIOLOGY

The true incidence of endometriosis is difficult to measure because the diagnosis can be accurately made only by direct visualization along with histologic sampling. It has been estimated that the prevalence of endometriosis in the general U.S. population is about 10%.[1]

The incidence also varies between the populations studied. In low-risk groups, such as women undergoing laparoscopic tubal ligation, a prevalence of 2% to 5% has been reported.[2] However, a study among low-risk Norwegian women revealed a much higher prevalence of 18%.[3] A similar prevalence was reported in a Hawaiian study.[4] On the other hand, in high-risk groups, such as infertility patients, a prevalence of 30% to 40% is not uncommon.[2, 5]

Houston and associates estimated the age-specific prevalence rates to be highest in the 35- to 45-year-old age group, with an overall incidence of endometriosis in the ages 15 to 50 years of 1.6 per 1000 woman-years.[6]

Several studies showed a preponderance of this disease in white women.[7, 8] However, once confounding variables were accounted for, this difference disappeared.[9] However, a racial predilection has been shown to exist in Asian women, who have an incidence twice as high as that of white women.[10]

Endometriosis is also believed to be more common in women who delay their first pregnancy and less common in the highly parous.[11] This protective nature of childbearing is thought to be secondary to decreased exposure to menstrual cyclicity.[12] In the same context, endometriosis is rarely seen in the postmenopausal age group, and its occasional occurrence usually is associated with or precipitated by exogenous hormone supplementation.[13, 14] The disease is also virtually absent in girls younger than 15 years of age without outflow tract obstruction.[15] This low prevalence in young and old age groups may be only apparent rather than real, because all endometriotic lesions may not have been appropriately searched for or appreciated in earlier studies.

In the older literature, a positive correlation seemed to exist between higher socioeconomic status and endometriosis.[8, 16–18] However, these findings may be due to a detection bias, and their validity is questionable.

Evidence of a genetic or familial tendency of endometriosis has been reported in the literature.[19, 20] Simpson and colleagues[21] showed that of patients with endometriosis, 5.8% of their female siblings older than 18 years of age and 8.1% of their mothers were similarly affected. Overall, about 7% of all first-degree relatives were affected.[21] A polygenic, multifactorial pattern of inheritance is most probable.

An association between several menstrual characteristics and endometriosis has been shown by Cramer and coworkers.[22] In their study, the average age at menarche in patients with endometriosis was significantly younger than in the control subjects. There also was an increase in risk for endometriosis with increasing menstrual pain, increased duration of flow, heavier flow, and decreased cycle length. The same study showed endometriosis to be less common among patients who started smoking before 17 years of age and smoked more than one pack per day. Patients who exercised regularly were also shown less likely to have endometriosis, presumably secondary to decreased endogenous estrogen levels. Surprisingly, weight was not found to be a risk factor, and taller women had less risk for endometriosis in this study.[22]

PATHOGENESIS

As stated earlier, the pathogenesis of endometriosis is still not fully elucidated. The literature is full of speculations and scientifically poorly supported theories. A multifactorial etiology may be the reason for such a diversity of postulates. In the following sections, some of the proposed theories along with supportive scientific evidence are presented.

Menstrual Dissemination

In the mid-1920s, Sampson[23] theorized that backflow of menstrual blood from the uterine cavity through the fallopian tubes could result in endometriosis. More than 60 years later, retrograde menstruation remains the most popular postulated mechanism for the initiation of endometriosis. Many observations and studies support this theory (Table 33–1).

The inherent characteristic of endometriotic tissue to survive in ectopic locations, such as the peritoneal cavity, has been well documented. In addition, the presence of viable endometrial cells has been demonstrated in the menstrual effluent.[24] Experimental evidence supports this theory as well. The viability of menstrually shed endometrium in the peritoneal cavity of rhesus monkeys was shown in ingenious experiments by Scott and associates in 1953.[25] These investigators redirected and attached the cervix through the posterior cul-de-sac and thus allowed the flow of spontaneous menses into the peritoneal cavity. Experimental implantation of endometrial implants into the peritoneum of castrated monkeys and their survival in the presence of exogenous hormonal support is further proof of the possibility of a similar mechanism in vivo.[26] The presence of endometrial cells in the peritoneal fluid in women has also been demonstrated at the time of laparoscopy.[27]

There is no doubt that uterine contents are capable of passing through the physiologic cornual sphincter and flowing in a retrograde manner into the pelvis. The presence of blood in the peritoneal fluid in all menstruating women, including those with endometriosis, is common.[28] (The frequency of retrograde flow alone, however, would not explain the presence of this disease in only some women and not others. Other factors must contribute to the predisposition of some women to develop this condition.) The anatomic distribution of endometrial implants lends further support to this theory, in that implants are most commonly found in the dependent portions of the pelvis, such as the cul-de-sac or the ovarian fossa. Similarly, the ovarian surface, being in close approximation to the fimbria, is frequently involved.[29] The increased incidence of endometriosis in women with menorrhagia and congenital or acquired outflow obstruction constitutes further evidence that retrograde dissemination could initiate or propagate the disease.[21, 30–32] Finally, the ability of endometrial tissue to attach and grow on ectopic areas is shown by the transplantation of such tissue in surgical scars.[33]

Despite relatively strong scientific support, it is clear that this pathogenetic mechanism is inapplicable to all presentations of endometriosis.

Hematogenous-Lymphatic Dissemination

Suspicion for a lymphatic or hematogenous spread of endometriosis has arisen secondary to the finding of implants in locations such as lymphatic channels, lymph nodes, the pulmonary system (e.g., the lungs),[34] muscle, skin, and even the heart.[35]

Experiments in rabbits have been able to demonstrate that finely diced rabbit endometrium injected into the animal's ear vein resulted in pulmonary implants of viable endometrial tissue.[36] This presents direct proof of hematogenous spread of viable endometrial tissue.

Iatrogenic Dissemination

The accidental deposition of endometrial tissue in ectopic sites during surgical procedures on the uterus can occur. Therefore, endometriosis in cesarean section scars in and under the skin is not uncommon.[37] In subhuman primates, the iatrogenic displacement of such tissue after repeated hysterotomies eventually leads to pelvic endometriosis. Cases of endometriosis involving only the bladder dome following cesarean section have also been reported.[38]

Metaplastic de Novo Transformation

Support for the theory of metaplasia as a mechanism for the development of endometriotic implants comes from experiments done by Merril in 1966.[39] Fragments of autologous rabbit endometrium placed inside millipore diffusion chambers, which allow the passage of chemical substances but do not exclude cellular material, were implanted subperitoneally in the pelvis. At various times, each area was excised, including the diffusion chamber and adjacent tissue. Endometrium-like epithelium and glands were observed in the connective tissue adjacent to the implants.[39] These experiments suggest that some unknown factors, secreted by endometrial tissue, are capable of inducing metaplastic changes in peritoneal mesothelium.

Other than the experimental findings discussed earlier, additional solid evidence for the metaplasia theory is lacking. Many characteristics of endometriosis do not support this theory: the absence of this disease in women with congenital agenesis of the uterus, the rare occurrence of implants outside the pelvis even though coelomic epithelium covers the entire abdominal surface, and the rare presence of endometriosis in postmenopausal women.[40] The sporadic reports of endometriosis in males having received huge doses of estrogens indirectly support this theory.

TABLE 33–1. Supportive Evidence for Menstrual Dissemination in the Pathogenesis of Endometriosis

Inherent capability of endometrial tissue to survive in ectopic locations

Retrograde flow of menstrual effluent well documented

Successful peritoneal transplantation of endometrial tissue in animal models

Anatomic distribution of endometriotic implants consistent with retrograde spillage

Increased incidence of endometriosis in women with outflow tract obstruction

Peritoneal Fluid Environment in Endometriosis

The local environment that surrounds the endometriotic implant in the peritoneal cavity is dynamic. The presence of "foreign" tissue attracts, presumably by chemotaxis, scavenger cells of the mononuclear family to the implantation site. The predominant cells in the peritoneal fluid, indeed, are mononuclear phagocytes, macrophages. The total numbers and the activational status of peritoneal macrophages are increased in patients with endometriosis.[41–47] The major function of peritoneal fluid macrophages probably is phagocytosis of cellular debris or "foreign" cells, such as sperm. Macrophages also are capable of secreting various substances, such as growth factors, cytokines, prostanoids, and complement,[48, 49] that may play a role in facilitating implantation and growth of endometrial cells or as mediators of infertility (Fig. 33–1). The role of such cytokines and growth factors in the pathophysiology of endometriosis is increasingly gaining significance. One such cytokine, interleukin-1, is a mediator of host inflammatory immune response. It induces prostaglandin (PG) synthesis,[50] T-cell proliferation, and stimulation of B-lymphocyte immunoglobulin production.[51] The increased level of such cytokines in peritoneal fluid of patients with endometriosis,[52–55] along with the deleterious effect they can have on developing embryos[53] and their stimulatory capacity of fibroblast proliferation and collagen deposition,[56] may suggest a role for these peptides in the pathophysiology of endometriosis.

The exact role the peritoneal fluid volume plays in endometriosis is still debated. A recent review of the literature[57] examined 17 studies with different cycle timing of collection. Five of those 17 studies showed increased volume, and 11 showed no change.[57] Of those, the largest study, which evaluated 113 patients with endometriosis compared with 136 control subjects, revealed increased peritoneal fluid volume throughout the menstrual cycle.[41] Cycle length and collection techniques may explain the discrepancies in these studies. Even if this increase in peritoneal fluid volume is proved, its role in the pathogenesis or pathophysiology of endometriosis is still unknown, because higher volumes are also present in women with unexplained infertility. However, patients with endometriosis who have high peritoneal fluid volumes have lower overall chances for pregnancy than those with lower volumes. A progestogen-associated endometrial protein has been shown to be present in increased levels in the peritoneal fluid of women with moderate to severe endometriosis.[58] The origin and role of this protein in the pathogenesis of endometriosis are unknown. Another partially characterized peritoneal fluid factor has been shown to interfere with ovum pick-up.[59] Peritoneal fluid derived from patients with endometriosis has also been shown to stimulate proliferation of stromal cells in culture.[60]

The role of prostanoids in the pathophysiology of endometriosis is even less clear. There are several sources of PGs in the peritoneal cavity, including macrophages,[46] peritoneal surfaces,[61] ovarian follicles,[62] and endometriotic implants.[63, 64] Again, studies are conflicting and contradictory. However, the following observations and findings are worth mentioning:

- Several studies have shown elevated levels of certain PGs, such as $PGF_{2\alpha}$, in animals with endometriosis.[65, 66]

A report in women, however, has shown lower levels of this prostanoid in endometriotic implants compared with eutopic endometrium.[67]

- There are conflicting reports about levels of $PGF_{2\alpha}$ and PGE_2 in peritoneal fluid of women with and without endometriosis. Some of these have failed to show any difference,[45, 68–70] whereas others have found elevated levels throughout the menstrual cycle[71] or only in the secretory part of the cycle.[72]
- Similar contradictory results have been obtained when levels of thromboxane A_2 and prostacyclin metabolites were measured in peritoneal fluid. Some have shown significantly elevated levels in women with endometriosis,[73–76] whereas others did not confirm these findings.[71, 77, 78]
- Studies in rabbits have shown $PGF_{2\alpha}$ to stimulate deoxyribonucleic acid synthesis and increased cell numbers of endometrial cells.[79]

These statements illustrate how conflicting the literature is in regard to the role of PGs in the pathophysiology of endometriosis. In theory, prostanoids would certainly help explain the etiology of pain in this disorder[80] and could be involved in providing a stimulus to the proliferation of endometrial cells. A role in the associated infertility is also plausible, as discussed in a later section.

The Immune System in Endometriosis

Several investigations and observations point toward some role of the immune system in the pathogenesis of endometriosis. However, many of the studies have conflicting results.

The following findings point to an association between endometriosis and the humoral and cell-mediated immune systems:

- Increased numbers of T and B cells in the peripheral blood and peritoneal fluid from women with endometriosis have been reported.[81]
- Immunoglobulin G (IgG) and IgA autoantibodies have been identified against endometrial tissues in the sera, peritoneal fluid, and cervical and vaginal secretions of women with endometriosis.[82–85] Similarly, antibodies have been found against subcellular elements or antigens, such as phospholipids.[86, 87]
- Alterations in cell-mediated immunity against autologous endometrial antigens have been described in experimental animal models.[88] In women with severe endometriosis, cytotoxicity assays demonstrated decreased target cell lysis compared with control subjects.[89]

In view of the accumulated information, it appears that different mechanisms integrated together may lead to the development of endometriosis. The initial inciting event, whether retrograde flow of menstrual debris, iatrogenic dissemination, or coelomic metaplasia, initiates a chain of events, assisted by an altered immune system, to culminate in the ectopic implant. Local peritoneal factors, including macrophage activity and secretory products, may contribute to the persistence of the disease. Putative growth factors can lead to the excess deposition of extracellular matrix or colla-

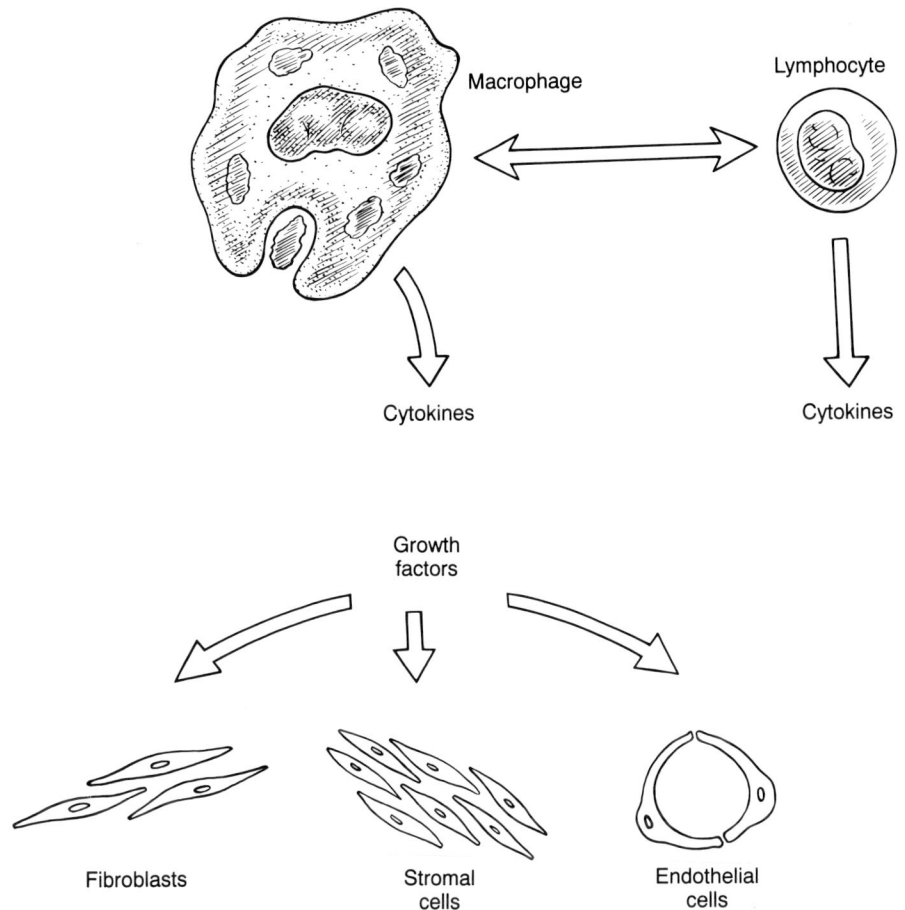

FIGURE 33–1. Role of macrophage and macrophage mediators in endometriosis.

gen, thereby forming fibrosis and adhesions, which are commonly present and an integral part of endometriosis.

IMPLANT CHARACTERISTICS

The histologic similarities between eutopic and ectopic endometrium are well known. The presence of endometrial glands surrounded by stromal cells is a hallmark of both, even though the phenotypic appearance of the endometriotic implants varies greatly depending on different histologic features. The prerequisite for histologic diagnosis of endometriosis is the presence of endometrial glands with either stromal elements or hemosiderin-laden macrophages, or preferably both. Many studies have shown a cyclic response, occasionally unpredictable, of the endometriotic implant to the hormonal changes of the menstrual cycle.[90, 91] Its dependency on estrogen for proliferation has also been shown in animal experiments.[26, 92] Despite the histologic resemblance, variations in the response to different hormonal milieus exist between eutopic and ectopic endometrium.[93, 94] Differences in the concentration of estrogen and progesterone receptors and in the expression of hydroxysteroid dehydrogenase enzyme have been shown between ectopic and eutopic endometrium in several studies.[95–97] These findings may explain why endometriotic tissue is unpredictable in its response to the cyclic hormonal changes.

PATHOPHYSIOLOGY OF INFERTILITY
(Table 33–2)

It is estimated that 30% to 40% of women with infertility have endometriosis,[98] and approximately 50,000 new cases will be diagnosed in the infertile population in the United States each year.[99] On the basis of epidemiologic calculations, Strathy and colleagues estimated the risk of infertility to be 20 times greater with endometriosis than without.[2]

The strongest data to suggest that endometriosis is associated with a lower probability of conception come from studies on women with azoospermic husbands undergoing therapeutic donor insemination.[100] On the other hand, some studies based on life table analysis of conceptions have concluded that mild endometriosis does not necessarily interfere with fertility.[101] Recent studies have actually suggested that women with minimal and mild endometriosis frequently conceive without specific therapy.[102, 103] Olive and coworkers,

TABLE 33–2. Pathophysiology of Infertility in Endometriosis

Mechanical interference
Hormonal/ovulatory dysfunction
Interference with implantation/embryogenesis
Interference with sperm function
Interference with fertilization
Interference with tubal function

from prospective data among infertile women, showed a monthly probability of conception of 5.7% for mild endometriosis and 3.2% for moderate disease without specific therapy.[104] One could argue, however, that the lack of efficacy of medical or surgical treatment in mild endometriosis reflects only the lack of any effective specific treatment modality. The issue is obviously not settled, and it appears that the stage of the disease is an important factor to consider when evaluating the association of infertility with endometriosis.

Mechanical Interference

It is not difficult to understand how severe endometriosis could interfere with fertility. The presence of extensive thick, dense adhesions and fibrosis can obviously interfere with ovum pick-up or tubal transport. Adhesions involving the surface of the ovaries can prevent exposure of the ovum, whereas those involving the fallopian tubes or the fimbria result in impaired capture and transport.

Hormonal and Ovulatory Dysfunction

Hormonal disturbances as a cause of infertility have been suggested by several investigators. Macrophages, for instance, have been shown to cause a decrease in granulosa cell progesterone production.[105] Because an increase in the total number of peritoneal macrophages in patients with endometriosis has been shown,[57] analogous intrafollicular macrophages may have adverse effects on local hormonal regulation.

Some studies have demonstrated an association between PGs and luteolysis.[106] An abnormal pattern of luteinizing hormone secretion has been demonstrated in patients with endometriosis.[107] The luteinized unruptured follicle syndrome was initially reported to occur in as many as 79% of patients with endometriosis,[108, 109] especially those with severe disease. Several other studies, however, have failed to corroborate these findings.[110–112] Abnormal levels of luteal phase progesterone have been found in patients with endometriosis by some investigators[107, 113, 114] and refuted by others.[115, 116] Similarly, elevated levels of prolactin concentrations have been reported in women with endometriosis.[113, 117]

An approximately 10% incidence of anovulation associated with endometriosis has also been shown in retrospective studies only.[118]

Because most results of these studies implicating an endocrine dysfunction as a cause of infertility are conflicting and contradictory, it is unlikely that such hormonal abnormalities play a major role in this disorder.

Interference with Implantation and Embryogenesis

An adverse effect of peritoneal fluid from patients with endometriosis has been shown in animal studies.[119]

PGs have been implicated as possibly interfering with implantation.[119] A possible mechanism is thought to be secondary to increased uterine contractility with resultant expul-

sion of the embryo. A deleterious effect of certain cytokines, such as interleukin-1, on the developing embryo in culture has also been shown.[53]

Some retrospective studies reported an increased incidence of spontaneous abortions in women with endometriosis.[120–123] Subsequent prospective studies have refuted such an association.[124, 125]

Interference with Sperm Function

Sperm phagocytosis by macrophages has been shown in animals[126] and humans.[127] Additional support for this theory comes from studies that show an increased incidence of sperm in the peritoneal fluid of patients without endometriosis compared with those with endometriosis.[128] Also, macrophages have been found in increased numbers in the fallopian tubes of women with endometriosis[129] compared with patients with tubal occlusion.[42]

Sperm function may also be influenced by secretory products of activated monocytes and macrophages, such as tumor necrosis factor-α, which has been shown to exert an adverse effect on sperm motility.[54, 130] In contrast, Halme and associates were unable to demonstrate any effect of peritoneal fluid from patients with endometriosis on sperm motility or on penetration of zona-free hamster ova.[131]

Interference with Fertilization

An abnormal in vitro fertilization rate of oocytes from patients with endometriosis has been demonstrated.[132] These studies raised the possibility of interference with oocyte function.

The increased volume of peritoneal fluid in patients with endometriosis, as shown by some,[57] along with detrimental constituents, has been postulated to interfere with fertilization. Animal studies in mice have shown a detrimental effect of the peritoneal fluid from women with endometriosis on sperm-ova interaction.[133] The possible mechanisms by which macrophages and their secretory products may interfere with sperm function or fertilization are summarized in Figure 33–2.

Interference with Tubal Function

Abnormal PG synthesis may possibly influence tubal transport. Studies in animals have shown accelerated ovum transport and reduced fertility with PGs.[134–136] Even though studies in humans have not confirmed such findings,[137] PGs could still have an important role in the reproductive pathophysiology in women.

The peritoneal fluid contains a diversity of components, including essentially all the serum proteins. A peritoneal fluid protein that interferes with ovum capture by the fimbria has been described.[59]

PRESENTATION

Phenotypic Appearance

The morphologic appearance of endometriotic implants varies greatly (Table 33–3 and Fig. 33–3 [see color section

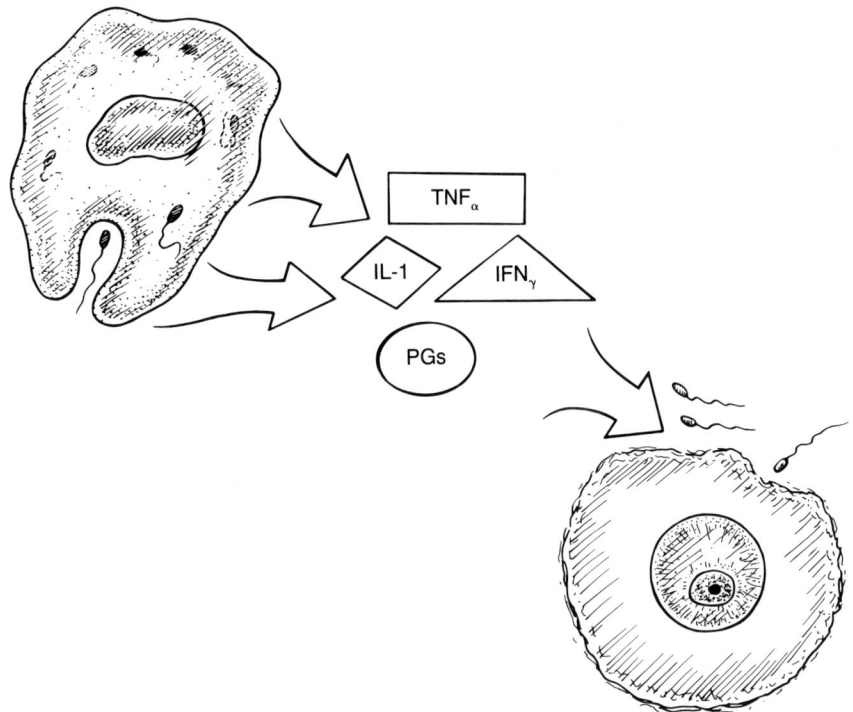

FIGURE 33–2. Possible mechanisms by which macrophages or their secretory products may interfere with reproductive processes. TNFα, tumor necrosis factor-α; IL-1, interleukin-1; PGs, prostanoids; IFN, interferon.

in the center of the book]). The spectrum ranges from the classic nodular implant, varying in color from white to blue or brown or black, to the red vesicular implants, which are characterized by prominent vascularization and usually appear singly or in clusters. Papular implants, which are small, whitish, yellow, or nonpigmented lesions enclosed in the subperitoneal tissue, have also been described.[138, 139] Jansen and Russell[139] performed 137 laparoscopic biopsies of nonpigmented peritoneal lesions in 77 patients. Eighty-five biopsy specimens showed endometrium-like glands or stroma. Nonpigmented lesions that were commonly endometriotic included white opacified peritoneum (endometriosis in 81%), red flamelike lesions (81%), and glandular lesions (67%).[139] The different morphologic appearances of these lesions probably represent different stages of the disease. The classic bluish-dark implant and deep infiltrating lesions are probably associated with later stages of the disease, when repeated in situ menstruation and fibrotic changes have occurred.[139a]

Endometriosis involving the ovaries can be superficial or present as cystic masses, varying in size, called *endometriomas.*[138] The term *chocolate cyst* has been given to these masses owing to the characteristic thick, brownish fluid content.

Few studies demonstrate any correlation between the phenotypic appearance of a lesion and symptoms, infertility, or

TABLE 33–3. Phenotypic Appearance of Endometriotic Implants

Adhesions
Nodular deep lesions
Superficial pigmented lesions
Superficial nonpigmented lesions
Peritoneal pockets
Cystic disease (endometrioma)

responsiveness to therapy. Koninckx and coworkers demonstrated a significant association between deep infiltrating lesions and pain.[140]

Anatomic Locations (Table 33–4)

Pelvic. Endometriosis most commonly involves the pelvic peritoneum in close proximity to the fallopian tube, the cul-de-sac, the ovaries, the fallopian tubes, and the uterosacral ligaments.[141, 142] Basically, any surface covered with mesothelium is a target for the endometriotic implant.

Urinary. Only about 1% of women with endometriosis have urinary tract involvement.[143] This involvement may include the bladder,[38] the ureters,[144, 145] or the kidneys.[142] Ureteral involvement, although a relatively rare phenomenon, has been reported in more than 120 cases.[146] In many of these, the diagnosis was made late because of lack of symptoms.

Gastrointestinal. Intestinal involvement is well documented, with an incidence ranging from 5% to 37% of patients with endometriosis.[147–149] Reports indicate that as many as 7% of cases of intestinal endometriosis occur in postmenopausal women.[147, 150, 151] Intestinal segments in the pelvis, such as the rectosigmoid, are the most commonly affected areas. Zwas and Lyon defined the anatomic distribution of involvement as follows: (1) rectosigmoid colon, 75% to 90%; (2) appendix, 3% to 18%; and (3) distal ileum, 2% to 16%.[152] Other studies documented a less than 1% appendiceal involvement.[153, 154] Rarely, endometriosis can affect intestinal organs such as the stomach,[155] pancreas,[156] transverse colon,[157] and anal canal.[158]

Thoracic-Pulmonary. There have been more than 17 reported cases of histologically proved thoracic endometriosis and more than 29 probable cases.[159] The mechanisms for the development of thoracic disease include endometrial emboli,

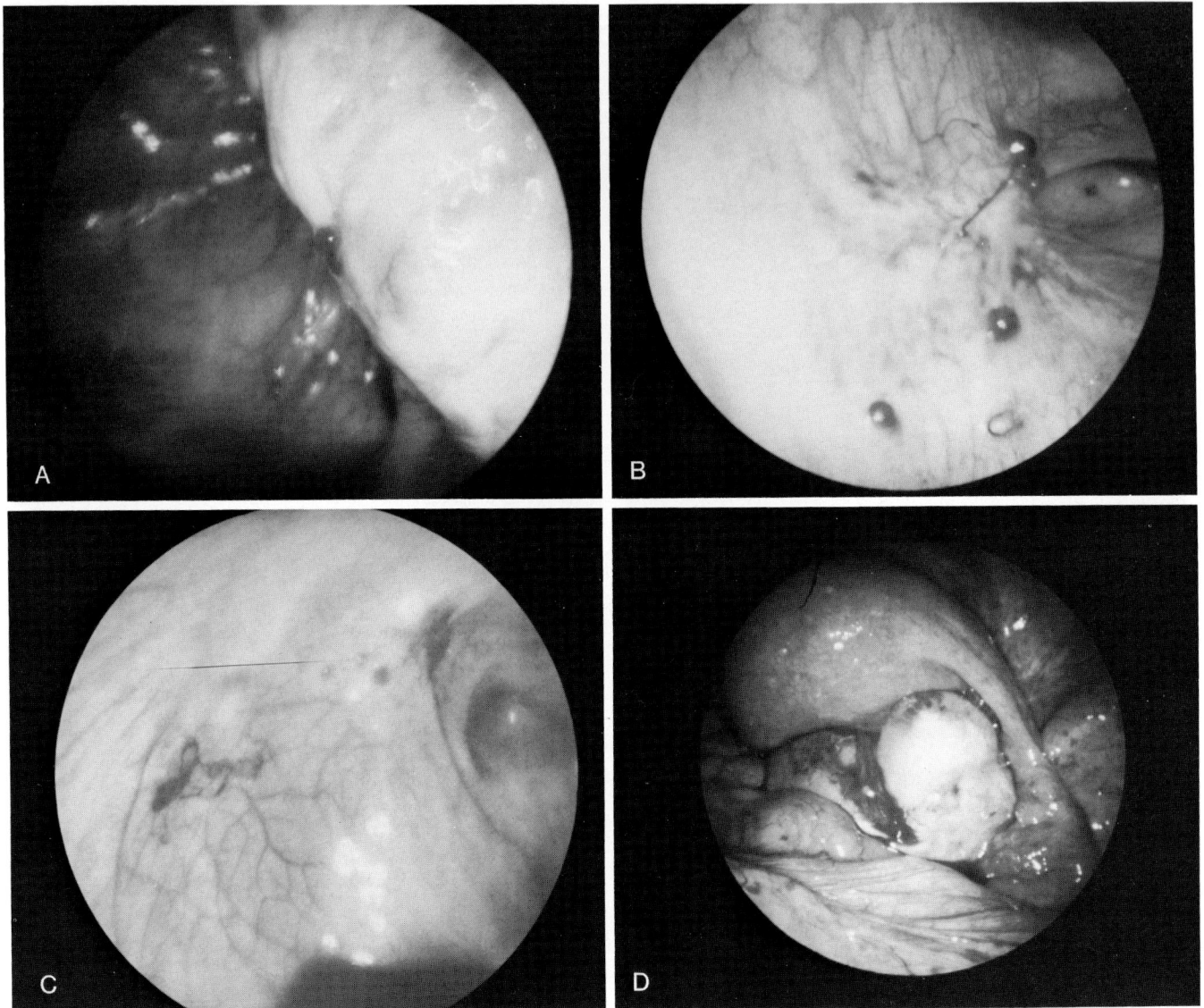

FIGURE 33–3. Examples of the gross appearance of endometriotic lesions. *A*, Adhesion from the ovarian fossa to an implant on the surface of the ovary. *B*, Superficial pigmented lesions. *C*, Peritoneal pocket and superficial pigmented lesions. *D*, Endometrioma of the ovary. (*A* to *D* courtesy of William R. Keye, Jr., M.D.)

contiguous dissemination through the diaphragm, or metaplasia. Congenital or diaphragmatic defects may lead to pulmonary involvement through contiguous migration.[160] Most thoracic endometriosis involves the right lung.

MISCELLANEOUS

Endometrial tissue has been identified in remote areas such as thigh muscle,[161] the nasal mucosa,[155] the inguinal canal,[162–164] the extraperitoneal portion of the round ligament,[164] incisional scars,[37, 165–169] within the sheath of the sciatic nerve,[170] the cerebrum,[171] and the heart.[172] Vulvovaginal or perineal involvement has also been reported,[173, 174] as well as lymphatic involvement, such as the inguinal nodes.[175]

Endometriosis occurring in men after estrogen exposure has been described in case reports, which obviously brings more uncertainty to the pathogenesis of this disorder.[176–178]

Symptomatology

Depending on the particular organ involvement, patients with endometriosis can have a multitude of presenting symptoms and signs (Table 33–5).

Pelvic. The classic symptoms associated with pelvic en-

TABLE 33–4. Common Anatomic Location of Endometriotic Implants

Pelvic	Gastrointestinal
Ovaries	Rectosigmoid
Cul-de-sac	Appendix
Uterosacral ligaments	Colon
Uterus	Small bowel
Fallopian tubes	Thoracic or pulmonary
Urinary	Parenchymal
Bladder peritoneum	Pleura
Ureters	

TABLE 33–5. Reported Symptoms Associated with Endometriosis	
Pelvic	Gastrointestinal
Dysmenorrhea	Abdominal pain
Dyspareunia	Diarrhea
Pelvic pain	Constipation
Urinary	Tenesmus
Flank pain	Hematochezia
Back pain	Pulmonary
Abdominal pain	Hemoptysis
Urgency	Scapular pain
Frequency	Catamenial chest pain

dometriosis include dysmenorrhea or pelvic pain and dyspareunia.[179, 180] Minimal or mild endometriosis may be associated with more severe symptoms than the more extensive lesions.[15] Thus, the severity of symptoms does not necessarily correlate with the extent of the disease. There are many possible explanations for the lack of such correlation. On one hand, in earlier studies on this subject, young nonpigmented lesions may have been missed, and sometimes these lesions may be particularly painful. On the other hand, the issue of pelvic pain is a complicated one, and often minimal (even questionable) lesions of endometriosis may be identified as the cause of pain even though it may actually be completely different (e.g., psychogenic). Dysmenorrhea characteristically starts a few days prior to menses and continues throughout the period. The pain is usually described as dull, in the lower abdomen, pelvis, or back, often with associated dyspareunia with deep penetration. The diagnosis of endometriosis in patients with pelvic pain, acute or chronic, or with severe dysmenorrhea longer than 6 months, has been reported to range between 12.5% and 32%.[18, 181] In another study, 41% of patients with endometriosis presented with abdominal pain or dysmenorrhea.[182] In some instances, these presenting symptoms lead to the diagnosis of congenital outflow tract obstruction in premenarcheal patients.[32]

Ovarian involvement with endometriomas can occasionally result in torsion or rupture and hemoperitoneum. Such patients may present with an acute abdomen and are obviously considered gynecologic emergencies.[30, 183, 184]

Ovarian disease may, in some instances, lead to anovulatory cycles, the mechanism of which is not understood. Therefore, anovulation as a presenting sign is possible.[118] Similarly, in some studies, women with endometriosis have been shown to have a higher incidence of galactorrhea and hyperprolactinemia.[117]

Infertility can obviously be the sole presenting symptom of endometriosis. Many studies have shown a high incidence of this disorder in infertile patients. The reported frequency ranges from 21% to 39%.[2, 185–188]

Premenstrual spotting as a presenting sign in endometriosis has been described.[139, 189] In one study, premenstrual spotting was reported to be present in 35% of patients with endometriosis.[189] The lack of clear definition of this symptom and of control groups weakens the significance of these studies, however.

Endometriosis may also mimic other pelvic conditions, and other forms of discomfort may be present. For example, many patients do not have pain that is cyclic. Others may complain only of bloating, backache, or gastrointestinal disturbances.

Urinary. Obstructive uropathy as a presenting symptom in endometriosis is occasionally seen. Some patients with this symptom have permanent loss of renal function with resultant renal failure.[142, 190] With the involvement of the ureters or the kidneys, many patients present with chronic flank or abdominal pain, edema, and, occasionally, hypertension. An intravenous pyelogram often establishes the diagnosis of ureteral obstruction and hydronephrosis.[142, 190] Although obstructive uropathy is most often observed in patients with extensive disease, with dense adhesions and fibrosis, it is not uncommon for it to occur with only minimal disease.[142, 191, 192]

Intrinsic ureteral involvement may lead to cyclic or persistent hematuria.[145] Vesical involvement results in complaints of dysmenorrhea, dysuria, urgency, and frequency, often related to the menstrual cycle.[38]

Gastrointestinal. The symptomatology of endometriosis involving the intestinal tract varies. The diagnosis requires a high index of suspicion. Physical examination is rarely revealing, although tenderness on palpation and nodularities are suggestive of the disease. Symptoms such as constipation, diarrhea, defecatory rectal pain, and hematochezia are not uncommonly seen.[193, 194] In one review, 40% of patients with bowel endometriosis complained of constipation and 17% of diarrhea.[152] Most patients show some association between symptoms and menstrual cycle. The most frequent complaint of patients with small bowel involvement is abdominal pain.[152] Invasive endometriosis of the terminal ileum with clinical features of Crohn's disease has been described.[195] Luminal obstruction[196] or perforation[197, 198] is a rare occurrence in severe cases. Patients with appendiceal disease may present with signs and symptoms of acute appendicitis.[150, 153, 199] Acute small bowel obstruction due to intussusception or volvulus has been reported.[147] Other studies have shown ileal obstruction in 0.8% of all surgically treated endometriosis cases.[200]

Thoracic-Pulmonary. Thoracic endometriosis can present in different ways depending on the severity and the location of the implants. The following associated signs and symptoms have been described[159, 201]:

- Pneumothorax or hemothorax
- Catamenial chest pain
- Scapular pain
- Hemoptysis
- Empyema
- Ascites

Asymptomatic lesions detected incidentally by radiographic examination are another mode of presentation.[202, 203]

Miscellaneous. As already stated, depending on the location, the endometriotic implant can have different expressions. For instance, endometriosis in the perineal body may be completely asymptomatic or present as a painful mass, noticeable only during menstruation.[204] The combination of endometriosis and ascites, albeit rare, has been described.[45, 205, 206] Referred pain in the groin, hip, or buttocks can also occur in certain cases.[164] Endometriosis in a rare location, the cerebrum, presents with perimenstrual headaches.[171]

Malignant Transformation

Malignant transformation of endometriosis has been described. The exact incidence is unknown. More than 200 cases of malignant tumors arising in foci of gonadal and extragonadal endometriosis have been reported. The ovary is the primary site in about 79% of the cases, whereas extragonadal sites represent 21%. Cases of adenocarcinoma arising in vaginal endometriosis have been described.[207] Endometrioid adenocarcinoma accounts for roughly 70% of the lesions.[208] However, cases of clear cell carcinoma and endometrioid stromal sarcomas arising in ovarian and extraovarian endometriosis have been reported.[209, 210]

The diagnosis of malignancy in endometriosis is made only when the tumor arises within the area or is contiguous with endometriosis. There should not be any evidence of invasion from another source. Whether endometriotic tissue preferentially undergoes malignant transformation is still to be proved. Endometriosis is such a common disease that it is not surprising that it can be coincidentally present with adenocarcinoma.

The prognosis of women with presumed malignant transformation is good, with a 67% 5-year survival for those with disease confined to the ovary and 100% 5-year survival for those with extragonadal disease confined to the site of origin.[208]

DIAGNOSIS (Table 33–6)

The gold standard for diagnosis of endometriosis is by visual inspection during laparoscopy confirmed by histology. With the variable phenotypic appearance of endometriotic implants, a high index of suspicion should be kept at all times and biopsies of suspected foci performed for confirmation.

The symptomatology on presentation provides the first hints toward the diagnosis of endometriosis. The constellation of symptoms such as dysmenorrhea and dyspareunia associated with infertility is not an uncommon finding. Uterosacral nodularity or a palpable adnexal mass on bimanual examination further supports the diagnosis.

Diagnostic laparoscopy provides an excellent means to both diagnose and treat endometriosis. The visualization and search for both pigmented and nonpigmented lesions should be performed in a systematic manner using the magnification provided by "near contact" laparoscopy to aid in the search.

One secondary probe at the pubic hairline on the side of the laparoscopist is usually needed for manipulation of pelvic organs, and live video is helpful for assistants in surgery. One should first inspect the anterior peritoneum and anterior cul-de-sac and both round and infundibulopelvic ligaments. One should then lift the uterus anteriorly away from the deep pelvis with the help of a uterine-controlling tenaculum attached to the cervix and inspect the posterior aspects of the uterus and the proximal tubes. The left adnexum is then lifted with a grasper in the secondary port, and all sides of the ovary and the distal tube are carefully inspected. Particular emphasis should be placed on visualization of the broad ligament under the ovary, and the path of the ureter should be inspected in close-up view. The right adnexum is then similarly inspected. At this point it is important to have the patient in maximal Trendelenburg position and to place the bowel loops into the upper abdomen to allow an unimpeded view of the deeper aspects of the pelvis, that is, the uterosacral areas and the cul-de-sac.

Because lesions in this area occasionally may be deep and not always visible even to the laparoscope, one useful technique at this point is to combine digital rectovaginal palpation with laparoscopic probing. This is done by using the laparoscopist's double-gloved index and middle finger rectovaginally to palpate the septum and the cul-de-sac while the assistant holds and directs the laparoscope. A simultaneous probing with a blunt instrument in the right hand from above can identify deep lesions that often are typically hard due to the presence of inflammatory tissue and scarring. This technique can be particularly useful if performed under sedation or local anesthesia in a patient with chronic pelvic pain to identify specific pain-eliciting lesions.

Special attention should be directed to peritoneal defects or pockets that have been shown to be associated with endometriosis.[211] These pockets can be everted by pulling up the deepest point with a grasper and a biopsy can be obtained with biopsy forceps through the laparoscope. Careful examination of nonpigmented lesions should also be performed.

In recent years, a cell-surface antigen, the CA-125, has emerged as a possible noninvasive means of following response to therapy. Its use as a diagnostic tool, however, is not recommended, because many other common conditions, such as inflammatory or infectious processes and cancerous lesions, are associated with elevated levels of this nonspecific marker.[212]

Various endometrial antibodies have been measured in the sera of patients with endometriosis to try to find a correlation.[85, 213, 214] Because of the many confounding variables, the accuracy of these tests remains suboptimal.

Ultrasonography as a diagnostic tool for endometriosis, in the absence of suspected pathology such as a pelvic mass, is not very sensitive or specific.[215] In the presence of an ovarian mass, it may be useful.

Computed tomography or magnetic resonance imaging usually is not helpful, except in special cases of ectopic implants in unusual locations.[216]

The intravenous pyelogram is a helpful ancillary diagnostic tool in certain cases of endometriosis, when involvement of the urinary tract is suspected. An intravenous or retrograde pyelogram may help localize the obstructed area. Occasionally, cystoscopy is diagnostic if the lesion extends through the bladder wall.

In cases of intestinal involvement, endoscopic or colonoscopic examination may reveal strictures, extrinsic compression, extramucosal masses, fixation, distortion, and occasional submucosal nodularities.[152] Barium enema may be helpful in cases of rectosigmoid endometriosis. Most common findings include external compression and filling defects. Luminal obstruction or strictures are also sometimes visualized.[152]

TABLE 33–6. Diagnostic Approaches in Endometriosis

History and physical examination
Pelvic examination
Laparoscopy/histology
Sonography
Intravenous pyelography and cystoscopy
Colonoscopy/barium enema
Computed tomography and magnetic resonance imaging

CONCLUSION

It is obvious that the pathogenesis of endometriosis is not fully understood. It is likely that this is a multifactorial disorder that involves the interplay of different physiologic systems. Evidence is accumulating that implicates the immune system, along with local peritoneal factors, in the propagation of this disease. The role of macrophages and their secretory products in the pathophysiology of this condition seems to be gaining support. Future studies will surely bring more insight into this ubiquitous disease and its pathophysiology.

REFERENCES

1. Goldman MB, Cramer DW. Current concepts in endometriosis. Prog Clin Biol Res 1989;323:17–23.
2. Strathy JH, Molgaard CA, Coulam CB. Endometriosis and infertility: a laparoscopic study of endometriosis among fertile and infertile women. Fertil Steril 1982;38:667–672.
3. Moen MH. Endometriosis in women at interval sterilization. Acta Obstet Gynecol Scand 1987;66:451–454.
4. Dodge ST, Humphrey RS, Miyazawa K. Peritoneal endometriosis in women requesting reversal of sterilization. Fertil Steril 1986;45:774–777.
5. Norwood GE. Sterility and fertility in women with pelvic endometriosis. Clin Obstet Gynecol 1960;3:456–471.
6. Houston DE, Noller RL, Melton LJ, et al. Incidence of pelvic endometriosis in Rochester, Minnesota, 1970–1979. Am J Epidemiol 1987;125:959–968.
7. Cavanagh WV. Fertility in the etiology of endometriosis. Am J Obstet Gynecol 1951;61:539–547.
8. Hasson HM. Incidence of endometriosis in diagnostic laparoscopy. J Reprod Med 1976;16:135–138.
9. Haney AF. The pathogenesis and etiology of endometriosis. In: Thomas E, Rock J, editors. Modern Approaches to Endometriosis. Norwell, MA: Kluwer Academic, 1991:3–21.
10. Miyazawa K. Incidence of endometriosis among Japanese women. Obstet Gynecol 1976;48:407–409.
11. Venter PF. Endometriosis. South Afr Med J 1980;57:895–899.
12. Olive DL, Hammond CB. Endometriosis and mechanism of infertility. Postgrad Obstet Gynecol 1986;5:1–12.
13. Molgaard CA, Golleck AL, Gresham L. Current concepts in endometriosis. West J Med 1985;143:42–46.
14. Ranney B. The prevention, inhibition, palliation, and treatment of endometriosis. Am J Obstet Gynecol 1975;123:778–785.
15. Ranney B. Endometriosis: pathogenesis, symptoms, and findings. Clin Obstet Gynecol 1980;23:865–874.
16. Meigs JV. Gynecology: endometriosis. N Engl J Med 1942;226:147–153.
17. Cavanagh WV. Fertility in the etiology of endometriosis. Am J Obstet Gynecol 1951;61:539–547.
18. Hasson HM. Incidence of endometriosis in diagnostic laparoscopy. J Reprod Med 1976;16:135–138.
19. Ranney B. Endometriosis: IV. Hereditary tendency. Obstet Gynecol 1971;37:734–737.
20. Frey GH. The familial occurrence of endometriosis. Am J Obstet Gynecol 1957;73:418–421.
21. Simpson JL, Elias S, Malinak LR, Buttram VC Jr. Heritable aspects of endometriosis: I. Genetic studies. Am J Obstet Gynecol 1980;137:327–331.
22. Cramer DW, Wilson E, Stillman RJ, et al. The relation of endometriosis to menstrual characteristics, smoking, and exercise. JAMA 1985;255:1904–1908.
23. Sampson JA. Peritoneal endometriosis due to menstrual dissemination of endometrial tissue into the peritoneal cavity. Am J Obstet Gynecol 1927;14:422–469.
24. Keetel WC, Stein RJ. The viability of the cast-off menstrual endometrium. Am J Obstet Gynecol 1951;61:440–442.
25. Scott RB, Te Linde RW, Wharton LR. Further studies of experimental endometriosis. Am J Obstet Gynecol 1953;66:1082–1099.
26. Dizerega GS, Barber DL, Hodgen GD. Endometriosis: role of ovarian steroids in initiation, maintenance, and suppression. Fertil Steril 1980;33:649–653.
27. Bartosik D, Jacobs SL, Kelly LJ. Endometrial tissue in peritoneal fluid. Fertil Steril 1986;46:796–800.
28. Halme J, Hammond MG, Hulka JF, et al. Retrograde menstruation in healthy women and in patients with endometriosis. Obstet Gynecol 1984;64:151–154.
29. Jenkins S, Olive DL, Haney AF. Endometriosis: pathogenetic implications of the anatomic distribution. Obstet Gynecol 1986;67:335–338.
30. Huffman W. Endometriosis in young teenage girls. Pediatr Ann 1981;10:44–49.
31. Olive DL, Henderson DY. Endometriosis and müllerian anomalies. Obstet Gynecol 1987;69:412–415.
32. Schifrin BS, Erez S, Moore JG. Teen-age endometriosis. Am J Obstet Gynecol 1973;116:973–980.
33. Ridley JH, Edwards KI. Experimental endometriosis in humans. Am J Obstet Gynecol 1958;76:783–789.
34. Javert CT. Pathogenesis of endometriosis based on endometrial homeoplasia, direct extension, exfoliation and implantation, lymphatic and hematogenous metastasis. Cancer 1949;2:399–409.
35. Ridley JH. A review of facts and fancies. Obstet Gynecol Surv 1968;23:1–24.
36. Hobbs JE, Borntnick AR. Endometriosis of the lungs. Am J Obstet Gynecol 1981;140:227–232.
37. Field CA, Banner EA, Symonds RE. Endometriosis of abdominal scar after cesarean section. Mayo Clin Proc 1962;37:12–15.
38. Buka NJ. Vesical endometriosis after cesarean section. Am J Obstet Gynecol 1988;158:1117–1118.
39. Merril JA. Endometrial induction of endometriosis across millipore filters. Am J Obstet Gynecol 1966;94:780–789.
40. Kempers RD, Dockerty MB, Hunt AB. Significant postmenopausal endometriosis. Surg Gynecol Obstet 1960;111:348–356.
41. Syrop CH, Halme J. Cyclic changes of peritoneal fluid parameters in normal and infertile patients. Obstet Gynecol 1987;69:416–418.
42. Halme J, Becker S, Wing R. Accentuated cyclic activation of peritoneal macrophages in patients with endometriosis. Am J Obstet Gynecol 1984;148:85–90.
43. Haney AF, Muscato JJ, Weinberg JB. Peritoneal fluid cell populations in infertility patients. Fertil Steril 1981;35:696–698.
44. Zeller JM, Henig I, Radwanska E, Dmowski WP. Enhancement of human monocyte and peritoneal macrophage chemiluminescence activities in women with endometriosis. Am J Reprod Immunol Microbiol 1987;13:78–82.
45. Halme J, Becker S, Hammond MJ, et al. Increased activation of pelvic macrophages in infertile women with mild endometriosis. Am J Obstet Gynecol 1983;145:333–337.
46. Halme J, Becker S, Haskill S. Altered maturation and function of peritoneal macrophages: possible role of pathogenesis of endometriosis. Am J Obstet Gynecol 1987;156:783–789.
47. Dunselman GA, Hendrix MG, Boukaert PX, Evers JL. Functional aspects of peritoneal macrophages in endometriosis of women. J Reprod Fertil 1988;82:707–710.
48. Werb Z. Macrophages. In: Stiles DP, Stobo JD, Wells JV, editors. Basic and Clinical Immunology. 6th edition. Norwalk, CT: Appleton and Lange, 1987:96.
49. Halme J, White C, Kauma S, et al. Peritoneal macrophages from patients with endometriosis release growth factor activity in vitro. J Clin Endocrinol Metab 1988;66:1044–1049.
50. Rossi V, Brevario F, Ghezzi P, et al. Interleukin-1 induces prostacyclin in vascular cells. Science 1985;229:174–176.
51. Falkoff RJ, Muraguchi A, Hong JX, et al. The effects of interleukin-1 on human B-cell activation and proliferation. J Immunol 1983;131:801–805.
52. Hill JA, Anderson DJ. Lymphocyte activity in the presence of peritoneal fluid from fertile women and infertile women with and without endometriosis. Am J Obstet Gynecol 1989;161:861–864.
53. Fakih H, Baggett B, Holtz G, et al. Interleukin-1: a possible role in the infertility associated with endometriosis. Fertil Steril 1987;47:213–217.
54. Eiserman J, Gast MJ, Pineda J, et al. Tumor necrosis factor in peritoneal fluid of women undergoing laparoscopic surgery. Fertil Steril 1988;50:573–579.
55. Halme J. Release of tumor necrosis factor-α by human peritoneal macrophages in vivo and in vitro. Am J Obstet Gynecol 1989;161:1718–1725.
56. Kauma S, Clark M, White C, Halme J. Production of fibronectin by peritoneal macrophages and concentration of fibronectin in peritoneal fluid from patients with or without endometriosis. Obstet Gynecol 1988;72:13–18.

57. Hurst BS, Rock JA. The peritoneal environment in endometriosis. In: Thomas E, Rock J, editors. Modern Approaches to Endometriosis. Norwell, MA: Kluwer Academic, 1991:79–96.

58. Joshi SG, Zamah NM, Raikar RS, et al. Serum and peritoneal fluid proteins in women with and without endometriosis. Fertil Steril 1986;46:1077–1082.

59. Suginami H, Yano K, Watanabe K, Matsuura S. A factor inhibiting ovum capture by the oviductal fimbriae present in endometriosis peritoneal fluid. Fertil Steril 1986;46:1140–1146.

60. Surrey E, Halme J. Effect of peritoneal fluid from endometriosis patients on endometrial stromal cell proliferation in vitro. Obstet Gynecol 1990;76:792–797.

61. Herman A, Claeys M, Moncada S, Vane JR. Biosynthesis of prostacyclin PG_{I_2} and 12-HETE by pericardium, pleura, peritoneum, and aorta of rabbit. Prostaglandins 1979;18:439–446.

62. Marsh JM, Le Maire WJ. Cyclic AMP accumulation and steroidogenesis in the human corpus luteum: effect of gonadotropins and prostaglandins. J Clin Endocrinol Metab 1974;38:99–106.

63. Moon YS, Jeung PCS, Yuen BH, Gomel V. Prostaglandin F in human endometriotic tissue. Am J Obstet Gynecol 1981;141:344–345.

64. Ylikorkala O, Viinikka C. Prostaglandins in endometriosis. Acta Obstet Gynecol Scand Suppl 1983;113:105–107.

65. Schenken RS, Asch RH. Surgical induction of endometriosis in the rabbit: effect on fertility and concentration of peritoneal fluid prostaglandins. Fertil Steril 1980;34:581–587.

66. Schenken RS, Asch RH, Williams RF, Hodgen GD. Etiology of infertility in monkeys with endometriosis: measurement of peritoneal fluid prostaglandins. Am J Obstet Gynecol 1984;150:349–355.

67. Vernon MW, Beard JS, Graves K, Wilson EA. Classification of endometriotic implants by morphologic appearance and capacity to synthesize prostaglandin F. Fertil Steril 1986;46:801–806.

68. Rock JA, Dubin NH, Ghodgnoukar RB, et al. Cul-de-sac fluid in women with endometriosis: fluid volume and prostanoid concentration during proliferative phase of cycle-day 8–12. Fertil Steril 1982;37:747–750.

69. Dawood MY, Khan-Dawood FS, Wilson L. Peritoneal fluid prostaglandins in women with endometriosis, chronic PID, and pelvic pain. Obstet Gynecol 1984;148:391–395.

70. Chacho KJ, Chacho MS, Andresen PJ, Scommegna A. Peritoneal fluid in patients with and without endometriosis: prostanoids and macrophages and their effect on the spermatozoa penetration assay. Am J Obstet Gynecol 1986;154:1290–1296.

71. Badawy SZA, Marshall L, Cuenca V. Peritoneal fluid prostaglandins in various stages of the menstrual cycle: role in infertile patients with endometriosis. Int J Fertil 1985;30:48–53.

72. DeLeon FD, Vijayakumar R, Brown M, et al. Peritoneal fluid volume, estrogen, progesterone, prostaglandin, and epidermal growth factor concentration in patients with and without endometriosis. Obstet Gynecol 1986;68:189–194.

73. Drake TS, O'Brien WF, Ramwell PW, Metz SA. Peritoneal fluid thromboxane B_2 and 6-keto-prostaglandin $F_{1\alpha}$ in endometriosis. Am J Obstet Gynecol 1981;140:401–404.

74. Drake TS, O'Brien WF, Ramwell PW. Peritoneal fluid prostanoids in unexplained infertility. Am J Obstet Gynecol 1983;147:63–64.

75. Koskimies AI, Tenhunen A, Ylikorkala O. Peritoneal fluid 6-keto-prostaglandin $F_{1\alpha}$, thromboxane B_2 in endometriosis and unexplained infertility. Acta Obstet Gynecol Scand Suppl 1984;123:19–21.

76. Ylikorkala O, Koskimies A, Laatikainen T, et al. Peritoneal fluid prostaglandins in endometriosis, tubal disorders, and unexplained infertility. Obstet Gynecol 1984;63:616–620.

77. Sgarlata CS, Hertelendy F, Mikhail G. The prostanoid content in peritoneal fluid and plasma of women with endometriosis. Am J Obstet Gynecol 1983;147:563–565.

78. Mudge TJ, James MJ, Jones WR, Walsh JA. Peritoneal fluid 6-keto-prostaglandin $F_{1\alpha}$ levels in women with endometriosis. Am J Obstet Gynecol 1985;152:901–904.

79. Orlicky DJ, Silio M, Williams C, et al. Regulation of inositol phosphate levels by prostaglandins in cultured endometrial cells. J Cell Physiol 1986;128:105–112.

80. Lundstrom V, Green K. Endogenous levels of prostaglandin $F_{2\alpha}$ and its main metabolites in plasma and endometrium of normal and dysmenorrheic women. Am J Obstet Gynecol 1978;130:640–646.

81. Badawy SZ, Cuenca V, Stitzel A, Tice D. Immune rosettes of T and B lymphocytes in infertile women with endometriosis. J Reprod Med 1987;32:194–197.

82. Marthur S, Peress MR, Williamson HO, et al. Autoimmunity to endo-

83. Marthur S, Chihal HJ, Homm RJ, et al. Endometrial antigens involved in the autoimmunity of endometriosis. Fertil Steril 1988;50:860–863.

84. Badawy SZ, Cuenca V, Stitzel A, et al. Autoimmune phenomena in infertility patients with endometriosis. Obstet Gynecol 1984;63:271–275.

85. Wild RA, Shivers CA. Antiendometrial antibodies in patients with endometriosis. Am J Reprod Immunol 1985;8:84–87.

86. Gleicher N, El-Roeiy A, Confino E, Friberg J. Abnormal autoantibodies in endometriosis: is endometriosis an autoimmune disease? Obstet Gynecol 1987;70:115–122.

87. El-Roeiy A, Dmowski WP, Gleicher N, et al. Danazol but not GnRH agonist suppresses autoantibodies in endometriosis. Fertil Steril 1988;50:864–871.

88. Dmowski WP, Steele RW, Baker GF. Deficient cellular immunity in endometriosis. Am J Obstet Gynecol 1981;141:377–383.

89. Steele RW, Dmowski WP, Marmer DJ. Immunologic aspects of human endometriosis. Am J Reprod Immunol 1984;6:33–36.

90. Roddick JW, Conkey G, Jacobs EJ. The hormonal response of endometrium in endometriotic implants and its relationship to symptomatology. Am J Obstet Gynecol 1960;79:1173–1177.

91. Schweppe KW, Wynn RM. Ultrastructural changes in endometriotic implants during the menstrual cycle. Obstet Gynecol 1981;58:465–473.

92. Bergqvist A, Jeppson S, Kullander S, Ljungberg O. Human uterine endometrium and endometriotic tissue transplanted into nude mice. Am J Pathol 1985;121:337–341.

93. Schweppe KW, Wynn RM, Beller FK. Ultrastructural comparison of endometriotic implants and eutopic endometrium. Am J Obstet Gynecol 1984;148:1024–1039.

94. Bergqvist A, Ljunberg O, Mythre E. Human endometrium and endometriotic tissue obtained simultaneously: a comparative histological study. Int J Gynecol Pathol 1984;3:696–703.

95. Bergqvist A, Rannevik G, Thorell J. Estrogen and progesterone cytosol receptor concentration in endometriotic tissue and intrauterine endometrium. Acta Obstet Gynecol Scand Suppl 1981;101:53–58.

96. Janne O, Kauppila A, Kokko E, et al. Estrogen and progestin receptors in endometriotic lesions: comparison with endometrial tissue. Am J Obstet Gynecol 1981;141:562–566.

97. Lyndrup J, Thorpe S, Glenthoj A, et al. Altered progesterone/estrogen receptor ratios in endometriosis: a comparative study of steroid receptors and morphology in endometriosis and endometrium. Acta Obstet Gynecol Scand 1987;66:625–629.

98. Kistner RW. Endometriosis in infertility. Clin Obstet Gynecol 1979;22:101–119.

99. Thomas EJ. Endometriosis and infertility. In: Thomas E, Rock J, editors. Modern Approaches to Endometriosis. Norwell, MA: Kluwer Academic, 1991:113–128.

100. Jansen RPS. Minimal endometriosis and reduced fecundability: prospective evidence from an artificial insemination by donor program. Fertil Steril 1986;46:141–143.

101. Portuendo JA, Echanojauregui AD, Herran C, et al. Early conception in patients with untreated mild endometriosis. Fertil Steril 1983;39:22–25.

102. Schenken RS, Malinak LR. Conservative surgery versus expectant management for the infertile patient with mild endometriosis. Fertil Steril 1982;37:183–186.

103. Seibel MM, Berger MJ, Weinstein FJ, et al. The effectiveness of danazol on subsequent fertility in minimal endometriosis. Fertil Steril 1982;38:534–537.

104. Olive DL, Stohs GF, Metzger DA, Franklin RR. Expectant management and hydrotubations in the treatment of endometriosis-associated infertility. Fertil Steril 1985;44:35–41.

105. Halme J, Hammond MG, Syrop CH, Talbert LM. Peritoneal macrophages modulate human granulosa luteal cell progesterone production. J Clin Endocrinol Metab 1985;16:912–916.

106. Wentz AC, Jones GS. Transient luteolytic effect of prostaglandin $F_{2\alpha}$ in the human. Obstet Gynecol 1973;42:172–181.

107. Cheeseman KL, Ben-Nun I, Chatterton RT, Cohen MR. The relationship of luteinizing hormone, pregnanediol-3-glucuronide and estriol-16-glucuronide in the urine of infertile women with endometriosis. Fertil Steril 1982;38:542–548.

108. Brosens IA, Koninckx PR, Corvelyn PA. A study of plasma progesterone, estradiol-17-β, prolactin, and LH levels, and of the luteal phase appearance of the ovaries in patients with endometriosis and infertility. Br J Obstet Gynecol 1978;85:246–250.

82 (cont.). metrium and ovary in endometriosis. Clin Exp Immunol 1989; 50:259–266.

109. Donnez J, Thomas K. Incidence of the luteinized unruptured follicle syndrome in fertile women and in women with endometriosis. Eur J Obstet Gynecol Reprod Biol 1982;14:187–190.

110. Dmowski WP, Rao R, Scommegna A. The luteinized unruptured follicle syndrome and endometriosis. Fertil Steril 1980;33:30–34.

111. Dhont M, Serryn R, Duvivier P, et al. Ovulation stigma and concentration of progesterone and estradiol in peritoneal fluid: relation with fertility and endometriosis. Fertil Steril 1984;41:872–877.

112. Holtz G, Williamson HO, Mathur RS, et al. Luteinized unruptured follicle syndrome in mild endometriosis: assessment with biochemical parameters. J Reprod Med 1985;30:643–645.

113. Hargrove JT, Abraham GE. Abnormal luteal function in endometriosis. Fertil Steril 1980;34:302.

114. Ayers JW, Birenbaum DL, Menon KM. Luteal phase dysfunction in endometriosis: elevated progesterone levels in peripheral and ovarian veins during the follicular phase. Fertil Steril 1987;47:925–929.

115. Pittaway DE, Maxson W, Daniell J, et al. Luteal phase defects in infertility patients with endometriosis. Fertil Steril 1983;39:712–713.

116. Balasch J, Vanrell JA. Mild endometriosis and luteal function. Int J Fertil 1985;30:4–6.

117. Hirschowitz JS, Soler NG, Worstman J. The galactorrhea-endometriosis syndrome. Lancet 1978;1:896–898.

118. Soules MR, Malinak LR, Bury R, Poindexter A. Endometriosis and anovulation: a coexisting problem in the infertile female. Am J Obstet Gynecol 1976;125:412–415.

119. Hahn DW, Carraher RP, Foldesy RG, McGuire JL. Experimental evidence for failure to implant as a mechanism of infertility associated with endometriosis. Am J Obstet Gynecol 1986;155:1109–1113.

120. Naples JD, Batt RE, Sadigh J. Spontaneous abortion rate in patients with endometriosis. Obstet Gynecol 1981;57:509–512.

121. Olive DL, Franklin RR, Gratkins LV. The association between endometriosis and spontaneous abortion. J Reprod Med 1982;27:333–338.

122. Petersohn L. Fertility in patients with ovarian endometriosis before and after treatment. Acta Obstet Gynecol Scand 1970;49:331–333.

123. Groll M. Endometriosis and spontaneous abortion. Fertil Steril 1984;41:933–935.

124. Pittaway DE, Vernon C, Fayez JA. Spontaneous abortion in women with endometriosis. Fertil Steril 1988;50:711–715.

125. Regan R, Braude PR, Tembath PL. Influence of past reproductive performance on risk of spontaneous abortion. Br Med J 1989;299:541–545.

126. Ball RY, Scott N, Mitchinson MJ. Further observations on spermiophagy by murine peritoneal macrophages in vitro. J Reprod Fertil 1984;71:221–226.

127. Muscato JJ, Haney AF, Weinberg JB. Sperm phagocytosis by human peritoneal macrophages: a possible cause of infertility in endometriosis. Am J Obstet Gynecol 1982;144:503–510.

128. Hoxsey RJ, Rao R, Scommegna A. Sperm recovery in peritoneal fluid of endometriosis versus normal infertile patients. Fertil Steril 1984;41:395–398.

129. Haney AF, Misukonis MA, Weinberg JB. Macrophages and infertility: oviductal macrophages as potential mediators of infertility. Fertil Steril 1983;39:310–315.

130. Hill JA, Haimovici F, Politch JA, Anderson DJ. Effects of soluble products of activated lymphocytes and macrophages (lymphokines and monokines) on human sperm motion parameters. Fertil Steril 1987;47:460–465.

131. Halme J, Hall JL. Effect of pelvic fluid from endometriosis patients on human sperm penetration of zona free hamster ova. Fertil Steril 1982;37:573–576.

132. Wardle PG, McLaughlin EA, McDermott A, et al. Endometriosis and ovulatory disorder: reduced fertilization in vitro compared with tubal and unexplained infertility. Lancet 1985;2:236–239.

133. Morcos RN, Gibbons WE, Findley WE. Effect of peritoneal fluid on in vitro cleavage of 2-cell mouse embryos: possible role in infertility associated endometriosis. Fertil Steril 1985;44:678–683.

134. Spilman CH, Beuving DC, Roseman TJ, Larion LJ. Effect of vaginally administered 15(S)-15-methyl PGF$_{2\alpha}$ on egg transport and fertility in rabbits. Proc Soc Exp Biol Med 1976;151:575–578.

135. Eddy CA. Ovum transport in the rhesus monkey following postovulatory intravaginal 15(S)-15-methyl prostaglandin F$_{2\alpha}$ methyl ester administration. Am J Obstet Gynecol 1980;137:966–971.

136. Salomy M, Goldstein PJ. Prevention of pregnancy in rabbits using vaginal application of PGF$_{2\alpha}$. Fertil Steril 1978;29:456–458.

137. Croxatto HB, Ortiz ME, Guiloff E, Ibarra A. Effect of 15(S)-15-methyl prostaglandin F$_{2\alpha}$ on human oviductal motility and ovum transport. Fertil Steril 1978;30:408–414.

138. Brosens IA. The endometriotic implant. In: Thomas E, Rock J, editors. Modern Approaches to Endometriosis. Norwell, MA: Kluwer Academic Publisher. 1991:21–31.

139. Jansen RPS, Russell P. Nonpigmented endometriosis: clinical, laparoscopic, and pathologic definition. Am J Obstet Gynecol 1986;155:1154–1159.

139a. Redwine DB: Age-related evolution in color appearance of endometriosis. Fertil Steril 1987;48:1062–1063.

140. Koninckx PR, Meuleman C, Demeyere S, et al. Suggestive evidence that pelvic endometriosis is a progressive disease, whereas deeply infiltrating endometriosis is associated with pelvic pain. Fertil Steril 1991;55:759–769.

141. Ranney B. Endometriosis. Obstet Gynecol Annu 1978;7:219–234.

142. Kane C, Drouin P. Obstructive uropathy associated with endometriosis. Am J Obstet Gynecol 1985;151:207–211.

143. Moore JG, Hibbard LT, Growdon WA, Schiffrin BS. Urinary tract endometriosis: enigmas in diagnosis and management. Am J Obstet Gynecol 1979;134:162–170.

144. Tan AK, Khan Z, Leiter E. Laparoscopy as a diagnostic aid in women with localized ureteral obstruction due to endometriosis. Urology 1980;16:47–50.

145. Reddy AN, Evans AT. Endometriosis of the ureters. J Urol 1974;111:474–480.

146. Bradford JA, Ernest WI, Warwick BG. Ureteric endometriosis: three case reports and a review of the literature. Aust NZ J Obstet Gynecol 1989;29:421–424.

147. Macafee CHG, Greer HLH. Intestinal endometriosis: a report of 29 cases—a survey of the literature. J Obstet Gynaecol 1960;67:539–555.

148. Williams TJ, Pratt JH. Endometriosis in 1,000 consecutive celiotomies: incidence and management. Am J Obstet Gynecol 1977;129:245–250.

149. Prystowsky JB, Stryker SJ, Ujiki GT, Poticha SM. Gastrointestinal endometriosis: incidence and indications for resection. Arch Surg 1988;123:855–858.

150. Tedeschi LG, Masand GP. Endometriosis of the intestines—a report of seven cases. Dis Colon Rectum 1971;14:360–365.

151. Williams C. Endometriosis of the colon in the elderly woman. Ann Surg 1963;157:975–979.

152. Zwas FR, Lyon DT. Endometriosis: an important condition in clinical gastroenterology. Dig Dis Sci 1991;36:353–364.

153. Langman J, Rowland R, Vernon-Roberts B. Endometriosis of the appendix. Br J Surg 1981;68:121–124.

154. Martin LFW, Tidman MK, Jamigson MA. Appendiceal intussusception and endometriosis. J Can Assoc Radiol 1980;31:276–277.

155. Luciano AA, Pitkin RM. Endometriosis: approaches to diagnosis and treatment. Surg Annu 1984;16:297–312.

156. Marchevsky AM, Zimmerman MJ, Aufses AH, Weiss H. Endometrial cyst of the pancreas. Gastroenterology 1984;86:1589–1591.

157. Meyers WC, Kelvin FM, Jones RS. Diagnosis and surgical treatment of colonic endometriosis. Arch Surg 1979;114:169–175.

158. Minvielle L, Vargas de la Cruz J. Endometriosis of the anal canal—presentation of a case. Dis Colon Rectum 1968;11:32–35.

159. Lester TH, Schumann WR, Goldstein GE. Thoracic endometriosis: a review and report of two cases. Am J Obstet Gynecol 1981;140:227–232.

160. Ripstein CB, Rohman M, Wallach JB. Endometriosis involving the pleura. J Thorac Surg 1959;37:464–471.

161. Schlicke CP. Ectopic endometrial tissue in the thigh. JAMA 1946;132:445–446.

162. Christopher F. Inguinal endometriosis. Ann Surg 1927;86:918–920.

163. Strasser ES, Davis RM. Extraperitoneal inguinal endometriosis. Am Surg 1977;43:421–422.

163. Qualiarello J, Coppa G, Bigelow B. Isolated endometriosis in an inguinal hernia. Am J Obstet Gynecol 1985;152:688–689.

164. Pelligrini VD Jr, Pasternak HS, Macaulay WP. Endometrioma of the pubis: a differential diagnosis of hip pain. J Bone Joint Surg 1981;63:1333–1334.

165. Tornquist B. Endometriosis in vaginal, vulvar and perineal scars. Acta Obstet Gynecol Scand 1949;29:485–488.

166. Chatterjee SK. Scar endometriosis: a clinicopathologic study of 17 cases. Obstet Gynecol 1980;56:81–84.

167. Kale S, Shuster M, Shangold J. Endometrioma in a cesarean scar. Am J Obstet Gynecol 1971;111:596–597.

168. Brenner C, Wohlgemuth S. Scar endometriosis. Surg Gynecol Obstet 1990;170:538–540.

169. Hembrick E, Abcarian H, Smith D. Perineal endometrioma in episiotomy incisions: clinical features and management. Dis Colon Rectum 1979;22:550–554.

170. Baker GS, Parsons WR, Welch JS. Endometriosis within the sheath of the sciatic nerve. J Neurosurg 1966;25:652–655.

171. Muse K. Clinical manifestations and classification of endometriosis. Clin Obstet Gynecol 1988;31:813–822.

172. Felson H, McGuire J, Wasserman P. Stromal endometriosis involving the heart. Am J Med 1960;29:1072–1076.

173. Prince LM, Abrams G. Endometriosis of the perineum: review of the literature and case report. Am J Obstet Gynecol 1957;73:890–893.

174. Trampuz V. Endometriosis of the perineum: a report of 5 new cases. Am J Obstet Gynecol 1962;84:1522–1525.

175. Schwarz OH. Endometriosis: a clinical and surgical review. Am J Obstet Gynecol 1938;36:887–891.

176. Martin JD Jr, Hanck AE. Endometriosis in the male. Ann Surg 1985;51:426–428.

177. Oliker AJ, Harris AE. Endometriosis of the bladder in a male patient. J Urol 1971;106:858–859.

178. Schrodt GR, Alcorn MO, Ibane ZJ. Endometriosis of the male urinary system: a case report. J Urol 1980;124:722–723.

179. Stevenson CS, Campbell CG. The symptoms, physical findings, and clinical diagnosis of pelvic endometriosis. Clin Obstet Gynecol 1960;3:441–455.

180. Buttram VC Jr. Consecutive surgery for endometriosis in the infertile female: a study of 206 patients with implications for both medical and surgical therapy. Fertil Steril 1979;31:117–123.

181. Kresch AJ, Seifer DB, Sachs LB, et al. Laparoscopy in 100 women with chronic pelvic pain. Obstet Gynecol 1984;64:672–674.

182. Melega C, Marchesini FP, Bellettini L, et al. Diagnostic value of laparoscopy in endometriosis and infertility. J Reprod Med 1979;29:101–104.

183. Ranney B. Endometriosis: II. Emergency operations due to hemiperitoneum. Obstet Gynecol 1970;36:437–442.

184. Pratt JH, Shamblin WR. Spontaneous rupture of endometrial cyst of the ovary presenting as an acute abdominal emergency. Am J Obstet Gynecol 1970;108:56–62.

185. Musich JR, Behrman SJ. Infertility laparoscopy in perspective: review of five hundred cases. Am J Obstet Gynecol 1982;143:293–299.

186. Stillman RJ, Miller LC. Diethylstilbestrol exposure in utero and endometriosis in infertile females. Fertil Steril 1984;41:369–372.

187. Taylor PJ, Leader A, George RE, et al. Correlations between laparoscopic and hysteroscopic findings in 497 women with otherwise unexplained infertility. J Reprod Med 1984;29:137–139.

188. Wood GP. Laparoscopic examination of the normal infertile woman. Obstet Gynecol 1983;62:642–643.

189. Wentz AC. Premenstrual spotting: its association with endometriosis but not luteal phase inadequacy. Fertil Steril 1980;33:605–607.

190. Slutsky JN, Callahan D. Endometriosis of the ureter can present as renal failure: a case report and review of endometriosis affecting the ureters. J Urol 1983;130:336–337.

191. Pollock HM, Will JS. Radiographic features of ureteral endometriosis. Am J Roentgenol 1978;131:627–630.

192. Yates-Bell AJ, Molland EA, Pryor JP. Endometriosis of the ureter. Br J Urol 1972;44:58–67.

193. Croom RD, Donovan ML, Schwesinger WH. Intestinal endometriosis. Am J Surg 1984;148:660–667.

194. Samper ER, Slagle GW, Hand AM. Colonic endometriosis: its clinical spectrum. South Med J 1984;77:912–914.

195. Harty RF, Kaude JV. Invasive endometriosis of the terminal ileum. South Med J 1983;76:253–255.

196. Leber RE, Hume HA. Endometriosis requiring colostomy and resection: a case report and review of the literature. Am J Proctol 1966;17:380–387.

197. Clement PB. Perforation of the sigmoid colon during pregnancy—a rare complication of endometriosis. Br J Obstet Gynecol 1977;84:548–550.

198. Ledley GS, Shenk IM, Heit HA. Sigmoid colon perforation due to endometriosis not associated with pregnancy. Am J Gastroenterol 1988;83:1424–1426.

199. Uohara JK, Kobara TY. Endometriosis of the appendix: report of twelve cases and review of the literature. Am J Obstet Gynecol 1975;121:423–426.

200. Venable JH. Endometriosis of the ileum: four cases with obstruction. Am J Obstet Gynecol 1972;113:1054–1055.

201. Griffith RD, Sedlak JB, Little WP. Diaphragmatic pain in pulmonary endometriosis. South Med J 1988;81:89–91.

202. Jelihouski T, Grant AF. Endometriosis of the lung. Thorax 1968;23:434–437.

203. Mobbs GA, Pfanner DW. Endometriosis of the lung. Lancet 1963;1:472–474.

204. Pollack R, Gordon PH, Ferenczy A, Tulandi T. Perineal endometriosis: a case report. J Reprod Med 1990;35:109–112.

205. Jenks JE, Artman IE, Hoskins WJ, et al. Endometriosis with ascites. Obstet Gynecol 1984;63:75s–77s.

206. Olubuyide IO, Adebajo AO, Adeleye JA, Solanke TF. Massive ascites associated with endometriosis in a Nigerian African. Int J Gynecol Obstet 1988;27:439–441.

207. Haskel S, Chen SS, Spiegel G. Vaginal endometrioid adenocarcinoma arising in vaginal endometriosis: a case report and literature review. Gynecol Oncol 1989;34:232–236.

208. Heaps JM, Nieberg RK, Berek JS. Malignant neoplasms arising in endometriosis. Obstet Gynecol 1990;75:1023–1028.

209. Hitti IF, Glasberg SS, Lubicz SL. Clear cell carcinoma arising in extravarian endometriosis: report of three cases and review of the literature. Gynecol Oncol 1990;39:314–320.

210. Baiocchi G, Kavanagh J, Wharton T. Endometrioid stromal sarcomas arising from ovarian and extraovarian endometriosis: report of two cases and review of the literature. Gynecol Oncol 1990;36:147–151.

211. Chatman DL, Zbella EA. Pelvic peritoneal defects and endometriosis: further observations. Fertil Steril 1986;46:711–714.

212. Giudice LC, Jacobs A, Pineda J, et al. Serum levels of CA-125 in patients with endometriosis: a preliminary report. Fertil Steril 1986;45:876–878.

213. Chihal HJ, Mathur S, Holtz GL, et al. An endometrial antibody assay in the clinical diagnosis and management of endometriosis. Fertil Steril 1986;46:408–411.

214. Kreiner D, Fromowitz FB, Richardson DA, et al. Endometrial immunofluorescence associated with endometriosis and pelvic inflammatory disease. Fertil Steril 1986;46:243–246.

215. Friedman H, Vogelzang RL, Mendelson EB, et al. Endometriosis detection by US with laparoscopic correlation. Radiology 1985;157:217–220.

216. Hricak H, Lacey C, Schiriok E, et al. Gynecologic masses: value of magnetic resonance imaging. Am J Obstet Gynecol 1985;153:31–37.

CHAPTER 34

Endometriosis: Medical Therapy

ROBERT L. BARBIERI

Endometriosis is the presence of tissue resembling endometrial glands or stroma outside of the uterus. Endometriosis lesions often involve the pelvic peritoneum, uterosacral ligaments, ovarian surface, or ovarian stroma. An evolving concept is that endometriosis lesions are both functionally and structurally heterogeneous. For example, Vernon and colleagues[1] demonstrated the functional heterogeneity of endometriosis implants. Vernon and colleagues[1] examined prostaglandin F production in endometriosis lesions classified as "red petechial" implants, "reddish brown intermediate" implants, and "dark brown powder burn" implants. The "red petechial" implants synthesized 200% to 300% more prostaglandin F per milligram of tissue than the other two types of implants. Histologic evidence also supports the heterogeneity of endometriosis lesions. In Figure 34–1, two endometriosis lesions are presented. In one lesion, the epithelium displays no evidence of cellular atypia. In the second lesion, cellular atypia is present. Endometriosis lesions displaying evidence of cellular atypia have increased malignant potential.[2] These functional and structural observations underscore the heterogeneity of endometriosis lesions. Given this heterogeneity, the following generalizations concerning the hormone dependency of endometriosis lesions should be interpreted with caution.

HORMONE DEPENDENCY OF ENDOMETRIOSIS LESIONS

The central dogma that guides the hormonal therapy of endometriosis is the belief that the sex steroids are major regulators of the growth and function of endometriosis lesions. Endometriosis lesions have intracellular estradiol, progesterone, and androgen receptors.[3, 4] Using an estrogen receptor monoclonal antibody, Bergqvist and associates[3] demonstrated that all endometriosis lesions studied (n = 31) had intracellular estradiol and progesterone receptors. In the lesions studied, the concentration of estradiol and progesterone receptors was 50% to 70% lower than in matched specimens of eutopic endometrium.[3] Androgen receptors are present in low concentration in endometriosis lesions, but the concentrations of androgen receptors are similar in lesions and matched endometrial samples.[4]

Both clinical and laboratory observations suggest that estradiol is the critical steroid hormone modulating the growth of endometriosis lesions. Clinical observations that support this concept include the following: (1) Endometriosis rarely occurs before menarche; (2) menopause, either surgical or natural, usually produces regression of endometriosis lesions; and (3) new cases of endometriosis occur rarely after the menopause, unless exogenous estrogens are being prescribed.

Laboratory models of experimental endometriosis indicate that estradiol is a critically important growth factor for endometriosis lesions. Bergqvist and colleagues[5] implanted human endometriosis lesions in the abdominal wall of nude mice. In a hypoestrogenic environment, the implanted endometriosis lesions demonstrated decreased glandular activity. If estradiol was given to the mice, the endometriosis lesions did not atrophy. Sharpe and coworkers[6] autotransplanted rat endometrium to the intestinal mesentery. The autotransplanted endometrium grew into cystic structures lined with endometrium. These experimental "endometriosis" lesions underwent regression in a hypoestrogenic state. If estradiol or progesterone was administered to the animals, the experimental endometriosis lesions did not atrophy. Interestingly, estradiol plus progesterone appeared to be additive in their ability to promote the growth of these endometriosis lesions.

In contrast to estrogen, much less is known concerning the effects of androgens and progestins on endometriosis lesions. The administration of the androgens testosterone propionate, methyltestosterone, and danazol to women with endometriosis can produce regression in lesions.[7, 8] Low-dose danazol and methyltestosterone can produce regression in lesions without interrupting ovulation or menses, suggesting that androgens can produce regression in endometriosis lesions in the presence of normal estradiol concentrations.[7, 8]

The role of progesterone and the synthetic progestins in the regulation of growth of endometriosis lesions remains controversial. The native steroid progesterone may support the growth of endometriosis lesions.[6, 9] In contrast, the syn-

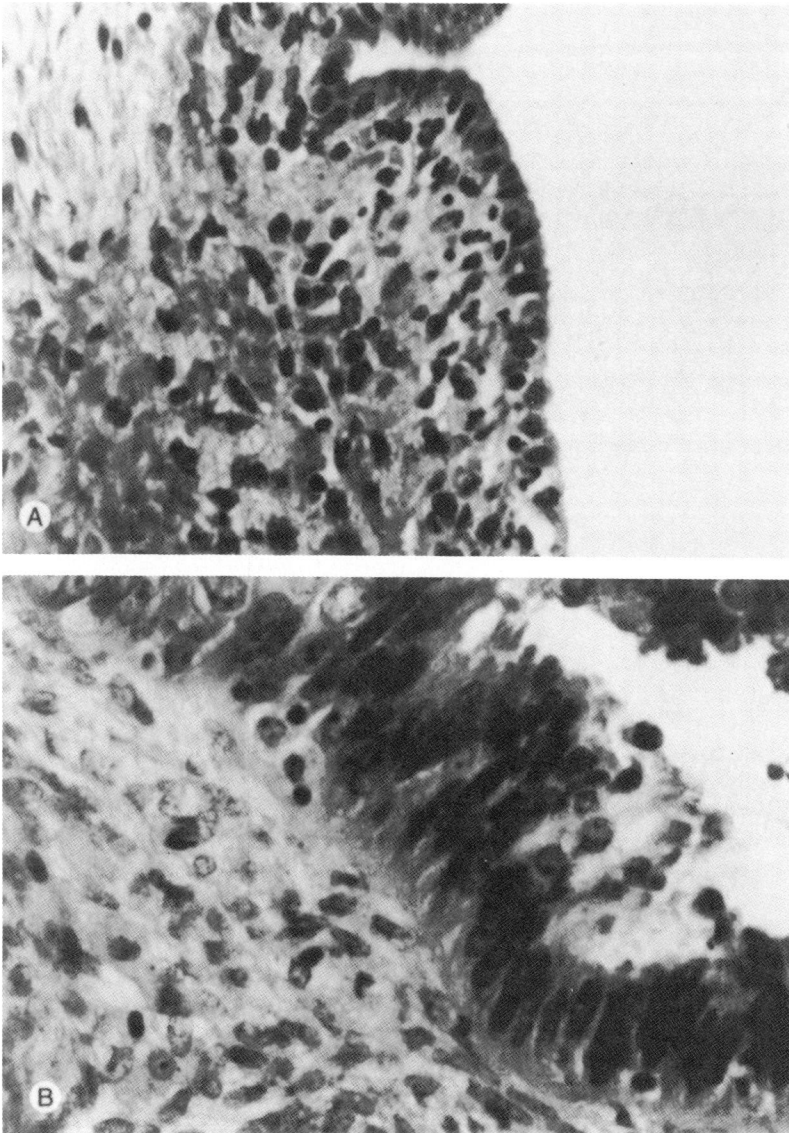

FIGURE 34–1. Photomicrographs of endometriosis lesions. *A*, Endometriosis lesions without architectural or cellular atypia. *B*, Atypical endometriosis with cellular crowding stratification tufting and nuclear enlargement. (From Chalas E, Chumas J, Barbieri RL, et al. Nucleolar organizer regions in endometriosis, atypical endometriosis, clear cell carcinoma and endometrioid carcinoma. Gynecol Oncol 1991; 40:260.)

thetic C-21 progestins (medroxyprogesterone acetate)[10] and the C-19 progestins (gestrinone) result in atrophy of endometriosis lesions.[11]

In simple terms, estrogens support the growth of endometriosis lesions, and androgens produce atrophy in endometriosis lesions. The polarity of response of endometriosis lesions to androgens and estrogens is the yin and yang on which most hormone therapy of endometriosis is based (Table 34–1). The gonadotropin-releasing hormone (GnRH) analogs nafarelin[12, 13] and leuprolide[14] can effectively produce a hypoestrogenic state and produce regression in endometriosis lesions. The synthetic androgen danazol produces a hyperandrogenic state that causes atrophy in endometriosis.[7] These agents are discussed in greater detail later.

ENDOMETRIOSIS AND INFERTILITY: CAUSE AND EFFECT?

The hypothesis that endometriosis causes infertility in humans has not been adequately tested. Experiments in rabbits, rats, and monkeys, however, suggest that advanced endometriosis is associated with infertility.[15–18] For example, Schenken and associates[17] examined the effects of surgically induced endometriosis on fertility in monkeys. Animals with surgically induced endometriosis and control animals with adipose tissue autografts were mated. Pregnancy rates were similar in control animals (42%) and animals with mild endometriosis (35%). Animals with moderate and severe endometriosis had reduced pregnancy rates (12%). Pelvic adhesions appeared to account, in part, for the reduction in fertility. Animals that had endometriosis and ovulated from an ovary with adhesions had a 0% per cycle pregnancy rate. Animals that had endometriosis and ovulated from an adnexa without adhesions had a 33% per cycle pregnancy rate. In addition, some of the animals with endometriosis appeared to have luteinized unruptured follicles, which accounted for a part of the reduction in fertility.

Women with endometriosis appear to have low fecundity. In normal couples, fecundity is in the range of 0.15 to 0.20 per cycle. For women with endometriosis, the fecundity per cycle is in the range of 0.05.[19–21] In one study, Toma and

TABLE 34–1. Steroid Hormone Manipulations Effective in the Treatment of Endometriosis

Hormonal State	Methods Available to Produce State	Typical Regimen (Reference)	Percent of Reduction in AFS Endometriosis Score	Percent of Patients with Improvement in Pain Symptoms	Side Effects
Hypoestrogenism	Oophorectomy GnRH analogs	Nafarelin (200 μg bid)[12]	45	80	Vasomotor symptoms, bone loss, headache, dry vagina, decreased libido
Hyperandrogenism	Danazol Methyltestosterone	Danazol (400–800 mg daily)[7]	50	75	Increased body muscle and mass, weight gain, hirsutism, acne, oily skin, deepening of voice
Hyperprogestational	Medroxyprogesterone Norethindrone Gestrinone	Medroxyprogesterone acetate (30–50 mg daily)[10]	68	85	Moliminal symptoms, bloating, mood changes, irregular uterine bleeding

AFS, American Fertility Society.

coworkers[21] evaluated fecundity in women with stage I and II endometriosis participating in a donor insemination program. The fecundity per cycle was 0.052 for stage I and 0.065 for stage II endometriosis. The fecundity per cycle for the control group was significantly higher (0.14, P<0.05). The observation that endometriosis is associated with *subfertility* does not necessarily imply that endometriosis causes subfertility. It is also possible that subfertility causes endometriosis. Evidence that treatment of endometriosis improves fecundity would strengthen the argument that endometriosis causes subfertility.

Data derived from retrospective studies of infertile women with endometriosis suggest that treatment of minimal endometriosis does not improve fecundity, but surgical treatment of severe endometriosis does improve fecundity. These data have been reviewed by this author in a previous publication and are briefly summarized subsequently.[22]

If minimal endometriosis causes infertility, it is reasonable to expect that effective therapy for minimal endometriosis should improve fecundity. Bayer and associates and Seibel and colleagues[19, 20] reported the first prospective, controlled randomized study of the effectiveness of danazol in the treatment of infertility associated with minimal endometriosis. Couples with 1 year of infertility were eligible for entry into the study after they completed a basic infertility evaluation, which included semen analysis, basal body temperature chart, postcoital test, hysterosalpingogram, and endometrial biopsy. Patients then underwent a diagnostic laparoscopy and tubal lavage. If Kistner stage I endometriosis[23] was observed, the patients were randomized to receive danazol or no treatment. The women who were randomized to the danazol treatment group received a regimen with a tapering dose of danazol: 800 mg daily for 2 months, 600 mg daily for 2 months, and 400 mg daily for 2 months. Patients were then observed for 12 months, either immediately after laparoscopy in the untreated group or after completion of danazol therapy in the treated group. A total of 37 patients were randomized to danazol treatment, and 36 were randomized to the no-treatment group. During the 12 months of follow-up, 35% of the danazol-treated women and 47% of the no-treatment group became pregnant; this difference was not statistically significant (Fig. 34–2). In conclusion, treatment of women with mild endometriosis with danazol did not improve fe-

cundity. Thomas and Cooke,[24] in a randomized study comparing gestrinone with placebo, observed similar results.

In a controlled trial, Fedele and coworkers[25] randomized 71 women with American Fertility Society (AFS) stage I or II endometriosis to receive hormonal treatment with the GnRH agonist analog buserelin (400 μg three times daily for 6 months), or to a group that received no treatment. Median follow-up was 17 months in the buserelin group and 18 months in the control group. The 1-year actuarial pregnancy rate was similar in both groups: buserelin 30%, control 37%. The 2-year actuarial pregnancy rate was also similar in both groups: buserelin 61%, control 61%. This study suggests that hormonal treatment of AFS stage I or II endometriosis with buserelin does not improve fecundity.

Data from nonrandomized studies support the conclusion of the randomized studies of Seibel and colleagues,[19, 20] Thomas and Cooke,[24] and Fedele and coworkers.[25] For example, in a retrospective review, Badawy and colleagues[26] observed that women with "mild" endometriosis (Acosta classification)[27] observed for 5 years had a 55% pregnancy rate if treated with danazol and a 90% pregnancy rate if they received no hormone treatment. Schenken and Malinak,[28] Garcia and David,[29] and Portuondo and colleagues[30] all observed that expectant management of women with mild endometriosis resulted in pregnancy rates of 75% (1 year of follow-up),[28] 65% (2 years of follow-up),[28] and 61% (2 years of follow-up).[29] No study suggests that surgical or hormonal treatment of infertile women with mild endometriosis results in better fertility rates than these retrospective studies demonstrate for expectant management. It should be noted, however, that a 65% pregnancy rate during a 2-year follow-up period indicates that mild endometriosis may be associated with lower than normal fecundability. It is possible that improved treatment modalities, yet to be developed, would be able to restore fecundability for these couples to the normal expected 90% to 95% cumulative pregnancy rate at 12 months of follow-up.

As noted earlier, experiments with monkeys demonstrate that severe endometriosis causes infertility. Clinical data support this observation. For example, Olive and Lee[31] retrospectively analyzed 130 infertile women treated with expectant management or surgery or both. In women with mild (Acosta classification[27]) or moderate endometriosis, expectant

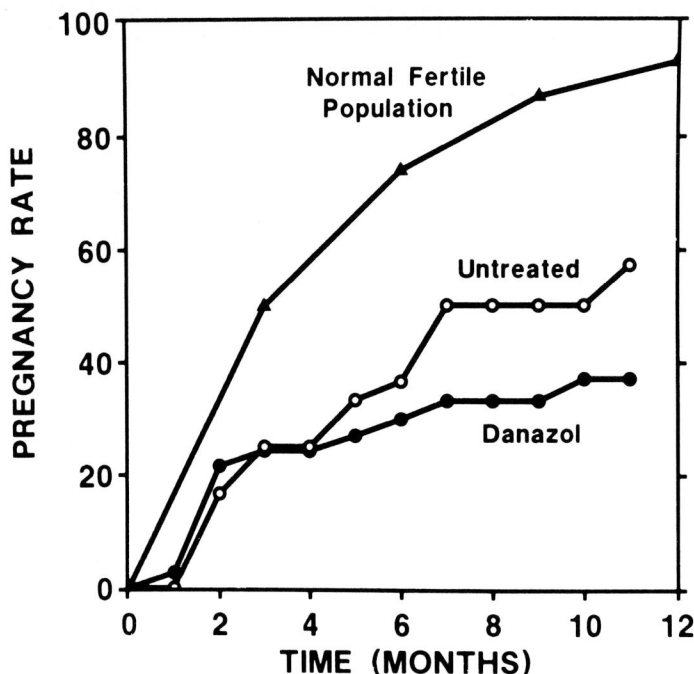

FIGURE 34–2. Cumulative pregnancy rates in danazol-treated and untreated patients with minimal endometriosis. The cumulative pregnancy rate in an ideal fertile population is also shown for comparison. (From Bayer SR, Seibel MM, Sattan DS, et al. The efficacy of danazol treatment for minimal endometriosis in an infertile population. J Reprod Med 1988; 33:179.)

management and surgical treatment resulted in similar fecundability. In contrast, in women with severe endometriosis, surgical treatment resulted in significantly enhanced fecundability as compared with expectant management. Of 32 women with severe endometriosis treated with expectant management, none became pregnant during 231 cumulative months of follow-up. Ten of 34 women with severe endometriosis became pregnant after surgical management during 702 cumulative months of follow-up. My assessment of the available data is that in women with minimal endometriosis and infertility, neither hormone therapy nor surgery is effective for improving fecundity. For women with advanced endometriosis and infertility, hormone therapy is not effective for improving fecundity, but surgical therapy may be effective.

Planning therapy for infertile women with endometriosis requires considerable clinical skill. Contributing to the difficulty of clinical decision making is that few randomized, controlled clinical trials have been completed dealing with endometriosis and infertility. An important clinical rule is to complete carefully the entire infertility evaluation and to search for all potential factors that contribute to each couple's fertility problem. The second most important clinical rule is that the primary therapy for advanced endometriosis associated with infertility is "conservative" surgery. The surgical treatment of endometriosis associated with infertility is reviewed by Morales and Murphy in Chapter 36. As noted previously, there is no definitive evidence that hormonal treatment of infertility caused by endometriosis improves fecundity. The main clinical indication for the use of hormonal therapy in women with endometriosis is to suppress pain symptoms.[7, 32, 33]

Five major options are currently available for the hormonal treatment of endometriosis: nafarelin, leuprolide, danazol, progestins, and estrogen-progestin. The clinical pharmacology of these agents has been examined in detail in previous publications[7, 32, 33] and is briefly reviewed next.

DANAZOL

Danazol is an isoxazole derivative of 17-ethinyltestosterone (Fig. 34–3). The pharmacology of danazol is best understood by examining its interaction with two classes of proteins: steroid hormone receptors and enzymes of steroidogenesis.

Steroid hormones produce biologic effects in steroid-responsive tissues by first binding to intranuclear steroid receptors. The interaction of a steroid with an intranuclear steroid receptor system can result in one of three possible outcomes: the steroid can *stimulate* the biologic response characteristic of the receptor system (agonist), it can *inhibit* the biologic effects typically seen after stimulation of the receptor system (antagonist), or it can produce a mixed pattern of agonist and antagonist effects. Danazol binds to androgen receptors and is an androgen agonist.[34] This is not surprising because danazol is a derivative of testosterone. Danazol binds to progesterone receptors and is a mixed progesterone agonist-antagonist. In some test systems, danazol produces progesterone-like effects (i.e., inducting secretory changes in estro-

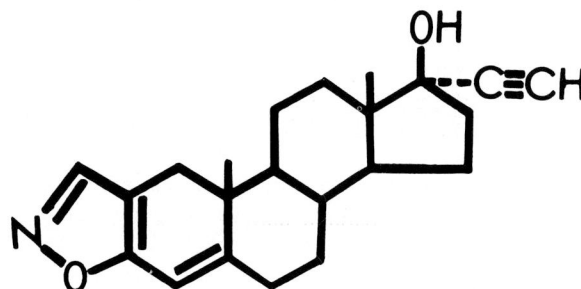

Danazol

FIGURE 34–3. Chemical structure of danazol. Danazol is an isoxazole derivative of ethinyltestosterone.

site of receptor
activation

Glu—His—Trp—Ser—Tyr
(1)   (2)   (3)   (4)   (5)

Gly
(6)

H₂N-Gly—Pro—Arg—Leu   site
(10)   (9)   (8)   (7)   of
cleavage

site of
cleavage

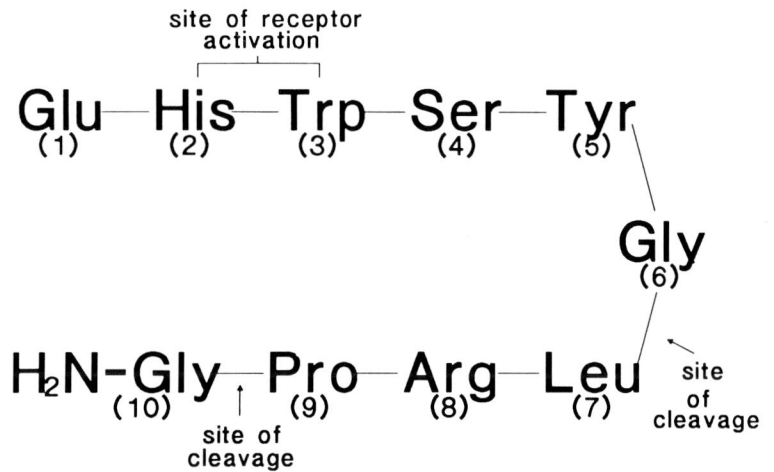

FIGURE 34–4. Chemical structure of the hypothalamic decapeptide gonadotropin-releasing hormone agonist.

gen-primed endometrium). In other test systems, danazol blocks the actions of progesterone. At pharmacologically "relevant" doses, danazol does not bind to estrogen receptors and has no estrogenic effects. Danazol also binds to sex hormone–binding globulin (SHBG), displacing testosterone from SHBG and resulting in a marked increase in the concentration of free testosterone.

Danazol inhibits multiple enzymes of steroidogenesis, including cholesterol cleavage enzyme, 3β-hydroxysteroid dehydrogenase-isomerase, 17α-hydroxylase, 17,20-lyase, and 17-ketosteroid reductase.[35] In women, these effects of danazol inhibit ovarian estrogen production. Danazol is efficacious in the treatment of endometriosis because it produces a high androgen/low estrogen environment, which results in atrophy of endometriotic implants (see Table 34–1).

Guidelines concerning the use of danazol continue to evolve. The following discussion highlights the areas of consensus and the breadth of disagreement concerning the use of the drug.[7] Most clinicians agree that patients with a suspected diagnosis of endometriosis must have confirmation of the diagnosis by laparoscopy or laparotomy before initiation of therapy. Danazol should be initiated at the completion of a normal menses. It is important that danazol not be administered to pregnant women; female pseudohermaphroditism is common in female offspring of mothers treated with danazol during the first and second trimesters of pregnancy.

Danazol is an effective contraceptive at doses of 400 to 800 mg/day (less than 1% incidence of ovulation). Patients with poor medication compliance, however, can become pregnant on these doses of danazol if they are taking the drug in an intermittent fashion. Therefore the use of a barrier contraceptive should be discussed with women taking danazol. Pregnancy testing and careful uterine examinations during danazol therapy ensure the early detection of an unplanned pregnancy.

Danazol in doses of 100 mg/day or greater produces pain relief in the majority of patients with endometriosis. Doses of 400 mg/day are required to induce amenorrhea reliably. Given these considerations and a desire to minimize costs, we start most patients on 200 mg danazol orally twice per day. Cessation of menses and measurement of serum estradiol concentrations are good clinical and laboratory monitors of danazol therapy. Dickey and colleagues[36] reported that during danazol treatment, there was a relationship between the mag-

nitude of suppression of serum estradiol and the successful treatment of endometriosis lesions. For example, complete remission of AFS class severe and moderate endometriosis required suppression of serum estradiol concentration to less than 22 and less than 41 pg/mL.

Initial trials investigating the efficacy of danazol evaluated a 6-month therapy regimen. This therapy interval need not be followed rigidly. For example, in the patient with advanced endometriosis who is scheduled for conservative laparotomy, a 12- to 24-week preoperative course of danazol is appropriate. For the patient with severe pain owing to endometriosis who does not desire pregnancy and is adamantly opposed to surgery, a 52- to 78-week course of danazol is not unreasonable if side effects are carefully monitored.

The major side effects seen with danazol therapy are (in decreasing order of frequency): weight gain, edema, decreased breast size, acne, oily skin, hirsutism, deepening of the voice, headache, hot flushes, changes in libido, and muscle cramps.[37] Significant weight gain (2 to 10 kg) is common.[7] In our experience, more than 75% of patients receiving danazol report one or more side effects.[37] Danazol is metabolized largely via hepatic mechanisms and has been reported to produce mild elevation in serum glutamic oxaloacetic transaminase and glutamic pyruvic transaminase.[38] Therefore in patients with hepatic dysfunction, danazol is relatively contraindicated.

GnRH ANALOGS: NAFARELIN AND LEUPROLIDE

During the 1980s, danazol was the primary hormonal agent used in the treatment of endometriosis. During the 1990s, the leading hormonal agents used to treat endometriosis are the GnRH analogs. GnRH is a hypothalamic decapeptide (Fig. 34–4) that controls the pituitary secretion of luteinizing hormone (LH) and follicle-stimulating hormone (FSH). In the follicular phase of the menstrual cycle, the hypothalamus releases one pulse of GnRH every 60 to 90 minutes into the portal circulation. The ability of GnRH to stimulate LH and FSH secretion is critically dependent on the frequency and amplitude of the GnRH pulse. If the GnRH pulse frequency is chronically slow or too fast, the pituitary does not secrete LH and FSH in response to the GnRH pulse.[39–41] A

TABLE 34–2. Effects of GnRH Analog on Estradiol Concentration, Reduction of Revised AFS Score, and Pain Relief in Women with Endometriosis

Article	No. of Subjects	Drug/Dose	Estradiol Concentration	Reduction in AFS Score	Pain Relief of Subjects
Henzl et al[12]	77	Nafarelin 400 μg intranasal for 6 months	28	43	73
	79	Nafarelin 800 μg intranasal for 6 months	15	42	77
Cirkel et al[47]	40	Buserelin acetate 300 μg 3 times a day intranasal for 6 months	28	51	—
LeMay et al[49]	10	Buserelin acetate 200 μg 2 times a day subcutaneously for 5 days, then 400 μg intranasal spray 3 times a day for 25 to 31 weeks	8	50	72
Dlugi et al[48]	52	Leuprolide acetate 3.75 mg IM every 4 weeks for 20 weeks	15	—	89
Shaw[50]	40	Goserelin 3.6 mg implant for 6 months	12.7	50	69.6

AFS, American Fertility Society.

continuous infusion of GnRH, through molecular mechanisms that are poorly understood, markedly decreases pituitary production of LH and FSH.[40]

Because much of the information in the GnRH signal is contained in the pulse frequency, GnRH has a short half-life (4 minutes). This insures that the pulse is clear and crisp. GnRH is metabolized by endopeptidases and carboxy-amide peptidases present in the pituitary circulation and pituitary gonadotrophs, which cleave the 6–7 and 9–10 peptide bonds.[42] By chemically altering the sixth amino acid, GnRH analogs that are resistant to cleavage by endopeptidases can be produced.[43] These GnRH analogs have a long half-life (2 to 4 hours) and are perceived by the pituitary as a continuous infusion of GnRH. Consequently, long-term administration of these GnRH analogs decreases LH and FSH secretion and causes a cessation of ovarian estrogen production.[44]

Two GnRH analogs are currently available for clinical application in the United States: leuprolide and nafarelin. Leuprolide is available as daily subcutaneous injections or as a monthly depot injection. Nafarelin is available as a nasal spray.

In a large, randomized clinical trial comparing the efficacy of danazol and nafarelin in the treatment of endometriosis, Henzl and colleagues[12] observed that both drugs produced symptomatic improvement in 80% of subjects and a 43% improvement in the revised AFS (rAFS) endometriosis score. Most of the side effects associated with nafarelin therapy were due to the hypoestrogenism. These side effects include hot flashes, headaches, mood changes, decreased libido, and vaginal dryness. Observations indicate that GnRH analogs can produce a decrease in vertebral bone density. For example, Dawood and colleagues[45] reported that 6 months of GnRH analog therapy with buserelin (1200 μg nasally per day) resulted in a 7% decrease in trabecular bone density. Six months after completing GnRH agonist therapy, the trabecular bone density remained 4% below pretreatment values. Similar losses in trabecular bone density during GnRH agonist therapy have been reported by Johansen and colleagues[46] using nafarelin and by Matta and colleagues[41] using buserelin. Interestingly, Matta and colleagues[41] reported that the bone loss was completely reversible once the GnRH analog was discontinued. The clinical impact of the GnRH analog-induced decrease in bone density in women of reproductive age remains to be fully characterized.

Multiple clinical trials suggest that GnRH agonists (1) suppress circulating estradiol concentrations, (2) reduce endometriosis disease activity as objectively measured by pretreatment and posttreatment laparoscopy, and (3) decrease pelvic pain.[12–14, 47–50] An important question that remains to be answered is: What precise estradiol concentration is required to suppress the activity of endometriosis lesions? A review of multiple studies suggests that estradiol concentrations of 15 pg/mL and 30 pg/mL are both efficacious in the treatment of endometriosis.[12, 47–50]

For example, regimens used by Henzl and colleagues[12] (nafarelin, 200 μg nasally twice a day) and Cirkel and associates[47] (buserelin, 300 μg nasally three times a day) both reduced the circulating estradiol to 30 pg/mL and reduced the rAFS endometriosis score by 43% and 51%. In addition, the regimen studied by Henzl and colleagues[12] reduced pelvic pain in 73% of patients. In contrast, Shaw[50] (goserelin, 3.6 mg implant every 4 weeks for 6 months), Dlugi and colleagues[48] (leuprolide acetate, 3.75 mg intramuscularly every 4 weeks), and Lemay and associates[49] (buserelin) studied regimens that reduced circulating estradiol concentrations to the range 8 to 15 pg/mL. These regimens produced a 50% decrease in the rAFS endometriosis score and decreased pelvic pain in 70% to 89% of subjects.[48–50] A direct comparison of these studies suggests that, on average, GnRH agonist regimens that produce circulating estradiol concentrations of 15 and 30 pg/mL are both efficacious in the treatment of endometriosis (Table 34–2). Logically a comparison of the side effects produced by estradiol concentrations of 15 pg/mL and 30 pg/mL becomes an important issue. When treating endometriosis by inducing a hypoestrogenic state, it may be best to use a regimen that produces the *minimal* degree of hypoestrogenism necessary to cause improvement in the pelvic pain. For many women, an estradiol concentration of 30 pg/mL is sufficient to cause atrophy of the endometriosis lesions.

PROGESTINS

Numerous progestins (medroxyprogesterone acetate [MPA], gestrinone, norethindrone acetate, and lynestrenol) have been used as single agents in the treatment of endometriosis. These agents produce an acyclic, hypoestrogenic environment by suppressing pituitary secretion of LH and FSH, which inhibits ovarian estrogen production. In addition, these agents have direct antiestrogenic actions on endometriosis lesions by binding to intracellular progesterone and androgen receptors. Synthetic progestins can be divided into two broad classes, the C-21 progestins, such as MPA, and the C-19 progestins, such as gestrinone. In general, the C-19 progestins have more androgenic effects (suppression of high-density lipoprotein cholesterol) than the C-21 progestins. Each of these agents is effective in the treatment of endometriosis.

Luciano and colleagues[10] reported one of the best designed and executed studies of the effects of MPA in the treatment of endometriosis. Twenty-one women with endometriosis were treated with oral MPA, 50 mg daily, for 4 months. Pretreatment and posttreatment laparoscopies indicated a 68% decrease in AFS score at the end of therapy. Eighty percent of patients had improvement in their symptoms of pelvic pain. Twenty percent of patients had irregular uterine bleeding. Biopsy of endometriosis implants at the completion of therapy demonstrated MPA-induced atrophic changes and pseudodecidual reactions in the implants. This study, although lacking a control group, strongly suggests that MPA is effective in the treatment of endometriosis. Of interest, MPA produced a significant decrease in circulating estradiol concentration from 80 to 46 pg/mL after 4 months of treatment. Some women treated with MPA had serum estradiol concentrations less than 20 pg/mL.

The effects of gestrinone, a C-19 progestin, on the treatment of endometriosis was investigated by Hornstein and associates.[11] Women with stage 2 or stage 3 endometriosis were randomized to receive 1.25 mg (group 1) or 2.5 mg (group 2) of gestrinone twice weekly. All women underwent laparoscopy before treatment and after 6 months of gestrinone treatment. In group 1, there was a 52% decrease in the AFS score. In group 2, there was a 63% decrease in the AFS score. The majority of patients had a decrease in their symptoms of pelvic pain during therapy. The major side effects were weight gain (mean increase of 2.1 kg), headache, palpitations, hirsutism, and irregular uterine bleeding. This study suggests that gestrinone is effective in the treatment of endometriosis.

COMBINED ESTROGEN-PROGESTIN REGIMENS

In 1959, Kistner[51] reported that combined estrogen-progestogen contraceptives were effective in the treatment of endometriosis when used in a *continuous* "pseudopregnancy" regimen. Long-term administration of a combination of estrogen and a progestin results in (1) suppression of LH and FSH, resulting in the absence of ovarian follicular development, and (2) decidualization of the endometrium. Pseudopregnancy regimens produce an acyclic hormone environment but do expose the endometriotic lesions to significant amounts of estrogen. Although most synthetic progestins have sufficient androgenic and progestational activity to block the effects of coadministered estrogen, in some patients the administered estrogen actually stimulates metabolic activity in endometriotic lesions. We do not recommend the use of pseudopregnancy for women with severe endometriosis.

One group of patients may be especially suitable candidates for pseudopregnancy treatment. Young women with severe incapacitating dysmenorrhea and minimal or mild endometriosis usually report marked improvement in their pain during "mini-pseudopregnancy" therapy. A typical "mini-pseudopregnancy" regimen consists of 15 weeks of continuous estrogen-progestin therapy (five packages of birth control pills), followed by a 1-week withdrawal of hormone therapy, again followed by 15 weeks of continuous estrogen-progestin therapy, and so forth. Using this regimen, a young woman with endometriosis who had 13 painful menses per year before therapy had approximately only three menses per year after starting therapy, resulting in significant symptomatic relief.[32]

COMBINED HORMONE THERAPY AND SURGERY FOR THE TREATMENT OF ENDOMETRIOSIS

Few randomized, prospective clinical trials are available that evaluate the efficacy of combined medical-surgical treatment of endometriosis. Conceptually, the benefits of preoperative hormone therapy are to (1) reduce the size of endometriomas, thereby facilitating surgical removal; (2) minimize the chance of spreading viable endometriosis tissue around the peritoneal cavity at the time of surgery; (3) suppress ovarian follicular development and corpus luteum formation so that a large follicle or corpus luteum is not traumatized at the time of surgery; and (4) minimize inflammation in the cul-de-sac to facilitate the dissection of an obliterated cul-de-sac. Potential benefits of postoperative hormone therapy include: Foci of endometriosis that remain at the completion of surgery are eradicated, and reseeding of endometriosis lesions is minimized by suppressing retrograde menstruation. Disadvantages to preoperative or postoperative hormone therapy include: Preoperative treatment may produce atrophy or shrinkage of lesions such that they cannot be identified at surgery, and hormone treatment may disturb postoperative healing of the peritoneum and ovary. Scientific data are not available to address these issues definitively. My recommendation is to use 1 to 2 months of preoperative hormone therapy if an endometrioma is to be resected or if an attempt is to be made to dissect an obliterated cul-de-sac. Postoperative hormone therapy should be limited to cases in which substantial lesions were still present at the completion of surgery.

The hormonal therapy of endometriosis continues to evolve. In the 1940s, high-dose testosterone and diethylstilbestrol regimens were the only hormonal agents available for the treatment of endometriosis. These agents, although efficacious, were associated with intolerable side effects. In the 1950s and 1960s, progestin only and continuous estrogen-progestin regimens became available. The 1980s saw the use of danazol as the major hormonal agent for the treatment of endometriosis. In the 1990s, the GnRH agonist analogs have become the most widely used agents for the treatment of endometriosis. A better understanding of the biology of endometriosis is sure to result in new and better therapeutic agents.

REFERENCES

1. Vernon MW, Beard J, Graves KL, et al. Classification of endometriotic implants by morphological appearance and capacity to synthesize prostaglandin F. Fertil Steril 1986; 46:801.

2. Chalas E, Chumas J, Barbieri RL, et al. Nuclear organizer regions in endometriosis, atypical endometriosis, clear cell carcinoma. Gynecol Oncol 1991; 40:260.

3. Bergqvist A, Feno M. Steroid receptors in endometriotic tissue and endometrium: assay with monoclonal antibodies. In: Genazzani AR, editor. Recent Research in Gynecologic Endocrinology. Vol 1. Carnforth, UK: Panthenon, 1989: 384.

4. Tamaya T, Motoyama T, Ohono Y. Steroid receptor levels and histology of endometriosis and adenomyosis. Fertil Steril 1979; 31:396.

5. Bergqvist A, Jeppsson S, Jullander S, et al. Human uterine and endometriotic tissue transplanted into nude mice. Am J Pathol 1985; 121:337.

6. Sharpe K, Bertero MC, Muse KN, et al. Spontaneous and steroid-induced recurrence of endometriosis after suppression by a gonadotropin-releasing hormone antagonist in the rat. Am J Obstet Gynecol 1991; 165:187.

7. Barbieri RL, Ryan KL. Danazol endocrine pharmacology and therapeutic applications. Am J Obstet Gynecol 1981; 141:453.

8. Hammond MG, Hammond CB, Parker RT. Conservative treatment of endometriosis externa: the effects of methyltestosterone therapy. Fertil Steril 1978; 29:651.

9. Dizerega GS, Barber DL, Hodgen GD. Endometriosis: role of ovarian steroid in initiation maintenance and suppression. Fertil Steril 1980; 33:649.

10. Luciano AA, Turksoy RN, Carleo J. Evaluation of oral medroxyprogesterone acetate in the treatment of endometriosis. Obstet Gynecol 1988; 72:323.

11. Hornstein MD, Gleason RE, Barbieri RL. A randomized double-blind prospective trial of two doses of gestrinone in the treatment of endometriosis. Fertil Steril 1990; 53:237.

12. Henzl MR, Corson SL, Moghissi K, et al. Administration of nasal nafarelin as compared with oral danazol for endometriosis. A multicenter double-blind comparative trial. N Engl J Med 1988; 318:485.

13. Rolland R, Van der Heijden PFM. Nafarelin versus danazol in the treatment of endometriosis. Am J Obstet Gynecol 1990; 162:586.

14. Miller JD. Leuprolide acetate for the treatment of endometriosis. In: Chadha DR, Buttran VC, editors. Current Concepts in Endometriosis. New York: Alan R. Liss, 1990: 337.

15. Hahn DW, Carraher R, Foldesy R, et al. Studies on the mechanism of infertility associated without endometriosis and the effect of LHRH agonist in an animal model for endometriosis. In: Labrie F, Belanger A, Dupont A, editors. LHRH and Its Analogues. New York: Elsevier, 1984:203.

16. Schenken RS, Asch RH. Surgical induction of endometriosis in the rabbit: effect on fertility and concentration of peritoneal fluid prostaglandins. Fertil Steril 1980; 34:581.

17. Schenken RS, Asch RH, Williams RF, et al. Etiology of infertility in monkeys with endometriosis: luteinized unruptured follicles, luteal phase defects, pelvic adhesions and spontaneous abortions. Fertil Steril 1984; 41:122.

18. Vernon MW, Wilson EA. Studies on the surgical induction of endometriosis in the rat. Fertil Steril 1985; 44:684.

19. Bayer SR, Seibel MM, Saffan DS, et al. Efficacy of danazol treatment for minimal endometriosis in infertile women: a prospective randomized study. J Reprod Med 1988; 33:179.

20. Seibel MM, Berger MJ, Weinstein FG, et al. The effectiveness of danazol on subsequent fertility in minimal endometriosis. Fertil Steril 1982; 38:534.

21. Toma SK, Stovall DW, Hammond MG. The effect of laparoscopic ablation or danazol on pregnancy rates in patients with Stage I or II endometriosis undergoing donor insemination. Obstet Gynecol 1992; 80:253.

22. Barbieri RL. Infertility aspects of endometriosis. In: Sciarra JJ, Droegemueller W, editors. Gynecology and Obstetrics. Philadelphia: JB Lippincott, 1991:1–17.

23. Kistner RW, Siegler AM, Behrman SJ. Suggested classification for endometriosis. Fertil Steril 1977; 28:1008.

24. Thomas EJ, Cooke ID. Successful treatment of asymptomatic endometriosis: does it benefit infertile women? Br Med J 1987; 194:1117.

25. Fedele L, Parazzini F, Radici E, et al. Buserelin acetate versus expectant management in the treatment of infertility associated with minimal or mild endometriosis: a randomized clinical trial. Am J Obstet Gynecol 1992; 166:1345.

26. Badawy SZA, Elbakry MM, Samuel F, et al. Cumulative pregnancy rates in infertile women with endometriosis. J Reprod Med 1988; 33:757.

27. Acosta AA, Buttram VC, Besch PK, et al. A proposed classification of pelvic endometriosis. Obstet Gynecol 1973; 42:19.

28. Schenken RS, Malinak LR. Conservative surgery versus expectant management for the infertile patient with mild endometriosis. Fertil Steril 1982; 37:183.

29. Garcia CR, David SS. Pelvic endometriosis: infertility and pelvic pain. Am J Obstet Gynecol 1977; 129:740.

30. Portuondo JA, Echanojauregui AD, Herran C. Early conception in patients with untreated mild endometriosis. Fertil Steril 1983; 39:22.

31. Olive DL, Lee KL. Analysis of sequential treatment protocols for endometriosis-associated infertility. Am J Obstet Gynecol 1986; 154:613.

32. Barbieri RL. Endometriosis. Curr Probl Obstet Gynecol Fertil 1989; 12:6–13.

33. Barbieri RL. Endometriosis 1990. Current treatment approaches. Drugs 1990; 39:502.

34. Barbieri RL, Lee H, Ryan KJ. Danazol binding to rat androgen, glucocorticoid, progesterone and estrogen receptors: correlation with biologic activity. Fertil Steril 1979; 31:182.

35. Barbieri RL, Canick JA, Makris A, et al. Danazol inhibits steroidogenesis. Fertil Steril 1977; 28:809.

36. Dickey RP, Taylor SN, Curole DN. Serum estradiol and danazol. I. Endometriosis response, side effects, administration interval, concurrent spironolactone and dexamethasone. Fertil Steril 1984; 42:709.

37. Barbieri RL, Evans, Kistner RW. Danazol in the treatment of endometriosis: analysis of 100 cases with a 4 year follow-up. Fertil Steril 1982; 37:737.

38. Holt JP, Keller D. Danazol treatment increases serum enzymes. Fertil Steril 1984; 41:70.

39. Conn PM, Crowley WF Jr. Gonadotropin releasing hormone and its analogues. N Engl J Med 1991; 324:93.

40. Knobil E. The neuroendocrine control of the menstrual cycle. Rec Prog Horm Res 1980; 36:53.

41. Matta WH, Shaw RW, Hesp R, et al. Reversible trabecular bone density loss following induced by hypoestrogenism with the GnRH analogue buserelin in premenopausal women. Clin Endocrinol 1988; 29:45.

42. Marks N, Stern F. Enzymatic mechanisms for the inactivation of luteinizing hormone-releasing hormone. Biochem Biophys Res Commun 1974; 61:1458.

43. Karten MJ, Rivier JE. Gonadotropin releasing hormone analogue design: structure-function studies toward the development of agonists and antagonists. Endocr Rev 1986; 7:44.

44. Friedman AJ. The biochemistry, physiology, and pharmacology of gonadotropin releasing hormone (GnRH) and GnRH analogues. In: Barbieri RL, Friedman AJ, editors. Gonadotropin Releasing Hormone Analogues. New York: Elsevier, 1991.

45. Dawood MY, Lewis V, Ramos J. Cortical and trabecular bone mineral content in women with endometriosis: effect of gonadotropin releasing hormone agonist and danazol. Fertil Steril 1989; 52:21.

46. Johansen JS, Riis BJ, Hassager C, et al. The effect of a gonadotropin releasing hormone analogue (nafarelin) on bone metabolism. J Clin Endocrinol Metab 1988; 67:701.

47. Cirkel U, Schweppe KW, Ochs H, et al. Effects of LHRH agonist therapy in treatment of endometriosis. In: Chadha DR, Willemsen WNP, editors. Gonadotropin Down-Regulation in Gynecological Practice. Vol 225. New York: Alan R. Liss, 1986:189.

48. Dlugi AM, Miller JD, Knittle J, et al. Lupron depot in the treatment of endometriosis: a randomized placebo controlled double blind study. Fertil Steril 1990; 54:419.

49. Le May A, Maheuz R, Faure N, et al. Reversible hypogonadism induced by a luteinizing hormone releasing hormone agonist (buserelin) as a new therapeutic approach for endometriosis. Fertil Steril 1983; 41:863.

50. Shaw RW. Goserelin-depot preparation of LHRH analogue used in the treatment of endometriosis. In: Chadha DR, Buttram VC, editors. Current Concepts in Endometriosis. Vol 323. New York: Alan R. Liss, 1990:383.

51. Kistner RW. The treatment of endometriosis by inducing pseudopregnancy with ovarian hormones: a report of 58 cases. Fertil Steril 1959; 10:539.

CHAPTER 35

Endometriosis: Surgical Therapy

ARLENE J. MORALES and ANA A. MURPHY

Endometriosis was first described by Rokitansky in 1860 and popularized after the publication of John Sampson's "Peritoneal Endometriosis due to Menstrual Dissemination of Endometrial Tissue into the Peritoneal Cavity" in 1927.[1] Despite the century that has passed since the first introduction, the pathophysiology of endometriosis remains elusive. This disease has generated much debate and stimulated controversy about its etiology, natural history, pathogenesis, and appropriate treatment.

Three common theories of its causes are (1) retrograde menstruation with subsequent implantation,[1] (2) coelomic metaplasia,[2, 3] and (3) hematogenous or lymphatic transport of endometrial tissue.[4] The most common cause is believed to be reflux menstruation, because the anatomic distribution is consistent with this pattern of development. Some data suggest a link between the duration of exposure to spontaneous menstruation and the genesis of endometriosis.[5] The presence of endometriosis in women with müllerian tract anomalies and an obstructed outflow tract lends further support to the theory of retrograde menstruation proposed by Sampson.[6, 7] However, none of these theories can adequately account for all cases of endometriosis. It is likely that there are several different types of endometriosis with different causes or, possibly, that any of the mechanisms just described can initiate endometriosis in a particular host with alterations in cellular immunity.[8]

The treatment of endometriosis is based on a combination of scientific observations, clinical experience, and personal opinion. Much of the data available do not support the current approaches used in the treatment of endometriosis. Our inability to treat endometriosis in the most effective and efficient fashion stems from our lack of fundamental knowledge of the biology and natural history of this disease. This is further compounded by the presence of several classification systems for the staging of endometriosis; an inadequate number of randomized, controlled, prospective clinical trials; and our lack of consistent use of appropriate statistical methods such as life table analysis. Current treatment of endometriosis is usually based on symptoms, either pain or infertility, rather than just the presence of disease. The evidence that endometriosis in its early stages is a causative factor in female infertility is controversial. Subsequently, its treatment, whether by a medical or surgical approach, is also not fully validated. There are several promising avenues of research in endometriosis, and we look forward in the near future to a better understanding of the pathophysiology of endometriosis that will allow a more logical therapeutic approach. This chapter focuses on the surgical therapy of endometriosis specifically in the infertile woman.

PREVALENCE

Although the prevalence of endometriosis in the general female population is unknown because of the need for a surgical diagnosis, it is thought to be a common gynecologic disorder. Estimates of its prevalence are based on assessments of women undergoing surgery for a variety of reasons. Endometriosis has been noted in 10% to 50% of patients undergoing gynecologic laparotomies, with a generally accepted range of 20% to 40%.[9, 10] One prospective investigation of the prevalence of endometriosis involved 1542 premenopausal white females who underwent gynecologic surgery for infertility, sterilization, pelvic pain, or dysfunctional uterine bleeding.[11] Endometriosis was noted in 21% of infertile women versus 6% of women undergoing sterilization. The prevalence of endometriosis among women undergoing hysterectomy for dysfunctional uterine bleeding was 25%, whereas the prevalence among women undergoing laparoscopy for pelvic pain was 15%.[11] There have been three prospective studies in infertile women in which the prevalence of endometriosis was between 21% and 38.5% of women with primary infertility, 13% of women with secondary infertility, and 5.2% of fertile women.[5, 11, 12] The prevalence of endometriosis diagnosed by laparoscopy in infertile women in retrospective series ranges from 5% to 33%.[13, 14] The prevalence of endometriosis among patients undergoing sterilization has ranged from 1% to 43%, with most less than 20%.[15, 16] Mild pelvic endometriosis is thought to be frequent; its prevalence in the fertile female population is thought to be close to 10%.[17] Several studies have confirmed that infertile women are 7 to 10 times more likely to have endometriosis than are their fertile counterparts.[18]

Laparoscopy is now an accepted, integral part of an infertility evaluation; as a result, endometriosis is more frequently diagnosed in infertile women than in the era prior to laparoscopy. With the identification of a noninvasive method for diagnosis of endometriosis, a better estimate of the prevalence of endometriosis in women of reproductive age could be ascertained.

NATURAL HISTORY

The natural history of endometriosis is poorly understood. Its biologic behavior and response to treatment are not predictable. Based on clinical experience, the disease is believed to progress in most untreated patients, although spontaneous regression occurs, especially in mild cases.[19, 20] Surgical and medical therapies are presumed to prevent a progression of disease but probably do not eliminate all disease, especially retroperitoneal and microscopic. Whether these forms of endometriosis impact on fertility rates is unknown.

Because of the need for surgery to diagnose endometriosis, there have been no studies of the natural history of asymptomatic endometriosis in women. A model in the monkey has shown significant deterioration with time in severe stages only.[21] There are only two published studies in which a second laparoscopy was performed in a group of infertile women with endometriosis receiving placebo. In the study by Thomas and Cooke,[22] 17 women receiving placebo were studied 6 months after the first laparoscopy: 4 were unchanged, 9 improved (4 of whom had no visible disease), and 8 became worse. In the study by Telimaa,[19] 10 of 20 women receiving placebo had no change in stage of disease, 4 women had progression of disease, and 3 women improved. In addition, three women became pregnant. In summary, in 38% of infertile women, the extent of endometriosis was unchanged, 32% had progression of their disease, and 30% improved with expectant management over 6 months. The population studied was not representative of all stages of endometriosis. The argument that the treatment of minimal to mild disease in the infertile woman is for prevention of disease progression is probably irrelevant to most women. The problem is that there are no known factors that identify those women in whom progression of disease will occur.

DISTRIBUTION

Endometriosis has been described in a variety of anatomic sites, but by far the most common site is the pelvis. Table 35–1 shows the percentage for the most common locations. The most frequent sites of endometriotic involvement are the ovaries, pelvic peritoneum, posterior cul-de-sac, uterosacral ligaments, medial broad ligaments, and bladder serosa.[23]

Endometrial implants are common in the posterior cul-de-sac. Puckered blackish-blue peritoneal lesions are the most commonly described gross lesions of endometriosis. Atypical or subtle appearances of peritoneal endometriosis have been described and are being increasingly recognized.[24, 25] The cul-de-sac may become obliterated as the posterior aspect of the cervix becomes adherent to the rectum. The uterosacral liga-

Type	Site	Number	Percent*
Ovarian	Ovary—one	285	55.2
	Ovary—both	127	24.6
Superficial and small spots on serosa	Diffuse scattered pelvic	171	33.1
	Uterine surface	73	14.1
	Tubal surface	71	13.7
	Posterior cul-de-sac	24	4.7
	Uterosacral ligaments	19	3.7
	Anterior cul-de-sac	11	2.1
	Omentum	3	0.6
	Round ligaments	2	0.4
	Broad ligaments	1	0.2
	Small intestine	1	0.2
	Appendix	7	1.4
Intra-abdominal nodules	Rectovaginal septum	8	1.6
	Rectovaginal septum with rectosigmoid involvement	20	3.9
	Rectovaginal septum with vaginal extension	9	1.8
	Sigmoidal	4	0.8
	Anterior cul-de-sac	2	0.4
	Anterior cul-de-sac with bladder involvement	5	1.0
	Tube	8	1.6
	Broad ligament	4	0.8
	Round ligament	3	0.6
Extraperitoneal	Cervix	13	2.5
	Inguinal	4	0.8
	Umbilical	4	0.8
	Incisional—ventral	4	0.8
	Incisional—vulval	1	0.2

TABLE 35–1. Location of Endometriosis

*Total amounts to over 100% because of multiple lesions.

From Williams T. Endometriosis. In: Thompson JD, Rock JA, editors. Te Linde's Operative Gynecology. 7th edition. Philadelphia: JB Lippincott, 1992:470.

ments can become involved with nodular endometriotic implants, causing puckering of these ligaments. The depth of infiltration of endometriosis is thought to be an important aspect in terms of persistence of disease and pain symptoms. Deep endometriotic lesions are more often associated with pelvic pain than are superficial lesions.[26, 27] Endometriosis may also involve the rectovaginal septum and possibly may penetrate the posterior vaginal wall.

Ovarian involvement can vary from superficial implants to large endometriomas that completely replace the ovary. The surface of an ovarian endometrioma may be brown or black from intracystic hemorrhage. The endometrioma may also reside deep within the ovary so that the ovarian surface appears normal. On rupture of ovarian endometriomas, the extruded material is usually brown, tenacious, and thick; thus, they are commonly called "chocolate cysts."

Gastrointestinal involvement commonly occurs. Endometriosis is the third most common benign tumor of the colon. The involvement is usually from the serosal surface toward the mucosa and only rarely invades the mucosal surface. Williams[28] reported involvement of the intestinal tract in 41% of 325 consecutive cases; 84% of those with intestinal endometriosis had involvement of the sigmoid.

Implants may appear in the anterior cul-de-sac as superficial peritoneal implants. These implants may continue onto the round ligaments. Endometriosis may course down along the round ligament and rarely appears at the insertion site in the inguinal ring.

Implants in the anterior cul-de-sac most likely are superficial but may invade the bladder mucosa. Involvement of the urinary tract appears to be less common than gastrointestinal involvement. In addition to possible bladder involvement, the ureters may become involved either directly or by compression. Scarring and obstruction of the ureter may ensue. Rarely, renal endometriosis has been reported.

Implants in abdominal scars are not infrequent. Episiotomy and laparoscopy scars are also areas possibly affected. Excision is both diagnostic and curative in these cases.

DIAGNOSIS AND STAGING

The definitive diagnosis of endometriosis requires direct visualization. There are no symptoms sufficiently specific that the medical history alone can be used to make the diagnosis. However, in some patients who are not operative candidates, the patient's response to empiric therapy may be helpful in establishing a tentative diagnosis. Some argue that pathologic evidence on biopsy in addition to direct visualization should also be required. Sampson's description[1] of the gross appearance of endometriosis is still relevant, although many other more subtle lesions have been recently described.

A variety of histologic patterns are possible with the diagnosis of endometriosis. Classically, both endometrial stroma and glands should be present. However, in an endometrioma, the lining may be so thinned that no recognizable endometrial glands are seen and only scattered stromal cells are present. Biopsy of the blackish-blue "powder burn" implants usually reveals inactive endometrial glands and stroma. Portuondo and coworkers[29] were able to confirm the diagnosis of endometriosis by biopsy in only 72% of patients because of technical difficulties. In addition to technical difficulties, as many as 15% of patients in one series had only nonpigmented biopsy-proven endometriosis.[24]

The visual diagnosis, however, is not entirely specific, lacks sensitivity, and is obviously dependent on the experience and knowledge of the surgeon. In the past decade, surgeons have gained an appreciation for the changes in color of endometriosis implants that occur during the menstrual cycle as well as their invasive nature and multiple morphologic presentations.[30, 31] The classic puckered, blackish powder-burn lesions are the easiest to see and are well recognized by gynecologists. The gross appearance of endometriosis ranges from clear to brown, from flat plaques to raised vesicles, and from fibrotic adhesions to peritoneal defects.[25] Because of the varied appearance of endometriosis lesions, other lesions such as fibrotic scars, epithelial inclusions, inflammatory cysts, and carbon residue from previous laser surgery can be easily mistaken for endometriosis.

Even for the most experienced laparoscopist, the diagnosis of endometriosis can be challenging. Variables affecting the laparoscopic diagnosis of endometriosis include the stage of endometriosis, the quality of the laparoscope and camera equipment, the surgeon's experience, the presence of adhesions, aspiration of peritoneal fluid for adequate visualization, ovarian blind puncture, and recognition of atypical lesions of endometriosis. In addition, the visual appearance of endometriosis can be misleading if the woman is under ovarian suppression.[32] Photography may also be inadequate for documentation owing to the subtle changes in color and hue of some endometriotic implants.[33] The invasive nature of endometriosis is commonly not appreciated. Although its associated lesion may appear superficial to the inexperienced surgeon, complete removal of these types of lesions may require deep dissection. Peritoneal "windows" are associated with endometriosis in 50% of cases.[34, 35]

Investigations using the scanning electron microscope have revealed polypoid, intraperitoneal, and retroperitoneal endometriotic lesions that do not fit the classic description. The small polypoid lesions have been described as being from 200 to 700 μ in diameter.[36] Women with unexplained infertility may even have microscopic implants of endometriosis in normal-appearing peritoneum.[37, 38] It is imperative that the reproductive surgeon be familiar with the many different appearances and locations of endometriosis.[39]

Although it is agreed that the diagnosis of ovarian endometriomas is highly valuable for correct staging of endometriosis, there is controversy about whether blind ovarian puncture is a useful method of detection in women who have slightly enlarged ovaries with normal ovarian surface color and architecture. Candiani and associates[40] reported a prospective study of 52 women with unexplained infertility and enlarged ovaries (maximum diameter of 3.5 to 5 cm). No ovarian surface abnormalities were noted. Ovarian puncture resulted in chocolate-colored aspirates containing degenerate blood and pigment containing histiocytes in 28 of 67 punctures performed in these 52 women. In 48% (25) of the 52 women, a diagnosis of endometriosis or an increase in endometriosis stage resulted after the ovarian puncture. Establishing the diagnosis of endometriosis based on retrieval of chocolate-type material is probably insufficient because this material may also be retrieved from an old hemorrhagic corpus luteum. There may be a role for blind ovarian puncture in women with infertility and enlarged ovaries, although we suggest that further study is needed. Vercellini and colleagues[41] studied the visual diagnosis of ovarian endometrioma at laparotomy in 245 women with ovarian cysts. The gross characteristics for the diagnosis of ovarian endometriomas were that there were no ovarian cysts larger than 12 cm in diameter; adhesions were present to the pelvic sidewall or posterior broad ligament, or both; powder burns were seen; superficial endometriosis with adjacent puckering on the surface existed; and tarry, thick, chocolate-colored fluid content was present. These criteria yielded a sensitivity of 97%, a specificity of 95%, and an accuracy of 96%.[41]

A new development in the diagnosis of endometriosis is laser-induced luminescence.[41a] The principle of this laser-induced luminescence is based on the inherent fluorescence of human tissue when exposed to certain wavelengths of light. In addition, certain drugs that concentrate in endometriotic implants can potentially be used as "photoenhancers" to increase fluorescence and enhance the detection and localization of endometriosis.[42] Preclinical animal in vivo studies have revealed that tamoxifen and possibly tetracycline compounds may be useful in identifying ectopic endometrium with laser-induced luminescence.

Laparoscopy is the procedure of choice for the diagnosis of endometriosis. The hallmark of an accomplished laparoscopist is a systematic approach to visualization of the pelvis. Whenever endometriosis is encountered, formal American Fertility Society (AFS) classification staging should be performed and recorded (Fig. 35–1). Prior to the 1970s, it was

THE AMERICAN FERTILITY SOCIETY
REVISED CLASSIFICATION OF ENDOMETRIOSIS

Patient's Name _____ Date _____

Stage I   (Minimal) · 1-5
Stage II (Mild)   · 6-15
Stage III (Moderate) · 16-40
Stage IV (Severe)   · >40
Total _____

Laparoscopy _____ Laparotomy _____ Photography _____
Recommended Treatment _____
_____
Prognosis _____

PERITONEUM	ENDOMETRIOSIS	<1cm	1-3cm	>3cm
	Superficial	1	2	4
	Deep	2	4	6
OVARY	R Superficial	1	2	4
	Deep	4	16	20
	L Superficial	1	2	4
	Deep	4	16	20

	POSTERIOR CULDESAC OBLITERATION	Partial	Complete
		4	40

	ADHESIONS	<1/3 Enclosure	1/3-2/3 Enclosure	>2/3 Enclosure
OVARY	R Filmy	1	2	4
	Dense	4	8	16
	L Filmy	1	2	4
	Dense	4	8	16
TUBE	R Filmy	1	2	4
	Dense	4*	8*	16
	L Filmy	1	2	4
	Dense	4*	8*	16

*If the fimbriated end of the fallopian tube is completely enclosed, change the point assignment to 16.

FIGURE 35–1. American Fertility Society revised classification of endometriosis. (From The American Fertility Society. Revised classification of endometriosis: 1985, Fertil Steril 1985; 43:351. Reproduced with permission of the publisher, The American Fertility Society.)

virtually impossible to evaluate or compare the results of surgical treatment because there were no uniform staging classifications. In an attempt to encourage the careful recording of operative findings and to standardize documentation of extent of disease, the AFS devised a staging form in 1979 that was revised in 1985 to correct design flaws.[43] This form was empirically derived by a committee of experienced clinicians. Use of this form is strongly encouraged so that results of therapies can be interpreted in light of standardized data. All studies on endometriosis now refer to this classification. However, there are several problems with the revised AFS classification system.[44, 45] This revised classification is weighted for ovarian involvement. Because there are no data on expectant management of ovarian endometrioma, it is unclear if the decreased fecundity of women with ovarian endometriomata is a result of the endometriosis or of the postoperative adhesions that frequently form after surgical treatment of the endometriosis. Scoring is based on gross visualization of disease, although it is well recognized that reproductive prognosis and pain symptoms are not related solely to the amount of disease present. Finally, the current classification does not take into account nonpigmented (a form of atypical) lesions or extraperitoneal endometriosis.

INDICATIONS FOR SURGERY

Typically, endometriosis presents with pelvic pain, adnexal mass, infertility, or some combination of these three signs or symptoms.

Pain

Dysmenorrhea and dyspareunia are common symptoms of endometriosis.[46] Dysmenorrhea is typically secondary and centrally located; however, pelvic pain can be lateral and chronic. Dyspareunia is also typically secondary and usually present with deep insertion. This symptom may result in a cycle in which there is decreased coitus because of the pain and resultant infertility because of lack of coitus. Pelvic pain is a consequence not only of a patient's perception but also of the anatomy of pelvic innervation and is usually not discretely localized. Bleeding may be present with defecation when the bowel is involved. The presence of these symptoms should prompt the clinician to consider the diagnosis of endometriosis, although these symptoms are neither specific nor always present.

The prevalence of laparoscopically diagnosed endometriosis in patients with chronic pelvic pain has ranged from 4% to 52%.[47] In 243 patients with endometriosis, 51.4% had nonprogressive dysmenorrhea, whereas only 9.1% reported progressive dysmenorrhea.[48] Clinical experience and published literature have shown a poor correlation of pain with AFS stage of endometriosis.[49, 50] Preoperative psychological evaluation does not improve this poor correlation.[51] The location of endometriotic implants has been thought to account for particular symptoms. Recent data suggest that the depth and volume of implants are also related to pain.[27] Deep infiltration of fibromuscular tissue has also been strongly correlated with pelvic pain.[26] A prospective trial of 94 women revealed a correlation between preoperative focal tenderness and the depth and volume of endometrial implants.[52] Specifically, the presence of disease in the cul-de-sac was strongly associated with tenderness on preoperative examination, but there was no correlation between tenderness on examination and stage of endometriosis.

The disparity between stage of endometriosis and pelvic pain remains unexplained. It may be that the more metabolically active endometriotic implants are more painful. The importance of implants' different secretory capacity of substances such as prostaglandin F resulting in pain is currently unknown.[53] The severity of the pelvic pain associated with endometriosis is generally cyclic and believed to be dependent on ovarian hormone secretion. Surgical removal of the ovaries or ovarian suppression usually results in pain improvement in the overwhelming majority of patients. Data are available that support the use of excision of pelvic endometriosis for the relief of pain.[35] It is assumed that ovarian endometriomas commonly rupture and leak and that this may cause peritoneal irritation and subsequent pain, but this hypothesis has not been well addressed.

In summary, conservative surgery, usually laparoscopy, is indicated in those women with chronic pelvic pain or progressive dysmenorrhea and dyspareunia not alleviated by simple medical therapy, such as nonsteroidal analgesics, for both diagnosis and possible treatment. Because stage of endometriosis and pain are so poorly correlated, a cogent argument can be made for surgical ablation of any endometriotic lesions present in the woman with pelvic pain.

Mass

Adnexal masses may be identified in patients who have ovarian endometriomas or extensive involvement of the broad ligament or bowel, or both, with endometriosis. On pelvic examination, cul-de-sac nodularity, pelvic tenderness, and induration as well as a fixed, retroverted uterus may be palpated. The pelvic mass with or without symptoms presents a diagnostic challenge.[54] The results of a 1991 survey by the American Association of Gynecologic Laparoscopists revealed that laparoscopic excision of unsuspected invasive cancer is an uncommon event (with an incidence of 0.04%).[55] Careful patient selection is imperative in the use of laparoscopy for an adnexal mass. Variables to be used in the assessment of patients include their age; pelvic examination findings, including mass size and ultrasound characteristics of the mass; and duration that the mass is present.

Size of mass has been correlated with malignancy. In 180 women, 1% of masses smaller than 5 cm, 11% of masses between 5 and 10 cm, and 72% of masses larger than 10 cm were malignant.[56] The following comments are limited to women of reproductive age. Unilateral masses that are cystic, unilocular with regular borders are likely to be benign, whereas masses with septae, papillations, solid areas, or irregular borders are suspect for malignancy. Endometriomas can be variable on ultrasound examination but usually have regular borders and perhaps slightly thickened and diffuse internal echoes, unless fresh hemorrhage is present. Masses that appear to be simple ovarian cysts, unilocular and clear with thin borders, may be followed for as long as 8 weeks because many of these spontaneously resolve. Persistence beyond this period or suspicion of other types of ovarian lesions should lead to surgical diagnosis. There are no set current criteria that will absolutely predict whether an ovarian lesion is ma-

lignant or benign preoperatively. One can at best hope to minimize this risk by careful and judicious selection of appropriate candidates for laparoscopic resection of pelvic masses.

In one series, laparoscopic management of 433 cystic adnexal masses in patients 9 to 88 years of age revealed 90 endometriomas, 5 ovarian cancers, and 4 borderline ovarian tumors. The rest were functional cysts, serous cysts, teratomas, mucinous cysts, or parovarian cysts.[57]

Infertility and Subfertility

A causal association of infertility and severe endometriosis has long been accepted.[58] In severe stages of endometriosis, adhesions and a distortion of the anatomic relationship between the fallopian tube and ovary are most likely involved. Extensive ovarian involvement may result in adhesions that affect tubo-ovarian motility and distort anatomic relations with subsequent impairment of ovum pickup. Ovarian involvement may also result in ovulatory disturbance.[59, 60] Although the relationship between severe endometriosis and infertility is accepted and can be readily understood, the not infrequent finding of mild disease in the fertile woman calls into question the causal association between mild endometriosis and infertility. There is no clear scientific evidence that mild endometriosis is causally related to infertility.[58, 61] When there are only a few scattered implants without disruption of ovum pickup, a causal association is difficult to explain. In the minimal to mild cases of endometriosis, the pathophysiology of endometriosis remains obscure. It seems that the reproductive potential of women with minimal to mild endometriosis is normal but that conceptions in these women occur with a significantly reduced frequency.[58] Women with minimal to mild endometriosis are generally thought to be "subfertile," that is, having a lower monthly fecundity rate than normal.

Several mechanisms have been proposed to explain the association between infertility and minimal to mild endometriosis, such as alterations in peritoneal fluid (increased volume, increased prostanoid content, increased macrophage activity), ovulatory dysfunction (anovulation and luteinized unruptured follicle), luteal phase defects, and disturbed implantations. Cul-de-sac endometriosis may also result in dyspareunia and subsequent decreased coital frequency. Ovarian endometriosis may result in ovulatory disturbances or produce an inflammatory response that may affect tubal function. Chronic salpingitis has been noted in 33% (29/87) of women with ovarian endometriosis undergoing salpingectomy.[62] Laparoscopy is part of a workup in patients with infertility. Other less invasive steps in an infertility evaluation should usually be undertaken first. The goal of the laparoscopy in the infertile woman is to assess the pelvis not only for endometriosis but also for other disorders such as adhesions that may impair fertility. In an infertile woman with symptoms suggestive of endometriosis, such as pain, a laparoscopy may be done earlier in the infertility evaluation to attempt to diagnose and alleviate the source of pelvic pain.

TREATMENT

The management of endometriosis remains controversial because little objective data are available to support the rational use of various forms of medical and surgical therapy. During the past several years, important strides have been made in emphasizing investigative principles in reproductive surgery. Three important advances include the use of the randomized clinical trial to compare therapies; uniformity in classification of diseases; and the use of the life table analysis to adjust for variable followup of patients, especially with respect to pregnancy rates.[63-65]

For practical purposes, endometriosis is considered to be a singular disease entity, although it has a wide range of clinical presentations. For a given woman's situation, there are several acceptable treatment choices; therefore, therapy should be individualized. The stage of endometriosis does not necessarily dictate therapy. If pain is the presenting complaint, surgery offers the most prompt and long-term chance of relief, especially with moderate and severe disease. Medical therapy may be used if pain recurs or persists. If infertility is the presenting complaint, the stage takes on greater weight. In patients with moderate to severe disease, surgery is usually the initial treatment after other aspects of the infertility evaluation are completed. For an infertile woman with minimal to mild disease, no surgical therapy has been shown to be as effective as expectant management. Medical therapy is rarely used for therapy in the infertile patient with minimal to mild endometriosis except when accompanied by pelvic pain. Although both medical and surgical approaches have been used in the treatment of women with infertility, there is relatively little information available on their comparative success. Some women present with combined symptoms of pain and infertility.

Expectant Management

Expectant management of endometriosis consists of observation without specific medical or surgical therapy. Once the diagnosis of endometriosis is confirmed by laparoscopy, no additional therapy specific for endometriosis is used; although obviously in the infertile women, other factors of infertility are corrected. The importance of expectant management, especially in infertile patients with mild to minimal disease, remains controversial in spite of several series reporting good success.[17, 66, 67] Observation after a thorough evaluation may be rewarding for the young subfertile patient with minimal to mild endometriosis. A pregnancy rate of 65% has been reported in one study of patients managed expectantly.[17] A 61% pregnancy rate has also been reported in women with mild endometriosis after 18 months of expectant management.[66] Schenken and Malinak[67] reported a similar success without treatment for minimal and mild endometriosis. The monthly fecundity rates observed by Olive and colleagues[68] in 34 women with mild endometriosis managed expectantly was only 5.7% versus 16.5% in the fertile population. In the absence of complete data, most gynecologists limit expectant management to 1 to 2 years depending on the age of the patient. The 5-year cumulative pregnancy rate in women with mild endometriosis treated by expectant management may be as high as 90%.[69]

Expectant management can also be justified because, albeit small, there are risks associated with surgery. There is a risk that peritoneal surfaces destroyed by surgery may be a nidus for new adhesion formation, which may in themselves cause

infertility and pain.[70] Therefore, some gynecologists withhold medical-surgical therapy for women with early stages of endometriosis unless pain symptoms are present. Despite the lack of evidence of a beneficial effect of active treatment of minimal to mild endometriosis, many gynecologists continue to actively treat asymptomatic disease in the infertile woman. Those who treat minimal and mild endometriosis suggest that although it may not change fertility rates, it may prevent progression of disease in some patients.[71]

It is the opinion of many gynecologic surgeons that surgical therapy for moderate to severe disease results in higher pregnancy rates than does expectant management. This opinion is likely based on their experience with the correction of mechanical problems often seen in severe endometriosis. Although there are data supporting expectant management of women with moderate endometriosis (pregnancy rate of 20% with a monthly fecundity rate of 2.9%), few pregnancies occur with expectant management of women with severe endometriosis, and none has yet been reported in the literature.[68, 72] Furthermore, medical therapy has not been shown to be efficacious in the treatment of infertility associated with endometriosis.[73-75] In addition, many patients favor aggressive surgical therapy because they do not want to delay their attempts to conceive for the 6 months of medical therapy. Finally, many of the side effects of medications used to treat endometriosis decrease the quality of life of the patient.

Conservative Surgical Therapy

Our surgical treatment of endometriosis is based on scientific information that is insufficient and clinical experience that is anecdotal.[76] As a result, many aspects of surgical therapy are controversial. For example, we do not know if it is important to remove small endometriotic implants or only large pigmented, penetrating lesions to improve fertility or decrease pain. Some data suggest that only deeply invasive lesions should be removed. The activity of an endometrial implant has been directly related to the depth of implantation, with deep implants being most active.[26] In addition, as Dargent[77] suggested, the destruction of certain implants can be more destructive than beneficial. Adhesions that may develop after the removal of superficial lesions may be more problematic than the lesions themselves. Finally, there is the observation that microscopic endometriosis may be present in visually normal peritoneum and that surgical therapy of endometriosis rarely removes all of the disease—conservative surgical therapy should be thought of as cytoreductive rather than curative.[38] Conservative surgical therapy encompasses all surgical treatments of endometriosis except castration and hysterectomy. The use of conservative surgical therapy is justified in all women in whom childbearing plans are not yet completed. Even in those women who have completed their childbearing, there may be a role for conservative surgical therapy, especially in the milder stages of endometriosis when surgical therapy can be accomplished laparoscopically with minimal morbidity. Definitive or curative surgical therapy is usually accomplished only by castration and removal of the hormonal stimulus to growth.

When to use conservative surgical therapy as primary therapy in infertile women with endometriosis remains controversial. Most would agree that in a woman with infertility in the presence of stages III to IV endometriosis with extensive adhesions and ovarian endometriomas, surgical therapy is the most appropriate initial treatment. The aim of the surgery should be to restore normal pelvic anatomy, decrease or eliminate pain, and excise or ablate gross lesions of endometriosis.[78] An aggressive surgical approach should be countered with microsurgical techniques such as gentle tissue handling to avoid trauma and subsequent adhesion formation. When endometriosis is first diagnosed in an infertile woman with pain who is 35 years of age, surgical therapy may be preferred so as not to wait 6 months for medical therapy.

There is great difficulty in comparing the results of surgical treatments of endometriosis. Although in some situations conservative surgery is superior to expectant management, no study has yet shown an advantage of conservative surgery versus expectant management based on monthly fecundity rates and life table analysis.[72]

GENERAL CONSIDERATIONS

Accurate knowledge of normal and abnormal anatomy, disease states, and their clinical implications provides the basis of good surgical judgment. Good surgical judgment in combination with good microsurgical technique provides optimum results.

Microsurgical Techniques. Microsurgical technique is the philosophy of gentle manipulation of tissue in an attempt to avoid tissue trauma. The weight of clinical and experimental evidence suggests that ischemia of the peritoneum that commonly occurs with macrosurgery results from inflammation, trauma, coagulation, or foreign materials and leads to adhesion formation secondary to a local failure of the intrinsic peritoneal fibrinolytic system.[79, 80] Thus, the philosophy of microsurgery is requisite for all reproduction-enhancing surgery in women, regardless of the mode of therapy (laparotomy or laparoscopy). The desired result is the restoration of normal pelvic anatomy and function. The basic tenets of microsurgery include magnification, meticulous hemostasis, prevention of tissue desiccation, avoidance of foreign material, minimal tissue handling, and use of nonreactive suture when necessary.

Strictly defined, the microsurgical technique demands the use of the operating microscope. However, Gomel[81] has broadened its definition to include surgery performed under magnification provided by loupes. Similar pregnancy rates have been obtained with the operating microscope and the loupes for microsurgical tubal anastomosis in a randomized clinical trial.[82] The laparoscope can magnify up to $10\times$, depending on its working distance, so it also may be included in this broadened definition.

Atraumatic technique includes gentle tissue handing, avoidance of foreign bodies (suture, clips) unless absolutely necessary, and delicate instruments. Precise hemostasis should be achieved with minimal trauma because coagulation and vaporization may cause ischemia. During laparotomy or laparoscopy, the tissue may desiccate. Frequent irrigation is necessary to prevent this from occurring.

Modalities. Whether surgery is done by laparotomy or laparoscopy, similar modalities of hemostasis and destruction of endometriotic implants can be used. None of these modalities has been shown to be superior, so the most important determinants are the surgeon's experience and the availability

of the modality. Martin and coworkers[39] estimated the median depth of penetration of endometriosis as 3 mm and found lesions larger than 5 mm in 25% of women; therefore, the modality used must be effective at these depths. Each modality has its particular depth of tissue penetration and so may have advantages as well as disadvantages based on perceived tissue penetration.

Electrosurgery is probably the most commonly used modality. Most electrosurgical units offer both unipolar and bipolar modes. Many instruments may be combined with unipolar electrosurgery, most commonly scissors, scalpels, and point coagulators. When monopolar cautery is used, the current passes from the generator through the instrument to the ground plate and back to the generator again. The advantage of bipolar electrosurgery is that current is passed between two insulated blades of an instrument, so that the tissue between the blades completes the circuit. Current can be delivered in the cutting (continuous high-energy waveform) or the coagulating (initial high-energy waveform, quick dissipation) mode.

Unipolar instruments (point coagulators, scissors, scalpels) allow greater versatility of tissue effects. Needle-tip electrosurgery is an accurate and inexpensive alternative to laser surgery. The main disadvantage of unipolar electrosurgery is that lateral tissue damage can occur as far as 3 to 5 cm away.[83] This is in contrast with bipolar electrosurgery, which induces only 1 to 2 cm of lateral tissue damage. At laparotomy, fine tissue forceps are available. However, the only currently available laparoscopic instruments are bipolar paddles and micro-bipolar paddles. Unfortunately, these cannot be used as microsurgical forceps. Because the power output of bipolar electrosurgery is only one third that of unipolar, the power density obtained is usually too low to cut tissue. With knowledge of electrosurgery's complications and limitations, it is a powerful tool for both laparoscopic and laparotomy approaches to endometriosis surgery.[84]

Thermocoagulation, developed in 1962 by Semm, involves tissue desiccation and coagulation by increasing the temperature through heat convection (as high as 100° to 120°C) and not by electrical current.[85] Its main disadvantage is the lack of available instruments for microsurgery. In addition, the tip of the thermocoagulation unit does not cool instantly, so unwanted tissue damage may occur if normal tissue is touched inadvertently.

Lasers (light amplification by stimulated emission of radiation) are the newest modality introduced to reproductive surgery. Although lasers are not necessary to perform endometriosis surgery, they have become a popular modality. As with each modality, there are advantages and disadvantages to its use. The rapid advances of this modality have occurred without any randomized clinical trials to test its efficacy. Although lasers are a promising surgical modality, good clinical results will occur only if proven and established principles of microsurgery and reproductive surgery are used.

Advantages of lasers include precise destruction of tissue with the potential for minimal adjacent tissue damage. In addition, several tissue effects that can be achieved include desiccation and coagulation and cutting, depending on time of exposure, spot size, wattage (power), and wavelength of the laser. For example, the carbon dioxide (CO_2) laser, which has a long wavelength, is best used for vaporization. Conversely, the neodymium: yttrium-aluminum-garnet (Nd:YAG) laser is best for coagulation. The ideal laser with variable wavelength has not yet been developed. It is imperative that the surgeon be thoroughly familiar with all aspects of the particular laser that he or she uses.

The laser beam can be reflected or carried through fiber optic cables. The only beam laser in use is the CO_2 laser. There are three fiber-propagated lasers: argon, potassium-titanyl-phosphate (KTP), and Nd:YAG. In general, the beam laser is used for vaporization, whereas the fiber-propagated lasers are best used for coagulation. The depth of tissue effect of the CO_2, argon, KTP, and Nd:YAG laser, respectively, is 0.1, 0.3 to 1, 0.3 to 1, and 3 to 4 mm.

The CO_2 laser is most commonly used for endometriosis surgery because most of the tissue damage is immediately obvious.[86, 87] When focused to a fine beam (high-power density), the laser can be used for cutting, and when the beam is defocused (low-power density), it can be used for limited coagulation. A variety of pulsed modes of the CO_2 laser have been developed to limit the time in which the laser is applied to the tissue and the extent of unwanted thermal damage. The disadvantage of the CO_2 laser includes the high degree of smoke production, the need for an articulating arm for beam transmission, and the inability of the laser to be transmitted through a fluid medium. The CO_2 laser coagulates poorly, and electrosurgery must always be available.

Because of selective absorption of hemoglobin-pigmented lesions, the argon and the KTP lasers have been advocated for use in endometriosis surgery.[88] The use of sapphire tips to control the scatter of laser for improved cutting, vaporization, and depth of penetration has been advocated, especially for the Nd:YAG laser.[89, 90] However, the sapphire tips are delicate, expensive, and easily damaged; their use in endometriosis surgery has been limited. Randomized, prospective studies comparing these wavelengths for the treatment of endometriosis have not been performed. The argon laser has potential use with excitation of hematoporphyrin in photodynamic therapy.[91]

The depth of penetration of an endometriotic lesion determines whether excision or vaporization is most appropriate, which emphasizes the importance of knowing the depth of penetration of the modality used. Deep lesions may need to be excised to appreciate fully their extent, whereas superficial lesions are easily vaporized and thermal damage is then limited. Carbon deposits excised at second-look laparoscopy have been reported to contain endometriosis deep to the surface carbon after initial vaporization.[92] With excision of endometriosis, the possibility of residual gross endometriosis being obscured by the carbon deposit is minimized.[35]

SURGICAL PROCEDURES

Peritoneal Disease. The goal in the treatment of superficial endometriosis is selective ablation or resection of visible endometriosis implants with preservation of surrounding healthy tissue.

Laparotomy. Conservative surgery has, by convention, referred to surgery by laparotomy, which may include lysis of adhesions, excision of endometrial implants and endometriomas, plication of uterosacral ligaments, anterior uterine suspension, presacral neurectomy, and appendectomy. Conservative resection of disease by laparotomy is most valuable in patients with extensive pelvic adhesions or large ovarian

endometriomas. In addition, deep involvement of the rectovaginal septum with fibrotic extension into the perirectal fossa, invasion of the bowel muscularis, and endometriotic infiltration in the region of the uterine vessels and ureter may be best approached through the open abdomen, depending on the skill of the surgeon. The general approach is through a transverse suprapubic incision. A Pfannenstiel incision is the most commonly used incision; however, a Maylard incision may be used if greater exposure is desired. Midline incisions are generally used if a large mass is present or a presacral neurectomy is planned. Endometriosis may be ablated or resected (Fig. 35–2). The techniques are the same regardless of mode of access to the pelvis. It is imperative for the surgeon to be thoroughly familiar with the modality he or she chooses. Sharp dissection with a scalpel or scissors is inexpensive, simple, and effective. There is no clinically significant lateral tissue damage; furthermore, any inadvertent tissue injury is usually immediately obvious. When using electrosurgery, the operator should grasp small implants between forceps to limit extent of damage. Lesions that are less superficial may benefit from the increased depth of penetration of this modality when compared with the CO_2 laser. Knowledge of the depth of tissue destruction achieved with each modality is important. The most effective method may differ depending on the type of lesion. The CO_2 laser is the most frequently used laser in endometriosis surgery because of its ability to vaporize superficial implants with little surrounding tissue damage. However, even when using the laser, it is important to delineate the course of the ureter prior to vaporization in the broad ligament and pelvic sidewall. Because no modality has been shown to be superior to another, the surgeon's experience and equipment available should dictate which modality is used.

Endometriosis may be associated with extensive adnexal adhesions. After a thorough exploration of the pelvis and upper abdomen, immobilizing adhesions may be divided during the preparatory part of the case. More precise excision may take place later. Adhesions should be excised at the origin and insertion points rather than just divided. It is important to identify structures such as the ureter that may be injured during dissection, especially when operating in the posterior cul-de-sac near the insertion of the uterosacral ligament. The ovaries are frequently adherent to the posterior broad ligament and sidewall and must be freed prior to treating ovarian endometriosis.

Laparoscopy. Laparoscopy is being used with increasing frequency as an operative tool. As with laparotomy, the goal in laparoscopic treatment of superficial endometriosis is selective ablation or resection of visible endometriosis implants with preservation of surrounding healthy tissue. Laparoscopy is ideal because visualization is improved, especially in the posterior cul-de-sac. In addition, laparoscopes provide some magnification that can aid the surgeon in identifying abnormalities of the peritoneal surface. The principles of conservative therapy, whether the surgery is done through a laparotomy incision or laparoscopy, are the same.

Small, superficial lesions can be coagulated using unipolar or bipolar cautery, thermocoagulated, or vaporized. The lesion should be picked up with forceps if possible to limit the area of surrounding damage. Endometriotic foci may be excised instead of ablated, especially if pathologic confirmation is desired. The small lesions are grasped and excised circum-

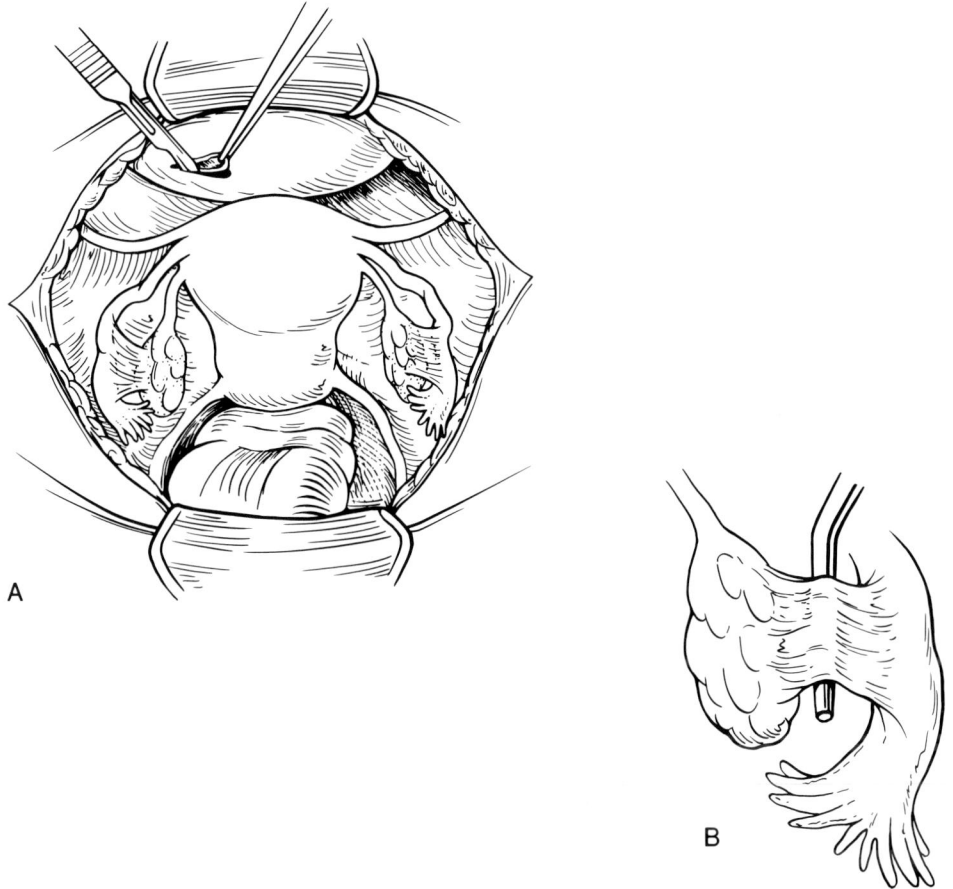

FIGURE 35–2. Excision or CO_2 laser vaporization of peritoneal implants. *A,* Superficial implants are vaporized using power densities between 1000 and 3000 W/cm², with a spot size of 0.8 to 1 mm or are cauterized with fine bipolar forceps. More extensive peritoneal disease is excised. Large defects may be closed with no. 5-0 or 6-0 polyglactin or polydioxanone sutures. *B,* Endometriosis may be associated with extensive adnexal adhesions. Wide adhesion bands may be retracted with a glass rod and excised with a microtip monopolar microelectrode. (Adapted from Helsa JS, Rock JA. Endometriosis. In: Rock JA, Murphy AA, Jones HW, editors. Female Reproductive Surgery. © 1992, the Williams & Wilkins Co., Baltimore.)

ferentially. With larger lesions, an incision is made in normal-appearing peritoneum. A blunt probe, hydrodissection, scissors, or laser may be used to separate the implant from the underlying normal tissue. Direct visualization of all involved areas and medial traction of sidewall peritoneum minimize tissue trauma. Peritoneal windows are associated with endometriosis and should be explored or excised. Ablation rather than excision of invasive implants may result in inadequate resection and a greater amount of ischemic damage to tissue. The choice of ablation or excision is based on the location of lesion, operator's skill, familiarity with the different modalities, and available instrumentation.

Frozen Pelvis/Obliterated Posterior Cul-de-Sac. When a surgeon encounters an obliterated posterior cul-de-sac, the goals of the patient must be reviewed. If pain management is the goal, complete gross dissection by en bloc resection may be undertaken.[93] Resection of deep posterior cul-de-sac nodules requires great expertise (Fig. 35–3). Vaginal removal of these implants combined with laparoscopy may be necessary. Retroperitoneal dissection may be aided by placement of a sponge forceps in the vagina and rectum for traction. If infertility is the main goal of the patient, the primary focus should be to restore normal anatomic relationships among the fallopian tubes, ovaries, and uterus.

Ovary. Endometriosis of the ovary is associated with subfertility.[43] Ovarian endometriomas, particularly those larger than 3 cm, are best approached surgically, because medical treatment alone has not been effective.[94–96] The best surgical technique for the management of ovarian endometri-

oma has yet to be defined. In the past, complete removal or destruction of the endometriotic cyst wall has been recommended, although recently, with the increase in popularity of laparoscopic surgery, drainage and medical therapy have been proposed as possible alternatives.

The diagnosis of ovarian endometrioma can sometimes be challenging when based on visual assessment alone. The differential diagnosis of an apparent ovarian endometrioma includes hemorrhagic corpus luteum, hemorrhagic follicular cyst, or other ovarian tumor, either benign or malignant. If there is any doubt about the diagnosis, a biopsy should be done. Some clinicians believe that a histologic diagnosis should always be obtained.[97] Because endometriomas were almost always excised when most endometriosis surgery was performed by laparotomy, the possibility of making a mistaken diagnosis at the time of surgery had few clinical implications. However, the same is not true when surgery is performed at laparoscopy because no pathologic specimen is usually obtained. In a prospective study, 52 suspected endometriomas were excised at laparoscopy.[98] Although 42 of these cysts contained dark-brown "chocolate" fluid, only 68% of these cysts were pathologically confirmed endometriomas. The most common other diagnosis was corpora lutea. Relying on the presence of chocolate fluid on aspiration of an ovarian cyst alone to diagnose ovarian endometrioma may be misleading. Using the expanded criteria of Vercellini, described under "Diagnosis and Staging," a laparoscopic surgeon can reliably diagnose an ovarian endometrioma at the time of surgery.

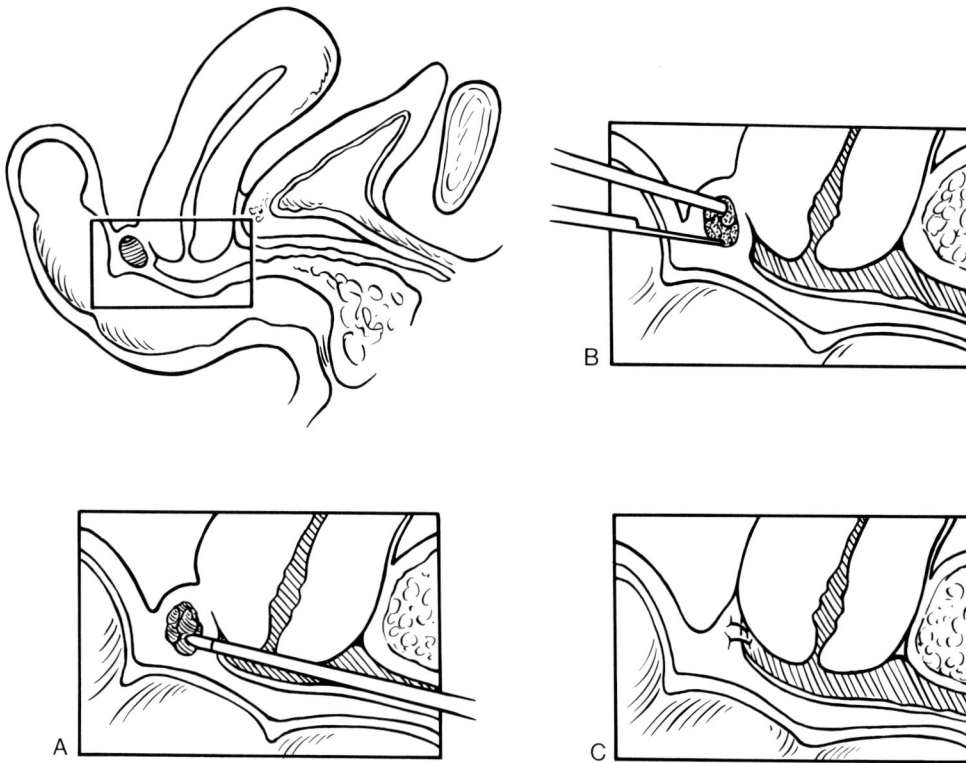

FIGURE 35–3. Deep laparoscopic dissection of the rectovaginal space, in combination with colpotomy, for the treatment of a large endometriotic nodule of the rectovaginal septum. *A,* Initial laparoscopic dissection of nodule. *B,* Completion of dissection via colpotomy incision. *C,* Suturing of the rectovaginal septum. (Adapted from Martin DC. Laparoscopic treatment of endometriosis. In: Azziz R, Murphy AA, editors. Practical Manual of Operative Laparoscopy and Hysteroscopy. New York: Springer-Verlag, 1992.)

Most ovarian endometriomas are amenable to a laparoscopic approach. Sulewski in 1980 first described fulguration of small (<1 cm) superficial endometriomas with unipolar coagulation.[99] Semm in 1980 described laparoscopic resection of ovarian endometriomas with coagulation of the base.[100] Reich and McGlynn in 1986 reported on the first large series of women with ovarian endometriomas treated laparoscopically.[101] Treatment ranged from drainage to fulguration of the cavity using the tip of the suction coagulator. The skill of the surgeon and the location and size of the endometrioma play a major role in defining the approach, either by laparotomy or laparoscopy.

Technique. Endometriomas should be resected with atraumatic technique and maintenance of the anatomic relationships between the fimbria ovarica and the utero-ovarian ligament. The ovary has a large propensity for adhesion formation; therefore, microsurgical techniques are especially important. Often, the lateral side of the ovary is adhered to the pelvic sidewall or posterior broad ligament. Fifty percent of subovarian adhesions will have associated endometriosis.[24] These adhesions should be excised or vaporized when possible to destroy endometriosis in the ovarian fossa. Small surface endometriomas may be ablated or coagulated laparoscopically. The excision of endometriomas smaller than 5 to 6 cm in diameter can often be easily accomplished through the laparoscope. Larger endometriomas may be difficult to handle through the laparoscope and may result in long operating times and an unacceptably high rate of bleeding or other complications.[102] Some clinicians prefer to resect very large endometriomas at laparotomy and argue that reconstruction of the ovary is important in these patients. However, there is suggestive evidence that less adhesion formation occurs following closure of ovarian defects by secondary in-

tention rather than by placement of sutures even with microsurgical technique.[103] Resection of large or multiple endometriomas presents a problem. Cortical incisions should be carefully placed so as to preserve the anatomic relationship of the utero-ovarian ligament and the ovarian fimbria. The fewest possible incisions should be made. Occasionally, a major portion of the ovary may be destroyed by endometriosis. After resection, only a small portion of the ovary may be left. Every effort should be made to preserve any ovarian tissue because pregnancies have been described in patients with little ovarian tissue.

Laparotomy. After the ovary is mobilized, it may be placed on a rubber platform for reconstruction. An elliptical incision is made above the thin ovarian cortex. The incision should be made in the axis of the ovary and in its most dependent area (Fig. 35–4A). This facilitates reconstruction of the ovary and ensures a more anatomic closure. The cyst may be separated from the cyst wall by developing a plane either bluntly or sharply (Fig. 35–4B). After the cyst wall has been completely separated from its adhesive attachments to the ovarian cortex, it may be "shelled out" without rupture. Occasionally, because of friability of the cyst wall, rupture may occur even with the gentlest technique. Surrounding the ovary with moist lint-free packs protects the pelvis from contamination if spillage occurs. After the cyst is removed, the dead space is obliterated with internal sutures placed as a pursestring, running lock, or interrupted no. 4-0 or 5-0 nonreactive suture (Fig. 35–4C to E). The ovarian cortex may be approximated with subcuticular sutures of no. 5-0 or 6-0 nonreactive suture or left unsutured if approximation has already been achieved (Fig. 35–4F). Suture on the surface should be avoided at all cost because of its adhesiogenic propensity.[104] If there is excessive redundant thin ovarian cortex, it may be

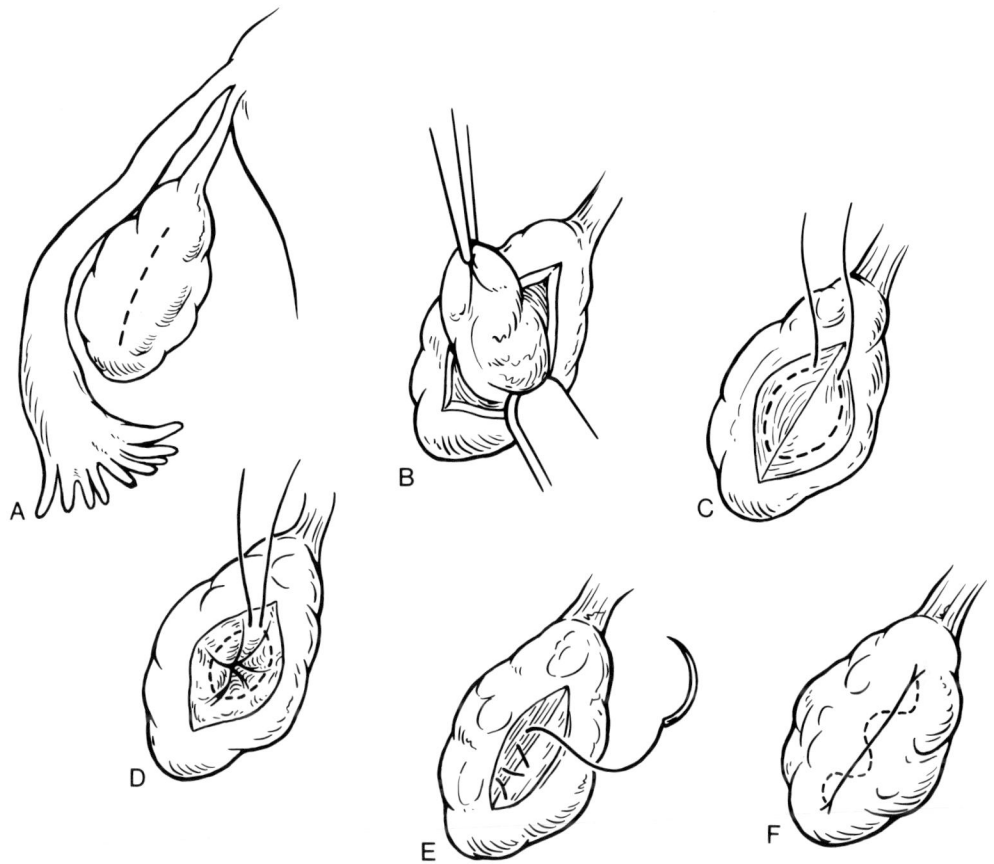

FIGURE 35–4. Excision of ovarian endometrioma through the open abdomen. *A,* The ovarian cortex is gently incised so as not to enter the endometrial cyst. The incision is made along the longitudinal axis of the ovary. *B,* The endometrioma is then peeled out with the blunt knife handle. *C* and *D,* The ovarian defect is obliterated with two layers of pursestring sutures of no. 4-0 absorbable nonreactive material. *E,* In the case of a deep defect, a more superficial running suture may be necessary before approximating the cortical edges with no. 5-0 nonreactive, delayed absorbable suture (*F*). (Adapted from Helsa J, Rock JA. Endometriosis. In: Rock JA, Murphy AA, Jones HW, editors. Endometriosis in Female Reproductive Surgery. © 1992, the Williams & Wilkins Co., Baltimore.)

trimmed. Generally, cortex should not be dissected off the ovary. The ovary most often resumes its normal shape and position if the appropriate incision has been made.

Laparoscopy. Several techniques of laparoscopic management of ovarian endometriomas have been recently investigated, from shelling out the cyst wall with traction or sharp dissection to ablation of the endometrioma cavity and aspiration with postoperative medical therapy.[105]

Prior to resection, the endometrioma is liberated from adhesions to the pelvic sidewall or other structures. Occasionally, the adhesions stabilize the ovary, and lysis of these adhesions is best performed after the endometrioma is removed. Careful attention should be paid to the course of the ureter, because the ovarian fossa is a common area for its damage. The endometrioma is stabilized with ancillary instruments and preferably placed on a shelf created by retrodisplacement of the uterus. The cyst is drained if rupture has not occurred. The endometrioma is opened with an incision in the most dependent portion and along the longitudinal axis (Fig. 35–5). The pseudocapsule is identified, and a plane of dissection developed. It is sometimes useful to make a perpendicular incision on one edge to identify the cyst wall. Atraumatic grasping forceps provide countertraction on the ovary. The cyst wall is grasped with claw or biopsy forceps, and the cyst wall usually peels off easily but sometimes requires blunt or sharp dissection. If the wall is not removed in its entirety, remaining areas should be coagulated or vaporized with electrocautery or laser.[106, 107] If one chooses to fenestrate the wall of the endometrioma, a large enough opening should be cut so that adequate inspection of the inner endometrial cyst wall can be accomplished. Great care

should be taken with dissection around the hilar vessels because bleeding from this area can be difficult to control laparoscopically.

Outcome. Correction of ovarian endometriomas by laparotomy versus laparoscopy is highly controversial, with most treatment outcomes for ovarian endometriomas reported in terms of successful treatment and rates of recurrence rather than pregnancy outcomes. Several groups have suggested the use of postoperative ovarian suppression.[108, 109]

Women with laparoscopically resected ovarian endome-

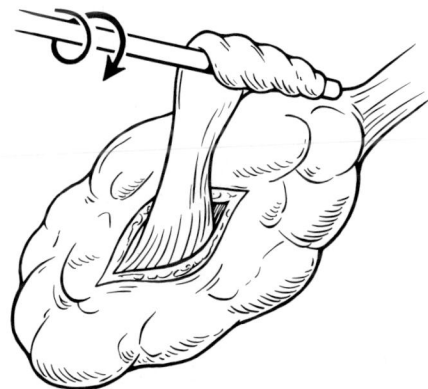

FIGURE 35–5. Resection of endometrioma cyst wall. To facilitate cyst enucleation, the cyst wall can be grasped with biopsy forceps and twisted while applying gentle traction, peeling the cyst wall from the underlying ovarian bed. (Adapted from Steinkamp MP, Azziz R. Laparoscopic ovarian and paraovarian surgery. In: Azziz R, Murphy AA, editors. Practical Manual of Operative Laparoscopy and Hysteroscopy. New York: Springer-Verlag, 1992.)

triomas have been reported to have higher pregnancy rates and fewer postoperative adhesions than those reported for laparotomy in the literature.[20] In patients treated with laparoscopic fenestration (in the dependent part) and aspiration of endometriomas followed by 6 to 10 months of medical therapy (danazol), 85% of women with endometriomas smaller than 3 cm in diameter had no residual endometriosis at second-look laparoscopy and 26% of those with endometriomas larger than 3 cm had only minimal residual endometriosis at second-look laparoscopy.[20] This study needs to be interpreted in light of the fact that no histologic proof of the diagnosis of ovarian endometrioma was offered; rather, these endometriomas were fenestrated and drained. Therefore, the diagnosis of hemorrhagic corpora lutea cannot be excluded. A prospective study of 33 women with moderate to severe stages of endometriosis and ovarian endometriomas treated with laparoscopic aspiration of cyst followed by treatment with gonadotropin-releasing hormone (GnRH) agonist for 3 months were compared with control subjects with no postoperative medical therapy.[109] There was no significant reduction in size of the ovarian endometriomas before laparoscopy and 6 month's followup or between the control group and the group treated postoperatively with medical therapy. The different results between these two studies[20, 109] may be explained in that the first[20] involved fenestration (making of a window) rather than aspiration alone and that the followup included a second-look laparoscopy in a few women.

There has been only one systematic study of the different laparoscopic techniques (complete excision with closure by second intention, stripping of lining, laser ablation of lining, drainage) of surgical treatments of endometriomas.[105] All women in this study were treated with postoperative medical (danazol) therapy and had a second-look laparoscopy 8 weeks after their initial surgery. There was a significant increase in periadnexal adhesions in the group of women undergoing excision (100%) versus the other three groups of women with no difference in recurrence of endometriosis (23% to 30%) between the four groups. Of interest is there were no recurrences of endometriomas in the excision group, but there was a 21% recurrence in the other three groups (none larger than 2 cm). Therefore, it appears that neither aspiration alone nor use of medical therapy alone is an efficacious treatment modality in women with ovarian endometriomas. The use of laparoscopic techniques that do not necessarily excise the ovarian endometrioma followed by medical therapy may be useful in some clinical scenarios, although the lack of histologic specimen precludes the exclusion of the lesion as a hemorrhagic corpus luteum. Early second-look laparoscopy in these patients reveals a low level of recurrence (15% to 20%) of endometriomas but an approximately 20% de novo adhesion formation and as much as a 40% to 82% recurrence rate of dense adhesions.[105, 110, 111] In these scenarios, the use of an early second-look laparoscopy for lysis of adhesions may be advocated.

Gastrointestinal. In a patient with endometriosis, gastrointestinal symptoms should be sought out preoperatively. Only a high degree of suspicion will elucidate a diagnosis. It has been estimated that as many as 50% of patients with severe endometriosis have some degree of bowel involvement.[112] The location of the bowel involvement is overwhelmingly in the area of the rectum or rectosigmoid colon.

In a report of outcome of 77 patients with deep colorectal endometriosis, most lesions were in the rectosigmoid colon with singular lesions in the ileum and cecum.[113] Symptoms such as constipation alternating with diarrhea, hematochezia, rectal pain, dyschezia, dyspareunia, and dysmenorrhea should alert the surgeon to possible bowel involvement. If present, a workup that may include a barium enema or sigmoidoscopy should be considered. These patients should have an outpatient bowel preparation prior to surgery if bowel endometriosis is suspected. Bowel resection should be considered in symptomatic patients and those with compromise of the bowel lumen. The approach to the treatment of bowel endometriosis has varied greatly; the tendency to avoid bowel resection has been due to the increased complication rates of this type of surgery without a known improved fertility outcome. Infertility is not thought to be affected by bowel endometriosis unless there is associated mechanical fallopian tubal obstruction. In patients with pain, the removal of bowel endometriosis is thought to be useful, but again this association is inconclusive. Whether these lesions will progress is also unknown.

Three percent to 5% of appendices are noted to be affected by endometriosis during surgery for endometriosis.[76] Thus, appendiceal endometriosis is a relatively uncommon finding, and incidental appendectomies should not be performed.

Large endometriotic implants of the bowel wall may protrude extensively into the lumen with minimal serosal manifestation. These lesions will not be detected preoperatively unless barium enema or colonoscopy is performed. Extensive lesions with luminal extension should undergo colonoscopy and biopsy to rule out adenocarcinoma. Preoperative preparation for bowel resection usually includes suppression with GnRH analogs or danazol for 3 months. Bowel preparation includes a mechanical cleansing and antibiotic therapy. Serosal and superficial endometriosis of the bowel may be resected by either excision or vaporization by laparoscopy or laparotomy. Laparotomy has been the standard of care for endometriosis involving the bowel wall. In most instances, this is still true. Deep colorectal involvement should undergo wedge or segmental bowel resection with end-to-end anastomosis. Rectal endometriosis may necessitate removal of uterosacral and vaginal tissue.

Technique. A full-thickness resection can be performed by either a disk or segmental resection with end-to-end anastomosis. Both descriptions of this procedure by laparotomy and, more recently, by laparoscopy have been published.[113, 114]

Outcome. Patients with extensive bowel disease generally are symptomatic. Resection of bowel disease is usually efficacious. Coronado and associates noted complete relief in 49.4% (38/77) of patients and an improvement in 39% who underwent full-thickness resection of the colon.[113] Postoperative febrile morbidity was 10.4% with no apparent anastomotic leaks. A 39.4% (13/33) term pregnancy rate was reported.

Urinary. Endometriosis of the urinary tract is usually limited to the bladder (superficial or deep involvement) and the ureters. Endometriosis involving the ureter is relatively uncommon, but at least 130 cases have been reported. Because of its intrapelvic course, the ureter is at risk of either intrinsic disease or extrinsic compression by adjacent endometriotic nodules. Extrinsic endometriosis presents four times more frequently than intrinsic involvement and is most likely to occur in the region of the ovarian fossa.[115] The ureters should always be identified prior to removal of sidewall endometriosis because its involvement with sidewall masses may be difficult to delineate. Renal damage can occur as the result of ureteral involvement, but it is commonly unilateral and rarely irreversible. However, ureteric endometriosis can remain asymptomatic for a long time and be found only incidentally at the time of surgery. Good surgical judgment must be used to decide if peritoneal or ureteral wall involvement exists. Likewise, the same is true of the bladder.

Technique. Involvement of peritoneum overlying the ureter is amenable to laparoscopic surgery. An incision is made in normal peritoneum. The peritoneum is pulled toward the midline, and the ureter is bluntly dissected from the peritoneum—it should be pushed away easily with a blunt probe or hydrodissection. Difficulty with this procedure may indicate involvement of the ureteral wall. Care should be taken not to disturb the periureteral vessels because this may lead to fistula formation. The lesion is then excised or vaporized. Superficial (serosa only) bladder involvement with endometriosis can be treated in the same fashion. This procedure may be accomplished either through laparoscopy or laparotomy. Involvement of the ureteral or bladder wall may require resection and reconstruction.

Uterine Suspension. Uterine suspension was often part of conservative surgery for moderate and severe endometriosis. With the increasing use of a laparoscopic approach to surgical therapy in infertile women with endometriosis, uterine suspension has been employed less often. The justification for this procedure is the prevention of postoperative adhesion formation by moving the uterus, especially a posterior or retroflexed one, away from the sigmoid and by elevating the fallopian tubes and ovaries away from the denuded peritoneal surfaces of the posterior cul-de-sac. There are many other techniques that decrease postoperative adhesion formation such as the use of microsurgery and adhesion barriers.

Technique. The most commonly used uterine suspension is the modified Gilliam suspension. In this procedure, a delayed absorbable traction suture is placed around the round ligament about 3 to 4 cm from the uterine cornua, and the uterus is elevated. The edge of the anterior rectus fascia is grasped by an Ochsner clamp at the level of the anterosuperior spine of the ilium to help separate it from the underlying rectus muscle. A Kelly clamp is used to grasp the peritoneal edge at the same level. The fascia at the lateral aspect of the rectus muscle is then pierced through to the underlying peritoneum where the Kelly clamp has been placed. The suture around the round ligament is brought out of the peritoneal cavity through the defect in the fascia, lateral to the rectus muscle. The loop of round ligament can then be sutured to the undersurface of the anterior fascia near the midline using permanent silk, care being taken not to encircle and then strangulate any part of the round ligament. This procedure is then repeated on the opposite side. The anatomic relationship of the fallopian tube to the ovary should be preserved during this procedure, and care should be taken to inspect the final position of the fallopian tube. Occasionally, the suspension needs to be taken down and a more satisfactory suspension performed. No gap or space should be left lateral to the suspension site. Finally, the fallopian tube should not be pulled up with the round ligament because it may become distorted or occluded.

This procedure has also been performed laparoscopically.[116] A trocar with cannula is inserted at the intended site on the lateral lower abdominal area approximately 5 cm lateral to the midline and 3 cm above the inguinal ligament. The anterior rectus fascia in this site is then tagged with a suture. The round ligament is grasped at a similar point, as described earlier, with laparoscopic forceps and elevated through the incision to the tagged anterior fascia. Particular attention needs to be paid to the subsequent anatomic location of the fallopian tubes. The round ligaments are sutured in place with the previously placed suture.

Outcome. No improvement in fertility rates has been shown when uterine suspension has been used as an adjunctive procedure at the time of laparotomy for endometriosis.[117, 118] The efficacy of this surgical procedure has not been evaluated separately from other procedures that usually accompany this surgery, and its value has been questioned.[119] In the reported results with a laparoscopic approach, the most frequent complication has been prolonged hospital stay for pain control. Of 80 women with deep dyspareunia and retrodisplaced uterus with no other pelvic pathology undergoing laparoscopic uterine suspension, 74 had reduction of symptoms while there were no reported ectopic pregnancies and 13 intrauterine pregnancies.[120] The only reported series specific to laparoscopic uterine suspension in women with endometriosis was done in combination with the destruction of endometriotic implants by a laser in 225 women with chronic pelvic pain.[121] Ninety-four percent of women reported a decrease in severity of pelvic pain, with 60% noting a complete resolution of pain. Attributing pain relief to the uterine suspension when destruction of implants and, in some patients, uterosacral nerve ablation were done can obviously not be defended. The conclusion of this report that increased monthly fecundity rates of early stages of endometriosis, which exceeded previously reported rates, were attributed to uterine suspension is seriously flawed. The use of uterine suspension, whether by laparotomy or laparoscopy, as an adjunctive procedure during surgery for endometriosis in infertile woman is obviously controversial and not of proven value.

Uterosacral Nerve Resection or Ablation. Laparoscopic uterosacral nerve ablation (LUNA) is a modification of the procedure described by Ruggi in 1899 and popularized by Doyle for the treatment of dysmenorrhea when conservative surgery is done.[122] Division of the uterosacral ligaments at or near their insertion into the posterior aspect of the uterine cervix should lead to the interruption of some sensory sympathetic fibers originating from T10 to L1 (inferior hypogastric plexus) and most of the parasympathetic components of the paracervical nerves originating from S1 to S3 or S4. Patients who complain of significant central dysmenorrhea have typically been identified as candidates for this procedure. It is unlikely to be of benefit to patients with lateral (adnexal) pain or pain of gastrointestinal or urinary origin. It is also contraindicated in patients with abnormal anatomy due to scarring or endometriosis and patients in whom identification of the uterosacral ligament and ureter is unclear.

Technique. This procedure has been adapted as an adjunctive procedure during laparoscopic surgery for dysmenorrhea.[123] If it is to be performed, it is paramount that the uterosacral ligaments be well identified as well as the course of the ureter and the uterine artery at the start of the surgery.

The uterus is anteverted with a uterine manipulator for maximum exposure. Applying pressure to the posterior uterus and cervix with a blunt probe can further define and expose the ligaments. Interruption can be performed with lasers or electrosurgery and scissors (Fig. 35–6). The extent of adjacent thermal damage is uncertain if electrosurgery is used. Although any type may be used, the KTP, argon, and Nd:YAG lasers provide better coagulation than the CO_2 laser and are preferred by some surgeons for this reason. Energy is applied to the ligament at its junction with the uterus until totally ablated. A 2- to 4-cm segment of each ligament should be vaporized to a depth of 1 cm. The posterior aspect of the uterus between the two uterosacral ligaments may be superficially vaporized to interrupt the sensory fibers crossing to the contralateral side.[124] With the use of unipolar or bipolar electrosurgery for coagulation, the ligament is usually transected sharply. It is imperative that the course of the ureter and uterine artery be well defined and that the uterosacral ligament be approached from its medial aspect to avoid injury to these structures.

Outcome. This procedure has no benefit in terms of increasing pregnancy rates and is used in conjunction with conservative resection of endometriosis in patients who complain of midline pelvic pain or dysmenorrhea. LUNA was reported to have a 50% to 70% success rate in relieving pain in uncontrolled short-term (1 year) studies.[125–127] Lichten and Bombard[127] published the only randomized, prospective, double-blind study of LUNA (bipolar cautery and transection) for the treatment of severe or incapacitating primary dysmenorrhea unresponsive to oral contraceptives and nonsteroidal anti-inflammatory agents. Nine of 11 women in the

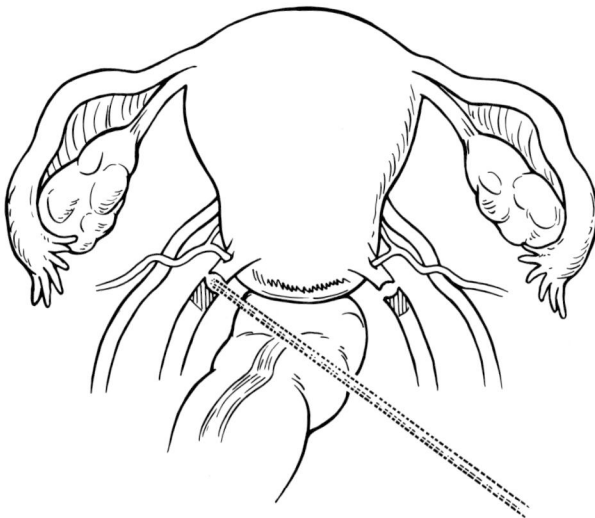

FIGURE 35–6. Laparoscopic uterosacral nerve ablation. The uterus should be displaced toward the anterior abdominal wall by an intrauterine manipulator. The uterosacral ligament is identified and followed to its insertion on the uterus. Laser energy is applied to the medial aspect of the ligament as its junction with the uterus until totally or partially ablated. Usually a 1.5- to 2-cm long × 1-cm deep area of vaporization through the ligament is required. A superficial **U**-shaped area of vaporization, connecting the two interrupted uterosacral ligament segments, may also be performed along the posterior aspect of the utero–cul-de-sac junction, which transects interconnecting fibers otherwise missed. (Adapted from Perry CP, Azziz R. Laparoscopic uterine nerve ablation, presacral neurectomy, and appendectomy. In: Azziz R, Murphy AA, editors. Practical Manual of Operative Laparoscopy and Hysteroscopy. New York: Springer-Verlag, 1992.)

treated group had significant relief of pain at 3 months, and 5 described complete relief from dysmenorrhea 1 year later. None of the control patients noted improvement. However, none of these patients had endometriosis. Uncontrolled, nonrandomized reports by Feste[126] and Donnez and Nicolle[125] described success rates of 71% and 50%, respectively, and included patients with primary dysmenorrhea as well as dysmenorrhea associated with endometriosis. How much of the improvement was secondary to resection of disease (endometriosis) versus LUNA cannot be determined. Although the cardinal ligaments and the pelvic floor musculature provide the major uterine support, the use of LUNA in two women with compromised pelvic uterine support resulted in uterine prolapse.[128] Other complications include hemorrhage, especially if the ablation is taken too far laterally or posteriorly. Deaths from unrecognized hemorrhage have been reported.[129] Long-term, well-designed studies are necessary to determine the efficacy and complication rate of this operation.

Presacral Neurectomy. Presacral neurectomy can be useful in the right patient for relief of midline pelvic pain. It can eliminate the midline uterine component of dysmenorrhea; however, there is no evidence that this procedure enhances fertility or reduces menstrual blood flow.[17, 130, 131]

Although presacral neurectomy is a procedure that does not enhance fertility, it may be a useful adjunct to conservative surgery for endometriosis in patients with midline pelvic pain or dysmenorrhea. The presacral nerve is the superior hypogastric plexus that supplies efferent stimulation to the viscera. It becomes the middle hypogastric plexus and passes over the bifurcation of the aorta and continues below the promontory of the sacrum (S1) before dividing into the right and left inferior hypogastric nerve. Unlike the LUNA, division of the presacral nerve does not include the parasympathetic nerves from S1 to S4 that form Frankenhauser's plexus. However, the addition of uterosacral nerve ablation (Doyle procedure) does not improve the efficacy of the presacral neurectomy.

Although most commonly performed at the time of laparotomy for extensive endometriosis, this procedure has been described by laparoscopy as well.[132–134] Unlike the uterosacral nerve ablation, this laparoscopic procedure requires significant surgical skill and should be performed only by surgeons with experience operating in the retroperitoneum.

Technique. Proper exposure is the first step in this procedure. The superior margin of dissection is the bifurcation of the aorta; the right margin, the right ureter, and common iliac artery; the left margin, the superior hemorrhoidal artery, and the inferior mesenteric, whereas the inferior margin is just below the division into the right and left inferior hypogastric plexus.

The peritoneum is opened longitudinally over the sacral promontory (Fig. 35–7A). Dissection of the areolar tissue and associated nerve fibers off the posterior aspect of the peritoneal flap may be accomplished sharply or with a Kitner sponge (Fig. 35–7B). The right ureter and common iliac artery are visualized and dissected free of areolar tissue. A right-angled clamp is useful to elevate the sheath and allow blunt dissection underneath. It is imperative that the middle sacral vessels be identified and left in place. Significant bleeding will be encountered if the middle sacral vein is injured. Moreover, the vessel may retract into the bone with disas-

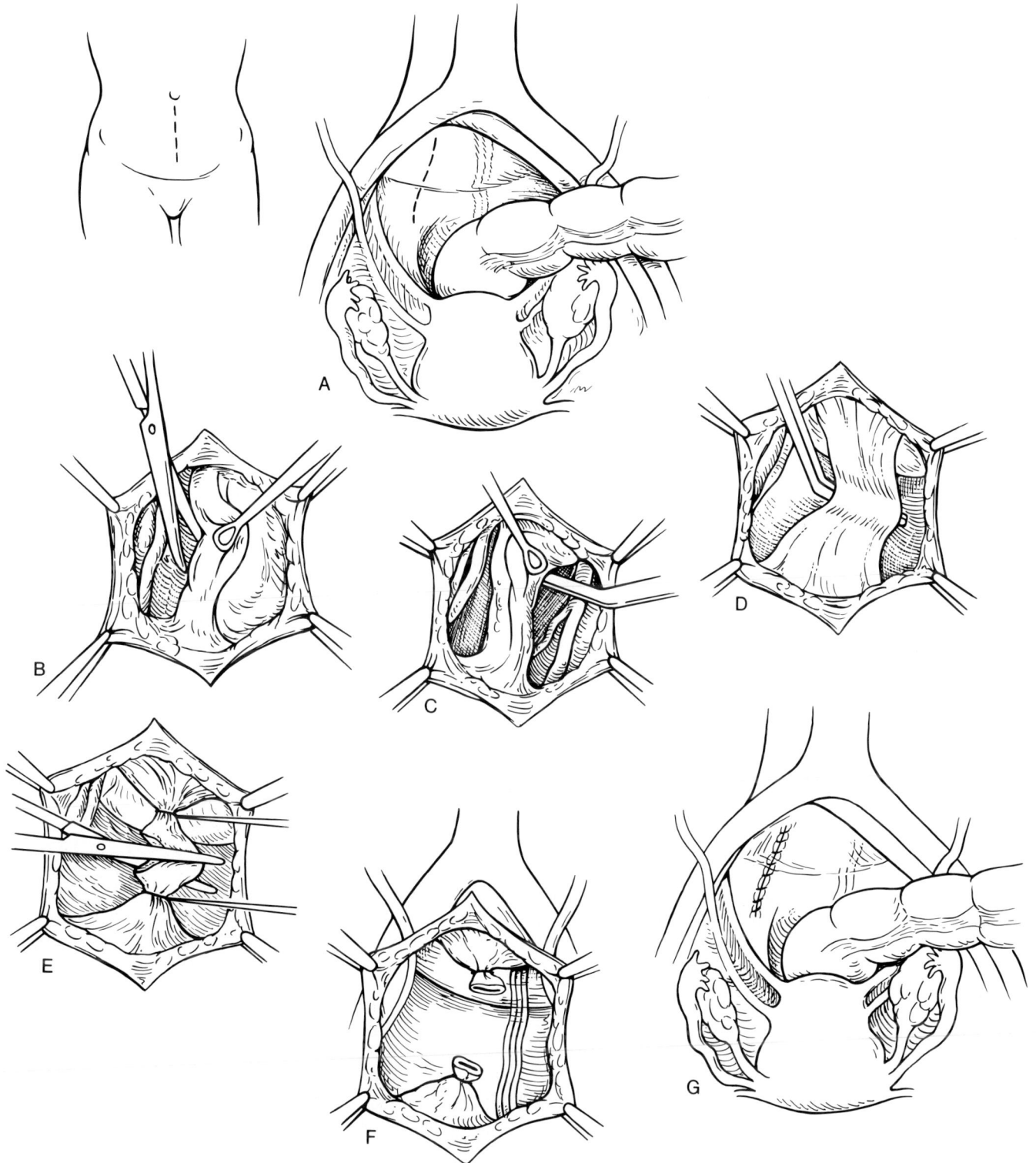

FIGURE 35–7. Presacral neurectomy: *A,* Location of incision in relation to anatomic landmarks. The descending colon is displaced superiorly and to the left for good exposure of the left margin of the hypogastric plexus. *B,* A Kitner sponge is used to dissect the areolar tissue medially and off the posterior aspect of the peritoneal flap. The right ureter may be easily identified. *C,* The areolar nerve–bearing tissue is dissected from the peritoneum on the left side, exposing the left internal iliac vessels and superior hemorrhoidal vessels. *D,* The plexus is isolated and elevated off the sacral promontory. *E,* An approximate 5-cm segment of plexus is isolated with no. 2-0 silk suture and excised. *F,* Relationship of pedicles of the excised nerve bundle with adjacent structures. *G,* Reperitonealization with no. 4-0 nonreactive absorbable suture. (Adapted from Helsa JS, Rock JA. Endometriosis. In: Rock JA, Murphy AA, Jones HW, editors. Female Reproductive Surgery. © 1992, the Williams & Wilkins Co., Baltimore.)

trous results. The use of a stainless-steel thumbtack to stem this type of hemorrhage has been described.[135] The dissection is carried out on the left with exposure of the superior hemorrhoidal vessels that remain on the peritoneum (Fig. 35–7C–G). The areolar tissue and nerves are then dissected medially. The plexus is elevated off the sacral promontory after isolation. The isolated plexus may be tied with no. 2-0 silk sutures and excised or separated using coagulation or clips. The peritoneum may be sutured or left open.

The boundaries for laparoscopic resection are exactly the same as those for laparotomy. Laparoscopically, the area may be approached from the umbilicus or the suprapubic area. At laparoscopy, placement of the patient in radical hysterectomy stirrups and a left lateral tilt is helpful in providing adequate exposure by displacing the bowel.

Outcome. There is no evidence that this procedure improves fertility.[130] Generally, complete resolution of midline pelvic pain is achieved in 58% to 70% of patients in retrospective series with variable followup lengths.[43, 136, 137] In the first randomized clinical trial of women with midline pelvic pain and severe endometriosis undergoing conservative surgery with or without presacral neurectomy, all patients undergoing presacral neurectomy noted a complete resolution of pelvic pain, and only 11.8% (2/17) noted recurrence of pain within the followup period (42 months).[138] These results contrast with the most recent randomized, controlled study of 71 women with moderate to severe endometriosis and midline dysmenorrhea undergoing conservative surgery with or without a presacral neurectomy.[132] Although preliminary results were encouraging, long-term followup revealed no difference in symptom relief between the two groups of women. In addition, 13 of 35 women who had a presacral neurectomy had worsened constipation, and 3 women complained of urinary urgency. The two most common complications of this procedure are vaginal dryness and constipation. Bladder atony may also be seen. All three symptoms usually resolve with time.

The first laparoscopic series reported only two failures in 25 patients with laparoscopic presacral neurectomy.[134] Followup in this series ranged from 6 to 27 months, and the only reported complication was a laparotomy for hemostasis. Most recently, a 94% (49/52) rate of pain relief in an uncontrolled study was noted in women undergoing laparoscopic vaporization of endometriosis and presacral neurectomy with a 1-year followup. No complications were noted.[133]

The value of either LUNA or presacral neurectomy when done as adjunctive procedures for pain relief in women with endometriosis has been questioned.[139] Additional studies are needed.

Outcome of Conservative Surgical Therapy

LAPAROTOMY

Overall, crude pregnancy rates following conservative laparotomy surgery for endometriosis are thought to be 60.7% for mild, 50% for moderate, and 39.2% for severe endometriosis.[58] Using the 1979 AFS classification, Olive and Haney[58] studied a total of 214 patients retrospectively. Monthly fecundity rates for mild (45/214), moderate (88/214), severe (66/214), and extensive (15/214) disease were 2.22%, 1.98%, 1.48%, and 1.46%, with an average of 1.82%.

Few studies have evaluated the effects of conservative surgery for endometriosis using modern statistical methods. The calculation of monthly fecundity rates or life table analysis is imperative in evaluating the efficacy of treatment after conservative surgery for endometriosis. Olive and Lee[72] retrospectively looked at 130 women with mild or moderate disease assigned to conservative versus expectant management.[72] Using Mantel-Byar analysis, the data revealed no significant overall increase in pregnancy rate with conservative surgical procedures. Stratification by degree of endometriosis noted no significant difference between mild and moderate disease. Conservative procedures appeared to be definitively therapeutic only in women with severe disease. However, the retrospective nature of this study limits the value of these results. Garcia and David[17] also noted in a retrospective study that among patients with minimal endometriosis, pregnancy rates were similar for surgery (64%) and expectant management (65%).[17] Additionally, in a retrospective study of 90 patients with mild pelvic endometriosis, Schenken and Malinak[67] compared patients treated surgically with those treated expectantly and found no difference in pregnancy rate or surgery-to-pregnancy interval. Moreover, at least in mild to moderate endometriosis, medical therapy does not appear to significantly improve pregnancy rates when compared with conservative surgery. Guzick and Rock[140] retrospectively examined 224 women with mild and moderate endometriosis using life table analysis. In this nonrandomized study, no difference in pregnancy rate was seen when medical (danazol) and conservative surgery treatment groups were compared. The results of life table analysis suggest that most patients with infertility "due to" endometriosis who will become pregnant after conservative therapy do so within the first 36 months after surgery.[141]

LAPAROSCOPY

The overall crude pregnancy rate for conservative surgery for mild endometriosis via laparoscopy (65% to 78%) is quite similar to the rates reported for conservative surgery by laparotomy (40% to 75%) (Tables 35–2 and 35–3). The results of CO_2 laser laparoscopy do not seem to differ from those reported for electrosurgery (44% to 75%) (see Table 35–2) or sharp excision.[99, 142–145] Martin and Vander Zwagg[92] reported a monthly fecundity rate of 2.8% to 3.3% with minimal and mild disease (stages I and II), whereas Nezhat and coworkers[146] reported a monthly fecundity rate of 6.5% and 6.7%, respectively. These data must be examined with caution in that prospective, randomized trials were not performed.

Several reports suggested that the laparoscopic treatment of moderate and severe endometriosis may be followed by a higher monthly fecundity rate than similar surgery performed at laparotomy. In a collected series of patients treated with the CO_2 laser at laparoscopy, a crude pregnancy rate of 50% was reported.[147] If pregnancy rates by stage are examined in women with endometriosis as an isolated factor, a 40% to 77% pregnancy rate is seen with moderate disease and monthly fecundity rates of 3% to 5.7%. In women with severe stages of endometriosis, a 35% to 73% pregnancy rate is noted with monthly fecundity rates of 3.3% to 5.6%.[106, 146, 147]

TABLE 35–2. Pregnancy Outcome in Patients with Endometriosis as Sole Factor for Infertility Treated by CO_2 Laser*

Year	Author	Minimal to Mild	Moderate No. (%)	Severe No. (%)	All No. (%)
1985	Feste[126]	31/44 (70)	10/14 (71)	1/2 (50)	42/60 (70)
1986	Martin[147]	9/13 (69)	6/11 (55)	8/10 (80)	23/34 (67)
1989	Nezhat et al[146]	28/39 (72)	60/86 (70)	80/118 (68)	168/243 (69)
1987	Paulsen and Asmar[142]	109/140 (78)	60/88 (68)	0/0	169/228 (74)
1988	Adamson et al[86]	31/47 (66)	7/11 (61)	0/2 (0)	39/65 (60)
	TOTAL	208/283 (73)	143/210 (68)	89/132 (67)	441/630 (70)

*All by American Fertility Society classification.

COMPARISON OF LAPAROSCOPY AND LAPAROTOMY

With the recent developments of refined laparoscopic instrumentation, optics, and video systems, the laparoscopic surgeon is more able to perform increasingly complex operative procedures. A recent retrospective review of the literature since 1975 to ascertain the superiority of laparotomy versus laparoscopy in improving pregnancy rates in women with endometriosis revealed similar complication rates between these two approaches.[148] In women with minimal and mild endometriosis, there was no evidence that either approach was more efficacious in improving fertility rates. In women with moderate to severe endometriosis, there was suggestive evidence that the use of the laser through the laparoscope may be superior to laparotomy in the treatment of infertility associated with endometriosis.[148] There have been two recent studies comparing the results of operative laparoscopy versus microsurgery at laparotomy in the treatment of endometriosis. Fayez and associates[149] reported a significantly better outcome with laparoscopy (58%) than with laparotomy (36%) in a group of patients operated on by the same surgeons. Their result can be interpreted either that laparoscopy is more efficacious than laparotomy or that these surgeons are more adept at laparoscopy. The second study by Chong and associates[150] compared the efficacy of CO_2 laser surgery by laparotomy versus laparoscopy in the treatment of infertility associated with severe endometriosis and reported comparable results between these two groups of women. There was extreme selection bias in that the surgeon whose expertise was in laparoscopy performed all the laparoscopy, and similarly, the surgeon whose expertise was microsurgery

performed all the laparotomies in this study. The value of this study, however, is that no difference in result could be noted when each surgeon employed their best technique. Monthly fecundity rates of 6.7% and a cumulative pregnancy rate of 70.5% were obtained for women with stages III and IV disease.

Recently, a large (n = 579) retrospective study (prospectively collected data set) compared pregnancy rates in women across all stages of endometriosis between no treatment, medical treatment, operative laparoscopy, and laparotomy using life table analysis.[151] The laparoscopic group pregnancy rates were equal to the no-treatment group pregnancy rates in all analyses and were significantly higher than the other treatment groups in several analyses. A subset of women (n = 258) with only endometriosis-related infertility was also analyzed between these four therapeutic modalities with similar results. The absence of an effect of operative laparoscopy may be due to the lack of sufficient statistical power in this study. The superiority of laparoscopy over laparotomy in this study could again be reflective of the singular surgeon or the technique.

The importance of the therapeutic efficacy of a no-treatment group, especially in the milder stages of endometriosis, must be emphasized. The argument for operative laparoscopy lies in the prevention of disease progression.[78] Given that there may be comparable efficacy between laparoscopy and laparotomy, the economic benefits take on great importance.

There is no question that laparoscopic surgery results in a significant reduction in hospital costs compared with laparotomy.[152] Azziz and coworkers[153] provided convincing evidence that recuperative time for even complex operative laparoscopy is shorter than for laparotomy. The only comparative

TABLE 35–3. Pregnancy Outcome in Patients with Endometriosis Treated by Conservative Laparotomy Surgery

Year	Author	Minimal to Mild No. (%)	Moderate No. (%)	Severe No. (%)	All No. (%)
AFS Classification					
1981	Rock et al[43]	28/45 (62)	48/88 (55)	39/81 (48)	115/214 (53)
1984	Gordts	8/20 (20)	42/99 (42)	20/57 (35)	70/176 (39)
Acosta Classification					
1986	Olive et al[58, 72]	5/11 (46)	22/43 (51)	10/34 (29)	37/88 (42)
1978	Schenken and Malinak[169]	32/42 (76)	12/36 (33)	6/21 (29)	50/99 (51)
1979	Buttram[117]	61/88 (69)	28/50 (56)	32/68 (47)	121/206 (59)
1983	Rantala[173]	26/44 (59)	22/39 (56)	18/46 (39)	66/129 (51)
	TOTAL	160/250 (64)	174/355 (49)	125/307 (40)	459/912 (50)

AFS, American Fertility Society.

study of economic cost specific to women with endometriosis revealed the total number of hospital days for the 60 women undergoing laparoscopy versus the 60 women undergoing laparotomy was 72 versus 258 days, respectively.[154] The total number of days of incapacitation for the two groups, respectively, were 216 and 1284, whereas the total cost of medical care was $223,260 versus $424,500, respectively.

In summary, the approach used in the infertile woman with moderate to severe endometriosis should primarily be decided based on the expertise of the surgeon. If the surgeon feels equally proficient in both approaches, the laparoscopic approach may provide economic and social benefits and similar results over laparotomy. The approach in the infertile woman with minimal to mild disease should be individualized. Expectant management definitively plays a role in the management of this stage but is modified by factors such as the age of the women, concurrent symptoms, and previous therapeutic approaches. If surgery is undertaken, a laparoscopic approach is usually indicated.

Definitive Surgical Therapy

The classic definition of definitive therapy is a hysterectomy with bilateral oophorectomy and removal of all endometrial implants. Definitive surgery for severe endometriosis (hysterectomy and bilateral salpingo-oophorectomy) is the only known "cure" for this disease. The decision to perform definitive surgery in a young woman is always a difficult one. The probability that symptoms will persist when only a hysterectomy is done with conservation of ovaries is unknown, and opinions vary widely on its likelihood. If a hysterectomy and oophorectomy are contemplated, issues of estrogen deprivation as it relates to bone metabolism and cardiovascular risks as well as estrogen replacement therapy and possible stimulation of endometrial implants must be discussed with the patient preoperatively. According to clinical experience, estrogen-progestin replacement therapy can be used with a negligible risk of recurrence of disease.[154] Indications for definitive surgery include intractable, incapacitating pelvic pain in a young woman who has failed medical and conservative surgical therapy. In a woman who has completed childbearing and has recurrence, definitive surgery may be entertained. With a variety of medical therapies available, and possible surgeries for pain control, the use of definitive therapy for endometriosis in the infertile women is rarely, if ever, needed.

Combined Medical and Surgical Therapy

Surgical and medical treatments of endometriosis are not mutually exclusive, and there is a role for combined therapy, although it is unclear. Both surgical and medical approaches have proved effective in relieving pain symptoms, yet neither has proven efficacious in nonmechanical, infertility-associated endometriosis. Although both surgical and medical therapy have been widely used in the treatment of women with infertility and endometriosis, there is relatively little information available on their comparative success.

There are two studies on the comparative success of preoperative versus postoperative medical therapy. The first study is a prospective, nonrandomized study of danazol ther-

apy alone and preoperative and postoperative therapy with danazol in patients with endometriosis. Assignment to treatment groups appeared biased; therefore, conclusions that could be made are that preoperative therapy with danazol resulted in a higher pregnancy rate than medical therapy alone in the mild stages and versus postoperative therapy in the severe stages.[162] The second study is a retrospective study in which monthly fecundity rates for women with endometriosis treated by laparoscopic CO_2 laser vaporization alone and with preoperative and postoperative therapy with danazol were compared.[87] No statistically significant differences between any treatment group were found.

PREOPERATIVE MEDICAL THERAPY

The argument for preoperative therapy has centered around facilitating surgical technique. Because a reduction in pelvic vascularization and inflammation is generally seen with medical therapy, theoretically this would allow easier dissection and subsequent higher pregnancy success and lower recurrence rates. In addition to this theoretical advantage, the infertile woman does not need to wait to attempt pregnancy after surgery. It has been suggested that the chances of conception are highest in the first year following conservative surgery.[156] Two surgeries are required: one for diagnosis and one for treatment after medical therapy.

The available data are conflicting on the advantages of preoperative medical therapy.[157] There are two reports on the use of danazol followed by conservative laparotomy in women with infertility and staged endometriosis, but both these reports have serious flaws, and no conclusions on efficacy can be made.[158, 159] In a study using a synthetic progestin, a 60% (21/35) pregnancy rate in patients with moderate endometriosis and a 47% (7/15) pregnancy rate in patients with severe endometriosis over 18 months was reported.[160] Unfortunately, no control group was studied.

POSTOPERATIVE MEDICAL THERAPY

Postoperative therapy is theorized to eliminate residual disease following surgery for endometriosis. Another advantage of postoperative medical therapy is that both diagnosis and treatment of endometriosis can occur during one surgical procedure. The main disadvantage of postoperative combination therapy is delaying attempts at pregnancy for several months when the efficacy of surgical therapy may be increased.[156] However, patients with persistent or recurrent pelvic pain may benefit from a combined surgical and medical treatment.

Only one study has found a striking advantage, 79% (15/19) pregnancy rate versus 30% (36/119) pregnancy rate over 31 months, of the use of postoperative medical (danazol) therapy compared with surgery (conservative laparotomy) alone.[161] This improvement in pregnancy rates with postoperative therapy has not been confirmed by other investigators.[162, 163]

There are no prospective studies combining surgery with preoperative GnRH analogs or on the influence of combination therapy on recurrences rates. Obviously, data are conflicting on the usefulness of combination therapy, whether preoperative or postoperative. Its role in the treatment of the infertile woman with endometriosis remains unknown and controversial.

RECURRENCE

It is generally believed that endometriosis will recur unless definitive surgery (bilateral salpingo-oophorectomy) is done. The time to recurrence is thought to be dependent on the stage of disease and completeness of resection at the time of initial surgery. Whether recurrence rates are truly recurrences or rather persistence of microscopic disease or nonpigmented lesions with progression is unknown. The ability to conceive is not thought to have an effect on recurrence rates.[161] The recurrence rate of endometriosis after conservative surgery ranges from 2% to 47%.[164, 165] Wheeler and Malinak,[166] using life table analysis, have noted that the cumulative recurrence rate of endometriosis is 13% in 3 years and 40% in 5 years. Using the 1979 AFS classification, Olive[167] studied a total of 214 patients retrospectively and noted recurrence rates for mild (45/214), moderate (88/214), severe (66/214), and extensive (15/214) disease of 31%, 25%, 38%, and 27%, respectively, with an average of 30%. Subsequent surgery became necessary in 13%, 11%, 14%, and 27% of this group, respectively, with an average of 14%. When conservative surgery was combined with medical therapy (danazol and GnRH agonist), the overall recurrence rate at 36 months was between 13.5% and 33%.[75, 158]

Repetitive Surgery

Because of the wide use of a conservative surgical approach (especially in the presence of adhesions and endometriomas) in the treatment of endometriosis, the issue of repetitive surgeries for recurrent symptoms has been examined. Several studies reported on followup after conservative reoperation for recurrence, the most recent being a large, prospective series by Candiani and associates.[61, 166, 168–171] In the prospective series of 42 women with infertility and pelvic pain and previous conservative laparotomy, 33% had stage IV and 59% had stage III endometriosis noted during the second conservative laparotomy.[61] Thirty-one women had combination medical and surgical therapy. Patients were followed for 41.8 ± 30.3 months. Pain symptoms reappeared during followup after the second surgery in 19% of women. Eight of 28 women attempting conception were successful, with a cumulative pregnancy rate at 27 months of 30.7%. A 20% to 47% crude pregnancy rate was reported in the three retrospective series.[166, 168, 170] Fourteen percent and 30% of patients underwent a third surgery because of recurrence of pain in two of the published series.[166, 172]

Redwine[145] reported on life table analysis of reoperation and persistent, recurrent disease in 359 women after conservative laparoscopic excision of endometriosis. Ninety-one women underwent reoperation within 1 to 10 years of their original surgery. The maximum cumulative rate of persistence-recurrence of disease was 19%, achieved in the fifth postoperative year. This recurrence rate is lower than most previously reported. Overall, the results corroborate the chronic and progressive course of endometriosis seen in some women. Even so, most women undergoing conservative surgery do not undergo repetitive surgery. Although progressive local invasion may occur, an aggressive advancement in disease stage is uncommon.

SUMMARY

In treating the infertile woman with endometriosis, many factors must be considered in selecting the appropriate mode of therapy. Endometriosis is best regarded as a chronic disease that can vary in symptoms over time. After the diagnosis of endometriosis is established, other factors such as stage of endometriosis, age of the patient, and symptoms of the patient need to be considered in developing a treatment plan. In cases of mechanical obstruction, such as can be found in stages III and IV endometriosis, the use of surgery is indicated and does improve the conception rate, whereas in the milder forms of endometriosis, a variety of options are available such as expectant management, operative laparoscopy, conservative laparotomy, and medical therapy. Assisted reproductive technologies (especially gamete intrafallopian tube transfer) should be considered in those patients who fail standard treatments. The next decade may yield new information about the pathophysiology of endometriosis that should lead to a more individualized and rational approach to therapy in the infertile woman.

REFERENCES

1. Sampson JA. Peritoneal endometriosis due to menstrual dissemination of endometrial tissue into the peritoneal cavity. Am J Obstet Gynecol 1927;14:422.
2. Batt RE, Smith RA. Embryologic theory of histogenesis of endometriosis in peritoneal pockets. Obstet Gynecol Clin North Am 1989;16:15.
3. Novak E. Significance of uterine mucosa in fallopian tubes with discussion of origin of aberrant endometrium. Am J Obstet Gynecol 1926;12:484.
4. Javert CT. Pathogenesis of endometriosis based on endometrial homeoplasia direct extension, exfoliation and implantation, lymphatic and hematogenous metastasis. Cancer 1949;2:399–410.
5. Mahmood TA, Templeton A. Prevalence and genesis of endometriosis. Hum Reprod 1991;6:544–549.
6. Olive DL, Henderson DY. Endometriosis and mild uterine anomalies. Obstet Gynecol 1987;69:412.
7. Pinsonneault O, Goldstein DP. Obstructing malformations of the uterus and vagina. Fertil Steril 1985;44:241–247.
8. Dmowski WP, Steele RW, Baker GF. Deficient cellular immunity in endometriosis. Am J Obstet Gynecol 1981;141:377–383.
9. Jeffcoate TA. Principles of Gynecology. London: Butterworth, 1975.
10. Williams T, Pratt JH. Endometriosis in 1000 consecutive celiotomies: incidence and management. Am J Obstet Gynecol 1977;129:245.
11. Mahmood TA, Templeton A. The relationship between endometriosis and semen analysis: a review of 490 consecutive laparoscopies. Hum Reprod 1989;4:782–785.
12. Verkauf BS. The incidence, symptoms and signs of endometriosis in fertile and infertile women. J Fla Med Assoc 1987;74:671.
13. Dunnigan NM, Jordan JA, Coughlan BM, Logan-Edwards R. One thousand consecutive cases of diagnostic laparoscopy. J Obstet Gynaecol Br Commonwealth 1972;79:1016–1024.
14. Musich JR, Behrman SJ. Infertilty laparoscopy in perspective: review of 500 cases. Am J Obstet Gynecol 1982;143:293–303.
15. Hasson HM. Incidence of endometriosis in diagnostic laparoscopy. J Reprod Med 1976;16:135–138.
16. Liu DTY, Hitchcock A. Endometriosis: its association with retrograde menstruation, dysmenorrhea and tubal pathology. Br J Obstet Gynaecol 1986;93:859–862.
17. Garcia CR, David SS. Pelvic endometriosis: infertility and pelvic pain. Am J Obstet Gynecol 1977;129:740–747.

18. Guzick DS. Clinical epidemiology of endometriosis and infertility. Obstet Gynecol Clin North Am 1989;16:43–59.

19. Telimaa S. Danazol and medroxyprogesterone acetate inefficacious in the treatment of infertility in endometriosis. Fertil Steril 1988;50:872.

20. Fayez JA, Collazo LM. Comparison between laparotomy and operative laparoscopy in the treatment of moderate/severe stages of endometriosis. Int J Fertil 1990;35:272–279.

21. Schenken RS, Williams RF, Hodgen GD. Effect of pregnancy on surgically induced endometriosis in cynomolgus monkeys. Am J Obstet Gynecol 1987;157:1392–1396.

22. Thomas EJ, Cooke ID. The impact of gestrinone on the course of asymptomatic endometriosis. Br Med J 1987;294:272.

23. Redwine DB. The distribution of endometriosis in the pelvis by age groups and fertility. Fertil Steril 1987;47:173.

24. Jansen RPS, Russel P. Non-pigmented endometriosis: clinical laparoscopic and pathologic definition. Am J Obstet Gynecol 1986;155:1154.

25. Stripling MC, Martin DC, Chatman DL, et al. Subtle appearance of pelvic endometriosis. Fert Steril 1988;49:427.

26. Cornillie FJ, Oosterlynk D, Lauweryns JM, Koninckx PR. Deeply infiltration pelvic endometriosis: histology and clinical significance. Fertil Steril 1990;53:978.

27. Koninckx PR, Meuleman C, Demeyere S, et al. Suggestive evidence that pelvic endometriosis is a progressive disease, whereas deeply infiltrating endometriosis is associated with pelvic pain. Fertil Steril 1991;55:759–765.

28. Williams T. Endometriosis. In: Mattingly RF, Thompson JD, editors. Te Linde's Operative Gynecology. Philadelphia: JB Lippincott, 1985:257–286.

29. Portuondo JA, Herrau C, Echanojaurequi AD, Riego AG. Peritoneal flushing and biopsy in laparoscopically diagnosed endometriosis. Fertil Steril 1982;38:538.

30. Dmowski WP. Pitfalls in clinical laparoscopic and histologic diagnosis of endometriosis. Acta Obstet Gynecol Scand Suppl 1984;123:611.

31. Dmowski WP. Visual assessment of peritoneal implants for staging endometriosis: do number and cumulative size of lesions reflect severity of a systemic disease? Fertil Steril 1987;47:382–384.

32. Evers JLH. The second-look laparoscopy for evaluation of the results of medical treatment of endometriosis should not be performed during ovarian suppression. Fertil Steril 1987;47:502.

33. Chatman DL, Zbella EA. Pelvic peritoneal defects and endometriosis: further observations. Fertil Steril 1986;46:711.

34. Chatman DL. Pelvic peritoneal defects and endometriosis: Allen-Masters syndrome revisited. Fertil Steril 1981;36:751.

35. Davis GD, Brooks RA. Excision of pelvic endometriosis with the carbon dioxide laser laparoscope. Obstet Gynecol 1988;72:816–819.

36. Vasquez G, Cornillie F, Brosens IA. Peritoneal endometriosis: scanning electron microscopy and histology of minimal pelvic endometriotic lesions. Fertil Steril 1984;42:696.

37. Bronsens I, Vasquez G, Gordts S. Scanning electron microscopy study of the pelvic peritoneum in unexplained infertility and endometriosis. Fertil Steril 1984;41:215.

38. Murphy AA, Green WR, Bobbie D, et al. Unsuspected endometriosis documented by scanning electron microscopy in visually normal peritoneum. Fertil Steril 1986;46:522.

39. Martin DC, Hubert GD, Levy BS. Depth of infiltration of endometriosis. J Gynecol Surg 1989;5:55.

40. Candiani GB, Vercellini P, Fedele L. Laparoscopic ovarian puncture for correct staging of endometriosis. Fertil Steril 1990;53:994.

41. Vercellini P, Vendola N, Bocciolone L, et al. Reliability of visual diagnosis of ovarian endometriosis. Fertil Steril 1991;56:1198–2000.

41a. Vancaillie TG, Hill RH, Tiehl RM, et al. Laser-induced fluorescence of ectopic endometrium in rabbits. Obstet Gynecol 1989;74:225–230.

42. Schenken RS, Vancaillie TG, Riehl RM, et al. New developments in diagnostic techniques. Prog Clin Bio Res 1990;323:137–149.

43. Rock JA, Guzick DS, Sengos C, et al. The conservative surgical treatment of endometriosis: evaluation of pregnancy success with respect to the extent of disease as categorized using contemporary classification systems. Fertil Steril 1981;35:131–137.

44. Groff TR. Classifications. In: Schenken RS, editor. Contemporary Concepts in Clinical Management. Philadelphia: JB Lippincott, 1989:145–167.

45. Weitzman FA, Buttram VC. Classification of endometriosis. Obstet Gynecol Clin North Am 1989;16:61–77.

46. Fedele L, Bianchi S, Bocciolone L, et al. Pain symptoms associated with endometriosis. Obstet Gynecol 1992;79:767–769.

47. Pittaway DE. CA-125 in women with endometriosis. Obstet Gynecol Clin North Am 1989;16:237.

48. Scott RD, Burt JH. Clinical experimental endometriosis: fifteen years' experience at University Hospital of Cleveland. South Med J 1962;55:129.

49. Fedele L, Parazzini F, Bianchi S, et al. Stage and localization of pelvic endometriosis and pain. Fertil Steril 1990;53:155–158.

50. Vercellini P, Fedele L, Molteni P, et al. Laparoscopy in the diagnosis of gynecologic chronic pelvic pain. Int J Gynecol Obstet 1990;32:261–265.

51. Stout AL, Steege JF, Dodson WC, Hughes CL. Relationship of laparoscopic findings to self-report of pelvic pain. Am J Obstet Gynecol 1991;164:73.

52. Ripps BA, Martin DC. Correlation of focal pelvic tenderness with implant dimension and stage of endometriosis. J Reprod Med 1992;37:620–624.

53. Vernon MW, Beard JS, Graves K, Wilson EA. Classification of endometriotic implants by morphologic appearance and capacity to synthesize prostaglandin F. Fertil Steril 1986;46:801–806.

54. Parker WH. Management of adnexal masses by operative laparoscopy: selection criteria. J Reprod Med 1992;37:603–606.

55. Hulka JF, Parker WH, Surrey M, Phillips J. Management of ovarian masses: AAGL 1990 survey. J Reprod Med 1992;37:599.

56. Granberg S, Wikland M, Jansson I. Macroscopic characterization of ovarian tumors and the relation to the histologic diagnosis: criteria to be used for ultrasound evaluation. Gynecol Oncol 1989;35:139.

57. Mage G, Canis M, Manhes H, et al. Laparoscopic management of adnexal cystic masses. J Gynecol Surg 1990;6:71.

58. Olive DL, Haney AF. Endometriosis-associated infertility: critical review of therapeutic approaches. Obstet Gynecol Surv 1986;41:538–555.

59. Thomas EJ, Lenton EA, Cooke ID. Follicle growth patterns and endocrinological abnormalities in infertile women with minor degrees of endometriosis. Br J Obstet Gynecol 1986;93:852.

60. Tummon IS, Maclin VM, Radwanska E, et al. Occult ovulatory dysfunction in women with minimal endometriosis and unexplained infertility. Fertil Steril 1988;50:716.

61. Candiani GB, Vercellini P, Fedele L, et al. Mild endometriosis and infertility: a critical review of epidemiologic data, diagnostic pitfalls, and classification limits. Obstet Gynecol Surv 1991;46:374–382.

62. Czernobilsky B, Silverstein A. Salpingitis in ovarian endometriosis. Fertil Steril 1978;30:45.

63. American Fertility Society. Revised American Fertility Society classification of endometriosis: 1985. Fertil Steril 1985;43:351.

64. Jones HW, Rock JA. The evaluation of surgical results. In: Jones HW, Rock JA, editors. Reparative and Constructive Surgery of the Female Genital Tract. Baltimore: Williams & Wilkins, 1983.

65. Tulandi T, Cherry N. Clinical trials in reproductive surgery: randomization and life-table analysis. Fertil Steril 1989;52:12–14.

66. Portuondo JA, Echanojaurregui AD, Herran D, Alijarte I. Early conception in patients with untreated mild endometriosis. Fertil Steril 1983;39:22.

67. Schenken RS, Malinak LR. Conservative surgery versus expectant management for the infertile patient with mild endometriosis. Fertil Steril 1982;37:183–186.

68. Olive DL, Stohs GF, Metzger DA, Franklin RR. Expectant management and hydrotubations in the treatment of endometriosis-associated infertility. Fertil Steril 1985;44:35–41.

69. Badaway SZ, Bakry MM, Samuel F, Dizer M. Cumulative pregnancy rates in infertile women with endometriosis. J Reprod Med 1988;33:757–760.

70. Diamond MP, Daniell JF, Feste J, et al. Adhesion formation and de novo adhesion formation after reproductive pelvic surgery. Fertil Steril 1987;47:864–866.

71. Mahmood TA, Templeton A. Pathophysiology of mild endometriosis: review of literature. Hum Reprod 1990;5:765–784.

72. Olive DL, Lee KL. Analysis of sequential treatment protocols for endometriosis-associated infertility. Am J Obstet Gynecol 1986;154:613.

73. Bayer SR, Siebel MM, Saffon DS. Efficacy of danazol treatment for minimal endometriosis in infertile women: a prospective randomized study. J Reprod Med 1988;33:181.

74. Hull ME, Moghissi KS, Magyar DFF, Haves MF. Comparison of different treatment modalities of endometriosis in infertile women. Fertil Steril 1987;47:40.

75. Fedele L, Bianchi S, Arcaini L, et al. GnRH agonists in the treatment of endometriosis. Acta Eur Fertil 1988;119:5–12.

76. Wilson EA. Surgical therapy for endometriosis. Clin Obstet Gynecol 1988;31:857.

77. Dargent D. General rules for surgery in treatment of endometriosis. Contrib Gynecol Obstet 1987;16:271–279.

78. Houston DE. Evidence for the risk of pelvic endometriosis by age, race, and socioeconomic status. Epidemiol Rev 1984;6:167–191.

79. Ellis H, Harrison W, Hugh TB. The healing of peritoneum under normal and pathologic conditions. Br J Surg 1965;52:471–476.

80. Ellis H. The cause and prevention of postoperative intraperitoneal adhesions. Surg Gynecol Obstet 1971;133:497–511.

81. Gomel V. Tubal reanastomosis by microsurgery. Fertil Steril 1977;28:59.

82. Rock JA, Bergquist CA, Kimball AW, et al. Comparison of the operating microscope and loupe for microsurgical tubal anastomosis: a randomized clinical trial. Fertil Steril 1984;41:229.

83. Riedel HH, Semm K. An initial comparison of coagulation techniques of sterilization. J Reprod Med 1982;27:261.

84. Eposito JM. The laparoscopist and electrosurgery. Am J Obstet Gynecol 1976;126:633.

85. Semm K. Pelviscopic technique of the triphasic treatment of endometriosis. In: Semm K, Greenblatt KR, Mettler L, editors. Genital Endometriosis in Infertility. New York: Thieme/Stratton, 1982:67–108.

86. Adamson GD, Lu J, Suback LL. Laparoscopic CO_2 laser vaporization of endometriosis compared with traditional treatments. Fertil Steril 1988;50:794.

87. Olive DL, Martin DC. Treatment of endometriosis associated infertility with CO_2 laser laparoscopy: the use of one- and two-parameter exponential models. Fertil Steril 1987;48:18.

88. Keye WR, Hansen LW, Astin M, et al. Argon laser therapy of endometriosis: a review of 92 consecutive patients. Fertil Steril 1987;47:208.

89. Corson SL, Unger M, Kwa D, et al. Laparoscopic laser treatment of endometriosis with the Nd:YAG sapphire probe. Am J Obstet Gynecol 1989;160:718–723.

90. Kojima E, Morita M, Otaka K, et al. YAG laser laparoscopy of ovarian endometriomas. J Reprod Med 1990;35:592.

91. Dougherty TJ. Photodynamic therapy. In: Shapshay SM, editor. Endoscopic Laser Surgery Handbook. New York: Marcel Dekker, 1987:424.

92. Martin DC, Vander Zwagg R. Excisional techniques for endometriosis with the carbon dioxide laser laparoscope. J Reprod Med 1987;32:752.

93. Redwine DB. Laparoscopic en bloc resection for the treatment of the obliterated cul-de-sac of endometriosis. J Reprod Med 1992;37:695–698.

94. Franssen AM, Kuer FM, Chadha DR, et al. Endometriois: treatment with gonadotropin-releasing hormone agonist buserelin. Fertil Steril 1989;51:401.

95. Schenken RS. Gonadotropin-releasing hormone analogs in the treatment of endometriomas. Am J Obstet Gynecol 1990;162:579.

96. Shaw RW, Fraser HM, Boyle H. Intranasal treatment with luteinising hormone–releasing hormone agonist in women with endometriosis. Br Med J 1983;287:1667.

97. Martin DC. Laparoscopic treatment of ovarian endometrioma. Clin Obstet Gynecol 1991;34:452–458.

98. Koninckx P, Muyldermans M, Moerman P, et al. CA-125 concentrations in ovarian "chocolate" cyst fluid can differentiate an endometriotic cyst from a cystic corpus luteum. Hum Reprod 1992;7:1314–1317.

99. Sulewski JM, Curcio FD, Brotinsky C, Stenger VG. The treatment of endometriosis at laparoscopy for infertility. Am J Obstet Gynecol 1980;138:128.

100. Semm K, Mettler L. Technical progress in pelvic surgery via operative laparoscopy. Am J Obstet Gynecol 1980;138:121.

101. Reich H, McGlynn F. Treatment of ovarian endometriomas using laparoscopic techniques. J Reprod Med 1986;31:577–584.

102. Daniell JF, Kurtz BR, Gurley LD. Laser laparoscopic management of large endometriomas. Fertil Steril 1991;55:692.

103. Brumsted JR, Deaton J, Lavigne E, et al. Postoperative adhesion formation after ovarian wedge resection with and without ovarian reconstruction in the rabbit. Fertil Steril 1990;53:723.

104. Wiskind AK, Toledo AA, Dudley AG, Zusmanis K. Adhesion formation after ovarian wound repair in New Zealand white rabbits: a comparison of ovarian microsurgical closure with ovarian nonclosure. Am J Obstet Gynecol 1990;163:1674.

105. Fayez JA, Vogel MF. Comparison of different treatment methods of endometriomas by laparoscopy. Obstet Gynecol 1991;78:660–665.

106. Canis M, Mage G, Manhes H, Pouly JL, et al. Laparoscopic treatment of endometriosis. Acta Obstet Gynecol Scand Suppl 1989;150:15–20.

107. Marrs RP. The use of potassium-titanyl-phosphate laser for laparoscopic removal of ovarian endometrioma. Am J Obstet Gynecol 1991;164:1622–1626.

108. Daniell JF, Christianson C. Combined laparoscopic surgery and danazol treatment for pelvic endometriosis. Fertil Steril 1981;35:521.

109. Vercellini P, Vendola N, Bocciolone L, et al. Laparoscopic aspiration of ovarian endometriomas: effect with gonadotropin-releasing hormone agonist treatment. J Reprod Med 1992;37:577–580.

110. Canis M, Mage G, Wattiez A, et al. Second-look laparoscopy after laparoscopic cystectomy of large ovarian endometriomas. Fertil Steril 1992;58:617–620.

111. Wood C, Maher P, Hill D. Diagnosis and surgical management of endometriomas. Aust N Z J Obstet Gyncaeol 1992;32:161–163.

112. Kistner RW: Endometriosis. In: McElin TW, Sciarra JJ, editors. Gynecology and Obstetrics. Hagerstown, MD: Harper & Row, 1981:1.

113. Coronado C, Franklin RR, Lotze EC, et al. Surgical treatment of symptomatic colorectal endometriosis. Fertil Steril 1990;53:411–416.

114. Nezhat C, Nezhat F, Pennington E. Laparoscopic proctectomy for infiltrating endometriosis of the rectum. Fertil Steril 1992;57:1129–1132.

115. Shook TE, Nyberg LM. Endometriosis of the urinary tract. Urology 1988;31:1–6.

116. Candy JW. Modified Gilliam uterine suspension using laparoscopic visualization. Obstet Gynecol 1976;47:242–243.

117. Buttram VC. Conservative surgery for endometriosis in the infertile female—a study of 206 patients: implications for both medical and surgical therapies. Fertil Steril 1979;31:117.

118. Buttram VC, Reiter RC. In: Surgical Treatment of the Infertile Female. Baltimore: Williams & Wilkins, 1985:81.

119. Mann WJ, Stenger VG. Uterine suspension through the laparoscope. Obstet Gynecol 1978;51:563–566.

120. Gordon SF. Laparoscopic uterine suspension. J Reprod Med 1992;37:615–616.

121. Ivey JL. Laparoscopic uterine suspension as an adjunctive procedure at the time of laser laparoscopy for the treatment of endometriosis. J Reprod Med 1992;37:757–765.

122. Doyle JB. Paracervical uterine denervation by transection of the cervical plexus for the relief of dysmenorrhea. Am J Obstet Gynecol 1955;70:11.

123. Frangenheim H, Kleindienst W. Chronic pelvic disease of unknown origin. In: Phillips JM, Keith L, editors. Gynecologic Laparoscopy. New York: Stratton, 1974:52.

124. Daniell JF. Fiberoptic laser laparoscopy. Baillieres Clin Obstet Gynecol 1989;3:545.

125. Donnez J, Nicolle M. CO_2 laser laparoscopic surgery: adhesiolysis, salpingostomy, laser uterine nerve ablations, and tubal pregnancy. Baillieres Clin Obstet Gynecol 1989;3:525.

126. Feste JR. Laser laparoscopy: a new modality. J Reprod Med 1985;30:413.

127. Lichten EM, Bombard J. Surgical treatment of primary dysmenorrhea with laparoscopic uterine nerve ablation. J Reprod Med 1987;32:37.

128. Good MC, Copas PR, Doody MC. Uterine prolapse after laparoscopic uterosacral transection. J Reprod Med 1992;37:995–996.

129. Hesla JS, Rock JA. Endometriosis. In: Rock JA, Murphy AA, Jones HA, editors. Female Reproductive Surgery. Baltimore: Williams & Wilkins, 1992.

130. Hernandez E, Sapp K, Rock JA. Danazol in the treatment of recurrent or persistent endometriosis: a preliminary report. Infertility 1981;4:29.

131. Polan ML, DeCherney A. Presacral neurectomy for pelvic pain in infertility. Fertil Steril 1980;34:557–560.

132. Candiani GB, Fedele L, Vercellini P, et al. Presacral neurectomy for treatment of pelvic pain associated with endometriosis: a controlled study. Am J Obstet Gynecol 1992;167:100–103.

133. Nezhat C, Nezhat F. A simplified method of laparoscopic presacral neurectomy for the treatment of central pelvic pain due to endometriosis. Br J Obstet Gynecol 1992;99:659–663.

134. Perez JJ. Laparoscopic presacral neurectomy results of the first 25 cases. J Reprod Med 1990;35:625.

135. Pastner B, Orr JW. Intractable venous sacral hemorrhage: use of stainless steel thumbtacks to obtain hemostasis. Am J Obstet Gynecol 1990;162:452.

136. Black WT. Use of presacral sympathectomy in the treatment of dysmenorrhea. Obstet Gynecol 1964;9:16.

137. Fliegner JR, Umstad MP. Presacral neurectomy—a reappraisal. Aust N Z J Obstet Gynecol 1991;31:76–79.

138. Tjaden BT, Schlaff WD, Kimball A, Rock JA. The efficacy of presacral neurectomy for the relief of midline dysmenorrhea. Obstet Gynecol 1990;76:86–91.

139. Vercellini P, Fedele L, Bianchi S, Candiani GB. Pelvic denervation for chronic pain associated with endometriosis: fact or fancy? Am J Obstet Gynecol 1991;1655:645–649.

140. Guzick DS, Rock JA. Estimation of a model of cumulative pregnancy following infertility therapy. Am J Obstet Gynecol 1981;140:573.

141. Jones HW, Rock JA. Endometriosis externa. In: Jones HW, Rock JA, editors. Reparative and Constructive Surgery of the Female Generative Tract. Baltimore: Williams & Wilkins, 1983.

142. Paulsen JD, Asmar P. The use of CO_2 laser laparoscopy for treating endometriosis. Int J Fertil 1987;32:237.

143. Hasson HM. Electrocoagulation of pelvic endometriotic lesion with laparoscopic control. Am J Obstet Gynecol 1979;135:115.

144. Murphy AA, Schlaff WD, Hassiakos D, et al. Laparoscopic cautery in the treatment of endometriosis-related infertility. Fertil Steril 1991;55:246.

145. Redwine DB. Conservative laparoscopic excision of endometriosis by sharp dissection: life table analysis of reoperation and persistent or recurrent disease. Fertil Steril 1991;56:628–634.

146. Nezhat C, Crowgey S, Nezhat F. Video laseroscopy for the treatment of endometriosis associated with infertility. Fertil Steril 1989;51:237–240.

147. Martin DC. CO_2 laser laparoscopy for endometriosis associated with infertility. J Reprod Med 1986;31:1089.

148. Gant NF. Infertility and endometriosis: comparison of pregnancy outcomes with laparotomy versus laparoscopic techniques. Am J Obstet Gynecol 1992;166:1072–1081.

149. Fayez JA, Collazo LM, Vernon C. Comparison of different modalities of treatment for minimal and mild endometriosis. Am J Obstet Gynecol 1988;159:927–932.

150. Chong AP, Luciano AA, O'Shaughnessy AM. Laser laparoscopy versus laparotomy in the treatment of infertility patients with severe endometriosis. J Gynecol Surg 1990;6:179.

151. Adamson GD, Hurd SJ, Pasta DJ, Rodriguez BD. Laparoscopic endometriosis treatment: is it better? Fertil Steril 1993;59:35–44.

152. Levine RL. Economic impact of pelviscopic surgery. J Reprod Med 1985;30:655.

153. Azziz R, Steinkampf MP, Murphy A. Postoperative recuperation: relation to the extent of endoscopic surgery. Fertil Steril 1989;51:1061–1064.

154. Luciano AA, Lowney J, Jacobs SL. Endoscopic treatment of endometriosis-associated infertility: therapeutic, economic, and social benefits. J Reprod Med 1992;37:573–576.

155. Dmowski WP, Radwanska E, Rana W. Recurrent endometriosis following hysterectomy and oophorectomy: the role of residual ovarian fragments. Int J Gynecol Obstet 1988;26:93–103.

156. Andrews WE, Larsen GD. Endometriosis: treatment with hormonal pseudopregnancy and/or operation. Am J Obstet Gynecol 1974;118:643.

157. Kettel LM, Murphy AA. Combination medical and surgical therapy for infertile patients with endometriosis. Obstet Gynecol Clin North Am 1989;16:167–179.

158. Barbieri RL, Evans S, Kistner RW. Danazol in treatment of endometriosis: analysis of 100 cases with a 4-year follow-up. Fertil Steril 1982;37:737–746.

159. Audebert AJM, Larrue-Charlus S, Emperaire JC. Endometriosis and infertility: a review of 62 patients treated with danazol. Postgrad Med J 1979;55:10.

160. Donnez J, Lemaire-Rubbers M, Karaman Y, et al. Combined (hormonal and microsurgical) therapy in infertile women with endometriosis. Fertil Steril 1987;48:239.

161. Wheeler JM, Malinak LR. Postoperative danazol therapy in infertility patients with severe endometriosis. Fertil Steril 1981;36:460.

162. Buttram VC, Reiter RC, Ward S. Treatment of endometriosis with danazol: a report of a 6-year prospective study. Fertil Steril 1985;43:353.

163. Hammond CB, Rock JA, Parker RT. Conservative treatment of endometriosis: the effects of limited surgery and hormonal pseudopregnancy. Fertil Steril 1976;27:756.

164. Ranney B. Endometriosis: I. Conservative operations. Am J Obstet Gynecol 1970;107:743.

165. Ranney B. Endometriosis: II. Complete operations. Am J Obstet Gynecol 1971;109:1137.

166. Wheeler JM, Malinak LR. Recurrent endometriosis: incidence, management, and prognosis. Am J Obstet Gynecol 1983;146:247–250.

167. Olive DL. Conservative surgery. In: Schenken R, editor. Conservative Surgery in Endometriosis. Philadelphia: JB Lippincott, 1988.

168. Evers JLH, Dunselman GAJ, Land JA, Bouckaert PX. Endometriosis: the management of recurrent disease. In: Shaw RE, editor. Endometriosis. Carnforth: Parthenon, 1990:93–105.

169. Schenken RS, Malinak LR. Reoperation after initial treatment of endometriosis with conservative surgery. Am J Obstet Gynecol 1978;131:416–424.

170. Wheeler JM, Malinak LR. Recurrent endometriosis. Contrib Gynecol Obstet 1987;16:13–21.

171. Tulandi T, Tommaso F, Kafka I. Second-look operative laparoscopy 1 year following reproductive surgery. Fertil Steril 1989;52:421–424.

172. Candiani GB, Fedele L, Vercellini P, et al. Repetitive conservative surgery for recurrence of endometriosis. Fertil Steril 1991;77:421–424.

173. Rantala ML, Kahnapaa KV, Koskimies AI, et al. Fertility prognosis after surgical treatment of pelvic endometriosis. Gynaecol Acta Obstet Scand 1983;62:11–14.

CHAPTER 36

Surgical Treatment of Diseases of the Ovary

JOSEPH S. SANFILIPPO
and STEPHEN R. LINCOLN

HISTORY

The year 1870 marked the earliest investigation regarding the cellular components of the ovary and the origin of primordial germ cells.[1] The thesis proposed that germ cells arise during embryonic development from the proliferation of germinal epithelium on the external surface of the gonad. This concept became a point of controversy when additional theories postulated that "the continuity of germ-plasm" associated with germ cells segregated before the formation of the actual ovarian organ system.[1] The current theory regarding migration of primordial germ cells to the gonadal ridge has been proposed by Franchi and coworkers.[1]

EMBRYOLOGY

Formation of the genital ridge is initially represented by coelomic epithelial thickening on the ventral-lateral aspect of the developing mesonephros in the area of the wolffian ducts.[2] Of interest, the midsection of this thickening is the area that ultimately becomes the actual gonad.[3] It is hypothesized that hypertrophy of the coelomic epithelium in the area of the genital ridge occurs as a direct result of the entry of the primordial germ cells.[4] The medulla of the undifferentiated gonad appears to give rise to the adult ovarian tissue. In the female, there seems to be more than one cycle of proliferation of cells. The first cycle gives rise to sex cords somewhat similar to those noted in the male during the stage of indifferent gonadal differentiation. Ultimately this proliferative cell mass elongates and becomes separated from the cortical regions of the gonad by what ultimately becomes the primary tunica albuginea. The medulla of the ovary becomes organized into radially arranged cords, which eventually come in contact with the mesonephric remnant. The development of the medulla appears to be independent of the presence of germ cells. A second proliferative cycle of surface epithelium gives rise to the ovarian cortex.[1]

SURGICAL ANATOMY

These bilateral pelvic organs, approximately 4 cm in length, 2 cm in width, and 8 mm in thickness and weighing up to 3.5 g, remain an integral part of every gynecologic examination and a source of a great deal of active research. The ovary lies in the ovarian fossa on the lateral wall of the pelvis. It is outlined by the external iliac vessels, the obliterated umbilical artery, and the ureter. It receives its blood supply from the ovarian artery, which is derived from the aorta. In addition, a second blood supply is derived from the uterine artery. Anastomoses occur in the mesovarium (Fig. 36–1). Blood from the mesovarium ultimately enters the hilum of the ovary. The ovarian veins emerge from the ovarian hilum and give rise to the pampiniform plexus. The ovarian vein, then established, runs parallel to the ovarian artery and ultimately empties into the inferior vena cava. The left ovarian vein empties into the left renal vein, whereas the right empties directly into the vena cava. The nerve supply is derived from the hypogastric and ovarian plexuses.

The location of the ovary appears to change, especially during the first pregnancy. It is displaced cephalad and never really returns to its original position. In the erect posture, the long axis of the ovary is vertical. The infundibulopelvic ligament is identified in the cephalad segment of the ovary adjacent to the fimbria ovarica; the ovarian branch of the iliac vessels is located in this ligament. The utero-ovarian blood supply is carried in the utero-ovarian ligament of the ovary, which lies within the broad ligament and contains a number of smooth muscle fibers. The medial surface of the ovary is covered by the fimbriated portion of the fallopian tube. The fimbria ovarica anchors the fimbriated portion of the fallopian tube and can be a burdensome site of bleeding if transected.

A number of embryologic remnants are found in the broad ligament in the area of the ovaries. Specifically the epoöphoron, a wolffian duct remnant, is noted in the mesosalpinx between the ovary and the fallopian tube. The paroöphoron is of similar origin and composed of scattered rudimentary

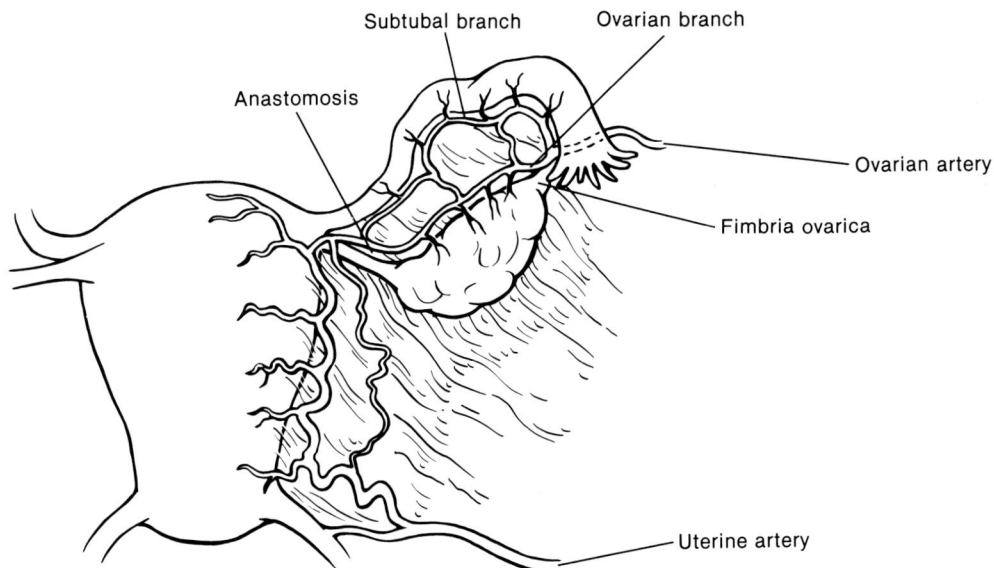

FIGURE 36–1. Vascular anatomy of the oviduct and ovary. Note cornual branch, subtubal vessels, and artery beside the fimbria ovarica. (From Hunt R. Atlas of Female Infertility Surgery. Chicago: Year Book, 1986.)

tubules also located in the broad ligament. In the fetus, the ovaries are located in the lumbar region near the kidneys and gradually descend into the pelvis.[5] In the adult, the ovary is composed of an outer cortical layer and inner stroma (Fig. 36–2). The latter is composed of connective tissue abundantly supplied with blood vessels. The former is composed of short connective tissue fibers with fusiform cells between (tunica albuginea).

PREMENARCHAL OVARY

Where does it all begin? Is a 46,XX genetic complement mandatory to have functional ovarian tissue? Sex determination most certainly is an active area of molecular biologic research and provides a host of new and intriguing data to enhance our understanding of ovarian physiology.

Continued investigation to determine the *testes-determining gene* in mammals is also an area of active research. In work published by McLaren,[5] a gene within a 35 kb region of the Y chromosome named the SRY gene was identified as the sex-determining region of the Y chromosome. It is not expressed in the developing ovary of mouse embryos, in which the testis-determining gene on the Y chromosome (Tdy) was known to be defective. SRY appears to be what is necessary to induce maleness. Development of the ovary may well be due to absence of the SRY gene apparatus.

Antenatal diagnosis of ovarian cysts can often prove to be a most challenging problem for the clinician as well as a source of significant anxiety for parents of the unborn child. In a retrospective study conducted by Garel and coworkers,[6] 29 ovarian cysts were identified in 27 patients over a 10-year period ending in 1990. The ovarian cysts were identified between 28 and 38 weeks of gestation. Ten of the infants ultimately underwent surgical treatment, eight immediately following birth and two at 5 and 7 months. All 10 cases revealed a benign histology consistent with a functional cyst;

however, torsion requiring oophorectomy occurred in six patients. In Garel's review of 257 patients in the literature, 69 cases of torsion were reported. The size of the cyst(s) and the ultrasonographic appearance are of paramount importance in clinical management.[7] Ovarian torsion occurs most often with ultrasonographic findings of fluid and debris, internal echos, and complex patterns. Serial ultrasonography appears to be most important in the continued evaluation and treatment decision making and prevention of unnecessary oophorectomy in this patient population. If the ovarian cyst is 4 cm or larger, the fetus becomes a candidate for percutaneous aspiration, especially in light of the concern for potential torsion of the adnexa.[8]

Follicular cysts have been reported in females aged 1 day to 17 years.[8] These cysts have been defined by Liapi and Evain-Brion[8] as ranging in diameter from 30 to 60 mm on ultrasonography; the cysts were all noted to "disappear" on follow-up ultrasonography. They may be associated with the onset of precocious pseudopuberty with premature thelarche. True precocious puberty results from reactivation of the hypothalamic-pituitary ovarian axis at the onset of thelarche (breast development) and adrenarche (pubic hair development), whereas precocious pseudopuberty results from extrapituitary secretion of gonadotropins or ovarian secretion of steroids independent of the pituitary axis. Abdominal pain may be an associated feature with ovarian cyst formation in the premenarchal age range. After 10 years of age, the primary presentation for an adnexal cystic mass is menstrual aberration or acute abdominal pain. In the series of 20 patients ranging from age 1 day to 17 years who were followed conservatively, 9 showed spontaneous disappearance of the ovarian cyst within 3 to 32 weeks.[9] Each patient in the series was noted to have a follicular cyst. Oophorectomy was necessary in eight patients because of torsion of a large adnexal mass; in seven, laparotomy was performed primarily out of concern for the underlying pathology. Ovarian cystectomy occurred in the remaining three patients. In general, a patho-

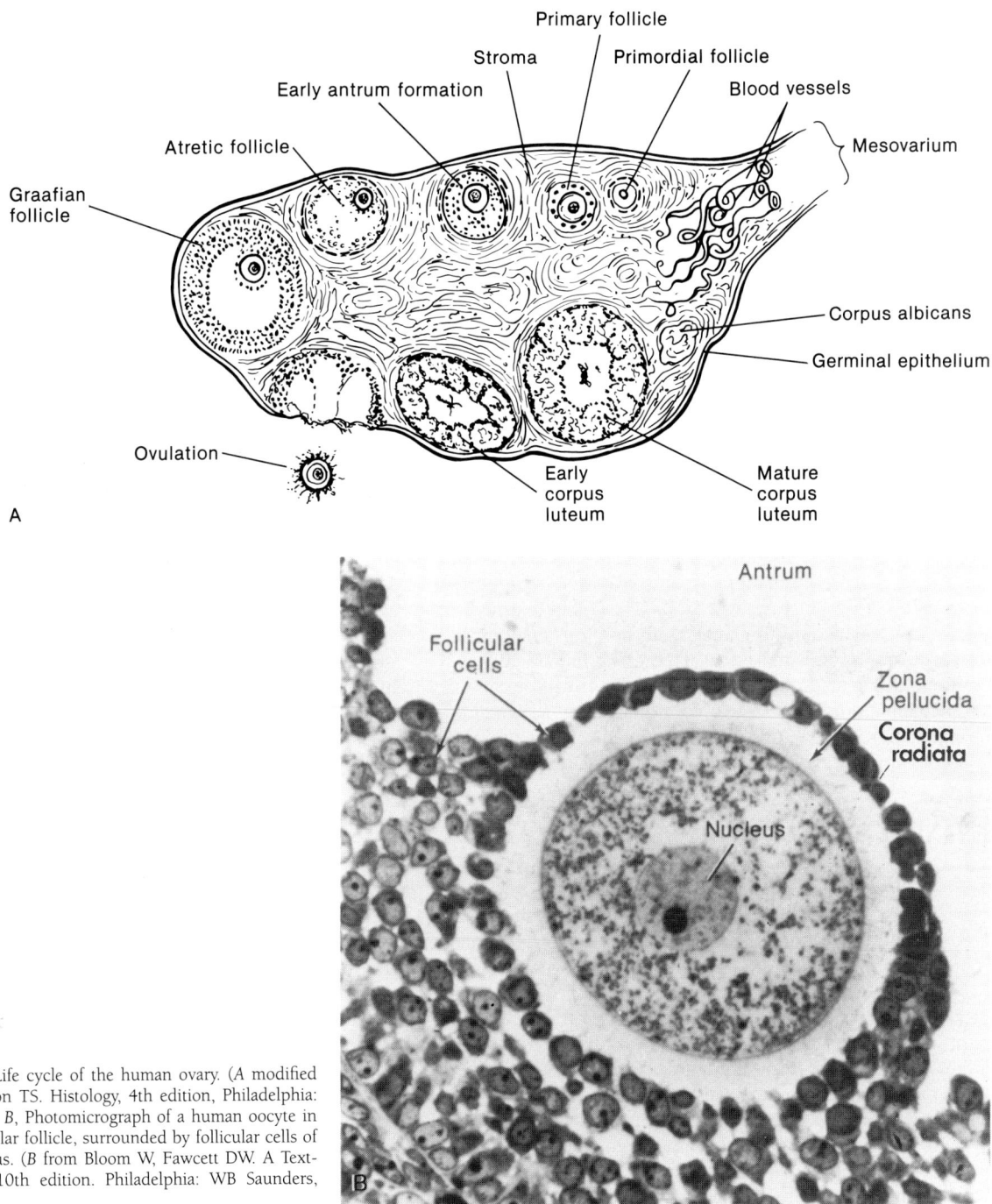

FIGURE 36-2. *A*, Life cycle of the human ovary. (*A* modified from Ham AW, Leeson TS. Histology, 4th edition, Philadelphia: JB Lippincott, 1968.) *B*, Photomicrograph of a human oocyte in a secondary or vesicular follicle, surrounded by follicular cells of the cumulus oophorus. (*B* from Bloom W, Fawcett DW. A Textbook of Histology, 10th edition. Philadelphia: WB Saunders, 1975.)

logic cyst was thought to be associated with a nonechogenic area 20 mm or larger. If the cyst is 55 mm or smaller, spontaneous resolution usually occurs.[9]

The formation of polycystic ovaries (PCO) in the premenarchal female is an intriguing phenomenon. PCO has been reported in a premenarchal girl of age 12 who presented with an abdominal-pelvic mass and virilization.[10] This large ovarian cyst was removed at laparotomy. Histologic diagnosis identified no evidence of an androgen-secreting tumor, and both ovaries had a polycystic appearance.

Gonadotropin-independent precocious (pseudoprecocious) puberty is associated with an ovarian source of hormone production; associated ovarian cysts and neoplasms

have been reported with this entity. Of special interest is the McCune-Albright syndrome because it is currently believed that the initial nidus for significant estrogen production begins at the ovarian level.[11]

The role of ultrasonography in management of ovarian masses in children has been reported by Thind and coworkers.[12] In a retrospective study, 16 female patients with ovarian cysts and neoplasms were evaluated over a 4-year period. Most ovarian cysts were benign, and conservative management with serial ultrasonography appeared to be appropriate. This population with cystic ovaries did not require surgical intervention. It was re-emphasized that, if there is a palpable, solid mass, a tissue diagnosis is mandatory. Masses associated with calcification demand a tissue diagnosis as well as masses associated with persistent pyrexia.

Ovarian dysgenesis primarily appears to correlate with a chromosomal abnormality. Turner's syndrome—45,X—trisomy 13, and trisomy 18 are the more common causes clinically encountered. In work published by Cuniff and coworkers,[13] all infants in the reported series were trisomies 13 or 18. Triploidy and 45,X were found to have a severe ovarian dysgenesis characterized by absence of primary oocytes.[13] In contrast, trisomy 21 patients as well as those with partial deletion or duplication of one other autosome demonstrated variable numbers of oocytes ranging from complete absence to a mild decrease in total oocyte number. The authors concluded that the attrition of germ cells in chromosomally abnormal infants is the result of faulty meiotic pairing and that perhaps ovarian dysgenesis is a more frequent finding in children with karyotype abnormalities than has been previously considered.

We now live in an age in which assisted reproductive technology is available for an individual with ovarian dysgenesis, enabling a woman to carry a child to term with use of ovum donation. In vitro fertilization and embryo transfer and gamete and zygote intrafallopian transfer have been reported in women with premature ovarian failure.[14] The treatment of infertility in agonadal individuals with chromosomal aberrations remains promising, especially as technologic advances continue to be made. In general, estradiol and progesterone supplementation allows one to coordinate the menstrual cycles and appropriately prepare the recipient uterine endometrium for implantation.

ENLARGED PREMENOPAUSAL OVARY

Evaluation and treatment of adnexal masses in reproductive-aged women set the stage for a plethora of viewpoints among gynecologic surgeons. When patients desire maximal reproductive function, the management of adnexal masses becomes even more delicate. The value of conservative surgical approaches must be weighed against the risks of malignant neoplasms and reduction of fecundity secondary to adhesion formation from any surgical procedure. Still there are a number of pathologic conditions of the ovary in which surgical approaches improve future fertility.

Before surgical assessment is undertaken, appropriate medical treatment and evaluation should be initiated. Transvaginal ultrasonography is rapidly becoming the standard of care in characterizing adnexal masses. The presence or absence of loculations, septations, solid components, and echogenic patterns of cystic fluid may aid the clinician in determining the nature of the adnexal mass. Specific dimensions of adnexal masses can also be obtained. Although the ideal screening marker for ovarian malignancy has yet to be elucidated, when ovarian malignancy is suspected, appropriate tumor markers (e.g., CA-125) should be obtained. Their limitations, however, should be kept in mind.

The management of adnexal cysts continues to evolve. Many have suggested hormonal ovarian suppression, such as with oral contraceptives, as the ideal method of inducing resolution of functional cysts.[15, 16] Despite lack of prospective, controlled studies to document the efficacy of this approach, this treatment seems to have become an accepted clinical practice. It is generally accepted that hormonal treatment does prevent formation of new functional ovarian cyst(s),[17] but there remains little evidence that these medications help resolve cysts that are already present. Work by Steinkampf and colleagues[18] demonstrated no improvement in the resolution of functional cysts induced with clomiphene citrate therapy by treatment with hormone suppression over those patients treated with observation alone.

A persistent adnexal mass in a premenopausal woman that has not responded to observation should have a tissue diagnosis. Consensus with respect to type of surgical approach is changing from laparotomy to laparoscopy, but the clinician must comply with guidelines.[19] Parker and Berek[20] have suggested preoperative ultrasonic criteria for laparoscopic management of cystic masses: less than 10 cm in diameter, distinct borders; no irregular or solid segment, thick septi, ascites, or matted bowel; and a normal CA-125. Diagnostic laparoscopy is then performed, allowing careful inspection of all pelvic organs. The tumor surface and presence or absence of adhesions and ascites are evaluated, and cyst fluid is aspirated and cytologically assessed. Cystectomy or removal of the cyst lining is carried out as outlined in the following section. If cystectomy cannot be performed, multiple biopsy specimens of the cyst wall (particularly any thickened areas) should be obtained. Further laparoscopic treatment of the mass, if necessary, follows when there is no evidence of malignancy.

The risk of ovarian malignancy should always be of concern to the physician and discussed with patients preoperatively. Review of the literature[21–23] suggests the risk of malignancy in a unilocular persistent ovarian mass, 10 cm or less, is approximately 2 to 3 per 1000 ovarian masses. Many oncologists remain concerned over the potential risk of poor prognosis after rupture of a cyst with ovarian carcinoma. Published work in 1973 did suggest a poorer prognosis if tumor rupture occurs intraoperatively[24]; subsequent studies by Dembo and coworkers,[25] however, clearly demonstrate that tumor rupture at laparotomy is not a significant predictor of survival rates. They noted grade of tumor, presence or absence of ascites, and significant tumor adherence to be of paramount importance as predictors of survival, whereas cyst rupture had little if any effect.[25] A similar study of the impact of rupture at laparoscopy has not yet been reported.

The advantages of the laparoscopic approach to ovarian surgery are several: It is usually an outpatient procedure, and when performed by a skilled laparoscopic surgeon is associated with a shorter recovery time, has lower total cost, and has fewer postoperative adhesions.[26, 27] Every operative laparoscopist, however, must be cognizant of his or her own abilities in pelviscopic surgery.[28]

SPECIFIC SURGICAL TECHNIQUES

A Word of Caution

This chapter emphasizes the operative laparoscopic approach, while the reader is referred to a number of well-established textbooks for details of the techniques of ovarian surgery. Technologic advances have allowed the gynecologic surgeon to approach many ovarian lesions endoscopically that traditionally were performed via laparotomy. Particularly in the case of the infertile patient, laparoscopy has become the procedure of choice for evaluation and treatment of the adnexal mass. Specific guidelines for laparoscopic ovarian surgery, however, have not been clearly defined, and poor preoperative assessment or patient selection may result in an inappropriate procedure and poor results. All patients who undergo laparoscopy for an adnexal mass should have preoperative sonographic evaluation. In addition, depending on the patient's age, as in the postmenopausal patient, CA-125 should be obtained. In the pediatric age group, human chorionic gonadotropin (hCG) and alpha-fetoprotein should be obtained. In the premenopausal patient, a confounding factor involves the fact that an elevation of CA-125 may be associated with endometriosis, acute pelvic inflammatory disease, or liver disease.[29] Clinical judgment must be used in the decision for a laparoscopic versus laparotomic approach. In either case, peritoneal washings should be obtained, the pelvis and upper abdomen should be explored, and any abnormal areas should be evaluated by biopsy. When any ovarian mass with external excrescences or suspicion for malignancy is discovered at laparoscopy, a laparotomy is indicated.

Cystectomy via Endoscopy

Many benign ovarian cysts may theoretically interfere with fertility by disruption of ovulation and ovum release; therefore associated fecundity should be improved after cystectomy. The goal of surgery is to remove the cyst while leaving as much functionally normal ovarian tissue as possible. An endoscopic approach may be preferred to reduce overall de novo adhesion formation, patient cost, and postoperative recovery time.[30] Endometriosis, mature teratomas, and benign adenomas currently constitute the majority of neoplasms that can be extirpated endoscopically.

Aspiration of the ovarian cyst should be undertaken initially. The ovary is held securely with an atraumatic grasping forceps, or alternatively the ovarian ligament is grasped and rotated to allow full visualization of the cyst. A fine needle attached to a syringe is inserted into the cyst with negative pressure on the syringe (Fig. 36–3), allowing aspiration of cyst fluid for cytologic evaluation. Subsequently a coagula-

tion system such as a unipolar needle or laser can be used to open the cyst, while having the suction-irrigator immediately available for placement into the cyst cavity. Care should be taken to minimize spillage of cyst contents. When the thick sebaceous content of a mature teratoma is encountered, copious amounts of irrigation (patient in reverse Trendelenburg position) on completion of the cystectomy is advisable. Ideally the cyst (or teratoma) is excised intact and can be placed in a pouch (e.g., Endopouch, Ethicon Inc., Somerville, NJ) and removed without spillage.

If the cyst is aspirated, however, the lining usually can be stripped from the ovary. The cyst opening is enlarged and the ovarian cortex grasped with a forceps at the edge of the incision. The cyst lining is then grasped with a second forceps so a traction-countertraction technique allows stripping of the cyst lining from the ovarian bed (Fig. 36–4). Often blunt dissection and hydrodissection (with a suction-irrigator) aids in completely excising the cyst wall. Occasionally it may be technically impossible to remove the entire cyst wall completely. In this circumstance, ablation of the adherent cyst wall with laser or electrocautery is recommended to prevent recurrence. Every effort to remove or ablate the cyst wall should be undertaken to decrease recurrence (Table 36–1). Once the cyst wall has been removed, the specimen is histologically evaluated; if it is at all suspicious for malignancy, a frozen section should be obtained.

Next all bleeding areas on the ovarian bed should be identified and controlled. Hemostasis usually can be obtained with laser ablation in a defocused mode for small capillary sites or electrocautery for larger bleeding areas. Once hemostasis is obtained, repair of the ovarian defect may be undertaken. The edges of the ovarian incision can be reapproximated with sutures (endoscopically). If the edges are in close proximity, however, suturing is not recommended. Preliminary data concerning second-look laparoscopy after cystectomy suggests that repair of the ovarian defect is rarely necessary because the ovary heals spontaneously and with decreased adhesion formation than when suturing is performed.[30, 31]

The presence of an ovarian cyst in the form of an endometrioma deserves further discussion. Work by Fayez and Vogel[32] compared four techniques of managing large *chocolate*

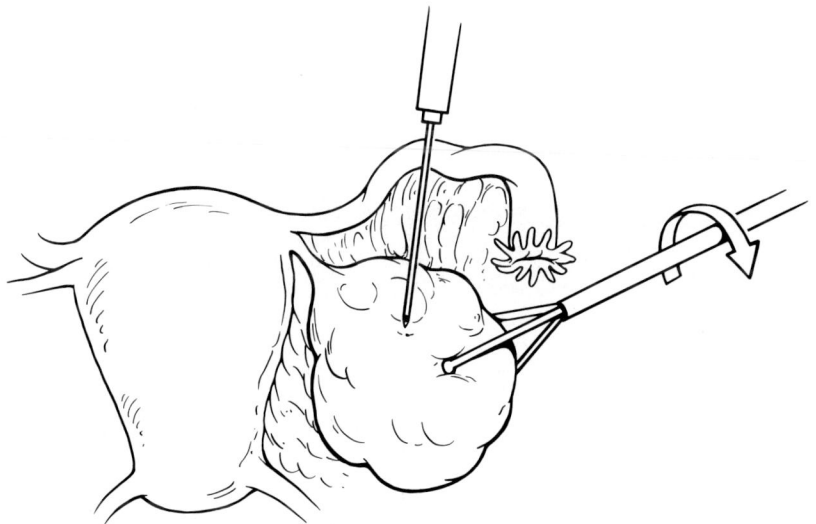

FIGURE 36–3. Fine-needle aspiration of ovarian cyst. (Modified from Hasson HM. Ovarian surgery. In: Sanfilippo JS, Levine RL, editors. Operative Gynecologic Endoscopy. New York: Springer-Verlag, 1989.)

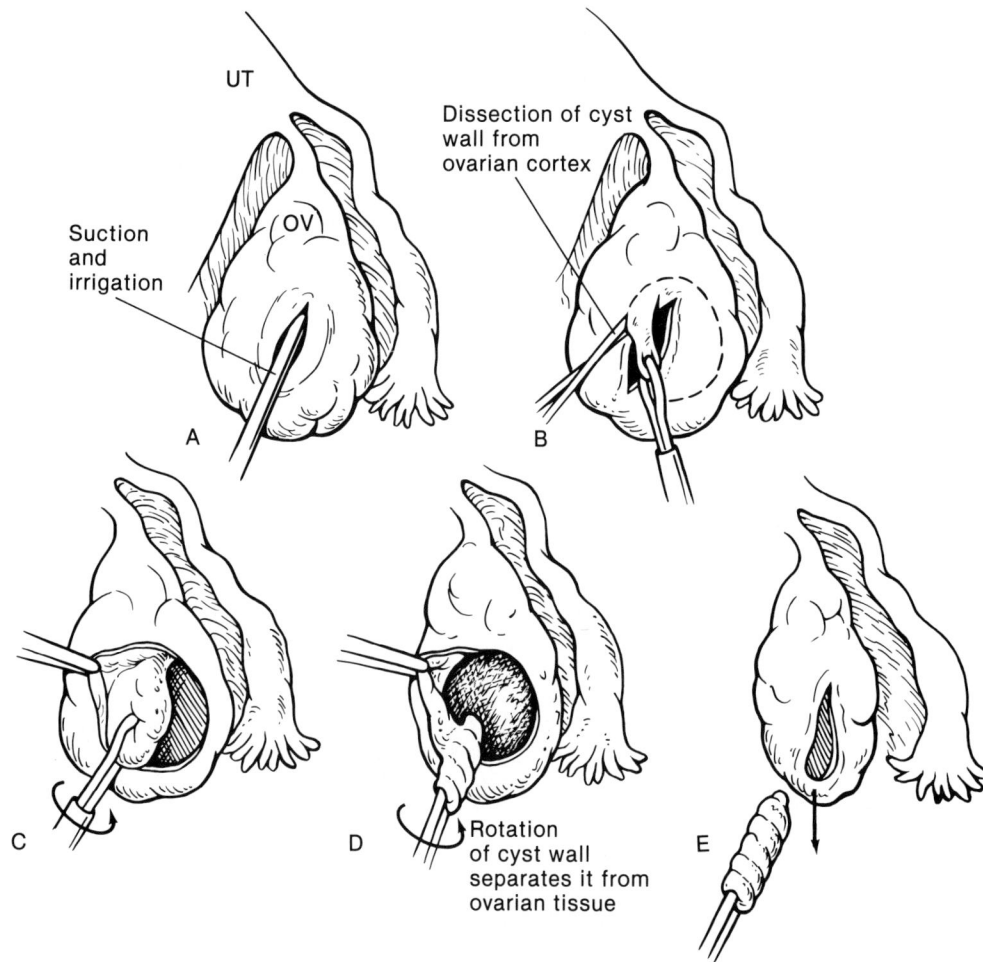

FIGURE 36–4. Removal of a small ovarian endometrial cyst through the laparoscope. *A*, After incision of the ovarian cortex, the contents of the endometrioma are removed with suction and irrigation. Ut, uterus; Ov, ovary. *B*, The plane between the ovary and the cyst wall is developed by using traction and twisting the forceps clockwise. *C*, The endometrial cyst wall is grasped with forceps. *D*, The cyst wall separates from the ovarian tissue using a twisting motion. The ovarian defect may be left open to heal by second intention or be closed with vertical mattress sutures. *E*, The cyst wall is removed. (*A* to *E* modified from Rock JA. Surgery for benign disease of the ovary. In: Thompson JD, Rock JA, editors. Te Linde's Operative Gynecology, 7th edition. Philadelphia: JB Lippincott, 1991:450.)

cysts laparoscopically, including complete excision, stripping of the lining, laser ablation (of the lining), or simple incision and drainage. Patients subsequently underwent second-look laparoscopy. The complete excision group was noted to have a significant increase in pelvic adhesions in all patients versus a 21% to 22% adhesion formation rate in the remaining categories. The authors suggested that incision and drainage may be preferred because this technique is simple and involves less tissue destruction. Histologic sections of endometriomas usually are composed of fibrous tissue and show no evidence of active endometrial implants; thus the authors concluded that removal was not necessary and may be detrimental. Still the possibility of carcinoma, albeit rare, must be considered, and a specimen for histologic evaluation should

be obtained. In the Fayez and Vogel series,[32] all patients received preoperative and postoperative ovarian suppression, and the incidence of recurrence of endometriomas at 8 weeks was not different (22% for stripping versus 21% for drainage). Long-term risks of recurrence, however, may be higher for drainage only as suggested by Hasson.[33] Until better data exist, we do not endorse simple drainage. We believe tissue diagnosis in the form of stripping the cyst lining or ovarian biopsy is required for histologic diagnosis.

Oophorectomy via Endoscopy

Oophorectomy in the infertile patient is rarely indicated, but the patient with chronic pelvic pain secondary to ovarian pelvic adhesions and endometriosis or in whom ovarian function is compromised may benefit from oophorectomy to prevent further adhesion formation.[34] Two methods of oophorectomy have been described for endoscopic procedures. Semm and Mettler[35] developed a loop ligation method involving placement of three pretied synthetic sutures (e.g., Endoloops, Ethicon, Inc.) over the ovarian pedicle (Fig. 36–5). Once the ligatures are securely in place, the pedicle is cut free and the tissue morcellated. The ovarian pedicle may be cauterized to ensure hemostasis if bleeding occurs.

The second method of oophorectomy involves separate identification, coagulation, and division of the infundibulo-

TABLE 36–1. Pelviscopic Surgical Treatment of Ovarian Endometriomas with and without Removal or Coagulation of the Cyst Lining

Treatment	Total No. of Patients	Pregnancy Occurred	Endometrioma Recurred
Fenestration with removal or ablation of cyst wall	13	5/5	1/13
Fenestration without removal or ablation of cyst wall	9	2/5	8/9

From Hasson HM: Ovarian surgery. In: Sanfilippo JS, Levine RL, editors. Operative Gynecologic Endoscopy. New York: Springer-Verlag, 1989:99.

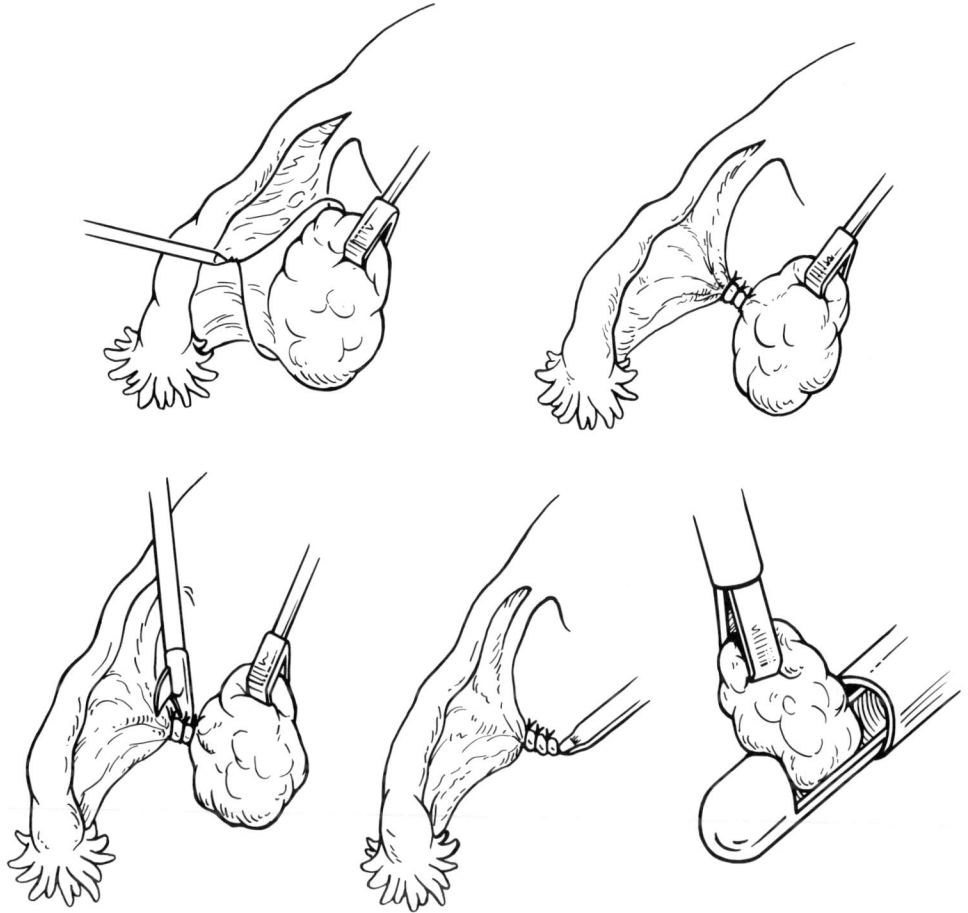

FIGURE 36–5. Oophorectomy using the three-ligature technique. After the ligatures are applied, the ovary is cut free, the stump is endo-coagulated, and the tissue is morcellated. (Modified from Levine RL. Instrumentation. In: Sanfilippo JS, Levine RL, editors. Operative Gynecologic Endoscopy. New York: Springer-Verlag, 1989.)

pelvic and utero-ovarian ligaments. As described by Reich,[36] bipolar electrocautery is used for hemostatic control of the ovarian and utero-ovarian vasculature before transection; the ovary can then be removed. Either technique is acceptable when the patient requires oophorectomy.

As previously noted, the Endopouch has been designed to reduce spillage of ovarian contents at oophorectomy via endoscopy (Fig. 36–6). The pouch can be placed through a second puncture site and the intact ovary freed and inserted into the pouch. The pouch can then be removed.

ADHESIOLYSIS

Adhesions within the pelvis and particularly around the ovary frequently are the result of an inflammatory process, which may be secondary to endometriosis, previous surgery, or infection. Ovarian adhesions interfere with ovum release and fallopian tube capture of the ovum. Adhesiolysis is best accomplished by first placing tension on all adhesions to visualize and characterize the nature of the lesions. Postinfectious adhesions are frequently thin and avascular and can be

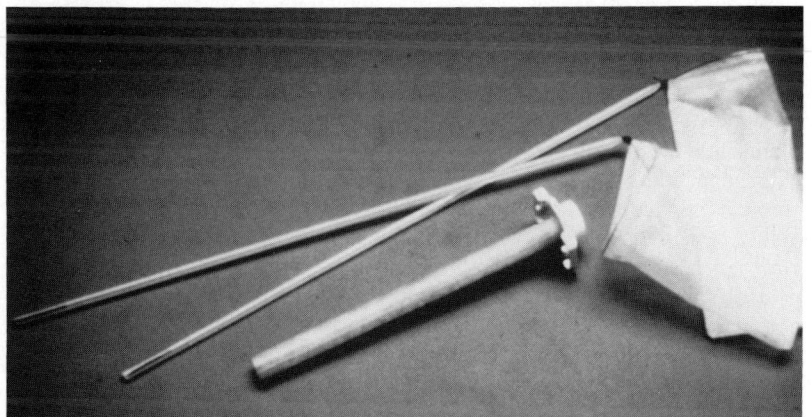

FIGURE 36–6. Endopouch. (Courtesy of Ethicon, Inc., Somerville, NJ.)

lysed with sharp scissors and blunt dissection. Postoperative adhesions usually are more dense and vascular, requiring hemostasis with coagulation before transection. The adhesion should be excised instead of transected, but this is not always feasible. Bowel or omental adhesions to the ovary present a more difficult challenge and should be endoscopically lysed with extreme caution.

A thorough knowledge of the anatomy of the fallopian tube and ovary is a prerequisite for laparoscopic adhesiolysis. One should avoid transection of the fimbria ovarica because this frequently results in bleeding and subsequent adhesion formation. The ureter runs in close approximation to the ovarian fossa, and adhesions on the posterior aspect of the ovary, as for example with endometriosis, may distort the normal anatomy predisposing to ureteral injury.[37]

As described by Cook and Rock,[34] laparoscopic lysis of adhesions must be a meticulous, delicate process with minimal trauma to the tissue and complete hemostasis. Technical difficulties may arise owing to limitations of the surgical field in laparoscopy as well as inability to palpate tissue. When vital structures involving the adhesion complex cannot be clearly identified before dissection, laparotomy is indicated. Second-look laparoscopy appears to play an increasing role in preventing postoperative adhesions.[38]

ENDOMETRIOSIS INVOLVING THE OVARY

The ideal approach to surgical management of endometriosis (in the absence of an endometrioma) continues to stir controversy. Haney[39] has challenged the concept of improved fecundity with any type of surgical treatment of minimal or mild stages of endometriosis. Well-controlled prospective studies to demonstrate improved pregnancy rates after medical (danazol, GnRH analog, oral contraceptives) or surgical (coagulation laser or excision) therapy is clearly needed.[40] Some researchers believe surgical intervention does improve pregnancy rates, even in minimal or mild stages.[41] Still others state that although endometriosis is a progressive disease, its mild form does not cause infertility. Therefore they believe that asymptomatic infertility patients may delay surgery until endometriosis becomes symptomatic.[42] An attempt at surgical therapy when endometriosis is diagnosed at laparoscopy is frequently pursued in the infertile patient, but one should be cognizant of the paucity of information proving increased fecundity.

When endometriosis is diagnosed as moderate or severe with possible mechanical obstruction of ovum release, surgical intervention appears appropriate. The techniques of ovarian cystectomy for endometriomas and ovarian adhesiolysis have been conveyed. When ectopic endometrial implants are identified, they may be treated by a variety of surgical techniques. Laparoscopy offers a feasible approach to surgical treatment, but laparotomy still has a place when the ability to dissect between tissue planes safely is lost or the clinician has limited pelviscopic experience.[34] The primary goal of surgical intervention is to remove both typical and atypical (clear and polypoid appearing) implants completely.[43] The goal can be accomplished with cautery, laser, or excision, with little apparent advantage to any one method. The deeper the implant, the more active the disease.[43] The

most deeply penetrating lesions are frequently associated with pain.[44] Whether the implant is removed by an energy source (electrocautery, electrocoagulation, or laser) or by excision, removal of the entire implant is recommended.

POLYCYSTIC OVARIAN SYNDROME

PCO, as first described (1935), encompasses a heterogenicity of symptoms associated with oligomenorrhea, hirsutism, obesity, and bilateral polycystic ovaries.[44] The variability of clinical presentations of PCO is emphasized in Table 36–2. The patient with PCO-like symptoms should be distinguished from other individuals with hirsutism and anovulation, such as patients with Cushing's syndrome, adult-onset congenital adrenal hyperplasia, ovarian or adrenal neoplasms, hyperprolactinemia, hyperthyroidism, and hypothyroidism.[44]

Intense investigation of the pathophysiology of PCO continues to reveal new concepts in the cause of this disease process. The precise cause initiating PCO remains unclear to this day. Rosenfield and associates[45] have focused on enzymatic defects in the adrenal and an exaggerated activation of 17,20-lyase and 17α-hydroxylase enzymatic activity. The cytochrome P-450 gene encodes these enzyme activities, and aberrant regulation of the gene may initiate PCO.[45] Adrenocorticotropic hormone (ACTH) stimulation after adrenal suppression results in hyperresponsiveness of adrenal androgen precursors.[46] Insulin resistance plays a key role in the development of PCO, and hyperinsulinemia, in turn, can result in decreased sex hormone–binding globulin, which is noted in PCO patients. Obesity, particularly centripetal, results in increased estrogens, androgens, and gonadotropins.[48] Whether obesity per se is an initiating or confounding element continues to be a subject of debate.

Regardless of the cause, the hallmark of PCO includes elevation of excess androgens and their precursor(s).[49] A detailed discussion of the intricate role of exaggerated GnRH release, ovarian growth factor proteins, decreased sex hormone–binding globulin, insulin, and insulin receptor defects is beyond the scope of this chapter, but the ultimate elevation of luteinizing hormone pulsatile release and intraovarian increase in androgens results in a chronic anovulatory state.

Before surgical management of PCO in the infertile patient is proposed, all medical modalities should be explored. Clo-

TABLE 36–2. Frequency of Clinical Manifestations of Proven Cases of Polycystic Ovary Syndrome (N = 1079)

Symptoms	Frequency (%)	
	Mean	Range
Obesity	41	16–49
Hirsutism	69	17–83
Virilization	21	0–28
Amenorrhea	51	15–77
Infertility	74	35–94
Functional bleeding	29	6–65
Biphasic basal temperature	15	12–40
Corpus luteum at operation	22	0–71

From Goldzieher JW, Green JA. The polycystic ovary: I. Clinical and histologic features. J Clin Endocrinol Metab 1962;22(Mar):325–338. © The Endocrine Society.

miphene citrate, an antiestrogen, is a well-established successful modality of treatment for inducing ovulation.[50] If clomiphene therapy alone fails to induce ovulation, addition of 0.5 mg dexamethasone may be considered if there is evidence for increased adrenal androgen production (increased dehydroepiandrosterone or its sulfate).[51, 52] Other researchers have shown that the addition of cyclic medroxyprogesterone acetate, 10 mg orally for 10 days, or progesterone, 50 mg intramuscularly for 5 days, may initiate ovulation in clomiphene-failure patients.[53, 54] Human menopausal gonadotropins have been successful in inducing ovulation and pregnancy, but the incidence of hyperstimulation in PCO patients is substantial.[55] Pulsatile administration of gonadotropin-releasing hormone is also successful in inducing ovulation in this patient population but only after the pituitary has been down-regulated with GnRH agonists.[56]

Once all attempts at medical management have been exhausted and there is continued failure to ovulate, surgical options may prove appropriate. Reports vary, but resumption of permanent ovulatory cycles (80% to 90%) and pregnancy rates (60%) are well described.[57] The risk of postoperative adhesion formation, however, has led to infrequent use of the classic wedge resection.[58, 59]

With the advent of laparoscopy, Gjonnaess[60] and others[3] have confirmed resumption of ovulation after electrocoagulation of cystic follicles in patients with PCO. Multiple points (5 to 20) 3 to 5 mm in diameter are cauterized along the ovarian cortex at the time of laparoscopy (Fig. 36–7). In a similar manner, multiple ovarian biopsies with resultant partial ovarian resection have produced successful results by Campo and associates[3] and Hasson.[33] Daniell and Miller[61] reported a series of 85 anovulatory patients treated by laparoscopic laser vaporization of multiple points on the ovary resulting in 100% ovulation rate and 58% pregnancy rate. A summary of the data is provided in Table 36–3.

Concern over postoperative adhesion formation even after a laparoscopic surgical approach in PCO patients relegates surgical therapy to those patients who fail to ovulate with medical management. Future studies on the long-term risks of pelvic adhesions and reduced fecundity currently must be

TABLE 36–3. Indication for Laser Laparoscopy in PCOD Patients	
Indication	**No. of Patients**
Failure to conceive after 6 months or more of ovulatory cycles on CC	47
Failure to ovulate on CC 150 mg plus hCG	38
Total	85

PCOD, polycystic ovary disease; CC, clomiphene citrate; hCG, human chorionic gonadotropin.

Adapted from Daniell JF, Miller W: Polycystic ovaries treated by laparoscopic laser vaporization. Fertil Steril 1989;51:232. Reprinted with permission of the publisher, The American Fertility Society.

evaluated as the role of second-look laparoscopy continues to evolve.

OVARIAN BIOPSY

The indications for ovarian biopsy in the infertile patient are relatively few and generally reserved for patients with developmental abnormalities or suspicious ovarian lesions. The benefit of biopsy from an otherwise anatomically normal-appearing ovary must be weighed against the risks of adhesion formation and hemorrhage. If ovarian biopsies are to be performed, the hilar region should be avoided because of the risk of hemorrhage.

Depending on the clinical circumstances, the primary amenorrheic infertility patient may be a candidate for ovarian biopsy. Evaluation of this tissue can help determine the presence of a mosaic Y chromosome not identified in peripheral blood, thus requiring gonadectomy. The presence of elevated gonadotropins with primordial follicles in ovarian stroma on biopsy is indicative of the gonadotropin-resistant ovary syndrome, and some researchers state that ovarian biopsy may be diagnostic as well as therapeutic.[62]

As previously discussed, the ovarian biopsy specimen is best obtained during an endoscopic procedure. The ovary is held securely with an atraumatic forceps (Fig. 36–8). A variety of endoscopic biopsy forceps can be used, allowing an adequate specimen to be obtained. Occasionally the ovarian cortex is difficult to penetrate or puncture. Bleeding can be a problem, but usually electrocautery is sufficient to achieve hemostasis. Rarely, endoscopic suturing is required to control bleeding. The risk of adhesions and hemorrhage must again be emphasized, so unnecessary biopsies should be avoided.

MANAGEMENT OF OVARIAN ECTOPIC PREGNANCY

Ovarian ectopic pregnancy is a rare event estimated to occur in 1 in 3600 to 7000 deliveries.[63, 64] Diagnostic criteria include (1) the fallopian tube intact and clearly separate from the ovary, (2) the gestational sac occupying the normal position of the ovary, (3) the sac connected to the uterus by the utero-ovarian ligament, and (4) ovarian tissue demonstrated in the wall of the sac. The presence of an intrauterine device may increase the incidence of ovarian ectopic pregnancy.[64]

At present, laparotomy and ovarian wedge resection ap-

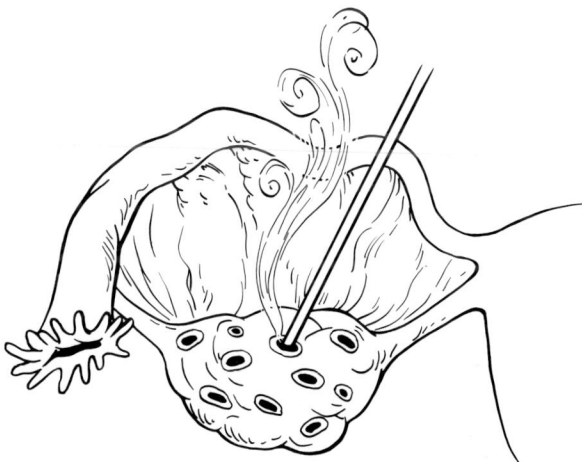

FIGURE 36–7. Vaporizing defects in the cortex of the ovary with the CO_2 laser for treatment of polycystic ovarian disease. (Reprinted from Female Patient: Vol. 14; 1989, [pgs. 69–83].)

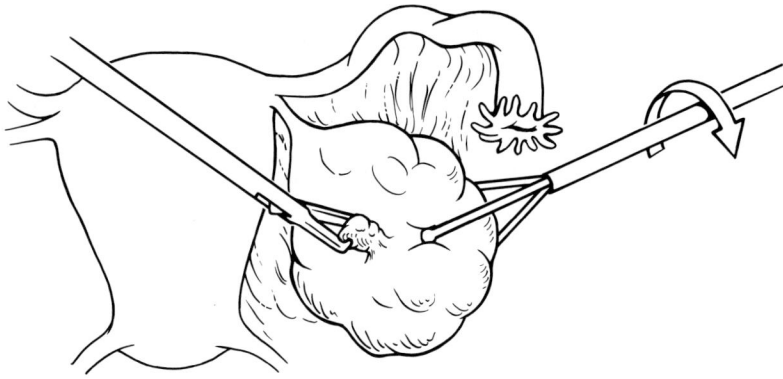

FIGURE 36–8. Ovarian biopsy. (Modified from Hasson HM. Ovarian surgery. In: Sanfilippo JS, Levine RL, editors. Operative Gynecologic Endoscopy. New York: Springer-Verlag, 1989.)

pear to be the standard of care, but inevitably a laparoscopic approach may be feasible. The ovary can be preserved by a conservative resection of the hemorrhagic portion, and rarely is oophorectomy necessary except for the case of severe hemorrhage. Hemoperitoneum and large blood loss, however, are frequently reported, and rapid surgical intervention is advised.[63]

ADNEXAL TORSION

Traditional teaching has recommended that when a diagnosis of torsed adnexa is established, oophorectomy should be performed out of concern for dislodging a thrombotic embolus by "untwisting" the adnexa. In a review of the literature, however, there were "no reported cases of a thrombotic embolus arising from the untwisted adnexa and thus, supportive of conservation of the adnexa rather than routine extirpation (except when necrotic) is the preferred method of treatment."[65] Thus the clinician perhaps has alternatives with respect to management of adnexal torsion. In one other study, representing a 35-year retrospective review of children with an ovarian lesion requiring surgical intervention, 21 of 51 children were noted to have unilateral ovarian torsion. The focus of the report was on adnexal torsion. Five of the torsed ovaries were microscopically normal. It was recommended that contralateral oophoropexy be performed when dealing with unilateral torsion.[66] Theoretically the process of torsion can be aborted by ovarian cystectomy.[67] In our experience, conservation of the ovary is most feasible in the patient who desires preservation of her childbearing capability and when there is evidence of viability of the adnexa with correction of the torsion. Oophoropexy ought to be considered if either adnexa is associated with a long suspensory ligament in an effort to prevent subsequent torsion.

Why torsion occurs is an interesting question. Evidence for excessive mobility secondary to congenitally long supportive ligaments has been reported.[68] Oophoropexy or shortening of the ligamentous support of the remaining functional ovary after torsion is recommended in an attempt to prevent subsequent torsion. It is possible that torsed edematous ovarian tissue may "convert" to a nonviable necrotic tissue, necessitating oophorectomy. Thus, careful postoperative follow-up is most important when a conservative approach is rendered. Endoscopic "unwinding" of a torsed ischemic hemorrhagic adnexa has been reported by Ben-Rafael and coworkers.[68] The authors conclude that laparoscopic "detorsion of ische-

mic adnexa is feasible." Subsequent oocyte formation occurred without damage secondary to the torsion of the ovary as noted on ultrasound study. Thus the conservative approach should be considered in women during their reproductive years and in every case in which malignancy can be ruled out. An additional 35 cases of laparoscopic management of adnexal torsion have been reported.[69] Early diagnosis and treatment appear to be most efficacious when a conservative approach is planned. Pelvic calcification and autoamputation of the adnexa has been reported in the adolescent.[70] Specifically the involved ovary was noted to have endometriosis on the cortex, and pelvic calcification and autoamputation of the involved right adnexa occurred.

Adnexal torsion has been noted in the neonate as the result of antenatal or neonatal ultrasonic assessment of ovarian cysts. Ovarian cysts are indeed a common incidental finding in term infants and can be large with associated dystocia, torsion, or rupture.[71, 72] Twelve neonates with ultrasound evidence of ovarian torsion were explored at 4 to 16 days of age.[71, 72] Ovarian torsion was confined to the right side in all patients.[73]

As stated, in the pediatric-aged group, adnexal torsion is rare and usually occurs on the right (84% of the time).[73] Normal adnexa can be involved with torsion (13 of 19 patients) as well as with adnexa involved in cyst formation (6 of 19). Indeed, *detorsion* with recovery of vascularization has been reported.[73] Most patients tend to present with lower abdominal pain of sudden onset. Of interest is that the average duration between first symptom and actual hospital admission is 5.2 days, with a mean delay of 30.2 hours between consultation and surgical intervention.[73] Eighty-four percent of patients in the pediatric age group with adnexal torsion present with nausea or vomiting accompanying the abdominal pain. A mass is palpable abdominally in only 42% of the patients.[73] Ultrasonography tends to be most instrumental in suspecting the diagnosis.

Conservative management of adnexal torsion in the adult should be considered intraoperatively. Laparoscopy is useful both for diagnosis and for treatment, but laparotomy can be undertaken if ideal conditions for operative laparoscopy do not exist. Once adnexal torsion is diagnosed, the organs are gently "untwisted" to assess ischemic lesions so further management can be decided on (Fig. 36–9). Gangrenous adnexa are not candidates for conservative treatment, and radical therapy should occur. Adnexa with no evidence of ischemia or with complete recovery of mildly ischemic lesions can be treated conservatively. The cause of the torsion is ascertained

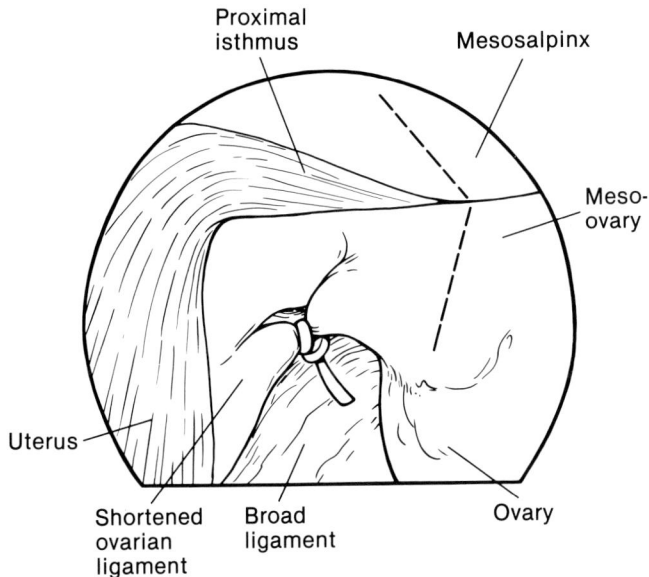

FIGURE 36–9. Laparoscopy for adnexal torsion. Initial laparoscopy: the uterine cornu and ovarian ligament after placement of the endosuture. The axis of torsion runs traversely, immediately lateral to the suture. This axis has been "broken" (*broken line*) by shortening of the ovarian ligament. (Modified from Vancaillie T, Schmidt EH. Recovery of ovarian function after laparoscopic treatment of acute adnexal torsion: a case report. J Reprod Med 1987: 32[7]:561.)

and subsequent treatment carried out. As previously stated, ovarian cysts and adnexal adhesions are frequent causes of torsion and should be treated via cystectomy and adhesiolysis as previously described. Congenitally aberrant attachments of the ovary can also result in torsion, and oophoropexy should be performed if recurrent torsion seems likely.

MANAGEMENT OF THE ECTOPIC OVARY AND OVARIAN REMNANT

The ectopic ovary was first reported in a stillborn female.[74] It has also been termed the *accessory ovary* and the *supernumerary ovary*. The latter two terms are quite imprecise, and perhaps the best terminology is that of *ovarian implants*. Under most circumstances, no specific management is indicated, but when identified, they should be documented in the operative report. Furthermore, neoplasms such as Brenner tumor have been reported in association with ectopic ovaries.[75] Indeed, neoplasms in ectopic ovaries are a rare phenomenon. The clinician must be cognizant that ectopic ovaries (accessory ovaries) are frequently small and often overlooked during definitive gynecologic surgical procedures, including diagnostic laparoscopy.

The ovarian remnant syndrome occurs in a patient who has had previous bilateral salpingo-oophorectomy; a segment of ovarian tissue remains to become associated with pelvic pain and not uncommonly dyspareunia. The ovarian remnant syndrome must be distinguished from the residual ovary syndrome, the latter in which ovaries were intentionally conserved during the prior surgical procedure. It often proves difficult with respect to both diagnosis and management. An incidence of 2.3% has been reported in patients undergoing previous hysterectomy.[76] Furthermore, malignant transfor-

mation was noted in 0.26%.[75,76] This incidence was compiled from a series of 35 patients retrospectively evaluated. The typical presentation is that of chronic pelvic pain. Intraoperatively, extensive pelvic adhesions are frequently noted, sometimes associated with ovarian cyst formation. A pelvic mass may be associated with the ovarian remnant. Often the initial gynecologic surgery is performed for endometriosis or pelvic inflammatory disease with incomplete excision of the ovaries.[77] Medical hormonal therapy usually is unsatisfactory, that is, with respect to pain relief, and surgical extirpation is required. In one other series of 27 patients evaluated over a 7-year period, all were noted to have a chief complaint of pelvic pain.[78] In addition, the majority (20 of 27) had a palpable mass. Unfortunately, the ovarian remnant syndrome can be associated with dense bowel adhesions, necessitating segmental bowel resection. In the series reported by Webb,[78] partial bladder resection was required.

Alternative treatment for ovarian remnant (residual) syndrome can include oophoropexy.[79] Recurrent endometriosis also has been reported in association with residual ovary fragment(s) in a series of seven patients with recurrent endometriosis after definitive surgery. The diagnosis was based on serum parameters (estradiol, follicle-stimulating hormone, and luteinizing hormones) indicative of ovarian hormone secretion by residual ovarian fragments. This series of patients appeared to respond to hormonal manipulation or pelvic irradiation. The authors concluded that small ovarian fragments may hypertrophy under increased gonadotropin stimulation. The surgeon must be aware of the potential for ureteral trauma during resection of the remnant tissue, and the patient must be appropriately counseled preoperatively. Intraoperative use of ureteral stents facilitates surgical extirpation.[80] Additionally, preoperative treatment with ovulation-inducing agents (clomiphene citrate or human menopausal gonadotropins) may aid in identification of remnant fragments.

SECOND-LOOK LAPAROSCOPY AFTER OVARIAN SURGERY

Second-look laparoscopy had its beginning in 1967 with the work of Swolin,[81] who first reported this surgical procedure. Subsequent work by Pittaway and coworkers[82] evaluated 23 infertility patients who had previously undergone bilateral wedge resection for PCO, oophorocystectomy, or resection of endometriomas. In their study, adhesions were graded both preoperatively and postoperatively and before and after laparoscopic lysis of adhesions on each ovary. At second-look laparoscopy, periovarian adhesions were noted in at least one ovary in all women. Pregnancy rates appeared to be affected by the underlying pathology. In the series of 23 patients, 22 desired pregnancy: Three of 3 in the wedge resection group conceived, 1 of 3 in the oophorocystectomy group, and 6 of 16 with endometriomas. This preliminary study indicated that ovarian surgery does produce significant adhesion formation, and second-look laparoscopy is an opportunity to reassess the pelvis, perform adhesiolysis, and communicate appropriate prognosis for the infertile couple. Of interest, second-look laparoscopies were performed from 4 to 6 weeks after the initial laparotomy. At this point in the recovery period, adhesions are theoretically less dense and easier to lyse.[31, 83] Nezhat and coworkers[28] evaluated 157 patients; there was total absence of de novo adhesion formation in those who underwent operative laparoscopy as noted at second-look laparoscopy 4 to 18 months after the initial surgical procedure.

One may conclude that second-look laparoscopy does appear to play a significant role, both from the therapeutic perspective, that is, adhesiolysis, and from the counseling aspect, to enable a patient to proceed along the lines of either assisted reproductive technology or subsequent tubal surgical intervention. De novo adhesion formation seems to occur less when the initial procedure is performed endoscopically.[84]

REFERENCES

1. Franchi LL, Mandl AM, Zuckerman S. The development of the ovary and the process of oogenesis. In: Zuckerman S, editor. The Ovary. Vol 1. New York: Academic Press, 1962:1–3.
2. Willier B. The embryonic development of sex. In: Allan E, editor. Sex and Internal Secretions. London: Bailliere Tindall & Cox, 1939:64.
3. Campo S, Garcea N, Caruso A, Siccardi P. Effective celioscopic ovarian resection in patients with polycystic ovaries. Gynecol Obstet Invest 1983; 15:213.
4. Brambell F. Ovarian changes. In: Parkes A, editor. Marshall's Physiology of Reproduction. Vol 1, Part 1. London: Longmans, Green & Co, 1956:397.
5. McLaren A. The making of male mice. Nature 1991; 350:96.
6. Garel L, Filiatrault D, Brandt M, et al. Antenatal diagnosis of ovarian cysts: natural history and therapeutic implications. Pediatr Radiol 1991; 21:182.
7. Grumbach MM, Styne DM. Puberty: Ontogeny, neuroendocrinology, physiology, and disordes. In: Wilson JD, Foster DW, editors. Williams Textbook of Endocrinology. Philadelphia, WB Saunders, 1982:1186.
8. Liapi C, Evain-Brion D. Diagnosis of ovarian follicular cysts from birth to puberty: a report of twenty cases. Acta Paediatr Scand 1987; 76:91.
9. Clarke C, Piesowicx A, Edmunds K, Grant D. Polycystic ovary syndrome in a virilized, premenarcheal girl. Arch Dis Child 1989; 64:1307.
10. Yen SCC. Chronic anovulation due to CNS-hypothalamic pituitary dysfunction. In: Yen SSC, Jaffe RB, editors. Reproductive Endocrinology—Physiology and Clinical Management. Philadelphia: WB Saunders, 1991:537.
11. Lee PA, Van Dop D, Migeon CH. McCune-Albright syndrome: long-term follow-up. JAMA 1986; 256:290.
12. Thind C, Carty H, Pilling D. The role of ultrasound in the management of ovarian masses in children. Clin Radiol 1989; 40:180.
13. Cuniff C, Jones KL, Benirschke K. Ovarian dysgenesis in individuals with chromosomal abnormalities. Hum Genet 1991; 86:552.
14. Hens L, Devroey P, Van-Waesberghe L, et al. Chromosome studies and fertility treatment in women with ovarian failure. Clin Genet 1989; 36:81.
15. Fuller ME. Oral contraceptive therapy for differentiating ovarian cysts. Postgrad Med 1971; 50:143.
16. Spanos WJ. Preoperative hormonal therapy of cystic adnexal masses. Am J Obstet Gynecol 1973; 116:551.
17. Vessey M, Metcalfe A, Wells C, et al. Ovarian neoplasms, functional ovarian cysts, and oral contraceptives. Br Med J 1987; 294:1518.
18. Steinkampf MP, Hammond KR, Blackwell RE. Hormonal treatment of functional ovarian cysts: a randomized, prospective study. Fertil Steril 1990; 54:775–777.
19. Seltzer VL, Maiman M, Goldstein S, et al. Clinical opinion: the role of laparoscopic surgery in the management of ovarian cysts. Unpublished data, 1991.
20. Parker WH, Berek JS. Management of selected cystic adnexal masses in postmenopausal women by operative laparoscopy. A pilot study. Am J Obstet Gynecol 1990; 163:1574.
21. Koonings PP, Campbell K, Mishell DR Jr, Grimes DA. Relative frequency of primary ovarian neoplasms: a ten year review. Obstet Gynecol 1989; 74:921.
22. Stein AL, Koonings PP, Schlaerth JB, et al. Relative frequency of malignant paraovarian tumors: should paraovarian tumors be aspirated? Obstet Gynecol 1990; 75:1029.
23. Lehmann-Wilkenbrock A, et al. A retrospective study of 169 cases.

Preoperative assessment of tumor dignity—a retrospective analysis of 1,016 ovarian tumors [abstr]. VII World Congress on Human Reproduction, Helsinki, Finland, 1990.
24. Webb MJ, Decker DG, Muissey E, Williams TJ. Factors influencing survival of stage I ovarian cancer. Am J Obstet Gynecol 1973; 116:222.
25. Dembo AJ, Davy M, Stenwig AE, et al. Prognostic factors in patients with stage 1 epithelial ovarian cancer. Obstet Gynecol 1990; 75:263.
26. Nezhat C, Winer WK, Cooper JD, Nezhat F. Endoscopic infertility surgery. J Reprod Med 1989; 34:127.
27. Gomel V. Salpingoovariolysis by laparoscopy and infertility. Fertil Steril 1983; 40:607.
28. Nezhat C, Nezhat FR, Metzger DA, Luciano AA. Adhesion reformation after reproductive surgery by videolaseroscopy. Fertil Steril 1990; 53:1008.
29. Niloff JM, Klug TL, St. John E, et al. Elevation of serum CA125 in carcinomas of the fallopian tube, endometrium and endocervix. Am J Obstet Gynecol 1984; 148:1057.
30. Nezhat C, Nezhat F. Postoperative adhesion formation after ovarian cystectomy with and without ovarian reconstruction [abstr]. 47th Annual Meeting of the American Fertility Society, Orlando, 1991.
31. Raj SG, Hulka JF. Second-look laparoscopy in infertility surgery: therapeutic and prognostic value. Fertil Steril 1982; 38:325.
32. Fayez JA, Vogel MF. Comparison of different treatment methods of endometriomas by laparoscopy. Obstet Gynecol 1991; 78:660.
33. Hasson HM. Ovarian surgery. In: Sanfilippo JS, Levine RL, editors. Operative Gynecologic Endoscopy. New York: Springer-Verlag, 1989:99.
34. Cook AS, Rock JA. The role of laparoscopy in the treatment of endometriosis. Fertil Steril 1991; 55:663.
35. Semm K, Mettler L. Technical progress in pelvic surgery by operative laparoscopy. Am J Obstet Gynecol 1980; 138:121.
36. Reich H. Laparoscopy oophorectomy and salpingoophorectomy in the treatment of benign tubo-ovarian disease. Int J Fertil 1987; 32:233.
37. Gomel V, James C. Interoperative management of ureteral injury during operative laparoscopy. Fertil Steril 1991; 55:416.
38. Dunaif A, Green G, Futterweit W, Dobrjansky A. A suppression of hyperandrogenism does not improve peripheral or hepatic insulin resistance in the polycystic ovary syndrome. J Clin Endocrinol Metab 1990; 70:699.
39. Haney AF. The risk/benefits of laparoscopic cautery for endometriosis. Fertil Steril 1991; 55:243.
40. Nowroozi K, Chase JS, Check JH, Wu CH. The importance of laparoscopic coagulation of mild endometriosis in infertile women. Int J Fertil 1987; 32:442.
41. Thomas EJ, Cooke ID. Impact of gestrinone on a course of asymptomatic endometriosis. Br J Gynaecol Obstet 1987; 294:272.
42. Koninckx PR, Meuleman C, Demeyere S, et al. Suggestive evidence that pelvic endometriosis is a progressive disease, whereas deeply infiltrating endometriosis is associated with pelvic pain. Fertil Steril 1991; 55:579.
43. Martin DC, Hubert GD, Vander Zwaag R, El-Zeky FA. Laparoscopic appearances of peritoneal endometriosis. Fertil Steril 1989; 51:63.
44. Yen SSC. Chronic anovulation caused by peripheral endocrine disorders. In: Yen SSC, Jaffe RB, editors. Reproductive Endocrinology. Philadelphia: WB Saunders, 1991:593.
45. Rosenfield RL, Barnes RB, Cara JF, Lucky AW. Dysregulation of cytochrome P450c17α as the cause of polycystic ovarian syndrome. Fertil Steril 1990; 53:784.
46. Lachelin GCL, Barnett M, Hopper G, et al. Adrenal function in normal women and women with polycystic ovary syndrome. J Clin Endocrinol Metab 1979; 49:892.
47. Burghen GA, Givens JR, Kitabchi AE. Correlation of hyperandrogenism with hyperinsulinemia in polycystic ovarian disease. J Clin Endocrinol Metab 1980; 50:113.
48. DeRidder CM, Bruning PF, Zonderland ML, et al. Body fat mass, body fat distribution, and plasma hormones in early puberty in females. J Clin Endocrinol Metab 1990; 70:888.
49. Siiteri PK, MacDonald PC. Role of extraglandular estrogen in human endocrinology. In: Greep RO, Astwooe E, editors. Handbook of Physiology: Endocrinology. Vol II. Washington, DC: American Physiological Society, 1973:615.
50. Hammond MG. Monitoring techniques for improved pregnancy rates during clomiphene ovulation induction. Fertil Steril 1984; 42:499.
51. Lobo RA, Paul W, March CM, et al. Clomiphene and dexamethasone in women unresponsive to clomiphene alone. Obstet Gynecol 1982; 60:497.
52. Daly DC, Walters CA, Soto-Albors CE, et al. A randomized study of dexamethasone in ovulation induction with clomiphene citrate. Fertil Steril 1984; 41:844.

53. Yen SSC, Vela CP, Ryan KJ. Effect of clomiphene citrate in polycystic ovary syndrome: relationship between serum gonadotropin and corpus luteum function. J Clin Endocrinol Metab 1970; 31:7.

54. Homburg R, Weissglas L, Goldman J. Improved treatment for anovulation in polycystic ovarian disease utilizing the effect of progesterone on the inappropriate gonadotropin release and clomiphene response. Hum Reprod 1988; 3:284.

55. Kelly AC, Jewelewicz R. Alternate regimens for ovulation induction and polycystic ovarian disease. Fertil Steril 1990; 54:195.

56. Filicori M, Flamigni C, Campaniello E, et al. The abnormal response of polycystic ovarian disease patients to exogenous pulsatile gonadotropin releasing hormone: characterization and management. J Clin Endocrinol Metab 1989; 69:825.

57. Goldzieher JW, Green JA. The polycystic ovary. I. Clinical and histological features. J Clin Endocrinol Metab 1962; 22:325.

58. Weinstein D, Polishuk WS. The role in which resection of the ovary is the cause for mechanical sterility. Surg Gynecol Obstet 1975; 141:417.

59. Taoff R, Taoff ME, Peyser MR. Infertility following wedge resection of ovaries. Am J Obstet Gynecol 1976; 124:92.

60. Gjonnaess H. Polycystic ovarian syndrome treated by ovarian electrocautery through the laparoscope. Fertil Steril 1984; 41:20.

61. Daniell JF, Miller W. Polycystic ovaries treated by laparoscopic laser vaporization. Fertil Steril 1989; 51:232.

62. Cohen J, Leal de Meirelles H. Fertilite apres biopsie ovarienne percoelioscopique. J Gynecol Obstet Biol Reprod (Paris) 1983; 12:73.

63. Grimes HG, Nosal RA, Gallagher JC. Ovarian pregnancy: a series of 24 cases. Obstet Gynecol 1983; 61:174.

64. Raziel A, Golan A, Pansky M, et al. Ovarian pregnancy: a report of 20 cases in one institution. Obstet Gynecol 1990; 163:1182.

65. Wagerman R, Williams R. Conservative therapy for adnexal torsion. A case report. J Reprod Med 1990; 35:833.

66. Shun A. Unilateral childhood ovarian loss: an indication for contralateral oophoropexy? Aust NZ J Surg 1990; 60:791.

67. Davis A, Feins N. Subsequent asynchronous torsion of normal adnexa in children. J Pediatr Surg 1990; 25:687.

68. Ben-Rafael Z, Bider D, Mashiach S. Laparoscopic unwinding of twisted ischemic hemorrhagic adnexa after in vitro fertilization. Fertil Steril 1990; 53:569.

69. Unage G, Canis M, Manhes H, et al. Laparoscopic management of adnexal torsion. A review of 35 cases. J Reprod Med 1989; 34:520.

70. Henry L, Rauh J, Burket R. Pelvic calcification and autoamputation of the uterine adnexa in an adolescent. J Adolesc Health Care 1988; 9:225.

71. Alrabeeah A, Galliana C, Giacomantonio M, et al. Neonatal ovarian torsion: report of 3 cases and review of the literature. Pediatr Pathol 1988; 8:143.

72. Nussbaum A, Sanders R, Hartman D, et al. Neonatal ovarian cyst: sonographic-pathologic correlation. Radiology 1988; 168:817.

73. Spigland N, Ducharme J, Yazbeck S. Adnexal torsion in children. J Pediatr Surg 1989; 24:974.

74. Lachman M, Berman M. The ectopic ovary. A case report and review of the literature. Arch Pathol Lab Med 1991; 115:233.

75. Heller DS, Harpaz N, Breakstone B. Neoplasms arising in ectopic ovaries: a case of Brenner tumor in an assessory ovary. Int J Gynecol Pathol 1990; 9:185.

76. Hwu Y, Wu C, Yang Y, Wang K. The residual ovary syndrome. Chung-Hua-I-Hsueh Tsa Chic 1989; 43:335.

77. Price F, Edwards R, Buchsbaum H. Ovarian remnant syndrome: difficulties in diagnosis and management. Obstet Gynecol Surv 1990; 45:151.

78. Webb M. Ovarian remnant syndrome. Aust NZ J Obstet Gynaecol 1989; 29:433.

79. Bukovsky I, Liftschitz Y, Langer R, et al. Ovarian residual syndrome. Surg Gynecol Obstet 1988; 167:132.

80. Hajj S, Mercer L. Retrograde dissection of the adnexa in residual ovary syndrome. Surg Gynecol Obstet 1987; 165:451.

81. Swolin K. Spontanheilung nach Querresektion der Tube Fallopi. Acta Obstet Gynecol Scand 1967; 46:219.

82. Pittaway DE, Daniel JF, Maxson WS. Ovarian surgery in an infertility patient as an indication for a short-interval second look laparoscopy: a preliminary study. Fertil Steril 1985; 44:611.

83. Surrey M, Friedman S. Second-look laparoscopy following reconstructive surgery for infertility. J Reprod Med 1982; 27:658.

84. Diamond MP, Daniell JF, Feste I, et al. Adhesion reformation and de novo adhesion formation after reproductive pelvic surgery. Fertil Steril 1987; 47:864.

Medical and Surgical Management of the Infertile Male

R. JEFFREY CHANG

CHAPTER 37

Pathophysiology of Male Infertility

ALVIN M. MATSUMOTO

Approximately 14% of couples are infertile and are unable to achieve a pregnancy after 1 year of unprotected intercourse.[1] It is estimated that a male factor is solely responsible for the inability to conceive in 20% to 30% and contributes to infertility in conjunction with a female factor in another 20% of infertile couples.[2, 3] Therefore, infertility occurs in approximately 6% of men in the reproductive age group, making it a common affliction and stressing the importance of investigating men in the evaluation of infertility.

Accurate diagnosis and appropriate management of male infertility require knowledge of the underlying pathophysiology. Unfortunately, in a majority of cases, the pathophysiologic mechanisms are unclear, and therefore male infertility is mostly idiopathic and untreatable. It is important to note, however, that although uncommon, some cases of male infertility may be successfully treated, and careful, systematic evaluation to identify treatable conditions is needed. For example, gonadotropin or gonadotropin-releasing hormone (GnRH) therapy often stimulates sufficient sperm production to induce or restore fertility in men with hypogonadotropic hypogonadism.

PHYSIOLOGY OF MALE FERTILITY

In men, fertility requires normal functioning and coordination of complex physiologic processes resulting in production, transport, and ejaculation of adequate numbers of normally functioning spermatozoa and deposition of sperm into the female genital tract at the appropriate time in relationship to ovulation. Thus the key processes required for the maintenance of normal male fertility (Fig. 37–1) are (1) the production of adequate numbers of spermatozoa by the testes (*spermatogenesis*), (2) the transport and maturation of spermatozoa produced in the testis through the male genital tract with the acquisition of normal motility and fertilizing capacity (*sperm transport and accessory gland function*), (3) adequate penile erection to complete intercourse and ejaculation (*erectile function*), (4) forward ejaculation of adequate numbers of spermatozoa (*ejaculation*), and (5) appropriate frequency and

timing of intercourse and delivery of adequate numbers of normally functioning motile sperm into the female genital tract to permit fertilization of an ovum (*coitus and functional sperm*). Each of these processes is under separate physiologic regulation, and disorders in any of these key functions may result in male infertility.

PATHOPHYSIOLOGY OF MALE INFERTILITY

An understanding of the physiologic requirements for normal fertility in men provides a logical and practical organizational framework for dealing with the causes of male infertility based on pathophysiology (Tables 37–1 to 37–6). Infertility in men may result from (1) *disorders of spermatogenesis* (see Table 37–2), (2) *disorders of sperm transport and accessory gland function* (see Table 37–3), (3) *erectile dysfunction* (see Table 37–4), (4) *disorders of ejaculation* (see Table 37–5), or (5) *coital disorders and disorders of sperm function* (see Table 37–6). The spectrum of disorders that cause male infertility together with those that reduce fertility in women emphasizes the heterogeneous nature of infertility and the need for an interdisciplinary approach to its evaluation and management, involving gynecologists, reproductive endocrinologists, urologists, and psychologists.

The vast majority (90%) of men with infertility have disorders of sperm production (see Table 37–1).[4, 5] Unfortunately, the cause of disordered spermatogenesis resulting in infertility in most men is not known (i.e., idiopathic oligozoospermia or azoospermia). Disorders of sperm transport and accessory gland function occur in about 6%, erectile dysfunction in 2%, disorders of ejaculation in 1%, and disorders of coitus and sperm function in 1% of unselected men with infertility (see Table 37–1).[4, 5] The prevalence of specific disorders within each category is highly dependent on the evaluating physician's type of practice and referral base. For example, reproductive endocrinologists are likely to see more men with hormonal disorders than urologists, who see more individuals with varicocele, erectile dysfunction, and ejaculatory disorders.

Certain conditions may cause infertility by more than one

All the material in this chapter is in the public domain, with the exception of any borrowed figures or tables.

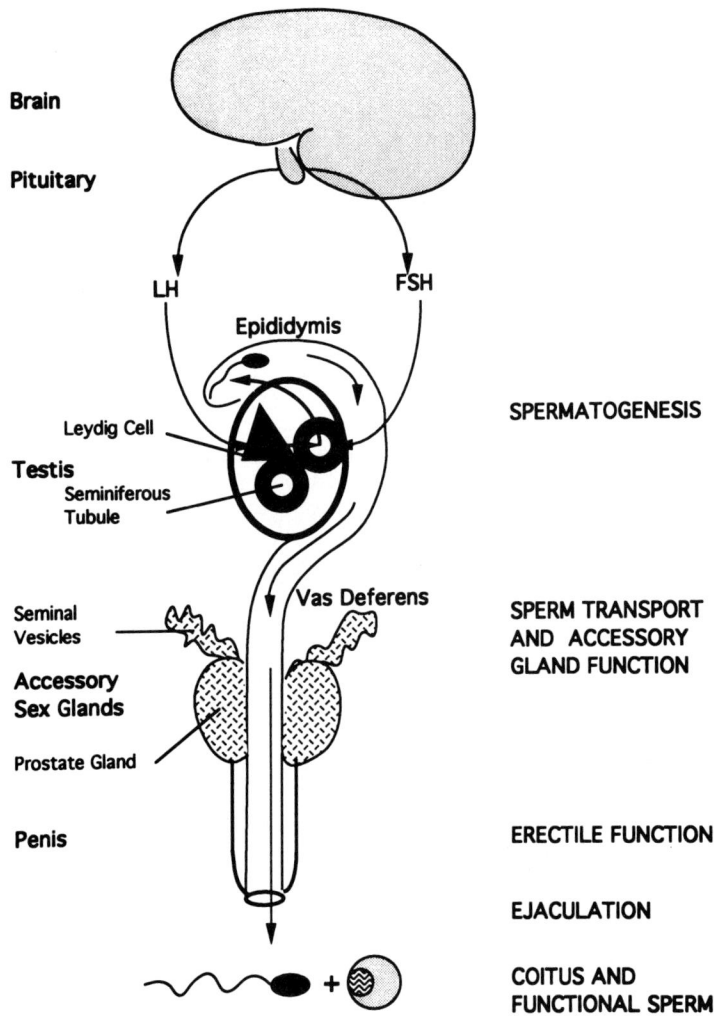

FIGURE 37–1. Schematic diagram of the normal physiology of male fertility. The key processes involved in maintenance of normal male fertility are normal spermatogenesis, sperm transport and accessory gland function, erectile function, ejaculation, and coitus and functional sperm.

pathophysiologic mechanism. For example, androgen deficiency resulting from either primary or secondary hypogonadism causes infertility by impairing spermatogenesis, impairing epididymal and accessory gland function, and causing erectile dysfunction and reduced libido. Men with spinal cord injury may have disordered sperm production, erectile function, or ejaculation, which may contribute to infertility. The relationship between some conditions, such as varicocele, antisperm antibodies, and male genital tract infections, and infertility are poorly understood. Although it is clear that they may be a cause of infertility in some men, these conditions may also be present in other individuals without causing infertility.

TABLE 37–1. Causes of Male Infertility

Disorders of spermatogenesis	90%
Primary hypogonadism	89%
Secondary hypogonadism	1%
Androgen resistance syndromes	0.1%
Disorders of sperm transport and accessory gland function	6%
Erectile dysfunction	2%
Disorders of ejaculation	1%
Coital disorders and disorders of sperm function	1%

Disorders of Spermatogenesis

PHYSIOLOGIC CONSIDERATIONS

The testis is composed of two distinct compartments: the *interstitial compartment,* containing *Leydig cells,* which produce testosterone, the major sex steroid hormone produced by the testis, and the *seminiferous tubule compartment,* containing *Sertoli cells* that envelope and nurture developing *germ cells,* which mature into spermatozoa.[6, 7] Because approximately 90% of the total testis volume is composed of seminiferous tubules, a significant reduction in testis size is likely to reflect reduced spermatogenesis.

Normal testicular function requires the action of the anterior pituitary gonadotropins, *luteinizing hormone* (LH) and *follicle-stimulating hormone* (FSH), which are both stimulated by the hypothalamic peptide, *GnRH.*[8–10] Hypothalamic neurons that secrete GnRH are regulated by numerous excitatory and inhibitory neurotransmitter and neuropeptide systems within the central nervous system (CNS) (e.g., noradrenergic, dopaminergic, serotoninergic, and endogenous opiate systems) as well as testicular feedback signals (primarily sex steroid hormones).[11–14]

Both LH and FSH are secreted into the circulation in an episodic fashion, in response to pulsatile secretion of

TABLE 37–2. Disorders of Spermatogenesis

Primary Hypogonadism
  Idiopathic oligozoospermia or azoospermia
  Congenital or developmental disorders
    Varicocele
    Cryptorchidism
    Klinefelter's syndrome
    Myotonic dystrophy
    Sertoli-cell–only syndrome
    Functional prepubertal castrate syndrome
    Noonan's syndrome
    Polyglandular autoimmune disease
    Down syndrome
    Complex genetic syndromes
  Acquired disorders
    Orchitis (e.g., mumps)
    Drugs (e.g., cytotoxic drugs, sulfasalazine, alcohol, marijuana, ketoconazole, cyclosporine, spironolactone(?), flutamide, histamine$_2$ receptor antagonist)
    Irradiation
    Hyperthermic injury
    Spinal cord injury
    Environmental toxins (e.g., DBCP)
    Surgical or traumatic castration/physical trauma
  Systemic disorders
    Hepatic cirrhosis
    Chronic renal failure
    Malignancy (e.g., Hodgkin's disease, testicular carcinoma)
    Vasculitis (periarteritis)
    Infiltrative disease (amyloidosis)
    Sickle cell disease
Secondary Hypogonadism
  Congenital or developmental disorders
    Hypogonadotropic eunuchoidism (Kallmann's syndrome)
    Hemochromatosis
    Complex genetic syndromes
  Acquired disorders
    Hypopituitarism (destructive or infiltrative pituitary disease)
    Hyperprolactinemia
    Androgen excess (testosterone, anabolic steroids, congenital adrenal hyperplasia, androgen-secreting tumors)
    Estrogen excess or progestogens
    Opiate-like/other CNS-active drugs
  Systemic disorders
    Glucocorticoid excess (Cushing's syndrome)
    Nutritional deficiency (e.g., malnutrition, anorexia nervosa)
    Acute and chronic stress or illness
    Massive obesity
Androgen Resistance Syndromes
  Reifenstein's syndrome
  Idiopathic oligozoospermia or azoospermia
  5α-reductase deficiency
  Celiac disease

DBCP, dibromochloropropane.

TABLE 37–3. Disorders of Sperm Transport and Accessory Gland Function

Ductal Obstruction
  Congenital defects of vas, seminal vesicles, or epididymis (e.g., cystic fibrosis)
  Young's syndrome
  Müllerian duct cyst
  Vasectomy
  Postinfectious obstruction of epididymis, seminal vesicles, or vas
Impaired Sympathetic Innervation of Ducts
  Spinal cord disease
  Sympathectomy or sympatholytic drugs
  Retroperitoneal lymphadenectomy
  Vasovasostomy
Epididymal and Accessory Gland Dysfunction
  Androgen deficiency or resistance
  Hyperthermic injury
  Genital tract infection (?)

TABLE 37–4. Causes of Erectile Dysfunction

Central Nervous System Disorders
  Psychiatric disturbance
    Emotional stress or performance anxiety
    Depression
    Major psychiatric illness
    Chronic medical illness
    Cardiac, respiratory, renal or liver disease
    Malignancy
    CNS-active drugs
    Centrally active antihypertensives
    Antidepressants
    Antipsychotics
    Sedative-hypnotics
    Alcohol
    Endocrine disorders
    Androgen deficiency or resistance
    Hyperprolactinemia
    Thyroid disease
    CNS diseases
    Temporal lobe or limbic system disorders
Spinal Cord Disease
  Spinal cord injury
  Multiple sclerosis
  Transverse myelitis
  Tumor
  Vascular compromise
  Epidural abscess
  Spinal stenosis or spina bifida
  Syphilis
Autonomic Nervous System Dysfunction
  Pelvic surgery
  Diabetic autonomic neuropathy
  Other peripheral neuropathies
Drugs Affecting Peripheral Erectile Response
  Anticholinergic drugs
  Antidepressants
  β-adrenergic antagonists
  Antihistamines
  Antihypertensive drugs
  Sympathomimetic agents
  α-Adrenergic agonists
Vascular Disease
  Distal aortoiliac disease
  Penile arterial disease (e.g., diabetes)
  Venous incompetence
Penile Abnormalities
  Peyronie's disease or chordee
  Micropenis
  Penile trauma
  Priapism

GnRH.[8–10] LH stimulates Leydig cell production of testosterone, which plays important roles in the development and maintenance of male sexual characteristics, functioning, and behavioral characteristics and the feedback regulation of gonadotropin secretion.[15] In addition, high intratesticular levels of testosterone stimulated by LH also regulate Sertoli cell function and play an important role in the initiation and maintenance of spermatogenesis.[16, 17] FSH stimulates Sertoli cell production of seminiferous tubule fluid, numerous proteins (e.g., androgen binding protein, transferrin, inhibin, clusterin, several growth factor–like proteins, and plasminogen activator), polyamines, and lactate, which are thought to be important in regulating germ cell development and spermatogenesis.[18] Other Sertoli cell products play an important

TABLE 37–5. Disorders of Ejaculation

Premature or Retarded Ejaculation
Retrograde Ejaculation
   Bladder neck surgery
      Prostatectomy
      Bladder neck incision
      Y-V urethrocystoplasty
   Sympathetic nervous system dysfunction
      Autonomic neuropathy (e.g., diabetes)
      Sympatholytic drugs or sympathectomy
      Retroperitoneal or abdominopelvic surgery
      Spinal cord injury
Reduced Ejaculation
   Androgen deficiency or resistance
   Sympathetic nervous system dysfunction
   Urethral abnormalities (e.g., stricture, hypospadias, epispadias)

role in the male internal genitalia (müllerian inhibitory hormone) and possibly in the feedback regulation of gonadotropin secretion (inhibin) and in paracrine regulation of Leydig cell function.[18, 19]

Spermatogenesis is the process of differentiation and maturation of *spermatogonia,* undifferentiated stem cells that line the basal or outer portion of the seminiferous tubule, into *spermatozoa.*[6] Some spermatogonia continuously undergo mitotic divisions to replenish the stem cell pool, whereas others become committed to further differentiation into spermatocytes that undergo *meiosis,* which occurs in the adluminal or inner portions of the seminiferous tubule. *Primary spermatocytes* undergo two meiotic divisions, initially forming *secondary spermatocytes* and then spermatids, which contain a haploid DNA and chromosomal complement. *Spermatids* undergo further maturation (*spermiogenesis*), involving nuclear changes, acrosome formation, flagellar development, and cytoplasmic redistribution, to form *spermatozoa.* In humans, completion of a full cycle of spermatogenesis takes approximately 74 days,[20] and daily sperm production from the human testis is about 120 million sperm per day.[21, 22] Sperm concentration in the ejaculate is extremely variable and ranges from 20 to 200 million/mL in normal men.[7, 23, 24]

Both LH and FSH stimulation of the testis are required for the initiation of sperm production at the time of puberty.[16, 25, 26] In animals, testosterone stimulated by LH induces spermatogonia to undergo meiosis and primary spermatocytes to complete meiosis, and FSH facilitates maturation of spermatids into spermatozoa during spermiogenesis.[17] The precise sites of action of gonadotropins on human spermatogenesis, however, are unclear. In patients with prepubertal hypogonadotropic hypogonadism, replacement of both gonadotropins is generally necessary to initiate spermatogenesis.[16, 25, 26]

In adults, normal levels of neither LH nor FSH are necessary for maintenance of spermatogenesis. Initiation and maintenance of spermatogenesis in men with hypogonadotropic hypogonadism acquired postpubertally can be achieved with LH replacement alone.[16, 25, 26] Furthermore, selective replacement of either LH or FSH results in stimulation of *qualitatively* normal sperm production in normal men with experimentally induced gonadotropin deficiency.[16, 25, 27–30] Replacement of both gonadotropins, however, is required for maintenance of *quantitatively* normal sperm production in these hypogonadotropic men.[16, 25, 31]

Disorders of spermatogenesis (see Table 37–2) may result

from either diseases that affect the testis primarily (*primary hypogonadism*) or disorders of the pituitary or hypothalamus that cause inadequate gonadotropin stimulation of the testis (*secondary hypogonadism*). In men with primary hypogonadism, deficiency in sperm production may occur in isolation or in conjunction with androgen deficiency. In primary hypogonadal men who have reduced sperm and androgen production, gonadotropin levels are increased as a result of diminished testicular negative feedback (i.e., *hypergonadotropic hypogonadism*). Men with isolated impairment of sperm production owing to primary testicular failure have selective elevation in FSH levels when germ cell loss is severe or normal gonadotropin levels with milder degrees of damage.[32, 33] Men with secondary hypogonadism usually have deficiency of both sperm and androgen production. These men have low or low-normal gonadotropin levels (i.e., *hypogonadotropic hypogonadism*). Because androgen action within the testis is required for spermatogenesis, *androgen resistance* may also result in impaired spermatogenesis and infertility. These men usually have high to high-normal serum testosterone and gonadotropin levels.

The distinction between primary and secondary hypogonadism has important clinical implications. With the exception of some men with varicocele or drug-induced testicular dysfunction, impaired spermatogenesis and infertility in the majority of men with primary hypogonadism are not treatable. In contrast, the testis is usually able to respond normally when given adequate gonadotropin stimulation in men with secondary hypogonadism. Therefore administration of gonadotropins or, in some instances, GnRH may stimulate sperm production and restore fertility in these men (Fig. 37–2). Furthermore, it is important to recognize that secondary hypogonadism may be caused by destruction of pituitary gonadotropin-secreting cells, for example, by a hypothalamic or pituitary tumor. In addition to causing gonadotropin deficiency and infertility, these tumors may be associated with mass effects (e.g., visual field defects or hydrocephalus). Pituitary tumors may also cause deficiency (e.g., panhypopituitarism) or hypersecretion (e.g., hyperprolactinemia, acromegaly, or Cushing's disease) of other anterior pituitary hormones.

PRIMARY HYPOGONADISM

Idiopathic Oligozoospermia or Azoospermia. The majority of men who present with infertility are found to have

TABLE 37–6. Coital Disorders and Disorders of Sperm Transport

Coital Disorders
   Infrequent intercourse
   Excessive intercourse or masturbation
   Poor timing in relationship to ovulation
   Premature withdrawal
Disorders of Sperm Function
   Sperm-toxic lubricants
   Sperm dysmotility
      Idiopathic asthenospermia
      Immotile cilia syndrome (Kartagener's syndrome)
      Protein carboxyl methylase deficiency
      Immunologic (antisperm antibodies)
      Idiopathic polyzoospermia (?)

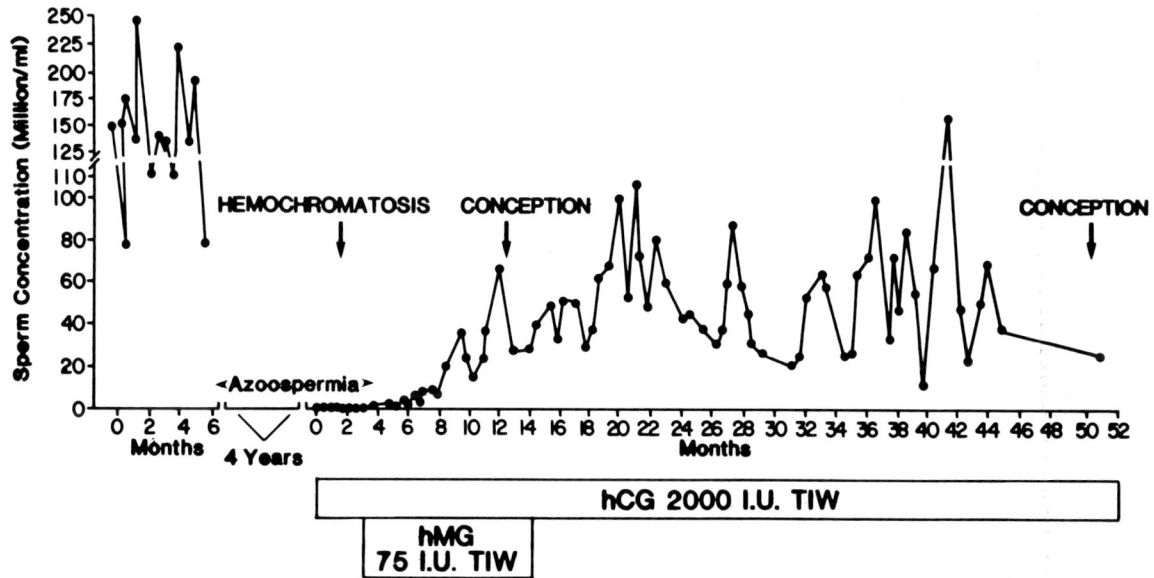

FIGURE 37–2. Sperm concentrations in a patient prior to and after the development of hemochromatosis and hypogonadotropic hypogonadism 4 years later. Spermatogenesis and fertility were restored with combined human chorionic gonadotropin (hCG) and human menopausal gonadotropin (hMG) therapy and maintained with hCG treatment alone for more than 3 years. TIW, three times per week. (From Matsumoto AM, Bremner WJ. Endocrinology of the hypothalamic-pituitary-testicular axis with particular reference to the hormonal control of spermatogenesis. Baillieres Clin Endocrinol Metab 1987;1:83.)

an isolated impairment of spermatogenesis with an identifiable cause: *idiopathic oligozoospermia* or *azoospermia.* In reports of conditions associated with male infertility, approximately 40% of men are found to have idiopathic oligozoospermia or azoospermia.[4, 5] *Varicocele,* a dilatation of the venous pampiniform plexus surrounding the spermatic cord (see later), is found in association with infertility in another 40% of men. It is probably not the cause of infertility in the majority of these men, however, because fertility is restored in at most 25% to 40% of *selected* men who undergo varicocele repair.[34] Therefore idiopathic oligozoospermia or azoospermia probably occurs in 70% to 80% of unselected men with infertility.[4, 5] Because male infertility is so common, occurring in up to 6% of men in the reproductive age group, idiopathic oligozoospermia or azoospermia represents the most common cause of male hypogonadism.

The pathophysiology of idiopathic oligozoospermia or azoospermia is likely to be heterogeneous. Serum testosterone and gonadotropin levels are usually normal. About 30% of men demonstrate selective elevation of serum FSH or exaggerated FSH response to GnRH administration.[32, 35] Some of these men with isolated FSH elevation are found to demonstrate a decreased frequency of pulsatile LH (and presumably GnRH) secretion,[36] and short-term pulsatile GnRH administration at an increased frequency lowers FSH levels.[37] Longer-term administration of GnRH, however, has not consistently improved sperm production or fertility,[38–41] and the pathophysiologic significance of the decreased pulsatile LH secretion remains unclear. Other investigators have found decreases in testosterone production rates despite normal serum testosterone levels in infertile men with selective FSH elevation.[42] Finally, some men with idiopathic oligozoospermia or azoospermia demonstrate androgen receptor abnormalities.[43, 44] These men are otherwise phenotypically normal males and have serum testosterone and LH levels that are high-normal to slightly elevated, suggesting mild androgen

resistance. Other investigators have not found androgen receptor defects in men with idiopathic oligozoospermia or azoospermia.[45, 46]

On testis biopsy, most men with idiopathic oligozoospermia or azoospermia demonstrate primarily two histologic patterns, which can occur in the same patient (Fig. 37–3; see color section in the center of the book): (1) a *maturation arrest* pattern, in which germ cell maturation is arrested at a specific stage of development, or (2) a *hypospermatogenesis* pattern, in which there is reduction in all germ cell elements with normal maturation.[5, 47] Interestingly, there is generally little to no peritubular hyalinization or seminiferous tubule sclerosis and no evidence of inflammatory cell infiltration,[5, 47] suggesting that testicular damage is neither severe nor irreversible. Although less common, peritubular hyalinization in conjunction with more severe degrees of germ cell loss can be observed. This is usually associated with elevated serum FSH levels and poor prognosis for fertility. Unfortunately, the mechanisms underlying diminished sperm production in these patients are not known. Therefore treatment regimens have been empiric and have not improved fertility compared with placebo-treated men, who have a fertility rate of approximately 25% in 1 year.[48]

Congenital or Developmental Disorders. *Varicocele* is a dilatation of the pampiniform plexus and internal spermatic vein that surrounds the spermatic cord and drains the testis. Varicoceles are found in approximately 40% of men who present with infertility.[4, 5] They are also present, however, in men with recently documented fertility.[49, 50] The incidence of varicocele in the general population is 10% to 15%, and as many as one half of these men have low sperm counts, abnormal morphology (nonspecific, *stress* pattern with increased percentage of tapered and amorphous forms) or reduced motility.[50–52] Most men with varicocele, including those with known recent fertility, demonstrate lower sperm counts and evidence of primary testicular dysfunction as ev-

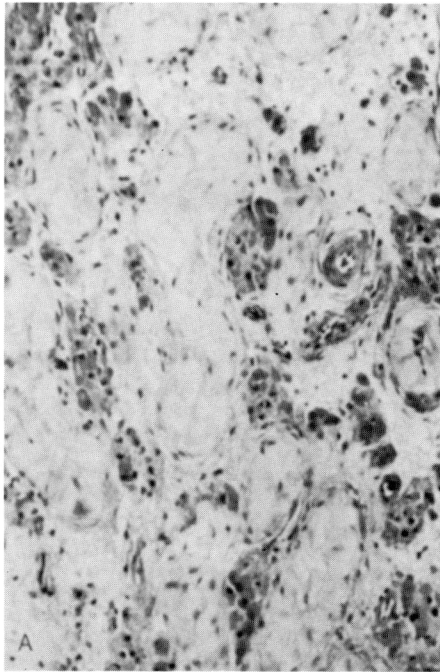

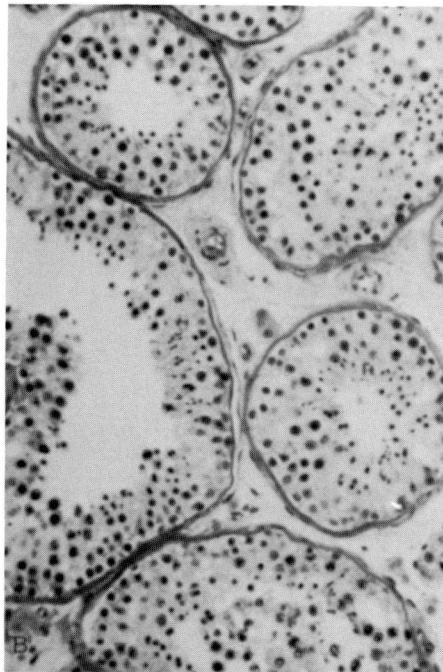

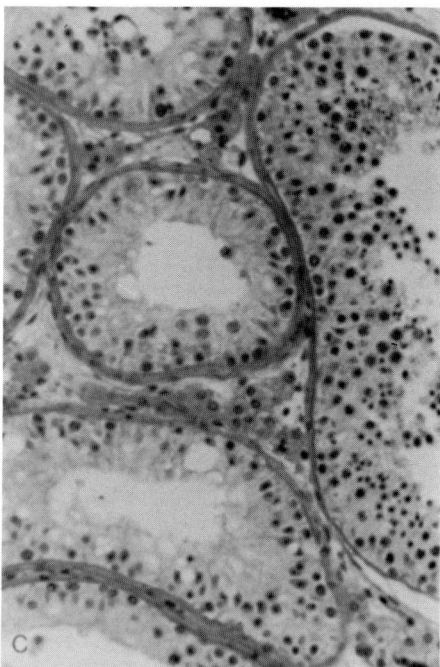

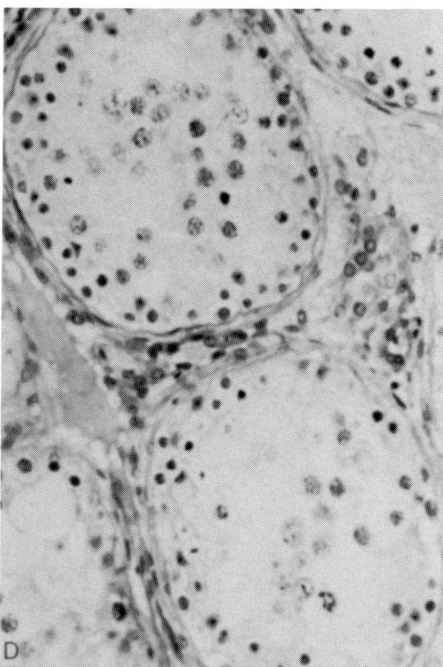

FIGURE 37–3. Testis biopsies from (A) a man with testicular damage from mumps orchitis. Note the severe germ cell loss and seminiferous tubule sclerosis with clumped Leydig cells in the interstitium; (B) an infertile man with idiopathic oligozoospermia, demonstrating a hypospermatogenesis pattern; (C) another infertile man with idiopathic oligozoospermia, demonstrating more severe hypospermatogenesis than that found in the previous man; and (D) an infertile male with idiopathic azoospermia, demonstrating a maturation arrest pattern with very few spermatids present. (Reprinted from Paulsen CA. In: Santen RJ, Swerdloff RS, editors. Male Reproductive Dysfunction: Diagnosis and Management of Hypogonadism, Infertility, and Impotence. New York: Marcel Dekker, 1986, p. 202 by courtesy of Marcel Dekker, Inc.)

idenced by elevated serum FSH levels or exaggerated gonadotropin responses to GnRH stimulation, compared with men without varicocele.[50] Therefore it is clear that varicocele is not uniformly associated with impaired fertility despite abnormal seminal fluid characteristics.

Approximately 90% of varicoceles occur on the left side, as a result of incompetent or absent valves in the left internal spermatic vein as it enters the left renal vein, which causes increased venous pressure in the spermatic vein and dilatation of the pampiniform plexus.[34] The mechanism by which varicocele may cause reduced fertility is unclear. The most likely explanation for infertility is that varicocele increases scrotal temperature, resulting in relative testicular and epididymal hyperthermia, which is known to impair spermatogenesis.[34, 53] Scrotal temperatures, however, may also be elevated in infertile men without detectable varicocele.[54]

Treatment of varicocele is usually surgical ligation of the internal spermatic vein high within the inguinal canal. The results of varicocele repair have been inconsistent, in part reflecting selection bias, differences in the degree of baseline testicular dysfunction, and differences in the evaluation of female factors. In the majority of uncontrolled reports of varicocele repair, semen quality is improved in about 50% to 70%, and pregnancy rate is approximately 25% to 40%.[34, 55]

Results of retrospective, controlled studies, however, are mixed and fail to find consistently a beneficial effect of varicocele repair on fertility.[34, 56–58] Without prospective, double-blind, randomized, controlled studies involving large numbers of men that demonstrate improved fertility with varicocele repair, the etiologic association between varicocele and infertility remains a question, and the value of varicocele repair remains controversial. In the absence of such studies and because of the general lack of other treatments for infertility associated with primary disorders of spermatogenesis, varicocele repair remains a useful therapeutic option.

Cryptorchidism results from a developmental failure of the testis to descend normally from the abdomen into the scrotum or from an obstruction to normal testicular descent.[59] Cryptorchid testes may be located in abdomen, inguinal canal, or high in scrotum. In contrast, *ectopic testes* are located in areas outside the normal pathway of testicular descent, for example, in the perineal, femoral, superficial inguinal, or suprapubic areas or in the opposite scrotum. Whether unilateral or bilateral, cryptorchidism is associated with reduced spermatogenesis and infertility and an increased risk of developing testicular carcinoma.[59–61] It is important to distinguish cryptorchid testes from *retractile testes,* which are located in the scrotum but may be retracted into the inguinal canal with minimal stimulation of the cremasteric reflex. Retractile testes are usually not associated with infertility or increased risk of testicular cancer,[62] although high retractile testes may demonstrate disordered spermatogenesis.[63]

The testes usually descend into the scrotum during the eighth month of gestation. Approximately 3% to 4% of full-term infants, however, may have cryptorchid testes that descend during the first year of life.[59] The prevalence of cryptorchidism in adults is about 0.3% to 0.4%.[59] Cryptorchidism is found in approximately 6% of infertile men.[4, 5]

Cryptorchidism is frequently associated with congenital disorders, especially those that cause hypogonadism or androgen resistance (e.g., functional prepubertal castrate syndrome, Noonan's syndrome, Klinefelter's syndrome, hypogonadotropic eunuchoidism, and Reifenstein's syndrome), suggesting an important role for androgens in the regulation of normal testicular descent.[59, 64] In these men, disordered spermatogenesis is caused, in part, by the associated androgen deficiency or resistance. Uncommonly, testicular descent is impeded by congenital defects that prevent development of normal intra-abdominal pressure (e.g., prune-belly syndrome) or that cause obstruction in the normal pathway of descent.[59] The majority of men with cryptorchidism do not have clinical androgen deficiency or resistance or predisposing congenital defects. In these men, the cause of cryptorchidism is unclear. Underlying developmental abnormalities of testis and gubernaculum (which pulls the testis into the scrotum during development), perhaps owing to mild gonadotropin and androgen deficiency during fetal life, are thought to contribute to the cause of cryptorchidism in these men.[65]

Infertile men with cryptorchidism usually demonstrate moderate-to-severe germinal cell degeneration with varying degrees of peritubular hyalinization.[66, 67] The degree of impairment of sperm production depends on the position and length of time the testis remained cryptorchid, with long-standing intra-abdominal testes showing the most severe germ cell loss.[66] Serum FSH is usually elevated, and gonadotropin responses to GnRH are usually exaggerated, consistent with primary testicular failure. Unless cryptorchidism is associated with a disorder that causes androgen deficiency or resistance, Leydig cell function is usually preserved, and serum testosterone and LH levels remain normal.

Disordered sperm production in men with cryptorchidism that is not associated with androgen deficiency or resistance results, in part, from increased testicular temperature.[68] Spermatogenesis, however, may also be defective in the normally descended testis of men with unilateral cryptorchidism.[60, 67, 69] Although they usually improve, sperm production and fertility remain reduced (and risk of malignancy remains increased) in men with nonobstructive cryptorchidism following orchiopexy performed during childhood.[59, 67, 70, 71] In contrast, men with cryptorchidism owing to obstruction from anatomic impediments to normal testicular descent have normal testicular function if orchiopexy is performed before puberty. These findings suggest that an underlying developmental abnormality of both testes may contribute to both the impaired spermatogenesis and the pathophysiology of abnormal testicular descent in men with cryptorchidism. Cryptorchid testes are also at increased risk to undergo testicular torsion, which may contribute to germ cell loss if not treated promptly.[59]

Klinefelter's syndrome is the most common cause of primary hypogonadism that results in impairment of both sperm and androgen production. It occurs in approximately 1 in every 400 to 500 men.[72, 73] Klinefelter's syndrome is characterized by small, firm testes; azoospermia; gynecomastia; varying degrees of testosterone deficiency and eunuchoidism; and elevated serum gonadotropins.[74–76] The underlying defect in this syndrome and its variants is the presence of one or a number of extra X chromosomes.

In classic Klinefelter's syndrome, the karyotype of all cells is XXY.[75] This results from either maternal or paternal meiotic nondisjunction during gametogenesis. Azoospermia is present in more than 95% of these men.[74, 76] Testis size is usually less than 2 cm in length (normal greater than 3.5 cm). Testis biopsy (Fig. 37–4; see color section in the center of the book) generally demonstrates an absence of spermatogenesis with severe seminiferous tubule sclerosis and hyalinization.[75, 76] It is hypothesized that the presence of an extra X chromosome shortens germ cell life span. This results in accelerated and progressive rate of germ cell loss during childhood, such that by adulthood most patients with Klinefelter's syndrome have lost their entire complement of germ cells. Infertility in classic and most variant forms is irreversible.

Total testosterone levels are reduced but range from below to within the normal range.[75, 77, 78] Because estradiol levels are often elevated, which results in increased sex hormone–binding globulin levels, free testosterone levels are low in most men with Klinefelter's syndrome.[77, 79] Serum gonadotropin, especially FSH, levels are elevated.[75, 77, 80] Despite biochemical evidence of Leydig cell dysfunction (i.e., low testosterone or elevated LH levels or both), affected individuals may not present with clinical androgen deficiency, and many escape diagnosis until they present with azoospermia in infertility clinics. Androgen replacement is effective in treatment of undervirilization but does not improve spermatogenesis or restore fertility.[76]

In *mosaic* Klinefelter's syndrome (XXY/XY), some cell lines

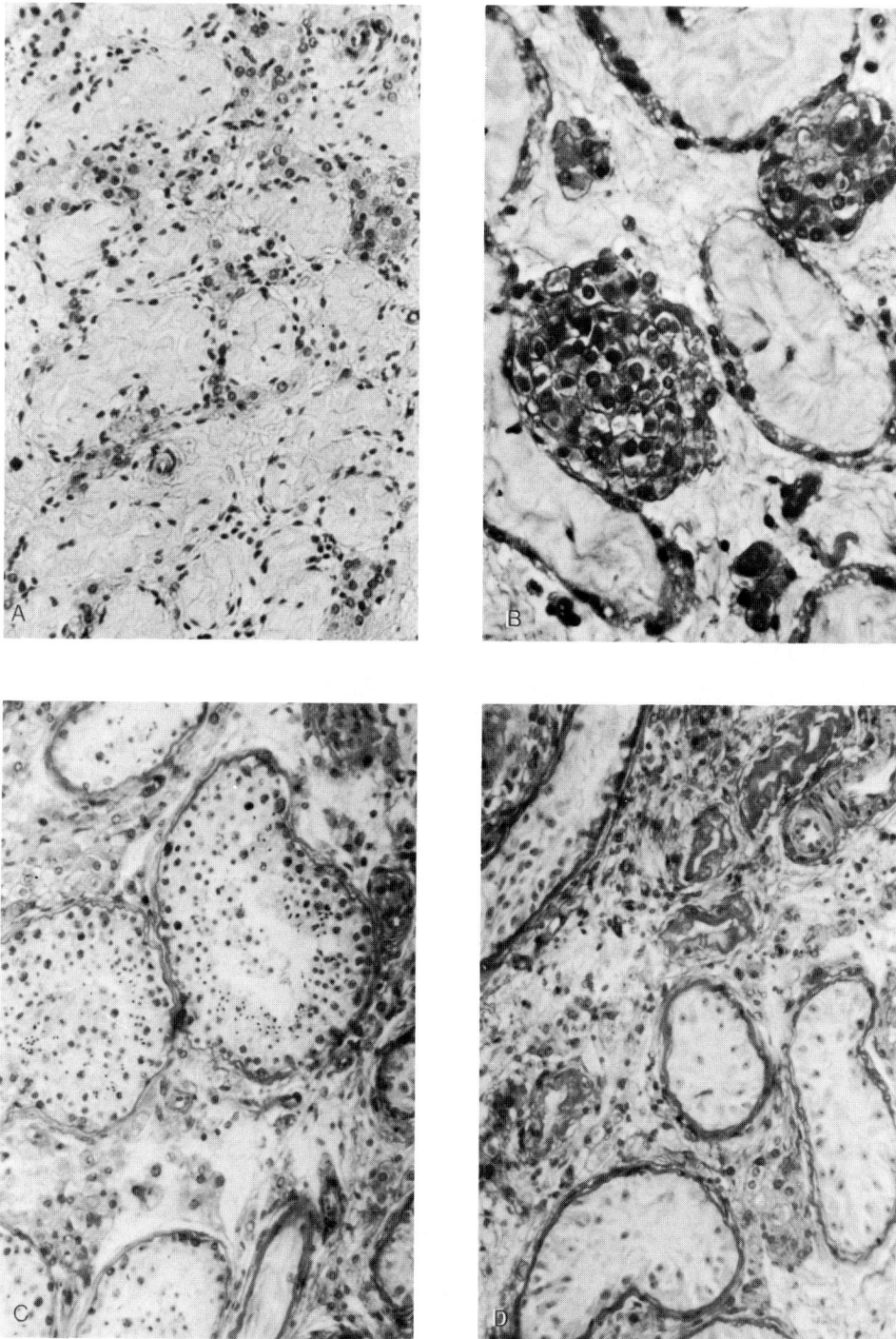

FIGURE 37-4. Testis biopsies from men with Klinefelter's syndrome, demonstrating (A) total sclerosis of seminiferous tubules and Leydig cells that are dispersed throughout the interstitium; (B) reticular fibers surrounding hyalinized seminiferous tubules and Leydig cells that are present in adenomatous clumps; (C) a variable pattern of germ cell damage with some seminiferous tubules showing active spermatogenesis; and (D) a variable pattern of germ cell loss with a mixture of hyalinized seminiferous tubules and tubules containing only Sertoli cells. (Reprinted from Paulsen CA. In: Santen RJ, Swerdloff RS, editors. Male Reproductive Dysfunction: Diagnosis and Management of Hypogonadism, Infertility, and Impotence. New York: Marcel Dekker, 1986, p. 201 by courtesy of Marcel Dekker, Inc.)

have an XXY, whereas others have an XY karyotype.[75, 76] Mosaicism results from mitotic nondisjunction after fertilization. Clinical manifestations in men with mosaic Klinefelter's syndrome are atypical. Testis size may be larger, and spermatogenesis and fertility may be present in rare individuals.[81] Variant syndromes characterized by more than two X chromosomes (*poly X syndromes*) are associated with more severe abnormalities than classic Klinefelter's syndrome.[82, 83] There is a higher incidence of mental retardation and somatic abnormalities, such as hypospadias, cryptorchidism, and skeletal abnormalities (e.g., proximal radioulnar synostosis) in poly X syndromes.[82, 83] Patients with the *XXYY syndrome* re-

semble classic Klinefelter's syndrome but are taller and have increased aggressive behavior.[84, 85] Finally, men with the *XX male syndrome* also resemble classic Klinefelter's syndrome but are shorter, have an increased incidence of hypospadias, and are not mentally retarded.[86] Most of these men probably have translocation of Y chromosomal material (carrying testis-determining genes) onto an X chromosome or autosome.[87]

Myotonic dystrophy is an autosomal dominant disorder characterized by prolonged contraction of skeletal muscles (myotonia), especially in the face, neck, and distal extremities, resulting in progressive muscle atrophy and weakness.[88] Associated abnormalities include cataracts, premature frontal balding, cardiac arrhythmias, mild mental deterioration, and primary hypogonadism. Testicular failure occurs in approximately 80% of affected men usually between 30 and 40 years of age.[89] The majority of men with myotonic dystrophy and testicular failure demonstrate isolated impairment of sperm production and infertility with normal androgen production. The severity of disordered spermatogenesis varies from complete loss of germ cells with seminiferous tubule sclerosis and peritubular hyalinization to more moderate defects in sperm production.[90] Serum FSH levels are nearly always elevated.[89] Clinical androgen deficiency is uncommon (occurring in only approximately 20%), but mild Leydig cell dysfunction with low normal testosterone and elevated LH levels is found more frequently.[89] The pathogenesis of testicular failure in myotonic dystrophy is not known. Androgen replacement therapy is indicated for men with low testosterone levels, although there is no evidence that it reverses or delays muscle atrophy and weakness. No treatment exists for the infertility associated with myotonic dystrophy.

Sertoli-cell–only syndrome or *germinal cell aplasia* is an uncommon disorder characterized on testicular biopsy (Fig. 37–5) by seminiferous tubules that are devoid of germ cells and contain only Sertoli cells.[91] There is little to no peritubular hyalinization and a normal number of Leydig cells in the interstitial compartment. Patients with Sertoli-cell–only syndrome present with azoospermia, elevated serum FSH levels, slightly smaller-than-normal size testes, and infertility that is irreversible.[32, 92] They usually have normal serum testosterone levels and are normally virilized. As many as 50% of men with Sertoli-cell–only syndrome, however, have mild or subclinical Leydig cell dysfunction, as evidenced by slightly elevated LH and reduced testosterone levels or blunted testosterone response to human chorionic gonadotropin (hCG) stimulation.[32, 92]

The histologic picture of Sertoli-cell–only syndrome is most commonly seen in men with idiopathic azoospermia. The most likely cause of this syndrome is congenital absence or early neonatal loss of germ cells perhaps owing to abnormal gonocyte migration or Sertoli cell function. Other disorders that cause severe seminiferous tubule damage, for example, cryptorchidism; mumps orchitis; or exposure to

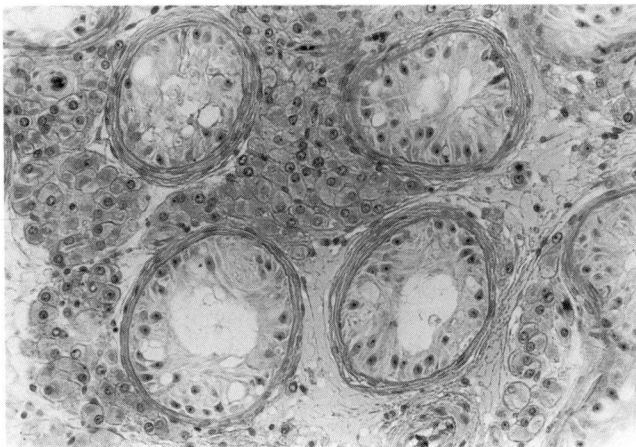

FIGURE 37–5. Testis biopsy from a patient with Sertoli-cell–only syndrome. Note the absence of germ cells and seminiferous tubules lined only with Sertoli cells. (From Paulsen CA. In: Williams RH, editor. Textbook of Endocrinology. 6th edition. Philadelphia: WB Saunders, 1981:315.)

cytotoxic drugs, irradiation, or toxins, may also result in a histologic pattern similar to that of Sertoli-cell–only syndrome.[32, 91] In these acquired causes, however, there is usually extensive peritubular hyalinization and seminiferous tubule sclerosis. Infertility in Sertoli-cell–only syndrome is irreversible.

Functional prepubertal castrate (or congenital anorchia) syndrome is a rare disorder characterized by severe prepubertal testicular failure and the complete absence of testicular tissue, occasionally associated with absent epididymides.[93] Otherwise normal internal and external genitalia without müllerian duct–derived structures and normally descended vas and spermatic blood vessels in the scrotum are present, suggesting that functioning testes were present during critical periods of fetal development (from 8 to 14 weeks' gestation). It is hypothesized that testicular damage (e.g., from bilateral testicular torsion in utero or autoimmune destruction) occurs after these critical developmental periods, during fetal or prepubertal life, resulting in degeneration of all or nearly all testis tissue.

Patients with this syndrome usually present with suspected bilateral cryptorchidism before puberty or sexual infantilism during adolescence or adulthood. The distinction between anorchia and bilateral cryptorchidism is important and can generally be made by determining the testosterone response to hCG administration. Although there are exceptions, usually men without testes do not respond to hCG, whereas those with functioning testes do.[94] Laparoscopy or surgical exploration is sometimes necessary to confirm the presence or absence of abdominal testes.

Serum testosterone levels are low, and gonadotropin levels are markedly elevated, both in the castrate range.[95] Men with congenital anorchia may be aspermic (i.e., without an ejaculate) before androgen treatment or azoospermic. Androgen therapy is needed to induce development of normal secondary sex characteristics and sexual function. Infertility in these men is irreversible.

Noonan's syndrome (male Turner's syndrome) is an autosomal recessive (rarely dominant) disorder in which genotypic XY males manifest clinical features similar to those of Turner's syndrome in girls. Typical features include short stature, webbed neck, typical facies (low hairline, hypertelorism, eye slant, ptosis, low-set ears, micrognathia, high-arched palate, and dental malocclusion), shieldlike chest, pectus excavatum, cubitus valgus, cardiovascular anomalies (pulmonic stenosis and atrial septal defect), mental retardation, and lymphedema.[96] Uncommonly a mosaic XO/XY cell line may be present in these men. Cryptorchidism is frequently present. Patients with Noonan's syndrome usually exhibit impairment of both sperm and androgen production. Testis biopsy reveals moderate-to-severe reduction of spermatogenesis, and these men usually have severe oligozoospermia or azoospermia, resulting in infertility that is not treatable.[83] Serum testosterone levels are low, and both FSH and LH levels are elevated, consistent with primary testicular failure.

Polyglandular autoimmune disease is a familial disorder characterized by autoimmune dysfunction of several endocrine organs and circulating organ-specific autoantibodies.[97] Specific autoimmune disorders that occur in conjunction with each other are Addison's disease, Hashimoto's thyroiditis, Graves' disease, insulin-dependent diabetes, ovarian failure, pernicious anemia, hypoparathyroidism, vitiligo, mucocutaneous candidiasis, hypopituitarism, and alopecia totalis. In contrast to ovarian failure, autoimmune testicular failure and antitesticular antibodies occur much less commonly in polyglandular autoimmune disease.[97] Leydig cell failure induced by the autoantibodies reduces testosterone production, which can impair spermatogenesis and contribute to infertility.

Down syndrome (trisomy 21) is associated with moderate-to-severe reduction in sperm production with normal to elevated gonadotropin levels.[98, 99] A number of rare *complex genetic syndromes,* for example, *Alström, ataxia telangiectasia, Sohval-Soffer, Weinstein,* and *Werner syndromes,* are associated with primary testicular failure.[100, 101] Although more commonly associated with hypogonadotropic (secondary) hypogonadism, the *Prader-Labhart-Willi* and *Laurence-Moon-Beidl* syndromes may also demonstrate primary hypogonadism.[100, 101]

Acquired Disorders. Because germ cell development requires active cell division, spermatogenesis is much more sensitive than Leydig cell function to external or environmental influences. As a result, most disorders causing acquired primary testicular failure result in isolated impairment of sperm production with normal androgen production.

Viral orchitis, most commonly due to *mumps,* is a common cause of acquired primary testicular failure. Approximately 15% to 25% of pubertal or adult males who acquire mumps infection develop painful, inflammatory orchitis, usually within a few days of parotitis.[102, 103] Although clinical orchitis is unilateral in most cases, degenerative changes in the clinically uninvolved testis have been observed. During the acute inflammatory phase of orchitis, germinal epithelium is sloughed, and the interstitium is severely edematous.[102–104] This is followed by progressive germ cell loss, seminiferous tubule sclerosis, and peritubular hyalinization resembling the histologic picture of Klinefelter's syndrome (see Fig. 37–3). Testicular atrophy occurs over a period of months to years.[102–104] Germ cells are lost directly as a result of viral injury and indirectly from ischemia secondary to testicular edema. The majority of men with previous bilateral mumps orchitis develop severe oligozoospermia or azoospermia and infertility that is irreversible.[105, 106] Serum FSH alone or, in some instances, both FSH and LH levels are elevated. In severe cases, Leydig cell failure and clinical androgen deficiency also develop following mumps orchitis,[107] and low serum testosterone levels require androgen replacement.

Orchitis and testicular failure may also be caused by other viral infections, such as *echovirus* and *arbovirus* infections, and granulomatous infections, such as *leprosy* and *tuberculosis.*[108, 109] Rarely, severe epididymo-orchitis caused by gonorrhea, *Chlamydia,* or gram-negative bacilli may result in testicular failure.

The principal *drugs* that cause primary testicular failure and infertility are *cytotoxic drugs,* for example, alkylating agents such as cyclophosphamide, which are used extensively for cancer chemotherapy and immunosuppressive therapy. When used in high dosages or in combination regimens, cytotoxic agents can induce severe germ cell damage to the extent that seminiferous tubules may be devoid of all germ cell elements (i.e., Sertoli-cell–only syndrome).[110, 111] Serum FSH levels are usually elevated. Serum testosterone and LH levels are usually unaffected. With severe testicular damage, however, both LH and FSH levels may be elevated.[112] *Sulfasalazine,* a drug used in the treatment of inflammatory bowel disease, may also cause an isolated impairment of spermatogenesis, oligozoospermia, and infertility.[113]

Other drugs can result in infertility primarily by producing androgen deficiency or by interfering with androgen action. Because androgens are required to maintain normal sperm production and sexual function, these drugs may contribute to the cause of infertility in some men. Examples of drugs that act in this way are *alcohol* and *marijuana,* frequently abused drugs that have direct inhibitory effects on testosterone production as well as sperm function[114, 115]; *ketoconazole,* an antifungal agent, and perhaps cyclosporine, an immunosuppressive agent, which inhibit testosterone biosynthesis[116, 117]; *spironolactone,* an aldosterone antagonist, which both inhibits synthesis and blocks action of androgens[118]; and *flutamide,* an androgen antagonist, and *histamine$_2$ receptor antagonists* (e.g., cimetidine), which primarily block androgen action.[119]

The human testis is exquisitely sensitive to ionizing *irradiation.* Exposure to irradiation usually occurs as a result of treatment regimens for malignancy (e.g., Hodgkin's disease, testicular carcinoma, or prostate cancer). The degree of germ cell damage and suppression of spermatogenesis depends on whether exposure occurs before or after puberty and the dosage and duration of exposure.[120, 121] Compared with prepubertal exposure, germ cell damage is more severe if irradiation occurs during or after puberty. As little as 15 rad of irradiation may significantly suppress sperm production, and 50 rad generally causes azoospermia in adults.[121, 122]

Sperm counts usually recover if adequate numbers of spermatogonia remain after irradiation. Doses of irradiation greater than 600 rad, however, usually produce complete and irreversible germ cell loss and result in permanent infertility.[121, 122] Doses greater than 800 to 1000 rad may also result in Leydig cell failure and androgen deficiency.[123] Despite testicular shielding, permanent germ cell damage and infertility can occur, especially when irradiation is used in conjunction with combination chemotherapy regimens in the treatment of malignancy (e.g., lymphoma). Banking of sperm before irradiation or chemotherapy should be considered in patients who may wish to father children at a later date. It should be recognized, however, that men with malignant disease (e.g., Hodgkin's disease or testicular cancer) may have testicular dysfunction before the institution of therapy.[124, 125]

As discussed previously, spermatogenesis is sensitive to temperature. Hyperthermic germ cell damage probably contributes to the pathophysiology of infertility in men with varicocele and cryptorchidism. *Hyperthermic injury* causes transient suppression of sperm production following an *acute febrile illness.*[68] This may contribute transiently to infertility in some men, but a more common problem is that low sperm counts following a fever may result in a falsely abnormal assessment of overall spermatogenesis during the evaluation of male infertility. Heat injury may also contribute to the suppression of spermatogenesis in men with *spinal cord injury,* whose scrotal temperature may be increased as a result of defective sympathetic nervous system thermoregulation.[126, 127]

Testicular damage and infertility may result from exposure to *environmental toxins.* Chemical agents that are toxic to the testis and suppress spermatogenesis are *dibromochloropropane* (DBCP), a nematocide; *carbon disulfide,* an industrial solvent; and metals, including *lead, cadmium,* and *mercury.*[128] These agents together with a large number of other chemicals (including cigarette smoke) that have been implicated as potential testicular toxins and as yet unidentified toxins may contribute significantly to the cause of infertility in some men.[129]

Obviously, bilateral *surgical or traumatic castration* or *physical trauma* with vascular compromise (e.g., testicular torsion) are also causes of primary infertility and androgen deficiency.

Systemic Disorders. Cirrhosis of the liver and chronic renal failure may cause impairments in both sperm and androgen production resulting in infertility. Although these disorders affect testicular function primarily by direct effects on the testis, they usually also cause abnormalities in gonadotropin secretion, perhaps from malnutrition or stress related to chronic illness. Thus patients with chronic liver and renal disease usually have both primary and secondary hypogonadism. This is probably the case to some extent in all of the systemic disorders described in this section that mostly cause primary testicular dysfunction.[130]

Testicular atrophy and histologic evidence of reduced spermatogenesis and peritubular fibrosis are present in approximately 50% of men with *hepatic cirrhosis*.[131] Testicular damage probably occurs to a large extent as a sequela of chronic alcohol abuse (with its associated nutritional deficiency), the most common cause of hepatic cirrhosis. Serum testosterone levels are usually low, estradiol levels are relatively increased, and gonadotropins are in the high-normal range to moderately elevated.[131, 132] The relatively high estradiol levels may contribute to the pathogenesis of gynecomastia (increased breast tissue) and testicular failure.

Chronic renal failure also causes reduction in both sperm and androgen production. Spermatogenesis and fertility are usually severely affected in most men with chronic renal failure.[133] Serum testosterone levels are usually reduced, and gonadotropin levels are increased, in part owing to reduced clearance rates.[133] The cause of testicular dysfunction is poorly understood but is probably multifactorial with contributions from nutritional (including zinc) deficiency, relative estrogen excess, hyperprolactinemia, and nondialyzable uremic toxins. Successful renal transplantation improves testicular function and fertility but does not completely normalize them, probably because of the immunosuppressive therapy that is required.[133]

For unclear reasons, men with advanced *malignancy*, for example, Hodgkin's disease or testicular cancer, may have low sperm counts or testosterone levels before therapy.[124, 125] Systemic *vasculitis* (e.g., periarteritis nodosa), *infiltrative disease* (e.g., amyloidosis), and *sickle cell disease* may cause primary testicular failure and infertility.[134–136]

SECONDARY HYPOGONADISM

Congenital or Developmental Disorders. *Hypogonadotropic eunuchoidism (Kallmann's syndrome)* is a congenital disorder characterized by isolated gonadotropin deficiency resulting in *eunuchoidism* (sexual infantilism and eunuchoidal body habitus) and *anosmia* or *hyposmia*, which occurs in about 80% of cases.[137, 138] These patients may also exhibit other midline defects (e.g., cleft lip or palate), skeletal abnormalities (e.g., short fourth metacarpals, syndactyly, craniofacial asymmetry), pes cavus deformity, abnormalities of brain function (e.g., cerebellar dysfunction or eye and mirror movement abnormalities), or cryptorchidism.[137–140] In the absence of associated abnormalities, Kallmann's syndrome can-

not be easily distinguished from constitutional delayed puberty. Spontaneous pubertal onset, which eventually occurs in the latter, is the most reliable way to differentiate these two disorders, both of which cause isolated hypogonadotropic hypogonadism. Kallmann's syndrome occurs as both sporadic and familial disorders and predominantly in men. In the familial forms, autosomal dominant transmission is most common, but X-linked recessive and autosomal recessive inheritance patterns have also been described in other kindreds.[141, 142]

Isolated gonadotropin deficiency in Kallmann's syndrome is caused by a defect in GnRH secretion, and long-term pulsatile administration of GnRH restores normal pituitary gonadotropin secretion.[9, 10] The degree of GnRH and gonadotropin deficiency and as a result the clinical presentation are variable. The majority of men with this syndrome have low-normal to undetectable LH and FSH levels (with undetectable or abnormally low spontaneous pulsatile gonadotropin secretion) and low serum testosterone levels.[143] Patients with classic Kallmann's syndrome present with infantile external genitalia and accessory sex organs, aspermia or azoospermia, and eunuchoidism, which is characterized by lack of a male hair pattern, high-pitched voice, poor muscular development, prepubertal fat distribution, and excessive long bone growth (due to delayed epiphyseal closure) as a result of prepubertal androgen deficiency.[137–140] Testis size and histology are prepubertal, reflecting the lack of gonadotropin stimulation (Fig. 37–6).[83] In the absence of cryptorchidism, there is no peritubular hyalinization. Infertility is not only due to impaired sperm production, but also may be related to severe prepubertal androgen deficiency, which results in the poorly developed accessory sex glands and deficient seminal fluid production as well as sexual dysfunction.

Less severe degrees of gonadotropin and GnRH deficiency occur in some patients. Men with *isolated LH deficiency* or *FSH deficiency* have variants of Kallmann's syndrome.[144–147] Depending on the severity of androgen deficiency, men with less severe gonadotropin (and presumably GnRH) deficiency have varying degrees of virilization. Spermatogenesis is impaired, however, and infertility is nearly uniformly present, even in those with relatively well-preserved FSH secretion, the so-called *fertile eunuch syndrome*.[144, 145]

In most cases, the cause of GnRH deficiency in Kallmann's syndrome is uncertain. No major mutations in the GnRH gene have been identified.[148] In an X-linked form of Kallmann's syndrome, disordered migration of GnRH neurons from the olfactory region to the hypothalamus has been observed.[149–151] It is unclear, however, whether this defect is the cause of GnRH deficiency in other forms of this probably heterogeneous disorder. Anosmia or hyposmia, which often accompanies gonadotropin deficiency in Kallmann's syndrome, is caused by defective development of the olfactory bulbs and tracts.[152] Therefore it is hypothesized that in most cases of Kallmann's syndrome, GnRH deficiency results from an absence of embryonic GnRH neurons located in the olfactory area.

Infertility in Kallmann's syndrome is potentially treatable. Androgen production and spermatogenesis may be stimulated, and fertility may be achieved by administration of gonadotropin or pulsatile GnRH therapy in men with Kallmann's syndrome.[10, 16, 25, 26] Usually, treatment with gonadotropins (i.e., hCG and human menopausal gonadotropin

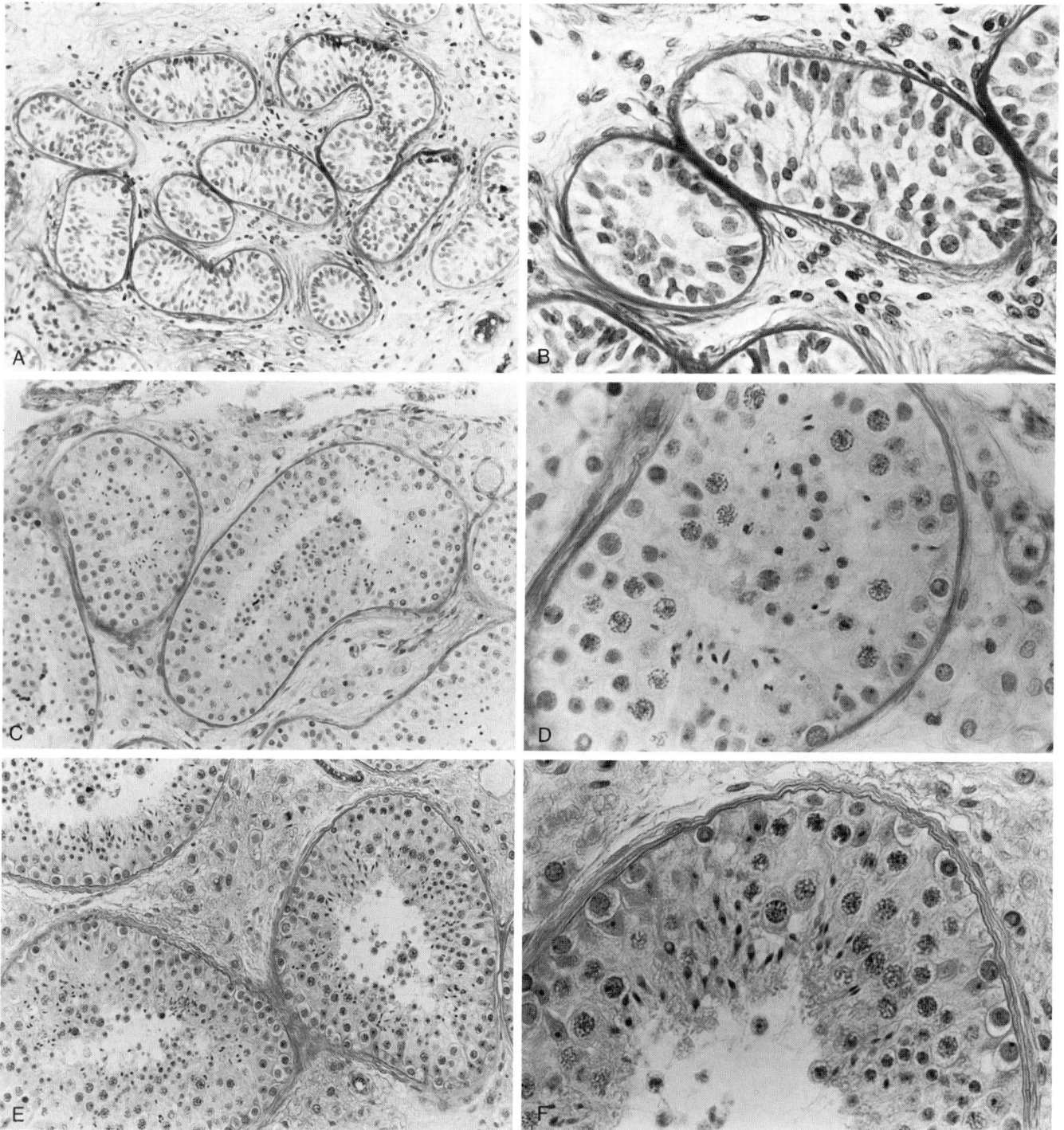

FIGURE 37–6. Sequential testis biopsies at low (left) and high (right) power from a man with hypogonadotropic eunuchoidism: (*A* and *B*) at presentation, prior to any treatment. Note the immature germinal epithelium and mesenchymal cells (precursors of Leydig cells) within the interstitium; (*C* and *D*) 59 weeks after human chorionic gonadotropin (hCG) therapy alone. Spermatogenesis is in progress, and all germ cell types can be detected, up to and including Sc and d spermatids; (*E* and *F*) 31 weeks after combined hCG and human menopausal gonadotropin treatment. Note the increase in numbers of all germ cells. Sperm counts at this time ranged from 10 to 13.6 million/mL. (From Paulsen CA. In: Williams RH, editor. Textbook of Endocrinology. 6th edition. Philadelphia: WB Saunders, 1981:333.)

[hMG] or FSH) is needed to stimulate sufficient sperm production to induce fertility (see Fig. 37–6).[10, 16, 25, 26, 153] In men with relative preservation of FSH secretion, however, sperm production may be stimulated with LH-like activity alone.[10, 16, 25, 26, 153] It should be recognized that an impairment of

testicular function may also exist in this disorder, as evidenced by the lack of uniformly normal testosterone and sperm production in response to gonadotropin stimulation in some men with Kallmann's syndrome.[26, 154–156] Poor testicular response to gonadotropins can be explained by the coexistence of cryptorchidism (especially if bilateral) in many of these men, but poor responses have also been observed in men with normally descended testes.[26, 154–156]

Hemochromatosis is a genetic disorder of mucosal iron transport that results in tissue parenchymal iron deposition, predominantly in liver, skin, pancreas, and heart. Iron overload within the pituitary gland causes isolated gonadotropin deficiency. Testicular atrophy and impairments of both androgen and sperm production occur in approximately 60% of men with this disorder.[157–159] Hypogonadism and infertility associated with hemochromatosis are usually treatable (see Fig. 37–2). Despite iron deposition within the testis, gonadotropin administration usually stimulates spermatogenesis and restores fertility.[16, 158, 159] Occasionally, therapy aimed at decreasing iron overload, such as frequent phlebotomy or chelation therapy with desferrioxamine, may restore normal gonadotropin secretion.[160] Pituitary gonadotropin responsiveness to GnRH is absent or markedly attenuated,[158, 159] and pulsatile GnRH therapy is generally not effective in treating the infertility caused by hemochromatosis. Pituitary iron deposition and hypogonadotropic hypogonadism may also occur in conditions requiring frequent blood transfusions, such as thalassemia.[161–163]

Gonadotropin deficiency may be present in a number of *complex genetic syndromes*, including the *Prader-Labhart-Willi, Laurence-Moon-Beidl, Lowe, familial cerebellar ataxia, steroid sulfatase deficiency, RUD, CHARGE,* and *LEOPARD* syndromes.[100, 101]

Acquired Disorders. *Hypopituitarism* may result from any destructive or infiltrative lesion of the hypothalamus or pituitary gland.[164, 165] These lesions may cause gonadotropin deficiency with or without deficiencies of other anterior pituitary hormones. Destructive processes involving the pituitary usually cause a sequential loss of hormone secretion. Gonadotropin and growth hormone secretion are usually lost before compromise of thyroid-stimulating hormone (TSH) release (which causes secondary hypothyroidism), which, in turn, usually occurs before diminished adrenocorticotropic hormone (ACTH) secretion (which causes secondary adrenal insufficiency). With severe destructive or infiltrative processes, all anterior pituitary function may be lost, resulting in *panhypopituitarism,* a life-threatening condition. Hypothalamic or high pituitary stalk lesions may destroy or compromise neurons that synthesize antidiuretic hormone (ADH) or arginine vasopressin, resulting in *diabetes insipidus.* Furthermore, pituitary adenomas causing hypogonadotropic hypogonadism may be functional and secrete excessive amounts of prolactin, growth hormone, or ACTH, which may cause clinical manifestations of hyperprolactinemia, acromegaly, and Cushing's disease. Finally, hypothalamic or pituitary lesions may cause *mass effects* (e.g., visual field defects) by impinging on vital brain structures. Therefore it is important to re-emphasize that infertility caused by gonadotropin deficiency may be the first clue to a mass lesion of the hypothalamus or pituitary and either deficiency or excessive secretion of other anterior pituitary hormones.

Specific destructive or infiltrative conditions that may cause hypopituitarism are *pituitary adenomas* (functional or nonfunctional), *suprasellar tumors* (e.g., craniopharyngioma, meningioma, optic glioma, or astrocytoma), *metastatic cancer, lymphoma, surgical removal or irradiation* of the pituitary gland, *trauma, vascular compromise* (e.g., infarction, apoplexy,

or vasculitis), *aneurysm or arteriovenous malformation, autoimmune hypophysitis, granulomatous disease* (e.g., tuberculosis, sarcoidosis, fungal disease, or histiocytosis X), *abscess,* and *transfusion-related iron overload.*[164, 165]

In hypopituitarism, both serum testosterone and sperm production are impaired, and gonadotropin levels are low or low normal. Infertility may be treated in these men with acquired hypogonadotropic hypogonadism by administration of gonadotropins. Often, treatment with LH-like activity (i.e., hCG) alone stimulates sufficient spermatogenesis to restore fertility in men who become gonadotropin deficient as adults.[10, 16, 25, 26, 153] In contrast, most men who acquire gonadotropin deficiency prepubertally usually require treatment with both LH-like and FSH-like activity to stimulate spermatogenesis.[10, 16, 25, 26, 153]

Elevated serum prolactin or *hyperprolactinemia* often causes hypogonadotropic hypogonadism resulting in infertility. A common cause of hyperprolactinemia is a *prolactin-secreting pituitary adenoma.* In men, these tumors are usually large (i.e., macroadenomas), and gonadotropin deficiency is caused in part by destruction of pituitary gonadotropin-secreting cells.[166, 167] Even in the absence of a destructive lesion in the pituitary, however, hyperprolactinemia has an inhibitory effect on GnRH and gonadotropin secretion and may cause secondary hypogonadism.[168] Other causes of elevated serum prolactin levels include *CNS-active drugs* (e.g., phenothiazines and other antipsychotics, opiates, sedative-hypnotics, stimulants, anesthetics, antiemetics, and antidepressants), *hypothyroidism, dopamine antagonist drugs* (e.g., metoclopramide), *antihypertensive drugs* (e.g., α-methyldopa, reserpine), *estrogens, renal failure, chest wall lesions,* or *nipple stimulation.*[167, 169] Treatment of the underlying cause of hyperprolactinemia (e.g., removal of prolactin-secreting pituitary adenoma or discontinuation of drugs that stimulate prolactin secretion) or administration of a dopamine agonist, such as bromocriptine, may restore normal gonadal function and fertility.[167, 170] In the unusual circumstance that hyperprolactinemia cannot be treated, these men would also respond to GnRH or gonadotropin therapy.[168, 171] It should be noted, however, that impotence, which may contribute to the infertility of hyperprolactinemia, may not be corrected until elevated prolactin levels are reduced.[167]

Sex steroid hormones (androgens, estrogens, and progestogens) inhibit endogenous GnRH and gonadotropin secretion, resulting in secondary testicular failure. *Androgen excess* suppresses both endogenous GnRH and gonadotropin secretion directly, causing suppression of testicular function. Despite suppression of LH and endogenous testosterone secretion, the secondary hypogonadism that is induced is manifested by isolated impairment of sperm production and infertility because androgen levels are maintained exogenously.[13, 172] Androgen excess may be caused by exogenous administration of androgens. Administration of *testosterone enanthate* and other androgenic compounds to normal men have been shown to suppress spermatogenesis effectively in male contraceptive development trials.[172, 173] *Androgenic anabolic steroids,* often in suprapharmacologic doses, have been used by elite athletes to enhance performance and have caused severe oligozoospermia or azoospermia.[174] Excessive endogenous androgen secretion may occur in men with *congenital adrenal hyperplasia* (e.g., 21-hydroxylase or 11β-hydroxylase deficiency) or with *testosterone-secreting tumors* (e.g., Leydig cell tumors).[175, 176]

Estrogen excess also suppresses gonadotropin secretion and causes secondary hypogonadism.[177] In contrast to the situation with androgen excess, both testosterone deficiency and impairment of spermatogenesis usually result.[178, 179] Estrogen excess may result from administration of estrogens or estrogenic substances (e.g., diethylstilbestrol administration in men with metastatic prostate cancer) or endogenous secretion from an estrogen-secreting neoplasm (e.g., feminizing adrenal carcinoma).[176, 180] Digoxin may increase estradiol and suppress LH and testosterone levels.[181] Administration of *progestogens* (e.g., medroxyprogesterone acetate for sleep apnea) or *opiate-like drugs* (e.g., morphine, methadone, and heroin) and other *CNS-active drugs* may also inhibit gonadotropins and testicular function.[182–185]

Systemic Disorders. A number of systemic disorders may cause secondary hypogonadism and impaired androgen and sperm production, which may contribute to the pathogenesis of infertility. *Glucocorticoid excess* or *Cushing's syndrome* suppresses endogenous GnRH and gonadotropin secretion and results in secondary testicular failure with infertility.[186, 187] The causes of Cushing's syndrome include chronic glucocorticoid therapy (most commonly), ACTH-secreting pituitary adenoma, ectopic ACTH syndrome, and glucocorticoid-secreting adrenal tumors (adenomas or carcinomas). *Nutritional deficiency* (e.g., *protein-calorie malnutrition* or *anorexia nervosa*) also inhibits GnRH and gonadotropin secretion and may cause secondary hypogonadism.[188, 189] Activation of the hypothalamic-pituitary-adrenal axis and malnutrition may both contribute to the suppression of GnRH and gonadotropin secretion and secondary hypogonadism associated with *acute and chronic stress and illness* (e.g., with *psychiatric disorders; malignancy; burns*; and *chronic cardiac, lung, liver, and kidney disease*).[124, 125, 190–199] In all of these disorders, diminished GnRH secretion is the major mechanism underlying the secondary testicular failure. Concomitant primary testicular dysfunction, however, may also be present in some men. Men with *massive obesity* may have low gonadotropin and testosterone levels and impaired spermatogenesis and infertility.[200]

ANDROGEN RESISTANCE SYNDROMES

Incomplete androgen resistance syndromes may present with underandrogenization and infertility in men with normal or nearly normal male external genitalia. These men may also have varying degrees of gynecomastia, hypospadias, and cryptorchidism. Some men with *Reifenstein's syndrome* and *idiopathic oligozoospermia or azoospermia* may present in this way.[43, 44, 201, 202] Serum testosterone levels are increased, and LH levels are usually elevated reflecting resistance to androgen action at the hypothalamic-pituitary level. Testis biopsy reveals a varying picture ranging from maturation arrest to germ cell aplasia.[43] More severe germ cell damage occurs in those men with associated cryptorchidism. The underlying molecular defects in many of these men with androgen resistance are genetic mutations in the androgen receptor gene, resulting in decreased androgen receptor number, stability, or function.[203]

Men with deficiency of 5α-reductase, the enzyme that converts testosterone to dihydrotestosterone (DHT), also exhibit partial androgen resistance.[204–206] At birth, patients with 5α-reductase deficiency have ambiguous genitalia and are usually raised as girls. At the time of puberty, however, increasing testosterone secretion from the testes overcomes the partial deficiency of 5α-reductase, and incomplete virilization occurs. Facial hair, acne, frontal balding, and prostate enlargement, which depend on DHT formation, remain conspicuously absent. Serum testosterone level is normal to slightly elevated, DHT concentration is reduced, and gonadotropin levels are slightly increased in these men. Spermatogenesis is impaired because testes are usually undescended, and these men are infertile.[207]

Men with *celiac disease* have a testicular dysfunction associated with a hormonal pattern that suggests androgen resistance, that is, elevated serum testosterone and LH concentrations.[208, 209]

Disorders of Sperm Transport and Accessory Gland Function

PHYSIOLOGIC CONSIDERATIONS

On completion of spermiogenesis, spermatozoa are released from the Sertoli cell into the lumen of the seminiferous tubule (*spermiation*) and transported into the *rete testis, ductuli efferentes,* and *caput epididymidis.* Newly formed spermatozoa are immotile, and transport through the excurrent duct system occurs as a result of tubular reabsorption of seminiferous tubule fluid, ciliary action of tubular epithelial cells, and spontaneous peritubular contractions.[210, 211]

During passage through the *epididymis,* spermatozoa undergo further maturation changes and acquire the ability to move and fertilize eggs.[212–214] In the caput epididymidis, spermatozoa are exposed to high concentrations of hydrogen, potassium and magnesium ions, carbonic anhydrase, glyceryl phosphorylcholine, L-carnitine, and sialic acid, and sodium and chloride ions and water are actively removed from luminal fluid.[210, 211, 215] In addition, several proteins secreted into the luminal fluid bind or are incorporated into the plasma membrane of spermatozoa and affect the motility of sperm (e.g., progressive motility sustaining factor).[210, 211, 216, 217] The changes in tubular fluid milieu are thought to play an important role in sperm maturation and transport. The exact mechanisms, however, are poorly understood. This lack of understanding of the mechanisms by which the epididymis affects sperm maturation and function represents a major impediment to further understanding of the pathophysiology of male infertility.

Maintenance of the epididymal structure and function is androgen dependent and requires *DHT,* which is actively synthesized from testosterone in epididymal cells by the action of the enzyme, 5α-reductase.[210, 211, 218] Movement of spermatozoa through the epididymis occurs as a result of ciliary action of efferent duct cells, hydrostatic pressure gradients, and peristaltic contractions of the epididymal duct.[210, 211] The transit time of sperm through the epididymis is approximately 12 days.[22, 219] Normal sperm maturation requires transit through the caput and corpus epididymidis and is complete on arrival in the cauda epididymidis, which is the major storage site of spermatozoa.[220] Sperm are stored in the cauda epididymidis for about 4 days, depending on the frequency of ejaculation. Sperm storage in the epididymis is sensitive to elevated temperature. Reduced epididymal sperm storage and function induced by increased local temperature may contribute to the infertility associated with varicocele. Infertility due to reduced or absent motility or abnormal sperm morphology or otherwise unexplained (idiopathic) infertility could potentially be attributable to epididymal dysfunction. At present, however, definitive evidence for this is lacking.

The *vas deferens* primarily serves to transport sperm from the epididymis to the urethra during ejaculation. As a result of the acidic, nutrient-deficient milieu, spermatozoa in the vas deferens are relatively dormant.[221] The ampulla of the vas deferens serves to store a significant number of spermatozoa before ejaculation. Sperm movement through the vas deferens occurs mainly at the time of ejaculation, when increased sympathetic nervous system activity stimulates peristaltic contractions of the smooth muscle layers of the vas, resulting in *emission* of sperm to the posterior urethra.[222] Loss of the sympathetic innervation, for example, after retroperitoneal lymphadenectomy or local damage following vasovasostomy, results in loss of sperm movement through the vas deferens and failure of emission.

The major physiologic role of the *seminal vesicles* and *prostate* is to produce the bulk of seminal plasma. Although sperm motility and function are affected by seminal plasma components, the precise relationship between specific accessory gland secretions and male fertility remains speculative. Thus the majority of infertile men with isolated defects in sperm motility (asthenospermia) or function remain idiopathic.

The *seminal vesicles* secrete fluid containing large amounts of fructose and phosphorylcholine and smaller amounts of prostaglandins, ascorbic acid, inositol, fibrinogen, ergothioneine, flavin, potassium, and amino acids.[223, 224] During ejaculation, after stored sperm are emptied from the vas deferens and the cauda epididymidis, the seminal vesicles empty their contents into the ejaculatory duct. In addition to contributing to the bulk ejaculated semen volume (50% to 80%), fructose secreted by the seminal vesicles is a primary source of energy for sperm.[225] Other seminal vesicle products are thought to play important roles in regulating motility and fertilizing capacity of ejaculated sperm and coagulation of semen.[223, 224]

The *prostate gland* secretes a more alkaline fluid containing citric acid, calcium, zinc, acid and alkaline phosphatase, spermine, diamine oxidase, amylase, lactate dehydrogenase, β-glucuronidase, plasminogen activator, a clotting enzyme, and a fibrinolysin (seminin).[223, 224] The physiologic roles of these products are poorly understood. Along with seminal vesicle products, prostatic secretions are thought to be important for coagulation and liquefaction of semen, survival of ejaculated spermatozoa, and acquisition of sperm motility and fertilizing capacity.[226]

The relatively alkaline nature of prostatic fluid is thought to play an important role in neutralizing the acidity of vas deferens fluid and female vaginal secretions after ejaculation, thereby enhancing sperm motility and fertilizing capacity. A clotting enzyme in prostatic fluid causes clotting proteins, including fibrinogen from seminal vesicle fluid, to form a coagulum.[225, 226] Within about 20 minutes, activation of prostatic proteases (including the kallikrein-like serine protease, prostate specific antigen (PSA), and fibrinolysin) results in liquefaction of the coagulum.[225, 226] After liquefaction, sperm become highly motile. Although sperm can live for many weeks in the male genital tract, once they are ejaculated in

semen their maximal life span is only 24 to 72 hours at body temperature.[227]

The male accessory sex organs depend on androgen, primarily DHT, for their development, growth, and function.[15, 223, 224] The vas deferens, seminal vesicles, and prostate gland are primarily regulated by sympathetic input from the hypogastric nerve, which originates from spinal cord level T12-L2.[223, 224] Sympathetic adrenergic fibers control smooth muscle contraction, whereas sympathetic cholinergic fibers regulate epithelial cell secretion from the accessory sex glands.[223, 224] The physiologic role of parasympathetic innervation of these glands is unclear.

Infertility may result from impaired sperm transport as a result of mechanical obstruction of the excurrent duct system or abnormal epididymal or accessory gland function (see Table 37–3). Although accessory sex glands are essential for fertility, problems of sperm transport are relatively uncommon, and identifiable abnormalities of accessory gland function are rare causes of clinical male infertility.

DUCTAL OBSTRUCTION

Obstruction of sperm transport from the testis to urethra results in azoospermia and infertility. Measurement of serum FSH levels may be helpful in differentiating obstructive azoospermia from azoospermia caused by severely impaired spermatogenesis.[32, 33, 228] Elevated FSH levels usually indicate severely disordered spermatogenesis and poor prognosis for fertility. Normal FSH levels are not helpful because they can occur with either obstructive azoospermia or seminiferous tubule failure.

Congenital defects of the vas deferens, seminal vesicles, and epididymis may obstruct sperm transport. These include *congenital absence of the vas and seminal vesicles,* which is most commonly due to wolffian duct agenesis associated with *cystic fibrosis* or less commonly occurring as an *isolated* malformation,[229, 230] and congenital malformations of the epididymis as a consequence of *in utero diethylstilbestrol exposure.*[231] In *Young's syndrome,* inspissated secretions within the vas and epididymis impede normal transport of sperm and result in azoospermia.[232] Consistent minor abnormalities of the sperm tail axoneme have also been found.[233] Both cystic fibrosis and Young's syndrome are also associated with recurrent respiratory tract (sinus and pulmonary) infections. *Müllerian duct cysts* may also cause bilateral obstruction of sperm transport.[234] The ejaculatory duct is a common site of obstruction associated with congenital wolffian or müllerian duct abnormalities.[235]

The most common cause of acquired obstruction of sperm transport is *vasectomy. Postinfectious obstruction of the epididymis, seminal vesicles, or vas* (e.g., secondary to tuberculosis, *Chlamydia,* or gonorrhea) may result in excurrent ductal obstruction, azoospermia, and infertility.[236, 237]

IMPAIRED SYMPATHETIC INNERVATION OF DUCTS

Damage to the sympathetic nervous system innervation of the excurrent ducts results in absence of epididymal and vas deferens contractions and loss of emission at the time of ejaculation. This may contribute to the cause of infertility associated with *spinal cord disease, sympathectomy or sympa-*

tholytic drugs, and *retroperitoneal lymphadenectomy.* Local injury to sympathetic nerves also leads to inadequate contraction of the excurrent ducts. This may contribute, in part, to the oligozoospermia that may occur after apparently successful *vasovasostomy.*

EPIDIDYMAL AND ACCESSORY GLAND DYSFUNCTION

Normal development and function of the epididymis and accessory glands depend on androgens. Thus it is likely that infertility associated with *androgen deficiency or resistance* is caused, in part, by epididymal, seminal vesicle, and prostate gland dysfunction. Storage of sperm in the cauda epididymidis is highly sensitive to elevated temperature. *Hyperthermic injury* of epididymal spermatozoa probably contributes to the infertility associated with varicocele and cryptorchidism. *Genital tract infections* involving the epididymis, prostate, and seminal vesicles are most commonly caused by *Neisseria gonorrhoeae, Chlamydia trachomatis, Ureaplasma urealyticum,* gram-negative bacilli, and *Mycobacterium tuberculosis.*[238, 239] It is hypothesized that these infections result in epididymal and accessory sex gland dysfunction and cause infertility. Except for infections that cause orchitis or excurrent duct obstruction (see earlier), however, a causal relationship between genitourinary infections and infertility has not been established.[238, 239]

Erectile Dysfunction

PHYSIOLOGIC CONSIDERATIONS

Penile erectile tissue consists of two dorsal corpora cavernosa and a ventral corpus spongiosum, which surrounds the urethra and forms the glans penis.[240, 241] The corpora are composed of numerous cavernous spaces lined by vascular epithelial cells separated by smooth muscle containing trabeculae. A fibrous tissue sheath surrounds each corpus (tunica albuginea), and all three corporal bodies are surrounded by a single fascia (Buck's fascia).

Penile erection is primarily a vascular event that is regulated by the nervous system, both by the brain and the parasympathetic and sympathetic nervous system. Erections are generated by two synergistic neural mechanisms: (1) *Reflexogenic erections* are induced by sensory stimulation of the penis and mediated by a sacral spinal cord reflex arc, and (2) *psychogenic erections* are induced by psychic stimulation from higher brain centers and mediated by both thoracolumbar and sacral spinal cord erection centers.[240–242]

In reflexogenic erections, sensory afferent impulses from the penis travel via the pudendal nerve to the sacral spinal cord erection center (S2-S4).[240–242] Efferent parasympathetic fibers return via the pelvic splanchnic nerve (nervi erigentes), which joins the pelvic plexus and reaches the penis via the cavernosal nerve. Efferent somatic fibers traveling in the pudendal nerve innervate the striated perineal muscles.

Sympathetic nerve fibers originate in the thoracolumbar spinal cord erection center (T12-L2), travel via the hypogastric nerve to the pelvic plexus, and also reach the penis via the cavernosal nerve.[240–242] In psychogenic erections, a variety of visual, tactile, auditory, and gustatory stimuli are received

in cortical and subcortical brain regions, integrated in the limbic system, and relayed via descending pathways to both the thoracolumbar and the sacral spinal cord erection centers. Penile erection is primarily but not exclusively controlled by the parasympathetic nervous system. Nerve fibers of the pelvic plexus also innervate the vas deferens, seminal vesicles, prostate, and bladder, serving to coordinate erection and antegrade ejaculation.[240–242]

The stimuli that induce psychogenic erections also stimulate *libido,* or sexual desire and drive. Therefore disorders that reduce libido are nearly always accompanied by erectile dysfunction or impotence. Libido is primarily regulated by psychological factors and to a variable degree by androgens.[242, 243]

Activation of the spinal cord erection centers results in corporeal trabecular smooth muscle relaxation and vasodilatation of cavernosal arterioles and sinusoids. The neurotransmitters that mediate these actions are poorly understood but probably involve cholinergic (acetylcholine) stimulation of secondary noncholinergic, nonadrenergic neurotransmitter systems (e.g., vasoactive intestinal peptide, neuropeptide Y, and endothelium-derived nitric oxide)[244–247] and inhibition of other neurotransmitter systems (primarily basal α-adrenergic constrictive tone).[248] With the relaxation of penile smooth muscle, blood flow into the corporal spaces increases and causes engorgement of the penis (i.e., tumescence). Expansion of the trabecular walls against the tunica albuginea impedes venous outflow from the penis, resulting in sustained tumescence (i.e., an erection).[241, 249] Contraction of the perineal (ischiocavernosus and bulbocavernosus) muscles by pudendal nerve stimulation increases cavernosal pressure to levels greater than systemic blood pressure, resulting in maximal penile rigidity.[249] Detumescence results from α-adrenergic vasoconstriction, which reduces arterial blood flow and penile smooth muscle relaxation, causing collapse of corporal trabeculae and increased venous outflow.[241, 249]

Impotence is a consistent inability to achieve or maintain an erection sufficient to complete intercourse and achieve *orgasm* (the pleasurable sensation at the climax of sexual activity).[240, 241] *CNS disorders, spinal cord diseases, autonomic nervous dysfunction, drugs that affect peripheral erectile response, vascular disease* (affecting either the arterial supply or venous drainage of the penis), and *penile abnormalities* may cause erectile dysfunction (see Table 37–4) and infertility by interfering with the ability to complete intercourse successfully.[240, 241] Furthermore, some CNS disorders (e.g., androgen deficiency) may also reduce libido, or interest and initiative, which may also contribute to the pathophysiology of infertility.

CENTRAL NERVOUS SYSTEM DISORDERS

Normal CNS functioning is necessary to maintain libido and potency. CNS disorders cause erectile dysfunction by interfering with central regulation of erectile function or erotic response in the brain. Thus most disorders of the CNS that cause impotence also reduce libido. They include varying degrees of *psychiatric disturbance* from *emotional stress* and *performance anxiety* to *major psychiatric illness,* such as major depression or psychotic disorders[250]; *chronic medical illness,* including chronic cardiac, respiratory, renal, and liver disease and malignancy[251, 252]; *CNS-active drugs* (e.g., *central antihy-*

pertensive, antidepressant, antipsychotic, and *sedative-hypnotic drugs* and *alcohol*)[253–256]; and *endocrine disorders,* especially *androgen deficiency, hyperprolactinemia, hyperthyroidism,* and *hypothyroidism.*[167, 243, 251, 257–259] Hyperprolactinemia causes impotence and diminished libido primarily by suppressing GnRH and gonadotropin secretion and inducing androgen deficiency. In many hyperprolactinemic men, however, testosterone replacement alone does not restore sexual function, and normal erectile function and libido do not return until prolactin levels are normalized, suggesting an independent effect of hyperprolactinemia on sexual functioning. In contrast to the CNS disorders already mentioned, some destructive or infiltrative *CNS diseases,* such as infarction or tumors, involving the limbic system or temporal lobe may cause impotence in the absence of reduced libido.[260–263]

SPINAL CORD DISEASE

Spinal cord diseases, such as *spinal cord injury, multiple sclerosis, transverse myelitis, tumor, vascular compromise, epidural abscess, spinal stenosis or spina bifida,* or *syphilis,* may cause erectile dysfunction, usually without diminished libido.[264–266] Patients with high spinal cord lesions in the thoracic or lumbar level (i.e., above the sacral spinal erection center [S2-S4]) generally retain the ability to have reflexogenic erections.[264] Psychogenic erections are possible in some men with spinal cord lesions below the thoracolumbar spinal erection center (T12-L2).[264]

AUTONOMIC NERVOUS SYSTEM DYSFUNCTION

Disorders affecting peripheral autonomic nervous system function may cause impotence and contribute to infertility by interfering with normal regulation of penile vascular and smooth muscle. *Pelvic surgery* (e.g., *abdominoperineal resection of the rectum, pelvic lymph node dissection, prostatectomy, aortoiliac bypass,* and *lumbar sympathectomy*) may disrupt autonomic innervation of the penis resulting in erectile dysfunction.[265, 267–271] *Diabetes* and other conditions causing *peripheral autonomic and sensory neuropathy* (e.g., *amyloidosis, vasculitis, arsenic or mercury exposure, vasculitis, renal failure, Shy-Drager syndrome, and acute intermittent porphyria*) may also cause impotence.[265, 272]

DRUGS AFFECTING PERIPHERAL ERECTILE RESPONSE

Drugs may cause erectile dysfunction by inhibiting penile smooth muscle relaxation and arterial vasodilation. Classes of medications that do this include *anticholinergic drugs, antidepressants, β-adrenergic antagonists, antihistamines,* and *antihypertensive drugs.*[253–256, 273] The mechanism of impotence reported with many antihypertensives (e.g., diuretics, calcium channel antagonists, and angiotensin-converting enzyme inhibitors) and other drugs is unclear. Other drugs, such as *sympathomimetic agents* and *α-adrenergic agonists,* result in premature detumescence by inducing arterial vasoconstriction.[248]

PERIPHERAL VASCULAR DISEASE

Distal aortoiliac obstruction from atherosclerotic vascular disease is a common cause of impotence, particularly in el-

derly men.[274–277] Atherosclerotic involvement of smaller distal *penile arteries* may also contribute to cause of erectile dysfunction in some men, for example, elderly men with *diabetes.* Both large and small vessel atherosclerotic disease together with peripheral autonomic neuropathy are major factors contributing to the high incidence of impotence (50%) in diabetic men.[278–280] Although atherosclerotic vascular disease is by far the most common, other causes of arterial obstruction (e.g., surgical trauma, radiation damage) may also cause impotence.[281, 282] Obstructive arterial disease causes erectile dysfunction by preventing sufficient blood flow into the penis to result in tumescence. Uncommonly, some men have an adequate arterial blood supply to initiate penile tumescense but are unable to maintain an erection because of penile *venous incompetence* resulting in premature detumescence.[283, 284]

PENILE ABNORMALITIES

Finally, abnormalities of the penis may interfere with the ability to achieve an erection sufficient to initiate or complete normal intercourse. Thus, *Peyronie's disease, chordee, micropenis, penile trauma,* and *priapism* may cause erectile dysfunction and compromise fertility.[252, 281, 285, 286] In addition to the anatomic abnormalities associated with these conditions, they may cause pain and interfere with normal intercourse.

Ejaculatory Disorders

PHYSIOLOGIC CONSIDERATIONS

During ejaculation, sympathetic nervous system activation of neurons located in thoracolumbar spinal cord (T12-L2) stimulates contraction of the cauda epididymidis, vas deferens, and ejaculatory ducts via the hypogastric nerve, resulting in movement of sperm into the posterior urethra (*emission*).[222, 241, 287, 288] Sympathetic activation that occurs via α-adrenergic receptors also stimulates seminal vesicle and prostate fluid secretion, which constitute the bulk of seminal fluid, and the internal urethral sphincter, which results in bladder neck closure and prevents retrograde ejaculation of sperm into the bladder. Emission is followed by reflex stimulation of neurons in the sacral spinal cord (S2-S4), which send somatic fibers in the pudendal nerve to the perineum and stimulate rhythmic contractions of the bulbocavernosus and ischiocavernosus muscles causing expulsion of semen from the urethra (i.e., *ejaculation*).[222, 241, 287, 288] Ejaculation normally occurs simultaneously with *orgasm,* the pleasurable experience associated with ejaculation, which is stimulated by ascending spinal cord pathways to the CNS. Both emission and ejaculation are also regulated by higher brain centers. Normal antegrade ejaculation requires normal sympathetic stimulation and contraction of the bladder neck muscles (internal urethral sphincter). Normal ejaculation produces 1.5 to 5.0 mL of semen.[7, 23, 24]

Premature, retarded, retrograde, or *reduced ejaculation* may result in infertility by interfering with the delivery of a normal number of sperm into the female genital tract (see Table 37–5).

PREMATURE OR RETARDED EJACULATION

Premature ejaculation is characterized by ejaculation occurring before or immediately on vaginal penetration, followed by a rapid loss of erection. The majority of men with this disorder have an underlying psychological disorder, for example, performance anxiety, unresolved marital difficulties, or emotional problems.[289] Rarely, organic disorders, such as prostatitis, multiple sclerosis, or spinal cord tumors, may cause premature ejaculation.[289, 290] *Retarded ejaculation* is a psychological disorder characterized by inability to ejaculate despite sexual desire, erection, and stimulation. Anxiety (e.g., related to fear of pregnancy or religious conflicts) is commonly associated with retarded ejaculation.[291, 292]

RETROGRADE EJACULATION

Retrograde ejaculation into the bladder occurs in conditions that disrupt the functional competence of the bladder neck during ejaculation. *Bladder neck surgery* commonly disrupts the muscles and innervation of the functional internal urethral sphincter. Thus, retrograde ejaculation occurs in 40% to 90% of men who have undergone transurethral and abdominal *prostatectomy*.[293, 294] It is much less common with transurethral *bladder neck incision*.[295] Men who had *Y-V urethrocystoplasty* performed during childhood may also demonstrate retrograde ejaculation.[296]

Normal antegrade ejaculation requires coordinated sympathetic nervous system stimulation of the epididymal and vas deferens contraction, accessory sex gland secretion, and bladder neck muscle contraction. Therefore *sympathetic nervous system dysfunction* may also cause retrograde ejaculation. Disorders that may disrupt the normal sympathetic innervation of the bladder neck and cause retrograde ejaculation include *autonomic neuropathy* (e.g., caused by diabetes),[265, 297] *sympatholytic drugs* (e.g., *antihypertensive, antipsychotic, antidepressant* medications) or *sympathectomy,*[253–256, 298, 299] *retroperitoneal or abdominopelvic surgery* (e.g., *retroperitoneal lymph node dissection, abdominal aortic aneurysm repair,* or *aortoiliac bypass*),[267, 268, 300, 301] and *spinal cord injury.*[264, 265, 302]

REDUCED EJACULATION

In severe prepubertal *androgen deficiency or resistance,* ejaculation may be markedly reduced or absent (aspermia) as a result of poorly developed and functioning accessory sex glands.[17, 223, 224] *Sympathetic nervous system dysfunction* (see earlier) may result in a failure of emission and result in reduced ejaculation, even in the absence of retrograde ejaculation.[253–256, 298, 299] Finally, *urethral abnormalities* (e.g., *strictures* or *trauma*) may cause reduced ejaculation as well as contribute to retrograde ejaculation,[303, 304] and rarely cause infertility. *Hypospadias* or *epispadias* may interfere with deposition of adequate amounts of sperm into the vagina.

Coital Disorders and Disorders of Sperm Function

PHYSIOLOGIC CONSIDERATIONS

Coital habits may affect delivery of normal sperm numbers into the vagina. Because sperm survival is approximately 2 days, the most effective frequency of intercourse to achieve fertility is every 2 days around the midcycle ovulatory peak.[305] This frequency improves the chances that adequate numbers of viable sperm will be present during the 12 to 24 hours that the ovum will be within the fallopian tube and be capable of being fertilized.

Normal forward motility is required for sperm transport through cervical mucus and the female genital tract and for penetration of the corona radiata and zona pellucida before fertilization of the ovum.[306] A normally functioning sperm tail (*cilium*) is required for normal forward propulsion of spermatozoa. The structure within the cilium that is responsible for the generation of movement is called the *axoneme.*[307] The structure of the axoneme, which is highly conserved throughout phylogeny, consists of nine outer pairs surrounding a central pair of microtubules composed of tubulin dimers, the so-called $9+2$ configuration.[307] Projecting from each outer microtubular pair are inner and outer *dynein arms,* which interact with adjacent pairs to produce bending of the cilium.[307] The dynein arms contain the magnesium-dependent ATPase (dynein), which provides the driving force for microtubules to slide against each other and produce wave-like cilial movement.[308, 309] *Nexin links* and *radial spokes* connect outer pairs with each other and with the central pair of microtubules and are important in modulating the waveform of movement.[308, 309]

As discussed in a previous section, acquisition of normal sperm motility requires transit through and exposure to the luminal milieu of the epididymis. The mechanism by which sperm acquire motility is unclear but may involve exposure to epididymal proteins (such as progressive motility sustaining factor) and the numerous biochemical changes that occur in the epididymis.[210, 211, 215–217, 310] Spermatozoa remain immotile in the cauda epididymidis until ejaculation occurs, when mechanical constraints on movement are removed, epididymal inhibitors are diluted, and sperm are exposed to seminal plasma, which contain substances that may enhance motility.[221] Normally the percentage of sperm that are motile in ejaculated semen samples is greater than 60%.[23, 24]

Ejaculated spermatozoa must undergo a poorly understood series of morphologic and physiologic changes known as *capacitation* followed by *acrosome reaction* to acquire the ability to fertilize ova.[311] Human sperm can be induced experimentally to undergo capacitation and fertilize human eggs in vitro.[312] The changes in sperm metabolism and membrane that occur during capacitation permit spermatozoa to undergo the subsequent acrosome reaction. The precise conditions and factors involved in regulating capacitation are unclear.

The acrosome is a membrane-bound structure covering the anterior portion of the sperm head. During the acrosome reaction, the outer membrane of the acrosome breaks down, resulting in release of hydrolytic enzymes and exposure of the inner acrosomal membrane, both of which are important for sperm penetration of the cellular and noncellular investments of the egg and binding to and fertilization of the ovum.[313, 314] The current use of in vitro fertilization for diagnosis of infertile men and treatment of infertile women has emphasized the clinical importance of understanding capacitation and the acrosome reaction.

Infertility may be caused by coital disorders that result in deposition of inadequate sperm numbers at an inappropriate time in relationship to ovulation or by disorders of sperm function, such as motility (see Table 37–6).

COITAL DISORDERS

Although defects in coital technique are rare causes of infertility, they are important because they are potentially reversible with proper education of the infertile couple. *Infrequent intercourse, excessive intercourse or masturbation, poor timing of intercourse in relationship to ovulation,* or *premature withdrawal of the penis* are common problems encountered in this category of disorders.[305] These coital habits all reduce the likelihood of fertility.

DISORDERS OF SPERM FUNCTION

The use of *sperm-toxic lubricants* may reduce the number of viable or functional sperm. For example, K-Y Jelly, Keri Lotion, and saliva inhibit sperm motility in vitro.[315–317] Although these substances probably do not cause infertility by themselves, they may contribute to reduced fertilizing capacity of sperm and are easily discontinued.

Sperm dysmotility is commonly found in infertile men, either in conjunction with oligozoospermia or in isolation. Care in the collection of semen is required to avoid artifactual reduction in sperm motility.[306] Such artifacts may be induced by exposure of semen to spermicidal containers or substances (e.g., soap or saliva) or cold or prolonged exposure to seminal plasma (i.e., an old sample). Isolated *asthenospermia* (<60% motile sperm) or *necrospermia* (no motile sperm) occurs infrequently in a general infertile male population (approximately 0.5%).[306] In the majority of cases, the cause of isolated sperm dysmotility is unclear (i.e., *idiopathic asthenospermia*).

The *immotile cilia syndrome* is an autosomal recessive disorder characterized by immotile sperm tails and cilia on respiratory epithelial cells, which cause infertility and chronic, recurrent sinopulmonary infections owing to impaired mucociliary clearance mechanisms.[318, 319] These men usually have severe asthenospermia or necrospermia. Approximately half of these men have Kartagener's syndrome, which is situs inversus, bronchiectasis, and chronic sinusitis.[318, 319] Rarely, sperm tail abnormality and infertility occur in isolation without respiratory tract problems.[320] The immotile cilia syndrome is caused by an underlying ultrastructural defect in the axoneme. A variety of defects have been found, but the most common abnormality causing immotile cilia in this syndrome is a genetic deficiency of the outer and inner dynein arms of the axoneme.[318, 319, 321] Ultrastructural axonemal abnormalities have also been found in sperm with limited or dyskinetic motility.[306] There is considerable variation in the axonemal structure in sperm from normal men.[322] Therefore the diagnosis of axonemal defects requires careful analysis of sperm ultrastructure (i.e., examination of adequate numbers of sperm and multiple cross sections per sperm).

Immotile sperm may also result from *protein-carboxyl methylase deficiency,* an enzyme that transfers methyl groups from S-adenosylmethionine to carboxyl groups of proteins.[323] This enzyme is found in high concentrations in the sperm tail and plays an important role in regulating cell motility, including that of spermatozoa.

Immunologic Disorders (Antisperm Antibodies). Antisperm antibodies may be found in the serum and semen of both fertile and infertile men.[324, 325] The exact role of these antibodies, however, in the pathophysiology of infertility is uncertain. Antibodies to the sperm surface may be induced by damage or disruption of the testis or genital tract[324–326] or may occur primarily without an inciting factor.[324, 325] In some men (e.g., with impaired fertility after vasectomy, genital tract infection, sperm agglutination), antisperm antibodies may impair sperm function (such as sperm motility and fertilizing capacity) and may contribute to infertility.[324, 325, 327, 328] Immunosuppressive therapy with glucocorticoids has been apparently successful in restoring fertility in some men with antisperm antibodies.[324, 325] The response, however, is not predictable, and the treatment is associated with significant risks.[329]

Idiopathic Polyzoospermia. Men with sperm counts greater than 250 million/mL have polyzoospermia. The cause of this rare disorder is unclear, but fertility may be reduced, and the incidence of fetal wastage may be increased.[330]

Acknowledgments

This work was supported by Department of Veterans Affairs Medical Research Funds and National Institutes of Health Grant HD12629.

REFERENCES

1. Mosher WD. Infertility: why business is booming. American Demographics 1987;9:42–43.
2. MacLeod J. Human male infertility. Obstet Gynecol Surv 1979;26:335–351.
3. Simmons FA. Human infertility. N Engl J Med 1956;255:1140–1146.
4. Greenberg SH, Lipshultz LI, Wein AJ. Experience with 425 subfertile male patients. J Urol 1978;119:507–510.
5. Baker HWG, Burger HG, deKretser DM, Hudson B. Relative incidence of etiological disorders in male infertility. In: Santen RJ, Swerdloff RS, editors. Male Reproductive Dysfunction: Diagnosis and Management of Hypogonadism, Infertility, and Impotence. New York: Marcel Dekker, 1986:341–372.
6. deKretser DM. Morphology and physiology of the testis. In: Becker KL, editor. Principles and Practice of Endocrinology and Metabolism. Philadelphia: JB Lippincott, 1990:928–937.
7. Matsumoto AM. The testis and male sexual function. In: Wyngaarden JB, Smith LH, Bennett JC, editors. Cecil Textbook of Medicine. 19th edition. Philadelphia: WB Saunders, 1991:1333–1350.
8. Santen RJ, Bardin CW. Episodic luteinizing hormone secretion in man: pulse analysis, clinical interpretation, physiological mechanisms. J Clin Invest 1973;52:2617–2628.
9. Bremner WJ, Fernando NN, Paulsen CA. The effect of luteinizing hormone-releasing hormone in hypogonadotropic eunuchoidism. Acta Endocrinol (Copenh) 1977;86:1–14.
10. Hoffman AR, Crowley WF Jr. Induction of puberty in men by long-term pulsatile administration of low-dose gonadotropin-releasing hormone. N Engl J Med 1982;3078:1237–1241.
11. Rasmussen DD, Liu JH, Wolf PL, Yen SSC. Gonadotropin-releasing hormone neurosecretion in the human hypothalamus: in vitro regulation by dopamine. J Clin Endocrinol Metab 1986;62:479–483.
12. Rasmussen DD, Gambacciani M, Swartz W, et al. Pulsatile gonadotropin-releasing hormone release from the human medial basal hypothalamus in vitro: opiate-mediated suppression. Neuroendocrinology 1989;49:150–156.
13. Matsumoto AM, Bremner WJ. Modulation of pulsatile gonadotropin secretion by testosterone in man. J Clin Endocrinol Metab 1984;58:609–614.
14. Winters SJ, Troen P. Evidence for a role of endogenous estrogen in hypothalamic control of gonadotropin secretion in men. J Clin Endocrinol Metab 1985;61:842–845.
15. Mooradian AD, Morley JE, Korenman SG. Biological actions of androgens. Endocr Rev 1987;8:1–28.

16. Matsumoto AM, Bremner WJ. Endocrinology of the hypothalamic-pituitary-testicular axis with particular reference to the hormonal control of spermatogenesis. Bailliere's Clin Endocrinol Metab 1987;1:71–87.

17. deKretser DM, McLachlan RI, Robertson DM, Wreford NG. Control of spermatogenesis by follicle stimulating hormone and testosterone. Bailliere's Clin Endocrinol Metab 1992;6:335–354.

18. Jegou B. The Sertoli cell. Bailliere's Clin Endocrinol Metab 1992;6:273–311.

19. Robertson DM, Risbridger GP, deKretser DM. The physiology of testicular inhibin and related proteins. Bailliere's Clin Endocrinol Metab 1992;6:355–372.

20. Heller CG, Clermont Y. Spermatogenesis in man: an estimate of its duration. Science 1963;140:184–186.

21. Amann RP, Howards SS. Daily spermatozoal production and epididymal spermatozoal reserves of the human male. J Urol 1980;124:211–215.

22. Amann RP. A critical review of methods for evaluation of spermatogenesis from seminal characteristics. J Androl 1981;2:37–58.

23. MacLeod J, Gold RZ. The male factor in fertility and infertility. II. Spermatozoan counts in 1000 men of known fertility and in 1000 cases of infertile marriage. J Urol 1951;66:436–449.

24. Belsey MA, Eliasson R, Gallegos AJ, et al, editors. World Health Organization: Laboratory Manual for the Examination of Human Semen and Semen-Cervical Mucus Interaction. Singapore: Press Concern, 1980.

25. Matsumoto AM. Hormonal control of human spermatogenesis. In: Burger H, deKretser D, editors. The Testis. New York: Raven Press, 1989:181–196.

26. Finkel DM, Phillips JL, Synder PJ. Stimulation of spermatogenesis by gonadotropins in men with hypogonadotropic hypogonadism. N Engl J Med 1985;313:651–655.

27. Bremner WJ, Matsumoto AM, Sussman AM, Paulsen CA. Follicle-stimulating hormone and spermatogenesis. J Clin Invest 1981;68:1044–1052.

28. Matsumoto AM, Karpas AE, Paulsen CA, Bremner WJ. Reinitiation of sperm production in gonadotropin-suppressed normal men by administration of follicle-stimulating hormone. J Clin Invest 1983;72:1005–1015.

29. Matsumoto AM, Paulsen CA, Bremner WJ. Stimulation of sperm production by human luteinizing hormone in gonadotropin-suppressed normal men. J Clin Endocrinol Metab 1984;59:882–887.

30. Matsumoto AM, Bremner WJ. Stimulation of sperm production by human chorionic gonadotropin after prolonged gonadotropin suppression in normal men. J Androl 1985;6:137–143.

31. Matsumoto AM, Karpas AE, Bremner WJ. Chronic human chorionic gonadotropin administration in normal men: evidence that follicle-stimulating hormone is necessary for the maintenance of quantitatively normal spermatogenesis in man. J Clin Endocrinol Metab 1986;62:1184–1192.

32. deKretser DM, Burger HG, Fortune D, et al. Hormonal, histological and chromosomal studies in adult males with testicular disorders. J Clin Endocrinol Metab 1972;35:392–401.

33. Leonard JM, Leach RB, Couture M, Paulsen CA. Plasma and urinary follicle-stimulating hormone levels in oligospermia. J Clin Endocrinol Metab 1972;34:209–214.

34. Howards SS. Varicocele. Infert Reprod Med Clin North Am 1992;3:429–441.

35. Baker HEG, Bremner WJ, Burger HG, et al. Testicular control of follicle-stimulating hormone secretion. Rec Prog Horm Res 1976;32:429–476.

36. Gross KM, Matsumoto AM, Southworth MB, Bremner WJ. Evidence for decreased luteinizing hormone-releasing hormone pulse frequency in men with selective elevations of follicle-stimulating hormone. J Clin Endocrinol Metab 1985;60:197–202.

37. Gross KM, Matsumoto AM, Berger RE, Bremner WJ. Increased frequency of pulsatile LHRH administration selectively decreases FSH levels in men with idiopathic azoospermia. Fertil Steril 1986;45:392–396.

38. Wagner TOF, von zur Muhlen A. Slow pulsing oligospermia: treatment by longtime pulsatile LHRH therapy. In: Wagner TOF, Filicori M, editors. Episodic hormone secretion: from basic science to clinical application. Hemelin, West Germany: TM Verlag, 1987:197–203.

39. Autlitzky W, Frick J, Hadziselimovic F. Pulsatile LHRH therapy in patients with oligozoospermic and disturbed LH pulsatility. Int J Androl 1989;12:265–272.

40. Bals-Pratsch M, Knuth UA, Honigl W, et al. Pulsatile GnRH-therapy does not improve seminal parameters despite decreased FSH levels. Clin Endocrinol (Oxf) 1989;30:549–560.

41. Matsumoto AM, Gross KM, Sheckter CB, Bremner WJ. The luteinizing hormone-releasing hormone pulse generator in men: abnormalities and clinical management. Am J Obstet Gynecol 1990;163:1743–1752.

42. Booth JD, Merriam GR, Clark RV, et al. Evidence for Leydig cell dysfunction in infertile men with a selective increase in plasma follicle-stimulating hormone. J Clin Endocrinol Metab 1987;64:1194–1198.

43. Aiman J, Griffin JE. The frequency of androgen receptor deficiency in infertile men. J Clin Endocrinol Metab 1982;54:725–732.

44. Morrow AF, Gyorki S, Warne GL, et al. Variable androgen receptor levels in infertile men. J Clin Endocrinol Metab 1987;64:1115–1121.

45. Eil C, Gamblin GT, Hodge JW, et al. Whole cell and nuclear androgen uptake in skin fibroblasts from infertile men. J Androl 1985;6:365–371.

46. Bouchard P, Wright F, Portois MC, et al. Androgen insensitivity in oligospermic men: a reappraisal. J Clin Endocrinol Metab 1986;63:1242–1246.

47. Coburn M, Wheeler T, Lipshultz LI. Testicular biopsy: its use and limitations. Urol Clin North Am 1987;14:551–561.

48. Sherins RJ, Brightwell D, Sternthal PM. Longitudinal analysis of semen of fertile and infertile men. In: Troen P, Nankin HR, editors. The Testis in Normal and Infertile Men. New York: Raven Press, 1977:473–488.

49. Fariss BL, Fenner DK, Plymate SR, et al. Seminal characteristics in the presence of a varicocele as compared with those of expectant fathers and prevasectomy men. Fertil Steril 1981;35:325–327.

50. Nagao RR, Plymate SR, Berger RE, et al. Comparison of gonadal function between fertile and infertile men with varicoceles. Fertil Steril 1986;46:930–933.

51. MacLeod J. Seminal cytology in the presence of varicocele. Fertil Steril 1965;16:735–757.

52. Rodriguez-Rigau LJ, Steinberger E. Varicocele and the morphology of spermatozoa. Fertil Steril 1981;35:325–327.

53. Takahara H, Sakatoku J, Cockett ATK. The pathophysiology of varicocele in male infertility. Fertil Steril 1991;55:861–868.

54. Mieusset R, Bujan L, Mondinat C, et al. Association of scrotal hyperthermia with impaired spermatogenesis in infertile men. Fertil Steril 1987;48:1006–1011.

55. Pryor JL, Howards SS. Varicocele. Urol Clin North Am 1987;14:499–513.

56. Nillson S, Edvinsson A, Nillson B. Improvement of semen and pregnancy rate after ligation and division of the internal spermatic vein: fact or fiction? Br J Urol 1979;51:591–596.

57. Baker HWG, Burger HG, deKretser DM, et al. Testicular vein ligation and fertility in men with varicocele. Br Med J 1985;291:1678–1680.

58. Vermeulen A, Vanderweghe M, Deslypere JP. Prognosis of subfertility in men with corrected or uncorrected varicocele. J Androl 1986;7:147–155.

59. Rajfer J. Congenital anomalies of the testis. In: Walsh PH, Gittes RF, Perlmutter AD, et al, editors. Campbell's Urology. 5th edition. Philadelphia: WB Saunders, 1986:1947–1968.

60. Hezmall HP, Lipshultz LI. Cyptorchidism and infertility. Urol Clin North Am 1982;9:361–369.

61. Benson RC, Beard CM, Kelalis PP, Kurland LT. Malignant potential of the cryptorchid testis. Mayo Clin Proc 1991;66:372–378.

62. Puri P, Nixon HH. Bilateral retractile testes—subsequent effects on fertility. J Pediatr Surg 1977;12:563–566.

63. Nistal M, Paniagua R. Infertility in adult males with retractile testes. Fertil Steril 1984;41:395–403.

64. Buyse M, Feingold M. Syndromes associated with abnormal external genitalia. In: Vallet HL, Porter IH, editors. Genetic Mechanisms of Sexual Development. New York: Academic Press, 1979:425–435.

65. Hutson JM, Williams MP, Fallat ME, Attah A. Testicular descent: new insights into its hormonal control. Oxf Rev Reprod Biol 1990;12:1–56.

66. Andersen H, Andreassen M, Quaade F. Testicular biopsies in cryptorchidism. Acta Endocrinol (Copenh) 1955;18:567–569.

67. Alpert PF, Klein RS. Spermatogenesis in unilateral cryptorchid testis after orchiopexy. J Urol 1983;129:301–302.

68. Kandeel FR, Swerdloff RS. Role of temperature in regulation of spermatogenesis and the use of heating as a method for contraception. Fertil Steril 1988;49:1–23.

69. Lipshultz LI, Caminos-Torres R, Greenspan CS, Synder PJ. Testicular function after orchiopexy for unilateral undescended testis. N Engl J Med 1976;295:15–18.

70. David G, Bisson JP, Martin-Boyce A, Ferneux D. Sperm characteristics and fertility in previously cryptorchid adults. In: Job JC, editor. Cryptorchidism. New York: Karger, 1979:187–194.

71. Krabbe S, Berthelsen JG, Volsted P, et al. High incidence of undetected neoplasia in maldescended testes. Lancet 1979;1:999–1000.

72. Maclean N, Harnden DG, et al. Sex chromosome abnormalities in newborn babies. Lancet 1964;1:286–290.

73. Paulsen CA, deSouza A, Yoshimura T, Lewis BM. Results of a buccal smear survey in noninstitutionalized adult males. J Clin Endocrinol Metab 1964;24:1182–1187.

74. Klinefelter HF Jr, Reifenstein EC Jr, Albright F. Syndrome characterized by gynecomastia, aspermatogenesis with a-Leydigism, and increased secretion of follicle-stimulating hormone. J Clin Endocrinol Metab 1942;2:615–627.

75. Paulsen CA, Gordon DL, Carpenter KW, et al. Klinefelter's syndrome and its variants: a hormonal and chromosomal study. Rec Prog Horm Res 1968;24:321–363.

76. Becker KL. Clinical and therapeutic experiences with Klinefelter's syndrome. Fertil Steril 1972;23:568–578.

77. Hseuh WA, Hsu TH, Federman DD. Endocrine features of Klinefelter's syndrome. Medicine 1978;57:447–461.

78. Gabrilove JL, Freiberg EK, Johnson MW. Testicular function in Klinefelter's syndrome. J Urol 1980;124:825–826.

79. Wieland RG, Zorn EM, Johnson MW. Elevated testosterone-binding globulin in Klinefelter's syndrome. J Clin Endocrinol Metab 1980;51:1199–1200.

80. Wang C, Baker HWG, Burger HG, et al. Hormonal studies in Klinefelter's syndrome. Clin Endocrinol (Oxf) 1975;4:399–411.

81. Laron Z, Dickerman Z, Zamir R, Galatzer A. Paternity in Klinefelter's syndrome. Arch Androl 1982;8:149–151.

82. Fraccaro M, Kaljser K, Lindsten J. A child with 49 chromosomes. Lancet 1960;2:899–902.

83. Bardin CW, Paulsen CA. The testes. In: Williams RH, editor. Textbook of Endocrinology. 6th edition. Philadelphia: WB Saunders, 1981:293–354.

84. Mudal S, Ockey CH, Thompson M, White LLR. The "double male": a new chromosomal constitution in the Klinefelter's syndrome. Lancet 1960;2:492.

85. Bloomington ZT, Delozier CD, Cohen MP, et al. Genetic and endocrine findings in a 48, XXYY male. J Clin Endocrinol Metab 1980;50:740–743.

86. Schweikert HU, Weissbach L, Leyendecker G, et al. Clinical, endocrinological, and cytological characterization of two 46, XX males. J Clin Endocrinol Metab 1982;54:745–752.

87. Andersson M, Page DC, de la Chapelle A. Chromosome Y-specific DNA is transferred to the short arm of X chromosome in human XX males. Science 1986;233:786–787.

88. Harper P. Myotonic Dystrophy. Philadelphia: WB Saunders, 1979.

89. Takeda R, Ueda M. Pituitary-gonadal function in male patients with myotonic dystrophy: serum luteinizing hormone, follicle stimulating hormone and testosterone levels and histological damage of the testis. Acta Endocrinol (Copenh) 1977;84:382–389.

90. Drucker WD, Blanc WA, Rowland LP, et al. The testis in myotonic dystrophy: a clinical pathologic study with a comparison with the Klinefelter syndrome. J Clin Endocrinol Metab 1963;23:59–75.

91. Rothman CM, Sims CA, Stotts CL. Sertoli cell only syndrome. Fertil Steril 1982;38:388–390.

92. Micic S, Ilic V, Micic M, et al. Endocrine profile of 45 patients with sertoli cell only syndrome. Andrologia 1983;15:228–232.

93. Aynsley-Green A, Zachmann M, Illig R, et al. Congenital bilateral anorchia in childhood: a clinical, endocrine and therapeutic evaluation of twenty-one cases. Clin Endocrinol (Oxf) 1976;5:381–391.

94. Ehrlich RM, Dougherty LJ, Tomashefsky P, Lattimer JK. Effect of gonadotropin in cryptorchidism. J Urol 1969;102:793–795.

95. Winter JSD, Faiman C. Serum gonadotropin concentrations in agonadal children and adults. J Clin Endocrinol Metab 1972;35:561–564.

96. Mendez HMM, Opitz JM. Noonan syndrome: a review. Am J Med Genet 1985;21:493–506.

97. Elder M, Maclaren N, Riley W. Gonadal antibodies in patients with hypogonadism and/or Addison's disease. J Clin Endocrinol Metab 1981;52:1137–1142.

98. Hsiang Y-HH, Berkovitz GD, Bland GL, et al. Gonadal function in patients with Down syndrome. Am J Med Genet 1987;27:449–458.

99. Johannisson R, Gropp A, Winking H, et al. Down's syndrome in the male: reproductive pathology and meiotic studies. Hum Genet 1983;63:132–138.

100. Castro-Magana M, Bronsther B, Angulo MA. Genetic forms of male hypogonadism. Urology 1990;35:195–204.

101. Rimoin DL, Schimke RN. The gonads. In: Rimoin DL, Schimke RN, editors. Genetic Disorders of the Endocrine Glands. St. Louis: CV Mosby, 1971:258–356.

102. Adamopoulos DA, Lawrence DM, Vassilopoulos P, et al. Pituitary testicular interrelationships in mumps orchitis and other viral infections. Br Med J 1978;1:1177–1180.

103. Beard CM, Benson RC Jr, Kelalis PP, et al. The incidence and outcome of mumps orchitis in Rochester, Minnesota. 1935–1974. Mayo Clin Proc 1977;52:3–10.

104. Gall EA. The histopathology of acute mumps orchitis. Am J Pathol 1947;23:637–651.

105. Werner CA. Mumps orchitis and testicular atrophy. II. A factor in male sterility. Ann Intern Med 1950;32:1075–1086.

106. Bartak V, Skalova E, Nevarilova A. Spermiogram changes in adults and youngsters after parotitic orchitis. Int J Fertil 1968;13:226–232.

107. Aiman J, Brenner PF, MacDonald PC. Androgen and estrogen production in elderly men with gynecomastia and testicular atrophy after mumps orchitis. J Clin Endocrinol Metab 1980;50:380–386.

108. Riggs S, Sanford JP. Viral orchitis. N Engl J Med 1962;266:990–993.

109. Morley JE, Distiller LA, Sagel J, et al. Hormonal changes associated with testicular atrophy and gynaecomastia in patients with leprosy. Clin Endocrinol (Oxf) 1977;6:299–303.

110. Schilsky RL, Lewis BL, Sherins RJ. Gonadal dysfunction in patients receiving chemotherapy for cancer. Ann Intern Med 1980;93:109–114.

111. Byrne J, Mulvihill JJ, Myers MH, et al. Effects of treatment on fertility in long-term survivors of childhood or adolescent cancer. N Engl J Med 1987;317:1315–1321.

112. Friedman NM, Plymate SR. Leydig cell dysfunction and gynaecomastia in adult males treated with alkylating agents. Clin Endocrinol (Oxf) 1980;12:553–556.

113. Birnie GG, McLeod TIF, Watkinson G. Incidence of sulphasalazine-induced male infertility. Gut 1981;22:452–455.

114. Van Thiel DH, Galaver JS. Hypothalamic-pituitary-gonadal function in liver disease with particular attention to the endocrine effects of chronic alcohol abuse. Prog Liver Dis 1986;8:273–282.

115. Kolodny RC, Masters WH, Kolodner RM, Toro G. Depression of plasma testosterone levels after chronic intensive marijuana use. N Engl J Med 1974;290:872–874.

116. Feldman D. Ketoconazole and other imidazole derivatives as inhibitors of steroidogenesis. Endocr Rev 1986;7:409–420.

117. Samojlik E, Kirschner MA, Ribot S, Szmal E. Changes in the hypothalamic-pituitary-gonadal axis in men after cadaver kidney transplantation and cyclosporine therapy. J Androl 1992;13:332–336.

118. Loriaux DL, Menard R, Taylor A, et al. Spironolactone and endocrine dysfunction. Ann Intern Med 1976;85:630–636.

119. Van Thiel DH, Gavaler JS, Smith WI Jr, Paul G. Hypothalamic-pituitary-gonadal dysfunction in men using cimetidine. N Engl J Med 1979;300:1012–1015.

120. Lushbaugh CC, Casarett GW. The effects of gonadal irradiation in clinical radiation therapy: a review. Cancer 1976;37:1111–1120.

121. Clifton DK, Bremner WJ. The effect of testicular X-irradiation on spermatogenesis in man: a comparison with the mouse. J Androl 1983;4:387–392.

122. Rowley MJ, Leach DR, Warner GA, Heller CG. Effect of graded doses of ionizing radiation on the human testis. Radiat Res 1974;59:665–677.

123. Shalet SM, Tsatsoulis A, Whitehead E, Read G. Vulnerability of the human Leydig cell to radiation damage is dependent upon age. J Endocrinol 1989;120:161–165.

124. Vigersky RA, Chapman RM, Berenberg J, Glass AR. Testicular dysfunction in untreated Hodgkin's disease. Am J Med 1982;73:482–486.

125. Hansen PV, Trykker H, Andersen J, Helkjaer PE. Germ cell function and hormonal status in patients with testicular cancer. Cancer 1989;64:959–961.

126. Perkash I, Martin DE, Warner H, et al. Reproductive biology of paraplegics: results of semen collection, testicular biopsy and serum hormone evaluation. J Urol 1985;134:284–288.

127. Hirsch IH, McCue P, Allen J, et al. Quantitative testicular biopsy in spinal cord injured men: comparison to fertile controls. J Urol 1991;146:337–341.

128. Schrag SD, Dixon RL. Occupational exposures associated with male reproductive dysfunction. Ann Rev Pharmacol Toxicol 1985;25:567–592.

129. Gagnon C. The role of environmental toxins in unexplained male infertility. Semin Reprod Endocrinol 1988;6:369–376.

130. Baker HWG. Testicular dysfunction in systemic disease. In: Becker KL, editor. Principles and Practice of Endocrinology and Metabolism. Philadelphia: JB Lippincott, 1990:971–975.

131. Baker HWG, Burger HG, deKretser DM, et al. A study of the endocrine manifestations of hepatic cirrhosis. Q J Med 1976;45:145–178.
132. Van Thiel DH, Lester R, Sherins RJ. Hypogonadism in alcoholic liver disease: evidence for a double defect. Gastroenterology 1974;67:1188–1199.
133. Handelsman DJ. Hypothalamic-pituitary gonadal dysfunction in renal failure, dialysis and renal transplantation. Endocr Rev 1985;6:151–182.
134. Shurbaji MS, Epstein JI. Testicular vasculitis: implications for systemic disease. Hum Pathol 1988;19:186–189.
135. Handelsman DJ, Yue DK, Turtle JR. Hypogonadism and massive testicular infiltration due to amyloidosis. J Urol 1983;129:610–612.
136. Abbasi AA, Prasad AS, Ortega J, et al. Gonadal function abnormalities in sickle cell anemia: studies in adult male patients. Ann Intern Med 1976;85:601–605.
137. Kallmann FJ, Schoenfeld WA, Barrera SE. The genetic aspects of primary eunuchoidism. Am J Ment Defic 1944;48:203–236.
138. Christensen RB, Matsumoto AM, Bremner WJ. Idiopathic hypogonadotropic hypogonadism with anosmia (Kallmann's syndrome). Endocrinologist 1992;2:332–340.
139. Lieblich JM, Rogol AD, White BJ, Rosen SW. Syndrome of anosmia with hypogonadotropic hypogonadism (Kallmann syndrome). Clinical and laboratory studies in 23 cases. Am J Med 1982;73:506–519.
140. Schwankhaus JD, Currie J, Jaffe MJ, et al. Neurologic findings in men with isolated hypogonadotropic hypogonadism. Neurology 1989;39:223–226.
141. Santen RJ, Paulsen CA. Hypogonadotropic eunuchoidism. I. Clinical study of the mode of inheritance. J Clin Endocrinol Metab 1973;36:47–54.
142. White BJ, Rogol AD, Brown KS, et al. The syndrome of anosmia with hypogonadotropic hypogonadism: a genetic study of 18 new families and a review. Am J Med Genet 1983;15:417–435.
143. Spratt DI, Carr DB, Merriam GR, et al. The spectrum of abnormal patterns of gonadotropin releasing hormone secretion in men with idiopathic hypogonadotropic hypogonadism: clinical and laboratory correlations. J Clin Endocrinol Metab 1987;64:283–291.
144. Faiman C, Hoffman DL, Ryan RJ, Albert A. The "fertile eunuch" syndrome: demonstration of isolated luteinizing hormone deficiency by radioimmunoassay technique. Mayo Clin Proc 1968;43:661–667.
145. Santen RJ, Leonard JM, Sherins RJ, et al. Short- and long-term effects of clomiphene citrate on the pituitary-testicular axis. J Clin Endocrinol Metab 1971;33:970–979.
146. Maroulis GB, Parlow AF, Marshall JR. Isolated follicle-stimulating hormone deficiency in man. Fertil Steril 1977;28:818–822.
147. Al-Ansari AA-K, Khalil TH, Kelani Y, Mortimer CH. Isolated follicle-stimulating hormone deficiency in men: successful long-term gonadotropin therapy. Fertil Steril 1984;42:618–626.
148. Weiss J, Adams E, Whitcomb RW, et al. Normal sequence of the gonadotropin-releasing hormone gene in patients with idiopathic hypogonadotropic hypogonadism. Biol Reprod 1991;45:743–747.
149. Schwanzel-Fukuda M, Bick D, Pfaff DW. Luteinizing hormone-releasing hormone (LHRH)-expressing cells do not migrate normally in an inherited hypogonadal (Kallmann) syndrome. Mol Brain Res 1989;6:311–319.
150. Franco B, Guioli S, Pragliola A, et al. A gene deleted in Kallmann's syndrome shares homology with neural cell adhesion and axonal pathfinding molecules. Nature 1991;353:529–536.
151. Legoulis R, Hardelin J-P, Levilliers J, et al. The candidate gene for the X-linked Kallmann syndrome encodes a protein related to adhesion molecules. Cell 1991;67:423–435.
152. Klingmuller D, Dewes W, Krahe T, et al. Magnetic resonance imaging of the brain in patients with anosmia and hypothalamic hypogonadism (Kallmann's syndrome). J Clin Endocrinol Metab 1987;65:581–584.
153. Burris AS, Rodbard HW, Winters SJ, Sherins RJ. Gonadotropin therapy in men with hypogonadotropic hypogonadism: the response to human chorionic gonadotropin is predicted by initial testicular size. J Clin Endocrinol Metab 1988;66:1144–1151.
154. Santen RJ, Paulsen CA. Hypogonadotropic hypogonadism. II. Gonadal responsiveness to exogenous gonadotropins. J Clin Endocrinol Metab 1973;36:55–63.
155. Ley SB, Leonard JM. Male hypogonadotropic hypogonadism: factors influencing response to human chorionic gonadotropin and human menopausal gonadotropin, including exogenous androgens. J Clin Endocrinol Metab 1985;61:746–752.
156. Burris AS, Clark RV, Vantman DJ, Sherins RJ. A low sperm concentration does not preclude fertility in men with isolated hypogonadotropic

hypogonadism after gonadotropin therapy. Fertil Steril 1988;50:343–347.
157. Stock AE, Martin FIR. Pituitary function in haemochromatosis. Am J Med 1968;45:839–845.
158. Iyer R, Duckworth WC, Solomon SS. Hypogonadism in idiopathic hemochromatosis. Arch Intern Med 1981;141:517–518.
159. Charbonnel B, Chupin M, Le Grand A, Guillon J. Pituitary function in idiopathic haemochromatosis: hormonal study in 36 male patients. Acta Endocrinol (Copenh) 1981;98:178–183.
160. Siemons LJ, Mahler CH. Hypogonadotropic hypogonadism in hemochromatosis: recovery of reproductive function after iron depletion. J Clin Endocrinol Metab 1987;65:585–587.
161. Schafer AI, Cheron RG, Dluhy R, et al. Clinical consequences of acquired transfusional iron overload in adults. N Engl J Med 1981;304:319–324.
162. DeSantis V, Vullo C, Katz M, et al. Induction of spermatogenesis in thalassemia. Fertil Steril 1988;50:969–975.
163. Vannasaeng S, Fucharoen S, Pootrakul P, et al. Pituitary function in thalassemic patients and the effect of chelation therapy. Acta Endocrinol (Copenh) 1991;124:23–30.
164. Imura H. Hypopituitarism. In: Imura H, editor. The Pituitary Gland. New York: Raven Press, 1985:501–525.
165. Dexter RN. Hypopituitarism. In: Becker KL, editor. Principles and Practice of Endocrinology and Metabolism. Philadelphia: JB Lippincott, 1990:160–171.
166. Carter JN, Tyson JE, Tolis G, et al. Prolactin-secreting tumors and hypogonadism in 22 men. N Engl J Med 1978;299:847–852.
167. Molitch ME. Pathologic hyperprolactinemia. Endocrinol Metab Clin North Am 1992;21:877–901.
168. Bouchard P, Lagoguey M, Brailly S, Schaison G. Gonadotropin-releasing hormone pulsatile administration restores luteinizing hormone pulsatility and normal testosterone levels in males with hyperprolactinemia. J Clin Endocrinol Metab 1985;60:258–262.
169. Hell K, Wernze H. Drug-induced changes in prolactin secretion: clinical implications. Med Toxicol 1988;3:463–498.
170. Segal S, Yaffe H, Laufer N, Ben-David M. Male hyperprolactinemia: effects on fertility. Fertil Steril 1979;32:556–561.
171. Luboshitzky R, Rosen E, Trestian S, Spitz IM. Hyperprolactinemia and hypogonadism in men: response to exogenous gonadotrophins. Clin Endocrinol (Oxf) 1979;11:217–223.
172. Matsumoto AM. Effects of chronic testosterone administration in normal men: safety and efficacy of high dosage testosterone and parallel dose-dependent suppression of luteinizing hormone, follicle-stimulating hormone and sperm production. J Clin Endocrinol Metab 1990;70:282–287.
173. World Health Organization Task Force on Methods for the Regulation of Male Fertility. Contraceptive efficacy of testosterone-induced azoospermia in normal men. Lancet 1990;336:955–959.
174. Schurmeyer T, Belkien L, Knuth UA, Nieschlag E. Reversible azoospermia induced by the anabolic steroid 19-nortestosterone. Lancet 1984;1:417–420.
175. Bonaccorsi AC, Adler I, Figueiredo JG. Male infertility due to congenital adrenal hyperplasia: testicular biopsy findings, hormonal evaluation, and therapeutic results in three patients. Fertil Steril 1987;47:664–670.
176. Freeman DA. Steroid hormone-producing tumors of the adrenal, ovary, and testes. Endocrinol Metab Clin North Am 1991;20:751–766.
177. Veldhuis JD, Dufau ML. Estradiol modulates the pulsatile secretion of biologically active luteinizing hormone in man. J Clin Invest 1987;80:631–638.
178. de la Balze FA, Mancini RE, Bur GE, Irazu J. Morphologic and histochemical changes produced by estrogens on adult human testes. Fertil Steril 1954;5:421–436.
179. Veldhuis JD, Sowers JR, Rogol AD, Dufau ML. Pathophysiology of male hypogonadism associated with endogenous hyperestrogenism: evidence for dual defects in the gonadal axis. N Engl J Med 1985;312:1371–1375.
180. Byar DP, Corle DK. Hormone therapy for prostate cancer: results of the Veterans Administration Cooperative Urologic Research Group studies. In: NCI Monographs. No. 7 (NIH publication no. 88-3005). Washington, DC: Government Printing Office, 1988:165–170.
181. Stoffer SS, Hynes KM, Jiany NS, Ryan RJ. Digoxin and abnormal serum hormone levels. JAMA 1973;225:1643–1644.
182. Heller CG, Moore DJ, Paulsen CA, et al. Effects of progesterone and synthetic progestins on the reproductive physiology of normal men. Fed Proc 1959;18:1057–1064.

183. Wang C, Chan V, Yeung RTT. The effect of heroin addiction on pituitary-testicular function. Clin Endocrinol (Oxf) 1978;9:455–461.

184. Smith CG, Asch RH. Drug abuse and reproduction. Fertil Steril 1987;48:355–373.

185. Brown WA, Laughren TP, Williams B. Differential effects of neuroleptic agents of the pituitary-gonadal axis in men. Arch Gen Psych 1981;38:1270–1272.

186. Luton J-P, Thieblot P, Valcke J-C, et al. Reversible gonadotropin deficiency in male Cushing's syndrome. J Clin Endocrinol Metab 1977;45:488–495.

187. MacAdams MR, White RH, Chipps BE. Reduction in serum testosterone levels during chronic glucocorticoid therapy. Ann Intern Med 1986;104:648–651.

188. Smith SR, Chhetri MK, Johanson AJ, et al. The pituitary-gonadal axis in men with protein-calorie malnutrition. J Clin Endocrinol Metab 1975;4:60–69.

189. Lemaire A, Ardaens K, Lepretre J, et al. Gonadal hormones in male anorexia nervosa. Int J Eating Dis 1983;2:135–144.

190. Spratt DI, Bigos ST, Beitens I, et al. Both hyper- and hypogonadotropic hypogonadism occur transiently in acute illness: bio- and immunoreactive gonadotropins. J Clin Endocrinol Metab 1992;75:1562–1570.

191. Hein K. The interface of chronic illness and the hormonal regulation of puberty. J Adolesc Health Care 1987;8:530–540.

192. McGrady AV. Effects of psychological stress on male reproduction: a review. Arch Androl 1984;13:1–7.

193. Chlebowski RT, Heber D. Hypogonadism in male patients with metastatic cancer prior to chemotherapy. Cancer Res 1982;42:2495–2498.

194. Plymate SR, Vaughan GM, Mason AD, Pruitt BA. Central hypogonadism in burned men. Horm Res 1987;27:152–158.

195. Wang C, Chan V, Tse TF, Yeung RTT. Effect of acute myocardial infarction on pituitary-testicular function. Clin Endocrinol (Oxf) 1974;9:249–253.

196. Semple PD'A, Beastall GH, Brown TM, et al. Sex hormone suppression and sexual impotence in hypoxic pulmonary fibrosis. Thorax 1984;39:46–51.

197. Bannister P, Handley T, Chapman C, Losowsky MS. Hypogonadism in chronic liver disease: impaired release of luteinizing hormone. Br Med J 1986;293:1191–1193.

198. Handelsman DJ, Dong Q. Hypothalamo-pituitary-gonadal axis in chronic renal failure. Endocrinol Metab Clin North Am 1993;22:145–161.

199. Wang C, Chan V, Yeung RTT. Effect of surgical stress on pituitary-testicular function. Clin Endocrinol (Oxf) 1978;9:255–266.

200. Strain GW, Zumoff B, Miller LK, et al. Effect of massive weight loss on hypothalamic-pituitary-gonadal function in obese men. J Clin Endocrinol Metab 1988;66:1019–1023.

201. Aiman J, Griffin JE, Gazak JM, et al. Androgen insensitivity as a cause of infertility in otherwise normal men. N Engl J Med 1979;300:223–227.

202. Wilson JD, Harrod MJ, Goldstein JL, et al. Familial incomplete male pseudohermaphroditism, type I: evidence for androgen resistance and variable clinical manifestations in a family with the Reifenstein syndrome. N Engl J Med 1974;290:1097–1103.

203. Griffin JE. Androgen resistance—the clinical and molecular spectrum. N Engl J Med 1992;326:611–618.

204. Walsh PC, Madden JD, Harrod MJ, et al. Familial incomplete male pseudohermaphroditism, type 2: decreased dihydrotestosterone formation in pseudovaginal perineoscrotal hypospadias. N Engl J Med 1974;291:944–949.

205. Imperato-McGinley J, Peterson RE, Gautier T, Strula E. Androgens and the evolution of male-gender identity among male pseudohermaphrodites and 5α-reductase deficiency. N Engl J Med 1979;300:1233–1237.

206. Andersson S, Berman DM, Jenkins EP, Russell DW. Deletion of the steroid 5α-reductase 2 gene in male pseudohermaphroditism. Nature 1991;354:159–161.

207. Johnson L, George FW, Neaves WB, et al. Characterization of the testicular abnormality in 5α-reductase deficiency. J Clin Endocrinol Metab 1986;63:1091–1099.

208. Farthing MJG, Edwards CRW, Rees LH, Dawson AM. Male gonadal function in coeliac disease. I. Sexual dysfunction, infertility, and semen quality. Gut 1982;23:608–614.

209. Farthing MJG, Rees LH, Boylan LM, Dawson AM. Male gonadal function in coeliac disease. 2. Sex hormones. Gut 1983;24:127–135.

210. Robaire B, Hermo L. Efferent ducts, epididymis, and vas deferens: structure, functions and their regulation. In: Knobil E, Neill JD, editors. The Physiology of Reproduction. New York: Raven Press, 1988:999–1080.

211. Yamamoto M, Turner TT. Epididymis, sperm maturation and capacitation. In: Lipshultz LI, Howards SS, editors. Infertility in the Male. 2nd edition. St. Louis: Mosby-Year Book, 1991:103–123.

212. Hinrichsen MJ, Blaquier JA. Evidence supporting the existence of sperm maturation in the human epididymis. J Reprod Fertil 1980;60:291–294.

213. Moore HDM, Hartman TD, Pryor JP. Development of the oocyte-penetrating capacity of spermatozoa in the human epididymis. Int J Androl 1983;6:310–318.

214. Cooper TG. In defense of a function for the human epididymis. Fertil Steril 1990;54:965–975.

215. Hinton BT. The epididymal microenvironment: a site of attack for a male contraceptive? Invest Urol 1980;18:1–10.

216. Sheth AR, Gunjikar AN, Shah GV. The presence of progressive motility sustaining factor (PMSF) in human epididymis. Andrologia 1981;13:142–146.

217. Blaquier J, Cameo MS, Dawidowski A, et al. On the role of epididymal factors in sperm maturation in man. In: Serio M, editor. Perspectives in Andrology. New York: Raven Press, 1989:37–44.

218. Tezon JG, Blaquier JA. The organ culture of human epididymal tubules and their response to androgens. Mol Cell Endocrinol 1981;21:233–242.

219. Rowley M, Teshima JF, Heller CG. Duration of transit through the human male ductular system. Fertil Steril 1970;21:390–396.

220. Amman RP, Howards SS. Daily spermatozoal production and epididymal spermatozoal reserves of the human male. J Urol 1980;124:211–215.

221. Turner TT, Howards SS. Factors involved in the initiation of sperm motility. Biol Reprod 1978;18:571–578.

222. Alm P. On the autonomic innervation of the human vas deferens. Brain Res Bull 1982;9:673–677.

223. Coffey DS. The biochemistry and physiology of the prostate and seminal vesicles. In: Harrison JH, Gittes RF, Perlmutter AD, et al, editors. Campbell's Urology. 4th edition. Philadelphia: WB Saunders, 1970:161–201.

224. Mawhinney MG, Tarry WF. Male accessory sex organs and androgen action. In: Lipshultz LI, Howards SS, editors. Infertility in the Male. 2nd edition. St. Louis: Mosby-Year Book, 1991:124–154.

225. Mann T. The Biochemistry of Semen and of the Male Reproductive Tract. New York: John Wiley, 1964.

226. Tauber CW, Zaneveld LJD. Coagulation and liquefaction of human semen. In: Hafez ESE, editor. Human Semen and Fertility Regulation in Men. St. Louis: CV Mosby, 1976:153–166.

227. Insler V, Glezerman M, Zeidel L, et al. Sperm storage in the human cervix: a quantitative study. Fertil Steril 1980;33:288–293.

228. Handelsman DJ. Azoospermia. Med J Aust 1992;157:149–152.

229. Holsclaw DS, Perlmutter AD, Jockin H, Scwachman H. Genital abnormalities in male patients with cystic fibrosis. J Urol 1971;106:568–574.

230. Wagenknecht LV, Lotzin CF, Sommer HJ, Schirren C. Vas deferens aplasia: clinical and anatomical features of 90 cases. Andrologia 1983;15:605–613.

231. Whitehead ED, Leiter E. Genital abnormalities and abnormal semen analyses in male patients exposed to diethylstilbestrol in utero. J Urol 1981;125:47–50.

232. Handelsman DJ, Conway AJ, Boylan LM, Turtle JR. Young's syndrome: obstructive azoospermia and chronic sinopulmonary infections. N Engl J Med 1984;310:3–9.

233. Wilton LJ, Teichtahl H, Temple-Smith PD, et al. Young's syndrome (obstructive azoospermia and chronic sinobronchial infection): a quantitative study of axonemal ultrastructure and function. Fertil Steril 1991;55:144–151.

234. Sharlip ID. Obstructive azoospermia or oligozoospermia due to mullerian duct cyst. Fertil Steril 1983;39:435–436.

235. Pryor JP, Hendry WF. Ejaculatory duct obstruction in subfertile males: analysis of 87 patients. Fertil Steril 1991;56:725–730.

236. Simon HB, Weinstein AJ, Pasternak MS, et al. Genitourinary tuberculosis: clinical features in a general hospital population. Am J Med 1977;63:410–420.

237. Berger RE. Acute epididymitis: etiology and therapy. Semin Urol 1991;9:28–31.

238. Fowler JE Jr. Infections of the male reproductive tract and infertility: a selected review. J Androl 1981;3:121–131.

239. Berger RE, Holmes KK. Infection and male infertility. In: Santen RJ,

Swerdloff RS, editors. Male Sexual Dysfunction: Diagnosis and Management of Hypogonadism, Infertility and Impotence. New York: Marcel Dekker, 1986:407–438.

240. Krane RJ, Goldstein I, Saenz de Tejada I. Impotence. N Engl J Med 1989;321:1648–1659.

241. Benson GS, McConnell J. Erection, emission, and ejaculation: physiological mechanisms. In: Lipshultz LI, Howards SS, editors. Infertility in the Male. 2nd edition. St. Louis: Mosby-Year Book, 1991:155–176.

242. deGroat WC, Steers WD. Neuroanatomy and neurophysiology of penile erection. In: Tanagho EA, Lue TF, McClure RD, editors. Contemporary Management of Impotence and Infertility. Baltimore: Williams & Wilkins, 1988:3–27.

243. Bancroft J. Reproductive hormones and male sexual function. In: Sitson JMA, editor. Handbook of Sexology. Amsterdam: Elsevier Science Publishers, 1988:297–315.

244. Benson GS, McConnell J, Lipshultz LI, et al. Neuromorphology and neuropharmacology of the human penis: an in vitro study. J Clin Invest 1980;65:506–513.

245. Ottesen B, Wagner G, Virag R, Fahrenkrug J. Penile erection: possible role for vasoactive intestinal peptide as a neurotransmitter. Br Med J 1984;288:9–11.

246. Adrian TE, Gu J, Allen JM, et al. Neuropeptide Y in the human male genital tract. Life Sci 1984;35:2643–2648.

247. Burnett AL, Lowenstein CJ, Bredt DS, et al. Nitric oxide: a physiologic mediator of penile erection. Science 1992;257:401–403.

248. Hedlund H, Andersson K-E. Comparison of the responses to drugs acting on adrenoreceptors and muscarinic receptors in human isolated corpus cavernosum and cavernous artery. J Auton Pharmacol 1985;5:81–88.

249. Lue TF, Tanagho EA. Physiology of erection and pharmacological management of impotence. J Urol 1987;137:829–836.

250. Smith AD. Psychological factors in the multidisciplinary evaluation and treatment of erectile dysfunction. Urol Clin North Am 1988;15:41–51.

251. Slag MF, Morley JE, Elson MK, et al. Impotence in medical clinic outpatients. JAMA 1983;249:1736–1740.

252. Korenman SG. Sexual dysfunction. In: Wilson JD, Foster DW, editors. Williams Textbook of Endocrinology. Philadelphia: WB Saunders, 1992:1033–1048.

253. Mitchell JE, Popkin MK. Antidepressant drug therapy and sexual dysfunction in men: a review. J Clin Psychopharmacol 1983;3:76–79.

254. Segraves RT, Madsen R, Carter CS, et al. Erectile dysfunction associated with pharmacological agents. In: Segraves RT, Schoenberg HW, editors. Diagnosis and Treatment of Erectile Disturbances: A Guide for Clinicians. New York: Plenum, 1985:22–63.

255. Smith PH, Talbert RL. Sexual dysfunction with antihypertensive and antipsychotic drugs. Clin Pharmacol 1986;5:373–384.

256. Wein AJ, Van Arsdalen KN. Drug-induced male sexual dysfunction. Urol Clin North Am 1988;15:23–31.

257. Kwan M, Greenleaf WJ, Mann J, et al. The nature of androgen action on male sexuality: a combined laboratory self-report study on hypogonadal men. J Clin Endocrinol Metab 1983;57:557–562.

258. Perryman RL, Thorner MO. The effects of hyperprolactinemia on sexual and reproductive function in man. J Androl 1981;5:233–242.

259. Pogach LM, Vaitukaitis JL. Endocrine disorders associated with erectile dysfunction. In: Krane RJ, Siroky MD, Goldstein I, editors. Male Sexual Dysfunction. Boston: Little, Brown, 1983:63–76.

260. Kalliomaki JL, Markkanen TK, Mustonen VA. Sexual behavior after cerebral vascular accident. Fertil Steril 1961;12:156–158.

261. Hierons R, Saunders M. Impotence in patients with temporal lobe lesions. Lancet 1966;2:761–763.

262. Coslett HB, Heilman KM. Male sexual function: impairment after right hemisphere stroke. Arch Neurol 1986;43:1036–1039.

263. Herzog A, Seibel M, Schomer D, et al. Reproductive endocrine disorders in men with partial seizures of the temporal lobe. Arch Neurol 1986;43:347–350.

264. Bors E, Comarr E. Neurological disturbances of sexual function with special reference to 529 patients with spinal cord injury. Urol Surv 1960;10:191–222.

265. Torrens MJ. Neurologic and neurosurgical disorders associated with impotence. In: Krane RJ, Siroky MB, Goldstein I, editors. Male Sexual Dysfunction. Boston: Little, Brown, 1983:55–61.

266. Valleroy ML, Kraft GH. Sexual dysfunction in multiple sclerosis. Arch Phys Med Rehabil 1984;65:125–128.

267. Whitelaw GP, Smithwick RH. Some secondary effects of sympathectomy: with particular reference to disturbance of sexual function. N Engl J Med 1951;245:121–130.

268. Kedia KR, Markland C, Fraley EE. Sexual function following high retroperitoneal lymphadenectomy. J Urol 1975;114:237–239.

269. Yeager ED, Van Heerden JA. Sexual dysfunction following proctocolectomy and abdominoperineal resection. Ann Surg 1980;191:169–170.

270. Walsh PC, Donker PJ. Impotence following radical prostatectomy insight into etiology and prevention. Urology 1982;19:259–262.

271. Lue TF, Zeinah SJ, Schmidt RA, Tanagho EA. Neuroanatomy of penile erection: its relevance to iatrogenic impotence. J Urol 1984;131:273–280.

272. Palmer JDK, Fink S, Berger RH. Diabetic secondary impotence: neuropathic factor as measured by peripheral motor nerve conduction. Urology 1986;28:197–200.

273. Papadopoulos C. Cardiovascular drugs and sexuality: a cardiologist's review. Arch Intern Med 1980;140:1341–1345.

274. Leriche A, Morel A. The syndrome of thrombotic obliteration of the aortic bifurcation. Ann Surg 1948;127:193–206.

275. Zorgniotti AW, Possi G, Padula G, Makovsky RD. Diagnosis and therapy of vasculogenic impotence. J Urol 1980;123:674–676.

276. Michal V. Arterial disease as a cause of impotence. Clin Endocrinol Metab 1982;11:725–748.

277. Michal V, Kovac I, Belan A. Arterial lesions in impotence: phalloarteriography. Int Angiol 1984;3:247–254.

278. Herman A, Adar R, Rubinstein Z. Vascular lesions associated with impotence in diabetic and nondiabetic arterial occlusive disease. Diabetes 1978;27:975–981.

279. McCulloch DK, Campbell IW, Wu FC, et al. The prevalence of diabetic impotence. Diabetologia 1980;18:279–283.

280. Kaiser FE, Korenman SG. Impotence in diabetic men. Am J Med 1988;85:147–152.

281. Sharlip ID. Penile arteriography in impotence after pelvic trauma. J Urol 1981;126:477–481.

282. Goldstein I, Feldman MI, Deckers PJ, et al. Radiation-associated impotence: a clinical study of its mechanism. JAMA 1984;251:903–910.

283. Ebbehoj J, Wagner G. Insufficient penile erection due to abnormal drainage of cavernous bodies. Urology 1979;13:507–510.

284. Tudoriu T, Bourmer H. The hemodynamics of erection at the level of the penis and its local deterioration. J Urol 1983;129:741–745.

285. Emond AM, Holman R, Hayes RJ, Serjeant GR. Priapism and impotence in homozygous sickle cell disease. Arch Intern Med 1980;140:1434–1437.

286. Van Arsdalen KN, Malloy TR, Wein J. Erectile physiology, dysfunction and evaluation. Part II: etiology and evaluation of erectile dysfunction. Monogr Urol 1983;4:165–185.

287. Newman HF, Reiss H, Northrup JD. Physical basis of emission, ejaculation and orgasm in the male. Urology 1982;19:341–350.

288. Murphy JB, Lipshultz LI. Abnormalities of ejaculation. Urol Clin North Am 1987;14:583–596.

289. Levine SB. Marital sexual dysfunction: ejaculation disturbances. Ann Intern Med 1976;84:575–579.

290. Williams W. Secondary premature ejaculation. Aust N Z Psychol 1984;18:333–340.

291. Munjack DJ, Kanno PH. Retarded ejaculation: a review. Arch Sex Behav 1979;8:139–150.

292. Hamer PM, Bain J. Ejaculatory incompetence and infertility. Fertil Steril 1986;45:384–387.

293. Lipshultz LI, McConnell J, Benson GS. Current concepts of the mechanisms of ejaculation: normal and abnormal states. J Reprod Fertil 1981;26:499–507.

294. Shaban SF. Treatment of abnormalities of ejaculation. In: Lipshultz LI, Howard SS, editors. Infertility in the Male. 2nd edition. St. Louis: Mosby-Year Book, 1991:409–426.

295. Heldlund H, Ek A. Ejaculation and sexual function after endoscopic bladder neck incision. Br J Urol 1985;57:164–167.

296. Ochsner MG, Burns E, Henry HH. Incidence of retrograde ejaculation following bladder neck revision as a child. J Urol 1970;104:596–597.

297. Greene LF, Kelalis PP. Retrograde ejaculation of semen due to diabetic neuropathy. J Urol 1968;98:693–696.

298. Buffum J. Pharmacosexology: the effects of drugs on sexual function: a review. J Psychoact Drugs 1982;14:5–44.

299. Kedia K, Markland C. The effect of pharmacological agents on ejaculation. J Urol 1975;114:569–773.

300. Weinstein MH, Machleder HI. Sexual function after aorto-iliac surgery. Ann Surg 1975;181:787–790.

301. McConnell JA, Benson GS, Wood J. Disturbance of autonomic fibers to pelvic/perineal viscera of the human male. Anat Rec 1978;190:475.

302. Lisenmeyer TA, Perkash I. Infertility in men with spinal cord injury. Arch Phys Med Rehabil 1991;72:747–754.

303. Dobrowolski Z, Piasecki Z, Augustyn M. Assessment of sexual efficiency in patients after the pull-through operation for stricture of the posterior urethra. J Urol 1982;128:703–704.

304. Paramo PG, Mertinez-Pineiro JA, De La Pena JJ, Paramo PS Jr. Andrological implications of congenital posterior urethral valves in adults: a case of retained ejaculation and review in western literature. Eur Urol 1983;9:359–361.

305. Sigman M, Lipshultz LI, Howards SS. Evaluation of the subfertile male. In: Lipshultz LI, Howards SS, editors. Infertility in the Male. 2nd edition. St. Louis: Mosby-Year Book, 1991:179–210.

306. McConnell JD. Abnormalities of sperm motility: techniques of evaluation and treatment. In: Lipshultz LI, Howards SS, editors. Infertility in the Male. 2nd edition. St. Louis: Mosby-Year Book, 1991:254–276.

307. Linck RW. Advances in the ultrastructural analysis of the sperm flagellar axoneme. In: Fawcett DW, Bedford JM, editors. The Spermatozoan. Baltimore: Urban & Schwarzenberg, 1979:99–115.

308. Satir R. Basis of flagellar motility in spermatozoa: current status. In: Fawcett DW, Bedford JM, editors. The Spermatozoan. Baltimore: Urban & Schwarzenberg, 1979:81–90.

309. Gibbons BH. Studies on the mechanism of flagellar movement. In: Fawcett DW, Bedford JM, editors. The Spermatozoan. Baltimore: Urban & Schwarzenberg, 1979:91–97.

310. Hoskins DD, Barndt H, Acott TS. Initiation of sperm motility in the mammalian epididymis. Fed Proc 1978;37:2534–2542.

311. Chang MC. The meaning of sperm capacitation: a historical perspective. J Androl 1984;5:45–50.

312. Perreault SD, Rogers BJ. Capacitation pattern of human spermatozoa. Fertil Steril 1982;38:258–260.

313. Bedford JM. Sperm capacitation and fertilization in mammals. Biol Reprod 1970; 2(suppl):128–158.

314. Nagae T, Yanagimachi R, Sviratava PN, Yanagimachi H. Acrosome reaction in human spermatozoa. Fertil Steril 1986;45:701–707.

315. Tagatz GE, Okagaki T, Sciarra JJ. The effect of vaginal lubricants on sperm motility and viability in vitro. Am J Obstet Gynecol 1972;113:88–90.

316. Tulandi T, Plouffe L Jr, McInnes RA. Effect of saliva on sperm motility and activity. Fertil Steril 1982;38:721–723.

317. Boyars SP, Corrales MD, Huzar G, DeCherney AH. The effects of Lubrin on sperm motility in vitro. Fertil Steril 1987;47:882–884.

318. Afzelius BA. A human syndrome caused by immotile cilia. Science 1976;193:317–319.

319. Afzelius BA, Mossberg B. The immotile-cilia syndrome including Kartagener's syndrome. In: Standbury JB, Wyngaarden JB, Fredricksen DS, et al, editors. The Metabolic Basis of Inherited Disease. 5th edition. New York: McGraw-Hill, 1983:1986–1994.

320. Wilton LJ, Teichtahl H, Temple-Smith PD, deKretser DM. Kartagener's syndrome with motile cilia and immotile spermatozoa: axonemal ultrastructure and function. Am Rev Respir Dis 1986;134:1233–1236.

321. Eliasson R, Mossberg B, Camner P, Afzelius BA. The immotile-cilia syndrome. N Engl J Med 1977;297:1–6.

322. Wilton LJ, Teichtahl H, Temple-Smith PD, deKretser DM. Structural heterogeneity of the axonemes of respiratory cilia and sperm flagella in normal men. J Clin Invest 1985;75:825–831.

323. Gagnon C, Sherins RJ, Phillips DM, Bardin CW. Deficiency of protein-carboxyl methylase in immotile spermatozoa of infertile men. N Engl J Med 1982;306:821–825.

324. Haas GG Jr. Male fertility and immunity. In: Lipshultz LI, Howards SS, editors. Infertility in the Male. 2nd edition. St. Louis: Mosby-Year Book, 1991:277–296.

325. Hendry WF. The significance of antisperm antibodies: measurement and management. Clin Endocrinol (Oxf) 1992;36:219–221.

326. Alexander NJ, Anderson DJ. Vasectomy: consequences of autoimmunity to sperm antigens. Fertil Steril 1979;32:253–260.

327. Haas GG Jr, Ausmanus M, Culp L, et al. The effect of immunoglobulin occurring on human sperm in vivo on the human sperm/hamster ova penetration assay. Am J Reprod Immunol Microbiol 1985;7:109–112.

328. Haas GG Jr. The inhibitory effect of sperm-associated immunoglobulins on cervical mucus penetration. Fertil Steril 1986;46:334–337.

329. Hendry WF. Bilateral aseptic necrosis of femoral heads following intermittent high dose steroid therapy. Fertil Steril 1982;38:120.

330. Glezerman M, Bernstein D, Zakut C, et al. Polyzoospermia: a definite pathologic entity. Fertil Steril 1982;38:605–608.

CHAPTER 38

Methods and Interpretation of Semen Analysis

JAMES W. OVERSTREET and
RUSSELL O. DAVIS

The semen evaluation is one of the most basic laboratory tests for clinical assessment of the infertile couple. The parameters of semen quality provide information on sperm production by the testis, patency and function of the male reproductive tract, activity of the accessory glands, and capability for ejaculation. Like most clinical laboratory tests, the purpose of this evaluation is detection of disease, in this case, male infertility. The absence of abnormal findings does not necessarily imply that the male is fertile, because traditional measurements of semen quality are relatively superficial, and their subjectivity and lack of standardization may result in unreliable values. Because of the variety of endpoints measured and the timing of this procedure in the infertility workup, semen analysis may provide the first indication that a male factor is contributing to the couple's infertility. The clinical usefulness of semen evaluation is improving rapidly as more objective, standardized methodology is introduced into practice and data become available from large-scale studies with defined populations of fertile and infertile men. In this chapter, we emphasize the methods of semen evaluation that we use in our laboratory and the approach that we take for interpretation of semen parameters. We also describe other methodology that is widely used in current clinical practice. The details of these laboratory procedures are also discussed in other reviews and handbooks.[1–6]

COLLECTION AND TRANSPORTATION OF SEMEN SPECIMENS

Variability in Semen Parameters

A single semen analysis is seldom adequate for even the most general assessment of a male's fertility status, and multiple evaluations are always required to establish quantitative parameters of semen quality. Longitudinal studies of fertile men have demonstrated significant day-to-day variability in semen parameters.[5, 7] Coefficients of variation for semen parameters may exceed 50% for normal semen[8] as well as for abnormal semen.[9] However, a considerable amount of this variation is probably technical and not due to biologic variability. There have been reports that human sperm concentration, total sperm number per ejaculate, and motile sperm concentration may vary with the season and are reduced during the summer.[10] Transient semen abnormalities also may be induced by infection, trauma, environmental stressors, or medications.[11, 12] Therefore, knowledge of clinical conditions such as viral infection or febrile illness, recreational practices such as alcohol, tobacco or drug use, and environmental exposures (such as contact with toxic chemicals and excess heat) is useful for interpretation of semen parameters. When there is a recent history of such conditions, followup semen evaluation may be appropriate after 2 to 3 months have elapsed to allow for a new cycle of spermatogenesis.[13] We obtain information on the medical, social, and occupational history of all men referred for semen evaluation. This information is provided in the answers to a brief questionnaire that is mailed to all patients and returned to the laboratory at the time of semen delivery.

Sexual Abstinence Prior to Semen Evaluation

The period of abstinence from ejaculation has been shown to have a significant effect on semen volume and sperm concentration and a lesser effect on sperm motility and morphology.[9, 14, 15] We request 48 to 72 hours of abstinence before a semen sample is collected for evaluation. The required period of abstinence is specified along with other instructions for collection and transportation of the specimen, which are mailed to the patient together with the health questionnaire.

This period of abstinence is more than adequate to replenish epididymal sperm reserves and provides a reasonable indication of testicular sperm production.[16] It cannot be assumed that the patient will comply with these instructions, and we also request that the actual period of abstinence be recorded on the questionnaire as well as the usual frequency of coitus for the couple. Because the standardized period of abstinence may not reflect the normal ejaculation frequency of the patient, in some instances it may be warranted to evaluate specimens at intervals that approximate the coital frequency of the couple.[17]

Collection of Semen

If possible, the clinical laboratory should provide a comfortable, private room for collection of semen specimens, and the patient should be informed that such a facility is available at the time the appointment is made for semen evaluation. Semen should be collected by masturbation into a wide-mouthed plastic container provided by the laboratory. Semen collection containers and all other laboratory plasticware should be tested regularly for cytotoxicity to spermatozoa. We routinely apply a simple sperm survival assay in which motile sperm are incubated with the test material for 24 hours and their motility is compared with that of an aliquot incubated in a standard low-toxicity control vessel. Semen collection at the laboratory avoids artifacts associated with semen aging and transportation, but some patients are unwilling to collect ejaculations on site. There is evidence that sexual stimulation before and during semen collection may affect ejaculation,[18] and stressful conditions during specimen collection could artificially lower semen quality. Semen-collection condoms are available for patients who are unwilling to collect the specimen by masturbation,[18] but contraceptive condoms should never be used because they are spermicidal. Semen collection by coitus interruptus should also be discouraged because of the risk of losing the sperm-rich first fraction of the ejaculate.

Occasionally, analysis of a split ejaculate[1, 19] may be requested by a referring physician. The split ejaculate is collected in two or more containers, and the patient is instructed to collect the first few drops of specimen into the first container. The first fraction usually contains the majority of spermatozoa and primarily prostatic fluid. The sperm motility in this fraction may also be superior to that in other fractions that are made up primarily of secretions from the seminal vesicles.[1, 19] Before the procedure of intrauterine insemination with washed spermatozoa became widely practiced, this method was used to provide a small volume of concentrated semen for cervical insemination.

In instances when no semen is produced in spite of orgasm or in cases of low semen volume, retrograde ejaculation may be suspected.[20] The diagnosis of retrograde ejaculation can be made by evaluation of a postejaculation urine specimen. The whole urine should be examined microscopically for spermatozoa, and, if necessary, a centrifugate can also be evaluated. When there is antegrade ejaculation, some spermatozoa normally will be present in the urine because of urethral contamination. However, large numbers of sperm in the urine indicate that a portion of the ejaculate is passing into the bladder. Following appropriate treatment to alkalin- ize the urine, these spermatozoa may be recovered for artificial insemination.[20]

Transportation of Semen

When semen specimens must be produced at home, they should reach the laboratory within 1 hour of collection. The instructions to the patient should specify that the laboratory will provide the container, and information should be given on how the specimen can be protected from extremes of heat and cold. We advise that the patient carry the container near the body in an inside pocket. In less temperate regions it is advisable to provide an insulated container for transportation of the semen specimen.

EVALUATION OF THE FRESH SEMEN SPECIMEN

Physical Characteristics of Semen

The semen should be evaluated macroscopically and microscopically as soon as it is received by the laboratory. Semen samples can be maintained in the laboratory at either room or body temperature, but microscopic observations should be carried out at body temperature (37°C) to avoid variability that may result from fluctuations in room temperature.[17] First, the specimen should be examined for the presence of a coagulum. It is important to distinguish semen coagulation and viscosity.[21] Most specimens are fully coagulated (clotlike) immediately after ejaculation and require 15 to 30 minutes for liquefaction to occur. As liquefaction takes place, the semen becomes increasingly fluid. Liquefaction should be confirmed microscopically, because partially liquified semen is not sufficiently homogeneous for analysis. Specimens that have not fully liquified within 1 hour are considered abnormal and may require special treatment.[21]

The sample should be thoroughly mixed before evaluation. Mixing can be accomplished by repeated pipetting with a transfer pipette, but care must be taken to avoid producing bubbles. Alternative methods for semen mixing include vigorous swirling, gentle vortex mixing, or stirring with a rod. The physical characteristics of the semen including its color and odor should be evaluated, although we do not routinely record these characteristics unless they are unusual. The semen is normally opaque and gray-white in color. A translucent appearance is associated with low sperm concentrations or azoospermia. Yellow, pink, or red coloration of the semen is abnormal and should be noted. Samples that smell of putrefaction or urine should be identified. Comments should also be made on other unusual conditions, such as specimen containers and condoms that were provided by the patient, and evidence of spillage. Semen pH can be measured by dropping a 10-μL aliquot of semen onto pH paper and is typically 7.2 to 7.8.[22]

The semen volume is measured using a 1-, 5-, or 10-mL disposable serologic pipette and pipette pump. The semen volume is recorded to the nearest 0.1 mL. The semen viscosity can be assessed during the process of determining semen volume. We assess the viscosity subjectively on a scale of 0 to 4 (Table 38–1). If more precision in viscosity measurement

Semen Parameter	Score				
	0	*1*	*2*	*3*	*4*
Semen viscosity	Waterlike	Increased, but forms drops from pipette	Forms thread from pipette	Forms thread >2 cm in length	Gel-like
Sperm agglutination	None	1 agglutinate per 3 20× fields	1 agglutinate per 2 20× fields	1 agglutinate per 20× field	—
Motility progression	Immotile sperm	Twitching sperm	Sluggish to fair progression	Good progression	Vigorous progression

TABLE 38–1. Subjective Assessments of Semen

is required, the rate can be measured at which drops are formed when the semen is allowed to flow from a 0.1-mL pipette.[22] If the semen viscosity is high, it may be necessary to reduce the viscosity before the semen can be analyzed. Viscosity reduction can usually be accomplished by aspirating the semen into and out of a hypodermic syringe fitted with a 15-gauge blunt needle.

Visual Assessment of Sperm Motility

We use phase-contrast microscopy for evaluation of sperm motility. To achieve a standard depth of preparation, sperm are observed in 20-μM-deep μ-Cell slides (Spectrum Technologies, Berkeley, California). It is possible to obtain an approximate standard depth of sperm suspension on an ordinary microscope slide by using standard volumes of semen and cover glass sizes.[3] A 7-μL aliquot of thoroughly mixed semen is transferred to each side of the prewarmed μ-Cell slide. A 20× objective lens and a 10× wide-field ocular with a 5-mM, 25-square (5 × 5) reticle grid (Kharmann Rulings, Inc., Manchester, New Hampshire) are used to view the sperm suspension. The percentage of motility is assessed on one side of the two-chambered slide at least 5 mM from the fluid boundary. At least five randomly selected microscopic fields are sampled. Motile and immotile sperm are scored with a hand counter in the five small squares on the top row of the ocular grid. Motile sperm are defined as any sperm with a moving flagellum, whether or not the sperm is progressive. At least 100 sperm are scored in this manner to determine the percentage of motility. This counting procedure is repeated in the second chamber of the μ-Cell slide, and the percentage of motility for this sperm suspension is determined. If the percentage of difference between the two values is 10% or greater, the mean of the two values is recorded as the percentage of motility. If the percentage of difference is more than 10%, a third 7-μL aliquot is counted in a new μ-Cell slide, and the median of the three values is recorded as the percentage of motility.

Forward progression is rated for the sperm suspension as a whole on a scale of 1 to 4, with a score of 1 being twitching sperm with no progression and a score of 4 being vigorous, progressively motile sperm (see Table 38–1). Sperm with sluggish to fair progression are scored as 2, and sperm with good progression are scored as 3. When progression falls between two categories, a half point is added, for example, 3.5. In our laboratory a score of 3 is required for "normal" progression. The subjective criteria for assessing sperm progression are learned by viewing videotapes of semen with

various sperm concentrations for which the sperm velocities have been previously measured.

Some semen evaluation methods assess sperm progression by counting the percentage of progressive sperm among the motile sperm in addition to counting the overall percentage of motility.[4] In our experience, these complex counting protocols cannot be carried out with acceptable precision. Other protocols calculate a "sperm drive" to quantify sperm progression. The time required for a spermatozoon to travel between two parallel lines in a hemocytometer chamber is measured, and the average value for 20 spermatozoa is expressed in s/0.05 mM.[6]

Although there are significant difficulties in standardizing subjective assessments of percentage of motility and progression, these measurements are extremely important, even when objective methods for sperm analysis are used. Visual assessment of the semen ensures a backup record of the semen quality and provides a frame of reference for interpretation of unusual or erroneous quantitative data; in some laboratories this may be the only assessment of sperm motion. Some semen evaluation protocols include repeated sperm motility assessments after 4 hours and again at 24 hours as a means of assessing sperm longevity.[6] However, under physiologic conditions, sperm do not remain in seminal plasma but migrate rapidly into cervical mucus. The postcoital test is therefore the most relevant means of assessing sperm longevity.[23]

Other Microscopic Observations

Following the assessment of sperm motility, sperm agglutination is assessed in the μ-Cell chambers. Any motile sperm that stick to one another by the head, midpiece, or tail are considered agglutinated. Immotile sperm clumps or motile sperm that are stuck to other cells or debris are not considered agglutinated. Agglutination is ranked on a scale of 0 to 3 (see Table 38–1). Agglutination scores of 3 or higher are considered significant. In other protocols the percentage of agglutinated sperm is counted, and it is considered abnormal when more than 10% are agglutinated.[3]

The semen specimen should also be evaluated with the 40× objective lens for the presence of epithelial cells, red blood cells, bacteria, and protozoa, which should be noted if present. Sperm morphology should also be assessed initially at this time. Although the sperm morphology is not assessed in detail, specific abnormalities such as coiled tails, duplicate forms, or headless flagella should be recorded, if prevalent. The presence of round cells is noted at this stage of the evaluation, but leukocyte and germinal cells cannot be differentiated with certainty by phase-contrast microscopy of unstained specimens. If spermatozoa are absent, the ejaculate should be centrifuged and the pellet examined for sperm. If no spermatozoa are observed in the centrifuged pellet, a qualitative test for fructose[2] should be performed. The absence of both spermatozoa and fructose in the semen is suggestive of congenital absence of the vas deferens.[24] A number of other biochemical tests can be performed on the semen,[25] but these tests are generally not considered to be part of the routine semen evaluation.

Measurement of Sperm Concentration

Sperm concentration traditionally has been measured using a hemocytometer.[3, 4] We do not favor this method because of the large dilutions that are required and the consequent effects on precision. The Makler chamber is also used widely for determination of sperm counts,[26] but we have found the precision of the μ-Cell to be approximately twice that of the Makler chamber. The protocol that we use for sperm counting with the μ-Cell is given in Table 38–2.

The manual measurement of sperm concentration is used to prepare the specimen for videorecording and to calibrate the computer-aided sperm analysis (CASA) instrument. Although the CASA instrument can be used to measure sperm concentrations automatically, errors are encountered when there are low or high sperm concentrations, significant sperm agglutination, or large amounts of seminal debris.[27] We have found that the manual count can be routinely obtained with a coefficient of variation of less than 10%. Therefore, we use the sperm concentration value from the manual count for the clinical report.

Automated Assessment of Sperm Motility

CASA technology is now applied widely for clinical assessment of sperm motion.[27] A number of objective methods for

---

TABLE 38–2. Protocol for Sperm Counting with a μ-Cell Chamber

1. 50-μL aliquots of sperm fixative solution (5 g $NaHCO_3$, 1 mL formalin, 100 mL H_2O) are placed in each of two 0.5-mL beakers.
2. 50-μL aliquots of well-mixed semen are added to each beaker of fixative.
3. The two fixed sperm suspensions are mixed by vortexing and are loaded into the two chambers of the μ-Cell counting chamber, respectively.
4. The 20× objective and the 5-mM, 25-square (5 × 5) reticle-fitted eyepiece are used to count the number of sperm in all 25 boxes of the grid.
5. The sperm concentration ($\times 10^6$/mL) is estimated by dividing the total number of sperm counted in the grid by the volume of the sperm suspension defined by the grid (area of the grid × depth of μ-Cell) and multiplying this number by 2.
6. If the estimated concentration is $\geq 20 \times 10^6$/mL, the number of sperm in six complete grids is counted for each chamber of the μ-Cell. If the estimated concentration is $<20 \times 10^6$/mL, the number of sperm in 12 complete grids is counted.
7. The final sperm concentration for each side of the μ-Cell is calculated as in step 5, by dividing the mean number of sperm counted per grid by the volume of the sperm suspension and multiplying this number by 2.
8. The percentage of difference between the two concentrations is determined, and if it is $\leq 10\%$, the mean value is recorded as the sperm concentration. If the percentage of difference is $>10\%$, steps 1–7 are repeated with a third aliquot of semen, and the median of the three values is recorded as the sperm concentration.

---

measuring sperm motility preceded CASA including time-exposure photomicrography,[28] multiple-exposure photomicrography,[29] and videomicrography.[30] Although such methods were used clinically, they never gained wide acceptance. The commercialization of CASA has resulted in the availability of a number of instruments, easy access to technical support, and greater awareness of the potential advantages of an automated approach to semen evaluation. Different CASA instruments employ different hardware and image-processing algorithms. However, when standard laboratory protocols are used for specimen preparation and recording, the differences in measurements between instruments are slight and unlikely to be clinically significant.[27] The technology of CASA and its application in both clinical and research settings has been reviewed recently.[27] A brief explanation of CASA technology is given here so that its application and limitations in current clinical practice can be appreciated.

CASA instruments digitize the electric signals that result from repeated video scans of a field of sperm. The sperm cell is recognized because of its optical contrast with the background, and its position (centroid) is calculated. A succession of centroids calculated over time defines the swimming trajectory of the sperm. The CASA instrument calculates a variety of movement characteristics from this trajectory. Subjectively, an observer may characterize sperm motion in terms of swimming speeds (e.g., "vigorous motion") and swimming patterns (e.g., "space-gaining motion"). CASA provides numbers that quantitate the vigor and pattern of movement on a per-sperm basis. The measure of sperm vigor that is used most frequently is the curvilinear velocity (VCL), which is defined as the average distance per unit time between successive positions of each centroid in the swimming path. The most reliable measure of sperm progression is the straight-line velocity (VSL), which is defined as the distance between the first and last centroids of the swimming path divided by the total elapsed time. CASA reports may also include values for linearity (LIN), which is defined as VSL/VCL and is a measure of the straightness of the swimming trajectory; amplitude of lateral head displacement (ALH), which measures the amplitude of variations in the swimming trajectory; and the mean angular displacement (MAD), which measures the turning angle of the sperm head. A number of other sperm movement parameters are measured by CASA instruments, including average path velocity, wobble, straightness, and beat-cross frequency.[27] The clinical value of CASA parameters is a focus of current research, and except for VSL, we do not include them in our clinical report.

The subjectivity and lack of precision in visual assessments of sperm motion[31, 32] have limited their usefulness in semen evaluation. CASA provides the capability to make such measurements objectively. However, limitations in both technology and biomedical knowledge currently restrict the clinical application of CASA to measurement of a relatively small set of sperm movement characteristics. With appropriate standardization of procedures and quality control, CASA can provide precise measurements of sperm concentration, percentage of motility, and sperm movement characteristics.[27] However, CASA is inaccurate in assessing semen samples with high and low sperm concentrations. Immotile sperm may not be distinguished from debris, and in specimens with low sperm concentrations, misclassification of debris may lead to significant errors. In specimens with high sperm concentrations, motile sperm frequently collide with other motile sperm, immotile sperm, and debris. The optical conjunctions that result from those collisions create artifacts in measurements of sperm concentration, percentage of motility, and sperm movement characteristics that cannot be avoided with contemporary CASA instruments.

The only workable approach for analysis of semen with high sperm concentrations is dilution of the specimen.[27] The requirement for semen dilution has raised a number of technical and biologic questions, many of which have not been resolved. It is clear that dilution has significant effects on sperm motility.[33] There has been debate concerning the appropriate medium for sperm dilution (homologous seminal plasma and phosphate-buffered saline are widely used) and whether all specimens should be diluted rather than those with high sperm concentrations alone.[27] Although semen dilution introduces an uncontrolled biologic variable, the value of obtaining quantitative, objective measurements of sperm movement outweighs any disadvantage.

The problems encountered in using a CASA instrument to measure the percentage of motility accurately, especially in undiluted specimens, outweigh its technical advantages, and we use the visually obtained percentage of motility in our clinical reports. The percentage of motility, as well as sperm velocity, is affected by dilution.[33] Moreover, the definition of a motile sperm as detected by the CASA instrument is not the same as that specified by most manual counting protocols. In the latter, sperm with any evidence of flagellar activity are usually classified as motile. CASA instruments, on the other hand, require that a sperm achieve a minimal progression (e.g., 10 μM/s) to classify it as motile.[27] The advantage of separately measuring the percentage of sperm with flagellar activity and the swimming speed of the moving sperm is hypothetical but is sufficiently supported by our clinical experience to justify continuation of the practice.

The laboratory procedures for semen preparation prior to analysis with the CASA instrument are critical for obtaining reliable information on sperm movement characteristics. The information obtained during visual evaluation of the specimen is used to prepare the semen for videorecording and to calibrate the CASA instrument during analysis. We use the following procedures to analyze sperm motion with the CellTrak-S instrument (Motion Analysis Corp., Santa Rosa, California):

1. If the sperm concentration is greater than 40×10^6/mL, 500 μL of semen are diluted with Dulbecco's phosphate-buffered saline at 37°C according to the dilution table shown in Table 38–3.

2. The diluted semen is mixed by gentle pipetting and is allowed to incubate at 37°C for 3 minutes before videotaping. Semen with sperm concentrations 40×10^6/mL or less are videotaped without dilution.

3. The semen is mixed again, and 7 μL is loaded into one of the 20-μM-deep μ-Cell chambers.

4. After drifting movements in the chamber have ended, the percentage of motility is determined by the visual method to provide information on motility changes resulting from dilution. If the percentage of difference between the percentage of motilities of the diluted and undiluted semen is 25% or less, the diluted semen is videotaped. If the percentage of difference is higher than 25%, the second chamber of the

TABLE 38–3. Dilution of Semen for Videotaping

Concentration	Dilution Ratio	DPBS Volume (μL)
40–80	1:1	500
80–120	1:2	1000
120–160	1:3	1500
160–200	1:4	2000
200–240	1:5	2500
240–280	1:6	3000
280–320	1:7	3500
320–360 etc.	1:8	4000

DPBS, Dulbecco's phosphate-buffered saline.

μ-Cell slide is loaded with diluted semen, and this second chamber is videotaped.

5. The 10× positive phase-contrast objective and a green filter are used for videotaping 10 microscopic fields for 7 seconds each. Fields with debris and agglutinated sperm are avoided, if possible. If the sperm concentration is less than 20×10^6/mL, 15 fields are taped. During videotaping the focus is adjusted so that the sperm heads are slightly out of focus, and the microscope illumination is adjusted to achieve maximum contrast between the sperm head and the background.

CASA is performed from the videotape rather than the live image. A brief description of the analysis procedures is given here. Additional details and references can be found in a recent review article.[27] The minimum threshold velocity is set at 10 μM/s, and the maximum threshold velocity is set at 250 μM/s. The ALH smoothing parameter is set to 5 data points. All specimens are digitized at 30 frames per second (fps) for 0.5 second, and the minimum number of frames to analyze is set to equal the maximum number of frames to analyze (e.g., 15 points when digitizing at 30 fps). The digitization threshold is set by turning on all four edges and tracking a motile sperm. The threshold is adjusted until the image is approximately equal in size to the motile sperm head. Three edges are then turned off, and analysis is carried out using only one edge. At least 100 motile sperm are analyzed, and 200 sperm are analyzed whenever possible.

ASSESSMENT OF SPERM MORPHOLOGY

Sperm morphology usually is assessed from seminal smears that are prepared at the time of semen evaluation and subsequently stained. This component of the semen evaluation is the least standardized and therefore is most likely to be performed improperly. Sperm morphology assessment is complicated by the variety of sperm sizes and shapes that are encountered in semen from fertile men as well as from subfertile men. The clinical evaluation of sperm morphology usually includes determination of the percentage of "normal" spermatozoa in the sample. Experimental data indicate that spermatozoa with visible anatomic defects are not functional cells,[34-36] and there are many clinical reports that associate defective sperm shapes with infertility (see later). However, the criteria that define a normal sperm are based on an aesthetically pleasing oval shape[37, 38] rather than biologic experiments or clinical data on fertility. It should not be surprising that there is substantial disagreement concerning metric standards for the normal spermatozoon.

The most widely applied criteria for normal sperm morphology are those of the World Health Organization (WHO), which originally provided metric standards for definition of normal sperm morphology as assessed on Papanicolaou-stained smears.[5] More recently, strict morphologic criteria for normal sperm have been shown by Kruger and Menkveld and their colleagues to be useful in predicting the success of in vitro fertilization.[39–42] Although the original WHO criteria and the strict criteria are based on similar metric standards for sperm head length and width, the strict criteria exclude many more sperm from the normal category because of subtle abnormalities in sperm head shape and staining properties.[39–42] Thus, semen from fertile men may have as few as 14% normal sperm by strict criteria in comparison with the 50% cutoff point for normal morphology by the original WHO criteria. Recently, the WHO revised its criteria for normal sperm morphology, recommending new metric standards and a stricter method of sperm classification.[4] According to the new WHO standards, the cutoff point for normal semen is 30% normal forms.[4] Reconciliation of the various criteria for normal sperm morphology is made more difficult by the subjective nature of the visual morphology assessment process, which contributes to the considerable variation that has been demonstrated within and between technicians and laboratories.[31, 43–45]

In view of the fundamental disagreements that exist in the definition of a normal sperm, it is not surprising that there is even less consensus on the definitions of particular types of sperm abnormalities. Most morphologic classification protocols assign abnormal sperm to one or more categories or types (e.g., tapered head, amorphous tail) based on defects that are observed in the shape of the head, midpiece, and tail.[2–4, 6, 22] Metric standards have been proposed for classifying abnormal sperm types,[46] but the process of type classification is largely subjective. Some investigators have proposed using a "teratospermia index," which is a measure of the average number of defects per sperm,[47] but others have expressed doubt as to the value of this approach because multiple defects in sperm are likely to be correlated.[48]

As closer attention is paid to sperm measurements, the method of sperm preparation assumes greater importance. Sperm dimensions are different on seminal smears in comparison with wet preparations,[49] and staining methods can affect cell classification.[50, 51] The greatest accuracy and precision in morphometric measurements are obtained when sperm are washed and resuspended to a standard concentration before slide preparation.[50]

The clinical application of objective metric standards for sperm morphology classification has been limited. One reason for this lack of progress has been the absence of laboratory equipment to facilitate morphometric evaluation of sperm. The practice of performing metric measurements on individual sperm with an eyepiece micrometer has been proposed,[40] but such an approach is not feasible for routine clinical evaluation. We have used video images for many years to aid in the process of manual sperm morphology assessment,[52] but this practice has not been widely applied. Recently, automated sperm morphometry analysis (ASMA) instruments have become commercially available. These instruments can provide objective data on sperm shapes analogous to the way in which CASA instruments quantitate sperm motility.[33, 50, 53, 54] However, it is likely that different ASMA instruments will produce different results[55] until image-processing hardware and classification algorithms are standardized.

We use videomicrography for manual assessment of sperm morphology to standardize the classification procedure and to minimize subjectivity. Sperm are assessed on Papanicolaou-stained seminal smears using a 100×, oil-immersion, bright-field objective lens and a 10× widefield ocular. Sperm images are transmitted simultaneously to a black-and-white monitor using a 6.7× photo ocular. Sperm tail and midpiece morphology are determined after visual inspection, and if necessary, measurements are made on the video screen. Sperm head morphology is determined with the aid of a transparent overlay calibrated with metric standards for sperm head length and width (Fig. 38–1). We use the original WHO criteria[5] and consider a sperm to be normal if the head is oval in shape with a smooth and symmetrical outline and a length of 3 to 5 μM and a width of 2 to 3 μM. The midpiece must be slender, less than 1 μM in width, and straight and regular in outline. It must be aligned to the longitudinal axis of the head and be 7 to 8 μM long. The tail must be slender, uncoiled, and at least 45 μM in length.

A hierarchical classification system is used for scoring sperm morphology (Fig. 38–2). Sperm are evaluated in detail only if they have a single head and tail. Sperm with multiple

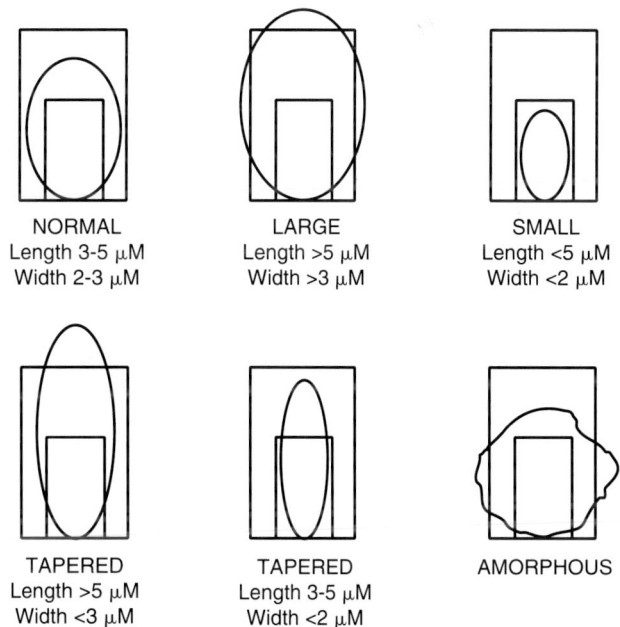

NORMAL
Length 3-5 μM
Width 2-3 μM

LARGE
Length >5 μM
Width >3 μM

SMALL
Length <5 μM
Width <2 μM

TAPERED
Length >5 μM
Width <3 μM

TAPERED
Length 3-5 μM
Width <2 μM

AMORPHOUS

FIGURE 38–1. A transparent overlay is drawn using a stage micrometer to determine the size of the boxes. The overlay is placed on the video screen so that the base of the sperm head is aligned with the bottom of the overlay. If the length and width lie between the two boxes, the classification is "normal." If the length and width lie outside of the outer box, the classification is "large." If the length lies within the inner box, the classification is "small." If the length lies outside the outer box and the width between the boxes, or if the length lies between the boxes and the width inside the inner box, the classification is "tapered." If the outline of the sperm head is irregular or asymmetrical, or both, the classification is "amorphous," regardless of the sperm dimensions. If the outline is smooth and symmetrical but the length lies between the boxes and the width lies outside the outer box, the classification is "amorphous."

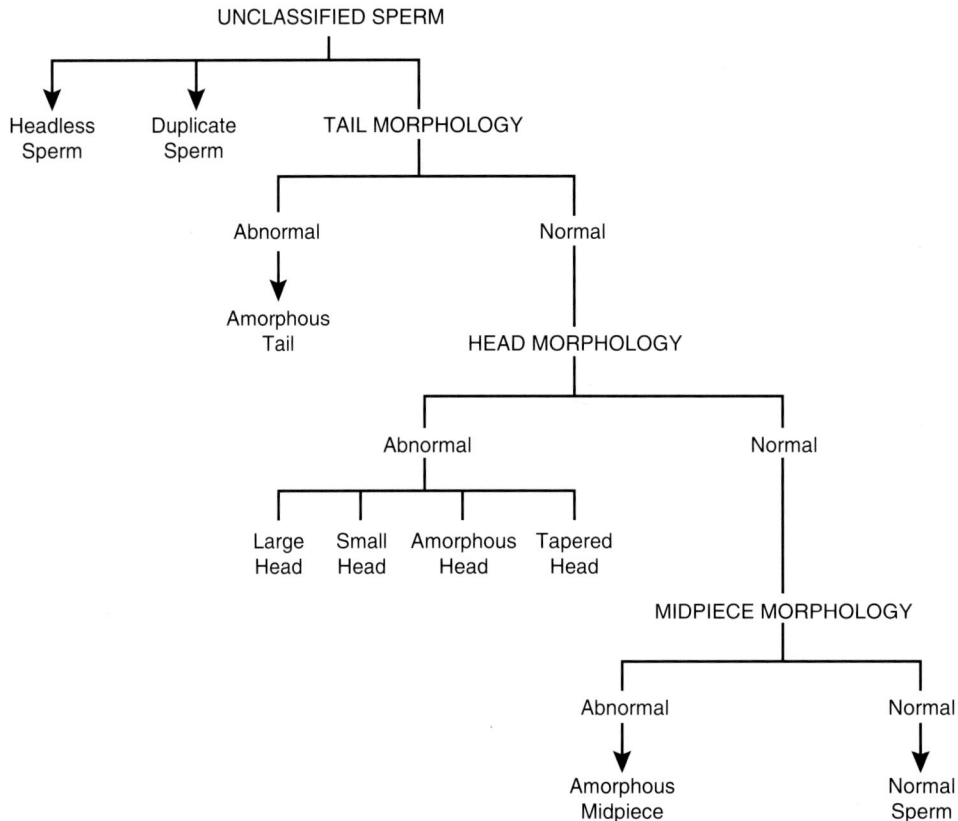

FIGURE 38–2. The classification system for scoring sperm morphology requires that a "normal sperm" have a normal head, midpiece, and tail. Abnormal sperm are assigned to only one category according to a classification system that evaluates tail morphology first, then head morphology, and, finally, midpiece morphology.

heads or tails, or both, are scored as "duplicate sperm" and sperm without heads (often referred to as "pinhead" sperm) are classified as "headless sperm." Sperm with any tail abnormality (coiled, shortened, broken) are classified as "amorphous tail" regardless of head or midpiece morphology. The rationale for primacy of tail morphology is that such sperm can be considered dysfunctional a priori, because absent or severely abnormal flagellar activity will likely result in failure of sperm transport to the site of fertilization or penetration of the oocyte. If the sperm tail is normal, the size and shape of the sperm head are considered. Sperm heads are classified as normal or abnormal with the aid of the video image and the transparent overlay. Sperm heads that are irregular in outline or asymmetrical, or both, are classified as "amorphous head." Sperm heads with smooth and symmetrical outlines are classified as "normal head," "large head," "small head," "tapered head," or "amorphous head" according to metric standards (see Fig. 38–1). Midpiece morphology is assessed last, and it is evaluated only for sperm with normal heads and tails. To be classified as normal, the sperm must be normal by all three criteria (head, midpiece, tail). One hundred consecutive sperm are scored in each of two randomly selected areas of the slide. If the percentage of difference between the percentage of normal sperm in the two areas is 15% or less, the mean of the two values is recorded as the percentage of normal morphology. If the percentage of difference is more than 15%, 100 sperm are scored in a third area of the slide, and the median of the three values is recorded as the percentage of normal morphology. The per-

centage of abnormal forms in each of the other categories (e.g., large head, amorphous tail) is calculated in the same way as the percentage of normal sperm; that is, either the mean or median value is used for the other categories, depending on whether 200 or 300 sperm were scored. The same approach with videomicrography and transparent overlays can also be used to analyze sperm morphology by strict criteria (e.g., the method proposed by Kruger and associates[41] or the revised method of the WHO[4]).

Human semen normally contains other cells in addition to sperm. Round cells that are observed in wet mounts of semen are often reported to be leukocytes. However, leukocytes cannot be identified with phase-contrast microscopy alone. The concentration of granulocytes in semen can be determined using peroxidase staining and hemocytometer counts,[4] but in the routine semen evaluation we estimate the leukocyte count on the Papanicolaou-stained seminal smear. The slide is scored for leukocytes using a $60\times$ bright-field objective and the $10\times$ wide-field ocular fitted with the 25-square reticle. Polymorphonuclear leukocytes are recognized by nuclear morphology, and the number of these cells in five fields (25 squares per field) is counted. The number of sperm cells in the same five fields is also counted. The concentration of leukocytes ($\pm 10^6$/mL) is then calculated using the following formula:

$$\text{Concentration of leukocytes} = \frac{\text{Total leukocytes in five fields}}{\text{Total sperm in five fields}} \times \text{Sperm concentration in semen}$$

According to the WHO, a leukocyte concentration greater

than 10[6]/mL is considered abnormal,[4] and we report the leukocyte concentration when it exceeds this value. Round cells that lack polymorphonuclear morphology may be immature germinal cells (spermatocytes, spermatids),[56] or they may be leukocytes. Positive identification of round cells in semen can be made using special staining procedures with monoclonal antibodies.[57]

QUALITY CONTROL OF LABORATORY METHODOLOGY

Quality control should be considered an essential element in the operation of every clinical laboratory. However, the requirement for formal quality control procedures in semen evaluation has been recent.[58] In general, quality control issues relate to (1) equipment, reagents, and media; (2) laboratory protocols and written instructions for all procedures; (3) laboratory reports and data analysis; (4) training, certification, and performance of personnel.[59]

Equipment should be well maintained, regularly calibrated, and monitored. In the andrology laboratory, such equipment includes microscopes and warming stages, video equipment and CASA instruments, incubators, balances, and centrifuges. Written records should be kept of all activities related to maintenance, monitoring, and calibration of instruments. All chemicals and media should be obtained, stored, and disposed of according to written procedures. Media preparation logs should be maintained, and quality control assays should be regularly performed for chemical activity and media toxicity.

Detailed written protocols should be maintained for every procedure carried out in the laboratory and should include information on controls, standards, calibration procedures, and limits for the particular test or assay. Protocols should include procedures for detection of errors and instructions or steps to be taken when errors are detected. Procedures must be in place to verify patent sample identity and to track patent samples in the laboratory.

Written reports to physicians should be generated in a timely manner and include quality control data and normal ranges. Data on positive and negative controls should be included in the report as appropriate (e.g., tests for fructose). Quality control data should be reviewed regularly by the laboratory staff, tolerance limits should be defined, and procedures should be in place to recognize unusual results.

The job requirements of all personnel should be described explicitly. Personnel should have appropriate training and certification for the tasks they perform. The chain of authority and responsibility should be clearly defined. Files should be kept of all laboratory errors, miscommunications, complaints, and adverse reactions. Approved biohazard protocols should be followed.

INTERPRETATION OF SEMEN PARAMETERS

Fertility Prediction on the Basis of Semen Parameters

A number of clinical approaches have been used to identify the minimum standards for fertile semen. One approach is to compare the results of semen evaluations in groups of fertile and infertile males. An early study of this type was by Macomber and Sanders in 1929,[60] and a number of data sets with 1000 or more subjects have been reported subsequently.[61–63] None of these studies have used modern methods of semen evaluation, and clinical definitions of the infertile populations have been inadequate (e.g., couples with female infertility factors were usually not excluded). Nevertheless, this body of literature has been used to justify the standards for normal semen quality that are used in most clinical laboratories.[2–4, 6]

A second approach to identifying standards for normal semen is to compare infertile couples who conceive with those who remain infertile during followup. Such a study was performed by Polansky and Lamb, who found no semen parameter predictive of conception in 1089 couples followed an average of 16 months after semen evaluation.[64] However, only one semen evaluation was used for prediction, and methods for assessment of sperm motility and morphology were subjective. Subjective semen evaluation methods were also used in the study of Dunphy and coworkers, who followed 739 patients and estimated 32-month pregnancy rates.[65] The predictive value of various semen parameters was tested using Cox's life table regression. In couples with a normal female partner and less than 4 years of infertility, the percentage of sperm with midpiece defects was the only predictive factor. For couples with more than 4 years of infertility, the most significant predictive factor was the concentration of motile sperm with sluggish or nonlinear motility (i.e., grade b by WHO criteria[5]), which is a biologically implausible result. Peng and associates selected 709 couples for followup study after excluding couples with known female infertility factors.[66] These investigators tested the ability of semen parameters to predict pregnancy-based receiver-operating characteristic curves. They found no clear threshold for either sperm concentration or the total number of motile sperm per ejaculate. The highest positive predictive values (75%) were associated with cutoff points at 5×10^6 sperm per milliliter and 5×10^6 motile sperm per ejaculate. The false-positive rates when these cutoff points were used were 4.3% for sperm concentration and 5.6% for total motile sperm per ejaculate. Bostofte and colleagues studied more than 1000 men and attempted to predict fertility from semen parameters using Cox's proportional hazards models.[67] These studies included a cohort of 765 men evaluated in 1950 and 1951 and a second group of 321 men evaluated between 1977 and 1985. The groups were followed up by questionnaire. The sperm concentration, the number of morphologically normal sperm, the number of motile sperm, and the quality of sperm motility all were significant when tested singly, and two factors were jointly predictive, that is, the percentage of morphologically normal sperm and the comparative sperm numbers with "good" or "poor" motility.[67]

The results of these followup studies are inconsistent, but most have provided evidence that parameters of semen quality are predictive of male fertility. A common shortcoming of these studies is the reliance on a single semen evaluation for prediction and the absence of objective methods for measurements of sperm motility and morphology. Future studies that address these problems may be more successful in fertility prediction.

Sperm Numbers

Until more fertility data become available from large-scale clinical studies, even objective semen parameters will have limited value in predicting male fertility and in detecting male infertility. In current practice, the results of semen evaluations can be used only to assign patients to broad clinical categories such as "normal," "marginal," or "abnormal" (Table 38–4). We use 20 to 250 × 10⁶/mL as a normal range for sperm concentration (see Table 38–4). The lower limit of 20 × 10⁶/mL is based primarily on the extensive clinical studies of MacLeod and Wang, which included data from more than 15,000 semen evaluations.[68] Although there is no biologic explanation for reduced fertility at high sperm concentrations, there is clinical evidence that reproductive performance is impaired when the sperm concentration exceeds 250 × 10⁶/mL.[69] MacLeod and Wang emphasized that sperm numbers alone provide limited information on fertility potential,[68] and there are several lines of indirect evidence that support this view. Men who are treated with contraceptive agents may remain fertile even when sperm concentration in the semen is less than 10⁶/mL.[70] Patients treated with exogenous gonadotropins for hypogonadotropic hypogonadism may become fertile with sperm counts of 10 × 10⁶/mL or less.[71] These data suggest that low sperm production is compatible with fertility as long as normal sperm cells are produced. Abnormal sperm function rather than insufficient sperm number is likely to be the primary cause of infertility even in men with low sperm counts. This idea is supported by experimental data that indicate that spermatozoa from infertile men may be dysfunctional even if they have no recognizable morphologic defects.[34–36] Nevertheless, sperm production is a valuable indicator of the function of the germinal epithelium and is an important measure of semen quality. In this sense, the total number of sperm per ejaculate is a more informative semen parameter than is sperm concentration. We consider 40 million sperm per ejaculate as the cutoff point for normal sperm numbers per ejaculate.

Semen Volume

Very large and very small semen volumes are associated with infertility,[72] and abnormality of semen volume alone may be a significant factor in particular types of male infertility. Low semen volume may be associated with retrograde ejaculation or partial blockage of the male reproductive tract and should be followed up with a urologic evaluation. Seminal plasma plays an important role in buffering the vaginal acidity that is detrimental to sperm survival.[73] Therefore, it is often useful to interpret abnormalities of semen volume in light of the results of a postcoital test. If the postcoital test result is normal, abnormalities of semen volume may have little clinical significance, provided total sperm numbers per ejaculate are adequate.

Sperm Motility

Although a few reports now have appeared on objective parameters of sperm motility in fertile and subfertile men,[74–76] the published clinical data are inadequate to establish a normal range of values. The range of values that we use has been established empirically in our laboratory. The lower limit for the percentage of motile sperm is 50%, although we consider sperm motilities in the range of 40% to 50% to be borderline. We report VSL as the measure of sperm progression, and its lower limit is set at 25 μM/s based on our previous experience with manual assessments of sperm swimming speed.[28, 30] Provisional normal values have also been established for VCL (>45 μM/s), LIN (>59), and MAD (>15 degrees).[77] We currently consider sperm motility to be normal overall when the percentages of motility and VSL reach or exceed the lower limits. We do not use other CASA parameters for clinical evaluation of semen, although these data are collected routinely for research purposes. Additional CASA parameters will be included in the clinical report when justified by our research findings or by published reports of other investigators.

Sperm Morphology

The criteria that we use for sperm morphology assessment are the original criteria of the WHO,[5] and 50% or greater normal sperm is the cutoff point for normal semen quality. There are two specific situations in which a knowledge of the types of abnormal sperm also may be useful in clinical assessment or therapy of subfertile males. One of these situations is the association of tapered sperm with varicocele, and the second is the finding of sperm with tail abnormalities in cases of epididymal dysfunction. Tapered sperm, together with amorphous sperm and immature sperm cells, were originally reported as characteristic of a stress pattern observed in the semen of men with varicoceles,[78] but other investigators subsequently were unable to confirm this association.[79–82] We used a retrospective case-control study design and metric standards for tapered sperm cells to evaluate sperm morphology in men with varicocele.[83] Cases and controls were matched for the percentage of motile sperm and the total number of sperm per ejaculate. Varicocele patients had significantly more tapered sperm, as defined by metric standards, than did patients with idiopathic infertility (36% versus 15%).[83] On the basis of these data, we recommend varicocelectomy for men with palpable varicoceles when there are more than 25% tapered sperm in the semen, even if the semen quality overall is borderline or within the normal range. Epididymal dysfunction may be associated with abnormalities of the sperm tail. Although there is no visible change in the morphology of the human sperm flagellum during epididymal passage, the flagellar axoneme is stabilized

TABLE 38–4. Classification of Semen Quality

Semen Parameter	Normal Semen Quality	Marginal Semen Quality	Abnormal Semen Quality
Semen volume (mL)	2–5*	1–2	<1
Sperm concentration (× 10⁶/mL)	20–250*	10–20	<10
Sperm motility (% motile)	>50	40–50	<40
Straight-line velocity (μM/s)	>25	20–25	<20
Sperm morphology (% normal)	>50	40–50	<40

*Values that exceed the upper range of normal may result in classification of the semen as marginal or abnormal.

during transport through the epididymis by formation of disulfide bonds.[84] Abnormalities of fluid and electrolyte transport in the epididymis may lead to hypo-osmotic conditions that result in coiling of the sperm tail with subsequent fixation of the tail in the coiled position by disulfide bonding. We have observed large numbers of sperm with coiled tails in the semen of men following vasovasostomy for vasectomy reversal, and these findings may be indicative of epididymal dysfunction secondary to prolonged vasal occlusion.[85]

Clinical Interpretation of Semen Parameters

As evaluated by contemporary laboratory methods, abnormal semen is a general and relatively nonspecific clinical sign of disordered spermatogenesis. It has been well established that parameters of sperm motility and morphology are correlated with one another and with parameters of sperm production.[8, 9, 22, 86–89] These close correlations may explain the reason that integrated parameters of semen quality that can be obtained by multiplication of individual parameters (e.g., total motile sperm per ejaculate) have not been shown to be better predictors of male fertility than single parameters alone.[66] On the other hand, measurements of multiple parameters on a per-sperm basis may have greater diagnostic value. Experimental studies have been carried out in which sperm motility and morphology were assessed simultaneously for individual cells.[35, 52, 90] Sperm with defective heads were more likely to be immotile than sperm without visible defects, and defective sperm, when motile, swam more slowly than sperm with normal head morphology.[35, 52] A similar relationship between abnormal sperm motility and morphology was observed in semen from fertile men and subfertile men.[35, 52] However, when only sperm with normal morphology were considered, the motility of such sperm was less vigorous in the semen of subfertile men than in the semen of fertile men.[35, 52] These data suggest that measurements of functional characteristics of sperm subpopulations (e.g., movement characteristics of morphologically normal sperm) may have clinical value in detecting male infertility. Unfortunately, such approaches cannot be applied routinely unless they are included in automated CASA instruments.

In current practice, the semen parameters are considered individually and are used to assign patients to clinical categories. In our institution, the following categories are used: (1) semen quality within normal limits, no evidence for infertility; (2) marginal semen quality, infertility is possible; and (3) abnormal semen quality, infertility is likely (see Table 38–4). Because of the multiplicity of semen parameters and normal variability in semen quality, it is not always possible to objectively assign a given patient to a clinical category. In general, when one or more semen parameters consistently falls within an abnormal or marginal range of values (e.g., marginal sperm concentration), the patient is assigned to the corresponding clinical category. Depending on individual variability, a number of semen evaluations may be required to classify a patient. When there is inconsistency in repeated evaluations, the patient is assigned to the clinical category that reflects the poorest semen parameters recorded. A urologic evaluation is recommended for all patients with marginal or abnormal semen quality. We recommend that the female partners of men with marginal semen quality be completely evaluated, including laparoscopy, before it is concluded that a male factor is contributing significantly to infertility. Even the patients with abnormal semen quality overall may have one or more semen parameters that are within the normal range. In our laboratory semen samples are frequently evaluated in which sperm morphology is the only parameter that is outside the normal range. Isolated abnormalities of sperm numbers and motility are more unusual. For the reasons previously discussed, men with low sperm concentrations but otherwise normal semen have a good prognosis for future fertility. Abnormalities of sperm motility may be a result of artifact induced by semen collection, transportation, or handling in the laboratory. The suspicion of artifact may be reinforced by information in the patient's questionnaire or in laboratory worksheets, but such findings always require confirmation by repeated evaluations.

Assessments of semen quality that are based on objective, quantitative data should be accurate in detecting infertility. However, in the absence of clinical studies that correlate such data with fertility endpoints, detection of male infertility by semen evaluation alone will remain problematic. Sperm function tests, such as tests of sperm–cervical mucus interaction, sperm penetration assays with zona-free hamster oocytes, and the hemizona assay,[9, 92] provide additional information on male fertility, but these tests have many of the same problems as the semen evaluation, for example, insufficient standardization and lack of rigorous assessment in fertility studies. As increasing emphasis is placed on standardization and quality control of all andrology tests, the information that is required for clinical interpretation of the semen evaluation as well as ancillary tests will also be forthcoming.

REFERENCES

1. Eliasson R, Lindholmer C. Distribution and properties of spermatozoa in different fractions of split ejaculates. Fertil Steril 1972;23:252.
2. Keel BA. The semen analysis. In: Keel BA, Webster BW, editors. CRC Handbook of the Laboratory Diagnosis and Treatment of Infertility. Boca Raton: CRC Press, 1990:27–69.
3. Mortimer D. The male factor in infertility: semen analysis. Curr Probl Obstet Gynecol 1985;8:4–87.
4. World Health Organization. WHO Laboratory Manual for the Examination of Human Semen and Sperm–Cervical Mucus Interaction. 3rd edition. Cambridge, England: Press Syndicate of the University of Cambridge, 1992.
5. World Health Organization. WHO Manual for the Examination of Human Semen and Semen–Cervical Mucus Interaction. 2nd edition. Cambridge, England: Press Syndicate of the University of Cambridge, 1987.
6. Zanaveld LJD, Jeyendran RS. Modern assessment of semen for diagnostic purposes. Semin Reprod Endocrinol 1988;6:324–337.
7. Overstreet JW. Assessment of disorders of spermatogenesis. In: Lockey JE, editor. Reproduction: The New Frontier in Occupational and Environmental Health Research. New York: Alan Liss, 1984:275–292.
8. Freund M. Interrelationships among the characteristics of human semen and factors affecting semen specimen quality. J Reprod Fertil 1962; 4:143–159.
9. Sherins RJ, Brightwell D, Sternthal PM. Longitudinal analysis of semen of fertile and infertile men. In: Troen P, Nankin HR, editors. The Testis in Normal and Infertile Men. New York: Raven Press, 1977:473.
10. Levine RJ, Mathew RM, Chenault CB, et al. Differences in the quality of semen in outdoor workers during summer and winter. N Engl J Med 1990;323:12–16.
11. MacLeod J. The significance of deviation in human sperm morphology in the human testis. Adv Exp Med Biol 1970;10:481.
12. Schrader SM. Occupational and environmental factors and male infertility. Infertil Reprod Med Clin North Am 1992;3:319–328.

13. Heller GC, Clermont Y. Kinetics of the germinal epithelium in man. Recent Prog Horm Res 1964;20:545.

14. Freund M. Effect of frequency of emission on semen output and an estimate of daily sperm production in man. J Reprod Fertil 1963;6:269–286.

15. Swartz D, Laplanche A, Jouannet P, David G. Within-subject variabilities of human semen in regard to sperm count, volume, total number of spermatozoa and length of abstinence. J Reprod Fertil 1979;57:391–395.

16. Amann RP. A critical review of methods for evaluation of spermatogenesis from seminal characteristics. J Androl 1981;2:37–60.

17. Freund M, Peterson RN. Semen evaluation and fertility. In: Hafez ESE, editor. Human semen and fertility regulation in men. St. Louis: CV Mosby, 1976:344–354.

18. Zavos PM. Seminal parameters of ejaculates collected from oligospermic and normospermic patients via masturbation and at intercourse with the use of a Silastic seminal fluid collection device. Fertil Steril 1985;44:517–520.

19. Singer R, Sagiv M, Barnet M, et al. Some characteristics of split human semen of various sperm densities. Andrologia 1982;14:260.

20. Thomas AJ Jr. Ejaculatory dysfunction. Fertil Steril 1983;39:445–454.

21. Overstreet JW. Semen liquefaction and viscosity problems. In: Tanagho EA, Lue TF, McClure RD, editors. Contemporary Management of Impotence and Infertility. Baltimore: Williams & Wilkins, 1988:311–312.

22. Eliasson R. Analysis of semen. In: Behrman SJ, Kistner RW, editors. Progress in Infertility. 2nd edition. Boston: Little, Brown, 1975:691–713.

23. Overstreet JW. Evaluation of sperm–cervical mucus interaction. Fertil Steril 1986;45:324–326.

24. Lipshultz LI, Howards SS. Evaluation of the subfertile man. In: Lipshultz LI, Howards SS, editors. Infertility in the Male. New York: Churchill Livingstone, 1983:187–206.

25. Glezerman MG, Bartoov B. Semen analysis. In: Insler V, Lunenfeld B, editors. Infertility. New York: Churchill Livingstone, 1986:243–271.

26. Makler A. The improved ten-micrometer chamber for rapid sperm count and motility evaluation. Fertil Steril 1980;33:337–338.

27. Davis RO, Katz DF. Operational standards for CASA instruments. J Androl 1993;14:385–394.

28. Overstreet JW, Katz DF, Hanson FW, et al. A simple, inexpensive method for objective assessment of human sperm movement characteristics. Fertil Steril 1979;31:162–172.

29. Makler A. A new multiple-exposure photography method for objective human spermatozoal motility determination. Fertil Steril 1978;30:192–199.

30. Katz DF, Overstreet JW, Samuels SJ, et al. Morphometric analysis of spermatozoa in the assessment of human male fertility. J Androl 1986;7:203–210.

31. Dunphy BC, Kay R, Barratt CLR, et al. Quality control during the conventional analysis of semen, an essential exercise. J Androl 1989;10:378–385.

32. Jequier AM, Ukome EB. Errors inherent in the performance of a routine semen analysis. Br J Urol 1983;55:434–436.

33. Davis RO, Boyers SP. The role of digital-image analysis in reproductive biology. Arch Pathol Lab Med 1992;116:351–363.

34. Franken DR, Oehninger S, Burkman LJ, et al. The hemizona assay (HZA): a predictor of human sperm-fertilizing potential in in vitro fertilization (IVF) treatment. J In Vitro Fertil Embryo Transfer 1989;6:44–50.

35. Morales P, Katz DF, Overstreet JW, et al. The relationship between the motility and morphology of spermatozoa in semen. J Androl 1988;9:241–247.

36. Morales P, Overstreet JW, Katz DF. Changes in human sperm motion during capacitation in vitro. J Reprod Fertil 1988;83:119–128.

37. Eliasson R. Standards for investigation of human semen. Andrologie 1971;3:49–64.

38. Freund M. Standards for the rating of human sperm morphology: a cooperative study. Int J Fertil 1966;11:97–118.

39. Kruger TF, Acosta AA, Simmons KF, et al. New method of evaluating sperm morphology with predictive value for human in vitro fertilization. Urology 1987;30:248–251.

40. Kruger TF, Acosta AA, Simmons KF, et al. Predictive value of abnormal sperm morphology in in vitro fertilization. Fertil Steril 1988;49:112–117.

41. Kruger TF, Menkveld R, Standler FSH, et al. Sperm morphologic features as a prognostic factor in in vitro fertilization. Fertil Steril 1986;46:1118–1123.

42. Menkveld R, Stander FSH, Kotze TJ, et al. The evaluation of morphological characteristics of human spermatozoa according to stricter criteria. Hum Reprod 1990;5:586–592.

43. Baker HWG, Clarke GN. Sperm morphology: consistency of assessment of the same sperm by different observers. Clin Reprod Fertil 1987;5:37–43.

44. Neuwinger J, Behre HM, Nieschlag E. Computerized semen analysis with sperm tail detection. Hum Reprod 1990;5:719–723.

45. Zaini A, Jennings MG, Baker HWG. Are conventional sperm morphology and motility assessments of predictive value in subfertile men? Int J Androl 1985;8:427–435.

46. Katz DF, Diel L, Overstreet JW. Differences in the movement of morphologically normal and abnormal human seminal spermatozoa. Biol Reprod 1982;26:566–570.

47. Jouannet P, Ducot B, Feneux D, et al. Male factors and the likelihood of pregnancy in infertile couples: I. Study of sperm characteristics. Int J Androl 1988;11:379–394.

48. Davis RO, Gravance CG. Consistency of sperm morphology classification criteria. J Androl 1993;15:88–91.

49. Katz DF, Overstreet JW. Sperm motility assessment by videomicrography. Fertil Steril 1981;35:188–193.

50. Davis RO, Gravance CG. Standardization of specimen preparation, staining, and sampling methods improves automated sperm-head morphometry analysis. Fertil Steril 1993;59:412–417.

51. Moruzzi JF, Wyrobek AJ, Mayall BH, Gledhill BL. Quantification and classification of human sperm morphology by computer-assisted image analysis. Fertil Steril 1988;50:142–152.

52. Overstreet JW, Price MJ, Blazak WF, et al. Simultaneous assessment of human sperm motility and morphology by videomicrography. J Urol 1981;126:357–360.

53. Davis RO, Bain DE, Siemers RJ, et al. Accuracy and precision of the CellForm-Human automated sperm morphometry instrument. Fertil Steril 1992;58:763–769.

54. Kruger TF, DuToit TC, Franken DR, et al. A new computerized method of reading sperm morphology (strict criteria) is as efficient as technician reading. Fertil Steril 1993;59:202–209.

55. Turner TW, Schrader SM. Sperm morphometry as measured by three different computer systems. J Androl 1988;9:45.

56. MacLeod J. Human male infertility. Obstet Gynecol Surv 1971;26:335.

57. Wolff H, Anderson DJ. Immunohistologic characterization and quantitation of leukocyte subpopulations in human semen. Fertil Steril 1988;49:497–504.

58. American Fertility Society. Guidelines for human embryology and andrology laboratories. Fertil Steril 1992;58:Suppl 1:1–16.

59. Muller CH. The andrology laboratory in assisted reproductive technologies program: quality assurance and laboratory methodology. J Androl 1992;13:349–360.

60. Macomber D, Sanders MR. The spermatozoa count. N Engl J Med 1929;200:981–984.

61. MacLeod J, Gold RZ. Semen quality in 1000 men of known fertility and 800 cases of infertile marriage. Fertil Steril 1951;2:115–139.

62. Rehan NE, Sobrero AJ, Fertig JW. The semen of fertile men: statistical analysis of 1300 men. Fertil Steril 1975;26:492–502.

63. Zuckerman Z, Rodriguez-Rigau LJ, Smith KD, Steinberger E. Frequency distribution of sperm counts in fertile and infertile males. Fertil Steril 1977;28:1310–1313.

64. Polansky FF, Lamb EJ. Do the results of semen analysis predict future fertility? A survival analysis study. Fertil Steril 1988;49:1059–1065.

65. Dunphy BC, Neal LM, Cooke ID. The clinical value of conventional semen analysis. Fertil Steril 1989;51:324–329.

66. Peng H-Q, Collins JA, Wilson EH, Wrixton W. Receiver-operating characteristics curves for semen analysis variables: methods for evaluating diagnostic tests of male gamete function. Gamete Res 1987;17:229–236.

67. Bostofte E, Bagger P, Michael A, et al. Fertility prognosis for infertile men: results of follow-up study of semen analysis in infertile men from two different populations evaluated by the Cox regression model. Fertil Steril 1990;54:1100–1106.

68. MacLeod J, Wang Y. Male fertility potential in terms of semen quality: a review of the past, a study of the present. Fertil Steril 1979;21:103–116.

69. Glezerman M, Bernstein D, Zakut CH, et al. Polyzoospermia—a definite pathological entity. Fertil Steril 1982;38:605–608.

70. Barfield A, Melo J, Coutinho E, et al. Pregnancies associated with sperm concentrations below 10 million/mL in clinical studies of a potential male contraceptive method, monthly depot medroxyprogesterone acetate and testosterone esters. Contraception 1979;20:121.

71. Burris AS, Clark RV, Vantman DJ, et al. A low sperm concentration does not preclude fertility in men with isolated hypogonadotropic hypogonadism after gonadotropin therapy. Fertil Steril 1988;50:343–347.

72. Dubin L, Amelar RD. Etiologic factors in 1294 consecutive cases of male infertility. Fertil Steril 1971;22:169.

73. Fox CA, Meldrum SJ, Watson BW. Continuous measurement by radiotelemetry of vaginal pH during human coitus. J Reprod Fertil 1973;33:69–75.

74. Mathur S, Carlton M, Ziegler J, et al. A computerized sperm motion analysis. Fertil Steril 1988;46:484–488.

75. Vantman D, Banks SM, Koukoulis G, et al. Assessment of sperm motion characteristics from fertile and infertile men using a fully automated computer-assisted semen analyzer. Fertil Steril 1989;51:156–161.

76. Vantman D, Koukoulis G, Burris AS, et al. Sperm motion characteristics in men with isolated hypogonadotropic hypogonadism treated with gonadotropin. Fertil Steril 1989;51:162–166.

77. Davis RO. The promise and pitfalls of computer-aided sperm analysis. Infertil Reprod Med Clin North Am 1992;3:341–352.

78. MacLeod J. Seminal cytology in the presence of varicocele. Fertil Steril 1965;16:735.

79. Ayodeji O, Baker HWG. Is there a specific abnormality of sperm morphology in men with varicoceles? Fertil Steril 1986;45:839–842.

80. Farris BL, Fenner DK, Plymate SR, et al. Seminal characteristics in the presence of a varicocele as compared with those of expectant fathers and prevasectomy men. Fertil Steril 1981;35:325–327.

81. Portuondo JA, Calabozo M, Echanojauregui AD. Morphology of spermatozoa in infertile men with and without varicocele. J Androl 1983;4:312–315.

82. Rodriguez-Rigau LJ, Smith KD, Steinberger E. Varicocele and the morphology of spermatozoa. Fertil Steril 1981;35:54–57.

83. Naftulin BN, Samuels SJ, Hellstrom WJG, et al. Semen quality in varicocele patients is characterized by tapered sperm cells. Fertil Steril 1991;56:149–151.

84. Bedford JM, Calvin H, Cooper GW. The maturation of spermatozoa in the human epididymis. J Reprod Fertil 1973; Suppl 18:199–213.

85. Pelfrey RJ, Overstreet JW, Lewis EL. Abnormalities of sperm morphology in cases of persistent infertility after vasectomy reversal. Fertil Steril 1982;28:112–114.

86. MacLeod J, Gold RZ. The male factor in fertility and infertility: III. An analysis of motile activity in the spermatozoa of 1000 fertile men and 1000 men in infertile marriage. Fertil Steril 1951;2:187–204.

87. MacLeod J, Gold RZ. The male factor in fertility and infertility: IV. Sperm morphology in fertile and infertile marriage. Fertil Steril 1951;2:394–414.

88. Mortimer D, Templeton AA, Lenton EA, et al. Semen analysis parameters and their interrelationships in suspected infertile men. Arch Androl 1982;8:165.

89. Singer R, Sagiv M, Segenreich E, et al. Motility, vitality and percentages of morphologically abnormal forms of human spermatozoa in relation to sperm counts. Andrologia 1980;12:92.

90. Makler A. Distribution of normal and abnormal forms among motile, non-motile, live and dead human spermatozoa. Int J Androl 1980;3:620.

91. Critser JK, Noiles EE. Bioassays of sperm function. Semin Reprod Endocrinol 1993;11:1–16.

92. Zanaveld LJD, Jeyendran RS. Sperm function tests. Infertil Reprod Med Clin North Am 1992;3:353–371.

CHAPTER 39

Tests of Sperm Function

RONALD L. URRY

OVERVIEW AND HISTORY

Traditionally, fertility tests until relatively recently have centered on the female because the responsibility for fertility and the "blame" for infertility were borne primarily by the female.[1] Theories on reproduction by notables such as Aristotle and William Harvey, despite their numerous scientific accomplishments, hypothesized primarily a female contribution to conception. Aristotle believed that the female always supplied the matter for creation, whereas the male provided the power of creation.[2] Harvey, the father of physiology, believed that coitus excited within the uterus a substance equivalent to a desire or imagination in the female brain that led to conception and did not require a significant contribution from the male.[1]

The role of sperm in conception became more clear with the brilliant observations by Van Leeuwenhoek, who, having taken an interest in the microscope, used it in 1696 to first describe what he called *animalcules* (sperm) from a dog ejaculate and described the attrition of the animalcules over a multinight period.[3] Eventually, a group known as the "Spermatists" led by Dr. Dalen Patious claimed that the individual is contained completely within the sperm and therefore the female serves merely as an incubator for human development (Fig. 39–1). A scientist who first applied the art of experimentation to the area of reproduction was Abbe Spallanzani, who obtained frog semen from which he separated the cells from the fluid with filter paper.[3] He then demonstrated that the fluid portion, when added to frog's eggs, did not result in fertilization. When he took the sperm portion and added it to eggs, fertilization and embryo development resulted. Unfortunately, he did not pay attention to the data and went along with previous theories to conclude that the fluid portion activated a live force within the egg and caused embryo development.

It took until the nineteenth century before the role of sperm became better defined with respect to conception. Prevost and Dumas reported that the absence of sperm was the single unifying factor that prevented breeding in elderly animals, mules, and birds outside the mating season.[1] These investigators concluded that the animalcules are important and that there exists a vital relationship between their presence in the reproductive organs and the fertilizing power of the animal. They also believed that sperm penetrates the ovum. Others such as Bischoff and Koliker believed that sperm just need to be in the general vicinity of the ovum for fertilization.[1]

Oskar Hertwig and Hermann Fol in 1876 supported the findings of Prevost and Dumas and further demonstrated that it is the union of the egg nucleus with the sperm nucleus that is necessary to produce a nucleus endowed with living forces.[1] The first test of sperm function, in the form of a semen analysis, was completed by Alois Lode.[4] He studied the treatise of Prevost and Dumas wherein the critical role of spermatozoa and fertility was established, and he then proceeded to measure sperm counts in nine men, on multiple occasions, over an extended period. No further counts were reported for the next 20 years. From these early beginnings and the observations and descriptions of sperm by the earlier-mentioned people, as well as numerous other investigators, extensive efforts have been undertaken to determine how best to evaluate the fertilization potential of sperm.

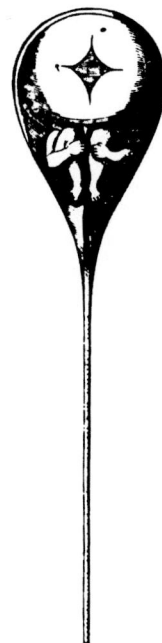

FIGURE 39–1. Spermatist's concept of the containment of the entire fetus within a sperm cell.

Methods to evaluate the biochemical characteristics of seminal fluid, determination of sperm concentration, motility, viability, sperm membrane function, sperm morphology, sperm penetration capacity, and zona-binding characteristics, in addition to mucus penetration capacity, and a range of metabolic and biochemical assays, all have been described for the last 90 years in an effort to better elucidate the fertility potential of sperm (Table 39–1). Although a great deal of controversy still exists as to which test gives the greatest relationship to fertility potential, several common threads connect the vast amount of published information on sperm function. This chapter outlines the various tests that have been used to attempt to describe sperm function and information about a given male's fertility potential. The discussion includes the methodology, efficiency, advantages, and disadvantages of each test. Essentially, the laboratory needs to provide information to the clinician regarding the likelihood of the sperm and the egg being able to get together at the site of fertilization and, further, the ability of the sperm to bind to and penetrate the egg on reaching it.

SEMEN ANALYSIS

A series of carefully conducted semen analyses produces information with respect to the ability of sperm to reach the site of fertilization. The semen analysis is discussed elsewhere and is not reviewed in this chapter.

Sperm Membrane Function

Sperm membrane structure and function can be determined by evaluating sperm viability and obtaining a hypo-osmolarity (HOS) score. Viable sperm with an intact membrane do not allow eosin to pass into the sperm head and

TABLE 39–1. Tests to Determine Sperm Function

Semen analysis
  Semen volume
  Semen viscosity
  Semen pH
  Sperm motility
  Sperm viability
  Sperm agglutination
  Sperm morphology
Sperm hypo-osmolarity
Sperm longevity test
Hemizona assay
Sperm penetration assay/in vitro fertilization
Acrosome reaction test
Semen/sperm biochemistry
  Acrosin
  ATP
  Creatine phosphokinase
  DNA
  O$_2$ uptake
  Protein-carboxyl methylase
  Hyalinuronidase activity
  α-Glucosidase
  Transferrin
Mucus-sperm testing
Antisperm antibody tests

ATP, adenosine triphosphate; DNA, deoxyribonucleic acid.

therefore the sperm appear white against a dark background. Sperm that have a structural membrane defect allow eosin to leak into the sperm, and these appear pink. Therefore, membrane structural integrity can be measured by the viability test. The HOS test measures physiologic function of the sperm membrane. These tests are described in the following section.

SPERM VIABILITY

The viability of sperm can be determined using relatively simple techniques.[5, 6] Sperm viability measurement is important because it allows the differentiation of necrospermic samples from samples with no sperm motility but where the sperm are live. More important, careful viability determination can serve as a cross-check on sperm motility with the number of dead-staining sperm often correlating with the number of nonmotile sperm. In addition, as mentioned earlier, the structural integrity of the sperm membrane can be determined because live sperm may allow leakage of the stain, thus staining dead, because of abnormal sperm membranes that indicate an underlying sperm defect. The defect may be caused by a variety of problems, including the attachment to the sperm of antisperm antibodies. Sperm viability is determined as follows[5–7]:

1. A 5% aqueous eosin solution is prepared by adding distilled water to 5 g of eosin Y and bringing to a total volume of 100 mL. This is stored at room temperature.

2. A 10% aqueous nigrosin solution is prepared by adding distilled water to 10 g of nigrosin to a total volume of 100 mL. This is stored at room temperature.

3. One drop of well-mixed seminal fluid (within 1 hour of collection) is placed on a warm (37°C) microscope slide.

4. To the drop of seminal fluid, add two drops of the 5% eosin solution and gently mix.

5. Add three drops of 10% nigrosin solution to the mixture of seminal fluid and eosin and gently mix.

6. Make a thin smear from the mixture, and place the slide on a warm (to touch) hot plate (30° to 37°C) until the smear is dry.

7. Count 100 to 200 total sperm, and report the dead sperm (pink) and the live sperm (white).

Sperm viability correlates with fertility with respect to both the number of viable sperm potentially available to reach the site of fertilization and to sperm with abnormal membranes and therefore abnormal function. Particular attention should be paid to a reverse-stain ratio where more sperm stain dead than are nonmotile in the sample, thus indicating a sperm membrane problem.

HYPO-OSMOLARITY MEASUREMENT

Along with the structural membrane integrity information of the sperm viability test, the HOS test gives information about the functional integrity of the sperm membrane. We have used this test as a routine part of our semen analysis for the past 5 years. This test appears to give different information about sperm membrane function than that given by the viability test,[8] although other reports show a good correlation between the two.[9, 10] The viability test appears to give information about sperm membrane function with respect to the

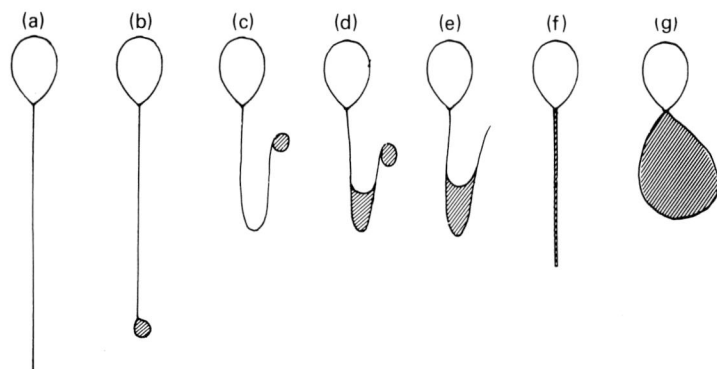

FIGURE 39–2. Diagrammatic representation of nonreacted (straight) and reacted (coiled) sperm tails using the hypo-osmolarity score assay. (From Jeyendran RS, VanderVen HH, Perez-Pelaez M, et al. Development of an assay to assess the functional integrity of the human sperm membrane and its relationship to other semen characteristics. J Reprod Fertil 1984;70:219–228.)

ability to transport fluids and probably other substances across the membrane. HOS values may be selectively altered by certain procedures. We have reported that cryopreservation, using different cryopreservation techniques, has different effects on viability and HOS, and these are selectively altered depending on the procedure used.[11] This also indicates that the tests give different information about sperm membrane function. The HOS test, like most other sperm tests, has given conflicting data with respect to its correlation with other tests of sperm function or fertility. Previous reports have suggested a strong correlation between the results of the HOS test and sperm concentration, motility, viability, and morphology.[9, 10] Additional reports did not find a correlation with any or many of the earlier discussed tests of sperm function. A number of studies have compared the HOS result with sperm penetration capacity or with the ability to fertilize human eggs. A close correlation between sperm penetration and HOS results has been found in several papers, whereas minimal or no relationship has been reported by other studies. Along with other indices of sperm function, it may correlate to the outcome of fertilization with in vitro fertilization (IVF) procedures.[12, 13] Another report found a relationship between acrosin activity, HOS, and infertility.[14]

We have found the HOS test particularly useful to predict sperm membrane damage, and when used in conjunction with the sperm viability, sperm motility, and sperm agglutination results, it can predict the clinical presence and effects of antisperm antibodies in the male, as discussed in the section on antibody measurement. The HOS value also appears to be changed by an increase in free radicals, as seen with an increase in the number of semen white blood cells. These changes in HOS caused by free radicals can be blocked by superoxide dismutase.[15] The HOS test can be determined as follows[8]:

1. Reagents are prepared as follows:
   a. Fructose solution (2.7 g in 100 mL of distilled water).
   b. Sodium citrate solution (1.47 g in 100 mL of distilled water).
   c. Prepare the HOS solution by adding 50 mL of the fructose solution to 50 mL of the sodium citrate solution and mix.
   d. Pipette 1 mL of the HOS solution into 5-mL polyethylene or polypropylene test tubes; cap and store for later use. The tubes can be stored at room temperature for short periods, refrigerated or frozen.
2. Add 0.1 mL of well-mixed seminal fluid to one of the HOS tubes from No. 1 and mix.
3. Incubate the reaction tube for 30 to 120 minutes at 37°C.
4. Terminate the reaction with two drops of formaldehyde.
5. Place a drop of the well-mixed solution on a microscope slide and coverslip. Observe the sample under phase contrast ($\times 400$) for coiling of the sperm tail (HOS-reacted sperm). Count 100 to 200 sperm per slide, and report the percentage of sperm with coiled and noncoiled tails on the slide (Fig. 39–2).

The test has been further refined to count specific types of tail coiling, and it has been shown that certain categories correlate better with sperm motility and sperm penetration than other patterns of coiling.[10] Additional attempts to modify and simplify the assay have included development of a water assay. This technique involves the incubation of sperm for only 5 minutes in distilled water instead of the solutions described earlier for longer periods.[16] A normal value for HOS is more than 55% to 60% reacted sperm per semen sample and an abnormal value is less than 50% reacted sperm. Samples with less than 40% reacted sperm particularly correlate with fertility problems.

Sperm Longevity Testing

The capacity of the motility of spermatozoa to survive incubation, under optimal conditions for an extended period, has been used for a variety of purposes. A bioassay measuring sperm longevity was used to evaluate the effects of several different plastics on sperm function.[17] This assay used sperm incubated over a 4-day period at room temperature under 5% carbon dioxide (CO_2) and compared final motility with initial motility after periods of incubation of the sperm in solutions with pieces of plastics and rubber. Another bioassay was described also evaluating one type of plastic syringe on sperm longevity that declined after exposure to the materials used in the syringe.[18]

More recently, sperm longevity was used to study male factor infertility as defined by defects in a semen analysis.[19] Also the study compared sperm longevity in sperm obtained through electrical ejaculation. Both male factor infertility and electrical-ejaculated sperm showed diminished sperm longevity compared with fertile controls. Another study reported a high correlation between sperm longevity over a 24-hour period and fertilization rates with IVF.[20] The correlation between the sperm longevity assay and fertilization was stronger than correlations between other traditional parameters of sperm function.

A recent review of our data evaluating sperm longevity found a correlation between longevity and both gamete intrafallopian transfer (GIFT) and IVF and pregnancy outcomes. The sperm longevity assay is accomplished as follows:

1. A sperm sample is obtained and allowed to liquefy at 37°C for 20 to 30 minutes. Sperm motility, viability, and HOS values are recorded.

2. The sperm sample is then mixed with the medium to be used in a ratio of two parts medium to one part semen. The sample is then centrifuged (washed) at 250g for 8 to 10 minutes.

3. The supernatant is discarded, and the pellet is resuspended in 0.5 to 2.5 mL of fluid. We currently use 8% pooled female preovulatory serum in the medium that provides a standard basis for the interpretation of test results. Higher volumes of medium are used for higher counts to prevent sperm association (clumping or agglutination) and provide adequate nutrients. Sperm motility is recorded after washing.

4. The sample is then placed in a 5% CO_2 incubator for 24 hours, the sample is mixed, and the sperm motility, viability, and HOS value recorded. The sample can be placed back into the incubator, and the earlier measurements can be obtained again at 48 hours, although we have found the 24-hour sample adequate for the test. Samples should not have a decline in progressive sperm motility of more than 30% to 40%. For example, if the progressive motility is 40% prior to the prolonged incubation, we like to see at least 25% to 30% progressive motility 24 hours after incubation.

5. Interpretation of the results needs to be correlated with data in a specific laboratory. In general, samples that have a substantial decline in progressive sperm motility within a 24-hour period are associated with a lower IVF rate and poorer fertility outcome.

Specimen Fertility Score

For many years researchers and clinicians involved with male fertility have searched for one number, from sperm function tests, that would have a reasonable correlation with male fertility potential. This factor has been elusive, and no one number, particularly from the type of information obtained with most sperm function tests, can give a perfect correlation with the prediction of fertility problems. The author has used a specimen fertility score for several years that has shown some correlation with the prediction of male fertility potential, as well as the outcome of IVF procedures (Table 39–2).[21] The score uses a scale that assigns points for progressive sperm motility, progressive motile sperm density, and sperm morphology. Points are added from the earlier

TABLE 39–2. Correlation of Semen Fertility Scores to Outcome of IVF Fertilization Rate and Pregnancy

Semen Fertility Score Range	IVF Fertilization Rate (%)	IVF Pregnancy Rate (%)
>25	>65	>30
<10	<20	<6*

*$P < 0.001$ compared to scores >25.
IVF, in vitro fertilization.

discussed categories, and then points are subtracted for sperm agglutination, semen viscosity problems, and the presence of white blood cells. The calculation is made as follows:

1. Points are given for the progressive sperm motility as follows:

Progressive Motility (%)	Points
>50	10
40–50	8
30–40	6
20–30	4
10–20	2
<10	0

2. Add to the above, points given for the progressive motile sperm concentration as follows:

Progressive Motile Sperm Density ($\times 10^6$)	Points
>60	10
60–80	8
40–60	6
20–40	4
10–20	2
<10	0

3. Add to the points above, points given for sperm morphology as follows:

Normal Heads (%)	Points
>70	10
60–70	8
50–60	6
40–50	4
20–40	2
<20	0

4. From the points obtained by adding Nos. 1, 2, and 3, subtract 1, 3, or 5 points, respectively, for the following:
   a. White blood cells (slight [1 point], moderate [2 points], severe [3 points]).
   b. Agglutination (slight, moderate, severe)
   c. Viscosity (slight, moderate, severe)
   d. HOS score (<60%, <50%, <40%)

5. The resulting number is the semen specimen fertility score.

Sperm Membrane Binding, Capacitation, and Penetration

HYPERACTIVATED SPERM MOTILITY

Hyperactivation of sperm is associated with a particular type of sperm motility and is probably related to capacitation.[22] Hyperactivation is defined as "an increased flagellar beat amplitude which is associated with a decrease in progressive sperm motility."[22] This type of motility in mammalian sperm is often circular in nature. The purpose of the motility is not completely understood, but it has been hypothesized to be useful to enable the sperm to cover a greater area of the oviduct lumen to enable the probability of the sperm contacting the egg, to facilitate migration through the oviduct, to provide the necessary force to prevent the sperm from attaching to the oviduct epithelium, to enhance penetration of the cumulus and zona pellucida, and to increase mixing of the surrounding fluid.[23] Observation of this type of motility is related to the ability of the sperm to capacitate.

Various types of sperm manipulation prior to use for advanced reproductive techniques must increase the ability of sperm to reach the egg but not enhance the premature initiation of the acrosome reaction, which might actually decrease the immediate ability of the sperm to reach the site of fertilization. Observation of hyperactivated motility may provide useful information on the relative capability of the sperm to reach and penetrate the egg.

HEMIZONA ASSAY

Since its description in 1988, the hemizona assay has been studied as an assay to determine the ability of sperm to bind to and penetrate an egg.[24, 25] Its potential usefulness remains uncertain pending more diverse study. In addition, because the assay uses human zona that are not available to most laboratories participating in the evaluation of sperm quality, it cannot be considered a serious assay for the determination of sperm function that can be adapted for widespread use.

The hemizona assay uses matched zona halves from a human egg to compare the binding of patient sperm to be tested with that of a comparable fertile control. The assay is accomplished as follows:

1. Immature human oocytes can be obtained from ovaries removed at autopsy, ovaries removed during surgery, or immature, unfertilized oocytes from patients undergoing IVF cycles.

2. The eggs are separated from the tissue and placed into a concentrated salt solution. The eggs are rinsed in culture medium and held with the aid of a micromanipulator. Under the microscope the micromanipulators are used to cut the zona into two equal halves. The matching hemizona are placed in the same drop of fluid.

3. Sperm are prepared from both proven fertile control groups and the patients to be tested. Sperm are prepared with the serum swimup technique, and approximately 250,000 control sperm are incubated with one of the matched hemizona. The remaining hemizona is incubated with patient sperm. The resulting sperm-zona mixture is incubated for approximately 4 hours.

4. The hemizona is thoroughly rinsed, and the number of sperm are counted that are bound to the zona. The hemizona assay index is calculated by dividing the number of test sperm bound to the hemizona by the number of control sperm bound to the hemizona and multiplying by 100.

Oocytes can be preserved by storage in concentrated salt solutions at 4°C. Recently, it was shown that eggs do better stored in liquid nitrogen and have better binding than eggs stored at 4°C.[26] It was also demonstrated that sperm binding to nonfertilized eggs from IVF cycles is better if the original IVF cycle has less than 50% fertilization. When fertilization was more than 50%, binding fell, and it appeared to be less accurate to use these eggs for binding studies. Binding to eggs not previously inseminated with sperm gave greater consistency in binding than previously inseminated but non-fertilized eggs.[26]

The hemizona assay has been reported to have a reasonable correlation to IVF outcome. In 95% of the IVF patients with fertilization failure, the hemizona index was less than 62%.[27] Recent studies have questioned the ability of the assay to discriminate which patients will fertilize with IVF. This study found substantial overlap between fertilization rates and the hemizona index.[28]

Other studies have demonstrated that the test can be altered by a variety of factors, including incubation of the zona with monoclonal antihuman sperm antibodies, which decreases the ability of sperm to bind to the zona.[29] Frozen-thawed sperm had lower binding ability than fresh sperm by approximately 30%. Overnight refrigeration of the sperm in egg yolk medium increased binding of the sperm and the hemizona index.[30] Other studies have reported that sperm morphology alterations decrease sperm binding to the intact zona and that the zona appears to be specific to binding morphologic normal sperm.[31]

The biggest drawback of the assay, as mentioned previously, is the lack of general availability of zona for use with the hemizona assay. In addition, more research is necessary to determine the exact role of the assay, if any, in the general testing of sperm function.

HAMSTER EGG–HUMAN SPERM PENETRATION ASSAY

There is no assay used to evaluate sperm function that has been studied more extensively or that remains more controversial than the sperm penetration assay (SPA). Although this assay has been given several names over the 17 years it has been used, most current studies use *SPA* when referring to the test. Differences in techniques used to complete the assay, the experience of the clinician completing the test, the use of frozen or fresh sperm, and the use of fresh or frozen hamster eggs all are areas that may cause increased variability and discrepancies when comparing results from one laboratory to another. Because the test has been studied and reviewed extensively, this chapter examines at length the techniques used to complete the assay, when it may be helpful, techniques that can be used to treat low penetration values, and the relationship of the SPA to the prediction of fertility, as well as prediction of the outcome of advanced reproductive techniques.

Generally, the sperm of one species cannot fertilize the eggs of another species. The specificity to fertilize appears to reside in the zona pellucida, although even after removal of the zona species specificity still persists in most species. Zona-free hamster ova, unlike those of most species, can be penetrated by the sperm of other species, including human sperm. This finding allowed development of an assay to test the penetration of human sperm.

Properties of sperm function measured by the evaluation of penetration capacity include sperm capacitation, acrosomal reaction, ability for membrane fusion, incorporation into the ooplasm, and the decondensation of the sperm chromatin. The ability of the sperm to penetrate does not measure the ability of sperm to fertilize exactly, and therefore penetration values are given, not fertilization values.

Techniques for Standard Sperm Penetration Assay. The techniques used to complete the hamster test are variable, but the original, standard technique is completed as follows (Fig. 39–3)[32]:

1. Hamster ova are obtained by injecting 7- to 12-week-old golden Syrian hamsters, on day 1 of estrus as determined by the presence of a vaginal viscous discharge, with 30 to

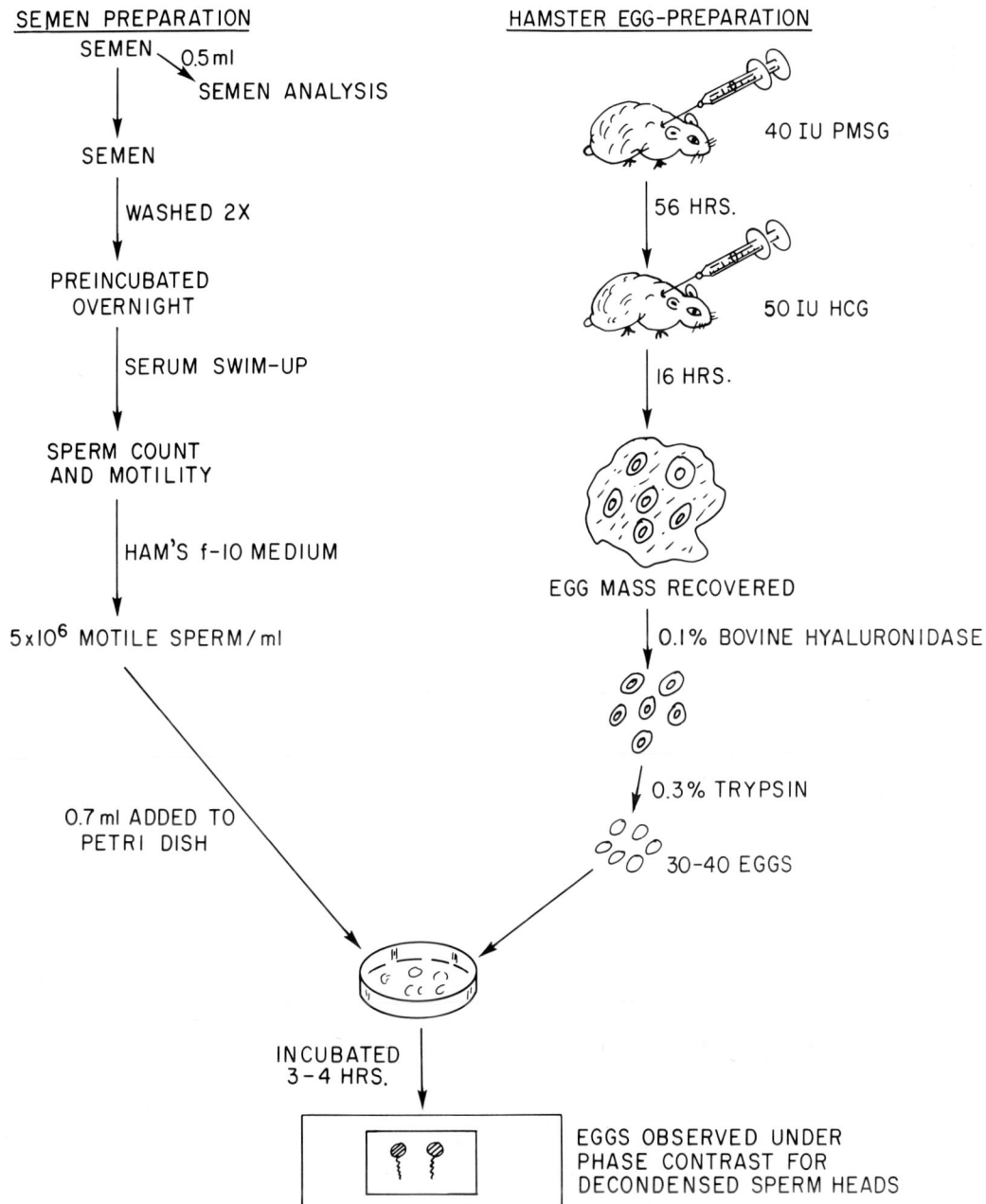

FIGURE 39–3. Procedure for the standard hamster egg–human sperm test to determine human sperm penetration capacity. PMSG, pregnant mare serum gonadotropin; HCG, human chorionic gonadotropin.

40 IU intraperitoneally (ip) of pregnant mare serum gonadotropin (PMSG). The animals are then injected with human chorionic gonadotropin (hCG, 30 to 40 IU, ip) 48 to 70 hours after the PMSG. The animals are then killed 16 to 18 hours later using saturated CO_2. Ova are obtained and processed as follows:

a. The oviducts are removed, and the cumulus mass containing the ova is identified in the swollen portion of each tube. The cumulus mass is removed and rinsed in Ham's F-10 medium or Biggers, Whitten, Whittingham (Bww) medium.

b. The ova are separated from the cumulus mass with 0.1% hyaluronidase and rinsed in medium.

c. The zona are removed with 0.1% trypsin and the ova are rinsed two to three times in medium.

d. A minimum of 25 to 40 eggs are added to sperm for each patient to be tested. Typically, 20 to 50 eggs can be obtained from each hamster stimulated as described earlier.

2. Sperm are processed by washing in protein-supplemented medium (8% pooled female preovulatory serum) at 250g for 10 minutes. The sperm were then resuspended and incubated in a humidified, 37°C, 5% CO_2 incubator overnight. The sperm are adjusted to a concentration of 5×10^6 progressively motile sperm per milliliter. Approximately 0.7 mL of the sperm suspension was placed in the center well of a 50 × 60-mm center well Petri dish (Falcon Plastics, Oxnard, California) to which 25 to 40 zona-free hamster eggs are added. Incubation times for the sperm can vary from only a few hours to 24 or more

hours. Studies have demonstrated more consistent results with longer (>20-hour) incubation times.[33]

3. Eggs and sperm are coincubated for 3 to 5 hours, after which time the eggs are removed, washed, and gently compressed under a coverslip packed on the edges with paraffin/petroleum jelly to determine if the eggs contain decondensed sperm heads (swollen heads associated with a sperm tail; Fig. 39–4). Observations are made with the aid of a phase-contrast microscope at 400× magnification. The percentage of ova penetrated is then reported. Additional observations, such as the mean number of spermatozoa per ovum and the relative number of sperm bound per egg, can also be reported. Appropriate controls are run with each assay.

Factors Affecting the Assay. Numerous factors can potentially alter the SPA and therefore contribute to increased variability or can at least alter the outcome of the results. The following factors have been reported to influence the outcome of the standard hamster assay: coital abstinence (>12 hours gives more consistent results),[34] length of time sperm are in contact with seminal fluid (increased time inhibits fertilization),[35] type of sperm preparation (sperm wash, serum swimup, Percoll gradient preparations give different penetration rates),[36] medium additions (increased penetration with human follicular fluid, test-yolk buffer, calcium ionophore, ions, energy sources), and pH.[37]

Modifications of the Standard Assay

"Challenge" Sperm Penetration Assay. One problem with the SPA has been the lack of ability to do anything about low penetration rates, other than to counsel the couple that this

may be one more factor in their fertility difficulty. Our laboratory began an intensive study in 1987 to evaluate the effectiveness of treatments designed to improve penetration capacity. These studies led to the development of a modified "challenge" SPA that allows us to determine the extent the penetration capacity can be improved with treatment. Early studies indicated that the largest improvements in the penetration capacity of sperm were achieved through refrigeration (plus test-yolk buffer incubation) of the sperm as well as heparin treatment and treatment of the sperm with calcium ionophore (Fig. 39–5). The use of refrigeration and calcium ionophore, the two most effective treatments, to treat sperm prior to testing resulted in the development of a modified SPA completed as follows[38]:

1. Ova are obtained and prepared as described earlier.

2. Fresh sperm to be tested are prepared by dividing the sample into two aliquots. One portion is mixed 1:1 with test-yolk buffer in a 15-mL conical sterile centrifuge tube that is placed in a beaker containing room temperature water, and then this is incubated a 4°C for 24 hours. At the end of the incubation period the mixture is warmed to 37°C, washed twice, adjusted to a 5×10^6 motile sperm per milliliter and incubated for 2 hours prior to use.

3. The remaining portion of the semen sample is washed twice and incubated at 37°C as described earlier. The sperm sample is adjusted to a concentration of 5×10^6 progressively motile sperm per milliliter. Approximately 0.7 mL of the sperm suspensions was added separately to the center well of a 50×60-mm Petri dish with 25 to 40 eggs as described earlier.

4. The percentage of eggs penetrated prepared with regu-

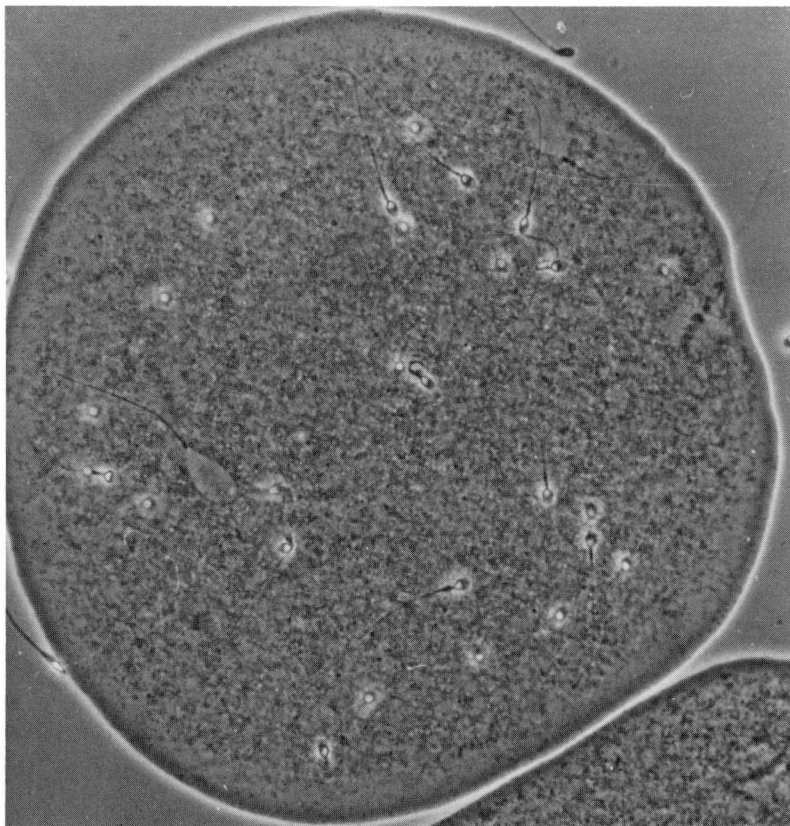

FIGURE 39–4. Zona-free hamster ova with two penetrated (swollen) sperm, each containing a tail. The smaller sperm are on the outside of the egg.

SEMEN PREPARATION

HAMSTER EGG–PREPARATION

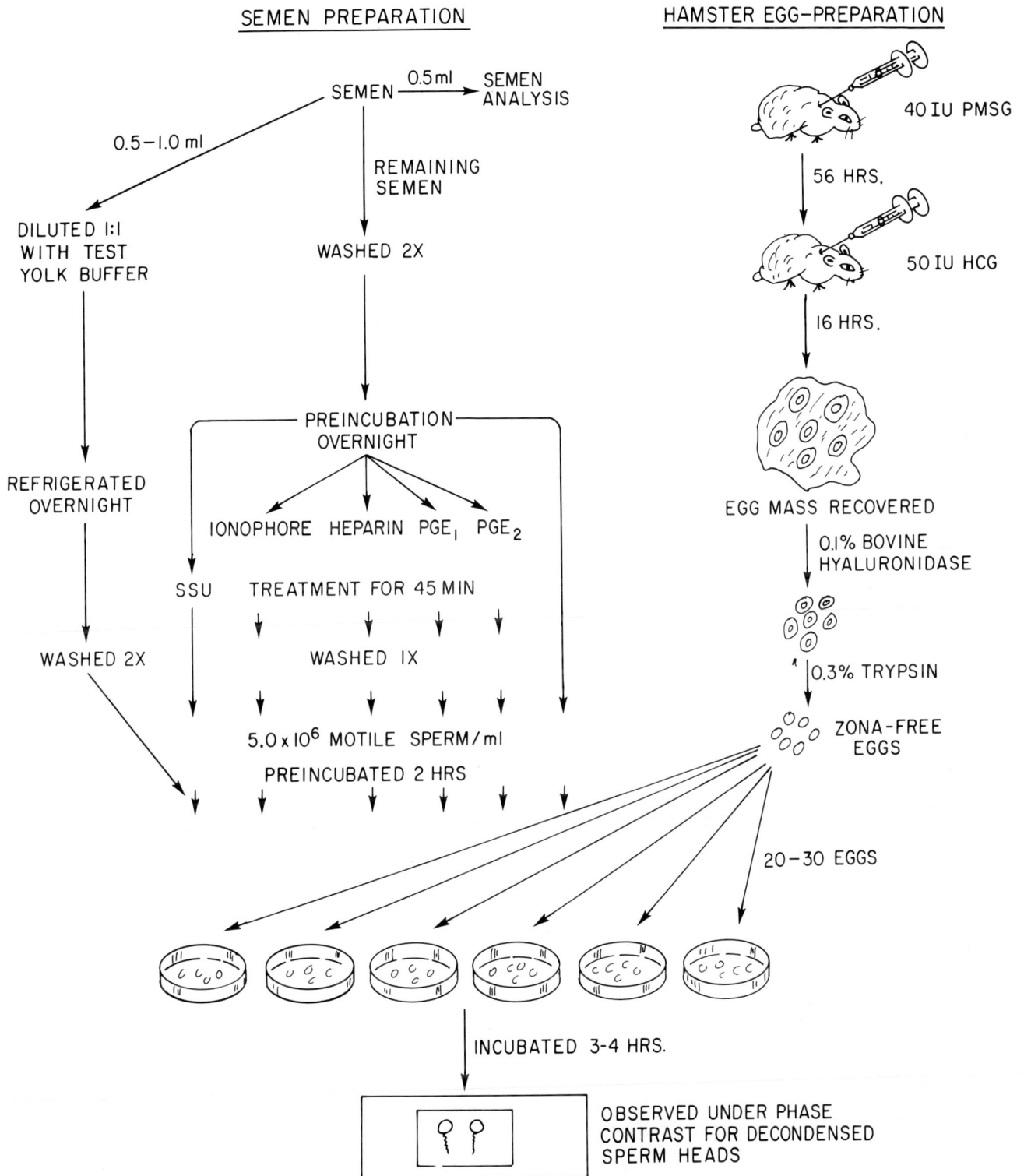

SEMEN $\xrightarrow{\text{0.5ml}}$ SEMEN ANALYSIS

0.5–1.0 ml

REMAINING SEMEN

DILUTED 1:1 WITH TEST YOLK BUFFER

WASHED 2X

REFRIGERATED OVERNIGHT

PREINCUBATION OVERNIGHT

IONOPHORE HEPARIN PGE$_1$ PGE$_2$

WASHED 2X

SSU TREATMENT FOR 45 MIN

WASHED 1X

5.0×10^6 MOTILE SPERM/ml

PREINCUBATED 2 HRS

40 IU PMSG

56 HRS.

50 IU HCG

16 HRS.

EGG MASS RECOVERED

0.1% BOVINE HYALURONIDASE

0.3% TRYPSIN

ZONA-FREE EGGS

20–30 EGGS

INCUBATED 3-4 HRS.

OBSERVED UNDER PHASE CONTRAST FOR DECONDENSED SPERM HEADS

FIGURE 39–5. Procedure for the challenge hamster egg–human sperm penetration assay. PGE, prostaglandin E; PMSG, pregnant mare serum gonadotropin; HCG, human chorionic gonadotropin.

lar, overnight incubation is recorded and compared with the percentage of ova penetrated by sperm treated overnight with refrigeration. Normal penetration is more than 15%, whereas in those samples with low penetration (<15%), we define a modest improvement with treatment to be an increase to

20% to 30%, a moderate improvement to 30% to 50% penetration, and a substantial improvement, to more than 50%.

5. Frozen sperm tested with the modified SPA are thawed, washed once, and incubated with 75 μM calcium ionophore (A23187) for 45 to 60 minutes. A control aliquot is incubated

without ionophore. The sperm were then washed and resuspended at a concentration of 5×10^6 motile sperm per milliliter and incubated at 37°C for 2 hours before the addition of zona-free ova as previously described. Interpretation of the results is as described earlier for fresh sperm.

The modified assay described earlier is useful in determining if a given person's SPA is normal and whether any of the earlier described treatments may be of benefit in treating the sperm prior to their use for inseminations or advanced reproductive techniques. For example, if a person's sperm penetration rate was less than 10% with nontreated sperm and this rate could be increased to 40% with refrigeration treatment, refrigeration would be used to prepare the sperm prior to use. We feel comfortable clinically using both refrigeration and heparin incubation to attempt to increase sperm penetration prior to use and have extensively studied their relationship to fertilization and pregnancy outcome when treating specific sperm penetration defects. It appears that specific sperm penetration defects can be identified and often treated, which appears to improve both fertilization and pregnancy rates.[38]

"Optimized" Sperm Penetration Assay. Although the standard hamster test, described earlier, is the most widely used version of the SPA, others have used a modified assay where it is expected that 100% of the eggs will be penetrated and the important measurement is the number of sperm that penetrate a given egg (sperm capacitation index). The assay is accomplished as follows[39]:

1. Sperm are prepared by allowing the sample to liquefy and then are diluted with an equal volume of room temperature, sterile test-yolk buffer and carefully mixed. This mixture is placed in room temperature water and placed into a refrigerator at 4°C. The sample is incubated for 42 hours.
2. The sample is removed from the refrigerator, and the pellet resuspended in warm medium (thermal shock). All sperm are centrifuged for 10 minutes at 600g. The sample is rewashed, and a swimup procedure is performed.
3. Hamster ova are obtained from previously superovulated hamsters as described earlier. Ova are added to 250,000 motile sperm prepared from the swimup. Controls are prepared from previously frozen and thawed sperm.
4. The number of penetrations per ova and the average number of penetrations for all ova counted are determined.

For all assays, fresh and frozen sperm can be used, as well as fresh and frozen hamster ova. These give similar rates in most reports.[40] The choice of a given technique is really laboratory specific. Our sperm penetration data appear to have a reasonable correlation to predicting fertility and fertilization rates, when used with other indices of sperm function, but we have had the same person doing the test for 17 years and have refined the techniques so that they are consistent in our laboratory. It would seem important for every laboratory to work with a particular technique enough to ensure it works consistently for that laboratory.

Additional Modifications. As mentioned previously, addition of human follicular fluid has been reported in a number of studies to increase penetration capacity. Incubation of sperm in test-yolk buffer was even more effective in increasing penetration capacity than was human follicular fluid.[37] A combination of test-yolk buffer and glass wool filtration increased the penetration capacity in a synergistic fashion.[41] Pentoxyfylline incubation also was reported to increase sperm penetration capacity in recent studies.[42] In addition, other modifications have been made to the assay, including development of a recent micro penetration assay useful for low sperm counts with a single ova.[43]

Correlation with Fertilization and Pregnancy Prediction

Relationship Between Sperm Parameters and Penetration. As discussed earlier, correlation of the results of the SPA to fertility remains controversial. In addition, correlation of traditional parameters of semen quality to sperm penetration capacity remains in dispute. Previous studies have suggested a relationship between the penetration capacity of sperm to the total motile oval count,[44] sperm count, motility, morphology,[45] HOS,[46] sperm velocity, tail beat cross-frequency,[47] subtle biochemistry defects,[48] and motile sperm density.[49] Other studies have reported minimal correlation between sperm penetration capacity and other indices of sperm function.[50] It appears that in most studies finding a correlation, the sperm morphology and the progressive motile sperm density have the best relationship to prediction of sperm penetration capacity.

Penetration Capacity and IVF Outcome. Numerous studies have evaluated the relationship of the sperm penetration assay to the outcome of IVF. Many studies, including evaluation of data from our IVF programs, indicate a reasonable prediction of IVF outcome using information from the SPA.[51] Also, in another study, the ability of sperm aspirated from the epididymis to fertilize human eggs correlated with their ability to penetrate modified hamster eggs.[52] Many reports indicate a high correlation of IVF in general with the SPA, whereas others report a correlation only to patients with tubal infertility and unexplained infertility and not those with oligoasthenospermia.[53] A few other studies report no correlation between IVF and data provided from the SPA.[54]

Pregnancy and Fertility. Many studies have also studied the usefulness of the SPA to predict subsequent fertility in patients. One study found that in combination with the HOS result, the SPA was 77.6% accurate in predicting patient fertility.[55] The SPA was predictive of increased pregnancy rates in oligospermic men and couples with unexplained infertility.[56] When the SPA was used with other semen data, such as sperm motility and motile sperm density, a strong correlation was found with future fertility.[49] Data from the SPA also appeared useful to predict which couples with unexplained infertility could benefit by using donor sperm.[57] Other studies do not report a correlation between the SPA and the prediction of fertility.[54]

Conclusions. The SPA is perhaps the most useful test to obtain at least some information about the potential fertilization capability of a given person's sperm. Used in conjunction with other indices of sperm function, it can provide information that should correlate to future outcome. The test is difficult to ensure consistency and must be optimized for a given laboratory. It will remain difficult to compare results from one laboratory to another, and therefore its use in a given program appears to be its most important role in the prediction of male fertility potential.

Acrosome Detection and Reaction

Sperm undergo biochemical changes over a several-hour period that results in hyperactivation of the sperm, defined as capacitation; this is a prerequisite for the acrosome reaction and for sperm to penetrate the zona. Freshly ejaculated sperm are not able to fertilize eggs without undergoing changes either in vitro or in the female tract. Although not completely understood, the process involves complex biochemical as well as physical changes in the sperm membrane, also resulting in changes in the metabolism of sperm. Capacitation appears to be reversible and involves the removal of sperm membrane surface proteins that can be subsequently replaced to "decapacitate" capacitated sperm.[58] Capacitation appears to occur over time and varies with respect to the amount of time it takes from one individual to another and between different samples from the same person. Seminal fluid contains proteins that act to coat the membrane surface and prevent capacitation. The process of capacitation involves loss of the decapacitating proteins on the surface of the sperm, a change in the negative charge on the sperm membrane, a change in membrane permeability with an increased efflux of cholesterol and an influx of unsaturated fatty acids, calcium ions, glucose, and oxygen thus resulting in hyperactivated motility. The process of capacitation is a prerequisite for the sperm to acrosome react. The ability of the sperm to acrosome react is measured primarily with the SPA.

It was shown recently that sperm can capacitate but do not acrosome react in the cervix of the female.[59] The acrosomal reaction appears to occur in vivo only as the sperm come in contact with the ovum. This reaction is defined as the morphologic alterations that lead to the dissolution of the sperm plasma membrane as well as the outer acrosomal membrane and acrosomal matrix. The acrosomal reaction appears to be induced by attaining a certain sperm calcium ion threshold concentration.[60] Addition of calcium to sperm incubated in calcium-free medium induces the acrosomal reaction. Likewise, addition of a calcium ionophore induces the sperm to acrosome react.[61] The ultrastructural description of the reaction includes swelling of the anterior part of the acrosomal cap, fusion of the plasma and outer acrosomal membrane, and disappearance of the plasma and outer acrosomal membrane, thus leaving the sperm head with one layer of a continuous inner acrosomal membrane.[62] This process results in sperm membrane permeability changes resulting in the release of acrosin, which is necessary for zona binding, penetration, and fertilization.

Therefore, the percentage of sperm that have already acrosome reacted, and the percentage of sperm that have the ability to acrosome react may be important measurements in detecting potential fertility difficulties. Because the presence of an acrosome in human sperm cannot be verified easily with normal sperm morphology stains and the light microscope, many studies of the acrosome have been accomplished with the aid of the electron microscope. Numerous studies have followed the course of the acrosomal reaction with the aid of the electron microscope. Because this is not practical for most laboratories, several techniques have been developed that enable use of the light microscope to verify the presence of an acrosome. This allows the laboratory to count the sperm with an intact acrosome versus those that are missing the acrosome. Techniques used to determine the presence of an acrosome are described in the following section.

TRIPLE-STAIN TECHNIQUE

The triple-stain technique enables evaluation of sperm viability along with the presence of the acrosome using the light microscope.[63] Because the acrosome is fragile and can break down with sperm death, it is important to determine if the sperm are live or dead when evaluating the presence of the acrosome. Live and dead sperm are counted using the vital stain trypan blue. The acrosomal and postacrosomal regions are differentiated by using the stains Rose bengal and Bismarck brown. Rose bengal specifically stains the acrosome, and absence of the stain on the sperm indicates the lack of the acrosome. One can, therefore, report the percentage of live sperm that are acrosome reacted and nonreacted, as well as the percentage of dead sperm reacted and nonreacted. The triple stain must be carefully completed and the sperm counted by an experienced observer to minimize the large degree of variability that is inherent in this type of assay. In addition, the stain must be carefully prepared using the same technique each time to minimize variation.

We use this technique along with a challenge test to evaluate both the initial and postchallenge percentage of live sperm from a given sample that have acrosome reacted. This allows us to determine how many sperm can be forced to acrosome react. The triple stain with the challenge test is accomplished as follows:

1. Sperm to be tested are washed, resuspended, and incubated for 4 to 24 hours and divided into two aliquots. One aliquot serves as the control while the other will be treated with calcium ionophore.

2. The treated aliquot is added to 100 μM of calcium ionophore (A23187) and incubated along with the control aliquot for 10 minutes at 37°C.

3. Sperm are washed, and each fraction is suspended in 1 mL of medium.

4. Each sample is diluted 1:1 with 2% trypan blue and incubated at 37°C for 15 minutes.

5. The sperm are washed twice and suspended in 1 mL of glutaraldehyde fixative and incubated at room temperature for 30 to 45 minutes.

6. The sperm are then washed three times and suspended in 0.5 mL of distilled water. A portion of each sperm sample (control and treated) is put on a microscope slide, smeared, and allowed to air dry.

7. Each slide is stained with 0.8% Bismarck brown for 5 minutes at 37°C. Wash the slides with distilled water for 5 to 10 seconds.

8. Stain each slide with 0.8% Rose bengal for 30 minutes at room temperature. Rinse each slide by dipping 5 to 7 times in 50% ethanol then 10–15 times in 95% ethanol and 20–25 times in 99% ethanol.

9. Slides are rinsed in clearing solution 10 to 15 times, and a coverslip is secured with mounting solution.

Interpretation of the results depends on the staining pattern of the sperm. Trypan blue is a viability stain, and the bottom half of the sperm head will stain blue-black if the sperm is nonviable. Bismarck brown is a counterstain so that viable sperm can be visualized. The bottom of a viable sperm head will stain clear to light brown. Rose bengal stains the acrosome. A nonacrosome-reacted sperm head will stain clear to light pink on the tip or distal half of the sperm head. At least 200 sperm are counted on each slide, and the percentage of sperm reacted without treatment is observed along with the percentage of sperm reacted that were treated with calcium ionophore. Studies continue to define the normal percentage of increase in fertile versus infertile men.

FLUORESCENCE TECHNIQUES

Another approach to the visualization of the acrosome involves the binding of fluorescence labels to a variety of materials that would selectively attach to the acrosome, thus allowing determination of which sperm contain an acrosome. Popular conjugates include the following.

Lectins. Lectins are plant proteins with a high affinity for specific sugar residues. These bind to both glycoproteins and glycolipids present in cell membranes and within the acrosomal contents. These lectins include pea, soybean, and wheat. The most common lectin used is pea (*Pisum sativum* agglutinin [PSA]).[64, 65] Using this technique, sperm are first stained with a viability stain (Hoechst 33258) to determine which of the viable sperm have an intact acrosome. Sperm are then treated with ethanol to permeabilize the acrosome receptors. These sperm are then smeared and dried on a microscope slide and stained with a drop of fluorescein isothiocyanate conjugated lectin. The slides are rinsed in distilled water, and the coverslip is mounted and the slides observed with a fluorescence microscope.

This assay works well if carefully performed, and in our hands gives results comparable with the triple-stain technique. Its disadvantage is that it cannot be used in the presence of cervical mucus or zona pellucida, both of which contain glycoproteins.

Chlortetracycline Fluorescence Assay. Chlortetracycline, when bound to calcium, binds to the sperm membrane and thus can be used to visualize the acrosomal region of the sperm with the aid of a fluorescence microscope.[66] This assay, developed to follow the time sequence of the acrosome reaction, is relatively simple, although care still needs to be used to ensure accuracy. It was shown to correlate with the assays described earlier.

Polyclonal Antisera. Sperm can be permeabilized with ethanol, dried on a microscope slide and incubated with antisera, washed, and combined with FITC conjugate.[67] This procedure is combined with Hoechst supravital stain to determine the acrosomal status of only the live sperm.

Monoclonal Antibodies. Monoclonal antibodies add specifically to the test by binding against specific acrosomal antigens.[68] Several groups have reported development of specific monoclonal antibodies against the acrosome. These include C 11 H, HS-19, HS-21, T5, T6, and T15.[66] Using these methods, sperm spreads in microwells are fixed with paraformaldehyde and washed, and the cells are exposed to the monoclonal antibody for 1 hour. The sperm are washed and then bound to an FITC-conjugated immunoglobulin and observed with a fluorescence microscope. As earlier, Hoechst stain is used to differentiate viable sperm.

Several reports describe the use of one or more of the earlier discussed techniques to determine the number of sperm that have acrosome reacted. The ability of sperm to acrosome react has been correlated with the ability of sperm to fertilize eggs with IVF.[65] It does appear that measurement of the presence of the acrosome and the ability of sperm, under challenge, to acrosome react can provide useful information to predict male fertility potential.[69]

Biochemical Measurement of Sperm Function

ACROSIN MEASUREMENT

Acrosin, a proteinase that is in the sperm acrosome, is necessary for normal penetration and fertilization. Acrosin is present as proacrosin, an inactive form, that becomes active before fertilization. Assays to determine acrosin have centered on the measurement of the quantity of acrosin present in a sperm sample or determination of the amount of acrosin activity. It would make sense that the amount of acrosin would not provide as meaningful information compared with the degree of acrosin activity. Acrosin activity measures the ability of proacrosin to be converted to acrosin. Because activity is the important event in the ability of sperm to fertilize, measurement of activity should provide more useful information on the ability of sperm to function normally.[70]

The amount of acrosin can be measured by extracting the acrosin and using immunologic techniques to determine the amount of the enzyme. Several techniques have been developed to measure acrosin activity in human sperm samples.[71, 72] Some assays are difficult and require large numbers of sperm or are difficult to quantitate. A simple technique has been reported that appears to overcome some of the shortcomings encountered while trying to determine acrosin activity.[72] Essentially, this technique removes proteinase inhibitors in seminal fluid that might interfere with acrosin activity by washing over Ficoll. Next, acrosin is removed from the sperm using a detergent that disrupts the acrosome and causes the release of acrosin. Proacrosin is converted to active acrosin by using a basic pH and a chromophobic substrate is used to quantitate the enzyme with the use of a spectrophotometer. This assay can be adapted with microtechniques to determine activity in samples under 2 million spermatozoa. To quantify acrosin activity, 1 IU of acrosin activity is defined as the quantity of enzyme that hydrolyzes 1 μM of substrate per minute at 23°C. The activity is expressed as micro-international units per million spermatozoa. Another recently described is a simple assay for measuring acrosin activity that involves placing sperm on a microscope slide containing a thin layer of gelatin and measuring the ability of the sperm to digest the gelatin, thus measuring the proteolytic activity of the sperm.[73] Although still primarily used for research studies, measurement of acrosin activity, similar to HOS, sperm penetration activity, sperm longevity studies, and hemizona binding may be useful to complete the overall picture of the true fertilization capacity of sperm from a given person. Several studies had found a correlation between the amount of acrosin activity and other parameters of semen quality, IVF outcome, and the prediction of future fertility.[74, 75] A few studies have found no correlation between acrosin activity and IVF outcome or other parameters of sperm function.[76] More research needs to be done to determine exact relationships of acrosin activity to future fertility.

ADENOSINE TRIPHOSPHATE MEASUREMENT

To enable the sperm to develop progressive sperm motility, the contractile filaments of the tail need energy to function. This energy is derived primarily from adenosine triphosphate (ATP), which is produced in the mitochondria of the sperm tail midpiece and then is transported to the flagellum. ATP is then converted by adenosine triphosphatase into adenosine diphosphate and adenosine monophosphate, during which time energy production results, which is used for filament contraction and sperm movement. Because ATP is necessary for sperm movement, and because progressive sperm motility correlates with male fertility, measurement of ATP may be useful to help predict male fertility potential. In fact, ATP levels have been shown to correlate with both quantitative progressive sperm motility as well as sperm concentration and have been reported to have a linear correlation with both parameters.[77–79] A decreased ATP level is associated with poor sperm motility, and thus its measurement when low motility is observed may be helpful to attempt to determine the reason for the motility defect.[78]

A popular, relatively easy and World Health Organization–recommended technique involves a chemoluminescence method that measures the ability of ATP to participate in the luciferine-luciferase reaction that is read in a luminometer as relative luminescence units.[80] It is important to understand that ATP is metabolized and decreases with time after ejaculation and therefore needs to be measured within 30 minutes to 1 hour after ejaculation.

Previous work has suggested a relationship between ATP concentration and sperm concentration, number of motile sperm per milliliter, progressive sperm motility, and progressive motile sperm concentration, and the SPA.[81] The relationship is linear between sperm concentration and ATP levels. Other studies did not find a relationship between ATP and sperm parameters.[82]

ATP levels have also been suggested to be useful to determine the fertility potential of frozen donor sperm.[83] Frozen donor sperm are inherently less successful in contributing to pregnancy than are fresh sperm. Anything that could be used to help further differentiate frozen sperm with a higher fertility potential from other samples with diminished potential would be extremely useful. Previous studies found that ATP levels could be used to predict which frozen samples would give a higher chance for pregnancy. Success was found to be able to be substantially improved by using ATP measurements versus motile sperm density, the standard determination to determine the fertility potential of a frozen sample.

ATP measurement was also found to be useful to predict IVF outcome.[83, 84] This is particularly true when the swimup ATP measurement was measured instead of the total semen ATP measurement. Low swimup ATP levels resulted in no or low fertilization rates.[77]

Therefore, measurement of ATP may help in gaining more information about a given person's sperm function and add to the ability to predict fertility potential.

CREATINE PHOSPHOKINASE ASSAY

Creatine phosphokinase (CK) is an important enzyme in the synthesis and transport of energy and may be a marker

for midpiece fertility. Creatine phosphate may increase sperm motility and velocity under certain circumstances; it shows an inverse correlation with sperm concentration; and its levels may correlate with the success of intrauterine insemination.[85] The measurement of CK, accomplished by fluorescence or electrophoresis techniques, is difficult and time consuming and is still primarily a research procedure. The isoforms of CK may further differentiate normal and abnormal sperm and are measured with electrophoresis.

DNA DETERMINATION

Deoxyribonucleic acid (DNA) status can be determined using the fluorochrome acridine orange (AO) coupled with microscopic fluorescence.[86] AO is reported to bind to double-stranded normal DNA, which results in green fluorescence, whereas red fluorescence occurs when AO binds to denatured, single-stranded DNA. A high percentage of green sperm supposedly indicates a large number of normal sperm, whereas a high percentage of red indicates abnormal or infertile sperm. The technique is relatively easy to accomplish. We have used the technique extensively and found that it is very fragile, sensitive to small changes, and variable. Therefore, results can be artificially created by minor alterations with the procedures. Various studies have reported conflicting results with respect to the usefulness of these methods to predict fertility problems.[86, 87] We have developed modifications for the technique to eliminate some of the variability. However, the technique still needs to be considered for research use only until additional studies can clarify its potential usefulness.

OTHER BIOCHEMICAL DETERMINATIONS

Numerous additional biochemical determinations have been used over the years in an attempt to better define sperm function and to predict male infertility. Almost any individual measurement has been, in one or more studies, reported to correlate to infertility. There is still no consensus that measurement of any additional factors would prove useful to predict subsequent male fertility. Additional measurements have included quantitative fructose, zinc, acid phosphatase, ions, prostaglandins, citric acid, lipids, polyamines, hormone levels, L-carnitine, glycerylphosphorycholine, oxygen uptake and metabolism, protein carboxylmethylase, oxygen-reactive species, hyaluronidase activity, α-glucosidase, and transferrin.

Mucus Penetration Capacity

The ability of sperm to penetrate thick fluids has been demonstrated in numerous studies to give information that allows a high correlation with subsequent fertility.[88] The ability of sperm to penetrate human cervical mucus generally correlates well with prediction of fertility, although some studies have reported poor mucus-sperm compatibility with standard tests while at the same time finding sperm in the peritoneal fluid at the time of laparoscopy.[89] The cervix has been reported to act as a sperm reservoir and can continue to supply sperm into the uterus for prolonged periods after intercourse.[90] Numerous techniques have been developed to evaluate the interaction of ovulatory cervical mucus with sperm. These include techniques that are described in the following section, including postcoital tests, mucus slide test, bovine cervical mucus–sperm test, and artificial mucus–sperm test.

EVALUATION OF MUCUS QUALITY

The first step to completing a mucus-sperm test is to evaluate the quality of the cervical mucus that will be used to complete the test. Poor-quality mucus cannot support adequate sperm function. Mucus quality is determined by rating its quantity and quality. A scoring system has been proposed to rate mucus.[91] The system uses five properties of cervical mucus related to the penetration capacity and survival and migration of sperm. These include the amount of mucus, spinnbarkeit (stretchability), ferning, viscosity, and cellularity. Each item receives a score of 0 to 3, with 3 representing the best quality. A maximum score of 15 indicates mucus that should be receptive to sperm, assuming no other hostile factors such as antisperm antibodies. The mucus should be collected and evaluated near the time of ovulation. Once the mucus to be used has been evaluated for quality, subsequent tests can be performed to determine mucus-sperm interaction.

POSTCOITAL TEST

The most common and popular way to determine mucus-sperm compatibility is the postcoital test.[91–93] This test is useful because it gives an idea of the ability of the sperm and mucus to interact under conditions that at least simulate natural intercourse. With this technique the couple has intercourse on the day of ovulation. The male is instructed to abstain from ejaculation for 2 to 5 days prior to the test. The woman is asked to come into the physician's office 2 to 8 hours after intercourse. Mucus is removed, evaluated for quality as indicated earlier, and then examined under the microscope. The test is occasionally performed 18 to 24 hours after intercourse, particularly if the initial postcoital test is normal and the couple still has unexplained infertility. At least two separate tests should be completed before making a final decision on the compatibility of the mucus and the sperm. After the mucus has been evaluated for quality, the mucus is observed microscopically for the numbers and motility of the sperm in the mucus. The tests should be evaluated by checking three areas in the female tract. The vaginal pool sperm are checked to make sure that seminal fluid was deposited into the *vagina*. A specimen is examined from the lower part of the *cervical canal*. Within a few hours after intercourse, there is a large accumulation of sperm in the lower part of the cervical canal (>25 motile sperm with forward motility). Observation of this area several hours after intercourse may indicate lower numbers of sperm. An *endocervical* sample can be obtained several hours after intercourse and one would expect to see more than 10 sperm with progressive motility. This should also be the result when checking this area with the longer test (18 to 24 hours after intercourse). One postcoital test is relatively worthless, particularly if it is poor. The test is useful if it is normal because it may indicate that the couple should be able to achieve pregnancy on their own, assuming all other factors are normal. However, a poor postcoital test result is not helpful.

This result may reflect a problem with sperm or mucus, or both. To eliminate the guesswork involved, we prefer the two-way mucus-sperm test described in the following section.

TWO-WAY MUCUS-SPERM TEST

Numerous tests have been developed that enable the clinician to get a better idea of the ability of mucus to interact with sperm other than just the postcoital test. After one or two poor postcoital test results, the mucus slide-sperm inhibition test is useful to try and identify the nature of the problem.[32] This test is completed by having the woman come in on the day of ovulation. The day of ovulation should not be estimated based on previous cycles but should be determined from more accurate tests such as luteinizing hormone urine measurement. Cervical mucus is recovered from the woman and placed on the center of a warm microscope slide. A drop of the male partner's sperm to be tested is placed on one side of the mucus, making sure that the mucus makes good contact with the sperm sample. A drop of fresh sperm, previously demonstrated to have normal mucus-sperm interaction, is placed on the other side of the mucus, also making sure to have an area of good contact between the sperm and mucus (Fig. 39–6). A 20 × 60-mm microscope slide cover is carefully placed on the slide, and the slide is maintained in a humidified 37°C incubator. The initial sperm numbers are estimated and quantitative motility is recorded. Motility and numbers are recorded for each sample in the drops outside the mucus. Every 20 minutes, for 2 hours, the sperm sample from each side is observed at the mucus-sperm interface to determine the sperm motility and relative numbers of sperm that have penetrated the mucus from each sample. This test is useful because it helps define where the problem resides with a poor test. For the sperm penetrating into the mucus, we like to see reasonable numbers of sperm in the mucus with at least 30% progressive sperm motility by 1 hour. If the husband's sperm and test sperm both penetrate well, one assumes that the couple should be able to have a chance of pregnancy with intercourse. If the test sperm penetrates well, and the husband's sperm does not, then it is assumed that the woman's fluids support sperm function but that something is going to have to be done to improve the motility of the husband's sperm. If both samples penetrate poorly, the woman should be checked for antisperm antibodies to make sure this is not the cause of the poor penetration. Alternatively, ovulatory mucus from a donor of proven fertility can be used in a four-way test to compare the interaction of male partner sperm and test sperm and can serve for a control penetration value. This four-way test is completed as described earlier for the two-way test.

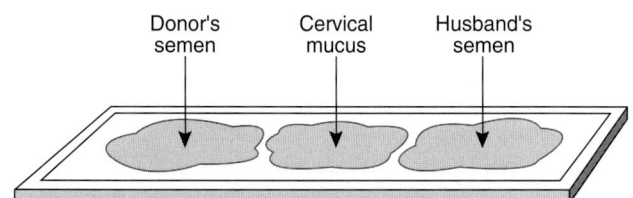

FIGURE 39–6. Representation of the mucus-sperm slide inhibition test to determine mucus-sperm compatibility.

We have not found frozen sperm useful to serve as the control sperm to evaluate the ability of sperm to penetrate cervical mucus. Frozen-thawed sperm have poor capability to penetrate cervical mucus and therefore are not helpful for this purpose.[40]

SPERM-MUCUS CAPILLARY TESTS

The sperm-mucus capillary test uses a rectangular capillary tube filled with the mucus to be tested. The tube can be filled with the human female's mucus to be tested, bovine cervical mucus, or artificial cervical mucus. After the tube is filled with mucus, the tube is inserted into a reservoir of sperm. We observe the tube every 30 minutes for 2 hours while the tube is incubated at 37°C. The test is evaluated by observing the motility of the sperm that have penetrated into the mucus and the penetration density at 1 to 4 and 4 to 5 cm from the semen reservoir.[94] The distance of the vanguard or most advanced sperm in the capillary can also be recorded. Control values can be obtained by taking another tube of the same mucus to be tested, and it is placed in a reservoir of test sperm. This tube is then observed as described earlier.

Bovine estrus cervical mucus has been used commercially as a substitute for human cervical mucus. Human sperm exhibit similar characteristics in bovine mucus compared with human mucus.[94] It should be understood that interpretation of these results is different than the tests described previously. This test describes the ability of sperm to interact with thick fluids but does not give information about the ability of a given male's sperm to interact with his female partner's mucus. Along with all of the other sperm tests described, it would seem reasonable to evaluate the ability of the sperm to swim through mucus, although we still prefer testing the woman's own mucus with her male partner's sperm, in addition to test sperm.

Similar to bovine mucus, artificial mucus can be manufactured in the laboratory to simulate human mucus and thereby determine the ability of sperm to swim through thick fluids.[95] We have used this to show a reasonable correlation of artificial mucus to bovine mucus, which in turn has a reasonable correlation with human mucus, but the manufacture of artificial mucus is extremely variable and sensitive, which makes it difficult to obtain consistent results.

Antisperm Antibodies

Antibodies and the measurement of antisperm antibodies have long been a staple of sperm function determination. The role of antibodies on sperm function and subsequent fertility remains controversial. Numerous studies have shown a substantial effect of antisperm antibodies on human sperm function and the prediction of fertility of a given male, whereas other studies have minimized the role of antibodies on fertility.[96–98] It is not surprising that there remains some controversy, because there are several different techniques to measure antibodies and to determine whether they are altering sperm function. We have found that clinical manifestations of significant antisperm antibodies in the male include sperm agglutination (differentiated from sperm clumping) in a definitive pattern, and poor sperm motility, including increased nonmotile sperm or increased immobilizing motility, and

poor sperm membrane function as evidenced by poor viability and low HOS scores.[99] The presence of this triple defect (motility, viability, and HOS) has a high correlation with the presence of antibodies in a given male. In fact, these are the criteria we currently use to determine if antibodies are having a clinical effect in a given person with antibodies. It is also well known that antibodies cause a sperm penetration defect, and this is another correlate of clinical effects of antibodies.[100]

Numerous techniques have been used to measure the levels of antisperm antibodies. These include macro- and micro-agglutination tests, immobilization tests, immunobead tests, radioimmunoassays, and a variety of enzyme-linked immunosorbent assays (ELISAs). All the techniques have advantages and disadvantages. We prefer an antibody profile on all patients tested for antibodies. This includes the Kibrick macroagglutination test, Isojima immobilization test, and the immunobead test with immunoglobin G (IgG), IgA, and IgM bound immunobeads. This profile, when done on both serum and seminal fluid, gives a high correlation to the clinical effects of antibodies on sperm function as well to the prediction of fertility problems in a given male.

SPERM MACROAGGLUTINATION

Sperm agglutination tests have been described by Franklin-Dukes, Friberg, and Kibrick. The Kibrick test is the most common test to determine the presence of sperm-agglutinating antibodies.[101] With this test sperm from a normal donor, who is negative for antibodies, is suspended in a gelatin mixture in small test tubes along with a portion of complement-inactivated serum or with seminal fluid from the patient to be tested. The tubes are carefully observed at 30 and 60 minutes. Appropriate positive and negative controls are used, and we like to have two independent observers read this assay. The tubes are observed for the formation of a flocculent precipitate. The control and positive samples are run at various dilutions to determine the concentration of antibodies in the fluid tested, and the results are reported as the last dilution tested that was positive. For example, dilutions can be made at 1:0, 1:4, 1:16, 1:64, and 1:256. The precipitate can be observed under the microscope to determine the pattern of sperm binding.

SPERM-IMMOBILIZING ANTIBODIES

Sperm-immobilizing antibodies can be determined with the technique described by Isojima.[102] With this technique, donor sperm are incubated with the serum or seminal fluid to be tested, along with complement obtained from a fresh rabbit, guinea pig, or human serum that is antibody free. The mixture is incubated and observed at 30 minutes and again at 60 minutes. A positive test for antibodies is determined to be a reduction in motility of at least 50% of the control motility at 60 minutes when compared with the negative control.

IMMUNOBEAD ASSAYS

Immunobead assays use microscopic immunobeads that allow detection of the class of immunoglobulins involved including IgG, IgA, and IgM.[103] These immunobeads can be incubated separately with the person's sperm to be tested after washing (direct test), and the mixture is incubated in a humidified chamber and a drop observed at 3 to 10 minutes. If antibodies are present, the antibodies bound to sperm membranes will bind with the antihuman immunoglobulins bound to the immunobeads. The percentage of sperm bound to the beads is recorded, and the location of the bead binding is noted, that is, sperm head, tail, midpiece, and tip of tail. With the direct test the patient's own sperm is tested and evaluated with the immunobeads. With the indirect test, the patient's heat-inactivated serum or the seminal fluid is incubated with donor's sperm for approximately 30 to 60 minutes, and then the washed sperm are incubated with the beads as described earlier. The indirect test is needed occasionally because of the lack of sufficient numbers of sperm in a given patient to be tested. Also, patients with high levels of antibodies often have such poor sperm motility that the sperm do not move well enough to pick up the beads with the direct test. There must be sperm motility for the immunobead test to allow the beads to bind to the antibodies on the sperm membrane. For this reason, we often utilize the indirect immunobead test although the direct may have a higher correlation to fertility.[104] We have found that an antibody profile of a given patient can best be determined by completing all three tests (Kibrick, Isojima, immunobead) on both the serum and seminal fluid. This gives the best idea of whether the patient has levels of antibodies that may be playing a role in the patient's infertility.

OTHER TYPES OF ANTIBODY TESTS

The other type of common assay to detect antisperm antibodies is the group of ELISA tests.[105] This test is nonsubjective and quantitative and is immunoglobulin specific as well as rapid and simple. We have not found the results from this assay to be as useful in correlating the results of antisperm antibodies with clinical findings of antibodies in the patient, but the assays have been widely used with several studies reporting a reasonable correlation with fertility prediction.

Conclusions

After a series of carefully conducted semen analyses, there remains several tests to evaluate the fertility potential of sperm and to predict male fertility potential. SPAs appear useful to diagnose penetration capability of sperm and perhaps to treat sperm penetration defects prior to their use with fertility-enhancing procedures. Sperm membrane function, sperm longevity, and mucus penetration tests help determine more subtle observations of sperm quality relating to the ability of sperm to reach and penetrate the egg. Sperm-binding tests have been helpful to predict fertilization rates with IVF. Determination of the ability of sperm to acrosome react may also predict the fertilization capability of a given person's sperm. Numerous biochemical markers may be helpful to further refine prediction capabilities of human male infertility. Last, antisperm antibody measurement, when appropriate, can help define the role of antibodies in a male's fertility problems.

There is no one assay or combination of assays that predicts, with 100% accuracy, a given male's fertility potential. Fertility is a complex event, and it is not surprising that isolated tests cannot perfectly describe a given person's prognosis. Nevertheless, multiple tests, carefully performed, will come the closest to aiding the medical team to assist the couple with fertility difficulties and to predict outcome for a given male.

REFERENCES

1. Spark RF. Evolving concepts of male fertility. In: The Infertile Male: The Clinician's Guide to Diagnosis and Treatment. New York: Plenum, 1988:3–7.
2. Lillie FR. The history of the fertilization problem. Science 1916;43:39–53.
3. Castellani C. Spermatozoan biology from Leeuwenhoek to Spallanzani. J Hist Biol 1973;6:37–68.
4. Lode A. Untersuchungen Uber die Zahlen-und Regenerationsverhaltnisse der Spermatozoiden bei Hund und Mensch. Ges Physiol 1891;L:278–292.
5. Berthelsen JG. Vital staining of spermatozoa performed by the patient. Fertil Steril 1981;35:86–89.
6. Dougherty KA, Urry RL, Cockett ATK. Supravital staining of spermatozoa: relationship of eosin concentration to the percentage of cells staining live. J Urol 1977;118:1008–1014.
7. Urry RL. Laboratory diagnosis of male infertility. Clin Lab Med 1985;5:355–370.
8. Jeyendran RS, VanderVen HH, Perez-Pelaez M, et al. Development of an assay to assess the functional integrity of the human sperm membrane and its relationship to other semen characteristics. J Reprod Fertil 1984;70:219–224.
9. Chan SY, Fox EJ, Chan MM, et al. The relationship between the human sperm hypoosmotic swelling test, routine semen analysis, and the human sperm zona-free hamster ovum penetration assay. Fertil Steril 1985;44(5):668–672.
10. Mordel N, Dano I, Epstein-Eldan M, et al. Novel parameters of human sperm hypo-osmotic swelling test and their correlation to standard spermatogram, total motile sperm fraction, and sperm penetration assay. Fertil Steril 1993;59(6):1276–1279.
11. Urry RL. Various techniques to cryopreserve sperm and their effects on sperm hypoosmolarity scores, viability and motility. Presented at the Pacific Coast Fertility Society Annual Meetings, Palm Springs, 1988.
12. Daya S, Gunby J, Kohut J. Semen predictors of in vitro fertilization and embryo cleavage. Am J Obstet Gynecol 1989;161:1284–1289.
13. Van der Ven HH, Jeyendran RS, Al-Hassani S, et al. Correlation between human sperm swelling in hypo-osmotic medium (hypo-osmotic swelling test) and in vitro fertilization. J Androl 1986;7:190–196.
14. Toda T, Sofikitis N, Miyagawa I, et al. The importance of the hypo-osmotic swelling test and acrosin activity assay for identifying subpopulations of idiopathic infertile men. Arch Androl 1992;29(3):219–224.
15. Gavella M, Lipovac V. Effect of leucocytes on the hypoosmotic swelling test of human sperm. Arch Androl 1993;30:55–61.
16. Lomeo AM, Giambersio AM. "Water-test": a simple method to assess sperm-membrane integrity. Int J Androl 1991;14:278–282.
17. Critchlow JD, Matson PL, Newman MC, et al. Quality control in an in vitro fertilization laboratory: use of human survival studies. Hum Reprod 1989;4(5):545–549.
18. de Ziegler D, Cedars MI, Hamilton F, et al. Factors influencing maintenance of sperm motility during in vitro processing. Fertil Steril 1987;48(5):816–820.
19. Denil J, Ohl DA, Hurd WW, et al. Motility longevity of sperm samples processed for intrauterine insemination. Fertil Steril 1992;58(2):436–438.
20. Franco JG, Mauri AL, Peterson CG, et al. Efficacy of the sperm survival test for the prediction of oocyte fertilization in culture. Hum Reprod 1993;8(6):916–918.
21. Urry RL. Correlation between sperm function and fertilization and pregnancy rates in infertile couples. Presented at the American Urology Association Annual Meeting, New Orleans, LA, 1990.
22. Burkman LJ. Hyperactivated motility of human spermatozoa during in vitro capacitation and implications for fertility. In: Gagnon C, editor. Controls of Sperm Motility: Biological and Clinical Aspects. Boca Raton, FL: CRC Press, 1990:303–330.
23. Katz DF, Drobnis EZ, Overstreet EZ, Overstreet JW. Factors regulating mammalian sperm migration through the female reproductive tract and oocyte vestments. Gamete Res 1989;22:443–448.

24. Burkman LJ, Coddington CC, Franken DR, et al. The hemizona assay (HZA): development of a diagnostic test for the binding of human spermatozoa to the human hemizona pellucida to predict fertilization potential. Fertil Steril 49:688–697, 1988.

25. Oehninger S, Coddington CC, Scott R, et al. Hemizona assay (HZA): assessment of sperm (dys) function and prediction of in vitro fertilization (IVF) outcome. Fertil Steril 1989;51:665–674.

26. Hammitt DG, Syrop CH, Walker DL, Bennett MR. Conditions of oocyte storage and use of noninseminated as compared with inseminated, non-fertilized oocytes for the hemizona assay. Fertil Steril 1993;60(1):131–136.

27. Burkman LJ, Coddington CC, Franken DR, et al. Development of a diagnostic test for the binding of human spermatozoa to the human hemizona pellucida to predict fertilization potential. Fertil Steril 1988;49:1988–1992.

28. Franken Dr, Acosta AA, Krueger TF, et al. The hemizona assay: its role in identifying male factor infertility in assisted reproduction. Fertil Steril 1993;59(5):1075–1080.

29. Coddington CC, Alexander NJ, Fulgham D, et al. Hemizona assay (HZA) demonstrates effects of characterized mouse antihuman sperm antibodies on sperm zona binding. Andrologia 1992;24(5):271–277.

30. Lanzendorf SE, Holmgren WJ, Jeyendran RS. The effect of egg yolk medium on human sperm binding in hemizona assay. Fertil Steril 1992;58(3):547–550.

31. Liu DY, Clarke GN, Lopata A, et al. A sperm–zona pellucida binding test and in vitro fertilization. Fertil Steril 1989;52(2):281–287.

32. Urry RL. Advances in diagnosing and treating sperm problems and reproductive techniques. In: Smith JA, editor. High-Tech Urology: Technologic Innovations and Their Clinical Applications. Philadelphia: WB Saunders, 1992:251–270.

33. Johnson JP, Alexander NJ. Hamster egg penetration: comparison of preincubation periods. Fertil Steril 1984;41:599–602.

34. Rogers BJ, Perreault SD, Bentwood BJ, et al. Variability in the human-hamster in vitro assay for fertility evaluation. Fertil Steril 1983;39(2):204–211.

35. Kanwar KC, Yanagimachi R, Lopata A. Effects of human seminal plasma on fertilizing capacity of human spermatozoa. Fertil Steril 1979;31:321–325.

36. Chan SY, Tucker MJ. Differential sperm performance as judged by the zona-free hamster egg penetration test relative to the differing sperm preparation techniques. Hum Reprod 1992;7:255–260.

37. Chan SY, Tucker MJ. Comparative study on the use of human follicular fluid or egg yolk medium to enhance the performance of human sperm in the zona-free hamster oocyte penetration assay. Int J Androl 1992;15:32–42.

38. Carrell DT, Bradshaw WS, Jones KP, et al. An evaluation of various treatments to increase sperm penetration capacity for potential use in an in vitro fertilization program. Fertil Steril 1992;57:134–138.

39. Smith RG, Johnson A, Lamb DJ, Lipschultz LI. Functional tests of spermatozoa. Urol Clin North Am 1987;14(3):451–462.

40. Urry RL, Carrell DT, Hull DB, et al. Penetration of zona-free hamster ova and bovine cervical mucus by fresh and frozen human spermatozoa. Fertil Steril 1983;39:690–694.

41. Holmgren WJ, Jeyendran RS. Synergistic effect of test–yolk buffer treatment and glass wool filtration of spermatozoa on the outcome of the hamster oocyte penetration assay. Hum Reprod 1993;8:425–427.

42. Lambert H, Steinleitner A, Eisermann J, et al. Enhanced gamete interaction in the sperm penetration assay after coincubation with pentoxifylline and human follicular fluid. Fertil Steril 1992;58:1205–1208.

43. Bronson RA, Oula A, Bronson SK. A microwell sperm penetration assay. Fertil Steril 1992;58:1078–1080.

44. Brandeis VT. Importance of total motile oval count in interpreting the hamster ovum sperm penetration assy. J Androl 1993;14:53–59.

45. Campana A, Gatti MY, Ruspa M, et al. Relationship between fertility, semen analysis, and human sperm penetration of zona-free hamster eggs. Acta Eur Fertil 1983;14:331–336.

46. Okada A, Inomata K, Matsuhashi M, et al. Correlation of the hypo-osmotic swelling test, semen score, and the zona-free hamster egg penetration assay in humans. Int J Androl 1990;13:337–343.

47. Fetterolf PM, Rogers BJ. Prediction of human sperm penetrating ability using computerized motion parameters. Mol Reprod Dev 1990;27:326–331.

48. Grunfeld L. Workup for male infertility. J Reprod Med 1989;34:143–149.

49. Leroy-Martin B, Saint-Pol P, Bouhdida M, Hermand E. Correlation of the penetration test of zona-free hamster oocytes and other sperm parameters: value of this test in evaluating male infertility. J Gynecol Obstet Biol Reprod Paris 1989;18:729–734.

50. Osser S, Wramsby H, Liedholm P. A comparison between the hamster egg penetration test and the seminal parameters in men of infertile couples. Int J Fertil 1988;33:207–211.

51. Nahhas F, Blumenfield Z. Zona-free hamster egg penetration assay: prognostic indicator in an IVF program. Arch Androl 1989;23:33–37.

52. Rojas FJ, La AT, Ord T, et al. Penetration of zona-free hamster oocytes using human sperm aspirated from the epididymis of men with congenital absence of the vas deferens: comparison with human in vitro fertilization. Fertil Steril 1992;58:1000–1005.

53. Margalioth EJ, Navot D, Laufer N, et al. Correlation between the zona-free hamster egg penetration assay and human in vitro fertilization. Fertil Steril 1986;45:665–670.

54. Kuzan FB, Muller CH, Zarutskie PW, et al. Human sperm penetration assay as an indicator of sperm function in human in vitro fertilization. Fertil Steril 1987;48:282–286.

55. Wang C, Chan SY, Ng M, et al. Diagnostic value of sperm function tests and routine semen analyses in fertile and infertile men. J Androl 1988;9:384–389.

56. Margalioth EJ, Feinmesser M, Navot D, et al. The long-term predictive value of the zona-free hamster ova–sperm penetration assay. Fertil Steril 1989;52:490–494.

57. Kremer J, Jager S. The significance of the zona-free hamster oocyte test for the evaluation of male infertility. Fertil Steril 1990;54:509–512.

58. Coetzee K, Swanson RJ, Kruger TF. Hamster zona-free oocyte spermatozoa penetration assay. In: Acosta AA, Swanson RJ, Ackerman SB, et al, editors. Human Spermatozoa in Assisted Reproduction. Baltimore: Williams & Wilkins, 1990;119–137.

59. Bielfeld P, Jeyendran RS, Zanefeld LJD. Human spermatozoa do not undergo the acrosome reaction during storage in the cervix. Int J Fertil 1991;36:302–306.

60. Murphy SJ, Rolden ERS, Yanagimachi R. Effects of extracellular cations and energy substrates on the acrosome reaction of precapacitated guinea pig spermatozoa. Gamete Res 1986;14:1–15.

61. Aitken RJ, Ross A, Hargreave T, et al. Analysis of human sperm function following exposure to ionophore A23187. J Androl 1984;5:321–326.

62. Nagae T, Yanagimachi R, Drivastava PN, Yanagimachi H. Acrosome reaction in human spermatozoa. Fertil Steril 1985;45:701.

63. Talbot P, Chacon RS. A triple-stain technique for evaluating normal acrosome reactions of human sperm. J Exp Zool 1981;215:201–208.

64. Cross NL, Morales P, Overstreet JW, Hanson FW. Two simple methods for detecting acrosome reacted human sperm. Gamete Res 1986;15:213–225.

65. Liu DY, Baker HWG. The proportion of human sperm with poor morphology but normal intact acrosomes detected with Pisum sativum agglutinin correlates with fertilization in vitro. Fertil Steril 1988;50:288–296.

66. Lee MA, Trucco GS, Bechtol KB, et al. Capacitation and acrosome reactions in human spermatozoa monitored by a chlortetracycline fluorescence assay. Fertil Steril 1987;48:649–658.

67. Bruckner D, Alexander NJ. Evaluation of the acrosome: immunological methods. In: Acosta AA, Swanson RJ, Ackerman SB, et al, editors. Human Spermatozoa in Assisted Reproduction. Baltimore: Williams & Wilkins, 1990;114–118.

68. Wolf DP, Boldt J, Byrd W, Bechtol KB. Acrosomal status evaluation in human ejaculated sperm with monoclonal antibodies. Biol Reprod 1985;31:1157–1168.

69. Aitken RJ, Thatcher S, Glasier AF, et al. Relative ability of modified versions of the hamster oocyte penetration test, incorporating hyper-osmotic medium or the ionophore A23187, to predict IVF outcome. Hum Reprod 1987;2:227–238.

70. Koukoulis G, Vantman D, Dennison Z, Sherins RJ. Consistently low acrosin activity in sperm of a subpopulation of men with unexplained infertility. J Androl 1988;9:46P.

71. Goodpasture JC, Zavos PN, Zaneveld LJD. Relationship of human sperm acrosin and proacrosin II correlations. J Androl 1987;8:267–276.

72. Kennedy WP, Kaminski JM, VanderVen HH, et al. A simple clinical assay to evaluate the acrosin activity of human spermatozoa. J Androl 1989;10:221–231.

73. Welker B, Bernstein GS, Diedrick K, et al. Acrosomal proteinase activity of human spermatozoa and relation of results to semen quality. Hum Reprod 1988;3:75–80.

74. Gerhard I, Frohlich E, Eggert-Kruse W, et al. Relationship of sperm

acrosin activity to semen and clinical parameters in infertile patients. Andrologia 1989;21:146–154.

75. DeJonge CJ, Tarchala SM, Rawlins RG, et al. Acrosin activity in human spermatozoa in relation to semen quality and in vitro fertilization. Hum Reprod 1993;8:253–257.

76. Wolf DP. Acrosomal status quantitation in human sperm. Am J Reprod Immunol 1989;20:106–113.

77. Comhaire F, Vermeulen L, Ghedira K, et al. Adenosine triphosphate in human semen: a quantitative estimate of fertilizing potential. Fertil Steril 1983;40:500–507.

78. Gerris J, Punjabi U, Delbeke L, et al. Luminometric measurement of ATP concentrations in human semen. Acta Eur Fertil 1987;18:25–28.

79. Comhaire FH, Vermeulen L, Schoonjans F. Reassessment of the accuracy of traditional sperm characteristics and adenosine triphosphate (ATP) in estimating the fertilizing potential of human semen in vivo. Int J Androl 1987;40:653–662.

80. Gottlieb C, Svanborg K, Eneroth P, Bygdeman M. Adenosine triphosphate in human semen: a study on conditions for a bioluminescence assay. Fertil Steril 1987;47:992–999.

81. Calamera JC, Quiros MC, Brugo S, et al. Adenosine 5'-triphosphate (ATP) concentration and acrosin activity in human spermatozoa: their relation with the sperm penetration assay (SPA). Andrologia 1986;18:574–580.

82. Chan SY, Wang C. Correlation between adenosine triphosphate and sperm fertilizing capacity. Fertil Steril 1987;47:717–719.

83. Comhaire FH, Vermeulen L, Hinting A, Schoonjans F. Biochemistry: ATP—accuracy of traditional sperm characteristics and ATP in assessing fertilizing potential of human sperm in vivo and in vitro. In: Acosta AA, Swanson RJ, Ackerman SB, editors. Human Spermatozoa in Assisted Reproduction. Baltimore: Williams & Wilkins, 1990:195–199.

84. Chan SY, Chan YM, Tucker MJ, et al. The diagnostic valve of seminal adenosine triphosphate (ATP) in an in vitro fertilization (IVF) program. Andrologia 1990;22:531–537.

85. Huszar G, Vigue L. Oligo/asthenospermia and the activities of creatine kinase and dynein ATPase in human sperm. American Fertility Society Annual Meeting, Toronto, 1986.

86. Tejada RI, Mitchell JC, Norman A, et al. A test for the practical evaluation of male fertility by acridine orange (AO) fluorescence. Fertil Steril 1984;42:87–91.

87. Ibrahim ME, Pedersen H. Acridine orange fluorescence as male fertility test. Arch Androl 1987;20:125–129.

88. Buxton CL, Southam AL. Cervical physiology. In: Human Infertility. New York: PB Hoeber, 1958.

89. Asch RH. Sperm recovery in peritoneal aspirate after negative Sims-Huhner test. Int J Fertil 1978;23:57–62.

90. Moghissi KS. Sperm–cervical mucus interaction. In: Keel BA, Webster BW, editors. Handbook of the Laboratory Diagnosis and Treatment of Infertility. Boca Raton, FL: CRC Press, 1990:149–165.

91. Moghissi KS. The cervix in infertility. Clin Obstet Gynecol 1979;22:27–35.

92. Davajan V, Kunitake G. Fractional in vivo and in vitro examination of postcoital cervical mucus in the human. Fertil Steril 1969;20:197–204.

93. World Health Organization. Laboratory Manual for Examination of Human Semen and Semen–Cervical Mucus Interaction. Cambridge: Cambridge University Press, 1987.

94. Schuttle B. Penetration ability of human spermatozoa into standardized bovine cervical mucus (Penetrak) in patients with normal and pathological semen samples. Andrologia 1987;19:317–326.

95. Urry RL, Middleton RG, Mayo D. A comparison of the penetration of human sperm into bovine and artificial cervical mucus. Fertil Steril 1986;45:135–140.

96. Witkin SS, David SS. Effect of sperm antibodies on pregnancy outcome in a subfertile population. Am J Obstet Gynecol 1988;158:59–65.

97. Grunfeld L. Workup for male infertility. J Reprod Med 1989;34:143–149.

98. Brannen-Brock LR, Hall JL. Effect of male antisperm antibodies on sperm fertility ability in vitro. Arch Androl 1985;15:15–19.

99. Urry RL, Carrell DT, Middleton RG. Antisperm antibodies: clinical evidence for the presence of and necessity for treatment of anti-sperm antibodies in the infertile male. Presented at The Western Section American Urological Association Annual Meeting, 1991.

100. Urry RL, Candle MR, Rote NS. Autoimmune infertility and recurrent abortion. In: Immunology in Obstetrics and Gynecology. Norwalk, CT: Appleton-Century-Crofts, 1985;77–106.

101. Kibrick S, Belding DL, Merrill B. Methods for the detection of antibodies against mammalian spermatozoa: II. A gelatin agglutination test. Fertil Steril 1952;3:430–438.

102. Isojima S, Li ST, Ashitaka Y. Immunologic analysis of sperm-immobilizing factor found in sera of women with unexplained sterility. Am J Obstet Gynecol 1968;101:677–684.

103. Clarke GN, Elliott PJ, Smaila C. Detection of sperm antibodies in semen using the immunobead test: a survey of 813 consecutive patients. Am J Reprod Immunol Microbiol 1985;7:118–126.

104. Clarke GN. Detection of antisperm antibodies using immunobeads. In: Keel BA, Webster BW, editors. Handbook of the Laboratory Diagnosis and Treatment of Infertility. Boca Raton, FL: CRC Press, 1990;177–192.

105. Cimino C, Barba G, Gusteila G, et al. An ELISA for antisperm antibody detection in serum: comparison w/TAT and SIT in serum, with MAR-test, immunobead test, and TAT in semen and with micro-SIT in cervical mucus. Acta Eur Fertil 1987;18:11–19.

CHAPTER 40

Medical Treatment of Male Infertility

CHRISTINA WANG and
RONALD S. SWERDLOFF

MANAGEMENT OF THE INFERTILE COUPLE

Infertility is a problem of the couple. The approach to the management of the infertile man includes the assessment and treatment of the female partner. We have reported in a study of patients attending a male infertility clinic that 17% of their female partners had ovulatory problems, 6% tubal disorders, and 8% endometriosis.[1] Treatment of correctable conditions in the woman frequently may lead to achievement of pregnancy despite the persistence of the male factor. It is imperative that the investigation and treatment strategy for the infertile couple be a coordinated effort by physicians attending the man (andrologists, urologists, endocrinologists) and those attending the female partner (gynecologists, reproductive endocrinologists).

MALE INFERTILITY EVALUATION

The evaluation of a male partner of an infertile couple includes detailed medical history, physical examination, semen analyses, and, in patients with azoospermia or severe oligospermia, measurements of serum levels of follicle-stimulating hormone (FSH), luteinizing hormone (LH), and testosterone.[2-4] The laboratory data are used to help identify the pathogenesis of the disorder and to provide guidance for therapy (Fig. 40–1). The methods and interpretation of the results of semen analyses are discussed in Chapter 38. Low serum FSH, LH, and testosterone levels associated with azoospermia indicate a hypothalamic-pituitary disorder. Serum prolactin level should be measured to exclude hyperprolactinemia. Other investigations should be directed to assess other anterior pituitary functions and to localize the lesion. High levels of FSH and LH in association with low testosterone and azoospermia or severe oligospermia point to pantesticular failure (dysfunction of Leydig cells, Sertoli cells, and germ cells). Isolated elevations of FSH associated with azoospermia or severe oligospermia indicate severe germinal epithelium damage and Sertoli cell dysfunction. This monotropic elevation of FSH may be due to the low levels of testicular secretion of inhibin and is a poor prognostic sign in a male patient with infertility. Combined elevations of LH and testosterone in the presence of normal or low FSH suggest that the gonadotropes are not sensitive to testosterone feedback and the presence of androgen resistance. In patients with normal hormone levels, normal-sized testes, and azoospermia, the diagnosis of genital tract obstruction and retrograde ejaculation must be excluded. Some patients with azoospermia and normal physical findings show significant disruption of spermatogenesis, most frequently germ cell arrest. In patients with oligospermia and normal hormonal levels, the clinical examination would have assessed the presence of a varicocele, and additional laboratory tests should be performed to exclude sperm autoimmunity (see Fig. 40–1).

Based on this information, the patient usually can be classified into one of the following common diagnostic categories (see Chapter 37): primary pantesticular failure (which occurs in about 10% to 15% of patients with male factor infertility), hypothalamic-pituitary dysfunction (1%), obstruction in the epididymis and vas deferens (8% to 10%), sperm autoimmunity (4% to 8%), sexual dysfunction (1%), and idiopathic causes (70% to 75%). Included in the last category are isolated germinal epithelium dysfunction presenting as azoospermia (no spermatozoa in ejaculate), oligospermia (low sperm concentration), asthenospermia (poor sperm motility), or teratozoospermia (increased percent of spermatozoa with abnormal morphology); patients with varicoceles or genital urinary tract infections; and a group of patients in whom no demonstrable abnormalities in semen analysis or hormonal assessment were found.[5-7]

MANAGEMENT OF MALE INFERTILITY

Depending on the probable diagnosis, a treatment category can usually be assigned (Table 40–1). The treatment cate-

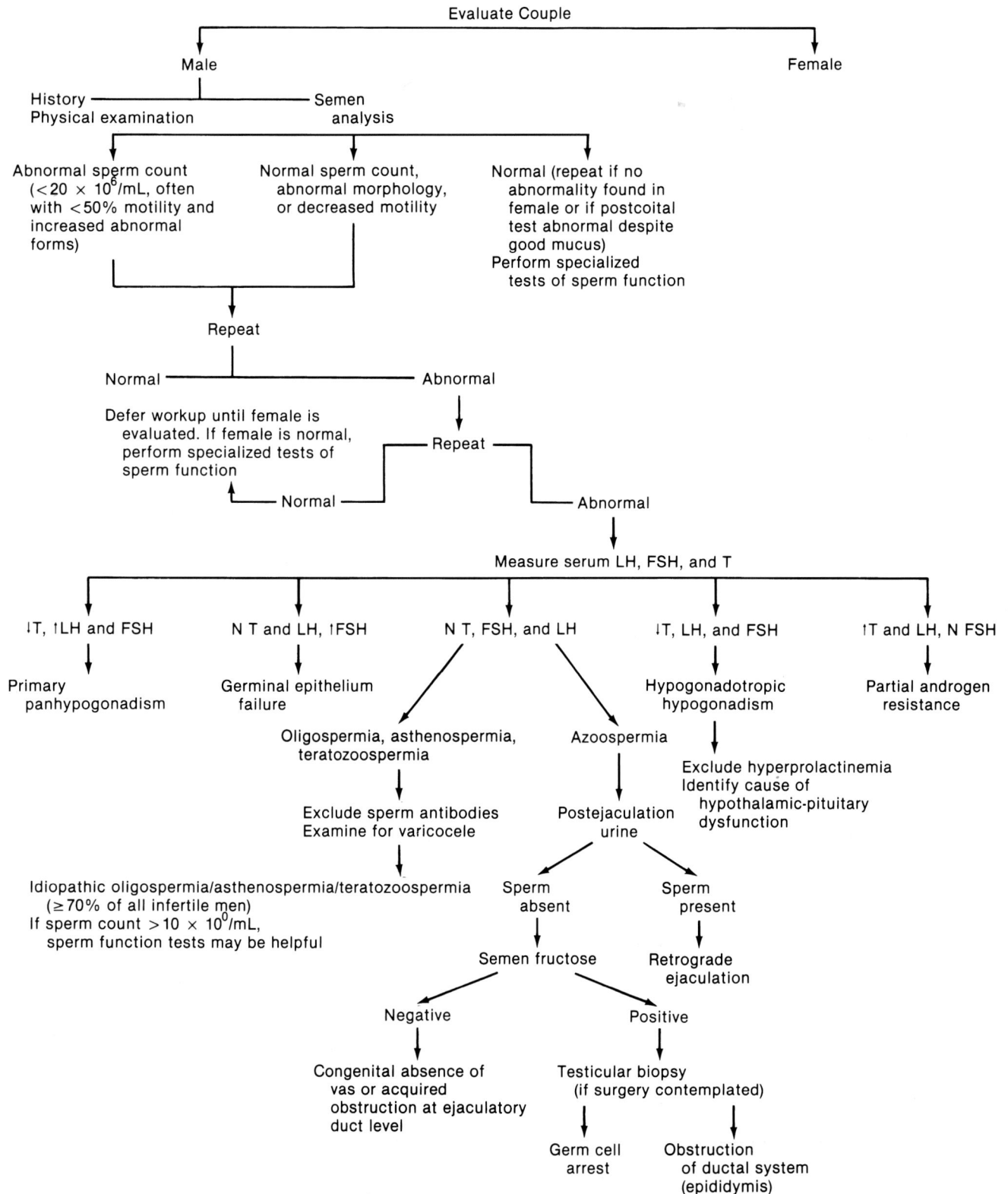

FIGURE 40–1. Evaluation of male infertility. T, testosterone; FSH, follicle-stimulating hormone; LH, luteinizing hormone; N, normal. (Adapted from Wang C, Swerdloff RS. Clinical and laboratory evaluation of male infertility. Am Assoc Clin Chem Endocrinol Metab 1992;10:9–15.)

TABLE 40–1. Treatment of Male Infertility

Category	Cause	Treatment
No treatment for infertility	Primary testicular failure	TDI or adoption Androgen replacement if indicated
Specific treatment	Hypogonadotropic hypogonadism Hyperprolactinemia Sexual dysfunction Obstructive azoospermia	Gonadotropins/GnRH Bromocriptine Counseling, AIH Vaso- or epididymovasostomy, microsurgical epididymal retrieval of spermatozoa for IVF

Value of treatment
  controversial/under investigation
	Varicocele
	
	Sperm autoimmunity
	Genital tract infection
	Idiopathic oligospermia, asthenospermia,
	  teratospermia, normozoospermia
		Varicocele ligation, ovarian hyperstimulation with
		  IUI, IVF
		Glucocorticoids, IVF
		Antibiotics
		Empiric treatment, IVF, ZIFT, micromanipulation

TDI, Therapeutic donor insemination; AIH, artificial insemination with husband spermatozoa; IUI, intrauterine insemination; IVF, in vitro fertilization; ZIFT, zygote intrafallopian transfer; GnRH, gonadotropin-releasing hormone.

gories can be classified into those in which no known treatment for infertility is available, specific treatment for infertility is appropriate, or the value of the treatment is still under evaluation or controversial. Surgical treatment, including those for varicocele, cryptorchidism, and obstructive azoospermia, is discussed in Chapter 42. Treatment of genital tract infections, sperm autoantibodies, and sexual dysfunction are discussed in Chapters 43, 44, and 45. The use of assisted reproductive technologies, including insemination with husband (AIH) or donor (DI) spermatozoa, in vitro fertilization (IVF), gamete or zygote intrafallopian transfer (GIFT or ZIFT), and gamete micromanipulation are discussed in Chapters 47, 48, 53, 54, and 60.

In this chapter, we focus on the medical management of male infertility, including specific therapies for hypothalamic-pituitary disorders and the empiric medical treatment strategies that have been administered to men with male factor infertility. We conclude with an algorithm outlining our recommendations for the management of male factor infertility.

NO KNOWN TREATMENT FOR INFERTILITY

Primary Testicular Disorder

In this category are included patients with chromosomal disorders (Klinefelter's syndrome and variants), testicular damage owing to infection (mumps, other viral infections), surgery, cryptorchidism, irradiation, drugs (chemotherapeutic agents), and toxins. These patients have persistent azoospermia, small testes, and elevated FSH. Their infertility is not treatable. The patients and their partners should be counseled regarding the options of therapeutic donor insemination (TDI) or adoption. In many patients with adult seminiferous tubule failure, isolated FSH increases are common. Some patients show impaired Leydig cell function associated with elevated LH and low testosterone levels. Those patients with low testosterone and high LH levels have androgen deficiency and should have testosterone replacement therapy because prolonged androgen deficiency leads to loss of bone and muscle mass, low hematocrit, and loss of sexual function. The patient should be advised that such treatment will not improve his sperm counts and correct the infertility.

The most commonly used androgens are testosterone esters, such as testosterone enanthate or cypionate. After an intramuscular injection of 200 (or 250) mg of testosterone enanthate, peak levels of testosterone are achieved within 1 to 3 days. The testosterone levels gradually decrease and reach baseline levels usually within 10 to 14 days (Fig. 40–2).[8] Most hypogonadal men respond well to 150 to 200 mg testosterone enanthate or cypionate once every 2 weeks. Occasionally, emotional changes and mood swings may occur preceding the injection. For these rare patients, 100 mg of testosterone enanthate can be administered every week. Although available in Europe, Asia, and Australia, testosterone undecanoate, an orally active testosterone ester, is not available in the United States. The drug is absorbed through the lymphatics, has a short duration of action, and must be taken several times per day. Another oral preparation, testosterone cyclodextrin, is still under development. Long-acting preparations of testosterone, such as testosterone encapsulated in

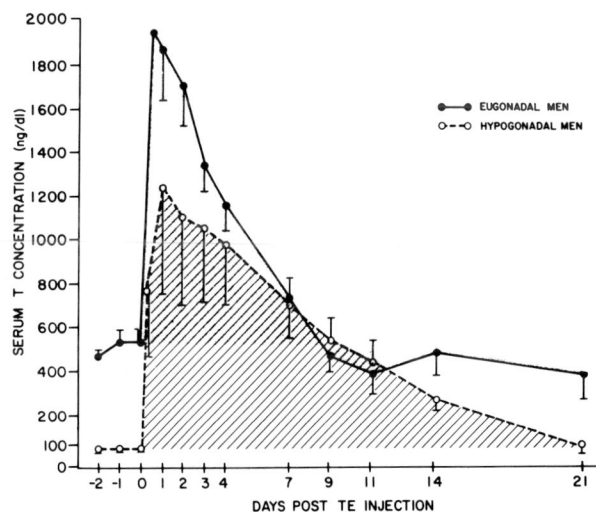

FIGURE 40–2. Mean and SE of testosterone (T) levels in eugonadal and hypogonadal men before and at various time intervals after an intramuscular injection of 200 mg of testosterone enanthate (TE). (From Sokol RZ, Palacios A, Campfield LA, Saul C, Swerdloff RS. Comparison of the kinetics of injectable testosterone in eugonadal and hypogonadal men. Fertil Steril 1982;37:425–30. Reproduced with permission of the publisher, The American Fertility Society.)

microcapsules or the long-acting testosterone ester, testosterone buciclate, can maintain normal testosterone levels in hypogonadal men for 10 to 12 weeks. The development of these long-acting preparations for treatment of the hypogonadal man will enable androgen replacement to be given in a more physiologic manner. Transdermal delivery systems of testosterone applied to scrotal skin leads to physiologic levels of testosterone and high 5α-dihydrotestosterone (DHT) levels. The pharmacologic significance of an elevated serum DHT-to-testosterone ratio is unknown. Further development with enhanced skin patches applied to nongenital skin may be required to decrease the DHT-to-testosterone ratios after application of these systems.[9-11]

Androgen Resistance Syndrome

A small proportion of infertile men with severe oligospermia or azoospermia have the features of androgen resistance syndrome.[12] These phenotypically normal men may present with gynecomastia and small testes. Laboratory investigations show high-normal to elevated LH, testosterone, and estradiol levels in the presence of normal FSH levels. Elevated estradiol levels are the result of the aromatization of high circulating levels of testosterone. The increased estrogen-to-androgen ratio may manifest clinically as gynecomastia. Diagnosis is confirmed by quantitative measurement or qualitative assessment of androgen receptors in skin fibroblasts obtained from genital skin. There is no specific treatment for infertility for these patients. Some men with partial androgen resistance may respond to high doses of testosterone.[13] A report showed that treatment with the antiestrogen, tamoxifen, in a man with classic features of incomplete androgen resistance syndrome led to an increase in FSH and improvement in semen quality and achievement of pregnancy in his partner.[14]

It has been suggested that a subtle form of incomplete androgen receptor deficiency may account for as many as 40% of men with idiopathic seminiferous tubule failure.[12, 15] These men have none of the features of classic androgen resistance, such as elevated LH in the presence of high testosterone levels. These studies have not been confirmed. Subsequent studies have demonstrated that androgen receptor levels are similar in fertile and infertile men.[16, 17] Moreover, the androgen receptor levels are similar in men with idiopathic oligospermia, cryptorchidism, or varicocele. Although a small subgroup of infertile men may have low androgen receptor levels, these men do not exhibit the clinical features of androgen resistance. They have normal LH and testosterone levels and can be fertile.[18] It is unlikely that abnormalities of the androgen receptor are the cause in the majority of patients with idiopathic oligospermia.

Structural Abnormality of Spermatozoa

In rare patients with total teratozoospermia (usually called globozoospermia) the ejaculates contain round-headed spermatozoa that are viable and motile but lack acrosome vesicles.[19, 20] These acrosomeless sperm heads do not bind or penetrate zona-free oocytes. Whether these abnormal spermatozoa can be directly microinjected into human oocytes to cause fertilization and subsequent cleavage and embryo de-

velopment has not yet been studied. Similarly, in the immotile cilia syndrome, in which all the spermatozoa are immotile owing to the absence of dynein arms in the sperm tails, the patients are infertile and have previously been classified as not treatable.[21] With the continued advancement and development of microinjection technology and gamete manipulation, it may be foreseeable in the future to inject tail-less human sperm heads directly into human oocytes to initiate pregnancy.

SPECIFIC THERAPY AVAILABLE FOR MALE INFERTILITY

Hypothalamic-Pituitary Disorders

Patients with hypothalamic-pituitary disorders are characterized by the association of hypogonadism with infertility. These patients have low serum FSH, LH, and testosterone levels. Organic causes, such as tumors and vascular, postinfective, surgical, postirradiation, or infiltrative lesions, should be excluded by radiologic investigations and treated appropriately. Other pituitary hormone deficiencies should be investigated and identified and appropriate hormone replacement given. Included in this group of patients with hypogonadotropic hypogonadism are those individuals with an idiopathic defect of gonadotropin-releasing hormone (GnRH) pulse generator. This defect can be isolated or associated with abnormal secretion of other hypothalamic hormones (such as growth hormone–releasing hormone and thyrotropin-releasing hormone). Isolated hypogonadotropic hypogonadism is often associated with anosmia or hyposmia (Kallmann's syndrome) and occasionally with other congenital midline defects, such as cleft palate and harelip. Multiple and frequent blood sampling in patients with hypogonadotropic hypogonadism may reveal an absence of pulsatile secretion of LH (which reflects absence of pulsatile GnRH secretion), sleep-entrained pulsatile LH secretion only (as in midpubertal children), or more subtle abnormalities in the amplitude or frequency of LH pulses.[22]

If fertility is not desired, the hypogonadism in these patients can be corrected with testosterone replacement therapy as discussed previously. When fertility is desired, stimulation of spermatogenesis can be achieved with gonadotropin or GnRH therapy. Prior treatment with testosterone therapy does not modify the subsequent responsiveness to gonadotropin therapy in terms of reinitiating spermatogenesis and fertility.[23, 24]

Gonadotropin therapy (Table 40–2) in the man is usually initiated with human chorionic gonadotropin (hCG, 1500 to 3000 IU) given intramuscularly two to three times per week for at least 6 months to stimulate testosterone secretion and initiate spermatogenesis. In some men, especially those with adult-onset hypogonadotropic hypogonadism, who previously have undergone normal puberty and adulthood, spermatogenesis can be reinitiated and maintained on hCG alone. In most patients with prepubertal onset of hypogonadotropic hypogonadism, addition of human menopausal gonadotropin (hMG, with FSH bioactivity), 37 to 150 units intramuscularly three times weekly, to the hCG therapy stimulates spermatogenesis, appearance of mature spermatozoa in the ejaculate, and fertility (Fig. 40–3). Before the initiation of gonadotropin

TABLE 40–2. Treatment of Hypogonadotropic Hypogonadism

Gonadotropins (intramuscular)

hCG 1500–3000 IU 2 or 3 × weekly for at least 6 months; if azoospermia persists, add

hMG 37–150 IU, 3 × weekly (once spermatogenesis is initiated, dose of hMG can be reduced to 37 IU or withdrawn)

GnRH Pulsatile administration with portable pump (intravenous or subcutaneous) 5–20 μg GnRH per pulse at 90–120-min intervals

hCG, Human chorionic gonadotropin; hMG, human menopausal gonadotropin; GnRH, gonadotropin-releasing hormone.

therapy, the female partner should be thoroughly assessed to exclude other causes of infertility. The treatment with hCG and hMG is continued until fertility is achieved. Frequently, pregnancy in the partner occurs when the sperm counts are considerably less than 20 million/mL (e.g., 5 to 10 million/mL). Once adequate spermatogenesis is initiated by hCG and hMG, hMG can be reduced or withdrawn.[25, 26] In most patients, the response is good, with the appearance of spermatozoa in the ejaculate after 6 to 18 months of therapy. It is important for the clinician and the patient to be aware that treatment with gonadotropins sometimes must be extended for up to 2 years before spermatogenesis is initiated. Patients with a prior history of cryptorchidism carry a poorer prognosis. Uncommonly, patients may develop antibodies to the hCG administered[27] and become resistant to treatment. Recombinant human FSH as well as human LH are under development and may replace hMG and hCG, respectively, for the induction of spermatogenesis.

Alternatively, patients with idiopathic hypogonadotropic hypogonadism can be treated with GnRH using portable, automatic-infusion pumps. Low physiologic doses, usually 5 to 20 μg per pulse (25 to 200 ng/kg), of GnRH are administered at 90- to 120-minute intervals subcutaneously or intravenously (see Table 40–2). Within 3 months of GnRH replacement, serum testosterone levels rise to the normal range in most men. Basal and GnRH-stimulated gonadotropins also increase to normal levels. With continued administration, spermatogenesis is stimulated, and fertility can be achieved. The ability of exogenous GnRH replacement to restore pituitary and testicular function to normal in patients with idiopathic hypogonadotropic hypogonadism confirms that this disorder is the result of an abnormal pattern of secretion of endogenous GnRH.[22] Rarely, patients fail to achieve normal pituitary and gonadal function because of the development of neutralizing antibody against GnRH.[28] The success rate in achieving fertility may be somewhat less with GnRH than with gonadotropin replacement therapy. Although more physiologic, pulsatile GnRH administration requires the patient to carry a portable pump with an indwelling catheter and may be more inconvenient for the patient. For these reasons, we recommend hCG and hMG as the therapeutic modality of choice for hypogonadotropic hypogonadism.

Hyperprolactinemia

Male patients with hyperprolactinemia usually present with sexual dysfunction, hypogonadism, and infertility. The diagnosis is made by the finding of elevated prolactin levels, often in association with low gonadotropin and testosterone levels. Drug-induced hyperprolactinemia should be excluded by history. In contrast to findings in women, most of the male patients with prolactinomas have macroadenomas. Treatment with bromocriptine must be individualized as to dose, but 2.5 mg three times per day often restores the prolactin levels to normal and shrinks the tumor mass.[29–31] In some patients with prolactinomas, serum gonadotropin and testosterone levels return to normal with bromocriptine administration, and spermatogenesis improves. In other patients, the tumor mass itself may have resulted in permanent dysfunction or loss of adjacent anterior pituitary cells secreting gonadotropin, and infertility persists even after correction of hyperprolactinemia. In patients with persistent hypogonadotropic hypogonadism, treatment with hCG and hMG is required for fertility, or testosterone combined with bromocriptine is necessary to correct the androgen deficiency.

NONSPECIFIC OR EMPIRIC THERAPY FOR MALE INFERTILITY

Special Problems Associated with Treatment of Male Infertility

There are many problems that are associated with the empiric treatment of idiopathic oligospermia, asthenospermia, and teratozoospermia. By definition, these are cases in which the pathophysiology of the infertility is unknown. In our experience, such patients belong to a heterogeneous group with different causes and have different degrees of injury to the germinal epithelium or disturbances of sperm maturation. Because this is true, empiric therapy is unlikely to be effective in a large percentage of patients.

Despite these reservations, multiple attempts have been made to develop new approaches to men with infertility of unknown cause. Analysis of therapeutic efficacy requires consideration of several factors. One factor is duration of treatment. Spermatogenesis in men is a highly regulated and orderly process and involves the development of the spermatogonium through mitosis, meiosis, and spermiogenesis to the mature spermatozoon. In the human, it takes about 72 days to achieve this maturation process when beginning from the earliest sperm precursors (spermatogonia).[32] Another 14 days is required for the spermatozoa to transverse the epididymis, vas deferens, and ejaculatory duct. For a potential therapy to affect spermatogenesis, the effect may not be seen in the semen sample until 90 days after the start of treatment. Consequently, new therapies that may affect early stages of spermatogenesis must be administered for at least 12 weeks and preferably 24 weeks before their effects can be adequately assessed.

A second consideration is ascertainment bias and the need for placebo-controlled trials. Individual semen analyses from a patient may be low, average, or high for a given individual. If the initial sperm count was low, an increase may be seen during "treatment" that is independent of the treatment provided. For example, in a double-blind, controlled study using erythromycin for treatment of low sperm motility, there were significant increases in sperm motility in both control and placebo groups. The selection of patients was based on low

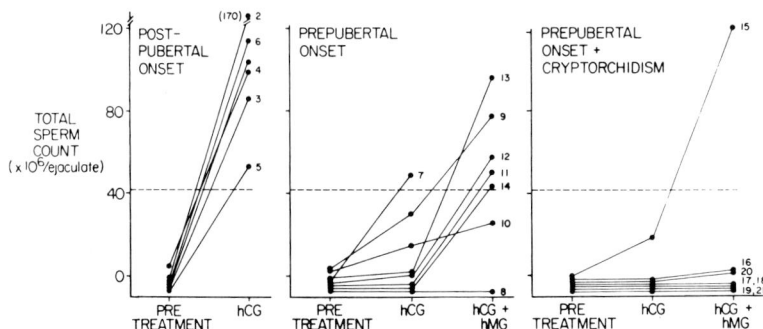

FIGURE 40–3. Effect of treatment with human chorionic gonadotropin (hCG) alone and in combination with human menopausal gonadotropin (hMG) on total sperm count. Pretreatment values are means of two determinations made before treatment; treatment values are means of the three highest determinations made during treatment. The *horizontal dashed line* represents the lower limit of normal. Numbers to the right of highest values denote patients listed in Table 1. In response to hCG alone, the sperm count increased to within the normal range in all 6 patients with postpubertal onset of hypogonadism but in only 1 of 15 with prepubertal onset ($P < 0.002$, contingency table analysis). In response to combined treatment, the count in the 14 other men with prepubertal onset increased to within the normal range in 5 of the 7 who had not had cryptorchidism but in only 1 of the 7 who had ($P < 0.05$). (Reprinted with permission from *The New England Journal of Medicine,* 313:654, 1985.)

sperm motility in the initial sample.[33] Similarly, in a double-blind, placebo-controlled trial with gonadotropins for severe oligospermia, both the placebo and the gonadotropin treatment group showed significant increases in sperm count during treatment.[34] The inherent variability of semen parameters highlights the importance of placebo-controlled trials in testing new agents for the treatment of male infertility.

Many studies reported in the literature have doubtful value because they are based on increases in semen quality or pregnancy rates in uncontrolled, poorly designed clinical trials. To conduct a controlled clinical trial for male infertility, Baker[35] proposed that the requirements should include the following: The prospective treatment should be promising, the subjects and their partners must be defined as completely as possible, all possible prognostic data should be collected, the subjects must be randomized to the treatment or placebo group,[36] there must be adequate numbers of subjects to allow meaningful statistical analyses, data should be analyzed by multiple regression,[37] and cumulative pregnancy rates should be calculated by life table analyses.[38]

Table 40–3 lists some of the empiric nonspecific therapies that have been used for the treatment of male infertility.[7, 39, 40] We discuss some of the more common therapies that have been tested in patients with idiopathic oligospermia, asthenospermia, and teratozoospermia, focusing on the more recently conducted placebo-controlled clinical trials.

TABLE 40–3. Empiric Medical Treatment for Idiopathic Oligozoospermia

Hormones	Others
GnRH	Kallikrein
Gonadotropins (hCG/hMG)	Pentoxifylline
Testosterone	Vitamin E (tocopherol)
Testosterone rebound	Andrenergic stimulants
Mesterolone	Amino acids
Antiandrogens	Antibiotics, anti-
Clomiphene citrate	inflammatory agents
Tamoxifen	Zinc
Aromatase inhibitor	
Testolactone	

GnRH, Gonadotropin-releasing hormone; hCG, human chorionic gonadotropin; hMG, human menopausal gonadotropin.

Gonadotropin-Releasing Hormone

Infertile men with severe oligospermia associated with monotropic increases in serum FSH are usually classified as having severe damage to seminiferous tubules. The prognosis in these patients is usually poor. Many of these patients with isolated increases in FSH have a decreased frequency of GnRH pulses. Short-term administration of pulsatile GnRH in physiologic doses (5 to 20 μg every 90 to 120 minutes) may lead to a progressive decrease in serum FSH levels into the normal range.[41, 42] These data suggest that changes in GnRH frequency may cause the changes in LH and FSH and may contribute to the defects in spermatogenesis in idiopathic oligozoospermia associated with selective elevation of FSH. Administration of pulsatile GnRH for 6 months to men with azoospermia or severe oligospermia and elevated FSH confirmed that FSH levels could be decreased and testosterone levels could be increased with GnRH pulsatile therapy. In some reports, however, the sperm concentrations in these patients did not improve after pulsatile GnRH therapy.[43, 44] Other groups have reported a stimulatory effect on sperm concentration by pulsatile GnRH therapy in men with severe or variable oligospermia with elevated FSH levels.[45, 46] Increases in sperm density and serum LH and a decrease in serum FSH were observed in patients with less severe germinal epithelium damage.[45] None of the studies included placebo-treated control subjects. As a consequence, no firm conclusions can be drawn. The use of pulsatile GnRH in patients with oligospermia and elevated FSH must be critically studied in double-blind, placebo-controlled trials before GnRH can be recommended for use in these patients with male infertility.

Gonadotropins

Gonadotropin replacement with hCG and hMG is highly successful in the treatment of male infertility secondary to hypothalamic-pituitary dysfunction. Based on these results, patients with idiopathic oligospermia have been treated with various combinations of gonadotropins despite obvious impairment in gonadotropin secretion. Improvement in sperm concentration and pregnancies in the partners have been reported after combined hCG and hMG or pure FSH therapy.[47–49] Once again, these results were based on uncontrolled studies. One placebo-controlled, double-blind trial of 39 men, randomly assigned to hCG (2500 IU twice a week) together with hMG (150 IU three times a week, 19 men) or placebo (same injections of saline, 20 men) treatment for 13 weeks, noted improvement in sperm concentrations in both the control and the hCG/hMG group. As discussed previously, this was due to inherent variability in sperm concentrations within each subject, with the treatment frequently started at the nadir of semen parameters. Treatment with either placebo or the active agent was associated with increasing sperm counts independent of the treatment (i.e., so-called regression toward the mean). Comparison with the placebo-treated controls showed that hMG/hCG had no significant effect on semen parameters.[34] The study showed that although gonadotropins were increased to above the physiologic range, sperm production was not improved. Because most oligospermic men do not have a deficiency of gonadotropins, gonadotropin treatment lacks a rational basis, has inconsistent results, and is not recommended at present for idiopathic male infertility.

The use of pure FSH in the treatment of severe oligospermia in the male partners of couples attending IVF programs was studied.[50] Although no significant improvement in semen parameters occurred after pure FSH treatment (150 IU three times a week for 3 months), there was a significant increase in fertilization rate in IVF (before FSH, 12% fertilization; after FSH, 49% fertilization). There were no pregnancies before FSH treatment and two pregnancies after FSH treatment. Although these preliminary results may be encouraging, one should note that the number of patients studied was relatively small (n = 36), the patients served as their own control based on data from a prior IVF cycle, there was no concurrent placebo control group, and improvement in fertilization was observed in vitro and not in vivo. A multicenter placebo-controlled trial to test the effectiveness of recombinant FSH improving fertility in male partners with severe oligospermia before an IVF cycle is being conducted to answer some of these questions.

Androgens

Testosterone enanthate given every week to normal men for about 3 to 4 months suppresses gonadotropins and leads to azoospermia in about 60% of the subjects. Heller and colleagues,[51] however, noted that in some oligospermic men, the suppression of spermatogenesis by testosterone was followed by recovery with substantial rebound in the sperm concentration. Since this early observation, several uncontrolled clinical trials have demonstrated that many infertile men who had been given *testosterone rebound therapy* (testosterone enanthate or cypionate, 100 to 200 mg every week) had variable increases in sperm count and pregnancy rates.[52–54] In some patients with severe oligospermia, the suppression of spermatogenesis persists for many months after testosterone withdrawal. In a placebo-controlled trial, we showed that testosterone enanthate, 100 or 200 mg every 2 weeks, did not improve sperm count or motility. There were no pregnan-

cies in either the placebo-treated or the testosterone-treated group.[55]

Other types of oral androgens, such as testosterone undecanoate, have also been used to treat idiopathic oligospermia. Testosterone undecanoate at the usual replacement dose (120 mg/day) resulted in improvement in semen parameters in one study but did not improve the pregnancy rate.[56] In another study, testosterone undecanoate (240 mg/day) was administered to men with idiopathic male infertility, but no changes in sperm characteristics were reported, and no improvement in pregnancy rate was observed.[57] High-dose testosterone therapy would seem to be illogical because suppression of LH and FSH and inhibition of spermatogenesis may occur.

Mesterolone (1α-methyl-5α-androstan-17β-ol-3-one, Proviron), a weak androgen that does not significantly suppress gonadotropins, has been widely used as empiric treatment for idiopathic oligospermia, especially in Europe. In a randomized, placebo-controlled trial involving more than 200 men, mesterolone increased semen parameters but did not improve pregnancy rates.[58] In other randomized, placebo-controlled studies, mesterolone did not significantly improve the results of semen analysis or pregnancy rates.[55, 59, 60] The World Health Organization[61] conducted a multicenter, double-blind, randomized study using two doses of mesterolone (75 or 150 mg/day) versus placebo in 157 infertile couples. Sperm concentration rose 3 months after the start of treatment in all groups, but the increase was greatest in the placebo-treated group and did not differ between the groups. There were no significant changes in sperm motility, viability, or morphology. The cumulative pregnancy rates were $11 \pm 5\%$ in the placebo, $12 \pm 5\%$ in the 75-mg-mesterolone, and $19 \pm 6\%$ in the 150-mg mesterolone groups. The pregnancy rates in the three groups did not differ significantly. Because of these findings, the World Health Organization is currently conducting a second multicenter trial comparing 150 mg mesterolone with placebo in seven centers, where 360 couples will be enrolled for study.[61] A preliminary report of a placebo-controlled trial with high-dose mesterolone (150 mg/day) showed that mesterolone had no advantage over placebo in improving sperm count, motility, and morphology or overall pregnancy rates.[62] Based on studies conducted to date, it is unlikely that mesterolone has any beneficial effects in patients with idiopathic male infertility.

Antiestrogens

Antiestrogens, by virtue of their ability to bind to estrogen receptors, lead to a decrease in negative feedback by estrogens on the reproductive hormone axis (predominantly on the hypothalamus). Thus administration of antiestrogen results in increases in GnRH secretion and elevations in serum FSH and LH levels. In concept, the increased LH stimulates intratesticular testosterone production and may improve spermatogenesis. This rationale is similar to that for gonadotropin treatment. Because of the inherent estrogenic activity of the antiestrogen clomiphene citrate, high dosages (200 to 400 mg/day) may lead to suppression of spermatogenesis. Lower dosages (25 to 50 mg/day) of clomiphene citrate have been reported to produce beneficial effects on semen parameters.[63] Numerous uncontrolled trials have reported variable increases in sperm concentration (0 to 80%) and pregnancy rates (0 to 90%) (for review, see reference[40]). Independent placebo-controlled trials of clomiphene citrate in oligospermic men have been performed by several groups. In some placebo-controlled studies, clomiphene citrate at 25 to 50 mg/day caused mild increases in sperm concentration without improving sperm motility and morphology.[55, 64] Pregnancy occurred in 10% and 28% of the patients receiving clomiphene citrate compared with 3% and 0% in the placebo groups. The responsiveness of the infertile men to clomiphene citrate, however, was variable. Pregnancy occurred mainly in the patients with mild or moderate oligospermia (more than 10 million per milliliter).[55, 64] In another study, clomiphene citrate did not enhance sperm fertilizing capacity as assessed by the zona-free hamster oocyte test.[65] In a more recent study comparing the effects of clomiphene citrate with placebo, no significant changes in the semen parameters or pregnancy in partners were noted.[66] The World Health Organization[67] conducted a multicenter, double-blind study of the effects of placebo versus clomiphene citrate in men with idiopathic oligospermia and was unable to document any significant improvement in pregnancy rates in patients treated with clomiphene citrate. From the available data, clomiphene citrate is not beneficial for patients with idiopathic oligospermia. Occasionally a patient may respond to 25 to 50 mg of clomiphene citrate given for 4 to 5 months. Unfortunately, it is not yet possible to identify which patient would respond to this treatment.

Because tamoxifen is an antiestrogen without demonstrable intrinsic estrogenic activity in men, it may have some advantage over clomiphene. Tamoxifen (20 mg/day) was reported to increase sperm concentrations in patients with mild or moderate oligospermia.[68] Subsequent placebo-controlled studies showed that therapy with tamoxifen in idiopathic male infertility had no significant effects on sperm count, motility, in vitro fertilizing capacity, or pregnancy rates in the partners.[69–71] In one of these trials,[69] the patients had mild oligospermia (sperm concentration averaging 17×10^6/mL). In our opinion, it is unlikely that tamoxifen will have any beneficial effect on spermatogenesis in most men with idiopathic oligospermia.

Aromatase Inhibitors

Because experimental studies have shown that excess estradiol can be directly toxic to the germinal epithelium and can decrease testosterone biosynthesis,[72, 73] decreasing estradiol production by aromatase inhibitors may improve spermatogenesis and fertility. The aromatase inhibitor testolactone (1 g/day) was shown to increase sperm counts and pregnancy rates in the partners in several uncontrolled studies.[74, 75] In a randomized, placebo-controlled, double-blind, cross-over trial, 25 subjects were given testolactone (2 g/day) or placebo for 8 months followed by cross-over to the other treatment for another 8 months. Testolactone led to small but significant increases in FSH, LH, and free testosterone levels and decreases in sex hormone–binding globulin levels, but sperm concentration, motility, and morphology remained unchanged. No pregnancy occurred in the placebo or in the testolactone group. The study documented that testolactone at that dose failed to maintain inhibition of the aromatase

enzyme over a protracted period of time and that this drug was not useful in idiopathic oligospermia.[76]

Phosphodiesterase Inhibitors

Phosphodiesterase inhibitors prevent the breakdown of cyclic adenosine monophosphate (AMP) and thus result in increased intracellular cyclic AMP. Because increases in cyclic AMP may cause increases in sperm motility,[77] these agents have been used to treat patients with oligoasthenospermia. Uncontrolled clinical trials suggested that pentoxifylline (a phosphodiesterase inhibitor), 400 mg three times per day, increases sperm motility and count.[78, 79] Subsequent placebo-controlled studies showed that pentoxifylline had no effect on semen parameters or fertility in patients with idiopathic oligoasthenospermia.[55]

Phosphodiesterase inhibitors, including pentoxifylline, have been used to treat spermatozoa in vitro before use of assisted reproductive technologies. These early studies showed some improvement in sperm motility and fertilization rate in semen samples from oligospermic men undergoing IVF.[80, 81] The results of these studies currently are being tested and must be confirmed by other groups.

Other Drugs

Many other drugs have been used for the treatment of idiopathic male infertility (see Table 40–3). Many of these therapies have no rational basis, whereas others may have some beneficial effect on sperm motility in in vitro studies.

Kallikrein stimulates the release of kinins, which may affect the smooth muscle contraction and vascular permeability. Kallikrein has been shown to have a stimulating effect on sperm motility in vitro.[82] Although several placebo-controlled studies with small numbers of men reported some beneficial effect on sperm motility, the actual sperm motility achieved after treatment remained below the normal range. Moreover, many of these subjects had normospermia.[82–84] These studies were not confirmed by others.[85]

Tocopherol (vitamin E), an antioxidant, has been reported to increase the efficacy of sperm penetration in vitro and improve zona-free hamster oocyte penetration tests, probably by reducing the generation of reactive oxygen molecules.[86] These agents, however, similar to the many others listed in Table 40–3, have not been critically assessed in clinical trials and cannot be recommended for use in the treatment of idiopathic male infertility.

Recommended Approach to the Management of Male Infertility

In patients with azoospermia, determination of serum hormone levels is essential for both diagnosis and management. For patients with severe germinal epithelium damage, germ cell arrest, or pantesticular failure, no treatment for their infertility is available. Testosterone replacement is essential for men with androgen deficiency. In patients with hypogonadotropic hypogonadism, testosterone replacement is given

Azoospermia

↓T,↑LH and FSH   N LH and T,↑FSH   N FSH, LH, and T   ↓FSH, LH, and T   ↓T and LH, N FSH

Primary
hypogonadism

Severe
germinal
epithelium
damage

Germ
cell
arrest

Obstructive
azoospermia

Retrograde
ejaculation

Partial
androgen
resistance

Testosterone
replacement

Epididymovasostomy or
vasovasostomy

Hypogonadotropic
hypogonadism

Microsurgical epididymal
aspiration of spermatozoa
and IVF or ZIFT

hCG/hMG
(GnRH)

No treatment
for infertility

Psychological
assessment,
medication,
electroejaculation,
and IUI

?High dose
T

DI or adoption

?Antiestrogen

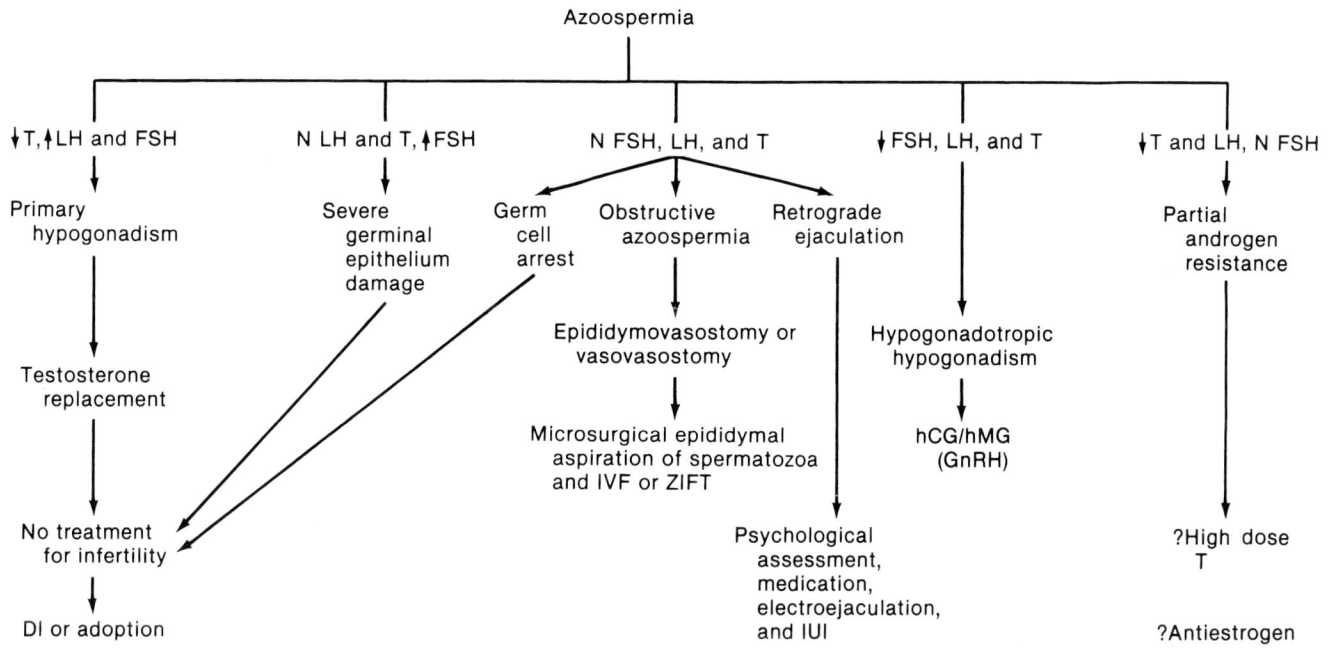

FIGURE 40–4. Schematic of approach to the management of a patient with azoospermia. T, testosterone; FSH, follicle-stimulating hormone; LH, luteinizing hormone; N, normal; IUI, intrauterine insemination; DI, donor insemination; IVF, in vitro fertilization; ZIFT, zygote intrafallopian transfer; GIFT, gamete intrafallopian transfer; GnRH, gonadotropin-releasing hormone; hCG, human chorionic gonadotropin; hMG, human menopausal gonadotropin.

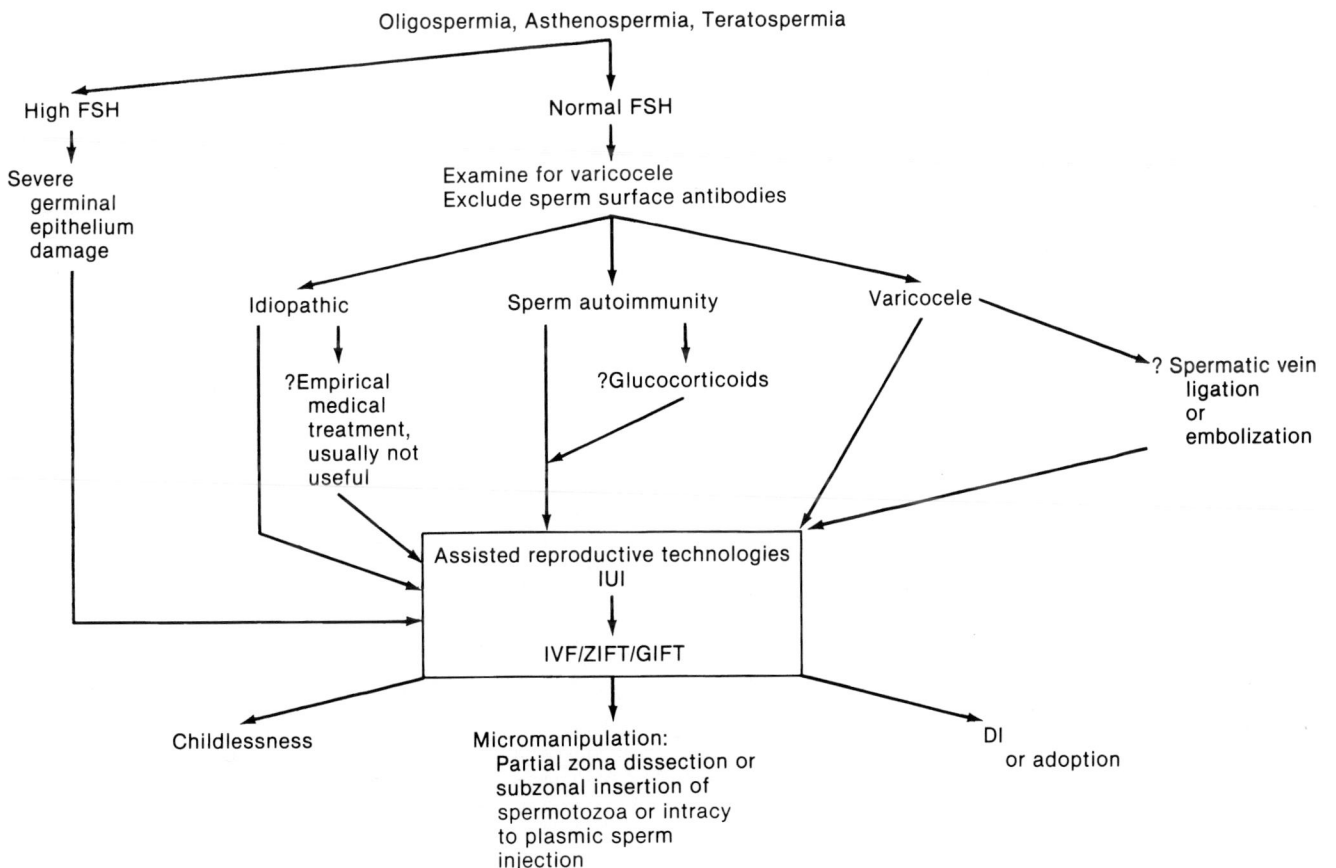

Oligospermia, Asthenospermia, Teratospermia

High FSH   Normal FSH

Severe
germinal
epithelium
damage

Examine for varicocele
Exclude sperm surface antibodies

Idiopathic   Sperm autoimmunity   Varicocele

?Empirical
medical
treatment,
usually not
useful

?Glucocorticoids

? Spermatic vein
ligation
or
embolization

Assisted reproductive technologies
IUI

IVF/ZIFT/GIFT

Childlessness   Micromanipulation:
Partial zona dissection or
subzonal insertion of
spermotozoa or intracy
to plasmic sperm
injection

DI
or adoption

FIGURE 40–5. Schematic of approach to the management of a patient with oligospermia, asthenospermia, or teratospermia. See Figure 40–4 for abbreviations.

until fertility is desired. The patients are then treated with hCG together with hMG (or pulsatile GnRH therapy) for induction of spermatogenesis. In the rare patient with androgen resistance, treatment with high-dose testosterone does not improve the spermatogenesis but may correct some of the features of hypogonadism. Treatment with antiestrogens is still considered experimental. Patients with obstructive azoospermia should be referred to urologists for corrective surgery (see Chapter 42), and those with retrograde ejaculation (see Chapter 45) require full neurologic assessment (Fig. 40–4).

For patients with oligospermia, asthenospermia, or teratozoospermia, serum FSH should be measured because elevated FSH levels usually indicate more severe dysfunction of the germinal epithelium. In these patients, the presence of a varicocele should be excluded by a careful physical examination, and sperm autoimmunity should be excluded by testing for sperm surface antibodies. Treatment of these conditions is discussed in subsequent chapters. Because empiric medical therapy has in general been proved to be of value in the management of idiopathic male infertility, there is little point in providing such therapy. Because these therapies have been discussed widely in publications on infertility, however, it is important to discuss the therapies with the couple and the reasons for withholding therapy. The possibility of intra-uterine insemination (IUI) with the male partner's spermatozoa and of IVF, ZIFT, or GIFT should then be discussed and offered to the couple. In the patient with severe oligospermia or failed IVF, ZIFT, or GIFT, the specialized techniques of micromanipulation to achieve fertilization and pregnancy, as a last resort, should also be discussed with the couple (Fig. 40–5). These maneuvers, however, are certainly experimental, and controlled trials documenting efficacy do not exist.

SUMMARY

Unless the infertile man has a treatable and identifiable cause of infertility, such as hypogonadotrophic hypogonadism, none of the medical treatment regimens has been proved to be clearly effective. The heterogeneous nature of the cause, the inherent variability of the degree of dysfunction of the germinal epithelium, and the lack of understanding of intra-testicular control of spermatogenesis make rational treatment of most male patients with infertility difficult. The assisted reproductive technologies, however, may provide some hope,[87, 88] based on the rationale that fewer motile, normal spermatozoa are required for fertilization in vitro. If the patient is severely oligozoospermic and, in particular, when sperm morphology is grossly abnormal, the success rate in IVF procedures is markedly decreased.[89, 90] The fertilization rate of human oocytes in vitro may be decreased to one half to one third compared with fertilization rates in couples with nonmale factor infertility (e.g., to less than 30%). In some of these patients, micromanipulation techniques, such as partial zona dissection, may be useful.[91, 92] Patients with severe impairment of sperm count (less than 5 million/mL), motility (less than 20%), or morphology (less than 10% normal) might be candidates for microinjection of spermatozoa into the perivitelline space or directly into the oocytes.[93, 94] Before such micromanipulation procedures are undertaken, however, the couple must be advised of the other options, such

as donor insemination and adoption. More importantly, the couples should be counseled on the low success rate of pregnancy and the even lower success rate of a "take-home baby" (probably less than 5%) with micromanipulation of gametes. These techniques are clearly experimental at this time. Because of these low success rates and the absence of any rational medical treatment, the physician's role in counseling the infertile couple remains important. The physician must discuss with the couple the probable diagnosis, the treatment options and alternatives, and frequently the poor prognosis even with the state-of-the-art assisted reproductive technologies. Most important of all, the physician must remain the infertile couple's primary counselor and resource for any problems, physical and emotional, associated with male factor infertility.

REFERENCES

1. Wang C, Chan SYW, Ng M, et al. Diagnostic value of sperm function tests and routine semen analysis in fertile and infertile men. J Androl 1988;9:384–389.
2. Swerdloff RS, Wang C, Kandeel FC. Evaluation of the infertile couple. Endocrinol Metab Clin North Am 1988;17:301–331.
3. Swerdloff RS, Wang C, Sokol RZ. Endocrine evaluation of the infertile male. In: Lipshultz LI, Howards SS, editors. Infertility in the Male. St. Louis: Mosby-Year Book, 1991:179–210.
4. Wang C, Swerdloff RS. Evaluation of testicular function. In: DeKretser D, editor. Bailliere' Clinical Endocrinology and Metabolism: The Testis. London: Bailliere Tindall, 1992:405–434.
5. Baker HWG, Burger HG. Male infertility. In: Steinberger E, Fraiese G, Steinberger A, editors. Reproductive Medicine. New York: Raven Press, 1986:187–197.
6. Burger HG, Baker HWG. The treatment of infertility. Palo Alto: Annual Reviews, Inc., 1987;38:29–46.
7. Wang C, Swerdloff RS. Male infertility: overview of current therapy. In: Boutaleb Y, Gzouli A, editors. The Treatment of Infertility. Carnforth: Parthenon, 1991:19–24.
8. Sokol RZ, Palacios A, Campfield LA, et al. Comparison of the kinetics of injectable testosterone in eugonadal men. Fertil Steril 1982;37:425–430.
9. Nieschlag E, Behre HM. Testosterone. Action, Deficiency, Substitution. Berlin: Springer Verlag, 1991.
10. Swerdloff RS, Wang C. Androgen replacement therapy. In: Bardin CW, editor. Current Therapy in Endocrinology and Metabolism. Philadelphia: BC Decker; 1991:683–694.
11. Wang C, Swerdloff RS. Androgens. In: Smith CM, Raynard AM, editors. Textbook of Pharmacology. Philadelphia: WB Saunders, 1991:683–694.
12. Aimen J, Griffin JE, Gazak JM, et al. Androgen insensitivity as a cause of infertility in otherwise normal men. N Engl J Med 1979;300:223–227.
13. Price P, Wass JAH, Griffin JE, et al. High dose androgen therapy in male pseudo hermaphroditism due to 5 α reductase deficiency and disorders of androgen receptor. J Clin Invest 1984;74:1496–1508.
14. Gooren L. Improvement of spermatogenesis after treatment with the antiestrogen tamoxifen in men with incomplete androgen insensitivity syndrome. J Clin Endocrinol Metab 1989;68:1207–1210.
15. Aiman J, Griffin JE: The frequency of androgen receptor deficiency in men. J Clin Endocrinol Metab 1982;54:725–732.
16. Bouchard P, Wright F, Portois MC, et al. Androgen insensitivity in oligospermic men: a reappraisal. J Clin Endocrinol Metab 1986;63:1242–1246.
17. Eil C, Gamblin GT, Hodge JW, et al. Whole cell and nuclear androgen uptake in skin fibroblasts from infertile men. J Androl 1985;6:365–371.
18. Morrow AF, Gyorki S, Warne GL, et al. Variable receptor levels in infertile men. J Clin Endocrinol Metab 1987;64:1115–1121.
19. Lalonde L, Langlais J, Antaki P, et al. Male infertility associated with round-headed acrosomeless spermatozoa. Fertil Steril 1988;49:316–324.
20. Syms AJ, Johnson AR, Lipschultz LI, Smith RG. Studies on human spermatozoa with round head syndrome. Fertil Steril 1984;42:431–437.
21. Eliasson R, Mossberg B, Camner P, Afzelius BA. The immotile-cilia

syndrome: a congenital ciliary abnormality as an etiologic factor in chronic airway infections and male sterility. N Engl J Med 1977;297:1–6.

22. Crowley WF, Filiconi M, Spratt D, Sandoro N. The physiology of gonadotropin-releasing hormone (GnRH) secretion in men and women. Rec Prog Horm Res 1985;41:473–531.

23. Burger HG, de Kretser DM, Hudson JB, Wilson JD. Effects of preceding androgen therapy on testicular response to human pituitary gonadotropin in hypogonadotropic hypogonadism: a study of three patients. Fertil Steril 1981;35:64–68.

24. Ley SB, Leonard JM. Male hypogonadotropic hypogonadism: factors influencing response to human chorionic gonadotropin, including prior exogenous androgens. J Clin Endocrinol Metab 1987;61:746.

25. Finkel DM, Phillips JL, Snyder PJ. Stimulation of spermatogenesis by gonadotropins in men with hypogonadotropic hypogonadism. N Engl J Med 1985;313:651–655.

26. Sherins RJ. Evaluation and management of men with hypogonadotropic hypogonadism. In: Garcia CR, Mastroianni L, Amelar RD, Dubin L, editors. Current Therapy in Infertility. Philadelphia: BC Decker, 1984:147–151.

27. Sokol RZ, McClure RD, Peterson M, Swerdloff RS. Gonadotropin therapy failure secondary to hCG induced antibodies. J Clin Endocrinol Metab 1981;52:929–933.

28. Santoro N, Fillconi M, Crowley WF. Hypogonadotropic disorders in men and women: diagnosis and therapy with pulsatile gonadotropin-releasing hormone. Endocr Rev 1986;7:11–23.

29. Molitch ME, Etton RL, Blackwell RE, et al. Bromocriptine as primary therapy for prolactin secreting macroadenomas: results of a prospective multicenter study. J Clin Endocrinol Metab 1985;60:698–705.

30. Thorner MO, Martin WH, Rogol AD, et al. Rapid regression of pituitary prolactinomas during bromocriptine treatment. J Clin Endocrinol Metab 1980;51:438–445.

31. Wang C, Lam KSL, Ma JTC, et al. Long-term treatment of hyperprolactinaemia with bromocriptine: effect of drug withdrawal. Clin Endocrinol 1987;27:363–371.

32. Heller CG, Clermont Y. Kinetics of the germinal epithelium in man. Rec Prog Horm Res 1964;20:545–571.

33. Baker HWG, Stratton WGE, McGowan MP, et al. A controlled trial of erythromycin for asthenospermia. Int J Androl 1984;7:383–388.

34. Knuth VA, Honigl W, Bals-Pratsch M, et al. Treatment of severe oligospermia with human chorionic gonadotropin: a placebo-controlled, double blind trial. J Clin Endocrinol Metab 1987;65:1081–1087.

35. Baker HWG. Development of clinical trails in male infertility research. In: Serio M, editor. Perspectives in Andrology. New York: Raven Press, 1989:367–374.

36. Altman DC. Randomization. Essential for reducing bias. Br Med J 1991;302:1481–1482.

37. Peterson HB, Kleinbaum DG. Interpreting the literature in obstetrics and gynecology. II. Logistic regression and other related issues. Obstet Gynecol 1991;78:717–720.

38. Olive DL. Analysis of clinical fertility trials: a methodologic review. Fertil Steril 1986;45:157–171.

39. Haidl G, Schill WB. Guidelines for drug treatment of male infertility. Drugs 1991;41:60–68.

40. Sigman M, Vance ML. Medical treatment of idiopathic infertility. Urol Clin North Am 1987;14:459–469.

41. Gross KM, Matsumoto AM, Berger RE, Bremner WJ. Increased frequency of pulsatile luteinizing hormone-releasing hormone administration selectively decreases follicle-stimulating hormone in men with idiopathic azoospermia. Fertil Steril 1986;45:392–396.

42. Honigl W, Knuth VA, Nieschlag E. Selective reduction of elevated FSH levels in infertile men by pulsatile LHRH treatment. Clin Endocrinol 1986;24:177–182.

43. Bals-Pratsch M, Knuth UA, Honigl W, et al. Pulsatile GnRH-therapy in oligozoospermic men does not improve seminal parameters despite decreased FSH levels. Clin Endocrinol 1989;30:549–560.

44. Matsumoto AM, Gross KM, Sheckter CB, Bremner WJ. The luteinizing hormone-releasing hormone pulse generator in men: abnormalities and clinical management. Am J Obstet Gynecol 1990;163:1743–1752.

45. Aulitzky W, Frick J, Hadziselimovic F. Pulsatile LHRH therapy in patients with oligozoospermia and disturbed LH pulsatility. Int J Androl 1989;12:265–272.

46. Wagner TOF, von zur Muhlen A. Slow pulsing oligospermia: treatment by long time pulsatile LHRH therapy. In: Wagner TOF, Filiconi M, editors. Episodic Hormone Secretion from Basic Science to Clinical Application. Hemelin: Verlag, 1987:197–225.

47. Homonnai ZT, Peled M, Paz GF. Changes in semen quality and fertility in response to endocrine treatment of subfertile men. Gynecol Obstet Invest 1978;9:244–255.

48. Lunenfeld B, Olchovsky D, Tadir Y, Alzerman M. Treatment of male infertility with human gonadotrophins: selection of cases, management and results. Andrologia 1979;11:331–336.

49. Schill WB, Jungst D, Unterburger P, Braun S. Combined hCG/hMG treatment in subfertile men with idiopathic normogonadotrophic oligozoospermia. Int J Androl 1982;5:467–477.

50. Acosta AA, Oehninger S, Ertunc H, Philport C. Possible role of pure human follicle-stimulating hormone in the treatment of severe male-factor infertility by assisted reproduction: preliminary report. Fertil Steril 1991;55:1150–1156.

51. Heller CG, Nelson WD, Hill IB, et al. Improvement in spermatogenesis following depression of the human testis with testosterone. Fertil Steril 1950;1:415–522.

52. Charny CW, Gordon JA. Testosterone rebound therapy: a neglected modality. Fertil Steril 1978;29:64–68.

53. Lamensdorf H, Compere D, Begley G. Testosterone rebound therapy in the treatment of male infertility. Fertil Steril 1975;26:469–472.

54. Rowley MJ, Heller CG. The testosterone rebound phenomenon in the treatment of male infertility. Fertil Steril 1972;23:498–504.

55. Wang C, Chan CW, Wong KK, Yeung KK. Comparison of the effectiveness of placebo, clomiphene citrate, mesterolone, pentoxifylline and testosterone rebound therapy for the treatment of idiopathic oligospermia. Fertil Steril 1983;40:358–365.

56. Pusch HH. Oral treatment of oligozoospermia with testosterone undecanoate: results of a double-blind placebo-controlled trial. Andrologia 21:76–82, 1989.

57. Comhaire F. Treatment of idiopathic testicular failure with high-dose testosterone undecanoate: a double blind pilot study. Fertil Steril 1990;54:689–693.

58. Mauss J. The results of the treatment of fertility disorders in the male with mesterolone or placebo. Arzneimittel-Forschung 1974;24:1338–1341.

59. Aafjes JH, van der Vijver JCM, Brugman FW, Schenck PE. Double-blind cross over treatment with mesterolone and placebo of subfertile oligozoospermic men, value of testicular biopsy. Andrologia 1983;15:531–535.

60. Hargreave TB, Kyle KF, Baxby K, et al. Randomized trial of mesterolone versus vitamin C for male infertility. Br J Urol 1984;56:740–744.

61. World Health Organization. Task Force on the Diagnosis and Treatment of Infertility. Mesterolone and idiopathic male infertility: a double-blind study. Int J Androl 1989;12:254–264.

62. Genis J, Comhaire F, Hellemars P, et al. Placebo-controlled trial of high-dose mesterolone treatment of idiopathic male infertility. Fertil Steril 1991;55:603–607.

63. Heller CG, Rowley NJ, Heller CV. Clomiphene citrate: a correlation of its effect on sperm concentration and morphology, total gonadotrophins, LH, estrogens and testosterone excretion and testicular cytology in normal men. J Clin Endocrinol Metab 1969;29:638–649.

64. Ronnberg L. The effect of clomiphene treatment on different sperm parameters in men with idiopathic oligozoospermia. Andrologia 1980;12:261–265.

65. Wang C, Chan SYW, Tang LCH, Yeung KK. Clomiphene citrate does not improve spermatozoal fertilizing capacity in idiopathic oligospermia. Fertil Steril 1985;44:102–105.

66. Sokol RZ, Steiner BS, Bustillo M, et al. A controlled comparison of the efficacy of clomiphene citrate in male infertility. Fertil Steril 1988;49:865–870.

67. World Health Organization. Special Programme of Research, Development and Research Training in Human Reproduction Annual Technical Report 1990. Geneva: World Health Organization, 1991:146–147.

68. Vermeulen A, Comhaire F. Hormonal effects of an antiestrogen, tamoxifen, in normal and oligospermic men. Fertil Steril 1978;29:320–327.

69. Ain Melk Y, Belisle S, Carmel M, Jean-Pierre T. Tamoxifen citrate therapy in male infertility. Fertil Steril 1987;48:113–117.

70. Torok L. Treatment of oligozoospermia with tamoxifen; open and controlled studies. Andrologia 1985;17:497–501.

71. Willis KJ, London DR, Bevis MA, et al. Hormonal effects of tamoxifen in oligospermic men. J Endocrinol 1977;73:171–178.

72. Ciaccio LA, Joseph AA, Kinel FA. Direct inhibition of testicular function in rats by estriol and progesterone. J Steroid Biochem 1978;9:1257–1259.

73. Samuels LT, Short G, Huseby RA. The effect of diethylstilbesterol on testicular 17α-hydroxylase and 17-desmolase activities in Balb/c mice. Acta Endocrinol 1964;45:487–497.

74. Dony JMJ, Smals AGH, Rolland R, et al. Effect of chronic aromatase inhibition by Δ^1-testolactone on pituitary-gonadal function in oligozoospermic men. Andrologia 1986;18:69–74.

75. Vigersky RA, Glass AR. Effect of testolactone on the pituitary-testicular axis in oligozoospermic men. J Clin Endocrinol Metab 1981;52:897–902.

76. Clark RV, Sherins RJ. Treatment of men with idiopathic oligozoospermic infertility using the aromatase inhibitor, testolactone. Results of a double-blinded randomized placebo-controlled trial with crossover. J Androl 1989;10:240–247.

77. de Turner EA, Aparicio NJ, Turner D, Schwarzstein D. Effect of two phosphodiesterase inhibitors, cyclic adenosine 3'5'-monophosphate and a β-blocking agent on human sperm motility. Fertil Steril 1978;29:328–331.

78. Aparicio NJ, Schwarzstein L, de Turner EA. Pentoxifylline by oral administration in the treatment of asthenozoospermia. Andrologia 1980;12:228–231.

79. Marrana P, Baraghini GF, Carani C, et al. Further studies on the effects of pentoxifylline on sperm count and sperm motility in patients with idiopathic oligoasthenospermia. Andrologia 1985;17:611–612.

80. Yovich JM, Edirisinghe WR, Cummins JM, Yovich JL. Preliminary results using pentoxifylline in a pronuclear stage tubal transfer (PROST) program for severe male factor infertility. Fertil Steril 1988;50:179–181.

81. Yovich JM, Edirisinghe WR, Cummins JM, Yovich JL. Influence of pentoxifylline in severe male factor infertility. Fertil Steril 1990;53:715–722.

82. Schill WB. Improvement of sperm motility in patients with asthenozoospermia by kallikrein treatment. Int J Fertil 1975;20:61–63.

83. Izzo PL, Canale D, Dianchi B, et al. The treatment of male subfertility with kallikrein. Andrologia 1983;16:156–161.

84. Micic S, Bila S, Ilic V, et al. Treatment of men with oligoasthenozoospermia and asthenozoospermia with kallikrein. Acta Eur Fertil 1985;16:51–54.

85. Comhaire F, Vermeulen L. Effect of high-dose oral kallikrein treatment in men with idiopathic subfertility: evaluation by means of in vitro penetration test of zona free hamster ova. Int J Androl 1983;6:168–172.

86. Aitken RJ, Clarkson JS. Significance of reactive oxygen species and antioxidants in defining the efficacy of sperm preparation techniques. J Androl 1988;9:367–376.

87. Cohen J, Edwards RG, Fehilly CB, et al. In vitro fertilization: a treatment for male infertility. Fertil Steril 1985;43:422–433.

88. Mahadevan MM, Trouson AO, Leeton JF. The relationship of tubal blockage, infertility of unknown cause, suspected male infertility and endometriosis to success of in-vitro fertilization and embryo transfer. Fertil Steril 1983;40:755–762.

89. Oehninger S, Acosta AA, Morshedi M, et al. Corrective measures and pregnancy outcome in in vitro fertilization in patients with severe sperm morphology abnormalities. Fertil Steril 1988;50:283–287.

90. Yates CA, Tronson AO, de Kretser DM. Male factor infertility and in vitro fertilization. In: Serio M, editor. IV International Congress of Andrology: Miniposters (Serono Symposium Review). Rome: Ares Serono, 1989: p 263.

91. Cohen J, Malter H, Fehilly C, et al. Implantation of embryos after partial opening of oocyte zona pellucida to facilitate sperm penetration. Lancet 1988;2:1–2.

92. Malter HE, Cohen J. Partial zona dissection of the human oocyte: a nontraumatic method using micromanipulation to assist zona pellucida penetration. Fertil Steril 1989;51:139–148.

93. Fishel S, Jackson P, Antinoni S, et al. Subzonal insemination for alleviation of infertility. Fertil Steril 1990;54:828–835.

94. Ng SC, Bongso A, Sathananthan H, Ratnam SS. Micromanipulation: its relevance to human in-vitro fertilization. Fertil Steril 1990;53:203–219.

CHAPTER 41

Surgical Treatment of Male Infertility

ALFRED SHTAINER and HARRIS M. NAGLER

Fifteen percent of American couples experience infertility.[1] Male factor infertility is found to be a contributing factor in approximately one half of these couples. Patients present to the gynecologist–reproductive endocrinologist and the urologist seeking consultation and advice concerning the therapy for each partner. It is imperative that both the gynecologist and the urologist be knowledgeable about the diagnostic and therapeutic options available to each.

Although obstruction of the reproductive tract leading to azoospermia is not the major cause of infertility, its diagnosis and treatment rely on sophisticated surgical techniques. Accurate diagnosis is essential and may allow for microsurgical reconstruction with dramatic results. A discussion of the diagnostic operative procedures, testicular biopsy, vasography, and scrotoscopy forms the first part of this chapter. Therapeutic modalities are then discussed. The microsurgical techniques that are presented permit successful reconstruction of an obstructed male reproductive tract due to congenital, iatrogenic, or purposeful (i.e., sterilization) causes. The varicocele remains a significant cause of infertility; the technique of varicocelectomy has undergone evolution to minimize its morbidity and to increase its effectiveness. These new modalities are reviewed. Finally, new techniques that have been developed to deal with unusual forms of obstruction such as ejaculatory duct obstruction and congenital vasal agenesis are reviewed.

TESTICULAR BIOPSY

Testicular biopsy has been widely used in the evaluation of male infertility since its introduction in 1940.[2] Although it has been used to evaluate patients with low sperm counts, it is primarily used in the diagnostic evaluation of the azoospermic patient to differentiate between testicular and posttesticular (obstructive) causes of infertility.[3] Testicular function can be indirectly assessed by the measurement of gonadotropin levels, which were first measurable in the urine and subsequently in serum samples. Gonadotropin determination has provided the practitioner with the ability to characterize male infertility as (1) hypogonadotropic, (2) hyper-

gonadotropic, or (3) normal gonadotropic (eugonadotropic). The significance of various gonadotropin levels has been determined by clinical correlation with testicular biopsies. These clinical studies led to the establishment of three major etiologic categories of male infertility: (1) pretesticular, (2) testicular, and (3) posttesticular.[4] Pretesticular causes of infertility are the result of inadequate hormonal stimulation of spermatogenesis. Testicular causes of infertility are the result of intrinsic testicular dysfunction and are characterized by elevated gonadotropin levels. Posttesticular abnormalities are the result of obstruction or dysfunction of the reproductive tract. Testicular biopsy is generally used in the diagnosis of the azoospermic male with normal gonadotropin levels (Fig. 41–1).

The indications for testicular biopsy were broad until the 1970 report of Garduno and Mehan.[5] Until then, testicular biopsies were performed in patients with (1) aspermia; (2) oligospermia; (3) abnormal sperm morphology; (4) abnormal sperm viability; and (5) abnormalities of the external genitalia. In this report, it was demonstrated that biopsies carried

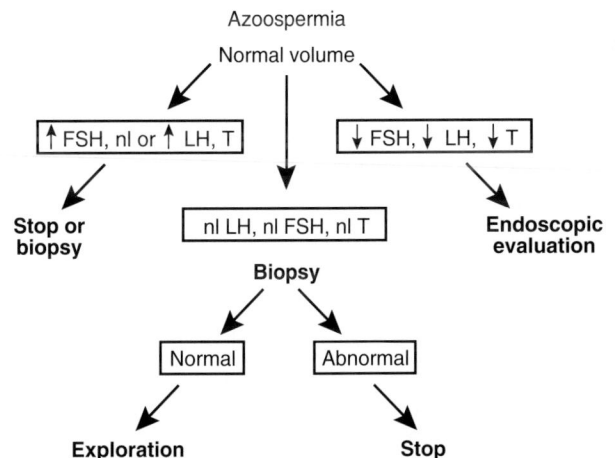

FIGURE 41–1. Evaluation algorithm. Indicating the role of testicular biopsy in the evaluation of the azoospermic patient. nl, normal; FSH, follicle-stimulating hormone; LH, luteinizing hormone; T, testosterone.

out in patients for reasons other than azoospermia did not reveal specific pathologic entities that affected the therapy that was subsequently rendered. Therefore, azoospermia was established as the principal indication for testicular biopsy.[4]

However, in recent years the indications for testicular biopsy have again been expanded owing to the work of Silber and Rodriguez-Rigau.[6] These authors highlighted the fact that partial (subclinical) epididymal obstruction may result in severe oligospermia. The diagnosis of partial epididymal obstruction is difficult to make and depends on detailed analysis of testicular biopsy material. Furthermore, a caveat to this broadening indication must be an awareness of the microsurgical skills of the urologic surgeon and his or her ability to repair epididymal obstruction. We do not advocate routinely performing a biopsy of oligospermic men unless the physical examination or history indicates that processes exist that may cause partial or unilateral obstruction of the reproductive system.[7] However, patients with counts of less than 1 million sperm per milliliter and normal gonadotropin levels may reasonably be subjected to testicular biopsy in an attempt to identify a subclinical epididymal obstruction.[4]

Many authors believe that testicular biopsy need not be done bilaterally. This belief is based on data suggesting that an adequate assessment of testicular function can be made by unilateral biopsy when the testes are not dissimilar.[8] Others have advocated bilateral biopsies when a difference in testicular size, a palpably absent vas deferens, or epididymal induration exists.[9] We advocate routine biopsy of both testes unless one is severely abnormal on routine physical examination. This practice has been reinforced by the finding of testicular inhomogeneity in apparently similar testes.[7, 10]

Surgical Technique

The "window" technique is widely employed for open testicular biopsy. The procedure is generally performed on an outpatient basis. Local, regional, or general anesthesia may be administered. Patients may be asked to prepare their scrotum with a gentle depilatory or shaving. Use of a depilatory may be particularly helpful if local anesthesia is to be used because shaving may heighten the patient's anxiety. The highly anxious patient may be given oral diazepam to take before arriving at the surgical outpatient unit.

Local anesthesia, 1% lidocaine hydrochloride and 0.25% bupivacaine, is used to infiltrate the scrotal skin demarcating the site of the transverse incision. The scrotal skin should be stretched tightly over the anterior surface of the testicle. Patients who are uncomfortable during the preparatory procedures may benefit from the administration of a cord block in addition to the infiltration of the scrotal skin.

A cord block is achieved by infiltration of 1% lidocaine hydrochloride both anterolateral and anteromedial to the spermatic cord as it crosses over the pubic tubercle after exiting from the inguinal canal via the external ring. The cord should not be infiltrated because this may injure the spermatic·vessels as well as result in intravascular infusion of the anesthetic agent (Fig. 41–2). Intravenous sedation with midazolam or diazepam may be beneficial.

Once satisfactory anesthesia has been established, the scrotum is grasped posteriorly, elevating and stabilizing the testicle against the stretched anterior scrotal wall. The testicle

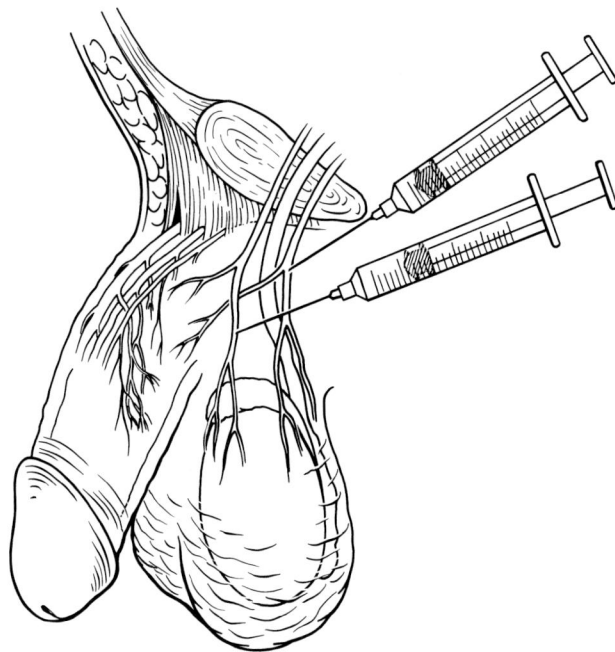

FIGURE 41–2. Cord block. The technique and anatomic landmarks for achieving adequate local anesthesia are demonstrated. (From Cohen MS, Warner RS. Needle biopsy of testes: A safe outpatient procedure. Urology. 1987; 29:279.)

should be stabilized throughout the procedure to minimize movement, which is often perceived as pain.

The skin is incised in a transverse direction between large cutaneous vessels that may appear in the scrotal skin. Biopsy of both testes may be accomplished through either separate incisions over each testicle (Fig. 41–3) or a single transverse incision traversing the median raphe and extending slightly over each hemiscrotum. The latter approach allows access to both hemiscrotal compartments through a single incision and shortens the operative time without compromising the quality of the biopsy tissue obtained.

The incisions are deepened through the dartos fascia until the tunica vaginalis is visualized. The epididymis is maintained in a posterior position throughout the procedure. Care should be taken in opening the tunica vaginalis. Several milliliters of clear, straw-colored fluid is generally released. Usually, the tunica albuginea of the testicle is immediately identifiable. This thick white covering should be identified with certainty to avoid inadvertent injury to the epididymis. If the tunica albuginea cannot be clearly identified, the testicle should be delivered through the scrotal incision. A stay suture of no. 4-0 chromic is placed into the tunica albuginea and tied (Fig. 41–4A). If the biopsy is being performed under local anesthesia, the patient must be warned that he may experience lower abdominal pain when this suture is placed. Dripping a local anesthetic agent onto the surface of the tunica albuginea may afford some benefit and should be done immediately on opening the tunica vaginalis. Once the stay suture has been placed, the needle is placed within the jaws of the needle holder to avoid inadvertent needle puncture. The stay suture stabilizes the testicle so that the anterior surface of the testicle and the subsequent biopsy site is maintained within the operative field. An incision is then made

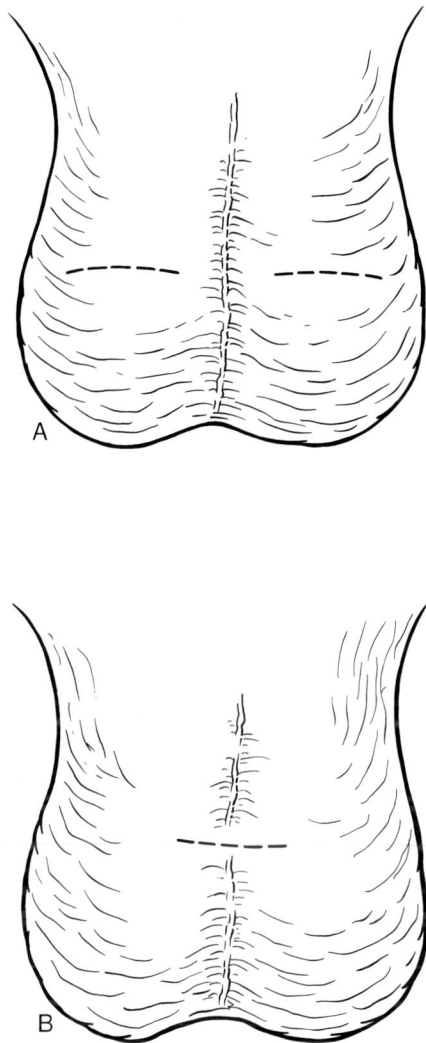

FIGURE 41–3. Scrotal incision. *A,* Bilateral transverse hemiscrotal incisions for testicular biopsies. *B,* Midline transverse incision allowing access to both hemiscrotal compartments for testicular biopsy.

transversely from the stay suture through the tunica albuginea. Immediately beneath the tunica albuginea is a rich anastomotic network of vessels, which may at times be visualized through the tunica. Care should be exercised to avoid these vessels because troublesome bleeding will result. Additionally, the incision should not extend into the testicular parenchyma because testicular architecture may become distorted. It is important to incise the entire thickness of the tunica albuginea. This allows the underlying testicular parenchyma to be extruded through the incision by gently squeezing the testicle with the hand that has been stabilizing it throughout the procedure (Fig. 41–4B).

The extruded seminiferous tubules are sharply excised using a "no-touch" technique. Using sharp iris scissors, tubules are cut and lifted away from the testicle in one motion. This technique maintains the integrity of the testicular parenchymal architecture. Again, in an attempt to minimize the trauma to the tissue while "passing off" the specimen, it is useful to have two sets of iris scissors on the operative field. Each set can then be immersed into the fixative rather than

picking up the specimen with forceps or attempting to shake the specimen free into the solution.

The surgeon must be aware that testicular architecture can be best preserved using either Bouin's or Zenker's solution. Formalin or formaldehyde should not be used because extensive shrinkage artifact will result and make accurate assessment of spermatogenesis difficult if not impossible.

When the biopsy has been completed, the tunica is closed in a running fashion using the previously placed stay suture. The underlying testicular parenchyma should not be incorporated into the closure. The scrotal incision is closed in two layers using no. 4-0 chromic catgut sutures. A collodion or Tegaderm dressing is applied to the wound. The patient is discharged and instructed to remain at bed rest and to place ice packs on the scrotum for the rest of the day. Most often, the patient is able to return to work the following morning.

Testicular Cytology

A limitation of the testicular biopsy as a diagnostic technique is its reliance on conventional pathologic interpretation of spermatogenesis. Histologic reporting is performed subjectively and is therefore often observer and experience dependent.[3]

Coburn and associates[11] have reported the use of two techniques to assess spermatogenesis that are based on the preparation of germinal epithelium for cytologic analysis: (1) the touch-imprint method and (2) cytocentrifuge preparations. In the touch-imprint method, a portion of testicular parenchyma obtained during an open biopsy procedure is touched to or gently moved across a microscopic slide with fine-tissue forceps. The slide is immediately fixed and stained with Papanicolaou or hematoxylin-eosin stain. Tailed spermatozoa should be readily apparent in the stained slide if spermatogenesis is complete. This technique permits the differentiation of late-maturation arrest from normal spermatogenesis, a diagnosis that may be difficult to discern with routine testicular histologic assessment. The other technique is a preparation of testicular cytology by cytocentrifuge. Testicular tissue is immersed in 1 mL of cold tissue-culture solution or saline. The specimen is then agitated gently for 30 seconds and removed from the solution. The cell-containing solution is centrifuged in a cytocentrifuge, depositing the cells on a glass slide that is then stained as described earlier. The tissue that has been removed can be placed in Bouin's solution for routine histologic assessment. The cytocentrifuge technique is slightly more cumbersome and may not be available in an operating room surgical pathology setting. However, because this technique is automated, it may avoid the variability that may be observed in the slide preparation using the touch-imprint technique.

The major advantage of these techniques is that they permit immediate and accurate assessment of spermatogenesis, allowing intraoperative decisions to be made with confidence. Frozen-section analysis of testicular histology is extremely difficult and unreliable. Further, as stated earlier, because these cytologic techniques clearly identify mature, intact spermatozoa, they are extremely useful in distinguishing late-maturation arrest from normal biopsy specimens. This distinction is often difficult on frozen or even permanent

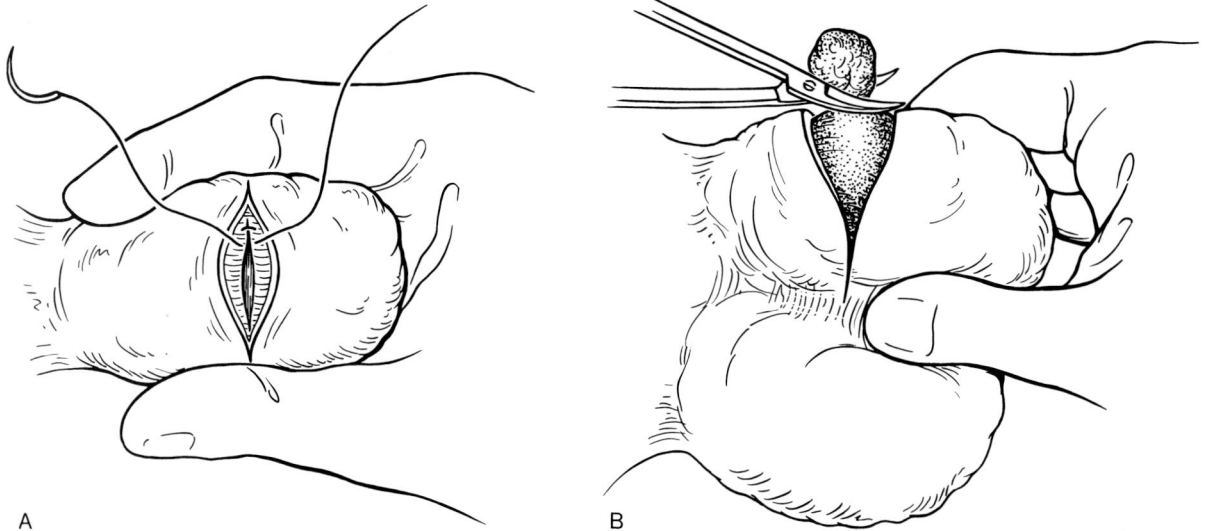

FIGURE 41–4. Window technique. *A,* A stay suture placed in the tunica albugina allows stabilization of the testes during the biopsy procedure. *B,* Once the tunica has been incised, the seminiferous tubules are extruded through the defect. They are then excised in a "no touch technique." (Modified from Nagler HM, Thomas AJ. Testicular biopsy and vasography in the evaluation of male infertility. Urol Clin North Am 1987; 14:167.)

sections. We no longer carry out any testicular biopsy without a concurrent cytologic preparation.

Needle Biopsy

Needle biopsy of the testes has been advocated in the evaluation of male infertility.[12–14] It is a rapid, simple, and inexpensive method. Additionally, it is safe and diagnostically accurate. In 1979, this technique was facilitated by a modification of the Tru-Cut biopsy needle (Fig. 41–5), making it shorter and easier to control.[15]

Following standard preparation of the scrotum, the skin overlying the anterior surface of testes is infiltrated with local anesthetic. Additional anesthesia is administered by grasping the spermatic cord above the testes and isolating the vas deferens. Lidocaine is injected both laterally and medially to the vas deferens, thereby anesthetizing the branches of the genitofemoral and ilioinguinal nerves. An identical cord block is carried out on the contralateral side to allow for bilateral testicular biopsies. After achieving adequate anesthesia, the assistant should grasp the testis, securing the epididymis posteriorly as described for the open biopsy technique. The appropriate stabilization of the testes and protection of the epididymis are more important with this technique because the structures will not be visualized at the time of the percutaneous biopsy.

The scrotal skin is punctured with a scalpel. With the obturator of the biopsy needle fully retracted to cover the specimen notch, the needle is passed through the scrotal incision. The underlying tunica albuginea is identified by a marked resistance to the passage of the needle. Increased pressure is required to traverse the tunica. Passage is appreciated by a characteristic "pop" as the needle enters the underlying testicular parenchyma. The cutting obturator is advanced while at the same time stabilizing the outer cutting sheath. The outer sheath is subsequently slid over the obtu-

rator to achieve the biopsy. The needle must be stabilized during this maneuver to prevent inadvertent advancement through the posterior aspect of the testicle and penetration of the epididymis. Subsequently, the needle is withdrawn in its entirety and opened by advancing the obturator. The specimen is removed and handled as described earlier in the section on surgical technique. Pressure should be applied directly to site of the puncture into the testicle. A suture may be placed to obtain skin hemostasis. We do not routinely

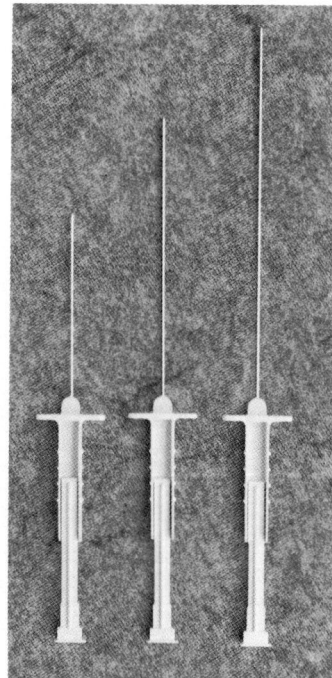

FIGURE 41–5. Tru-Cut soft tissue biopsy needles. (Courtesy of Baxter Healthcare Corporation, Valencia, CA. Tru-Cut is a registered trademark of Baxter Healthcare Corporation.)

employ prophylactic antibiotics unless there is an intercurrent indication. Infrequent complications include hematomas and transient orchialgia.

As with any biopsy technique, patients should be at bed rest for 12 to 24 hours. Ice packs applied to the scrotum minimize discomfort and swelling. Limited activity may be resumed according to the patient's comfort level. Patients should continue to wear a scrotal support until comfortable without one.

Although this technique is reported to provide a specimen adequate for pathologic diagnosis, spermatid count, tissue culture, and toxicology,[15] Kaufman and Nagler commented on its potential limitations, including small sample volume and associated distortion of tubular histology.[3] If necessary, standard open biopsy may be performed for definitive histologic diagnosis.

In 1989, Rajfer and Binder used a spring-loaded biopsy gun (Biopty gun; Fig. 41–6) to carry out testicular biopsies in seven men.[16] The preparation and technique for this procedure were identical to those described earlier for percutaneous biopsy techniques. The Biopty gun with the "loaded" needle can be operated with one hand and the testicle stabilized by the opposite hand. The needle tip punctures the scrotal skin, which is stretched tautly over the surface of the underlying testicle. Gentle pressure is applied to puncture the tunica albuginea and enter the testicular parenchyma. The gun is aimed at an angle so that the needle trajectory will be from lateral to medial. The epididymis is avoided by stabilizing it posteriorly. Additional samples can be obtained if necessary. The cutting groove of the standard Biopty gun used by Rajfer and Binder was 22 mm; the biopsy needle was 18 gauge. No complications were observed in this small group.[16]

The relative merits of various biopsy techniques can be debated. All biopsy techniques may be performed under local anesthesia, but the percutaneous needle biopsy techniques require no surgical tools other than the biopsy needle. This allows the clinician to carry out a biopsy in the office setting with relative ease. We continue to perform standard open window biopsies to ensure the quality of the specimen. The indications for testicular biopsy have not changed because of the relative ease of the procedure. Biopsies should only be performed when the information that may be obtained will alter the therapy offered to a patient (Fig. 41–7).

Flow Cytometry

The value of the biopsy techniques discussed earlier is dependent on histologic interpretation of the specimens obtained. Routine evaluation of testicular biopsy tissue is time consuming and subjective and permits only qualitative assessment of cellular defects. Deoxyribonucleic acid (DNA) flow cytometry is a rapid and reproducible technique that allows an objective, quantitative assessment of spermatogenesis.[3, 17–19] This analytic method distinguishes cell populations on the basis of the DNA content of individual cells. Testicular tissue is particularly well-suited for evaluation by this technique based on several factors. First, testicular parenchyma can be easily dispersed into a single-cell suspension. Second, normal spermatogenesis includes both mitotic and meiotic events that provide cells with diploid (2N), tetraploid (4N), and haploid (1N) chromosomal content. Therefore, normal spermatogenesis can be defined on the basis of an optimal ratio between populations of cells within each of these ploidy compartments. Alteration in these ploidy relationships may indicate disordered spermatogenesis.

ASPIRATION BIOPSY FOR FLOW CYTOMETRY

Testicular needle aspiration may be performed with or without local anesthesia. Because the technique is extremely rapid and a 20-gauge needle is used, we generally infiltrate only the skin overlying the aspiration site. The testicle is stabilized as described for routine testicular biopsy. The needle attached to a 10-mL syringe is plunged deep into the testicular parenchyma. At that moment, negative pressure is applied to the syringe and the needle is withdrawn. Immediately on withdrawal of the needle, propidium iodide (PI), a DNA fluorochrome, is aspirated into the syringe. The cellular debris is thus rinsed from the syringe and flushed into a collection tube.

Flow Cytometry Technique. A single-cell suspension of the aspirated specimens suitable for flow cytometric analysis

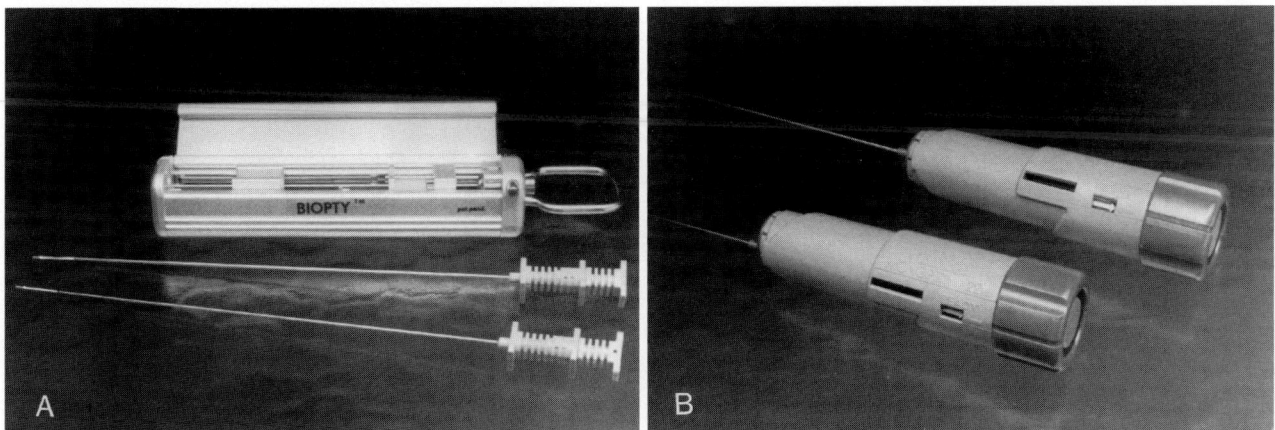

FIGURE 41–6. Spring-loaded biopsy equipment. *A,* Biopty gun. *B,* Monopty gun. (*A* and *B* courtesy of Bard Urological Division, Covington, GA.)

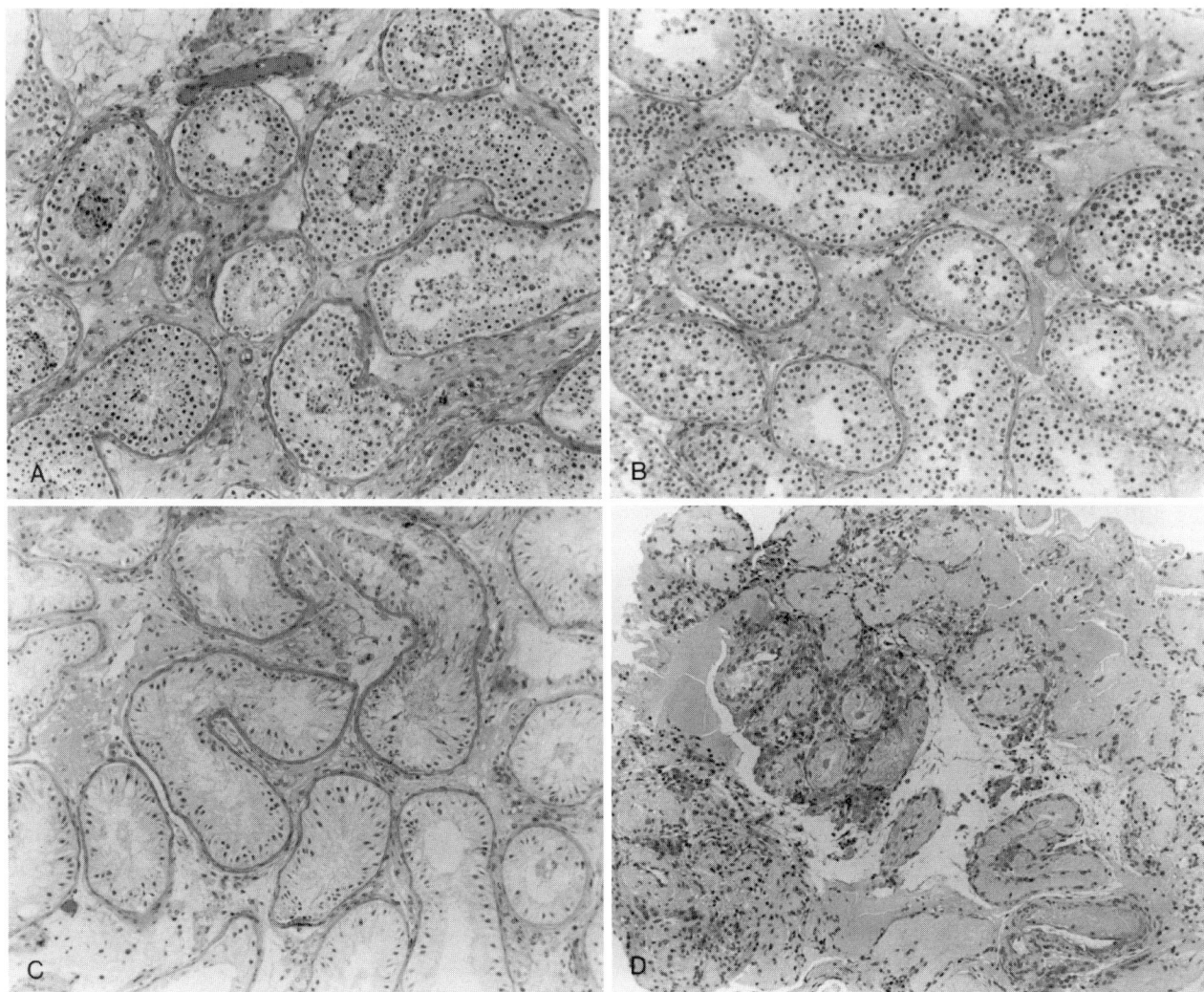

FIGURE 41–7. Representative testicular histologic patterns. *A,* Normal spermatogenesis. *B,* Maturation arrest. *C,* Sertoli-cell–only syndrome. *D,* Testicular hyalinization (Klinefelter's syndrome).

is created by mechanical dispersion. The PI-stained cell suspension is passed single file through the argon laser beam of the flow cytometer, which causes excitation of the stained DNA and elicits a fluorescent emission. The emitted signal is converted to an electrical impulse, which is measured, processed, and transformed into a DNA histogram. Each peak on the histogram, a ploidy compartment, represents a cell population with a specific DNA content. A reference sample of known diploid cells (PI-stained lymphocytes) is used for the identification of the generated ploidy peaks. Our studies with testicular flow cytometry demonstrated excellent correlation between the single-cell suspensions obtained using the aspiration technique and open testicular biopsy techniques.[3] Furthermore, constant flow cytometric relationships characteristic of specific histologic diagnoses were identified. The established ploidy relationships generated from flow cytometric analysis allow one to make appropriate therapeutic decisions in the azoospermic patient. However, this technique does not allow for the differentiation of abnormal spermatogenesis and obstruction in the oligospermic patient.

DNA flow cytometric analysis may provide the clinician with a convenient and effective means of quantifying sper-

matogenesis in the infertile male. In 1990, Hellstrom and associates showed that flow cytometric analysis provided a more reliable evaluation of spermatogenesis than did routine histology because of the improved sampling afforded by the technique.[20] Although this method does not provide information regarding tubular or interstitial morphometry, it appears to permit appropriate management decisions in the treatment of the azoospermic male.

Summary

Open testicular biopsy and touch preparation remain essential components of the evaluation of the azoospermic male. Newer techniques and modification have not decreased the value of this procedure.

VASOGRAPHY

Diagnostic seminal vesiculography, or vasography, was initially carried out by Belfield in 1913.[21] Actually, therapeutic vasography with the injection of various medications into the vas deferens in an attempt to treat "chronic vesiculitis" preceded diagnostic vasography by 8 years.[22] Several large series have been reported using this form of therapy.[23, 24] In 1935, Boreau published a beautifully illustrated textbook and atlas of seminal vesiculography.[25] Until this time, all attempts at vasography were carried out by surgically isolating and incising the vas. Subsequently, the technique of retrograde vasography performed cystoscopically became popularized. The ejaculatory ducts were cannulated and radiographic contrast media instilled.[26] In spite of the vast superiority of the current endoscopic equipment, the technique of retrograde vasography has been all but abandoned in recent years because of the intrinsic difficulty of the retrograde approach and the fact that most vasography is carried out at the time of reconstructive surgery.[27] Operative vasography allows for excellent delineation of the vas deferens, seminal vesicles, and ejaculatory ducts. The structures have been minimized by the advent of microsurgical techniques and less caustic (hydrophilic) contrast material.

Indication

The only indication for vasography is in the evaluation of the azoospermic patient. The procedure allows the physician to identify the presence or absence of obstruction of the vas or ejaculatory duct(s).[25] Vasography is performed at the time of definitive surgical exploration and reconstruction.

The adoption of a stepwise approach had been dictated by the inability to obtain adequate assessment of testicular histology from frozen-section analysis. The advent of the touch-imprint or cytocentrifuge preparations (see the section on testicular biopsy) has allowed the clinician to make accurate intraoperative assessments of spermatogenesis and appropriate intraoperative therapeutic decisions. In instances when there is a clear indication of obstruction on the basis of physical examination or history, the surgical procedure may include biopsy, vasography, and reconstruction all at the same sitting.

It is best to perform this radiologic examination at the time of anticipated reconstruction. Vasography and the required scrotal transgression result in adhesions and scarring, which needlessly make later corrective surgery more difficult.[27]

Technique

When vasography is anticipated, the surgeon should be certain that the patient is positioned in such a manner that a radiographic cassette can easily be placed beneath the pelvis. A single x-ray exposure should visualize the lower abdomen and entire genital area.

The optimal technique for entering the vas deferens at the time of vasography is controversial. Belfield described the instillation of contrast medium through a vasotomy using a blunt needle.[28] The vasotomy should traverse only one third the circumference of the vasa; this allows for adequate closure after vasography (Fig. 41–8A). Currently, microsurgical closure of the incision is recommended to prevent subsequent sperm leakage and possible iatrogenic scarring and obstruction. A longitudinal incision in the vas has been advocated by some authors. It is hypothesized that this technique preserves the vasal blood supply and facilitates closure.

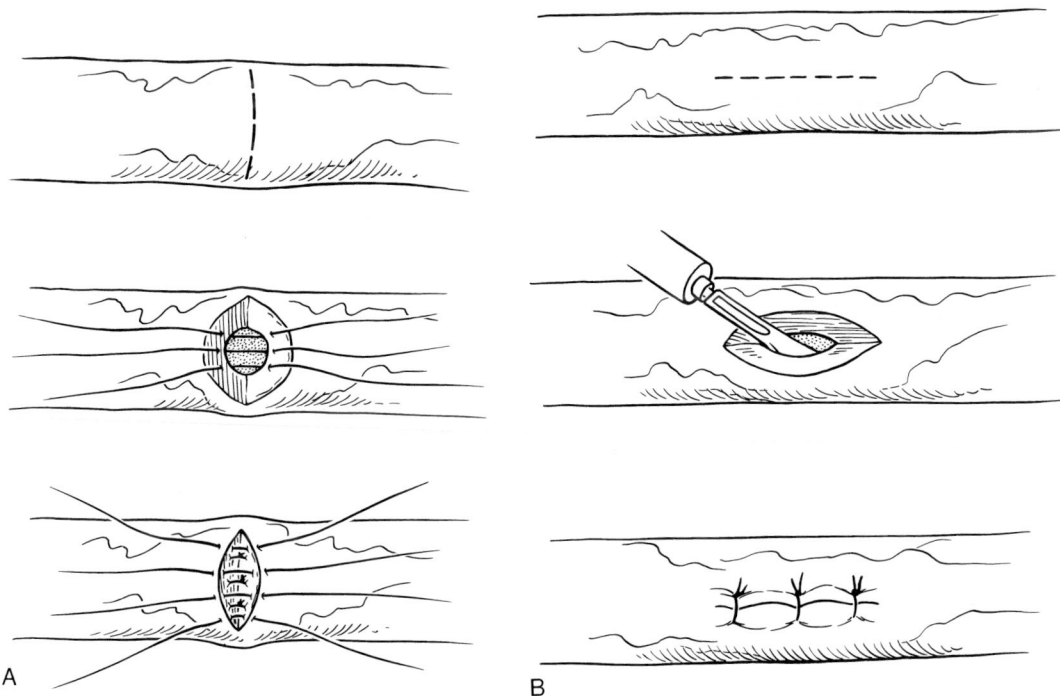

FIGURE 41–8. Vasotomy for vasography. *A,* Transverse incision. A transverse vasotomy should not exceed approximately one third of the vasal diameter. This permits successful and rapid closure using microsurgical techniques. *B,* Longitudinal incision. A longitudinal incision enters the vasal lumen without traversing vasal vessels and nerves. Closure can be accomplished using microsurgical techniques.

The incision may be adequately closed with a single layer of no. 9-0 nylon sutures incorporating only the muscular layer and excluding the mucosa (Fig. 41–8B). Direct vas puncture may be the least traumatic technique for vasography; however, it is difficult to perfect this technique. Multiple punctures may be required to enter the vasal lumen and therefore result in significant tissue damage and resultant obstruction. Direct-puncture vasography has been reported to cause scarring in experimental animals.[29]

Vasography should be carried out only at the time of attempted reconstruction. Local anesthesia is obtained by infiltrating the perivascular tissues as the vas is stabilized. The vas is then grasped with a vas-grasping (Fig. 41–9) or towel clamp. A 0.5-cm longitudinal skin incision is made and carried through the vasal adventitia. The vasal vessels should be preserved. A Vesi-loop is then passed beneath the vas. A 30-gauge lymphangiogram needle (no. 6657, Becton Dickinson & Co., Rutherford, NJ) is then passed through the vasal wall into the lumen. A second loop may be passed 0.5 cm distal to the first to achieve better vasal stabilization. There should be no resistance or extravasation during the injection. If none is encountered, formal vasography is performed with a 10-mL syringe and a dilute solution of Renografin-60 and saline (1:1). If resistance is met, either the needle is inappropriately positioned or there is distal obstruction. No further contrast medium should be instilled, and a radiograph should be obtained. The application of excessive pressure in an obstructed system may lead to reflux of contrast medium toward the testicle and result in epididymal damage.

If a formal vasotomy is made, the surgeon should pay special attention to the contents of the vas. The presence or absence of fluid must be noted. If fluid is present, it should be analyzed microscopically. The presence of sperm indicates obstruction distal (abdominal) to the vasostomy site (see the section on vasovasostomy surgical technique).

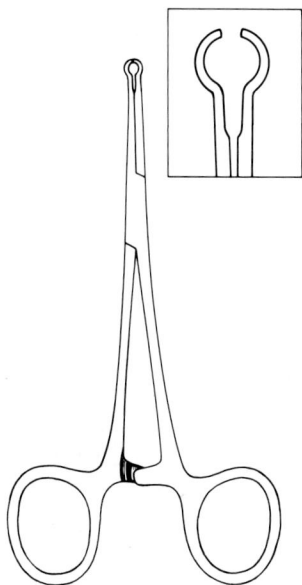

FIGURE 41–9. Vas fixation clamp. The vas may be stabilized or grasped using a towel clip or a vas fixation clamp as employed in the no-scalpel vasectomy technique. (From Li S, Goldstein M, Zhu J, Huber D. The no-scalpel vasectomy. J Urol 1991; 145:341–344, © American Urological Association.)

Visualization of the vasa, seminal vesicles, and ejaculatory ducts at the time of vasography may be enhanced by instilling air into the urinary bladder before exposing the radiograph. Furthermore, the anatomy of the ejaculatory ducts is more clearly delineated by tilting the x-ray tube approximately 30 degrees from perpendicular toward the patient's feet. This has the effect of "opening" the pelvis and exposing the anatomy that would otherwise be obscured by overlying bony and soft tissue densities.

Purposeful attempts at visualization of the epididymis may lead to inadvertent injury secondary to rupture of the delicate epididymal tubule. If the vas deferens is proved patent from the convoluted vas deferens to and including the ejaculatory ducts, the obstruction must lie between the testis and the tail of the epididymis. The site of obstruction is determined by exploration of the epididymis, as described later (see the section on vasoepididymostomy surgical technique).

Interpretation of Vasograms

The lumen of the vas deferens is approximately 0.4 mm in the unobstructed state. It will appear pencil thin as it follows its normal anatomic course through the inguinal canal. Turning medially and caudally at the level of the internal ring, it courses behind the bladder as it forms the ampulla, joining with the seminal vesicle and tapering into the fine ejaculatory duct. There should be bilateral symmetry. There should be no dilation throughout its course, and all components should be fully visualized to exclude obstruction. Additionally, contrast medium can be visualized entering the bladder (Fig. 41–10). Absence of contrast medium in the bladder may indicate ejaculatory duct obstruction.

Congenital anomalies, such as absence of the seminal vesicles and seminal vesicle cysts, may also be recognized. Acquired vasal obstruction may be the result of iatrogenic injury or inflammatory processes such as tuberculosis (Fig. 41–11).[30]

Interpretation of vasography may at times be complicated. To the less experienced urologist, the authors highly recommend Boreau's excellent text, which demonstrates both normal and pathologic anatomy of the vas deferens, epididymis, and seminal vesicles.[31]

SCROTOSCOPY

Scrotoscopy, or the endoscopic examination of the scrotal contents, is a new procedure that lacks significant literature or descriptions. Shafik designed a scrotoscope for the diagnosis and treatment of intrascrotal lesions.[32] This initial instrument, manufactured by the Arab Organization for Industrialization in Cairo, Egypt, is similar to standard endoscopic equipment and consists of a 5.5-mm sheath, telescope (30-degree, oblique), obturator, and accessories.

Suggested applications for the scrotoscope include biopsies and excision of masses in the spermatic cord, testis, and epididymis. It also has been used for venography of the pampiniform plexus and vasography.

Scrotoscopy may be performed as an outpatient procedure with either local or general anesthesia. Local anesthesia is achieved by a cord block in combination with direct infiltra-

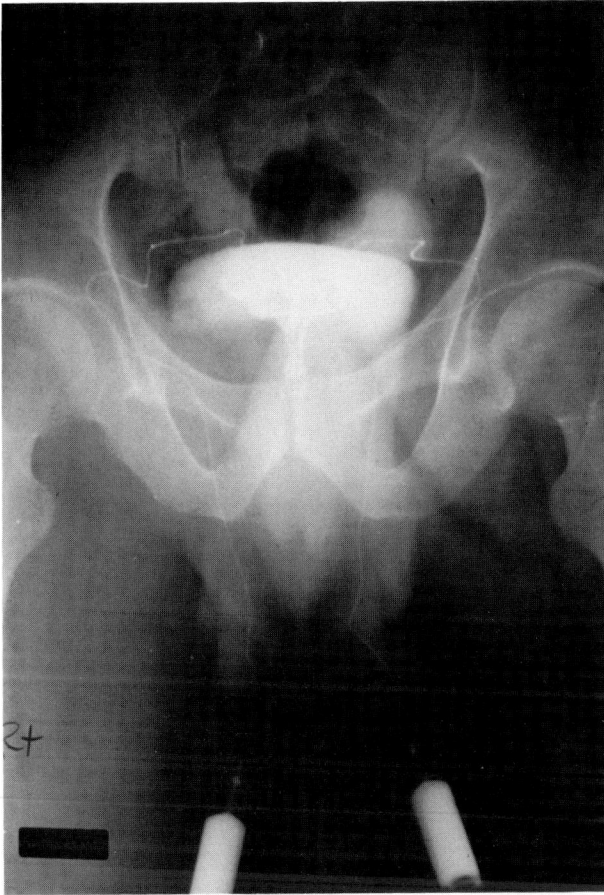

FIGURE 41–10. Normal vasogram. Contrast medium is seen filling vasa, seminal vesicles, and ejaculatory ducts. Contrast medium is also seen entering the bladder, indicating patency of the ejaculatory ducts.

in this country. Although the indications have yet to be well delineated, we are actively pursuing the development of this technique. It does appear to hold promise because of its minimally invasive nature.

VARICOCELECTOMY

The varicocele, an abnormal dilation of the scrotal portion of the pampiniform plexus–internal spermatic venous system draining the testicle, is considered the most common treatable cause of male infertility. In spite of its prominent position in the urologist's armamentarium, the varicocele continues to be surrounded by questions and controversies. The cause, pathophysiology, treatment, and even the significance of the varicocele continue to be debated.

Varicoceles have been reported to be present in as many as 15% of normal males; in contrast, the incidence in the infertile population has been reported to be 19% to 41%.[33, 34] Thus, it is clear that although not all men with varicoceles will be infertile, a significant percentage of infertile men will have a varicocele. The disparity between the incidence of the varicocele in normal men and infertile men may, in part, exist because varicoceles may have a progressively deleterious impact on spermatogenesis. Therefore, the "snapshot in time" that is provided by evaluating the semen of a young male with a varicocele may appear different from that of the same person later in life.[35] Further, it has been hypothesized that varicoceles may require the presence of a cofactor to exert their detrimental effect on sperm production.[36] This may explain the variable effect of the varicocele from individual to individual.

tion of the scrotal skin at the puncture site. This technique should not be used in the presence of skin infections. Shafik[32] used this technique in the presence of acute intrascrotal infection without complications and did not believe that this is a contradiction.

As previously described, a small incision (5 mm) is made in the skin and superficial fascia. A liter of normal saline in a closed system is connected to the inflow valve of the sheath. The sheath with the blunt obturator in place is passed through the incision. Thereafter, the scrotum is distended with 40 to 60 mL of saline. The testis, epididymis, and spermatic cord are examined from the anterior, posterior, and both lateral aspects. Using the scrotoscope, biopsies are performed blindly through the sheath after removal of the telescope. Alternatively, an additional sheath may be placed, allowing biopsies to be performed under direct visual guidance. Patients receive postoperative antibiotics and are advised to wear a scrotal support for 2 or 3 days.

We have used a modified short ureteroscope for scrotoscopy (Fig. 41–12). The tunica vaginalis is distended by drip saline infusion via a percutaneously placed angiocatheter under local anesthesia. After distention of the tunica vaginalis, this instrument is introduced into the space, allowing visualization of the testicle and epididymis. Videoendourologic techniques are used to facilitate this procedure.

This is a new technique that has not been used extensively

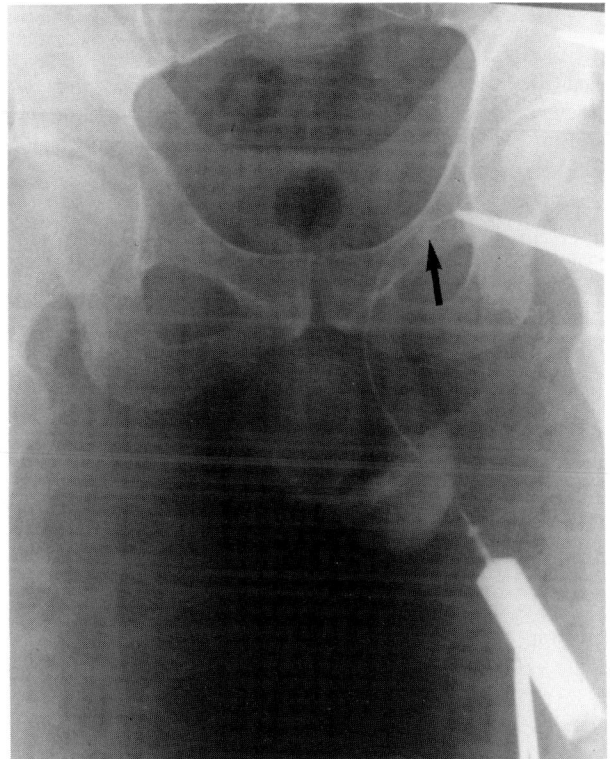

FIGURE 41–11. Abnormal vasogram. Vasogram demonstrating obstruction (*arrow*) within the inguinal canal resulting from pediatric herniorrhaphy.

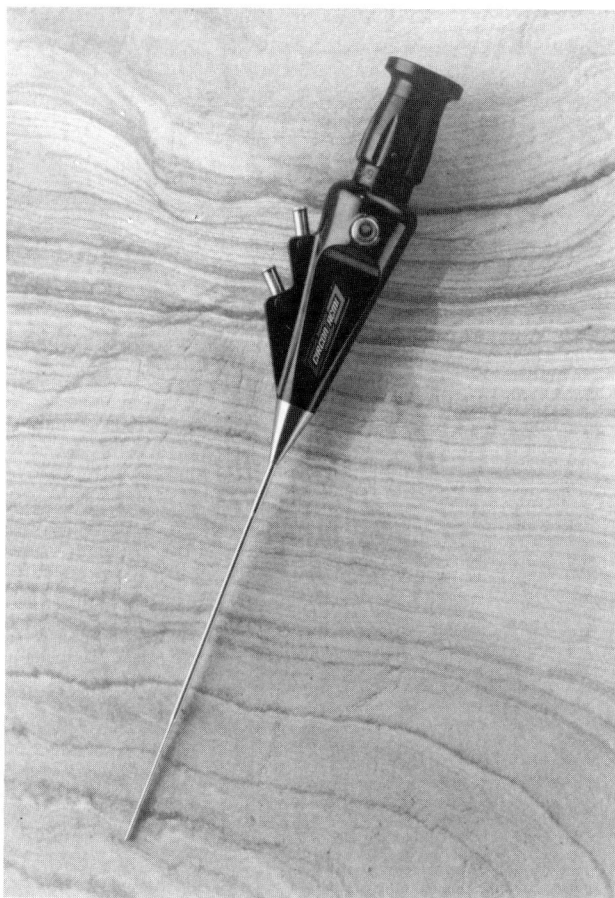

FIGURE 41–12. Short ureteroscope used for scrotoscopy. (Courtesy of Circon ACMI, Marlton, NJ.)

Although there have been controlled studies indicating that varicocelectomy has no beneficial effect on fertility rates, a review of the published uncontrolled studies encompassing thousands of infertile patients treated with varicocelectomy demonstrated the beneficial effect of varicocelectomy.[37] Approximately 50% to 80% of patients experience improved semen parameters, and 30% to 40% of patients initiated a pregnancy after varicocelectomy.[38] Furthermore, the controlled study of Okuyama and associates indicated that the untreated varicocele in the adolescent was associated with worse semen parameters and smaller testes than a control population that received no intervention.[39] Fertility was not studied. This indicates that varicocelectomy results in improvement in testicular function or a cessation of the deterioration that may accompany the varicocele.

Historical Perspective

Celsius first recognized the impact of dilated spermatic veins on the testicle. He observed the association of the varicocele and ipsilateral testicular atrophy.[40] In the "modern" era, varicoceles were noted to be associated with a decrease in the "secreting powers of the gland" by Curling in 1856.[41] He further speculated a potential relationship with male infertility. Barwell also observed that the ipsilateral testes of patients with a varicocele were small and soft.[42] Barwell car-

ried out the initial attempts at varicocele "ligation" by placing a wire loop around the dilated scrotal veins and noted normalization of the testicular consistency.[42] Bennet demonstrated the therapeutic value of varicocele ligation when he observed improved seminal parameters in a patient after bilateral varicocelectomy.[43] The *New England Journal of Medicine* published the report of Macomber and Sanders, which described an oligospermic subfertile patient who underwent varicocelectomy and subsequently became normospermic and fertile.[44] It was not until the report of Tulloch that the varicocele became established as a leading cause of male factor infertility.[45] It was then that the causal relationship between varicocelectomy and pregnancy became established.[46, 47]

ETIOLOGY OF THE VARICOCELE

The pathogenesis of the varicocele remains enigmatic. Most theories of "varicocelegenesis" explain the predominance of the left-sided varicocele. The unifying theme of these theories is that there is increased hydrostatic pressure within the left internal spermatic system. The mechanisms of this increased pressure include (1) the increased length (8 to 10 cm) of the left internal spermatic vein (ISV) as compared with the right; (2) the perpendicular insertion of the left ISV into the left renal vein as compared with the oblique insertion of the right ISV into the vena cava; and (3) compression of the left renal vein between the aorta and the superior mesenteric artery.[48] Shafik and Bedeir[49] demonstrated that the ISV in men with varicocele was associated with increased intraluminal hydrostatic pressure when compared with that of nondilated ISVs. The mean ISV pressure in subjects with varicoceles was reported to be greater than that in the control group.

Ahlberg and associates studied the ISV system in cadavers.[50] All cadavers with varicoceles had an absence of valves within the ISV, whereas cadavers without varicoceles were found to have numerous valves within the ISV.[40, 50]

It has become apparent that varicoceles are present bilaterally far more commonly than had been previously appreciated. Some authors reported bilateralism in as many as 69% of patients.[51] Although we do not observe such a high incidence of bilateralism, it is clear that the incidence is far higher than the 10% incidence reported historically. This observation led us to reevaluate the existent theories of varicocelegenesis. Perhaps a simple teleologic and evolutionary theory is most appropriate. Humans were designed to walk on four legs, not two. The assumption of the upright position will in certain instances overcome the competence of valvular or antireflux mechanisms within the ISVs. Because of the considerations outlined earlier, this occurs more frequently on the left side, but it may also occur on the right side. The simple assumption is that the valves within the ISV system are incompetent or absent.

Pathophysiology

Although many hypotheses have been proposed to explain the mechanism by which the varicoceles may adversely affect spermatogenesis, none of these theories has been proven to be operative. A thorough discussion of these hypotheses is beyond the scope of this chapter, but several theories are outlined. Currently, abnormal testicular thermoregulation secondary to a disrupted thermal exchange apparatus (i.e., the pampiniform plexus) is widely believed to be a significant factor in the pathophysiology of the varicocele. Abnormal thermoregulation may disrupt the hormonal homeostatic mechanisms that are required to support spermatogenesis. Experimental and clinical data do not support the hypothesis that toxins reflux down the ISV from the renal and adrenal veins.[52] Studies using gonadotropin-releasing hormone stimulation have indicated subtle alterations in the testicular response to stimulation.[53–55]

Diagnosis

PHYSICAL EXAMINATION

The principal method used for the diagnosis of the varicocele remains the physical examination. Careful examination of the scrotum and its contents should be carried out in a warm room with the patient in the supine and upright positions. A large varicocele may be easily visualized as a vermiform bluish discoloration of the scrotal skin appreciated superior to the testicle (Fig. 41–13). Large varicoceles have been described as feeling like "a bag of worms" on palpation. Dubin and Amelar proposed a simple, useful grading system for assessing the size of varicoceles.[46] Grade III (large) varicoceles are visible through the scrotal skin; grade II (moderate) varicoceles are easily palpable. Grade I (small) varicoceles are palpable only when the patient performs a Valsalva maneuver.

ADJUNCTIVE DIAGNOSTIC TESTS

Because varicocele has continued to be associated with male factor infertility, many techniques have been created and designed to aid in its diagnosis. These modalities have the potential to be used on a "witch hunt" for varicoceles. We believe that these modalities should be reserved to confirm the clinical diagnosis of the varicocele.

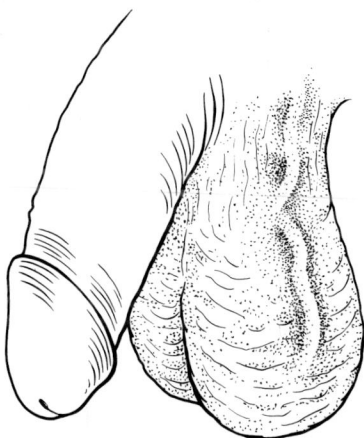

FIGURE 41–13. A large varicocele (grade III) or dilation of the pampiniform plexus is readily apparent through the scrotal skin. (Modified from Nagler HM, Zippe CD. Varicocele: current concepts. In: Lipschultz LI, Howards SS, editors. Infertility in the Male. St. Louis: Mosby-Year Book, 1991:313.)

Doppler Examination. The pencil-probe Doppler (9 mHz) stethoscope is a relatively inexpensive instrument that can be used to confirm reflux in a clinically suspected varicocele. Reflux can be auscultated or, as described by Greenberg and associates, visually displayed.[56, 57] The patient is examined in the upright position. Ultrasound conducting gel is applied to the upper aspect of the scrotum. There should be complete acoustical silence prior to having the patient perform a Valsalva maneuver. If one is auscultating the testicular artery at the time the Valsalva maneuver is performed, altered blood flow may be incorrectly attributed to a varicocele. A reflux associated with the varicocele can be appreciated as a venous "rush" during the maneuver.

The Doppler stethoscope should not be used to screen subfertile patients with oligospermia for subclinical varicoceles. Hirsh and colleagues[58] demonstrated Valsalva-induced, Doppler-positive reflux in 83% of the left spermatic veins and 59% of right spermatic veins of 118 patients without clinical varicoceles. There was no difference between the infertile and fertile men. Because of the high incidence of Valsalva-induced reflux, many authors advocate assessing reflux during quiet respiration. Using this method, Hirsh and colleagues found a varicocele pattern in 88% of patients with a clinical varicocele, whereas only 18% of patients without a varicocele showed the same pattern.[58] When Doppler studies were compared with internal spermatic venography, Doppler grading of venous reflux did not distinguish between competent and incompetent spermatic veins.[59] Thus, the Doppler should be used only as an adjuvant technique to confirm physical finding consistent with a varicocele.

Although we do not screen all infertile men with a Doppler stethoscope, we do examine clinically normal contralateral cord structures in the presence of a clinical varicocele. This is the only circumstance in which we search for "subclinical reflux." If a subclinical varicocele is appreciated, it is treated at the same time as the coexistent clinical varicocele. This approach is based on the observation that altered blood flow after varicocelectomy may unmask a subtle underlying contralateral venous anomaly and result in formation of a clinical varicocele.[60, 61]

Venography. Retrograde spermatic venography is generally regarded as the most sensitive, although the most invasive, method for diagnosis of the varicocele (Fig. 41–14*A* and *B*). Unfortunately, the relative lack of specificity of this technique limits it usefulness. Venography demonstrates reflux down the ISV system in virtually 100% of patients with clinical varicoceles.[62] However, reflux also has been reported in 60% to 70% of infertile patients without a palpable varicocele.[63] Netto and associates demonstrated venographic reflux in 58% of men with varicoceles and abnormal semen, in 58% of men with varicoceles and normal semen, and in 33% of a normal control group.[64]

Several explanations have been offered for this high degree of sensitivity and the marginal degree of specificity. During venography, inadvertent placement of the venographic catheter tip beyond the valvular mechanism of the ISVs bypasses the antireflux mechanism of the vein and results in the false appearance of a varicocele. Additionally, if excessive force is used to inject the contrast medium at the time of venography, reflux can be demonstrated even when there is a normal ISV.[65]

The invasive nature of this test and the ambiguity resulting

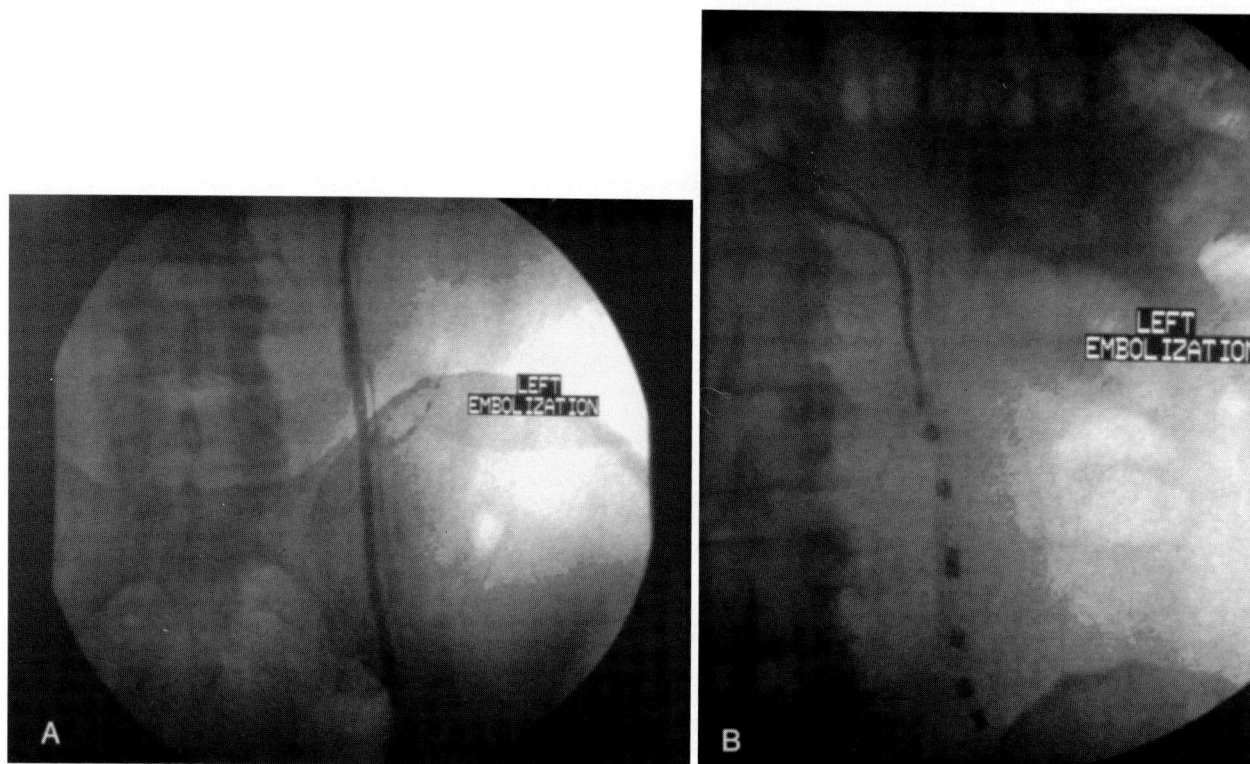

FIGURE 41–14. *A,* Venography demonstrating reflux from the renal vein into the internal spermatic venous system. *B,* Coils are positioned within the internal spermatic vein. After embolization, reflux is prevented.

from its relative lack of specificity have relegated venography to a role of therapeutic intervention. In the diagnosis and treatment of the recurrent or persistent varicocele after attempted varicocelectomy, venography can be both diagnostic and therapeutic. If abnormal reflux is identified using this technique, veno-occlusion is accomplished with either sclerosing agents,[66] Gianturco coils,[67] or detachable balloons (see later).[68, 69]

Additional Diagnostic Techniques. Scrotal contact thermography has been used to detect the elevated temperatures associated with the varicocele. Many authors have advocated the diagnostic value of this technique.[70, 71] Hirsh and coworkers demonstrated scrotal thermography to be as accurate as Doppler flow studies in detecting varicoceles.[58] However, Mieusset and associates demonstrated increased scrotal temperatures in infertile men without varicoceles.[72] Thus, although one cannot rely solely on scrotal thermography in the diagnosis of varicoceles, it may be used as an adjunctive test only to confirm the clinical impression.

Radionuclide technetium pertechnetate scintigraphy has been employed to detect varicoceles. However, this technique has not been widely embraced. This procedure is used to demonstrate abnormal pooling of radionuclide within the scrotum, indicating abnormal blood flow within the dilated pampiniform plexus.[73]

Surgical Treatment

Surgical varicocelectomy remains the cornerstone of varicocele therapy. Successful therapy must completely disrupt venous drainage via the ISV system without compromising

the internal spermatic artery, the vas deferens with its blood supply, or the lymphatics of the spermatic cord. Although three basic surgical approaches have been described, many modifications exist.

THE SCROTAL APPROACH

The *scrotal approach* should not be employed. Because of the complexity of the pampiniform plexus within the scrotum, this approach is doomed to fail. The rich anastomotic network of the pampiniform plexus makes complete ligation of all branches exceedingly time consuming and improbable. Arterial damage and resultant testicular ischemia are likely, because of the need for multiple sites of division and ligation. This technique is best avoided and is mentioned only for historical review.

RETROPERITONEAL APPROACH (MODIFIED PALOMO TECHNIQUE)

The retroperitoneal approach, or modified Palomo technique (Fig. 41–15*A*), exposes the ISV within the retroperitoneum prior to its coalescence with the spermatic cord structures and entrance into the inguinal canal. This technique requires general or regional anesthesia because of retraction on the peritoneum and abdominal musculature. A transverse abdominal incision is made medial to the anterosuperior iliac spine. The subcutaneous tissues are traversed, exposing the external oblique fascia, which is incised in the direction of its fibers (Fig. 41–16*A*). The underlying internal oblique muscle is bluntly spread and retracted (Fig. 41–16*B*). The retroperitoneum is thus entered slightly superior to the internal in-

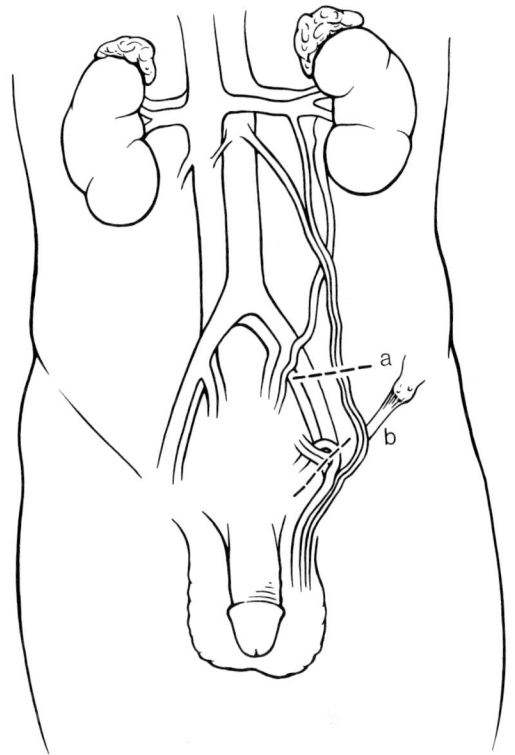

FIGURE 41–15. Incisions used for the retroperitoneal approach (a) and the standard inguinal approach (b).

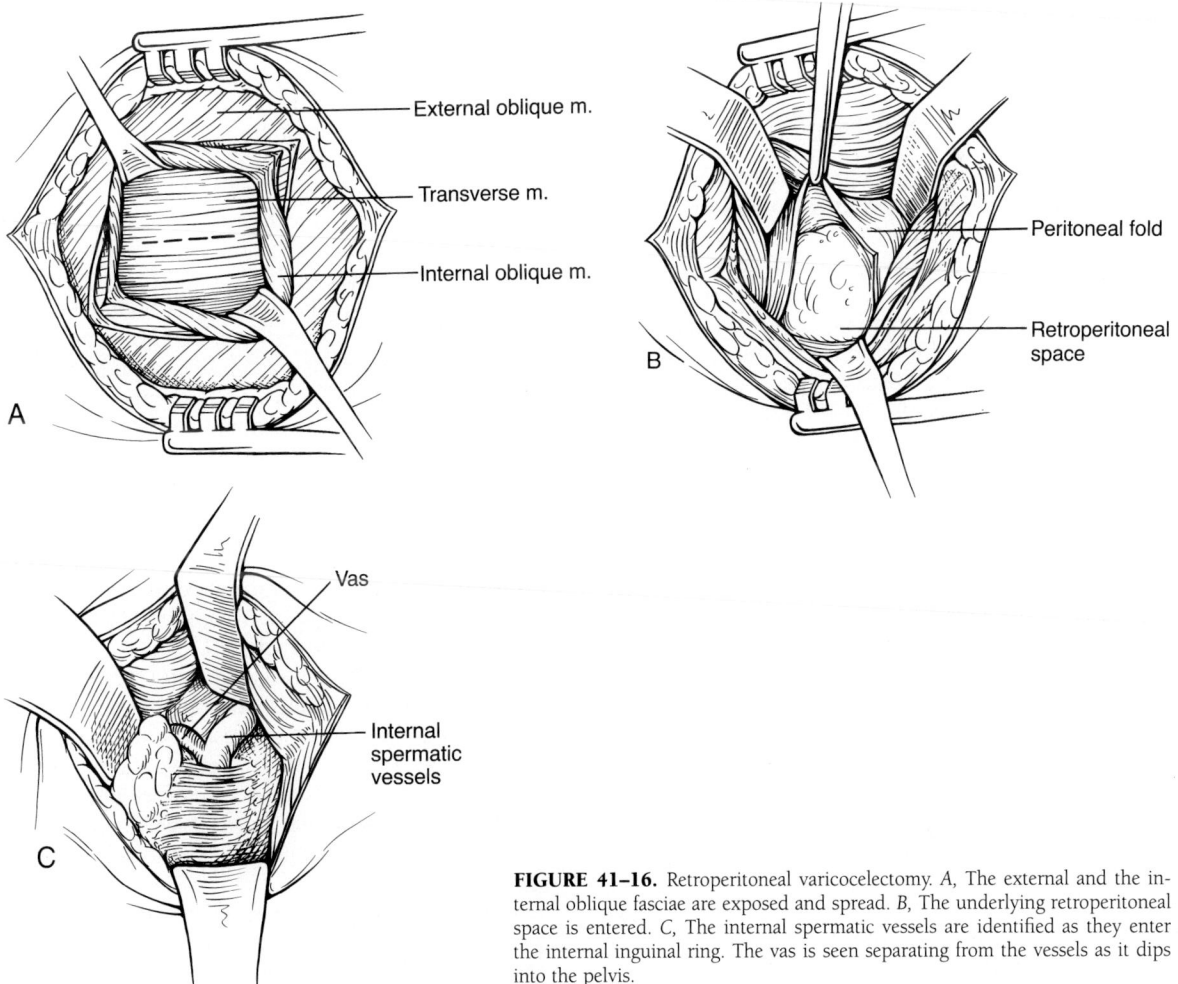

External oblique m.

Transverse m.

Internal oblique m.

A

Peritoneal fold

Retroperitoneal space

B

Vas

Internal spermatic vessels

C

FIGURE 41–16. Retroperitoneal varicocelectomy. *A,* The external and the internal oblique fasciae are exposed and spread. *B,* The underlying retroperitoneal space is entered. *C,* The internal spermatic vessels are identified as they enter the internal inguinal ring. The vas is seen separating from the vessels as it dips into the pelvis.

guinal ring, and the dilated ISVs are encountered (Fig. 41–16C). At this level the vas deferens can be identified separating from the cord structures and dipping deep into the pelvis. Identification of the vas is helpful in confirming that the encountered vessels are indeed the ISVs. Gentle traction on the testicle also aids in this process. The testicular artery is then identified visually or with the aid of an intraoperative Doppler. The spermatic veins are then identified, divided between clamps, and ligated with silk sutures. The spermatic vein should be traced in a cephalad direction to minimize the need for the division of multiple, more proximal tributaries. Although Palomo described ligating the internal spermatic artery and veins,[74] most authors believe that the artery should be identified and preserved.

The Palomo technique has the theoretical advantage of dividing the spermatic vein at a more cephalad level (distally along the course of the vessel). This should reduce the number of tributaries encountered, thus facilitating the surgery and increasing the likelihood that the entire incompetent venous system will be interrupted. Additionally, this approach may permit the interruption of spermatic venous communication between right and left varicoceles, as described by Etriby and colleagues.[75] This technique has been advocated by Cockett and coworkers.[76] A disadvantage of this technique is the inability to identify and ligate the external cremasteric vessels. These vessels have been implicated as a cause of recurrent and persistent varicoceles following varicocelectomy.[68] This technique is advantageous in patients with previous inguinal surgery: The surgeon can avoid the violated inguinal region and inadvertent injury to the testicular artery and ilioinguinal nerve.

INGUINAL APPROACH (MODIFIED IVANISSEVICH TECHNIQUE)

The inguinal approach, as described by Ivanissevich,[77] exposes the ISVs within the inguinal canal. This approach offers several anatomic advantages when compared with the other approaches discussed. The spermatic vein coalesces as it approaches the internal inguinal canal; ligation at this level can be generally accomplished with minimal difficulty, with only one or two large vessels being identified. This approach also allows for identification of large external cremasteric vessels that may contribute to the varicocele.[48]

Either an oblique or transverse incision may be used (see Fig. 41–15B). The location of the incision is determined by identifying the external inguinal ring by invaginating the scrotal skin. This is approximately two fingerbreadths above the symphysis pubis at the lateral edge of the scrotum. The incision is extended through Scarpa's fascia until the external oblique aponeurosis is encountered and incised in the direction of its fibers (Fig. 41–17A). Care is taken not to injure the underlying ilioinguinal nerve. The fascia can be safely incised by making a small stab through the fascia and then inserting a closed Metzenbaum scissors through the defect. The scissors are slid down to the external ring while the tips of the scissors are elevated against the undersurface of the fascia. The scissors are then rotated 90 degrees, exposing the groove between the two blades; this groove is used as a guide for the knife to incise the fascia. The fibers of the fascia should be clearly visualized; if the nerve is inadvertently "picked up" by the scissors tips, it will be readily visualized

beneath the fascia. In this instance, the maneuver is repeated until the surgeon is confident that the nerve is protected. The spermatic cord is then mobilized at the level of the pubic tubercle with peanut dissectors (Fig. 41–17B). A Penrose drain is passed beneath the cord and is used to elevate the cord from the canal. The ilioinguinal nerve should be identified and separated from the spermatic cord by passing it beneath the previously placed Penrose drain. Optical loupe magnification is used during the exploration and dissection of the spermatic cord. This aids in the identification of the spermatic artery, lymphatic channels, and all venous structures.

The cremasteric fascia is incised. Troublesome oozing may be encountered from the cremasteric fibers. Bipolar forceps should be used to achieve hemostasis. On exposing the spermatic vessel bundle, one should attempt to identify the artery by visual inspection and intraoperative Doppler ultrasonography (Fig. 41–17C).[78] When identified, a Vesi-loop is used to isolate the artery while the cord exploration continues. All venous channels are isolated and ligated with a nonabsorbable suture. A representative segment is excised. Great care is taken to identify even small venous channels, which may be cauterized with bipolar forceps. The vas deferens is identified and its vasculature preserved. Lymphatic channels should be identified and spared to minimize the incidence of hydrocele formation after varicocelectomy. When all veins have been identified, attention is redirected to the artery and surrounding veins encircled by the Vesi-loop. Meticulous dissection allows the surgeon to remove the rich anastomotic network of veins surrounding the spermatic artery. Optical magnification, intraoperative Doppler, and topical application of a vasodilator (papaverine) aid in the identification and preservation of the testicular artery. When the artery has been cleared of the surrounding veins, its pulsations are immediately apparent.

After the spermatic cord has been fully explored, the Penrose drain is repositioned so that the ilioinguinal cord and the spermatic cord are both encompassed by the drain. Upward traction exposes the floor of the inguinal canal, which is inspected for any external cremasteric veins. These veins perforate the canal and drain into the pudendal vein and, ultimately, the saphenous vein. These veins should be identified because they may contribute to recurrent varices in a small proportion of patients.[48] The external abdominal oblique is closed with a continuous no. 3-0 chromic suture and the subcutaneous layer is approximated with interrupted 3-0 plain catgut. A subcuticular absorbable closure is used.

Modifications of the Inguinal Approach

Subinguinal Approach. In this approach described by Marmar and coworkers, the spermatic cord is approached as it exits from the external inguinal ring; thus, the external oblique fascia is not incised.[79] Although Marmar and coworkers described the use of sclerosing agents at the time of surgical exploration to ensure the obliteration of all venous collateral circulation and reduce the incidence of varicocele recurrence, this technique has not been adopted by most authors. However, the subinguinal incision has been used by other authors.

Subinguinal Approach and Delivery of the Testicle. Goldstein and associates have described the use of the subinguinal approach and the deliverance of the testicle from the scrotum

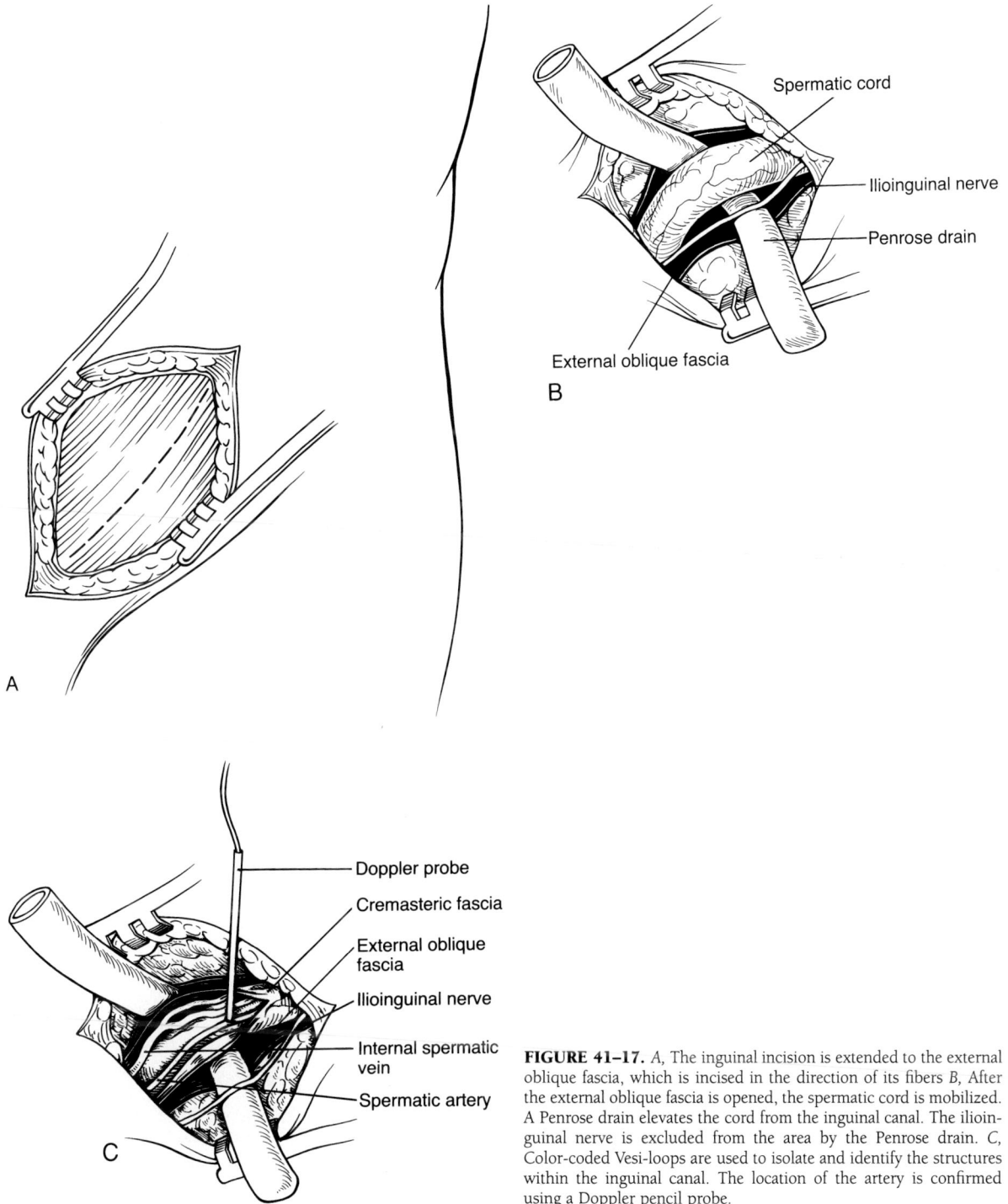

FIGURE 41-17. *A,* The inguinal incision is extended to the external oblique fascia, which is incised in the direction of its fibers *B,* After the external oblique fascia is opened, the spermatic cord is mobilized. A Penrose drain elevates the cord from the inguinal canal. The ilioinguinal nerve is excluded from the area by the Penrose drain. *C,* Color-coded Vesi-loops are used to isolate and identify the structures within the inguinal canal. The location of the artery is confirmed using a Doppler pencil probe.

via this incision.[80] The authors claim that this approach allows the ligation of gubernacular vessels, which may provide collateral circulation to the varicocele and result in recurrence if not ligated. In this study optical magnification is provided by an operating microscope, although the dissection of the cord is as described earlier.

LAPAROSCOPIC VARICOCELECTOMY

Recent years have seen an explosion of "minimally" invasive surgical procedures using laparoscopic techniques (Fig. 41–18). The proponents of this approach report reduced postoperative morbidity and analgesic use. Several reports of laparoscopic varicocelectomy have appeared in the literature. Mehan and colleagues performed ISV ligation via the laparoscope in 22 patients with hypofertility believed, at least in part, due to a varicocele.[81] Standard laparoscopic instrumentation was used. No major or significant operative complications were experienced. Operative time varied from 75 to 105 minutes; all these procedures were done bilaterally. The authors reported that the magnification provided by the laparoscope enabled identification and preservation of the testicular artery. Two to five vessels were ligated. All surgery was performed on an ambulatory basis, and patients returned to work within 72 hours. No recurrence was documented by routine clinical criteria. Sixty percent of the patients treated in this fashion experienced statistically significant improvement in one or more semen parameters. No significant morbidity was observed in this study, although minor complications were noted. Complications specific to laparoscopy included shoulder pain lasting 48 hours (two patients) and pneumoscrotum (one patient).

Other reports have not found reduced morbidity from laparoscopic varicocelectomy. Many investigators believe that the standard extraperitoneal approach to varicocelectomy should not be replaced with an intraperitoneal procedure that has the potential for severe morbidity and potential mortality. The potential seriousness of laparoscopy for genitourinary surgery was recently reviewed by Kavoussi and colleagues.[82] Additionally, the laparoscopic approach to varicocelectomy

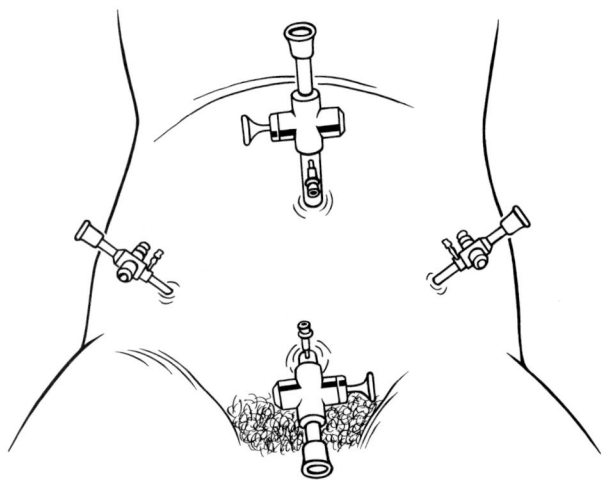

FIGURE 41–18. Laparoscopic varicocelectomy. The puncture sites for laparoscopic varicocelectomy are indicated. (Adapted from Winfield HN. Suddenly, urology takes up the laparoscope. Contemp Urol 1991; 3:70.)

does not provide access to the external cremasteric vessels, which may contribute to varicoceles in 49.5% of patients.[83] The efficacy, safety, and benefits of laparoscopic varicocelectomy have yet to be demonstrated.

Complications of Varicocele Therapy: Surgical and Venographic

There are few serious complications after varicocelectomy. Certainly, one of the most troubling is recurrence or persistence of the varicocele. The recurrence rate after surgical therapy has been reported to be between 0% and 20%.[33] In 1977, Dubin and Amelar[51] reported on 986 patients who underwent "standard" inguinal varicocelectomy. In this series, only one patient was noted to have a recurrent varicocele postoperatively. With the use of the magnified approach outlined earlier, the recurrence rate in our patients is 1.5%. Goldstein and coworkers recently reported a recurrence rate of 0.6% using an operative microscope to accomplish varicocelectomy.[80] The recurrence after venographic techniques is reported to be between 2% and 12%.[84] In a review of varicocelectomy techniques, Pryor and Howards assessed nine reports of venographic occlusion.[33] They noted that not all attempts at venographic occlusion are accomplished owing to the inability to either enter or identify the varicocele. These technical failures occurred in 0% to 71% of veno-occlusive attempts. In addition, there was an additional 5% recurrence rate. Thus, the overall success rate for these 900 attempted venographic occlusions was 69%. Although not all of these patients technically had a recurrence of their varicocele, they did undergo an unsuccessful procedure. This significant percentage indicates that venographic varicocelectomy may be less efficient than standard operative techniques. When compared with magnified varicocelectomy techniques, venographic techniques become even less attractive.

There are complications that are specific to the various techniques. Surgical repair may be accompanied by hydrocele formation 3%, epididymitis (less than 1%), and, rarely, wound infections.

Injury to the ilioinguinal nerve may occur with the approaches that violate the inguinal region. Testicular atrophy is a serious but extremely rare complication that occurs as a result of damage to the spermatic artery. The newer techniques emphasize the identification of the artery using optical magnification techniques, and, thus, this rare complication should become even rarer.

Prognosis: Infertility

Although the efficacy of varicocelectomy continues to be challenged by some, it continues to be thought of as the leading surgically correctable cause of male infertility. Pryor and Howards assembled 15 studies evaluating the success of varicocele surgery in 2466 patients.[33] The overall reported pregnancy rate was 43% (range of 24% to 53%). These studies had no rigorous scientific control and were not well-designed controlled studies. Several controlled studies have been reported that refute and support the effectiveness of varicocelectomy. There have been only six controlled studies investigating the effectiveness of varicocelectomy in treating male factor infertility. Unfortunately, these are not prospective, blinded, or randomized studies. The studies of several investigators demonstrated improved seminal parameters and pregnancy rates in patients treated with varicocelectomy as compared with those not receiving varicocelectomy.[85, 86] However, other reports did not demonstrate a beneficial effect.[37, 87] Furthermore, Nilsson and coworkers indicated that varicocelectomy had a deleterious effect on fertility.[88] Okuyama and associates carried out a controlled, prospective study evaluating the effectiveness of varicocelectomy on semen parameters.[39] In this study, adolescents with varicoceles were either surgically corrected or observed. The semen analysis in those who had undergone surgical correction was of a "higher" quality after completion of sexual maturation than in those simply observed. Unfortunately, the response to varicocelectomy is unpredictable and variable. Marks and associates attempted to identify prognostic factors for response to varicocelectomy.[89] The absence of testicular atrophy was found to indicate a good prognosis; 56% of patients with normal testicular size established pregnancies compared with a 33% pregnancy rate in patients with testicular atrophy. Patients with initial total sperm counts of 50 million or higher were significantly more likely to initiate a pregnancy after varicocelectomy. Thirty percent of patients with preoperative sperm motility of less than 60% produced pregnancies. An elevation in follicle-stimulating hormone (FSH) level was, as expected, a poor prognostic indicator; only 25% of patients with an elevation in FSH level achieved pregnancies, whereas 46% of the patients with normal FSH levels did initiate pregnancies.

Attempts have been made to correlate the size of the varicocele and response to varicocelectomy. Dubin and Amelar initially reported that varicocele grade (size) did not influence the response to varicocelectomy.[46] Tinga and colleagues subsequently studied the relationship between the varicocele size and prognosis and reported that men with moderate varicoceles and abnormal semen parameters can experience improved semen characteristics postoperatively.[90] In contrast, men with small varicoceles had a chance of experiencing a deterioration of semen parameters postoperatively. No correlation was observed between the varicocele size and the pregnancy rates after varicocelectomy. Recently, Steckel and coworkers[91] reported a positive correlation between increasing varicocele grade and seminal abnormalities. These authors observed that men with larger varicoceles were likely to have poorer preoperative semen parameters and experienced greater improvement postoperatively.

A double-blind, prospective study of patients with varicoceles, comparing those treated surgically with those treated by observation alone, would be ideal. However, it is difficult to withhold surgical intervention when studies have indicated that scrotal varicoceles result in impaired testicular function.

VASOVASOSTOMY

It is estimated that 1 million men undergo vasectomy or vasal ligation for voluntary sterilization in the United States each year. It is among the most common of all urologic procedures performed in this country.[92] In 1982, more than 15% of all couples using contraception relied on sterilization of the male partner.[93]

Although appropriate prevasectomy counseling includes the fact that vasectomies are to be considered irreversible, many patients subsequently seek vasectomy reversal. There are many reasons why a person seeks reversal of vasectomy. Most commonly, patients have been divorced and are either remarried or contemplating remarriage. Infrequently, the death of a spouse or child leads to attempted vasovasostomy.

Recent studies have demonstrated an apparent association between vasectomy and the development of prostate carcinoma.[94] Although these disturbing studies require validation, they may result in an increased demand for vasectomy reversal. However, the American Urological Association, in a statement issued on February 17, 1993 in response to these studies,* stated, "Since the relationship between vasectomy and prostate cancer is unproven, . . . the mechanism . . . is unknown—we do not recommend reversal of vasectomy."

Before the advent of improved operative techniques, instruments, and optics, successful vasectomy reversal was the exception rather than the rule. The widespread use of microsurgical techniques and the awareness of microsurgical principles have made vasectomy reversal a highly successful procedure, with sperm returning to the ejaculate (technical success) in more than 90% of patients.

Although one thinks of vasectomy reversal as a modern phenomenon, the first reported successful vasovasostomy was performed by Quinby in 1919. He used a stent of a strand of silkworm gut that was removed after 10 days. The modern era of vasovasostomies began when O'Connor reported the results of a survey of urologists who reported having performed 420 vasovasostomies.[95] The patency rate (defined as the presence of sperm in the ejaculate) was approximately 35%. In 1973, Derrick and associates reported a similar survey in which 1630 vasovasostomies were performed with a similar patency rate. The pregnancy rate for this series was 19%.[96]

Initial attempts at vasovasostomy were carried out using macroscopic (nonmagnified) techniques. Phadke and Phadke reported an individual series using a macroscopic technique with a nylon stent.[97] The pregnancy rate in this series was 55%. It was recognized early in the history of vasovasostomies that mucosal alignment was of paramount importance. This realization encouraged the use of stents, which provide the theoretical advantage of aligning the mucosal lumen. Nonabsorbable stents were exteriorized through a separate puncture site in the vas wall. This puncture point may have led to a secondary point of obstruction owing to scar and sperm granuloma formation.

Middleton and other researchers reported two large series of macrosurgical unstented vasovasostomies.[98, 99] The results as reported by Middleton were better than those reported in the initial surveys as discussed earlier. The recognition that macroscopic vasovasostomies did not allow for reliable juxtaposition of the mucosa led to widespread use of loupes for magnification. Patency rates ranged from 63% to 92% in several large series. The pregnancy rates were reported to be as high as 57%.[100–102] Attempts to improve on the results of loupe magnification vasovasostomies resulted in the combination of loupe techniques with stenting procedures. Patency

---

*Policy Statement of the American Urological Association developed by a committee composed of Drs. S. S. Howards, P. C. Walsh, J. T. Grayhack, and D. S. Coffey and endorsed by the Executive Committee, January 1993.

rates as high as 84% have been reported with this combination. Pregnancy rates as high as 70% were achieved.[100, 103-105]

The true modern era of vasovasostomy was heralded by the reports of Owen[106] and Silber,[107] who concurrently developed a two-layer microsurgical vasovasostomy. This technique allowed exact mucosal alignment without the need for stenting. Silber reported a 91% patency rate in 42 patients.[107] These patency rates were higher than those reported for all other techniques with the single exception of the report by Shessel and colleagues using a stented loupe-magnified approach.[103] Sharlip carried out a single-surgeon study comparing a two-layer microsurgical vasovasostomy and a one-layer anastomosis.[108] He reported essentially identical results. In a 20-year experience with 624 patients, Lee demonstrated a slight but not significant advantage of the two-layer anastomosis over a one-layer one in terms of the return of sperm to the ejaculate (91% versus 89%) and pregnancy (52% versus 50%).[109] Both microscopic techniques were superior to the macroscopic technique, which resulted in an 84% patency and 35% pregnancy. Most reports using a two-layer anastomosis have confirmed the superiority of the microsurgical technique compared with the macrosurgical and loupe-magnified vasovasostomy technique. However, the pregnancy rates do not seem to reflect the improved patency rates. Macroscopic techniques require no specialized training, but microscopic vasovasostomy requires that the surgeon acquire a certain level of expertise in the use of the operating microscopic and microsurgical skills.[110] The experience of the operating surgeon seems to be the most significant variable determining successful outcome.[111] Vasovasostomy is used for vasectomy reversal; however, these techniques are used in the reconstruction of iatrogenic, inflammatory, and congenital causes of obstruction.

Surgical Technique

As with any microsurgical procedure, the operating table must be prepared to allow surgeons to sit with their legs positioned comfortably beneath the surgical field. We employ an extension that positions the patient's pelvis away from the table pedestal.

Platforms should be created that allow the surgeon's arms to rest comfortably. We employ an additional set of armboards brought in alongside the table to accomplish this (Fig. 41-19). The reader is referred to microsurgical texts for descriptions of instrumentation.

Vasovasostomy may be performed under local, regional, or general anesthesia. When the site of vasectomy is easily identified, the surgeon may choose to simply exteriorize the vasal ends through a small vertical incision. This approach is most easily accomplished when a large sperm granuloma exists or metal clips were used during vasectomy. On the other hand, if the vasectomy site is not palpable, the testicle, within the intact tunica vaginalis, may be delivered via a vertical scrotal incision. After adequate mobilization of the vas above and

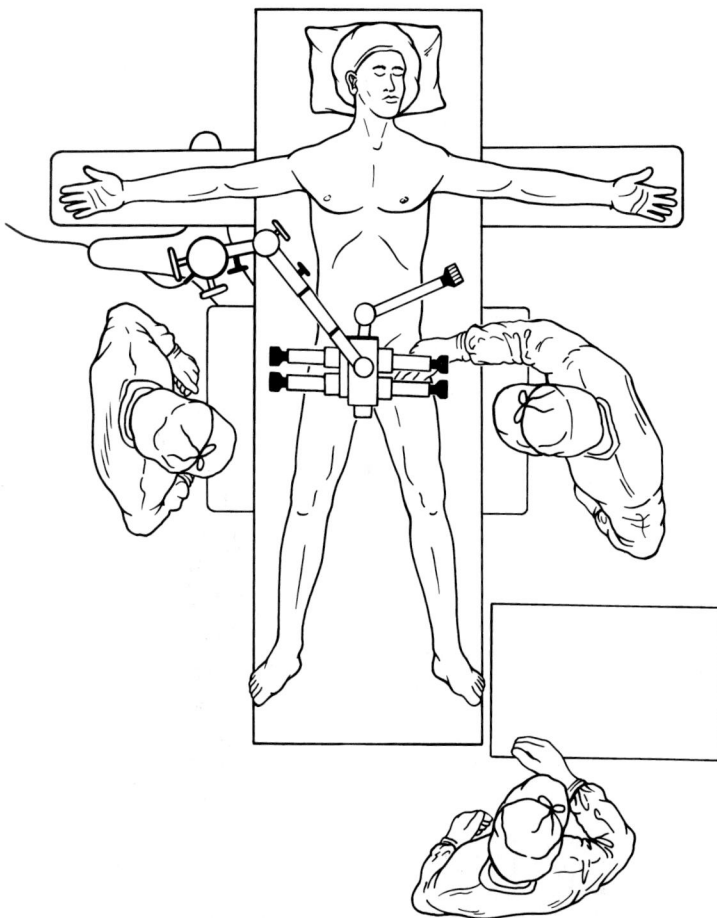

FIGURE 41-19. Table setup. This overhead view demonstrates the use of two sets of armboards. The first set is for the patient's arms. The second set, at the level of the patient's pelvis, forms a stable platform for the surgeon and assistant's arms. The position of the surgeon, assistant, operating microscope, and scrub nurse is illustrated.

below the vasectomy site, place each vasal end on a tongue blade and sharply incise with a Beaver ophthalmic scalpel. Care should be taken to make this incision perpendicular to the long axis of the vas to ensure the roundest vasal lumen and concentric muscular wall. Although it is not necessary to excise the vasectomy site, this may at times facilitate the anastomosis. The testicular vas is serially transected until fluid is obtained. A small angiocatheter is used to aspirate the fluid, which is then microscopically assessed under a phase contrast. If sperm are visualized, a vasovasostomy is performed. If copious fluid without sperm is observed, attention is redirected to the contralateral side and the fluid is reexamined later for the presence of sperm.

Before carrying out a vasovasostomy, the surgeon should confirm the patency of the abdominal or distal vas. After gentle dilation of the abdominal vas with a microsurgical forceps, a 24-gauge angiocatheter is introduced. Approximately 5 mL of dilute methylene blue is instilled. If more than gentle pressure is required to instill this fluid, distal obstruction may exist. If this is the case, formal radiologic vasography as described earlier should be carried out. This is generally not required during the routine vasectomy reversal case. After instillation of methylene blue is accomplished, the bladder is catheterized with a 16 F red rubber catheter. The return of blue-stained urine confirms the patency of the distal reproductive ducts. On the contralateral side, saline instillation can be used to establish distal patency. It is essential that the perivascular vasculature be preserved during the dissection and mobilization of the vas deferens. Hemostasis must be obtained with a bipolar cautery to prevent extensive thermal injury.

When the proximal (testicular) and the distal (abdominal) vasal ends have been mobilized, patency confirmed, and sperm identified, they are placed in a vas approximator clamp (Fig. 41–20). There must be sufficient length of vas to

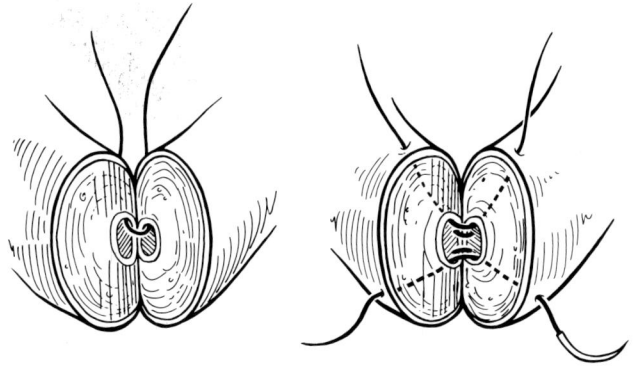

FIGURE 41–21. Modified one-layer anastomosis. This cross-sectional diagram demonstrates the position and relationship of the full-thickness sutures and the intervening muscle reinforcing sutures.

allow a tension-free anastomosis. If insufficient length of the vas is obtained, additional maneuvers may be necessary (see later). Care should be taken to ensure that the vas is not being twisted as it is being positioned in the clamp. This can be avoided by observing the location of the vasal vessels in relation to the vasal wall. The perivascular adventitia is trimmed to expose a clean muscular layer. This dissection should be limited to avoid devascularization of the anastomotic site. The application of methylene blue to the cut surface of the vas enhances the visibility of the mucosal surface. A sterile piece of colored plastic background material placed under the clamp provides contrast with the suture and enhances visibility.

SELECTION OF TECHNIQUE

As described earlier, microsurgical techniques appear to provide better results than macrosurgical techniques. We believe that these represent the current standard of care and therefore limit our discussion to the various microsurgical techniques that are currently employed.

One-Layer Microsurgical Vasovasostomy. In the modified one-layer anastomosis, a no. 9-0 suture is initially passed through the entire thickness of either the proximal or distal vas deferens from the outside in. This suture incorporates the serosa, muscularis, and mucosa of the vas. On the opposite side of the anastomosis, the suture is passed from inside to outside—again incorporating all layers of the vas. The suture is tied with the knot on the outside. Three or four additional sutures are placed similarly dividing the circumference of the vas into equal segments (Fig. 41–21). Thereafter, additional sutures are placed between each of the original sutures. This reinforcing layer of sutures does not enter the lumen and only incorporates the muscular wall of the vas. It is important to be certain that all quadrants of the vas are sutured. This can be ensured by rotating the approximating clamp 180 degrees to visualize the posterior aspect of the anastomosis. Hemostasis should be confirmed prior to removing the approximating clamp. The clamp should be carefully removed to prevent disruption of the anastomosis. The inner aspect of the scrotal wall should be examined for bleeding points. This later maneuver is particularly important if the testicle had been delivered from the scrotum to achieve the anastomosis.

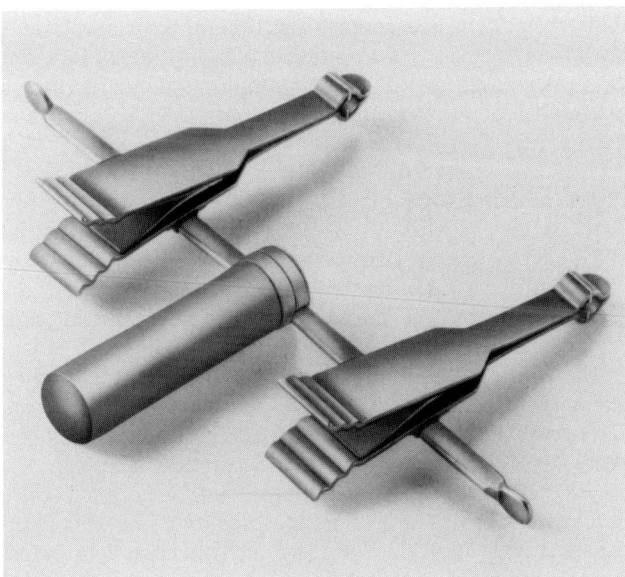

FIGURE 41–20. Vas-approximating clamp. A vas approximator (Microspike) is demonstrated. The spikes secure the vas. The hinge folds and exposes the entire vasal cross section, thus facilitating the anastomosis. (Courtesy of ASSI—Accurate Surgical and Scientific Instruments Corporation, Westbury, NY.)

The testis and epididymis are then returned to the scrotum and the dartos muscle and skin are closed in layers.

Two-Layer Microsurgical Vasovasostomy. The preparation of the vas for a two-layer vasovasostomy is identical to that required for one-layer anastomoses. The anastomosis is commenced with the approximator clamp in the bent position. This permits clear visualization of what will be the posterior muscular wall of the vas as well as the mucosal lumen.

Sutures are placed at the 5 and 7 o'clock positions, creating a posterior muscular wall (Fig. 41–22). These sutures are no. 9-0 nylon and incorporate only the muscular layer of the vas on each side. The knots are tied on the outside; one is left long. This suture acts as a marker for the posteriormost aspect of the anastomosis and allows the surgeon to flip the vas to examine it circumferentially. After these initial muscular sutures are in place, the mucosal anastomosis is begun. A double-armed short 10-0 nylon is used. The initial mucosal suture is placed at 6 o'clock between the previously placed muscular sutures. The mucosal sutures should approximate the mucosa and exclude completely intervening muscle. Thereafter, additional mucosal sutures are placed and tied at the 4 and 8 o'clock positions. The knots must be on the outside. The "tails" should be short so that they do not protrude into the vasal lumen. The anterior sutures are placed at 10 and 2 o'clock; these are left untied until the anteriormost suture at 12 o'clock is placed. They are tied sequentially in the order they were positioned. The vas approximator should be straightened before tying the suture. This facilitates mucosal approximation. Care must be taken to be certain that the anterior sutures do not inadvertently incorporate the posterior wall of the anastomosis. After completion of the mucosal anastomosis, the remainder of the muscular wall is anastomosed. This is accomplished with 8 to 10 sutures of 9-0 nylon positioned between the underlying

mucosal sutures. It is important that these sutures do not incorporate the mucosal anastomosis. The clamp can be positioned and flipped (rotated along the long axis of the vas) to facilitate completion of the anastomosis circumferentially. The posterior aspect of the anastomosis is most likely to be "neglected," and care should be taken to be certain that sutures are placed in proximity to the "long" posterior suture that was placed at the beginning of the anastomosis.

Before removing the vas from the approximator clamp, no. 4-0 chromic sutures placed through perivascular tissue may be used to remove any tension from the anastomosis. Hemostasis is secured with bipolar electrocautery. The wound is irrigated and then closed in two layers with interrupted 4-0 chromic sutures.

Treatment of Large Vas Deferens Defects

Occasionally, at the time of vasovasostomy, the surgeon is faced with a long segment of damaged or absent vas. This may be the result of a "vigorous" vasectomy, electrocautery damage to the vas, or iatrogenic injury at the time of unrelated inguinal or scrotal surgery. Treatment of large defects of the vas deferens has been described by Gilis and Borovikov.[112] By rerouting the normal anatomic course of the vas, additional length may be achieved. In cadavers, these authors demonstrated that as much as 14 cm of vasal length could be acquired by rerouting maneuvers. These have not been widely employed. Buch and Woods demonstrated in cadavers that retroperitoneal mobilization of the vas deferens resulted in a 5.83 ± 0.65-cm increase in available vasal length.[113] The combination of retroperitoneal mobilization with rerouting of the vas throughout the inguinal floor at the level of the external ring may provide sufficient length to permit reconstruction of the vas when there has been extensive iatrogenic damage.

Crossed transseptal vasovasostomy/vasoepididymostomy has been reported by several authors to achieve reconstruction when there is a solitary functioning testicle without a reconstructible vas and a contralateral vas without a functioning testicle (Fig. 41–23). These procedures allow the surgeon to establish one intact functioning unit.[114, 115]

New Techniques

There have been many modifications of the techniques used to achieve vasovasostomies. Some are simply tricks that may facilitate the procedure; others are new approaches to achieving an anastomosis.

The feasibility of laser-executed anastomoses has been extensively investigated.[116, 117] Both the neodymium:YAG and carbon dioxide lasers have been used. These modalities have been advocated because of their theoretical simplicity and speed.[118] However, these techniques still require successful mucosal apposition and therefore provide minimal theoretical advantage. Muscular "welding" after mucosal anastomosis may decrease the total operative time. These techniques, although attractive, have not been widely embraced in clinical practice.

Fibrin-tissue glue has been investigated as a replacement for sutured anastomosis. Again, this technique does not ob-

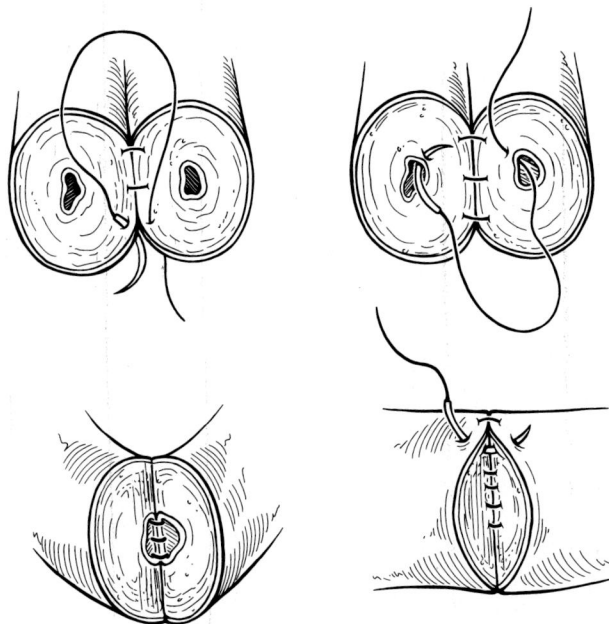

FIGURE 41–22. Two-layer anastomosis. *A,* Initial placement of posterior wall muscular sutures. *B,* Initiation of mucosal anastomosis. *C,* Completion of the posterior aspect of the mucosal anastomosis. *D,* Completion of the mucosal anastomosis and placement of the muscular sutures.

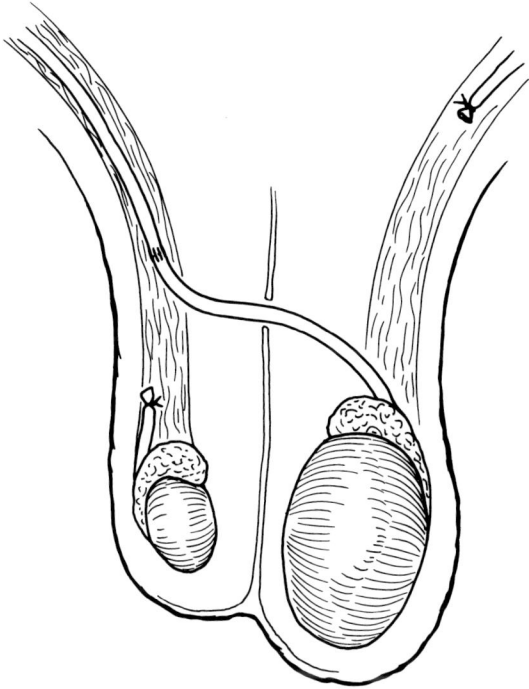

FIGURE 41–23. Crossed-septal anastomosis. One possible map for rerouting of a vas that is associated with a nonfunctional testes to a functional testes. (Modified from Goldstein M. Surgery of male infertility and other scrotal disorders. In: Walsh PC, Retik AB, Stamey TA, Vaugham ED Jr, editors. Campbell's Urology. 6th edition. 1992:3130.)

viate the need for suture placement, but as in the case of laser, it may diminish both the surgical time and operative skill required.[119] This approach had been eschewed because of the requirement for pooled fibrin and the associated risk of transmitted diseases. Recently, a technique has been described for generating autologous fibrin glue that avoids this potential drawback.[120] This approach remains investigational.

Prognostic Factors

It is generally accepted that the success rate of vasovasostomy, as measured by pregnancy, is inversely related to the interval since vasectomy. Silber reported return of sperm to the ejaculate in only 47% of patients who had undergone vasectomy longer than 10 years prior to vasovasostomy, whereas 91% of those undergoing reversal within 10 years of vasectomy had return of sperm to their ejaculate.[107] As reported by the Vasovasostomy Study Group, the deterioration in success appears to be gradually progressive rather than abrupt alterations at specific intervals.[121]

As discussed earlier, the fluid in the testicular portion of the vas should be examined at the time of vasovasostomy. The characteristics of this fluid may have prognostic significance. If no fluid is obtained or if no sperm are seen in the fluid, epididymal obstruction should be suspected (see the section on vasoepididymostomy). The Vasovasostomy Study Group examined the impact of the characteristics of the intraoperative vas fluid on the operative success. With or without the presence of sperm in the fluid, increasing degrees of creaminess (watery, opalescent, and creamy) had an inverse effect on subsequent success.[121] Silber also observed that when no sperm were present in the vas fluid, the presence of

clear and colorless fluid was associated with a better prognosis.[122]

Sperm granuloma at the vasectomy site may prevent epididymal damage by preventing pressure buildup by venting, or releasing, access pressure from the testicle. This has been referred to as a *pop-off valve*. Silber reported that the presence of a sperm granuloma ensured the presence of sperm within the vas at the time of vasectomy reversal no matter how long since vasectomy, whereas in the absence of a sperm granuloma, the longer the interval of obstruction, the less likely sperm would be present.[107]

Complications

The complications associated with reconstructive procedures are similar to those associated with any scrotal surgery. These include scrotal hematoma, swelling, or infection. In general, we do not employ a drain postoperatively; however, if oozing is noted, we do not hesitate to place one and remove it the following day. Infections have not been a problem, and antibiotics are not routinely employed.

Testicular atrophy may be the result of injury to the spermatic artery. This is a rare complication and is more likely to occur when there has been a previous attempt at microsurgical reconstruction. Hemostasis intraoperatively is obtained with a bipolar cautery to reduce the amount of tissue injury and avoid inadvertent damage to the testicular artery.

Microsurgical vasovasostomy is the current standard of care. The specific technique used is determined by the surgeon's preference. New modalities under investigation are yet to be proven to be of benefit.

Reconstruction After Failed Vasovasostomy

Persistent azoospermia after vasovasostomy is indicative of failure. This may be the result of technical failure or unrecognized epididymal obstruction at the time of initial reconstruction. As discussed earlier, a small but significant number of men undergoing vasovasostomy continue to be azoospermic. These patients may benefit from another attempt at vasal reconstruction; however, it is important that they are counseled appropriately. The surgeon should attempt to ascertain the cause of the failure from the prior operative report. Specifically, the findings of the intraoperative vasal fluid should be noted. The absence of fluid within the vas or the absence of sperm within the fluid at the time of initial reversal indicates the probable need for vasoepididymostomy, whereas the presence of sperm in the fluid may indicate that a repeat vasovasostomy may be indicated. If the operative report does not describe the vasal fluid, one should assume that a vasoepididymostomy will be required. As discussed, vasoepididymostomy is technically more difficult and is associated with a lower technical and functional success rate (i.e., pregnancy) compared with vasovasostomy. The patient must be apprised of this prior to any reattempt at vasectomy reversal (see the later section on prognosis).

TECHNICAL CONSIDERATIONS

In repeat reversal attempts, the scrotal contents are delivered through a vertical incision in the scrotum. The site of the prior anastomosis is identified. A vasotomy is made proximal to this site, and the fluid is examined microscopically. If sperm are present just proximal to the anastomosis, obstruction is almost certainly at the site of the prior anastomosis. However, more distal obstruction may exist if patency was not demonstrated at the time of the previous surgery. Distal patency should be assessed by the instillation of saline or formal vasography.

If obstruction is demonstrated at the prior anastomosis, it should be excised and reanastomosis performed using meticulous microsurgical technique. If sperm are not identified proximal to the prior anastomosis, epididymal obstruction exists. This finding does not preclude the possibility of distal obstruction and, therefore, patency must be demonstrated prior to proceeding with vasoepididymostomy. If the anastomotic site is patent, vasoepididymostomy is performed without disturbing the previous anastomosis. However, if the site is not patent, the vas distal to the initial vasovasostomy may be mobilized and used for the vasoepididymostomy. Great care must be exercised to preserve the vascular supply to the vas in secondary vasovasostomies.

PROGNOSIS

The results of repeat vasectomy reversal are affected by the procedure required. The Vasovasostomy Study Group reported a 75% technical success rate in 199 evaluable patients.[121] When bilateral vasovasostomy was performed in this group, 102 of 121 (84%) of the patients had sperm return to the ejaculate. Only 12 of 28 (43%) of the patients undergoing bilateral vasoepididymostomy experienced return of sperm to the ejaculate. The pregnancy rates were 53% and 15%, respectively. Although patients should be offered repeat attempts at vasectomy reversal, they should have realistic expectations.

VASOEPIDIDYMOSTOMY

Although the epididymis is the first portion of the conduit system for the transport of sperm, it is more than a pipeline. The epididymis is a poorly understood organ with complex functions related to sperm storage, maturation, and transport.[123] In the in vivo situation, it appears that spermatozoa require passage through at least a portion of the epididymis to gain motility and the ability to fertilize. The mechanisms by which sperm gain these functions within the epididymis have not been delineated, nor is it clear how much of the epididymis or whether specific portions of the epididymis are required for the maturation of spermatozoa.[124] Although early studies suggested that sperm maturation is completed in the cauda epididymidis, subsequent studies indicated that fertilizing capacity is gained within the proximal corpus epididymidis.[125, 126] Recently, sperm from the most proximal portions of the epididymis and efferent tubules have demonstrated the capacity to fertilize ova in vitro.[127] Extrapolation from in vitro to in vivo data may not accurately represent the functional significance of different portions of the epididymis. The results of microsurgical reconstruction procedures indicate that sperm that traverse greater portions of the epididymis are functionally superior. It is this observation that makes understanding the function of the epididymis of such great clinical importance. The distal or cauda epididymides serve

as a storage reservoir capable of containing more than 400 million sperm in the fertile male.[128] It is clear that epididymal function is complex and contributes to sperm motility, maturation, and storage.

In spite of the fact that the physiology of the epididymis has not been clearly delineated, at the time of microsurgical reconstruction of the obstructed epididymis, the surgeon should attempt to preserve as much of the epididymis as possible. Epididymal obstruction can be the result of (1) congenital anatomic abnormalities of the vas and epididymis; (2) inflammatory processes; or (3) vasal obstruction. Obstruction of the vas results in increased intratubular epididymal pressures. This increased pressure will, at times, cause the epididymal tubule to rupture or "blow out"—this will be the site of obstruction. Epididymitis from infectious organisms such as Neisseria gonorrhoeae, Mycobacterium tuberculosis, and Chlamydia trachomatis is frequently cited as a cause of obstructive azoospermia.[129, 130]

Epididymal obstruction is discovered in two clinical settings. The first is the azoospermic male undergoing evaluation for infertility. (The algorithm for this evaluation is outlined in the section on testicular biopsy.) Epididymal obstruction is often suspected because of the patient's history or physical examination. However, the diagnosis of epididymal obstruction can be made only at the time of definitive surgical exploration of the azoospermic male. The second clinical setting is the patient undergoing vasectomy reversal. This patient is also diagnosed as having epididymal obstruction at the time of surgical exploration; however, the vasectomy patient does not undergo the evaluation as outlined for the nonvasectomy azoospermic patient.

In the azoospermic male with proven spermatogenesis, the absence of vasal sperm indicates epididymal obstruction. In the vasectomy reversal patient, the absence of fluid in the testicular portion of the vas indicates epididymal obstruction. The presence of fluid without sperm may or may not be associated with epididymal obstruction. Investigators have studied the prognostic significance of the physical characteristics of vasal fluid that is devoid of sperm. Clear, copious fluid or fluid with sperm heads is associated with a good prognosis for the return of sperm following vasovasostomy. A poor prognosis is associated with the absence of fluid or thick, pasty fluid.[131, 132] If the latter is found, epididymal obstruction should be suspected and treated. The decision to proceed with vasoepididymostomy should also be tempered by the recognition of one's microsurgical skills and the ability to perform this difficult procedure successfully.

Vasoepididymostomy Techniques

Macroscopic and three main types of microscopic vasoepididymostomy have been described: microsurgical single-tubule, end-to-end (Silber technique), and end-to-side tubule anastomoses.

MACROSCOPIC TECHNIQUE

The advent of microsurgical techniques has resulted in the abandonment of macrosurgical vasoepididymostomy.[123] Macrosurgical vasoepididymostomy relied on the creation of a fistula between incised epididymal tubules and a spatulated vas deferens. This technique is mentioned only for completeness because it does not represent the standard level of care. The epididymal tunic and the underlying epididymal tubule are incised, releasing the fluid from the obstructed system. The vas is then spatulated longitudinally and sutured to the edge of the epididymal tunic. This technique relies on the formation of a controlled fistula between the epididymal and the vasal lumina. Its major advantage is its ease; its disadvantage is its lack of success. Additionally, the most distal point of epididymal obstruction could not be identified. This technique should no longer be used to treat epididymal obstruction.

MICROSURGICAL SINGLE-TUBULE ANASTOMOSIS

The use of the operating microscope enabled the development of techniques that allow for direct anastomosis of the vasal lumen to the epididymal lumen. Silber is generally credited with the development of a tubule-specific vasoepididymostomy.[133] The relative reliability of this technique, when compared with macroscopic techniques, has resulted in its widespread use and modification.[134, 135]

END-TO-END VASOEPIDIDYMOSTOMY (SILBER TECHNIQUE)

In the end-to-end vasoepididymostomy (Silber technique), the testicle is delivered from the scrotum when a vasoepididymostomy is anticipated. The vas is identified and isolated. A vasotomy is performed as described in the section on vasography. The vasal lumen is assessed for the presence or absence of fluid. Fluid, if present, is analyzed. Vasal and ejaculatory duct patency is confirmed by either dye (methylene blue) or radiologic studies. When the decision to proceed with vasoepididymostomy has been made, the tunica vaginalis is opened, exposing the epididymis. The epididymis is then visually inspected. Obstruction is associated with dilated tubules, which are generally easily appreciated through the tunica of the epididymis. An abrupt transition is often noted between dilated and empty tubules, indicating the point of obstruction. The tail of the epididymis is mobilized by dividing its attachment to the testes. The epididymis is then transected serially from the distalmost portion proceeding to the caput. The cut surface is examined for the presence of a tubule that effluxes fluid. If fluid is encountered, it is examined for the presence of sperm. The cut surface of the epididymis will have many "lumen"; however, only the proximal lumen (i.e., the lumen that is in continuity with the proximal epididymal tubule) will continue to drain sperm-containing fluid. Meticulous hemostasis is required to identify the draining lumen. The cephalad progression must be methodical until the appropriate lumen is identified and marked with a no. 10-0 nylon suture. (This marking suture will facilitate the subsequent anastomosis.) The transected abdominal vas is then approximated to the epididymal tunic. Approximately four double-armed 10-0 nylon sutures are placed within the epididymal tubule (Fig. 41–24). These are then placed inside-out through the vasal mucosa and tied serially. Care must be taken to tie all knots on the outside. The vas wall is then sutured to the epididymal tunic with interrupted 9-0 nylon sutures.[131–133, 136, 137] This completes a two-layer end-to-

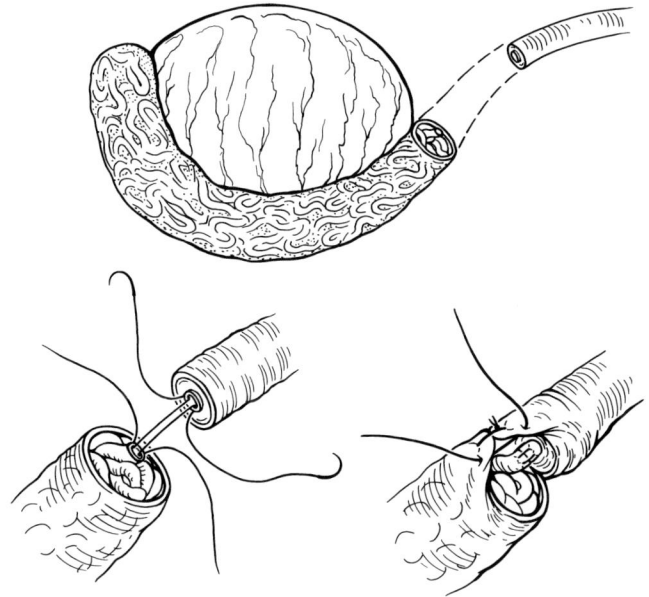

FIGURE 41–24. End-to-end vasoepididymostomy. *A,* The distal epididymis has been transected. The "proximal" epididymal tubule is identified by the persistent drainage of sperm-containing fluid. *B,* Double-armed no. 10-0 nylon sutures are placed in the lumen of the epididymal tubule and then through the vasal mucosa. These are tied sequentially with the knots on the outside *C,* A second layer of no. 9-0 nylon sutures approximates vasal adventitia and tunica of the epididymis, thus completing a watertight anastomosis. (Modified from Goldstein M. Surgery of male infertility and other scrotal disorders. In: Walsh PC, Retik AB, Stamey TA, Vaughan ED Jr, editors. Campbell's Urology. 6th edition. 1992:3114.)

end vasoepididymostomy. Routine microsurgical principles must be adhered to.

Although Silber reported excellent results with this technique, it is difficult and tedious. Hemostasis of the transected epididymis is difficult to obtain, and identification of the "proximal" tubule is cumbersome.[134, 135] This technique, however, should be recognized as an important contribution to the reconstruction of the obstructed epididymis.

END-TO-SIDE TUBULE ANASTOMOSIS

The assessment and initial preparation for the end-to-side tubule anastomosis technique are the same as for the end-to-end anastomosis. Again, the epididymis is examined with the operating microscope to identify the presumed point of obstruction. When dilated tubules are visualized beneath the epididymal tunic, a small window is then created. If the tunica is not thickened, the underlying tubule may be inadvertently entered. This is an annoying and troublesome complication that should be avoided. Once the tunica window has been created, underlying tubules are readily visualized. The epididymis should be grasped between the surgeon's forefinger and thumb; gentle pressure aids in the identification of a tubule. The tubule is then cleared of surrounding tissue. It is important that appropriate attention is paid to this detail, because it will facilitate both the opening of the tubule and the anastomosis.

At this point, the previously prepared vas deferens is approximated to the epididymal window with two no. 9-0 nylon sutures. These sutures will form the posterior wall of the anastomosis. Only after these sutures have been placed should the epididymal tubule be opened. Methylene blue should be applied to the prepared tubule and an ellipse made with sharp microsurgical scissors. At times, an ultrasharp microsurgical knife may be used.

Immediately on opening the epididymal tubule, a no. 10-0 nylon suture is used to mark the edge of the lumen. The previously placed methylene blue aids in the identification of the wall: The lumen appears white; the wall blue. Fluid is aspirated into a syringe with an angiocatheter and assessed for the presence of sperm. If sperm are found, three or four additional double-armed 10-0 nylon sutures are placed. These sutures are then passed inside out through the vasal mucosa (Fig. 41–25). They are tied sequentially with the knots on the outside. The outer layer of the anastomosis is completed with 9-0 nylon sutures from the vasal wall to the epididymal tunica, thus completing a two-layer end-to-side vasoepididymostomy.

We prefer the end-to-side vasoepididymostomy technique. Because it avoids transection of the epididymis, hemostasis is not problematic, and identification of sperm-containing epididymal tubules is facilitated. Furthermore, one can be certain that the anastomosis is carried out to the "proximal" tubule because this technique does not disrupt the epididymal tubule.

Results

As with vasovasostomy, success can be measured in terms of patency (i.e., return of sperm to the ejaculate) or, more appropriately, of pregnancy. Patency has been reported to be between 50% and 70%.[138] Silber reported a 78% patency rate

when anastomosis was performed at the corpus epididymidis.[139] Pregnancy rates are not as encouraging and are reported to vary between 15% and 30%.[138] It has been also noted that the greater the length of epididymis that the sperm traverse, the higher the pregnancy rate. Silber reported a 72% pregnancy rate for "patent" vasoepididymostomies performed at the level of the corpus epididymidis, whereas the pregnancy rate for patent anastomoses at the level of the caput was 43%.[139] Vasoepididymostomy is a technically demanding procedure that can be associated with a reasonable degree of success.

TRANSURETHRAL RESECTION OF EJACULATORY DUCT OBSTRUCTION

Ejaculatory duct obstruction is an uncommon form but a readily treatable cause of obstruction of the male reproductive tract. It has been reported to occur in 3% to 7.4% of infertile men.[140, 141] Historically, the diagnosis of ejaculatory duct obstruction was made on the basis of intraoperative vasography. However, widespread use of transrectal ultrasonography and its ability to detect abnormalities of the ejaculatory duct apparatus has resulted in an apparent increased incidence of this diagnosis. Treatment of distal or ejaculatory duct obstruction is through transurethral surgery.[142]

Etiology

Obstruction of the ejaculatory duct apparatus may be the result of either congenital-embryologic or acquired abnormalities. Congenital midline retroprostatic and retrovesical

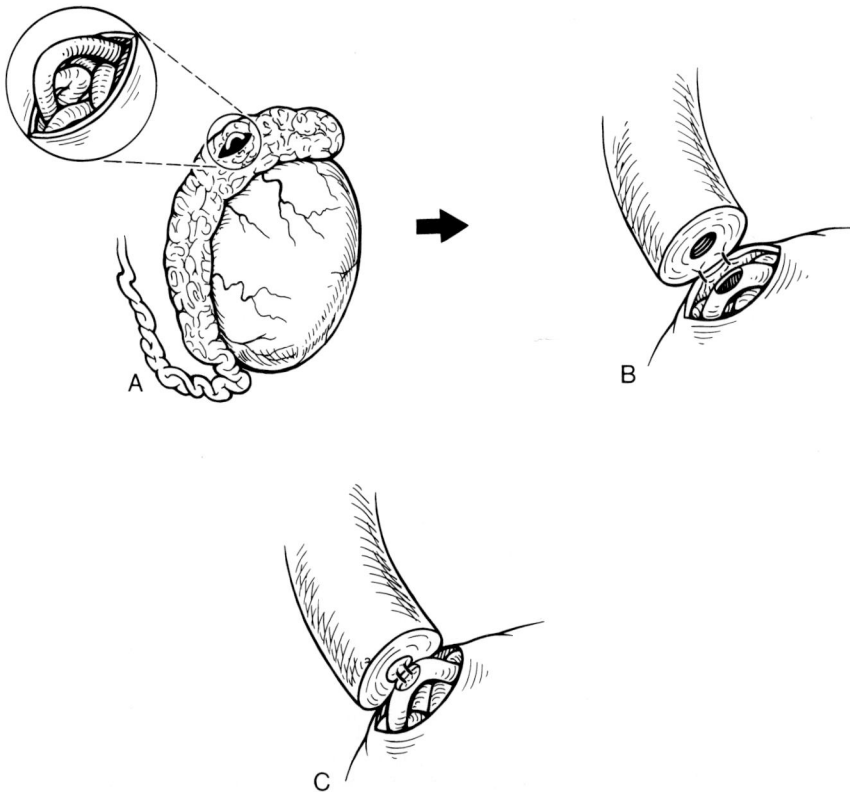

FIGURE 41–25. End-to-side vasoepididymostomy. A, The tunica overlying a dilated epididymal tubule is opened. This creates a window to expose the dilated tubule. B, The muscular wall of the vas is sutured to the tunica of the epididymis, creating the posterior wall of the vasoepididymostomy. C, No. 10-0 nylon sutures are placed in the epididymal tubule for the mucosal anastomosis. Knots should be outside the lumen.

cysts that communicate with the vasa and seminal vesicles may cause ejaculatory duct obstruction.[143] Aspiration of these cysts reveals sperm-containing fluid if spermatogenesis is present. Intraprostatic "cysts" that contain sperm have been classified as ejaculatory duct diverticula and are wolffian duct in origin. Midline müllerian cysts that may cause obstruction of the ejaculatory ducts do not communicate with the ejaculatory ducts. Müllerian cysts cause obstruction by compression of the ejaculatory ducts. These cysts are devoid of sperm when aspirated or entered endoscopically.[144]

Acquired obstructions are common and may account for a significant portion of patients with ejaculatory duct obstruction. This form of obstruction is the result of inflammatory processes of the posterior urethra, such as prostatitis, tuberculosis, and gonococcal urethritis.[145]

Urethral trauma or instrumentation resulting from indwelling urethral catheters, urethral foreign bodies, or transurethral surgery can also produce ejaculatory duct obstruction.[146]

Diagnosis

Bilateral ejaculatory duct obstruction has classically been suspected in the patient with fructose-negative azoospermia associated with a low ejaculate volume. The patient who is suspected of having ejaculatory duct obstruction as the cause of fructose-negative azoospermia should have normal testicular size and bilaterally palpable vas deferens. The patient with absent vas deferens may also present with fructose-negative azoospermia. However, in this situation the fructose-negative azoospermia is secondary to the absence of the seminal vesicles and the vasa rather than an obstruction of the ejaculatory duct; therefore, it is important that the presence of the vasa be confirmed by physical examination. Addition-

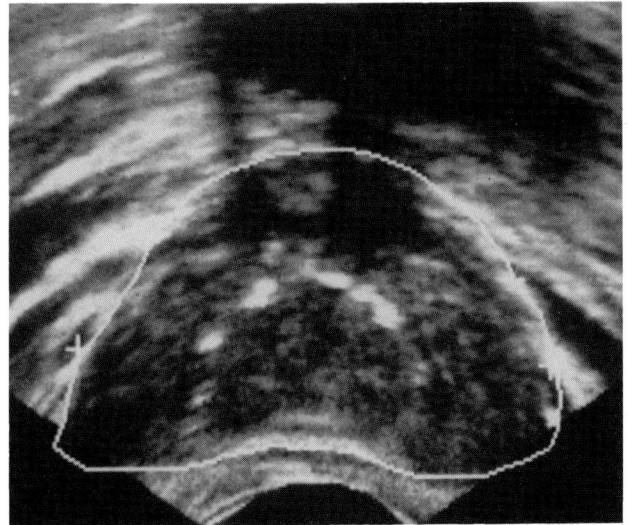

FIGURE 41–27. Axial view from a transrectal ultrasonographic examination demonstrating a midline cystic structure with a hyperechoic cystic wall.

ally, retrograde ejaculation should be ruled out by examining an immediate postejaculatory urine specimen (Fig. 41–26).[147] Recently, it has been appreciated that patients with severe oligospermia and a low ejaculate volume may have partial ejaculatory duct obstruction.

When the diagnosis of ejaculatory duct obstruction is suspected on the basis of the parameters just described, transrectal ultrasonography is performed. This modality allows for the accurate assessment of the size of the seminal vesicles and ejaculatory ducts as well as abnormalities such as cystic structures and digitation of the ejaculatory duct (Fig. 41–27). Preoperative transrectal ultrasonography may also determine the site of obstruction and allow the surgeon to determine whether the obstruction is amenable to transurethral resection (TUR). In some instances the site of obstruction is beyond the confines of the prostate, and TUR of the prostate would be of no benefit.[148]

Although vasography has traditionally been used to make the diagnosis of ejaculatory duct obstruction, this modality is now rarely required if the diagnosis is suspected. Some authors have suggested the use of testicular biopsy in these patients.[149] However, we do not perform testicular biopsy if ejaculatory duct obstruction is clearly demonstrated ultrasonographically and the patient has normal testicles and endocrinologic studies and a negative past history.[150]

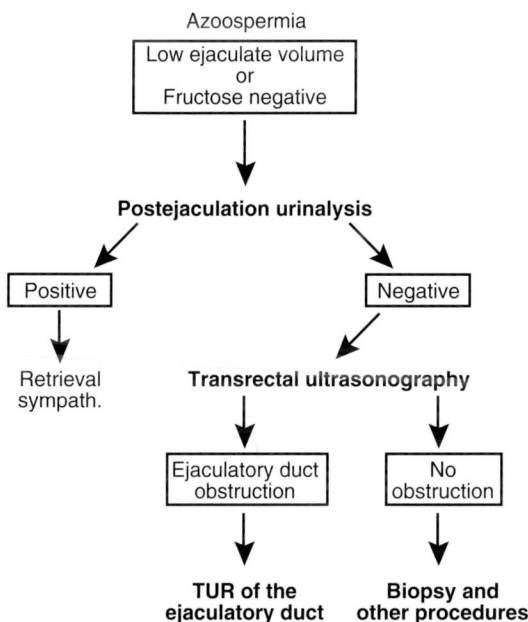

FIGURE 41–26. Diagnostic algorithm outlining the approach to the patient with low ejaculate volume or fructose-negative azoospermia (see text for explanation).

Surgical Technique

The technique of TUR of the ejaculatory ducts involves unroofing the distal ends of the ducts as they lie within the posterior portion of the prostate gland lateral to the verumontanum. Patients are placed in the dorsal lithotomy position as if being prepared for transurethral prostatectomy. An O'Connor drape is placed within the rectum to permit digital guidance during the resection. Although earlier reports describe two separate incisions, lateral and proximal to the verumontanum, we resect the proximal portion of the verumontanum (Fig. 41–28).[146, 150] If the obstruction is distal, the

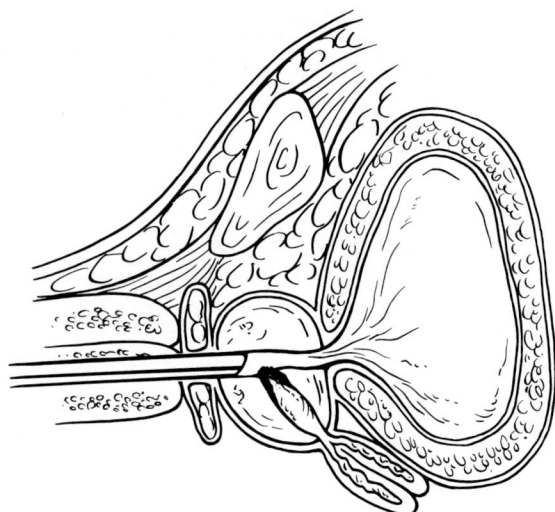

FIGURE 41–28. Schematic sagittal view of a prostate with a midline cyst causing ejaculatory duct obstruction. The obstruction is relieved by resecting the proximal verumontanum and continuing posteriorly and toward the bladder neck until the cyst is entered.

dilated ejaculatory ducts may be entered immediately. If not, the resection is continued toward the bladder neck and posteriorly until efflux of seminal fluid is seen emanating from the unobstructed ejaculatory ducts. Palpation through the rectum is used throughout the procedure to ensure the integrity of the rectum and attempt to express seminal vesicle contents as the resection proceeds. Care must be taken to avoid penetrating the prostatic capsule or injuring the bladder neck or external urethral sphincter. Injury to the bladder neck may result in retrograde ejaculation; external urethral sphincteric injury may result in urinary incontinence.

Patients are catheterized for 24 hours postoperatively. Terazosin is initiated postoperatively to facilitate urination.

Complications

As discussed earlier, the major complications of TUR of the ejaculatory ducts relate to injury of adjacent structures. Because most of the patients undergoing this procedure are young men with small prostate glands, great care must be taken to avoid injury of the bladder neck, external sphincter, or rectal wall. Epididymitis may result from any urethral instrumentation. Accordingly, it is generally believed that disruption of the normal ejaculatory duct apparatus may be associated with an increased incidence of epididymitis. Because many patients experience difficulty urinating postoperatively, we routinely discharge patients on terazosin for 1 week. Long-term complications include the potential for fibrosis and reobstruction of the ejaculatory duct. Therefore, in the oligospermic patient, a complete explanation of therapeutic alternatives should be given to the patient before this form of therapy is used.

Results

Goldwasser and associates have emphasized that the prognosis for patients with ejaculatory duct obstruction varies with the cause of the obstruction.[150] In their series, congenital obstruction treated by transurethral surgery resulted in normal sperm counts in 71% of the patients and pregnancies in 57%. Acquired obstruction not associated with genital tract infection resulted in normal sperm counts in 50% of patients. In contrast, obstruction caused by genital infections was associated with a poor prognosis, and none of their patients achieved normal sperm counts or pregnancy.[146]

We have found that the cause of ejaculatory duct obstruction is often unclear. Of 24 patients treated with TUR of the ejaculatory ducts, 22 have experienced either an increase in semen volume or concentration/count, or both.[151]

Although the response to TUR of ejaculatory duct obstruction is variable, the response can be quite dramatic. The patient with low-ejaculate, fructose-negative azoospermia may have essentially normal semen parameters postoperatively. Semen parameters may improve sufficiently to allow other therapies to be employed. Because there are potentially significant complications associated with this therapy, patients must be fully apprised of the risks and alternatives.[146]

ALLOPLASTIC SPERMATOCELE

Many forms of obstructive azoospermia exist that are not amenable to corrective surgery. Nonremedial obstruction may be due to congenital vasal agenesis, vasal atresia, failed prior reconstruction, or anejaculation secondary to procedures such as retroperitoneal lymph node dissection. Common to these conditions are normal testicular sperm production and abnormal sperm delivery.[152] It has long been appreciated that sperm may be retrieved from naturally forming spermatoceles.[153] Therefore, early attempts were made to create spermatoceles from which sperm could be retrieved and used for insemination procedures. Unfortunately, these early efforts using human tissues had minimal success.[154–159] Early attempts at creating reservoirs relied on the use of human tissue.

Because of the relative lack of success using autologous tissue, artificial spermatoceles were developed. These reservoirs have been termed *alloplastic spermatoceles.*

Kelami and associates[160] first used silicone prostheses in pigs. The devices were installed on 22 caput epididymides and 47 cauda epididymides. Two established pregnancies were reported in their series of 10 inseminations with sperm from alloplastic spermatoceles.

In 1981, a human pregnancy was achieved after implanting 18 prostheses in 14 patients.[161] Kelami determined that 3 to 5 days' postimplantation was the optimal time for aspiration. All devices became occluded between 1 week and 6 months after implantation. Unfortunately, most efforts to use alloplastic spermatoceles have met with limited or no success.[162–169]

In 1992, Moni and colleagues[170] described a procedure called a *Moni's window.* This procedure created a window between the obstructed epididymal tubule and the tunica vaginalis space. Sperm accumulated in this potential space and was then aspirated for insemination. Four patients underwent a Moni's window procedure: all had sperm on aspiration, and one couple achieved a pregnancy.

Surgical Technique

The techniques used to create alloplastic spermatoceles vary with the device implanted. In general, the microsurgically incised tubule is sutured to the epididymal tunica in an attempt to maintain a patent ostium for drainage into the reservoir. A new device (designed by a collaborative group) is based on the principle of suturing the edge of the tubule directly to the device. The preliminary animal data have been encouraging.[170a]

Moni's window technique sutures the edge of the epididymal tubule to the visceral surface of the tunica vaginalis. Thus, the entire space of the tunica vaginalis (i.e., between the parietal and visceral surfaces) becomes a spermatocele, and aspirations are initiated 4 to 6 weeks postoperatively. The validity of this approach has yet to be confirmed.

The optimal timetable for spermatocele aspiration has not been established. Individual investigators have established arbitrary schedules. None of these techniques has proved reliable. In Moni's window procedure, aspirations are initiated 4 to 6 weeks postoperatively.

Conclusion

The low pregnancy rate of 7.7% and term delivery rate of 4.4% achieved from 130 artificial spermatocele implantations in 91 patients[167] suggests that other techniques are necessary to achieve conception for men with congenital vasal agenesis.

MICROSCOPIC EPIDIDYMAL SPERM ASPIRATION

Congenital absence of vas deferens has been reported to account for approximately 10% of noniatrogenic obstructive azoospermia.[171] This anatomic abnormality precludes reconstruction procedures. Surgeons have been able to acquire sperm from natural or alloplastic spermatoceles for use in insemination. Although there have been pregnancies reported with this technique, the results have been unsatisfactory. No therapy could be afforded to these patients, who had normal testes and spermatogenesis, until microsurgical techniques were used to acquire sperm from the epididymis that were then used for in vitro fertilization.

Microsurgical epididymal sperm aspiration (MESA) was first described in 1985. Initially, this technique was used in the treatment of patients with secondary obstructive azoospermia.[172] In 1988 Silber and coworkers used this procedure to treat males with bilateral vasal agenesis.[173]

Patient Evaluation

Because both the male and female undergo invasive procedures when MESA is used, it is important that a thorough preliminary evaluation is carried out. As indicated earlier, MESA may be used for the treatment of nonreconstructible acquired or congenital obstructive azoospermia. The diagnosis of congenital obstruction secondary to congenital vasal agenesis is easily rendered: These patients have, in general, normal testicular size; the vas is not palpable; the epididymis is only partially formed and may be globular in configuration; and endocrinologic studies are normal. It is imperative that both the male and female partner undergo genetic counseling because of the high incidence of heterozygosity for the genes of cystic fibrosis in patients with congenital vasal agenesis (see later).[174] If the diagnosis is certain, no other evaluation of the male is required. Hollander and associates[175] recommended performance of testicular biopsy prior to MESA. Although this was our practice initially in patients with congenital vasal agenesis, we no longer perform biopsies when the patient's testicular examination and hormonal assessment are normal. However, the patient undergoing MESA for other causes of presumed obstructive azoospermia requires the appropriate evaluation of azoospermia as indicated by physical examination, history, and laboratory studies.

The female partner must undergo appropriate evaluation before in vitro fertilization is initiated. This is guided by history, physical examination, and the results of preliminary laboratory studies.

CONGENITAL VASAL AGENESIS AND CYSTIC FIBROSIS: GENETIC EVALUATION

Kaufman and colleagues first reported an apparently healthy adult with bilateral vasal agenesis who was subsequently diagnosed as having cystic fibrosis.[176] It was suggested that men with bilateral vasal agenesis be suspected of having cystic fibrosis. Oates and coworkers reported that 55% of men with congenital agenesis of the vas were carriers of cystic fibrosis, whereas only 4% of control patients were heterozygous for cystic fibrosis.[174] Recently, Patrizio and associates reported the genetic testing of the parents and offspring of patients with congenital vasal agenesis.[177] They demonstrated that 56% of the patients were positive for at least one of the cystic fibrosis mutations. Six of 18 parents studied were also positive, and 3 of 10 offspring were found to be carriers of cystic fibrosis mutations. These observations emphasize the importance of genetic screening.

Technique

The reproductive endocrinologist and urologic surgeon establish a target date for MESA. Current stimulation protocols allow for excellent coordination and timing. Different MESA teams have had differing approaches to the "order" of the procedures. Should egg retrieval precede sperm retrieval, or vice versa? Because it is rare that either of these procedures will be unsuccessful in acquiring gametes, we have chosen to proceed with egg retrieval first, because an unnecessary epididymal aspiration may cause damage and potentially preclude subsequent aspirations. In a recent review by Belker and coworkers, only 11% of attempted aspirations yielded no sperm or sperm inadequate for ovum insemination.[178]

Scrotal contents are brought out through a longitudinal scrotal incision, the tunica vaginalis is opened, and the testicle and epididymis are exposed. Using the operating microscope, the tunica of epididymis is incised with microscissors, thus exposing the dilated epididymal tubules. We use a mi-

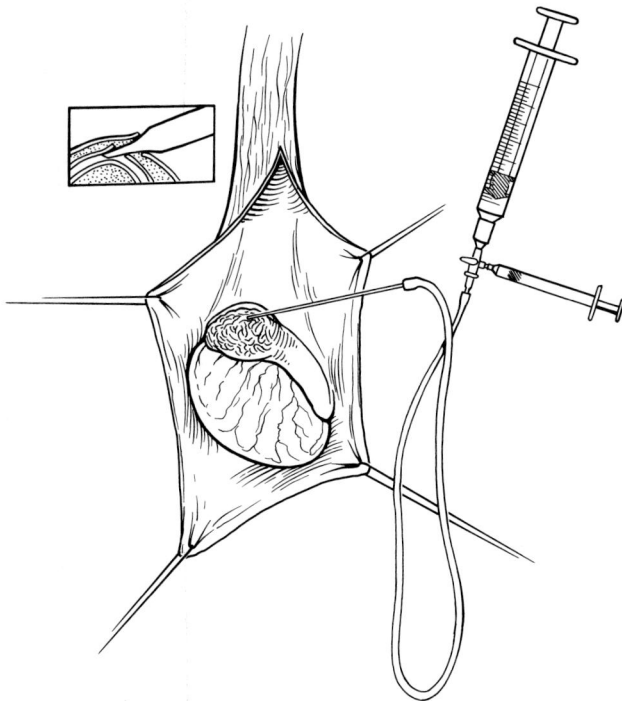

FIGURE 41–29. A sharpened micropipette (250–350 μ) with attached tubing and aspiration syringe is used to microsurgically puncture the epididymal tubule for MESA. (Modified from Goldstein M. Surgery of male infertility and other scrotal disorders. In: Walsh PC, Retik AB, Stamey TA, Vaughan ED Jr, editors. Campbell's Urology. 6th edition. 1992:3138.)

cropipette system as described by Schlegel to retrieve sperm from the epididymis.[179] This allows direct puncture of the epididymal tubule and aspiration of the contents without contamination (Fig. 41–29). The aspirating micropipette is preloaded with HEPES buffer or a suitable culture medium. Care should be taken to maintain the pH of the medium. This preloading permits the surgeon to flush the sperm-containing fluid into an appropriate chamber containing additional fluid for immediate assessment by laboratory personnel.

It is imperative to ensure the presence of motile sperm. If none is found, more proximal aspirations are attempted. Once the area of motile sperm is located, the sperm-containing fluid is patiently aspirated. The epididymal fluid and buffer medium are transported to an in vitro fertilization laboratory for processing. Standard ovum insemination or micromanipulation is performed.

The epididymal tubules are closed with no. 10-0 nylon sutures. The tunica is closed with 9-0 nylon sutures. This microsurgical closure minimizes scarring that may interfere with repeat MESA procedures. Belker and colleagues reported that 12% of 193 MESA attempts were repeat MESA procedures.[178] The scrotum is closed in the standard fashion.

Results

Historically, it has been thought that sperm must traverse the epididymis to mature and acquire fertilization potential.[180–184] This dogma was the result of basic laboratory ex-

perimental studies and clinical observations of the results after microsurgical vasoepididymostomy.[183] The recent success of MESA procedures clearly indicates that epididymal sperm are capable of fertilization under in vitro conditions.[184] Although sperm that have not traversed the epididymis are capable of fertilization under these conditions, one cannot assume that epididymal function is not required for fertilization in vivo. The requirements for fertilization may be different under in vitro fertilization conditions. Furthermore, the congenitally abnormal epididymis may express different functions within different segments when compared with the normal epididymis. Therefore, it is not possible to assess normal epididymal physiology on the basis of the in vitro function of sperm from the pathologic congenitally obstructed epididymis. Silber and colleagues reported a fertilization rate of 60% and clinical pregnancy rate of 31%.[184] Seven deliveries and three miscarriages were reported for a live birth rate of 21.9% per cycle. Other authors have not experienced similar results. Belker and coworkers reviewed MESA in 219 patients at 22 centers in the United States.[178] The overall fertilization rate was reported to be 33%; the pregnancy rate per center ranged from 9% to 33%. Micromanipulation techniques have shown that epididymal sperm lacking motility may have fertilization capacity,[185] and in the future this may improve pregnancy rates. MESA is an exciting, extremely expensive, labor-intensive new technique that provides a form of therapy for couples with a previously untreatable condition. Couples must undergo appropriate genetic counseling and be aware of the emotional and financial risks before embarking on this form of therapy.

CONCLUSION

The evaluation and treatment of male factor infertility rely on the appropriate use of the diagnostic and therapeutic techniques discussed in this chapter. Some of these techniques are in evolution and represent significant advances. They also highlight the need for appropriate cooperation and collaboration between the gynecologist/reproductive endocrinologist in the treatment of the infertile couple.

REFERENCES

1. Lipshultz LI, Howards SS. Evaluation of the subfertile man. In: Lipshultz LI, Howards SS, editors. Infertility in the Male. New York: Churchill Livingstone, 1983.
2. Charny CW: Testicular biopsy: its value in male sterility. JAMA 1940;115:1429.
3. Kaufman DG, Nagler HM. Aspiration flow cytometry of the testes in the evaluation of spermatogenesis in the infertile male. Fertil Steril 1987;48(2):287.
4. Nagler HN, Thomas AJ. Testicular biopsy and vasogram in the evaluation of male infertility. Urol Clin North Am 1987;14(1):167.
5. Garduno A, Mehan DJ. Testicular biopsy findings in patients with impaired fertility. J Urol 1970;104:871.
6. Silber SJ, Rodriguez-Rigau LJ. Quantitative analysis of testicular biopsy: determination of partial obstruction and prediction of sperm count after surgery for obstruction. Fertil Steril 1981;36:480.
7. Krause I, Nagler HM. The role of bilateral testicular biopsies in the evaluation of infertile males. New York Academy of Medicine Valentines Essay Contest, 1992.
8. Posinovec J. The necessity for bilateral biopsy in oligo- and azoospermia. Int J Fertil 1976;21:189.

9. Ibrahim AA, Awad HA, El-Haggar S, et al. Bilateral testicular biopsy in men with varicocele. Fertil Steril 1977;28:663.

10. Lipshultz LI, Howards SS, McClure RD, et al. When and how to do a testis biopsy and vasogram. Contemp Urol 1990;7:45.

11. Coburn M, Wheeler TM, Lipshultz LI. Cytological examination of testis biopsy specimens [Abstract]. Presented at the Annual Meeting of the American Fertility Society, Birmingham, Alabama, 1986:122.

12. Cohen MS, Frye S, Warner RS, et al. Testicular needle biopsy in diagnosis of infertility. Urology 1984;24:439.

13. Nseyo UO, Englander LS, Huben RP, et al. Aspiration biopsy of testis: another method for histologic examination. Fertil Steril 1984;42:281.

14. Hendricks FB, Lambird PA, Murphy GP. Percutaneous needle biopsy of the testes. J Small Animal Pract 1979;20:219.

15. Cohen MS, Warner RS. Needle biopsy of testes: a safe outpatient procedure. Fertil Steril 1979;29(3):279.

16. Rajfer J, Binder S. Use of Biopty gun for transcutaneous testicular biopsies. J Urol 1989;142:1021.

17. Thorud E, Clausen OPF, Abyholm T. Fine-needle aspiration biopsies from human testes evaluated by DNA flow cytometry. Flow Cytometry IV, Proceedings of the Fourth International Symposium on Flow Cytometry, Voss, June 4–8, 1979. Universiteterforlaget, New York: Columbia University Press, 1980.

18. Pfitzer P, Gilbert P, Rolz G, et al. Flow cytometry of human testicular tissue. Cytometry 1982;3:116.

19. Chan SL, Lipshultz LI, Schwartzendruber D. DNA flow cytometry: a new modality for quantitative analysis of testicular biopsies. Fertil Steril 1984;41:485.

20. Hellstrom WJ, Tesluk H, Deitch AD, et al. Comparison of flow cytometry to routine testicular biopsy in male infertility. Fertil Steril 1990;35(4):321.

21. Witten DM, Myers GH, Utz DC. Clinical Urography. 4th edition. Philadelphia, WB Saunders, 1977:76.

22. Belfield WT. Pus tubes in the male seminal. JAMA 1905;44:1277.

23. Pereira A. Roentgen interpretation of vesiculograms. Am J Radiol 1953;69:361.

24. Vestby GW. Vaso-seminal vesiculography in hypertrophy and carcinoma of the prostate with special reference to the ejaculatory ducts. Acta Radiol Suppl (Stockh) 1960;2:199.

25. Boreau J. Les Images des Voies Seminales. Basel: S Karger, 1935.

26. Merricks JW. The modern conception of the diagnosis and treatment of the seminal vesicles with roentgenographic visualization of these organs by catheterization of ejaculatory ducts. New Int Clin 1940;2:193.

27. Nagler HM, Thomas AJ. Testicular biopsy and vasography in the evaluation of male infertility. Urol Clin North Am 1987;14(1):167.

28. Belfield WT. Vasostomy-radiography of the seminal ducts. Surg Gynecol Obstet 1913;16:569.

29. Gordon JA, Clahassey EB. Evaluation of stricture formation as a complication of vasopuncture and vasography in the guinea pig. Fertil Steril 1978;29:180.

30. Mygind HB. Urogenital tuberculosis in the human male: vesiculographic and urethrographic studies. Dan Med Bull 1960;7:13.

31. Boreau J. Images of the Seminal Tracts. Paris: S Karger, 1974.

32. Shafik A. The scrotoscope: a new instrument for examining the scrotal contents. Br J Urol 1990;65:209.

33. Pryor JL, Howards SS. Varicocele. Urol Clin North Am 1987;14:499.

34. Saypol DC, Lipshultz LI, Howards SS. Varicocele. In: Lipshultz LI, Howards SS, editors. Infertility in the Male. New York: Churchill Livingstone, 1983:299.

35. Gorelick JI, Goldstein M. Loss of fertility in men with varicocele. Fertil Steril 1993;59(3):613.

36. Peng BCH, Tomashefsky P, Nagler HM. The cofactor effect: varicocele and infertility. Fertil Steril 1990;54(1):143.

37. Vermeulen A, Vanderweghe M, Deslypere JP. Prognosis of subfertility in men with corrected and uncorrected varicocele. J Androl 1986;7:147.

38. Nagler HM, Zippe CD. Varicocele: current concepts. In: Lipshultz LI, Howards SS, editors. Infertility in the Male. 2nd edition. St. Louis: Mosby-Year Book, 1991:313.

39. Okuyama M, Nakamura M, Namiki M, et al. Surgical repair of varicocele at puberty: preventive treatment for fertility improvement. J Urol 1988;139:562.

40. Kaufman DG, Nagler HM. The varicocele: concepts of pathophysiology—present and future. World J Urol 1986;4:88.

41. Curling TB. A Practical Treatise on the Disease of the Testis and of the Spermatic Cord and Scrotum. Philadelphia: Blanchard & Lea, 1856.

42. Barwell R. One hundred cases of varicocele treated by the subcutaneous wire loop. Lancet 1885;1:978.

43. Bennet WH. Varicocele, particularly with reference to its radical cure. Lancet 1889;1:261.

44. Macomber D, Sanders MB. The spermatozoa count: its value in the diagnosis, prognosis, and treatment of sterility. N Engl J Med 1929;200:981.

45. Tulloch WS. A consideration of sterility factors in the light of subsequent pregnancies: subfertility in the male. Trans Edinburgh Obstet Soc 1952;59:29.

46. Dubin L, Amelar RD. Varicocele size and results of varicocelectomy in selected subfertile men with varicocele. Fertil Steril 1970;21:606.

47. Dubin L, Amelar RD. Varicocelectomy as therapy in male infertility: a study of 504 cases. Fertil Steril 1975;26:217.

48. Coolsaet BL. The varicocele syndrome: venography determining the optimal level for surgical management. J Urol 1980;124:833.

49. Shafik A, Bedeir G. Venous tension patterns in cord veins in normal and varicocele individuals. J Urol 1980;123:383.

50. Ahlberg NE, Bartkey O, Chidekel N. Right and left gonadal veins: an anatomical and statistical study. Acta Radiol Diagn 1966;4:517.

51. Dubin L, Amelar RD. Varicocelectomy: 986 cases in a 12-year study. Urology 1977;10:446.

52. Al Juburi A, Pranikoff K, Dougherty KA, et al. Alteration of semen quality in dogs after creation of varicocele. Urology 1979;13:535.

53. Hudson RW, Perez-Marrero RA, Crawford VA, et al. Hormonal parameters in incidental varicoceles and those causing infertility. Fertil Steril 1976;45:692.

54. Hudson RW, Crawford VA, McKay DE. The gonadotropin response of men with varicoceles to a four-hour infusion of gonadotropin-releasing hormone. Fertil Steril 1981;36:633.

55. Hudson RW, Perez-Marrero RA, Crawford VA, et al. Hormonal parameters in men before and after varicocelectomy. Fertil Steril 1985;43:905.

56. Greenberg SH, Lipshultz LI, Morganroth J, et al. The use of Doppler stethoscope in the evaluation of varicoceles. J Urol 1977;117:296.

57. Greenberg SH, Lipshultz LI, Wein AJ. A preliminary report on "subclinical varicocele" diagnosis by Doppler ultrasonic stethoscope: examination and initial results of surgical therapy. J Reprod Med 1979;22:77.

58. Hirsh AV, Cameron KM, Tyler JP, et al. The Doppler assessment of varicoceles and internal spermatic vein reflux in infertile men. Br J Urol 1980;53:50.

59. Hirsh AV, Kellet M, Robertson G, et al. Doppler flow studies: venographic technique in the evaluation of fertile and subfertile males. Br J Urol 1980;52:560.

60. Amelar RD, Dubin L. Right varicocelectomy in selected infertile patients who have failed to improve after left varicocelectomy. Fertil Steril 1987;47:833.

61. Ayodeji O, Baker HWG. Is there a specific abnormality of sperm morphology in men with varicoceles? Fertil Steril 1986;45:839.

62. Ahlberg NE, Bartley O, Chidekel N, et al. Phlebography in varicocele scroti. Acta Radiol (Diagn) 1966;4:517.

63. Narayan P, Gonzales R, Amplatz K. Varicocele and male subfertility. Presented at the Annual Meeting of the American Fertility Society, Houston, Texas, March 1980.

64. Netto NR Jr, Lemos GC, DeGoes GM. Varicocele: relation between anoxia and hypospermatogenesis. Int J Fertil 1977;22:174.

65. Nadel SN, Hutchins GM, Albertson PC, et al. Valves of the spermatic vein: potential for misdiagnosis of varicoceles by venography. Fertil Steril 1984;41:479.

66. Seyferth W, Jecht E, Zeitler E. Percutaneous sclerotherapy of varicoceles. Radiology 1981;139:335.

67. Morag B, Rubenstein ZJ, Goldwasser B, et al. Percutaneous venography and occlusion in the management of spermatic varicoceles. Am J Radiol 1984;143:635.

68. Murray RR Jr, Mitchell SE, Kadir S, et al. Comparison of recurrent varicocele anatomy following surgery and percutaneous balloon occlusion. J Urol 1986;135:286.

69. Walsh PC, White RI Jr. Balloon occlusion of the internal spermatic vein for the treatment of varicoceles. JAMA 1981;246:1701.

70. Comhaire F, Monteyne R, Kunnen M. The value of scrotal thermography as compared with selective retrograde venography in the internal

spermatic vein for the diagnosis of "subclinical" varicocele. Fertil Steril 1976;27:694.

71. Pochaczevsky R, Lee WJ, Mallet E. Management of male infertility: roles of contact thermography, spermatic venography, and embolization. Am J Radiol 1986;147:97.

72. Mieusset R, Bujan L, Mondinat LA, et al. Association of scrotal hyperthermia with impaired spermatogenesis in infertile men. Fertil Steril 1987;48:1006.

73. Wheatley JK, Fajman WA, Witten FR. Clinical experience with the radioisotope varicocele scan as a screening method for the detection of subclinical varicoceles. J Urol 1982;128:57.

74. Palomo A. Radical cure of varicocele by a new technique: preliminary report. J Urol 1969;61:604.

75. Etriby AA, Ibrahim AA, Mahmoud KD, et al. Subfertility and varicocele: I. Venogram demonstration of anastomosis sites in subfertile men. Fertil Steril 1975;26:1013.

76. Cockett ATK, Takihara H, Cosentino MJ. The varicocele. Fertil Steril 1984;41:1.

77. Ivanissevich O. Left varicocele due to reflux: experience with 4,470 cases in forty-two years. J Int Coll Surg 1960;34:742.

78. Wosnitzer M, Roth JA. Optical magnification and Doppler ultrasound probe for varicocelectomy. Urology 1983;22:24.

79. Marmar JL, De Benedictis TJ, Praiss D. The management of varicoceles by microdissection of the spermatic cord at the external inguinal ring. Fertil Steril 1985;43:583.

80. Goldstein M, Gilbert BR, Dicker A, et al. Microsurgical inguinal varicocelectomy with delivery of the testes: an artery and lymphatic sparing technique. J Urol 1992;148:1808.

81. Mehan DJ, Andrus CH, Parra RO. Laparoscopic internal spermatic vein ligation: report of a new technique. Fertil Steril 1992;58(6):1263.

82. Kavoussi LR, Sosa E, Chandhoke P, et al. Complications of laparoscopic lymph node dissection. J Urol 1993;149:322.

83. Chehval MJ, Purcell MH. Varicocelectomy: incidence of external spermatic vein involvement in the clinical varicocele. Urology 1992;39:573.

84. Murray RR Jr, Mitchell SE, Kadir S, et al. Comparison of recurrent varicocele anatomy following surgery and percutaneous balloon occlusion. J Urol 1986;135:286.

85. Rodriguez-Netto N Jr, Fahrani EP, Lemos GC. Varicocele: clinical or surgical treatment? Int J Fertil 1984;29:164.

86. Newton R, Schinfeld JS, Schiff I. The effect of varicocelectomy on sperm count, motility, and conception rate. Fertil Steril 1980;34:250.

87. Baker HWG, Burger HG, Dekretzer DM. Testicular vein and fertility in men with varicoceles. Br Med J 1985;291:1678.

88. Nilsson S, Edvinsson A, Nilsson B. Improvement of semen and pregnancy rate after ligation of the internal spermatic vein: fact or fiction? Br J Urol 1979;51:591.

89. Marks JL, McMahon R, Lipshultz LI. Predictive parameters of successful varicocele repair. J Urol 1986;136:609.

90. Tinga DJ, Jager S, Bruignen SL, et al. Factors related to semen improvement and fertility after varicocele operation. Fertil Steril 1984;41:404.

91. Steckel J, Dicker AP, Goldstein M. Relationship between varicocele size and response to varicocelectomy. J Urol 1993;149:769.

92. Montie JE, Stewart BH. Vasovasostomy: past, present, and future. J Urol 1974;112:111.

93. Pratt WF, Mosher WD, Bachrach CA, et al. Understanding U.S. fertility: findings from the National Survey of Family Growth, Cycle III. Pop Bull 1985;39(5):1.

94. Giovannucci E, Tosteson TD, Speizer FE, et al. A retrospective cohort study of vasectomy and prostate cancer in U.S. men. JAMA 1993;269(7):878.

95. O'Connor VJ. Anastomosis of vas deferens after purposeful division for sterility. JAMA 1978;136:162.

96. Derrick FC, Yarbrough W, D'Agostine J. Vasovasostomy: results of questionnaire of members of the American Urological Association. J Urol 1973;110:556.

97. Phadke GM, Phadke AG. Experience in the reanastomosis of the vas deferens. J Urol 1967;97:888.

98. Middleton RG, Henderson D. Vas deferens reanastomosis with splints and without magnification. J Urol 1978;119:763.

99. Middleton RG, Urry RL. Vasovasostomy and semen motility. J Urol 1980;123:518.

100. Wagenknecht LV, Kosterhalfen H, Schirren C. Microsurgery in andrologic urology: I. Refertilization. J Microsurg 1980;1:370.

101. Fallon B, Miller RK, Gerber W. Nonmicroscopic vasovasostomy. J Urol 1981;126:361.

102. Kessler R, Freiha F. Macroscopic vasovasostomy. Fertil Steril 1981;36:531.

103. Shessel FS, Lynne CM, Politano VA. Use of exteriorized stents in vasovasostomy. Urology 1981;17:163.

104. Urquhart-Hay D. A low-power magnification technique of reanastomosis of the vas. Br J Urol 1981;53:466.

105. Redman JF. Clinical experience with vasovasostomy utilizing absorbable intravasal stent. Urology 1982;20:59.

106. Owen ER. Microsurgical vasovasostomy: A reliable vasectomy reversal. Aust NZ J Surg 1977;47:305.

107. Silber SJ. Microscopic vasectomy reversal. Fertil Steril 1977;28:11.

108. Sharlip ID. Vasovasostomy: comparison of two microsurgical techniques. Urology 1981;17:347.

109. Lee HY. A 20-year experience with vasovasostomy. J Urol 1986;136:413.

110. Yarbro ES, Howards SS. Vasovasostomy. Urol Clin North Am 1987;14(3):515.

111. Nagler HM. Unpublished data, 1987.

112. Gilis J, Borovikov AM. Treatment of vas deferens large defects. Int Urol Nephrol 1989;21(6):627.

113. Buch JP, Woods T. Retroperitoneal mobilization in the complex vasovasostomy. Fertil Steril 1990;54(5):931.

114. Fujioka H, Matsui T, Doi Y, et al. Microsurgical transvasovasostomy. Acta Urol Jpn 1990;36:367.

115. Lizza EF, Marmar JL, Schmidt SS. Transseptal crossed vasovasostomy. J Urol 1985;134:1131.

116. Jain KK, Gorsich W. Repair of small vessels with the neodymium-YAG laser: a preliminary report. Surgery 1979;85:684.

117. Quigley MR, Bailes JE, Kwaan HC. Microvascular anastomosis using the milliwatt CO_2 laser. Laser Surg Med 1985;5:357.

118. Gilbert PT, Beckert R. Laser-assisted vasovasostomy. Lasers Surg Med 1989;9:42.

119. Weiss JN, Mellinger BC. Fertility rates with delayed fibrin glue vasovasostomy in rats. Fertil Steril 1992;57(4):908.

120. Neiderberger C, Ross LS, Mackenzie B Jr, et al. Vasovasostomy in rabbits using fibrin adhesive prepared from a single human source. J Urol 1993;149(1):183.

121. Belker AM, Thomas AJ, Fuchs EF. Results of 1,469 microsurgical vasectomy reversals by the Vasovasostomy Study Group. J Urol 1991;145:505.

122. Silber SJ. Epididymal extravasation following vasectomy as a cause of failure of vasectomy reversal. Fertil Steril 1979;31:309.

123. Thomas AJ. Vasoepididymostomy. Urol Clin North Am 1987;14(8):527.

124. Marshall FF, Chang T, Vindivich D. Microsurgical vasoepididymostomy to corpus epididymis in treatment of inflammatory obstructive azoospermia. Urology 1987;30(6):565.

125. Hinrichsen MJ, Blaquier JA. Evidence supporting the existence of sperm maturation in the human epididymis. J Reprod Fertil 1980;60:291.

126. Moore HDM, Hartman TD, Pryor JP. Development of the oocyte-penetrating capacity of spermatozoa in the human epididymis. Int J Androl 1983;6:310.

127. Silber SJ, Ord T, Balmaceda J, et al. Congenital absence of the vas deferens: the fertilizing capacity of human epididymal sperm. N Engl J Med 1990;323(26):1788.

128. Howards SS. The epididymis, sperm maturation, and capacitation. In: Lipshultz LI, Howards SS, editors. Infertility in the Male. New York: Churchill Livingstone, 1983:121.

129. Hagner FR. The operative treatment of sterility in the male. JAMA 1955;107:1851.

130. Hanley HG. The surgery of male infertility. Ann R Coll Surg 1955;17:159.

131. Silber SJ. Reversal of vasectomy and the treatment of male infertility: role of microsurgery, vasoepididymostomy and pressure-induced change of vasectomy. Urol Clin North Am 1981;8:53.

132. Silber SJ. Microsurgery for vasectomy reversal and vasoepididymostomy. Urology 1984;23:505.

133. Silber SJ. Microscopic vasoepididymostomy: specific microanastomosis to the epididymal tubule. Fertil Steril 1978;30:565.

134. Fogdestam I, Fall M, Nilsson S. Microsurgical epididymovasostomy in the treatment of occlusive azoospermia. Fertil Steril 1986;46:925.

135. Wagenknecht LV. Ten years' experience with microsurgical epididymostomy: results and preposition of a new technique. J Androl 1985;6:26.
136. Silber SJ. Epididymal extravasation following vasectomy as a cause for failure of vasectomy reversal. Fertil Steril 1979;31:309.
137. Silber SJ. Vasoepididymostomy to the head of the epididymis: recovery of normal spermatozoal motility. Fertil Steril 1980;34:149.
138. Goldstein M. Surgery of male infertility and other scrotal disorders. In: Walsh PC, Retik AB, Stamey TA, Vaughan ED Jr, editors. Campbell's Urology, 6th edition. Philadelphia: WB Saunders, 1992:3114.
139. Silber SJ. Results of microsurgical vasoepididymostomy: role of epididymis in sperm maturation. Hum Reprod 1989;4(3):298.
140. Dubin L, Amelar RD. Etiologic factors in 1294 consecutive cases of male infertility. Fertil Steril 1971;22:496.
141. Wagenknecht LV. Obstruction in the male reproductive tract. In: Brain J, Schill WB, Schwarzstein L, editors. Treatment of Male Infertility. Berlin: Springer-Verlag, 1982:221.
142. Lipshultz LI, Howards SS. Surgical treatment of male infertility. In: Lipshultz LI, Howards SS, editors. Infertility in the Male. New York: Churchill Livingstone, 1983:343.
143. Elder JS, Mostwin JL. Cyst of the ejaculatory duct/urogenital sinus. J Urol 1984;132:768.
144. Shabsigh R, Lerner S, Fishman I, et al. The role of transrectal ultrasonography in the diagnosis and management of prostatic and seminal vesicle cysts. J Urol 1989;141:1206.
145. Amelar RD, Dubin L. Ejaculatory duct obstruction. In: Amelar RD, Dubin L, editors. Current Therapy of Infertility. Trenton: BC Decker, 1982:80.
146. Carson CC. Transurethral resection for ejaculatory duct stenosis and oligospermia. Fertil Steril 1984;41:482.
147. Keiserman WM, Dubin L, Amelar RD. A new type of retrograde ejaculation: report of three cases. Fertil Steril 1974;25:1071.
148. Porch PP Jr. Aspermia owing to obstruction of distal ejaculatory duct and treatment by transurethral resection. J Urol 1978;119:141.
149. Belker AM. Microsurgical repair of obstructive causes of male infertility. Semin Urol 1984;2:91.
150. Goldwasser BZ, Weinerth JL, Carson CC III. Ejaculatory duct obstruction: the case for aggressive diagnosis and treatment. J Urol 1985;134:964.
151. Mitchnick EI, Medley NE, Nagler HM. Unpublished data, 1992.
152. Ross LS, Prins G. Alloplastic spermatoceles: a 5-year experience. J Urol 1986;136:410.
153. Ludvik W. Artificial spermatocele persisting for 14 years. J Urol 1990;144:992.
154. Hanley H. The surgery of male subfertility [Hunterian lecture]. Ann R Coll Surg Engl 1955;17:159.
155. Schoysman R. La creation d'un spermatocele artificiel dans les agenesies du canal deferent. Bull Soc Belge Gynecol Obstet 1968;38:307.
156. Schoysman R, Drouart JM. Proges recents dans la chirurgie de la sterilite masculine et feminine. Acta Chir Belg 1972;71:261.
157. Schoysman R. Commentaire sur la revue par Cognat et Guillaud. Andrologie 1973;5:43.
158. Schoysman R. Exploration and treatment of obstructions and infections in the seminal duct and accessory genital glands: surgical procedures. In: Proceedings of the International Congress of Andrology, Barcelona, 1976.
159. Rubin SO. Congenital absence of the vas deferens. Scand J Urol Nephrol 1975;9:94.
160. Kelami A, Rohloff D, Affeld K, et al. Alloplastic spermatocele: insemination from epididymal reservoir. Urology 1977;10:310.
161. Kelami A. Kelami-Affeld alloplastic spermatocele and successful human delivery. Urol Int 1981;36:368.
162. Wagenknecht L, Holstein AF, Schirren C. Tierexperimentelle unteruchungen zur bildung einer kunsstlichen spermatocele. Andrologia 1975;7:273.
163. Wagenknecht LV, Weitze KH, Hoppe LP, et al. Microsurgery in andrologic urology: II. Alloplastic spermatocele. J Microsurg 1980;1:428.
164. Wagenknecht LV, Weitze KH, Hoppe LP, et al. New development in surgical andrology: alloplastic spermatocele. Invest Urol 1980;17:432.
165. Jiminez-Cruz JF. Artificial spermatocele. J Urol 1980;123:885.
166. Marmar JL, De Benedictis TJ, Praiss DE. Clinical experience with an artificial spermatocele. J Androl 1984;5:304.
167. Ross LS, Prins GS. Alloplastic spermatoceles: five-year experience. J Androl 1985;6(Suppl 1):102.
168. Yoshida H, Naitoh Y, Imamura K. Implantation of artificial spermatocele with cup-shaped silicone prosthesis to excretory azoospermia. J Androl 1985;6(Suppl 1):97.
169. Yoshida H, Migamoto K, Yoshida T, et al. Implantation of artificial spermatoceles with cup-shaped prosthesis for excretory azoospermia and chemical management of aspirated spermatozoa. J Androl 1986;7:220.
170. Moni VN, Lalitha PA. Moni's window operation: a new surgical technique to create a sperm reservoir in congenital vasal agenesis. J Urol 1992;148:843.
170a. Grantmyre JE, Thomas AT, Falk RM, et al. Development of a new alloplastic spermatocele demonstrating successful sperm retrieval in an animal model. Submitted for publication.
171. Belker A, Jimenez-Cruz JF, Kelami A, et al. Alloplastic spermatocele: poor sperm motility in intraoperative epididymal fluid contraindicates prosthesis implantation. J Urol 1986;136:408.
172. Temple-Smith PD, Southwick GJ, Yates CA, et al. Human pregnancy by in vitro fertilization (IVF) using sperm aspiration from the epididymis. J In Vitro Fertil Embryo Transf 1985;2(3):119.
173. Silber SJ, Balmaceda J, Borrero C, et al. Pregnancy with sperm aspiration from the proximal head of the epididymis: a new treatment for congenital absence of the vas deferens. Fertil Steril 1988;50(3):525.
174. Oates RD, Anguiano A, Milunsky A, et al. Bilateral congenital absence of the vas (CAV) and cystic fibrosis (CF): a genetic association? [Abstract]. Presented at the 47th Annual Meeting of the American Fertility Society, Orlando, 1991:S4.
175. Hollander MB, Carter MD, Lipshultz LI. Microscopic epididymal sperm aspiration (MESA). Personal communication, 1993.
176. Kaufman D, Schulman II, Nagler HM. Cystic fibrosis presenting in a 45-year-old man with infertility. J Urol 1986;136:1081.
177. Patrizio P, Asch RH, Handelin B, et al. [Abstract]. Presented at the Annual Meeting of the American Fertility Society, New Orleans, November 2–5, 1992.
178. Belker AM, Oates RD, Goldstein M, et al. Results in the United States with sperm microaspiration retrieval techniques and assisted reproductive technologies: the Sperm Microaspiration Retrieval Techniques Study Group. Personal communication, 1993.
179. Schlegel P. Male Reproduction/Urology. Presented at the Annual Meeting of the American Urologic Association Meeting, Toronto, June 1991.
180. Amann RP. Function of the epididymis in bulls and rams. J Reprod Fertil 1987;34(Suppl):115.
181. Cooper TG. In defense of a function for the human epididymis. Fertil Steril 1990;54(6):965.
182. Orgebin-Crist MC. Studies of the function of the epididymis. Biol Reprod 1969;1:155.
183. Schoysman RJ, Bedford JM. The role of the human epididymis in sperm maturation and sperm storage as reflected in the consequences of epididymovasostomy. Fertil Steril 1986;476:293.
184. Silber SJ, Ord T, Balmaceda J, et al. Congenital absence of the vas deferens: the fertilization capacity of human epididymal sperm. N Engl J Med 1990;323:1788.
185. Olar TT, La Nassa J, Dickey RP. Fertilization of human oocytes by microinjection of human sperm aspirated from the caput epididymis of an individual with obstructive azoospermia. J In Vitro Fertil Embryo Transf 1990;7(3):160.

CHAPTER 42

Infection and Male Infertility

RICHARD E. BERGER

Pelvic inflammatory disease with its resultant tubal obstruction is a common, well-documented, potentially preventable cause of female infertility. The role of infections in causing infertility in men is much less clear. Although symptomatic genitourinary infections caused by sexually transmitted diseases (STDs) are common in men of the reproductive age group, the role of either symptomatic or asymptomatic infection in male infertility has been the subject of great debate. Genital infection in animals is known to be an important cause of veterinary infertility.[1] Unfortunately, in men, infection-induced infertility has been much more difficult to document. Furthermore, much confusion exists between the presence of inflammation in seminal or prostatic fluid and actual infection. Often inflammation has been assumed to mean infection where none has been documented. Methods have been developed to localize genital infection in men, and culture methods are available to determine the possible infectious causes of genital inflammation. These methods seldom have been used in studies of infectious causes of male infertility. In this chapter, I review the syndromes of symptomatic male genital infection and then discuss information available relating infections to male infertility.

GONOCOCCAL URETHRITIS

Urethritis may be divided into (1) gonococcal urethritis and (2) nongonococcal urethritis (NGU). Gonococcal urethritis is caused by the gram-negative diplococcus, *Neisseria gonorrhoeae*. Gonococcal urethritis usually becomes symptomatic immediately but may take up to 3 months to manifest itself.[2] Gonococcal urethritis is acquired during intercourse. The risk of acquiring gonococcal urethritis during a single episode with an infected partner appears to be approximately 17%.[3] The risk increases with the number of sexual contacts. Transmission to the man may occur from vaginal or oropharyngeal contact. Symptoms include a purulent urethral discharge and burning on urination. Typically, 40% to 60% of contacts with individuals with known gonorrhea are asymptomatic.[4, 5] Without treatment, symptomatic gonorrhea usually improves. The man, however, may remain a carrier

and be potentially infectious.[6] Gonococcal urethritis may be prevented by the regular use of condoms. Most men, however, still do not use this protection even in the acquired immunodeficiency syndrome (AIDS) era.[7] Moreover, resistant strains of gonorrhea are common owing to the widespread, indiscriminate use of prophylactic antibiotics.[2]

Diagnosis is made by the intraurethral insertion of a calcium alginate (Calgiswab, Inolex) swab at least 1 hour after the patient has last urinated. Cotton swabs are bactericidal.[8] Swabs should be rolled gently on a slide, heat fixed, air dried, and examined immediately with Gram stain. A Gram stain makes the diagnosis with 99% specificity and 95% sensitivity.[9] The swab should then be plated onto Thayer-Martin and New York City media. There are a number of serologic and fluorescent tests available. These, however, are not usually necessary.[10, 11]

Gonococcal urethritis was first successfully treated in the 1940s with penicillin. Resistance, however, has steadily increased. The gonococcus acquired a plasmid for penicillinase production in 1976 making some strains totally resistant.[5] The summary of current Centers for Disease Control and Prevention (CDC) recommendations for treatment of gonorrhea is listed in Table 42–1, but recommendations may change as new resistant strains are identified. Ceftriaxone (250 mg intramuscularly) is currently the recommended drug of choice. Because of concomitant chlamydial infection in 30% of men with gonococcal urethritis, treatment with a tetracycline derivative is also recommended.

NONGONOCOCCAL URETHRITIS

Along with herpes simplex 2 and genital warts, NGU is one of the faster increasing STDs. The morbidity and complications of NGU are equal to and perhaps even greater than those of gonococcal urethritis. NGU is probably the most common genitourinary infection in reproductive-aged men. The most dangerous cause of NGU is *Chlamydia trachomatis*.[12–14] Chlamydia can be isolated from the urethra in 25% to 60% of heterosexual men with NGU, 4% to 35% of men with gonorrhea, and 0 to 7% of men seen in STD clinics

TABLE 42–1. Treatment of Gonococcal Urethritis in Men*

Treatment	Advantages	Disadvantages
Ceftriaxone, 250 mg IM	Effective against PPNG	
Spectinomycin, 2 g IM once	Effective against PPNG	
Ciprofloxacin, 500 mg IM once	Effective against PPNG	
Norfloxacin, 800 mg orally once	Effective against PPNG	
Cefuroxime axetil, 1 g orally once with probenecid, 1 g	Effective against PPNG	
Ceftizoxime, 500 mg IM once	Effective against PPNG	
Amoxacillin, 3 g orally with probencid, 1 g	Effective against PPNG	Not effective against PPNG

*All patients must be treated with Doxycycline, 100 mg bid for 2 days to treat coexisting *Chlamydia* infection. Erythromycin, 500 mg 4 times a day for 7 days, or erythromycin ethylsuccinate may be substituted in patients who cannot take tetracycline (e.g., pregnant women).

PPNG, penicillinase-producing *Neisseria gonorrhoeae*.

Modified from Centers for Disease Control. 1989 Sexually transmitted disease treatment guidelines. MMWR 1989; 381:1–43.

TABLE 42–2. Etiology of Sexually Transmitted Nongonococcal Urethritis

	Acute*	Persistent†	Recurrent‡
Chlamydia trachomatis	30–50%	0%	0–5%
Ureaplasma urealyticum	30–40%	40–50%	10–20%
Neither	20–30%	50–60%	70–80%
Trichomonas vaginalis	1–2%	5–10%	1–2%
Herpes simplex virus	1–2%	5–10%	0%
Yeasts	Rare	Rare	Rare
Gardnerella vaginalis	Rare	Rare	Rare
Staphylococcus saprophyticus	Rare	?Never	?Never
Corynebacterium genitalium	Rare	?Never	?Never
Others	?	?	?

*Acute nongonococcal urethritis (NGU) = Less than 1 month's duration, without prior treatment for that episode.

†Persistent NGU = Persists unchanged or only minimally improved at the end of 1 week of tetracycline.

‡Recurrent NGU = Recurs within 6 weeks of starting treatment, without intercourse with a new or untreated partner.

From Bowie WR. Nongonococcal urethritis. Urol Clin North Am 1984; 11:55.

without symptoms of urethritis.[15] Asymptomatic infections occur in 50% of male contacts of women with cervical chlamydial infection.[16] Up to 80% of female sexual contacts of men with *C. trachomatis* also have *C. trachomatis* isolated. Postgonococcal urethritis may develop in men with gonococcal urethritis treated with penicillin who have concomitant chlamydial infections.

Twenty percent to 50% of men with NGU have infections with *Ureaplasma urealyticum*. The role of *U. urealyticum* in the cause of NGU is difficult to determine because genital colonization with this organism in symptomatic or asymptomatic men is directly proportional to the number of previous sexual partners. In patients with three to five partners, specimens in 40% of men and 70% of women contain ureaplasma.[17] In men with few sexual partners, no history of urethritis, and negative chlamydia cultures, the rate of isolation of ureaplasma is significantly higher than in those with positive chlamydial cultures.[18] Urethritis also persists in a group of chlamydia-positive and ureaplasma-positive men who are treated with antibiotics to which only chlamydia is sensitive.[19] Differential treatment studies have confirmed the role of *U. urealyticum*.[20]

In twenty percent to 30% of cases, the cause of urethritis has not been determined (Table 42–2). Smoking may be an independent risk factor for the development of NGU.[21] Uncircumcised men are more likely to have NGU than circumcised men.[22] Hernandez and colleagues[23] found oral sex to be significantly associated with chlamydia-negative, ureaplasma-negative NGU.

The incubation period for NGU is usually 1 to 5 weeks. Longer incubations occur. Common symptoms are dysuria and discharge.

Diagnosis of NGU requires the demonstration of urethritis and exclusion of infection with *N. gonorrhoeae*. Men suspected of having urethritis should be examined after 4 hours of urinary continence. Finding more than four polymorphonuclear leukocytes per field in five 1000-power oil immersion fields makes the diagnosis of urethritis. Finding 15 or more polymorphonuclear leukocytes in five random 400-power fields on spun sediment of first-void urine also confirms the finding of urethritis.[24, 25] If urethritis is highly suspected but initial examination is negative, the patient should be examined before voiding in the morning. Urethral cultures for *C. trachomatis* should be used when available. Cultures for *U. urealyticum* are of no value in the evaluation of an individual with urethritis owing to the high rate of colonization in normal, sexually active men. The current CDC recommendations for treatment of NGU are based on chlamydial infection and are given in Table 42–3 but may change with time if resistance emerges. Although quinolones adequately treat gonococcal infections, they are less effective in chlamydial infections.[26] Response to therapy is best in men with *C. trachomatis* infection and worst in men with neither *C. trachomatis* nor *U. urealyticum*. Treatment of sexual partners of men with gonococcal and nongonococcal urethritis is indicated to prevent recurrent disease in the man and infection in the partner.

TABLE 42–3. Management of Nongonococcal Urethritis

Investigation
  Careful physical examination
  Demonstrate a polymorphonuclear leukocyte response—Gram stain or first voided urine sediment
  Exclude *Neisseria gonorrhoeae* infection—Gram stain ± culture
  Reassess in the morning before voiding if necessary
Initial Management of NGU if diagnosed
  Seven days of treatment with tetracycline, 500 mg qid, or minocycline or doxycycline, 100 mg twice daily, or erythromycin, 500 mg qid for 7 days
  Treat partner(s) appropriately
Management of persistent or recurrent NGU
  Question about compliance and re-exposure
  Examine carefully for less usual causes of urethritis
  Demonstrate urethritis
  Treat any specific cause that can be elucidated
  If a specific etiology is not found or *Ureaplasma urealyticum* is present, treat with erythromycin base, 500 mg qid for 14 days

NGU, Nongonococcal urethritis.

Modified from Bowie WR. Nongonococcal urethritis. Urol Clin North Am 1984; 11:55.

		TABLE 42–4. Etiology of Acute Epididymitis					
	Total No. of Men	**Age <35 Years** **No./Total (%)**			**Age >35 Years** **No./Total (%)**		
		Gonococcus (%)	*Chlamydia trachomatis* (%)	*Escherichia coli* (%)	*Gonococcus* (%)	*Chlamydia trachomatis* (%)	*Escherichia coli* (%)
Berger et al, 1989[61]	23	0/13 (0)	10/13 (77)	0/13 (0)	0/10 (0)	8/10 (80)	0/10 (0)
Berger et al, 1979[52]	50	7/34 (21)	16/34 (47)	1/34 (3)	0/16 (0)	1/16 (6)	12/16 (75)
Berger et al, 1987[148]	51	9/51 (18)	19/51 (37)	6/51 (12)*			
Hawkins et al, 1986[149]	40	2/27 (19)	13/27 (48)	0/27 (0)	3/13 (23)	2/13 (15)	3/13 (23)
Scheibel et al, 1983[150]	52	1/31 (3)	13/31 (42)	0/31 (0)	0/13 (0)	0/13 (0)	6/13 (46)
Kristensen et al, 1984[151]	16	4/16 (25)	14/16 (88)				
Kojima et al, 1988[152]	45	3/30 (10)	21/30 (70)	0/30 (0)	0/15 (0)	0/15 (0)	7/15 (47)
Grant et al, 1987[153]	54	2/42 (5)	13/42 (31)	1/42 (2)	0/12 (0)	1/12 (8)	8/12 (67)
De Jong et al, 1988[155]†	25	1/13 (8)	11/13 (85)	1/13 (80)	0/12 (0)	1/12 (8)	10/12 (23)
Melekos et al, 1988[156]‡	21		6/11 (55)	4/11 (36)		1/10 (10)	7/10 (70)

*Six of nine homosexual men had coliform infection: one other had infection with *Haemophilus influenzae*. None of 42 heterosexual men had coliform infection.

†Forty subjects were evaluated; 25 had a single organism identified.

‡Cutoff between younger and older men was age 40.

ORCHITIS AND EPIDIDYMITIS

Infections causing destruction of testicular substance or occlusion of the transport tubules for spermatozoa may lead directly to male infertility. In mumps, testicular involvement occurs in 30% of males who are above the age of 10. Before that age, orchitis rarely accompanies mumps. Bilateral orchitis occurs in one third of men, and one third of these develop azoospermia. Serum follicle-stimulating hormone (FSH) is often elevated, and the testicle may be atrophic or fibrotic.[27]

Mycobacterium tuberculosis may infect both the testicle and the epididymis. Abdel and Morsy[28] found that men with tuberculosis often had abnormalities of the epididymis. Mycobacterium also frequently involves the testicle and leads to infertility.[29] Lepromatous leprosy is the only type of leprosy associated with orchitis.[30]

Epididymitis has been associated with bacteria such as *N. gonorrhoeae*, *C. trachomatis*, *U. urealyticum*, Enterobacteriaceae, and a number of mycobacteria. Rarely, members of the herpesvirus groups and fungi have also been associated with epididymitis. Epididymitis also usually involves the testicle and may lead to testicular atrophy. Wolin[31] performed testicular biopsies on men with epididymitis and found 20 of 28 to have decreased spermatogenesis and 9 of 28 to have testicular inflammation. Nilsson and associates[32] performed aspiration biopsies on testicles of men with acute epididymitis and found that 16 of 20 showed inflammatory cells in the testicle. Subsequent testicular atrophy was in direct proportion to initial inflammation and occurred in two thirds of men. Ludwig and Haselberger[33] followed 46 patients with unilateral epididymitis from 8 days to 1 year. Two thirds were found to have oligospermia. Twenty-eight percent had long-term abnormalities in their semen analysis. Krishnan and Heal[34] found enlargement of the seminal vesicle on the side of the epididymis in 75% of cases indicating seminal vesicular as well as epididymal involvement. Osegbe[35] found that only 40% of men with a history of epididymitis had semen samples considered adequate for conception. Twenty-six percent had permanent azoospermia, and 33% had permanent oligospermia with counts less than 10 million. Of 225 azoospermic men, Micic[36] found that 63% had obstruction in the

epididymis. Campbell[37] noted that 40% of patients with unilateral epididymitis secondary to gonorrhea were sterile. Pelouze[38] found that 11% of patients with gonococcal urethritis were sterile, 24% of men with unilateral epididymitis were sterile, and 42% of men with bilateral epididymitis were sterile.

Damage to the epididymis or testicle on one side could effect overall fertility by producing sperm autoimmunity. Minimal or subclinical epididymitis could affect epididymal function without causing obstruction. Damage to the testicle from torsion[39, 40] causes contralateral testicular abnormalities. Hendry and associates[41] described 32 patients who had unilateral vasal or epididymal obstruction. Eighty-one percent of these men had antisperm antibodies. He also found that 37% of infertile men with antisperm antibodies had vasal or epididymal obstruction. Kessler and associates[42] showed that unilateral vasal occlusion in mice could lead to infertility by producing sperm autoimmunity.[43] Rumke and others[44, 45] have suggested that vas deferens or epididymal obstruction can be detected in 50% of men with sperm antibodies. Bandhauer and Marberger[46] found that 9 of 48 men with unilateral epididymitis had sperm antibodies. Bietz[47] found toxic changes in the contralateral testicle in patients 150 to 250 days after onset of unilateral epididymitis. Animal models in rats and monkey have been developed and may be used to study the effect of epididymitis on infertility.[48, 49]

The most common causes of epididymitis in young men are the sexually transmitted pathogens, *C. trachomatis* and *N. gonorrhoeae* (Table 42–4). Jalil and associates[50] isolated *U. urealyticum* in the epididymitis of a 28-year-old man, suggesting that *U. urealyticum* may also be a cause of epididymitis. Although urethritis usually coexists with epididymitis, men are generally unaware of the discharge.[51, 52]

Coliform infection associated with bacteriuria also may cause epididymitis. Diagnosis of epididymitis is made by Gram stain and culture of urethra to detect gonococcal and nongonococcal urethritis and culture of midstream urine to detect bacteriuria. Although epididymitis is relatively common in developed countries, it and its sequelae appear even more common in developing countries. In some parts of sub-Saharan Africa, where gonorrhea and chlamydia infections often go untreated, epididymitis may be a leading cause of infertility.[53, 54] Treatment for epididymitis is outlined in Table 42–5.

PROSTATITIS

Symptomatic prostatitis syndromes have been classified as (1) acute bacterial prostatitis, (2) chronic bacterial prostatitis, (3) nonbacterial or idiopathic prostatitis, and (4) prostatodynia. Prostatitis may also be asymptomatic.[55]

Acute bacterial prostatitis usually presents with fever, bacteriuria, difficulty urinating, and a tender, enlarged prostate. The agents causing acute prostatitis are usually the coliform bacteria, *Pseudomonas*, and enterococcus. Acute bacterial prostatitis also can be caused by untreated gonococcal infection. The pathogen causing acute prostatitis can almost always be cultured from the urine or urethra. Prostatic massage is not necessary to make the diagnosis and may precipitate bacteremia.[55, 56]

Chronic bacterial prostatitis is characterized by relapsing bladder infection. It is relatively uncommon, constituting less than 10% of all cases. Chronic bacterial infections within the prostate are resistant to treatment and may only suppress the organism. When treatment ceases, the organism may reemerge from the prostate to infect the bladder.[55] The diagnosis of chronic bacterial prostatitis is made by prostatic localization cultures (also known as four-glass urine cultures) as described by Meares and Stamey.[57] The first-void specimen (BV$_1$) (the first 10 to 15 ml of urine passed) is collected. This specimen shows maximum urethral contamination. Next the patient passes 50 to 100 ml of urine, and about 10 ml is collected during this void. This represents a midstream collection (BV$_2$). A rectal examination and prostatic massage are then performed, and expressed prostatic secretions (EPS) are collected from the urethra. The patient is then asked to void 10 to 15 ml, which is called the postmassage specimen (BV$_3$). The diagnosis is made by finding at least 1 log higher count of pathogenic bacteria in the BV$_3$ or EPS as compared with the BV$_1$. Prostatic secretions usually show numerous white blood cells. The upper limit of normal is 10 white blood cells per 400 hpf or 1000 cells per cubic millimeter on hemocytometer count of the EPS. Biochemical abnormalities of prostate secretions are also common.[57] Zinc concentrations are low. Levels correlate with the antimicrobial properties of

EPS.[58] The pH of prostatic fluid, which is usually acidic, is also alkaline, with an average pH of 8.32.[58] Local immunity in EPS to urinary pathogens can be demonstrated in chronic bacterial prostatitis. Serum antibody titers to bacterial specific antigens are elevated and decrease with treatment. Antigen-specific secretory immunoglobulin IgA in EPS also correlates with disease activity.[59]

In chronic idiopathic prostatitis, there is inflammation in EPS but no identifiable infection. These patients complain of dysuria, perineal pain, testicular pain, groin discomfort, urgency, nocturia, and sometimes hematospermia or ejaculatory pain.[57]

Anderson and Weller[60] found 4543 ± 650 leukocytes/mm^3 in EPS of patients with symptoms of idiopathic prostatitis versus 887.88 ± 11 leukocytes in controls without symptoms ($P < 0.001$). Berger and coworkers[61] also found that more patients with symptoms of prostatitis than controls without symptoms had greater than 1000 white blood cells/mm^3 in the prostatic secretions. Others have found, however, a poor correlation of symptoms to the presence of leukocytes.[62] Although none of the common bacterial urinary pathogens can be localized to the prostate in men with idiopathic prostatitis, commensal bacteria, such as *Staphylococcus epidermidis* and streptococci, are often isolated.[63] Berger and coworkers[61] found no difference, however, in the isolation of these organisms in cases and controls. Local IgA to these commensal bacteria has been shown to be absent,[64] and up to 70% of asymptomatic volunteers can have commensal bacteria isolated to the prostate by four-glass urine cultures.[61]

Sexually transmitted organisms have been implicated in the cause of idiopathic prostatitis. *C. trachomatis* causes up to 50% of nongonococcal urethritis and therefore is a likely candidate to cause nonbacterial prostatitis. Berger and coworkers[3] were unable to isolate chlamydia from 40 men with symptoms of chronic bacterial prostatitis. Måardh and colleagues[65] concluded, from a study of 53 men with nonbacterial prostatitis, that chlamydia was an extremely rare cause. Bruce and associates,[66] however, studied 70 men with chronic prostatitis and found 50% to have early morning urine specimens positive for *C. trachomatis* by immunofluorescence. There is some inconclusive evidence that the prostate as well as the urethra may be involved in men with acute chlamydial urethritis. Nilsson and associates[67] found that 26 of 96 men with chlamydia-positive NGU and greater than 20 white blood cells per high-power field in EPS also had chlamydia in the expressed prostatic secretions. EPS is, however, by necessity contaminated with urethral secretions, and any culture results must be interpreted with caution. Poletti and associates[68] was able to isolate chlamydia from transrectal prostatic aspirates in men with symptoms of urethritis and prostatitis. These cases, however, differ in that most men with symptoms of nonbacterial prostatitis do not have the symptoms of urethritis.

U. urealyticum is a possible etiologic agent in chronic idiopathic prostatitis. Weidner and coworkers[69] found *U. urealyticum* to localize to the prostate in 36 of 137 men with symptomatic nonbacterial prostatitis. After treatment with tetracycline, 30 of the patients were free of ureaplasma and 23 were free of symptoms. Persistence of ureaplasma was related to coexistent infection in the patient's sexual partner. Weidner and coworkers[69] concluded that ureaplasma was the

---

TABLE 42–5. Treatment of Acute Epididymo-orchitis

Epididymo-orchitis secondary to bacteriuria
  Urine culture and sensitivity
  Prompt administration of broad-spectrum antimicrobial (e.g., tobramycin, trimethoprim/sulfamethoxazole, quinolone antibiotic)
  Bedrest and scrotal evaluation
  Strongly consider hospitalization
  Evaluate for underlying urinary tract disease
Epididymo-orchitis secondary to sexually transmitted urethritis
  Gram stain of urethral smear
  Administer: ceftriaxone, 250 mg and tetracycline, 500 mg orally qid for at least 10 days, or doxycycline, 100 mg orally bid for at least 10 days
  Bedrest and scrotal elevation
  Examine and treat sexual partners

Adapted from Berger RE. Urethritis and epididymitis. Semin Urol 1983; 1:143.

etiologic agent in 9% of men with the symptoms of nonbacterial prostatitis.[69]

ASYMPTOMATIC BACTERIAL COLONIZATION OF THE GENITOURINARY TRACT AND MALE INFERTILITY

Although acute symptomatic infections of the epididymis and testicle may cause infertility, the role of asymptomatic infection is far from clear. Few studies on the roles of infections and inflammation on male infertility have been well controlled. Comparisons have been made between groups of men attending fertility clinics who were stratified based on single semen analysis, which is an unreliable indicator of fertility. Other studies have equated seminal inflammation with infection without culture documentation. Furthermore, the origin of leukocytes in the semen has seldom been determined. Leukocytes could come from the urethra, prostate, seminal vesicle, epididymis, or testicles. Studies using localization cultures to establish the origin of bacteria in semen, such as those used in studies of symptomatic chronic bacterial prostatitis, are lacking. Sometimes the presence of biochemical abnormalities in the semen and prostatic secretions has been used to infer the presence of prostatic infection because these abnormalities are found in chronic bacterial prostatitis. The actual relationship, however, of such bio-chemical abnormalities to asymptomatic seminal colonization, inflammation, and fertility is poorly defined.

Several investigators have tried to relate asymptomatic coliform infection to male infertility. Harrison and Johnson[70] found gram-negative bacteria in the semen in 29 of 100 men with abnormal semen but in no men with normal semen. Toth and Lesser[71] were unable to isolate *Escherichia coli* from semen of 30 fertile men. They did, however, isolate *E. coli* in 2% of infertile men with no history of genitourinary infection and 11% of infertile men with a history of prostatitis or urethritis. Ulstein and colleagues[72] examined age-matched fertile and infertile men with four-glass localization cultures. Gram-negative organisms were found in only those with abnormal semen. Berger and coworkers,[61] however, found no difference in coliform colonization bacteria and infertile men and controls. *E. coli*, when added to sperm in quantities of 10^7 or greater, can decrease motility. A motility-decreasing factor has been isolated from *E. coli* filtrates.[73, 74] Comhaire and associates[74] found that acid phosphatase was decreased in the semen of men with coliform bacteria. Whether coliform colonization causes male infertility is still not clear. It is infrequent.

Most investigators have not found gram-positive commensal organisms to be associated with male infertility.[75-78] It is noteworthy that gram-positive organisms from different portions of split ejaculate may differ, suggesting that bacteria may originate from different reproductive glands.[79] Alternatively, different antibacterial factors may be present in different parts of the split ejaculate. Bacterial counts may actually

TABLE 42–6. Correlations of Seminal Fluid Analysis, Sperm Penetration Assay, and Sperm Autoimmunity with Cigarette Smoking, Marijuana Use, and Alcohol Use

	Cigarette Use		Marijuana Use			Alcohol Use (ounces/week)		
	Smokers	Nonsmokers	Users	Nonusers	None	<2	3–30	>30
No. patients	22	142	10	132	27	82	46	8
Sperm penetration assay in median % penetration (range)	2.5* (0–57)	8 (0–92)	7 (0–14)	7 (0–75)	12 (0–67)	8 (0–92)	7 (0–92)	4.5 (0–40)
Sperm count (× 10^6/ml)†	66.7 ± 53.0	68.1 ± 68.4	68.1 ± 78.3	63.3 ± 62.5	55.2 ± 51.4	75.3 ± 68.5	63.8 ± 73.3	69.0 ± 50.0
% Oval sperm†	74.0 ± 16.9	68.7 ± 16.7	79.4 ± 8.2	69.8 ± 16.6	67.4 ± 21.6	68.9 ± 16.0	71.2 ± 14.3	67.2 ± 20.4
% Motile sperm†	45.6 ± 22.2	44.6 ± 24.7	62.8 ± 21.5‡	40.8 ± 24.3	42.7 ± 25.6	41.6 ± 22.4	51.2 ± 24.9	45.6 ± 31.2
Median leukocytes/100 sperm (range)	6§ (0–20)	3 (0–52)	10‖ (3–52)	4 (0–39)	5 (0–20)	3 (0–16)	3 (0–52)	10¶ (2–18)
% Agglutinating antibody (prevalence)	18 (4/22)	18 (25/140)	10 (1/10)	20 (26/131)	26 (7/27)	20 (16/80)	11 (5/46)	12 (1/8)
% Immobilizing antibody (prevalence)	5 (1/20)	14 (17/123)	0 (0/9)	14 (17/123)	23 (6/26)	12 (8/66)	7 (3/42)	12 (1/8)
% Serum cytotoxic antibody (prevalence)	29 (4/14)	24 (14/59)	12 (1/8)	26 (17/65)	0 (0/11)	31 (10/32)	24 (6/26)	50 (2/4)
% Semen cytotoxic antibody (prevalence)	8 (1/12)	12 (5/42)	0 (0/7)	13 (6/47)	11 (1/9)	21 (4/19)	4 (1/22)	0 (0/4)

*Mann-Whitney test $P = 0.05$.
†Mean ± standard deviation.
‡Mann-Whitney test $P = 0.006$.
§Mann-Whitney test $P = 0.02$.
‖Mann-Whitney test $P = 0.007$.
¶Kruskal-Wallis test $P = 0.01$.
From Close CE, Roberts PL, Berger RE. Cigarettes, alcohol and marijuana are related to pyospermia in infertile men. J Urol 1990;144:900–903. © American Urological Association, Inc.

increase as semen is diluted. This is possibly due to an antimicrobial effect of the zinc on bacterial growth.[58] It is possible that increased bacterial counts may actually be attributed to decreased bacteriostatic effects of semen and represent accessory gland dysfunction rather than actual infection. Although there seems to be little evidence relating seminal inflammation to present gram-positive colonization, there is perhaps a relationship to infection in the past.[71] Morton[80] found the highest seminal white blood cell counts in men with histories of genital infections.

Inflammation in semen or EPS is not always, or even often, caused by infection.[74, 81] Berger and colleagues[61] found no difference in the bacteriology of semen or four-glass urine cultures in men with symptomatic prostatitis, idiopathic infertility, or controls, although the men with idiopathic prostatitis had more leukocytes. Hillier and associates[82] cultured semen samples for aerobes, anaerobes, and mycoplasmas. They found no correlation of cultures with the parameters of semen analysis, number of white blood cells, or sperm penetration assay (SPA). Cumming and associates[83] found that granulocyte elastase levels, which correlate with inflammation, did not correlate with anaerobic or aerobic bacterial growth from the seminal plasma of infertile men. Guillet-Rosso and coworkers[84] found a reduction of pregnancy rate per cycle in in vitro fertilization with increasing amounts of any bacteria in the semen. If these findings are confirmed, it may indicate that bacterial counts are important in in vitro fertilization. They did not, however, address the primary cause of infertility in the couple. Persson and coworkers[85] suggested that high concentrations of uridine and xanthine in seminal plasma could crystallize out and constitute the first step in the development of prostatitis. Gattuccio and colleagues[86] found a correlation between the presence of a varicocele and genital inflammation. They suggested that the cause of inflammation could include venous congestion of the pelvis, resulting in anoxic inflammation of the prostate. Close and associates[87] found a relationship to alcohol intake and cigarette smoking to seminal inflammation (Table 42–6). Cigarette smoking was also related to poor hamster SPAs. Perhaps toxic effects from substances can produce seminal inflammation. Prostatic inflammation might decrease the immunosuppressive activities of prostatic components and alter the relationship of secretions of the seminal vesicle and prostate, leading to sperm dysfunction.[88–90] Some investigators have found that there is an inverse relation between the number of leukocytes and the concentration of zinc in the semen of men with bacterial prostatitis and in men with idiopathic prostatitis.[91–93] They have inferred that men with idiopathic prostatitis also have infection. This inference, however, has not been proved. Electron microscopic evidence by Hughes and associates[94] showed that 57 of 144 infertile men had large numbers of leukocytes in the semen. White blood cells from 35 of these 57 men contained bacteria, whereas white blood cells in the remaining 22 men contained only phagocytized spermatozoa. Pathogenic bacteria were isolated from only two men in each group. Koehler and associates[95] noted that sperm phagocytosis was common in the semen of infertile men. Maroni and coworkers[96] and Clark and Klebanoff[97] found that normal spermatozoa could interact with serum or plasma to generate C5A, a potent chemotactic factor derived from the fifth component of the complement. Pandya and Cohen[98] found that spermatozoa created leukocytosis in cervical mucus after artificial insemination. Therefore, under certain conditions, sperm are capable of attracting leukocytes in semen.

Bacteria may affect semen quality by using important substances, inducing sperm phagocytosis, stimulating antibodies, causing inflammation, decreasing secretory function of the accessory sex glands, or damaging the gonads or adnexa.[99] Inflammation in seminal secretions without infection can also affect sperm function. Berger and colleagues[100] found abnormal sperm function as measured by the in vitro hamster penetration test (SPA) correlates with the number of leukocytes in this semen. There was an 8.7 times risk of an abnormal SPA with at least one leukocyte per 100 sperm as compared with those with less than one leukocyte per 100 sperm (Fig. 42–1). They found no correlation with the number of leukocytes and the number or concentration of bacteria in the semen. Maruyama and colleagues[101] found that adding leukocytes to the semen of fertile donors decreased sperm penetration values. Supernatants of white blood cells added to sperm also decreased SPA scores (Fig. 42–2). When white cells were removed by physical means, the SPA scores improved. Berger and others[61, 100] found that the number of white blood cells was inversely related to sperm count and motility. These findings were confirmed by Wolff and associates[102] (Fig. 42–3). Wolff and Anderson[103] furthermore found that high numbers of T lymphocytes were related to decreased sperm velocity (Fig. 42–4). They found higher num-

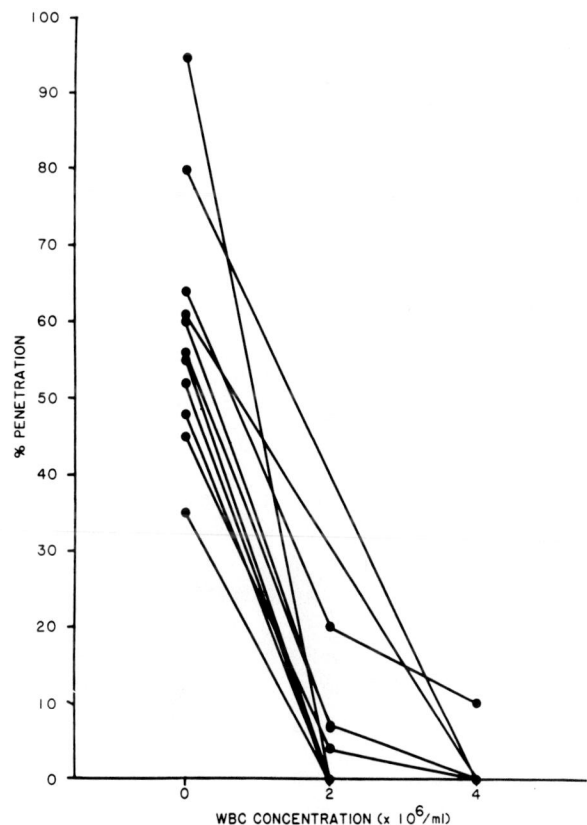

FIGURE 42–1. Effect of white blood cell (WBC) addition prior to preincubation on the percentage of eggs penetrated by spermatozoa from individual semen samples. (From Maruyama DK, Hale RW, Rogers BJ. Effects of white blood cells on the in vitro penetration of zona free hamster eggs by human spermatozoa. J Androl 1985;6:130.)

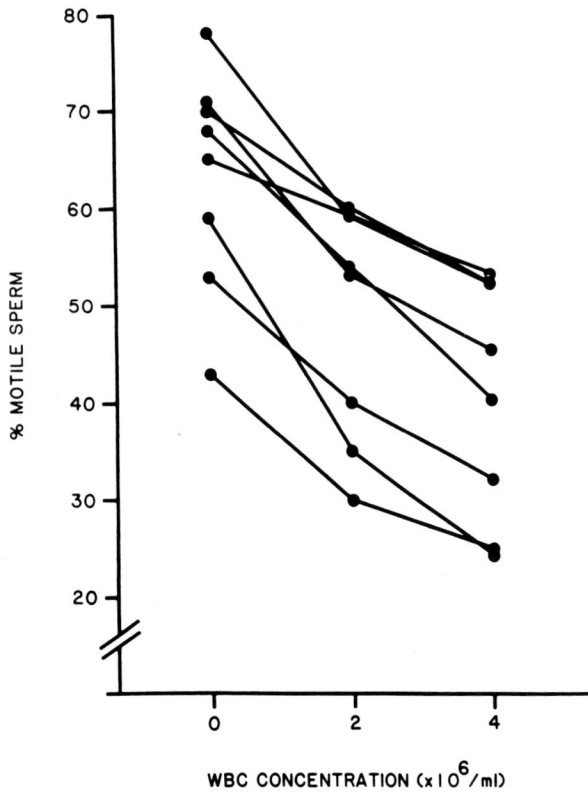

FIGURE 42–2. Percentage of motile spermatozoa following preincubation with prepared white blood cells (WBCs). (From Maruyama DK, Hale RW, Rogers BJ. Effects of white blood cells on the in vitro penetration of zona free hamster eggs by human spermatozoa. J Androl 1985;6:131.)

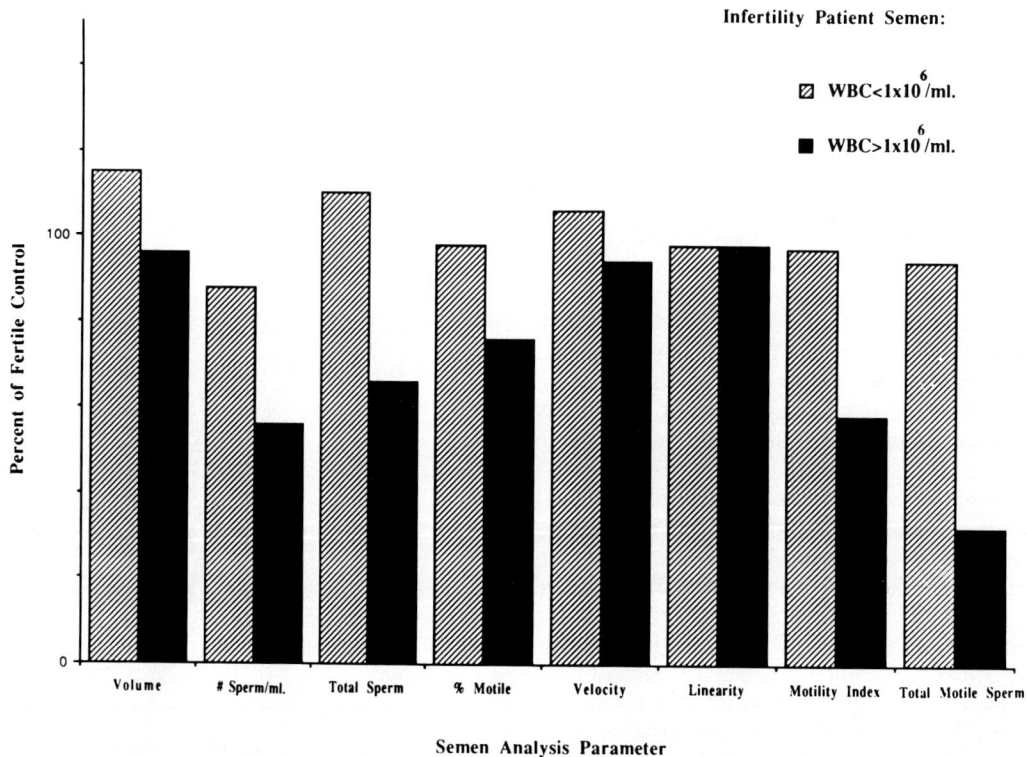

FIGURE 42–3. Reduction of semen parameters in infertility patients with high total white blood cell (WBC) per ejaculate. Group medians of semen parameters in infertility patients with high numbers (>3 × 10⁶ WBC/ejaculate; n = 44) and low numbers (<3 × 10⁶ WBC/ejaculate; n = 135) of WBC are expressed as a percentage of the respective medians in the fertile control group (n = 15). WBC were identified by the monoclonal antibody anti-Hle-1. (From Wolff H, Politch JA, Martinez A, et al. Leukocytospermia is associated with poor semen quality. Fertil Steril 1990;53:531. Reproduced with permission of the publisher, The American Fertility Society.)

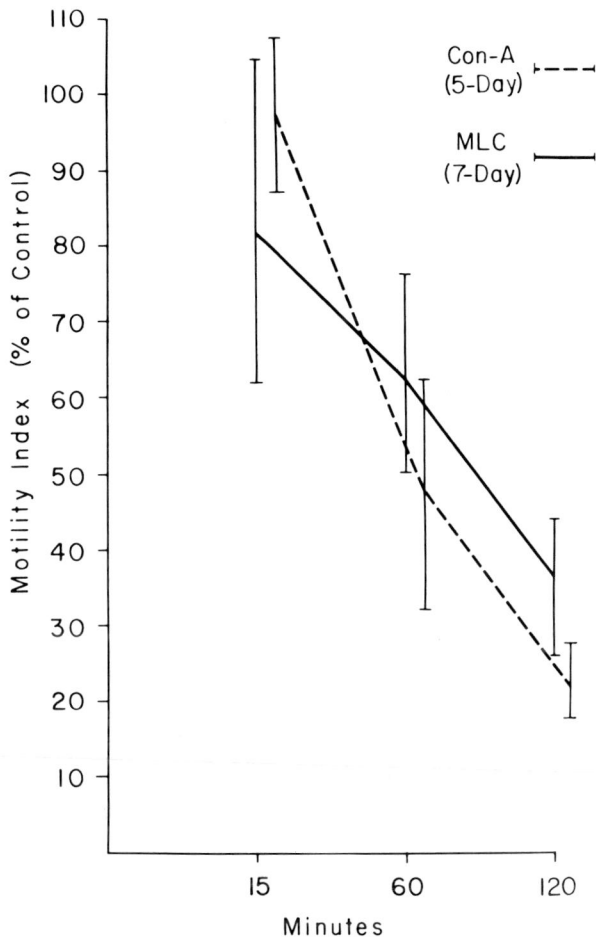

FIGURE 42–4. Effect of concanavalin A (Con-A) and mixed lymphocyte culture–activated lymphocyte supernatants on the index of sperm motility. (From Hill JA, Haimovici F, Politch JA, et al. Effects of soluble products of activated lymphocytes and macrophages [lymphokines and monokines] on human sperm motion parameters. Fertil Steril 1985;47:460–465. Reproduced with permission of the publisher, The American Fertility Society.)

bers of granulocytes, monocytes, macrophages, and lymphocytes in infertile as opposed to fertile groups of men. Shy and coworkers[104] found that the presence of pyospermia, defined as six or more white blood cells per 100 sperm, was associated with continued infertility as compared with those without white blood cells. Sixty-five percent of men without white blood cells had pregnancies after 4 or more years versus 17% of men with more than six white blood cells (Fig. 42–5).

Although it would seem simple to identify leukocytes in semen, this may not be so. Care must be taken to differentiate leukocytes from the other round cells. Immature sperm can easily be confused with lymphocytes. A number of methods have been developed to differentiate leukocytes from immature sperm.[105–108] Couture and coworkers[105] used a combined Brian-Leishman stain to differentiate white blood cells from immature sperm. Peroxidase staining has been used to identify leukocyte peroxidase and differentiate granulocytes from nonseparated spermatocytes.[109] The development of monoclonal antibodies to leukocyte subsets has led to the use of these antibodies and the identification of leukocytes in the semen. Wolff and coworkers[102] found that patients with high concentrations of monocytes and macro-

phages had significantly reduced ejaculate volume. He also found that patients with high numbers of T lymphocytes had decreased sperm velocity. El and coworkers,[109] however, found no lymphocytes in a group of infertile men. Some investigators have suggested that there also could be cross-reactivity with some of the immature sperm with monoclonal antibodies specific for leukocytes.[110] To circumvent some of the problems in identifying leukocytes histologically, some authors have tried to use leukocyte products, such as granulocyte elastase, in semen to identify inflammation. Wolff and coworkers[102] found that the levels of granulocyte elastase correlated significantly with number of white blood cells, total sperm number, and total motile sperm number. Jochum and associates[111] also found seminal plasma elastase to correlate with number of bacteria on stained semen samples and on number of round cells in the semen.

UREAPLASMA UREALYTICUM AND MALE INFERTILITY

Many investigators have addressed the role of *U. urealyticum* in both male and female infertility. The role of this organism, however, still remains uncertain. *U. urealyticum* has been implicated as a causative factor in male infertility for several reasons: (1) Semen analysis abnormalities have been found to be more common among culture-positive infertile men than among culture-negative infertile men in some studies; (2) some case control studies have shown higher frequencies of isolation of *U. urealyticum* in infertile men than in controls, although few of these studies have applied appropriate matching to their controls; (3) some treatment studies have shown improved semen analysis or fertility in men treated with antibiotics to which ureaplasma are sensitive.

Although *U. urealyticum* has been strongly implicated in nongonococcal urethritis, this has only been because of rigorous methodologic techniques. These include epidemiologic studies using carefully matched cases and controls (especially in relationship to sexual activity and past STDs), the use of quantitative cultures, a definition of a subset of urethritis not

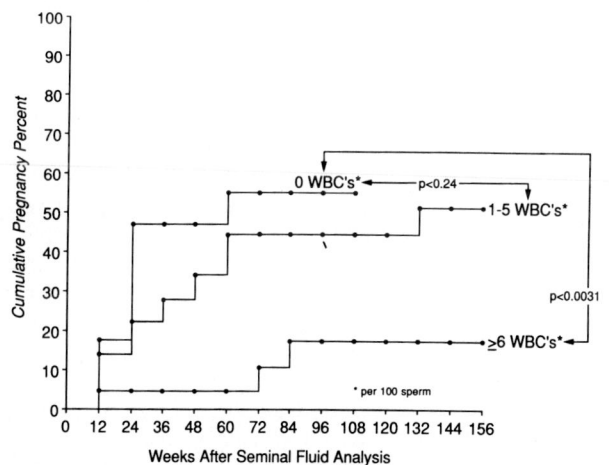

FIGURE 42–5. Three-year cumulative pregnancy percentages according to white blood cells (WBCs)/100 spermatozoa for men from infertile couples (n = 74) without female infertility factor. (Reprinted with permission from the American College of Obstetricians and Gynecologists [Obstetrics and Gynecology, 1988;71:688].)

associated with pathogens such as *C. trachomatis*, experimental inoculation, and controlled therapeutic trials comparing antibiotics with and without activity against ureaplasma. Most of these methods have yet to be applied to assess the role of ureaplasma in male infertility. This is especially important because ureaplasma is common in the sexually active population. The presence of ureaplasma in a symptomatic or asymptomatic man is directly proportional to the number of sexual partners. Therefore in any individual case of urethritis or infertility, it is impossible to assess the significance of a positive ureaplasma culture clinically.

Changes in semen analysis in men with ureaplasma infection has been reported by several authors. Toth and coworkers[112] found fuzzy and coiled tails in 70% of men colonized with ureaplasma and 19% of men not colonized. Men with ureaplasma more often had a history of genital infection. He did not differentiate between the role of ureaplasma and the role of past infection. Fowlkes and associates,[113] with electron microscopy, found increased numbers of sperm with coiled tails in ureaplasma-positive men and were able to identify ureaplasma in the sperm head and midpiece. He also found decreased semen volume, decreased sperm counts, poor morphology, and decreased motility in culture-positive patients. Grossgebauer and Hennig[114] demonstrated ureaplasma in the heads of spermatozoa in a man with symptoms of urethritis. Swenson and associates[115] found decreased sperm motility in ureaplasma-positive patients. Valvo and coworkers[116] found the semen pH to be greater in the ureaplasma-positive than in ureaplasma-negative patients possibly because of the urease enzyme present in ureaplasma. They also found greater numbers of white cells in ureaplasma-positive men than ureaplasma-negative men. They found, however, no other semen analysis difference between culture-positive and culture-negative men.[117, 118] Berger and colleagues[100] found no differences in the rate of recovery of *U. urealyticum* in men with normal or abnormal sperm function as measured by the in vitro hamster assay (SPA). Shalhoub and coworkers[119] found no difference in the semen analysis, SPA, or bovine cervical mucus penetration in ureaplasma-positive and ureaplasma-negative men. Hargreave and coworkers[120] found no association with ureaplasma culture and agglutinating sperm antibodies. Guillet-Rosso[84] found that any positive semen culture, including ureaplasma, seems to have a negative effect on the results of in vitro fertilization.

Case control data have also implicated ureaplasma in male infertility. Friberg and Knarpe[121] recovered *U. urealyticum* in 81% of men and 91% of women in infertile couples and 22% of pregnant women and 20% of their male partners. Stray-Pedersen and coworkers[122] confirmed this finding. De Louvois and colleagues,[123] however, found no difference in the incidence of ureaplasma colonization among fertile and infertile men. No studies have compared ureaplasma isolation rates among fertile and infertile subjects while adjusting or controlling for sexual experience and other variables. Cassell and associates[124] did a multivariable risk analysis among infertile couples. They found ureaplasma isolation from the woman to be highly correlated with a diagnosis of male factor infertility. He defined male factors as two or more subfertile semen analyses or a history of chronic prostatitis, although he did not define chronic prostatitis. A significantly higher percentage of cervical infection was found in those couples with a diagnosis of male factor infertility than in any other

diagnosis (74%). Eighty-seven percent of couples who had male factor infertility also had other factors related to infertility.

Numerous antibiotic trials have been aimed at the eradication of *U. urealyticum* in infertile couples. Most, however, are not placebo controlled or randomized or involve only a short duration of therapy. Some studies have shown a positive effect on treatment of infertility, whereas others have not. Toth and associates[125] followed patients for 3 years after treatment with doxycycline. Pregnancy occurred in 60% of couples in whom ureaplasma had been eradicated and in 5% of those in whom it persisted. Toth and associates postulated that the isolation of ureaplasma after treatment could be attributed to doxycycline resistance but did not document this.

U. urealyticum is a known pathogen of the male urethra and does cause urethritis. Weidner and colleagues,[126] in a large study of symptomatic prostatitis using quantitative cultures, found 10^3 colony formations in semen to discriminate infection and noninfection by ureaplasma. He also found a negative correlation between the number of ureaplasma and zinc concentration in semen. Unfortunately, such quantitative descriptions of number of ureaplasma in semen or expressed prostatic secretions in infertile patients are lacking. Audring and associates[127] formed a rat model for ureaplasma that showed that the bacteria actually got into the seminiferous tubules. Jalil and others[50] isolated ureaplasma in the epididymis of a 28-year-old man with acute epididymitis. More studies are needed using the latest techniques in semen analysis, semen histology, and epidemiology to determine if ureaplasma has a role in male infertility.

THE ROLE OF CHLAMYDIA IN MALE INFERTILITY

There is little doubt that *C. trachomatis* infection, by causing obstructive epididymitis, may lead to azoospermia and male infertility. Because chlamydia urethral infection is extremely prevalent, chlamydia could be a common cause of male infertility. Probably less than 1% of men with urethral infection, however, get epididymal infection. Because chlamydia is a sexually transmitted organism and can cause cervicitis and salpingitis in women, infection in men can certainly lead to a couple's infertility via salpingitis and tubal obstruction. In men presenting with infertility, however, it appears that chlamydial infection is extremely rare.[61, 128, 129, 130] In men with the symptoms of prostatitis and urethritis, Poletti and coworkers[68] found that chlamydia could be isolated to the prostate by transrectal aspiration in 10 of 33 men. Soffer and colleagues[131] actually found chlamydia to be more frequent in normal men than in men with abnormalities in semen analysis. Suominen and colleagues,[132] however, found significantly higher seminal fluid antichlamydia IgA levels in infertile men (51.1%) versus fertile men (23.2%) ($P < 0.01$). Wolff and coworkers[133] found granulocyte elastase to be increased in infertile men with *C. trachomatis* antibody. They did not obtain cultures for chlamydia. Close and associates[43] found no relationship of past exposure to *C. trachomatis* with SFA or SPA but did find a relationship to the presence of serum agglutinating antibody (Table 42–7).

It appears that *C. trachomatis* may infect the prostate as

TABLE 42–7. Correlations of Parameters of Male Fertility with Past Exposure to *C. trachomatis* in 270 Infertile Men

	C. trachomatis–antibody* titer ≥16 (n = 16)	*C. trachomatis*–antibody* titer <16 (n = 254)	P
History of nonspecific urethritis (%)	3/11 (27)	7/141 (5)	0.03
Median number of sexual partners in lifetime	11.5 (n = 4)	3.0 (n = 74)	0.007
No. with agglutinating antibody (geometric) (mean titer) (%)	8/16 (1:21) (50%)	41/249 (1:25) (16%)	0.003

*Micro-immunoflorescence antibody titer ≥ or IgG is considered seropositive.
From Close CE, Wang SP, Roberts P, Berger RE. The relationship of infection with *Chlamydia trachomatis* to the parameters of male fertility and sperm autoimmunity. Fertil Steril 1987; 48:880–883. Reproduced with permission of the publisher, The American Fertility Society.

well as the epididymis and that this infection could have long-term effects on prostate function or prostate inflammation. It appears that most men with infertility and seminal inflammation either with symptomatic or asymptomatic prostatitis do not have active chlamydia infection.

INFECTION AND SPERM AUTOIMMUNITY

Many authors have found sperm-directed autoantibodies to be related to male infertility.[44, 45] IgG or IgM antibodies may be found in blood. IgA antibodies are found in semen only and reflect locally produced secretory IgA. Vasectomy and vasal or epididymal obstruction lead to the generation of antisperm antibodies.[134, 135] With obstruction, macrophages migrate into the vas and epididymis and carry sperm with them into the lymph nodes. Because infection of the vas and epididymis may cause obstruction, it is possible that such obstruction may be related to subsequent male infertility even if only found unilaterally. Experimentally, ligation of one vas deferens in the mouse may produce autoimmunity and subsequent infertility.[42] Bandhauer and Marberger[46] found that 9 of 48 men with unilateral epididymitis subsequently developed sperm antibodies. Hendry and coworkers[41] found that among 32 patients with unilateral epididymal obstruction, 81% had antibodies to sperm. They estimated that 37% of infertile men with antisperm antibodies have evidence of vasal or epididymal obstruction. Soffer and coworkers[131] found increased antisperm antibody activity in men with any positive semen culture, whether it be ureaplasma or any other bacteria.

Hargreave and colleagues[136] found that ureaplasma colonization in men was unrelated to the presence of sperm autoimmunity. Micic[36] found no significant relationship between genitourinary tract infection, inflammation, and sperm autoimmunity. Hargreave and colleagues[120] found no difference between fertile men and men attending an STD clinic in the incidence of sperm antibodies. Witkin and Toth,[137] however, found a higher incidence of sperm antibodies in prostatitis patients than in controls. Barratt and associates[138] found that there was a preponderance of helper inducer T cells in the ejaculate of men with antibodies as opposed to suppressor/cytotoxic cells in men without antibodies.

Although there is probably a relationship between vasal obstruction and development of antibodies in male infertility,

it is not clear how frequently this phenomenon occurs or if it is treatable. The relationship of prostatitis to sperm autoimmunity is even less clear.

TREATMENT OF INFLAMMATION AND INFECTION IN MALE INFERTILITY

Methodologic problems have made the interpretation of treatment studies of inflammation and infection of male infertility difficult (Table 42–8). Some investigators have studied only those patients with idiopathic infertility. Others have studied oligospermic patients, whereas still others have studied men who have specific bacterial isolations from semen cultures. Some have tried to study men with white blood cells in the semen. Criteria for success in treatment have also varied and include improved counts, motilities, decreased white blood cells, and pregnancy. Few studies have used the special stains needed to differentiate immature sperm from white blood cells. None have controlled for effects of past infection. No studies, thus far, have controlled for effects of some toxic exposures.[104] Many studies have used tetracycline to treat *U. urealyticum*. It is interesting to note that tetracyclines directly affect leukocyte migration and phagocytosis and therefore may affect white cell function and numbers independently of their antibiotic effect.[139–141] Berger and colleagues[142] gave doxycycline to infertile men who had increased leukocyte concentrations and poor sperm function by the hamster penetration test (SPA). SPAs of these men improved, and they had more pregnancies than an untreated but poorly controlled group. It is possible that a subset of men, based on sperm dysfunction as identified by the hamster penetration test, may benefit from tetracycline therapy. It is entirely unclear, however, if this is due to the antibiotic effect. Studies are needed that assess sperm function before and after treatment. Moreover, it is not known whether both male and female partners should be treated.

Comhaire and associates[143] performed a double-blind, placebo-controlled study using doxycycline in men with prostatic inflammation. They followed these patients for 175 months. They found no differences between the patient and control groups in SFA or pregnancy. Interestingly, both motility and morphology showed improvement in both groups. Also, white cells disappeared in both groups. It is possible that the evaluation and treatment process themselves, including advice about toxic exposures and coital frequency, may

TABLE 42–8. Review of Therapy Trials for Male Infertility					
Reference	Treatment	Female Criteria	Male Criteria	Faults of Study	% Pregnancies
Knudsin et al[157]	Demeclocycline, 150 mg for 10 days	Unexplained infertility *Ureaplasma*	Normal seminal fluid analysis *Ureaplasma*	Uncontrolled Patient selected on basis of *Ureaplasma* Short treatment	15/36 (42%)
Quesada[158]	Antibiotics 59 with antisperm antibodies 50 without antisperm antibodies	Normal	Sole contributor to infertility	Uncontrolled No definitive treatment Mixed bacterial infection and nonbacterial inflammation Mixed symptomatic and asymptomatic	6.8% with antibodies 24% without antibodies
Sokol[164]	10 weeks, methenamine mandelate	None	15 WBC/HPF semen	Treatment with methenamine mandelate No definitive treatment Uncontrolled	5/28 (18%)
Harrison et al[163]	Doxycycline, 100 mg for 28 days Placebo No treatment	Ovulating Patent tubes	No oligospermia	Short-duration therapy Not randomized? Small number studied	5/30 (17%) 4/28 (14%) 5/30 (17%)
Matthews et al[159]	Doxycycline, 100 mg for first 10 days of each cycle for 6 months No treatment	Ovulating Patent tubes	Normal seminal fluid analysis	Randomized? No placebo	13/62 (18%) 10/42 (24%)
Idriss[160]	Tetracycline, 2 g/day for 14 days No treatment	Ovulating Open tubes	Normal seminal fluid analysis	Not consecutive or randomized Short treatment No placebo	10/24 (42%) 23/71 (32%)
Taymor[161]	Tetracycline, 2 g for 10 days Untreated	*Ureaplasma* present	*Ureaplasma*	No placebo Short treatment Nonrandomzied	10/24 (42%) 17/67 (25%)
Khatanee and Decker[162]	Demeclocycline, 150 mg Untreated	No demonstrable abnormality	No criteria	Untreated controls from gynecology clinic population and not all trying to conceive	31/68 (46%) 19/62 (30%)

WBC, white blood cell.

have been the important factor in decreasing white cells in semen independent of drug treatment.

Although prolonged treatment with antibiotics has been advocated by some, there may be problems with this approach. Several authors have found that antibiotics have an adverse effect on testicular function. Sulfasalazine, commonly used in ulcerative colitis, decreases sperm counts.[144] Several investigators have found that tetracycline and its derivatives cause testicular atrophy in animals and may decrease sperm counts in men.[145–147] Cephalosporins, penicillins, and trimethoprim also decreased spermatogenesis.[150] It is interesting that in the doxycycline treatment study by Berger and coworkers,[52] all pregnancies took place in the first month after therapy. Continued therapy did not increase pregnancy rate. It is possible that short-term therapy is beneficial, whereas longer courses of antibiotics cause problems with sperm production. Obviously, much more effort is needed in this area.

REFERENCES

1. Branny J, Zerabala M. Some characteristics of viruses isolated from bull semen and their possible pathogenicity. Br Vet J 1970;127:88–92.
2. Harrison WO. Cefaclor in the treatment of uncomplicated gonococcal urethritis. Postgrad Med J 1979;55:85.
3. Greenberg SH. Male reproductive tract sequelae of gonococcal and nongonococcal urethritis. Arch Androl 1979;2:317–319.
4. Crawford G, Knapp JS, Hale J, et al. Asymptomatic gonorrhea in men. Science 1937;196:1352.
5. John J, Donald WH. Asymptomatic urethral gonorrhea in men. Br J Vener Dis 1978;54:322–323.
6. McCutchan JA. Gonorrhea and nongonococcal urethritis. In: Braude AI, editor. Medical Microbiology and Infectious Disease. Philadelphia: WB Saunders, 1981:1201–1210.
7. Hooper RR, Wiesner PJ, Harrison WO, et al. Cohort study of venereal disease. 1. Risk of transmission from infected women to men. Am J Epidemiol 1978;108:136–144.
8. Kellogg DS, Holmes KK, Hill GA. Cumitech 4: laboratory diagnosis of gonorrhea. Washington, DC: American Society for Microbiology, 1976.
9. Granato PA, Schneible-Smith C, Weiner LB. Use of New York City medium for improved recovery on N. gonorrhoeae from clinical specimens. J Clin Microbiol 1981;13:963–968.
10. Harrison WO. Gonococcal urethritis. Urol Clin North Am 1984; 11:45–53.
11. Stamm WE. Diagnosis of *Neisseria gonorrhoeae* and *Chlamydia trachomatis* infections with antigen detection methods. Diagn Microbiol Infect Dis 1986;4(3 suppl):93S–99S.
12. Lassus A, Paavonen J, Kousa M, et al. Erythromycin and lymecycline treatment in Chlamydia-positive and Chlamydia-negative nongonococcal urethritis: a partner-controlled study. Acta Derm Venereol 1979;59:278–281.
13. Bowie WB, Wang SP, Alexander ER, et al. Etiology of nongonococcal urethritis: evidence for *C. trachomatis* and *U. urealyticum*. J Clin Invest 1977;59:735–742.
14. Ripa KT, Mårdh P-A, Thelin I. *Chlamydia trachomatis* urethritis in men attending a venereal disease clinic: A culture and therapeutic study. Acta Derm Venereol 1978;58:175–179.
15. Schacter J. Chlamydial infections. N Engl J Med 1978;298:423.
16. Thelin I, Wenstrom AM, Mårdh PA. Contact tracing in patients with genital chlamydial infection. Br J Vener Dis 1980;56:259–262.

17. Taylor-Robinson D, McCormack WM. The genital mycoplasmas. N Engl J Med 1980;302:1003–1010.
18. Bowie WR, Pollock HM, Forsyth PS, et al. Bacteriology of the urethra in normal men and men with nongonococcal urethritis. J Clin Microbiol 1977;6:482–488.
19. Stimson JB, Hale J, Bowie WR, Holmes KK. Tetracycline resistant *Ureaplasma urealyticum:* a cause of persistent urethritis. Ann Intern Med 1981;94:192.
20. Bowie WR, Floyd JF, Miller V, et al. Differential response of chlamydial and ureaplasma-associated urethritis to sulfafurazole (sulfisoxazole) and aminocyclitols. Lancet 1976;2:1276–1278.
21. Pessione F, Dolivo M, Casin I, et al. Sexual behavior and smoking: risk factors for urethritis in men. Sex Transm Dis 1988;15:119–122.
22. Smith GL, Greenup R, Takafuji ET. Circumcision as a risk factor for urethritis in racial groups. Am J Pub Health 1987;77:452–454.
23. Hernandez AI, Alvarez DC, Gili M, et al. Oral sex as a risk factor for Chlamydia-negative nongonococcal urethritis. Sex Transm Dis 1988;15:100–102.
24. Bowie WR. Etiology and treatment of nongonococcal urethritis. Sex Transm Dis 1978;5:27–33.
25. Swartz SL, Kraus SJ, Herrmann KL, et al. Diagnosis and etiology of nongonococcal urethritis. J Infect Dis 1978;138:445–454.
26. Bowie WR, Yu JS, Jones HD. Partial efficacy of clindamycin against *Chlamydia trachomatis* in men with nongonococcal urethritis. Sex Transm Dis 1986;13:76–80.
27. Candel S. Epididymitis in mumps, including orchitis: further clinical studies and comments. Ann Intern Med 1951;34:20–36.
28. Abdel RM, Morsy F. Genitourinary mycobacteria in infertile Egyptian men. Fertil Steril 1990;54:713–717.
29. Ibrahiem AA, Awad HA, Metawi BA, Hamada TA. Pathologic changes in testis and epididymis of infertile leprotic males. Int J Lepr Other Mycobact Dis 1979;47;44–49.
30. El SS, El HH, Abdel FA, et al. Testicular and epididymal involvement in leprosy patients, with special reference to gynecomastia. Int J Dermatol 1976;15:52–58.
31. Wolin LH. On the etiology of epididymitis. J Urol 1971;105:531–533.
32. Nilsson S, Obrant KO, Persson PS. Changes in the testis parenchyma caused by acute nonspecific epididymitis. Fertil Steril 1968;19:748–757.
33. Ludwig VG, Haselberger J. Epididymitis and fertilat: Behandlungsergebnisse bei akuter unspezifischer epididymitis. 1977;95:397–399.
34. Krishnan R, Heal MR. Study of the seminal vesicles in acute epididymitis. Br J Urol 1991;67:632–637.
35. Osegbe DN. Testicular function after unilateral bacterial epididymoorchitis. Eur Urol 1991;19:204–208.
36. Micic S. Incidence of aetiological factors in testicular obstructive azoospermia. Int J Androl 1987;10:681–684.
37. Campbell MS. Surgical pathology of epididymitis. Ann Surg 1928;88:98–111.
38. Pelouze PS. Epididymitis in Gonorrhea in the Male and Female. Philadelphia: WB Saunders, 1941:141.
39. Chakraforty J, Jhunjhunwala J. Experimental unilateral torsion of the spermatic cord in guinea pigs. Effects on the contralateral testes. J Androl 1982;3:117–123.
40. Krarup T. The testes after torsion. Br J Urol 1978;30:43–46.
41. Hendry WF, Parslow JM, Stedronska J, Wallace DMA. The diagnosis of unilateral testicular obstruction in subfertile males. Br J Urol 1982;54:774–779.
42. Kessler DL, Smith WD, Hamilton MS, Berger RE. Infertility in mice after unilateral vasectomy. Fertil Steril 1985;43:308–312.
43. Close C, Wang S-P, Berger RE. Relationship of sperm autoimmunity to *C. trachomatis* infection in infertile men. Fertil Steril 1974;25:393–398.
44. Rumke PH, Van Amstad N, Messer EN, Bezemer PD. Prognosis of fertility of men with sperm agglutinins in the serum. Fertil Steril 1974;25:393–398.
45. Rumke PH, Hellinga G. Autoantibodies against spermatozoa in sterile men. Am J Clin Pathol 1959;32:357–363.
46. Bandhauer K, Marberger H. Spermagglutinins in diseases of the epididymis. 5th World Congress on Fertility and Sterility, Chicago, IL, 1966:781.
47. Bietz O. Fertilitatsuntersuchungen bei des unspezifichen epididymitis. Hauturzt 1959;10:134–135.
48. Kuzan FB, Patton DL, Allen SM, Kuo CC. A proposed mouse model for acute epididymitis provoked by genital serovar E, Chlamydia trachomatis. Biol Reprod 1989;40:165–172.
49. Hackett RA, Huang TW, Berger RE. Experimental *E. coli* epididymitis in rabbits. Urology 1988;32:236–240.
50. Jalil N, Doble A, Gilchrist C, Taylor RD. Infection of the epididymis by Ureaplasma urealyticum. Genitourin Med 1988;64:367–368.
51. Watson RA. Gonorrhea and acute epididymitis. Milit Med 1979;144:785–786.
52. Berger RE, Alexander ER, Harnisch JP, et al. Etiology, manifestations and therapy of acute epididymitis: Prospective study of fifty cases. J Urol 1979;121:750–754.
53. Arya OP, Tuder SR. Correlates of venereal disease and fertility in rural Uganda. Presented at the Medical Society for the Study of Venereal Disease, Malta, 1975.
54. Osegbe DN, Amaku EO. The causes of male infertility in 504 consecutive Nigerian patients. Int Urol Nephrol 1985;17:349–358.
55. Meares EM. Prostatitis syndromes: New perspectives about old woes. J Urol 1980;123:141–147.
56. Meares EM, Burbalras GA. Prostatitis, bacterial, non-bacterial and prostatodynia. Semin Urol 1983;1:146–154.
57. Meares EM, Stamey TA. Bacteriologic localization patterns in bacterial prostatitis and urethritis. Invest Urol 1968;5:492–518.
58. Fair WR, Cordonnier JJ. The pH of prostatic fluid: A reappraisal and therapeutic implications. J Urol 1978;120:695–698.
59. Shortliffe LMD, Wehner N, Stamey TA. The detection of a local prostatic immunologic response to bacterial prostatitis. J Urol 1981;125:509–515.
60. Anderson RW, Weller C. Prostatic secretion leukocyte studies in nonbacterial prostatitis (prostatosis). J Urol 1979;121:292–294.
61. Berger RE, Krieger JN, Kessler D, et al. Case-control study of men with suspected chronic idiopathic prostatitis. J Urol 1989;141:328–331.
62. Cumming JA, Dawes J, Hargreave TB. Granulocyte elastase levels do not correlate with anaerobic and aerobic bacterial growth in seminal plasma from infertile men. Int J Androl 1990;13:273–277.
63. Meares EM. Bacterial prostatitis vs prostatosis, a clinical and bacteriological study. JAMA 1973;224:1372–1375.
64. Centifano VM, Drylie DM, Dearddourff SL, Kaufman HE. Herpes virus type 2 in the male genitourinary tract. Science 1972;178:318–319.
65. Måardh P-A, Ripa KT, Colleen S, et al. Role of *Chlamydia trachomatis* in non-acute prostatitis. Br J Vener Dis 1978;54:330–334.
66. Bruce AW, Chadwick P, Willet WS, O'Shaughnessy M. The role of chlamydiae in genitourinary disease. J Urol 1981;126:625–629.
67. Nilsson S, Obrant KO, Persson PS. Changes in the testis parenchyma caused by acute nonspecific epididymitis. Fertil Steril 1968;19:748–757.
68. Poletti F, Medici MC, Alinovi A, et al. Isolation of Chlamydia trachomatis from the prostatic cells in patients affected by nonacute abacterial prostatitis. J Urol 1985;134:691–693.
69. Weidner W, Brunner H, Krause W. Quantitative culture of *Ureaplasma urealyticum* in patients with chronic prostatitis or prostatosis. J Urol 1980;124:622–625.
70. Harrison KL, Johnson DK. Chronic asymptomatic genital tract infection and semen quality. Pathology 1979;11:289–292.
71. Toth A, Lesser ML. Asymptomatic bacteriospermia in fertile and infertile men. Fertil Steril 1981;36:88–91.
72. Ulstein M, Capell P, Homes KK, Paulsen CA. Nonsymptomatic genital tract infection and male infertility. In: Esem G, editor. Human Semen and Fertility Regulation in Men. St. Louis: CV Mosby, 1976:355–362.
73. Paulson JD, Polakoski KL. A glass wool column procedure for removing extraneous material from the human ejaculate. Fertil Steril 1977;28:178–181.
74. Comhaire F, Vershraegen G, Vermeulen L. Diagnosis of accessory gland infection and its possible role in male infertility. Int J Androl 1980;3:32–45.
75. Harrison KL, Johnson DK. Chronic asymptomatic genital tract infection and semen quality. Pathology 1979;11:289–292.
76. Ulstein M, Capell P, Holmes KK, Paulsen CA. Nonsymptomatic genital tract infection and male infertility. In: Hafez ESE, editor. Human Semen and Fertility Regulation in Men. St. Louis: CV Mosby, 1976:355–362.
77. Rehewy MSE, Hafez ESE, Thomas A, Brown WJ. Aerobic and anaerobic bacterial flora in semen from fertile and infertile groups of men. Arch Androl 1979;2:263–268.
78. Moberg PJ, Eneroth P, Ljung A, Nord CE. Bacterial growth in samples from cervix and semen from infertile couples. Int J Fertil 1979;24:157–165.
79. Eneroth A, Wadstrom L, Moberg PJ, Nord CE. Bacterial growth in samples from cervix and semen from infertile couples. Int J Fertil 1979;24:157–165.
80. Morton RS. White cell counts in human semen. Br J Vener Dis 1968;44:72–74.

81. Svendsen M. Leukocytes and bacteria in human semen. J Pathol Bacteriol 1960;60:131–135.

82. Hillier SL, Rabe LK, Muller CH, et al. Relationship of bacteriologic characteristics to semen indices in men attending an infertility clinic. Obstet Gynecol 1990;75:800–804.

83. Cumming JA, Dawes J, Hargreave TB. Granulocyte elastase levels do not correlate with anaerobic and aerobic bacterial growth in seminal plasma from infertile men. Int J Androl 1990;13:273–277.

84. Guillet-Rosso F, Fari A, Taylor S, et al. Systemic semen culture and its influence on IVF management. Br J Obstet Gynaecol 1987;94:543–547.

85. Persson BE, Sjoman M, Niklasson F, Ronquist G. Uridine, xanthine and urate concentrations in prostatic fluid and seminal plasma of patients with prostatitis. Eur Urol 1991;19:253–256.

86. Gattuccio F, Di TD, Romano C, et al. Urogenital inflammations: aetiology, diagnosis and their correlation with varicocele and male infertility. Acta Eur Fertil 1988;19:201–208.

87. Close CE, Roberts PL, Berger RE. Cigarettes, alcohol and marijuana are related to pyospermia in infertile men. J Urol 1990;144:900–903.

88. Vallely PJ, Sharrard RM, Rees RC. The identification of factors in seminal plasma responsible for suppression of natural killer cell activity. Immunology 1988;63:451–456.

89. Quayle AJ, Kelly RW, Hargreave TB, James K. Immunosuppression by seminal prostaglandins. Clin Exp Immunol 1989;75:387–391.

90. Mukhopadhyay NK, Saha AK, Smith W, et al. Inhibition of neutrophil and natural killer cell function by human seminal fluid acid phosphatase. Clin Chim Acta 1989;182:31–40.

91. Colleen S, Mårdh P-A, Schytz A. Magnesium and zinc in seminal fluid of healthy males and patients with non-acute prostatitis with and without gonorrhea. Scand J Urol Nephrol 1975;9:192–197.

92. Caldamone AA, Dougherty KA, Cockett ATK. Monitoring zinc concentration in seminal plasma during treatment of prostatitis and infertility. Surg Forum 1981;32:644–646.

93. Caldamone AA, Emilson LBVC, Al-Juburi A, Cockett ATK. Prostatitis: Prostatic secretory dysfunction affecting fertility. Fertil Steril 1980;34:602–603.

94. Hughes L, Ryder TA, McDenzie ML, et al. The use of transmission electron microscopy to study nonspermatozoal cells in semen. In: Frajese G, Hafez ESE, Conti C, Fabrini C, editors. Oligozoospermia: Recent Progress in Andrology. New York: Raven Press, 1981:65–75.

95. Koehler JK, Berger RE, Karp LE. Spermophagy. In: Hafez ESE, Kenemans P, editors. Atlas of Human Reproduction. Berlin: MSP Press, 1983:213–218.

96. Maroni MS, Symon DNK, Wilkinson PC. Chemotaxis of neutrophil leukocytes towards spermatozoa and seminal fluid. J Reprod Fertil 1972;28:359–368.

97. Clark RA, Klebanoff SJ. Neutrophil mediated tumor cytotoxicity. Role of peroxidase system. J Exp Med 1975;141:1442–1447.

98. Pandya IJ, Cohen J. The leukocytic reaction of the human uterine cervix to spermatozoa. Fertil Steril 1985;43:417–421.

99. Megory E, Zuckerman H, Shoham Z, Lunenfeld B. Infections and male fertility. Obstet Gynecol Surv 1987;42:283–290.

100. Berger RE, Karp LE, Williamson RA, et al. The relationship of pyospermia and seminal fluid bacteriology to sperm function as reflected in the sperm penetration assay. Fertil Steril 1982;37:557–564.

101. Maruyama DK, Hale RW, Rogers BJ. Effects of white blood cells on the in vitro penetration of zona free hamster eggs by human spermatozoa. J Androl 1985;6:127–135.

102. Wolff H, Politch JA, Martinez A, et al. Leukocytospermia is associated with poor semen quality. Fertil Steril 1990;53:528–536.

103. Wolff H, Anderson DJ. Male genital tract inflammation associated with increased numbers of potential human immunodeficiency virus host cells in semen. Andrologia 1988;20:404–410.

104. Shy K, Stenchever MA, Muller CH. Sperm penetration assay and subsequent pregnancy: a prospective study of 74 infertile men. Obstet Gynecol 1988;71:685–690.

105. Couture M, Ulstein M, Leonhard J, Paulsen CA. Improved staining method for differentiating immature germ cells from white blood cells in human seminal fluid. Andrologia 1976;8:61–66.

106. Endz AW. A rapid staining method for differentiating granulocytes from "germinal cells" in Papanicolaou-stained semen. Acta Cytol 1974;18:2–7.

107. Phadke AM. Neutral red supravital staining for cellular elements in the semen. Andrologia 1978;10:80–84.

108. Riedd HH. Techniques for the detection of leukospermia in human semen. Arch Androl 1980;5:287–293.

109. El DM, Hargreave TB, Busuttil A, et al. Identifying leukocytes and leukocyte subpopulations in semen using monoclonal antibody probes. Urology 1986;28:492–496.

110. Mathur S, Goust JM, Williamson HO, Fudenberg HH. Cross-reactivity of sperm and T lymphocyte antigens. Am J Reprod Immunol 1981;1:113–118.

111. Jochum M, Pabst W, Schill WB. Granulocyte elastase as a sensitive diagnostic parameter of silent male genital tract inflammation. Andrologia 1986;18:413–419.

112. Toth A, Swenson CE, O'Leary WM. Light microscopy as an aid in predicting ureaplasma infection in human semen. Fertil Steril 1978;39:586–691.

113. Fowlkes DM, Dooher GB, O'Leary WM. Evidence by scanning electron microscopy for an association between spermatozoa and T-mycoplasmas in men of infertile marriage. Fertil Steril 1975;26:1203–1222.

114. Grossgebauer K, Hennig A. Ureaplasma-infected human sperm in infertile men. Arch Androl 1984;12(suppl):35–41.

115. Swenson CE, Toth A, O'Leary WM. *Ureaplasma urealyticum* and human infertility: correlation of infection with alterations in seminal parameters. Fertil Steril 1979;31:660–665.

116. Valvo JR, Caldamone AA, Hipp S, et al. Elevated seminal pH and *Ureaplasma urealyticum*. J Androl 1982;3:144–148.

117. Desai S, Cohen MS, Kratamee M, Leiter E. Ureaplasma urealyticum (T-mycoplasma) infection: does it have a role in male infertility? J Urol 1980;124:469–471.

118. Cintron RD, Wortham JWE, Acosta A. The association of semen factors with the recovery of *Ureaplasma urealyticum*. Fertil Steril 1981;36:648–652.

119. Shalhoub D, Abdel LA, Fredericks CM, et al. Physiological integrity of human sperm in the presence of Ureaplasma urealyticum. Arch Androl 1986;16:75–80.

120. Hargreave TB, Harvey J, Elton RA, McMillan A. Serum agglutinating and immobilising sperm antibodies in men attending a sexually transmitted diseases clinic. Andrologia 1984;16:111–115.

121. Friberg J, Knarpe H. Mycoplasma in semen from fertile and infertile men. Andrologia 1974;6:45–46.

122. Stray-Pedersen B, Eng J, Mannsaker Reikvan T. Uterine T-mycoplasma colonization in reproductive failure. Am J Obstet Gynecol 1978;130:307–311.

123. de Louvois J, Blades M, Hurley R, et al. Frequency of mycoplasma in fertile and infertile couples. Lancet 1974;1:1073–1075.

124. Cassell GH, Younger JB, Brown MB, et al. Microbiologic study of infertile women at the time of diagnostic laparoscopy. N Engl J Med 1983;308:502–505.

125. Toth A, Lesser ML, Brooks C, Labriola D. Subsequent pregnancies among 161 couples treated for T-mycoplasma genital tract infections. N Engl J Med 1983;308:505–507.

126. Weidner W, Krause W, Schiefer HG, et al. Ureaplasma infections of the male urogenital tract, in particular prostatitis, and semen quality. Urol Int 1985;40:5–9.

127. Audring H, Klug H, Bollmann R, et al. Ureaplasma urealyticum and male infertility: an animal model. II. Morphologic changes of testicular tissue at light microscopic level and electron microscopic findings. Andrologia 1989;21:66–75.

128. Hellstrom WJ, Schachter J, Sweet RL, McClure RD. Is there a role for Chlamydia trachomatis and genital mycoplasma in male infertility? Fertil Steril 1987;48:337–339.

129. Bennett AH, Hipp SS, Alford LM. Pyosemia and carriage of chlamydia and ureaplasma in infertile men. J Urol 1982;128:54–56.

130. Ruijs GJ, Kauer FM, Jager S, et al. Is serology of any use when searching for correlations between *Chlamydia trachomatis* infection and male infertility? Fertil Steril 1990;53:131–136.

131. Soffer Y, Ron ER, Golan A, et al. Male genital mycoplasmas and Chlamydia trachomatis culture: its relationship with accessory gland function, sperm quality, and autoimmunity. Fertil Steril 1990;53:331–336.

132. Suominen J, Gronroos M, Terho P, Wichmann L. Chronic prostatitis, *Chlamydia trachomatis* and infertility. Int J Androl 1983;6:405–413.

133. Wolff H, Neubert U, Zebhauser M, et al. Chlamydia trachomatis induces an inflammatory response in the male genital tract and is associated with altered semen quality. Fertil Steril 1991;55:1017–1019.

134. Ansbacher R, Keung-Yeung K, Wurster JC. Sperm antibodies in vasectomized men. Fertil Steril 1972;23:640–643.

135. Linnet L, Hjort T. Sperm agglutinins in seminal plasma and serum after vasectomy. Correlation between immunological and clinical findings. J Exp Immunol 1977;30:413–420.

136. Hargreave TB, Torrance M, Young H, Harris AB. Isolation of *Urea-*

plasma urealyticum from seminal plasma in relation to sperm antibody levels and sperm motility. Andrologia 1982;14:223–227.

137. Witkin SS, Toth A. Relationship between genital tract infections, sperm antibodies in seminal fluid, and infertility. Fertil Steril 1983;40:805–808.

138. Barratt CL, Harrison PE, Robinson A, Cooke ID. Antisperm antibodies and lymphocyte subsets in semen—not a simple relationship. Int J Androl 1990;13:50–58.

139. Belsheim J, Gnarpe H, Persson S. Tetracyclines and host defense mechanisms: interference with leukocyte chemotaxis. Scand J Infect Dis 1979;11:141–145.

140. Forsgren A, Schmeling D. Effects of antibiotics on chemotaxis of human leukocyte chemotaxis. Scand J Infect Dis 1979;11:141–145.

141. Forsgren A, Gnarpe H. The effect of antibacterial agents on the association between bacteria and leukocytes. Scand J Infect Dis 1982;33:115–120.

142. Berger RE, Smith D, Critchlow CW, et al. Improvement in the sperm penetration (hamster ova) assay (SPA) results after doxycycline treatment of infertile men. J Androl 1983;4:126–130.

143. Comhaire FH, Rowe PJ, Farley TM. The effect of doxycycline in infertile couples with male accessory gland infection: a double blind prospective study. Int J Androl 1986;9:91–98.

144. D'Arcy PF. Drug interactions and reactions update. Drug Intell Clin Pharm 1982;16:218–221.

145. Deichmann WB, Bernal E, Anderson WAD, et al. The chronic oral toxicity of oxytetracycline HCl and tetracycline HCl in the rat, dog, and pig. Indust Med Surg 1964;33:787–806.

146. Desau FI, Sullivan WJ. A two-year study of the toxicity of chlortetracycline hydrochloride in rats. Toxicol Appl Pharm 1961;3:654–677.

147. Timmermans L. Influence of antibiotics on spermatogenesis. J Urol 1974;112:348–349.

148. Berger RE, Kessler D, Holmes KK. The etiology and manifestations of epididymitis in young men: correlations with sexual orientation. J Infect Dis 1987;155:1341–1343.

149. Hawkins DA, Taylor-Robinson D, Thomas BJ, Harris JR. Microbiological survey of acute epididymitis. Genitourin Med 1986;62:342–344.

150. Scheibel JH, Anderson JT, Brandenhoff P, et al. Chlamydia trachomatis in acute epididymitis. Scand J Urol Nephrol 1983;17:47–50.

151. Kristensen JK, Scheibel JH. Etiology of acute epididymitis presenting in a venereal disease clinic. Sex Transm Dis 1984;11:32–33.

152. Kojima H, Wang SP, Kuo CC, Grayston JT. Local antibody in semen for rapid diagnosis of Chlamydia trachomatis epididymitis. J Urol 1988;140:528–531.

153. Grant JB, Costello CB, Sequeira PJ, Blacklock NJ. The role of *Chlamydia trachomatis* in epididymitis. Br J Urol 1987;60:355–359.

154. Doble A, Taylor-Robinson D, Thomas BJ, et al. Acute epididymitis: a microbiological and ultrasonographic study. Br J Urol 1989;63:90–94.

155. De Jong Z, Pontonnier F, Plante P, et al. The frequency of Chlamydia trachomatis in acute epididymitis. Br J Urol 1988;62:76–78.

156. Melekos MD, Asbach HW. The role of chlamydiae in epididymitis. Int Urol Nephrol 1988;20:293–297.

157. Knudsin RB, Horneth HW, Kosasu TX. T-mycoplasma associated human infertility: results of treatment. In: Abstracts of the Annual Meeting of the American Society for Microbiology, 1974.

158. Quesada EM, Dukes CD, Dee GH, Franklin RR. Genital infection and sperm agglutinating antibodies in infertile men. J Urol 1968;99:106–108.

159. Matthews CD, Clupp KH, Tonsing JA, Cox LW. T-Mycoplasma genital infection. The effects of dycycline therapy on human unexplained infertility. Fertil Steril 1978;30:98–102.

160. Idress WM, Patton WC, Taylor ML. On the etiologic role of *Ureaplasma urealyticum* (T-mycoplasma) infection in infertility. Fertil Steril 1978;30:293–296.

161. Taymor ML. Mycoplasma infection. In: Taymore ML, editor. Infertility. New York, Grune & Stratton, 1978:126.

162. Khatanee NA, Decker WH. Recovery of genital mycoplasmas from infertile couples using New York City medium. Infertility 1978;1:155–166.

163. Harrison RF, Blades M, Dehouvon J, Huylley R. Doxycycline treatment and human infertility. Lancet 1975;1:605–607.

164. Sokol S, Jacobson CB, Derrick FC. Use of methenamine hippurate in male infertility. Urology 1975;6:59–62.

CHAPTER 43

Immunology of Spermatozoa

JOHN E. GOULD

Antisperm antibodies are now a well-established cause of male infertility. Although this relationship was suggested more than 30 years ago, a precise description of this association is lacking. Current basic science research is improving our understanding of the complex relationship between infertility and the immune system. Approximately 10% to 30% of men with unexplained infertility are thought to have immunologic factors involved, underscoring the importance of this research.

Immunity to sperm is a relative, not absolute, cause of infertility.[1] The reason for this relativity is that the immune response is qualitatively and quantitatively complex. For example, the relationship of antisperm antibody presence to infertility is complicated by many factors: concentration of antibodies present, percent of sperm cells bound, isotype (e.g., IgG, IgA), locations of antibody binding on sperm cells, body fluid containing the antibodies (serum versus semen), the type of assay used to detect the antibodies, and complement titers in the female reproductive tract.[2–5] In this context, it is easy to understand why antisperm antibodies are only a relative risk factor for infertility. Considerable current research activity is attempting to define the importance of these variables.

BLOOD-TESTIS BARRIER

Sperm cell production begins at puberty long after the immune system has matured and learned to recognize self from nonself. The process of spermatogenesis results in the expression of new sperm surface antigens.[6] The new antigens are isolated from the immune system by a blood-testis barrier. This barrier is anatomically defined as a series of tight junctions between neighboring Sertoli cells, which separate the adluminal spaces of the seminiferous tubules from the basal area.[7] The new antigens on sperm cells do not normally develop until the developing sperm cell enters the adluminal compartment; they are not present on spermatogonia. Therefore it is widely accepted that the function of the blood-testis barrier is to prevent the new foreign antigens from contacting

elements of the immune system. It is believed that the sequestration from the immune system continues along the epididymis, vas deferens, and urethra, but the exact nature of this isolation barrier is not as well characterized.

The acquisition of foreign sperm surface antigens is a complex process. The addition or alteration of sperm surface antigens is thought to occur in the seminiferous tubules and the epididymis. The functions and characteristics of the surface antigens are not known. It is known that the ability of sperm to undergo capacitation usually requires sperm transit through the epididymis.[8] One might presume that the surface antigens involved in sperm capacitation compose some of these foreign antigens. Epididymal proteins involved in the acquisition of sperm motility might similarly represent some of these foreign antigens.

Conditions that disrupt the blood-testis barrier are associated with antisperm antibodies. Historical risk factors include testicular trauma, torsion, tumor, ductal obstruction (including vasectomy), previous infection or inflammation, and otherwise unexplained infertility.[9, 10] Laboratory risk factors for antisperm antibodies include sperm agglutination on semen evaluation, an abnormal postcoital test in the presence of good-quality mucus and a normal semen evaluation, and fertilization failure as in a negative sperm penetration assay or failed in vitro fertilization. An abnormal postcoital test may also indicate the presence of antisperm antibodies in the cervical mucus. The postcoital test may show no sperm in good-quality mucus or sperm stuck in the mucus with a "shaking" type of motion.[11]

Potential sites for sperm contact with the immune system include the rete testis and efferent ducts. The tight junctions between cells lining these areas appear to be weak.[6] In addition, T suppressor cells are abundant in between the epithelial cells in the rete testis, epididymis, vas deferens, seminal vesicles, and prostatic acini.[12] The ratio of T suppressor to T helper cells in this environment and the magnitude of antigenic leak may be important factors in immune infertility. Further evidence for rete testis involvement in antigen leakage comes from the experimental allergic orchitis model, in which passive transfer of leukocytes activated by testicular antigens produces an orchitis in the recipient animal.[13] Furthermore, immune complexes can be observed outside the efferent ducts following vasectomy in rhesus monkeys.[6]

Witkin[14] has proposed three possible mechanisms for sperm antibody formation that involve genital tract immune suppressor functions. First, a decrease in the T suppressor cell numbers or activity might potentiate immune response to sperm surface antigens. Second, if genital tract fluids are deficient in soluble factors that modulate suppressor cell activity (e.g., interferons, prostaglandins), sperm antibody formation may occur. Third, there is evidence that spermatozoa and developing sperm cells are capable of suppressing immune responses.[15, 16] Factors that alter sperm-induced immunosuppression might therefore be important in modulating immune responses to sperm.

Antisperm antibodies develop in the serum of approximately two thirds of men who have undergone a vasectomy.[17, 18] Although serum IgG has been shown to be a good predictor of sperm surface antibodies,[19] the biologic relevance of antisperm antibodies in serum to fertility impairment is controversial. Alexander[20] showed diminished fertility in vasectomized men with sperm agglutinating antibodies in serum, whereas Silber[21] found no such correlation.

PATHOPHYSIOLOGY

Data are quickly accumulating on the role of antisperm antibodies in infertility. Evidence suggests that sperm survival and migration through the female reproductive tract may be impaired by sperm surface antibodies, possibly by macrophage phagocytosis and complement-mediated cytotoxicity.[22, 23] Complement proteins have been identified in cervical mucus and follicular fluid.[24] Ultrastructural studies of antibody-bound human sperm do not show significant alteration of acrosomal morphology, suggesting that this is not an important mechanism of infertility.[25] Numerous studies have shown that sperm surface antibodies impair the sperm-egg interactions.[26] Additional potential sites of damage include the process of sperm development and maturation in the testis and epididymis. Putative processes that might be impaired by sperm surface antibodies include penetration of cervical mucus and sperm motility, sperm transport to the oviduct, capacitation, the acrosome reaction, penetration of the cumulus oophorus and zona pellucida, fusion with the vitellus, and embryogenesis.[1, 11]

The immunoglobulin class and location of binding to the sperm cell surface appear to be important pathophysiologic characteristics. For example, IgM is rarely found in significant concentrations in semen, and its significance in serum is unknown.[27] IgA appears to be an important inhibitor of cervical mucus penetration, whereas IgG does not appear to exclude sperm significantly from cervical mucus.[3]

Clarke and coworkers[26] showed that high levels of IgA immunoglobulins on the sperm surface significantly impaired fertilization rates. When the male patient had 80% or more of his motile sperm covered with IgG or IgA, overall fertilization rates were only 27%. In nine male patients with sperm-surface antibodies but in whom less than 80% of motile sperm were coated with IgA antibodies, the fertilization rate was 72%. Higher fertilization rates were observed in patients even if the IgG surface binding was quite high. The

authors did not observe any problems with subsequent implantation and pregnancy. Subsequent work by Junk and colleagues[28] indicated that fertilization rates in in vitro fertilization cycles are reduced only if both IgA and IgG antibodies are present together, but no effect was observed when only one of the two isotypes was present. A subsequent study by Mandelbaum and coworkers[29] involved 40 couples in in vitro fertilization cycles in whom antisperm antibodies were present in serum, semen, and follicular fluid. In this study, antibodies to the sperm tail tip did not adversely affect fertilization rates. Head-directed antisperm antibodies did not affect fertilization rates if they were observed in semen or male serum, but head-directed antibodies detected in female serum reduced fertilization rates. A similar detrimental effect was observed when head-directed antibodies were found in follicular fluid.

A detrimental effect of female circulating antisperm antibodies on in vitro fertilization has been shown.[30, 31] This emphasizes the importance of screening for antisperm antibodies in female sera before in vitro fertilization cycles regardless of the indication for in vitro fertilization. Clarke and associates[30] showed higher fertilizations in in vitro fertilization cycles in which the antibody-positive serum was replaced by antibody-negative serum.

The precise mechanism by which antibodies impair sperm-egg interactions is unclear. Presumably the surface antibodies cover or alter important sperm surface proteins. For example, penetration of the zona pellucida requires tight binding between the spermatozoa and the zona surface.[32] The binding is thought to involve specific receptors between the zona surface and specialized sperm-head regions. Blockage of these zona receptors could produce fertilization failure.[33, 34] Sperm surface antibodies may also interfere with fusion of sperm with hamster vitelli,[35, 36] and it is presumed that fusion with the human vitellus might be similarly impaired.

Monoclonal antibodies have been used to help define the molecular mechanisms of immunologic infertility. For example, an IgM monoclonal antibody (H6-3C4) has been produced by fusing mouse myeloma cells with lymphocytes from an infertile female patient. This antibody is one of several responsible for complement-dependent immobilization (Isojima assay). Using this antibody, researchers have found that an internal lactosaminoglycan is a specific site for sperm-immobilizing antibody binding and may be the molecular basis for infertility in women who possess this antibody.[37] Monoclonal antibodies have also been used to characterize the antibodies and antigens that result in sperm agglutination and immobilization[38] as well as those following vasectomy.[39] Riedel and coworkers[40] have looked at the effect of specific monoclonal antisperm antibodies on penetration rates of hamster ova. Monoclonal antibody technology is also used to characterize white blood cell types in semen; certain types of leukocytes are associated with poor semen quality. This relationship is not thought to be based on immunologic phenomena.[41]

DIAGNOSTIC TESTS

There are a wide variety of tests available to detect the presence of antisperm antibodies.[1] Comparisons of these tests continue to comprise significant current research effort. It is important to realize that the various tests provide different information on antisperm antibodies.

Sperm agglutination tests are based on the principle that large, multivalent isotypes, such as IgM or secretory IgA, may be able to cross-link large numbers of sperm. In its simplest form, the agglutination test comprises a mixing of test serum with sperm cells and performing a microscopic evaluation of sperm clumping after 1- to 2-hour incubation at 37°C. The agglutination tests are known by several different names, including the tube-slide agglutination test (Franklin-Dukes), the tray agglutination test (Friberg), and gelatin agglutination test (Kibrick). False-positive results are possible with all of these agglutination techniques because bacteria and nonimmunoglobulin proteins in semen and serum may cause significant sperm agglutination. A variation of these tests is the mixed agglutination reaction, which was designed to detect antibodies directly on the sperm cells (no serum added). In this test, a mixture of human red blood cells with IgG on their surface and test sperm cells are combined with a rabbit anti-IgG. A mixed agglutination of blood cells and sperm cells is indicative of sperm surface IgG. The ensuing agglutination is macroscopic and does not allow for a determination of the proportion of sperm with antibodies or the sperm surface regional specificity.

The *sperm immobilization test* (Isojima) is based on the principle that sperm cells with surface antibodies, in the presence of complement, lose their ability to move. This test may recapitulate a mechanism of immunologic infertility because complement is present in the female reproductive tract and may interfere with the progression of antibody-coated sperm. False-positive results are rare, and this test therefore has high specificity. A disadvantage to the sperm immobilization test is a lack of sensitivity. IgA, which does not fix complement, is not detected. Head-directed antibodies may also go undetected because even in the presence of complement, such antibodies may not impair motility.

Indirect immunofluorescence is another method to detect antibody-bound sperm. A fluorescent label is attached to an antihuman antibody. When this antibody recognizes sperm surface antibodies, fluorescence is observed under fluorescence microscopy. This test is sensitive, as false-negative results are uncommon. The location of the antibody on the sperm surface can also be determined. False-positive results are encountered because the methodology allows internal sperm antigens to be released. Internal sperm antigens are not thought to be related to immunologic infertility. A variation on this idea is the *radiolabeled antiglobulin assay*. Here the antihuman immunoglobulin is labeled to a radioisotope, and the washed sperm suspension is counted for residual radioactivity. False-positive results are possible here, again owing to internal antigens released from dead cells. When this test is applied to motile cells, such as in a swimup preparation, it is highly specific and sensitive. It does not give information on the regional specificity of binding or on the proportion of sperm that are antibody bound.

The *enzyme-linked immunosorbent assay* is a calorimetric assay for antisperm antibodies. An enzyme is linked to an antiglobulin, which recognizes sperm surface antibodies. When the enzyme is placed in the presence of its substrate, a color change develops, which is measured photometrically. The methods involved in this assay may expose internal antigens or damage surface antigens; therefore false-positive and false-negative results may occur.

The *immunobead test* is now widely used and readily available. In this test, polyacrylamide beads are linked to isotype-specific rabbit antihuman antibodies. Immunobeads bind to the sperm surface, where antibodies are found, and under light microscopy, the regional specificity is determined. Immunobeads therefore may be used to indicate the immunoglobulin class and its location on the sperm surface. The beads are used both as a direct test of sperm surface antibodies and as an indirect test of serum antibodies after a passive transfer to donor sperm cells. Passive transfer of antibodies to donor sperm is also possible using follicular fluid, cervical mucus, and seminal plasma. False-positive results are low with this test, but false-negative results may occur in that only motile sperm cells are tested.

Bio-Rad Laboratories, which makes immunobeads, also introduced the SpermCheck Assay, which is now being used in some centers.[42] The SpermCheck assay system comes with immunoglobulin-coated latex beads and positive and negative controls. The kit also contains ready-to-use buffer reagents and is therefore essentially ready to use. The immunoglobulin isotypes are mixed together so the class of immunoglobulin present cannot be determined.

TREATMENT

Treatment for male immunologic infertility is currently suboptimal. The search for a simple, inexpensive method for overcoming the detrimental effects of sperm-surface antibodies has yet to be found. The treatment modalities that have been investigated constitute four broad categories: barrier methods, steroids, in vitro sperm processing techniques, and assisted reproductive technologies.

The use of condoms to prevent female sensitization to sperm antigens has been advocated,[9, 43] but the effectiveness of this therapy has been questioned.[44] The use of intrauterine insemination for women with serum antisperm antibodies has been advocated,[45] although the study was not controlled.

The use of steroids for treating male immunologic infertility is controversial.[46–51] Haas and Manganiello[48] studied 43 men with sperm-surface antibodies in a double-blind, placebo-controlled study of methylprednisolone. The protocol established by the authors did seem to decrease sperm-surface IgG, but sperm-surface IgA and serum IgG antisperm antibodies were not affected. There was no demonstrable improvement in either semen parameters or pregnancy rates with the methylprednisolone regimen.

A beneficial effect of steroid treatment was suggested by Hendry and colleagues[49] in an uncontrolled study. Two different steroid regimens were used in 47 infertile men with serum antisperm antibodies. The authors provided data suggesting improved sperm count, decreased antibody titers, and improved fecundity in steroid-treated men, but the lack of controls makes the data difficult to interpret. A later study by Hendry and colleagues[50] involved 43 subfertile men with serum antibodies in a double-blind, cross-over trial using prednisolone, 20 mg twice daily, on menstrual cycle days 1 through 10 followed by 5 mg on days 11 and 12, for a total of 9 months. The authors reported nine pregnancies in the prednisolone group and two pregnancies in the placebo group. The difference in the two groups was observed only after 6 months of treatment, and the authors suggested that

Immunology of Spermatozoa

some studies may be faulted for short-term treatment protocols.

De Almeida and associates[51] failed to show a beneficial effect of corticosteroid therapy in a small, randomized, double-blind study. Ten infertile men with serum and seminal plasma antibodies were randomized to receive prednisolone or placebo. The treatment protocol had no significant effect on serum antibody levels or semen characteristics. The prednisolone group was seen to have a slight decrease in the seminal antibody titer. Although rare, the devastating complications of steroid use, such as aseptic necrosis of the hip, mandate careful and judicious use.[52]

Conceptually a simple in vitro technique to alter or remove sperm-surface antibodies would offer an attractive treatment option for couples with immunologic infertility. One such processing technique that has been investigated is the use of proteolytic enzymes. Pattinson and coworkers[53] investigated the effects of subtilisin, chymotrypsin, trypsin, and papain. Although some of these agents had a beneficial effect on sperm disagglutination, there was a concomitant impairment of sperm-mucus interaction or zona-free hamster egg penetration.[54] Trypsin seemed to improve penetration of zona-free hamster eggs but did not improve sperm-mucus interaction. Bronson and associates[55] showed that an IgA protease can be used to improve in vitro sperm–cervical mucus penetrating ability.

In vitro immunoabsorption techniques to select antibody-free motile sperm have been investigated.[56, 57] Kiser and associates[57] attempted to allow sperm to swim out of an immunobead mixture, but the overlying buffer had few sperm. Magnetic isolation of sperm carrying surface antibodies resulted in a population of sperm with markedly diminished motility. Passage of sperm through a column of dextran beads seemed to provide the best population of motile sperm with improved function as measured by the sperm penetration assay. Magnetic separation techniques were also used by Foresta and colleagues[58] with some in vitro success. Magnetic microspheres were used to separate sperm cells with surface antibodies from sperm without antibodies. The technique seemed to produce a population of sperm with diminished surface antibody activity. The authors did not apply this technique clinically and did not entertain the possibility that the magnetic technique was physically removing surface antibody molecules.

The use of a discontinuous Percoll gradient has been described[59] in an uncontrolled study. The authors obtained semen samples from patients with known sperm-surface antibodies and processed the sperm through a discontinuous Percoll gradient. The resulting sperm population had a reduced level of immunobead binding.

Elder and coworkers[60] provided data that suggested an improved fertilization and conception rate when antibody-positive semen was collected into a small volume of medium containing 50% serum. The study was retrospective and was not controlled. It was presumed that the serum inhibited the binding of antibodies to the sperm surface.

We have shown that immunobeads (Bio-Rad, Richmond, CA) can be used to lower the proportion of sperm bound with antisperm antibodies.[61] Our data show that coincubation of immunobeads with sperm results in a decrease in the number of sperm bound to immunobeads. The decreased binding results from a transference, at least part, of the anti-

sperm antibody from the sperm to the immunobead.[62] These data may provide the basis for a new sperm-processing technique that, coupled with intrauterine insemination, could offer a new treatment option for male immunologic infertility.

In vitro fertilization has been used successfully in couples with male immunologic infertility with an average pregnancy rate of 14%.[63] Data suggest that embryo cleavage seems to progress normally if fertilization occurs using sperm with surface antibodies.[28, 64] Studies by Clarke and associates[26] do not demonstrate that fertilization impairment is related to the location of the antisperm antibodies on the sperm surface, as one might predict. Microinjection technology may offer hope in the future for couples who fail in vitro fertilization therapy.[65]

FUTURE DIRECTIONS

The complexities of the immune system are only beginning to be defined, and the interactions of the component parts are as intricate as any biologic systems known. The characterization of the immunologic response to sperm cells as well as the consequences and treatment of that response will remain a central focus of infertility research for years to come. The future may bring innovative application of immunologic principles to the treatment of infertility. It would be reasonable to speculate that selected surface antibodies may enhance various aspects of sperm function. At least one report has shown improved penetration of zona-free hamster eggs by antibody-bound sperm compared with antibody-free sperm.[66] Application of specific monoclonal antibodies may someday provide treatment for certain types of male infertility. In the future, manipulation of the immune system may allow for sophisticated molecular level therapeutics that may benefit patients with a wide range of infertility diagnoses.

1. Bronson R, Cooper G, Rosenfeld D. Sperm antibodies: their role in infertility. Fertil Steril 1984;42:171.
2. Hellstrom WR, Overstreet JW, Samuels SJ, Lewis EL. The relationship of circulating antisperm antibodies to sperm surface antibodies in infertile men. J Urol 1988;140:1039–1044.
3. Clarke GN. Immunoglobulin class and regional specificity of antispermatozoal autoantibodies blocking cervical mucus penetration by human spermatozoa. Am J Reprod Immunol Microbiol 1988;16:135–138.
4. Menge AC, Beitner O. Interrelationships among semen characteristics, antisperm antibodies, and cervical mucus penetration assays in infertile human couples. Fertil Steril 1989;51:486–492.
5. Eggert-Kruse W, Christmann M, Gerhard I, et al. Circulating antisperm antibodies and fertility prognosis: a prospective study. Human Reprod 1989;4:513–520.
6. Alexander NJ, Anderson DJ. Immunology of semen. Fertil Steril 1987;47:192–205.
7. Gilula NB, Fawcett DW, Aoki A. The Sertoli cell occluding junctions and gap junctions in mature and developing mammalian testis. Dev Biol 1976;50:142.
8. Overstreet JW. Human sperm function: acquisition in the male and expression in the female. In: Santen RJ, Swerdloff RW, editors. Male Reproductive Function. New York: Marcel Dekker, 1986;29–47.
9. Franklin RR, Dukes DC. Antispermatozoal antibody and unexplained infertility. Am J Obstet Gynecol 1964;89:6.
10. Haas GG. Antibody-mediated causes of male infertility. Urol Clin North Am 1987;14:539.
11. Haas GG. Immunologic male infertility. Infert Reprod Med Clin North Am 1992;3:413.

12. El-Demiry MIM, Hargreave TB, Busuttil A, et al. Lymphocyte subpopulations in the male genital tract. Br J Urol 1985;47:769.

13. Tung KSK, Yule TD, Mahi-Brown CA, et al. Distribution of histopathology and Ia positive cells in actively induced and passively transferred experimental autoimmune orchitis. J Immunol 1987;138:762.

14. Witkin SS. Mechanisms of active suppression of the immune response to spermatozoa. Am J Reprod Immunol Microbiol 1988;17:61.

15. Hurtenback U, Shearer GM. Germ cell-induced immune suppression in mice. Effect of inoculation of syngeneic spermatozoa on cell-mediated immune responses. J Exp Med 1982;155:1719.

16. Hurtenback U, Morgenstern F, Bennett D. Induction of tolerance in vitro by autologous murine testicular cells. J Exp Med 1980;151:827.

17. Shulman S, Zappi E, Ahmed U, et al. Immunologic consequences of vasectomy. Contraception 1972;5:269.

18. Fuchs EF, Alexander NJ. Immunologic considerations before and after vasovasostomy. Fertil Steril 1983;40:497.

19. Hellstrom WJG, Overstreet JW, Samuels SJ, Lewis EL. The relationship of circulating antisperm antibodies to sperm surface antibodies in infertile men. J Urol 1988;140:1039–1044.

20. Alexander NJ. Antibody levels and immunologic infertility. In: Isojima S, Billington WE, editors. Reproductive Immunology 1983. Amsterdam: Elsevier Science Publishers, 1983:207–212.

21. Silber SJ. The relationship of abnormal semen parameters to pregnancy outcome. In: Seibel MM, editor. Infertility: A Comprehensive Text. Norwalk, CT: Appleton & Lange, 1990:149–155.

22. Schumacher GFB. Immunology of spermatozoa and cervical mucus. Human Reprod 1988;3:289.

23. Cohen J, Werrett DJ. Antibodies and sperm survival in the female tract of the mouse and rabbit. J Reprod Fertil 1975;42:301.

24. Price RJ, Boettcher B. The presence of complement in human cervical mucus and its possible relevance to infertility in women with complement-dependent sperm-immobilizing antibodies. Fertil Steril 1979;32:61.

25. Bronson RA, Cooper GW, Phillips DM. Effects of anti-sperm antibodies on human sperm ultrastructure and function. Human Reprod 1989;4:653–657.

26. Clarke GN, Lopata A, McBain JC, et al. Effect of sperm antibodies in males on human in vitro fertilization (IVF). Am J Reprod Immunol Microbiol 1985;8:62–66.

27. Rumke P. The origin of immunoglobulins in semen. Clin Exp Immunol 1974;17:287.

28. Junk SM, Matson PL, Yovich JM, et al. The fertilization of human oocytes by spermatozoa from men with antispermatozoal antibodies in semen. J In Vitro Fert Embryo Transfer 1986;3:350–352.

29. Mandelbaum SL, Diamond MP, DeCherney AH. Relationship of antisperm antibodies to oocyte fertilization in in vitro fertilization-embryo transfer. Fertil Steril 1987;47:644.

30. Clarke GN, Lopata A, Johnston WIH. Effect of sperm antibodies in females on human in vitro fertilization. Fertil Steril 1986;46:435.

31. Mandelbaum SL, Diamond MP, DeCherney AH. Relationship of antibodies to sperm head to etiology of infertility in patients undergoing in vitro fertilization/embryo transfer. Am J Reprod Immunol 1989;19:3.

32. Bleil JD, Wasserman PM. Sperm-egg interactions in the mouse: sequence of events and induction of the acrosome reaction by a zona pellucida glycoprotein. Dev Biol 1983;95:317.

33. Bronson RA, Cooper GW, Rosenfeld DL. Sperm-specific isoantibodies and autoantibodies inhibit the binding of human sperm to the human zona pellucida. Fertil Steril 1982;38:724.

34. Tsukui S, Noda Y, Yano J, et al. Inhibition of sperm penetration through human zona pellucida by antisperm antibodies. Fertil Steril 1986;46:92.

35. Dor J, Rudak E, Aitken RJ. Antisperm antibodies: their effect on the process of fertilization studies in vitro. Fertil Steril 1981;35:535.

36. Haas GG, Sokoloski JE, Wolf DP. The interfering effect of human IgG antisperm antibodies on human sperm penetration of zona-free hamster eggs. Am J Reprod Immunol 1980;1:40.

37. Gill TJ. Human antisperm antibodies. Immunol Today 1989;10:91.

38. Batova I, Kameda K, Hasegawa A, et al. Monoclonal antibody recognizing an apparent peptide epitope of human seminal plasma glycoprotein and exhibiting sperm immobilizing activity. J Reprod Immunol 1990;17:1–16.

39. Ben KL, Hamilton MS, Alexander NJ. Vasectomy-inducted autoimmunity: monoclonal antibodies affect sperm function and in vitro fertilization. J Reprod Immunol 1988;13:73–84.

40. Riedel HH, Wellnitz K, Lehmann-Willenbrock E. Effect of monoclonal antisperm antibodies on the penetration rates of human spermatozoa in zona pellucida-free hamster oocytes. J Reprod Med 1990;35:128–132.

41. Wolff H, Politch JA, Martinez A, et al. Leukocytospermia is associated with poor semen quality. Fertil Steril 1990;53:528.

42. McClure RD, Tom RA, Watkins M, Murthy S. SpermCheck: a simplified screening assay for immunological infertility. Fertil Steril 1989;52:650.

43. Haas GG. Immunologic infertility. Obstet Gynecol Clin North Am 1987;14:1069.

44. Isojima S, Li TS, Ashitaka Y. Immunologic analysis of sperm immobilizing factor found in sera of women with unexplained infertility. Am J Obstet Gynecol 1968;101:677.

45. Margalloth EJ, Sauter E, Bronson RA, et al. Intrauterine insemination as treatment for antisperm antibodies in the female. Fertil Steril 1988;50:441.

46. Shulman JF, Shulman S. Methylprednisolone treatment of immunologic infertility in the male. Fertil Steril 1982;38:591.

47. Hendry WF, Stedronska J, Parslow J, et al. The results of intermittent high dose steroid therapy for male infertility due to antisperm antibodies. Fertil Steril 1981;36:351.

48. Haas GG Jr, Manganiello P. A double-blind, placebo-controlled study of the use of methlyprednisolone in infertile men with sperm-associated immunoglobulins. Fertil Steril 1987;47:295–301.

49. Hendry WF, Stedronski J, Hughes L, et al. Steroid treatment of male subfertility caused by antisperm antibodies. Lancet 1979;2:498–501.

50. Hendry WF, Hughes I, Scammell G, et al. Comparison of prednisolone and placebo in subfertile men with antibodies to spermatozoa. Lancet 1990;335:85.

51. De Almeida M, Feneux D, Rigand C, Jouannet P. Steroid therapy for male infertility associated with antisperm antibodies. Results of a small randomized clinical trial. Int J Androl 1985;8:111.

52. Hendry WF. Bilateral aseptic necrosis of the femoral heads following intermittent high dose steroid therapy. Fertil Steril 1982;38:120.

53. Pattinson HA, Mortimer D, Curtis EF, et al. Treatment of spermagglutination with proteolytic enzymes. I. Sperm motility, vitality, longevity and successful disagglutination. Human Reprod 1990;5:167.

54. Pattinson HA, Mortimer D, Taylor PJ. Treatment of spermagglutination with proteolytic enzymes. II. Sperm function after enzymatic disagglutination. Human Reprod 1990;5:174.

55. Bronson RA, Cooper GW, Rosenfeld DL, et al. The effect of an IgA$_1$ protease on immunoglobulins bound to the sperm surface and sperm cervical mucus penetrating ability. Fertil Steril 1987;47:985.

56. Bronson RA, Cooper GW, Rosenfeld D. Use of freeze-thawed sonicated human sperm as an in vitro immunoabsorbent. Am J Reprod Immunol 1982;2:162.

57. Kiser GC, Alexander NJ, Fuchs EF, Fulgham DL. In vitro immune absorption of antisperm antibodies with immunobead-rise, immunomagnetic, and immunocolumn separation techniques. Fertil Steril 1987;47:466.

58. Foresta C, Varotto A, Caretto A. Immunomagnetic method to select human sperm without sperm surface-bound autoantibodies in male autoimmune infertility. Arch Androl 1990;24:221.

59. Grundy CE, Robinson J, Gordon AG, Hay DM. Selection of an antibody-free population of spermatozoa from semen samples of men suffering from immunological infertility. Human Reprod 1991;6:593.

60. Elder KT, Wick KL, Edwards RG. Seminal plasma anti-sperm antibodies and IVF: the effect of semen sample collection into 50% serum. Human Reprod 1990;5:179–184.

61. Gould JE, Brazil CK, Overstreet JW. Sperm-immunobead binding decreases with in-vitro incubation. Fertil Steril 1994;62:167–171.

62. Gould JE, Ordorica RC. Removal of sperm surface antibodies using immunobeads. Abstract presented at the American Fertility Society 48th Annual Meeting, New Orleans, 1992.

63. Haas GG. Male infertility and immunity. In: Lipshultz LI, Howards SS, editors. Infertility in the Male. St. Louis: Mosby-Year Book, 1991:287–290.

64. Clarke GN, Elliott PJ, Smaila C. Detection of sperm antibodies in semen using the immunobead test: a survey of 813 consecutive patients. Am J Reprod Immunol Microbiol 1985;7:118–123.

65. Lamb DJ, Stockton JD, Lipshultz LI. New roads to fertility: manipulation of gametes provides the possibility of fertilization for more infertile couples. Contemp Urol 1991;3:32.

66. Bronson R, Cooper G, Rosenfeld D. Ability of antibody-bound sperm to penetate zona-free hamster ova in vitro. Fertil Steril 1981;36:778–783.

CHAPTER 44

Sexual and Ejaculatory Dysfunction as a Cause of Male Infertility

SAMUEL T. THOMPSON,
STANTON C. HONIG, and
LARRY I. LIPSHULTZ

Sexual dysfunction, sometimes overlooked as a cause of male infertility, is the sole cause of infertility in 5% of couples.[1, 2] Sexual dysfunction includes impotence, premature ejaculation, retrograde ejaculation, lack of ejaculation, failure of intromission, unfavorable timing of intercourse, too-frequent masturbation, and aberrant sexual behavior. Although unfavorable timing of intercourse was reported as the most frequent cause of male infertility in one of the largest studies ever published, impotence was the cause in 2.1% of couples.

Impotence in the infertile couple may be situational, psychogenic, or organic. Situationally impotent men have satisfactory spontaneous intercourse but are unable to maintain an erection under the stressful circumstances of timed coitus necessary to initiate a pregnancy. Psychogenically impotent men achieve nocturnal erections and are able to masturbate to obtain a semen sample but cannot achieve adequate erections for intercourse. Psychogenic impotence may represent an advanced, continuing form of situational impotence. Hormonal alterations, diabetes mellitus, and spinal cord injuries (SCIs) are among the organic causes of impotence in men in the fertility age group. This chapter discusses the evaluation and treatment of men with ejaculatory dysfunction as well as psychogenic and organic impotence.

IMPOTENCE

Psychogenic Impotence

Attempting to initiate a pregnancy may create psychosexual conflict and stress in a couple's relationship through the demands of timed intercourse; masturbation to produce multiple semen samples for analysis; and complicated, costly, and invasive testing. This stress can lead to tension, guilt, anxiety,

depression, anger, feelings of inferiority or uselessness, and often sexual dysfunction in the infertile couple.[3–5]

Physicians may not recognize sexual dysfunction if they do not obtain a detailed sexual history from both partners. Because couples seldom volunteer information about their sexual inadequacies, sympathetic questioning often is required to elicit it. Physicians can rule out organic impotence using the medical history, physical examination, and objective evidence of nocturnal erections, such as Rigiscan and snap-gauge testing.

Behavior-oriented sex therapy is an effective treatment for psychogenic impotence. The goals of sex therapy are to decrease the performance anxiety that inhibits men from attaining an erection and to promote an adequate level of stimulation by encouraging noncoital sexual activity. Sensate focus exercises decrease anxiety and guilt and allow for a slow, progressive return of potency by emphasizing the couple's mutual enjoyment of noncoital activity.[6] Reported success rates range from 35% to 85%.[7] Some men receiving medical or surgical treatment for organic impotence also benefit, both before and after treatment, from sex therapy.

Organic Impotence

HORMONAL ALTERATIONS

Hormonal alterations are caused by abnormalities of hypothalamic-pituitary function, primary gonadal abnormalities, and defective androgen synthesis or action. The causes, signs, and symptoms of hypothalamic-pituitary dysfunction and primary gonadal dysfunction are detailed in Tables 44–1 and 44–2.

Treatment of *hypothalamic-pituitary dysfunction* depends on the cause. The congenital hypogonadotropic syndromes, such as Prader-Willi, are usually recognized at birth and treated

TABLE 44–1. Abnormalities of Hypothalamic-Pituitary Function

Congenital Types

Isolated gonadotropin (FSH, LH) deficiency or Kallmann's syndrome
  Absence of GnRH causes lack of LH and FSH secretion; otherwise, anterior pituitary function is intact. Serum FSH and LH levels are low
  Patients present with microphallus, cryptorchidism, or delay in sexual maturation
Isolated LH deficiency or fertile eunuch
  Patients present with eunuchoid proportions, various degrees of virilization, and gynecomastia. Serum LH and testosterone levels are low normal. FSH levels are normal
Congenital hypogonadotropic syndromes
  All have multiple associated somatic findings
  Include Prader-Willi, Laurence-Moon-Biedl, Alstrom's, and familial cerebellar syndromes
Idiopathic prepubertal panhypopituitarism
  Deficiency of all pituitary hormones

Acquired Types

Pituitary insufficiency secondary to tumors, infarction, iatrogenic damage (surgery, radiation), or infiltrative or granulomatous processes
  Before puberty, presents with growth retardation and adrenal and thyroid insufficiency
  After puberty, presents with *decreased libido, impotence,* and *infertility,* and in advanced cases may present with headache, visual field abnormalities, and deficiency of thyroid and adrenal hormones.
Elevated exogenous and endogenous hormones (androgens, estrogens, glucocorticoids, thyroid, and growth hormones) suppress endogenous pituitary gonadotropins and lead to secondary testicular failure
Hyperprolactinemia secondary to pituitary adenoma, medications, or idiopathic causes
  Patients present with loss of *libido, impotence,* galactorrhea, gynecomastia, and *infertility* with elevated prolactin and low testosterone levels
Hemochromatosis presents with testicular dysfunction and may be related to iron deposition in the pituitary or the testicle

FSH, Follicle-stimulating hormone; LH; luteinizing hormone; GnRH, gonadotropin-releasing hormone.

with hormone replacement therapy before they affect fertility. In disorders such as Kallmann's syndrome, in which endogenous gonadotropin-releasing hormone (GnRH) is lacking and the pituitary is normal, pulsatile administration of exogenous GnRH stimulates the production of follicle-stimulating hormone (FSH) and luteinizing hormone (LH). In cases of impaired pituitary function secondary to tumor, damage to the pituitary, or the presence of excessive amounts of end-organ hormones that cause negative feedback, such as anabolic steroids, exogenous LH and FSH preparations are required to restore libido, fertility, and potency. Treatment of hyperprolactinemia is directed toward the etiologic process, such as a pituitary adenoma or decreased dopamine neurotransmitter activity.

In a patient newly diagnosed with hypogonadotropic hypogonadism, testosterone is usually administered to achieve virilization quickly. Although testosterone treatment should not be used to stimulate spermatogenesis in these patients, its use does not reduce the chance of subsequently inducing spermatogenesis by GnRH or human chorionic gonadotropin (hCG)/human menopausal gonadotropin (hMG) treatment. For patients with pituitary insufficiency, gonadotropin replacement is achieved with injections of hCG and hMG. Therapy is initiated with hCG, 1500 to 2500 IU twice a week for 4 to 8 weeks to stimulate Leydig cell function. Thereafter, hMG, 37.5 to 150 IU three times a week, is added. Therapy is continued until sperm appear in the ejaculate and pregnancy is attained.

In patients with Kallmann's syndrome or idiopathic hypogonadotropic hypogonadism, either GnRH or hCG/hMG treatment may be used. GnRH is administered subcutaneously in a pulsatile fashion using portable infusion pumps. The initial dose is 5 μg/pulse with pulse intervals of 120 minutes. The pulse dose may be increased to 20 μg according to serum levels of LH, FSH, and testosterone. Treatment is continued until the appearance of sperm and occurrence of pregnancy. At least 1 year is needed for an adequate trial of treatment.[8]

Normal testis size and sperm counts are not always achieved using GnRH and hCG/hMG treatment regimens.[9–11] Even the subnormal numbers of sperm produced, however, are often sufficient to initiate pregnancies. Gonadotropin administration is effective for the induction of spermatogenesis and in one study resulted in a pregnancy rate of 85%.[12] Pulsatile GnRH therapy and hCG/hMG are comparably effective because either therapy can be used initially in patients with hypogonadotropic hypogonadism or as an alternative if the response to one treatment regimen is inadequate.

Hyperprolactinemia is accompanied frequently by hypogonadism and less frequently by galactorrhea. The only clue to the presence of hyperprolactinemia may be reduced libido or impotence. Bromocriptine has been favored for treatment of idiopathic hyperprolactinemia or when pituitary microadenomas are the cause. If a macroadenoma is detected on computed tomography (CT) scan or magnetic resonance imaging (MRI), surgical ablation and radiation treatment are also options depending on the size of the lesion.

Severe, irreversible testicular failure is frequently secon-

TABLE 44–2. Primary Gonadal Abnormalities

Chromosomal abnormalities
  Klinefelter's syndrome (classically XXY) presents with decreased androgenicity; gynecomastia; small, firm testes; elevated FSH and LH, low-normal testosterone, elevated TeBG, low free testosterone, and elevated estrogen levels; and azoospermia
  XX disorder is a variant of Klinefelter's syndrome similar in presentation but with the addition of hypospadias and short stature
  Noonan's syndrome is the male counterpart of Turner's syndrome and has a similar presentation (short stature, webbed neck, low-set ears, cubitus valgus, ocular abnormalities, and cardiovascular abnormalities)
  Laboratory abnormalities include decreased testicular function and elevated serum FSH and LH levels
Bilateral anorchia (vanishing testes syndrome) is thought to be caused by intrauterine testicular torsion or trauma
  Patients present with sexual immaturity, eunuchoid proportions, and impalpable testes
  Laboratory studies include elevated FSH and LH and low testosterone levels, and normal karyotype
Gonadotoxins include chemotherapeutic agents, radiation, alcohol, cimetidine, ketoconazole, spironolactone, cyproterone, marijuana, heroin, methadone, and occupational exposure to lead and some pesticides (dibromochloropropane)
Gonadal injury such as orchitis, trauma, and iatrogenic injury
Systemic diseases
  Uremic patients present with decreased libido, impotence, gynecomastia, and altered spermatogenesis
  Hepatic cirrhosis patients have impotence, testicular atrophy, and gynecomastia with mildly elevated LH and FSH as well as low testosterone levels
  Sickle cell disease patients have delayed sexual maturity, impaired skeletal growth, and reduced testicular size suggestive of hypogonadism, but hormonal evaluation can be variable

FSH, Follicle-stimulating hormone; LH; luteinizing hormone; TeBG, testosterone-estradiol–binding globulin.

dary to a chromosomal or congenital cause of *primary hypogonadism* (see Table 44–2). Severe bilateral testicular trauma or infection can also permanently injure the testicles. Depending on the extent of testicular damage, infertility can result, and treatment of reduced libido with androgen replacement is indicated.

The goal of androgen replacement in impotence secondary to hypogonadism is the maintenance of serum testosterone in the physiologic range. Oral testosterone preparations should not be used because they have poor and erratic absorption rates and present the potential for hepatotoxicity.[13] The long-acting parenteral esters, testosterone cypionate and enanthate, are the drugs of choice for replacement therapy in male hypogonadism. The dosage regimen for hypogonadal men is 150 to 200 mg of testosterone cypionate or testosterone enanthate intramuscularly every 2 weeks.[14] Self-reported measures of libido, nocturnal erections, and potency increased with treatment of hypogonadal men,[15, 16] and studies using objective measures, such as those of nocturnal penile tumescence, have shown an increase in sleep-related erections.[17] A transdermal testosterone delivery system in which patches containing 10 or 15 mg of testosterone are applied to the scrotum daily is under study. Of the few men treated, many have had a prompt increase in serum testosterone and dihydrotestosterone levels as well as improvement in libido and erections.[18-20] Larger, long-term studies are needed for this promising method of treatment.

Side effects of parenteral testosterone therapy are rare but may include breast tenderness and gynecomastia secondary to peripheral aromatization of testosterone to estradiol and slight increases in erythrocyte and leukocyte concentrations as a result of the stimulation of erythropoietin. Weight gain, acne, and increased oiliness of the skin are also reported.[14] Although testosterone therapy does not cause prostate cancer, this malignancy is androgen dependent, and consequently men with prostate cancer are not candidates for testosterone therapy. In addition, men older than 40 years of age who are receiving testosterone therapy should undergo yearly digital rectal examination, prostate-specific antigen measurement, and transrectal ultrasonography.

Hypogonadism secondary to gonadal toxins is frequently reversible with discontinuation of the harmful agent. Although these agents (see Table 44–2) disrupt spermatogenesis, they rarely affect Leydig cell function to such a degree that impotence or reduced libido becomes clinically manifested.

Hypogonadism secondary to systemic illness probably has a multifactorial origin. Impotence, decreased libido, and altered spermatogenesis associated with uremia have been treated with successful renal transplantation.[14] Hypogonadism secondary to hepatic cirrhosis may be treated with testosterone replacement. Patients with sickle cell disease sometimes have hypogonadism and erectile dysfunction but are candidates for androgen replacement.

Congenital defects in *androgen synthesis* are rare and present at birth with ambiguous genitalia. *Androgen resistance* syndromes are disorders in which 46 XY males with bilateral testes fail to develop as phenotypically normal men. Complete discussion of these syndromes is beyond the scope of this chapter, but patients with these disorders frequently have undescended testicles and are sterile.

DIABETES MELLITUS

Forty percent to 60% of diabetic patients suffer from erectile dysfunction.[21] They also may have decreased sperm motility and density, abnormal morphology, and generally increased seminal plasma abnormalities,[22] although the exact mechanism is unknown. A study by Dinulovic and Radonjic[23] demonstrated no significant differences in serum FSH, LH, total testosterone, estradiol, and dihydroepiandrosterone concentrations in diabetic patients with and without impotence. Average prolactin concentrations, however, were significantly increased in a majority of patients with decreased libido, and the mean free testosterone levels were significantly decreased in a majority of patients with organic causes of erectile dysfunction.[23] Despite the hormonal alterations found in diabetics with erectile dysfunction, somatic and autonomic neuropathy have been implicated as the main causative factors in diabetic impotence.[24] Treatment of these patients has focused on injection of vasoactive agents because this therapy is particularly effective in patients with neuropathic causes of impotence.

SPINAL CORD DISORDERS

SCIs and multiple sclerosis frequently occur in men of the reproductive age group, and the disease processes may affect erectile function. Erections in patients with SCIs can be psychogenic or reflexogenic. Psychogenic erections are independent of cutaneous stimulation and are initiated by imagination, visual simulation, and perception of a potential sexual situation and maintained by the absence of inhibitory factors, such as stress, anxiety, depression, relationship conflicts, and cognitive interferences. Psychogenic erections are possible only in SCI patients with a lower motor neuron or spinal lesion below T12. Approximately 26% of patients with complete lower motor neuron lesions have psychogenic erections, and coitus is successful in 65% to 70% of this group.[25] Reflexogenic erections occur by stimulation of the genitalia, pelvic viscera, or surrounding skin below the level of the spinal lesion. A suprasacral SCI unmasks the spinal reflex mechanism whereby tactile stimulation produces an erection. Ninety-three percent of patients with complete upper motor neuron lesions have reflexogenic erections, and approximately 72% of this group can complete coitus successfully.[25] Patients with complete thoracic or cervical spinal cord lesions cannot achieve psychogenic erections. Multiple sclerosis is associated with erectile dysfunction in 26% to 75% of patients and affects many young men interested in achieving fertility. The cause of erectile dysfunction is thought to be secondary to the demyelinating process of this disease.

Pharmacologic injection therapy is the most effective treatment of erectile dysfunction in patients with spinal cord diseases. Virag and associates[26] noted a 93% success rate in patients with neurogenic impotence. The use of penile prostheses in SCI patients has demonstrated a higher erosion and infection rate compared with its use in those with other causes of erectile dysfunction.[27]

TREATMENT OF ORGANIC IMPOTENCE

Treatments of organic causes of impotence include the use of vacuum erection devices, pharmacologic injection therapy, implantation of penile prostheses, and, infrequently, vascular surgery of the penis.

Vacuum Erection Devices. Vacuum erection devices are external appliances with three components: a vacuum chamber that fits over the penis and forms an airtight seal against the skin of the pubis, a pump that creates negative pressure within the chamber, and a constrictor or tension band that slips off the base of the vacuum chamber and traps the blood in the engorged penis to maintain an erection-like state. Because the constrictor band remains on the penis during intercourse and prevents antegrade ejaculation, these devices are not recommended for patients attempting to initiate a pregnancy.

Pharmacologic Injection Therapy. Over the last decade, self-administered intracavernosal injection of vasoactive agents has been an important advance in therapy for impotence. The vasoactive agents have been selected either to relax the corporeal smooth muscle directly or to block adrenergic tone. Combining several vasoactive agents in a single injection increases the response of the corporeal smooth muscle and minimizes the side effects of the individual agents by reducing the dose of each agent. The most commonly used agents are papaverine and prostaglandin E_1; direct smooth muscle relaxants; and phentolamine, an α-blocking agent. These agents are commonly combined in dosages such as that described by Bennett and colleagues[28] (Table 44–3). The therapeutic goal of pharmacologic injection therapy is to create an erection rigid enough to achieve vaginal penetration and complete satisfactory intercourse.

The first step in a pharmacologic injection program is for the patients to understand and sign a detailed informed consent that explains the known complications of therapy and possible long-term side effects. Some patients should not be offered this therapy. Among them are men with poor manual dexterity or poor visual acuity or those in whom a transient hypotensive episode might have a deleterious effect, such as patients with a history of cardiovascular disease or transient ischemic attacks. In addition, patients with psychiatric disease or potential for abuse or misuse of this form of therapy should be excluded from treatment.

Next the proper dose of the vasoactive agent must be determined. Patients are injected initially with low doses, which are increased incrementally. Dosages determined in the physician's office are commonly decreased by the patient at home because he is in a sexually stimulating environment.

Patients must be instructed in the proper technique for

TABLE 44–4. Penile Prosthesis

Malleable Devices

Small-Carrion: Semirigid, silicone only (Mentor Corporation, Goleta, CA)
AMS600: Semirigid, stainless steel wire core (American Medical Systems, Minneapolis, MN)
Mentor: Semirigid, silver wire core (Mentor Corporation, Goleta, CA)
Duraphase II: Semirigid (Dacomed Corporation, Minneapolis, MN)

Inflatable Devices

Two-Piece Devices—Combined Pump, Reservoir, and Cylinders: GFS Mark II (Mentor Corporation, Goleta, CA)
Three-Piece Devices—Pump, Reservoir, and Cylinders:
  AMS 700 (American Medical Systems, Minneapolis, MN)
  AMS Ultrex (American Medical Systems, Minneapolis, MN)
  Mentor Alpha 1 (Mentor Corporation, Goleta, CA)
Self-Contained—Cylinders, Pump, and Reservoir as One Piece: Dynaflex (American Medical Systems, Minneapolis, MN)

self-injection. They are taught to draw up the solution and to inject it into the corpora with a 27- to 30-gauge needle and a 1-mL insulin syringe using sterile technique. The patients must also compress the injection site for 3 minutes after injection to prevent the formation of a hematoma. Patients should use no more than two to three injections per week and should alternate sides of the penis for injection.

It is important that patients are aware of potential side effects of treatment, the two most important of which are prolonged erection and localized fibrotic changes of the corpora cavernosum. Priapism is seen in 2.3% to 15% of patients during the dose determination phase[29] but occurs in fewer than 1% of patients performing self-injection. Patients need to know that if their erection lasts more than 4 hours, they must call their physician and undergo intracavernosal injection of a reversal agent. Painless fibrotic nodules of the penis can lead to penile curvature, and their occurrence has been reported in 1% to 60% of patients.[30, 31] Systemic side effects are rare but include vasovagal episodes and elevation of liver function tests.

Penile Prosthesis. The purpose of the penile prosthesis is to provide penile rigidity sufficient for intercourse. The various malleable and inflatable prostheses that are available are listed in Table 44–4. Penile implants should be considered only if the less invasive treatments are not appropriate or if patients do not respond to these treatments. Success of the surgery partially depends on appropriate counseling of both patients and their partners. Patients should be told that an inflatable prosthesis is a mechanical device that has a finite life span and will eventually wear out if used extensively. They should be assured that if a mechanical problem develops, a new prosthesis or prosthetic component can be implanted. Implantation of a prosthesis does not affect the patient's ability to have an orgasm and ejaculate, and it does not increase the length of the penis nor improve a deteriorating marital relationship.

Patients undergoing prosthesis implantation should be informed of the potential complications as well as their frequencies and sequelae. The risk of infection in one large series was 2.7%,[32] with increased rates in poorly controlled diabetics. The reoperative rate for penile prosthetic surgery has been reported to be 14% to 44%,[33] with a decreased rate in newer series.[34] More than 90% of patients report satisfaction after penile prosthesis surgery.[35]

Evaluation of individual penile prostheses and discussion

TABLE 44–3. Combination of Pharmacologic Erection-Inducing Agents

Components	Dosage
Papaverine	75 mg
Phentolamine	2.5 mg
Prostaglandin E_1	2.5 μg
Total Volume	4.25 mL

Standard dose is 0.25 mL, which contains 4.4 mg papaverine, 0.15 phentolamine, and 1.5 μg prostaglandin E_1

From Bennett AH, Carpenter AJ, Barada JH. An improved drug combination for a pharmacologic erection program. J Urol 1991; 146:1564–1565. © American Urological Association, Inc., 1991.

of the various surgical techniques are beyond the scope of this chapter but have been reviewed by Goldstein and Krane.[36]

Vascular Surgery. Vascular surgery for the treatment of impotence consists of procedures for arterial revascularization and procedures for correcting corporeal veno-occlusive dysfunction. Because these procedures are indicated for a select group of impotent men, patient selection is important.

Microsurgical arterial revascularization is used to bypass an obstruction of the arterial inflow to the penis. Young men with discrete lesions in the pudendal artery, common penile artery, or both resulting from pelvic or perineal trauma have the highest success rates for this procedure. Older men with diffuse atherosclerotic disease of the hypogastric arterial system have a poor success rate and should be excluded from this operation. The revascularization procedure described by Goldstein and Krane[36] uses the epigastric artery anastomosed end-to-side or end-to-end to the dorsal artery, the dorsal vein, or the cavernosal artery of the penis or a saphenous vein bypass to the dorsal artery. The success rate of this procedure is 31% to 80%.[36] Complications include minor loss of sensation, loss of erectile length, and rarely glans hypervascularization.[37]

Patients with veno-occlusive dysfunction can be reliably identified with dynamic infusion cavernosometry and cavernosography. The underlying cause of the veno-occlusive dysfunction remains unclear, but as the role of the cavernosal smooth muscle in producing veno-occlusion becomes more apparent,[38] the efficacy of ligating penile veins to correct the veno-occlusive dysfunction comes into question. Patients with veno-occlusive dysfunction have been treated with crural plication, ligation of the deep dorsal vein of the penis, ligation of the cavernosal veins, spongiolysis, or combinations of these. Short-term success rates of 28% to 76% have been reported.[36] Complications of these procedures have included decreased penile sensation and shortened penile length.[37] More recent long-term follow-up has revealed a disappointing 24% sustained potency rate if vein ligation was the only treatment for impotence. Vein ligation for the treatment of impotence apparently is more successful in a subgroup of men who have site-specific venous leak secondary to trauma.[39]

Summary

Impotence is often an unsuspected cause of male infertility because of the patient's unwillingness to volunteer information and the physician's failure to cover this important part of the infertile couple's history. Erectile dysfunction is often caused by psychogenic factors, such as the stress of an extensive infertility evaluation. Organic factors, such as hormonal alterations, diabetes, and spinal cord disorders, can produce impotence in young men that interferes with fertility. Behavior-oriented sexual therapy, hormonal treatment, pharmacologic injection therapy, and implantation of a penile prosthesis are highly successful forms of treatment for erectile dysfunction of differing causes. Surgical repair of the vascular system of the penis is also successful in a select subgroup of patients. Research is underway to address the causes of impotence at the molecular level and devise new treatment strategies.

EJACULATORY DYSFUNCTION

Patients with ejaculatory dysfunction are a small but important subset of infertile men. Basic and clinical research with these unique patients has resulted in a greater understanding of the pathophysiology of ejaculatory dysfunction and improved treatment outcomes.

Anatomy and Physiology of Seminal Emission and Ejaculation

The anatomy and physiology of the dynamic, well-timed process of erection and ejaculation are discussed in Chapter 37. Figures 44–1 and 44–2 summarize the neurologic pathways that mediate seminal emission and antegrade ejaculation. Ejaculation is a complex process by which semen is deposited in the vagina during intercourse through seminal emission, bladder neck closure, and antegrade ejaculation of semen. A detailed review of this process has been published by Seftel and coworkers.[25]

Tactile stimulation of the glans penis sends sensory afferent nerve transmission via the sensory division of the pudendal nerve through the spinal cord to the cerebral cortex. Dopaminergic-mediated cerebral input controls transmission down the anterolateral spinal columns via efferent sympathetic fibers that traverse the *ejaculatory coordination center* in the spinal cord (level T10–L3). Long preganglionic fibers continue through the hypogastric nerve (without synapsing) and synapse with short adrenergic postganglionic nerve fibers near the end organs (epididymis, vas deferens, seminal vesicles, vasal ampulla, and prostate). Stimulation of these nerves causes seminal emission and bladder neck closure, which deposit semen in the posterior urethra.

Antegrade ejaculation is controlled by the somatic nervous system. Sensory afferents from the glans penis travel through the pudendal nerve to the cerebral cortex, travel down the spinal cord, and synapse in the S2 to S4 region. Somatic efferents then exit the spinal canal and travel through the motor branch of the pudendal nerve to stimulate the bulbospongiosus, ischiocavernosus, and pelvic floor musculature. The rapid, rhythmic contractions of these muscles result in projectile propulsion of the previously deposited semen in an antegrade direction through the urethra. Interruptions of the normal anatomic and physiologic processes cause ejaculatory dysfunction.

Evaluation of Patients with Ejaculatory Dysfunction

Physicians should approach patients with ejaculatory dysfunction as they would any subfertile man because abnormalities in sperm production, maturation, and transport may also be present. This is especially true in SCI patients, because testis biopsy studies in these patients have shown abnormalities in sperm production.[40–44] A thorough history, physical examination, hormone profile, laboratory evaluation (including analyses of semen and postejaculatory urine, if possible) and adjunctive diagnostics, such as scrotal and transrectal ultrasonography, are often important in the evaluation of these patients.

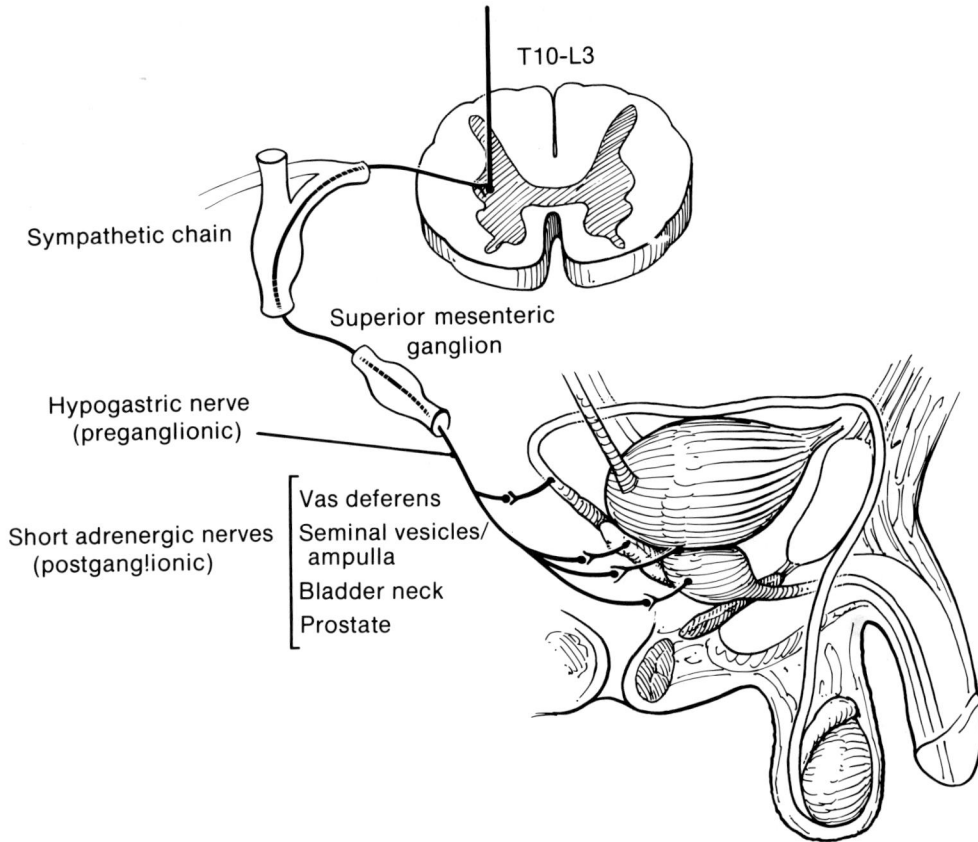

FIGURE 44–1. Innervation of the emission apparatus. (From Shaban SF, Lipshultz LI. Electroejaculation. In: Rajfer J, editor. Common Problems in Infertility and Impotence. Chicago: Year Book Medical, 1989.)

The interview should start with a review of the couple's fertility history. Pregnancies, including spontaneous abortions and terminations of pregnancy, either as a couple or with others, should be recorded. This is especially important in patients with acquired ejaculatory dysfunction because defining the premorbid status of the patient aids in the evaluation.

The history should include risk factors for male infertility and ejaculatory disturbances. Infections of the genital organs,

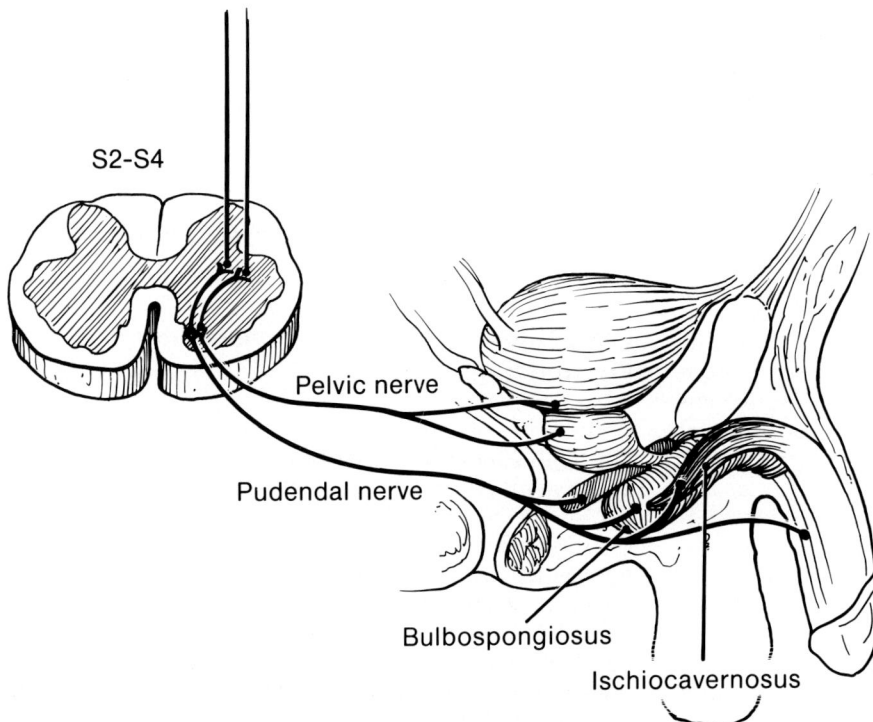

FIGURE 44–2. Innervation of the ejaculatory apparatus. (From Shaban SF, Lipshultz LI. Electroejaculation. In: Rajfer J, editor. Common Problems in Infertility and Impotence. Chicago: Year Book Medical, 1989.)

that is, bladder, prostate, and epididymis, may lead to infertility or subfertility. This is especially significant in SCI patients because they are at high risk for genitourinary infections resulting from bladder dysfunction. Congenital problems, such as a myelomeningocele, bladder exstrophy/epispadias, posterior urethral valves, or ureteroceles, can affect bladder neck function and cause retrograde, dry, or dribbling ejaculation.[45–47]

Acquired systemic illnesses may affect the ejaculatory process. Diabetes mellitus can cause erectile dysfunction, retrograde ejaculation, or anejaculation. The ejaculatory defect is thought to be a result of a peripheral neuropathy affecting sympathetic nerves. In these patients, calcification of the vasa and seminal vesicles may interfere with semen transport. Neurologic conditions, such as multiple sclerosis, may involve many levels of the spinal cord as well as ejaculation. Tumors of the spinal cord rarely cause ejaculatory dysfunction.

Assessing the level and duration of injury helps counsel SCI patients with regard to the probable success of different treatments. A history of bladder function and any corresponding treatment should be obtained.

A thorough history of medical treatment is particularly important in patients with idiopathic ejaculatory dysfunction. Drugs that have been implicated in causing ejaculatory dysfunction are listed in Table 44–5. Most of the medications listed have psychotropic or α-sympatholytic properties.[48, 49]

Previous surgery may have caused ejaculatory disturbances by processes listed in Table 44–6. Surgery can cause denervation of the sympathetic nerves controlling ejaculation or interfere with the normal physiology of emission and bladder neck closure through disruption of the normal anatomy in the posterior urethra. Acquired urethral and bladder problems may also lead to ejaculatory dysfunctions. Urethral stricture disease,[50] previous bladder neck Y-V plasty,[45] prostate surgery,[51] and surgical treatment of some of the congenital problems already mentioned[46] can result in dry, dribbling, or retrograde ejaculation. Transurethral resection of the prostate frequently causes retrograde ejaculation, whereas transurethral incision of the prostate infrequently results in retrograde ejaculation.[51] Y-V plasty was a common treatment for ureteral reflux and "neurogenic bladder" dysfunction in the 1960s. Men who underwent this procedure are now in their

reproductive years and may present with ejaculatory disturbances. Specifically reviewing the details of previous urethral, bladder neck, and prostate surgery may aid in the subsequent diagnosis and treatment of related ejaculatory dysfunction.

Prior surgery also may affect innervation of seminal emission. Any surgical procedures that involved dissection near the aortic bifurcation may damage the hypogastric plexus and cause ejaculatory problems. These include retroperitoneal lymph node dissection (RPLND) for testis cancer, lymphoma or any retroperitoneal tumor, abdominopelvic bowel surgery, sympathectomy, and radical bladder and prostate surgery. In cancer patients, a complete record of adjuvant treatment (chemotherapy, radiation, hormonal manipulation) helps in assessing potential causes of infertility.

It is important to determine whether the patient has a "dry," dribbling, or normal antegrade ejaculation. Patients with retrograde ejaculation usually have normal orgasms associated with a dry, dribbling, or low-volume antegrade ejaculate. Ejaculatory duct obstruction, which also can result in a low-volume ejaculate, is not discussed in this chapter.

The next step in the evaluation is a complete physical examination. The general habitus and secondary sex characteristics should be assessed. Specific attention to the genitourinary organs is important for patients with SCI because many have both testicular and epididymal abnormalities. Because SCI patients spend most of their day in a sitting position, many have testicular atrophy associated with elevated scrotal temperature.[52] Because a history of epididymal infections is common in these patients, they should be examined for epididymal induration and associated epididymal occlusion. A digital rectal examination, performed to assess rectal tone, prostatic abnormalities, and any rectal pathology, is particularly important if rectal probe electroejaculation (RPE) is anticipated. A good neurologic assessment in SCI patients is important to determine the likelihood of success with vibratory stimulation. Brindley[53] reported that vibratory stimulation always failed in patients whose hips did not undergo reflex flexion when the soles of the feet were scratched, indicating damage of the L2–S1 spinal level.

Laboratory testing is also important. Determination of serum FSH concentration is helpful in assessing the overall

TABLE 44–5. Drugs That Affect Ejaculation

Antihypertensives	**Others**
Phenoxybenzamine hydrochloride	Alcohol
Phentolamine	Baclofen
Prazosin	Chlordiazepoxide
Terazosin	Σ-Aminocaproic acid
Thiazides	Methadone
	Naproxen
Antipsychotics	
Chlorpromazine	
Chorprothixene	
Haloperidol	
Perphenazine	
Thioridazine	
Trifluoperazine hydrochloride	
Pargyline	
Phenelzine sulfate	

Modified from Murphy JB, Lipshultz LI. Abnormalities of ejaculation. Urol Clin North Am 1987; 14:588.

TABLE 44–6. Causes of Ejaculatory Dysfunction

Neurogenic Factors	**Anatomic Abnormalities**
Central nervous system	*Congenital*
Spinal cord injury (trauma)	Ureterocele
Transverse myelitis	Extrophy/epispadias
Multiple sclerosis	Posterior urethral valves
Myelomeningocele	*Acquired*
Peripheral nerve injury or dysfunction	Transurethral resection of the prostate
Retroperitoneal lymph node dissection (testis cancer, lymphoma)	Transurethral incision of the prostate
Diabetes mellitus	Open prostatectomy
Abdominopelvic colorectal surgery	Y-V plasty
Abdominal vascular surgery	Urethral stricture disease
Radical prostate/bladder surgery	Bladder neck incision
Sympathectomy	Radical prostate/bladder surgery
Drugs	Surgery complication
	Idiopathic
	Psychogenic (?)

state of the germinal epithelium. The seminal vesicles are androgen-dependent organs and account for 80% of the ejaculate volume. Measurement of serum testosterone concentrations helps to identify a hypogonadal state that might be associated with a low ejaculate volume. Examination of post-ejaculate urine determines the presence of retrograde ejaculation in the patient who may be normospermic, oligospermic, or azoospermic. Typically, retrograde ejaculation is associated with low-volume normospermia or oligospermia. Three cases of antegrade azoospermia associated with significant retrograde ejaculation, however, have been reported.[54] If no sperm are present in a wet-mount urine sample, centrifugation of the specimen is necessary to rule out low-density retrograde ejaculation.

Additional procedures may contribute to the diagnosis and help establish a regimen for treatment of ejaculatory dysfunction. Transrectal ultrasonography is a minimally invasive diagnostic test that may detect abnormalities of the prostate, posterior urethra, and bladder neck—defects that might account for ejaculatory abnormalities. Cystoscopy can identify specific, treatable abnormalities of the bladder neck or urethra. These abnormalities include urethral stricture disease, mild posterior urethral valves, and ureteroceles resulting in incomplete closure of the bladder neck.

A complete evaluation of the patient's partner is especially important because many couples require an assisted reproductive technique, such as intrauterine insemination (IUI) or in vitro fertilization (IVF), to achieve a pregnancy. These procedures are expensive and it is cost effective to screen the woman for any abnormalities that might jeopardize success.

Treatment of Patients with Retrograde Ejaculation

The cause of retrograde ejaculation determines the therapeutic approach.[55] The initial goal of therapy is to convert retrograde ejaculation to antegrade ejaculation and thus allow the couple to achieve a pregnancy with natural, timed intercourse. Patients taking medications that influence ejaculatory function should discontinue usage if possible. In patients with idiopathic retrograde ejaculation, cystoscopy is indicated to rule out pathology that might affect antegrade passage of semen or result in abnormal bladder neck closure. An anatomic urethral abnormality, such as a urethral stricture, should be treated to restore normal semen transport.[126a]

Patients with retrograde ejaculation associated with neurogenic disorders often respond to medical therapy. The two most commonly used drugs are imipramine hydrochloride and pseudoephedrine hydrochloride.[56] Imipramine potentiates stimulation of adrenergic synapses by blocking the active uptake of norepinephrine from the extracellular fluid into the cytoplasm at postganglionic nerve terminals.[57] Pseudoephedrine is an α-sympathomimetic agent that directly increases the intrasynaptic concentration of norepinephrine at postganglionic fibers by allowing its transport from the cytoplasm to the extracellular fluid.[58] We usually begin with pseudoephedrine hydrochloride 60 mg orally four times a day for 2 weeks. If there is no improvement, we add imipramine 25 to 50 mg orally twice a day. Because the side effects are minimal, these drugs should be tried as an initial treatment in patients with retrograde ejaculation as a result of

peripheral nerve injury or dysfunction. Patients with a history of RPLND or other surgery resulting in injury to the hypogastric plexus may improve on sympathomimetic medications.[59–61] Diabetics are less likely to respond, but several cases of return of antegrade ejaculation in this population have been reported.[62–64] In general, patients with anatomic abnormalities of the posterior urethra and bladder neck resulting from earlier surgery do not respond to medical therapy. Success with the processed retrograde semen specimens in conjunction with assisted reproductive techniques has minimized the need for open surgical correction of retrograde ejaculation (such as Young-Dees bladder neck repair).[58, 65, 66] In a few instances, ejaculation with a full bladder has been reported to result in antegrade ejaculation.[67, 68] Although this therapy usually is not successful, a trial in some patients with retrograde ejaculation may be warranted.

If medical therapy does not produce an antegrade ejaculate, other methods of treatment are indicated. The mainstay of treatment is retrieval of an optimized postejaculatory urine specimen.[69] After the urine specimen is processed to remove the seminal plasma, IUI is performed. If this is not successful or if the semen quality is poor, a more advanced reproductive technique, such as gamete intrafallopian transfer (GIFT) or IVF, may be employed.

Success with this procedure in conjunction with IUI,[70, 71] IVF, and GIFT[73] has been reported often. Testing of ovulation with urine ovulation kits, transvaginal ultrasonography, or both is important to determine optimal timing for insemination.

Bladder Preparation to Optimize Retrograde Specimen

To optimize the quality of the specimen obtained from retrograde ejaculation, it is necessary to improve the environment of the bladder for sperm survival. Alkalization of the urine to a urine pH higher than 7 is recommended. This level usually is achieved with an increased fluid intake in conjunction with a course of sodium bicarbonate, 650 mg orally four times a day, 24 to 48 hours before the procedure. Because these patients often have a history of urinary tract infections, a urine culture is recommended 1 week before the procedure. If infection is present, antimicrobial treatment is begun 5 days before the procedure. If the urine culture is sterile, prophylactic antimicrobial treatment of one or two doses of ciprofloxacin, 500 mg orally, is given on the evening before and the morning of the procedure. Immediately before ejaculation, a sterile catheter lubricated only with sperm-washing media is passed into the bladder. The bladder is emptied and then irrigated with 60 to 100 mL of this buffered solution. We use a mixture of 100 mL of modified human tubal fluid medium with HEPES buffer, penicillin G, streptomycin sulfate, and 24 mL of modified sperm wash with albumin (Irvine Scientific, Santa Ana, CA). Approximately 30 mL of this solution is left in the bladder, and the catheter is removed. Masturbation or an assisted ejaculatory procedure (vibratory stimulation or electroejaculation) is performed, and the retrograde specimen may be collected on the next void (within 20 minutes) or, if urination is not possible, with repeat catheterization. Options for sperm use after retrieval are listed in Table 44–7.

TABLE 44–7. Options for Sperm Management After Retrieval by Assisted Ejaculatory Procedures

Cryopreservation
Intravaginal/cervical placement
Natural cycle/intrauterine insemination
Hyperstimulation/intrauterine insemination (clomiphene citrate or Pergonal)
In vitro fertilization
In vitro fertilization/micromanipulation

Treatment of Patients with Anejaculation

Anejaculation is the inability to produce an ejaculate in an antegrade or retrograde fashion. The causes of these disorders are listed in Table 44–6. In most patients, the cause is organic, usually a neurogenic injury; however, patients with idiopathic anejaculation have been reported, some of whom have extremely strong religious beliefs that have resulted in a psychological barrier to ejaculation.

The initial approach to treatment of anejaculation in humans was through trials of chemical stimulation. Attempts have been made to stimulate seminal emission and ejaculation with acetylcholinesterase inhibitors. The mechanism of action is unclear, but these chemicals have been postulated to cause a direct stimulation of the spinal ejaculatory center.[73]

Spira[74] first reported the use of intrathecal neostigmine to induce ejaculation in a T6 paraplegic. Semen of good quality was obtained, and artificial insemination resulted in a pregnancy. Guttmann and Walsh[75] used this technique on 134 patients and reported successful ejaculation in 59%. One patient, however, died of a cerebral hemorrhage resulting from hypertension associated with severe autonomic dysreflexia. More recently, a similar nonfatal complication resulted after a 0.3-mg intrathecal injection of neostigmine.[76] Subcutaneous injection of physostigmine, which crosses the blood-brain barrier, has been used in conjunction with masturbation to induce ejaculation without complications.[77] With the subcutaneous approach, good-quality semen has been obtained,[78] a pregnancy has been reported,[79] and side effects have been minimal and controlled by pretreatment with a peripheral anticholinergic agent. Because of the major complications described and the availability of other less invasive procedures, however, this mode of therapy has generally been abandoned in the United States.

MEDICAL THERAPY

Seminal emission is controlled by the sympathetic nervous system. The preganglionic nerves are cholinergic and originate in the ejaculatory coordination center (T10 to L3). The postganglionic nerves are adrenergic, and neural transmission is mediated with norepinephrine as they synapse near the end organs (epididymis, vas deferens, seminal vesicles, vasal ampulla, and prostate). Theoretically, increasing the concentration of neurotransmitter at the postganglionic site may improve ejaculatory capability in patients with anejaculation. Sympathomimetic drugs have been used with variable success in this capacity.

The two drugs most commonly used to treat anejaculatory men are pseudoephedrine hydrochloride (Sudafed) and imipramine hydrochloride. We usually begin with pseudoephed-

rine hydrochloride 60 mg orally four times a day, for 2 weeks. If there is no improvement, we add imipramine, 25 to 50 mg orally twice a day. The greatest success with these medications in the anejaculatory patient has been in patients with peripheral nerve dysfunction, such as patients with diabetes or surgical injury to the hypogastric plexus. Both α-sympathomimetic drugs[80–82] and imipramine[80] have been used in an attempt to improve semen quality in anejaculatory patients with testis cancer after RPLND. Proctor and Howards[82] described marginal improvement in semen quality with several oral α-sympathomimetic drugs, but no pregnancies resulted in this study. Lynch and Maxted[83] reported two pregnancies initiated by a patient similarly treated with ephedrine sulfate, 75 mg. This medication produced a subjectively judged improvement in semen volume, but no objective data on semen quality were recorded. The most striking response to medication was reported by Kelly and Needle,[80] who described the serendipitous finding of increased ejaculate volume and increased semen concentration in an aspermic post-RPLND patient treated with imipramine for depression. This finding was reversed by discontinuing the medication. One year later, the patient was treated for a cold with pseudoephedrine with a "similar sudden return of ejaculation." These medications have also been reported to convert dry or dribble ejaculation to antegrade or retrograde ejaculation.[60, 61]

In SCI patients, we do not routinely start with a trial of medical therapy. If vibratory stimulation and electroejaculation are unsuccessful, however, we treat SCI patients with both α-sympathomimetics (pseudoephedrine hydrochloride, 60 mg orally four times a day) and imipramine (50 mg orally twice a day) for 2 weeks and repeat these procedures before we proceed to other more invasive modalities.

PENILE VIBRATORY STIMULATION

If medical therapy is unsuccessful, a trial of penile vibratory stimulation is recommended.[83] This procedure is most successful in SCI patients with lesions above the ejaculatory coordination center at T10 to L3. If an intact reflex arc is present from S2 to S4 to the ejaculatory coordination center, both seminal emission and antegrade ejaculation can occur. Penile vibratory stimulation should be attempted in SCI patients of all levels because some patients have incomplete lesions with intact nerve fibers leading to the ejaculatory coordination center. Because these patients are susceptible to autonomic dysreflexia, pretreatment with nifedipine (10 mg sublingually) is necessary for those who have a history of episodic hypertension. The procedure usually is performed in an office setting where blood pressure can be monitored. If successful, the vibratory stimulation procedure causes seminal emission and antegrade ejaculation because both peripheral sympathetic and somatic nerves are intact and stimulated during this procedure. Sometimes retrograde ejaculation occurs, so bladder preparation, as described previously, is necessary. Vibratory stimulation is rarely, if ever, successful in nonneurogenic patients, but a successful result has been reported in one patient with idiopathic anejaculation.[84]

After the buffered medium has been placed in the bladder, the frenular surface of the penis is stimulated with a penile vibrator. If erection and subsequent ejaculation do not occur within 3 to 5 minutes, the vibrator is moved to a different area on the glans penis, and the vibration procedure is continued. Patients sometimes have specific "trigger points" on the glans penis that stimulate ejaculation, and these should be recorded for future procedures. The specific vibrator frequency should be 60 to 100 Hz with a peak-to-peak amplitude of 1.6 to 2.5 mm.[85] Better results have been reported with vibratory stimulation in patients with lesions above L1 with a higher frequency and lower amplitude vibrator.[86] Usually, antegrade ejaculation is preceded by erection and contractions of the skeletal muscles of the abdomen and lower extremities. Because of bladder neck insufficiency, retrograde ejaculation sometimes occurs, so catheterization is required after the procedure. If skeletal muscle contraction occurs but antegrade ejaculation does not, recatheterization of the bladder is recommended to rule out retrograde ejaculation before an attempt with rectal probe electroejaculation is initiated.

The first reported case of semen retrieval by penile vibratory stimulation was performed by Sobrero and colleagues[87] in 1965 in a patient with primary anorgasmia and by Comarr[88] in 1970 in an SCI patient. Francois and associates[89] reported that 72% of SCI patients undergoing vibratory stimulation produced an ejaculate, and 14% initiated a pregnancy. In 1984, Brindley[53] reported his results of 93 SCI patients undergoing vibratory stimulation. Semen was obtained in 59% of patients who were at least 6 months past injury, but only 9% responded if the interval since the injury was less than 6 months. In this study, seven couples initiated pregnancies using vibratory stimulation in conjunction with vaginal (six couples) or cervical (one couple) insemination. Oates and Staskin[90] reported that 52% of SCI patients, mostly those with high thoracic or cervical SCI, responded to vibratory stimulation. Because semen quality is variable in these patients, IUI usually is the first assisted reproductive technique used to achieve a pregnancy. Vibratory stimulation in conjunction with IVF, however, has been successful as well.[91]

RECTAL PROBE ELECTROEJACULATION

If medical therapy and vibratory stimulation are unsuccessful, a trial of RPE is warranted. When vibratory stimula-

tion is performed, both seminal emission and antegrade ejaculation occur, but with electroejaculation, only seminal emission follows. Electrical stimulation of the vasal ampullae, prostate, seminal vesicles, vas deferens, and epididymis results in deposition of semen within the posterior urethra. This fluid must be milked out of the posterior urethra or retrieved if directed in a retrograde direction.

Electrical stimulation to induce seminal emission was used first in veterinary medicine by Gunn[92] and was subsequently used for animal breeding.[93–95] The early veterinary equipment was primitive and has been significantly improved for application in humans. RPE in men was first reported by Horne and colleagues[96] in 1948. Three of 18 patients undergoing this procedure produced motile sperm after prostatic massage. Significant improvements in equipment and technology continued, but it was not until 1975, in Australia, that the first pregnancy was achieved using sperm obtained with RPE in conjunction with IUI.[97] In this instance, semen was again obtained after prostatic massage. Unfortunately, the neonate died on its first day of life as a result of complications of transposition of the great vessels. Francois and associates[89] subsequently reported the first viable pregnancy in a series of 31 anejaculatory patients treated with RPE. This initiated the current era of success with this technique.

The procedure can be performed without anesthesia in SCI patients who have no sensation, but otherwise it requires a light general anesthesia. We have found that muscle-relaxing agents may inhibit the emission reflex and thus discourage their use during anesthesia.[98] If these agents are used, a return of the muscle twitch is necessary before the procedure. The RPE is performed with the patient in either the dorsolithotomy or the lateral decubitus position. The patient undergoes the preliminary protocol for urine alkalization, bladder wash, and antimicrobial prophylaxis previously described. After the patient is catheterized, a digital examination is performed, and the Model 10-12 electroejaculator probe is inserted into the rectum with the electrodes oriented anteriorly. Upward parallel pressure is exerted on the anterior rectal wall near the seminal vesicles. A schematic of this procedure is shown in Figure 44–3. The initial stimulation is at 5 V.

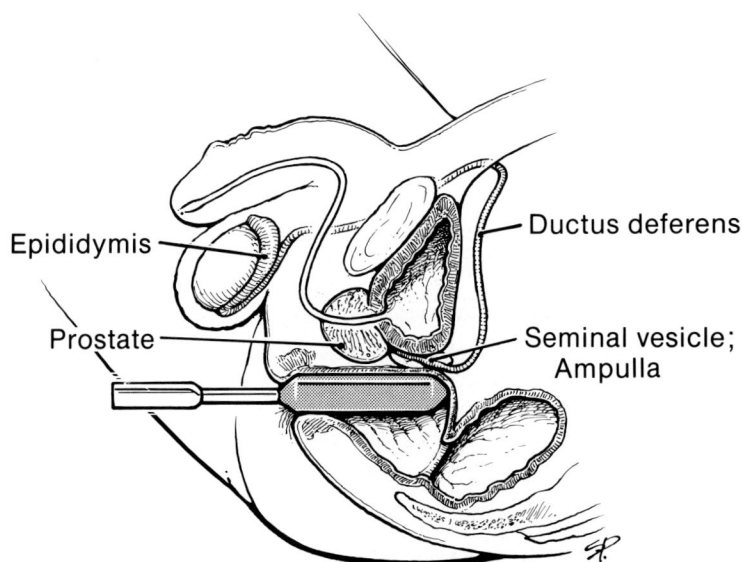

Epididymis

Prostate

Ductus deferens

Seminal vesicle; Ampulla

© Baylor College of Medicine 1987

FIGURE 44–3. Sagittal view showing rectal probe placement. (From Shaban SF, Seager SWJ, Lipshultz LI. Clinical electroejaculation. Med Instrum 1988;22[2]:78. Reprinted with permission of the publisher, The Association for the Advancement of Medical Instrumentation, Arlington, Virginia.)

Subsequently a series of stimulations of increasing voltages using two stimulations for each voltage increment with each stimulation lasting approximately 2 to 4 seconds is performed, with a return each time to a baseline of 5 V until emission occurs or the temperature of the probe reaches 40°C. An assistant is present with a sterile cup near the penis to retrieve the specimen once seminal emission has occurred. As emission occurs, the penile urethra is milked to collect the complete specimen. The probe is removed, and the bladder is recatheterized to retrieve any retrograde specimen. The rectum is examined for injury with anoscopy.

Urinary infection and retention have been seen after RPE. Minor rectal bleeding is not uncommon, but significant rectal injury is extremely rare. One case of rectal perforation requiring a temporary colostomy has been reported. Autonomic dysreflexia is common in patients with high thoracic and cervical lesions but in most cases is easily prevented or controlled during the procedure with sublingual nifedipine. In instances of severe dysreflexia, the stimulus should be removed and the procedure terminated. In these patients, general anesthesia must be used.

Results of successful treatment with RPE are summarized in Table 44–8. Since the initial success of Thomas,[97] Francois,[89] and David,[99] more than 100 pregnancies have been achieved with RPE in the United States. This success has been with natural cycle IUI,[53, 89, 97, 99–104] hyperstimulation IUI,[105, 106] IVF,[105, 107, 108] GIFT,[105] and IVF with micromanipulation,[106] as shown in Table 44–8. RPE has been successful in patients with SCI, peripheral nerve injury or dysfunction, and idiopathic ejaculatory dysfunction.

Sperm retrieval should be possible in more than 90% of patients.[98] In refractory cases, the status of the germinal epithelium can be assessed by testis biopsy because these patients may also have primary testicular abnormalities. Examination of the epididymis may reveal epididymal induration from earlier infection resulting in epididymal occlusion.

Semen generally has normal or high sperm concentration with low motility and decreased forward progression, and pregnancy rates continue to be from 10% to 30% (see Table 44–8). Because of these findings, research has been directed toward identifying specific abnormalities and improving semen quality.

Denil and coworkers[109] evaluated the functional characteristics of semen obtained by RPE using cervical mucus penetration testing and the zona-free hamster sperm penetration assay. Although no statistical analysis was performed, the RPE sperm showed impaired penetration through cervical mucus, impaired survivability in overnight culture, and impaired sperm penetration assay results compared with donor sperm.

Antisperm antibodies do not appear to affect the fertility of these patients significantly. Denil and coworkers[109] reported that 31 of 32 specimens tested negative for antisperm antibodies with the direct immunobead test. In this study, 13.5% (19 of 22) of patients had serum antisperm antibodies in RPE-obtained specimens, whereas previous studies reported a 37.5% (3 of 8) incidence.[110]

Certain factors may be predictive of better semen quality. In a study by Ohl and associates,[111] quality of sperm was related to the level of injury, with the highest sperm concentrations obtained from patients with thoracic-level injuries. In addition, the sperm concentration and motility were higher in the group with injury at the thoracic level than in the group with injury at the cervical and lumbar levels. Bladder management also affected the success of RPE. Patients whose bladders were managed with intermittent catheterization fared best, whereas those whose bladders were managed with an indwelling catheter or voiding with Credé or reflex voiding fared worst. Factors such as age and interval between injury and RPE did not seem to affect the quality of semen obtained. These judgments, however, were based on observation because statistical analysis was not performed.[111]

The reason for the poor quality of semen obtained by RPE in patients with neurogenic ejaculatory dysfunction is unclear but probably is complex. Several possible explanations are listed in Table 44–9.

Primary sperm production in SCI patients has been shown to be abnormal by testis biopsy.[40, 43, 44] Although many of these patients have fathered children, histologic changes, most notably hypospermatogenesis, have been found on histologic testis examination.

Ductal system denervation has been suggested as the cause of the poor quality of semen in these patients. This role may be manifested at any level of denervation, that is, testis, epididymis, vas deferens, vasal ampulla, seminal vesicle, and

TABLE 44–8. Pregnancies Achieved with Sperm Obtained After Rectal Probe Electroejaculation

Date	Author	Cause	No. of Patients	Percentage with Ejaculate	Sperm Placement	Pregnancies
1975	Thomas[97]	SCI–T12	1	100	Natural AI	Yes, but died
1977–1978	David[99]	SCI	16	25	Natural AI	Yes, 1
1978–1979	Francois[89]	SCI–T6	1	80	Natural AI	Yes, healthy
1984	Brindley[53]	SCI	154	63	Natural IUI	Yes, 11
1988	Bennett[100]	RPLND	1	100	Natural AI	Yes, 1
1989	Bennett[101]	SCI	37	59	IUI and IVF	Yes, 4
1988	Shaban[103]	SCI/RPLND	30	79	IUI	Yes, 2
1989	Stewart[104]	Idiopathic	1	100	Natural AI	Yes, 1
1990	Randolph[108]	SCI/RPLND	7	100	IVF/GIFT	Yes, 2 (1 live birth)
1990	Blank[107]	Gunshot wound, not SCI	1	100	IVF/ZIFT	Yes, 1
1991	Lucas[102]	SCI/DM	12	75	AI	Yes, 1
1991	Ohl[105]	RPLND	24	87	Clomid, IUI/IVF	Yes, 7
1992	Toledo[106]	SCI/RPLND	10	100	Hyperstimulation, IUI, IVF/micromanipulation	Yes, 1 IUI, 2 IVF/ micromanipulation (no live birth)

SCI, Spinal cord injury; AI, artificial insemination; IUI, intrauterine insemination; RPLND, retroperitoneal lymph node dissection; IVF, in vitro fertilization; GIFT, gamete intrafallopian transfer; ZIFT, zygote intrafallopian transfer; DM, diabetes mellitus.

TABLE 44–9. Hypotheses to Explain Poor Quality of Semen Obtained by Electroejaculation in Patients with Neurogenic Ejaculatory Dysfunction

Primary testicular abnormality
Denervation resulting in abnormal sperm maturation
Functional obstruction of the ductal system
Electrical current–induced injury to the sperm during rectal probe
    electroejaculation procedure

prostate. Theoretically, injury to the innervation of the testicle could result in an abnormal testicular milieu (such as growth factor suppression) resulting in decreased sperm production. More likely, however, primary epididymal dysfunction is present. This theory is based on evidence of epididymal abnormalities produced in an experimental rat model when inferior mesenteric plexus ablation was performed. In their experiment, Billups and colleagues[112] showed that epididymal weight increased, and the number of sperm in the cauda epididymis increased, suggesting either a functional obstruction or a primary epididymal maturation problem. Additionally, computerized testing of sperm motility comparing inferior mesenteric plexus–ablated rat epididymal sperm with vasectomized rat epididymal sperm showed decreased sperm motility in the inferior mesenteric plexus–ablated rats. This suggests that the primary motility disorder of epididymal sperm was more likely related to a primary denervation effect on the epididymis than to an obstruction.[113]

Clinical evidence does exist for a functional obstruction of the ductal system in these patients. In the presence of a functional obstruction, a higher quality sperm would be expected from areas more proximal in the ductal system. In their series of obstructive azoospermia patients treated with microscopic sperm aspiration, Honig and coworkers[114] included five anejaculatory patients whose sperm were obtained from the proximal ductal system. Semen quality was good in these patients, and two pregnancies were achieved using sperm aspiration in conjunction with IVF.[114] In addition, Colpi and colleagues[115] used a sperm washout technique to obtain more proximal sperm from an anejaculatory patient in whom RPE was unsuccessful. The sperm used in conjunction with GIFT resulted in a pregnancy for this T12 paraplegic and his partner.[115] Honig and coworkers[114] reported on a series of anejaculatory patients who underwent repeated multiple sequential RPE over a short interval. The authors showed an improvement in sperm motility in 54% of cases and improved forward progression in 75% of cases when a second procedure was performed shortly after the first (6 to 72 hours). These reports of improved semen quality and pregnancies resulting from sperm obtained more proximally in the ductal system lend support to the hypothesis that a functional obstruction occurs in some patients with neurogenic ejaculatory dysfunction.

Denervation of the seminal vesicles and prostate may produce an abnormal biochemical milieu for semen. Hirsch and associates[116] reported on the biochemical characteristics of semen obtained via RPE and compared them with chemistry of normal controls. There was a lower level of fructose, glutamic oxaloacetic transaminase, and alkaline phosphatase and a higher level of chloride present in the RPE-obtained specimens.[116] The significance of these findings is unclear but may represent denervation-related abnormalities that could affect semen quality.

Finally, decreased sperm motility and poor functional characteristics of RPE-obtained sperm could result from electrical current–related injury to spermatozoa at the time of the procedure. Using an in vitro RPE model, Witt and others[117] showed no change in sperm motility or forward progression in sperm exposed to electrical current of similar amperage and voltage used in RPE. Honig and colleagues[119] used the same model and assessed functional characteristics of sperm before and after exposure to electrical current. There was no difference in cervical mucus penetration, strict morphology of spermatozoa, or penetration of zona-free hamster oocytes between these groups. Other in vitro studies have suggested that electrical current has a detrimental effect on semen parameters,[46a, 120, 121] but it is unclear whether electrical current plays a major role in the poor quality of semen obtained by RPE.

FUTURE DIRECTIONS

Semen quality may be optimized in two ways. First, it may be optimized by obtaining higher quality sperm from the patient. Second, semen may be improved in the laboratory by sperm-enhancing agents that improve sperm motility, forward progression, and functional ability. Research is underway in both areas.

The functional obstruction hypothesis suggests that retrieval of sperm more proximally in the ductal system may result in better quality sperm. Use of repeated sequential electroejaculations over a short interval,[120, 122, 123] proximal vasal washout techniques,[115] and microscopic vasal or epididymal sperm aspiration[88, 90, 114] has been reported. Microscopic vasal sperm aspiration in anejaculatory men was reported first by Bustillo and Rajfer[124] and subsequently by Berger and colleagues.[125] In these cases, the sperm obtained were used in conjunction with artificial insemination, and one pregnancy was achieved.[90] Most recently, this technique has been applied in conjunction with IVF by Honig and coworkers[114] to five anejaculatory men, all of whom achieved fertilization. Two couples achieved pregnancies.

The second approach to improving semen quality involves treatment of sperm with sperm-enhancing agents after the production of the specimen. Sikka and Hellstrom[126] added different concentrations of pentoxifylline and caffeine to RPE-obtained sperm to improve sperm motility. They showed that these agents improved percent motility, curvilinear velocity, and straight-line velocity. In one patient, the semen was used in conjunction with GIFT, and a pregnancy and live birth were achieved.

On the technologic horizon, Brindley and coworkers[127] reported on implantation of hypogastric nerve stimulators in eight anejaculatory patients (seven with SCI; one with primary anorgasmia). He was able to obtain good quality sperm in six of eight patients. Five pregnancies and two live births were reported. Significant pain, however, was noted with stimulation in two patients. Future refinements in equipment may allow performance of painless in vivo stimulation. Laparoscopic implantation of hypogastric nerve stimulators has been performed without complication in animals,[128] but their use in humans should be considered experimental.

It is hoped that the continuing application of technology

to improve semen quality will increase the overall pregnancy rate in this special group of male infertility patients.

REFERENCES

1. Dubin L, Amelar RD. Sexual causes of male infertility. Fertil Steril 1972;23:579–582.
2. Rantala M, Koskimies AI. Sexual behavior of infertile couples. Int J Fertil 1988;33:26–30.
3. Boyarsky S, Boyarsky R. Psychogenic factors in male infertility: a review. Med Aspects Hum Sex 1983;17:86h–86q.
4. Kedem P, Milkulincer M, Nathanson YE. Psychological aspects of male infertility. Br J Med Psychol 1990;63:73–80.
5. Mahlstedt PP. The psychological component of infertility. Fertil Steril 1985;43:335–346.
6. Masters WH, Johnson VE. Human Sexual Inadequacy. Boston: Little, Brown, 1970.
7. LoPiccolo J, Stock WE. Treatment of sexual dysfunction. J Consult Clin Psychol 1986;54:158–160.
8. Nieschlag E. Care of the infertile male. Clin Endocrinol 1993;38:123–133.
9. Liu L, Banks SM, Barmnes KM, et al. Two-year comparison of testicular responses to pulsatile gonadotropin-releasing hormone and exogenous gonadotropins for the inception of therapy in men with isolated hypogonadotropic hypogonadism. J Clin Endocrinol Metab 1988;67:1140–1145.
10. Saal W, Happ J, Cordes U, et al. Subcutaneous gonadotropin therapy in male patients with hypogonadotropic hypogonadism. Fertil Steril 1991;56:319–324.
11. Schopohl J, Mehltretter G, von Zumbusch R, et al. Comparison of gonadotropin-releasing hormone and gonadotropin therapy in male patients with idiopathic hypothalamic hypogonadism. Fertil Steril 1991;56:1143–1150.
12. Lunenfeld B, Berezin M, Sack J, et al. Gonadotropic therapy in men with gonadotrophic insufficiency results, tolerance and follow-up of children fathered by these patients. In: Menchini GF, Fabris W, Pasini W, et al, editors. Therapy of Andrology. Boston: Medica, 1982:13–21.
13. Wilson JD, Griffin JE. The use and misuse of androgens. Metabolism 1984;33:1052–1058.
14. McClure RD. Endocrine evaluation and therapy of erectile dysfunction. Urol Clin North Am 1988;15:53–64.
15. Davidson JM, Carmargo CA, Smith ER. Effects of androgen on sexual behavior in hypogonadal men. J Clin Endocrinol Metab 1979;48:955–958.
16. Salmimies P, Kockott G, Pirke KM, et al. Effects of testosterone replacement on sexual behavior in hypogonadal men. Arch Sex Behav 1982;11:345–353.
17. Cunningham GR, Hirshkowitz M, Korenman SG, et al. Testosterone replacement therapy and sleep-related erection in hypogonadal men. J Clin Endocrinol Metab 1990;70:792–797.
18. Ahmed SR, Boucher AE, Manni A, et al. Transdermal testosterone therapy in the treatment of male hypogonadism. J Clin Endocrinol Metab 1988;66:546–551.
19. Carey PO, Howards SS, Vance ML. Transdermal testosterone treatment of hypogonadal men. J Urol 1988;140:76–79.
20. McClure RD, Oses R, Ernest ML. Hypogonadal impotence treated by transdermal testosterone. Urology 1991;37:224–228.
21. Miccoli R, Giampietro D, Tognarelli M, et al. Prevalence and type of sexual dysfunction in diabetic males: a standardized clinical approach. J Med 1987;18:305.
22. Tesone M, Ltalle LBS, Foglia VG, et al. Diabetes and male reproduction. In: Paulson JD, Negro-Vilar A, Lucena E, et al, editors. Andrology: Male Fertility and Sterility. Orlando: Academic Press, 1986:85.
23. Dinulovic D, Radonjic G. Diabetes mellitus/male infertility. Arch Androl 1990;25:277–293.
24. Campbell IW. Diabetic autonomic neuropathy. Br J Clin Pract 1976;3:153.
25. Seftel AD, Oates RD, Krane RJ. Disturbed sexual function in patients with spinal cord disease. Neurol Clin North Am 1991;9(3):757–778.
26. Virag R, Sussman H, Floresco J, et al. Late results on the treatment of neurogenic impotence by self-intracavernous-injection (SICI) of vasoactive drugs. World J Urol 1987;5:166.
27. Collins KP, Hackler RH. Complications of penile prosthesis in spinal cord injury patients. J Urol 1987;140:984.
28. Bennett AH, Carpenter AJ, Barada JH. An improved drug combination for a pharmacologic erection program. J Urol 1991;1564–1565.
29. Zentgraf M, Baccouche M, Junemann KP. Diagnosis and therapy using papaverine and phentolamine. Urol Int 1988;43:65.
30. Levine SB, Althof SE, Turner LA, et al. Side effects of self-administration of intracavernous papaverine and phentolamine for the treatment of impotence. J Urol 1989;141:54–57.
31. Padma-Nathan H, Goldstein I, Payton TR, et al. Intracavernosal pharmacotherapy: the pharmacologic erection program. World J Urol 1987;5:160–170.
32. Montague DK. Periprosthetic infections. J Urol 1987;138:68–69.
33. Kessler R. Surgical experience with inflatable penile prosthesis. J Urol 1980;124:611–613.
34. Furlow WL, Goldwasser B, Gundian JC. Implantation of model AMS 700 penile prosthesis: long term results. J Urol 1988;139:741–743.
35. Malloy TR, Wein AJ, Carpiniello VL. Reliability of AMS 700 inflatable penile prosthesis. Urology 1986;27:385–387.
36. Goldstein I, Krane RJ. Diagnosis and therapy of erectile dysfunction. In: Walsh PC, Retik AB, Stamey TA, et al, editors. Campbell's Urology. Philadelphia: WB Saunders, 1991:3033–3070.
37. Levine FJ, Goldstein I. Vascular reconstructive surgery in the management of erectile dysfunction. Int J Impotence Res 1990;2:59–78.
38. Lerner SE, Melman A, Christ GJ. A review of erectile dysfunction: new insights and more questions. J Urol 1993;149:1246–1255.
39. Penson DF, Seftel AD, Krane RJ, et al. The hemodynamic pathophysiology of impotence following blunt trauma to the erect penis. J Urol 1992;148:1171–1180.
40. Bors E, Engle ET, Rosenquist RC. Fertility in paraplegic males: a preliminary report of endocrine studies. J Clin Endocrinol 1950;10:381–398.
41. Chapelle P-A, Roby-Brami A, Yakovleff A, et al. Neurological correlations of ejaculation and testicular size in men with a complete spinal cord section. J Neurol Neurosurg Psychiatry 1988;51:197–202.
42. Linsenmeyer TA, Perkash I. Infertility in men with spinal cord injury. Arch Phys Med Rehabil 1991;72:747–754.
43. Perkash I, Martin DE, Warner H, et al. Reproductive biology of paraplegics: results of semen collection, testicular biopsy and serum hormone. J Urol 1985;134:284–288.
44. Stemmermann GN, Weiss L, Auerbach O, et al. A study of the germinal epithelium in male paraplegics. Am J Clin Pathol 1950;20:24–34.
45. Ochsner MG, Burns E, Henry HH II. Incidence of retrograde ejaculation following bladder neck revision as a child. J Urol 1970;104:596–597.
46. Páramo PG, Martinez-Piñeiro JA, De La Peña JJ, et al. Andrological implications of congenital posterior urethral valves in adults. A case of retained ejaculation and review in Western literature. Eur Urol 1983;9:359–361.
46a. Hellstrom WJ, Aertker MW, Wang R, et al. The detrimental effects of electrical current on the motion parameters of normal sperm. Fertil Steril 1991;(suppl):S81.
47. Reilly JM, Oates RD. Preliminary investigation of the potential fertility status of postpubertal males with myelodysplasia. J Urol 1992; 147:251A.
48. Blair JH, Simpson GM. Effect of antipsychotic drugs on reproductive functions. Dis Nerv Syst 1966;27:645–647.
49. Kedia K, Markland C. The effect of pharmacologic agents on ejaculation. J Urol 1975;114:569–573.
50. Vijayan P, Sundin T. Island patch urethroplasty: effects on urinary flow and ejaculation. Br J Urol 1983;55:69–72.
51. Hedlund H, Ek A. Ejaculation and sexual function after endoscopic bladder neck incision. Br J Urol 1985;57:164–167.
52. Brindley GS. Deep scrotal temperature and the effect on it of clothing, air temperature, activity, posture and paraplegia. Br J Urol 1982;54:49–55.
53. Brindley GS. The fertility of men with spinal injuries. Paraplegia 1984;22:337–348.
54. Keiserman WM, Dubin L, Amelar RD. A new type of retrograde ejaculation: a report of three cases. Fertil Steril 1974;25:1071–1072.
55. Sandler B. Idiopathic retrograde ejaculation. Fertil Steril 1979;32:474–475.
56. Stockamp K, Schreiter F, Altwein JE. Alpha-adrenergic drugs in retrograde ejaculation. Fertil Steril 1974;25:817–820.
57. Idem. Functional anatomy of synaptic transmission. Anesthesiology 1968;29:643.
58. Von Euler US. Synthesis, uptake and storage of catecholamine in adrenergic nerves: the effects of drugs, catecholamine. In: Blaschko H,

Muscholl E, editors. Handbook of Experimental Pharmacology. Berlin: Springer-Verlag, 1972:186.

59. Brooks ME, Sidi A. Treatment of retrograde ejaculation using imipramine [letter to the editor]. Urology 1981;18:633.

60. Narayan P, Lange PH, Fraley EE. Ejaculation and fertility after extended retroperitoneal lymph node dissection for testicular cancer. J Urol 1982;127:685–688.

61. Nijman JM, Jager SA, Boer PW, et al. The treatment of ejaculation disorders after retroperitoneal lymph node dissection. Cancer 1982;50:2967–2971.

62. Brooks ME, Berezin M, Braf Z. Treatment of retrograde ejaculation with imipramine. Urology 1980;15:353–355.

63. Ellenberg M, Weber H. Retrograde ejaculation in diabetic neuropathy. Ann Intern Med 1966;65:1237–1246.

64. Stewart BH, Bergant JA. Correction of retrograde ejaculation by sympathomimetic medication: preliminary report. Fertil Steril 1974; 25:1073–1074.

65. Abrahams JI, Solish GI, Boorjian P, et al. The surgical correction of retrograde ejaculation. J Urol 1975;114:888–890.

66. Middleton RG, Urry RL. The Young-Dees operation for the correction of retrograde ejaculation. J Urol 1986;136:1208–1209.

67. Crich JP, Jequier AM. Infertility in men with retrograde ejaculation: the action of urine on sperm motility, and a simple method for achieving antegrade ejaculation. Fertil Steril 1978;30:572–576.

68. Templeton A, Mortimer D. Successful circumvention of retrograde ejaculation in an infertile diabetic man. Case report. Br J Obstet Gynaecol 1982;89:1064–1065.

69. Riesner C. The etiology of retrograde ejaculation and a method for insemination. Fertil Steril 1961;12:488–492.

70. Fuselier HA Jr, Schneider GT, Ochsner MG. Successful artificial insemination following retrograde ejaculation. Fertil Steril 1976;27:1214–1215.

71. Thiagarajah S, Vaughan ED Jr, Kitchin JD III. Retrograde ejaculation: successful pregnancy following combined sympathomimetic medication and insemination. Fertil Steril 1978;30:96–97.

72. Vernon M, Wilson E, Muse K, et al. Successful pregnancies from men with retrograde ejaculation with the use of washed sperm and gamete intrafallopian tube transfer (GIFT). Fertil Steril 1988;50:822–824.

73. Otani T, Kondo A, Takita T. A paraplegic fathering a child after an intrathecal injection of neostigmine: a case report. Paraplegia 1985;23:32–37.

74. Spira R. Artificial insemination after intrathecal injection of neostigmine in a paraplegic. Lancet 1956;270:670–671.

75. Guttmann L, Walsh JJ. Prostigmine assessment test of fertility in spinal man. Paraplegia 1971;9:39–51.

76. Ushiyama T, Kusano S, Shibuya K, et al. The side effect of prostigmine test for male paraplegic. Proceedings of the 19th Annual Meeting of the Japanese Paraplegic Society, Fukuota, 1984:75.

77. Chapelle P-A, Blanquart F, Puech AJ, et al. Treatment of anejaculation in the total paraplegic by subcutaneous injection of physostigmine. Paraplegia 1983;21:30–36.

78. Jesionowska H, Hemmings R. Good-quality semen recovered from a paraplegic man with physostigmine salicylate treatment. A case report. J Reprod Med 1991;36:167–169.

79. Blockmans D, Steeno O. Physostigmine as a treatment for anejaculation with paraplegic men. Andrologia 1988;20:311–313.

80. Kelly ME, Needle MA. Imipramine for aspermia after lymphadenectomy. Urology 1979;13:414–415.

81. Lynch JH, Maxted WC. Use of ephedrine in post-lymphadenectomy ejaculatory failure. A case report. J Urol 1983;129:379.

82. Proctor KG, Howards SS. The effect of sympathomimetic drugs on postlymphadenectomy aspermia. J Urol 1983;129:837–838.

83. Schellen TMCM. Induction of ejaculation by electrovibration. Fertil Steril 1968;19:566–569.

84. Wheeler JS Jr, Walter JS, Culkin DJ, et al. Idiopathic anejaculation treated by vibratory stimulation. Fertil Steril 1988;50:377–379.

85. Brindley GS. Reflex ejaculation under vibratory stimulation in paraplegic men. Paraplegia 1981;19:299–302.

86. Sonksen J, Biering-Sorensen F, Kristensen JK. Penile vibratory ejaculation in men with spinal cord injury. J Urol 1993;149:437A.

87. Sobrero AJ, Stearns HE, Blair JH. Technique for the induction of ejaculation in humans. Fertil Steril 1965;16:765–767.

88. Comarr AE. Sexual function among patients with spinal cord injury. Urol Int 1970;23:134–168.

89. Francois N, Maury M, Jouannet D, et al. Electro-ejaculation of a complete paraplegic followed by pregnancy. Paraplegia 1978–1979; 16:248–251.

90. Oates RD, Staskin DR. Vibratory stimulation of ejaculation in the spinal cord injured male. Presented at the American Fertility Society Annual Meeting, San Francisco, 1989.

91. Elliot S, Szasz G, Zouves C. The combined use of vibrostimulation and in vitro fertilization: successful pregnancy outcome from a retrograde specimen obtain from a spinal cord injured male. J In Vitro Fertil Embryo Transfer 1991;8:348–352.

92. Gunn RM. Fertility in sheep: artificial production of seminal ejaculation and characteristics of the spermatozoa contained therein. Council for Scientific and Industrial Research Bulletin 1936;94:1.

93. Dziuk PJ, Graham EF, Donrek JD, et al. Some observations in collections of semen from bulls, goats, boars and rams by electrical stimulation. Vet Med 1954;49:455.

94. Seager SW, Wild DE, Platz C. Semen collection by electroejaculation and artificial vagina in over 100 species of animals. Proceedings of the 9th International Congress on Reproduction, 1980:571.

95. Seager SW. The breeding of captive wild species by artificial methods. Zool Biol 1983;2:235.

96. Horne HW, Paull DP, Munro D. Fertility studies in the human male with traumatic injuries of the spinal cord and cauda equina. N Engl J Med 1948;239:959–961.

97. Thomas RJS, McLeish G, McDonald IA. Electroejaculation of the paraplegic male followed by pregnancy. Med J Aust 1975;2:798–799.

98. Lipshultz LI, Witt MA, Grantmyre JE. Electroejaculation. Infertil Reprod Med Clin North Am 1992;3:455–467.

99. David A, Ohry A, Rozin R. Spinal cord injuries: male infertility aspects. Paraplegia 1977–1978;15:11–14.

100. Bennett CJ, Seager SW, Vasher EA, et al. Sexual dysfunction and electroejaculation in men with spinal cord injury: review. J Urol 1988;139:453–457.

101. Bennett CJ, Ohl DA. Electroejaculation after retroperitoneal lymph node dissection. In: Lytton B, Catalona WJ, Lipshultz LI, et al, editors. Advances in Urology. Vol 2. Chicago: Year Book Medical, 1989:85–95.

102. Lucas MG, Hargreave TB, Edmond P, et al. Sperm retrieval by electroejaculation. Preliminary experience in patients with secondary anejaculation. Br J Urol 1991;67:191–194.

103. Shaban SF, Oates RD, Lipshultz LI. Experience with rectal probe electroejaculation in 30 patients. 44th Annual Meeting of the American Fertility Society, Reno. 1988; Fertil Steril (Suppl) P-014.

104. Stewart DE, Ohl DA. Idiopathic anejaculation treated by electroejaculation. Int J Psychiatry Med 1989;19:263–268.

105. Ohl DA, Denil J, Bennett CJ, et al. Electroejaculation following retroperitoneal lymphadenectomy. J Urol 1991;145:980–983.

106. Toledo AA, Tucker MJ, Bennett JK, et al. Electroejaculation in combination with in vitro fertilization and gamete micromanipulation for treatment of anejaculatory male infertility. Am J Obstet Gynecol 1992;167:322–326.

107. Blank W, Batzofin J, Tran C, et al. The use of electroejaculation and zygote intrafallopian transfer to achieve a pregnancy after a major gunshot wound to the abdomen: a unique application. Fertil Steril 1990;54:950–952.

108. Randolph JF Jr, Ohl DA, Bennett CJ, et al. Combined electroejaculation and in vitro fertilization in the evaluation and treatment of anejaculatory infertility. J In Vitro Fertil Embryo Transfer 1990;7:58–62.

109. Denil J, Ohl DA, Menge AC, et al. Functional characteristics of sperm obtained by electroejaculation. J Urol 1992;147:69–72.

110. Hirsch IH, Sedor J, Callahan HJ, et al. Systemic sperm autoimmunity in spinal-cord injured men. Arch Androl 1990;25:69–73.

111. Ohl DA, Bennett CJ, McCabe M, et al. Predictors of success in electroejaculation of spinal cord injured men. J Urol 1989;142:1483–1486.

112. Billups KL, Tillman S, Chang TSK. Ablation of the inferior mesenteric plexus in the rat: alteration of sperm storage in the epididymis and vas deferens. J Urol 1990;143:625–629.

113. Billups KL, Tillman S, Chang TSK. Reduction of epididymal sperm motility after ablation of the inferior mesenteric plexus in the rat. Fertil Steril 1990;53:1076–1082.

114. Honig SC, Dubay A, Oates RD. Successful microscopic sperm aspiration and pregnancies in patients with obstructive azoospermia/severe oligoasthenospermia. J Urol 1992;147:398A.

115. Colpi GM, Nigri L, Stamm J, et al. Full term pregnancy obtained with sperm recovered by seminal tract washout from an anejaculatory man [letter]. J Urol 1992;148:1266–1267.

116. Hirsch IH, Jeyendran RS, Sedor J, et al. Biochemical analysis of electroejaculates in spinal cord injured men: comparison to normal ejaculates. J Urol 1991;145:73–76.

117. Witt MA, Grantmyre JE, Lomas M, et al. The effect on semen quality

of the electrical current and heat generated during rectal probe electro-ejaculation. J Urol 1992;147:747–749.

118. Linsenmeyer T, Wilmot C, Anderson RU. The effects of the electroejac-ulation procedure on sperm motility. Paraplegia 1989;27:465–469.

119. Honig SC, Lomas M, Grossman S, et al. Functional character of in vitro electroejaculation. Accepted for Presentation at the American Fertility Society Annual Meeting, Montreal, 1993.

120. Honig SC, Amar L, Thompson ST, et al. Repeated sequential rectal probe electroejaculation in a short interval improves semen quality in anejaculatory men. J Urol 1993;149:437A.

121. Sikka SC, Wang R, Fussell EN, et al. Morphological evaluation of human sperm after in vitro stimulation by electric current. Fertil Steril 1992;(suppl):S115.

122. Gross AJ, Michl UH. Functional characteristics of sperm obtained by electroejaculation [letter]. J Urol 1993;149:380.

123. Siösteen A, Forssman L, Steen Y, et al. Quality of semen after repeated ejaculation treatment in spinal cord injury men. Paraplegia 1990; 28:96–104.

124. Bustillo M, Rajfer J. Pregnancy following insemination with sperm aspirated directly from vas deferens. Fertil Steril 1986;46:144–145.

125. Berger RE, Muller CH, Smith D, et al. Operative recovery of vasal sperm from anejaculatory men: preliminary report. J Urol 1986; 135:948–949.

126. Sikka SC, Hellstrom WJG. The application of pentoxifylline in the stimulation of sperm motion in men undergoing electroejaculation. J Androl 1991;12:165–170.

126a. Virupannavar C, Tomera F. An unusual case of retrograde ejaculation and a brief review of management. Fertil Steril 1982;37:275–276.

127. Brindley GS, Sauerwein D, Hendry WF. Hypogastric plexus stimulators for obtaining semen from paraplegic men. Br J Urol 1989;64:72–77.

128. Hübner WA, Trigo-Rocha F, Schmidt RA, et al. Laparoscopic implanta-tion of electrodes for stimulation of the hypogastric nerve and the vas deferens in dogs. J Urol 1993;149:624–626.

CHAPTER 45

Sperm Cryopreservation

DON P. WOLF

Normal human sperm, when appropriately processed and protected, retain viability during freezing, prolonged exposure to extremely low temperatures, and thawing. This process of sperm cryopreservation provides the basis for both husband or homologous insemination (TI) and for the use of quarantine donor semen (heterologous) in therapeutic insemination (TDI), an established medical procedure with worldwide application.

Many early endeavors in cryobiology, dating back as far as 100 years, employed sperm as experimental cells based on their availability (ease of collection), readily apparent measure of cellular integrity (motility), number, and small size. This was advantageous for andrology and future clinical application because it led to the development of successful sperm cryopreservation protocols. However, many of the principles of cryobiology were overlooked during these early studies, reflecting in part the uniqueness of the sperm cell, that is, its relatively low water content and high surface-to-volume ratio. Moreover, the high cell number in semen meant that fertility retention was possible in the face of very low survival levels. The successful cryopreservation of larger, more hydrated cells awaited the development of an appreciation for the importance of cooling and warming rates and seeding for intracellular ice crystal formation. As a case in point, protocols for the cryopreservation of mammalian embryos were not developed until the 1970s. It is also noteworthy that the empirically derived protocols currently available for human semen, developed in large measure from experience with domestic animal sperm, do not often apply with the same degree of success to the semen of other mammalian species.[1]

The routine cryopreservation of human semen became a reality only after the serendipitous discovery of the cryoprotective properties of glycerol by Polge and coworkers in 1949.[2] This observation, that sperm motility could be recovered following semen storage at low temperature in glycerol, raised the question of whether such cells retained fertilizing capacity; that is, did freezing affect the ability of sperm to fertilize the egg and induce normal embryonic development? An answer to this question was provided in 1953 when pregnancies were reported in patients inseminated with sperm previously frozen and stored on dry ice ($-78°C$).[3] A decade later the liquid nitrogen vapor technique for the freezing of human semen, with subsequent storage at $-196°C$,

was introduced with additional reports of pregnancy success.[4]

To answer the more demanding question of whether deoxyribonucleic acid damage occurred during cryopreservation, it was necessary to accrue large numbers of offspring produced with frozen-thawed semen. After some 24,000 births worldwide, survey data summarized by Sherman[5] gave a 1% incidence of abnormal progeny and a 13% incidence of spontaneous abortions, with both values well within the range associated with the use of nonfrozen sperm. It has even been suggested that cryopreservation "freezes out defective sperm," resulting in lowered frequencies of birth defects and spontaneous abortions following TDI with frozen donor sperm.[6] Cryoinduced damage detected by chromosomal assessment has also been directly evaluated on sperm that fused with and were decondensed by the ooplasm of zona-free hamster eggs.[6] Cryopreservation did not affect the frequencies or types of chromosomal abnormalities in the sperm from 10 normal men.

APPLICATIONS IN HUMAN REPRODUCTIVE MEDICINE

Cryopreservation associated with homologous insemination is often considered before surgical, chemical, or radiologic therapy that endangers the donor's reproductive integrity. This is a common practice, for instance, *before* medical treatments for malignant disease, because alkylating and other chemotherapeutic agents cause azoospermia in most treated adult males with only a small likelihood that these men will eventually recover spermatogenesis after therapy is discontinued. As an extension to this approach, feasibility studies have also been conducted on semen collection and cryopreservation *during* chemotherapy with encouraging results,[7] which should prove beneficial to men who do not complete the banking process before therapy is begun.

Another application of cryopreservation concerns "fertility insurance" for the vasectomy candidate. The high probability that antisperm antibodies will form postvasectomy with implications for fertility and the relatively high cost of vasovasostomy, make the banking of semen prior to vasectomy an attractive alternative for some men.

Semen banking is also of value in the treatment of infertility via the assisted reproductive technologies. Men who anticipate problems in collecting a sample during in vitro fertilization or gamete intrafallopian transfer can bank a sample in advance of the procedure for use in the event a freshly collected ejaculate is unobtainable.

Attempts to accumulate sperm by freezing multiple ejaculates from the oligospermic patient are usually unsuccessful because abnormal semen specimens tolerate cryopreservation poorly. In view of this limitation, the low rate of success, and the necessity of collecting and preparing multiple specimens, this approach is not recommended. Parenthetically, two or three ejaculates can be collected over a 24-hour period, processed, and stored at ambient temperature with the option of combining samples for intrauterine insemination (IUI).

Cryopreservation is essential to TDI because the risk of infectious disease transmission must be minimized by sample quarantine. TDI can be used when genetic problems exist in the husband, severe semen abnormalities are present, the patient is single, or as a backup in the assisted reproductive technologies.

FACTORS AFFECTING SPERM CRYOSURVIVAL

The principal determinants in cell survival following freezing include size, shape, hydration state, and membrane permeability properties. In fact, the cell response can be predicted, given information on its permeability coefficient, surface area, the osmotic gradient between outside and inside, and the temperature.[8] A discussion of additional factors as they relate specifically to sperm cryosurvival follows.

Maturation Stage at Storage

Motile sperm represent the cells of interest for cryopreservation, which is normally accomplished in the presence of seminal plasma. Prior to acquiring fertilizing ability, these cells must undergo a final maturation step called *capacitation*, which occurs during sperm transit in the female reproductive tract or following sperm processing in vitro. Thus, the motile, seminal sperm population available for cryopreservation is in a noncapacitated state. In view of the increased use of washed sperm for IUI, protocols for the cryopreservation of washed, capacitating sperm would be of interest. At least one such approach has been reported.[9]

Sperm Processing

Semen should be allowed to liquefy for 30 to 60 minutes prior to cryoprotectant addition. The mechanism of action of cryoprotectants, which includes a lowering of the freezing point of the solution and cellular dehydration, is incompletely understood. Glycerol is more effective in buffering the effects of low temperature on human sperm than is dimethyl sulfoxide or propanediol even though the latter cryoprotectants also dehydrate and lower the solution freezing point. Parenthetically, these latter two cryoprotectants are preferred

in the cryopreservation of human one- to eight-cell stage embryos. Although there are scattered reports of human sperm banking in the absence of glycerol, most freezing is done in the presence of a final concentration of glycerol in the 5% to 10% range, often in the presence of various extenders, such as hen's egg yolk and citrate, to name a few. A systematic evaluation of several commonly employed buffers and extenders can be found in an article by Prins and Weidel.[10]

Temperature Shock, Seeding, and Cooling Rate

Temperature shock or damage induced in sperm during cooling to the freezing point is often limiting in the successful low-temperature storage of domestic animal sperm.[1] Such damage may reflect transition changes in membrane lipids that are critical to cell survival. Human sperm do not experience temperature shock.[11]

Seeding, or the induction of ice crystal formation in supercooled mixtures during cryopreservation, is critical to survival of large, hydrated cells such as eggs and embryos but is not commonly included in sperm freezing protocols. In a report by Critser and coworkers,[12] seeding resulted in only modest enhancements in sperm cryosurvival.

The use of optimum cooling rates is also critical to cryosurvival for many cell types because it influences the extent and rate of dehydration; however, human sperm are tolerant of a wide range of cooling rates from 0.5° to 50°C/min.

Duration of Storage

The biochemical processes that occur in cells stored in liquid nitrogen are negligible, with the major risk of storage damage restricted to the accumulated exposure to cosmic radiation. Hundreds of years may be required before radiation damage becomes significant.[8] Nevertheless, the evidence or bias persists that a decline in sperm survival occurs over time of storage. If such a decline occurs, it may reflect improper storage, for instance, transient but repeated exposure to ambient temperature during sample accessing. The judicious recommendation would therefore be that storage time is limited, perhaps to 10 years.

Temperature of Storage

Semen storage at −80° to −85°C, in a mechanical freezer, may be as efficacious as storage in liquid nitrogen at −196°C based on motility recovery.[13] Despite this finding, long-term semen storage usually is conducted at −196°C in liquid nitrogen. The use of dry ice at −135°C for shipping is not recommended, because sample contact with the refrigerant cannot always be ensured.

Warming Rate

Frozen semen samples are tolerant of a wide range of warming rates. Normally, samples are thawed at ambient temperature or in a 37°C water bath.

Semen Quality

With human sperm, initial semen quality is probably the most significant single factor in determining cryosurvival. This empirically derived conclusion probably simply reflects the fact that highly viable cell populations are more capable of surviving the insults of cryopreservation than are their less viable counterparts. This is consistent with the generally accepted notion that patients with abnormal semen parameters cryopreserve poorly. On the high end of the quality spectrum, however, this relationship is not so obvious, because even pregnancy-proven donors show wide variations in sperm cryosurvival.[14]

CRYOSURVIVAL

Although no entirely satisfactory laboratory method is available for measuring cryosurvival, the process is routinely assessed by postthaw motility scores, determined in the presence of cryoprotectant. The premise, of course, is that the easily measured parameter of motility is reflective of fertility. A minimum standard of 50% survival of the initial motile sperm population is expected.

The kinetics of motility loss after thawing and cryoprotectant removal (stress test) can also be used in quality evaluation. To conduct a stress test, sperm are washed free of cryoprotectant and then incubated in an appropriate medium at 37°C for as long as 24 hours. Computer-assisted semen analysis can be used to quantitate changes in individual sperm trajectories induced by freeze-thawing. Cryoprotectant addition and removal alone without freezing induces only minor changes in the percentage of motile cells and in the averaged individual parameters of motility such as curvilinear and straightline velocity, linearity, amplitude of lateral head displacement, and beat-cross frequency. In contrast, freezing is usually associated with an immediate decline in the percentage of motile cells and time-dependent declines in curvilinear velocity and in the mean amplitude of lateral head displacement. Within 24 hours of thawing, the percentage of cryopreserved sperm that retain motility is low (10%) compared with a greater than 50% survival in nonfrozen controls. This increased lability of cryopreserved sperm carries obvious implications for the timing of therapeutic insemination.

A stress test can also be conducted, postthaw, on the sample before processing, that is, measured in the presence of cryoprotectant at 37°C. Holt and coworkers[15] used such an approach over a 3.5-hour incubation in a comparison of two groups of TI donors, those with presumed high versus low fecundity. The mean (SEM) velocities for the groups at 0 time were 65.9 (1.8) and 50.4 (3.2) and, after 3.5 hours, 42.1 (2.1) and 24.7 (5.7), respectively. The conclusion was reached that, despite the absence of significant differences in prefreeze semen parameters, the velocity differences measured postthaw in washed sperm were correlated with fertility estimates.

With domestic animals, cryodamage is often monitored not only by motility measures but also by quantitative assessments of acrosomal status.[1] Because acrosomal and plasma membrane damage also appear as sequelae of human sperm cryopreservation,[13, 16] this approach should be considered

clinically. Indirect immunofluorescence assays for this purpose are readily available.[17]

The sperm penetration assay has been used by Critser and coworkers[12] to evaluate cryosurvival; however, this assay is cumbersome and impractical as a routine test for large sample numbers.

CRYOPRESERVATION OF HUMAN SPERM

Several itemized semen freezing protocols have been published by Sherman.[18] The following protocol is from the Oregon Health Sciences University; however, several general comments are appropriate before considering the detailed procedure. As indicated earlier, glycerol is the cryoprotectant of choice for mammalian sperm cryopreservation; however, glycerol toxicity at high concentrations has been described.[19] Direct addition of glycerol to semen is possible but at the risk of sperm damage induced by the localized high glycerol concentrations that can occur. Consequently, special attention should be devoted to mixing with the direct addition approach. The final glycerol concentration may also contribute to cryosurvival,[20] as can the presence or absence of extenders. The latter are available commercially. Several culture media have been used in human semen cryopreservation, and although a comparative study expressing preferences is available,[10] medium requirements are probably of limited concern given adequate pH stability, ionic composition, and energy sources. The protein additive used may be of comparable importance.

The use of biologic, controlled-rate freezers for human sperm cryopreservation has led to the suggestion that slow freezing may result in improved motility recoveries.[21, 22] Nevertheless, many programs still use a fast-freezing protocol in liquid nitrogen vapor.

In the detailed protocol that follows, the ratio of semen to cryoprotectant has been adjusted from 1:1 to 3:1 to increase sperm concentration, thereby reducing storage volume. This is a test yolk medium with a liquid nitrogen vapor freezing procedure modified from an Irvine Scientific bulletin dated 11/14/88. A list of materials with possible suppliers is included in Table 45–1.

Precautions

Semen is a biologic hazard and may contain infectious agents. Discard all waste by hospital-accepted protocols. Glycerol is viscous, and accurate measurement requires patience, care, and cleanliness. After loading glycerol into the measuring pipette, be sure to carefully wipe the outside of the pipette with a clean tissue before addition to the extender or sample. Alternatively, add glycerol on the basis of weight instead of volume. Be aware of the hazards of working with liquid nitrogen and its vapor because severe burns can result. Additionally, asphyxiation can result if large spills occur in poorly ventilated areas. Wear gloves and goggles for protection, and work in a well-ventilated area.

TABLE 45–1. Sperm Cryopreservation Materials and Suppliers

Materials	Source
Freezing medium-TEST yolk buffer (TYB) with glycerol stored at −20°C	Irvine Scientific, Santa Ana, CA
Glycerol C₃H₅ (OH)₃	American Scientific Products, McGaw Park, IL
Specimen collection container: size 4 oz (118 mL)	Baxter Scientific, McGaw Park, IL
Disposable sterile 15 mL conical plastic centrifuge tubes, Falcon No. 2095	Becton Dickinson, Oxnard, CA
Disposable sterile 1 mL serologic pipettes, Falcon No. 7521	Becton Dickinson, Oxnard, CA
Disposable sterile Pasteur pipette (washed glass); 5¾ in., No. 13-678-20B	Fisher Scientific, Pittsburgh, PA
Disposable sterile 3-mL syringes and 20-gauge needles	Monoject, Division of Sherwood Medical, St. Louis, MO
Laminar flow hood—vertical flow	Baker Company, Sanford, ME
Water bath	Baxter Scientific, McGaw Park, IL
Gloves, pharmaseal	Baxter Scientific, McGaw Park, IL
Nunc Cryotubes, 3-66656	Cryogenics Northwest, Seattle, WA
Sharpies permanent marker; black, fine-point	Sanford Corporation, Bellwood, IL
Labels, colored tape	Baxter Scientific, McGaw Park, IL
Adjustable pipettes, Gilson Pipetman, P-20 and P-100	Rainin Instrument Company, Emeryville, CA
Microman positive displacement pipette-M50	Rainin Instrument Company, Wolburn, MA
Disposable tips; Clean-Pak-S presterilized pipette tips, No. RT-20s	Rainin Instrument Company, Emeryville, CA
Wands (canes); cane for holding cryotubes, No. A-2	Cryogenics Northwest, Seattle, WA
Cryogenic refrigerators (freezer or tanks); storage units for semen, embryos, or biological samples at liquid nitrogen temperatures	Cryogenics Northwest, Seattle, WA, or Minnesota Valley Engineering, New Prague, MN
Dewar; wide-mouth liquid nitrogen storage unit, LD series	Cryogenics Northwest, Seattle, WA
Kimwipes	Kimberly-Clark Corporation, Roswell, GA
Hemacytometer; bright-line hemacytometer	Reichert-Jung, Cambridge Instruments, Inc., Buffalo, NY
Liquid nitrogen	Polar, Portland, OR

Semen Collection

The sperm donor should abstain sexually for 24 to 72 hours but not more than 5 days prior to producing an ejaculate to be cryopreserved. A short abstinence period is associated with reduced counts, whereas samples collected after prolonged abstinence typically show reduced motility and morphology.

Procedure

1. Make up TEST-modified cryoprotectant (giving 29.6% glycerol) just before use by adding 1 mL of glycerol (100%) to 4 mL of commercially available TEST Yolk Buffer with glycerol (12%). Measure the glycerol carefully. After addition of glycerol, thoroughly wash the inside of the pipette by aspirating the TEST-modified cryoprotectant mixture in and out of the pipette. This mixture can be filter sterilized with a 0.45 µL filter. A 1:4 dilution of this stock will give a final glycerol concentration of 7.4%.

2. Allow semen to liquefy for 30 minutes at 37°C. Note that samples with high viscosity may require the additional step of repeated pipetting with a sterile Pasteur pipette or passage through an 18-gauge needle to reduce viscosity and to ensure thorough mixing.

3. After thorough mixing, transfer the entire sample using a sterile serologic pipette to a prelabeled sterile 15-mL conical tube. Measure and record the volume.

4. Remove aliquots using a positive displacement pipette (2 × 10 µL) for analysis. Determine the count and motility. Note any abnormalities.

5. Samples from *donors*: record semen information on a sperm donation record form (Fig. 45–1), including date, donor number, and donation number. Samples from *patients*: record name, medical record number, and semen information on a patient cryopreservation form (Fig. 45–2).

6. Determine the amount of cryoprotectant to be added using a ratio of three parts of semen to one part of cryoprotectant.

7. Add, at ambient temperature, the predetermined amount of cryoprotectant drop by drop using a sterile serologic pipette. Mix well by gently pipetting up and down. Do not vortex.

8. Label Nunc Cryotubes with a permanent marker as follows (Fig. 45–3): Place the tube so that the screw top is to the left as you write in the label area. For the *donor* sample, write the donor (always four digits); under that, write the donation number (three digits); below that, write the vial number (two digits starting with 01, 02, and so forth). For *patients,* write the name, medical record number, and date on the Nunc Cryotube, again having the screw cap to your left as you write in the label area.

9. Transfer the sample to prelabeled Nunc Cryotubes. Fill the cryotube with no more than 90% of the tube's volume to permit sample expansion during freezing. Be sure the cryotube screw cap is tightened normally; overtightening distorts the seal and risks leakage. Be sure that the thread of the cryotube screw cap is completely dry before closing; liquid drops impair the seal in liquid nitrogen. Always set up a vial to be thawed for test thaw results. This vial can be filled with only 0.5 mL.

10. Place the cryotubes/vials at the top of the wand at the first clip located just below the labeling area. Use one wand for each vial.

11. Place the wands upside down and completely submerged in an ambient temperature bath. (A 600-mL plastic beaker can be used filled with 600 mL of water.)

12. Transfer the bath (plastic beaker) containing the wands to a 4°C refrigerator for 1.5 hours to allow slow cooling of the sperm and cryoprotectant mixture (−0.2°/min).

13. After the 4°C exposure, transfer the wands (right side up) to a Dewar flask or similar insulated jar containing enough liquid nitrogen so that the vials are 2 to 4 in. above the liquid nitrogen level. Leave the wands and vials suspended in the vapors for 30 to 45 minutes.

14. To avoid exposure to room temperature, work in the vapors of a wide-mouth Dewar flask containing liquid nitrogen. Transfer the vials from each donor or patient to prelabeled wands for permanent storage in a liquid nitrogen tank

OHSU Andrology Lab

Sperm Donation Record

DATA ENTRY
entered in bank.dbf_____
entered in donate.dbf____
post-thaw entered_____

DONOR NO._____

DONATION NO._____

DATE OF DONATION_____   FREEZING PROTOCOL: TEST, TEST-MODIFIED
                                                    circle one

SEMEN DATA

    INITIAL: Vol(ml):____   Count:_____   Motility:_____ %

        IS SAMPLE ADEQUATE?_____

    POST-THAW: Vol(ml):____   Count:_____   Motility:_____ %

        Total Motile/ml:_____   Total Motile/Vial:____

        FREEZE THAW TEST SUCCESSFUL(Y/N):_____

ABNORMAL MOTILE FORMS	Kinked	Pinhead	Looped	Other
%				

LOCATION/# OF SPECIMENS/VIALS

_____ CRYOPRESERVATION

    # of Vials:_____   Volume/Vial:_____mls

Spec#	Tank	Bucket	Wand	
____	____	____	____	For Tanks 1-5, all specimens will be listed under one wand #;
____			____	
____			____	
____			____	For Tanks 6-11, each specimen
____			____	has its own wand
____			____	(i.e., slot #)
____			____	

_____ CONTROL (circle: SPA, IBT, ABS, RES, OTH)

_____ RESEARCH

_____ DISCARD

_____ OTHER
_____

_____ TOTAL SPECIMENS OBTAINED

wp\forms\blue.she

FIGURE 45-1. Sperm donation record form.

OREGON HEALTH SCIENCES UNIVERSITY

Andrology/Embryology Labs
(503) 494-8261

Date:
Unit No.:
Name:
Birthdate:

PATIENT CRYOPRESERVATION RECORD

Referring Physician: _____   Contact's Name: _____

Indication: Vasectomy, Cancer, IVF, TIH, Misc., Known Donor, GIFT

Freeze Date:_____   Indication:_____

FRESH SEMEN DATA, FREEZE ___ | POST-THAW SEMEN DATA, FREEZE ___
Volume:_____ Viscosity:_____
Count:_____ Morphology:____ %
   Motility:____%
   Forward Progression:_____
   Round Cells:_____

   Count:_____
   Motility:_____
   Forward Progression:_____
   Total Motile per ml: _____
   Motile Morphology (% normal)

VIAL #	TANK	BUCKET	WAND	Volume/Vial	Usage Date	T.M./Vial
___	___	___	___	___	___	___
___	___	___	___	___	___	___
___	___	___	___	___	___	___
___	___	___	___	___	___	___
___	___	___	___	___	___	___

Freeze Date:_____   Indication:_____

FRESH SEMEN DATA, FREEZE ___ | POST-THAW SEMEN DATA, FREEZE ___
Volume:_____ Viscosity:_____
Count:_____ Morphology:____ %
   Motility:____%
   Forward Progression:_____
   Round Cells:_____

   Count:_____
   Motility:_____
   Forward Progression:_____
   Total Motile per ml: _____
   Motile Morphology (% normal)

VIAL #	TANK	BUCKET	WAND	Volume/Vial	Usage Date	T.M./Vial
___	___	___	___	___	___	___
___	___	___	___	___	___	___
___	___	___	___	___	___	___
___	___	___	___	___	___	___
___	___	___	___	___	___	___

Freeze Date:_____   Indication:_____

FRESH SEMEN DATA, FREEZE ___ | POST-THAW SEMEN DATA, FREEZE ___
Volume:_____ Viscosity:_____
Count:_____ Morphology:____ %
   Motility:____%
   Forward Progression:_____
   Round Cells:_____

   Count:_____
   Motility:_____
   Forward Progression:_____
   Total Motile per ml: _____
   Motile Morphology (% normal)

VIAL #	TANK	BUCKET	WAND	Volume/Vial	Usage Date	T.M./Vial
___	___	___	___	___	___	___
___	___	___	___	___	___	___
___	___	___	___	___	___	___
___	___	___	___	___	___	___

FIGURE 45–2. Patient cryopreservation record form.

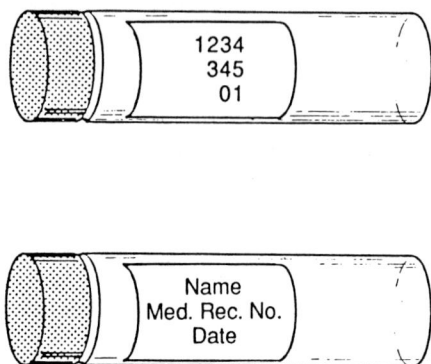

FIGURE 45–3. Cryotube labeling system for Oregon Health Sciences University sperm bank. *Upper*, Donor sample. *Lower*, Patient sample.

or freezer. For *donors,* place vial number one at the bottom of the wand and work upward, ending with vial number six at the top. Use more wands, if needed, that have been prelabeled with the same wand number. For *patients,* place the vials on prelabeled wands starting at the bottom and work to the top of the wand.

15. Place all vials in preassigned liquid nitrogen tank/freezer for storage. Test vials can be thawed at a later time to determine the number of total motile sperm per vial.

16. Record the number of vials (excluding test vial) and their location in the storage container (the bucket or drawer number; the wand number or slot number in the drawer) on the appropriate donor or patient form.

17. Log donor and patient information into the computer.

Quality Assurance

Trial thaw values for donors should contain a minimum of 30 million motile sperm per sample (sample size may vary but will usually be 1 mL). All sperm banking activities must be supported by extensive record keeping. An example of a specimen-usage record form is presented in Figure 45–4.

Thawing Frozen Semen

Check the aluminum cane to make sure that you have the correct number of vials and that the cane is marked with the correct patient name or donor identification number. *Most important, never expose frozen vials to room temperature until you are ready to thaw the vial, and never use an inadequately identified sample.*

To thaw a vial, remove the cane with the desired vial from the tank, remove the vial from the cane, and simply let the vial stand at room temperature until thawing is complete, generally 10 to 20 minutes. Thawing may be hastened by holding the vial in your hand, or exposure to warm, body temperature water. Vials just removed from liquid nitrogen will be extremely cold and should not come in contact with bare skin.

When the vial is completely thawed, unscrew the cap and aspirate the contents into your insemination device or pipette in the event you are going to process the sample before insemination. You should check sperm motility under the

microscope to ensure that sperm have survived the freezing process. Be sure the sample has warmed to ambient temperature before assessing motility, and also examine the motile sperm population for morphologic abnormalities. A minimum of 30% of the cells should be progressively motile.

PRACTICAL APPLICATION OF SEMEN CRYOPRESERVATION

The monthly fecundity, or probability of conception, for TDI is a function of a large number of parameters that are beyond the scope of this chapter (see Chapter 47). In general, cycle fecundities, as established in the 1970s and 1980s with fresh donor semen using an intracervical route of insemination, were in the range of 15% to 20%. With the transition to the exclusive use of quarantined, cryopreserved semen, expectations and realizations have declined, although several reports are available citing results within the fresh semen range quoted earlier when multiple intracervical inseminations are performed.[15, 23] Moreover, when studies have been conducted comparing intracervical insemination with IUI, the latter is clearly superior in a single timed insemination with donor semen or the washed sperm from semen.[24, 25]

Because of the increased lability of cryopreserved sperm, the method employed in sperm preparation for IUI is critical. In the protocol detailed here, a simple wash by repeated centrifugation-resuspension is used. However, it is recognized that less damaging methods to separate motile sperm from semen and cryoprotectant are desirable. In a recent study, Percoll-separated sperm showed decreased motility, viability, and acrosomal integrity in comparison with sperm washed with or without Sephadex filtration.[26]

Proceeding on the supposition that cryopreserved sperm are at a disadvantage in fertilization in part because of their low swimming speed and inability to generate the minimum thrust required to penetrate cervical mucus or the zona pellucida, or both, strategies designed to stimulate motility have been attempted.[27] These authors tested caffeine, pentoxifylline, 2-deoxyadenosine, cyclic adenosine monophosphate, relaxin, adenosine, kallikrein, and calcium and concluded that cryopreserved sperm were consistently stimulated (velocity or percentage of motile sperm) only by caffeine, pentoxifylline, and 2-deoxyadenosine. When these chemical stimulants were examined in greater detail, pentoxifylline treatment was concluded to be superior. However, the efficacy of motility stimulants used either acutely or chronically has yet to be established.

Patient Semen

A major concern in homologous TI is when and how much semen to freeze. The success of the freezing process varies between individuals as well as potentially between semen samples, and expectations are lowered when male factors are present. The recommendation for a person to proceed with cryopreservation is, thus, most appropriately made following a trial freeze. Based on the postthaw recovery of motile sperm, conception rates for the current technology and individual needs and time constraints, the patient, with the advice of his physician, can decide how many samples to freeze.

B [ ]   Specimen #:_____   Usage Type: [ ] AIDIUI [ ] AIDTBW   Name:_____
F [ ]   Location: [ ] OHSU   [ ] OHOT   [ ] _____   Med Rec #:_____
S [ ]   [ ] NOOT [ ] LSHP   [ ] SHIP   _____(MD)   N₂ (liq): [ ] YES

B [ ]   Specimen #:_____   Usage Type: [ ] AIDIUI [ ] AIDTBW   Name:_____
F [ ]   Location: [ ] OHSU   [ ] OHOT   [ ] _____   Med Rec #:_____
S [ ]   [ ] NOOT [ ] LSHP   [ ] SHIP   _____(MD)   N₂ (liq): [ ] YES

B [ ]   Specimen #:_____   Usage Type: [ ] AIDIUI [ ] AIDTBW   Name:_____
F [ ]   Location: [ ] OHSU   [ ] OHOT   [ ] _____   Med Rec #:_____
S [ ]   [ ] NOOT [ ] LSHP   [ ] SHIP   _____(MD)   N₂ (liq): [ ] YES

B [ ]   Specimen #:_____   Usage Type: [ ] AIDIUI [ ] AIDTBW   Name:_____
F [ ]   Location: [ ] OHSU   [ ] OHOT   [ ] _____   Med Rec #:_____
S [ ]   [ ] NOOT [ ] LSHP   [ ] SHIP   _____(MD)   N₂ (liq): [ ] YES

B [ ]   Specimen #:_____   Usage Type: [ ] AIDIUI [ ] AIDTBW   Name:_____
F [ ]   Location: [ ] OHSU   [ ] OHOT   [ ] _____   Med Rec #:_____
S [ ]   [ ] NOOT [ ] LSHP   [ ] SHIP   _____(MD)   N₂ (liq): [ ] YES

B [ ]   Specimen #:_____   Usage Type: [ ] AIDIUI [ ] AIDTBW   Name:_____
F [ ]   Location: [ ] OHSU   [ ] OHOT   [ ] _____   Med Rec #:_____
S [ ]   [ ] NOOT [ ] LSHP   [ ] SHIP   _____(MD)   N₂ (liq): [ ] YES

B [ ]   Specimen #:_____   Usage Type: [ ] AIDIUI [ ] AIDTBW   Name:_____
F [ ]   Location: [ ] OHSU   [ ] OHOT   [ ] _____   Med Rec #:_____
S [ ]   [ ] NOOT [ ] LSHP   [ ] SHIP   _____(MD)   N₂ (liq): [ ] YES

B [ ]   Specimen #:_____   Usage Type: [ ] AIDIUI [ ] AIDTBW   Name:_____
F [ ]   Location: [ ] OHSU   [ ] OHOT   [ ] _____   Med Rec #:_____
S [ ]   [ ] NOOT [ ] LSHP   [ ] SHIP   _____(MD)   N₂ (liq): [ ] YES

B [ ]   Specimen #:_____   Usage Type: [ ] AIDIUI [ ] AIDTBW   Name:_____
F [ ]   Location: [ ] OHSU   [ ] OHOT   [ ] _____   Med Rec #:_____
S [ ]   [ ] NOOT [ ] LSHP   [ ] SHIP   _____(MD)   N₂ (liq): [ ] YES

B [ ]   Specimen #:_____   Usage Type: [ ] AIDIUI [ ] AIDTBW   Name:_____
F [ ]   Location: [ ] OHSU   [ ] OHOT   [ ] _____   Med Rec #:_____
S [ ]   [ ] NOOT [ ] LSHP   [ ] SHIP   _____(MD)   N₂ (liq): [ ] YES

B [ ]   Specimen #:_____   Usage Type: [ ] AIDIUI [ ] AIDTBW   Name:_____
F [ ]   Location: [ ] OHSU   [ ] OHOT   [ ] _____   Med Rec #:_____
S [ ]   [ ] NOOT [ ] LSHP   [ ] SHIP   _____(MD)   N₂ (liq): [ ] YES

B [ ]   Specimen #:_____   Usage Type: [ ] AIDIUI [ ] AIDTBW   Name:_____
F [ ]   Location: [ ] OHSU   [ ] OHOT   [ ] _____   Med Rec #:_____
S [ ]   [ ] NOOT [ ] LSHP   [ ] SHIP   _____(MD)   N₂ (liq): [ ] YES

B [ ]   Specimen #:_____   Usage Type: [ ] AIDIUI [ ] AIDTBW   Name:_____
F [ ]   Location: [ ] OHSU   [ ] OHOT   [ ] _____   Med Rec #:_____
S [ ]   [ ] NOOT [ ] LSHP   [ ] SHIP   _____(MD)   N₂ (liq): [ ] YES

Insemination Location   Usage Types
OHSU - on campus, OHSU phys   AIDIUI - intrauterine
OHOT - on campus, non-OHSU phys   AIDTBW - to be washed elsewhere
NOOT - off campus   AID - cervical
LSHP - shipment, local   IVF, GIFT - in vitro fert, gamete intrafal xfer
SHIP - shipment   OTH - other

Record Keeping: B = Billed; F = Patient's File; S = Spec List (del from bank)   Page Complete (initial):_____
wp\forms\yellow.sheet   rev 9/91

FIGURE 45-4. Frozen specimen usage record form.

In general, the recommendation is made that a minimum of 20 million motile sperm be provided, postthaw, per TI. Semen samples of average or better quality will yield this number per vial, three vials per ejaculate. Male factor patients seldom produce these levels. If IUI is selected as the route of insemination, larger sperm numbers are required postthaw because sperm washing is only approximately 50% efficient. The recommended number of inseminations to perform per cycle is one or two, and the recommended route of insemination is IUI because of generally higher pregnancy rates.[25] Assuming 12 vials, at 25 million or more motile sperm per vial postthaw were frozen, 12 cycles of cervical and 4 to 6 cycles of IUI at one insemination per cycle could be conducted.

Donor Semen

Guidelines for the use of semen in TDI have been established by the Centers for Disease Control and Prevention, the American Fertility Society, and the American Association of Tissue Banks. A detailed description of the management of a donor insemination program can be found in Chapter 47. Of course, the major impetus behind the relatively recent but widespread cryopreservation of human semen is the risk of infectious disease transmission. The human immunodeficiency and hepatitis viruses (B and non-A, non-B, or C) can, along with a number of other infectious agents, be transmitted heterosexually. In 1986,[28] fresh donor semen use in TDI was recommended as long as the donor was seronegative initially, did not belong to any of the high-risk groups, and was seronegative at 6-month intervals. However, in 1988[29] and again in 1990,[30] the American Fertility Society revised its guidelines to mandate the exclusive use of frozen semen that had been quarantined for 180 days. Thus, semen collected from a donor who was seronegative initially could not be released for TDI until the sample had been held for at least 180 days and the donor had been retested and found to be seronegative for HIV. This recommendation revolutionized the TDI process and, in the time frame of 1988 to 1990, many TDI programs could not be sustained for lack of quarantined sperm.

Sperm Banks

Quarantined donor semen may be purchased from a number of sperm banks, a listing of which is maintained by the American Fertility Society in Birmingham, Alabama. The American Association of Tissue Banks also maintains a list of member banks. Policies vary between banks regarding (1) provision of samples to single versus married women; (2) shipping across state lines; (3) method of payment and fees; (4) the minimum number of motile sperm provided per insemination unit; (5) semen packaging, that is, straws versus cryovials; (6) provision of samples directly to the recipient versus to the physician; (7) donor qualifications and screening; and (8) the release of nonidentifying donor characteristics.

Donor information that is usually provided by the bank includes physical characteristics such as height, weight, hair and eye color, and blood type. Racial and ethnic background information is also included and, occasionally, family medical history, educational attainment, intellectual quotient, religion, occupation, and interests or hobbies.

Donor-recipient matching can be based on the recipient's response to a questionnaire but commonly includes consideration of the physical characteristics listed earlier plus blood type, Rh factor, and race. Sperm from donors representing widely diverse backgrounds or characteristics are accessible through the collective sperm banking activity in the United States. Samples may be shipped in liquid nitrogen transport tanks by overnight or two-day delivery using one of several available express carriers. Dry ice transport is not considered as reliable and, therefore, is not recommended. Advance notice to sperm banks is judicious when timed inseminations are conducted and local liquid nitrogen storage is unavailable.

Quality Control and Assurance

A quality control and quality assurance program is essential to the delivery of high-quality medical care. General laboratory guidelines or standards are available that also apply to the andrology/sperm banking laboratory, for example, the Joint Commission on Accreditation of Hospitals and Healthcare Organizations or the College of American Pathologists. Currently, a joint program from the American Fertility Society and the College of American Pathologists accredits human embryology and andrology laboratories. In so doing, this program addresses the unique activities of these specialty laboratories. Most notable of the unique quality assurance features in human sperm cryopreservation is the need to quarantine semen and to conduct trial thaws on banked specimens for use in a TDI program. In the latter case, an aliquot from each semen sample (ejaculate) stored in the sperm bank is set aside, subjected to the same cryopreservation protocol as the banked specimen, and, prior to release of any sample for insemination, thawed for a quality check. Only samples with trial thaws meeting acceptable, pre-established postthaw thresholds can be released for use. Both prefreeze and postthaw semen parameters should be included along with identifying information for all specimens leaving the laboratory for therapeutic use.

TROUBLESHOOTING SEMEN CRYOPRESERVATION

Cryopreservation technologies require a high degree of precision, and problems capable of influencing outcome can arise during any phase of the procedure. Generalized concerns involving storage containers, cryoprotectants, freezing machines if used, cooling or warming rates, and cryoprotectant removal have been discussed adequately by Kuzan and Quinn.[31] Additionally, in sperm cryopreservation, low postthaw motilities or fecundities may reflect microbial contamination of the initial sample, transient but repeated exposure to room temperature during storage, and improper handling after thawing and processing.

Acknowledgments

The author acknowledges the secretarial and editorial skills of Patsy Kimzey. This work was supported in part by National Institutes of Health Grant RR00163, Publication No. 1892 of the Oregon Regional Primate Research Center.

REFERENCES

1. Watson PF. Artificial insemination and the preservation of semen. In: Lamming GE, editor. Marshall's Physiology of Reproduction. Volume 2: Reproduction in the Male. 4th edition. New York: Churchill Livingstone, 1990:747–869.

2. Polge C, Smith AU, Parkes AS. Revival of spermatozoa after vitrification and dehydration at low temperatures. Nature 1949;164:666.

3. Bunge RG, Sherman JK. Fertilizing capacity of frozen human spermatozoa. Nature 1953;172:767–768.

4. Sherman JK. Improved methods of preservation of human spermatozoa by freezing and freeze-drying. Fertil Steril 1963;14:49–64.

5. Sherman JK. Current status of clinical cryobanking of human semen. In: Paulson JD, Negro-Vilar A, Lucena E, Martini L, editors. Andrology: Male Fertility and Sterility. Orlando: Academic Press, 1986:517–547.

6. Martin RH, Chernos JE, Rademaker AW. Effect of cryopreservation on the frequency of chromosomal abnormalities and sex ratio in human sperm. Mol Reprod Dev 1991;30:159–163.

7. Carson SA, Gentry WL, Smith AL, Buster JE. Feasibility of semen collection and cryopreservation during chemotherapy. Hum Reprod 1991; 6:992–994.

8. Mazur P. Freezing of living cells: mechanisms and implications. Am J Physiol 1984;247:C125–C142.

9. Katz DF. Freeze preservation of isolated populations of highly motile human spermatozoa. In: David G, editor. Human artificial insemination and semen preservation. New York: Plenum Press, 1980:557–563.

10. Prins GS, Weidel L. A comparative study of buffer systems as cryoprotectants for human spermatozoa. Fertil Steril 1986;46:147–149.

11. Sherman JK. Temperature shock in human spermatozoa. Proc Soc Exp Biol Med 1955;88:6–7.

12. Critser JK, Huse-Benda AR, Aaker DV, et al. Cryopreservation of human spermatozoa: I. Effects of holding procedure and seeding on motility, fertilizability, and acrosome reaction. Fertil Steril 1987;47:656–663.

13. Mahadevan M, Trounson AO. Effect of cooling, freezing and thawing rates and storage conditions on preservation of human spermatozoa. Andrologia 1984;16:52–60.

14. Beck WW Jr, Silverstein I. Variable motility recovery of spermatozoa following freeze preservation. Fertil Steril 1975;26:863–867.

15. Holt WV, Shenfield F, Leonard T, et al. The value of sperm swimming speed measurements in assessing the fertility of human frozen semen. Hum Reprod 1989;4:292–297.

16. Cross NL, Hanks SE. Effects of cryopreservation on human sperm acrosomes. Hum Reprod 1991;6:1279–1283.

17. Wolf DP. Acrosomal status quantitation in human sperm. Am J Reprod Immunol 1989;20:106–113.

18. Sherman JK. Cryopreservation of human semen. In: Keel BA, Webster BW, editors. CRC Handbook of the Laboratory Diagnosis and Treatment of Infertility. Boca Raton: CRC Press, 1990:229–259.

19. Critser JK, Huse-Benda AR, Aaker DV, et al. Cryopreservation of human spermatozoa: III. The effect of cryoprotectants on motility. Fertil Steril 1988;50:314–320.

20. Hammitt DG, Walker DL, Williamson RA. Concentration of glycerol required for optimal survival and in vitro fertilizing capacity of frozen sperm is dependent on cryopreservation medium. Fertil Steril 1988;49:680–687.

21. Serafini P, Marrs RP. Computerized-staged freezing technique improves sperm survival and preserves penetration of zona-free hamster ova. Fertil Steril 1986;45:854–858.

22. Taylor PJ, Wilson J, Laycock R, Weger J. A comparison of freezing and thawing methods for the cryopreservation of human semen. Fertil Steril 1982;37:100–103.

23. Centola GM, Mattox JH, Raubertas RF. Pregnancy rates after double versus single insemination with frozen donor semen. Fertil Steril 1990;54:1089–1092.

24. Byrd W, Bradshaw K, Carr B, et al. A prospective randomized study of pregnancy rates following intrauterine and intracervical insemination using frozen donor sperm. Fertil Steril 1990;53:521–527.

25. Patton PE, Burry KA, Thurmond A, et al. Intrauterine insemination outperforms intracervical insemination in a randomized, controlled study with frozen, donor semen. Fertil Steril 1992;57:559–564.

26. Drobnis EZ, Zhong CQ, Overstreet JW. Separation of cryopreserved human semen using Sephadex columns, washing, or Percoll gradients. J Androl 1991;12:201–208.

27. Hammitt DG, Bedia E, Rogers PR, et al. Comparison of motility stimulants for cryopreserved human semen. Fertil Steril 1989;52:495–502.

28. American Fertility Society. New guidelines for the use of semen donor insemination: 1986. Fertil Steril 1986;46(Suppl 2):95S–110S.

29. American Fertility Society. Revised new guidelines for the use of semen-donor insemination. Fertil Steril 1988;49:211.

30. American Fertility Society. New guidelines for the use of semen donor insemination: 1990. Fertil Steril 1990;53(Suppl 1):1S–13S.

31. Kuzan FB, Quinn P. Cryopreservation of mammalian embryos. In: Wolf DP, editor. In Vitro Fertilization and Embryo Transfer: A Manual of Basic Techniques. New York: Plenum Press, 1988:301–347.

CHAPTER 46

Sperm Preparation and Homologous Insemination

WILLIAM BYRD

Insemination with the husband's sperm is now a widely applied technique for the treatment of infertility caused by male factor, cervical factor, and immunologic abnormalities. It has also been used to treat patients with unexplained infertility. Various methods of insemination exist, which are defined by the source of sperm—husband or donor—and where in the reproductive tract sperm are deposited. When sperm are obtained from the husband, the procedure has been referred to as *artificial insemination by husband* (AIH). Correspondingly, when sperm are obtained from someone other than the husband, it is referred to as *artificial insemination by donor* (AID) or *therapeutic donor insemination* (TDI). The latter term (TDI) is growing in acceptance so as to distinguish the procedure from the disease acquired immunodeficiency syndrome (AIDS). In a sense, AID and TDI both are inaccurate. The insemination is not "artificial," and it is "therapeutic" only if pregnancy results. Perhaps the term *assisted insemination* would be a more accurate description.

Insemination can be performed intravaginally using the whole (entire) or a split (a portion of) ejaculate, intracervically (intracervical insemination [ICI]) or pericervically with an unprocessed ejaculate or washed spermatozoa. The deposition of spermatozoa at any point superior to the internal os is considered intrauterine insemination (IUI). Deposition of sperm directly into the fallopian tubes would be transuterotubal insemination (TUTI). Direct deposit of sperm into the peritoneal cavity is called *direct intraperitoneal insemination* (DIPI). The choice of technique or where sperm will be deposited depends largely on the clinical indications for infertility.

Of the available insemination procedures, IUI has received the most recent attention and implementation. The increased use of this technique has been fueled by the development of improved sperm preparation techniques that have resulted in part from the growth of human in vitro fertilization (IVF). The dramatic increase in the past 5 years in the number of IUIs performed and reported in the literature can be seen in Figure 46–1. Other factors that have contributed to the growing use of IUI have been the ability to predict ovulation with simple home-use luteinizing hormone (LH)-test kits, the use of supraovulation regimens with adequate monitoring,

and the technical development of transfer catheters. Although the popularity of IUI has grown since the first review of the procedure by Mastroianni and associates,[1] questions remain concerning its efficacy. Bypassing the cervical barrier with IUI results in significantly higher pregnancy rates than does ICI in most published studies.[2–10] However, some studies have reported little or no difference between the two techniques.[11, 12] These discrepancies are due to lack of objective analyses of pregnancies resulting from IUI. As in many medical procedures, the end result used to measure success (e.g., pregnancy) is based on a series of interactions, each of which may have a number of variables affecting it. Often overlooked is the fact that many couples entered into IUI

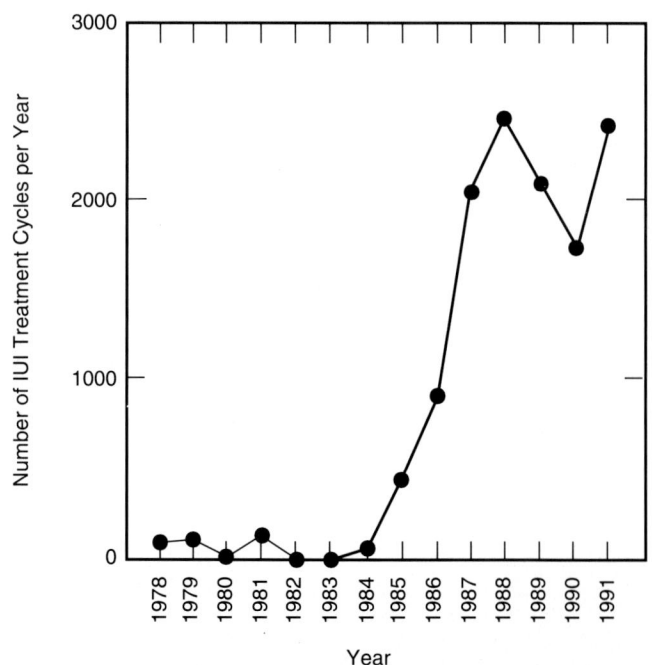

FIGURE 46–1. The number of reported intrauterine insemination (IUI) treatment cycles reported in the literature. The data were compiled from references in Tables 46–3 through 46–5.

study protocols have had previous cycles of treatment or surgery and varied lengths of infertility. There are notable differences in the literature as to the method of sperm preparation, the timing of insemination, the number of inseminations per cycle, the clinical indication for IUI, and the presence or absence of agents that cause multiple follicular development. In addition, studies often fail to identify types of pregnancy: clinical, biochemical, ongoing, or term.

The paucity of prospective, randomized studies has raised specific questions about the reported success rates. A prospective approach would encompass the following (but would not be limited to): (1) a rigorous definition of the type of infertility, examination of the couple, and the type of infertility treated; (2) randomization of the couple into study protocols and the use of some type of control; (3) control of treatment cycles and elimination of unprotected intercourse to exclude pregnancies that are not treatment related; (4) proper documentation of the quantity and quality of semen or sperm deposited; (5) documentation of insemination and the time of ovulation; (6) documentation of follicular stimulation, if any; and (7) documentation of pregnancy and outcome. Most studies, however, do not meet these standards, or they lack a proper control group.

INDICATIONS AND RATIONALE FOR INSEMINATION

Indications and Rationale for Intracervical Insemination

Although IUI has been shown to be superior to ICI in prospective trials,[8, 13] there is still a clinical role for the less complex technique of ICI. Normal intercourse and ICI both have the same result, that is, placement of sperm into the cervical region. Therefore, the indications for ICI would seem to be restricted to conditions when normal deposition of sperm cannot take place, including anatomic defects such as hypospadias, impotence or sexual dysfunction such as vaginismus or dyspareunia, or donor insemination. Studies using fresh donor sperm have shown that a couple should experience pregnancy rates of 8% to 17% per treatment cycle and approximately 60% of all couples should conceive after 6 months of treatment.[14, 15]

Indication and Rationale for Intrauterine Insemination

The rationale for IUI is the same as for gamete intrafallopian transfer (GIFT) or IVF; that is, it increases the number of gametes at the site of fertilization. Normally, there is a mechanical-immunologic filtering effect by the cervical mucus. At a microscopic level, the cervical mucus appears to be a loose network of fibers with fluid-filled interstitial spaces. These spaces are small compared with the sperm so that sperm must be motile to push their way through the mucus.[16] Cervical mucus limits the passage of motile spermatozoa, filters out the nonmotile cells and debris, and prevents the passage of seminal plasma into the uterus. Studies by Settlage and colleagues[17] indicated that only about 0.1% of

sperm placed in the upper vagina are present in the cervical canal 1 hour after insemination. Mortimer and Templeton[18] demonstrated a reduction in sperm numbers along the reproductive tract of five to six orders of magnitude. Direct deposition of motile spermatozoa into the reproductive tract can reverse this situation and thus increase the chances for successful fertilization.

The indications for IUI have been reviewed by Nachtigall and coworkers,[19, 20] Allen and associates,[21] Moghissi,[22] Pardo and Bancells,[23] and Taylor and Kredentser[24] and are summarized in Table 46–1. IUI may be applied to three categories of infertile couples, as discussed in the following paragraphs.

One of the most frequent indications for IUI and the most widely argued is *male factor infertility*, including conditions such as oligospermia, asthenospermia, teratozoospermia, retrograde ejaculation, diabetes, and neurologic disease. It appears that IUI has a definite superiority to ICI when there is a compromised sperm sample such as in oligospermia.[2] When male factor couples were stimulated with clomiphene citrate or human menopausal gonadotropins (hMG), there was a 1.2% pregnancy rate per treatment cycle with ICI compared with a 7.3% pregnancy rate per treatment cycle with IUI.[2] Byrd and associates[8] compared IUI and ICI success rates with frozen donor sperm in a prospective study. Frozen donor sperm was shown to have a lowered fecundity when compared with fresh sperm. The researchers found that there was a 9.7% pregnancy rate with IUI versus 3.9% with ICI. These data point out a higher pregnancy rate when IUI is used with these infertility factors.

The second indication for IUI is *cervical factor*, when some deficiency in the cervical mucus limits the transport of sperm, there is an anatomic defect of the cervix, or storage of sperm in the cervical mucus effectively results in a barrier to sperm. The defect in mucus may be due to the loss of mucous-producing glands by surgery, anatomic changes in the cervix, or "hostile" cervical mucus. Hostile cervical mucus limits or prevents sperm motility and survival within the endocervical canal, which may be due to immunologic infer-

---

TABLE 46–1. Indications for IUI

I. Normal semen analysis
  A. Anatomic male causes
    1. Retrograde ejaculation
      a. Surgery
      b. Trauma
      c. Systemic disease
      d. Medications
  B. Female causes
    1. Cervical stenosis, conization, cauterization, diethylstilbestrol exposure
    2. Deficiencies in cervical mucus
    3. Defects in sperm transport or survival
  C. Coital dysfunction
    1. Impotence
    2. Premature ejaculation
    3. Vaginismus
  D. Unexplained infertility
II. Abnormal semen analysis
  A. Oligospermia
  B. Asthenospermia
  C. Volume disorders
  D. Immune-mediated disorders
  E. Multiple male factor disorders
III. Frozen donor or husband sperm

tility, infection, or some chemical alteration of the cervical mucus.

The third indication is a *transport problem* or a similar problem in the fallopian tubes preventing sperm from reaching the oocyte. These situations would necessitate the use of IUI, TUTI, or DIPI. Overall, one would expect that the highest success rates after bypassing the cervix would be experienced in couples with cervical factor or male factor. Whether or not there is a treatment-related effect is discussed in greater detail subsequently.

SPERM PREPARATION

The human ejaculate is a mixture of motile, nonmotile, and dead spermatozoa as well as different types of seminal components such as debris, prostaglandins, and micro-organisms. In 1957, initial attempts at AIH-IUI used unwashed semen in which the sperm was concentrated by centrifugation.[1] In this study group of 29 patients receiving IUI, one patient conceived (3.4%), whereas five patients complained of abdominal cramps. When cervical or vaginal inseminations were performed with nontreated sperm, there was a pregnancy rate of 6.4% to 9.7%. The authors of this study concluded that AIH-IUI for male factor couples was fruitless and that vaginal insemination with nontreated sperm was the most successful procedure. In 1976, Dixon and colleagues[25] treated a series of 158 patients with cervical cap or ICI who had male factor, immunologic, or unexplained infertility. They noted a 9.5% pregnancy rate following treatment. However, there was an 18% pregnancy rate in nontreatment cycles. These early reports painted a rather bleak picture for the successful use of AIH for male factor infertility. With the advent of human IVF programs, there was renewed interest in washed sperm preparations, which were soon used in IUI programs.

Sperm Separation Techniques

During natural intercourse, approximately 100 million sperm are normally deposited in the vagina, with only a few million actually passing through the cervical mucus.[17] Of these millions of sperm, only a few hundred can actually be found at the site of fertilization. Any element that interferes with sperm deposition and transport decreases the probability of fertilization.

To increase the chances of fertilization, the cervical barrier is bypassed and IUI performed with a sperm preparation composed of viable, motile sperm free of seminal plasma and debris. A variety of methods have been developed to separate motile sperm from semen. The most commonly used sperm isolation techniques described here involve washing and centrifugation, which may result in some damage to the sperm.[15, 26, 27] Also, many motile sperm remain in the supernatant after centrifugation, thus reducing the efficiency of recovery of motile sperm. A variety of different media have been used successfully for IUI preparations. All media are isotonic saline solutions that are buffered to a pH favorable to sperm and supplemented with serum or albumin. An ideal isolation technique would be rapid, inexpensive, and isolate all motile sperm without damaging them. A recent concern[28] is that the

more traditional methods for preparation of sperm may lead to iatrogenic damage to sperm. Aitken and Clarkson[27] have shown that centrifugal force generates production of reactive oxygen species that may damage sperm and impair their fertility potential.

GLASS-WOOL FILTRATION

Paulson and coworkers[29] first described a glass-wool column that reduced the amount of debris and concentrated the number of motile spermatozoa. The liquefied specimen is placed on top of a column consisting of a 5-in. glass Pasteur pipette filled with loosely packed glass-wool fibers and collected in tubes. This procedure is relatively fast, requiring only about 10 minutes for filtration. However, there is some evidence of structural damage to spermatozoa,[30] and glass fibers may contaminate the inseminating mixture. Using a modified technique, Jeyendran and associates[31] found that spermatozoa recovered from the column retain the functional integrity of their membranes after filtration. The rate of recovery of motile sperm from this technique is high (Table 46–2). The sperm population recovered after filtration is functionally superior to the original ejaculate in the penetration of zona-free hamster oocytes.[32] Katayama and colleagues[33] found that filtration of sperm resulted in a higher percentage of fertilized oocytes than did the swimup procedure in a human IVF program. This technique has been used successfully to isolate sperm from samples with high viscosity. Despite its apparent high recovery rates, this technique has not been widely used for IUI.

Sperm Preparation Technique. The glass-wool column is prepared by filling a 5¾ in. Pasteur pipette with glass-wool fiber (borosilicate glass, Pyrex). Borosilicate glass is preferred because it has greater strength and resistance to breakage. About 40 to 50 mg of borosilicate glass wool is used to loosely pack the column. The liquefied sample (as much as 2.5 mL) is applied directly to the column. As the sample passes through the mesh of glass wool, debris and nonmotile sperm are trapped in the fibers. Because there is no buffer applied to the column, the recovery of sperm and fluid in the effluent is variable. This sample still requires simple washing to remove the spermatozoa from the seminal plasma contaminants.

ALBUMIN COLUMNS

Ericsson and associates[34] described the use of human serum albumin columns to separate progressively motile

---

TABLE 46–2. Efficiency of Different Sperm Isolation Techniques	
Technique	**Percentage of Motile Cells Recovered (%)**
Sperm wash	28–59
Swimup	6–18
Percoll gradients	17–70
Albumin gradients	13–60
Glass-wool filtration	50
Hyaluronic acid swimup	12–18
Nycodenz gradients	39
Sephadex columns	50

sperm from nonmotile forms and debris. A small volume of semen sample (0.5 mL) is diluted with 10% serum and is placed on a small column containing medium supplemented with 7.5% albumin on a discontinuous gradient. The mixture is incubated for 60 to 120 minutes, and then the motile sperm can be recovered from the bottom of the column. Glass and Ericsson[35] first used this procedure for a case of sperm-agglutinating antibodies; however, no pregnancy was achieved in this report. Dmowski and colleagues[36] introduced a modification of this technique. Semen was diluted (1:1 with medium) and centrifuged; the sperm pellet was resuspended; and then motile sperm were isolated on two-step albumin gradients. Although albumin gradients have a good yield of sperm (see Table 46–2), their use appears to be limited to a sperm sex selection technique.

Sperm Preparation Technique. Semen is diluted with Tyrode's medium (1:1), and sperm and other debris are isolated by centrifugation. The pellet is resuspended in Tyrode's medium to a final concentration of 100×10^6 sperm/mL. There are several variations to the separation technique. However, one simple approach is to add 0.4 mL of a 15% albumin solution (15% bovine serum albumin in Tyrode's medium) to a heat-sealed Pasteur capillary pipette. A layer of 3% to 6% albumin in medium (0.8 mL) is then layered over the denser medium. After the gradient is formed, 0.5 mL of resuspended sperm suspension is layered over the albumin. The sperm migrate downward into the albumin gradients over the next 30 to 60 minutes. This enriched portion of spermatozoa can then be recovered from the albumin, washed in Tyrode's medium, and used for insemination.

WASHED SPERMATOZOA

The most widely used technique of preparing sperm for IUI is dilution of semen with buffered saline or culture media followed by centrifugation at 300 to 800g to concentrate spermatozoa. This approach was first described by Hanson and Rock.[37] Although this technique eliminates or dilutes the effect of the seminal plasma, motile and nonmotile sperm, particulate matter, and possibly bacteria are included in the material to be inseminated. There is a moderately good yield of motile cells (see Table 46–2). The overall success of washed sperm in other IUI programs has been previously published.[15, 23] The overall pregnancy rate for washed sperm according to a review by Pardo and Bancells[23] was 23% per couple, regardless of the type of infertility experienced by the couple.

Sperm Preparation Technique. The ejaculate is allowed to liquefy for at least 30 minutes prior to analysis and preparation. The ejaculate is transferred to a conical centrifuge tube and is thoroughly mixed before an aliquot is taken for analysis. Three volumes of medium are then added to every one volume of sperm (Fig. 46–2A). If a male factor is present, it is important to reduce the overall volume of sperm and medium in each tube. Volumes exceeding 6 to 8 mL have a correspondingly poor recovery of spermatozoa[15] because relatively lower g forces are used and spermatozoa will remain in the column of medium. Specimens in which there are high volumes of sperm and medium present require splitting of the mixture into smaller aliquots (2 to 3 mL maximum) in several centrifuge tubes to enhance the yield of sperm. Following centrifugation, sperm and medium are then thoroughly mixed in the tube and centrifuged at 200g for 5 to 10 minutes. The total percentage of sperm that can be recovered increases if higher centrifugal forces are used; however, collection of sperm at these higher g forces results in increased damage to the sperm.[15] Following centrifugation, the overlaying supernatant is removed by aspiration, and the pellet is resuspended in 2 mL of medium. The pellet/medium are resuspended and centrifuged again at 200g for 5 to 10 minutes. The final pellet is resuspended in 0.5 mL of medium if the pellet is to be used immediately for insemination.

SWIMUP METHOD

The earliest method of separating motile from nonmotile sperm and cellular debris was the sperm-rise of Drevius[38] or the swimup of Lopata and associates.[39] This technique involved layering medium directly on semen samples. Spermatozoa in the seminal plasma could migrate into a culture medium. Following 30 to 90 minutes of incubation, the upper "buffy" coat or layer is removed and motile cells are recovered form this layer. The presence of small amounts of seminal plasma generally requires a centrifugation and resuspension step at this point. Variations of this technique include a preliminary wash step followed by the migration step. Swimup migration methods are noted for low rates of recovery of motile cells (see Table 46–2).[39, 40] The percentage of morphologically normal forms using this technique increases from 53% normal in washed samples to 80.8% normal forms in the swimup.[40] All the abnormal forms decrease, with the exception of microcephalic sperm.[40] The use of swimup populations of sperm in IUI has been reviewed by Kerin and Byrd[15] and Pardo and Bancells.[23] In the review by Pardo and Bancells,[23] the swimup preparation had a pregnancy rate per couple of 16% in 521 couples.

Sperm Preparation Technique. The washed pellet recovered in Figure 46–2A is gently mixed, then carefully overlayed with 1 to 3 mL of culture medium (Fig. 46–2B). The centrifuge tube is then incubated at 37°C for 30 to 90 minutes before recovery of the overlying supernatant containing motile sperm. Incubating the tube in a slant rack so that the tube is tilted at a 45- to 60-degree angle creates a greater surface area of medium over the pellet and a better recovery of motile sperm. The percentage of recovery of motile sperm is influenced by the size of the pellet, the quality of the sperm, and the time of incubation allowed for sperm to swim into the medium. Splitting single pellets into several tubes, followed by swimup, also increases the yield of motile spermatozoa. After the final supernatant fraction is recovered and gently mixed, an aliquot is taken for analysis of count and motility of the spermatozoa.

DISCONTINUOUS OR CONTINUOUS GRADIENT SYSTEMS

A modified colloidal silica medium for density gradient separation of cells was developed in 1977 by Pertoft and colleagues.[41] This technique was used by Gorus and Pipeleers[42] to fractionate human spermatozoa according to their progressive motility by centrifuging fresh semen samples on continuous Percoll (Pharmacia AB, Uppsala, Sweden) gradients. Percoll is diluted with culture medium to make solutions in the 40% to 90% Percoll range. These solutions are

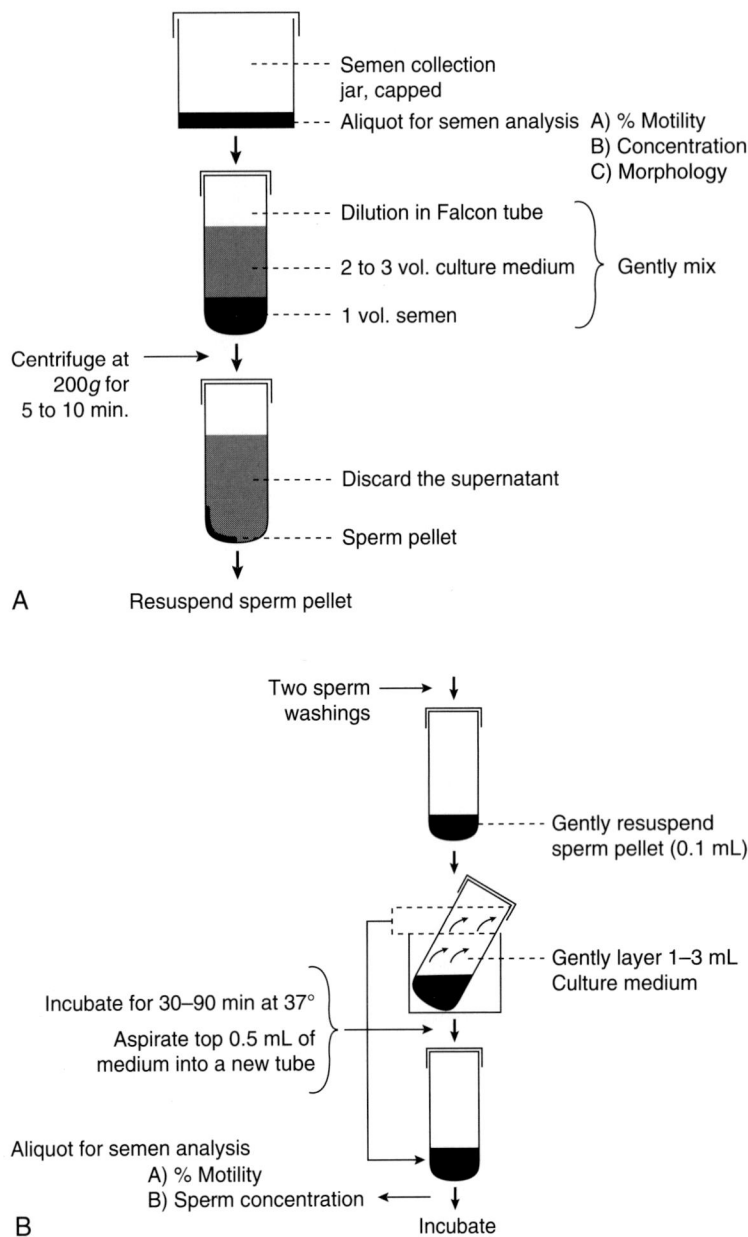

FIGURE 46–2. *A*, Simple sperm washing. *B*, Sperm wash and swimup.

then layered on top of each other to form either discontinuous or continuous gradients, and then the semen sample is layered on top of the Percoll gradients and centrifuged. Following centrifugation, the more progressively motile spermatozoa are found distributed in the higher-density fractions in the bottom of the tube. However, one drawback to such an application is that it requires a final wash in Percoll-free physiologic medium to remove colloidal silica particles from the sample. There is also the possibility of endotoxin contamination. The separation of sperm on Percoll has been shown to remove bacterial contamination,[43] and it selects for morphologically normal forms of spermatozoa.[44] Although this method has proved its efficacy in selecting motile sperm for IUI,[23, 45–48] the percentage of recovery of motile sperm is somewhat low (see Table 46–2). The factors regulating the recovery of spermatozoa are the density of the spermatozoa, sperm motility, the centrifugal force used, and the final vol-

ume of Percoll gradients.[49] The use of Percoll gradients can increase the yield of motile cells with normal morphology at least twofold. There does not appear to be any advantage to using Percoll gradients to isolate fresh spermatozoa over the widely used swimup techniques in prospective studies that examine the pregnancy rates.[50]

Another density gradient material used for sperm isolation is Nycodenz (Nycomed Diagnostics, Oslo, Norway). Nycodenz is an iodinated organic molecule dissolved in TRIS buffer. One study[51] showed that Nycodenz gradients can be used effectively to isolate motile sperm from oligoasthenospermic males. Both of these density gradient techniques have been shown to improve sperm function as measured by the zona-free hamster egg bioassay.[52, 53]

Sperm Preparation Technique. One simple method for the preparation of Percoll gradients for isolation of motile spermatozoa from nonmale factors is to prepare isotonic Percoll using a concentrated 10× medium containing HEPES buffer. Isotonic Percoll can be prepared by mixing one part of 10× HEPES–based buffer with nine parts of Percoll (0.3 mL:2.7 mL). The Percoll is then diluted with medium, and the different concentrations can be used to make discontinuous or continous gradients. To prepare a discontinuous gradient, a 4-mL Percoll gradient is prepared by first mixing 1.2 mL of HEPES medium with 0.8 mL of isotonic Percoll (40%). A denser 80% Percoll fraction is made with 0.4 mL of HEPES medium and 1.6 mL of isotonic Percoll. The 40% Percoll fraction is then carefully layered over the 80% fraction. Fresh or frozen-thawed semen can then be layered directly over the 40% gradient (Fig. 46–3). Although this sperm can be washed first prior to isolation in Percoll, it is inadvisable because additional centrifugation steps may induce even more damage to the spermatozoa, particularly frozen-thawed specimens. The sperm–Percoll gradient is then centrifuged at 600g for 20 to 30 minutes. Following centrifugation, there should be three layers in the tube: (1) a layer on top of the 40% gradient consisting mainly of seminal plasma components, cells, and debris; (2) a fraction of sperm enriched in more motile spermatozoa at the interface of the 40% and 80% gradient; and (3) at the bottom of the 80% gradient, an enriched pellet of highly motile spermatozoa. This pellet is resuspended in 1 to 2 mL of medium and centrifuged for 5 to 10 minutes at 200g to dilute out and remove some of the Percoll. After centrifugation, the pellet can be resuspended in 0.5 mL of medium for immediate use or stored at 37°C for future use. A small aliquot can be taken out for analysis of the spermatozoa.

SPERM MIGRATION: FICOLL AND HYALURONIC ACID

A modification of the swimup technique is to overlay the semen sample with Ficoll (Pharmacia AB, Uppsala, Sweden) or hyaluronic acid (Sperm Select, Pharmacia AB, Uppsala, Sweden).[54] Both of these techniques create a gradient-density interface at the surface, and only actively motile spermatozoa can swim across it. The advantage of Sperm Select is that it tries to mimic cervical mucus in composition. Sperm selected in this fashion may have decreased oxidative damage.[28] More-

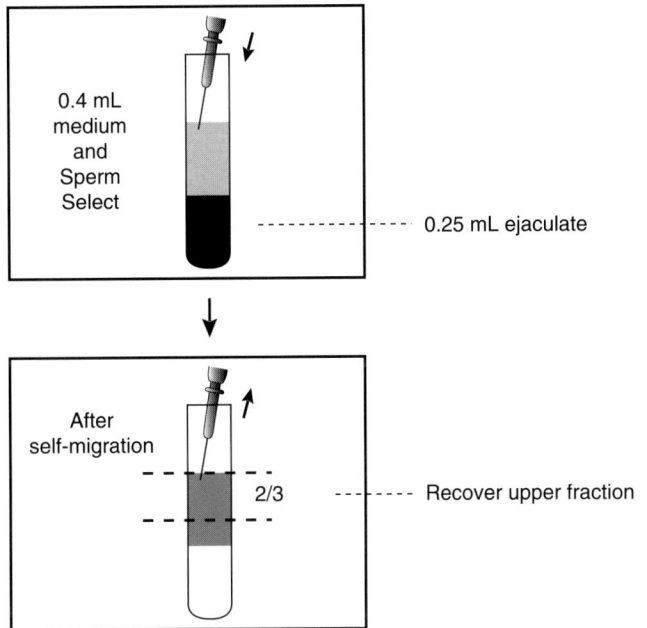

FIGURE 46–4. Isolation of motile sperm on hyaluronic acid (Sperm Select).

over, the sample can be directly inseminated, but then sperm must be motile for sperm to be recovered.

Sperm Preparation Technique. The medium for separation is prepared by adding Ham's F-10 or Earle's medium to a stock solution of Sperm Select to a final concentration of 1 mg/mL. The stock solution has a concentration of 2 mg/mL in phosphate buffer. The medium is equilibrated in a 5% carbon dioxide (CO_2) atmosphere and should have a pH of 7.4 and an osmolarity of 282 mOsm/L following equilibration. An aliquot of the sperm specimen (0.25 mL) is added to a Pasteur pipette that is closed at one end (Fig. 46–4). The sample is then overlayed with 0.4 mL of Sperm Select medium. The pipette is incubated in 5% CO_2 in air at 37°C for 60 minutes. After incubation, the upper two thirds of the medium containing motile spermatozoa is then gently aspirated and transferred to a sterile tube.

SEPHADEX COLUMNS

Sephadex columns have been used to separate motile cells from semen.[55–57] The advantage of the column separation technique is its rapid separation of motile cells, usually requiring about 15 minutes. However, a subsequent centrifugation step is still required to remove seminal plasma.

Sperm Preparation Technique. Prepared columns of Sephadex can be purchased commercially. Although these columns can also be prepared in the laboratory, they must be sterilized prior to separation of patient's sperm, and their results may not be as consistent. The dry beads in the plugged column are first hydrated with medium containing 0.3% human serum albumin (Fig. 46–5). The filter pad that prevents redistribution of beads during shipping is removed with a Pasteur pipette, and the pipette is then used to remove any bubbles in the column. After the dry beads in the column have been exposed to medium for at least 10 minutes, the medium is allowed to flow out the column until there is only

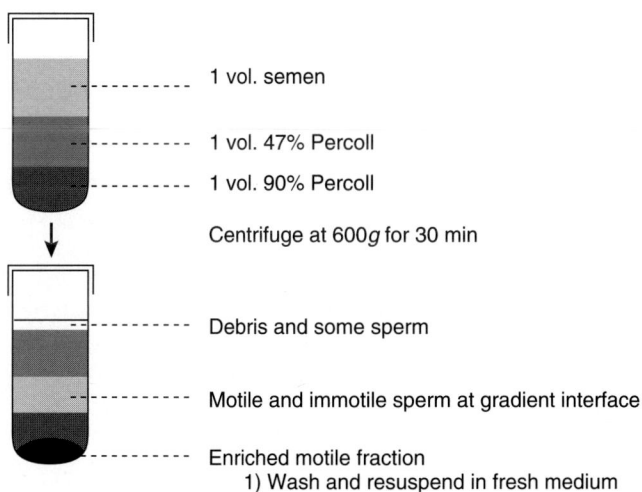

FIGURE 46–3. Isolation of motile sperm on a Percoll gradient.

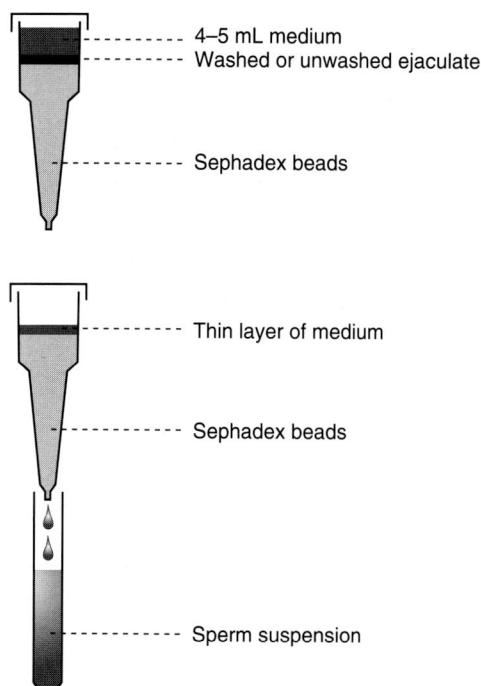

FIGURE 46–5. Isolation of motile sperm on Sephadex columns (Sperm Prep).

a thin layer of medium on top of the column, and the column is then plugged again. A washed or unwashed ejaculate can then be added directly to the top of the column. Highly viscous samples have to be washed or diluted prior to separation because clogging of the column will occur. The sperm specimen is then overlayed with 4 to 5 mL of medium. The medium and sperm suspension in the column are then allowed to run into a conical centrifuge tube. The sperm suspension containing sperm and seminal plasma components is then washed once by centrifugation at 200g for 5 to 10 minutes. The resulting pellet is then resuspended in 0.5 mL of medium containing 0.3% human serum albumin and is ready for insemination.

SUMMARY

It is difficult to determine which sperm separation method or technique should be used. The lack of standardization and the heterogenous patient populations in published studies make this decision difficult. The occurrence of pregnancies that are independent of treatment and the lack of properly controlled studies add to the confusion. The recovery rate within a technique still is highly dependent on sperm motility for several of these techniques; therefore, some male factors may not do well. Another confounding factor is that conventional semen analysis of volume, sperm density, and motility does not appear to differ between conception and nonconception cycles.[58] It is expected that the introduction of computer-aided sperm analysis (CASA) would be able to provide more discrimination between fertile and nonfertile donors. One recent study[59] has been able to distinguish between fertile and nonfertile donors in TDI donor based on CASA. Conventional semen parameters and functional assays such as the sperm penetration assay have been of little use in

discriminating between fertile and nonfertile donors. Other assays of interest might be the use of more sophisticated techniques for quantitating biochemical lesions in the sperm such as creatine kinase,[60] which might point out more subtle defects in sperm functions that influence pregnancy outcome. All the commonly used techniques have been examined and are associated with good pregnancy rates in the literature.

Physiologic Capacitation of Spermatozoa and Stimulation of Motility

In vivo, there is a separation of motile sperm from the seminal plasma that allows capacitation to occur.[61] It is known that long-term exposure to seminal plasma has a deleterious effect on sperm and reduces the ability of sperm to penetrate cervical mucus[61] and zona-free hamster oocytes.[62] There is a physiologic need for capacitation or maturation of sperm in vitro or in vivo because they are incapable of fertilizing an oocyte until this event has occurred.[63] Once sperm have undergone capacitation, they can undergo a change in motility referred to as *hyperactivation*, which is believed to be a prerequisite to fertilization.[64] The necessity for capacitation in vitro prior to IUI has not yet been established. The short time of incubation (60 to 120 minutes) seen in most sperm isolation techniques would not allow enough time for large numbers of sperm to undergo capacitation.[65] Sperm populations seem to undergo capacitation somewhat asynchronously for 24 hours, with most sperm requiring at least 6 hours.[65] Once inseminated in the reproductive tract, the sperm should be able to complete the capacitation process, which begins after physical isolation of the sperm from seminal plasma.

Several attempts have been made at improving the functional quality of the sperm to be inseminated. Phosphodiesterase inhibitors such as caffeine have been used in an effort to increase the number of progressively motile spermatozoa available for insemination,[66, 67] but any improvement in motility has not been consistently noted.[56, 68] Pentoxifylline, another phosphodiesterase inhibitor, improved the counts of total motile and total progressive spermatozoa in patients with oligospermia and asthenospermia.[69, 70] Blumenfeld and Nahhas[71] showed that sperm pretreated with follicular fluid gave a statistically significant increase in the pregnancy rate when compared with nontreated sperm in a prospective trial of IUI.

EFFICACY OF IUI IN VARIOUS CATEGORIES

The effectiveness of treatment of infertility disorders is easily assessed by the pregnancy rates per treatment cycle or per patient. The interpretation of these results with respect to IUI is clearly handicapped by a lack of control groups. To interpret the literature, we must make generalizations. Although cycle fecundity clearly indicates the degree of success of that treatment, we know that even with abnormal sperm counts spontaneous pregnancy may occur.[72] We can also assume that the probability of conception is dependent on the underlying disorders.

TABLE 46–3. Male Factor: Literature Survey of IUI Results					
	Number of Patients	Number of Treatment Cycles	Average Number of Treatment Cycles/Patient	Pregnancy Rate/Patient	Pregnancy Rate/Cycle
All cases: reference numbers 2, 4, 6, 7, 11, 35, 36, 58, 69, 71, 76, 78, 79, 81–108	2080	7039	3.4 ± 1.2	21.7	6.4
Unstimulated cycles	986	3451	3.5 ± 1.1	19.8	5.7
Stimulated + unstimulated cycles	581	1862	3.1 ± 1.1	22.9	7.1
Stimulated cycles	513	1726	3.4 ± 1.3	23.9	7.1

IUI, intrauterine insemination.

Spontaneous Pregnancy

The underlying assumption in the analysis of any treatment is that the likelihood of pregnancy without treatment is negligible. In the absence of proper controls and prospective, randomized studies, one of the confounding problems in interpretation of IUI data is the spontaneous pregnancy rate. The incidence of spontaneous pregnancies is inversely related to the duration of infertility in a couple. Collins and coworkers[73] reported a spontaneous or treatment-independent pregnancy rate of 23% in a group of untreated infertile couples. The rate of pregnancy in a 3-year followup was 63% in couples with less than 2 years of infertility, which decreased to 27% if these couples had experienced 4 or more years of infertility.[73] Aafjes and associates[72] reported that about 20% of all couples will achieve pregnancy independent of treatment within 3 years, if the initial duration of infertility is less than 2 years. Nachtigall[20] reported in a review that of 408 couples undergoing AIH, 18% achieved pregnancy in treatment cycles, whereas 14% of the couples became pregnant in spontaneous cycles who did not conceive with AIH. However, these patients may not represent the typical infertility patient seen in most assisted reproductive technology programs. A survey of some studies[8, 58, 74–79] with 787 patients undergoing IUI revealed a 24.1% pregnancy rate per patient during treatment cycles and a 2.2% spontaneous pregnancy rate per patient for nontreatment pregnancies.

Male Factor

The definitions of male factor in the IUI literature are highly variable. Some authors state merely that a male factor is present; others use their own standards for male factor; still others use the World Health Organization guidelines.[80] If the sperm from a male factor patient are placed in the uterus (assuming that these sperm are fertile), IUI should increase the chance of fertilization. However, many reports have criticized the use of homologous IUI for treatment of male factor.[11, 12, 22]

A survey of the IUI literature on male factor is seen in Table 46–3.[2, 4, 6, 7, 10, 11, 26, 35, 36, 58, 69, 71, 76, 78, 79, 81–108] Because there is little standardization between the different studies on male factor, it was decided to average all the data and then divide them into stimulated, nonstimulated cycles and studies in which both stimulated and nonstimulated data were reported together. The overall pregnancy rate for all couples with male factor was 21.7% (range of 0 to 57.1%) and a pregnancy rate per treatment cycle of 6.4% (range of 0 to 20.5%). Ovulatory cycles in which gonadotropins or clomiphene citrate were used did not appear to significantly improve the pregnancy rate per couple or per treatment cycle.

Female Factor

With respect to female factors, the role of IUI in the treatment of cervical factor and unexplained infertility seems to be more accepted in the literature. If cervical mucus is absent or hostile to sperm, bypassing it with IUI would appear to be a natural treatment. The use of IUI for treatment of unexplained infertility is changing because this patient group is declining[109] probably owing to better diagnostic techniques in reproductive endocrinology and laparoscopy. A summary of results of IUI for female factor and unexplained infertility is shown in Table 46–4. Unexplained infertility is often reported with female factor, and it is included in Table 46–4. The overall pregnancy rate for female factor or unexplained infertility, or both, following IUI was 24.9% (range of 0 to 75%), and the pregnancy rate per treatment cycle was 9.1% (range of 0 to 35.3%). There did not appear to be a significant increase in pregnancy rates following treatment with gonadotropins or clomiphene citrate. This group was further broken down into women who had identified cervical factor,[46, 47, 69, 74, 75, 77, 83, 84, 86, 91, 95, 101, 102, 108, 112–118] or endometriosis[46, 69, 86, 91, 107, 108, 119] or couples with unexplained infertility

TABLE 46–4. Female Factor/Unexplained: Literature Survey of IUI Results					
	Number of Patients	Number of Treatment Cycles	Average Number of Treatment Cycles/Patient	Pregnancy Rate/Patient	Pregnancy Rate/Cycle
All cases: reference numbers 3, 6, 7, 10, 69, 71, 75, 76, 78, 79, 83, 84, 86–93, 95–99, 101, 103, 105, 106	1911	5198	2.7 ± 1.0	24.9	9.1
Unstimulated cycles	797	2327	2.9 ± 1.0	27.6	9.5
Stimulated + unstimulated cycles	454	1250	2.6 ± 0.9	22.7	8.2
Stimulated cycles	660	1621	2.5 ± 1.2	23.0	9.4

IUI, intrauterine insemination.

(Table 46–5).[3, 86, 88, 91, 95, 101, 102, 108, 110–114] Although this significantly reduced the number of studies, with cervical factor the pregnancy rate per couple was 28.7% overall (20 studies, range 0 to 100%). However, it was clear that the group with identified endometriosis (without regard for the severity of the disease) had the lowest pregnancy rate per patient overall with 17.9% (range of 0 to 29%). There seemed to be some improvement with follicular stimulation followed by IUI, but this was not statistically significant. There were insufficient data to present the pregnancy rates per treatment cycle for this group.

Immunologic Infertility

Immunologic infertility is probably the least understood of all the factors that influence fertility of the couple. The presence of antibodies in the woman's serum or on the man's sperm is presumed to confer a relative infertility or delay until the time of conception. In the man, the antibodies can be found in the sera or the seminal plasma and coating the spermatozoa. In the woman, these antibodies can be found in the cervical mucus or sera. The reporting of success or failure in this group is burdened by the number of different sperm antibody assays in use. Some clinicians believe that as many as 10% to 20% of women with unexplained infertility may have sperm antibodies.[120, 121] In our infertility practice, a recent study[122] showed that 11.2% of all women tested (n = 812) had immunoglobulins G and A and antibodies in their serum that exceeded 25% and that this figure was 21.2% positive for all men tested. A large portion of these patients had been referred with a diagnosis of male factor. Prior to immunobead testing, it was not possible to gather precise data on the location of antibodies on the sperm and the antibody types.[123] Even when the immunobead assay is used,

there is no standard agreement on what constitutes a "positive" or "negative" result. In addition, the location of the antibodies on the sperm may functionally alter their fertility. When antisperm antibodies are directed against the head of the sperm, this may markedly reduce or prevent the sperm from penetrating zona-free hamster eggs.[124]

Data on immunologic infertility and IUI are provided in Table 46–6.[69, 83, 86, 115, 125] The lower pregnancy rates per couple probably represent a higher cutoff for antibody-positive patients. It would appear from the larger study by Margalloth and colleagues[125] that human gonadotropin stimulation certainly improves the chances of pregnancy on a couple or treatment cycle basis. The exact mechanism by which hMG stimulates the pregnancy rate in these women is unknown. It has been suggested that the high estrogen levels somehow lower the number of antisperm antibodies and the complement in the reproductive tract.[125]

SPONTANEOUS OVULATION VERSUS SUPEROVULATION FOR IUI

Preliminary studies suggest that a combination of hMG administered to the female to induce superovulation and IUI is superior to IUI or hMG alone. Most prospective studies show an increase in pregnancy rates in which IUI is compared with IUI with hMGs with or without clomiphene citrate.[92, 111, 126, 127] This trend is not as easily seen in the summaries in Tables 46–3 to 46–5. However, these data (in the tables) represent an average of all studies and may not be representative of the data that a prospective, randomized trial might provide.

SPERM NUMBERS AND TIMING OF INSEMINATION

Number of Motile Sperm Required for IUI

Successful pregnancies have been established following IUI with fewer than 500,000 motile sperm in the inseminating volume.[58, 79, 86] However, a review of the literature makes it seem probable that the chances of pregnancy following IUI with fewer than 1 million motile sperm is quite low.[12, 58, 79, 86, 103, 128–130] In general, there is an increase in the pregnancy rate with increasing numbers of motile sperm inseminated (Fig. 46–6).[15, 128, 130] There does not appear to be an advantage to inseminating more than 20 million motile cells from either fresh or frozen-thawed specimens; at concentrations of fewer than 5 million motile sperm, there is a decrease in the pregnancy rate per cycle. However, in the case of women stimulated with hMG, two studies suggested different results. Shelden and coworkers[128] found that there is a dramatic increase in the pregnancy rate when more than 20 million motile cells are used, whereas Horvath and associates[130] could not demonstrate a difference in the pregnancy rate in these women when sperm concentrations ranging from 1 million to 100 million motile sperm were used for insemination.

In severe male factor, one should consider the possibility of pooling sequential ejaculates. A recent report by Tur-Kaspa

	Number of Patients	Pregnancy Rate/Patient
TABLE 46–5. Cervical Factor, Endometriosis, and Unexplained Infertility: Literature Survey of IUI Results		
Cervical Factor		
All cases: reference numbers 46, 47, 69, 74, 75, 77, 83, 86, 91, 95, 101, 102, 108, 112–116	359	28.7
Unstimulated cycles	183	32.4
Stimulated + unstimulated cycles	86	33.7
Stimulated cycles	90	16.7
Endometriosis		
All cases: reference numbers 46, 69, 86, 91, 107, 108, 119	151	17.9
Unstimulated cycles	60	13.3
Stimulated + unstimulated cycles	29	10.3
Stimulated cycles	62	25.8
Unexplained		
All cases: reference numbers 3, 86, 88, 91, 95, 101, 102, 108, 110–114	180	25.0
Unstimulated cycles	62	24.1
Stimulated + unstimulated cycles	29	17.2
Stimulated cycles	89	28.1

IUI, intrauterine insemination.

TABLE 46–6. Summary of Results of IUI with Immunologic Infertility (Sperm Antibodies)

Reference	Number of Patients	Percentage Per Patient	Pregnant/ Cycle	Average Number of IUI Cycles	Stimulation Protocol
Toffle et al,[115] 1985	9	11.1	—	—	Mixed
Confino et al,[83] 1986					
Male	8	25.0	6.6	3.7	None
Female	10	40.0	10.5	3.8	None
Byrd et al,[86] 1987	15	6.7	—	—	None
Margalloth et al,[125] 1988	67	13.4	3.2	4.3	None
	20	30.0	7.0	4.3	CC
	28	39.3	10.8	3.6	hMG
Yovich and Matson,[69] 1988					
Male	14	35.7	18.5	1.9	Mixed
Female	19	36.8	17.1	2.2	Mixed

IUI, intrauterine insemination; CC, clomiphene citrate; hMG, human menopausal gonadotropin.

and colleagues[131] suggested that there is no significant difference between two sequential ejaculates. Two samples collected within 4 hours may be pooled and used for IUI.

Timing of Insemination

Spermatozoa placed in the uterus normally migrate rapidly into the fallopian tubes and peritoneal cavity.[18, 132] This creates an effective dilution without cervical release, as with ICI. There is evidence that endometriosis and sperm antibodies may cause deleterious effects on sperm. Because the survival time of spermatozoa is not precisely known and ovulation cannot always be documented, insemination should be performed as close as possible to the time of ovulation, and timing of ovulation during natural or spontaneous cycles is required. The most commonly used methods for timing during natural or spontaneous cycles are basal body temperature, cervical mucus scores, quantitative and qualitative urinary LH concentrations, and ultrasound (US) monitoring.

The detection of LH in urine or serum has been aided by the development of rapid LH kits. Urinary LH assays based on monoclonal antibodies have been used effectively to monitor ovulatory cycles. An advantage of urinary LH assays is that they measure a pool of LH collected over time. Based on published studies,[8, 15] the optimal time for insemination is the day after the LH rise. We have previously published a time for IUI in a single-cycle insemination in which ovulation occurred about 15.8 ± 2.6 hours after the LH peak or about 30 to 33 hours after the LH rise in urine.[15]

Follicular rupture following stimulation by hMG is rarely synchronous and may occur within 24 to 72 hours with human chorionic gonadotropin (hCG).[91] Silverberg and co-workers[133] recently compared single IUIs with a regimen employing two IUIs in patients undergoing follicular stimulation with hMG. They found a significant increase in the pregnancy rate per treatment cycle (52%) with two inseminations compared with the 8.7% pregnancy rate per cycle observed after one IUI. It is possible that the greater success rate may have resulted from multiple ovulation over several hours. The authors speculate that the preovulatory IUI performed at 18 hours post-hCG may be more important than the postovulatory IUI. Data from natural cycles suggest that inseminations performed just prior to ovulation result in an enhanced pregnancy rate.[8]

Timing must be considered not only in respect to the individual cycle but also with respect to the total number of cycles performed on each patient. Most pregnancies following IUI occur within the first three treatment cycles.[15] It would seem logical therefore to restrict IUI to six cycles or less. In our own program, we find that most pregnancies occur within four cycles in both our husband and donor populations. In Figure 46–7, we examined the outcome of 791 cycles of IUI performed with frozen-thawed donor sperm. Timing of insemination was determined by a quantitative urinary LH assay performed in the laboratory on at least two or three samples per day. We found that the highest percentage of pregnancies occurred within the first three cycles of treatment.

Intrauterine Catheters

Catheters used for IUI should be nontoxic, contain little dead space, and be capable of being passed through the

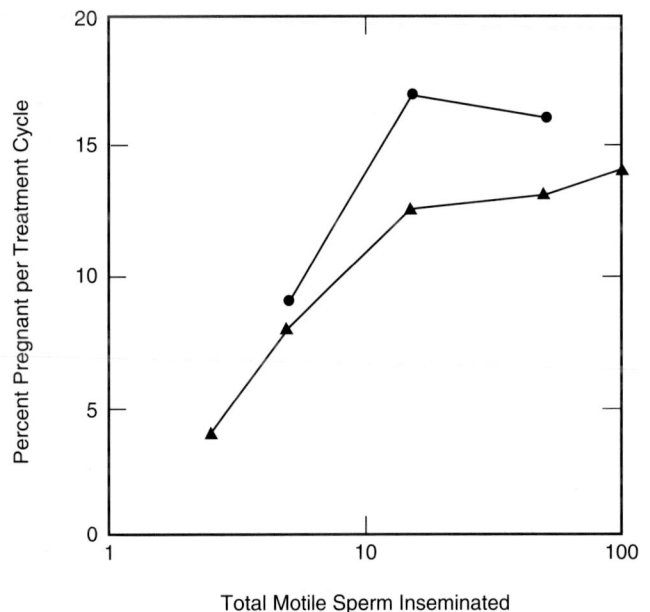

FIGURE 46–6. The influence of the numbers of motile sperm inseminated and the pregnancy outcome per treatment cycle. These data were gathered from cycles when there was a single insemination. The *solid triangles* represent fresh husband's sperm. The *solid circles* represent cycles in which frozen-thawed donor sperm was used for insemination. X axis: log of total motile sperm inseminated $\times\ 10^{-3}$. (Data from references 8, 15, and 86.)

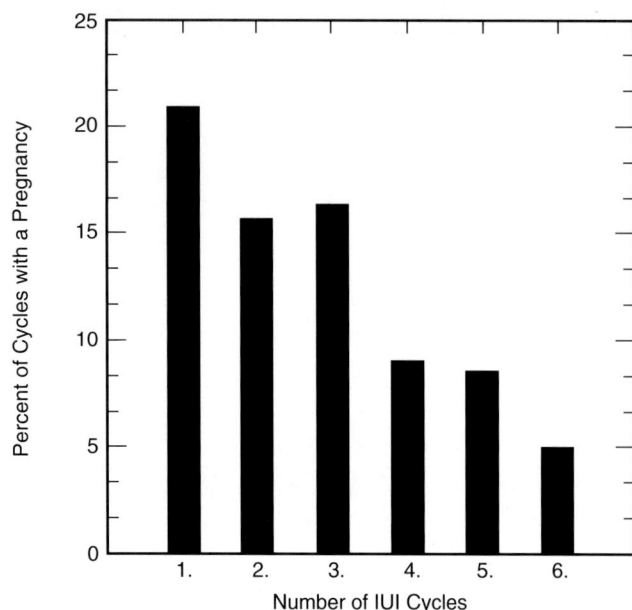

FIGURE 46–7. Percentage of each intrauterine insemination (IUI) cycle ending in a pregnancy in a donor insemination program using frozen-thawed sperm. Data are from 791 cycles of donor insemination that was timed by quantitative urinary luteinizing hormone.

cervix without causing any pain or trauma. There are a variety of catheters available for use[15]; however, none appear to be associated with a higher pregnancy rate. Because each catheter has its particular advantage, physicians may choose the one they are most comfortable using. In our experience, the Tom Cat catheter has proved reliable and economical to use.

TRANSUTEROTUBAL AND INTRAPERITONEAL INSEMINATION

Direct Intraperitoneal Injection

DIPI was first reported by Forrler and associates[134, 135] and has been applied in cases of cervical factor, severe male factor, unexplained infertility, and endometriosis.[127, 134–141] In this procedure, a needle attached to a syringe is passed through the posterior fornix under US guidance into the pouch of Douglas. After the needle tip is confirmed to be in the peritoneal cavity, washed spermatozoa are injected. This should facilitate the transport of sperm to the peritoneal cavity, a site they are known to reach following insemination.[18] The purported advantage to this technique is bypassing the cervical mucus and uterine secretions.

If this procedure proves to be efficacious in the treatment of certain types of infertility, it would represent a less expensive alternative to GIFT. However, in a prospective trial by Dooley and colleagues,[138] DIPI had a much lower pregnancy rate compared with GIFT. However, all GIFT patients were stimulated with hMG, whereas only some of the DIPI cycles were stimulated, which could have resulted in a lower pregnancy rate. The exposure of sperm to the peritoneal fluid in some women may have a negative effect. Forrler and coworkers[135] noted that no pregnancies occurred in women whose peritoneal fluid had a negative effect on sperm in vitro. It is also possible that DIPI may result in an activation of the immune system and the development of sperm antibodies.

An examination of the literature (Table 46–7) suggests that DIPI has no advantage over IUI based on pregnancy rates per couple or treatment cycle. Cycle fecundity correlates with increasing sperm concentrations, as was seen with IUI.[141] Pregnancies have been reported with inseminations of 100,000 to 200,000 sperm.[135, 141] However, in the presence of cervical stenosis or any factor that would interfere with normal IUI, DIPI may prove to be a viable alternative to IUI or GIFT.

Transuterotubal Insemination

It is possible to guide a catheter with the use of US through the cervical canal and into the uterotubal junction. Spermatozoa can be directly injected into the fallopian tubes. Whether intratubal insemination will prove to be superior to IUI has yet to be shown. The feasibility of this technique has been demonstrated by Jansen and associates,[142] who catheterized the fallopian tubes via the vagina and introduced sperm into them. Using transvaginal sonography, a 5.5 Fr Teflon outer catheter was passed through the cervix and into the uterine cavity on the side of the dominant follicle. A soft 2 Fr inner catheter was passed 3 to 4 cm past the uterotubal junction. Following placement of the catheter in the fallopian tube, 30 µL of sperm was introduced. In this initial study, there was a reported 12% pregnancy rate per treatment cycle.[142]

POSSIBLE RISKS OF IUI

Infection

Micro-organism contamination can be commonly found in semen, and it is possible that the presence of these organisms in the specimen may contribute to a decrease in the fertilization rate.[43, 102, 143] Micro-organisms have been isolated by laparoscopy from the peritoneal fluid of women undergoing IUI.[144] Micro-organisms that have been reported to be transmitted by artificial insemination include *Neisseria gonorrhoeae*,[145] *Trichomonas vaginalis*,[146] *Streptococcus*,[146] *Ureaplasma*,[118] hepatitis B,[147] herpesvirus,[148] and human immunodeficiency virus.[149] In most reported cases of transmission, donor insemination was performed by intravaginal insemination or ICI. Indeed, many of them were performed prior to the recommendations of the American Fertility Society for screening of donors prior to use of their semen for donor insemination.[150] In a review of 38 studies, Sacks and Simon[151] examined more than 3267 reports of women who had undergone IUI. There were only six reported cases of infections, giving an incidence of 1.83 infectious complications per 1000 women. These infection rates were not altered by semen washing with antibiotics or the administration of prophylactic antibiotics to the women. It is apparent that infection rates following IUI are low and that the administration of prophylactic antibiotics to the patient is not justified.

TABLE 46–7. Therapeutic Insemination: DIPI Versus IUI or Intercourse

Reference	Procedure	Number of Patients	Number of Treatment Cycles	Percent Pregnant/ Couple (%)	Percent Pregnant/ Treatment Cycle (%)
Forrler et al,[135] 1986	DIPI ± hMG or CC	40	56	20.0	14.3
Curson & Parsons,[137] 1987	DIPI + CC / hMG	10	—	10.0	—
Dooley et al,[138] 1988	DIPI + hMG or CC	33	51	9.0	5.9
	GIFT + hMG	36	42	33.3	28.6
Menard et al,[136] 1988	DIPI + hMG ± CC	105	171	20.0	12.3
Crosignani et al,[139] 1990	Intercourse + CC	—	—	2.7	—
	IUI + CC	—	—	12.5	—
	DIPI + CC	—	—	17.5	—
Evans et al,[127] 1991	Intercourse + hMG/CC	56	63	—	3.1
	IUI + hMG/CC	—	56	—	3.5
	DIPI + hMG/CC	—	84	—	11.9
Campos-Liete et al,[140] 1982	Intercourse + hMG or CC	26	25	16.0	16.0
	DIPI + hMG or CC	—	25	0	0
Turhan et al,[141] 1992	DIPI + CC/hMG/FSH				
	Male factor	50	118	34.0	14.4
	Cervical factor	16	19	37.5	31.6
	Unexplained infertility	45	92	46.6	22.8

DIPI, direct intraperitoneal insemination; hMG, human menopausal gonadotropin; CC, clomiphene citrate; GIFT, gamete intrafallopian transfer; FSH, follicle-stimulating hormone.

Pain or Uterine Cramping

There have been several reports in the literature of cramping after IUI. Allen and colleagues[21] reported severe cramps in 6% to 17% of patients. Isolating sperm from the seminal plasma and reducing the volume of the insemination sample to less than 0.5 mL should decrease this problem.

Spontaneous Abortion

The rate of spontaneous abortion in patients undergoing IUI has ranged from 0 to 75% in reported series.[19–21, 50] The generally accepted rate of spontaneous abortion in the first 20 weeks is 15% in couples who have not undergone assisted reproductive techniques. Earlier summaries of spontaneous abortion rates following artificial insemination reported an average rate of approximately 26%.[20, 21] A more recent survey of the spontaneous abortion rate following artificial insemination is seen in Table 46–8.[2, 23, 36, 46, 50, 69, 74–77, 83, 86, 88, 91, 104, 115, 129, 152–154] It appears that the spontaneous abortion rate is approximately twice as high following IUI. Whether this apparent higher abortion rate is related to infertility factors or to ascertainment bias is unknown.

Development of Antisperm Antibodies

IUI has been suggested as a treatment for immunologic infertility. Antibodies may interfere with the motility of sper-

matozoa within the cervical mucus[155]; interrupt capacitation, sperm attachment, or penetration of the zona pellucida or plasma membrane of the oocyte[123, 156, 157]; cause complement-mediated sperm cytotoxicity[158]; or enhance phagocytosis of sperm by macrophages. Although the treatment of infertility caused by sperm antibodies remains controversial, couples with low to moderate levels of antibodies present in the male or female are able to achieve pregnancy (see Table 46–6). Data from Margalloth and coworkers[125] using the indirect Immunobead Test (BioRad, Richmond, CA) suggest that there is a significant decrease in the pregnancy rate when more than 50% of the sperm have antibodies bound to the head. High levels of antibody binding to the tail do not decrease the pregnancy rate as much, perhaps because the cervical barrier has been bypassed. Conception rates in these women with antisperm antibodies can also be compromised by other infertility factors.[125]

One question raised about the safety of placement of large numbers of spermatozoa into the uterine cavity is whether such therapy can lead to the development of sperm antibodies.[122, 159] Several factors are thought to prevent the formation of an immune response in women, including the cervical filtration of sperm, the phagocytosis of sperm, and the presence of immunosuppressive substances in the seminal fluid. The induction of immunity to sperm in women who have measurable antibody titers or those who have not been previously sensitized to sperm has been examined.[103, 159–162] Several studies have focused on measuring antibody levels in women who were either positive or negative for sperm antibodies over several cycles of IUI.[103, 161]

TABLE 46–8. Therapeutic Insemination: Spontaneous Abortion Rate*

Stimulation Protocol	Number of Cycles	Number Pregnant	Number Aborted	Percentage Aborted (%)
Spontaneous	1181	90	28	31.1
Spontaneous or stimulated	4195	252	62	24.6
hMG and/or CC	1402	185	52	28.1

*All cases: references 2, 23, 36, 46, 50, 69, 74–77, 83, 86, 88, 91, 104, 115, 129, 152–154.

Such studies find little or no evidence to support the hypothesis that sperm antibody levels as measured by indirect immunobead testing increase after gonadotropin stimulation and IUI. Two separate groups have reported the development of some antibodies in approximately 10% of the women undergoing IUI. However, there is some question as to the clinical significance of these findings. Goldberg and associates[161] suggested that there is no significant induction of antisperm antibody production in unsensitized women or women with low titers of sperm antibodies. Friedman and colleagues[160] suggested that the presence of antisperm antibodies in the male partner or the number of IUI cycles does not increase the risk of a woman developing antisperm antibodies following IUI. It is difficult to correlate the presence of a "positive" sperm antibody assay and clinical outcome. There are different levels of sperm antibodies that are considered positive in different laboratories. In the absence of control groups not undergoing IUI and long-term followup of antibody levels, more data may be required before a final conclusion can be made.

Multiple Pregnancies

The rate of spontaneous occurrence of twins is 1.05% to 1.35% of all births and that of triplets is 0.01% to 0.017%.[163] The increased number or incidence of multiple pregnancies after follicular stimulation with clomiphene or gonadotropins is probably due to the increased number of oocytes available for fertilization.

Following IUI in cycles stimulated with gonadotropins, multiple gestation rates of 5% to 27% have been reported.[78, 92, 106, 108, 128, 130, 165] In one study, multiple gestation was linked to the total number of motile cells inseminated. Shelden and coworkers[128] reported a high risk of multiple pregnancies when more than 20 million motile sperm were inseminated. However, Dodson and associates[108] could not determine or successfully predict which patients would be more inclined to have a multiple pregnancy. They examined peak estradiol concentration, the number of follicles larger than 10 mm in diameter on the day of hCG administration, and the total number of motile cells inseminated. Indeed, Friedman[164] published a case report of a woman with only one follicle larger than 15 mm and numerous small follicles with hMG stimulation who became pregnant with sextuplets following IUI.

SUMMARY

IUI has been used empirically in the past for the treatment of various types of infertility. The data presented suggest that there is a therapeutic benefit from IUI, particularly for women with cervical factor. This assumes that appropriate sperm selection techniques are used, that there are adequate numbers of motile cells inseminated, and that insemination is timed within a few hours of ovulation.

Male subfertility has been the most controversial indication for IUI. Although the pregnancy rate of IUI in the presence of male factor and endometriosis is low, the procedure should not be rejected outright without considering the cost effectiveness when compared with GIFT and IVF. In cases of male factor when more than 1 million motile sperm can be harvested and in cases of cervical hostility, unexplained infertility, and antisperm antibodies, IUI should provide a higher pregnancy rate than the pregnancy rate that would occur spontaneously (especially with superovulation). The literature suggests that the use of clomiphene citrate alone in ovulatory women does not improve pregnancy rates with IUI. The indications are that no more than six cycles of IUI should be attempted.

There are still many questions regarding IUI, but the use of the technique has been firmly established. This technique should continue to be a safe, noninvasive procedure that can be used to treat infertility in most couples trying to achieve pregnancy.

REFERENCES

1. Mastroianni L Jr, Laberge JL, Rock J. Appraisal of the efficacy of artificial insemination with husband's sperm and evaluation of insemination techniques. Fertil Steril 1957;8:260–266.
2. Cruz RI, Kemmann E, Brandeis VT, et al. A prospective study of intrauterine insemination of processed sperm from men with oligoasthenospermia in super ovulated women. Fertil Steril 1986;46:673–677.
3. Irvine DS, Aitken RJ, Lees MM, Reid C. Failure of high intrauterine insemination of husband's semen. Lancet 1986;2:972–973.
4. Kerin J, Quinn P. Washed intrauterine insemination in the treatment of oligospermic infertility. Semin Reprod Endocrinol 1987;5:23–33.
5. Urry R, Middleton R, McGavin S. A simple and effective technique for increasing pregnancy rates in couples with retrograde ejaculation. Fertil Steril 1986;46:1124–1127.
6. Friedman A, Haas S, Kredentser J, et al. A controlled trial of intrauterine insemination for cervical factor and male factor: a preliminary report. Int J Fertil 1989;34:199.
7. te Velde, van Kooy R, Waterreus J. Intrauterine insemination of washed husband's spermatozoa: a controlled study. Fertil Steril 1989;51:182–185.
8. Byrd W, Bradshaw K, Carr B, et al. A prospective randomized study of pregnancy rates following intrauterine and intracervical insemination using frozen donor sperm. Fertil Steril 1990;53:521–527.
9. Martinez AR, Bernardus RE, Voorhorst FJ, et al. Intrauterine insemination does and clomiphene citrate does not improve fecundity in couples with infertility due to male or idiopathic factors: a prospective, randomized, controlled study. Fertil Steril 1990;53:847–853.
10. Kirby CA, Flaherty SP, Godfrey BM, et al. A prospective trial of intrauterine insemination of motile spermatozoa versus timed intercourse. Fertil Steril 1991;56:102–107.
11. Hughes EG, Collins JP, Garner PR. Homologous artificial insemination for oligoasthenospermia: a randomized controlled study for comparing intracervical and intrauterine insemination. Fertil Steril 1987;48:278–281.
12. Ho P, Poon I, Chan S, Wang C. Intrauterine insemination is not useful in oligoasthenospermia. Fertil Steril 1989;51:682–684.
13. Patton PE, Burry KA, Novy MJ, Wolf DP. A comparative evaluation of intracervical and intrauterine routes in donor therapeutic insemination. Hum Reprod 1990;5:263–265.
14. Bradshaw KD, Guzick DS, Grun B, et al. Cumulative pregnancy rates for donor insemination according to ovulatory function and tubal status. Fertil Steril 1987;48:1051–1054.
15. Kerin J, Byrd W. Supracervical placement of spermatozoa: utility of intrauterine and tubal insemination. In: Soules MR, editor. Controversies in Reproductive Endocrinology and Infertility. New York: Elsevier, 1989:183–204.
16. Katz DF, Drobnis EZ, Overstreet JW. Factors regulating mammalian sperm migration through the female reproductive tract and oocyte investments. Gamete Res 1989;22:443–469.
17. Settlage DSF, Motoshima M, Tredway DR. Sperm transport from the external cervical os to the fallopian tubes in women: a time and quantitation study. Fertil Steril 1973;24:655–661.
18. Mortimer D, Templeton AA. Sperm transport in the human female reproductive tract in relation to semen analysis characteristics and time of ovulation. J Reprod Fertil 1982;64:401–408.

19. Nachtigall RD, Faure N, Glass RH. Artificial insemination of husband's sperm. Fertil Steril 1979;32:141–147.
20. Nachtigall RD. Indications, techniques, and success rates for AIH. Semin Reprod Endocrinol 1987;5:5–9.
21. Allen NC, Herbert CM, Maxson WS, et al. Intrauterine insemination: a critical review. Fertil Steril 1985;44:569–580.
22. Moghissi KS. Some refections on intrauterine insemination. Fertil Steril 1986;32:141–147.
23. Pardo M, Bancells N. Artificial insemination with husband's sperm (AIH): techniques for sperm selection. Arch Androl 1989;22:15–27.
24. Taylor PJ, Kredentser JV. Washed intrauterine insemination: indication and success. Int J Fertil 1989;34:378–384.
25. Dixon RE, Buttram VC Jr, Schum CW. Artificial insemination using homologous semen: a review of 158 cases. Fertil Steril 1976;27:647–654.
26. Tarlatzia BC, Bontis J, Kolibianakis EM, et al. Evaluation of intrauterine insemination with washed spermatozoa from the husband in the treatment of infertility. Hum Reprod 1991;6:1241–1246.
27. Aitken RJ, Clarkson JS. Cellular basis of defective sperm function and its association with the genesis of reactive oxygen species by human spermatozoa. J Reprod Fertil 1987;81:459–469.
28. Mortimer D. Sperm preparation techniques and iatrogenic failures of in vitro fertilization. Hum Reprod 1991;6:173–176.
29. Paulson JD, Polakoski K, Leto S. Further characterization of glass wool column filtration of human semen. Fertil Steril 1979;32:125–126.
30. Sherman JK, Paulson JD, Liu KC. Effect of glass wool filtration on ultrastructure of human spermatozoa. Fertil Steril 1981;36:643–647.
31. Jeyendran RS, Perez-Pelaez M, Crabo BG. Concentration of viable spermatozoa for artificial insemination. Fertil Steril 1986;45:132–134.
32. Rana N, Jeyendran RS, Holmgren WJ, et al. Glass wool–filtered spermatozoa and their oocyte penetrating capacity. J In Vitro Fertil Embryo Transfer 1989;6:280–284.
33. Katayama KP, Stehlik E, Jeyendran RS. In vitro fertilization outcome: glass wool–filtered sperm versus swim-up sperm. Fertil Steril 1989;52:670–672.
34. Ericsson RJ, Langevin CN, Nishino M. Isolation of fraction rich in human Y sperm. Nature 1973;246:421–424.
35. Glass RH, Ericsson RJ. Intrauterine insemination of isolated motile sperm. Fertil Steril 1978;29:535–539.
36. Dmowski WP, Gaynor L, Lawrence M, et al. Artificial insemination homologous with oligospermic semen separated on albumin columns. Fertil Steril 1979;31:58–62.
37. Hanson FM, Rock J. Artificial insemination with husband's sperm. Fertil Steril 1951;2:162–174.
38. Drevius L-O. The "sperm-rise" test. J Reprod Fertil 1971;24:427–429.
39. Lopata A, Patullo MJ, Chang A, James B. A method for collecting motile spermatozoa from human semen. Fertil Steril 1976;27:677–684.
40. Russell LD, Rogers BJ. Improvement in the quality and fertilization potential of a human sperm population using the rise technique. J Androl 1987;8:25–33.
41. Pertoft H, Rubin K, Kjellen L, et al. The viability of cells grown or centrifuged in a new density gradient medium, Percoll (TM). Exp Cell Res 1977;110:449–454.
42. Gorus FK, Pipeleers DG. A rapid method for the fractionation of human spermatozoa according to their progressive motility. Fertil Steril 1981;35:662–665.
43. Bolton VN, Warren RE, Braude PR. Removal of bacterial contaminants from semen for in vitro fertilization or artificial insemination by the use of buoyant density centrifugation. Fertil Steril 1986;46:1128–1132.
44. Pousette A, Akerlof E, Rosenborg L, Fredricsson B. Increase in progressive motility and improved morphology of human spermatozoa following their migration through Percoll gradients. Int J Androl 1986;9:1–13.
45. Iizuka R, Kaneko S, Kobanawa K, et al. Semen by Percoll density gradients and its application to AIH. Arch Androl 1988;20:117–124.
46. Lalich RA, Marut EL, Prins GS, Scommegna A. Life table analysis of intrauterine insemination pregnancy rates. Am J Obstet Gynecol 1988;158:980–984.
47. Pardo M, Barri P, Bancells N, et al. Spermatozoa selection in discontinuous Percoll gradients for use in artificial insemination. Fertil Steril 1988;49:505–509.
48. Tanphaichitr N, Agulnick A, Seibel M, Taymor M. Comparison of the in vitro fertilization rate by human sperm capacitated by multi-tube swim-up and Percoll gradient centrifugation. J In Vitro Fertil Embryo Transfer 1988;5:119–122.
49. Velez de la Calle JF. Human spermatozoa selection in improved discontinuous Percoll gradients. Fertil Steril 1991;56:737–742.
50. Tredway DR, Chan P, Henig I, et al. Effectiveness of stimulated menstrual cycles and Percoll sperm preparation in intrauterine insemination. J Reprod Med 1990;35:103–108.
51. Gellert-Mortimer ST, Clark GN, Baker HWG, et al. Evaluation of Nycodenz and Percoll density gradients for the selection of motile human spermatozoa. Fertil Steril 1988;49:335–341.
52. Berger T, Marrs RP, Moyer DL. Comparison of techniques for selection of motile spermatozoa. Fertil Steril 1985;43:268–273.
53. Serafini P, Blank W, Tran C, et al. Enhanced penetration of zona-free hamster ova by sperm prepared by Nycodenz and Percoll gradient centrifugation. Fertil Steril 1990;53:551–555.
54. Wikland M, Wik O, Steen Y, et al. A self-migration method for preparation of sperm for in-vitro fertilization. Hum Reprod 1987;3:191–195.
55. Graham EF, Vasquez IA, Schmehl MKL, Evensen BK. An assay of semen quality by use of Sephadex filtration. Int Cong Animal Reprod Artificial Insem 1976;8:896–899.
56. Weeda AJ, Cohen J. Effects of purification or split ejaculation of semen and stimulation of spermatozoa by caffeine on their motility and fertilizing ability with the use of zona-free hamster ova. Fertil Steril 1982;37:817–822.
57. Drobnis EZ, Zhong CQ, Overstreet JW. Separation of cryopreserved human semen using sephadex columns, washing or Percoll gradients. J Androl 1991;12:201–208.
58. Kerin JFP, Peek J, Warnes GM, et al. Improved conception rate after intrauterine insemination of washed spermatozoa from men with poor quality semen. Lancet 1984;1:533–535.
59. Marshburn PB, McIntire D, Carr BR, Byrd W. Spermatozoal characteristics from fresh and frozen donor semen and their correlation with fertility outcome after intrauterine insemination. Fertil Steril 1992;58:179–186.
60. Huzar G, Vigue L, Corrales M. Sperm creatine phosphokinase activity as a measure of sperm quality in normospermic, variable spermic, and oligospermic men. Biol Reprod 1988;38:1061–1066.
61. Kanwar KC, Yanagimachi R, Lopata A. Effects of human seminal plasma on the fertilizing capacity of human spermatozoa. Fertil Steril 1979;31:321–327.
62. Wolf DP, Sokoloski JE. Characterication of the sperm penetration assay. J Androl 1982;3:445–451.
63. Byrd W. Fertilization, embryogenesis and implantation. In: Carr BR, Blackwell RE, editors. Textbook of Reproductive Medicine. New York: Appleton and Lange, 1992:1–16.
64. Yanagimachi R. Mechanisms of fertilization in mammals. In: Mastrioanni L, Biggers JD, editors. Fertilization and Embryonic Development in Vitro. New York: Plenum Press, 1981:81–182.
65. Byrd W, Tsu J, Wolf DP. Kinetics of spontaneous and induced acrosomal loss in human sperm incubated under capacitating and noncapacitating conditions. Gamete Res 1989;22:109–122.
66. Schoenfeld C, Amelar RD, Dubin L. Stimulation of ejaculated human spermatozoa by caffeine: a preliminary report. Fertil Steril 1973;24:772–775.
67. Harrison RF. Insemination of husband's semen with and without the addition of caffeine. Fertil Steril 1978;29:532–535.
68. Dougherty KA, Cockett ATK, Urry RL. Caffeine, theophylline and human sperm motility. Fertil Steril 1976;27:541–545.
69. Yovich JL, Matson PL. The treatment of infertility by the high intrauterine insemination of husband's washed spermatozoa. Hum Reprod 1988;3:939–943.
70. Yovich JL, Aitken J, Yovich JM, et al. In vitro pentoxifylline improves the fertilization rate of oligospermic and asthenozoospermic males. 7th Annual Meeting of the European Society Human Reproduction and Embryology, 1991:141a.
71. Blumenfeld Z, Nahhas N. Pretreatment of sperm with human follicular fluid for borderline male infertility. Fertil Steril 1989;51:863–868.
72. Aafjes JH, Vijver JCM, Schenck PE. The duration of infertility: an important datum for the fertility prognosis of men with semen abnormalities. Fertil Steril 1978;30:423–425.
73. Collins JA, Wrixon W, Janes LB, Wilson EH. Treatment-independent pregnancy among infertile couples. N Engl J Med 1983;309:1201–1206.
74. DiMarzo SJ, Rakoff JS. Intrauterine insemination with husband's washed sperm. Fertil Steril 1986;46:470–475.
75. Quagliarello J, Arny M. Intracervical versus intrauterine insemination: correlation of outcome with antecedent postcoital testing. Fertil Steril 1986;46:870–875.

76. Huzar G, DeCherney A. The role of intrauterine insemination in the treatment of infertile couples: the Yale experience. Semin Reprod Endocrinol 1987;5:11–32.

77. Kemmann E, Bohrer M, Shelden R, et al. Active ovulation management increases the monthly probability of pregnancy occurrence in ovulatory women who receive intrauterine insemination. Fertil Steril 1987;48:916–920.

78. Horbay GLA, Cowell CA, Casper RF. Multiple follicular recruitment and intrauterine insemination outcomes compared by age and diagnosis. Hum Reprod 1991;6:947–952.

79. Karlstrom PO, Bakos O, Bergh T, Lundkvist O. Intrauterine insemination and comparison of two methods of sperm preparation. Hum Reprod 1991;6:390–395.

80. World Health Organization. Laboratory Manual for the Examination of Human Semen and Semen–Cervical Mucus Interaction. Cambridge: Cambridge University Press, 1987.

81. Harris SJ, Milligan MP, Masson GM, Dennis KJ. Improved separation of motile sperm in asthenospermia and its application to artificial insemination homologous (AIH). Fertil Steril 1981;36:219–221.

82. Francavilla F, Catignani P, Romano R, Fabbrini A. Treatment of infertile couples by intrauterine artificial insemination homologous (AIH) of motile sperm collected by swim-up in human serum. Acta Eur Fertil 1985;16:411–414.

83. Confino E, Friberg J, Dudkiewicz AB, Gleicher N. Intrauterine inseminations with washed human spermatozoa. Fertil Steril 1986;46:55–60.

84. Hull ME, David D, Magyar DO, et al. Experience with intrauterine insemination for cervical factor and oligospermia. Am J Obstet Gynecol 1986;154:1333–1338.

85. Thomas EJ, McTighe L, King H, et al. Failure of high intrauterine insemination of husband's semen. Lancet 1986;2:693–694.

86. Byrd W, Ackerman GE, Carr BR, et al. Treatment of refractory infertility by transcervical intrauterine insemination of washed spermatozoa. Fertil Steril 1987;48:921–927.

87. Makler A. Washed intrauterine insemination in the treatment of idiopathic infertility. Semin Reprod Endocrinol 1987;5:35–43.

88. Melis GB, Paoletti AM, Strigini F, et al. Pharmacologic induction of multiple follicular development improves the success rate of artificial insemination with husband's semen in couples with male-related or unexplained infertility. Fertil Steril 1987;47:441–445.

89. Szollosi J, Szilagyi I, Daru J, Sas M. Intrauterine insemination with washed sperm. Arch Androl 1989;23:71–76.

90. Francavilla F, Romano R, Santucci R, Poccia G. Effect of sperm morphology and motile sperm count on outcome of intrauterine insemination in oligozoospermia and/or asthenozoospermia. Fertil Steril 1990;53:892–897.

91. Irianni FM, Acosta AA, Oehninger S, Acosta MR. Therapeutic intrauterine insemination (TII): controversial treatment for infertility. Arch Androl 1990;25:147–167.

92. Chaffkin LM, Nulsen JC, Luciano AA, Metzger DA. A comparative analysis of the cycle fecundity rates associated with combined human menopausal gonadotropin (hMG) and intrauterine insemination (IUI) versus either hMG or IUI alone. Fertil Steril 1991;55:252–257.

93. Friedman AJ, Juneau-Norcross M, Sedensky B, et al. Life table analysis of intrauterine insemination pregnancy rates for couples with cervical factor, male factor, and idiopathic infertility. Fertil Steril 1991;55:1005–1007.

94. Hoing LM, Devroey P, Van Steirteghem AC. Treatment of infertility because of oligoasthenoteratospermia by transvcervical intrauterine insemination of motile spermatozoa. Fertil Steril 1986;45:388–391.

95. Wiltbank MC, Kosasa S, Rogers B. Treatment of infertile patients by intrauterine insemination of washed spermatozoa. Andrologia 1985;17:22–30.

96. Yovich JL, Matson PL. Pregnancy rates after high intrauterine insemination of husband's spermatozoa or gamete intrafallopian transfer. Lancet 1986;2:1287.

97. McGovern P, Quagliarello J, Arny M. Relationship of within-patient semen variability to outcome of intrauterine insemination. Fertil Steril 1989;51:1019–1023.

98. Adamson GD, Subak LL, Boltz NL, McNulty MA. Failure of intrauterine insemination in a refractory infertility population. Fertil Steril 1991;56:361–363.

99. Yavetz H, Mosek A, Yogev L, et al. Intrauterine insemination in subfertile couples. Andrologia 1990;22:29–33.

100. Tarlatzis BC, Bontis J, Kolibianakis EM, et al. Evaluation of intrauterine insemination with washed spermatozoa from the husband in the treatment of infertility. Hum Reprod 1991;6:1241–1246.

101. Sher G, Knutzen VK, Stratton CJ, et al. In vitro sperm capacitation and transcervical intrauterine insemination for the treatment of refractory infertility: phase I. Fertil Steril 1984;41:260–264.

102. Hewitt J, Cohen J, Fehilly CB, et al. Seminal bacterial pathogens and in vitro fertilization. J In Vitro Fertil Embryo Transfer 1985;2:105–108.

103. Sunde A, Kahn J, Molne K. Intrauterine insemination. Hum Reprod 1988;193:97–99.

104. Bolton VN, Braude PR, Ockenden K, et al. An evaluation of semen analysis and in-vitro tests of sperm function in the prediction of the outcome of intrauterine AIH. Hum Reprod 1989;4:674–679.

105. Mansour RT, Serour GI, Aboulghar MA. Intrauterine insemination with washed capacitated sperm cells in the treatment of male factor, cervical factor and unexplained infertility. Asia-Oceania J Obstet Gynaecol 1989;15:151–154.

106. Allegra A, Volpes A, Coffaro F, et al. Superovulation with buserelin and gonadotropins dramatically improves the success rate of intrauterine insemination with husband's washed semen. Acta Eur Fertil 1990;21:191–195.

107. Dodson WC, Haney AF. Controlled ovarian hyperstimulation and intrauterine insemination for treatment of infertility. Fertil Steril 1991;55:457–467.

108. Dodson WC, Whitesides DB, Hughes CL Jr, et al. Superovulation with intrauterine insemination in the treatment of infertility: a possible alternative to gamete intrafallopian transfer and in vitro fertilization. Fertil Steril 1987;48:441–444.

109. Pepperell RJ, McBain JC. Unexplained infertility; a review. Br J Obstet Gynaecol 1985;92:569–575.

110. Serhal PF, Katz M. Intrauterine insemination. Lancet 1987;1:53.

111. Serhal P, Katz M, Little V, Woronowski H. Unexplained infertility; the value of Pergonal superovulation combined with intrauterine insemination. Fertil Steril 1988;49:602–606.

112. Emperaire JC, Verdaguer S, Meulet-Girard Y, Audebert AJM. Insemination intrauterine de sperm capacite: efficacite conceptionnelle comparee dans differents types d'infertilite du couple. J Gynecol Obstet Biol Reprod 1988;17:387–395.

113. Sueldo C, Hovel L, Gocke C. Intrauterine insemination for the treatment of infertility. Infertility 1986;9:217–244.

114. Perino A, Cimino C, Catinella E, et al. In vitro sperm capacitation and intrauterine insemination (IVC-insem): a simple technique for the treatment of refractory infertility unrelated to female organic pelvic disease. Acta Eur Fertil 1986;17:325–331.

115. Toffle RC, Nagel TC, Tagatz GE, et al. Intrauterine insemination: the University of Minnesota experience. Fertil Steril 1985;43:743–747.

116. Baerthlein WC, Muechler EK, Chaney K. Simplified sperm washing techniques and intrauterine insemination. Obstet Gynecol 1988;71:277–279.

117. Glezerman M, Bernstein D, Insler V. The cervical factor of infertility and intrauterine insemination. Int J Fertil 1984;29:16–19.

118. Barrett JC, Marshall J. The role of conception on different days of the menstrual cycle. Popul Studies 1969;23:378–384.

119. Dodson WC, Hughes CL, Haney AF. Multiple pregnancies conceived with intrauterine insemination during superovulation: an evaluation of clinical characteristics and monitored parameters of conception cycles. Am J Obstet Gynecol 1989;159:382–385.

120. Haas GG. Immunologic infertility. Obstet Gynecol Clin North Am 1987;14:1069–1085.

121. Menge AC. Clinical immunologic infertility: diagnostic measures, incidence of antisperm antibodies. In: Dhindsa DS, Schumacher GFB, editors. Immunologic Aspects of Infertility and Fertility. New York: Elsevier, 1980:205.

122. Kutteh WH, McAllister D, Byrd W, Mestecky J. Antisperm antibodies: present knowledge and new horizons. Molec Androl 1992;4:183–193.

123. Bronson RA, Cooper GW, Rosenfeld DL. Sperm antibodies: their role in infertility. Fertil Steril 1984;42:171–183.

124. Bronson RA, Cooper GW, Rosenfeld DL. Complement-mediated effects of sperm head–directed human antibodies on the ability of human spermatozoa to penetrate zona-free hamster eggs. Fertil Steril 1983;40:91–95.

125. Margalloth EJ, Sauter E, Bronson RA, et al. Intrauterine insemination as treatment for antisperm antibodies in the female. Fertil Steril 1988;50:441–446.

126. Corson SL, Batzer FR, Gocial B, Maislin G. Intrauterine insemination and ovulation stimulation as treatment of infertility. J Reprod Med 1989;34:397–406.

127. Evans J, Wells C, Gregory L, Walker S. A comparison of intrauterine

insemination, intraperitoneal insemination, and natural intercourse in superovulated women. Fertil Steril 1991;56:1183–1187.

128. Shelden R, Kemmann E, Bohrer M, Pasquale S. Multiple gestation is associated with the use of high sperm numbers in the intrauterine insemination specimen in women undergoing gonadotropin stimulation. Fertil Steril 1988;49:607–610.

129. Tucker MJ, Wong CJY, Chang YM, et al. Intrauterine insemination as frontline treatment for non-tubal infertility. Asia-Oceania J Obstet Gynaecol 1990;16:137–143.

130. Horvath P, Bohrer M, Shelden R, Kemmann E. The relationship of sperm parameters to cycle fecundity in superovulated women undergoing intrauterine insemination. Fertil Steril 1989;52:288–294.

131. Tur-Kaspa I, Dudkiewicz A, Confino E, Gleicher R. Pooled sequential ejaculates: a way to increase the total number of motile sperm from oligospermic men. Fertil Steril 1990;54:906–909.

132. Moghissi KS. Sperm migration through the human cervix. In: Insler V, Bettendorf G, editors. The Uterine Cervix in Reproduction. Stuttgart: Georg Thieme, 1977:146–165.

133. Silverberg KM, Johnson JV, Olive DL, et al. A prospective, randomized trial comparing two different intrauterine insemination regimens in controlled ovarian hyperstimulation cycles. Fertil Steril 1992;57:357–361.

134. Forrler A, Dellenbach P, Nisand I, et al. Direct intraperitoneal insemination in unexplained and cervical infertility. Lancet 1986;1:916–917.

135. Forrler A, Badoc E, Moreau L, et al. Direct intraperitoneal insemination: first results confirmed. Lancet 1986;2:1468.

136. Menard A, Moreau L, Arbogast E, Dellenbach P. Intraperitoneal insemination: a new method of treatment of various types of sterility. Rev Fr Gynecol Obstet 1988;83:625–627.

137. Curson R, Parsons J. Disappointing results with direct intraperitoneal insemination. Lancet 1987;1:112.

138. Dooley M, Lim-Howe D, Savvas M, Studd JWW. Early experience with gamete intrafallopian transfer (GIFT) and direct intraperitoneal insemination (DIPI). J Royal Soc Med 1988;81:637–639.

139. Crosignani PG, Ragni G, Lombroso Finzi GC, et al. Intraperitoneal insemination—simple and effective treatment for male and unexplained infertility: results of 164 cycles. Presented at the II Joint Centre d'Etude et de Conservation du Sperme Humain–European Society for Human Reproduction and Embryology Meeting, Milan, Italy, 1990.

140. Campos-Liete E, Insull M, Kennedy SH, et al. A controlled assessment of direct intraperitoneal insemination. Fertil Steril 1992;57:168–173.

141. Turhan NO, Artini PG, D'Ambrogio G, et al. Studies on direct intraperitoneal insemination in the management of male factor, cervical factor, unexplained and immunological infertility. Hum Reprod 1992;7:66–71.

142. Jansen RPS, Anderson JC, Radonic I, et al. Pregnancies after ultrasound-guided fallopian insemination with cryostored donor semen. Fertil Steril 1988;49:920–922.

143. Busolo F, Zanchet R, Lanzone E, Cusinato R. Microbial flora in semen of asymptomatic infertile men. Andrologia 1983;16:269–275.

144. Stone S, de la Maza L, Peterson E. Recovery of microorganisms from the pelvic cavity after intracervical or intrauterine artificial insemination. Fertil Steril 1986;46:61–65.

145. Fiumara NJ. Transmission of gonorrhea by artificial insemination. Clin Obstet Gynecol 1980;23:667–682.

146. Kleegman SJ. Therapeutic donor insemination. Conn Med 1967;31:705–713.

147. Berry WR, Gottesfeld RL, Alter HJ, Wierling JM. Transmission of hepatitis B virus by artificial insemination. JAMA 1987;257:1079–1081.

148. Moore DE, Ashley RL, Zarutskie PW, et al. Transmission of genital herpes by donor insemination. JAMA 1989;261:3441–3443.

149. Stewart GJ, Cunningham AL, Driscoll GL, et al. Transmission of human T-cell lymphotropic virus type III (TLV-III) by artificial insemination by donor. Lancet 1985;2:581–585.

150. American Fertility Society: Revised new guidelines for the use of semen-donor insemination. Fertil Steril 1988;49:211.

151. Sacks PC, Simon JA. Infectious complications of intrauterine insemination: a case report and literature review. Int J Fertil 1991;36:331–339.

152. Chiu TTY, Tam PPL, Mao KR. Pregnancies established by intrauterine insemination with washed spermatozoa. Asia-Oceania J Obstet Gynecol 1987;4:467–471.

153. Belker AM, Cook CI. Sperm processing and intrauterine insemination for oligospermia. Urol Clin North Am 1987;14:597–607.

154. Kobayashi T, Sato H, Kaneko S, et al. Intrauterine insemination with semen of oligozoospermic men: effectiveness of the continuous-step density gradient centrifugation technique. Andrologia 1991;23:251–254.

155. Jager S, Kremer J, de Wilde-Janssen IW. Are sperm immobilizing antibodies in cervical mucus an explanation for a poor post-coital test? Am J Reprod Immunol 1984;5:56–61.

156. Alexander NJ. Antibodies to human spermatozoa impede sperm penetration of cervical mucus or hamster eggs. Fertil Steril 1984;41:433–439.

157. Tsukui S, Noda Y, Yano J, et al. Inhibition of sperm penetration through human zona pellucida by antisperm antibodies. Fertil Steril 1986;46:92–96.

158. Price RJ, Boettcher B. The presence of complement in human cervical mucus and its possible relevance to infertility in women with complement-dependent sperm-immobilizing antibodies. Fertil Steril 1979;32:61–64.

159. Kremer J. A new technique for intrauterine insemination. Int J Fertil 1979;24:53–56.

160. Friedman AJ, Juneau-Norcross M, Sedensky B. Antisperm antibody production following intrauterine insemination. Hum Reprod 1991;6:1125–1128.

161. Goldberg JM, Haering PL, Friedman CI, et al. Antisperm antibodies in women undergoing intrauterine insemination. Am J Obstet Gynecol 1990;163:65–68.

162. Moretti-Rojas I, Rojas FJ, Leisure M, et al. Intrauterine inseminations with washed human spermatozoa does not induce formation of antisperm antibodies. Fertil Steril 1990;53:180–182.

163. Schenker JG, Yarkoni S, Granat M. Multiple pregnancies following induction of ovulation. Fertil Steril 1981;35:105–123.

164. Friedman AJ. Sextuplet pregnancy after human menopausal gonadotropin superovulation and intrauterine insemination: a case report. J Reprod Med 1990;35:113–115.

165. Houatta O, Lahteenmaki P, Kurunmaki H, et al. Direct intraperitoneal or intrauterine insemination and superovulation in infertility treatment: a randomized study. Fertil Steril 1990;54:339–341.

CHAPTER 47

Therapeutic Donor Insemination

SANDER S. SHAPIRO

Artificial insemination with donor sperm (AID), also known as *therapeutic donor insemination* (TDI), is the oldest and most widely applied form of assisted reproductive technology. It has been estimated that as many as 24,000 conceptions occurred in the United States during 1987 (the most recent year for which data are available) as a result of this therapeutic process.[1] A general acceptance of AID has developed over the past 40 years, and a legal framework to define its results has begun to appear.[2] Nevertheless, AID application, methodology, efficiency, and outcome vary immensely among therapists. A fundamental understanding of artificial insemination in its many aspects will promote attainment of the individual practitioner's goals as one applies this technology.

HISTORICAL BACKGROUND

Although the notion of cellular organization within living organisms did not develop until the seventeenth century, a semen factor required for fertilization was recognized in earliest history. Hebrew text from the Roman era implied that a woman might become pregnant after exposure to semen deposited in public bath water.[3] Arabian tribesmen of the fourteenth century also understood the relationship between semen and conception. In that society both enhancement[4] and sabotage[5] of equine blood lines were undertaken by placing semen-soaked cloth in the vaginas of brood mares. By the eighteenth century, organized attempts at breeding through the opportune application of semen were being made; first in fish (Jacobi, 1765) and, shortly thereafter, in mammals (Spallanzani, 1785).[4] Spallanzani's success at impregnating poodle dogs was widely disseminated and led to a host of successful artificial impregnations in various mammalian species.

In the sixteenth century Eustachius is said to have advised the wife of a physician to permit digital manipulation following coitus in an effort to introduce semen into the cervix.[4] However, the first attempt to overcome human infertility by artificial insemination is usually credited to John Hunter, who injected semen from a hypospadic man into the vagina of the man's wife, thereby attaining a pregnancy.[6] Systematic attempts to treat infertility by this technique were not described until 1866. Then, a New York physician, J. Marion Sims, reported attainment of a pregnancy in an infertile woman with cervical stenosis and uterine retroversion in whom he performed intrauterine insemination with her husband's semen.[7] His publication describing the procedure engendered a great deal of interest and inspired a host of efforts at intrauterine insemination with husband's semen. Reports on this subject, predominantly from Europe, continued to appear until World War II. Sims, himself, after failing to attain a pregnancy in 55 inseminations in an additional five women, abandoned the procedure.[7]

AID was carried out surreptitiously late in the last century.[8] William Pancoast, a physician at Jefferson Medical College in Philadelphia, having identified azoospermia as the cause of a couple's infertility, proceeded to inseminate the wife with semen from a medical student while she was anesthetized and without either her or her husband's knowledge. When this event and the subsequent pregnancy were revealed in a medical periodical 25 years later, they provoked substantial discussion among the medical fraternity.[8] By this time, however, others were actively treating azoospermic infertility by donor insemination.[9] Dickinson in New York is recognized as an early advocate and teacher of AID.[10] During the first decades of the present century, procedural guidelines and a legal framework for donor insemination began to take shape.[11, 12] Therapy at this time frequently included placing at least a portion of the specimen within the uterus[13] and sometimes involved the splitting of an ejaculate to accommodate several recipients. By 1940 more than 3500 births from AID could be documented in the United States.[14]

After World War II, articles in the medical literature reflected a broadening acceptance of and interest in donor insemination. Whether this was the result of a change in public attitudes toward the process or a lack of adoptable babies remains unclear. However, by the late 1950s, a substantial body of literature, including a number of large AID series, had accumulated.[15] It was at this time that the protective action of glycerol on cells undergoing freezing was first noted.[16] That finding enabled the successful cryopreservation of sperm and sperm banking as originally suggested 100 years earlier by Montegazza.[17] Although rapidly developed by Sherman,[17] Behrman and Ackerman,[18] and others, the methodology for cryopreservation was not employed widely by practitioners in the United States. Resistance to the use of frozen semen stemmed from the absence of a centralized medical organization within the country and a recognition that fresh semen provided a more efficient means of obtaining pregnancies. In contrast, Europeans, especially the French, accepted sperm cryopreservation and organized their AID programs around the new technology.[19, 20]

Appearance of the highly virulent human immunodeficiency virus (HIV) in the 1980s precipitated a reevaluation of insemination practices within the United States and other countries where fresh semen was the primary vehicle.[21] In 1988 the extent and mortality of this epidemic, that is spread by contact with bodily fluids, forced the adoption of a national policy prescribing the exclusive use of frozen-quarantined semen obtained from serologically negative donors.[22] The result has been a widespread use of semen from commercial cryobanking facilities and a more intense search for ways to optimize pregnancy rates obtained with cryopreserved sperm. It has also meant a change in the procedure's name from AID to one that was favored by an early advocate, Sophi Kleegman. Now, to avoid confusion with acquired immunodeficiency syndrome (AIDS), the procedure is more often referred to as TDI.

INDICATIONS FOR THERAPEUTIC DONOR INSEMINATION

There are only a few generally accepted indications for TDI (Table 47–1). Most often (95% of cases) the procedure is performed because of male factor infertility.[1] Less frequently, overcoming a genetic problem (1% to 3%) or attaining unmarried motherhood (4%) is the objective (Table 47–2). Among the infertile group, almost two thirds have outright azoospermia, either constitutional or iatrogenic. Oligospermia or depressed motility, or both, account for the other third.[23] Men with fewer than 20×10^6 sperm per milliliter in their ejaculate or a motility of less than 50% are considered to have abnormal semen. Yet many men eventually impregnate their mates despite such handicaps.[24] Recognition of this phenomenon and the uncertainty in predicting the

TABLE 47–2. Frequency of Indicated Therapeutic Donor Insemination

	University of Michigan[18] Circa 1960*,† (%)	University of Wisconsin[61] Circa 1985†,‡ (%)
Azoospermia	76	55
Vasectomy		21
Failed vasectomy reversal		4
Oligospermia	19	35
Rh incompatibility	3	
Subfertility	1	2
Genetic	1	3
Ejaculatory failure		4

*Among 208 women receiving therapeutic donor insemination.
†Center did not provide insemination to unmarried women.
‡Among 427 women who conceived by therapeutic donor insemination.

likelihood of pregnancy for an individual[25] has led authorities to caution against the liberal use of TDI for relative male factor infertility.[5] There is no consensus as to which parameters to use as indicators for TDI in oligospermia and other semen defects.[26] Most centers request that a medical evaluation and trial of therapy be undertaken by the male partner before attempting pregnancy by TDI. A thorough evaluation of the female partner is justified because numerous studies have shown that these women often have compromised reproductive potential.[27–32] In addition, a relatively longer trial at natural conception (usually ≥3 years) is suggested. Both of these strategies are supported by the finding that a substantial (17%) fraction of oligospermia couples having TDI pregnancies will become pregnant again without artificial insemination.[23] In vitro fertilization (IVF) can also be considered when the extent to which sperm are functionally handicapped cannot be determined.

The oldest and, for a time, most frequent genetic indication for TDI was Rh incompatibility coupled with a past history of erythroblastosis. The availability of prophylactic immunoglobulin therapy reduced the appearance of this problem and has practically eliminated requests for TDI on this basis. Inheritable diseases continue to be the impetus for a small (0.8%), but increasing, fraction of donor insemination.[33] At least one third of U.S. physicians performing TDI have done so on occasion for genetic reasons.[34] Autosomal dominant disorders (such as myotonic dystrophy), chorea, von Recklinghausen's disease, a number of osseous conditions (such as achondroplasia and osteogenesis imperfecta), several forms of blindness, and certain malformations in the male patient direct couples' attention to the alternative of donor insemination. This type of situation (60% of genetically indicated inseminations) accounts for about one fourth of genetic TDI.[33] Similarly, couples who have given birth to an autosomal recessive–affected infant (such as cystic fibrosis, phenylketonuria, Tay-Sachs disease, sickle cell disease, congenital adrenal hyperplasia, and Werdnig-Hoffmann disease) or persons affected by multifactorial genetic problems (such as diabetes mellitus and asthma) may seek TDI rather than undertake the path of prenatal diagnosis and selective abortion. The complexity of these problems, the variance in their expression, and the improving potential for prenatal diagnosis as well as treatment dictate that therapists make provision for patient education and counseling. People may

TABLE 47–1. Indications for Therapeutic Donor Insemination

Azoospermia
  Pathologic
  Postvasectomy
Severe oligospermia
  Should be unresponsive to medical therapy
  Associated with infertility of >3 year's duration
Genetic disease
  Rh incompatibility with past fetal loss
  Dominantly inherited disease in one member of the couple; with full
    disclosure of alternatives provided through genetic counseling
  Recessive disease in previous conceptions; with full disclosure of
    alternatives provided through genetic counseling
  Multifactorial genetically determined disease
Ejaculatory disturbances unresponsive to treatment, or recovery of sperm
  that have the fertility potential to fertilize an oocyte
Unmarried women

have an ill-informed view of their options or a misguided concept of the outcome that will result from natural conception. In addition, those couples using donor semen as a means of avoiding autosomal recessive homozygosity or the manifestations of multifactorial inherited disease need to be aware of the limitations to which such problems can be investigated and ruled out during the donor selection process. For example, most autosomal recessive disorders are rare so that a couple may choose to accept the remote chance of having an affected child by TDI rather than take the 1 in 4 risk inherent in their carrier status. On the other hand, when the carrier state is common, as in cystic fibrosis, the potential parents must understand that without testing the donor for carrier status they risk a 1 in 88 chance of having an affected child if the mother is a carrier. Men who have an X-linked recessive disorder will not transmit their disorder to sons but will provide the gene to all their daughters. The prospect of producing unaffected gene carriers rarely encourages affected men to opt for TDI. Ultimately, the decision to use TDI is a subjective one that must be made by the affected family. The responsibility of ensuring full and accurate disclosure falls to the TDI therapist. However, as illustrated in the national survey of 1979, many physicians performing artificial insemination are poorly equipped to offer genetic counsel.[34] Fortunately, couples who are faced with genetic problems that make TDI a tenable option frequently come to therapy by way of a trained genetic counselor.[35] Those who do not should be directed to an appropriate specialist when complex genetic issues need to be explored.

In the past, some couples would be encouraged to accept TDI as a means of circumventing infertility of undetermined causes or therapeutically unresponsive habitual abortion. Emergence of advanced reproductive technologies beyond TDI has diminished the use of donor insemination in these situations. There are still, nevertheless, a few instances in which an apparently normal husband's sperm fails even at the level of IVF. In these circumstances a trial of TDI may be justified, provided that the couple has been fully informed of the alternatives.[36] In the past, immune infertility identified by the presence of sperm antibodies was occasionally treated by TDI after specific immunologic therapies had failed. Now, with IVF and gamete intrafallopian transfer (GIFT) having proved effective for this autoantibody problem, TDI is seldom applied.

The most rapidly increasing reason for using donor insemination is pregnancy outside of marriage. Although only about 10% of TDI practitioners observed this indication in 1977, more than 30% performed inseminations on unmarried women in 1987. This use of donor insemination is not, strictly speaking, a medical one. There is nothing in the law that directly prohibits unmarried women from seeking this service.[37–39] There is also a great variance of opinion concerning the ethics of this form of TDI within the medical community.[40, 41] It, therefore, seems reasonable to leave decisions about the insemination of unmarried women to each individual practitioner until such time as the public makes its wishes known more concretely through legislation.[39]

Contraindications to TDI are relatively few and are, to some degree, dependent on individual practitioner bias.[42] Presence of an autosomal dominant inheritable disease in a candidate may be considered an absolute contraindication to donor insemination by some practitioners. For others such a situation might merely indicate the need for more thorough genetic counseling. Lack of or incomplete understanding of the role played by generational genetics, as well as nurturing on the physical and intellectual outcome of any pregnancy, could cause a practitioner to hesitate in offering therapy. Any suggestion of coercion on the part of either the recipient or her husband is also a reason to reappraise plans for TDI. Absence of a heterosexual or a legally recognized partnership is, for some, reason to deny therapy.

Severely debilitating or progressive disease in the male partner limiting his future parental role may be disconcerting to some physicians. Others will see this situation as one requiring clarification in the minds of the couple and suggest counseling to ensure the parents clear comprehension of their future. Debilitating disease in the recipient may also be a reason for delay or refusal of therapy. When a disease has the potential to worsen during pregnancy or to endanger pregnancy outcome, expert advice, consultation, and specific therapy may be undertaken before insemination is initiated. The implications of maternal age on spontaneous abortion[23, 43] and fecundability rates ($\hat{f}$) should be discussed with older TDI candidates including perimenopausal women. The individual therapist needs to consider the extent to which the patient understands the issue and the likelihood of successful outcome. Finally, TDI may be requested solely for psychological reasons. Such requests require a sorting out that is best approached through professional consultation and extended discussion with the patient. Those who choose to participate in therapy for marginal indications will do well to document their efforts to clarify the therapy and its alternatives with the requesting couple.

Patient Evaluation

In all cases it behooves the treating physician to perform a complete history and physical examination. Attention should be directed toward identifying factors that may have an effect on potential fecundity.[44] Prolonged, unsuccessful attempts at pregnancy with a past partner, mild or moderate oligospermia in the present partner, a history of pelvic inflammatory disease or abdominal surgery, and symptoms of endometriosis suggest the need for further diagnostic testing and may alter the physician's therapeutic plan. A history of irregular menstrual cycles or amenorrhea requires evaluation and eventual therapy. Because timing is important to success in TDI, assurance of regular ovulatory cycles enhances the chances for early pregnancy.

Another historical area, that of genetic burden, is often overlooked by TDI therapists. A well-designed questionnaire to seek out potentially harmful genetic carrier states should be given to every potential semen recipient.[45–47] In this way one may avoid inducing an increase in the genetic load of children conceived through TDI. A woman who has multiple allergies, for instance, should not be paired with a donor who has a similar polygenic medical history. Women with family histories of autosomal recessive diseases (such as phenylketonuria, congenital adrenal hyperplasia, and cystic fibrosis) ought to be given an opportunity to be tested for the heterozygous state and, if positive, matched to a similarly tested but negative donor.[48] The same approach should be used in women from a defined population recognized to exhibit a high frequency of a specific trait (such as sickle cell anemia and Tay-Sachs disease).[49]

The complete battery of standard diagnostic tests performed to evaluate infertility is seldom undertaken as part of the initial evaluation. Some centers accept a biphasic basal body temperature (BBT) graph or a luteal phase progesterone determination as sufficient evidence of normal ovulation. Others demand normal histology in an endometrial biopsy that additionally ensures the absence of a luteal phase defect. There is also some disagreement as to the necessity of evaluating tubal status before beginning inseminations. Some require a hysterosalpingogram (HSG) on all candidates, whereas others perform this test selectively.[50, 51] Retrospective evaluation of an HSG series from a group of TDI patients at one center produced abnormal findings in only 4 of 89 studies, with one half of the women that had an abnormal test attaining pregnancy within the first six treatment cycles.[52] The authors of this study argued that pretreatment HSGs were not justified on the grounds of either economy or enhanced fecundity. They proposed that tubal patency studies be delayed until after six treatment cycles in all but those with a history suggestive of tubal disease.

Few therapists routinely carry out diagnostic laparoscopy on women requesting donor insemination because of an absolute male factor problem unless there is a history suggesting peritoneal or tubal disease.[53] These studies, although prognostically helpful, are quite expensive, involve risk, and have a low likelihood of demonstrating pelvic disease when done at this juncture.[51]

Laboratory tests that are usually considered as routine for candidate evaluation include Rh type and rubella titer. Should the applicant be found Rh negative, an attempt can be made to match with an Rh-negative donor (as is required by statute in New York City). However, when an Rh-negative donor with other characteristics that are desired cannot be found, availability of Rh immunoglobulin limits the potential of sensitization from exposure to an Rh-positive donor.

Testing recipient candidates for infectious disease is carried out routinely, more as a defensive legal matter than for public health purposes. Those seeking TDI have a very low incidence of active venereal disease. For example, at the University of Wisconsin Infertility Clinic, there has been just one positive cervical culture for *Neisseria gonorrhoeae* from among the last 1100 candidates' samples and no positive luetic serologic studies from this same group. Nevertheless, hepatitis B and C, HIV, *Chlamydia trachomatis*, cytomegalovirus, and *Ureaplasma urealyticum* all are sought in this population. Recommendations on candidate screening are provided by the American Fertility Society (AFS).[54]

Some therapists require that couples seeking TDI undergo a psychological evaluation. Those who endorse this procedure believe that it affords an additional conduit by which to inform candidate couples about TDI and a means to ensure that they have thoroughly considered their decision.[55, 56] Advocates readily admit that such interviews screen only for the most blatant psychiatric problems. More dynamic psychiatric testing is generally considered unwarranted because the capacity to screen for future good parenting capabilities is dubious. More often, TDI practitioners omit specific psychological counseling sessions, believing that a comprehensive medical infertility evaluation by the therapeutic team will provide all of the information and insight required. The rela-

tively low rate of divorce among TDI parents suggests that this group tends to self-select for marital stability.[23] Moreover, TDI couples interviewed after having established their families did not regret the absence of preinsemination psychological counseling.

PREPARATION FOR THERAPEUTIC DONOR INSEMINATION

A formal conference should be undertaken once the initial evaluation has been completed but before therapy commences. An informed consent document should then be signed and witnessed. This paper should state that both husband and wife request the performance of AID and that they are aware of the alternatives to insemination and the more common complications that may arise (including maternal infection and birth defects). The consent should state the source of semen (local or from a commercial source) and clarify the therapist's role in selection of a suitable donor. It should also affirm confidentiality for the donor's identity (unless he has waived this right) and pledge the couple's future cooperative efforts to inform the therapist about the outcome of any resultant pregnancy. Prototype informed consent forms are available from several sources, including the AFS.[54] However, every practitioner and institution must modify these forms to comply with their particular practice and state statutes.

Once acceptance into an insemination program has occurred, the goal of both the therapist and the patient is pregnancy. Rates of success similar to those reported for couples attempting conception through coitus[10, 57–59] are, in fact, attained with routinely administered donor insemination.[13, 60–62] It appears that simple measures are all that is required; freshly ejaculated semen containing normal numbers of motile sperm placed on the cervix or in the uterus on several occasions over the period of expected ovulation have repeatedly produced pregnancies at rates corresponding to those recorded for natural intercourse. Neither method of placement[13, 63] nor exact time for insemination seems to matter appreciably.[50] The numbers of sperm in a single ejaculate provide such numerical redundancy, and their capacity for prolonged viability within the female genital tract such temporal redundancy, that pregnancy readily occurs in the healthy, unencumbered woman.[64] This is not automatically the case when cryopreserved semen is routinely used. Extensive experience by a host of therapists has shown the limited capacity of cryopreserved sperm to effect pregnancy (Table 47–3).[65] The diminished pregnancy rate observed with use of cryopreserved donor sperm is more important now that AIDS has made exclusive use of cryopreserved, quarantined sperm necessary. The abandonment of fresh semen has provoked a reappraisal of the protocols used for donor insemination. Variations in donor recruitment, specimen preparation, insemination site, and timing all are undergoing critical evaluation. At present, it is unclear whether the success rates reported with fresh semen can be economically attained using cryopreserved specimens. Practitioners must critically appraise available methodologic and technical options in relation to cost and success rate to establish their own particular treatment scheme.

		TABLE 47–3. Frozen Semen: Comparison Studies for Insemination Timing			
Study	**Year**	**Number of Patients**	**Number of Cycles**	**% $\hat{f}$**	**Protocol Comparison**
Leader et al[66]	1985	20	95	5 and 10.8	Ultrasound timed vs. multiple inseminations
Barratt et al[67]	1989	54	230	4 and 7	LH timed vs. standard
Kossoy et al[68]	1989	54	110	13.4 and 11.6	LH timed vs. standard
Centola et al[69]	1990	99	213	6 and 21	LH timed, one vs. two inseminations
Federman et al[92]	1990	60	264	12.3 and 5.3	LH timed vs. standard
Odem et al[70]	1991	113	437	6 and 13	LH timed vs. standard

$\hat{f}$, fecundability rate; LH, luteinizing hormone.

TIMING ARTIFICIAL INSEMINATION

In natural cycles the timing of intercourse is not terribly crucial to the achievement of pregnancy. Evidence from several sources, including experience with IVF, suggests that the optimal fertilization window for human ova is limited to the 12 to 24 hours following ovulation. The capacity of sperm to remain motile and functional within the female genital tract has been shown to extend well beyond 48 or even 72 hours.[71] This capability, together with a frequency of intercourse exceeding once in 96 hours, guarantees that sperm will be available for fertilization whenever a ripe ovum appears. Similarly, cervical capacity for sperm maintenance permits successful insemination at 48-hour intervals when using fresh semen. However, the functional life span of cryopreserved sperm is substantially less than that of fresh specimens (Fig. 47–1).[72–75] Thus, insemination intervals must be shortened or timed more precisely to ensure pregnancy rates like those attainable with fresh specimens. Daily or even twice-daily insemination with cryopreserved specimens could ensure the presence of functionally capable sperm within the upper female genital tract whenever ovulation occurs.[76] This strategy, however, would be expensive and require that more time be devoted to the effort than is acceptable to most patients.

An alternative method is to identify ovulation accurately and schedule inseminations accordingly.[77, 78] In women with normal luteal function, that event occurs about 14 days before the onset of the next menses. However, because of variation in the length of most women's menstrual cycles, every-other-day insemination over a 3- or 5-day interval was a commonly adopted protocol for fresh semen administration. The near universal use of frozen specimens since 1989 has heightened interest in various methods of monitoring the menstrual cycle in the hope that either fewer inseminations per cycle or better rates of pregnancy might be obtained.[79, 80]

BBT charts offer substantive, although limited, retrospective evidence with which to evaluate insemination timing.[81, 82] Errors in the way patients record their temperatures, therapist interpretation of charts, and variability in the relationship between periovulatory events and BBT changes can occur. Thus, it is not surprising that when BBT charts from successful single insemination cycles were evaluated, only 21% of the inseminations occurred on the day of temperature nadir.[83] Furthermore, like maintenance of a menstrual calendar, this timing technique offers limited prospective help in identifying the day or hour of ovulation.[84] A relatively simple means of predicting ovulation can be accomplished by serial observation of cervical mucus—the Insler scoring system.[85] This system provides a fairly accurate, prospective indication

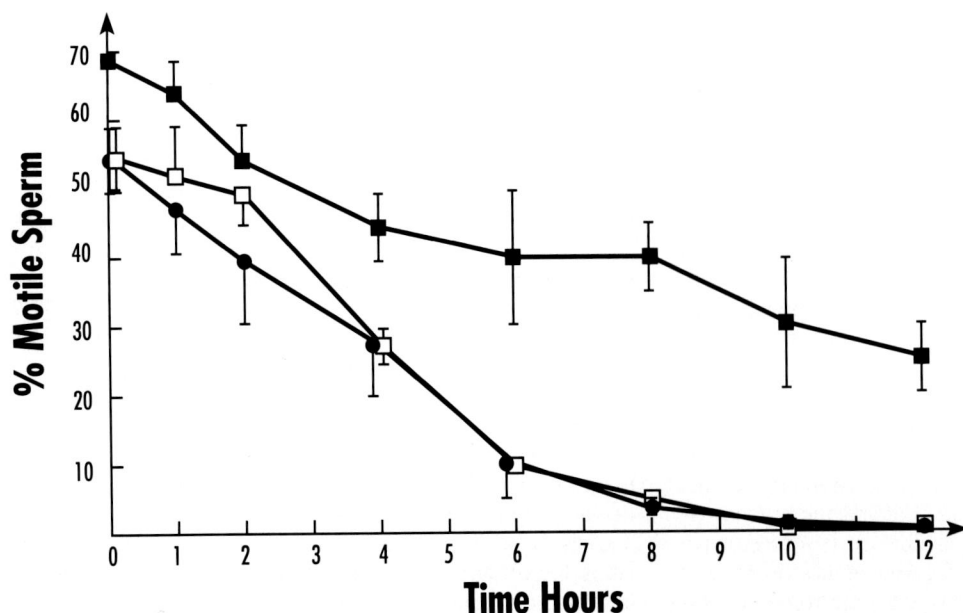

FIGURE 47–1. Survival of fresh (*solid square*) and postthaw (*solid circle* and *open square*) human sperm. (Modified from Friberg J, Gemzell C. Sperm-freezing and donor insemination. Int J Fertil 1977; 22:148–154.)

of impending ovulation; however, it is not universally effective and requires that the patient make daily office visits for as long as a week.[66] To predict or identify ovulation with sufficient temporal accuracy to provide for efficient insemination, more sophisticated technologic methods are required.

Serial ultrasound measurements of the ovaries can identify whether ovulation has occurred but are not helpful in predicting the time of ovulation, primarily because of the wide range of diameters at which rupture occurs.[86] For this reason ultrasound has proved satisfactory only as a general means of telling when to begin inseminations and when to stop them.[79, 87] Its cost and the time expenditure necessary to gain optimal advantage have also limited its incorporation into standard insemination protocols.

The most promising current means of predicting ovulation is by determining the luteinizing hormone (LH) surge.[82, 84, 88] Urinary assays, which can be performed at home by the patient, seem to offer an inexpensive, minimally time-consuming way to foretell the day of ovulation.[86, 89] Because the half-life of LH in serum is short (about 20 minutes), the amount detected in a urine sample usually accurately reflects the level in serum over the collection period.[90, 91] It is important to remember that single daily assays can, like serum assays, provide misleading or inaccurate information as to the exact time of ovulation.

Attempts at incorporating urine LH assays into the timing protocol for TDI have given variable and less than enthusiastic results.[80] In one study that compared a single insemination timed to the day after the urinary LH surge with two inseminations, with timing dictated by past temperature graphs, an increased efficiency, reflected in substantial cost savings, was demonstrated.[92] However, in another similar study, contrary results were obtained.[70] Failure to substantially increase the success rate for TDI in these and other comparative studies[67, 68] has been disheartening. Yet, the less than exciting results of these studies may reflect the choice of insemination timing rather than the limits of the assay protocol. Presently, the optimal time for insemination with frozen sperm is unknown. Moreover, when once-a-day LH assays are used predictively, the time of ovulation may be off by as much as 24 hours. Doubling the frequency of assay and performing inseminations on both the day of and the day after the LH surge might provide substantially improved pregnancy rates. Results similar to those obtained with fresh semen have been obtained using just such a protocol in one small study.[69] Obviously, more testing is needed to determine the extent to which pregnancy rates can be improved by precise timing of insemination. The best available alternatives seem to be to use urinary LH assays with inseminations on two successive days or to continue with timing protocols that rely on BBT charting and accept pregnancy rates that are significantly lower than those obtained with fresh semen (Tables 47–3 and 47–4).[61]

INSEMINATION PROTOCOLS

After all preliminary testing is completed, consent permits signed, and the patient's orientation completed, plans for insemination are made. Based on past menstrual history, a time for either performing inseminations or beginning urinary LH assays is chosen. Ideally, patients should have access

TABLE 47–4. Comparison of Fresh Versus Frozen Semen Fecundability Rates (F's)

Study	Year	Number of Patients	Number of Cycles	$\hat{f}$
Frozen Semen f*				
Steinberger and Smith[93]	1973	59	372	9.7
Friedman[94]	1977	227	947	9.5
Bromwich et al[95]	1978	214	1,610	5.0
Leeton et al[96]	1980	514	1,500	15.2
Richter et al[97]	1984	381	1,200	5.0
Iddenden et al[98]	1985	20	150	8.6
Bordson et al[99]	1986	120	165	10.3
Gillet et al[100]	1986	82	318	18.2
Hammond et al[101]	1986	155	591	9.0
Brown et al[61]	1988	125	566	10.4
LeLannou and Lansac[102]	1989	4,900	23,192	8.3
Keel and Webster[103]	1989	209	917	4.8
Wong et al[104]	1989	227	984	10.0
DiMarzo et al[105]	1990	113	371	5.9
Hogerzeil et al[195]	1991	362	2,159	10.9
Fresh Semen f				
Multiple Insemination Protocol				
Kleegman[13]	1954	16	376	19.4
Haman[63]	1954	177	677	19.7
Behrman[107]	1959	168	625	20.0
Glezerman[62]	1981	270	1152	19.8
Aiman[60]	1982	116	368	21.0
Brown et al[61]	1988	163	559	27.4
Single Insemination Protocol				
Meeks et al[108]	1986	80	309	14.8
Bordson et al[99]	1986	120	165	11.5
Foss and Hull[31]	1986	116	800	11.7
Edvinsson et al[51]	1990	1,336	7,125	11.6

*Standard protocols.

to therapy 7 days a week.[60] If the patient is to schedule several inseminations based on her menstrual cycle length, she is instructed to make her upcoming appointments early in the cycle. If results of an LH assay are to dictate insemination timing, the patient is instructed to begin urinary testing about 3 days before the anticipated hormone rise.

Most routine TDI is carried out in a suitable gynecologic examining room. A prepared semen specimen is placed inside the external cervical os while the patient is in lithotomy position. This is usually done with a syringe attached to a sort of cannula (Fig. 47–2) or directly from the straw in which it was stored. Frozen specimens almost always have a volume of less than 1 mL. Nevertheless, some portion of the specimen may spill over the cervix onto the speculum or posterior vaginal fornix. It remains to be determined whether this small portion of a frozen specimen is functionally lost or is capable of contributing to pregnancy.[109] A cervical cap may be used to hold the specimen in close proximity to the cervix. When whole ejaculates were used, some evidence was produced to suggest that advantage could be gained by this maneuver.[107, 110] Similar studies are not available for frozen specimen TDI. Early therapists frequently placed fresh semen directly into the uterus but eventually abandoned the practice because their patients frequently experienced painful uterine contractions.[13] Those practitioners who continued the practice limited the intrauterine portion of fresh ejaculate insemination to about 0.1 mL.[51, 97] Most recently, some clinicians using frozen samples have returned to the practice of depositing whole frozen specimens within the uterus. Results from

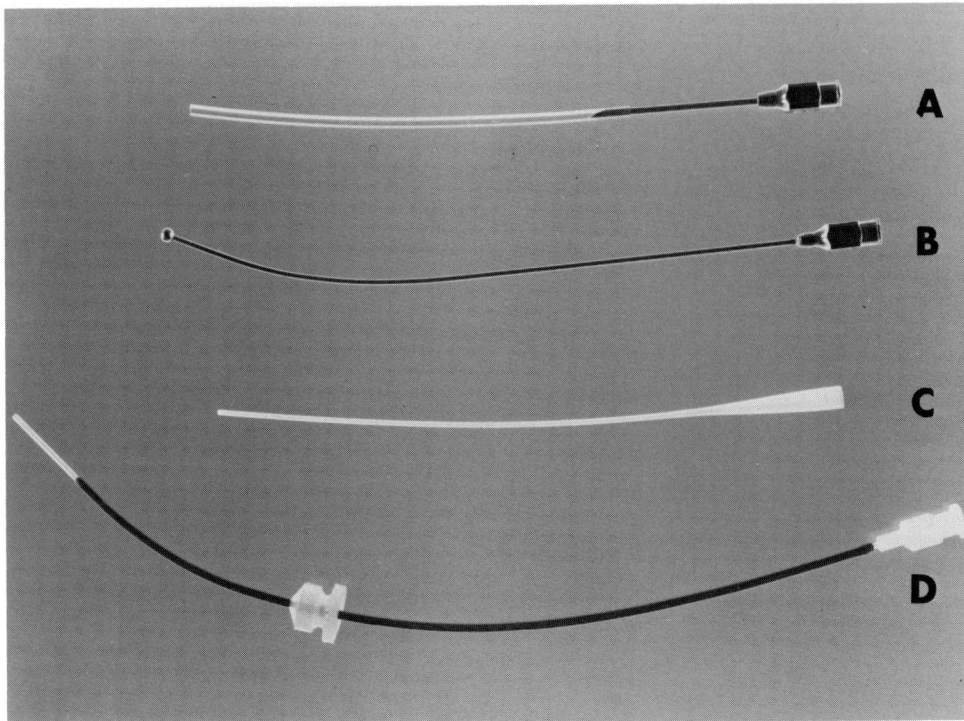

FIGURE 47-2. Commonly used instruments for intracervical (*A* and *B*) and intrauterine (*C* and *D*) sperm delivery. *A*, An 18-gauge spinal needle with a modified blunt tip. *B*, A standard 16-gauge needle with an extension of polyethylene tubing. *C*, Tomcat commercial thin plastic catheter (Sherwood Medical, St. Louis, MO). *D*, Shapiro intrauterine insemination set (Cook Ob/Gyn, Spencer, IN), including adjustable depth indicator.

this practice have been anecdotally positive. To place greater numbers of sperm within the uterus, methods of separating viable gametes from seminal fluid have been employed (see Chapter 46). Sperm are either diluted and centrifuged out of the fluid (sperm washing), layered by centrifugation, and allowed to swim into an overlying media (swimup) or placed in a column adjacent to media into which they may migrate (filtration).[111, 112] Only a few reports have appeared in which separated sperm preparations have been used for TDI.[7, 113–115] When fresh semen intracervical insemination (ICI) was compared with washed fresh semen intrauterine insemination (IUI) in a randomly assigned protocol, $\hat{f}$ (18.5% versus 14.85%) were not found to be statistically different.[115] However, at another center a similar study using frozen semen produced an $\hat{f}$ of 3.9% with frozen semen preparations delivered intracervically and an $\hat{f}$ of 9.7% when washed specimens were placed in the uterus. This difference in $\hat{f}$ was statistically different even though the rate for ICI was inexplicably low.[69] The same investigators were subsequently able to show statistically improved results by changing their wash medium from Ham's F-10 ($\hat{f} = 9.8\%$) to human tubal fluid medium ($\hat{f} = 17.5\%$).[113] An uncontrolled trial has also posted a remarkable $\hat{f}$ (24%) using frozen-swimup–prepared specimens.[7] These optimistic results should encourage additional exploration to further improve methods for TDI-IUI and to determine whether the increased administrative costs can be justified through sufficiently greater $\hat{f}$.[113] Expressed concerns about inducing antisperm antibodies through this route of insemination seem unjustified based on experience with homologous ICI.[116] More radical delivery systems using specially prepared specimens have also been attempted. Intraperitoneal deposition of sperm has produced pregnancies but has not undergone sufficiently critical appraisal to allow judgment as to its efficacy in TDI.[117] Deposition of sperm within the fallopian tubes by transcervical catheter has also been accomplished, but reports on its effectiveness have been contradictory.[118, 119]

After specimen application, the patient is asked to remain recumbent for a short time before she becomes active. There are no published data that document an optimal length of recumbency—10 to 20 minutes is usually stipulated.[120] Cervical caps have been used to eliminate this waiting period and free up examining rooms in some clinics. Concern has been expressed that the semen from infertile males may adversely affect the success of TDI. In one study, husband's seminal plasma was shown to frequently cause sperm agglutination-immobilization.[121] A subsequent clinical trial by the same authors showed greater $\hat{f}$ with TDI when subjects refrained from intercourse during the insemination period.[122] However, in another small (34-participant) clinical trial, mixing of donor and husband semen failed to show a harmful effect of this practice.[123]

COMPUTING THERAPEUTIC SUCCESS

Pregnancy is obviously the hallmark of success in TDI. For many years success was expressed simply as a pregnancy rate (number of pregnancies per number of patients undertaking TDI).[107, 124, 125] Each women who began therapy was included in the denominator of that fraction. This failed to take into account any variations in duration of treatment. Pregnancy rates tended to convey an underestimation of success because patients who dropped out of therapy after only a few cycles were considered as failures and given equal weight with those patients that underwent many therapy cycles. When a series had a particularly high early dropout rate, it would have a correspondingly low success rate. Alternatively, programs that did not include early dropouts in their computation overestimated pregnancy rates.[50, 124] Comparative statistics between series and between groups within a series were misleading because of this anomaly. During the past decade a computational improvement has been introduced through use of the concept of $\hat{f}$.[126] This term is computed as the number of pregnancies achieved divided by the number of insemination cycles undertaken during therapy and is usually expressed for each individual cycle in a series. It can also be tabulated for the whole series. Computations of $\hat{f}$ are unaffected by the number of dropouts or the time at which patients stop therapy.[127] Each therapeutic cycle is treated as an event that is either a success or a failure. Assumptions about matters such as changes in pregnancy rate over time can easily be evaluated by comparing $\hat{f}$ in individual treatment cycles (first, second, and so on) of a series. Fecundability rates derived from experience can be used to suggest the probability of success in future therapeutic efforts. Life table analysis is easily applied to fecundability data and provides an estimate of the cumulative probability for therapeutic success.[62] Comparative statistical methods also can be applied with greater rigor than before insemination data were compiled in the form of $\hat{f}$.[27]

A glance at the literature demonstrates the presence of sufficient tabular data to determine $\hat{f}$ for many published series. In the 1950s overall $\hat{f}$ of 19%,[13] 20%,[63] and 20%[107] were described for series using fresh ejaculate inseminations. Corresponding first-cycle rates for these series were 29%, 27%, and 15%. Recently, similar $\hat{f}$ have been attained using multiple insemination protocols[60, 97, 111] and much lower ones when only one fresh insemination was undertaken per cycle.[51, 108]

Fecundability rates for series that have used frozen semen have been substantially lower than those incorporating fresh semen (see Table 47–4). In the largest reported series, that of the French consortium CECOS, overall $\hat{f}$ for more than 16,000 pregnancies was 8%.[102] Individual clinics reporting large series have produced $\hat{f}$ of 10%[92] and 12%.[31] Over the whole frozen semen literature, $\hat{f}$ generally ranged from 5% to 12%.[101, 105] The marked contrast between success rates with fresh and frozen specimens clearly indicates that there is room for improvement when stored specimens are used.

DONOR SELECTION AND MONITORING

Although many practitioners obtain donor semen exclusively from commercial sources, all should be aware of the guidelines, procedures, and issues involved in these efforts. Donors in the CECOS program are usually married and fathers. They frequently are recruited by infertility couples seeking therapy and are not remunerated monetarily for their efforts.[33] In the United States most donors are single medical or college students who receive payment for their specimens. (In several states, payment could be interpreted as forbidden under an organ transplant law.[34]) Donors should be in good health with a low probability of passing infections or genetic diseases. Guidelines for the selection of donors have been formulated by CECOS,[36] the AFS,[54] and the American Association of Tissue Banks.[128] Although these are not obligatory, they establish standards that are both well thought out and provide a quasi-legal imprimatur.

An upper age limit of 35 years has been suggested in recognition of the rising incidence of chromosomal mutations with paternal age.[129, 130] In practice, however, most donors are considerably younger. None of the advisory medical bodies that have produced guidelines specifically require a minimum level of intelligence or education. Semen specimens should contain more than 50 million sperm per milliliter with more than 50% progressive motile and less than 30% to 40% abnormal morphology. Dependence on traditional parameters to establish minimal requirements for semen acceptability does not ensure fertility.[60, 65, 131] No currently available laboratory measure of sperm function provides this information, but sperm motion analysis may offer hope as a predictive instrument.[132, 133] The question of whether $\hat{f}$ can be substantially improved by identifying "high" fertility donors remains unanswered. The striking $\hat{f}$ that have been attained with fresh semen suggest that intrinsic characteristics that allow for sustained function after cryopreservation will, in all likelihood, prove more important to successful insemination.[132] Just the same, methods that can identify the low fertility donor without resorting to "field trials" will be welcome.[114, 134] After storage, specimens ought to have higher than 50% cryosurvival. These are minimum standards that, for reasons to be discussed, are considerably lower than those in actual use by most cryopreservation laboratories.[50, 135] Present semen criteria, although low, are nevertheless difficult to meet.[136] Ejaculate quality in industrialized countries appears to be declining, and only a fraction of those who volunteer consistently meet these criteria for semen quality.[136–138] In one donor program, 21% of donors were rejected on the basis of initial semen characteristics[139] and in another 53%.[140] A substantial fraction (about 20%) are also rejected because, despite adequate initial semen quality, they fail to meet cryosurvival requirements. This experience has caused most centers to analyze several ejaculates from each volunteer before proceeding to a more complete donor evaluation. Some centers, on the other hand, prefer to obtain a brief genetic history before doing semen testing even though that interview excludes only 3% of potential donors.[140]

At most cryopreservation centers a thorough history, physical examination, and laboratory testing are undertaken only after semen quality and cryosurvival are demonstrated. Two crucial significant aspects of a potential donor are his genetic-family background and any history of possible exposure to infectious diseases. Persons receiving periodic blood or blood product transfusions, illicit drug users, and those who have participated in homosexual activities are at high risk for HIV infection and are excluded from donating semen. Active donors may be required to sign a disclaimer of such activities periodically. Although not a guarantee that the donor will refrain from these activities, a disclaimer heightens his awareness.[141] Medical and genetic histories can be taken with the aid of a written questionnaire but should include a personal interview by a health care worker with the training, skills, and medical knowledge to elicit and identify pertinent factors from the volunteer's family history.[35, 142] It should not be assumed that medical students or other health care providers are sufficiently knowledgeable to screen themselves for genetic disease.[143] Specific, inclusive questions about first-degree and second-degree family members must be directed to all potential volunteers. Men with an autosomal dominant or X-linked disorder should be excluded from the donor pool. The same is true for those who either are affected by autosomal recessive disease or are potential carriers of these disorders. The donor should be free of any significant diseases having a known major genetic component.[45] Their family history should be documentable so that they are not suspected of being the carrier of an autosomal recessive gene. When the ethnic or racial background suggests the prevalence of a particular autosomal recessive disease, such as thalassemia in those of Mediterranean descent, Tay-Sachs disease in those descended from eastern European Jews, and sickle cell disease in blacks, specific testing must be carried out.[49] First-degree and second-degree relatives of potential donors should be historically free of nontrivial congenital malformations and known Mendelian disorders (such as Huntington's chorea, retinitis pigmentosa, multiple colon polyposis, and severe atherosclerotic disease at a young age). At physical examination particular attention is directed to recognition of nontrivial malformations in the donor, such as cleft lip, clubfoot, or hypospadias, which have a relatively high rate of occurrence in offspring. Physical signs of significant Mendelian abnormalities (such as albinism, neurofibromatosis, and hypercholesterolemia) are also sought. In this way, the possibility that a donor will contribute to the children's genetic burden can be limited. The likelihood that all children conceived with donor sperm will be made free of significant inheritable disorders, however, is zero.[45] This fact must be communicated to potential TDI couples.

There is considerable disagreement in the literature about the need for extensive, formalized genetic screening and karyotyping of potential donors. A documented lack of genetic sophistication on the part of infertility specialists has been used to encourage formal participation of geneticists in donor screening.[34] However, the extent to which this problem has been addressed in the medical press and the publication of genetic guidelines has done much to diffuse concern.[47, 144] Nevertheless, discrepancies have been found between the rate that donors self-report genetic disorders and genetic counselors actively identify these disorders.[145] Merely asking a potential donor or recipient whether they or family members have a genetic disorder has been found to be insufficient. For this reason, use of a comprehensive questionnaire in the screening process is advised.[45-47] Rejections based on genetic criteria are far less frequent than those based on semen characteristics—between 2% and 30%.[136, 140, 145, 146] The low rate of rejection (28% overall) that has been recorded for CECOS volunteers may relate to the requirement that these men already have fathered a normal child.[102]

Most donor centers do not routinely perform karyotyping on volunteers.[50, 136] None of the major advisory bodies with published standards require chromosomal evaluation. The likelihood of identifying an abnormality requiring rejection, coupled with monetary cost, has discouraged this practice.[144, 147] In those centers that have routinely performed karyotyping of potential donors, 2% to 3% are rejected because of abnormal findings.[136, 146, 147]

Currently, the number of children fathered by each donor is limited to diminish the potential for consanguinity in the next generation. Should the restriction on numbers of offspring from a single donor diminish as more widespread distribution of semen specimens by commercial semen banks occurs, the cost constraints that inhibit karyotypic and carrier state testing will decrease. The availability of karyotype data to TDI centers can, in addition to weeding out potential

chromosomal problems, provide medicolegal support should an untoward outcome occur.[73] In the future, molecular biologic techniques will undoubtedly be developed that will allow for more inclusive testing of potential donors (e.g., the autosomal gene defect for familial breast cancer). The result will be greater expense and increased rejection rates. With each new test the question of cost versus outcome will need to be reconsidered.[48] It also will become necessary to consider testing the potential recipient as adjunct to testing the donor. Because every person carries several mutant genes, unencumbered donors will not be found. It therefore may eventually become common to match donor and recipient so as to avoid homozygous states.

In addition to meeting the standards for semen quality and genetic background, each donor must undergo initial and ongoing screening for infectious diseases (Table 47-5). Despite the remarkable history donor insemination programs have had for minimizing passage of infectious diseases, there is near unanimity of opinion concerning the need for screening donors and semen samples.[148] Both fresh and frozen semen have the capacity to transmit a host of bacterial, viral, and other infectious agents.[77] Pregnancy complications (abortion, chorioamnionitis, prematurity), perinatal infection, and maternal infection can result. Infants can experience blindness, deafness, developmental anomalies, as well as neurologic defects as a result of intrauterine infection. Maternal infection can result in future infertility, general debility, and even death. As a result, recommended initial donor testing includes serologic tests for syphilis, serum hepatitis B, cytomegalovirus, and HIV. Urethral cultures for *N. gonorrhoeae* and *C. trachomatis* are also required. Screening for herpes simplex virus, Mollicutes species, and *Trichomonas vaginalis* have been recommended but are not part of the AFS guidelines.[135, 149] Additional screening includes that portion of the initial physical examination involving observation of the external genitalia. Evidence of warts, ulcers, or vesicles indicates the need for further testing and probable rejection.

Once past the initial phase of testing, donors are retested at a minimum of 6-month intervals. Practically, the requirement that all semen remain in quarantine for 6 months and

---

TABLE 47-5. Microbiologic Testing of Donors

Initial screen
  Urethral culture:
    Neisseria gonorrhoeae
    Chlamydia trachomatis
  Semen culture
    *Mycoplasma hominis**
    *Ureaplasma urealyticum**
  Serology
    HIV
    Treponema pallidum
    Hepatitis B
    Cytomegalovirus
    Herpes simplex virus*
  Semen examination
    Trichomonas vaginalis
Periodic testing
  Perform at 6-month intervals
  Release semen for use only after 6-month quarantine and a repeat HIV
    antibody determination that is negative

*American Fertility Society optional tests.
HIV, human immunodeficiency virus.

that a repeat HIV antibody test demonstrate seronegativity makes it necessary that each donor be tested at periodic intervals while they are active contributors. Many centers also choose to test every ejaculate that they process for gonorrheal and chlamydial infection. The AFS does not directly address screening after a donor changes sexual partners, but this situation ought to be approached by a complete rescreening within 3 months. It is for this reason that some centers require donors to sign monthly statements that address the question of new partners and homosexual activity. Although not totally effective, this measure should help minimize the presence of high-risk men in donor programs.[141] At some point in the recruitment and evaluation process, each donor should be given an overview of the clinic's activities. He should be told the reasons for predonation abstinence and for concern about exposure to multiple partners, clinic policy with regard to records and anonymity, and the sociolegal implications of his charitable activity. The donor's attention should also be directed to the psychological implications of fathering anonymous children. In addition, there should be ample opportunity for the donor to have his concerns and questions answered before he signs the agreement under which his sperm will be dispensed.

Donor Matching

There is no universally accepted protocol for assigning donors to couples requesting TDI. Practically, however, most couples desire assurance that the child will resemble the husband. Therefore, centers catalog their donors as to race, general coloring (skin, hair, eyes), and body build.[51] Most centers do not attempt to match for ABO blood group, preferring to expend their limited matching capacities on other characteristics.[34] Some provide brief bibliographies and pictures to allow for selection. It is important that the expectations of potential TDI couples be explored thoroughly before treatment is begun. When the specifics of a couple's requests for matching cannot be met, a frank discussion of the problem should be provided. Requests that are extremely specific and seemingly inappropriate may indicate a lack of acceptance of the couple's situation or totally misplaced expectations that signal need for more in-depth counseling.

When possible, Rh-negative women should receive semen from similarly negative donors. If a woman has a multifactorial genetic disease or a family history of an autosomal recessive disease, efforts to further clarify the donor's genetic burden must be carried out. The limited extent to which problems such as cystic fibrosis and phenylketonuria can be avoided should be understood by every requesting couple.

Cryopreserved Sperm

Frozen semen $\hat{f}$ are lower than those for fresh semen (see Table 47–4). The reasons for this discrepancy have not been clearly determined. Two factors that may be important are the abbreviated life span experienced by frozen-thawed sperm and the diminished numbers currently used for insemination. Experience with IVF suggests that ova maintain a capacity for fertilization for less than 24 hours following ovulation. This limitation dictates that sperm be available

during a narrow window of opportunity. The considerably longer life span of fresh sperm, plus their capacity to remain viable within the female genital tract, provides for substantial temporal tolerance. Inseminations performed at 2-day intervals over periods of expected ovulation guarantee that functionally capable sperm will be present during the critical period. More frequent inseminations may be necessary to ensure the presence of similar numbers of frozen-thawed sperm at the required time.[69, 78] Alternatively, more precise identification of the time of ovulation may permit single inseminations to be successful with greater frequency.

Studies of insemination efficiency in several mammalian species suggest that there is a critical number of sperm needed to attain maximal $\hat{f}$. Average ejaculate for these species contains several-fold more sperm than appear to be required (Fig. 47–3).[150, 151, 152] The smallest population of human sperm, in either fresh or frozen insemination samples, needed to match natural $\hat{f}$ is not known.[153] The common practice of placing a whole fresh ejaculate within a woman's genital tract ensures that sufficient numbers of sperm are available. Frozen semen inseminations, on the other hand, usually involve only a fraction of the ejaculate. Moreover, the lost motility that results from cryopreservation, together with the dilutional effect that occurs with addition of extender, brings about a further decline in viable insemination numbers. Most inseminations of cryopreserved sperm involve a volume of between 0.25 and 1 mL. Whereas whole ejaculates contain from 60 million to 500 million motile sperm, frozen inseminations usually provide only 10 million to 50 million motile gametes. Retrospective analyses of large insemination series have generally shown a positive correlation between the numbers of motile sperm inseminated and $\hat{f}$,[154, 155] although exceptions have been noted.[104] In the French national program, $\hat{f}$ were 7% with less than 40% postthaw motility and 17% when motility was more than 65%.[19] Data from these studies do not allow identification of the optimal number of sperm for insemination. Collectively, these and other reports suggest that the minimum number of sperm that will provide maximal fecundity is somewhere above 25 million.[18, 51, 61]

To furnish greater numbers of motile sperm using presently available freezing technologies, it is necessary to (1)

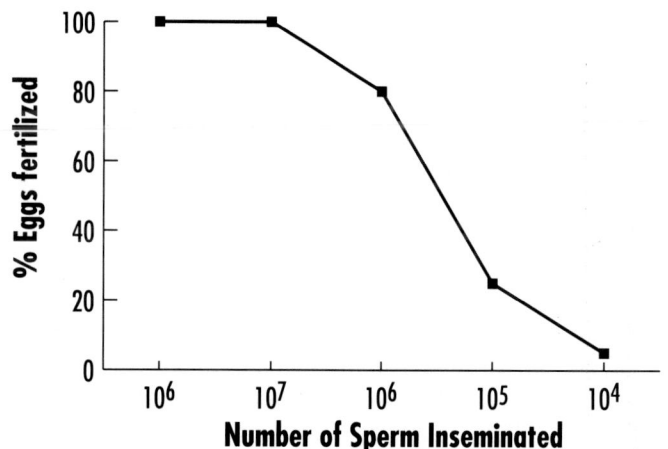

FIGURE 47–3. Effect of the number of spermatozoa inseminated into the pig uterus 6 hours before ovulation. (Adapted from Polge C. Fertilization in the pig and horse. J Reprod Fertil 1978; 54:461–470.)

recruit donors with extremely high sperm concentrations, (2) limit semen dilution by using more concentrated extenders, or (3) inseminate with larger sample volumes. Recruitment of sufficient numbers of volunteers is a difficult, ongoing task.[141] Significantly raising the minimal ejaculate concentration that is required of potential donors is impractical.[156] Few centers could meet substantially higher requirements.[134, 144, 157] A more likely approach might be to minimize the volume of extender that is added to ejaculates during preparation for freezing. One formulation that provides a 1:3 mixture of extender to semen has been tried clinically. In that series, an 18% $\hat{f}$, the most successful frozen semen rate reported to date, was attained.[100] Whether similarly high success rates can be achieved at other centers using this extender formulation remains to be determined. Clinical trials employing larger sample volumes are also needed before such a strategy can be generally advocated.[158] Commercial sperm banks that produce multiple specimens from each ejaculate attempt to provide between 10 and 30×10^6 motile sperm in each therapeutic unit. The number of sperm provided and the type of guarantee that is offered can usually be found within each company's sales literature.

Record Keeping

Standard clinical records should be maintained on every woman undergoing TDI. In addition, specific notations concerning certain factors that are peculiar to this therapeutic modality are also advisable. For example, BBT charts that additionally contain information about ovulatory drug use, LH monitoring, and dates of insemination provide an easy way to reconstruct each TDI series. These forms should be collected on a monthly basis and placed in the patient's chart to avoid loss. The identity of the donor used during each treatment cycle ought to be recorded. When there are concerns about maintaining anonymity, this can be done in code. The father of each pregnancy is then recorded in a manner that provides for recovery of the information at a date in the distant future. This effort will necessitate a log that the individual practitioner can pass forward on retirement. If the source of semen is local, the number of pregnancies accountable to each donor also must be determined. In this way a limit can be enforced on each donor's productivity.[54] Similar constraints should be imposed on donors from commercial sperm banks.

There are two major reasons for maintaining records about TDI conceptions. Should there be an infant born with a congenital abnormality or an inheritable metabolic disease, identification and removal of that donor's samples from the donor pool are required. Accurate records and single-donor insemination cycles are necessary for this determination to be possible. Donor notification about possible genetic abnormalities has been a more controversial subject. Because many practitioners are unaware of their TDI infants' health status, they do not have to face this dilemma. Those who do must consider the psychological burden that they place on a young man who is not married and may not yet be contemplating parenthood. Some authorities have recommended that the donor not receive such information.[159] Others, after canvasing their donor pool, believe that full disclosure is both desired by and in the best interest of these volunteers.[160]

Later, the determination of paternity may be desired in situations with the potential for consanguineous marriage (this situation has actually occurred[161]). Although both the mathematics of population interactions[162] and a policy of limiting donor productivity (AFS recommends a limit of 10 pregnancies per donor), make future consanguinity unlikely, the capacity to investigate that possibility should be available to all TDI offspring. This opinion concerning long-range record maintenance is not universally accepted. In fact, some therapists routinely destroy their records in an effort to ensure anonymity.[1, 163] The AFS, while recognizing that an ideal method of long-term record maintenance is not available, recommends that donor portfolios be maintained and that confidential access remain available to TDI offspring. In some states, legislative provision has been made for such records.[164] In those instances when donors have been queried about the release of personal information to the TDI couple or child, they generally have been agreeable. Their identity is the only piece of information that they would deny to the family.[159, 160, 165, 166] In advocating long-term record maintenance, there is the implicit presumption that TDI offspring will be informed of their origins; however, this may be an erroneous assumption. A followup study of 187 children who had reached school age found only one that had been given this information.[23] In another investigation of TDI parents, 86% said they did not intend to tell their child despite the fact that most had told some family member or peer about the therapy.[167] Clearly, there is a clash of opinions between public observers and TDI participants on this issue. Interested professionals (psychiatrists, sociologists, lawyers, and others) think that disclosure of TDI origins is desirable.[168] Some observers believe that donor identity should be made available to TDI children.[165] In Sweden, legal enforcement of this opinion has severely restricted the number of donor volunteers. Similar results would undoubtedly occur in the United States and other countries should laws require disclosure. This prediction is based on the finding that most donors, although agreeable to the communication of medical and social histories, are opposed to disclosure of their identity.[165] As long as TDI couples remain resistant to providing information about origin to their offspring, the issue of donor anonymity is unlikely to assume major significance.

At those centers that maintain their own semen supplies, a record of each donor's fecundability should be kept. Because all donors have high-quality semen, as judged by semen analysis, and because donors are known to vary widely in fecundity, the rate that they provide pregnancies to a TDI program must be monitored as part of an overall quality assurance program. Donors that fail to produce at least one pregnancy within a fixed number of insemination cycles may then be removed from further participation.[169] Analysis of one large donor series found that eliminating those that failed to produce a pregnancy within 12 cycles would have removed more than half of the donors with an $\hat{f}$ of less than 5%.[134]

STRATEGIES FOR FAILED TDI

Analysis has shown that $\hat{f}$ for TDI with frozen sperm remain fairly constant over the first 7 to 12 cycles of therapy (Fig. 47–4).[27, 31, 50, 56, 64] This has led most practitioners to

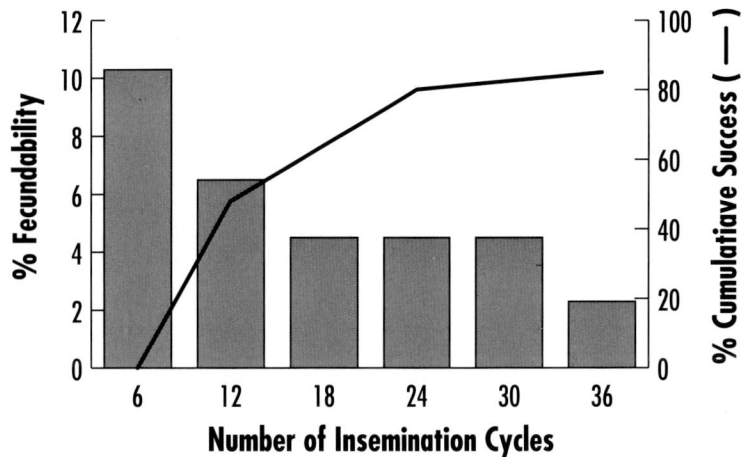

FIGURE 47–4. The fecundability rate *(bars)* and theoretical cumulative success rate *(solid line)* in women who undertook therapeutic donor insemination using frozen semen. (Modified from LeLannou D, Lansac J. Artificial procreation with frozen donor semen: experience of the French Federation CECOS. Hum Reprod 1989; 4:757–761; by permission of Oxford University Press.)

delay assessment of female reproductive capacity until a minimum of six unsuccessful treatment cycles has occurred. Then, the evaluation of the patient should be essentially identical to that of any infertile woman. Ovulatory function, internal genital anatomy, cervical function, and immune reproductive status ought to be evaluated.[170] When it is necessary to undertake ovulation induction, one can usually expect that the time to conception will be longer even though the likelihood of pregnancy is not reduced.[158, 171–173] Problems that require more extensive diagnostic efforts, such as laparoscopically identified pelvic disease, must await a decision to actively seek out specific causes of female infertility. Mild to moderate pelvic adhesions can be removed with an acceptable probability of eventually attaining pregnancy.[34, 60, 61, 92] Removal of extensive adhesion is not as likely to be productive. The course to be taken with minimal endometriosis is less certain.[174] Because there is substantial reason to doubt the culpability of these lesions in infertility, the value of continuing a standard TDI protocol following their discovery and destruction remains dubious.[175] Only two small studies have directly addressed the possible effect that endometriosis exerts on TDI.[176, 177] A retrospective analysis of one large TDI series found that although women with endometriosis had greater fecundability than those with other confounding pelvic factors, their success rate was considerably lower than that of women without other infertility factors.[28] Because the alternatives to standard TDI are much more expensive and because negating the import of minimal endometriosis leaves the woman without a demonstrable cause of infertility, it is reasonable to advocate another series of inseminations. This is especially the case when ablation of the endometrial lesions was undertaken at the time of laparoscopy.[110] When severe pelvic disease, which has a low probability for correction, is found, the alternative to TDI becomes IVF with donor sperm.[102] Although complex and expensive, it is an acceptable modality for many couples. Although advocated as a last resort by most clinics, a few observers have actually suggested that all TDI candidates who fail to become pregnant during their first 12 cycles of insemination resort to this form of assisted reproductive technology.[56]

When an evaluation fails to identify the cause of unsuccessful TDI, it is reasonable to attempt a second series of insemination, preferably using another donor. Should a second series fail and the cause of failure remains undetermined, only a limited group of options is available. Standard insemination routines can be continued despite the well-recognized deterioration in fecundability that occurs following 12 failed cycles. Alternatively, two other therapeutic modalities deserve consideration. Both are applied routinely in the treatment of general infertility that has no identifiable cause. Homologous IUI, coupled to controlled ovarian hyperstimulation, has been scrutinized extensively and appears to be effective for this purpose.[178, 179] Moreover, heterologous IUI has shown promise as an initial delivery form for TDI so that there is reason to suppose intrauterine deposition of washed, cryopreserved sperm following controlled ovarian hyperstimulation might provide an effective, albeit expensive, alternative to continued standard therapy.[113, 114, 180] To date, however, a critical clinical appraisal of this regimen has not been published. A second alternative is GIFT, which has been shown to effectively treat women after failed TDI.[181, 182] In a series of 106 women who had previously undergone 1073 cycles of fresh-semen TDI, there were 55 clinical pregnancies following 103 completed GIFT procedures. Such promising results deserve attention and attempts at duplication using cryopreserved semen specimens.

THERAPEUTIC DONOR INSEMINATION OUTCOME

The degree to which TDI is successful in producing pregnancy depends primarily on two general variables: the specific methodologies employed and the fecundity of those undergoing therapy. Because most reports that provide $\hat{f}$ involve unselected female populations, those rates reflect the effectiveness of the particular regimen used. With frozen semen these rates have been between 5% and 12%, for the most part (see Table 47–4). However, when subgroups segregated according to the women's status are evaluated, $\hat{f}$ are often widely divergent. For instance, women whose husbands are azoospermic produce higher $\hat{f}$ than women with oligospermic partners.[27, 29, 44] Women older than 30 years of age have progressively lower pregnancy rates,[44, 183] and those who require medical induction of ovulation produce lower rates than those who ovulate regularly.[78, 171] Information about published $\hat{f}$ for a definable subgroup is often helpful in counseling people who are considering TDI and in formulating the most efficient therapeutic strategy for a particular situation.[28]

Although the success rates of various programs have been reported in detail, birth outcome from these TDI pregnancies is poorly documented. Spontaneous abortion rates are known to be the same as those recorded for naturally conceived pregnancies: about 16% in 25-year-old women and rising to 40% among women in their 40's.[23, 43] The distribution of first-trimester and second-trimester losses is also comparable, as are complications of the third trimester and delivery.[23]

The incidence of congenital anomalies is similar in TDI children to naturally conceived children.[23, 144] In a series of 481 TDI infants from a single clinic, 22 major and 41 minor congenital anomalies were documented. This frequency is comparable to that found in longitudinal study of general populations.[183] There have also been reports suggesting a higher rate of trisomy among TDI offspring, but this was not confirmed in the one comprehensive study of a large TDI series.[23, 184] Overall, it would appear from the available data that TDI children, as a group, are not physiologically distinguishable from their counterparts. There is therefore no compeling reason to require genetic or sonographic evaluations of these fetuses. Claims that they have superior intelligence are based on limited data accumulation.[185] The degree to which parental social and educational levels may influence these findings has not been explored. The one major difference that has been found between products of natural and TDI conceptions is their sex distribution. Pooled data suggest a sex ratio of about 0.99 (male/female) from TDI as compared with 1.06 for the general population.[186] Whether this difference results from an effect of insemination timing or some other influence is unknown. Significant differences in sex ratios have been suggested but not conclusively found when fresh and frozen semen results were compared.[23]

When surveyed, both physicians and parents express satisfaction about the course and outcome of TDI.[23, 187–190] Marital difficulties resulting from TDI efforts and their outcome seem less frequent.[131] In fact, the rate of divorce among couples with infants gained through heterologous insemination is less than that found in a matched population.[23]

Despite the widespread acceptance of TDI and its beneficial results, there are some vocal critics of the manner in which organized medicine has carried out this reproductive service.[191, 192] These people, both participants in TDI and observers, urge that the procedure be demedicalized. There are those who wish to recruit their own donor, either out of distrust of the medical community or a desire to maintain an ongoing association with him. Others gravitate to nonmedical insemination to avoid the antiseptic, impersonal quality that they perceive as inherent in the clinical process or in an effort to gain a more participatory role. Single women and especially lesbians have taken to self-insemination because, in some instances, medical therapists refuse to participate in their attempts to become pregnant.[1] Some social activists have urged this course for all insemination recipients out of a belief that cost containment and public empowerment will result.[192]

Much of the do-it-yourself effort preceded the onset of the HIV epidemic. Then, people would recruit their own donors, educate themselves through counterculture literature or trips to the medical library, and perform the insemination with fresh semen.[191] In the gay community, a network, of sorts,

came into being that provided both know-how and semen. For some participants in this alternative route to insemination, issues such as donor health, genetics, and anonymity became as real as they are for the medical community. Most of these people, finding the issues and the effort to deal with them more time consuming or complex than anticipated, turned to the expertise of the medical community. Others, either by ignoring what they believed to be peripheral questions, or by seriously investigating them, got to the central theme and attained pregnancy. As the threat of HIV infection came to awareness and fresh semen could not longer be considered as acceptable, commercial sperm banks became the source of specimens. Although most banks do not provide donor names, the ability to self-inseminate continues to provide a sense of participation and empowerment that is attractive to some. Technical expertise as is necessary can be gained as demonstrated by the success of a home insemination program in The Netherlands.[106] There, after individualized clinic instruction of participants, a randomized study showed that pregnancies could be attained at home with equal celerity.

LEGALITY AND ETHICS OF THERAPEUTIC DONOR INSEMINATION

Public approval for TDI programs has increased over the past 100 years. Broad segments of society recognize the procedure as a personally acceptable means of overcoming infertility or circumventing genetic morbidity.[193] Early court decisions that left the child's legitimacy in question have been resolved by legislation and a host of judicial opinions. The AFS has appraised the procedure and expressed neither legal nor ethical reservations. There are, however, organized religions as well as people who oppose efforts at conception by other than natural means. In the United States, a decision to participate as a donor, recipient, or practitioner is left to the individual.

There are now 35 states that recognize the legitimacy of children born to consenting, married couples as a result of TDI. Statutes generally assume (explicitly or implicitly) that this service has taken place under the supervision of a licensed physician. Parental rights and obligations are apportioned equally between husbands and wives. Some (17) of the states recognize the donor and explicitly deny him parental rights and obligations.[194] A few stipulate the type of screening (infectious disease, genetic) that must be carried out on each donor.[161] There are also provisions in many states concerning the reporting of TDI and the manner in which confidentiality will be maintained.[37] Generally, in the United States a physician who provides TDI services to married couples and who follows good medical practice, as set down by recognized medical agencies, is acting in concert with established law. However, because the law concerning heterologous artificial insemination is not uniform, it would be prudent for every medical practice to review the local law before embarking on TDI. When this service is provided to individuals or nontraditional family groups, major legal uncertainties and a great deal of state-to-state variation are encountered. In most states there is neither legislation nor legal precedent that addresses the issues that may arise.

Legal and ethical issues concerning heterologous donor

insemination, both real and fabricated, abound.[37, 39] The medical community has, for historical and functional reasons, assumed that society entrusts this form of reproductive therapy to its supervision.[193] By and large this appears to be the case as divined from publicly expressed sentiment, legislative decree, and judicial pronouncement. There is, nevertheless, a vocal minority that wants TDI to become a "do-it-yourself" technology.[192] Because little legislation addresses the consequences of nontraditional TDI, individual practitioners and interested professional organizations prescribe the standards of practice. Nontraditionalists object to many of the practice policies that directly affect donor and recipient. This is especially true of those women who wish to become pregnant outside of legally recognized marriage. Although a majority of physicians refuse to provide this service, a substantial minority currently do offer TDI to unmarried women.[1] Legal experts generally believe that physicians are within the law when administering TDI to unmarried females. They also believe that physicians have the right to refuse participation because of personal, moral, or ethical concerns.[191] This may not be so for governmental institutions; in the only case to be judicially processed, a single woman sued a state medical school, claiming that its refusal of single women desiring insemination violated her constitutional rights. This suit was settled before the court was able to rule, with the school agreeing to provide unmarried women with equal service.

Legislative bodies have been slow to address the many legal ambiguities that might be created by nontraditional TDI. Until they do, practitioners will do well to carefully consider the implications of providing this form of fertility therapy beyond the traditional recipient population.

REFERENCES

1. Shapiro S, Saphire D, Stone W. Changes in American AID practice during the past decade. Int J Fertil 1990; 35:284–291.
2. Albert M, the Editorial Board. Medical technology and the law. Harvard Law Rev 1990;103:1519–1676.
3. Friberg J, Gemzell C. Sperm-freezing and donor insemination. Int J Fertil 1977; 22:148–154.
4. Rohelder H. Test Tube Babies: A History of the Artificial Impregnation of Beings. New York: Panurge Press, 1934.
5. Finegold W. Artificial Insemination. Springfield, IL: Charles C Thomas, 1964:5–25.
6. Home E. An account of the dissection of an hermophrodite dog. To which are prefixed some observations on hermaphrodites in general. Phil Trans London 1799; 89:157.
7. Sims JM. Clinical Notes on Uterine Surgery. Birmingham: Gryphon Editions, 1990.
8. Gregoire AT, Mayer RC. The impregnators. Fertil Steril 1965; 16:130–134.
9. Kleegman S. Artificial donor insemination. Med Aspect Hum Sex 1970; 4:85–111.
10. Guttmacher A. Factors affecting normal expectancy of conception. JAMA 1956; 161:855–860.
11. Cary W. Experience with artificial impregnation in treating sterility. JAMA 1940; 114:2183–2187.
12. Seymour F. Viability of spermatozoa in the cervical canal. JAMA 1936; 106:1728.
13. Kleegman S. Therapeutic donor insemination. Fertil Steril 1954; 5:7–32.
14. Seymour F, Koener A. Artificial insemination: present status in the United States as shown by a recent survey. JAMA 1941; 116:2747–2749.
15. Potter R. Artificial insemination by donors: analysis of seven series. Fertil Steril 1958; 9:37–53.
16. Polge C, Smith A, Parkes A. Revival of spermatozoa after vitrification and dehydration at low temperatures. Nature 1949; 164:666.
17. Sherman J. Research on frozen semen: past, present, and future. Fertil Steril 1964; 15:485–499.
18. Behrman S, Ackerman D. Freeze preservation of human sperm. Am J Obstet Gynecol 1969; 103:654–661.
19. David G, Czyglik F, Mayaux M, et al. Artificial insemination for frozen sperm: protocol, method of analysis, and results for 1188 women. Br J Obstet Gynecol 1980; 87:1022–1028.
20. Hansen K, Nielsen N, Rebbe H. Artificial insemination in Denmark by frozen donor semen supplied from a central bank. Br J Obstet Gynaecol 1979; 86:384–386.
21. Ulstein M. Fertility, motility, and penetration in cervical mucus of freeze-preserved human spermatozoa. Acta Obstet Gynecol Scand 1973; 52:205–210.
22. Centers for Disease Control. Semen banking, organ and tissue transplantation and HIV antibody testing. MMWR 1988; 37:58–59.
23. Amuzu B, Laxova R, Shapiro S. Pregnancy outcome, health of children, and family adjustment after donor insemination. Obstet Gynecol 1990; 75:899–905.
24. Zuckerman Z, Rodriguez-Rigau L, Smith KD, et al. Frequency distribution of sperm counts in fertile and infertile males. Fertil Steril 1977; 28:1310–1314.
25. Bostofte E. Prognostic parameters in predicting pregnancy. Acta Obstet Gynecol Scand 1987; 66:617–624.
26. Mortimer D, Lenton E. Distribution of sperm counts in suspected infertile men. J Reprod Fertil 1983; 68:91–96.
27. Albrecht B, Cramer D, Schiff I. Factors influencing the success of artificial insemination. Fertil Steril 1982; 37:792–797.
28. Chauhan M, Barratt C, Cooke S, et al. Differences in the fertility of donor insemination recipients: a study to provide prognostic guidelines as to its success and outcome. Fertil Steril 1989; 51:815–819.
29. Emperiare J, Gauyere-Soumire, Audebert A. Female fertility and donor insemination. Fertil Steril 1982; 37:90–93.
30. Formigli L, Formigli G, Gottardi L. Artificial insemination by donor results in relation to husband's semen. Arch Androl 1985; 14:209–211.
31. Foss G, Hull M. Results of donor insemination related to specific male infertility and unsuspected female infertility. Br J Obstet Gynaecol 1986; 93:275–278.
32. Kovacs G, Leeton J, Matthews C, et al. The outcome of artificial insemination compared to the husband's fertility status. Clin Reprod Fertil 1982; 1:295–299.
33. Federation C, Matter J, LeMarc B. Genetic aspects of artificial insemination by donor (AID): indications, surveillance and results. Clin Genet 1983; 23:132–138.
34. Curie-Cohen M, Luttrell L, Shapiro S. Current practice of artificial insemination by donor in the United States. N Engl J Med 1979; 300:585–590.
35. Karp L. Artificial insemination: a need for caution. Am J Med Genet 1981; 9:179–181.
36. Jalbert P, Leonard C, Selva J, et al. Genetic aspects of artificial insemination with donor semen: the French CECOS Federation Guidelines. J Med Genet 1989; 33:269–275.
37. Andrews L. Ethical and legal aspects of in vitro fertilization and artificial insemination by donor. Urol Clin North Am 1987; 14:633–642.
38. Doherty D. Contemporary medical ethics: would Hypocrates approve or even understand? Postgrad Med 1985; 77:212–216.
39. Fletcher J. Artificial insemination in lesbians. Arch Intern Med 1985; 145:419–420.
40. Editorial. Women without men. Nature 1991; 350:96.
41. McGuire M, Alexander N. Artificial insemination of single women. Fertil Steril 1985; 43:182–184.
42. Freedman B, Taylor P, Wonnacott T, et al. Non-medical selection criteria for artificial insemination and adoption. Clin Reprod Fertil 1987; 5:55–66.
43. Virro M, Shewchuk A. Pregnancy outcome in 242 conceptions after artificial insemination with donor sperm and effects of maternal age on the prognosis for successful pregnancy. Am J Obstet Gynecol 1984; 148:518–524.
44. Barratt C, Chauhan M, Cooke I. Donor insemination: a look to the future. Fertil Steril 1990; 54:375–387.
45. Smith P. Selection against genetic defects in semen donors. Clin Genet 1984; 26:87–108.
46. Timmons MC, Rao K, Sloan C, et al. Genetic screening of donors for artificial insemination. Fertil Steril 1981; 35:451–458.
47. Verp M. Genetic issues in artificial insemination by donor. Semin Reprod Endocr 1987; 5:59–68.

48. ten Kate L, te Meerman G, Buys C. Effectiveness of prevention of cystic fibrosis by artificial insemination by donor can be markedly improved by DNA analysis of sperm donors. Am J Med Genet 1989; 32:148–149.

49. Johnson WQ, Schwartz R, Chutorian A. Artificial insemination by donors: the need for genetic screening. N Engl J Med 1981; 304:755–757.

50. Corson S. Factors affecting donor artificial insemination rates. Fertil Steril 1980; 33:414–422.

51. Edvinsson A, Forssman L, Milsom I, Nordfors G. Factors in the infertile couple influencing the success of artificial insemination with donor semen. Fertil Steril 1990; 53:81–87.

52. Nach D, Haning R, Shapiro S. Value of hysterosalpingogram prior to donor artificial insemination. Fertil Steril 1979; 31:378–380.

53. Goss D. Current status of artificial insemination with donor semen. Am J Obstet Gynecol 1975; 122:246–249.

54. American Fertility Society. New guidelines for the use of semen donor insemination: 1990. Fertil Steril 1990; 53 (Suppl 1):10s–13s.

55. David A, Avidan D. Artificial insemination donor: clinical and psychologic aspects. Fertil Steril 1976; 27:528–532.

56. Kovacs G, Baker G, Burger H, et al. Artificial insemination with cryopreserved donor semen: a decade of experience. Br J Obstet Gynaecol 1988; 95:354–360.

57. Miller J, Williamson E, Glue J. Fetal loss after implantation—a prospective study. Lancet 1980; 2:554–556.

58. Peek J, Gilchrist S, Kelso M, et al. Comparison of three cryoprotective solutions for human semen. Clin Reprod Fertil 1982; 1:301–305.

59. Vessey M, Wright N, McPherson K, Wiggins P. Fertility after stopping different methods of contraception. Br Med J 1978; 1:265–267.

60. Aiman J. Factors affecting the success of donor insemination. Fertil Steril 1982; 37:94–99.

61. Brown C, Boone W, Shapiro S. Improved cryopreserved semen fecundability in an alternating fresh-frozen artificial insemination program. Fertil Steril 1988; 50:825–827.

62. Glezerman M. Two hundred and seventy cases of artificial donor insemination: management and results. Fertil Steril 1981; 35:180–187.

63. Haman J. Results in artificial insemination. J Urol 1954; 72:557–563.

64. Behrman S. Artificial insemination. Clin Obstet Gynecol 1979; 22:245–253.

65. Shapiro S. Strategies for improving the outcome of therapeutic donor insemination. Infertil Reprod Med Clin North Am 1992;3:469–485.

66. Leader A, Wiseman D, Taylor P. The prediction of ovulation: a comparison of the temperature graph, cervical mucus score, and realtime pelvic ultrasound. Fertil Steril 1985; 43:385–388.

67. Barratt C, Cooke S, Chauhan M. A prospective, randomized controlled trial comparing urinary luteinizing hormone dipsticks and basal body temperature charts with timed donor insemination. Fertil Steril 1989; 52:394–397.

68. Kossoy L, Hill G, Parker R, et al. Luteinizing hormone and ovulation timing in a therapeutic donor insemination program using frozen semen. Am J Obstet Gynecol 1989; 160:1169–1172.

69. Centola G, Mattox J, Raubertas R. Pregnancy rates after double versus single insemination with frozen donor semen. Fertil Steril 1990; 54:1089–1092.

70. Odem R, Durso N, Long C, et al. Therapeutic donor insemination: a prospective randomized study of scheduling methods. Fertil Steril 1991; 55:976–982.

71. Gould J, Overstreet J, Hanson F. Assessment of human sperm function after recovery from the female reproductive tract. Biol Reprod 1984; 31:888–894.

72. Critser J, Arneson B, Aaker D, et al. Cryopreservation of human spermatozoa: II. Postthaw chronology of motility and of zona free hamster ova penetration. Fertil Steril 1987; 47:980–984.

73. Fribert J. Survival of human spermatozoa after freezing with different techniques. In: David G, Price W, editors. Human Artificial Insemination and Semen Preservation. New York: Plenum Press, 1980:167–174.

74. Keel B, Black J. Reduced motility longevity in thawed human spermatozoa. Arch Androl 1980; 4:213–215.

75. Keel B, Karow A. Motility characteristics of human sperm, nonfrozen and cryopreserved. Arch Androl 1980; 4:205–212.

76. Jacobs L, Ory S. Changes in artificial insemination regimens for male factor infertility. Clin Obstet Gynecol 1989; 32:586–597.

77. Mascola L, Geenan M. Screening to reduce transmission in semen used for artificial insemination. N Engl J Med 1986; 314:1354–1359.

78. Smith K, Rodriguez-Rigau L, Steinberger E. The influence of ovulatory dysfunction and timing of insemination on the success of artificial insemination donor (AID) with fresh or cryopreserved semen. Fertil Steril 1981; 36:496–502.

79. Marinho A, Sallam H, Goessens L, et al. Real-time pelvic ultrasonography during the periovulatory period of patients attending an artificial insemination clinic. Fertil Steril 1982; 37:633–638.

80. Shapiro S. Can timing improve therapeutic donor insemination fecundability? Fertil Steril 1991; 55:869–871.

81. Bauman J. Basal body temperature: unreliable method of ovulation detection. Fertil Steril 1981; 36:729–733.

82. Newill R, Katz M. The basal body temperature chart in artificial insemination by donor pregnancy cycles. Fertil Steril 1982; 38:431–438.

83. Schwartz D, Mayaux M, Martin-Boyce A, et al. Donor insemination: conception rate according to cycle day in a series of 821 cycles with a single insemination. Fertil Steril 1979; 31:226–229.

84. Morris N, Underwood L, Easterling W. Temporal relationship between basal body temperature nadir and luteinizing hormone surge in normal women. Fertil Steril 1976; 27:780–783.

85. Insler V, Melmed H, Eichenbrenner I, et al. The cervical score: a simple semiquantitative method for monitoring of the menstrual cycle. Int J Gynaecol Obstet 1972; 10:223–227.

86. Vermesh M, Keltzky O, Davajan V, et al. Monitoring techniques to predict and detect ovulation. Fertil Steril 1987; 47:259–265.

87. Saaranen M, Suhonen M, Saarikoski S. Ultrasound in the timing of artificial insemination with frozen donor semen. Gynecol Obstet Invest 1986; 22:140–144.

88. Corson G, Ghazi D, Kammann E. Home urinary luteinizing hormone immunoassays: clinical applications. Fertil Steril 1990; 53:591–601.

89. Younger J, Boots L, Coleman C. The use of a one-day luteinizing hormone assay for timing of artificial insemination in infertility patients. Fertil Steril 1978; 30:648–653.

90. Kerin J, Warnes G, Crocker J, et al. 3-hour urinary radioimmunoassay for luteinizing hormone to detect onset of preovulatory LH surge. Lancet 1980; 2:430–431.

91. Martinez F, Trounson A, Besanko M. Detection of the LH surge for AID, AIH, and embryo transfer using twice daily dip stick assay. Clin Reprod Fertil 1986; 4:45–53.

92. Federman C, Dumesic D, Boone W, et al. Relative efficiency of therapeutic donor insemination using a luteinizing hormone monitor. Fertil Steril 1990; 54:489–492.

93. Steinberger E, Smith K. Artificial insemination with fresh or frozen semen. JAMA 1973; 223:778–783.

94. Friedman S. Artificial donor insemination with frozen semen. Fertil Steril 1977; 28:1230–1233.

95. Bromwich P, Kilpatrick M, Newton J. Artificial insemination with frozen stored donor semen. Br J Obstet Gynecol 1978; 85:641–644.

96. Leeton J, Selwood T, Trounson A. Artificial donor insemination frozen versus fresh semen. Aust NZ Obstet Gynaecol 1980; 20:205–207.

97. Richter M, Haning R, Shapiro S. Artificial donor insemination fresh versus frozen semen: the patient as her own control. Fertil Steril 1984; 41:277–280.

98. Iddenden D, Sallam H, Collins W. A prospective randomized study comparing fresh semen and cryopreserved semen for artificial insemination by donor. Int J Fertil 1985; 30:54–56.

99. Bordson B, Ricci E, Dickey R, et al. Comparison of fecundability with fresh and frozen semen in therapeutic donor insemination. Fertil Steril 1986; 46:466–469.

100. Gillet W, Cameron M, MacKay-Duff M. Pregnancy rates with artificial insemination by donor: the influence of the cryopreservation method and coexistent infertility factors. NZ Med J 1986; 99:891–903.

101. Hammond M, Jordan S, Sloan C. Factors affecting pregnancy rates in a donor insemination program using frozen semen. Am J Obstet Gynecol 1986; 155:480–485.

102. LeLannou D, Lansac J. Artificial procreation with frozen donor semen: experience of the French Federation CECOS. Hum Reprod 1989; 4:757–761.

103. Keel B, Webster B. Semen analysis data from fresh and cryopreserved donor ejaculates: comparison of cryoprotectants and pregnancy rates. Fertil Steril 1989; 52:100–105.

104. Wong A, Ho P, Kwan M, et al. Factors affecting the success of artificial insemination by frozen donor semen. Int J Fertil 1989; 34:25–29.

105. DiMarzo S, Huang J, Kennedy J, et al. Pregnancy rates with fresh versus computer-controlled cryopreserved semen for artificial insemination by donor in a private setting. Am J Obstet Gynecol 1990; 162:1483–1490.

106. Hogerzeil H, Hamerlynck J, Amstel N, et al. Results of artificial insem-

ination at home by the partner with cryopreserved donor semen: a randomized study. Fertil Steril 1988; 49:1030–1035.

107. Behrman S. Artificial insemination. Fertil Steril 1959; 10:248–258.
108. Meeks G, McDonald J, Gookin K, et al. Insemination with fresh donor semen. Obstet Gynecol 1986; 68:527–530.
109. Shields F. Artificial insemination as related to the male. Fertil Steril 1950; 1:271–280.
110. Bergquist C, Rock J, Miller J, et al. Artificial insemination with fresh donor semen using the cervical cap technique: a review of 278 cases. Obstet Gynecol 1982; 60:195–199.
111. Glass R, Ericsson R. Intrauterine insemination of isolated motile sperm. Fertil Steril 1978; 29:535–538.
112. Lopata A, Patullo M, Chang A, et al. A method of collecting motile spermatozoa from human semen. Fertil Steril 1976; 27:677–684.
113. Byrd W, Ackerman G, Bradshaw K. Comparison of bicarbonate and HEPES-buffered media on pregnancy rates after intrauterine insemination with cryopreserved donor sperm. Fertil Steril 1991; 56:540–546.
114. Byrd W, Bradshaw K, Carr B. A prospective, randomized study of pregnancy rates following intrauterine and intracervical insemination using frozen donor sperm. Fertil Steril 1990; 53:521–527.
115. Patton P, Burry K, Novy M, et al. A comparative evaluation of intracervical and intrauterine routes in donor therapeutic insemination. Hum Reprod 1990; 5:263–265.
116. Goldberg J, Haering P, Friedman C, et al. Antisperm antibodies in women undergoing intrauterine insemination. Am J Obstet Gynecol 1990; 163:65–68.
117. LaSala G, Torelli M, Valli F, et al. Birth after direct intraperitoneal insemination with frozen semen of donor. Acta Eur Fertil 1988; 9:37–39.
118. Brooks J, Mortimer D, Taylor P. Failure of hysteroscopic insemination of the fallopian tube in synchronized cycles. Int J Fertil 1988; 33:353–361.
119. Jansen R, Anderson J, Radonic I, et al. Pregnancies after ultrasound-guided fallopian insemination with cryostored donor semen. Fertil Steril 1988; 49:920–922.
120. Sulewski J, Eisenberg F, Stenger V. A longitudinal analysis of artificial insemination with donor semen. Fertil Steril 1978; 29:527–531.
121. Quinlivan W, Sullivan H. Spermatozoa antibodies in human seminal plasma as a cause of failed artificial donor insemination. Fertil Steril 1977; 28:1082–1083.
122. Quinlivan W. Therapeutic donor insemination: results and causes of nonfertilization. Fertil Steril 1989; 32:157–160.
123. Freidman S. Artificial insemination with donor semen mixed with semen of the infertile husband. Fertil Steril 1980; 33:125–128.
124. Dixon R, Buttram V. Artificial insemination using donor semen: a review of 171 cases. Fertil Steril 1976; 27:130–134.
125. Portnoy L. Artificial insemination (AID): experiences with its use in eighty barren marriages. Fertil Steril 1956; 7:327–340.
126. Olive D. Analysis of clinical fertility trials: a methodologic review. Fertil Steril 1986; 45:157–171.
127. Cramer D, Walker A, Schiff I. Statistical methods in evaluating the outcome of infertility therapy. Fertil Steril 1979; 32:80–86.
128. American Association of Tissue Banks. Standards for Tissue Banking. Washington, DC: 1989.
129. Bordson B, Leonardo V. The appropriate upper age limit for semen donors: A review of the genetic effects of paternal age. Fertil Steril 1991; 56:397–401.
130. Friedman J. Genetic disease in the offspring of older fathers. Obstet Gynecol 1981; 57:745–749.
131. Banks A. Aspects of adoption and artificial insemination. In: Behrman S, Kistner R, editors. Progress in Infertility. Boston: Little Brown, 1968.
132. Holt W, Shenfield F, Leonard T, et al. The value of sperm swimming speed measurements in assessing the fertility of human frozen semen. Hum Reprod 1989; 4:292–297.
133. Irvine D, Aitken R. Predictive value of in vitro sperm function tests in the context of an AID source. Hum Reprod 1986; 1:539–545.
134. McGowan M, Gordon Baker H, Kovacs G, et al. Selection of high-fertility donors for artificial insemination programmes. Clin Reprod Fertil 1983; 2:269–274.
135. Hummel W, Talbert L. Current management of a donor insemination program. Fertil Steril 1989; 51:919–930.
136. Mathews C, Ford J, Peek J, et al. Screening of karyotype and semen quality in an artificial insemination program: acceptance and rejection criteria. Fertil Steril 1983; 40:648–654.
137. Bendvold E. Semen quality in Norwegian men over a 20-year period. Int J Fertil 1989; 34:401–404.
138. Leto S, Frensilli F. Changing parameters of door semen. Fertil Steril 1981; 36:766–770.
139. Schroeder-Jenkins M, Roghmann S. Causes of donor rejection in a sperm banking program. Fertil Steril 1989; 51:903–906.
140. Chauhan M, Baratt C, Cooke S, et al. A protocol for the recruitment and screening of semen donors for an artificial insemination by donor programme. Human Reprod 1988; 3:873–876.
141. Tyler J, Dobler K, Driscoll G, et al. The impact of AIDS on artificial insemination by donor. Clin Reprod Fertil 1986; 4:305–317.
142. Urry P, Middleton R, Jones K, et al. Artificial insemination: a comparison of pregnancy rates with intrauterine versus cervical insemination and washed sperm versus swim-up sperm preparations. Fertil Steril 1988; 49:1038–1040.
143. Adamson D. Comments. Am J Obstet Gynecol 1990; 162:1489.
144. Verp M, Cohen M, Simpson J. Necessity of formal genetic screening in artificial insemination by donor. Obstet Gynecol 1983; 62:474–479.
145. Timmons M, Rao K, Sloan C, et al. Genetic screening of donors for artificial insemination. Fertil Steril 1981; 35:451–456.
146. Selva J, Albert L, Auger A, et al. Genetic screening for artificial insemination by donor (AID). Clin Genet 1986; 29:389–396.
147. MarPerez M, Marina S, Egozcue J. Karyotype screening of potential sperm donors for artificial insemination. Hum Reprod 1990; 5:282–285.
148. Strickler R. Transmission of disease during artificial insemination. N Engl J Med 1986; 315:1290.
149. Greenblatt R, Handsfield H, Sayers M. Screening therapeutic insemination donors for sexually transmitted disease: overview and recommendations. Fertil Steril 1986; 46:351–364.
150. Baker R, Dzuik P, Norton H. Effect of volume of semen, number of sperm, and drugs on transport of sperm in artificially inseminated gilts. J Anim Sci 1968; 27:88–93.
151. Sullivan J. Sperm numbers required for optimum breeding efficiency in cattle. In: Third Technical Conference on Artificial Insemination and Reproduction, sponsored by National Association of Animal Breeders, Chicago, IL, 1970:1.
152. Polge C. Fertilization in the pig and horse. J Reprod Fertil 1978; 54:461–470.
153. Marmar J, Praiss D, DeBenedictes T. An estimate of fertility potential of the fractions of the split ejaculate in terms of the motile sperm count. Fertil Steril 1979; 32:202–205.
154. David G, Czyglik F, Mayaux M, et al. The success of AID and semen characteristics: study of 1489 cycles and 192 ejaculates. Int J Androl 1980; 3:613–619.
155. Nielsen N, Risum J, Brogaard Hansen K, et al. Obtained pregnancies by AID using frozen semen in relation to specific qualities of the semen. Gynecol Obstet Invest 1984; 18:147–151.
156. Risum J, Nissen U, Grogaard Hansen K, et al. Evaluation of the quality variations of ejaculates from individual donors for establishing a quality control scheme. Gynecol Obstet Invest 1984; 17:149–156.
157. Yavetz H, Yogev L, Homonnai Z, et al. Prerequisites for successful human sperm cryobanking: semen quality and prefreezing holding time. Fertil Steril 1991; 55:812–816.
158. Paenvain E, Barlese E, Sauna F. Artificial insemination with donor cryopreserved semen: importance of the volume of semen and influence of ovulatory dysfunction. Acta Eur Fertil 1989; 20:90–95.
159. Danks D. Genetic considerations. In: Wood C, Leeton J, Kovacs G, editors. Artificial Insemination by Donor. Melbourne, Australia: Brown, Prior, Anderson, 1980:94.
160. Kovacs G, Clayton C, McGowan P. The attitudes of semen donors. Clin Reprod Fertil 1983; 2:73–75.
161. Andrews J. Reproduction and genetics. In: MacDonald M, Kaufman R, Carpon A, et al, editors. Treatise on Health Care Law. Vol. 4. New York: Time Mirror, 1991.
162. Curie-Cohen M. The frequency of consanguinous matings due to multiple use of donors in artificial insemination. Am J Hum Genet 1980; 32:589–600.
163. Loy R, Seibel M. Therapeutic insemination. In: Seibel M, editor. Infertility: A Comprehensive Text. Norwalk, CT: Appleton & Lange, 1990:199.
164. Bayslon M. A medical advancement in search of a legal theory: artificial insemination by donor and the law. Semin Reprod Endocrinol 1987; 5:69–76.
165. Mahlstedt P, Probasco K. Sperm donors: their attitudes towards providing medical and psychosocial information for recipient couples and donor offspring. Fertil Steril 1991; 56:747–753.
166. Rowland R. Attitudes and opinions on an artificial insemination by donor programme. Clin Reprod Fertil 1983; 2:249–259.

167. Klock S, Maier D. Psychology factors related to donor insemination. Fertil Steril 1991; 56:489–495.

168. Matot J, Gustin M. Filiation and secrecy in artificial insemination with donor. Hum Reprod 1990; 5:632–633.

169. Thorneycroft I, Bustillo M, Marik J. Donor fertility in an artificial insemination program. Fertil Steril 1984; 41:144–145.

170. Broekhuizen F, Haning R, Shapiro S. Laparoscopic findings in twenty-five failures of artificial insemination. Fertil Steril 1980; 34:351–355.

171. Bradshaw K, Guzick D, Grun B, et al. Cumulative pregnancy rates for donor insemination according to ovulatory function and tubal status. Fertil Steril 1987; 48:1051–1054.

172. Dalrymple J, Smith P, Shuter B, et al. Reduced pregnancy rates in AID women with unsuspected ovulatory failure. Clin Reprod Fertil 1983; 2:27–32.

173. Kemmann E, Pasquale S. Timing and frequency of artificial insemination in women under menotropin therapy. Fertil Steril 1985; 44:271–273.

174. Thomas E, Cooke I. Successful treatment of endometriosis: does it benefit infertile women? Br Med J 1987; 294:1117–1119.

175. Seibels M. Does minimal endometriosis always require treatment? Contemp Obstet Gynecol 1989; 34:27–39.

176. Jansen R. Minimal endometriosis and reduced fecundability: prospective evidence from an artificial insemination by donor program. Fertil Steril 1986; 46:141–143.

177. Rodriguez-Escudero F, Neyro J, Corcostegui B, et al. Does minimal endometriosis reduce fecundity? Fertil Steril 1988; 50:522–524.

178. Dodson W, Haney A. Controlled ovarian hyperstimulation and intrauterine insemination for treatment of infertility. Fertil Steril 1991; 55:457–467.

179. Kemmann E, Bohrer M, Sheldon R, et al. Active ovulation management increases the monthly probability of pregnancy occurrence in ovulatory women who receive intrauterine insemination. Fertil Steril 1987; 48:916–920.

180. Serhal P, Katz M, Little V, et al. Unexplained infertility: value of Pergonal superovulation combined with intrauterine insemination. Fertil Steril 1988; 49:602–606.

181. Asch R, Balmaceda J, Ellsworth L, et al. Preliminary experience with gamete intrafallopian transfer (GIFT). Fertil Steril 1986; 45:366–371.

182. Formigli L, Coglitore M, Roccio C, et al. One hundred and six gamete intra-fallopian transfer procedures with donor semen. Hum Reprod 1990; 5:549–552.

183. Holmes L. Congenital malformations. In: Berman RE, Vaughan V, editors. Nelson's Textbook of Pediatrics. 13th edition. Philadelphia: WB Saunders, 1987:268–269.

184. Forse R, Ackman C, Fraser F. Possible teratogenic effects of artificial insemination by donor. Clin Genet 1985; 28:23–26.

185. Iizuka R, Sawada Y, Nishina N, et al. The physical and mental development of children born following artificial insemination. Int J Fertil 1968; 13:24–32.

186. Alfredsson J. Artificial insemination with frozen semen: sex ratio at birth. Int J Fertil 1984; 29:152–155.

187. Baird W, Schmidt G, Williams S, et al. Cryopreserved donor semen: a laboratory comparison of five commercial sperm banks. Presented at the Annual Meeting of The American Fertility Society, San Francisco, CA. Abstract No. 0–043, 1989.

188. Clayton C, Kovacs G. AID offspring: initial follow-up study of 50 couples. Med J Aust 1982; 1:338–339.

189. Leeton J, Backwell J. A preliminary psychological follow-up of parents and their children conceived by artificial insemination by donor (AID). Clin Reprod Fertil 1982; 1:307–310.

190. Warner M. Artificial insemination review after thirty-two years' experience. NY State J Med 1974; 74:2358–2361.

191. Noble E. Having Your Baby by Donor Insemination: A Complete Resource Guide. Boston: Houghton Mifflin, 1987.

192. Wikler D, Wikler N. Turkey-baster babies: the demedicalization of artificial insemination. Milbank Q 1991; 69:5–50.

193. Rawson G. Human artificial insemination by donor and the Australian community. Clin Reprod Fertil 1985; 3:1–19.

194. Harvard J. Developments—medical technology and the law. Harvard Law Rev 1990; 103:1519–1537.

195. Hogerzeil H, Stevenhagen C, Oosting H, Hamerlynck JV. Daily insemination with cryopreserved donor semen is more effective than alternate-day insemination. Int J Fertil 1991; 36:281–286.

SECTION SIX

Assisted Reproductive Technologies

MICHAEL R. SOULES

CHAPTER 48

Glossary of Terminology for Assisted Reproductive Technologies and Early Embryonic Development

MICHAEL R. SOULES

The assisted reproductive technologies (ARTs) have been developed, tested, and applied over a relatively short span of time (since 1978). Many variants on the basic in vitro fertilization methodology have been introduced, and some have withstood the test of time. The proliferation of these procedures has led to a new lexicon of names and acronyms in the medical literature. Part I of this glossary describes the currently accepted procedures among the ARTs and the recommended acronym for each. In many instances other acronyms have been used for the same procedures. The authors of these chapters were polled, and the terms and acronyms presented represent a consensus among them.

The common theme among the ARTs is manipulation of gametes in the treatment of infertility. The union of gametes resulting in embryos has made the basic steps of embryo development a part of clinical medicine. Because these steps and stages of embryo development are new to clinical medicine, they have been listed in Part II of this glossary.

PART I.
Assisted Reproductive Technologies Glossary of Terms and Acronyms

DESCRIPTION	TERM	ACRONYM
Infertility treatment procedures that have in common the manipulation of oocytes, spermatozoa, and/or embryos	Assisted reproductive technologies	ART
Laboratory culture of aspirated oocyte(s) and spermatozoa followed by transcervical embryo transfer	In vitro fertilization Embryo transfer	IVF ET
Direct placement of aspirated oocyte(s) and spermatozoa into fallopian tube(s)	Gamete intrafallopian transfer	GIFT
Ovulation induction with monitoring in normal ovulatory women with the intent to induce multiple ovarian follicles	Controlled ovarian hyperstimulation	COH

Table continued on following page

PART I.

Assisted Reproductive Technologies Glossary of Terms and Acronyms
Continued

DESCRIPTION	TERM	ACRONYM
Ovulation induction combined with timed intrauterine insemination	Controlled ovarian hyperstimulation/intrauterine insemination	COH/IUI
Separation of spermatozoa from seminal fluid with suspension in buffer or culture media and insemination into the cervix, uterus, fallopian tube, or peritoneal cavity	Intracervical insemination Intrauterine insemination Intratubal insemination Intraperitoneal insemination	ICI IUI ITI IPI
Insemination with donor sperm	Donor insemination	DI
Laboratory culture of aspirated oocytes with spermatozoa followed by direct placement of fertilized zygote(s) or embryos into fallopian tube(s)	Zygote intrafallopian transfer Tubal embryo transfer	ZIFT TET
Insemination of a normal fertile woman for the purpose of conceiving a child and relinquishing it to an infertile couple	Surrogate mother	—
Transfer of embryo(s) to a normal fertile woman for the purpose of carrying a child and relinquishing it to an infertile couple	Gestational surrogate mother	—
Freezing of pronuclear concepti, zygote(s), and embryo(s) followed by storage in liquid nitrogen	Cryopreservation of pronuclear embryo(s) Cryopreservation of embryo(s)	CPN CPE
Uterine or tubal transfer of thawed pronuclear stage, zygote(s), or embryos	Frozen embryo transfer	FET
Insemination of a normal fertile woman followed by uterine flushing of an embryo and embryo transfer to an infertile woman	Ovum transfer	OT
Laboratory culture of aspirated oocytes from a donor woman followed by sperm/oocyte (in vitro fertilization) culture or placement of sperm/oocyte mixture into the fallopian tube (gamete intrafallopian transfer)	Oocyte donation	OD

PART II.
Glossary of Early Embryonic Staging Terminology

Blastocyst

The mammalian conceptus in the postmorula state. It resembles the blastula in that it has a fluid-filled cavity. It differs in that its surface layer is not exclusively embryoblast but is mainly or entirely trophoblast; in addition, it also has an eccentric embryoblast and is not limited to one germ layer. Attached to the inner surface of the trophoblast is an inner cell mass from which the embryo develops (*see* Free Blastocyst).

Conceptus

The derivatives of a fertilized oocyte at any stage of development from fertilization to birth; includes extraembryonic membranes, as well as the embryo, or fetus. The products of conception; all structures that develop from the zygote, both embryonic and extraembryonic.

Early-Cleavage-Stage Conceptus

The conceptus from the two-cell stage until the embryonic stage (*see* Embryo). The early-cleavage period ends at approximately 14 days after fertilization with development of the primitive streak. Often referred to as the *embryo* or *pre-embryo*.

Egg

Oocyte—the female gamete.

Embryo

The stage of the organism after development of the primitive streak; persists until major organs are developed. Once the neural groove and the first somites are present, the embryo is considered formed. In the human, the embryonic stage begins at approximately 14 days after fertilization and encompasses the period when organs and organ systems are coming into existence.

Fertilized Oocyte

An oocyte that has been penetrated by a spermatozoon; strictly, one in which gamete plasma membranes have become confluent. The stage before pronuclei are formed. Penetration of the oocyte usually occurs within 3 hours of insemination.

Fetus

The developing conceptus after the embryonic stage; the fetal period begins at the end of the 8th postovulatory week when more than 90% of the more than 4500 "named" structures of the adult body have appeared. The fetal period persists until birth.

Free Blastocyst

The unattached (nonimplanted) mass of cells after development of the blastocystic cavity. In mammals these cells have already differentiated into trophoblastic and embryonic cell lines.

Gamete

The oocyte or the spermatozoon; a mature haploid reproductive cell; any cell that, on union with another cell, results in the development of a new individual.

Immature Oocyte

An oocyte with chromosomes at Prophase I, a germinal vesicle–bearing oocyte.

Intermediate Oocyte

An oocyte with chromosomes at Metaphase I, characterized by the absence of both a first polar body and a germinal vesicle.

Mature Oocyte

An oocyte with chromosomes at Metaphase II, characterized by the presence of a first polar body.

Table continued on following page

PART II.
Glossary of Early Embryonic Staging Terminology *Continued*

Metaphase I Oocyte

An oocyte with chromosomes at Metaphase I of maturation, characterized by the absence of both a first polar body and a germinal vesicle. An oocyte at an intermediate stage of maturation.

Metaphase II Oocyte

An oocyte with chromosomes at Metaphase II of maturation, characterized by the presence of a first polar body. A fully mature oocyte. A secondary oocyte.

Morula

The 16-cell stage upward until blastocyst formation; the stage commonly observed between 72 and 96 hours after insemination. Some authors believe that the term *morula* is historically inappropriate for mammals.

Oocyte

The female gamete from inception of the first meiotic division until fertilization. In oogenesis, a cell that develops from an oogonium.

Oogonium

The cell that gives rise to the primary oocyte during oogenesis. Oogonia proliferate by mitotic division during early fetal life.

Ovum

A female gamete or germ cell; an oocyte. The term *ovum,* which has been used for such disparate structures as an oocyte and a 3-week embryo, has no scientific usefulness.

Pre-embryo

The conceptus during early-cleavage stages until the development of a single primitive streak at which point for the first time biologic individuation is ensured. This occurs at approximately 14 days after fertilization.

Prezygote

The penetrated oocyte that displays pronuclei and the second polar body; a pronuclear-stage conceptus. The stage of development before syngamy when the term *zygote* is appropriate. Some authors refer to this stage as an *ootid.*

Primary Oocyte

The oocyte (enlarged oogonium) formed in the ovary before birth. Primary oocytes begin the first meiotic division before birth, but completion of prophase does not occur until after puberty.

Pronuclear-Stage Oocyte

The penetrated oocyte, which displays pronuclei and the second polar body. The stage of development before syngamy; some authors describe this stage as the *ootid* or *prezygote.* Pronuclei are commonly observed 10 to 20 hours after sperm and oocyte are united.

Prophase I Oocyte

An oocyte with chromosomes at Prophase I of maturation, characterized by a germinal vesicle.

Secondary Oocyte

The oocyte after completion of the first meiotic division and arrest at metaphase of the second meiotic division. Also called a *mature oocyte* or *metaphase II oocyte,* this is the stage commonly associated with ovulated specimens or those collected from mature follicles for in vitro fertilization. The secondary oocyte is characterized by a first polar body and no nucleus.

PART II.
Glossary of Early Embryonic Staging Terminology *Continued*

Syngamy

The active union of two gametes in fertilization to form a zygote; the process of reorganization and pairing of maternal and paternal chromosomes in the zygote after pronuclear membrane breakdown.

Zygote

The one-cell stage after pronuclear membrane breakdown and before the first cleavage. This stage is characterized by maternal and paternal chromosomes assuming positions on the first cleavage spindle and, thus, lacks a nucleus. Commonly observed 18 to 24 hours after insemination.

Adapted from Veeck LL. Glossary of Staging Terms (Appendix A). In: Atlas of the Human Oocyte and Early Conceptus. Volume 2, p 405; © 1991, the Williams & Wilkins Co., Baltimore.

BIBLIOGRAPHY

Dorland's Illustrated Medical Dictionary. 26th edition. Philadelphia: WB Saunders, 1981.

Moore KL. The Developing Human. 3rd edition. Philadelphia: WB Saunders, 1982.

O'Rahilly R, Muller F. Developmental Stages in Human Embryos. Publication No. 637. Washington, DC: Carnegie Institute of Washington, 1987.

Stedman's Medical Dictionary. 25th edition. Baltimore: Williams & Wilkins, 1990.

Steen EB. Dictionary of Biology. Savage, MD: Barnes and Noble Books, 1971.

Veeck LL. Atlas of the Human Oocyte and Early Conceptus. Volume 1. Baltimore: Williams & Wilkins, 1986.

Veeck LL. Atlas of the Human Oocyte and Early Conceptus. Volume 2. Baltimore: Williams & Wilkins, 1991.

CHAPTER 49

History of In Vitro Fertilization

HOWARD W. JONES, JR.

Many times, clinical advances have eventuated because the clinician was familiar with developments that occurred at the research bench or from experiments in the animal house. The story of the clinical application of the process that has become known as *in vitro fertilization* (IVF) is an example extraordinaire of the benefits of the synergism of the fundamental and of the clinical.

However, the melding of the basic and applied was preceded by a number of independent observations at the mammalian subprimate level, which resulted from experiments that seemed to have been undertaken, not with a view to human clinical application, but from curiosity about arresting questions concerning reproduction in the mammal. The key questions were (1) can a mammalian egg be fertilized extracorporally, that is, in vitro, and will the egg so fertilized continue to develop? and (2) is it possible to transfer an early-developing conceptus from one animal to another and have it continue to grow in its adoptive uterus?

As might be expected, the first serious clinical application of what we now know as IVF was attempted by a clinician before the required basic studies had matured and several elementary requirements were unknown, such as the required pH and osmolality, and the result therefore failed.

Thus, it is necessary to begin with the basics. The first clear attempt to fertilize a fresh mammalian egg in vitro seems to have been recorded by Schenk in 1880.[1] His motive seemed to be entirely scientific curiosity. This took place in an era when laboratory techniques had developed to a point where fertilization could be profitably investigated. Thus, in the interval of 1878 to 1880, studies on fertilization in convenient laboratory marine animals, such as the sea urchin and the starfish, were worked out.

Schenk, in 1880 as just mentioned, tried to fertilize in vitro the oocytes of mammalian rabbits and guinea pigs.[1] The trial was a failure, and no wonder. Physiologic saline was not invented by Locke until 1901, 21 years after Schenk, and there was, at that time, no concept of the importance of the concentration of hydrogen ions.[2] We now know that mammalian eggs in fertilization require a steady osmolality and pH. Progress in in vitro research had to await an understanding of these basic factors.

It is curious that somewhat earlier than this, discussions were going on about the site in the mammalian reproductive tract where fertilization occurs. In 1847, Whitehead wrote:

Various opinions are entertained respecting the precise point at which the two elements of germination are brought into contact; some have stated that the spermatic animalcule has been found to have traversed the full length of the fallopian canal, while the ovule was still contained within the cavity of the corpus embryotum. In other instances, their communication has been witnessed in the course of the tube, sometimes near its inner extremity or even after the ovule has been deposited in the cavity of the uterus. The last named situation, it has been concluded, is that at which impregnation is probably always effected under normal circumstances, but the occasional occurrence of extrauterine fetation proves that fertilization may take place at any point between the ovarium and the uterus.[3]

About this same time, problems in the human that prevented the reproductive process from functioning were also discussed. For example, Fleetwood Churchill in 1846 wrote:

The fallopian tubes may be congenitally deficient or imperforate, although such cases are extremely rare. Their canal may be obliterated from acute or chronic inflammation, or their fimbriated extremities may become adherent to the ovaries. Even though not imperforate, yet the canal may be filled with adventitious matter. In all of these cases sterility is the consequence.[4]

It was to be almost exactly 100 years before the unsuccessful experiment of Schenk in 1880 was to become a successful experiment that led to the bypassing of the fallopian tubes that Churchill described in such a final and definitive way. For it was in 1978 that Steptoe and Edwards solved the problems of both Schenk and Churchill with the birth of Louise Brown.[5]

During this 100-year period, many workers contributed many points to make the system work.

In 1891, Walter Heape demonstrated that fertilized rabbit ova could be flushed from the fallopian tube and successfully transferred to a surrogate mother.[6] Heape's motivation was quite unrelated to any therapeutic application but was designed to examine the relative importance of maternal environment and genetic inheritance on certain characteristics. Nevertheless, this demonstration was a giant step in making possible the in vitro process as we know it.

In 1930, Gregory Pincus, at that time working at the School of Agriculture at Cambridge University, published a description of his first experiments on in vitro fertilization in the rabbit.[7] These experiments were unsuccessful, as none of the ova exposed to sperm and transplanted into the fallopian tube produced any offspring. Nevertheless, Pincus returned to Harvard and, with Enzmann, studied in vitro fertilization again. The results were published in 1934.[8] They thought that they had, in fact, succeeded. However, in the experiment, oocytes and sperm were mixed together and then transferred to the fallopian tubes, following which young were born, having characteristics of the genetic mother as opposed to the surrogate mother. We now understand that these eggs were transferred *not* having been fertilized in vitro, but probably fertilized in the fallopian tubes of the surrogate mother. Thus, Pincus and Enzmann did in the rabbit what is currently done in the human under what is called the gamete intrafallopian transfer (GIFT) procedure.

About this time, an extraordinary literary event occurred. In 1931, Aldous Huxley wrote his novel, *Brave New World*, which was published in 1932.[9] In this novel, Huxley realistically described the technique of in vitro fertilization as we now know it. The principal difference in the novel is that the embryo was allowed to develop entirely in tubes by a process that Huxley labeled *exogenesis*, which, at the present time, remains scientifically unattainable. It is interesting that in the Foreword to a new printing of *Brave New World* in 1950, Huxley describes the theme of the novel in the following words:

The only scientific advances to be specifically described are those involving the application to human beings of the result of future research in biology, physiology, and psychology. A book about the future can interest us only if its prophecies look as though they might conceivably come true.[9]

As we now know, some of Huxley's prophecies have come true, at least in part. After returning to Boston, Gregory Pincus worked with John Rock, a practicing gynecologist at Harvard, on a number of different projects. Very likely because of Rock's association with Pincus and because of the novel *Brave New World*, Rock decided that the time had come to attempt to fertilize human eggs in vitro to overcome some of the fertility problems he was dealing with daily. During World War II, in association with Miriam Menken, a Fellow, Rock retrieved more than 800 eggs from women on whom he was operating for a variety of conditions, some 138 of which were exposed to spermatozoa in vitro.[10] By today's standards, the maturational state of these eggs was crudely estimated. It is likely that they were maturationally heterogenous, because the timing of harvest in relation to ovulation was quite imprecise.

Menken and Rock thought that they had observed cleavage in three eggs[10]; however, no transfers were attempted. In retrospect, it is likely that instead of fertilization and cleavage, these eggs exhibited fragmentation, which is a relatively common experience in this type of work. In any case, after 4 years of work and only trivial success, Rock abandoned the project as impossible. In those preinstitutional research review board days, there seems to have been no social or ethical discussion of the project. Incidentally, Rock went on to take on a serious macrosocial problem—human overpopulation. He contributed mightily to the solution of this problem by introducing the contraceptive pill.

The problem of in vitro fertilization of the mammalian egg was tentatively solved in France in 1954 and definitively in the United States in 1959. Charles Thibault, working in Paris, also achieved fertilization in the rabbit.[11] However, Thibault was content to observe pronuclei and extrusion of the second polar body as proof of fertilization.

Working at the Worcester Foundation, which had meanwhile been established by Pincus, a young Chinese investigator named M. C. Chang was able to clearly solve the problem in the rabbit.[12] Chang, only to prove fertilization, transferred the concepti to rabbits of a different strain and was rewarded by the birth of rabbits of the original strain, thus proving that fertilization in vitro had in fact occurred. In the 1959 paper,[12] he emphasized this proof of in vitro fertilization and seemed to have had little interest in and did not mention the aspect of transfer, which Chang probably thought had been settled by the previous work of Heape.

Nevertheless, the discovery that Chang made was without, it seems, the understanding that he had observed an overwhelming point, that is, that oocytes fertilized in vitro were capable of developing if transferred into the uterus and producing live normal young.

After Chang's demonstration of the feasibility of fertilization in vitro in the rabbit, many other workers applied the techniques to other species—the mouse, the rat, and other laboratory animals. Among those who worked with the mouse was Robert Edwards, a young English biologist at Cambridge. He was basically a mouse geneticist interested in immunology who had succeeded in making the in vitro fertilization process work in this laboratory animal. In 1964, or perhaps before, Edwards thought that the process could be applied to the human and that it should be possible to solve the problems that had frustrated Rock 20 years earlier. Edwards was working at Cambridge University where, at that time, no medical school existed. Therefore, he had little access to human material. In attempting to find a place where human eggs might be available, he came as a Fellow to Johns Hopkins Hospital in 1965 at the time when ovarian wedge resection for polycystic ovary disease was a common procedure. In the wedges of removed tissue, Edwards was usually able to find 20 to 30 oocytes. With this material, Robert Edwards had access to a large number of human oocytes. He thought that the problem that had frustrated workers like Rock was that the concept of capacitation of sperm was not understood until it was elucidated by Chang in the 1950s. Therefore, in the 1965 effort, all measures were taken to try to capacitate sperm. The behind-the-scenes details of these efforts were reported by Jones in 1991 in a Festschrift for Edwards.[13] As with Menken and Rock's work, there seemed to be a few instances of fertilization but little evidence of cleavage. These 1965 results were published in the *American Journal of Obstetrics and Gynecology* in 1966.[14] Edwards returned to Cambridge, where he continued to work in the laboratory and where the potential for clinical application was opened by virtue of the introduction of the laparoscope into clinical practice. This was done in Great Britain by Patrick Steptoe, who met Edwards for the first time in the spring of 1968. From then, Steptoe worked with Edwards for some 10 years before all aspects of the in vitro fertilization system was made to work satisfactorily with the birth of Louise Brown in 1978, although there had been an ectopic pregnancy previously, probably from in vitro fertilization.[5] Interestingly enough, Klein and Palmer in 1960 had attempted to aspirate oocytes from the ovary, did harvest some, but apparently dropped the project without attempting anything further.[15] Edwards and Steptoe, in their initial work, succeeded in achieving a second pregnancy, which resulted in the birth of a boy in 1979. Following this, because of the necessity of Steptoe to retire from the National Health Service owing to age—he was 65 years old—they had to discontinue their work until the establishment of a private facility—Bourn Hall—in 1981.

Meanwhile, in Australia, Professor Carl Wood, together with Dr. Alex Lopata, a reproductive physiologist, had begun work on the same type of project in 1972 at Monash University.

However, a group at the University of Melbourne, under the direction of Dr. Ian Johnston, also began work on the in vitro fertilization concept. Dr. Lopata served as Reproductive Physiologist to this group; he also provided service to his Monash group until later replaced by Dr. Alan Trounson. It turned out that the University of Melbourne group had the first baby: Candice Reed, born in June 1980.[16]

The story of how in vitro fertilization came to the United States involves a considerable number of personal details that are included here only because (1) they are illustrative of how programs of this kind come about; (2) friends and associates have found them of interest; and (3) because of the unexpected spinoff into the world of ethics and public policy. There were undoubtedly other groups in the United States hard at work on such a project, but these details have never been published.

On June 30, 1978, Dr. Georgeanna Jones, according to the rules of The Johns Hopkins University, retired at the end of the academic year as Professor of Gynecology and Obstetrics and Director of the Division of Reproductive Endocrinology, after having held that position for 40 years. Dr. Howard W. Jones, Jr., had been required to retire 2 years previously but had been allowed to continue on the University premises as Professor Emeritus for the simple reason that Dr. Howard and Dr. Georgeanna had occupied the same office for many, many years, using a partners' desk. Dr. Howard was able to "sponge" a space in the hospital by virtue of his wife's professorial position for the last 2 years at Johns Hopkins.

Dr. Mason C. Andrews, of the new medical school in Norfolk, the Eastern Virginia Medical School, who had trained with Dr. Howard Jones on the house staff at Johns Hopkins immediately after World War II, renewed his invitation to join the faculty at Norfolk. This invitation was accepted with enthusiasm, and the plan was to stay 2 years for the purpose of establishing a Division of Reproductive Endocrinology in the Department of Obstetrics and Gynecology, of which Mason Andrews was Chairman.

On the day that the Joneses moved into Norfolk, July 28, 1978, Louise Brown, the first test tube baby in the world, was born in Oldham, England. A newspaper reporter of the *Norfolk Ledger Star* invited Dr. Andrews to comment on this curious English event. Dr. Andrews did so, but said that the Joneses, who were joining the Department, knew Dr. Edwards and might have some special comments to make. As a result, the reporter, Julia Wallace, interviewed the Joneses as the moving men were bringing boxes into their new house in Norfolk. At the end of the interview, she asked what seemed to be a flip question, inquiring "could this be done in Norfolk?". Believing it to be a flip question, she received a flip answer.

"Of course," said Dr. Howard.

Whereupon she said: "What would it take?"

"A little money," replied Dr. Howard.

In the write-up in the *Norfolk Ledger Star* the next day, the reporter quoted the Joneses as saying that this could easily be done in Norfolk, provided there was a little money.

A curious thing then happened. Dr. Georgeanna Jones had a telephone call from a patient who had been sent to Baltimore from Norfolk by Dr. Mason C. Andrews because of a reproductive problem. The patient had been rewarded by a child and she called to say that she was amazed to know that we were moving to Norfolk, that we were certainly welcome; she also noted that we said that we could use a little money. She offered to talk about this, and as a result, 48 hours later there was a conference in our home, with the furniture still in disarray, between the prospective donor (who has wished to remain anonymous to this day), Mr. Henry Clay Hofheimer (then Chairman of the Foundation of the Eastern Virginia Medical School), Dr. Mason C. Andrews, and the Joneses, during which it was agreed that a gift, which turned out to be very modest in terms of gifts of this kind, would be forthcoming if the program of in vitro fertilization could be established.

Although the Joneses had not planned to start a program of in vitro fertilization on joining the faculty in Norfolk, the proposal was not as far off base as it might appear to have been. As previously mentioned in this account, in 1965, Dr. Robert Edwards, who later teamed up with Mr. Patrick Steptoe to be responsible for the birth of Louise Brown, had actually been a Fellow at Johns Hopkins. That effort in 1965 to fertilize human eggs was unsuccessful, largely because of naiveté regarding the biology of fertilization.

Subsequent to this initial attempt, Drs. Georgeanna and Howard had occasion to visit Dr. Edwards' laboratory in Cambridge from time to time when they were in the United Kingdom. When Dr. Edwards was in this country, he visited in Baltimore on occasion. We had followed his work carefully and, after the birth of Louise Brown, called him from our office in the Norfolk General Hospital to congratulate him on this event.

Thus, we were not without knowledge of Dr. Edwards' efforts and, indeed, thought that it would be possible to do it in Norfolk, although we realized that he had been at it some 13 years, from the beginning of his human egg experience at Johns Hopkins until the successful application of his concept.

By the fall of 1978, after the Joneses conferred with the authorities at the Medical School and the hospital, a decision was made to go ahead with the project. The Dean of the Medical School, Dr. Jerry Holman, was enthusiastic and was able to provide a faculty position for a young investigator to help with the project. Dr. Mason C. Andrews, the Department Chairman, was enthusiastic from the first, and his support and guidance, particularly with persuading the Dean to create the faculty positions, was a key factor in our efforts. The anonymous $5000 gift from Dr. Georgeanna's patient was used for the purchase of special equipment and other items needed for the project. Dr. Jairo Garcia from Columbia, South America, a former Fellow in Reproductive Endocrinology under Dr. Georgeanna at Johns Hopkins, had coincidentally written and expressed a hope that somehow or other he could return to the States, so that we were able to offer him the position that had been created by the Dean. One other full-time member of the Department in Norfolk was Dr. Anibal Acosta, also a former Fellow in Reproductive Endocrinology at Johns Hopkins, and when the Joneses arrived in Norfolk in 1978, was one of the two full-time members of the Department in addition to Dr. Andrews. Dr. Acosta was knowledgeable in andrology and was enthusiastic about participating in the new venture. Dr. Acosta's studies of the male in assisted reproduction have been basic to the success of the program and have resulted in the publication of two key volumes on the subject.[17, 18] The Embryology Laboratory was organized from the Laboratory of Cytogenetics, which had come along with the Joneses to Eastern Virginia Medical School from Johns Hopkins, where a Cytogenetics Laboratory had been established by grant and other funds raised by Dr. Howard. Newly hired in the laboratory when it opened in 1978 was Lucinda Veeck, who had just graduated from a medical technology course at Norfolk General Hospital. After participating in cytogenetics for some months, she was offered the opportunity to transfer to the new effort and has become a leading embryologist in this developing field. Her definitive work, *Atlas of the Human Oocyte and Early Conceptus*,[19] appeared in 1986, and the second companion volume of the same title *Atlas of the Human Oocyte and Early Conceptus II*,[20] appeared in 1991.

There were several weeks and months of planning. Although I knew Dr. Edwards quite well, I knew Mr. Steptoe only slightly. Nevertheless, Dr. William C. Andrews, the brother of Mason C. Andrews, and himself a practicing gynecologist with a special interest in infertility in Norfolk, knew Mr. Steptoe quite well, with the result that in December 1978, Patrick Steptoe visited Norfolk and offered to give us consultative advice about our effort. Although Edwards and his colleagues had published from time to time reports of his efforts at in vitro fertilization, there had been no systematic report of the step-by-step protocol that had been followed by the birth of Louise Brown. Such a publication did not occur until September 1980, in the *British Journal of Obstetrics and Gynaecology*.[21] During Mr. Steptoe's visit to Norfolk in December 1978, he indicated that the Royal College of Obstetricians and Gynaecologists was going to have a private scientific meeting in January 1979, at which time the process and results would be described in great detail. He invited me to attend. Getting to England in January is not as easy as it is in some other months owing to uncertainties of the weather, and cancellation of plane flights ended up with a required trip on the Concorde to be in London at the appointed time. Edwards and Steptoe were generous in their advice, and they suggested several things, most of which were wrong, not intentionally, of course, but because of the state of knowledge. They said we should use the natural cycle for retrieval rather than a stimulated cycle, because they had tried gonadotropin stimulation for almost 100 cycles without success.

They said we should use a very small needle for aspiration. They said there should be a minimal time between the harvest of the egg and its insemintion—there was 90 seconds in the case of Louise Brown. We now know that all this advice was wrong. The stimulated cycle is generally used and is far superior to the natural cycle. A needle of suitable internal diameter has been developed, and we know that the egg most often needs to be matured in vitro for a few hours before insemination is efficient, unless the egg just happens to be mature at the time of harvest. In short, Edwards and Steptoe were lucky after more than 100 failures. On the successful effort, there happened to be a concurrence when everything was correct.

Meanwhile, in Norfolk, things were progressing well so that we thought that it would be possible to do some preliminary studies on patients prior to an actual harvest attempt by the end of 1979. The hospital had cooperated beautifully, having assigned an unused delivery room on the obstetric unit for the egg harvest procedures and converted an adjacent utility room into the embryology laboratory. The reconstruction for our purposes had been complete by about September 1979.

At this point, one of the hospital administrators had a concern. Mr. Glen Mitchell, the Chief Hospital Administrator, pointed out that, according to the Virginia State regulations then in force, any hospital initiating a new program needed to have a certificate of need prior to the initiation of the program. In view of the fact that this was a new program, he thought that the hospital should obtain such a certificate. He pointed out that this was a routine matter, believed there should be no problem, and thought it could be granted administratively, that is to say, without a general public hearing. We were advised that we did not need to be present at the time the application was made.

Much to the surprise of the administrator and to us, at the time the administrative application was made, there were a number of protesters who had been alerted by reading the agenda of issues before the State Board, which grants the certificates of need. Because of these protesters and their protests, a certificate of need by the administrative process was denied, but it was stated that an application with a full-scale public hearing could be entered. This hearing was scheduled for Halloween Day, 1979, in the auditorium of the Health Department of the city of Norfolk, where such hearings were normally held. The hearing began at 2:00 P.M. and lasted until 8:00 P.M. Because of the previous protests, it stimulated wide public interest. For example, the three major television networks were present, as were reporters from the print news media. The Eastern Virigina medical students became interested and were somehow organized by a person who, to this day, remains unknown to me, to march en masse (approximately 150 people) to the hearing auditorium in the Public Health Building adjacent to the medical complex. The medical students occupied essentially all of the seats by 1:30 P.M., and when the busloads of protesters began to arrive, there was only limited seating available for them. The Fire Department allowed only so many people in the auditorium, with the result that many protesters and others milled around outside of the building. Because we knew that the opposition would be organized, it was necessary to have a certain organization in favor of the project. Several distinguished speakers were brought from the outside—Dr. Roy Parker, Professor and Chairman of Obstetrics and Gynecology at Duke University and then President of the American College of Obstetricians and Gynecologists, spoke in favor of the project. So did Dr. John Biggers, Professor of Physiology at Harvard University and an old friend from Johns Hopkins. So did the Right Reverend Bishop Heath Light of the Episcopal Diocese of Southwestern Virginia, with headquarters at Roanoke, as did Rabbi Lawrence Foreman of Norfolk, and several others.

After due consideration and several subsidiary hearings, the certificate of need was granted in early 1980.

During the several days and weeks occupied by the hearings before the Commission for the Certificate of Need, I requested to appear before the Board of Directors of the Norfolk General Hospital and before the Commissioners of the Eastern Virginia Medical School. To each of these bodies, I explained that I regretted that I was causing some possible embarrassment to the hospital and the school, that the controversy that arose was quite a surprise, that it had not occurred to us that we were doing anything that could be considered unethical, and that we regarded the whole project as an attempt to extend therapy to those patients with infertility who could not be helped by methods that were then in vogue. I went on to explain to the hospital board and the Medical School Board that, if they were uncomfortable with the position in which everyone found themselves, it would be relatively easy at that point to discontinue the in vitro effort, and I offered to withdraw from the field. I requested, however, that if the boards felt that we should continue, their support should be of a long-term nature, because there would undoubtedly be some hills and valleys along the way.

After suitable discussion, the boards of each institution unanimously supported the project, suggested that we should go on, and from that time, there has never been a wavering of support by the board of either the hospital or the medical school.

As previously mentioned, the hospital had already completed construction of the Embryology Laboratory that was to be adjacent to the dedicated delivery room prior to the application for a certificate of need. When it became apparent that there was some difficulty with the certificate, it was decided to seal the Embryology Laboratory, and so this was closed and sealed with masking tape so that it would not be generally known that construction was undertaken before the matter of the certificate of need was resolved. It was unsealed only several months later in February 1980, just before the program was set to begin.

THE STRUGGLE FOR PREGNANCY

During the almost 1 year occupied by planning and the gathering of personnel, equipment, and space, the Australians, after working for about 5 years, had been successful in having their first baby delivered in June 1980. A single egg had been obtained in a natural cycle by laparoscopy and transferred at the eight-cell stage. As mentioned before, the principals who were involved were Professor Carl Wood at Monash University and Dr. Alex Lopata, their reproductive physiologist, although the baby was born at the University of Melbourne on the clinical service of Dr. Ian Johnston. It happened that I knew Professor Carl Wood quite well, having visited his clinic on at least two previous occasions, so that

during our year of planning, we had the pleasure of having a visit from Professor Wood in Norfolk, as well as from Dr. Lopata. Furthermore, Dr. Anibal Acosta of our staff visited Melbourne. We therefore believed that we had, on a personal basis, the necessary information to begin, although as I mentioned previously, nothing had been published in the peer review scientific literature either from England or Australia. We therefore began in March 1980, on the basis of advice we had from our friends overseas, to use the natural cycle, to use a small needle for laparoscopic harvest, and to inseminate the egg as promptly as possible. To make a predication as to when ovulation might occur with the use of a natural cycle, it was necessary to observe the patient's serum estradiol and luteinizing hormone (LH) levels with quick assays, both of which had been recently developed. It was then necessary to time the laparoscopy 2 or 3 hours before the expected ovulation. This meant that the operating room needed to be prepared to function at any time, day or night, 7 days a week.

When it became known, because of the publicity surrounding the hearings associated with the certificate of need, that an in vitro fertilization program was being organized, there was a flood of patients in the Norfolk area and elsewhere asking to be considered. This also caught us by surprise, because we had anticipated beginning slowly among suitable patients in our own infertility practice. After determining that it was necessary to obtain a certificate of need to conform to the state regulations covering new medical procedures, it seemed to follow that it should be necessary and appropriate to go to the Institutional Review Board. Thus, it was necessary to adopt some criteria and to develop a consent form. The criteria seemed rather straightforward; thus, we said that the patients had to be generally healthy, that the male had to be normal, that the woman had to be normally menstruating and have a normal uterus, and that the couple had to be younger than 35 years of age. In addition, not included in the consent form, was our own agreement among the teams that all patients had to have bilateral salpingectomies. This was adopted to be certain that in the event a pregnancy occurred, we would not have the slightest doubt that it was due to the in vitro process. Finally, in view of the fact that we were in a "fishbowl," we thought it would be appropriate to list as a criterion that we would accept only married couples. Curiously enough, this last criterion was the only thing questioned by the Institutional Review Board. One of the minority members on the board said that if we adopted that criterion, it would keep out many couples of the minority group. Therefore, the criterion was changed to couples with a stable relationship.

With the approval of the school and the hospital authorities, it was decided that there would be no professional fee charged until some time in the future, if and when the system was demonstrated to be workable. However, the hospital and the medical school did make a rather modest charge, which was calculated to be on an "out-of-pocket" basis, which did not include any item of the professional staff salary.

In spite of the fact that we told prospective patients that this was an experimental procedure, that there was no record of whether it would work, they did not seem to be deterred. On thinking about this, this was perhaps not unexpected, as the patients indeed were self-selected and knew from the publicity associated with the effort that it was a scientific venture.

In March 1980, there was a very heavy, wet snowstorm in Norfolk. Almost 36 inches of snow fell. On the second night of the snow, it happened that a patient was judged about to ovulate, and we scheduled her for laparoscopy at midnight. However, because of the snowstorm, there was considerable delay in gathering together the staff members of the team, as well as the patient, and it was about 3:00 A.M. before it was possible to carry out the laparoscopy. To the great disappointment of all, when we finally got to the laparoscopy, it was realized that the patient had already ovulated. We, of course, could not possibly see the egg, although we could see the stoma in the ovary, but it was thought that it might be possible to irrigate the ovary and the cul-de-sac and to suck out the fluid through a large suprapubic trocar and perhaps recover the egg in that way. This was done by inserting a 5-mm aspirating cannula suprapubically. It seemed unlikely that so tiny an object could be found by such a gross technique, but the competent Lucinda Veeck in the Embryology Laboratory did spot the egg. We all had an opportunity, probably for the first time ever, to observe under the microscope a spontaneously ovulated human egg. The most striking thing was that the egg, which measured about 100 μ in diameter, was surrounded by a huge, beautiful corona radiata. The corona, of course, had previously been described in animal eggs, but the striking thing was to measure the full diameter of the human corona. The egg, with the corona, measured about 500 μ in its shorter axis and as much as 1000 μ in its longest. This meant that the small needle that we had been using could not possibly accommodate the egg with its corona without either shearing off the corona or greatly compressing it. On the basis of this snowy night observation, a new needle was immediately designed measuring 2.2-mm internal diameter, with a cross-section area some four times larger than the small needle. With this new and improved needle, our efficiency of obtaining eggs greatly improved. I cite this as but an example of the sputtering development that characterized the early stages of the in vitro program.

During 1980, we made 41 attempts to obtain an egg in natural cycles; however, eggs were obtained in only 19 patients and transfer occurred 13 times. There were no pregnancies.

During the break for the Christmas holidays in 1980, there was understandable discouragement on the part of the members of the team. It seemed obvious that something needed to be changed. When the program was initiated, we had stated to the boards of the hospital and the medical school that we would give ourselves 3 years to see if we could make the system work. After all, it had taken some 13 years for the system to be devised in Great Britain, and we knew that the Australians had worked for more than 5 years. At the Christmas break, 1980, we had been at it for almost 1 year. There were still 2 years to go, but something had to change. Dr. Georgeanna had had considerable experience with ovulation induction using human menopausal gonadotropins in anovulatory women. It had *always* been used previously in anovulatory women. This was the technique that Edwards and Steptoe had used almost 100 times in ovulatory women and told us it would not work because the patients always had a short luteal phase. The explanation for this shortness was not to be explained for several years, but it is now understood.[22, 23] Nevertheless, it seemed curious that gona-

dotropin stimulation worked in anovulatory patients and could not be made to work in normal menstruating women. After thinking through the matter during the Christmas holidays, it was decided that beginning with patients in 1981, we would in fact use human menopausal gonadotropin for the recruitment of multiple eggs in spite of Edwards' advice to the contrary. Dr. Georgeanna did not think that Edwards, who was acting as the endocrinologist for the English crew, had used the gonadotropins in an appropriate way. In fact, she had a lively discussion with him about this matter on one occasion when we visited Edwards' laboratory in Cambridge. Her comments were highly technical and complicated, but her basic concern was that far too high a dose of gonadotropin was being used and that in the normal menstruating woman, a rather gentler stimulation was probably indicated.

When we started in 1981, the gentle stimulation of two ampules of menopausal gonadotropin per day seemed to be working quite well and we were harvesting three or four eggs from a single patient in contrast with the single egg, which we sometimes had recovered in the natural cycle. But still, among the first six cases, we did not obtain a pregnancy.

In the early part of May 1980, Dr. Georgeanna was invited to Paris to address a medical group about the function of the corpus luteum, a favorite topic of hers. It was decided that we would stop by Cambridge in response to an open invitation we had from Edwards and Steptoe to drop in whenever we could. We spent an entire day with them in the operating theater and in the laboratory. In the evening, when we were back in our hotel room, I called Norfolk and spoke to Jairo Garcia and told him I was puzzled by the fact that we did not have a pregnancy, because I did not see Edwards and Steptoe doing anything different from what we were doing. He replied that he thought we might have a pregnancy. A patient by the name of Judy Carr, whom I had transferred a few days before leaving Norfolk for Europe, was 2 days overdue. She was the 13th patient to receive gonadotropin stimulation. She did not live in Norfolk, and he was arranging to have a pregnancy test done, the results of which would be known in 2 days. We promised to call him when we got to Paris, where we were headed the next morning.

On arrival at the Sofitel Bourbon, our hotel in Paris, there was a message to call the Norfolk office. The news was great—the pregnancy test was positive. We decided to celebrate by having the most expensive meal available at a small family-style Left Bank restaurant that we had discovered while spending a month in Paris in 1979 as visiting scholars at Le College de France.

During the several days of the Parisian scientific meeting, we disclosed our information to a few of our close French friends and discovered that the team of Prof. Jacques Salat-Baroux, which had also been working in the in vitro field, had the year before had a pregnancy which had miscarried early. Their pregnancy had caused quite a stir in the media. Dr. Jean Cohen, who told us of this event, thought that the miscarriage might have been caused by the anxiety of the patient caused by the publicity associated with the event. He highly recommended that our pregnancy be concealed from the media.

In view of the fact that we had been very much working "in a goldfish bowl" beginning with the certificate of need process, wherein even the details of our medical changes such as the shift from the natural cycle to gonadotropin stimulation were recorded in the press, it seemed unlikely that we could conceal this pregnancy from the media. On the return flight across the Atlantic, I wrote a draft of a statement that I proposed to make to the media.

We arrived back in Norfolk on Mother's Day, 1981. We were met at the airport by Dr. Jairo Garcia with a Mother's Day greeting of congratulations and best wishes, and the pregnancy basal body temperature chart of Judy Carr that demonstrated her pregnancy. Dr. Mason C. Andrews and the public relations people of the medical school and hospital had also been considering what to do about the situation. There was general unanimity that it would not be possible to conceal the pregnancy but that we would try to withhold the name of the pregnant patient. We would request the media not to attempt to pursue the matter, saying that we were sure the media would not wish to feel responsible for an untoward event that might happen to the patient in the event that she were identified. We were of the opinion that an active investigative reporter could, in fact, trace the patient if enough people in the medical school or hospital were quizzed. A news conference was called, and a simple announcement of a pregnancy was made. It was stated that the patient had had a bilateral salpingectomy, that the pregnancy could not have been caused by anything other than the procedure that was carried out, and that, at the time of the announcement, the pregnancy was continuing. Anonymity for the patient was requested, pointing out to the press that they certainly would not like to be a party to causing a miscarriage. Of course, it seemed unlikely that stress per se could cause a miscarriage, but in view of the French experience, we took their advice with regard to publicity. The media acted very responsibly. The matter was reported in the newspaper; no effort was made to identify the patient; but the media easily calculated that, if all went well, the baby would be born sometime around Christmas 1981.

Roger and Judy Carr were residents of Westminster, Massachusetts, a small town not far from Worcester, and within an hour's drive of Boston. The question arose as to where the baby should be delivered. After discussing the many options, it was decided by the Carrs that she would be delivered in Norfolk and that she would be taken care of by Dr. Andrews. As already indicated, her identity would be concealed, and on the several prenatal visits that she made to Norfolk, I usually met her at the airport, took her to the Omni Hotel, where she was registered under a fictitious name to further obscure her true identity.

It was decided that she should reside continuously in Norfolk for 4 weeks before the expected date of delivery, and on about the first of December 1981, she moved into an apartment in Virginia Beach under an assumed name.

Dr. Andrews was concerned about the size of the fetus, and it was decided to deliver Judy by elective cesarean section, which was scheduled for 7:30 A.M. on December 28, 1981.

Because of the smallness of the baby, there was considerable concern on the part of Dr. Andrews and me that the baby might be abnormal. For this reason, on Christmas Day, after having had Christmas dinner with Judy and Roger Carr at the home of Dr. and Mrs. Garcia, I wrote out a statement to be used in the event it was found that the baby had a serious abnormality at cesarean section. In this projected press re-

lease, I indicated that we had experienced a tragic disappointment, that we would protect the name of the prospective parents, that we had every hope that the two other patients who were pregnant and progressing in our program had normal pregnancies, but that this would obviously have to be determined later.

Fortunately, it was not necessary to use this press release, and after arrival home from the hospital after the birth of Elizabeth Carr, this "worst case" news release was torn up and thrown away.

Sometime during that summer of 1981, I had received a telephone call from Southampton, England. The caller introduced himself as Gordon Stevens, a producer with IBC, the private broadcasting network of Great Britain. He said that he represented Peter Williams, one of their principals, and that they were interested in knowing whether we would allow them to come to America to film the activities of our in vitro program. He went on to explain that he had heard about the Norfolk program from news clips of the Halloween hearing and he offered the name of Bob Edwards as a reference, because they had made a similar film about the work of Edwards and Steptoe at Oldham, where Louise Brown was born. I told Mr. Stevens that I would be glad to consider the matter, that it happened that we were going to be in England later in 1981 and that I could meet with him and Peter Williams and discuss the matter further. It turned out that Stevens and Williams did not know we had a pregnancy when they first contacted us. Arrangements were made to have dinner together. This dinner conversation resulted in a visit to Norfolk by Gordon Stevens and an agreement to film our program. A British team consisting of six people came to Norfolk, first in November 1981 and again in December 1981, to film the work and anxieties of the program and, as it turned out, the birth of Elizabeth Jordan Carr, our first baby.

That film was originally broadcast on the Public Broadcasting System as a part of the *Nova* program and was aired on January 17, 1982.

The birth of Elizabeth Carr turned out to be more of a media event than anyone had anticipated. At a news conference at 11:00 A.M. on the day of her birth, there were a number of media people present. It was announced at that time that, because the baby had been born by cesarean section, it would not be possible to introduce the Carrs or the baby to the public. However, it was stated that if all went well, a second news conference would be held 3 days later, at which Mr. and Mrs. Carr and Elizabeth would be introduced. This was a major, major event that resulted in numerous invitations to make public appearances for all members of the team and was exceedingly time consuming, to say the least. Fortunately, it occurred during the Christmas holiday break, which was least disruptive to our routine schedule.

A SUIT FOR LIBEL

At the time of the original hearing for a certificate of need, there was considerable media interest in the events in Norfolk. A news clipping service identified more than 100 editorials in papers across the country dealing with the subject. With one exception, there was editorial support for the project. The exception was the local Norfolk newspaper.

From time to time during 1980 and 1981, a newspaper article, editorial, or a letter to the editor would appear in the local paper denigrating the work that was being done. On two or three occasions, it was called to our attention that some of the statements being made in the paper might be libelous, and if we wished to attempt to stop these articles and letters to the editor, it might be necessary to take legal action against the newspaper. This certainly seemed far fetched.

Five days after the birth of Elizabeth Carr, there was still another editorial in the newspaper. This editorial stated that the doctors at the in vitro clinic would not allow an abnormal baby to be born because the patients had to sign an agreement to have the pregnancy terminated if it was determined to be abnormal. We happened to know that the editor who wrote this editorial had been informed that the statement was probably untrue and should be checked prior to publication. This was not done. In actuality, the statement was not true.

A Norfolk lawyer, Mr. Robert Nusbaum, a long-time friend of Dr. Andrews, called this editorial to our attention and said that it had all the necessary legal points for libel, that if we were ever going to enter suit, now was the time to do it. It was his opinion that it was unlikely that the constant haranguing of the paper would cease unless they were forced to do so by legal action. After considerable discussion among the principals involved, namely Drs. Andrews, Acosta, Garcia, and Joneses, it was decided that such action would be taken. Accordingly, in early 1982, a suit was filed by Dr. Georgeanna against the newspaper for libel.

It would be a long, long story to detail the numerous depositions, consultations, conferences, and so forth, that ensued from this action. The trial was set for March 1983.

Just before the trial, Dr. Georgeanna and I were visited by two prominent Norfolk citizens, who said that they were quite aware of the suit, that they were afraid the suit would result in considerable divisiveness in the community, and that they wondered if we would allow them to attempt to act as intermediaries between the newspaper and the plaintiffs. To this we agreed.

This arrangement resulted in a favorable settlement. The principals had agreed going into the suit that, in the event we received any award, we would turn the money over to the Foundation for use in research. The newspaper printed an apology and provided a sum of money that supported our research over the next couple of years.

AN INVITATION TO THE VATICAN

In early 1984, we were surprised to receive a letter from Dr. Carlos Chagas of Rio de Janeiro, Brazil. He explained that he was President of the Pontifical Academy of Sciences and inquired if we would be available to attend a conference "in the Vatican Garden" in November 1984 concerning the moral status of in vitro fertilization. He went on to explain that, if we were agreeable, an official invitation from the Vatican would be forthcoming. He further went on to explain that our role would be to explain to the assembled moral theologians the scientific steps in the in vitro process.

In due course, the invitation was received and the group gathered in the Pontifical Academy of Science in the Vatican in November 1984. In addition to the Joneses, there were three other gynecologists—one was Prof. Rene Frydman of the University of Paris. The other two were Professors of Gynaecology at the University of Rome, but they attended only the first of eight sessions. At that time, there was no in vitro program in Italy. These Roman gynaecologists were there as symbolic representatives of the medical profession, and specifically, of the gynaecological and obstetrical faculties in Rome. There was a total of 12 people in attendance, there being a number of moral theologians from within the Vatican.

Dr. Georgeanna recognized early on that the concern of the moral theologians was not entirely with in vitro fertilization, but with contraception, because the issues involved, namely interference with the reproductive process, were, from a moral theological point of view, essentially the same question. At the beginning of the conference, we were told by Prof. Chagas that we should speak frankly, that the purpose was to develop the truth, that the conversations would be recorded, that the transcript would be circulated to the members of the Working Party for accuracy, and that a document would be prepared for the use of the Holy Father, who was considering the question of the licitness of in vitro fertilization, and by implication, other methods of assisted reproductive technology.

The first 2 days of the conference were devoted to the technical aspects of in vitro fertilization, in which the theologians quizzed the doctors after an exposition of the process. The latter part of the conference was a moral theological discussion about the licitness of the process. Toward the end of the conference, it became clear that there was general support for declaring that in vitro fertilization was an ethically acceptable process. There was one dissenter, namely Msgr. Carlos Caffari. Msgr. Caffari was President of the John Paul II Institute for Marriage and the Family, an appointment he received from the Pope. He steadfastly maintained that in vitro fertilization was illicit, because in vitro fertilization resulted in conception outside the bonds of conjugal love. In short, the natural process of sexual intercourse was not used. In summarizing the conference, Prof. Chagas noted that among those present, with one exception, there was a general agreement that the process should be considered licit. Prof. Chagas made an impassioned appeal to Msgr. Caffari that if he could not agree with this, at least in the name of charity, to please remain silent.

It is interesting, and probably significant, that a transcript of this conference was never circulated to the members present, as was planned. Furthermore, insofar as this attendant is aware, no document seems to have ever been produced.

In May 1987, 2 1/2 years after the conference, the "Instruction on Respect for Human Life in its Origin and on the Dignity of Procreation" (Donum Vitae) was issued by the Congregation for the Doctrine of Faith of the Vatican. This document held that in vitro fertilization and other methods of assisted reproductive technology were illicit for the reason advanced by Msgr. Caffari at the time of the ill-fated Vatican conference.

It is within the realm of possibility that the absence of a document from the Working Party of the Pontifical Academy was not by chance.

IN VITRO FERTILIZATION AND SOCIETY

The story of how in vitro fertilization first came to the United States has been set forth in some detail to indicate that the launching of this particular project required a response not only to unexpected, nonexistent, or erroneous scientific data but also to unexpected public exposure, to a very negative reaction by a segment of the population, and to moral theological questions in an unaccustomed forum. Thus, it became necessary to devote precious time to learning about things such as discovery, interrogatories, and depositions, and other words and procedures common to our judicial system, and to devote other equally precious time to being tutored in how to solve the ethical calculus, as well as in the cultural and religious attitudes bearing on the ancient question of when does life begin and the moral status of nascent human life.

Thus, in vitro fertilization began a new chapter in the biology of early human reproduction and required participation in the discussion attempting to develop a consensus about matters that heretofore seem to have been the domain of philosophers and moral theologians. Both the scientific and social aspects of in vitro fertilization continue to evolve.

REFERENCES

1. Schenk SL. Das Säugethierei künstlich befruchtet ausserhalb des Mutterthieres. Mittheilungen aus dem Embryologischen Institut der Wien IX Band, 1880.
2. Locke FS. Die wirking der metalle des blutplasmas und verschiedener zucker auf das isolarte säugetierherz. Zentralbl Physiol 1901; 14:670–972.
3. Whitehead J. On the causes and treatment of abortion and sterility. London: Churchill, 1847:402.
4. Churchill F. On the Theory and Practice of Infertility. 2nd edition. Philadelphia: Lea & Blanchard, 1846:157.
5. Steptoe PC, Edwards RG. Birth after the reimplantation of a human embryo. Lancet 1978; 366:2.
6. Heape W. Preliminary note on the transplantation and growth of mammalian ova within a uterine foster mother. Proc R Soc 1891; 48:457–458.
7. Pincus G. Observations on the living eggs of the rabbit. Proc R Soc Lond [Biol] 1930; 107:132–169.
8. Pincus G, Enzmann EV. Can mammalian eggs undergo normal development in vitro? Proc Natl Acad Sci U S A 1934; 20:121–122.
9. Huxley A. Brave New World. New York: Harper & Row, 1932.
10. Menken I, Rock J. In vitro fertilization and cleavage of human ovarian eggs. Am J Obstet Gynecol 1948; 55:440–451.
11. Dauzier L, Thibault C, Wintenberger S. La fecondation in vitro de l'oeuf de la lapine. Comptes Rendus Academie des Sciences 1954; 238:844–845.
12. Chang MC. Fertilization of rabbit ova in vitro. Nature 1959; 184:466–467.
13. Jones HW Jr. In the beginning there was Bob. Hum Reprod 1991; 6(1):5–7.
14. Edwards RG, Donahue RP, Baramki TA, Jones HW Jr. Preliminary attempts to fertilize human oocytes matured in vitro. Am J Obstet Gynecol 1966; 96:192–200.
15. Klein R, Palmer R. Technique de préelèvement des ovules humaines par ponction folliculaire sans calioscopie. Comptes Rendus Société de Biologie 1961; 155:1919–1921.
16. Lopata A, Johnston IWH, Hoult IJ, Spiers AI. Pregnancy following intrauterine implantation of an embryo obtained by fertilization of a preovulatory egg. Fertil Steril 1980; 33:117.
17. Acosta A, Swanson RJ, Ackerman SB, et al. Human Spermatozoa in Assisted Reproduction. Baltimore: Williams & Wilkins, 1991.
18. Menkveld R, Oettle EE, Kruger TF, et al. Atlas of Human Sperm Morphology. Baltimore: Williams & Wilkins, 1991.
19. Veeck L. Atlas of the Human Oocyte and Early Conceptus. Baltimore: Williams & Wilkins, 1986.
20. Veeck L. Atlas of the Human Oocyte and Early Conceptus. Volume 2. Baltimore: Williams & Wilkins, 1991.
21. Edwards RG, Steptoe PC, Purdy JM. Establishing full-term human pregnancies using cleaving embryos grown in vitro. Br J Obstet Gynaecol 1980; 87:737–768.
22. Jones GS. Corpus luteum composition and function. Fertil Steril 1990; 54(1):21–26.
23. Jones GS. Luteal phase defect: review of pathophysiology. Curr Opin Obstet Gynecol 1991; 3(5):641.

CHAPTER 50

Controlled Ovarian Hyperstimulation and Intrauterine Insemination

A. F. HANEY

Most couples seeking infertility care are not faced with sterility of one partner but have a relative lowering of their monthly likelihood of conception, or cycle fecundity. The most applicable term for this situation is *subfertility,* and spontaneous treatment-independent pregnancies certainly occur with predictable regularity, albeit at a low frequency.[1, 2] The generally accepted cycle fecundity of ostensibly normal couples approaches 15% to 20%, whereas the cycle fecundity of "infertile" couples, defined as those who do not conceive in 12 months without contraception, is as low as 1% to 3%.[3, 4] For all couples, the natural age-related decline in fertility also is present regardless of the cause of their reproductive problems. This "biologic clock" is a significant issue for many couples, paralleling the demographic trend toward later marriage and childbearing.[5, 6]

Many infertile couples do not have effective treatment options in the absence of a clear understanding of the mechanisms of their reproductive failure. Many share the following common features: (1) no mechanical distortion of the female pelvic viscera, regardless of the presence of some pelvic pathology, such as minimal endometriosis and filmy pelvic adhesions; (2) no obvious male factor as defined by a semen analysis within the range associated with normal fertility, despite the absence of proven paternity; and (3) ovulation as evidenced by a clinical marker of luteinization, such as elevated serum progesterone levels, biphasic basal body temperature charts, follicular collapse on ultrasonography, and in-phase secretory endometrial biopsies. Examples of frequently made diagnoses in this category of infertile couples include luteal phase defect, cervical factor, oligo-asthenospermia, luteinized unruptured follicle syndrome, and minimal endometriosis. For all practical purposes, these couples have idiopathic, or unexplained, infertility, at least based on the standard of having an unequivocally effective treatment option available. As a consequence, patients and their physicians have gradually focused their efforts on newer options such as assisted reproductive technologies, which may offer a nonspecific enhancement of cycle fecundity. The real issue is when these options can be used in a cost-effective manner.

The number of assisted reproductive technologies available as well as their use have dramatically increased since the birth of Louise Brown in 1978 from in vitro fertilization and embryo transfer (IVF-ET). A diverse array of technical approaches to assisted reproduction have rapidly proliferated despite the federal government absolving itself of a responsible role in basic and clinical research. As a consequence, clinical development of these newer treatments has been essentially experiential, supported by the patient's own discretionary income. These factors make assessing the relative efficiency of newer technologies difficult to characterize. In addition, without external funding of this clinical research, accurately quantifying the rate of success of these individual therapies will take an extended period to accomplish.[7] Controversy will continue to surround the atmosphere of entrepreneurism in which they are currently applied.[8, 9]

Controlled ovarian hyperstimulation combined with intrauterine insemination of capacitated sperm (COH-IUI) has recently been used to treat a subset of couples infertile in the absence of mechanical compromise of the pelvic viscera, in whom no other efficacious treatment options exist (Fig. 50–1).[10–12] This approach has four potential advantages over simply awaiting the infrequent spontaneous conception, that is, expectant management. These include (1) increasing the numbers of oocytes available for fertilization; (2) increasing the levels of follicular and luteal phase gonadal steroids; (3) optimizing the likelihood of gamete interaction with viable oocytes and sperm virtually guaranteed to be simultaneously present in the female genital tract; and (4) providing large numbers of capacitated sperm at the site of fertilization in the distal fallopian tubes. Many of these features are common to the more invasive oocyte retrieval technologies such as IVF-ET, gamete intrafallopian transfer (GIFT), and zygote intrafallopian transfer (ZIFT).[10] The major difference with COH-IUI is that the normal fallopian tubes can be antici-

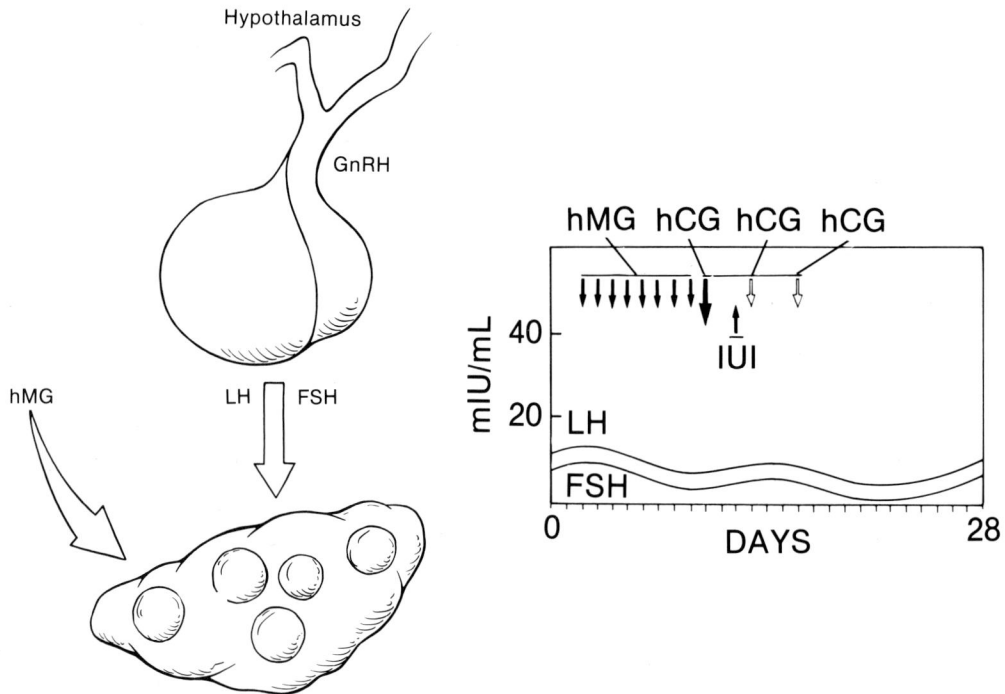

FIGURE 50–1. Schematic diagram of controlled ovarian hyperstimulation/intrauterine insemination (IUI). The administration of human menopausal gonadotropin (hMG) in the early follicular phase of a normally ovulatory woman augments the total amount of gonadotropin stimulation. This results in a larger cohort of follicles achieving dominant follicle status. The midcycle surge of luteinizing hormone (LH) is typically blocked by the higher levels of follicular regulatory peptides, released by the larger number of follicles. A surrogate LH surge is provided by an initial injection of human chorionic gonadotropin (hCG). The timing of the triggering dose of hCG may vary, depending on the rate of follicular development as measured by follicular diameter and the serum estradiol level. Approximately 36 hours after the hCG injection, multiple ovulations will occur and, as a consequence, a greater number of oocytes will be available for fertilization than under physiologic conditions. The IUI is timed to coincide with the appearance of oocytes in the ampullary portion of the fallopian tubes. Supplemental doses of hCG are administered early in the luteal phase to maintain the corpus luteum until the hCG from a pregnancy assumes this function in conceptive cycles. FSH, follicle-stimulating hormone; GnRH, gonadotropin-releasing hormone.

pated to function appropriately and no surgical procedures are required to collect oocytes. Although the physiology of oocyte capture by the fimbriated end of the fallopian tube is still largely unstudied, there are no known human diseases or syndromes that impair oocyte collection without alteration of the tubes' appearance with peritubular adhesions or obstruction.

WHO ARE APPROPRIATE CANDIDATES?

For many infertility diagnoses, there are no clearly efficacious treatments available based on the "gold standard" of adequately designed randomized clinical trials. There are various reasons for this state of affairs. Some treatments have not undergone rigorous documentation because their simplicity and low risk and the lack of significant expense have encouraged an empiric approach. Therapies in this category include progesterone vaginal suppositories and clomiphene citrate for the treatment of luteal phase defects as well as mucolytic agents to improve the quality of cervical mucus. Other complicated treatments lack randomized trials because they are complex, invasive, and expensive. These features, coupled with the federal government's lack of research support for clinical trials, require infertile couples to spend their own discretionary income to determine which of the newer therapeutic options will be most cost effective.

The initial suggestion that COH-IUI might be efficacious was based on the occasional pregnancies observed in women in IVF-ET programs when the oocyte retrieval was canceled because of poor follicular recruitment and IUI substituted in an effort to salvage some benefit from the cycle. This therapy quickly became a popular therapeutic option because of the relatively lower cost, the avoidance of oocyte retrieval and laparoscopy, and a cycle fecundity comparable with the other assisted reproductive technologies.[10–12] COH-IUI represents a therapy applicable to a wide variety of infertility diagnoses with no significant mechanical distortion of the pelvic viscera (Table 50–1). In addition, when other factors associated with low fecundity are present but are deemed insufficient to account for the failure to conceive, such as minimal adnexal adhesions and minimal endometriosis, these couples will also be candidates for COH-IUI.

TABLE 50–1. Diagnostic Clinical Categories of Infertility Considered as Candidates for COH-IUI

Cervical factor infertility	Minimal endometriosis
Oligo-asthenospermia	Uncharacterized immunologic infertility
Luteal phase defect	"Idiopathic" or "unexplained" infertility
Luteinized unruptured follicles	

COH-IUI, controlled ovarian hyperstimulation combined with intrauterine insemination of capacitated sperm.

PROPOSED MECHANISMS OF ENHANCED FERTILITY WITH COH-IUI

In couples with long-standing infertility in the absence of mechanical distortion of the pelvic viscera, the cause of their reproductive failure often remains speculative. Similarly, the mechanism of the enhanced cycle fecundity with COH-IUI in any individual couple remains uncertain. Current interest focuses on the functional characteristics of sperm, the quality of cervical mucus, and the subtle defects in ovulation. These possibilities cannot be readily separated by the currently available diagnostic tests, and COH-IUI would be anticipated to improve all three simultaneously. Other, as yet undefined, fertility-lowering factors may also be present and account for the failure of COH-IUI to be successful in all couples in this category.

The major reduction in sperm density physiologically occurs with the passage of sperm from the vaginal pool through the cervix and into the uterus.[13] Normally, the liquid portion of the ejaculate (seminal fluid) remains in the vagina after coitus, with entry into the uterus being prevented by the viscosity of the cervical mucus. Only the most mobile sperm enter the cervix. Following coitus, several hundred million sperm are typically deposited in the vagina, but only 0.1% of these sperm are present in the cervix in the initial hour after vaginal deposition.

The few sperm that traverse the cervix appear in the oviducts in less than 5 minutes after vaginal insemination.[14] It has been estimated that only 1 in 14 million motile sperm deposited in the vagina ever reaches the site of fertilization, the ampullary portion of the fallopian tube.[14] The number of sperm reaching the upper portion of the female genital tract is thus likely to be proportional to the total number deposited in the vagina. It is logical to consider that any procedure, such as IUI, that facilitates sperm entry into the female genital tract will have a beneficial effect on the number of sperm in the distal fallopian tube and, hence, the likelihood of fertilization. This is particularly true when abnormally low numbers of motile sperm are present in the ejaculate, such as in oligo-asthenospermia. The monitoring used in COH allows optimal timing of the insemination of large numbers of capacitated sperm, potentially compensating for an unrecognized male factor.

There seems little doubt that the cervical mucus serves a physiologic function by facilitating the entry and providing a reservoir for sperm in the female genital tract. However, there is no consensus on a valid method for detection of fertility problems involving cervical mucus factors. As a consequence, the diagnosis of cervical factor infertility remains one of the most contentious of the current fertility diagnoses. The postcoital test has been the traditional method of identifying a putative cervical factor. Women with persistently low numbers of motile sperm identified in qualitatively and quantitatively normal cervical mucus have been considered to have a mucus problem. IUI bypasses the cervical mucus entirely and would presumably eliminate this factor as a cause of infertility. Additionally, it can be anticipated that when human menopausal gonadotropin (hMG) is employed for COH, the cervical mucus production would be optimal, because the serum levels of estradiol will be substantially higher because of the larger number of mature follicles developed.

Many women conceiving with COH-IUI may have unrecognized ovulatory or luteal dysfunction. These problems would be corrected with COH analogous to women with hypogonadotropic hypogonadism in whom the efficacy of hMG in inducing ovulation and establishing pregnancies is excellent. Similar to the higher follicular phase levels of estradiol, the luteal phase progesterone levels are elevated substantially higher than those produced by a single corpus luteum after the hMG therapy. The experience has been similar when hMG has been used for COH in normally ovulating women in IVF-ET and GIFT. These features would suggest that any unrecognized ovulatory or luteal dysfunction would be overridden by COH.

For couples with either idiopathic infertility or minimal endometriosis, there is no well-defined pathophysiologic mechanism for their infertility.[15] As a consequence, the basis by which COH-IUI enhances the cycle fecundity in these couples should be considered nonspecific. In these couples COH-IUI may improve the cycle fecundity only in proportion to the increase in the number of mature oocytes released and the capacitated sperm inseminated. Similarly, infertile women in the older reproductive age group (older than 35 years of age) may have a low cycle fecundity entirely on the basis of the natural age-related decline in fertility.[16] As their cycle fecundity is not zero but simply reduced (perhaps on the basis of oocyte quality), increasing the numbers of oocytes available for fertilization with COH-IUI over a short period should increase the probabilities of a viable conception. Because the fecundity of these "older" women is rapidly declining, COH-IUI may represent their most cost-effective option for establishing a pregnancy.

INTRAUTERINE INSEMINATION

The introduction of semen or one of its constituents into the uterine cavity has been used in attempts to treat infertility for more than 100 years.[17–21] The use of IUI reduces the normal attrition of sperm as they ascend through the female genital tract and thus guarantees large numbers of capacitated sperm at the site of fertilization in the distal ampulla of the fallopian tube. This is similar to what is accomplished in IVF-ET and GIFT, when higher sperm densities are used during the oocyte incubation (IVF) or placed retrograde in the fallopian tube (GIFT). However, after IUI, the sperm are physiologically capacitated by their passage through the genital tract.

IUI is a distinctly nonphysiologic process because the normal entry of sperm into the female genital tract involves sperm penetration through the cervical mucus. The filtering effect of cervical mucus serves to reduce the numbers of sperm, selecting only the fraction with the highest motility, and initiates capacitation. In earlier studies the use of the raw ejaculate was abandoned because of problems of severe uterine contractions and the risk of infection.[18] Subsequently, in attempts to avoid these problems, reduction in inseminate volume, use of only a portion of the split ejaculate, and dilution and freezing the semen with egg-yolk buffer prior to insemination were advocated. With the advent of IVF-ET, methods to effectively separate the sperm from the liquid portion of the ejaculate while monitoring viability became available,[22] enabling satisfactory performance of IUI.[23]

The impact of IUI alone in enhancing cycle fecundity of couples with a significant male factor remains unsettled.[24, 25] In trials of couples with spontaneous ovulatory cycles with IUI (timed by the detection of endogenous luteinizing hormone [LH] surges) using a control group of similarly timed coitus, improved pregnancy rates in couples with oligospermia were noted.[26, 27] Another nonrandomized trial demonstrated an improved pregnancy rate as well.[28] However, other studies, both randomized[29, 30] and nonrandomized,[22, 23, 31–37] did not find improved fecundity; therefore, there is a lack of confidence in the use of IUI alone in couples when the only identifiable infertility factor is oligo-asthenospermia.[24, 25]

Theoretically, this subset of couples with oligo-asthenospermia as their only infertility factor may be appropriate candidates for a trial of IUI. Whether the use of additional tests of sperm function (such as computerized sperm motion analysis, interspecies sperm penetration assays, and anti-sperm antibodies) will help select appropriate candidate couples for IUI is also unknown. A study using the zona-free hamster egg penetration assay in an attempt to differentiate 16 normal men from 19 with poor oocyte penetration yielded a cycle fecundity of 0.13 in the normal men and only 0.02 in those with abnormal egg penetration tests.[38] Further data are required before this or other screening tests are recommended for accurate predictions of the likelihood of success with IUI in couples whose only identifiable factor is oligo-asthenospermia.

SPERM PREPARATION FOR INTRAUTERINE INSEMINATION

Semen should be collected by masturbation after a minimum of 36 hours of ejaculatory continence and delivered to the andrology laboratory within 30 minutes of collection. The sample should be collected in a sterile glass or plastic container and maintained at room temperature. After liquefaction (typically 25 to 30 minutes), the semen is diluted in an equal volume of physiologic medium. The diluted sperm preparation is centrifuged at 150g for 10 minutes, the supernatant discarded, the pellet resuspended in 2 mL of medium and the centrifugation step repeated. The loose pellet is then suspended in 0.2 to 0.4 mL of medium for insemination. Immediate IUI is optimal, but if a delay is anticipated, the sample should be kept in an incubator in a humidified atmosphere of 5% carbon dioxide in air at 37°C until the actual insemination. An aliquot should be removed for assessing the sperm density and motility and the presence of white blood cells as well as to evaluate the quantity and quality (e.g., motility) of the sperm inseminated.[10, 39]

An alternate approach to sperm preparation is to overlay the washed sperm pellet with fresh physiologic medium and incubate this for 1 or 2 hours under standard culture conditions. This allows the highly motile fraction to "swim up" into the supernatant, and this can be used for the insemination.[26, 27, 37, 40, 41] Similarly, centrifugation through a discontinuous Percoll gradient[41–43] or an albumin column[31, 44] can be performed and this fraction used for insemination. No differences could be discerned in a randomized trial comparing the swimup separation with the discontinuous Percoll gradient method in women undergoing COH-IUI.[41] Overall, no differences in pregnancy rates have been attributed to these

different sperm preparation methods, but some clinicians prefer the Percoll technique because it yields a greater number of motile sperm and reduces the amount of debris present in the inseminate.

The optimal medium for sperm separation has not emerged, but ideally it should allow survival of the maximum number of morphologically normal motile sperm. A variety of media have been used, and they should be tested individually under the conditions in which they are to be used to ensure optimal results. Ham's F-10 is most commonly used, but other media successfully employed for this purpose include BWW, Earle's, and Dulbecco's modified essential media, and even plain phosphate-buffered saline. The addition of some protein to the medium is usually preferred to maintain a high level of sperm motility, and these sperm preparations are typically supplemented with antibiotics such as penicillin and streptomycin.

The protein source can vary from the recipient or her partner's serum to commercially available human serum albumin to fetal cord serum. All serum supplements should be heat inactivated before use (typically heated to 60°C for 30 to 60 minutes). Because a number of diseases can be transmitted by serum, when autologous serum is not used for media supplementation, steps to minimize the infectious risk should be taken comparable with those required for blood transfusion (such as screening for human immunodeficiency virus and hepatitis). The medium should be demonstrated to support sperm survival for extended periods under culture conditions (e.g., hours), fertilization and early embryo growth in vitro. Furthermore, the medium should not cause uterine contractions. The media used for fertilization in IVF-ET programs would seem ideal for this purpose.

TIMING OF INSEMINATION

There is no substantive evidence that, in a normal couple with an appropriate frequency of coitus, timing intercourse to coincide with ovulation has any significant impact on the likelihood of pregnancy in that cycle. The length of time sperm survive in the female genital tract is dependent on the phase of the menstrual cycle. In the late-follicular phase with a predominantly estrogenic milieu, it can be anticipated that the female genital tract will harbor motile sperm for 2 to 5 days. As a consequence, coital timing is not a significant issue in the probability of conception for most couples. IUI, however, is a nonphysiologic means of sperm entry, and the optimal timing and number of IUI have not been determined.

Coitus should continue at whatever frequency is typical for the couple during the hMG stimulation, including the evening of the human chorionic gonadotropin (hCG) release, to ensure that, if a premature LH surge occurs, sperm will be present in the female genital tract in the periovulatory interval.

No data have been systematically collected on the survival characteristics of sperm at various levels in the female genital tract after IUI. However, IUI increases the percentage of women with sperm in the peritoneal fluid when the insemination occurred 2 hours prior to laparoscopy.[45] It is likely that the length of sperm survival in the genital tract is altered by bypassing the cervical reservoir, but the specific survival time in the female genital tract after IUI remains to be characterized. Judging from the experience with IVF-ET, the ideal timing for IUI should be 36 to 40 hours after the ovulating dose of hCG, ensuring that sperm and oocytes are present simultaneously in the distal fallopian tubes. It is not likely that sperm will survive if they pass on through the fallopian tubes into the peritoneal cavity, because they are immobilized in the peritoneal fluid[46–48] and phagocytized by peritoneal macrophages.[49]

Approximately 20% of women undergoing COH will initiate an LH surge prior to the triggering dose of hCG and thus have ovulations occur prior to the IUI. Because the typical COH-IUI cycle does not use a gonadotropin hormone–releasing hormone (GnRH) agonist to prevent an endogenous LH surge, earlier and multiple inseminations have been advocated to maximize the cycle fecundity. In contrast with IVF-ET, the patient's own fallopian tubes should collect the oocytes, and sperm viability is generally thought to last at least 24 hours, so multiple inseminations are not likely to be a critical issue. The IUI can be performed 24 hours after the hCG trigger if there is any suggestion that a premature LH surge has occurred based on a slowing of the rate of rise of estradiol levels in serum.

Typically, a single insemination is recommended approximately 36 hours after the hCG dose that initiates ovulation. A single randomized study using two inseminations at 24 and 48 hours after the ovulating dose of hCG compared with a single insemination 36 hours after the hCG found a higher cycle fecundity with multiple inseminations per cycle.[50] More data are required to demonstrate a clinically significant difference between coitus at the time of the triggering dose of hCG and a single insemination at 36 hours versus two inseminations.

INTRAUTERINE INSEMINATION TECHNIQUE

Depending on operator preference, the IUI can be performed with any number of narrow-gauge catheters with different diameters, lengths, and degrees of rigidity. A 5 Fr vessel catheter or a Tomcat catheter, comparable with those used for ET, will usually prove satisfactory. The patient is placed in the dorsal lithotomy position, a standard bivalve speculum is inserted, and the cervix is visualized. An antiseptic cleansing of the cervix may be used, but no data are available to indicate whether this maneuver alters the low rate of infection after IUI.

The insemination volume is limited by the intrinsic volume of the uterine cavity and, typically, 0.2 to 0.4 mL is used. In preparation for IUI the sperm concentrate is drawn into the catheter. The catheter is inserted through the cervix with the media delivered into the uterine corpus. A tenaculum is occasionally required when a narrow or circuitous endocervical canal is encountered. Rarely, a paracervical block is necessary, which may indicate pathologic cervical stenosis. Knowing the position of the uterus (flexion and version) beforehand is essential for an easy insemination. The insemination should be done slowly while the catheter is rotated slowly and withdrawn to minimize the endometrial trauma and bleeding that may reduce sperm viability. A small amount of the sperm concentrate may reflux through the cervix because of the relatively small volume of the endometrial cavity. Reflux does

not seem to alter the likelihood of conception and should not be considered as a reason for failure of a cycle of COH-IUI.

With experience, the IUI can be accomplished with minimal discomfort and is usually described by the patient as comparable with the sensation of undergoing a Pap smear. If perceptible cramping follows the insemination, a reevaluation of the sperm separation technique should be made as previously noted. Alternatively, the insemination technique itself may cause uterine contractions, particularly when the cervix is narrow and the procedure is difficult.

In the absence of a male factor, an improvement in cycle fecundity with the addition of IUI to COH has not been unequivocally established, but several studies suggest this may be true.[51–53] It is likely that a subset of couples will derive a benefit, whereas in the remainder, the mechanism of enhanced fertility is independent of the IUI. Currently, there is no method available to reliably identify the couples that will benefit from the addition of IUI. Because generally IUI is neither technically difficult nor painful, carries a low risk, and is relatively inexpensive, there has been little incentive for couples to participate in randomized trials of COH in which they might not undergo IUI. When large controlled clinical trials in well-defined clinical groups comparing COH with and without IUI are performed, the value of the IUI itself can be quantified. Only then will the optimal role for IUI and the ideal subset of infertile couples to receive this therapy be identified.

RISKS OF INTRAUTERINE INSEMINATION

Insemination of fresh semen into the endometrial cavity has several potentially serious complications.[54] The seminal plasma contains prostaglandins that have potent uterine contractile properties, limiting the volume of freshly ejaculated semen that can be used for IUI. "Washing" semen, that is, separating the liquid from the cellular components, allows placement of only the sperm suspended in nonirritating medium directly into the uterus, avoiding the prostaglandins in the semen.[23]

Because freshly ejaculated semen is not sterile, pelvic infection is a constant concern,[37, 54–57] particularly because asymptomatic prostatitis with varying degrees of pyospermia is common. It is prudent to view a drop of the separated sperm sample microscopically before every IUI to exclude the presence of significant numbers of round cells. If significant numbers of round cells are present, the sample should not be used for IUI. Typically, if an infection is present in the male genital tract, there are numerous round cells (leukocytes) present per high power field. Alternatively, the couple should be encouraged to have coitus to allow the cervical mucus to filter out the seminal microbial flora but still permit entry of the highly motile sperm into the female genital tract.

Studies in which culture of the sperm suspension after separation from the freshly ejaculated semen was performed revealed a marked reduction in the number of positive cultures, and these findings probably mitigate against infections. This is true for virtually all the separation techniques.[58–60] Studies performed to evaluate the impact of the different sperm separation techniques on the number of bacteria isolated from the final sperm suspension suggest that the swimup method is superior to the traditional washing technique. The use of a double-column discontinuous Percoll gradient reduces the number and spectrum of bacteria isolated, particularly the organisms found on the skin and the urethra. However, *Escherichia coli*, which represent common genital tract pathogens, was not completely eliminated by this method.[60]

Despite these precautions, pelvic infections may rarely occur after IUI. It is likely that many of these infections represent the activation of quiescent genital infections rather than new infections. The infection rate after IUI is likely comparable with the low rate of pelvic infection after endometrial biopsy or hysterosalpingography (lower than 1 in 500 procedures). The reason for the low rate of infection with this technique remains to be determined, but clearly little risk is encountered with IUI. Preparing the sperm suspension by the traditional washing technique did not eliminate the colonization of the peritoneal fluid by micro-organisms 2 to 4 hours after IUI.[61] Furthermore, the organisms encountered correlated with those cultured from the semen rather than those in the vagina, suggesting the source of contamination was the sperm suspension rather than contamination by the technique of insemination. Based on these data, some centers use prophylactic antibiotics around the time of the IUI (tetracycline, 250 mg, four times a day for 4 days or doxycycline, 100 mg, two times a day for 2 days), despite the absence of available data supporting the use of antibiotics in this setting.[30, 62] There is a more general willingness to use them in high-risk patients, that is, those with a history of pelvic inflammatory disease. Because of the extremely low rate of infection with IUI,[11] it probably will not be possible to evaluate the effectiveness of these antibiotic regimens until large numbers of patients are treated in controlled trials.

The female reproductive tract is not an immunologically protected site, and it is theoretically possible that the increased numbers of sperm entering with IUI may represent a large enough antigenic burden to generate an immune response that is not encountered with the smaller numbers of sperm entering after natural coitus. As a consequence, it has been a matter of interest to determine the incidence of antisperm antibodies before and after IUI. A study reported that fewer than 5% of women had antibodies after IUI using relatively imprecise tests of sperm agglutination and immobilization as well as the immunobead assay.[63] In another study, antisperm antibodies were detected with no higher frequency in women after COH when IUI was added to the regimen.[64] It has been suggested that women undergoing IUI may already have low levels of antisperm antibodies before treatment that may be increased by the insemination. Using the sperm agglutination test, other investigators found that the titer dilutions increased in 5 women after IUI; however, in the 15 women with negative agglutination assays initially, none were positive following the inseminations.[65] The clinical significance of any increase in the antisperm antibody titer is unclear, and, indeed, the issue of immune infertility remains one of the most controversial in all of reproductive medicine.

CONTROLLED OVARIAN HYPERSTIMULATION

The primary cycle fecundity–enhancing effect of COH is likely due to the increase in the number of oocytes released in a given cycle. The ovulation induction regimens suggested for use have included clomiphene citrate, hMG-hCG, clomiphene citrate and hMG-hCG, and hMG-hCG after pretreatment with a GnRH agonist.[11] No well-designed comparative trials have been performed to determine if one regimen is superior to another. Anecdotal evidence, coupled with the lower cycle fecundity observed with clomiphene citrate–induced ovulations in women with polycystic ovary syndrome, suggests that this method of COH, although less costly, yields a somewhat lower cycle fecundity than when the COH is induced with hMG. This is not surprising based on the potentially adverse effect of clomiphene citrate on the estrogen-responsive tissues in the genital tract, such as the cervical mucus, endometrium, and fallopian tubes. Finding the optimal cost-effective approach for COH that maximizes the cycle fecundity with acceptable risks for the different subsets of the infertile population is the next challenge in this area.

Luteal support is generally used, but without the benefit of controlled clinical trials demonstrating an improvement in the pregnancy rate. Supplemental hCG injections are most frequently used (2500 IU) the third and sixth days after the ovulating dose of hCG. Alternatively, progesterone injections and vaginal suppositories have also been used. Mid-luteal serum progesterone levels in hMG-hCG–stimulated cycles are well above those observed in natural cycles. Paradoxically, these women frequently have a shortened luteal phase, and this is returned to the usual 14 days with luteal support. This supplement usually does not prolong the luteal phase beyond 14 or 15 days in the absence of a pregnancy. Whether the conception rate is improved with luteal support, however, remains a controversial issue and requires a large clinical trial for resolution.

For standard COH-IUI, a hMG-hCG regimen comparable with that used for IVF-ET is commonly used (Table 50–2). The typical GnRH agonist pretreatment is not necessary as the timing of the IUI is not as critical as oocyte retrieval and a premature LH surge has not been to shown to decrease the pregnancy rate. In a randomized trial using hMG-hCG for the COH with and without pretreatment with GnRH agonist, no differences in the clinical pregnancy rates or the degree of stimulation were noted.[66] The hMG requirement was predictably increased with the use of a GnRH, and unless convinc-

---

TABLE 50–2. Typical Human Menopausal Gonadotropin Stimulation Protocol for COH-IUI

Protocol	Day of Cycle														
	1	2	3	4	5	6	7	8	9	10	11	12	13	14	15
hMG*	−	+	+	+	+	+	+	+	−	−	−	−	−	−	−
Monitoring†	−	−	−	−	−	−	+	+	+	−	−	−	−	−	−
hCG‡	−	−	−	−	−	−	−	−	^	−	−	^	−	−	^
IUI§	−	−	−	−	−	−	−	−	−	−	−	*	−	−	−

*Dosage depends on the age and weight of the patient.
†Vaginal ultrasonography and serum estradiol determination.
‡5000–10,000 IU intramuscularly as the surrogate LH surge when adequate follicular size is attained and 2500 IU intramuscularly on days 3 and 6 after the initial dose of hCG.
§Coitus should be encouraged during hMG administration injection. A single IUI is performed 36–40 h after the initial hCG injection.
COH-IUI, controlled ovarian hyperstimulation combined with intrauterine insemination of capacitated sperm; hMG, human menopausal gonadotropin; hCG, human chorionic gonadotropin; LH, luteinizing hormone.

ing data in a larger randomized study are forthcoming, there appears to be no advantage of the addition of GnRH agonist to the COH regimen. Alternatively, clomiphene citrate–hMG may offer some advantage in selected couples, reducing the dose of hMG required to achieve optimal stimulation. Clomiphene citrate stimulates an early follicular rise in the endogenous gonadotropins, whereas hMG provides an increase in exogenous gonadotropins later in the stimulation course. The relatively high late follicular phase estradiol levels may be sufficient to overcome any competitive antagonism attributable to the clomiphene citrate.

Compared with IVF-ET, it is advisable to lower the maximum number of dominant preovulatory follicles acceptable for COH-IUI because when the follicles are not going to be aspirated, the risk of a clinically significant hyperstimulation syndrome may be higher. The potential for excessive follicular recruitment is significant with any regimen, even clomiphene citrate alone, and the couple must accept an inherent risk associated with any COH. No single regimen has been uniformly found superior to another. Physicians should simply choose the ovulation induction regimen with which they have the most experience and individualize the dosage for each patient, being prepared to cancel cycles when unanticipated excessive follicular recruitment occurs.

RISKS OF CONTROLLED OVARIAN HYPERSTIMULATION

COH is not without its potential hazards; the most obvious ones are multiple gestation and severe ovarian hyperstimulation. These risks have also been reported with hMG-induced COH used in other types of assisted reproductive technologies.[67] These problems are not entirely avoidable because the greater the degree of follicular stimulation, the greater the likelihood of pregnancy and the higher the incidence of complications. Accordingly, a balance must be struck between the risks and the benefits for every patient in every cycle. There remain unexplained cycle-to-cycle and patient-to-patient variations in response to COH that must be considered. Only with substantial experience will the clinician be able to adequately counsel the couple regarding what constitutes appropriate stimulation for the maximum cycle fecundity yet represents an acceptable level of risk. Fully informed couples who have a good therapeutic relationship with their physicians will be better able to tolerate a cancellation of a COH cycle when the risks are prohibitive.

As most of the couples interested in this treatment have either not had children or have few, a twin gestation is often viewed as a more desirable outcome than a singleton pregnancy and sometimes even a triplet pregnancy does not evoke a negative response. By contrast, quadruplet pregnancies and beyond[68] should be avoided because they represent a major medical hazard for the mother, as well as a high rate of extremely premature deliveries with all the potential sequelae.[69]

Although both multiple gestation and the hyperstimulation syndrome are related to the degree of follicular recruitment, there appears to be a dichotomy of these risks with the age of the female partner. The endocrinology of follicular development, given a fixed number of follicles, appears independent of maternal age, whereas the likelihood of fertilization and embryo survival is inversely related to the age of the woman. As a consequence, these two inherent risks are not parallel and should be considered separately for each patient. A lower magnitude of both risks can be achieved with careful monitoring of the rise in the serum estradiol level and the number and size of ovarian follicles. There is no specific level of estradiol or number of large preovulatory and small follicles that can guarantee these adverse outcomes will not occur, regardless of maternal age.[70]

The multiple gestation risk is difficult to accurately predict because these patients have been repetitively ovulating for many years without conception. However, when pregnancy does occur, the risk of multiple gestation has been reported to range between 5% and 27%,[11, 71, 72] roughly comparable with those reported for the other assisted reproductive technologies.[73] Although this is undoubtedly related to the number of follicles recruited, the relationship is complex and likely involves the mechanism of infertility, the age of the woman, and other unidentified factors affecting fertilization and embryo development. When multiple pregnancy occurs, selective fetal reduction,[74] although not a palatable option for some couples, represents an alternative chosen by many, given the perinatal morbidity and mortality risks associated with premature deliveries common with multiple gestations. There exists no fail-safe method to use COH-IUI without some risk of triplet pregnancy and beyond, and couples should not undergo COH-IUI unless they are prepared to deal with these possible outcomes.

Some degree of ovarian hyperstimulation is inevitable because multiple corpora lutea will be present—hyperstimulation is an exaggeration of the physiologic ovarian enlargement associated with normal pregnancy. However, there are serious maternal complications with the full-blown hyperstimulation syndrome, including stroke, renal failure, cardiopulmonary compromise, and even death.[75] The severe form of hyperstimulation is rare in women undergoing COH-IUI.[11] This is likely due to the fact that the patients are spontaneously ovulatory, and this limits the number of recruitable follicles when exogenous gonadotropins are administered in the follicular phase. At this point in the cycle, the normal processes of follicular recruitment and selection have already begun, and the cohort of small follicles that are candidates to become the dominant follicle are already reduced somewhat. Anovulatory women pose a much greater risk for hyperstimulation, particularly those with estrogenized anovulation, that is, polycystic ovary syndrome. Careful documentation of the woman's ovulatory status thus becomes of paramount importance prior to initiation of the COH. If, despite the physician's best efforts, severe hyperstimulation syndrome occurs, it should be treated in a similar fashion as with anovulatory patients undergoing hMG therapy for ovulation induction.

OUTCOMES OF PREGNANCIES AFTER COH-IUI

The outcomes of pregnancy resulting from a cycle of COH-IUI appear to be comparable with those observed with other forms of infertility therapy (Table 50–3).[11] On initial inspection, there appears to be a high rate of spontaneous first-trimester pregnancy loss. However, when one takes into consideration the higher average maternal age of the infertile

TABLE 50–3. Outcome of Pregnancies Established by COH-IUI at Duke University Medical Center[11]

Pregnancy Outcome	Pregnancy Outcome / Total No. (%) of Pregnancies
Chemical pregnancy	10/112 (9)
Spontaneous abortion	12/112 (11)
Ectopic pregnancy	10/112 (9)
Delivery of viable infants	81/112 (81)
Multiple gestations (102 viable pregnancies)	
Single	76/102 (74)
Twins	19/102 (19)
Triplets	5/102 (5)
Quadruplets	2/102 (2)

COH-IUI, Controlled ovarian hyperstimulation combined with intrauterine insemination of capacitated sperm.

population undergoing this therapy and the high degree of early pregnancy detection, the spontaneous abortion rate does not appear to be significantly elevated over what would be anticipated with other infertility therapies. Similarly, the relatively high frequency of ectopic pregnancies may appear to be excessive. This may be true when the incidence of ectopic pregnancy is compared with the rate experienced by normally fertile women, but relatively high rates of ectopic pregnancy are the rule for infertile couples, probably secondary to subtle degrees of asymptomatic tubal disease, such as previous mild salpingitis. Whether there is any increased risk for ectopic pregnancy associated with the higher level of gonadal steroids or distortion of the fallopian tubes by the large ovaries remains uncertain. It is advisable to attempt early documentation of the location of any pregnancy by vaginal-probe ultrasonography and remain aware that, with the multiple ovulations associated with COH-IUI, heterotopic pregnancy occurs more frequently.

ANTICIPATED RESULTS OF COH-IUI

Cycle fecundity approaching that of normally fertile couples has been observed in many subsets of the infertile population treated with COH-IUI (Table 50–4).[11, 53] The underlying assumption is that any pregnancy that occurs in a treated cycle is treatment dependent. Although the spontaneous pregnancy rate is quite low in this population, the cycle fecundity without treatment is not zero.[1–4] Therefore, some of the apparent COH-IUI "successes," that is, conceptions during a cycle of COH-IUI, are undoubtedly treatment independent. However, it is unlikely that treatment-independent pregnancies contribute more that 1% to the cycle fecundity given the fact that the couples have experienced long intervals of infertility (typically longer than 36 months) and the average age of the female partner is in the mid-thirties in most series, and considering the failure of prior therapies. The term *treatment associated* includes both the spontaneous and treatment-dependent conceptions in these cycles. Whether pregnancies in cycles between COH treatment cycles are more frequent remains speculative, but the high levels of estradiol associated with hMG may affect the cohort of follicles destined for development in subsequent cycles. Only with an adequately large clinical trial including an untreated control group will the exact number of treatment-

dependent conceptions be reliably quantified for a specific population of infertile couples.

The reported success rates with COH-IUI vary significantly between different centers. These disparate findings are likely the result of several factors, including patient selection biases inherent at the individual centers, even when the couples have been carefully evaluated. The degree of COH also likely influences the outcome. The extent of COH used depends on the risks of hyperstimulation and multiple pregnancy the couple is willing to accept. Data are rapidly accumulating for individual clinical diagnoses, and the protocols used for COH are becoming more standardized. The anticipated results in experienced hands can be generally classified according to clinical categories (see Tables 50–1 and 50–4).

Male Factor Infertility

One of the most frequently identified, if imprecise, categories selected for COH-IUI is male factor infertility. The reported results of COH-IUI in the treatment of male factor infertility are presented in Table 50–5. The varying definitions of what constitutes a significant male factor complicates comparison of the different studies. These data do not address the efficacy of IUI by itself, because a timed coital control group was not included for comparative purposes. Similarly, as many of the couples undergoing hMG for COH had previously failed to conceive with clomiphene citrate with or without IUI, these are not comparable study populations. The overall fecundity of 0.09 in the hMG group is quite respectable, considering the length of the infertility and the variably defined male factor infertility in this heterogeneous population of infertile couples.

Idiopathic Infertility

Infertility in the absence of clear-cut anatomic or functional abnormalities has been termed *idiopathic* or *unexplained*. Approximately 10% to 20% of couples seeking infertility care have been given this diagnosis. Undoubtedly, these couples are not of normal fertility and have one or more

TABLE 50–4. Therapeutic Success of COH-IUI by Diagnostic Category[11, 53]

Diagnostic Category	No. of Pregnancies/ No. of Cycles	Cycle Fecundity
Male factor[11]	13/85	0.15
Adnexal adhesions[11]	13/131	0.10
Endometriosis[11, 53]	68/498	0.14
Minimal[11, 53]	45/280	0.16
Mild[11, 53]	14/143	0.10
Moderate[11]	9/51	0.18
Severe[11]	0/14	—
Leiomyomata uteri[11]	5/72	0.07
Idiopathic[11, 53]	21/133	0.16
Cervical factor[11, 53]	9/37	0.24
Other[11]	6/46	0.13
Total	135/1002	0.13

COH-IUI, controlled ovarian hyperstimulation combined with intrauterine insemination of capacitated sperm.

TABLE 50–5. Reported Results of COH-IUI in Male Factor Infertility

	No. of Patients	No. of Pregnancies/ No. of Cycles	Cycle Fecundity
Clomiphene Citrate Cycles			
Blumenfeld et al[76]	13	5/43	0.12
Bolton et al[77]	29	5/158	0.03
Hewitt et al[78]	36	3/64	0.05
Total	78	13/265	0.05
hMG Cycles			
Blumenfeld et al[76]	8	4/32	0.13
Cruz et al[79]	48	7/96	0.07
Horvath et al[55]	39	6/175	0.07
Sher et al[39]	4	1/4	0.25
Sunde et al[80]	40	8/56	0.14
Dodson and Haney[11]	39	13/85	0.15
Chaffkin et al[51]	—	17/111	0.15
Total	—	56/559	0.10

COH-IUI, controlled ovarian hyperstimulation combined with intrauterine insemination of capacitated sperm; hMG, human menopausal gonadotropin.

unidentified fecundity-lowering factors. There is a significant spontaneous "cure" rate of unexplained infertility, with as many as 60% of couples conceiving within 2 years of completing their infertility investigation.[1,2,81] However, the confounding impact of the age-related fertility decline undoubtedly lowers the outlook for many couples with long-term infertility, motivating them to seek therapeutic options beyond expectant management. Although couples with unexplained infertility are relatively simple to categorize diagnostically, they likely represent a heterogeneous collection of reproductive problems and, hence, no single therapy would be expected to be uniformly effective. COH-IUI has been used extensively in this group of patients, and the treatment-associated cycle fecundity appears to be optimal in this clinical population, approaching that of normal fertile couples (Table 50–6).

Endometriosis

The pathophysiologic mechanisms of the infertility associated with endometriosis remain to be established.[86] Recent investigations have centered on alterations in tubal function, macrophage and natural killer cell function, an inadequate luteal phase, and the unruptured luteinized follicle syndrome. In women with endometriosis, no single mechanism has been confirmed to be responsible for the failure to conceive in the absence of mechanical compromise of the pelvic viscera. These couples can essentially be considered to have idiopathic infertility, because no therapy directed toward the ectopic implants, such as surgical destruction and excision and medical suppression, has been shown to improve fecundity.[15] Many authors have not separated the patients sufficiently by diagnostic category to be able to isolate endome-

TABLE 50–6. Reported Results of COH-IUI in Idiopathic Infertility

	No. of Patients	No. of Pregnancies per No. of Cycles	Cycle Fecundity
Clomiphene Citrate Cycles			
Blumenfeld et al[76]	5	4/10	0.40
Hewitt et al[78]	9	1/12	0.08
Total	14	5/22	0.23
hMG Cycles			
Blumenfeld et al[76]	3	2/7	0.29
Serhal et al[82]	15	6/19	0.32
Dickey et al[83]	5	2/5	0.40
Sher et al[39]	5	2/5	0.40
Sunde et al[80]	11	1/15	0.07
Dodson et al[11]	57	17/116	0.15
Hurst et al[53]	—	4/17	0.24
Chaffkin et al[51]	—	15/46	0.33
Total	—	49/230	0.21
hMG Cycles Without IUI			
Welner et al[84]	97	12/388	0.03
Wang and Gemzell[85]	6	3/13	0.03
Chaffkin et al[51]	—	1/18	0.05
Hurst et al[53]	—	4/7	0.29
Total	—	16/419	0.04

COH-IUI, controlled ovarian hyperstimulation combined with intrauterine insemination of capacitated sperm; hMG, human menopausal gonadotropin.

triosis and thereby evaluate the effect of COH-IUI in this category. When this was done in a single large study, the cycle fecundity was virtually identical to that observed with unexplained infertility (see Table 50–4).

Cervical Factor Infertility

IUI may optimally use the placement of sperm in situations when a cervical factor is thought to be present regardless of whether the cause of the problem is immunologic, the intrinsic quality of the cervical mucus, or the presence of endocervicitis. In women characterized simply as having cervical factor infertility, the use of IUI alone has not consistently improved cycle fecundity.

In nonrandomized clinical series, the cycle fecundity has been reported as increased, slightly improved, or poor with IUI alone.[23, 28, 33, 87–90] In a study with a crossover design comparing natural coitus with IUI, no pregnancies were observed with coitus, whereas a cycle fecundity of 0.16 was observed with IUI.[29, 30] In a single nonrandomized trial, IUI with COH appeared to be superior to IUI alone in women with a purported cervical factor.[37] A significant problem with all these studies is the lack of a uniformly accepted standard definition of cervical factor infertility (including the detection of antisperm antibodies).

There remains a considerable range of opinion considering the number of sperm in cervical mucus that are predictive of fertility. Most available studies do not contain appropriate control groups, so any treatment-dependent enhancement of the cycle fecundity cannot be reliably quantified and the relative values of the IUI and COH cannot be separated. Nevertheless, COH-IUI remains a frequently used therapy for presumptive cervical factor infertility, more because of the absence of other viable alternatives rather than the demonstration of therapeutic efficacy.

Luteal Phase Defect

There seems to be widespread acceptance of the existence of an inadequate luteal phase, but a great deal of controversy surrounds the frequency of this phenomenon in fertile women and its pathophysiologic relationship with infertility.[91–95] There are no large randomized clinical studies supporting the use of therapies specifically directed toward the corpus luteum (progesterone supplementation and clomiphene citrate). As a result, these couples may be appropriately considered to have unexplained infertility. COH-IUI has been justified for the treatment of couples with the endocrinologic findings of lowered luteal progesterone secretion because of the elevated luteal progesterone levels with COH.[10, 11] The results appear to parallel those of women in the idiopathic category. The mechanism of any benefit remains uncertain because hMG-hCG without supplemental luteal hCG can be associated with a shortened luteal phase despite the higher than normal luteal progesterone levels.[96, 97] This effect can be reversed with luteal phase support, which is often used.

Immunologic Infertility

Of all the infertility diagnoses, none has engendered more debate as to its relevance to human reproduction than so-called "immunologic" infertility.[98, 99] The group most often identified is the couple in whom antisperm antibodies are identified in the female partner after an abnormal postcoital test. Although reduced numbers of sperm at the site of fertilization have been assumed on a theoretical basis in these patients, this has not been confirmed by direct observation of the sperm numbers in the fallopian tubes. In a single nonrandomized study, the cycle fecundity appeared to be improved when COH was included with IUI.[100] There is virtually no objective data directly testing the efficacy of COH-IUI in this group, despite the obvious logic of avoiding antisperm antibodies in cervical mucus by IUI.

Peritoneal Factor Infertility

The rationale for the use of COH-IUI in this group of couples is that the increased number of oocytes released will provide a greater opportunity for oocyte collection and, potentially, the larger ovary will be physically closer to the fimbria. To justify selection of this therapeutic option over IVF-ET, the fallopian tubes must be patent and the degree of tubal damage or adnexal adhesions mild. Women who have undergone reparative surgery for more severe disease, such as hydrosalpinges, would not be good candidates for COH-IUI and should be encouraged to consider IVF-ET if they do not conceive after surgery. Only two studies of COH-IUI have used this approach, and both have noted relatively favorable cycle fecundities (approximately 10%).[10, 101] Further effort is required to accurately characterize the extent of tubal damage and adnexal adhesions that is optimally treated by this technique.

OPTIMAL COH-CYCLE CHARACTERISTICS

When recommending COH-IUI as a therapy, it is important to determine the optimal stimulation pattern and number of cycles to maximize the cost effectiveness of this therapy and help guide management decisions. As both the cycle fecundity and complications of COH are likely proportional to the degree of follicular development, this involves a balance between risk and benefit.

Number of Cycles

COH-IUI is an expensive and emotionally stressful treatment, and undoubtedly there are patients in whom this therapy will not be effective. Therefore, the optimal number of COH-IUI cycles to attempt before abandoning this form of therapy is a critical issue. A model to help make this decision is normal pregnancy. For some number of months, the likelihood of pregnancy is constant and the pregnancies are randomly distributed. However, the cycle fecundity subsequently declines as the normal couples are rapidly removed

TABLE 50–7. Influence of the Number of COH-IUI Cycles on Cycle Fecundity[11]

Treatment Cycle Number	No. of Pregnancies/ No. of Cycles	Cycle Fecundity
1	50/371	0.14
2	34/225	0.15
3	12/117	0.10
4	11/58	0.19
5	2/21	0.10
6	1/12	0.08

COH-IUI, controlled ovarian hyperstimulation combined with intrauterine insemination of capacitated sperm.

from the population attempting pregnancy. The response to COH-IUI is likely comparable with treatment-dependent pregnancies being randomly distributed in the first several treatment cycles, with a constant cycle fecundity that becomes progressively lower as the couples who conceive with this therapy are removed from the population undergoing treatment. Although pregnancies certainly occur beyond the initial several cycles, the percentage drops off dramatically. There are little data to address this issue, but what are available (Table 50–7) suggest that three to four is a reasonable number of COH-IUI cycles to undergo before considering other therapeutic options.[11]

Quality of the Follicular Stimulation

Although the overall quality of follicular development is difficult to assess accurately, it unquestionably influences the outcome. In general, the greater the number of preovulatory follicles stimulated, the greater the likelihood of pregnancy. The two most significant measures of the adequacy of COH are the number of dominant follicles and the serum estradiol concentration attained on the day hCG is administered. There appears to be a critical minimal level of follicular[11] stimulation required to enhance the cycle fecundity with COH-IUI (two or more follicles and more than 500 pg of estradiol; Table 50–8). Beyond this threshold level, there appears to be little advantage in cycle fecundity, with greater degrees of COH that serve only to increase the risks of multiple gestation and severe ovarian hyperstimulation. The estradiol levels used for clinical decisions must be validated for each center, because they vary with the assay used.

Length of Stimulation

In a similar fashion, there is a minimum number of days of hMG associated with an increase in cycle fecundity. If the ovulation-initiating dose of hCG is given before cycle day 8, the likelihood of pregnancy is very low, probably because of an inadequate interval for oocyte maturation. There is no advantage, however, to prolonging the stimulation beyond day 9, once optimal preovulatory follicular development has been achieved.

Number of Sperm Inseminated

Theoretically, the number of sperm inseminated should influence the cycle fecundity as it applies to the number of

TABLE 50–8. Influence of the Degree of Stimulation (COH) on the Cycle Fecundity in COH-IUI[11]

Measure of Follicular Stimulation	No. of Pregnancies per No. of Cycles	Cycle Fecundity
Estradiol Level on the Day of hCG Administration (pg/mL)		
0–500	14/159	0.09
501–1000	45/233	0.19
1001–1500	29/135	0.22
1501–2000	9/42	0.21
>2000	5/19	0.26
Number of Follicles		
1	8/85	0.09
2	20/120	0.17
3	16/123	0.13
4	20/132	0.15
5	16/85	0.19
6	16/74	0.21
7	5/38	0.13
8	7/63	0.11

COH-IUI, controlled ovarian hyperstimulation combined with intrauterine insemination of capacitated sperm; hCG, human chorionic gonadotropin.

oocytes ovulated. However, there are scant data to address this issue, with a wide variety of sperm separation techniques used and no standardization in counting methodology. Because IUI is a nonphysiologic method of sperm entry, there is no basis for assuming the pattern of sperm distribution or longevity in the female genital tract after IUI will mirror that after normal coitus. When using the typical double-washing technique, there appears to be no enhancement of pregnancy with COH-IUI when more than 1 million sperm are inseminated (Table 50–9).[11] Only when comparative trials are performed with the different washing techniques in well-defined clinical populations will the optimal sperm separation techniques be apparent. No evidence suggests one separation technique is superior to another. Each physician should choose a separation technique based on the optimal number of motile sperm remaining after separation in their clinical setting.

Influence of Age and Duration of Infertility

Although the age of the male does not seem to significantly influence the outcome of infertility therapy until after age 50, the age of the female partner has a more dramatic impact (Table 50–10).[11] There is little question that when the

TABLE 50–9. Influence of the Number of Motile Sperm Inseminated in COH-IUI on the Cycle Fecundity[11]

No. of Motile Sperm Inseminated	No. of Pregnancies/ No. of Cycles	Cycle Fecundity
<1 × 10^6	0/17	0
1.1–5 × 10^6	10/58	0.17
5.1–10 × 10^6	9/65	0.14
10.1–20 × 10^6	10/95	0.11
>20 × 10^6	78/481	0.16

COH-IUI, controlled ovarian hyperstimulation combined with intrauterine insemination of capacitated sperm.

TABLE 50–10. Influence of the Female Partner's Age on Cycle Fecundity in COH-IUI[11]		
Female Partner's Age (yr)	No. of Pregnancies/ No. of Cycles	Cycle Fecundity
21–25	7/28	0.25
26–30	27/154	0.18
31–35	59/387	0.15
36–40	14/147	0.10
>40	2/38	0.05

COH-IUI, controlled ovarian hyperstimulation combined with intrauterine insemination of capacitated sperm.

woman is older than 35 years of age, there is a reduced likelihood of success with the use of any infertility therapy, including COH-IUI. Similarly, the duration of infertility is a related issue that appears to have less of an effect. With 1 to 2 years of infertility, the cycle fecundity is 0.16, whereas for 3 to 5 years, it is 0.15, and for longer than 5 years of infertility, 0.13.[11] Although these inherent factors should not be the sole basis for denying treatment for women in the latter reproductive years, it is appropriate to explain these factors to candidate couples so that they have realistic expectations.

SUMMARY

Substantial controversy remains regarding the pathophysiologic mechanisms of reproductive failure for a variety of infertility diagnoses for which no clearly efficacious therapies exist. Many of these couples who are candidates for COH-IUI share in common a male component with seminal fluid parameters within the range in which pregnancies are observed, spontaneous normal ovulation, and no significant mechanical distortion of the pelvic viscera. Examples of couples in this category are those with minimal to mild endometriosis, the milder degrees of oligo-asthenospermia, luteal phase defects, cervical factor, luteinized unruptured follicle syndrome, and immunologic infertility.

When the infertility is of many years' duration and all attempts at empiric therapy have failed, many of these couples have been referred for the newer reproductive technologies such as IVF-ET, GIFT, and ZIFT as their last option. All these techniques involve some form of COH and higher numbers of capacitated sperm at the site of fertilization, as well as oocyte retrieval. COH-IUI offers the appropriately selected infertile couple a comparable cycle fecundity to these more complex therapies without the expense and invasiveness of oocyte retrieval. As stated by Dr. Robert G. Edwards, "These [the results of COH-IUI] are the controls for IVF and GIFT."[102] They suggest that a substantial percentage of the conceptions attributed to oocyte retrieval in IVF-ET, GIFT, and ZIFT may actually be the result of the increased numbers of oocytes provided by COH and the increased numbers of capacitated sperm at the site of fertilization. COH-IUI is an attractive initial therapeutic alternative to the retrieval technologies of IVF, GIFT, and ZIFT, reducing the expense and avoiding the oocyte retrieval risks of IVF-ET, including that of laparoscopy when gametes or embryos are transferred into the oviducts.

The use of COH-IUI has dramatically increased in the past several years despite the absence of data comparing it directly with the more invasive and expensive retrieval technologies. Establishment of the ideal clinical population for whom COH-IUI is the best treatment and the optimal treatment cycle characteristics awaits controlled prospective trials in carefully defined infertile populations.

REFERENCES

1. Collins JA, Wrixon W, Janes LB, Wilson EH. Treatment-independent pregnancy among infertile couples. N Engl J Med 1983;309:1201–1206.
2. Haney AF, Hughes CL, Whitesides DB, Dodson WC. Treatment-independent, treatment-associated, and pregnancies after additional therapy in a program of in vitro fertilization. Fertil Steril 1987;47:634–638.
3. Lenton EA, Weston GA, Cooke IA. Long-term follow-up of the apparently normal couple with a complaint of infertility. Fertil Steril 1977;28:913–919.
4. Templeton AA, Penney GC. The incidence, characteristics, and prognosis of patients whose infertility is unexplained. Fertil Steril 1982;37:175–182.
5. Robinson GE, Garner DM, Gare DJ, Cranford B. Psychological adaptation to pregnancy in childless women more than 35 years of age. Am J Obstet Gynecol 1987;156:328–333.
6. Newcomb WW, Rodriquez M, Johnson JWC. Reproduction in the older gravida: a literature review. J Reprod Med 1991;36:839–845.
7. Haney AF. What is efficacious infertility therapy? Fertil Steril 1987;48:543–545.
8. Blackwell RE, Carr BR, Chang RJ, et al. Are we exploiting the infertile couple? Fertil Steril 1987;48:735–739.
9. Wallach EE. Gonadotropin treatment for the ovulatory patient—the pros and cons of empiric therapy for infertility. Fertil Steril 1991;55:478–480.
10. Dodson WC, Whitesides DB, Hughes CL, et al. Superovulation with washed intrauterine insemination in the treatment of infertility: a possible alternative to gamete intrafallopian transfer and in vitro fertilization. Fertil Steril 1987;48:441–445.
11. Dodson WC, Haney AF. Controlled ovarian hyperstimulation and intrauterine insemination for treatment of infertility. Fertil Steril 1991;55:457–467.
12. Corsan GH, Kemmann E. The role of superovulation with menotropins in ovulatory infertility: a review. Fertil Steril 1991;55:468–477.
13. Mortimer D, Templeton AA. Sperm transport in the human female reproductive tract in relation to semen analysis characteristics and time of ovulation. J Reprod Fertil 1982;64:401–408.
14. Settlage DSF, Motoshima M, Treadway DR. Sperm transport from the external cervical os to the fallopian tubes in women: a time and quantitation study. Fertil Steril 1972;24:655–661.
15. Olive DL, Haney AF. Endometriosis-associated infertility: a critical review of therapeutic approaches. Obstet Gynecol Surv 1986;41:538–555.
16. Stein ZA. Reviews and commentary—a woman's age: childbearing and child rearing. Am J Epidemiol 1985;121:327–342.
17. Sims JM. Clinical Notes on Uterine Surgery with Special Reference to the Management of the Sterile Condition. New York: William Wood, 1866.
18. Hanson FM, Rock J. Artificial insemination with husband's sperm. Fertil Steril 1951;2:162–174.
19. Barwin BN. Intrauterine insemination with husband's semen. J Reprod Fertil 1974;36:101–106.
20. Beck WW Jr. Two hundred years of artificial insemination [Editorial]. Fertil Steril 1984;41:193–195.
21. Cohen MR. Intrauterine insemination. Int J Fertil 1962;7:235–240.
22. Marrs RP, Vargyas JM, Saito H, et al. Clinical applications of techniques used in human in vitro fertilization research. Am J Obstet Gynecol 1983;146:477–481.
23. Confino E, Friberg J, Dudkiewicz AB, Gliecher N. Intrauterine inseminations with washed human spermatozoa. Fertil Steril 1986;46:55–60.
24. Allen NC, Herbert CM III, Maxson WS, et al. Intrauterine insemination: a critical review. Fertil Steril 1985;44:569–580.
25. Moghissi KS. Some reflections on intrauterine insemination. Fertil Steril 1986;46:13–15.

26. Kerin JFP, Peek J, Warnes GM, et al. Improved conception rate after intrauterine insemination of washed spermatozoa from men with poor quality semen. Lancet 1984;1:533–534.

27. Kirby CA, Flaherty SP, Godfrey BM, et al. A prospective trial of intrauterine insemination of motile spermatozoa versus timed intercourse. Fertil Steril 1991;56:102–107.

28. Bryd W, Ackerman GE, Carr BR, et al. Treatment of refractory infertility by transcervical intrauterine insemination of washed spermatozoa. Fertil Steril 1987;48:921–927.

29. te Velde ER, van Kooy RJ, Waterreus JJH. Intrauterine insemination of washed husband's spermatozoa: a controlled study. Fertil Steril 1989;51:182–185.

30. Ho P-C, Poon IML, Chan SYW, Wang C. Intrauterine insemination is not useful in oligoasthenospermia. Fertil Steril 1989;51:682–684.

31. Dmowski WP, Gaynor L, Lawrence M, et al. Artificial insemination homologous with oligospermic semen separated on albumin columns. Fertil Steril 1979;31:58–62.

32. Harris SJ, Milligan MP, Masson GM, Dennis KJ. Improved separation of motile sperm in asthenospermia and its application to artificial insemination homologous. Fertil Steril 1981;36:219–221.

33. Hull ME, Magyar DM, Vasquez JM, et al. Experience with intrauterine inseminations for cervical factor and oligospermia. Am J Obstet Gynecol 1986;154:1333–1338.

34. Yovich JL, Matson PL. Pregnancy rates after high intrauterine insemination of husband's spermatozoa or gamete intrafallopian transfer. Lancet 1986;2:1287.

35. Thomas EJ, McTighe L, King H, et al. Failure of high intrauterine insemination of husband's semen. Lancet 1986;2:693–694.

36. Hughes EG, Collins JP, Garner PR. Homologous artificial insemination for oligoasthenospermia: a randomized, controlled study comparing intracervical and intrauterine techniques. Fertil Steril 1987;48:278–281.

37. Corson SL, Batzer FR, Gocial B, Maislin G. Intrauterine insemination and ovulation stimulation as treatment of infertility. J Reprod Med 1989;34:397–406.

38. Wiltbank MC, Kosasa S, Rogers B. Treatment of infertile patients by intrauterine insemination of washed spermatozoa. Andrologia 1985;17:22–30.

39. Sher G, Knutzen BK, Stratton CJ, et al. In vitro sperm capacitation and transcervical intrauterine insemination for the treatment of refractory infertility: phase I. Fertil Steril 1984;41:260–264.

40. Galle PC, McRae MA, Colliver JA, Alexander JS. Sperm washing and intrauterine insemination for cervical factor, oligospermia, immunologic infertility, and unexplained infertility. J Reprod Med 1990;35:116–122.

41. Remohi J, Gastaldi C, Parrizio P, et al. Intrauterine insemination and controlled ovarian hyperstimulation in cycles before GIFT. Human Reprod 1989;4:918–920.

42. Gellert-Mortimer ST, Clark GN, Baker HWG, et al. Evaluation of Nycodenz and Percoll density gradients for the selection of motile human spermatozoa. Fertil Steril 1988;49:335–341.

43. Pardo M, Barri PN, Bancells N, et al. Spermatozoa selection in discontinuous Percoll gradients for use in artificial insemination. Fertil Steril 1988;49:505–509.

44. Glass RH, Ericsson RJ. Intrauterine insemination of isolated motile sperm. Fertil Steril 1978;29:535–538.

45. Weathersbee PS, Werlin LB, Stone SC. Peritoneal recovery of sperm after intrauterine insemination. Fertil Steril 1984;42:322–323.

46. Oak MK, Chantler EN, Vaughan-Williams CA, Elstein M. Sperm survival studies in peritoneal fluid from infertile women with endometriosis and unexplained infertility. Clin Reprod Fertil 1985;3:297–303.

47. Burke RK. Effect of peritoneal washings from women with endometriosis on sperm velocity. J Reprod Med 1987;32:743–746.

48. Soldati G, Piffaretti-Yanez A, Campana A, et al. Effect of peritoneal fluid on sperm motility and velocity distribution using objective measurements. Fertil Steril 1989;52:113–119.

49. Muscato JJ, Haney AF, Weinberg JB. Sperm phagocytosis by human peritoneal macrophages: a possible cause of infertility in endometriosis. Am J Obstet Gynecol 1982;144:503–510.

50. Silverberg KM, Johnson JV, Olive DL, et al. A prospective, randomized trial comparing two different intrauterine insemination regimens in controlled ovarian hyperstimulation cycles. Fertil Steril 1992;57:357–361.

51. Chaffkin LM, Nulsen JC, Luciano AA, Metzger DA. A comparative analysis of the cycle fecundity rates associated with combined human menopausal gonadotropin (hMG) and intrauterine insemination (IUI) versus either hMG or IUI alone. Fertil Steril 1991;55:252–257.

52. Evans J, Wells C, Gregory L, Walker S. A comparison of intrauterine insemination, intraperitoneal insemination, and natural intercourse in superovulated women. Fertil Steril 1991;56:1183–1187.

53. Hurst BS, Tjaden BL, Kimball A, et al. Superovulation with or without intrauterine insemination of the treatment of infertility. J Reprod Med 1992;37:237–241.

54. Mastroianni L, Laberge JL, Rock J. Appraisal of the efficacy of artificial insemination with husband's sperm and evaluation of insemination technics. Fertil Steril 1957;8:260–266.

55. Horvath PM, Bohrer M, Shelden RM, Kemmann E. The relationship of sperm parameters to cycle fecundity in superovulated women undergoing intrauterine insemination. Fertil Steril 1989;52:288–294.

56. Yovich JL, Matson PL. Treatment of infertility by the high intrauterine insemination of husband's washed spermatozoa. Hum Reprod 1988;3:939–943.

57. Horvatta O, Kurunmaki H, Titinen A, et al. Direct intraperitoneal or intrauterine insemination and superovulation in infertility treatment: a randomized study. Fertil Steril 1990;54:339–341.

58. Kuzan FB, Hillier SL, Zarutskie PW. Comparison of three wash techniques for the removal of micro-organisms from semen. Obstet Gynecol 1987;70:836–839.

59. Kaneko S, Oshio S, Kobanawa K, et al. Purfication of human sperm by a discontinuous Percoll density gradient with an inner column. Biol Reprod 1986;35:1059–1063.

60. Bolton VN, Warren RE, Braude PR. Removal of bacterial contaminants from semen for in vitro fertilization or artificial insemination by the use of buoyant density centrifugation. Fertil Steril 1986;46:1128–1132.

61. Stone SC, de la Maza LM, Peterson EM. Recovery of microorganisms from the pelvic cavity after intracervical or intrauterine artificial insemination. Fertil Steril 1986;46:61–65.

62. Tredway DR, Chan P, Henig I, et al. Effectiveness of stimulated menstrual cycles and Percoll sperm preparation in intrauterine insemination. J Reprod Med 1990;35:103–108.

63. Moretti-Rojas I, Rohas FJ, Leisure M, et al. Intrauterine inseminations with washed human spermatozoa does not induce formation of antisperm antibodies. Fertil Steril 1990;53:180–182.

64. Horvath PM, Beck M, Bohrer MK, et al. A prospective study on the lack of development of antisperm antibodies in women undergoing intrauterine insemination. Am J Obstet Gynecol 1989;160:631–637.

65. Kremer J. A new technique for intrauterine insemination. Int J Fertil 1979;24:53–56.

66. Dodson WC, Walmer DK, Hughes CL Jr, et al. Adjunctive leuprolide therapy does not improve cycle fecundity in controlled ovarian hyperstimulation and intrauterine insemination of subfertile women. Obstet Gynecol 1991;78:187–190.

67. Friedman CI, Schmidt GE, Chang FE, Kim MH. Severe ovarian hyperstimulation following follicular aspiration. Am J Obstet Gynecol 1984;150:436–437.

68. Friedman AJ. Sextuplet pregnancy after human unopposed gonadotropin superovulation and intrauterine insemination. J Reprod Med 1990;35:113–115.

69. Petrikovsky BM, Bintzileos AM. Management and outcome of multiple pregnancy of high fetal order: literature review. Obstet Gynecol Surv 1989;44:578–584.

70. Dodson WC, Hughes CL Jr, Haney AF. Multiple pregnancies conceived during superovulation: an evaluation of clinical characteristics and monitored parameters of conception cycles. Am J Obstet Gynecol 1988;159:382–385.

71. Shelden R, Kemmann E, Bohrer M, Pasquale S. Multiple gestation is associated with the use of high sperm numbers in the intrauterine insemination specimen in women undergoing gonadotropin stimulation. Fertil Steril 1988;49:607–610.

72. Schenker JG, Yarlini S, Granat M. Multiple pregnancies following ovulation induction. Fertil Steril 1981;35:105–123.

73. Medical Research International and the Society for Assisted Reproductive Technology, The American Fertility Society. In vitro fertilization-embryo transfer in the United States: 1988 results from the IVF-ET Registry. Fertil Steril 1990;53:13–20.

74. Berkowitz RL, Lynch L, Chitkara Y, et al. Selective reduction of multifetal pregnancies in the first trimester. N Engl J Med 1988;318:1043–1047.

75. Golan A, Ron-El R, Herman A, et al. Ovarian hyperstimulation syndrome: an update review. Obstet Gynecol Surv 1989;44:430–440.

76. Blumenfeld Z, Nahhas F. Pretreatment of sperm with human follicular fluid for borderline male infertility. Fertil Steril 1989;51:863–868.

77. Bolton VN, Braude PR, Ockenden K, et al. An evaluation of semen analysis and in vitro tests of sperm function in the prediction of the outcome of intrauterine AIH. Hum Reprod 1989;4:674–679.

78. Hewitt J, Cohen J, Krishnaswamy V, et al. Treatment of idiopathic infertility, cervical mucus hostility, and male infertility: artificial insemination with husband's semen or in vitro fertilization? Fertil Steril 1985;44:350–355.

79. Cruz RI, Kemman E, Brandeis VT, et al. A prospective study of intrauterine insemination of processed sperm from men with oligoasthenospermia in superovulated women. Fertil Steril 1986;46:673–677.

80. Sunde A, Kahn J, Molne K. Intrauterine insemination. Hum Reprod 1988;3:97–99.

81. Barnea ER, Holford TR, McInnes DRA. Long-term prognosis of infertile couples with normal basic investigations: a life table analysis. Obstet Gynecol 1985;66:24–26.

82. Serhal PF, Katz M, Little V, Woronowski H. Unexplained infertility—the value of Pergonal superovulation combined with intrauterine insemination. Fertil Steril 1988;49:602–606.

83. Dickey RP, Olar TT, Taylor SN, et al. Relationship of follicle number, serum estradiol, and other factors to birth rate and multiparity in human menopausal gonadotropin–induced intrauterine insemination cycles. Fertil Steril 1991;56:89–92.

84. Welner S, DeCherney AH, Polan ML. Human menopausal gonadotropins: a justifiable therapy in ovulatory women with long-standing idiopathic infertility. Am J Obstet Gynecol 1988;158:111–117.

85. Wang CF, Gemzell C. Pregnancy following treatment with human gonadotropins in primary unexplained infertility. Acta Obstet Gynaecol Scand 1979;58:141–146.

86. Metzger DA, Haney AF. Endometriosis: Etiology and pathophysiology of infertility. Clin Obstet Gynecol 1988;31:801–812.

87. White RM, Glass RH. Intrauterine insemination with husband's semen. Obstet Gynecol 1976;47:119–121.

88. Quaglirello J, Arny M. Intracervical versus intrauterine insemination: correlation of outcome with antecedent post-coital testing. Fertil Steril 1976;46:870–875.

89. Glezerman M, Bernstein D, Insler V. The cervical factor of infertility and intrauterine insemination. Int J Fertil 1984;29:16–19.

90. Arny M, Quagliarello J. Semen quality before and after processing by a swim-up method: relationship to outcome of intrauterine insemination. Fertil Steril 1987;48:643–648.

91. Jones GS. The luteal phase defect. Fertil Steril 1976;27:351–356.

92. Daly DC, Walters CA, Soto-Albors CE, Riddick DH. Endometrial biopsy during treatment of luteal phase defects is predictive of therapeutic outcome. Fertil Steril 1983;40:305–310.

93. Davidson BJ, Thrasher TV, Seraj IM. An analysis of endometrial biopsies performed for fertility. Fertil Steril 1987;48:770–774.

94. Davis OK, Berkeley AS, Naus GJ, et al. The incidence of luteal phase defect in normal, fertile women determined by serial endometrial biopsies. Fertil Steril 1989;51:582–586.

95. Balasch J, Vanrell JA. Corpus luteum insufficiency and fertility: a matter of controversy. Hum Reprod 1987;2:557–567.

96. Olson JL, Rebar RW, Schreiber JF, Vaitukaitis JL. Shortened luteal phase after ovulation induction with human menopausal gonadotropin and human chorionic gonadotropin. Fertil Steril 1983;39:284–291.

97. Laatikainen T, Kurunmaki H, Koshimies A. A short luteal phase in cycles stimulated with clomiphene citrate and human menopausal gonadotropin for in vitro fertilization. J In Vitro Fertil Embryo Trans 1988;5:14–17.

98. Smarr SC, Wong R, Hammond MG. Effect of therapy on infertile couples with antisperm antibodies. Am J Obstet Gynecol 1988;158:969–973.

99. Bronson R, Cooper G, Rosenfeld D. Sperm antibodies: their role in infertility. Fertil Steril 1984;42:171–183.

100. Margalloth EJ, Sauter E, Bronson RA, et al. Intrauterine insemination as treatment for antisperm antibodies in the female. Fertil Steril 1988;50:441–446.

101. Aboulghar MA, Mansour RT, Serour GI. Ovarian superovulation in the treatment of infertility due to peritubal and periovarian adhesions. Fertil Steril 1989;51:834–837.

102. Edwards RG. Comments during Symposium on New Reproductive Technologies. Washington, DC: National Academy of Sciences, 1989.

CHAPTER 51

In Vitro Fertilization

OWEN K. DAVIS and ZEV ROSENWAKS

In vitro fertilization (IVF) and related assisted reproductive technologies (ART) have attained a preeminent role in the management of infertility. The first successful human pregnancy following IVF was reported in 1978.[1] Currently in the United States alone, in excess of 5600 live deliveries per year result from ART procedures,[2] more than 3200 following IVF.

This chapter provides an overview of IVF with regard to applications, techniques, and outcome. Other ART procedures, including gamete intrafallopian transfer (GIFT), zygote intrafallopian transfer (ZIFT), and tubal embryo transfer (TET) are covered elsewhere in this text.

INDICATIONS

Tubal Factor

Approximately 25% of infertility is attributable to tubal disease. Although pregnancy rates may exceed 60% following microsurgical reversal of tubal ligation, surgical correction of more significant tubal pathology is far less successful, for example, in cases of distal tubal obstruction, severe pelvic adhesive disease, two-site tubal occlusion, or previously failed tubal surgery.

Although infertility following bilateral salpingectomy is an absolute indication, IVF should also be considered as primary therapy in instances of poor-prognosis tubal disease and in cases in which surgery has been unsuccessful. Examples of poor-prognosis tubal disease include two-site occlusion, large diameter (>3 cm) hydrosalpinx with absent fimbria, and frozen pelvis. At most centers, patients with tubal factor infertility compose the largest single diagnostic category. Outcome for these patients is favorable, with clinical pregnancy rates exceeding 25% per embryo transfer (ET) at successful programs.

Endometriosis

Infertility is a major potential consequence of endometriosis. Although the putative etiologic role of minimal-to-mild disease is now in question, moderate and severe endometriosis clearly contribute to reproductive failure. The pathophysiology of endometriosis-induced infecundity is poorly understood but may include distortion of pelvic anatomy owing to adhesion formation, local augmentation of prostanoid production, or increased numbers of activated peritoneal macrophages.

Standard management of endometriosis includes surgical ablation (excision, fulguration, or vaporization) and hormonal suppression with a variety of pharmacologic agents, including danazol, gonadotropin-releasing hormone (GnRH) agonists, and progestagens. When infertility fails to respond to conventional measures (e.g., no conception within a year of treatment), IVF offers success rates comparable to those seen in couples with tubal infertility. Although patients with severe endometriosis have been reported to fare less well, possibly owing to the recovery of fewer or poorer quality oocytes, evidence suggests that IVF success rates may be relatively unaffected by the stage of disease.[3]

Male Factor

Approximately 40% of infertile couples are diagnosed with a primary male factor. One or more semen analyses should be performed early in the infertility evaluation. Normal parameters on conventional analysis include a sperm concentration greater than 20×10^6/mL, motility greater than 50%, and greater than 30% normal forms. Kruger and colleagues[4] have proposed an alternate system of strict morphologic analysis, which appears to be highly predictive of IVF outcome. Single or more frequently multiple abnormalities may be detected on semen analysis, including low concentration (oligospermia), impaired motility (asthenospermia), and a low proportion of normal forms (teratospermia). Andrologic evaluation of the affected man may uncover a surgically correctable lesion (varicocele, obstructive disease) or immunologic, infectious, environmental, or endocrine factors. Male factor infertility is frequently idiopathic. If primary treatment of the male partner is unsuccessful, therapeutic insemination with split ejaculates or washed intrauterine insemination (IUI) may be helpful, especially when performed in conjunction with controlled ovarian hyperstimulation (COH). Such therapy is, however, often unsuccessful in cases of a severe male factor.

ART, and IVF in particular, has become increasingly useful in the management of refractory male factor infertility. The ability to add a high density of motile sperm to multiple oocytes in a small volume of culture medium enhances the likelihood of fertilization. Furthermore, IVF can serve as a diagnostic maneuver, insofar as gamete interaction and fertilization can be directly observed and assessed. Microsurgical fertilization techniques (discussed later in this chapter and elsewhere in this text) may further improve the chances of fertilization in cases of previously documented fertilization failure or in cases in which sperm quality is so poor as to predict a low probability of fertilization with conventional (zona-intact) IVF. Ultimately, fertilization failure despite aggressive therapy may direct a couple to therapeutic donor insemination.

As might be expected, fertilization rates are reduced in male factor IVF cases, resulting in embryo transfer rates of approximately 50% at most units. Per transfer pregnancy rates are nonetheless similar to those in other diagnostic groups when fertilization is achieved. Specific semen analysis variables do correlate with IVF outcome in individual cases, although no parameter short of azoospermia is absolute. Low numbers of recoverable, rapidly motile sperm ($<1.5 \times 10^6$) indicate a poor prognosis for success following insemination of zona-intact oocytes.[5] Severe teratospermia ($<4\%$ normal forms by strict morphologic analysis) also reduces the probability of fertilization. Increased numbers of inflammatory cells in the semen (leukospermia) may impede IVF results and mandates seminal culture and appropriate antibiotic therapy. The hamster egg penetration test (HEPT) correlates with fertilization potential in the man and to some extent with IVF outcome; the value of this assay as a screening test for IVF is limited, however, because fertilization and pregnancy may be seen even in the context of a 0% HEPT score.

One additional specific instance in which IVF should be considered are cases in which the male partner has cryobanked sperm before antineoplastic therapy for malignant neoplasia. Chemotherapy and radiation therapy frequently result in irreversible azoospermia. In such cases, the supply of pretherapy cryopreserved sperm is limited and often of poor quality.[6] IVF may be considered as primary therapy or if artificial insemination with a portion of the banked sperm has failed. Pregnancies have been reported following IVF using cryobanked sperm from men with lymphoma[7] and testicular carcinoma.[8]

Idiopathic Infertility

Idiopathic infertility is a diagnosis of exclusion applied to approximately 10% of infertile couples in the event that a thorough evaluation uncovers no identifiable cause. A complete workup must include, at minimum, semen analysis, postcoital testing, hysterosalpingography or endoscopic evaluation of pelvic anatomy, and documentation of ovulatory sufficiency. Ancillary diagnostic procedures may include cervical/seminal fluid cultures, antisperm antibody testing, and HEPT.

The treatment of idiopathic infertility is empiric. Controlled ovarian hyperstimulation combined with washed, intrauterine inseminations (COH/IUI) may be undertaken before consideration of ART.[9] IVF pregnancy rates for those couples are good, generally exceeding those for patients with pure tubal factor infertility. IVF may be of diagnostic value in

such cases because a failure to achieve fertilization may unmask an intrinsic gamete defect.

Immunologic Infertility

Immunologic infertility may initially be suggested by an abnormal postcoital test, typically manifested by the presence of immotile or "shaking" sperm, or may be detected by routine antisperm antibody testing in the evaluation of apparently unexplained infertility. Antisperm antibodies can be identified in semen, serum, or cervical mucus, most commonly by means of the direct or indirect Immunobead test for isotype-specific, sperm-coating antibodies. Other assays include tests for complement-dependent serum cytotoxic antibodies and serum agglutinating antibodies. Treatment options range from washed IUIs, with or without COH, to immunosuppression. The efficacy of immunosuppressive doses of corticosteroids has not been established, and risks and side effects can be significant (including aseptic necrosis of the femoral heads).

IVF pregnancy rates for couples with immunologic infertility appear comparable to the general ART population. When female circulating antisperm antibodies are identified, maternal serum should be excluded from the fertilization medium, and an alternative protein source used (e.g., Plasmanate). When antibodies are detected in the seminal fluid, ejaculation directly into medium may diminish sperm binding before the processing of the sample.

In Utero Diethylstilbestrol Exposure

Once widespread, the use of diethylstilbestrol (DES) in pregnancy was abandoned once the link between in utero DES exposure and the subsequent development of clear cell adenocarcinoma of the vagina and cervix was established. The extensive use of this medication through 1971 has had a lasting impact on the reproductive potential of so-called DES daughters, who are at a significantly increased risk for pregnancy loss from repetitive miscarriage, ectopic gestations, cervical incompetence, and preterm labor. The degree of risk is to some degree proportionate to the severity of uterine abnormalities identified by hysterosalpingography (e.g., T-shaped/hypoplastic uterus, uterine strictures), but all exposed patients should be considered to be high risk. It is less clear whether DES exposure per se is a cause of primary infertility. Clinical pregnancy rates in DES-exposed women who require IVF are similar to those seen in patients with a tubal factor,[10] but live birth rates are depressed owing to the increased likelihood of fetal wastage. Many IVF centers replace a smaller number of embryos in DES-exposed patients to minimize the risk of multifetal gestation in this high-risk population. Close surveillance in early pregnancy is mandatory, so as to detect a possible extrauterine gestation.

PATIENT SELECTION

Patient screening is an essential component of the ART process and is intended both to determine the appropriateness of therapy (has the infertility evaluation been complete, have other reasonable therapeutic options been considered/exhausted?) and to tailor the IVF treatment regimen to the individual couple's needs. Screening and selection criteria vary from program to program owing to differences both in clinical experience and in philosophy.

In general, both partners should be healthy, and maternal contraindications to pregnancy should be excluded. The IVF process, including risks, physical and emotional stresses, and cost, should be reviewed with prospective patients. Center-specific success rates should be presented and interpreted, with attention to the given couple's clinical situation (e.g., diagnosis, age). Most centers offer psychological counseling and support to couples who might benefit from these services.

Age of the female partner is a major determinant of IVF success; women over 40 years of age have a poorer prognosis than their younger counterparts.[11] The 1991 U.S. IVF Registry reported an overall delivery rate *per retrieval* (nonmale factor) of only 8% for women older than 40 years, in contrast with an 18% success rate for women under 40. The statistics for each cycle started are even grimmer, given the 25% cancellation rate in older patients.[2] Many IVF programs have established age limits (typically older than 40 to 42 years) determined by their local clinical experience. The diminished probability of viable pregnancy following IVF-ET in women over 40 results from both reduced implantation rates and an increased risk of miscarriage (60%).[11] Clinical experience with donor eggs suggests that it is oocyte senescence (decreased ovarian reserve) rather than the aging uterine environment that is primarily responsible for the age-related decline in IVF success.[12] Ovarian reserve, a reflection of the "biologic age" of the oocytes and follicular apparatus, can be assessed by the measurement of baseline peripheral follicle-stimulating hormone (FSH) and estradiol (E_2) levels in the early follicular phase (day 3). An elevated day 3 FSH[13] or E_2[14] level may be indicative of incipient ovarian failure and a reduced chance for success following IVF-ET. Along similar lines, it has also been suggested that dynamic testing with clomiphene citrate (clomiphene challenge test) may uncover subtle degrees of occult ovarian failure if an exaggerated rise in the FSH level results.[15]

At the initial consultation, IVF candidates should undergo a thorough review of their infertility workup and prior therapy, including a detailed examination of any previous IVF or ovarian stimulation cycles. Physical examination of the female partner should include, at minimum, bimanual assessment of uterine size and position, generally with performance of a uterine sounding or trial transfer, to determine the depth of the uterine cavity and the potential ease or difficulty of eventual ET. Papanicolaou smears and appropriate cervical cultures (e.g., *Chlamydia, Mycoplasma/Ureaplasma*) may be obtained at the time of pelvic examination. Hysterosalpingogram films or hysteroscopic photographs should be examined to rule out clinically significant intrauterine pathology, such as multiple or large filling defects (submucous myomata, polyps, synechiae) or a müllerian fusion defect that could impede blastocyst implantation or increase the risk of subsequent spontaneous abortion and preterm labor. Significant (especially fundal, e.g., >1 cm) filling defects or congenital uterine malformations suggested by radiography should be further pursued with hysteroscopy (and, where appropriate, laparoscopy) and surgically corrected. Although data are

sparse regarding the precise impact of fibroids, polyps, and so forth on implantation and pregnancy outcome, most clinicians concur on the importance of a relatively normal uterine lumen at the time of ET.

The IVF andrology laboratory should perform a complete semen analysis, including a wash and sperm separation procedure (e.g., swim-up, Percoll gradient centrifugation), in an effort to detect a possible male factor and to determine an optimal sperm extraction technique for the individual patient. Further testing, such as seminal fluid culture or assay for antisperm antibodies, may be indicated by findings on routine semen analysis. If sperm quality is sufficiently poor as to prognosticate a high risk for fertilization failure, options including microsurgically assisted fertilization should be considered and discussed with the couple before their treatment cycle.

OVARIAN STIMULATION

The first successful human IVF pregnancy resulted from a single oocyte retrieved in a spontaneous menstrual cycle.[1] Although this approach permitted the natural selection of a mature ovum by endogenous mechanisms, the clinical inefficiency of single embryo replacement hampered pregnancy rates. Moreover, natural cycle IVF can be a cumbersome technique, requiring round-the-clock hormonal monitoring to identify the onset of the luteinizing hormone (LH) surge, with the potential for oocyte retrieval at any hour of the day or night. Although some clinicians have evinced a renewed interest in natural cycle IVF, most programs routinely use one or a number of ovarian stimulation protocols to achieve multifollicular recruitment; pregnancy rates improve as the number of transferred concepti is increased.

Clomiphene Citrate

The use of clomiphene as a single agent for ART is now infrequent, owing to the recovery of only one or two oocytes per cycle. Further, this approach was complicated by a high cancellation rate (25% to 40%) owing to a poor response or premature LH surge. Typically, clomiphene was administered at a dose of 50 to 150 mg for 5 to 7 days, starting between the second and fifth day of the menstrual cycle. Cycle monitoring entailed serial sonograms and serum E_2 and LH levels. Near the time of follicular maturity, the frequency of serum or urine sampling was increased (every 3 hours) in an effort to detect the onset of the LH surge, with oocyte harvest 24 to 26 hours later. As an alternative, intramuscular human chorionic gonadotropin (hCG) could be administered once the lead follicle attained a mean diameter of greater than 17 mm, with oocyte recovery 34 to 36 hours after.

Combination Clomiphene/Human Menopausal Gonadotropin

The coadministration of human menotropins (human menopausal gonadotropin [HMG]) with clomiphene citrate enhanced multifollicular recruitment, leading to an increase in the number of embryos transferred and improved pregnancy rates. Concurrent and sequential dosing schedules have been used. In concurrent regimens, the clomiphene is initiated on cycle day 4 or 5, 50 to 150 mg for 5 days; hMG is administered concurrently, at a dose of 1 or 2 ampules daily, and may be continued after the course of clomiphene therapy is completed. Sequential regimens consist of a 5-day course of clomiphene followed by an additional 3 to 5 days of hMG.

Cycle monitoring consists of serial sonographic follicular studies and daily serum E_2 determinations. Spontaneous LH surges can occur, mandating frequent serum or urinary LH measurements once follicular development is advanced. When the lead follicles have achieved a mean diameter of greater than 17 to 18 mm, hCG is administered at a dose of 5000 to 10,000 IU to effect final maturation of the oocytes. Oocyte recovery is undertaken 34 to 36 hours later. If a spontaneous LH surge occurs in the presence of adequate follicular development, hCG may be given to augment the surge, with retrieval timed according to the onset of the endogenous rise in LH. One major disadvantage of combined clomiphene/hMG is the potential for a nighttime oocyte retrieval, given the significant propensity for spontaneous ovulation.

Pure Gonadotropin Protocols

Gonadotropin-only ART regimens were developed on the premise that gonadotropins represent a more physiologic approach to controlled ovarian hyperstimulation, avoiding some of the potentially detrimental effects of clomiphene on oocytes and endometrial development.[16] Currently available menotropin preparations include hMG, formulated in ampules containing 75 IU each of FSH and LH, and purified FSH, consisting of 75 IU of FSH with less than 1 IU of LH per ampule. Highly purified FSH and recombinant gonadotropin preparations are currently under investigation and should become commercially available in the near future.

Menotropin therapy is generally started at a daily dose of 2 to 4 ampules, intramuscularly, on the second or third day of the menstrual cycle, in an effort to maximize the recruitment of follicles from the "gonadotropin-sensitive" pool. Estradiol levels are obtained daily, with concurrent sonographic surveillance once the E_2 concentration exceeds a threshold level, usually by cycle day 6. The timing of the hCG injection is determined by a combination of variables, including lead follicular diameter, absolute E_2 level and the pattern of E_2 rise, and follicular growth. hCG is administered at a dose of 5000 to 10,000 IU once the lead follicles have achieved a mean diameter of greater than 14 to 16 mm, with the E_2 level typically exceeding 400 to 500 pg/mL. Timing is critical; if hCG is given prematurely, immature oocytes are obtained, and if given late, the oocytes may be predominantly postmature. Oocyte retrieval is performed in approximately 34 to 36 hours. Given the relatively infrequent occurrence of spontaneous LH surges in pure gonadotropin cycles (<10%), round-the-clock LH monitoring is not required, although daily LH measurements close to the time of hCG administration may permit timely intervention if a spontaneous surge is detected.

Gonadotropin may be administered in different formulations and dosage schedules. hMG or purified FSH can be given alone or in combination. The daily dosage of gonadotropin may be fixed, progressively increased, or tapered, as dictated both by protocol and individual response. We have preferred a tapering regimen, with the highest dose of menotropins (between 4 and 6 ampules/day) given on cycle days 3 and 4 and thereafter reduced, in a stepwise fashion, to 2 ampules over the succeeding few days. This clinical approach has been supported by experiments in the monkey, which have suggested that step-down regimens result in more synchronous folliculogenesis.[17] Gonadotropin may be withheld for 1 day before hCG administration ("coasting") once a threshold lead follicular diameter (approximately 14 to 15 mm) and E_2 level have been attained; this is our general practice in non–gonadotropin-releasing hormone (GnRH) agonist cycles.

It should be emphasized that no single approach optimizes outcome for all patients, and stimulation protocols should be adaptable to individual requirements. A given woman's response profile tends to be consistent from cycle to cycle on a given protocol, and this provides a rational basis for modifying subsequent regimens. Patients may be classified, according to peak E_2 level, as high, intermediate, or low responders; this pattern of response is predictive of IVF outcome.[18] Patients with a high response achieve greater numbers of oocytes and embryos for transfer and enjoy higher pregnancy rates when compared with low responders. A review of more than 1300 IVF cycles at Cornell, between January 1990 and December 1991, revealed that high responders (mean peak E_2 greater than 2000 pg/mL) had an ongoing pregnancy rate of 41% per replacement, whereas low responders (mean peak E_2 level less than 400 pg/mL) displayed a 19.6% success rate.

In a given stimulation cycle, cancellation before oocyte retrieval should be considered when the ovarian response predicts a sufficiently poor prognosis for success. An IVF cycle may be aborted for lack of response (E_2 less than 100 pg/mL after 5 days of menotropin therapy), a falling E_2 level on 2 consecutive days, a 20% to 30% drop in the E_2 concentration the morning after hCG injection, or failure to recruit more than one mature follicle. Although various investigators have reported a direct correlation between implantation rates and sonographically measured endometrial thickness, we have seen acceptable pregnancy rates even when endometrial thickness is less than 9 mm and therefore do not use this parameter as a criterion for cycle cancellation.

Pulsatile Gonadotropin-Releasing Hormone

The administration of pulsatile GnRH to normally ovulating women can effect multiple follicular development, and this has had some limited application in IVF.[19] GnRH may be given as 10-μg intravenous pulses, at an interval of 1 to 2 hours, via a portable, automated infusion pump. Monitoring of follicular growth is performed as with other stimulation regimens. Oocyte harvest may be scheduled either after a spontaneous LH surge or after hCG administration, as in natural cycle IVF. Although pregnancies have been reported, this approach is probably more cumbersome than menotropin therapy and confers no distinct advantages.

Gonadotropin-Releasing Hormone Analogs

A number of potent, long-acting GnRH agonists have been synthesized over the past several years. Amino acid substitutions at positions 6 and 10 of the native GnRH molecule reduce its susceptibility to degradation by endopeptidases and enhance the binding affinity of the hormone to its gonadotrope receptor. Initially, administration of a GnRH agonist results in a surge of gonadotropin release from the anterior pituitary; within a few days, prolonged GnRH receptor occupancy leads to pituitary desensitization and down-regulation and, consequently, a state of reversible hypogonadism.

When initially applied to IVF, adjunctive GnRH agonist therapy was intended to improve outcome for women with a previous poor response, for example, a history of premature LH surge or premature luteinization resulting either in cycle cancellation or the recovery of poor-quality oocytes. More recently, it has been suggested that routine administration of GnRH agonist in stimulation protocols leads not only to decreased cancellation rates and greater convenience, but also, more importantly, to an overall improvement in ART success rates.[20] A meta-analysis of randomized, controlled trials examining the efficacy of adjunctive GnRH agonist for ART supports its routine use. In this study, the overall clinical pregnancy rate per cycle commenced and per transfer was significantly improved after GnRH agonist treatment for IVF (common odds ratios of 1.8 and 1.4).[21] The specific mechanism of this enhancement may entail an improvement in oocyte and embryo quality, perhaps via suppression of bioactive LH, or an increase in the numbers of oocytes recovered. A study lends support to the latter contention; analysis of 294 gonadotropin-only and 449 gonadotropin/GnRH agonist cycles at Cornell revealed a significant increase in the average numbers of oocytes retrieved and embryos transferred in GnRH agonist cycles, whereas no significant difference in fertilization rates or per embryo implantation or delivery rates was observed.[22]

In the United States, the most widely used GnRH agonist for ART is leuprolide acetate, although experience with nafarelin acetate has been gaining. Leuprolide is generally administered in a single daily subcutaneous dose of 0.5 to 1.0 mg, commencing either in the midluteal phase of the preceding cycle (long protocol) (Fig. 51–1) or day 2 or 3 of the follicular phase (short or "flare" protocol). In the long protocol,

ovarian suppression is achieved by the onset of menses, before the start of menotropin therapy. In the "flare" approach, the agonist phase of GnRH agonist therapy synergizes with the exogenous gonadotropins before eventual pituitary suppression.[23] The short regimen has the advantage of reducing both the duration of therapy and the total dosage requirement for gonadotropin. Although both approaches have their proponents, a meta-analysis of adjunctive GnRH agonist for IVF failed to detect a significant difference in cancellation or pregnancy rates between the two protocols.[21] When a GnRH agonist is used for ovarian stimulation, exogenous luteal support with progesterone or hCG is particularly important to avoid luteal insufficiency in the peri-implantation period.

Current evidence supports the routine use of GnRH agonist as a beneficial adjunct in IVF stimulation regimens. Disadvantages of GnRH agonist coadministration include increased duration of therapy and cost owing to an augmented dosage requirement for menotropins, potential oversuppression of patients with impaired ovarian reserve (e.g., predicted by an elevated baseline FSH level), a possibly increased risk of developing ovarian hyperstimulation syndrome in high responder patients, and ovarian cyst formation.[24]

Ovarian Stimulation of the Difficult Patient

Patients with a poor response to controlled ovarian hyperstimulation fall into two distinct categories: low responders and overresponders. Low responders achieve peak E_2 levels of less than 300 to 500 pg/mL, yield low numbers of oocytes and embryos, and have lower pregnancy rates than average responders. In many cases, a low response to COH is attributable to diminished ovarian reserve (advanced biologic ovarian age), as discussed previously. In some instances, the low-responder does not manifest clinical evidence of incipient ovarian failure (e.g., a high FSH level), and the reason for the poor response is generally elusive. Some low-responder patients with normal baseline FSH levels may be found to have circulating gonadotropin antibodies.[25] One intuitive approach to COH of the low responder is to increase the dosage of administered menotropins. In one report, however, high-dose FSH therapy (6 ampules/day) in a group of low responders failed to change significantly peak E_2 levels, numbers of mature oocytes retrieved, or the number of embryos replaced.[26]

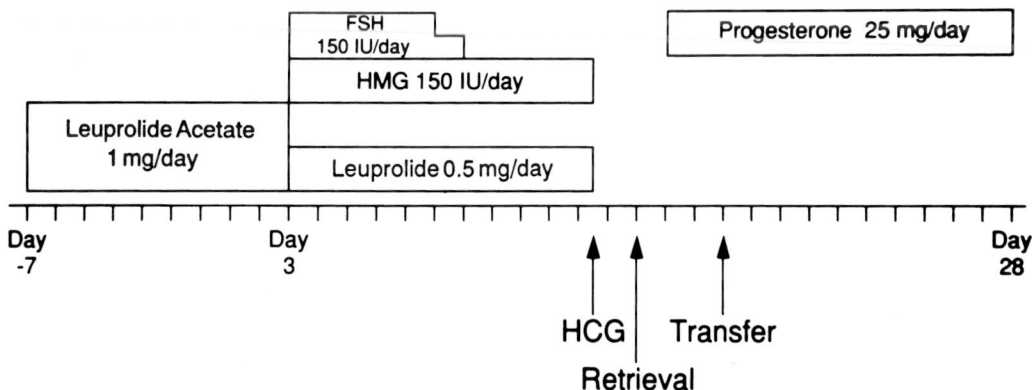

FIGURE 51–1. Example of long gonadotropin-releasing hormone (GnRH) agonist protocol with step-down gonadotropin stimulation. FSH, follicle-stimulating hormone; HMG, human menopausal gonadotropin; HCG, human chorionic gonadotropin.

Our experience has also indicated the limited utility of increasing gonadotropin dosage in these cases. In older women and poor responders with relatively normal day 3 FSH levels, however, we have seen a significant improvement in E_2 levels and clinical pregnancy rates when the standard dosage of leuprolide is halved (unpublished data). A novel adjunct in the treatment of low-responder patients is the use of exogenous growth hormone (GH) or growth hormone–releasing hormone (GHRH), predicated on evidence that insulin-like growth factor 1 (IGF-1) appears to act synergistically with gonadotropins in the facilitation of a number of ovarian functions, including the induction of LH receptors, aromatase activity, progesterone synthesis, and inhibin production. In an early report, pharmacologic doses of GH were found to enhance the ovarian response of women who were relatively resistant to menotropin therapy.[27] Another study was unable to document any beneficial impact of adjunctive GH treatment in poor responders undergoing IVF.[28] Any clear-cut benefit of GH or GHRH in the management of low-responder patients remains to be established.

Although high-responder patients enjoy better overall success rates than their low responder counterparts, exaggerated ovarian sensitivity to stimulation (e.g., seen in some young patients or women with polycystic ovary syndrome [PCOS] or elevated LH to FSH ratios) substantially increases the risk of severe ovarian hyperstimulation syndrome (OHSS) and may actually impair implantation rates owing to the adverse impact of a markedly elevated luteal phase E_2 to progesterone ratio. Hyperresponsive patients generally benefit from a reduced dose of gonadotropin (e.g., 2 ampules/day), attaining lower peak E_2 levels, reduced E_2 to progesterone ratios, and higher ongoing pregnancy rates.[29] Whether the use of purified FSH for ovulation induction in high responders with elevated LH to FSH ratios confers any advantage is open to question; a study comparing the efficacy of pure FSH versus hMG for IVF in patients with PCOS demonstrated no significant difference.[30] We have obtained encouraging results in high responders with a combined approach to ovarian suppression entailing pretreatment with an oral contraceptive preparation followed directly by GnRH agonist administration and low-dose menotropins.

Natural Cycle In Vitro Fertilization

Although efficient in stimulating multifollicular development, COH for IVF presents certain disadvantages, including increased per cycle cost, risk of OHSS and multiple gestations, and possibly diminished endometrial receptivity.[31] A meta-analysis further suggests a possible association between treatment with fertility drugs (unspecified) and the subsequent development of ovarian carcinoma in nulligravid women.[32] In part for these reasons, a renewed enthusiasm for natural cycle IVF has been expressed by some practitioners. Paulson and associates[33] reported a 12% ongoing pregnancy rate per retrieval following monitored natural cycle IVF in 46 normo-ovulatory patients. Others have combined natural cycle IVF with intravaginal gamete coculture to reduce cost further, with a reported success rate of 10% per retrieval.[34]

IVF in the natural cycle is unlikely to be an appropriate option for couples with a severe male factor because increasing the numbers of oocytes maximizes the potential for fertil-

ization. Further, the cost-effectiveness of unstimulated IVF varies between programs and depends on relative per cycle success rates, including the potential to transfer cryopreserved "excess" embryos at a later date following stimulated cycles.

TECHNIQUE OF OOCYTE RETRIEVAL

Oocyte recovery is performed 34 to 36 hours after the administration of hCG, which is given to stimulate the resumption of meiosis, with extrusion of the first polar body. For the first several years after the inception of human IVF, laparoscopic follicular aspiration was the dominant method of oocyte retrieval and still finds application in related procedures such as GIFT. Ultrasound-guided techniques, first developed to permit oocyte recovery in cases in which the ovaries were inaccessible to the laparoscope (e.g., severe pelvic adhesions), have since become the standard practice in IVF, owing to refinement in instrumentation and operator experience.

Laparoscopic Oocyte Retrieval

In general, successful laparoscopic retrieval requires visual access to a minimum of 50% of the total ovarian surface area. At some centers, pretreatment laparoscopies were undertaken to document ovarian accessibility in patients suspected of having significant pelvic adhesive disease.

Laparoscopic oocyte recovery is a surgical procedure that usually requires general anesthesia with endotracheal intubation. The procedure may be performed using a two- or three-puncture approach, with an intraumbilical site for abdominal insufflation and laparoscope placement and one or more lower abdominal incisions for additional instrumentation. The aspirating apparatus consists of a Teflon-lined needle (single or double lumen, the latter for ease of flushing) with an internal diameter of 1 to 2.2 mm, designed to permit efficient evacuation of the follicles while minimizing trauma to the oocyte-cumulus complex, connected via sterile tubing to a Falcon tissue culture tube or trap. The trap contains a small volume of buffered culture medium to neutralize the effects of any aspirated carbon dioxide on the pH of the collected follicular fluid. The entire aspirating apparatus should be toxicity tested, generally with a mouse embryo system, to ensure nontoxicity to embryos. Suction is provided by the application of a negative pressure of 100 to 120 mm Hg to the trap, controlled either manually or via a foot pedal for ease of operation.

At the start of the procedure, the pelvis is quickly inspected. Increased cul-de-sac fluid, when noted, may indicate ovulation, and it should be promptly aspirated in an effort to retrieve the oocyte(s) before equilibration with the carbon dioxide gas phase. The ovaries are then stabilized with atraumatic forceps, either by grasping the utero-ovarian ligaments or by wedging the ovaries against the pelvic sidewall, with care to avoid follicular rupture. The aspirating needle may be inserted either through the operating channel of the laparoscope or through an accessory cannula. Follicle puncture is performed at an avascular site midway between the base and dome of the follicle, with the application of suction at the

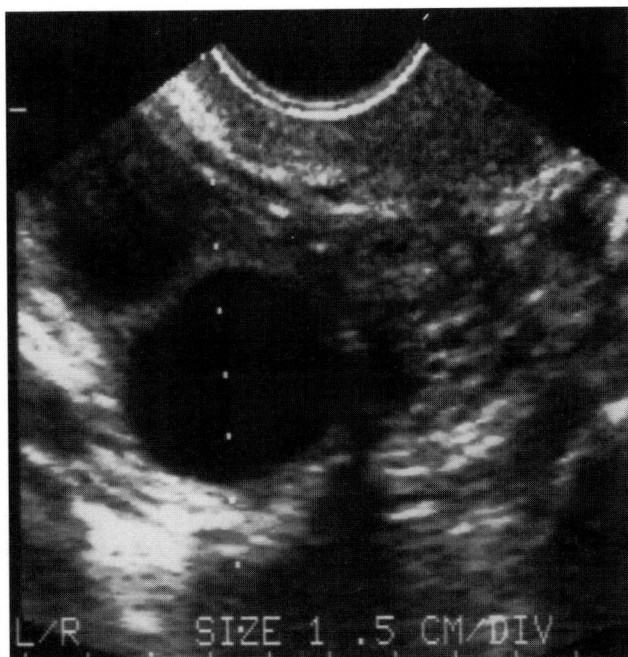

FIGURE 51–2. Sonographic image of follicle at oocyte recovery.

moment of puncture, to avoid excessive aspiration of carbon dioxide. There is no evidence that the carbon dioxide pneumoperitoneum affects the pH of *intact* follicles for up to 1 hour of exposure. The tip of the needle may be manipulated so as to "curette" the inner wall of the follicle as it collapses, to dislodge the oocyte. Following complete aspiration, the suction is cut off before withdrawing the needle from the follicle, again to minimize the aspiration of carbon dioxide. The system is then flushed with culture medium to recover any oocyte retained in the needle or tubing. The needle may be left in the follicle in case the oocyte is not identified in the initial aspirate, to facilitate flushing and reaspiration. All follicles are thus emptied, and the procedure is terminated.

Ultrasound-Guided Oocyte Retrieval

Ultrasound-guided follicle puncture was first described in 1981.[35] Abdominal or endovaginal sonography is performed, and the aspirating needle may be introduced into the ovary via the percutaneous-transvesical, transurethral-transvesical, or direct transvaginal route, either "freehand" or more commonly with a fixed needle guide. Transvaginal follicle aspiration using a transvaginal transducer was first reported in 1983,[36] and has become the dominant approach worldwide, essentially superseding laparoscopic oocyte harvest. The procedure is performed with the patient in the dorsal lithotomy position. Vaginal preparation consists of a wash with an antiseptic cleanser (e.g., povidone-iodine) followed by copious saline irrigation or saline lavage alone; although most antiseptics are toxic to oocytes/embryos, thorough vaginal lavage following application effectively eliminates detrimental effects. Although regional (e.g., epidural) or general anesthesia may be used, intravenous sedation/analgesia is adequate for most transvaginal egg retrievals. Although the efficacy of routine antibiotic prophylaxis has not been established, some

authors recommend its use;[37] although remarkably infrequent, postretrieval pelvic infection can be severe, occasionally resulting in adnexal abscess formation.[38]

The transvaginal ultrasound probe, which houses a high-frequency transducer (e.g., 7 MHz), is introduced into the vagina with an affixed needle guide. After a brief inspection of the pelvis, the follicles are located, and each is in turn aligned with the puncture line on the monitor screen (Fig. 51–2). The aspirating needle, the tip of which is machine-scored to enhance sonographic visibility, is advanced into the center of the follicle along the shortest path (Fig. 51–3). As with laparoscopic retrievals, a negative pressure of 100 to 120 mm Hg is applied to the needle at the instant of follicle puncture. Follicular collapse is readily visualized on the monitor, and the needle may be used to curette the follicle. An effort is made to align several follicles in the same plane so as to minimize the number of needle insertions through the vaginal wall and into the ovary. As each follicle is emptied, the needle may be advanced into the next follicle, removed and flushed with medium to recover any oocyte(s) retained in the line or kept in place for possible flushing and reaspiration of the follicle should an oocyte not be identified in the follicular fluid. In cases in which an increased volume of cul-de-sac fluid is observed, especially if egg recovery is low, peritoneal fluid may be aspirated to look for additional oocytes.

Ultrasound-directed oocyte recovery has all but replaced laparoscopic procedures owing to a number of significant advantages: (1) Oocytes may be easily retrieved in cases in which the ovaries may be inaccessible to the laparoscope owing to severe pelvic adhesions, (2) transvaginal follicle puncture has lower potential morbidity and a decreased recovery time, (3) general anesthesia is not required, (4) oper-

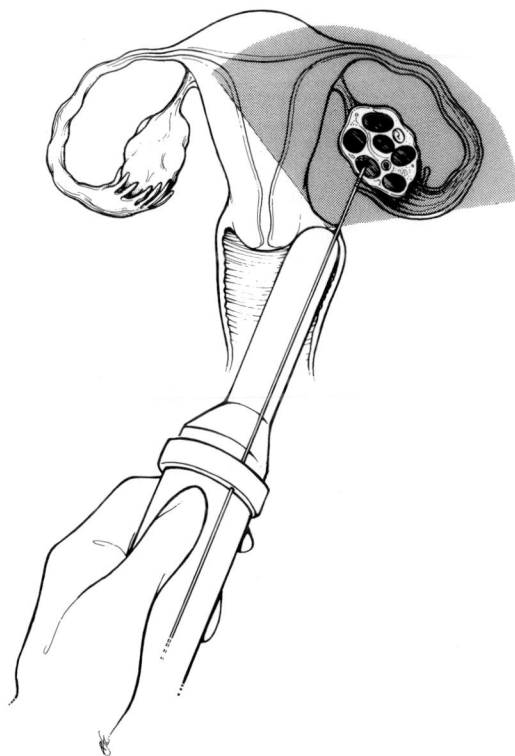

FIGURE 51–3. Ultrasound-guided transvaginal aspiration.

ative time is reduced, and (5) a carbon dioxide pneumoperitoneum is unnecessary, eliminating concerns regarding changes in follicular pH. Laparoscopy, however, remains the dominant technique in ART procedures entailing tubal cannulation (GIFT, ZIFT), may be useful in cases in which ART is programmed to coincide with a diagnostic pelviscopy, and may rarely be necessary in the event of a failed transvaginal procedure (e.g., in a woman with highly mobile ovaries).

CLASSIFICATION OF OOCYTE MATURITY

The determination of oocyte maturity by the embryologist is imperative because it allows the calculation of an appropriate preinsemination interval for each egg. Further, this classification permits improved timing of hCG administration in future cycles, especially in cases in which predominantly immature or postmature/atretic oocytes are recovered.

Oocyte evaluation is performed with a dissecting or inverted microscope. Grading is based on the appearance of the oocyte-corona-cumulus complex, including specific characteristics, such as the degree of mucification and dispersal of the corona radiata and cumulus and the presence or absence of the nuclear membrane (germinal vesicle) or first polar body. A mature oocyte manifests extensive dispersal of the surrounding granulosa cells with an expanded cumulus and corona radiata. The zona pellucida is distinct, and the ooplasm is clear. Identification of the first polar body documents that an oocyte is in metaphase II. An intermediate oocyte displays a slightly more dense corona and a dispersed cumulus but lacks both a nuclear membrane and polar body (metaphase I). An immature ovum is surrounded by a compact corona and only a few cell layers in the cumulus. A grossly immature oocyte manifests an intact germinal vesicle. The presence of a dark, irregular ooplasm is characteristic of an atretic oocyte. Nuclear grading may refine the assessment provided by simple inspection of the oocyte's investments but generally requires mechanical or enzymatic stripping of the cumulus and corona to visualize the ooplasm better.

Preovulatory oocytes are preincubated for 2 to 8 hours before insemination; immediate insemination yields lower fertilization rates. Oocytes of intermediate maturity may benefit from 12 to 24 hours of preincubation and immature oocytes from 22 to 36 hours of in vitro maturation.

OOCYTE INSEMINATION AND CULTURE

Rigorous quality control is essential to the operation of a successful IVF laboratory. Instruments, media, and plasticware must all be regularly tested for potential embryo toxicity, usually by means of a two- to four-cell mouse embryo assay. This discussion provides a broad overview of insemination and culture procedures used in the IVF process; details of these techniques vary between programs.

The male partner produces a semen sample just before or shortly after the oocyte retrieval. The ejaculate may be obtained in a sterile plastic jar by masturbation or occasionally by means of a Silastic condom. In cases in which situational impotence or anejaculation are anticipated, it is advisable to cryopreserve one or more samples in advance of the actual

ART procedure in the event that a fresh sperm sample is not obtainable. If the male partner harbors known antisperm antibodies in his seminal fluid, ejaculation directly into culture medium may decrease sperm binding.

The semen is first allowed to liquify at room temperature, which takes approximately 30 minutes. The sample is then washed to remove the seminal plasma; the semen is diluted with insemination medium containing 7.5% to 10% heat-inactivated serum or other protein source. The mixture is centrifuged, the supernatant is discarded, and the sperm pellet is resuspended in fresh medium. The wash is generally performed twice. One or more sperm separation procedures are then performed in an effort to enhance the quality of the sample. One technique is the sperm "swim-up," which consists of layering medium over the sperm pellet and allowing the actively motile sperm to rise into the medium over 30 to 60 minutes; the highly motile fraction is then pipetted off. Sperm may also be separated by means of Percoll gradient centrifugation. In selected cases, the addition of a chemical agent, such as pentoxifylline, may enhance sperm motility in vitro.

The sperm sample is subsequently incubated at 37°C in 5% carbon dioxide for approximately 1 hour. The incubation of sperm and oocytes is generally performed in Falcon culture dishes in a suitable medium such as Earl's Balanced Salt Solution or Human Tubal Fluid supplemented with a protein source, that is, maternal serum, fetal cord serum, or a commercial preparation such as Plasmanate. Maternal serum should be avoided in cases of a female immunologic factor (circulating antisperm antibodies). We prefer gamete coincubation in droplets of culture medium under sterile mineral oil, which provides a stable, consistent microenvironment. Following an interval of preincubation appropriate to their degree of maturity, the oocytes are then inseminated with a density of approximately 150,000 motile sperm per egg. In male factor cases, the concentration of added sperm may be increased to as high as 500,000/oocyte to enhance the probability of fertilization. The remaining sperm may be saved in an incubator for subsequent insemination of the less mature oocytes or for reinsemination procedures in the event of failed fertilization (in our experience, however, implantation and ongoing pregnancy rates appear to be reduced following the transfer of reinsemination-fertilized oocytes).

The gametes are coincubated in the fertilization medium for 12 to 18 hours in an incubator that maintains a temperature of 37°C in an atmosphere containing 5% carbon dioxide and a relative humidity of 98%. The embryologist examines the oocytes after this interval to check for fertilization, which is evidenced by the identification of two pronuclei (male and female) or extrusion of the second polar body. It is at the pronuclear stage that possible polyspermic fertilization can be documented (fertilization by more than one sperm), marked by the presence of more than 2 pronuclei; a polyploid embryo might otherwise escape detection and may cleave normally. The incidence of polyspermy following fertilization of zona-intact oocytes is approximately 10% and may be attributable to excessive sperm density or oocyte postmaturity or immaturity. When the zona pellucida is breached by one of the newer microsurgical fertilization techniques (discussed subsequently), the incidence of polyspermy is significantly increased.[39] Overall fertilization rates exceed 80% for mature oocytes but are typically reduced to

50% to 60% for immature oocytes and may be further compromised in male factor cases. More than 85% of fertilized oocytes subsequently cleave.

The resulting embryos are transferred to growth medium containing a higher concentration of serum or other protein source (10% to 20%) and are incubated for another 24 to 60 hours before transfer. Healthy embryos cleave to the four- to eight-cell stage 36 to 48 hours after insemination; however, normal pregnancies can follow the transfer of slowly dividing embryos. Embryo "quality" is assessed, before replacement by the application of morphologic criteria, including symmetry and shape of the blastomeres, extent of cytoplasmic fragmentation, and cell number. It has been proposed that the percentage variation in zona thickness is predictive of implantation rates,[40] and this finding has, in part, led to the development of assisted hatching (see later). Prediction of embryonic viability remains an inexact science, however, despite refinements in embryo grading, including the use of videocinematography; "poor-quality" embryos may implant and result in healthy offspring.

Zona Micromanipulation

Severe sperm abnormalities may preclude fertilization with conventional IVF. Microsurgical techniques aimed at assisting the fertilization process have therefore been developed and have proved effective even with sperm concentrations under 1×10^6 and in cases of prior fertilization failure. Oocyte micromanipulation enables sperm to traverse the barrier posed by the zona pellucida.

The least invasive microfertilization technique facilitates the entrance of sperm into the perivitelline space via the creation of a physical gap in the zona. This gap may be chemically "drilled" with acidic Tyrode's solution[41] or mechanically incised. The most successful variant of this procedure is partial zona dissection (PZD), a technique that led to the first human pregnancies following microsurgical fertilization.[42] This mechanical approach has the advantage of avoiding the deleterious effects of exposing the oocyte to an acidic solution. The oocyte is first shrunk away from the zona pellucida in an hyperosmolar sucrose solution, to minimize the likelihood of trauma to the oolemma. Using a micromanipulator, the oocyte is then stabilized with a suction micropipette, and a glass microneedle is used to incise the zona surgically. The incidence of oocyte injury following PZD is under 4%. The zona-dissected oocyte is then inseminated using routine IVF procedures.

An alternative microfertilization technique entails the direct insertion of sperm beneath the zona (subzonal insertion).[43] This method can be applied in cases of marked oligospermia or asthenospermia because only a few motile sperm are required for each oocyte. Successful PZD requires a relatively greater motile sperm density because the sperm have to "find" and traverse the gap in the zona.

The most invasive, and newest, technique is intracytoplasmic sperm injection, which involves the direct microinjection of a single, immobilized sperm into the ooplasm. Increasing experience with this procedure has demonstrated efficacy even in the most severe male factor cases, with a negligible incidence of polyspermy.

There are several risks inherent in oocyte micromanipula-

tion. The most significant is an increase in polyspermic fertilization rates, particularly following PZD or subzonal insertion. The zona pellucida is the principal block to polyspermy, and techniques that breach the zona tend to undermine this protective function. The rate of polyspermic fertilization is less than 10% following insemination of zona-intact eggs but rises to 25% following PZD for male factor. Enucleation procedures have been developed to remove supernumerary male pronuclei,[44] but these techniques will not be clinically useful until a reliable method for distinguishing paternal from maternal pronuclei is realized.[45] Other potential risks of zona micromanipulation include the extrusion and loss of blastomeres through large holes and the invasion of the embryos by bacteria or inflammatory cells. Cohen and associates[46] demonstrated that the administration of a brief course of oral antibiotics and a glucocorticoid (methylprednisolone) in the peritransfer period enhances the implantation rates of zona-manipulated embryos, and this is a component of our standard protocol.

A novel and promising application of zona micromanipulation has been the development of assisted hatching of embryos before replacement, in an effort to improve implantation rates.[47] Based on the observations that (1) embryos displaying reduced zona thickness implanted more frequently than those with thick zonae[40] and (2) microsurgically fertilized embryos with gaps in their zonae have higher implantation rates than zona-intact embryos, Cohen and coworkers[46] surmised that otherwise viable embryos with thick zonae might fail to hatch in utero, which is a prerequisite for blastocyst implantation. In the first prospective, randomized clinical trial of assisted hatching, replacement of zona-intact embryos was compared with transfer of embryos with gaps created via PZD; per embryo implantation rates were significantly improved in the hatched group (22% versus 13% in the controls).[48] This technique has since been modified by the use of zona drilling with acid Tyrode's solution to permit the creation of larger holes in the zonae. Randomized, controlled trials at Cornell have shown that assisted hatching is most helpful when selectively applied to embryos demonstrating thick zonae (>15 μm) and in women older than 38 years.[49] This latter finding suggests that advanced biologic age may impart physical or chemical changes in the zona, thus decreasing the efficiency of implantation.

EMBRYO TRANSFER

Embryo replacement can be successfully performed anywhere from 1 to 3 days following oocyte harvest, with embryos ranging from the 1- to 12-cell stage. Pronuclear stage embryos are generally replaced in tubal transfer procedures (e.g., ZIFT).

Success rates improve as the number of embryos transferred is increased; beyond three to four embryos, however, the risk of multiple gestation can increase sharply, particularly in younger women (<34 years). The number of transferred embryos is therefore restricted, permitting cryopreservation of "excess" embryos for future use.

Except in cases of tubal cannulation, ET is a nonsurgical, transcervical technique. A number of different transfer catheters are commercially available. They are manufactured with nontoxic plastic and differ with respect to length, caliber (generally 3.5 to 5 French), location of the distal port (end versus side loading), and degree of stiffness and memory. Some catheters are designed for direct insertion through the cervix, whereas others include a rigid introducer or outer sheath.

The patient is usually positioned in the dorsal lithotomy position for ET, although some programs use the knee-chest position for women with an anteverted uterus. There is no evidence that positioning per se affects outcome. A sterile speculum is inserted into the vagina, and the cervix is thoroughly cleansed with culture medium to remove excess cervical mucus and vaginal discharge (Fig. 51–4). When difficulty is encountered in negotiating the cervical canal, different maneuvers may be attempted, including the use of a more rigid catheter or an introducer sheath, readjusting the speculum or the patient's position, and application of a tenaculum to straighten the uterine axis.

In the adjacent embryology laboratory, the embryos are then loaded together into a sterile transfer catheter in a small volume of transfer medium (20 to 50 μL), containing a relatively high concentration of serum or other protein source (up to 50% to 75%). The catheter is often marked at a length approximately 1 to 2 cm short of the depth of the patient's uterine cavity, as previously determined by sounding in the office.

The loaded catheter is then delivered to the physician, who threads it atraumatically through the cervix and toward the uterine fundus; the embryos are gently injected using a small (e.g., tuberculin) syringe attached to the proximal end of the catheter. Care is taken to minimize the possibility of endometrial trauma at the time of transfer because even small amounts of fresh bleeding appear to reduce pregnancy rates.[50] After the transfer, the catheter is returned to the embryologist for inspection under a dissecting microscope and flushing with medium in an attempt to identify any retained embryos. If retained embryos are found, they are reloaded and replaced; this does not appear to reduce implantation rates significantly if performed atraumatically.[50] If the catheter is clean, the patient is transferred to a holding area, where she remains recumbent, generally for a period of at least 30 minutes, before discharge.

MANAGEMENT OF THE LUTEAL PHASE

Monitoring of the luteal phase may be limited to a single serum β-hCG determination 2 weeks after oocyte retrieval (exogenous hCG from the preretrieval injection is usually cleared within 9 days). Some centers subscribe to a more intensive protocol of luteal surveillance, including serial assay of E_2, P_4, and β-hCG concentrations. The absolute values and patterns of luteal hormone levels can be predictive of outcome because serum E_2 and P_4 values exhibit a significant rise in the late luteal phase of conception cycles. Indeed, one report suggests that luteal phase E_2 patterns may be more predictive of pregnancy viability than β-hCG levels.[51]

Although the importance of natural cycle luteal phase defect as a cause of infertility has been questioned by the finding of a similar histologic incidence in fertile women who underwent serial biopsies,[52] exogenous luteal support in ART cycles is the general practice owing to concerns that ovarian hyperstimulation may lead to a suboptimal, nonphysiologic endocrine milieu. Nonetheless, although most clinicians agree that luteal support is necessary in GnRH agonist cycles, it remains to be established whether routine, empiric supplementation is advantageous when GnRH agonists are not used. The rationale for luteal support derives from evidence that the incidence of luteal insufficiency is increased in women treated with ovulation-inducing agents[53] and concerns that the act of follicular aspiration may disrupt a sufficient volume of granulosa cells to impair luteal steroidogenesis. The latter contention would appear doubtful because

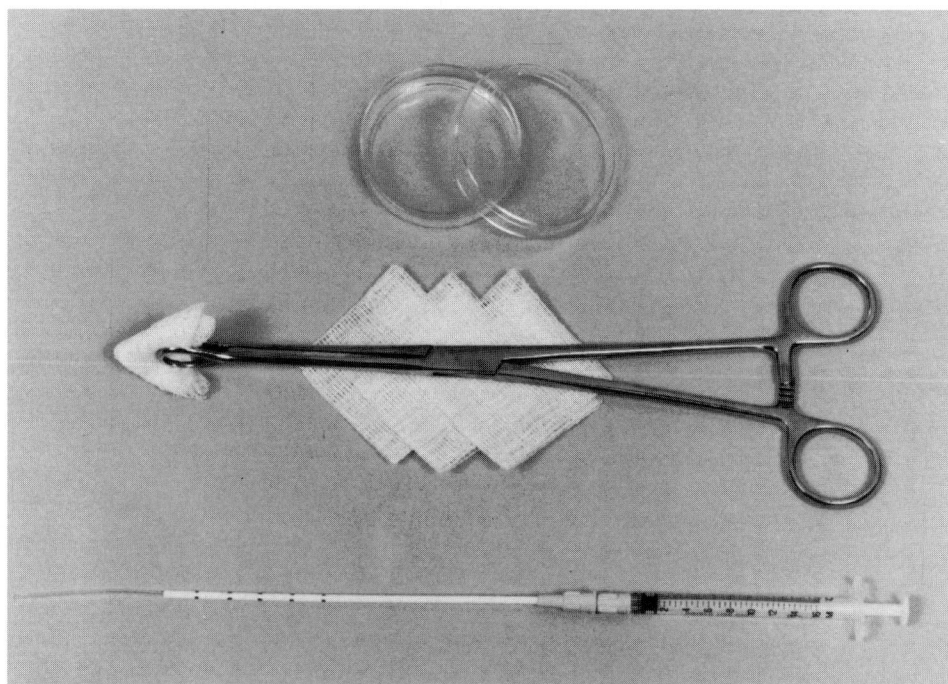

FIGURE 51–4. Setup for transcervical embryo transfer.

peak luteal E_2 and P_4 levels following IVF tend to exceed significantly those seen in the natural cycle, owing to the presence of multiple corpora lutea. One study described a high incidence of histologic luteal phase defect in canceled IVF cycles,[54] although this may not be entirely representative of more satisfactory stimulation cycles that culminate in ET.

Exogenous progesterone supplementation is usually initiated on the day following oocyte recovery. Progesterone may be administered intramuscularly, via vaginal suppositories, or less commonly in oral capsules. We favor intramuscular progesterone in oil, 25 to 50 mg/day, the higher dose for patients with markedly elevated peak follicular phase E_2 levels (>1500 to 2000 pg/mL), in an effort to promote a more physiologic luteal P_4 to E_2 ratio. Some programs support the luteal phase with additional injections of hCG, but this approach may increase the risk of developing OHSS.[55]

After a successful IVF-ET cycle, pregnancy is initially documented by a positive hCG titer 12 to 14 days after retrieval. Serial hCG measurements are performed subsequently, to document a reassuring rate of rise (doubling time of approximately 36 to 48 hours). Endovaginal sonography is performed 4 to 5 weeks after retrieval to demonstrate viability (fetal heart motion) and single versus multiple gestation. An abnormal rise in hCG titer or high-risk history for ectopic pregnancy may prompt earlier sonographic evaluation; in a normal pregnancy, an intrauterine sac can usually be discerned by vaginal ultrasonography once the β-hCG level reaches approximately 1000 mIU/mL (2nd International Standard hCG). Luteal support is discontinued once fetal heart activity is seen.

PREGNANCY OUTCOME FOLLOWING IN VITRO FERTILIZATION

Any discussion of IVF outcome and success rates mandates a strict definition of terms. A *pregnancy* can refer to anything from an early preclinical loss to a live delivery. The term *biochemical* pregnancy refers to implantation identified by the transient production of hCG, with early abortion before sonographic documentation. A *clinical* pregnancy progresses, at a minimum, to a stage where the gestational sac and fetal heart motion can be visualized. At any given point in time, *ongoing* pregnancies are comprised of currently viable gestations and successfully delivered neonates. Just as the numerator in a *success rate* requires strict definition, so to does the denominator. Pregnancy rates may be expressed per stimulation commenced, per egg retrieval, or per embryo transfer. We recommend that success rates be expressed as deliveries (or ongoing pregnancies) per transfer or retrieval but believe that per embryo implantation rates are most useful for rigorous comparison of specific techniques.

The 1991 U.S. IVF-ET Registry (215 clinics) recorded overall clinical pregnancy (intrauterine sac[s] documented by ultrasonography) and delivery rates of 19.1% and 15.25% following 20,914 oocyte retrieval procedures.[2] IVF efficiency can perhaps be more rigorously assessed by calculating per embryo implantation rates, a more accurate reflection of the quality of a given unit's methodology.

Overall, 20% of clinical IVF pregnancies are lost, most as first-trimester spontaneous abortions. In women over 40 years of age, this figure can exceed 50%. These pregnancy wastage rates exceed those following spontaneous conceptions in the general population and may be secondary to an adverse effect of supraphysiologic E_2 and E_2-to-P_4 ratios on endometrial development, an increased incidence of genetically abnormal oocytes and embryos following COH, or simply close surveillance of an inherently higher risk population. The 1991 IVF-ET Registry reported a 5.5% ectopic pregnancy rate,[2] which exceeds the 1% risk in the general population. The incidence of heterotopic gestations following IVF far exceeds the 1:30,000 risk in spontaneous pregnancies, owing to the transfer of multiple embryos.[56] Cervical[57] and abdominal[58] pregnancies have also been reported following IVF. A high index of suspicion coupled with early sonographic evaluation is therefore warranted in all pregnancies following ART.[59]

The most commonly encountered complication of IVF-ET is multiple gestation. According to the 1991 U.S. Registry, 30% of deliveries following IVF were multiple; 25% were twins, 4.8% triplets, and 0.2% higher-order multiple gestations.[2] Multifetal pregnancies pose a significantly increased risk of preterm labor and delivery, with the potential for serious sequelae in the offspring. This risk is greatest for high-order multiple gestations; the average length of gestation for triplets and quadruplets is 33 and 29 weeks.[60] Ultrasound-guided transabdominal multifetal pregnancy reduction offers an alternative to couples with high-order multiple gestations.[61]

Infants born after ART appear not to be at increased risk for congenital malformations or other perinatal morbidity, when controlling for maternal age and multifetal pregnancies, as compared with spontaneously conceived children. Although the 1991 U.S. IVF-ET Registry cited an incidence of 1.5 congenital defects per 100 neonates, incomplete reporting (owing in part to lack of follow-up) limits the validity of this figure.[2]

EMBRYO CRYOPRESERVATION

The first human pregnancy following transfer of a cryopreserved and thawed embryo was reported by Trounsen and colleagues[62] in 1983. Once novel, this technology has become fully integrated into the standard practice of IVF.

Embryo cryopreservation was developed in response to the potentially large numbers of oocytes and embryos that result from multifollicular stimulation. "Excess" embryos were previously either discarded, which was inefficient at the very least, or transferred with the attendant risk of high-order multiple gestation; selective insemination of only a portion of recovered oocytes could not insure an adequate number of embryos for transfer and wasted normal oocytes. The ability to cryopreserve and store embryos permits the insemination of all retrieved eggs, thus maximizing the probability of obtaining an optimal number of concepti for replacement in the same cycle, with the option of banking excess embryos for transfer in a future natural cycle. In successful units, embryo cryopreservation improves the efficiency of IVF, increasing the cumulative pregnancy rate per oocyte retrieval procedure.[63]

Human embryos can be frozen at virtually any developmental stage, from zygote (pronuclear) to blastocyst. Specific freezing and thawing protocols vary according to embryonic stage. Cellular dehydration is required, to minimize damage that can result from intracellular ice crystal formation during freezing and thawing. Cryoprotectants are agents used to replace cellular water, thus protecting the embryos from the potentially lethal effects of freezing. The choice of a particular cryoprotectant is dictated by the embryonic stage, owing to differences in cell membrane permeability. Propanediol is generally used for pronuclear and two-cell embryos, dimethyl sulfoxide (DMSO) for 4- to 12-cell embryos, and glycerol for blastocyts. The cryoprotectant is added, usually at room temperature, by pipetting the embryos through gradually increasing concentrations of the agent. The embryos are then sealed, either in glass ampules or plastic straws, and cooled to a relatively high subzero temperature for seeding (crystallization). The temperature is slowly reduced at a closely regulated rate in a controlled biologic freezer (capable of cooling in increments of 0.1 to 0.5°C per minute), cooling the embryos to a temperature of between −30°C to −80°C before they are plunged into liquid nitrogen (−196°C). Thawing, in essence, reverses this process. The embryos are gradually warmed and rehydrated and are then cultured for an interval before transfer.

Transfer of thawed embryos is usually performed in the natural cycle; synchronization of embryonic and endometrial "age" is achieved with close monitoring of serum or urine LH levels to pinpoint ovulation. Anovulatory women may be treated with ovulation-inducing agents to permit transfer of thawed embryos. As an alternative, ovarian function can be suppressed with a GnRH agonist and endometrial maturation stimulated with an exogenously administered regimen of estrogen and progesterone, similar to that used in donor egg IVF.

Approximately 50% to 70% of thawed cryopreserved embryos survive the process. In general, only those embryos retaining at least half of their original blastomeres are transferred. Success rates after replacement of thawed embryos improve with increasing numbers of embryos frozen, with decreasing degree of cytoplasmic fragmentation and if a pregnancy resulted from a "fresh" transfer of sibling embryos in the original treatment cycle. A major morphologic determinant of improved prognosis in thawed embryos is cell-to-cell adherence; poor cell-to-cell adherence correlates with reduced implantation rates.[64] Of the 4225 thawed ET procedures recorded in the 1991 U.S. IVF-ET Registry, the clinical pregnancy and delivery rates were 13.2% and 10.2%.[2] In some series, implantation rates of as high as 14% to 15% per thawed, replaced embryo have been reported.[65]

The world experience with cryopreservation of human oocytes has been considerably more limited, with only a few reported pregnancies.[66] Oocyte freezing techniques are analogous to those used in embryo cryopreservation. One major concern with oocyte freezing is the risk of microtubule depolymerization, which could result in damage to the mitotic spindle. Such injury could cause chromatid nondisjunction at the time of fertilization, resulting in aneuploidy. Research in this area is therefore proceeding with caution.

Cryopreservation technology is not limited to the storage of "excess" embryos, however. Embryo freezing can be used as an adjunct to GIFT procedures (if simultaneous IVF is performed), permitting future embryo replacement. Frozen embryos can be used to facilitate synchronization in donor egg IVF. In addition, women requiring chemotherapy or radiation for malignant neoplasia may elect to undergo pretreatment IVF with embryo cryopreservation, given their high risk for iatrogenic ovarian failure.

REFERENCES

1. Steptoe PC, Edwards RG. Birth after reimplantation of a human embryo. Lancet 1978;2:366.
2. Society for Assisted Reproductive Technology, The American Fertility Society. Assisted reproductive technology in the United States and Canada: 1991 results from the Society for Assisted Reproductive Technology generated from The American Fertility Society Registry. Fertil Steril 1993;59:956.
3. Feldberg D, Davis O, Grifo J, et al. Severity of endometriosis does not impact on pregnancy success after in vitro fertilization. Presented at the 7th World Congress on In Vitro Fertilization and Assisted Procreation, Paris, 1991:264.
4. Kruger TF, Acosta AA, Simmons KF, et al. Predictive value of abnormal sperm morphology in in vitro fertilization. Fertil Steril 1988;49:112.
5. van Uem JFHM, Acosta AA, Swanson RG, et al. Male factor evaluation in in vitro fertilization: Norfolk experience. Fertil Steril 1985;44:375.
6. Sanger WG, Armitage JO, Schmidt MA. Feasibility of semen cryopreservation in patients with malignant disease. JAMA 1980;244:789.
7. Davis OK, Bedford JM, Berkeley AS, et al. Pregnancy achieved through in vitro fertilization with cryopreserved sperm from a man with Hodgkin's lymphoma. Fertil Steril 1990;53:377.
8. Rowland GF, Cohen J, Steptoe PC, Hewitt J. Pregnancy following in vitro fertilization using cryopreserved semen from a man with testicular teratoma. Urology 1985;26:33.
9. Dodson WC, Whitesides DB, Hughes CL, et al. Superovulation with intrauterine insemination in the treatment of infertility: a possible alternative to gamete intrafallopian transfer and in vitro fertilization. Fertil Steril 1987;48:441.
10. Muasher SJ, Garcia JE, Jones HW. Experience with diethylstilbestrol-exposed infertile women in a program of in vitro fertilization. Fertil Steril 1984;42:20.
11. Romeu A, Muasher SJ, Acosta AA, et al. Results of in vitro fertilization attempts in women 40 years of age and older: the Norfolk experience. Fertil Steril 1987;47:130.
12. Sauer MV, Paulson RJ, Lobo RA. A preliminary report on oocyte donation extending reproductive potential to women over 40. N Engl J Med 1990;323:1157.
13. Scott RT, Toner JP, Muasher SJ, et al. Follicle-stimulating hormone levels on cycle day 3 are predictive of in vitro fertilization outcome. Fertil Steril 1989;51:651.
14. Licciardi FL, Liu H-C, Berkeley AS, et al. Day 3 estradiol levels as prognosticators of pregnancy outcome in in vitro fertilization, both alone and in conjunction with day 3 FSH levels. Presented at the 38th Annual Meeting of the Society for Gynecologic Investigation, San Antonio, 1991:169.
15. Navot D, Rosenwaks Z, Margolioth EJ. Prognostic assessment of female fecundity. Lancet 1987;2:645.
16. Jones GS. Update in in vitro fertilization. Endocr Rev 1984;5:62.
17. Abbasi R, Kenigsberg D, Danforth D, et al. Cumulative ovulation in human menopausal gonadotropin/human chorionic gonadotropin-treated monkeys: 'step-up' versus 'step-down' dose regimens. Fertil Steril 1987;47:1019.
18. Rosenwaks Z, Muasher SJ, Acosta AA. Use of hMG and/or FSH for multiple follicle development. Clin Obstet Gynecol 1986;29:148.
19. Shaw RW, Ndukwe G, Imoedemhe D, et al. Stimulation of multiple follicular growth for in vitro fertilization by administration of pulsatile luteinizing hormone-releasing hormone during the midfollicular phase. Fertil Steril 1986;46:135.
20. Meldrum DR, Wisot A, Hamilton F, et al. Routine pituitary suppression with leuprolide before ovarian stimulation for oocyte retrieval. Fertil Steril 1989;51:455.
21. Hughes EG, Fedorkow DM, Daya S, et al. The routine use of gonadotropin-releasing hormone agonists prior to in vitro fertilization and gamete intrafallopian transfer: a meta-analysis of randomized controlled trials. Fertil Steril 1992;58:888.
22. Liu H-C, Lai Y-M, Davis O, et al. Improved pregnancy outcome with gonadotropin releasing hormone agonist (GnRH-a) stimulation is due to the improvement in oocyte quantity rather than quality. J Assisted Reprod Genet 1992;9:338.

23. Garcia JE, Padilla SL, Bayati J, Baramki TA. Follicular phase gonadotropin-releasing hormone agonist and human gonadotropins: a better alternative for ovulation induction in in vitro fertilization. Fertil Steril 1990;53:302.
24. Ron-El R, Herman A, Golan A, et al. Follicle cyst formation following long-acting gonadotropin-releasing hormone analog administration. Fertil Steril 1989;52:1063.
25. Meyer WR, Lavy G, DeCherney AH, et al. Evidence of gonadal and gonadotropin antibodies in women with a suboptimal ovarian response to exogenous gonadotropin. Obstet Gynecol 1990;75:795.
26. Karande VC, Jones GS, Veeck LL, Muasher SJ. High-dose follicle-stimulating hormone stimulation at the onset of the menstrual cycle does not improve the in vitro fertilization outcome in low-responder patients. Fertil Steril 1990;53:486.
27. Homburg R, Eshel A, Abdalla HI, et al. Growth hormone facilitates ovulation induction by gonadotropins. Clin Endocrinol 1988;29:113.
28. Shaker AG, Fleming R, Jamieson ME, et al. Absence of effect of adjuvant growth hormone therapy on follicular responses to exogenous gonadotropins in women: normal and poor responders. Fertil Steril 1992;58:919.
29. Scott RT, Rosenwaks Z: Ovulation induction for assisted reproduction. J Reprod Med 1989;34:1.
30. Tanbo T, Dale PO, Kjekshus E, et al. Stimulation with human menopausal gonadotropin versus follicle-stimulating hormone after pituitary suppression in polycystic ovarian syndrome. Fertil Steril 1990;53:798.
31. Paulson RJ, Sauer MV, Lobo RA. Embryo implantation after human in vitro fertilization: importance of endometrial receptivity. Fertil Steril 1990;53:870.
32. Whittemore AS, Harris R, Itnyre J, The Collaborative Ovarian Cancer Group. Characteristics relating to ovarian cancer risk: collaborative analysis of twelve U.S. case-control studies. II. Invasive epithelial ovarian cancers in white women. Am J Epidemiol 1992;136:1184.
33. Paulson RJ, Sauer MV, Francis MM, et al. In vitro fertilization in unstimulated cycles: the University of Southern California experience. Fertil Steril 1992;57:290.
34. Taymor ML, Ranoux CJ, Gross GL. Natural oocyte retrieval with intravaginal fertilization: a simplified approach to in vitro fertilization. Obstet Gynecol 1992;80:888.
35. Lenz S, Lauritsen G, Kjellow M. Collection of human oocytes for IVF by ultrasonically guided follicular puncture. Lancet 1981;1:1163.
36. Gleicher N, Friberg J, Fullan N, et al. Egg retrieval for in-vitro fertilization by sonographically controlled vaginal culdocentesis. Lancet 1983;2:508.
37. Meldrum DR. Antibiotics for vaginal oocyte aspiration [editorial]. J In Vitro Fert Embryo Transf 1989;6:1.
38. Howe RS, Wheller C, Mastroianni LJ, et al. Pelvic infection after transvaginal ultrasound-guided ovum retrieval. Fertil Steril 1988;49:726.
39. Cohen J, Malter H, Talansky B, et al. Gamete and embryo micromanipulation for infertility treatment. Semin Reprod Endocrinol 1990;8:290.
40. Cohen J, Inge KL, Suzman M, et al. Videocinematography of fresh and cryopreserved embryos: a retrospective analysis of embryonic morphology and implantation. Fertil Steril 1989;51:820.
41. Gordon JW, Talansky BE. Assisted fertilization by zona drilling: a mouse model for correction of oligospermia. J Exp Zool 1986;239:347.
42. Cohen J, Malter H, Fehilly C, et al. Implantation of embryos after partial opening of oocyte zona pellucida to facilitate sperm penetration. Lancet 1988;2:162.
43. Ng SC, Bongso TA, Ratman SS, et al. Pregnancy after transfer of multiple sperm under the zona. Lancet 1988;2:790.
44. Malter HE, Cohen J. Embryonic development after microsurgical repair of polyspermic human zygotes. Fertil Steril 1989;52:373.
45. Wiker S, Malter HE, Wright G, et al. Recognition of paternal pronuclei in human zygotes. J In Vitro Fert Embryo Transf 1990;7:33.
46. Cohen J, Malter H, Elsner C, et al. Immunosuppression supports implantation of zona pellucida-dissected human embryos. Fertil Steril 1990;53:662.
47. Cohen J. Assisted hatching of human embryos. J In Vitro Fert Embryo Transf 1991;8:179.
48. Cohen J, Wright G, Malter H, et al. Impairment of the hatching process following IVF in the human and improvement of implantation by assisting hatching using micromanipulation. Hum Reprod 1990;5:7.
49. Cohen J, Alikani M, Trowbridge J, et al. Implantation enhancement by selective assisted hatching using zona drilling of human embryos with poor prognosis. Hum Reprod 1992;7:685.
50. Leonard G, Berkeley A, Alikani M, et al. Difficulty of embryo transfer and IVF pregnancy outcome. Presented at the 7th World Congress on In Vitro Fertilization and Assisted Procreation, Paris, 1991:394.
51. Liu H-C, Davis O, Berkeley A, et al. Late luteal estradiol patterns are a better prognosticator of pregnancy outcome than serial beta-human chorionic gonadotropin concentrations. Fertil Steril 1991;56:421.
52. Davis OK, Berkeley AS, Naus GJ, et al. The incidence of luteal phase defect in normal fertile women determined by serial endometrial biopsies. Fertil Steril 1989;51:582.
53. Kubik CJ: Luteal phase dysfunction following ovulation induction. Semin Reprod Endocrinol 1986;4:293.
54. Graf MJ, Reyniak JV, Battle-Mutter P, et al. Histologic evaluation of the luteal phase in women following follicle aspiration for oocyte retrieval. Fertil Steril 1988;49:616.
55. Herman A, Ron-El R, Golan A, et al. Pregnancy rate and ovarian hyperstimulation after luteal human chorionic gonadotropin in in vitro fertilization stimulated with gonadotropin-releasing hormone analog and menotropins. Fertil Steril 1990;53:92.
56. Dimitry ES, Subak-Sharpe R, Mills M, et al. Nine cases of heterotopic pregnancies in 4 years of in vitro fertilization. Fertil Steril 1990;53:107.
57. Bayati J, Garcia JE, Dorsey JH, Padilla SL. Combined intrauterine and cervical pregnancy from in vitro fertilization and embryo transfer. Fertil Steril 1989;51:725.
58. Oehninger S, Kreiner D, Bass MJ, et al. Abdominal pregnancy after in vitro fertilization and embryo transfer. Obstet Gynecol 1988;72:499.
59. Rein MS, DiSalvo DN, Friedman AJ. Heterotopic pregnancy associated with in vitro fertilization and embryo transfer: a possible role for routine vaginal ultrasound. Fertil Steril 1989;51:1057.
60. Caspi E, Romen J, Schreyer P, et al. The outcome of pregnancy after gonadotropin therapy. Br J Obstet Gynaecol 1976;83:967.
61. Lynch L, Berkowitz RL, Chitkara U, et al. First-trimester transabdominal multifetal pregnancy reduction: a report of 85 cases. Obstet Gynecol 1990;75:735.
62. Trounsen AO, Mohr L. Human pregnancy following cryopreservation, thawing and transfer of an eight-cell embryo. Nature 1983;305:707.
63. Cohen J, DeVane GH, Elsner CW, et al. Cryopreservation of zygotes and early cleaved human embryos. Fertil Steril 1988;49:283.
64. Cohen J, Wiemer KE, Wright G. Prognostic value of morphologic characteristics of cryopreserved embryos: a study using videocinematography. Fertil Steril 1988;49:827.
65. Wright G, Wiker S, Elsner C, et al. Observations on the morphology of pronuclei and nucleoli in human zygotes and implications for cryopreservation. Hum Reprod 1990;5:109.
66. Chen C. Pregnancy after human oocyte cryopreservation. Lancet 1986;1:884.

CHAPTER 52

Gamete Intrafallopian Transfer

JOSE P. BALMACEDA, ALEJANDRO MANZUR, and
RICARDO H. ASCH

PHYSIOLOGIC BASES

In human reproduction, the fallopian tubes have three well-recognized functions that, chronologically, are as follows: (1) ovum pickup, (2) site of fertilization, and (3) transportation of the embryo or unfertilized egg. Gamete intrafallopian transfer (GIFT) is an assisted reproductive technology (ART) that bypasses only the first of these functions by placing oocytes and sperm directly into the ampullary region of the fallopian tube. Through these means, in vivo fertilization is ideally obtained, and the early embryo is consequently transported to the endometrial cavity in a physiologic manner.

Most of the knowledge about human oocyte transportation comes from the original contributions of Croxatto and Diaz and others.[1, 2] The investigators studied healthy, ovulatory multiparous women undergoing elective bilateral salpingectomy for sterilization purposes. The surgery was scheduled at different intervals following the luteinizing hormone (LH) peak. Both fallopian tubes were segmentally ligated into four compartments before being removed, and the endometrial cavities were concomitantly flushed by a transfundal approach. The presence and localization of the unfertilized egg was correlated with time after ovulation. These investigators concluded that human ovulation occurs approximately 17 hours after LH peak. Ovum pickup is rapid, because the first ova recovered from the fallopian tubes were found 24 hours after the LH peak. During the next 72 hours, the oocyte remains in the ampullary portion of the tubes. The ovum/embryo traverses the isthmus in a rather short period because the earliest egg recovered from the endometrial cavity was approximately 80 hours after ovulation (96 hours after LH peak) (Fig. 52–1).

Another important contribution was made by Buster and coworkers[3] while performing human embryo transfers. Five days after the LH peak, the authors performed a uterine lavage in oocyte donors who had previously undergone a single artificial insemination in the periovular interval. The recovered embryos were transferred to the endometrial cavi-

ties of synchronized recipients. The investigators observed that most pregnancies occurred when a blastocyst stage embryo was collected from the uterine cavity, suggesting that chronology of entrance and the stage of embryo development are significant variables affecting the chances of implantation. Finally, there is indirect evidence from mice studies[4] and human in vitro fertilization (IVF) practice[5] that mature human oocytes are fertilizable only within the first 24 hours after follicular extrusion, a fundamental aspect to be considered while performing GIFT.

The theoretical advantages of IVF are to allow embryo development in the protective ambiance of the tube, entering the endometrial cavity in a natural way, and thereby increasing the chances of implantation.

INDICATIONS

The technique developed by Asch and colleagues[6] in 1984 followed extensive research performed in primates by these investigators. It was proposed as a simplified alternative to in vitro fertilization–embryo transfer (IVF-ET) for all nontubal causes of infertility. It quickly became apparent, however, that in cases of severe male factor (low sperm count or motility) or immunologic infertility, the results with GIFT were disappointing.[7]

Today the main indications for GIFT are unexplained infertility and endometriosis in patients having at least one normal fallopian tube. Other conditions in which GIFT has proved to be useful are (1) mild male factor, (2) failure of previous donor artificial insemination cycles, (3) iatrogenic pelvic adhesions, (4) cervical factor, and (5) oocyte donation in premature ovarian failure patients.

TECHNICAL ASPECTS

A controlled ovarian hyperstimulation regimen with gonadotropin derivatives is performed in every patient enrolled

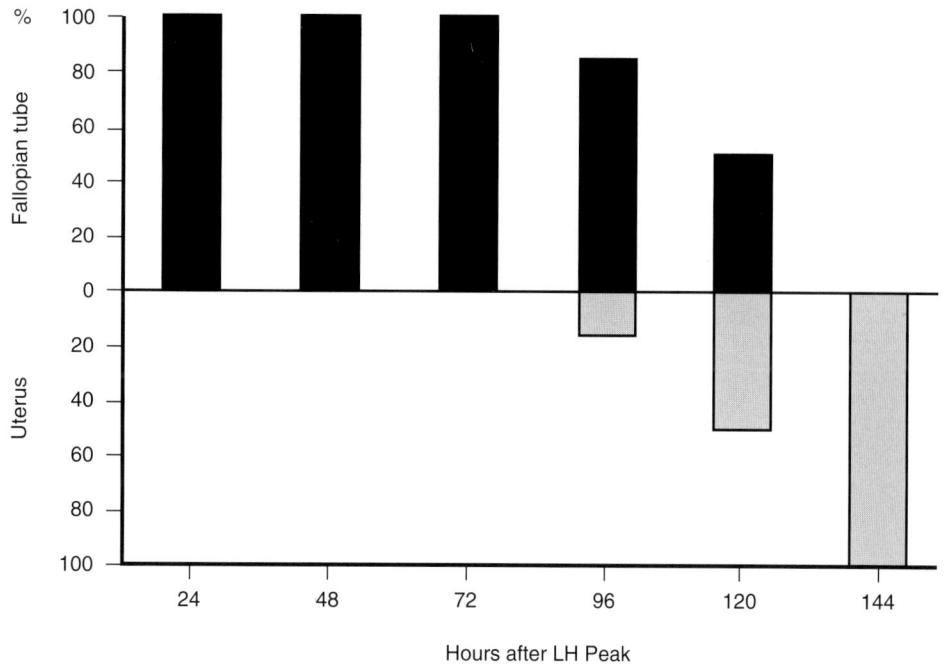

FIGURE 52–1. Distribution of ova in the human genital tract at various times following the luteinizing hormone (LH) peak. (From Ortiz ME, Croxatto HB. Distribution of ova in the human genital tract at various times following LH peak. Presented at the Serono Symposia, Newport Beach, CA, November 6–10, 1988.)

for a GIFT cycle (Fig. 52–2). Better results in terms of number and quality of oocytes retrieved have been obtained with pituitary down-regulation with gonadotropin-releasing hormone (GnRH) agonists.[8] Once two or more follicles have reached a mean diameter of 20 to 22 mm, measured by serial transvaginal ultrasonography, human chorionic gonadotropin (hCG), 10,000 IU, is administered intramuscularly. Cancella-

tion of the cycle is discussed with the patients whenever less than two follicles fail to reach the above measurements. The oocyte retrieval is scheduled 34 to 36 hours after the hCG injection. The follicular aspiration can be achieved either laparoscopically, as was originally described,[9] or transvaginally with sonographic guidance. The latter has become the method of choice in modern infertility practice[10, 11] because

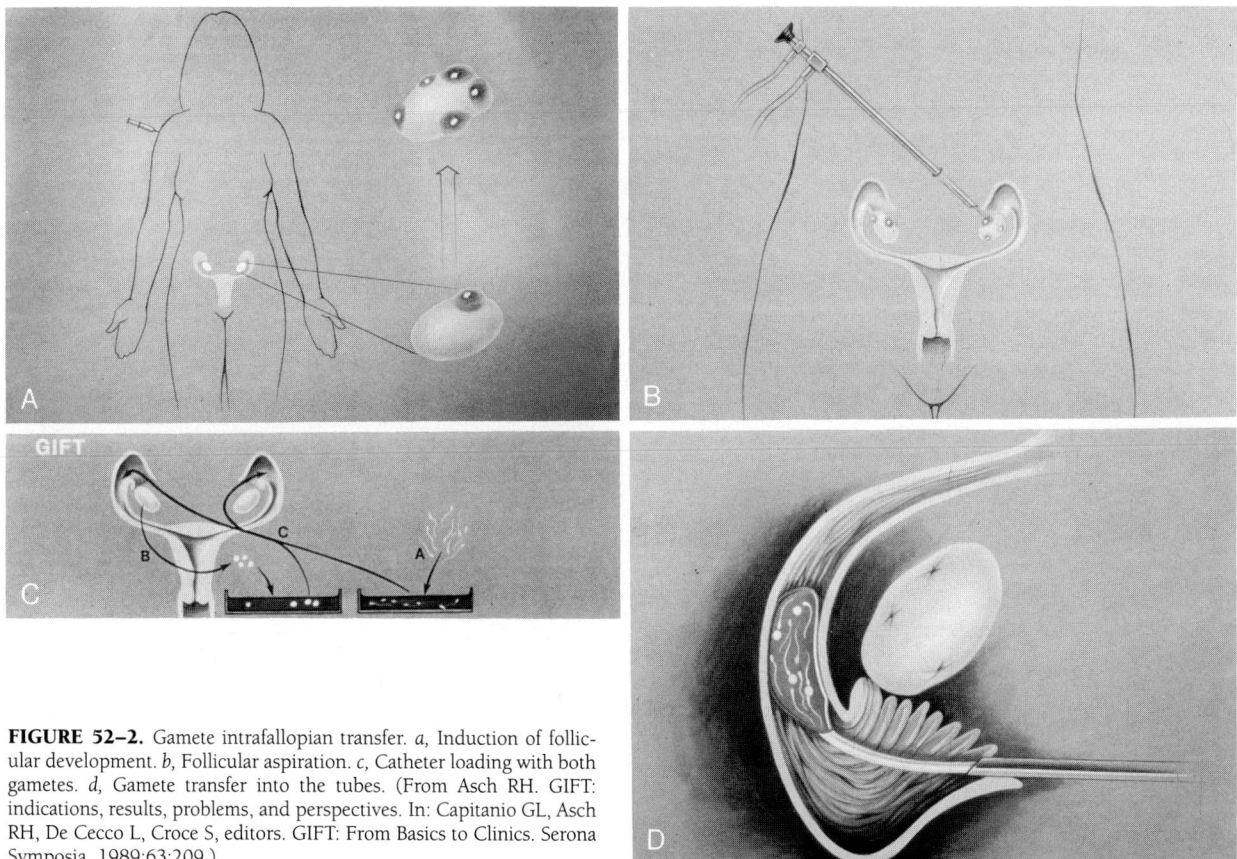

FIGURE 52–2. Gamete intrafallopian transfer. *a,* Induction of follicular development. *b,* Follicular aspiration. *c,* Catheter loading with both gametes. *d,* Gamete transfer into the tubes. (From Asch RH. GIFT: indications, results, problems, and perspectives. In: Capitanio GL, Asch RH, De Cecco L, Croce S, editors. GIFT: From Basics to Clinics. Serona Symposia, 1989;63:209.)

it is easier to perform, allows better visualization of the follicles, does not require general anesthesia, and permits assessment of oocyte quality before doing laparoscopy. Our current practice is to aspirate every follicle seen with the ultrasonography no matter the size. As stated later, extranumerary oocytes are fertilized in vitro and frozen.

Two hours before the oocyte recovery, the male partner, whose semen analysis has previously been considered acceptable for a GIFT treatment, produces a semen sample by masturbation. A 3-day abstinence period is recommended for a standard non–male factor GIFT; otherwise, up to 7 days are required for mild or moderate male factor cases. The sample is allowed to liquefy and is then examined for count, motility, and morphology. After doing so, the seminal plasma is removed by washing the sperm with culture medium. Finally, by a swimup[12] or Percoll gradient technique,[13] the most motile fraction of the sperm is separated and used for the transfer. The standard procedure for a non–male factor case uses between 300,000 and 700,000 motile sperm. In general, the lower the count of normal form and motility after the wash, the higher the number of sperm injected into the tube, although there are no fixed formulas. The total volume of fluid injected should not be over 30 μL, to avoid reflux from the ampullary portion back to the peritoneal cavity.

selected, sperm and oocytes are loaded into a special Teflon catheter that can be easily threaded through the fimbriated end of the fallopian tube. In our current practice, we use a 50-cm, 5-French Marrs catheter (Cook, Spencer, IN), which we consider easy to handle. There are many other catheters available, none of them clearly superior to the rest, so surgeons should choose them according to their preference.

ransfer itself can be accomplished either by laparoscopy or by minilaparotomy. Similar results are reported with either route (we recommend physicians rely on their experience at the moment of choosing one of the methods). Laparoscopic transfer has the advantage of prompt postoperative recovery, with minor discomfort for the patient, and is actually considered the method of choice. Minilaparotomy offers an accurate transfer of gametes into the tube and is especially indicated in patients with pelvic adhesions or multiple abdominal surgeries, in whom laparoscopic approach could be risky owing to persistent adhesions.

The laparoscopic technique requires a standard two-puncture laparoscopy, plus a third puncture for the catheter sheath. The third puncture is usually performed in one of the patient's flanks, 2 to 3 cm below the umbilical incision. For right-handed surgeons, the patient's right side is generally chosen, unless the elected tube has its fimbriated end pointing to the midline. The correct positioning of the catheter is critical in determining ease of cannulation, and whenever possible, an ideal parallel situation should be achieved between the axis of the catheter and the opening offered by the fimbriated ostium.

The decision of which tube will be cannulated is based on anatomic findings and accessibility at the time of doing the procedure. Bilateral tubal transfers do not offer any advantage over single transfers, as demonstrated by Yee and associates[14] and Haines and O'Shea.[15] Moreover, using only one tube reduces the operating time and avoids potential damage to the contralateral tube at the moment of catheterization.

The depth of penetration of the catheter into the tube is recommended to be at least 3 cm.[14] A 32% pregnancy rate (number of patients with positive β-hCG/total number of patients transferred) was reported when this condition was achieved, as opposed to only 16.7% in those who did not, and their results were independent of the total number of eggs transferred or whether one or both tubes were used.[14] Visible markers on the tip of the catheter facilitate determining the degree of penetration.

After the content has been expelled, the catheter is removed and inspected by the biologist to be certain that the gametes were transferred. An intracervical insemination is optionally performed once the transfer has been done.[16] The reason for the insemination is to ensure a more constant flowing of spermatozoa toward the tube. Theoretically, this should increase oocyte-sperm interaction and enhance the chances of fertilization. We have incorporated this procedure to our current practice of GIFT.

After the GIFT is performed, the patient spends an average of 2 hours in the recovery room. She is then discharged, needing bed rest for the following 3 days. Sexual abstinence is recommended for at least 1 week after the transfer.

Finally, some form of luteal phase support is routinely used in GIFT patients. Although seriously questioned initially, since the advent of extensive use of GnRH analogs for controlled ovarian hyperstimulation, we consider it necessary. The treatment can be achieved with daily progesterone (intramuscular, intravaginal, or sublingual) or with hCG, but this last form of luteal support has been associated with a higher incidence of symptomatic ovarian hyperstimulation.[17] If a β-hCG test performed 2 weeks after the transfer is positive, the luteal phase support can be maintained for 4 to 6 more weeks depending on pregnancy evaluation.

RESULTS AND VARIABLES THAT AFFECT THE SUCCESS OF GAMETE INTRAFALLOPIAN TRANSFER

The first multinational collaborative report on GIFT involved 2092 cases and was published in 1987.[7] Most of the participating centers achieved similar results, suggesting that this was a reproducible technique. The overall pregnancy rate for GIFT was 28.7%, a value clearly superior to IVF-ET results published during the same period. Nevertheless, there were significant differences depending on the cause of infertility (Table 52–1). The lowest success rates were reported

TABLE 52–1. Gamete Intrafallopian Transfer Results from a Multinational Cooperative Study

Etiology	No. Cases	No. Clinical Pregnancies	Percentage
Unknown	796	247	31
Endometriosis	413	132	32
Male factor	397	61	15
Tuboperitoneal	210	61	29
Failed artificial insemination	160	66	41
Cervical factor	68	19	28
Oocyte donation	18	10	56
Immunologic	30	5	16
Total	2092	601	28.7

From Asch RH, GIFT: indications, results, problems, and perspectives. In: Capitanio GL, Asch RE, De Cecco L, Croce S, editors. GIFT: From Basics to Clinics. Serono Symposia, 1989; 63:209.

TABLE 52–2. National Registry Results Achieved with Gamete Intrafallopian Transfer

Country	Year	Procedures (No.)	Clinical Pregnancy Rate (%)
United States	1988	3080	21.0
Australia	1988	2653	27.5
United Kingdom	1989	2840	20.8
France	1987–1989	2042	21.3
Total		10615	22.6

From Testart J, Plachot M, Madelbaum J, et al. World collaborative report on IVF-ET and GIFT: 1989 results. Hum Reprod 1992; 7:362; by permission of Oxford University Press.

for male factor (15% pregnancy rate) and immunologic factor (16% pregnancy rate), and the highest were obtained among oocyte donation recipients and women with previous failed assisted inseminations with donor sperm (56% and 41% pregnancy rates). Once pregnancy had been achieved, 79% progressed to third-trimester delivery, 17% had a first-trimester abortion, and 4% had an ectopic pregnancy. The best results were again reported for the oocyte donation group, with a 90% delivery rate.

An international collaborative report on IVF-ET and GIFT for 1989 has been published by Testart and coworkers.[18] The study involved 500 centers in the IVF-ET survey and 341 centers in the GIFT survey. The clinical pregnancy rate (number of patients with gestational sacs/total number of patients transferred) and "take home baby rate" (number of patients delivering living neonates/total number of patients transferred) per procedure were significantly lower for IVF compared with GIFT (16.4% and 11.9% versus 27.5% and 20.2%). The proportion of multiple pregnancies was similar in both groups (25.7% for IVF and 26.9% for GIFT).

Cohen,[19] in 1991, reported the results obtained with GIFT during the years 1987 through 1989 at the four main national registries in the United States, Australia, United Kingdom, and France. Table 52–2 illustrates his findings. The clinical pregnancy rate for GIFT cycles fluctuated between 20.8% and 27.5%, whereas for IVF, it was only 13% to 16.8% in those same countries. The last report from the U.S. IVF-ET Registry for 1990 showed a 22% overall "take home baby rate" per GIFT cycle, compared with 14% for IVF.[20]

We might be tempted to conclude from these results that GIFT offers a better success rate in the treatment of infertility than does IVF. Nevertheless, we must remember that they represent two different populations that cannot be directly compared. There is also a wide variation in IVF-ET results as

well as the patient selection criteria from clinic to clinic. In that sense, it is more valuable to compare results obtained by a single group of investigators because it decreases the differences between laboratories and clinicians. Unfortunately, results published in the literature appear contradictory, some clearly favoring tubal transfers[21, 22] and others preferring intrauterine embryo transfer.[23, 24] We think that those publications need to involve a larger number of patients to reach statistical differences and should differentiate their results obtained by age groups. As we attempt to demonstrate later, age is an important variable to consider.

The rates of congenital malformations and chromosomal abnormalities associated with GIFT are 3.1% and 2.1%.[20] These figures are similar to what is published for other ART procedures and, when corrected for patients' age, do not represent a significant variation from the normal population. It is still not clear if it is the influence of the GIFT technique itself or the selective population treated that explains the slightly increased incidence of abnormalities reported.

If we consider GIFT as a technique that mimics the natural process of in vivo fertilization, it appears obvious that quality of oocytes in terms of maturity may have an important effect on the outcome. This fact was originally demonstrated by Balmaceda and coworkers[25] while working with nonhuman primates (*Macaca fascicularis*). The authors performed GIFT in two groups of primates, one receiving only mature oocytes and the others only immature oocytes. The genital tract of the animals was flushed 24 hours after the transfer, looking for the presence of gametes or embryos. Not a single embryo was recovered from the group that received only immature oocytes, and the oocytes showed advanced signs of degeneration without evidence of maturation. The group that received mature oocytes showed a fertilization rate of 37%, which is significantly lower than the one obtained in vitro for the same quality of eggs. Later on, Guzick and associates,[26] analyzing 218 human GIFT cycles, reported a 39.6% pregnancy rate when up to five mature oocytes were transferred compared with 16.5% when only immature eggs were used. The authors concluded that oocyte quality is even more important than the number of oocytes transferred for the success of a GIFT procedure.

A frequent subject of controversy is the optimal number of oocytes to transfer. The decision needs to balance the chances of achieving pregnancy with the risk of multiple implantation. There are many publications indicating that the clinical pregnancy rate is increased with the number of oocytes transferred.[14, 20, 26, 27] These figures go as low as 6.3% for one oocyte to as high as 41% for four oocytes transferred. Results of the 1601 GIFT cycles recorded through the U.S. Registry during 1990 are shown in Table 52–3. In this report, the

TABLE 52–3. Number of Oocytes Transferred and Gamete Intrafallopian Transfer Outcome—United States: 1990 Results from the IVF-ET Registry

No. of Oocytes Transferred	Clinical Pregnancy Rate (%)	Delivery Rate (%)	Multiple Delivery Rate (%)
≤3	34/296 (11)	27/296 (9)	4/296 (1.4)
4	157/527 (30)	129/527 (24)	42/527 (8)
5–6	187/574 (33)	146/574 (26)	49/574 (8.5)
≥7	87/204 (43)	58/204 (28)	26/204 (12.7)
Total	465/1601 (29)	260/1601 (22.5)	121/1060 (7.6)

Adapted from Medical Research International, Society for Assisted Reproductive Technology (SART), The American Fertility Society. In vitro fertilization–embryo transfer (IVF-ET) in the United States: 1990 results from the IVF-ET Registry. Fertil Steril 1992; 57:15–24. Reproduced with permission of the publisher, The American Fertility Society.

TABLE 52–4. Comparative Results of Gamete Intrafallopian Transfer and In Vitro Fertilization According to the Age of the Female Partner

		GIFT/IVF				
Age Group	No. Transfers	Clinical Pregnancy Rate (%)	Ectopic Pregnancy Rate (%)	SAB (%)	Deliveries (%)	Multiple Deliveries (%)
<25	18/27	11.1/25.9	0/0	50/28.6	0/18.5	0/0
25–29	200/436	34/20.2	4.4/6.8	8.8/18.2	30/16.1	12.5/5.1
30–34	634/1331	36/23.7	5.7/7.6	15.8/15.9	28.9/19.3	10.1/5.6
35–39	532/1256	26.7/19.4	5.6/4.5	17.6/22.2	20.5/14.8	6.2/3.7
>40	214/350	16.8/10.9	2.8/7.9	38.9/28.9	8.9/6.6	1.4/1.7
Total	1599/3405	29.8/20	5.3/6.3	17.2/19	23.2/16	7.8/4.4
		P <.000001	NS	NS	P <.000001	NS

Modified from Medical Research International, Society for Assisted Reproductive Technology (SART), The American Fertility Society. In vitro fertilization–embryo transfer (IVF-ET) in the United States: 1990 results from the IVF-ET Registry. Fertil Steril 1992; 57:15. Reproduced with permission of the publisher, The American Fertility Society.

pregnancy rate achieved when three or less oocytes were transferred was significantly lower than when four or more oocytes were used. An acceptable 8% multiple delivery rate (number of patients having multiple deliveries/total number of patients retrieved) was obtained when four oocytes were used, compared with the higher 12.7% rate when transferring more than six oocytes. Penzias and colleagues[27] reported the outcome of 399 GIFT cycles and observed a threefold increase in the pregnancy rate for women receiving four or more oocytes compared with those who received three or less. These authors did not find a statistical difference in the pregnancy rate in patients receiving five, six, seven, or eight oocytes. Weckstein and associates[28] reported that it is beneficial to transfer four or five oocytes with GIFT, but oocytes in excess of five should be inseminated in vitro and the resulting embryos cryopreserved for future transfers to avoid excessively high multiple-pregnancy rates. An obvious alternative is to discard supernumerary oocytes, if the patient does not desire cryopreservation. In our center, each patient signs a consent form before undergoing the oocyte retrieval, choosing among the following possibilities: IVF and cryopreservation, oocyte donation for research, or discarding the oocytes.

Alam and coworkers[29] have published a 52.5% total cumulative pregnancy rate from one GIFT cycle, when all the consecutive frozen embryo transfers considered were to the same patient who had a previous failed GIFT. The authors made a mathematical calculation based on an additional 9.1% pregnancy rate achieved with frozen embryo transfers cycles, when using the remaining sibling embryos from the fresh GIFT procedure. These results certainly improve the pregnancy rate per procedure and avoid the need of another controlled ovarian hyperstimulation cycle for the patient.

The age of the patient is probably the most important variable to consider when choosing the number of oocytes to transfer. It has been consistently demonstrated that there is a natural decline in women's fertility with increasing age.[30] This issue becomes apparent in women older than 35 years of age and is definitely marked in patients older than 40 years of age. It is interesting to note that GIFT is the ART procedure that achieves the best results in this older group of women. Table 52–4 compares results achieved by GIFT and IVF according to women's age. Craft and colleagues[31] reviewed 1071 GIFT cases, finding a pregnancy rate that varied between 33.5% and 40.2% for different age groups of patients younger than 40 years old. In the over-40-year-old group,

the pregnancy rate was only 19.2%, and the multiple-pregnancy rate was significantly lower than in younger patients (16.2% versus 29%). The authors reported only one case of multiple pregnancy greater than twins from a total of 193 cycles studied in women older than 40, even when all oocytes retrieved were transferred. Guzick and associates[26] concluded that the chances of pregnancy, particularly multiple ones, are significantly reduced in patients over 40, despite the number of oocytes transferred.

Defective oocytes, rather than poor endometrial receptivity, may explain the decrease in women's fertility with aging. This hypothesis has been well documented with the oocyte donation programs, in which we have achieved a 57.9% pregnancy rate when transferring oocytes from young donors to poor-responder or complete ovarian failure recipients.[32] Cohen and coworkers[33] have postulated that zona pellucida hardening is the main cause of dysfunctional oocytes in older women. These authors performed IVF with assisted zonal hatching in women with poor implantation and normal fertilization rates. They observed a significant positive effect with this technique only in women over age 38, concluding that assisted zonal hatching should be offered only to that particular age group.

Lastly, another critical point that must be evaluated before recommending GIFT to an infertile couple is the relevance of individual sperm parameters. Sperm motility and morphology seem to be the most important ones, having an independent impact on the chances of pregnancy, as illustrated in Table 52–5. Guzick and colleagues,[26] analyzing 218 GIFT

Table 52–5. Semen Quality and Pregnancies with Gamete Intrafallopian Transfer in Two Studies

Authors	Sperm		% Pregnancies
Guzick et al[26]	Motility	<20%	6.7
		>30%	31.9
	Normal morphology	<50%	10.9
		>50%	35.8
Wiedemann et al[34]	Motility and normal morphology	<30%	23.3
		>30%	43.2

cycles performed in our center, showed a fivefold increase in pregnancy rate when motility was over 30% and a threefold increase when 50% of the spermatozoa demonstrated normal morphology. The total sperm count did not have a significant effect when added to this analysis. The latter fact has a logical basis because GIFT overcomes, in part, numerical problems of a semen analysis by placing a higher number of motile sperm directly into the ampulla. Nevertheless, the technique cannot overcome a major functional problem, such as low motility or abnormal morphology.[34]

CONCOMITANT DIAGNOSTIC LAPAROSCOPY AND GAMETE INTRAFALLOPIAN TRANSFER

Laparoscopy has become a popular, efficient method for the evaluation and treatment of a subfertile woman. It is especially indicated once male factor and ovulatory dysfunctions have been ruled out. Besides giving accurate anatomic information concerning the internal genital organs, it is considered the only reliable way to diagnose pelvic endometriosis.

A clear tendency to perform therapeutic operative procedures during diagnostic laparoscopy has occurred within the last few years. The most common operative procedures are adhesiolysis, ovarian cyst aspirations, and fulguration of endometriotic implants.

Combining diagnostic laparoscopy and GIFT is certainly an attractive idea for reducing cost and discomfort for the patients. The first clinical experience was reported in 1989 by Pampiglione and colleagues,[35] working with women who received clomiphene citrate for ovarian stimulation. Eighty-one percent of the patients responded adequately to the therapy, and 24% became pregnant. Gindoff and colleagues[36] reported similar results using human menopausal gonadotropin (hMG) and hCG in 33 patients undergoing a combined laparoscopy-GIFT. Twenty-one of the patients were found to have adhesions or endometriosis, and of these, 19 received concurrent therapeutic operative endoscopy in addition to the oocyte retrieval. The authors concluded that by using laparoscopy, it was possible to provide important diagnostic information, to attempt therapeutic measures, and to achieve good pregnancy rates.

Johns,[37] in a larger series of 62 patients, corroborated those statements, using clomiphene citrate to induce ovulation in patients with combined diagnostic and operative laparoscopy and GIFT.

Table 52–6 summarizes the aforementioned findings, plus our own experience with an ongoing study.[38] Using clomiphene citrate alone, we have achieved an acceptable 35%

TABLE 52–6. Results of Concomitant Diagnostic Laparoscopy and Gamete Intrafallopian Transfer

Authors	No. Patients	No. Clinical Pregnancies	Clinical Pregnancy Rate (%)
Pampiglione et al[35]	21	5	23.8
Johns[37]	62	15	24.6
Gindoff et al[36]	15	4	26.7
Balmaceda et al[38]	20	7	35.0
Total	118	31	26.3

TABLE 52–7. Ultrasound-Guided Transcervical Gamete Intrafallopian Transfer

Authors	Year	No. of Cycles	Pregnancies
Jansen & Anderson[39]	1989	10	1
Anderson & Jansen[40]	1989	7	1
Bustillo & Schulman[41]	1989	17	1
Hazout[42]	1989	18	1
Lucena et al[43]	1989	7	3/1*
Anderson et al[44]	1990	44	8/1*
Total		103	15/2*
Pregnancy rate/ectopic pregnancy rate			14.6/13.3%

*Ectopic pregnancies.

clinical pregnancy rate (7 of 20) with only one spontaneous abortion observed thus far. Nevertheless, we had already canceled eight patients owing to premature ovulation, which is certainly an inconvenience in patients without prior pituitary down-regulation (GnRH agonist treatment). We do not recommend gonadotropin therapy because the greater follicular development and consequently the larger ovarian sizes achieved with those protocols may impair the complete visualization of the pelvic organs.

TRANSCERVICAL GAMETE INTRAFALLOPIAN TRANSFER

The classic transabdominal techniques of GIFT, even though reproducible and highly accurate, require general anesthesia and the use of hospital facilities (e.g., post anesthesia care unit). Therefore a transcervical approach to the fallopian tubes represents a simplified, less expensive alternative.

At least three different methods of gaining access to the tubes have been described: ultrasound-guided catheterization, hysteroscopy, and blind transcervical gamete tubal transfer.

Jansen and Anderson[39] in 1987 described, for the first time, the catheterization of the fallopian tubes via a transcervical approach. These authors used a system of sliding catheters under ultrasound guidance. Since then, these and other investigators have reported a larger experience, in an effort to improve the technique itself as well as to use it for intratubal insemination, gamete, and embryo tubal transfers. Table 52–7 shows the latest reports in the literature for ultrasound-guided GIFT. In general, the results are clearly inferior, in terms of pregnancy rates, to those achieved by transabdominal tubal transfers, and the ectopic pregnancy rate (number of ectopic pregnancies/total number of patients becoming pregnant with the method) appears unacceptably high compared with classic GIFT (13.3% versus 4% to 5%). The wide variation of results obtained by different groups of investigators poses a serious question concerning the reproducibility of the method.

Hysteroscopic tubal catheterization allows a better visualization of the tubal ostium and a more precise estimation of the depth of catheter insertion into the fallopian tube. Nevertheless, the experience with this type of transfer is limited. Kururmaki and associates[45] reported two pregnancies out of nine cases of hysteroscopic zygote intrafallopian transfer in 1990. A year later, the first hysteroscopic GIFT series was

TABLE 52–8. Transcervical Catheterization of the Fallopian Tubes (Tactile Method)

Authors	Year	Procedure	No. of cycles	Pregnancies
Bauer et al[47]	1989	TEST	16	4
Lisse and Sydow[48]	1990	GIFT	44	10
Ferraiolo et al[49]	1991	GIFT	26	7/1*
Risquez et al[50]	1990	TEST	28	5/2*
Total			114	26/3*
Pregnancy rate/ectopic pregnancy rate				22.8/11.5%

*Ectopic pregnancies.
TEST: tubal embryo stage transfer; GIFT; gamete intrafallopian transfer.

published by Seracchioli and associates,[46] achieving a 26% pregnancy rate (13 of 50). The authors proposed hysteroscopy as an alternative method for patients with pelvic adhesions, in whom translaparoscopic transfer may be difficult to perform. Whether prolonged exposure of the tubal microenvironment to carbon dioxide or direct endometrial trauma will limit the efficacy of this technique remains to be determined. It is possible that new fiberoptic systems might significantly improve the results achieved with hysteroscopic GIFT.

Bauer and colleagues[47] reported 16 cases of blind transcervical tubal embryo transfers using the Jansen-Anderson intrafallopian insemination set (K-JIT 1000, Cook, Australia). The authors obtained four pregnancies and were able to catheterize the tubes in all but one of the patients. Later on, the same group reported a larger experience with transcervical tubal embryo transfers in cases of male factor infertility, with an optimistic 31% pregnancy rate (29 of 95). Lisse and Sydow[48] reported the first GIFT series using this method in 1991. Their results as well as those from other authors are illustrated in Table 52–8. Although the results are still too preliminary to draw definite conclusions, the tactile tubal catheterization method appears promising, and it may represent a reliable alternative to conventional GIFT techniques.

CONCLUSIONS

At present, GIFT is definitely a reliable therapeutic option for treating infertile patients with patent fallopian tubes and should be especially considered in older infertile women (age 40 or older). The ability to cryopreserve supernumerary embryos increases the efficiency of the technique. Therefore GIFT should be performed in a center that offers a complete array of ART procedures, such as IVF and embryo cryopreservation. Correct patient selection criteria are obviously of major relevance in the outcome of GIFT, as in other ART procedures.

The method of choice for performing GIFT is still laparoscopy, but simplified techniques, such as transcervical catheterization of the fallopian tubes, may represent an attractive alternative for selected patients.

Combined diagnostic/operative laparoscopy and GIFT is certainly an option for a limited group of patients, with acceptable results in experienced hands.

REFERENCES

1. Croxatto HB, Ortiz ME, Diaz S, et al. Studies on the duration of egg transport by the human oviduct. II. Ovum location at various intervals following luteinizing hormone peak. Am J Obstet Gynecol 1978; 132:629.
2. Diaz S, Ortiz ME, Croxatto HB. Studies on the duration of ovum transport by the human oviduct. III. Time interval between the luteinizing peak and recovery of ova by transcervical flushing of the uterus in normal women. Am J Obstet Gynecol 1980;137:116.
3. Buster JE, Bustillo M, Rodi IA, et al. Biologic and morphologic development of donated human ova recovered by nonsurgical uterine lavage. Am J Obstet Gynecol 1985;153:211.
4. Longo FJ. Changes in the zones pellucidae and plasmalemma of aging mouse eggs. Biol Reprod 1981;25:399.
5. Moore KL, Persaud TVN. The beginning of human development. In: The Developing Human. Clinically Oriented Embryology. 5th edition. Philadelphia: WB Saunders, 1993:14.
6. Asch RH, Ellsworth LR, Balmaceda JP, Wong PC. Pregnancy following translaparoscopic gamete intrafallopian transfer (GIFT) Lancet 1984; 2:1034.
7. Asch RH. GIFT: indications, results, problems, and perspectives. In: Capitanio GL, Asch RE, De Cecco L, Crose S, editors. GIFT: From Basics to Clinics. Serono Symposia Publications, 1989;63:209.
8. Hughes EG, Fedorkow DM, Daya S, et al. The routine use of gonadotropin releasing hormone agonists prior to in vitro fertilization and gamete intrafallopian transfer: a meta-analysis of randomized controlled trials. Fertil Steril 1992;58:888.
9. Steptoe PC, Edwards RG. Birth after reimplantation of a human embryo. Lancet 1978;2:366.
10. Wiseman DA, Short WB, Pattinson HA, et al. Oocyte retrieval in an in vitro fertilization–embryo transfer program: comparison of four methods. Radiology 1989;173:99.
11. Feichtinger W. Current technology of oocyte retrieval. Curr Opin Obstet Gynecol 1992;4:697.
12. Asch RH, Balmaceda JP, Ellsworth LR, Wong PC. Preliminary experiences with GIFT (gamete intrafallopian transfer). Fertil Steril 1986; 45:366.
13. Bolton VN, Braude PR. Preparation of human spermatozoa for in vitro fertilization by isopycnic centrifugation on self generating density gradients. Arch Androl 1984;13:167.
14. Yee B, Rosen GF, Chacon RR, et al. Gamete intrafallopian transfer: the effect of the number of eggs used and the depth of gamete placement on pregnancy initiation. Fertil Steril 1989;52:639.
15. Haines CJ, O'Shea RT. Unilateral gamete intrafallopian transfer: the preferred method? Fertil Steril 1989;51:518.
16. Tucker MJ, Wong CJ, Chan YM, et al. Postoperative artificial insemination: does it improve GIFT outcome? Hum Reprod 1990;5:189.
17. Araujo E Jr, Felix C, Bernardini L, et al. Luteal phase support for assisted reproductive technology: a prospective randomized study of human chorionic gonadotropin versus intramuscular progesterone. 41st Annual Meeting of the Pacific Coast Fertility Society, Indian Wells, CA, 1993:0–013.
18. Testart J, Plachot M, Madelbaum J, et al. World collaborative report on IVF-ET and GIFT: 1989 results. Hum Reprod 1992;7:362.
19. Cohen J. The efficiency and efficacy of IVF and GIFT [edit.]. Hum Reprod 1991;6:613.
20. Medical Research International Society for Assisted Reproductive Technology (SART), The American Fertility Society. In vitro fertilization embryo transfer (IVF ET) in the United States 1990 results from the IVF ET Registry. Fertil Steril 1992;57:15.
21. Asch RH. Uterine versus tubal embryo transfer in the human. Comparative analysis of implantation, pregnancy and live birth rates. Ann N Y Acad Sci 1991;626:461.
22. Mills MS, Eddowes HA, Cahill DJ, et al. A prospective controlled study

of in-vitro fertilization, gamete intra-fallopian transfer and intrauterine insemination combined with superovulation. Hum Reprod 1992;7:190.

23. Tanbo T, Dale PO, Abyholm T. Assisted fertilization in infertile women with patent fallopian tubes. A comparison of in-vitro fertilization, gamete intrafallopian transfer and tubal embryo stage transfer. Hum Reprod 1990;5:255.

24. Hammitt DG, Syrop CH, Hahn SJ, et al. Comparison of concurrent pregnancy rates for in-vitro fertilization-embryo transfer, pronuclear stage embryo transfer and gamete intrafallopian transfer. Hum Reprod 1990;5:947.

25. Balmaceda JP, Heitman T, Borrero C, Asch R. In vivo versus in vitro oocyte maturation in a primate animal model. Proceedings, Annual Meeting of the American Fertility Society, Toronto, Canada, 1986:5.

26. Guzick DS, Balmaceda JP, Ord T, Asch RH. The importance of egg and sperm factors in predicting the likelihood of pregnancy from gamete intrafallopian transfer. Fertil Steril 1989;52:795.

27. Penzias AS, Alper MM, Oskowitz SP, et al. Gamete intrafallopian transfer: assessment of the optimal number of oocytes to transfer. Fertil Steril 1991;55:311.

28. Weckstein LN, Jacobson A, Galen DI. The role of cryopreservation in gamete intrafallopian transfer and zygote intrafallopian transfer. Assist Reprod Rev 1992;2:2.

29. Alam V, Weckstein L, Ord T, et al: Cumulative pregnancy rate from one gamete intrafallopian transfer (GIFT) cycle with cryopreservation of embryos: A practical mathematical calculation. Hum Reprod 1993;8:559.

30. Federation CECOS, Schwartz D, Mayaux MJ. Female fecundity as a function of age. N Engl J Med 1982;306:404.

31. Craft I, Brindsen P. Alternatives to IVF: The outcome of 1071 first GIFT procedures. Hum Reprod 1989;4(Suppl 8):29.

32. Balmaceda JP, Alam V, Roszjtein D, et al. Embryo implantation rates in oocyte donation: a prospective comparison of tubal versus uterine transfers. Fertil Steril 1992;57:362.

33. Cohen J, Alikani M, Trowbridge J, Rosenwaks Z. Implantation enhancement by selective assisted hatching using zona drilling of human embryos with poor prognosis. Hum Reprod 1992;7:685.

34. Wiedemann R, Noss U, Hepp M. Gamete intrafallopian transfer in male subfertility. Hum Reprod 1989;4:408.

35. Pampiglione JS, Bolton VN, Parsons JH, Cambell S. Gamete intrafallopian transfer combined with diagnostic and operative infertility: a treatment for infertility in a district hospital. Hum Reprod 1989;4:786.

36. Gindoff PR, Hall JL, Nelson LM, Stillman RJ. Efficacy of assisted reproductive technology during diagnostic and operative infertility laparoscopy. Obstet Gynecol 1990;75:299.

37. Johns A. Clomiphene citrate-induced gamete intrafallopian transfer with diagnostic and operative laparoscopy. Fertil Steril 1991;56:311.

38. Balmaceda JP, Gonzales J, Benardini L. Gamete and zygote intrafallopian transfers and related techniques. Curr Opin Obstet Gynecol 1992;4:743.

39. Jansen RPS, Anderson JC. Catheterization of the fallopian tube from the vagina. Lancet 1987;2:309.

40. Anderson JC, Jansen RPS. Ultrasound guided catheterization of the fallopian tube for the non-operative transfer of gametes and embryos. Proceedings of the 6th World Congress In Vitro Fertilization and Alternative Assisted Reproduction, Jerusalem, 1989:80.

41. Bustillo M, Schulman JD. Transcervical ultrasound guided intrafallopian placement of gametes, zygotes and embryos. J In Vitro Fertil 1989;6:321.

42. Hazout A. Transcervical intrafallopian transfer of zygotes. Oral presentation. Proceedings of the 6th World Congress In Vitro Fertilization and Alternate Assisted Reproduction, Jerusalem, 1989.

43. Lucena E, Ruiz JA, Mendoza JC, et al. Vaginal intratubal insemination (VITI) and vaginal GIFT, endosonographic technique: early experience. Hum Reprod 1989;4:658.

44. Anderson JC, Jansen RPS, Radonic I, et al. Gamete intrafallopian transfer without anesthesia in the treatment of infertility. Hum Reprod 1991;6(Suppl 1):126.

45. Kururmaki H, Ratsula K, Lahteermaki A, Hovatta O. Hysteroscopic zygote intrafallopian transfer. Abstract of the 2nd Joint ESCO-ESHRE Meeting, Milan, Italy, 1990. Hum Reprod 1990;(Suppl 5):99.

46. Seracchioli R, Possati G, Bafaro G, et al. Hysteroscopic gamete intrafallopian transfer: a good alternative in selected cases to laparoscopic intrafallopian transfer. Hum Reprod 1991;6:1388.

47. Bauer O, Diedrich K, Ven VDH, et al. Transvaginal tubal-embryo-stage-transfer (TV-TEST). Proceedings of the 6th World Congress In Vitro Fertilization and Alternate Assisted Reproduction, Jerusalem, 1989:31.

48. Lisse K, Sydow P. Transvaginal gamete intrafallopian transfer. Abstract of the II joint ESCO-ESHRE Meeting. Hum Reprod 1990;(suppl 5):99.

49. Ferraiolo A, Croce S, Anserini P, et al. "Blind" transcervical transfer of gametes in the fallopian tube: A preliminary study. Hum Reprod 1991;6:537.

50. Risquez F, Boyer P, Rolet F, et al. Retrograde tubal transfer of human embryos. Hum Reprod 1990;5:185.

CHAPTER 53

In Vitro Fertilization with Donor Oocytes

CECILIA L. SCHMIDT-SAROSI

Assisted reproduction technology (ART) programs directed at establishing pregnancies with oocyte donations have been relatively quite successful in terms of per cycle pregnancy rate. Oocyte donation has also been integral to our expanding insight into endometrial development, the "window of implantation," and the hormonal requirements of early embryonic support.[1] Most importantly the advent of oocyte donation has provided an opportunity to carry and deliver a baby to a whole cohort of women formerly denied such an experience.

EARLY HISTORY: OVUM TRANSFER

Early attempts at donor ovum–recipient transfer involved in vivo insemination and subsequent fertilization of volunteer oocyte donors and were based on the physiologic assumption that an embryo most commonly arrives in the endometrial cavity on day 18 or day 19 of an idealized menstrual cycle, day 14 denoting the day of the luteinizing hormone (LH) surge.[1] Nonsurgical recovery of these early conceptuses was coupled with synchronization of a recipient's natural cycle LH surge and the donor's LH peak within 2 days. A female donor was inseminated with the infertile woman's husband's semen on the day of or after the LH peak. Five to 7 days later, the early conceptus was lavaged from the uterus of the donor with a transcervical double-lumen catheter. Although the procedure was first described by Seed and Seed[2] in 1980, it was not until 1985 that Buster and associates[3] reported two pregnancies. The efficiency of this recovery method, however, remained suboptimal, and the risk of an unwanted pregnancy was always present for the egg donor. Other risks included the transmission of sexually transmitted diseases or potentially human immunodeficiency virus (HIV) to the donor with the insemination or to the recipient via the conceptus. Also the donor could choose to forego the uterine flush and keep the pregnancy from this form of embryo transfer. Therefore nonsurgical lavage of a uterus for removal of a fertilized embryo is not as attractive an alternative as current oocyte donation programs.

CONTEMPORARY OOCYTE DONATION VIA IN VITRO FERTILIZATION METHODS

Instead, using current oocyte donation methods, oocytes are better collected and fertilized via conventional in vitro fertilization (IVF) methods. Particularly, controlled ovarian hyperstimulation (COH) enhances the number of oocytes retrieved, and ultrasound-guided follicular puncture[4] maximizes recovery of oocytes from the donor in the least invasive manner. In contrast to autologous IVF, COH of the donor does not jeopardize receptivity of the maturing endometrium by superphysiologic steroid levels. Neither exaggerated preaspiration estradiol (E_2) levels nor potential antiestrogenic effects of clomiphene citrate are a concern. Therefore, appropriate use of human menopausal gonadotropins (hMG) alone[5] or in combination with clomiphene citrate[6] can be tailored to the donor's ovulatory status. Furthermore, the addition of a gonadotropin-releasing hormone (GnRH) agonist to the regimen before gonadotropin stimulation[7, 8] has the triple advantage of decreasing cycle cancellation, reducing premature luteinization, and facilitating synchronization of the donor and the oocyte donation recipient.

Intrinsic to the establishment of a gestation in a woman without ovarian function is the procedure of embryo transfer.[9] In addition to the technical aspects of delivering two- to eight-cell embryos into a properly prepared uterine cavity, timing of the embryo transfer becomes critical. As is apparent in the following discussions, this synchronization of donor and oocyte preparation for optimal embryo transfer is best accomplished by tailoring standard regimens to the individual participants.

INDICATIONS FOR OOCYTE DONATION

Realizing that the technical expertise for successful oocyte donation is currently available, criteria for using this clinical tool have come under scrutiny. As recommended in the 1993

"Guidelines for Gamete Donation" published by the American Fertility Society, the primary indication for donor oocytes is premature menopause, attributable to ovarian failure or surgical removal of the ovaries, or gonadal dysgenesis.[10] Other accepted indications include avoiding transmission of a genetic defect, increasing the chance of pregnancy establishment in women with "declining fertility," and enhancing the success rate in women with poor oocyte quality after autologous oocyte retrieval.

As is obvious in the remainder of this chapter, oocyte donation can successfully be offered to women beyond their natural reproductive years. Because no significant body of data exists on pregnancy and its outcome in women older than 45 years of age, a thorough examination, including psychological evaluation, cardiovascular assessment, and high-risk obstetric consultation, should precede acceptance into an oocyte donation program.

SELECTION OF OOCYTE DONORS

Debate continues over the source of egg donation: anonymous versus known. Those proponents of using an anonymous donor cite both the precedent of anonymous semen donation and the reluctance of most practitioners to perform insemination with a known or related semen donor. Use of a known oocyte donor, however, simplifies recruitment and screening because the woman usually volunteers and her medical and social history are known to the couple. In either case, the long-term psychological ramifications of either choice remain unknown.

Screening of the donor should always include minimal genetic evaluation as detailed in the 1993 American Fertility Society guidelines.[10] In essence, this focuses on the elimination of family history and personal obstetric history suggestive of chromosomal abnormalities or of possible multigenic aberrancies. Similarly, infectious screening has been delineated in these recommendations as including exclusion of individuals at high risk for HIV (drug users or partners of drug users or of bisexual men) and serologic tests for syphilis, serum hepatitis B and hepatitis C, cervical gonorrhea, cervical *Chlamydia trachomatis*, and HIV-1 and HIV-2.

Satisfying both minimal genetic screening and the state's legal age statute without bypassing the age of 34 years is mandatory for an anonymous donor. Flexibility in these areas, however, with a donor identified by the couple is based on appropriate informed consent and acknowledgement of an increased risk of chromosomal problems. Again, difficulty recruiting anonymous donors justifies this practice. An alternative solution to this dearth of donors is to use supernumerary oocytes retrieved from a woman undergoing IVF. This donation, however, may defray the costs to the IVF couple but may deny them a potential pregnancy from cryopreservation of their extra embryos. Furthermore, the fecundity of eggs from infertile women may not be equal to that of fertile, or potentially fertile, donors. Hence, transfer of oocytes from an infertile woman undergoing autologous IVF to an infertile oocyte recipient is fraught with ethical dilemmas.

CONTROLLED OVARIAN HYPERSTIMULATION OF DONOR SYNCHRONIZED TO RECIPIENT

The specific regimen of COH chosen should reflect the experience of the ART team in manipulating the time of oocyte aspiration within a limited number of days. The recipient should be at day 15 to 17 of her replacement protocol, that is, day 1 to 3 of progesterone therapy, when the donor undergoes oocyte retrieval. The premature ovarian failure (POF) patient's schedule can be calculated from the usual length of the donor's cycle and expected menses. For instance, human chorionic gonadotropin (hCG) is typically administered on the evening of the menstrual cycle days 9 to 11 in an hMG induction.[1] Follicular monitoring of the donor with both LH urine kits and ultrasonography have been quite instrumental in predicting menses. Alternatively, ovarian suppression of the donor with a GnRH agonist permits coordination of the initiation of hMG with that of estrogen in the recipient. As described in one regimen with a GnRH agonist–suppressed donor, the recipient starts hormone replacement 16 days before the anticipated retrieval date.[11] To align further the timing of embryo transfer with the fourth day of progesterone exposure, adjustments can be made in the length of the follicular phase when necessary such that progesterone is started in the recipient on the day after hCG is given to the donor (Fig. 53–1). Other regimens have included suppressing the donor's cycle with oral contraceptives. No one design for synchronization has been shown to be superior.

HORMONE REPLACEMENT IN THE RECIPIENT

As seen in Tables 53–1 to 53–3, replacement regimens have previously been described that permit successful implantation and development of embryos transferred to patients suffering from premature menopause. These regimens use pharmacologic amounts of oral or transdermal vaginal E_2 (i.e., amounts markedly larger than those produced by the ovary during the menstrual cycle). Progesterone is administered by vaginal suppositories or injections during the last 2 weeks of the replacement cycle.

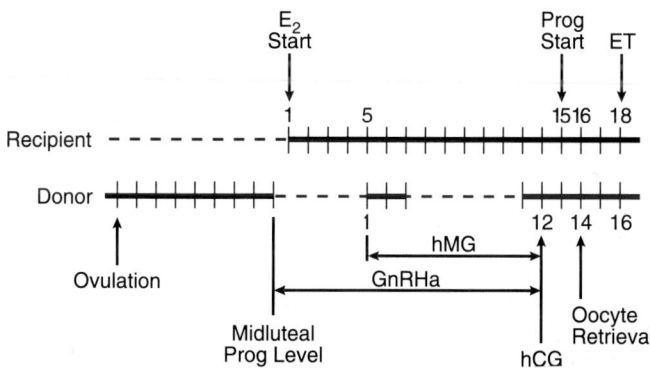

FIGURE 53–1. Synchronization of oocyte donor and embryo recipient on a gonadotropin-releasing hormone agonist (GnRHa) with exogenous estrogen and progesterone (Prog) protocol. hMG, human menopausal gonadotropins; hCG, human chorionic gonadotropin; ET, embryo transfer; E_2, estradiol.

TABLE 53–1. Estrogen Replacement Regimens in Oocyte Donation Recipients Throughout the Cycle and Subsequent Pregnancy

Study	Oral Estradiol (E₂)	Nonoral E₂	Duration of Treatment	Duration of Treatment After Embryo Transfer
Lutjen et al, 1984[29]	2–8 mg/day E₂ valerate	—	12 weeks	10 weeks
Feichtinger & Kemeter, 1985[48]	1–12 mg/day E₂ valerate	—	12 weeks	10 weeks
Navot et al, 1986[18]	1–24 mg/day E₂ valerate	—	11–16 weeks	9–14 weeks
Rosenwaks, 1987[1]	3–10 mg/day micronized E₂	Vaginal E₂ "rings"	13 weeks	11 weeks
DeZiegler et al, 1988[13]	—	0.05–12.0 mg/day transdermal E₂	9 weeks	7 weeks
Sauer et al, 1990[45]	1–6 mg/day micronized estradiol	—	18 weeks	16 weeks
Navot et al, 1991[16]	—	0.2–0.4 mg/day transdermal E₂ before positive hCG	—	—

hCG, human chorionic gonadotropin.

Estrogen Replacement

The need for higher amounts of oral E_2 is engendered by the transformation to estrone (E_1) by the digestive mucosa or inactivation during the first passage through the liver. Individual differences in intestinal or hepatic metabolism may be responsible in part for the variations in endometrial histology reported with regimens using oral E_2. Rosenwaks[1] described the use of the micronized E_2: 4 mg/day on days 6 to 9, 6 mg/day on days 10 to 13, and 4 mg/day on days 14 to 28 with modification as necessary. An alternate regimen used E_2-impregnated polysiloxane vaginal rings to create a highly individualized estrogenic milieu and required two to three preparatory cycles.[12]

We postulated that the administration of E_2 through a nonoral, nonvaginal route, such as transdermal, could achieve more predictable serum levels of E_2 and more reliable histologic transformation of the endometrium.[11, 13] This ultimately could improve the implantation rate of embryos transferred in oocyte donation patients. We therefore designed a new hormone replacement regimen for oocyte donation patients undergoing IVF–embryo transfer (ET) with donated oocytes. Amounts of E_2 similar to those normally produced by the ovary were administered transdermally. The dose was modified to duplicate the changes in the production of E_2

observed throughout the menstrual cycle (see Table 53–2). From day 15 to day 28, progesterone was administered with vaginal suppositories as depicted in Table 53–2.[11, 13, 14]

As we expected, transdermal administration of E_2 induced a dose-related increase in serum E_2 and, to a lesser extent, in serum E_1. This resulted in patterns of serum E_1 and E_2 levels that were similar to those seen in normal menstrual cycles. The administration of 0.4 mg of E_2/24 hours resulted by day 13 in serum levels of E_2 and E_1 of 250 ± 23 pg/mL and 135 ± 31 pg/mL, mean ± SEM. These induced E_2 levels closely mimicked E_2 levels observed during the preovulatory rise of E_2 when the production rate of E_2 by the ovary is approximately 0.4 mg/24 hours.

In contrast with the oral estrogen regimens that result in high E_1 levels (up to 1580 ± 345 pg/mL on day 14), transdermal E_2 was associated with maximum E_1 levels of 174 ± 8 pg/mL on day 14. Estradiol levels were 86 ± 16 pg/mL with the oral route at this time in the replacement cycle. Furthermore, the hepatic markers, sex hormone–binding globulin, thyroid-binding globulin, and renin substrate, were elevated with the oral preparation but not with the transdermal route.[12] These findings have been substantiated by other groups.[15]

Navot and colleagues[16, 17] have shown that variable lengths of follicular phases, as defined by duration of estrogen exposure, have been associated with ongoing pregnancies. A follicular phase spectrum has been spanned from a short 5 days of estrogen exposure (short follicular phase) to a long 35 days of estrogen stimulation (long follicular phase) before progesterone initiation. Although not significantly different, pregnancy rates were slightly higher after the long follicular phases (13 of 33; 39.4%) compared with those after short follicular phases (8 of 27; 29.6%). Hence the search continues for the optimal estrogen replacement regimen.

Progesterone Replacement

Progesterone delivered via vaginal suppositories or intramuscular injection can provide adequate progesterone levels. Although the exact doses of progesterone and the route of administration of progesterone may vary between programs, the overall profiles of administration are quite similar. As shown in Table 53–3, the initiation of progesterone defines day 15 of the cycle. Earlier renditions of this protocol en-

TABLE 53–2. Physiologic Replacement Regimens

Hormone Preparation	Schedule of Administration	Dosage (mg/24 hr)
Transdermal Estradiol (E₂) and Intramuscular Progesterone (P) in Oil		
Transdermal E₂	Day 1 (AM)–day 7 (AM)	0.1*
	Day 7 (AM)–day 11 (PM)	0.2
	Day 11 (PM)–day 15 (AM)	0.4
	Day 15 (AM)–day 18 (PM)	0.3
	Day 18 (PM)–day 25 (PM)	0.2
P in oil	Day 15 through day 28	50
Oral Estradiol (E₂) and Intramuscular Progesterone (P) in Oil		
Oral micronized E₂	Day 1–day 5	1
	Day 6–day 9	2
	Day 10–day 13	6
	Day 14–day 28	2
P in oil	Day 15	50
	Day 16–day 28	100

*Each 0.1 mg/24 h dose denotes a 0.1-mg patch replaced every 3½ days on a staggered schedule.

TABLE 53–3. Progesterone Therapy in Oocyte Donation Recipients from the Embryo Transfer Period* and into the Subsequent Pregnancy

Study	Progesterone Suppositories (Intravaginal)	Progesterone in Oil (Intramuscular)	Duration of Treatment After Embryo Transfer
Lutjen et al, 1984[29]	—	50–200 mg/day from embryo transfer	17 weeks
Feichtinger & Kemeter, 1985[48]	—	25–200 mg/day	10 weeks
Navot et al, 1986[18]	—	25–200 mg/day	16–20 weeks
Rosenwaks, 1987[1]	75–150 mg/day	25–50 mg/day after positive β-hCG	Midtrimester
DeZiegler et al, 1988[13]	50–150 mg/day	50 mg/day after positive β-hCG	10 weeks
Sauer et al, 1990[45]	—	50–100 mg/day	16 weeks
Navot et al, 1991[16]	—	50–150 mg/day	—

*See Table 53–4 for exact timing of embryo transfer after initiation of progesterone.
β-hCG, Beta-human chorionic gonadotropin.

tailed an increase in progesterone from 25 mg on day 15 and day 16 of the cycle to a plateau of 50 mg on day 17.[11, 13]

Trial Cycle of Hormone Replacement Therapy

A customary practice for most oocyte donation programs has been to monitor estrogen and progesterone replacement in a "mock cycle" before the actual donation cycle. Serum levels of E_2 and progesterone are evaluated and compared with at least one endometrial biopsy specimen. Navot and coworkers[18] found tubular glands with subnuclear vacuolization on day 17 of the cycle and glands with intraluminal secretion and edematous stroma with spiral arterioles on day 22 in other cycles. Similarly, Rosenwaks[1] studied early-to-midluteal biopsy specimens and late day-26-to-27 biopsy specimens in separate estrogen/progesterone replacement cycles. Consistently, early endometrial gland development appeared to lag behind stromal changes in the former biopsy specimens but seemed to "catch up" in the latter ones. Rosenwaks[1] postulated that glands may require prolonged exposure to a lower threshold of progesterone to achieve prompt and timely secretory changes. Using our progesterone replacement regimen (see Table 53–2), histologic dating of endometrial sampling on day 26 showed agreement within 1 day with menstrual dating in 24 of 24 cases.[13] Serial ultrasonographic evaluation of the endometrium under this E_2/progesterone regimen echoed the close alignment with

spontaneous cycles.[19] Once again, however, as with estrogen, there may not be an ideal dosage regimen of progesterone for a controlled endometrial environment. By varying the duration of exposure to progesterone before ET, Navot and coworkers[16] observed implantation between luteal day 1 (normalized cycle day 15 or the day of progesterone initiation) to luteal day 6 (normalized cycle day 20 or the sixth day of progesterone administration). No length of progesterone exposure was statistically found to correlate with enhanced endometrial receptivity.

Based on these experimental results, on the predictable decidualization of late biopsy specimens, and on the success rate of oocyte donation regardless of earlier luteal biopsy histology, established programs are moving toward foregoing "mock cycles." Instead, oocyte recipients are closely monitored over the days preceding the actual embryo transfer.

PREGNANCIES RESULTING FROM DONATED OOCYTES

It is quite evident that optimal rates of pregnancy, superior to those of autologous IVF cycles, occur when 2- to 16-cell embryos are replaced between days 17 and 19, the third to fifth day of progesterone exposure. A registry of conceptions and births from donor oocytes does not formally exist. A summary of published cases is presented in Table 53–4. Although this "window of transfer" may be extended to day 16 in accord with these data, further delineation of this

TABLE 53–4. In Vitro Fertilization of Donated Oocytes: Relationship of Day of Transfer to Pregnancy

Study	Day of Transfer Normalized to Day 15 as First Day of Progesterone Administration	Pregnancy Rates		
		Pregnancy/Transfer	*%*	*% Viable Pregnancy*
Lutjen et al, 1984[29]	16–18	6/31	19	13
Feichtinger & Kemeter, 1985[48]	17	1/4	25	15
Navot et al, 1986[18]	16–21	2/8	25	25
Navot et al, 1988[7]	17–19	11/30	37	30
	20–24	1/12	8	0
DeZiegler et al, 1988[13]	18	6/9	67	33
1988 IVF-ET Registry, 1990[43]	—	51/158	32	23
Sauer et al, 1990[45]	18	13/22	59	55
Navot et al, 1991[16]*	15–20	33/60	55	35
	16	9/13	69	62

*Excess oocytes from infertile women undergoing in vitro fertilization.

optimal uterine interval for ET and implantation in women requires further investigation of both simple[20, 21] and better understood protocols.[16, 17, 22] Furthermore, transfer of multiple embryos and of better quality, first-choice embryos may further improve these rates.

This latter point must be again emphasized because many oocyte donation clinics using "excess oocytes" from IVF cycles of infertile patients have lower pregnancy rates.

In the first 39 women who underwent IVF-ET of donated oocytes at UMDNJ–New Jersey Medical School, 15 conceived (unpublished data). Each recipient had provided her own donor, a relative or friend. All oocytes were retrieved by transvaginal ultrasound–guided follicular aspiration[13] and fertilized with the recipient's husband's sperm. A maximum of four embryos were transferred 48 hours later on day 18 of the replacement cycle, the fourth day of progesterone exposure. Extra embryos were cryopreserved. After a positive hCG titer was identified, transdermal administration of E_2 was progressively increased up to 1.5 mg/24 hours (15 of the 0.1 µg patches) over the subsequent 10 days. This was accomplished by having the patient wear up to 15 of the 0.1 µg patches. Each patch was changed every 3½ days, but the patches were divided into two groups with overlapping schedules. Specifically, 50% of the patches would be replaced on Monday morning and Thursday night, whereas the other 50% would be changed on Tuesday night and Saturday morning. The E_2 delivery rate was then maintained as constant by changing 50% of the patches. Replacement of the transdermal system was staggered to avoid excessive fluctuation in serum levels of E_2. When E_2 levels surpassed 1600 pg/mL, by 43 days after ET, transdermal administration of E_2 was gradually withdrawn. Similarly, 50 mg intramuscular progesterone in the morning was coupled with 100 mg vaginal suppository at night from the time of the positive hCG. Progesterone was discontinued at approximately 12 weeks of gestation, about 2 weeks after cessation of exogenous E_2. Of the 15 pregnancies from 39 donor oocyte retrievals, 8 delivered at term, 2 delivered at 35 weeks, 1 delivered triplets at 34 weeks, 3 underwent spontaneous first-trimester abortions, and 1 suffered a second-trimester abortion. These results parallel those of other nonanonymous donor oocyte programs[23, 24] and anonymous programs.[25, 26]

A closing debate on the establishment of pregnancy from oocyte donation focuses on the role of gamete intrafallopian transfer (GIFT). One report showed six clinical pregnancies in eight cycles.[27] In a prospective, randomized series of zygote intrafallopian transfer (ZIFT) versus IVF-ET of these embryos,[28] no significant difference in pregnancy rates was observed. Because this is not necessarily more successful than a simple transcervical transfer of embryos engendered from donated oocytes, final judgment of the efficacy of GIFT of donated oocytes or ZIFT of donated oocyte embryos need be reserved for larger series.

DEBATE ON THE HORMONAL MAINTENANCE OF AN EARLY INTRAUTERINE GESTATION

Maintenance of early pregnancy was effected in each of the protocols by estrogen and progesterone levels, which may, in actuality, be pharmacologic in dosage and prolonged in administration (see Tables 53–1 and 53–3). Lutjen and coworkers[29] continued E_2 until 12 weeks of pregnancy and progesterone injections until the 19th week based on an observed rise in endogenous steroids. Similarly, Navot and coworkers[18] believed that exogenous estrogen was mandatory up to the 11th week and exogenous progesterone until the 18th to 22nd week of pregnancy. Through data on luteectomies in the first trimester, however, Csapo and coworkers[30] showed that placental steroid production could support pregnancies without exogenous progesterone provided that the corpus luteum was removed beyond 50 to 60 days of pregnancy. Hence, the maintenance protocols at several different institutions have been individualized to allow lower doses of E_2 and progesterone for shorter periods of time. In fact, a study of five patients given lower, constant doses of E_2 and progesterone was directed at early detection of placental steroidogenesis. A significant increase was noted in E_2 secretion during week 7 and in progesterone production during week 9, with linear increase in both noted from weeks 6 and 7 onward. This proposed in vivo model suggests that placental progesterone production by week 9 accounts for placental maintenance of pregnancy in the face of removal of the corpus luteum.[31]

The "compulsive" nature of the pregnancy replacement regimens in use seek to mimic the steroidal secretions of the corpus luteum of pregnancy in a physiologic manner until the precise moment when the placenta assumes responsibility. This rigidity has been tempered by several venues of experiments. First, multiple case reports of estrogen/progesterone supplementation truncated at 5 to 7 weeks after ET[32] and of women neglecting to take their prescribed estrogen[33] have attested to the forgiving nature of the implanted embryo. Second, growth factors produced by trophoblastic tissue,[34] by the ovary (relaxin),[14] and by the maternal pituitary (growth hormone) are intertwined in the developing system.[35] We reported that both relaxin and growth hormone were higher in 17 normal pregnancies in women with corpora lutea, dated from intrauterine insemination or timed intercourse, compared with 10 pregnancies in women with ovarian failure who had received donated oocytes and exogenously administered estrogen and progesterone. Interestingly, these aluteal women exhibited higher levels of estrogen throughout the first trimester of pregnancy and no detectable relaxin.[14, 35] Furthermore, early pregnancy is shrouded by such enigmatic substances as inhibin and hCG,[36] and implantation is poorly understood.[37, 38] Despite the absence of these hormones and growth factors, however, pregnancies conceived through oocyte donation do not evidence a detrimental outcome.

FROZEN EMBRYO TRANSFERS: NATURAL CYCLE VERSUS CONTROLLED ENDOMETRIUM

The divorce of the endometrial milieu and stimulated oocyte maturation effected by oocyte donation is further emphasized by frozen-thawed ETs. In both these offshoots of IVF-ET technology, the endometrium into which embryos are placed has not been immediately subjected to the same pharmacologic concentrations of E_2 and progesterone that accompanied the oocyte development.

As we have seen, oocyte donation, marked by a highly successful pregnancy rate, couples prepared endometrium with oocytes from noninfertile women. Using several different steroidal replacement schema of oral or nonoral E_2 and intramuscular progesterone, viable pregnancy rates hover around 30% in most oocyte donation programs (see Table 53–4).

Instead of the two optimal factors of oocytes from a donor not plagued by infertility and a more natural host endometrium, transfer of previously frozen embryos focuses on the single beneficial factor of a receptive endometrium. Although the same woman who served as superovulated oocyte donor will become the embryo recipient, temporally separated replacement of the supernumerary embryos highlights a more undisturbed endometrial environment. In fact, modeled on oocyte donation regimens, either ovulation induction or ovarian suppression with a GnRH agonist followed by steroidal preparation can prepare the endometrium for frozen-thawed ET. Hence, the debate to be now opened is whether a natural or artificial endometrium can better ensure implantation and pregnancy after a transfer of previously frozen embryos.

The day of planned transfer has remained controversial. In spontaneous cycles, timing has been scheduled by using urine LH surge detection to tract impending ovulation and early luteal phase or by calculating progesterone exposure.[11] Furthermore, the oligo-ovulatory or anovulatory woman has posed an interesting dilemma: synchronization in the face of an estrogen-laden endometrial milieu. In lieu of ovulation induction with clomiphene citrate or hMG,[39] GnRH agonist ovarian suppression can be followed by physiologic steroidal replacement regimens to effect a receptive endometrial environment.[11, 40] The GnRH agonist is used to produce a medical oophorectomy, to convert the patient into one similar to a POF patient, and then to administer estrogen and progesterone according to efficacious oocyte donation protocols.

Based on our successful experience with oocyte donation at UMDNJ–New Jersey Medical School (Fig. 53–2), we first described this new approach to cryopreserved-thawed ETs using a GnRH agonist with exogenous estrogen and progesterone. This regimen can be used in the woman with recalcitrant ovarian dysfunction who has previously undergone an IVF cycle in which cryopreserved embryos have been obtained.

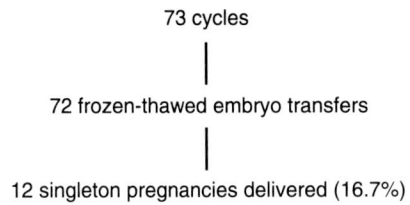

FIGURE 53–3. Outcome of first 73 cycles in which women received gonadotropin-releasing hormone agonist and exogenous estrogen and progesterone at the University of Medicine and Dentistry of New Jersey–New Jersey Medical School. Each patient underwent transfer of previously frozen embryos from oocytes retrieved during an autologous in vitro fertilization cycle.

tained. In our protocol, after attainment of ovarian suppression, women receive steroidal replacement with previously frozen embryos in a fashion prospectively synchronized with the fourth day of progesterone administration. Of the first 73 such cycles, a viable pregnancy rate of 16.7% was achieved in a group of women formerly demonstrating a 0% success rate after natural cycle transfer of frozen-thawed embryos (Fig. 53–3). It may be that the natural cycle in the infertile woman may not embody the perfect endometrial environment. Therefore, using GnRH agonist with a controlled endometrium must be compared with frozen-thawed embryo transfers performed in spontaneous cycles. Although ovarian suppression with estrogen and progesterone preparation of the endometrium constitutes a successful preparation for cryopreserved-thawed ETs in women with ovulatory dysfunction, the question of preference in the normally ovulating woman remains unanswered.

Furthermore, using this model, the role of progesterone in creating the receptive endometrium can be explored. We reported high pregnancy rates when embryos frozen with 1,2-propanediol were thawed and transferred on the fourth day of progesterone administration during hormonally programmed cycles. It can be argued that the total amount of progesterone, rather than the duration of exposure, may be the integral factor to pregnancy establishment. In 12 women with ovarian failure treated with transdermal and oral estrogens for 2 weeks, Salat-Baroux and associates[41] reported four pregnancies when cryopreserved-thawed embryos were replaced on the second day of progesterone supplementation with 20-mg vaginal suppositories. Endometrial biopsies performed on day 21 or day 22 of a "mock treatment cycle" had been found to be in phase in each of the pregnant women. Hence, the relationship between a physiologic endometrium and an optimal dosage and duration of administration of progesterone remains unclear. In fact, simplified regimens of minimal estrogen exposure followed by and coupled with a critical exposure to progesterone may be optimal.

To separate the effects of these nonphysiologic periovulatory steroid concentrations on the oocyte versus on the endometrium, we compared the periovulatory milieu of oocytes that would be transferred only after freezing and thawing in a natural or in an estrogen/progesterone controlled cycle. We hypothesized that the high E_2 milieu from which the supernumerary oocytes had been harvested was not detrimental to the oocytes or to the resultant embryos slated for cryopreservation and eventual transfer. Peak E_2 levels had reached over 7000 pg/mL in cycles from which oocytes were retrieved and embryos were frozen for future transfer.[42] There was no

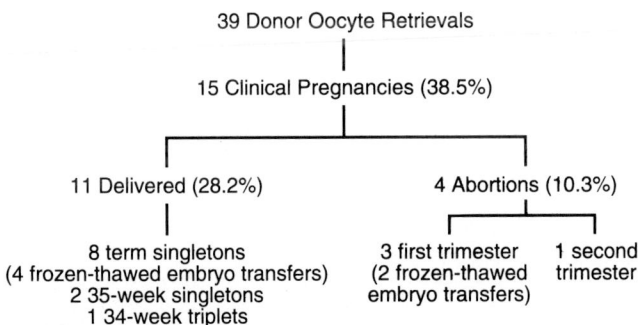

FIGURE 53–2. Results of first 39 oocyte retrieval cycles at the University of Medicine and Dentistry of New Jersey–New Jersey Medical School. Embryos were transferred whether fresh or after a freeze-thaw procedure.

significant difference between mean E_2 levels in those retrieval cycles that resulted in pregnancies after a later frozen-thawed ET and those that did not. Of 138 frozen-thawed ETs after 83 IVF and 9 oocyte donation cycles, 21 pregnancies translated into a 15.2% pregnancy rate/frozen-thawed ET. It is impressive that these embryos had been exposed as oocytes to levels of E_2 with a mean of 3000 pg/mL in the natural and steroid controlled cycles and 2000 pg/mL in the oocyte donation cycles. Hence, we could not demonstrate a direct detrimental effect of "nonphysiologic," elevated levels of E_2 on an embryo's ability to implant and remain viable. The ramifications of such pharmacologic steroid levels on endometrium, however, still remain to be elucidated.

EFFECT OF OVARIAN VERSUS UTERINE AGE

The poor fecundity in older women[43] and the correlation of elevated follicle-stimulating hormone (FSH) levels with poor folliculogenesis and ART outcome has focused on the cohort of aging oocytes as the key to this escalating infertility. Hence, protocols designed originally for the ovarian failure patient and the ovulatory dysfunctional woman have been adapted to the elderly infertility patient. Meldrum and co-workers[44] showed that pregnancy rates were affected directly by the age of the woman undergoing oocyte retrieval and not the age of the uterus. Thirteen donor oocyte cycles, in which the donor had a mean age of 30.8 years and the recipient had a mean age of 38.8 years, evidenced an overall pregnancy rate of 62% compared with 25 women (mean age 37.9 years) undergoing IVF-ET with a success rate of 28%. Therefore, oocyte donation into a controlled endometrial environment reversed the decline in embryo viability associated with increasing age. Sauer and associates[45] supported these conclusions by reporting five viable pregnancies in seven women, 40 to 44 years old, with ovarian failure after oocyte donation/steroidal endometrial preparation. As mentioned earlier, the outermost limit of age for an oocyte recipient has not been determined. Rather, we recommend thorough patient evaluation before such an assisted conception.

To emphasize the relative importance of *ovarian age* versus *uterine age*, incidental reports have appeared of pregnancies in surrogate gestational mothers who have been synchronized to the oocyte retrieval with clomiphene citrate/hCG[46] or hMG/hCG.[47] It is generally agreed that the quality of the embryos transferred, be they fresh or frozen-thawed, is best related to the oocyte donor's age and previous fertility and is the determining factor in establishing pregnancy.

SUMMARY

The entity of ovarian failure encompasses a substantial population of young and aging women who face the rigors of appropriate diagnosis and reversal of hypoestrogenicity. Through oocyte donation programs, such a woman, previously denied a pregnancy and childbirth, is granted a fulfilling experience. The door is now open to treat other manifestations of inadequate oocyte development, genetic or hormonal in derivation. In return, a greater insight has been, and will continue to be, gained into the relative contributions of ovarian function, oocyte chronology, and uterine milieu in implantation and gestational viability.

REFERENCES

1. Rosenwaks Z. Donor eggs: their application in modern reproductive technologies. Fertil Steril 1987;47:895–909.
2. Seed RG, Seed RW. Artificial embryonation: a progress report on human embryo transfer. Fertil Steril 1980;33:236–237.
3. Buster JE, Bustillo M, Rodi IA, et al. Biologic and morphologic development of donated human ova recovered by nonsurgical uterine lavage. Am J Obstet Gynecol 1985;153:211–217.
4. DeZiegler D, Baylor A, Colon J, et al. Precautions recommended for transvaginal ultrasound. Presented at the 43rd Annual Meeting of the American Fertility Society, Reno, 1987, Abstract No. 170.
5. Rosenwaks Z, Mauasher SJ, Acosta AA. Use of hMG and/or FSH and multiple follicle development. Clin Obstet Gynecol 1986;29:148–157.
6. Quigley MM, Maklad NF, Wolf DP. Comparison of two clomiphene citrate dosage regimens for follicular recruitment in an in vitro fertilization program. Fertil Steril 1983;40:178–182.
7. Navot D, Droesch K, Liu H-C, et al. Efficacy of human conception in vitro related the window of implantation. Presented at the 35th Annual Meeting of the Society of Gynecologic Investigation, Baltimore, 1988, Abstract No. 419.
8. Serafini P, Stone B, Kerin J, et al. An alternate approach to controlled ovarian hyperstimulation in "poor responders": pretreatment with a gonadotropin-releasing hormone analog. Fertil Steril 1988;40:90–95.
9. Schmidt CL. Techniques of embryo transfer. In: Wolf DP, Quigley MM, editors. Human In Vitro Fertilization and Embryo Transfer. New York: Plenum Press, 1984;327–340.
10. American Fertility Society: Guidelines for gamete donation, 1993. Fertil Steril 1993; Supplement 1:57–59.
11. Schmidt CL, DeZiegler D, Gagliardi CL, et al. Transfer of cryopreserved-thawed embryos: the natural cycle versus controlled preparation of the endometrium with gonadotropin-releasing hormone agonist and exogenous E2 and progesterone (GEEP). Fertil Steril 1989;42:609–616.
12. Steingold K, DeZiegler D, Reznikow S, et al. Comparison of transdermal to oral E2 administration on hepatic biochemical markers in women with premature ovarian failure in preparation for oocyte donation. Presented at the 35th Annual Society of Gynecologic Investigation, Baltimore, 1988, Abstract No. 161.
13. DeZiegler D, Gagliardi C, Matt D, et al. Successful transdermal E2 and vaginal progesterone regimen for in vitro fertilization and embryo transfer (IVF-ET) of donated oocytes in premature ovarian failure. Presented at the 35th Annual Meeting of the Society for Gynecologic Investigation, Baltimore, 1988, Abstract No. 160.
14. Johnson MR, Abdalla H, Allman ACJ, et al. Relaxin levels in ovum donation pregnancies. Fertil Steril 1991;56:59–61.
15. Droesch D, Navot D, Scott R, et al. Transdermal estrogen replacement in ovarian failure for ovum donation. Fertil Steril 1988;50:931–934.
16. Navot D, Bergh PA, Williams M, et al. An insight into early reproductive processes through the in vivo model of ovum donation. J Clin Endocrinol Metab 1991;72:408–441.
17. Navot D, Scott RT, Droesch K, et al. The window of embryo transfer and the efficiency of human conception in vitro. Fertil Steril 1991;55:114–118.
18. Navot D, Laufer N, Kopolovic J, et al. Artificially induced endometrial cycles and establishment of pregnancies in the absence of ovaries. N Engl J Med 1986;314:806–811.
19. Hung TT, Ribas D, Tsuiki A, et al. Artificially induced menstrual cycle with natural E2 and progesterone. Fertil Steril 1989;51:968–971.
20. Leeton J, Rogers P, Cameron I, et al. Pregnancy results following embryo transfer in women receiving low-dosage variable-length estrogen replacement therapy for premature ovarian failure. J In Vitro Fert Embryo Trans 1989;6:232–235.
21. Serhal PF, Craft IL. Ovum donation—a simplified approach. Fertil Steril 1987;48:264–269.
22. Navot D, Anderson TL, Droesch K, et al. Hormonal manipulation of endometrial maturation. J Clin Endocrinol Metab 1989;68:801–807.
23. Sauer MV, Paulson RJ, Macaso TM, et al. Establishment of a nonanonymous donor oocyte program: preliminary experience at the University of Southern California. Fertil Steril 1989;52:433–436.
24. Sauer MV, Paulson RJ, Macaso TM, et al. Oocyte and pre-embryo donation to women with ovarian failure. Fertil Steril 1991;55:39–43.

25. Frydman R, Letus-Konirsch H, DeZiegler D, et al. A protocol for satisfying the ethical issues raised by oocyte donation: the free, anonymous, and fertile donors. Fertil Steril 1990;53:666–672.
26. Leeton J, Freeman L, King C, et al. Successful pregnancy in an ovulating recipient following the transfer of two frozen-thawed embryos obtained from anonymously donated oocytes. J In Vitro Fert Embryo Trans 1988;5:22–24.
27. Asch RH, Balmaceda JP, Ord T, et al. Oocyte donation and gamete intrafallopian transfer in premature ovarian failure. Fertil Steril 1988;49:263–267.
28. Balmaceda JP, Rotsztein DA, Ord T, et al. Embryo implantation rates in oocyte donation: a prospective comparison of tubal versus uterine transfers. Presented at the 38th Annual Meeting of the Society for Gynecologic Investigation, San Antonio, 1991, Abstract No. 14.
29. Lutjen P, Trounson A, Leeton J, et al. The establishment and maintenance of pregnancy using in vitro fertilization and embryo donation in a patient with primary ovarian failure. Nature 1984;307:174–175.
30. Csapo AI, Pulkkinen MO, Wiest WG. Effects of luteectomy and progesterone replacement therapy in early pregnant patients. Am J Obstet Gynecol 1973;115:759–765.
31. Scott R, Navot D, Droesch K, et al. A unique human in vivo model for studying early placental steroidogenesis and pregnancy maintenance. Presented at the 35th Annual Meeting of the Society of Gynecologic Investigation, 1988, Abstract No. 420.
32. Rosenberg S. Ovum donation by sisters in ovarian failure: simplified priming and early withdrawal of exogenous support. J In Vitro Fert Embryo Trans 1989;6:228–231.
33. Kapetanakis E, Pantos KJ. Continuation of donor oocyte pregnancy in menopause without early pregnancy support. Fertil Steril 1990;54:1171–1173.
34. Hofmann GE, Anderson TL. Immunohistochemical localization of epidermal growth factor receptor during implantation in the rabbit. Am J Obstet Gynecol 1990;162:837–841.
35. Emmi AM, Gagliardi CL, Schmidt CL, et al. The relationship between peripheral relaxin and growth hormone concentrations in early pregnancy. J Clin Endocrinol Metab 1991;72:1359–1363.
36. Santoro N, Schneyer A, Abraham J, Schmidt CL. Pituitary, placental and luteal gonadotropin and inhibin secretion and early pregnancy in women without corpora lutea. Presented at the 73rd Annual Meeting of the Endocrine Society, Washington, D.C., 1991, Abstract No. 1515.
37. Cohen J, Malter H, Elsner C, et al. Immunosuppression supports implantation of zona pellucida dissected human embryos. Fertil Steril 1990;53:662–665.
38. Wiemer KE, Cohen J, Wiker SR, et al. Coculture of human zygotes on fetal bovine uterine fibroblasts: embryonic morphology and implantation. Fertil Steril 1989;42:503–508.
39. Frydman R, Forman RG, Belaisch-Allart J, et al. An assessment of alternative policies for embryo transfer in an in vitro fertilization-embryo transfer program. Fertil Steril 1988;50:466–470.
40. Dale PO, Tanbo T, Kjekshus E, Abyholm T. Pregnancy after transfer of cryopreserved embryos in clomiphene citrate resistant polycystic ovarian syndrome. Fertil Steril 1990;53:362–364.
41. Salat-Baroux J, Cornet D, Alvarez S, et al. Pregnancies after replacement of frozen-thawed embryos in a donation program. Fertil Steril 1988;49:817–821.
42. Wolf SA, Shintay EP, Gagliardi CL. E2 levels during in vitro fertilization are not predictive of pregnancy outcome after subsequent cryopreserved-thawed embryo transfer. Presented at the 46th Annual Meeting of the American Fertility Society, Washington, D.C., 1990, Abstract No. P-032.
43. Medical Research International and the Society for Assisted Reproductive Technology, The American Fertility Society. In vitro fertilization-embryo transfer in the United States: 1988 results from the IVF-ET Registry. Fertil Steril 1990;53:13–20.
44. Meldrum DR, Hamilton F, Marr B, et al. Oocyte donation increases the proportion of embryos implanting and reverses the age-related decline of fertility. Presented at Pacific Coast Fertility Society Meeting, Scottsdale, Arizona, 1990, Abstract No. A17.
45. Sauer MV, Paulson RJ, Lobo RA. A preliminary report on oocyte donation extending reproductive potential to women over 40. N Engl J Med 1990;323:1157–1160.
46. Michelow MC, Berstein J, Jacobson MJ, et al. Mother-daughter in vitro fertilization triplet surrogate pregnancy. J Vitro Fert Embryo Trans 1988;5:31–34.
47. Testart J, Lassalle B, Forman R, et al. Factors influencing the success rate of human embryo freezing in an in vitro fertilization and embryo transfer program. Fertil Steril 1987;48:107–112.
48. Feichtinger W, Kemeter P. Pregnancy after total ovariectomy achieved by ovum donation. Lancet 1985;2:722–723.

CHAPTER 54

Extended Techniques in Assisted Reproductive Technologies

ERIC S. SURREY and JOHN F. KERIN

This chapter describes and critically assesses the indications, techniques, and reported results associated with several of the assisted reproductive technologies that have not yet reached widespread use or acceptance. These include zygote intrafallopian transfer (ZIFT), tubal embryo transfer (TET), transcervical cannulation of the fallopian tubes for delivery of gametes and zygotes, direct intraperitoneal deposition of gametes, ovum transfer, and gestational surrogacy or "host womb."

ZYGOTE INTRAFALLOPIAN TRANSFER AND TUBAL EMBRYO TRANSFER

Technique

Reported national average pregnancy rates have been consistently higher for gamete intrafallopian transfer (GIFT) than for in vitro fertilization/embryo transfer (IVF/ET) procedures.[1] Although these data are derived from patients with different causes of infertility and may not be strictly comparable, one possible cause for this difference has been attributed to the placement of gametes at the physiologic site of fertilization in the ampullary portion of the fallopian tube during GIFT. This presumably allows for synchronized transport of the early-stage cleaved embryo from the distal fallopian tube to the uterine cavity (see Chapter 52). In addition, the hormonal and mitogenic milieu of the tubal lumen may be more advantageous to embryo development than that of the gamete laboratory. Other factors contributing to this discrepancy may include differences in the types of patients assigned to each treatment group. Patients with severe male or immunologic factor infertility have generally been treated with IVF/ET as opposed to GIFT. The inability to document or assist in the fertilization process in vitro represents a major drawback to placing unfertilized gametes into the fallopian tube in these cases.

The development of ultrasound-guided oocyte aspiration

techniques has allowed investigators to combine the advantages inherent in both of these procedures: the intratubal transfer of oocytes or zygotes fertilized in vitro. Early animal and human work suggested the potential efficacy of ZIFT.[2, 3] An increasing experience with ZIFT as a treatment for infertility has been accumulated over the last 3 years. The ability both to document and to enhance fertilization before zygote transfer makes ZIFT an ideal procedure for couples with male and immunologic factors as causes for their infertility.[3–7] Others have also used this form of therapy for other causes of refractory nontubal infertility, including endometriosis and unexplained infertility.[8–11] The absence of at least one normal patent fallopian tube is an *absolute contraindication* to performing this procedure. Potential indications for ZIFT are listed in Table 54–1.

Controlled ovarian hyperstimulation regimens that have been used for ZIFT are similar to those used for IVF/ET and GIFT with concomitant monitoring of follicular development by ultrasonography and endocrinologic parameters. Oocyte retrieval is performed transvaginally under ultrasound guidance as previously described (see Chapter 52). Oocytes are cultured and subsequently inseminated in vitro as is described elsewhere in this text (see Chapter 56). Fertilization can be further assisted in cases of severe oligoasthenospermia or high antisperm antibody titers using various media additives, sperm concentrations, and micromanipulation tech-

---

TABLE 54–1. Indications for Zygote Intrafallopian Transfer/Tubal Embryo Transfer

One normal patent fallopian tube
Male factor
Immunologic factor
Endometriosis (?)
Unexplained infertility (?)
Prior gamete intrafallopian transfer failures (?)
Prior in vitro fertilization failures (?)
Oocyte donation

---

niques as indicated.[3, 5, 12] Once normal fertilization is confirmed 18 hours after insemination, zygote transfer is planned. Transfer of zygotes has been generally performed by transfimbrial tubal cannulation in a manner similar to that of GIFT using a multipuncture laparoscopic or less frequently minilaparotomy approach (Fig. 54–1). The zygotes are gently deposited at a depth of 2 to 4 cm from the distal tubal ostium using the same catheters as those described for GIFT procedures (see Chapter 52). Techniques for transcervical cannulation of the fallopian tube are discussed subsequently.

The ideal time for transfer has not been clearly defined. Initial studies involved the intratubal transfer of pronuclear-stage zygotes, 18 to 24 hours after insemination.[3, 4, 7, 8, 11, 13–15] More recently, other investigators have allowed for confirmation of further early embryonic development in vitro and transferred cleaved embryos 40 to 50 hours postinsemination.[6, 10, 13, 14, 16] This latter procedure is separately described as TET. Aside from confirming embryo cleavage, the TET procedure allows patients an additional 24-hour interval for recovery from the initial oocyte aspiration procedure. As discussed subsequently, there have been no controlled compar-ative studies assessing the relative efficacy of these two times for transfer.

Results

Interpretation of reported pregnancy rates achieved with ZIFT procedures is extremely confusing. The 1991 registry report of the Society for Assisted Reproductive Technology documents a 24.4% overall clinical pregnancy rate and 19.7% ongoing pregnancy rate per retrieval.[1] These data are somewhat lower than rates reported for GIFT procedures. Unfortunately, results from both TET and ZIFT procedures are combined with no differentiation made for diagnosis or age-related success.

Success rates reported by individual investigators for laparoscopic ZIFT and TET are displayed in Tables 54–2 and 54–3. Data derived from transcervical transfer are discussed subsequently. Of 638 ZIFT cycles reported, a mean ongoing pregnancy rate per cycle of 32% was reported. Of only 141 reported TET cycles, a mean clinical pregnancy rate per cycle

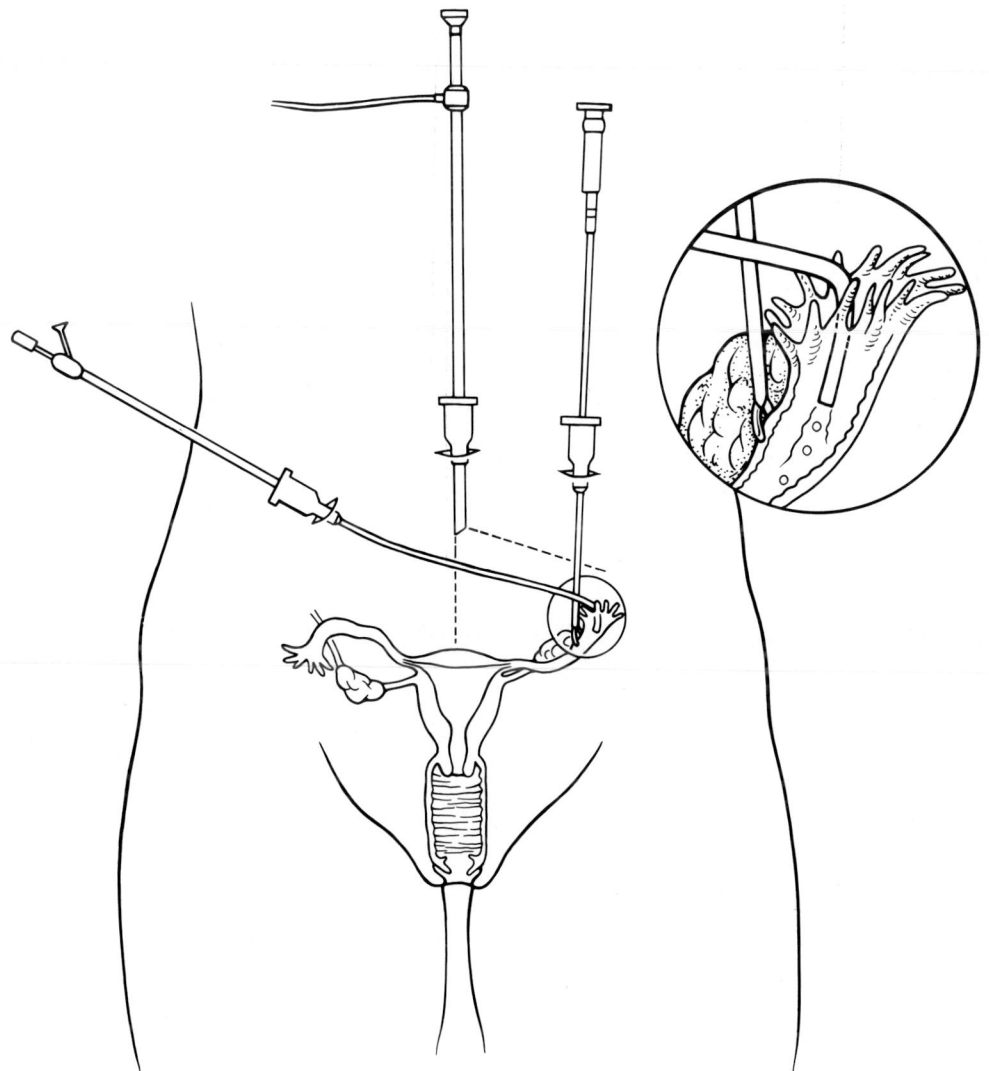

FIGURE 54–1. Laparoscopic trans-fimbrial tubal embryo transfer. (Modified from Bauer O, Diedrick K, van der Ven H, et al. The transvaginal tubal transfer: a new treatment in male infertility. Ann NY Acad Sci 1991; 626:468.)

TABLE 54–2. Laparoscopic Zygote Intrafallopian Transfer Outcome (Pronuclear Stage Embryos)

Author	Cycles (N)	Diagnosis	Ongoing Pregnancy/Cycle (%)	Ectopic Pregnancy	Study Design
Yovich et al[4]	55	Male	9 (32)	NR*	Nonrandomized
	8	Immunologic	3 (38)		Control: prior cycle
	4	Oocyte donation	2 (50)		
	15	Failed GIFT, DI	6 (0)		
Balmaceda et al[6]	123	Immunologic, male Failed GIFT	30 (24)	1	Nonrandomized Control: prior cycle
Yovich et al[5]	9	Male	5 (56)	NR	Nonrandomized Control: prior cycle
Hamori et al[8]	31	Unexplained	9 (29)	0	Nonrandomized Control: prior cycle
	8	Male	2 (25)		
	3	Endometriosis	1 (33)		
Devroey et al[9]	54	Unexplained	23 (43)	0	Uncontrolled
Palermo et al[7]	42	Male	11 (26)	0	Uncontrolled
Cummins et al[14]	46	Prior poor responders	13 (78)	NR	Nonrandomized Control: prior cycle
Tanbo et al[10]	73	Nontubal infertility	33 (45)	NR	Prospective nonrandomized Control: IVF, GIFT, TET in other patients
Pool et al[11]	132	Nontubal infertility	53 (40)	4	Prospective nonrandomized Control: IVF, GIFT, TET in other patients
Chang et al[12]	1	Male	1 (100)	0	Case report
Toth et al[17]	34	Male, endometriosis unexplained, PCO	9 (26)	0	Prospective nonrandomized Control: IVF in other patients
TOTAL	638		204 (32)		

*NR = not reported.

GIFT, Gamete intrafallopian transfer; DI, donor insemination; IVF, in vitro fertilization; TET, tubal embryo transfer; PCO, polycystic ovary syndrome.

of 37% was reported. Unfortunately, interpretation of these data is extremely difficult given the mixture of indications, stimulation regimens, transfer techniques, and study designs used. Most of these investigations are nonrandomized and uncontrolled or, at best, controlled only by patients' previous failed response to IVF/ET or GIFT. In one prospective study in which 150 patients with either male factor or unexplained infertility were randomly assigned to IVF/ET, TET, or GIFT, pregnancy rates were not significantly different among the treatment groups.[10] This finding was substantiated by Toth and coworkers.[17] In contrast, others have reported significantly higher success rates with ZIFT or TET in comparison to IVF/ET in nonrandomized series.[4, 11, 15] In an uncontrolled study, Yovich and coworkers[13] described equivalent success rates for GIFT as for TET/ZIFT when results for GIFT cycles

were adjusted for the fertilization rates achieved with IVF/ET and ZIFT/TET. Clinical pregnancy rates, however, were significantly higher for tubal versus intrauterine transfer. We are aware of no controlled investigation comparing the relative efficacy of TET versus ZIFT.

The relationship between number of zygotes transferred and pregnancy has been indirectly addressed by some observers. Yovich and coworkers[13] reported that although the clinical pregnancy rate for ZIFT plateaued with transfer of two embryos, a plateau was not reached with GIFT until four oocytes were transferred. These findings were confirmed by Palermo and associates[7] in managing couples with both unexplained and male factor infertility. This phenomenon could be accounted for by failed intratubal fertilization.

Tubal transfer of early-stage embryos represents a tech-

TABLE 54–3. Laparoscopic Tubal Embryo Transfer (Cleaved Embryos)

Author	Cycles (N)	Diagnosis	Clinical Pregnancy/Cycle (%)	Ectopic Pregnancy	Study Design
Yovich et al[13]	3	Oocyte donation	3 (100)	1	Case reports
Balmaceda et al[6]	16	Male	6 (38)	0	Uncontrolled
Cummins et al[14]	16	Prior poor responders	3 (19)	NR*	Nonrandomized Control: prior cycle
Tanbo et al[10]	42	Unexplained, male, endometriosis	16 (38)	NR	Prospective nonrandomized Control: GIFT, IVF, ZIFT in other patients
Rotsztejn et al[16]	11	Oocyte donation	9 (82)	0	Uncontrolled
Bauer et al[37]	53	Male	15 (28)	NR	Nonrandomized Control: Transcervical TET in other patients
TOTAL	141		52 (37)		

*NR = not reported.

GIFT, Gamete intrafallopian transfer; IVF, in vitro fertilization; ZIFT, zygote intrafallopian transfer; TET, tubal embryo transfer.

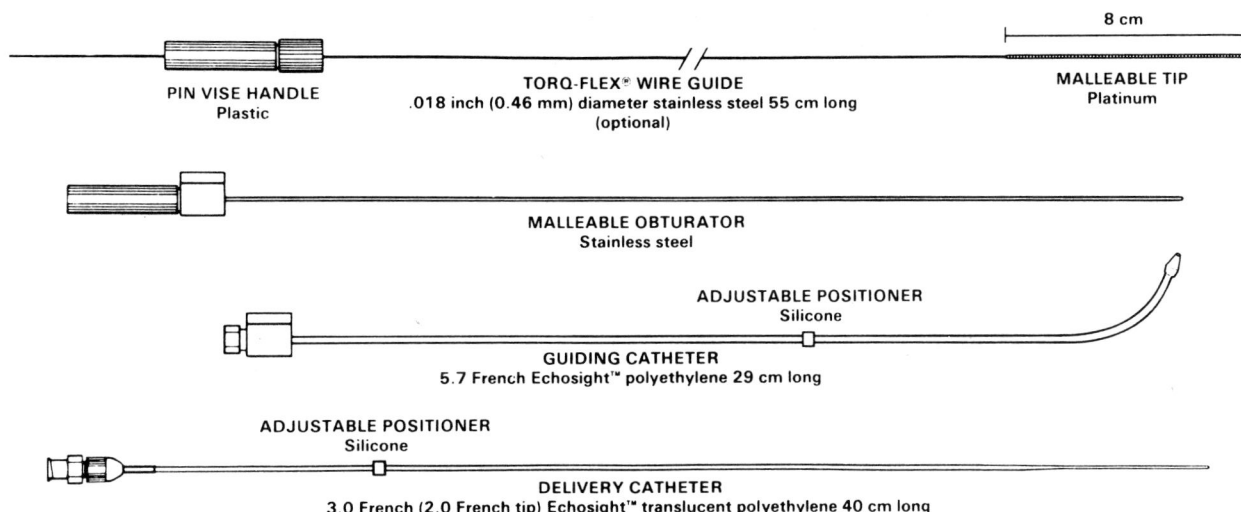

FIGURE 54–2. Jansen-Anderson tubal catheterization set. (Courtesy of Cook Ob/Gyn, Spencer, IN.)

nique with great theoretic advantage. Couples who require assisted extracorporeal fertilization may benefit by replacement of these zygotes into the more physiologic environment of the normal fallopian tube. A lack of well-designed prospective, randomized, controlled studies comparing ZIFT with the more traditional GIFT and IVF/ET procedures has tempered the initial, highly encouraging reports. In addition, the relative merit of TET versus ZIFT has not been well addressed to date. One inherent drawback of these procedures, the need for laparoscopic zygote transfer under general anesthesia 24 to 48 hours after initial oocyte aspiration, might be eliminated with perfection of transcervical approaches to zygote placement.

TRANSCERVICAL CANNULATION OF THE FALLOPIAN TUBE—A NEW WAY TO DEPOSIT GAMETES OR EMBRYOS?

Technique

Transcervical fallopian tube cannulation techniques for the tubal placement of sperm and embryos were first described by Jansen and coworkers in 1988.[18–20] These less invasive "nonsurgical" methods for gamete and embryo tubal placement are attempting to challenge more traditional laparoscopic and minilaparotomy-directed transfimbrial tubal placement techniques. Data that suggest that carbon dioxide pneumoperitoneum and general anesthetic agents exert deleterious effects on embryo and oocyte quality[21, 22] make this minimally invasive approach particularly attractive should it prove to be at least as successful as more invasive methods. Although theoretically more attractive, it still remains to be seen if tactile, ultrasound-guided, or endoscopic-guided techniques could provide a more accurate and successful means of tubal cannulation for gamete or embryo placement. An evaluation of current instrumentation, techniques, and pregnancy rates is presented here.

A coaxial system using a "malleable obturator" to curve and direct a "guiding catheter" toward the uterotubal ostium (UTO), under ultrasound guidance, and then replacing the

obturator with a smaller tubal gamete or embryo "delivery catheter" was first described by Jansen and coworkers.[18–20] Minor but important improvements in these insemination sets have been made by placing a small flared end on the "guiding catheter" for its smoother entry toward and into the UTO. The addition of polyethylene material has made the catheter more echogenic to enhance sonographic visualization. A torque-flex wire has also been included for cannulation of the tube as necessary. The "delivery catheter" has been lengthened by 5 to 40 cm with a proximal outside diameter of 3 Fr (1 mm), which tapers down to 2 Fr (0.6 mm) for its distal 4 to 5 cm yielding easy access into the medial one third of the fallopian tube. Details of the design of the current Jansen-Anderson Insemination Set (Cook OB/GYN, Spencer, IN) are displayed in Figure 54–2. A variety of other tubal coaxial cannulation systems have been developed. Examples of some of these systems are the Spirtos Coaxial Catheter Set for gamete transfer (Cook OB/GYN), Cook Hysteroscopic Insemination Catheter Set (Cook OB/GYN), Royal Women's Coaxial Catheter Set (Cook OB/GYN), and the Fallopian Tube Catheter Set (Labotect, GmbH, Gottingen, Germany).

Transcervical access to the fallopian tube has been successfully achieved using several modalities, including using ultrasound, endoscopic, and tactile guidance (Table 54–4). Transabdominal ultrasound imaging using a half to full bladder window technique can be used to guide the echogenic guiding catheter into the UTO. Unfortunately, use of abdominal ultrasound imaging even with a half-full bladder is inherently uncomfortable for the patient, especially with prolonged procedures. This discomfort can be reduced and image quality can be significantly enhanced with the use of vaginal ultrasound transducers. The transvaginal imaging technique for transcervical tubal catheterization as originally described by

TABLE 54–4. Techniques for Transcervical Tubal Catheterization

Ultrasonography: abdominal, transvaginal
Hysteroscopy
Falloposcopy
Tactile

Jansen and Anderson is demonstrated in Figure 54–3. The small delivery catheter can be gently fed into the tube for a depth varying from 2 to 6 cm. Catheter position in the tube can be confirmed by injecting air bubbles, which are echogenic. If the placement is satisfactory, an inner catheter containing sperm, sperm and oocytes, or embryos suspended in a minimal volume of medium is advanced to the ampullary-isthmic junction (approximately 3 cm) and the contents expelled. Hughes and colleagues[23] were able to demonstrate that successful coaxial cannulation of the fallopian tube could be successfully performed using transvaginal ultrasound appearance of the guide catheter in conjunction with the tactile sensation of a smooth passage of the inner catheter.[22] They confirmed 12 of 16 (75%) successful tubal cannulations at immediate postprocedure laparoscopy with the catheter reaching an average of 3.3 cm into the tube. A coaxial catheter system has been described with a small metal pellet in the distal tip of the inner delivery catheter and side opening proximal to this tip (Cook OB/GYN, "Echo-tip" catheter). The catheter "echo" tip can be seen entering the tube using either abdominal or vaginal ultrasound techniques. With successful cannulation, the transfer catheter is noted to have an S-shaped configuration without kinking.

Although vaginal ultrasound transducers afford enhanced image quality, simultaneous manipulation of an ultrasound transducer and coaxial catheter system within the vagina can be rather awkward. As a result, several investigators have used a "tactile" method for tubal cannulation using modifications of intrauterine embryo transfer techniques.[24–28] We have used a Teflon-coated prototype catheter (Cook Ob/Gyn)

with a 13-cm proximal shaft having an outer diameter of 6 Fr (7 mm) for negotiating the uterine cavity (Fig. 54–4).[28] The distal 0.6 cm is tapered down to 3 Fr (1 cm) and precurved by hand. This Teflon catheter is of the correct consistency to maintain a precurved bend and follow the natural angle of the uterine cavity without injury. Once the curvature of the endocervical canal is negotiated, the catheter is gently and gradually turned through an arc of 60 to 90 degrees as it is advanced into either the right or left "uterotubal gutter" and into the ostium by tactile sensation. Graduated markings on the shaft indicate placement at distances of 7, 8, 9, 10, and 11 cm. In 80% of cases in our experience, the small precurved distal end of the catheter slips into the tube to a depth of 1 to 3 cm with minimal to no discomfort. At a point of 2.5 to 3 cm from the UTO, the tubal lumen is at its narrowest and may be an appropriate point to inseminate a 0.2-mL volume of washed spermatozoa. For tubal oocyte, sperm, or embryo placement, an inner 2 Fr (0.6 mm) delivery catheter can be fed through the outer guide catheter and placed close to or beyond the ampullo-isthmic junction. The optimal site for gamete and zygote placement is still unknown. Similarly, whether this optimal site is different for oocyte, sperm, or embryo deposition has not been determined.

During hysteroscopically directed falloposcopy procedures that involve similar coaxial tubal cannulation techniques, we have observed that the UTO is active, particularly during the periovular period (see Chapter 25). The UTO frequently undergoes rhythmic contractions, which last 2 seconds and convert to spasmodic episodes lasting 8 to 15 seconds when

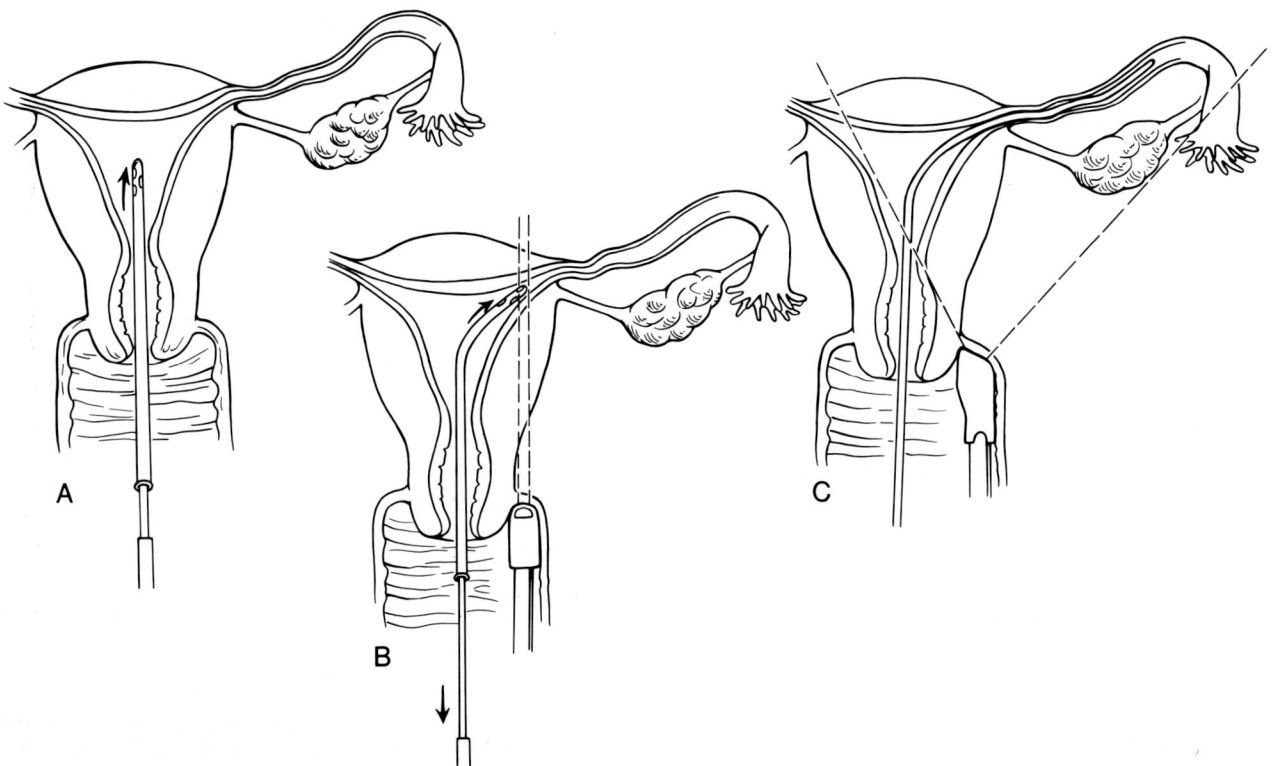

FIGURE 54–3. Ultrasound-guided fallopian tube catheterization: Jansen-Anderson technique. *A*, The cannula is guided through the endocervical canal into the endometrial cavity with the obturator advanced. *B*, The obturator is withdrawn, and the cannula is advanced to the uterotubal ostium. The transducer is in the sagittal plane. *C*, The catheter is advanced through the cannula to the ampulloisthmic junction. The transducer is in the transverse plane. (From Jansen RPS, Anderson JC. Catheterization of the fallopian tubes from the vagina. Lancet 1987; 2:309.)

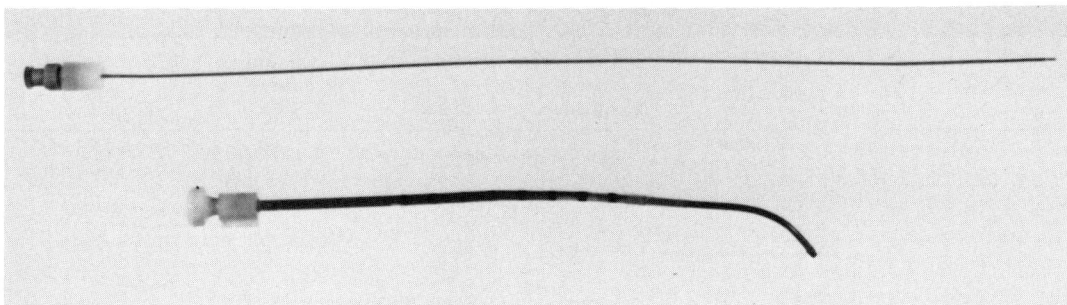

FIGURE 54–4. Prototypic tubal cannulation set (Cook OB/GYN) employed for ITT. *Upper*, Precurved transuterine catheter 30-cm long with a 2-mm distal outside diameter (OD) and control expansion of 3-mm OD at the tip. The shaft has markings to the 14-cm point. *Lower*, Tubal Echo-tip insemination catheter (Cook, Ob/Gyn) with 40-cm length; smooth, rounded leading end; side opening proximal to the tip; and an OD of 0.6 mm. (From Oei ML, Surrey ES, McCaleb B, Kevin JF. A prospective randomized study of pregnancy rates following transuterotubal and intrauterine insemination. Fertil Steril 1992; 58:167–171. Reproduced with permission of the publisher, The American Fertility Society.)

cannulation is difficult or if the ostium is deliberately probed with a stiff wire guide or cannula. Tubal spasm may be a reason why attempts at blind cannulation of the tube may occasionally prove to be painful, difficult, or fail altogether. If forceful probing is attempted, temporary or permanent ostial or luminal damage may potentially occur. As a result, hysteroscopic-directed cannulation of the UTO using coaxial techniques under direct visualization may provide a greater margin of safety.[30] Similarly, falloposcopic confirmation of the exact location of the UTO, the distance to the ampullary-isthmic junction from the UTO, and the absence of any cornual or luminal pathology may prove to be particularly useful before gamete or embryo transfer.[29, 31]

Theoretic risks of tubal cannulation procedures include those of infection, ectopic pregnancy, tubal trauma or perforation, vasovagal reactions, and development of antisperm antibodies. It is reassuring to note that the incidence of increase in antisperm antibody titers in women undergoing intrauterine insemination (IUI) is extremely low.[32] This phenomenon has not been assessed with intratubal insemination (ITI) or transcervical GIFT. Our experience with ITI, however, confirmed a minimal incidence of vasovagal symptoms and no evidence of tubal infection.[28] The incidences of ectopic pregnancy with transcervical GIFT and ZIFT appear to be only minimally increased over those reported with laparoscopic approaches, although the numbers presented are extremely small (Tables 54–5 and 54–6).

Results

Interpretation of results achieved with ITI, GIFT, and ZIFT is fraught by a lack of controlled studies. In their initial description of ITI, Jansen and associates[18] documented successful tubal catheterization using ultrasound guidance in 40 of 50 cycles with a cycle conception rate of 6 of 50 (12%). Clinical pregnancy rates ranging from 11% to 23% per cycle have been reported by other investigators in small series using either ultrasound-guided or tactile techniques.[26, 33, 34] Patients were treated for a variety of indications with many different controlled ovarian hyperstimulation regimens, which makes results difficult to interpret. In a controlled, prospective, randomized cross-over study of 414 cycles comparing both ultrasound-directed and tactile transuterine tubal insemination with IUI, Oei and coworkers[28] were unable to

demonstrate a significant difference in cycle outcome between the two methods.

Jansen and Anderson[20] and Bustillo and colleagues[35] initially described successful transcervical GIFT and TET procedures in 1988. Since that time, a limited number of preliminary studies reporting success with these procedures have been reported in peer-review journals. The results of these investigations are presented in Tables 54–5 and 54–6. Once again, these studies are marked by a lack of randomization and controls. Indications for these procedures have been variable as have been the techniques. In the majority of investigations, gametes or zygotes have been transferred to a single fallopian tube. All the retrograde GIFT studies were uncontrolled, with three using ultrasound-guided and one tactile catheterization techniques. The clinical pregnancy rate per cycle initiated was 28%, with 17% of these pregnancies becoming ectopic. These pregnancy rates are comparable to those reported for laparoscopic GIFT procedures, although the ectopic pregnancy rates are somewhat higher using a transcervical approach.

Results of nine published investigations assessing transcervical intratubal zygote placement included seven using cleaved embryos (TET), 1 using pronuclear-stage embryos (ZIFT), and one using both techniques are summarized in Table 54–6. No studies were randomized, and a variety of indications were used. Catheterization was performed using ultrasound, tactile, and hysteroscopic guidance. The largest series reported consisted of 105 cycles in patients with male factor infertility and described pregnancy rates comparable to those achieved in 53 cycles of other patients undergoing laparoscopic TET.[37, 42] Two other investigators used results of concomitant IVF cycles in other patients as controls.[38, 39] The mean overall clinical pregnancy rate per cycle in these reports presented in Table 54–6 was 60 of 134 (26%) with three ectopic pregnancies (5%). Overall, these results are generally comparable to those reported for laparoscopically guided transfimbrial zygote placement (see Tables 54–2 and 54–3).

Avoidance of exposure to general anesthesia and avoidance of multiple invasive procedures are significant advantages of transcervical approaches to tubal cannulation. To date, however, the best techniques and instrumentation system for tubal gamete and zygote placement have not been established. From sparse preliminary data, retrograde GIFT and ZIFT procedures appear to be relatively equivalent to more conventional techniques, although this has to be definitively

TABLE 54–5. Transcervical Gamete Intrafallopian Transfer

Author	Cycles (N)	Diagnosis	Technique	Catheter	Clinical Pregnancy/Cycle (%)	Ectopic (%)	Study Type
Lucena et al[34]	7	Unexplained, endometriosis	Ultrasound	Cook	3 (42)	1 (33)	Uncontrolled
Ferraiolo et al[27]	40	Unexplained, tubal, pelvic, endometriosis	Tactile	Med-Italia	7 (11)	1 (14)	Uncontrolled
Lucena et al[36]	16	Male, unexplained, failed DI, ovulatory factor	Ultrasound	Cook	7 (44)	1 (14)	Uncontrolled
Bustillo et al[35]	1	Unexplained	Ultrasound	Cook	1 (100)	0	Case report
TOTAL	64				18 (28)	3 (17)	

DI, donor insemination.

demonstrated. The unfortunate lack of well-designed prospective, randomized, controlled studies has further hampered adequate assessment of these extremely exciting and minimally invasive techniques.

INTRAPERITONEAL GAMETE TRANSFER

In an effort to enhance pregnancy rates while minimizing cost, several investigators have attempted to place gametes into the peritoneal cavity in the pouch of Douglas.[43–49] It has been postulated, but not proved, that progress of sperm toward the ampulla of the fallopian tube might be compromised in patients with unexplained infertility. Entry of sperm into the tube through the fimbriated end might allow for more direct access to the oocyte in the distal ampulla according to these hypotheses. It has therefore been proposed that an intraperitoneal pool of sperm in the cul-de-sac could serve as an ideal reservoir for tubal pick-up. Forrler and coworkers[45] described a technique of direct intraperitoneal insemination (IPI) in patients with unexplained and cervical factor infertility. After clomiphene citrate/human chorionic gonadotropin–controlled ovarian hyperstimulation, a small volume of washed sperm was introduced into the peritoneal cavity by culdocentesis, with 3 of 10 patients subsequently conceiving. Conflicting results, however, have been reported by

other investigators.[46–48] Two prospective, randomized crossover trials have been reported that compare pregnancy rates among patients treated with controlled ovarian hyperstimulation and subsequent IUI, direct IPI, and timed intercourse.[47, 48] Both groups of investigators demonstrated that IUI and IPI were superior to timed intercourse alone. However, Campos-Liete and coworkers[49] found no benefit of IPI over timed intercourse in a prospective, randomized, controlled study. Evans and colleagues[47] additionally noted a significantly increased pregnancy rate in patients receiving IPI over IUI, particularly for couples with unexplained infertility. In contrast, Hovatta and coworkers[48] could find no difference between these two groups. The need for larger-scale controlled trials to resolve this issue is clear.

Mason, Sharmas and others[43, 50] reported a series of 11 patients with unexplained infertility who underwent ultrasound-guided peritoneal oocyte and sperm transfer. After controlled ovarian hyperstimulation with clomiphene citrate, human menopausal gonadotropins, and human chorionic gonadotropin, oocyte aspiration was performed under ultrasound guidance using a transabdominal-transvaginal route. Oocytes and sperm were subsequently placed into the pouch of Douglas. Four of nine patients who underwent oocyte aspiration conceived, with three pregnancies ongoing. Subsequently, Gentry and colleagues[44] described a similarly successful procedure under transvaginal ultrasound guidance.

TABLE 54–6. Transcervical Zygote Intrafallopian Transfer/Tubal Embryo Transfer

Author	Cycles (N)	Diagnosis	ZIFT/TET	Technique	Catheter	Clinical Pregnancy/Cycle (%)	Ectopic Pregnancy (%)	Study Type
Jansen et al[19]	5	Male, endometriosis, tubal	ZIFT (4) TET (1)	Ultrasound	Cook	1 (20)	0	Uncontrolled
Scholtes et al[38]	38	Unexplained, male	ZIFT	Ultrasound	Cook	8 (21)	0	Nonrandomized Controls: IVF cycles in other patients
Risquez et al[40]	51	Male, endometriosis, tubal, unexplained	TET	Tactile	Ingenor	5 (10)	2 (40)	Uncontrolled
Yovich et al[39]	17	Pelvic, failed GIFT, male, ovum donation	TET	Ultrasound	Cook	3 (17)	1 (33)	Nonrandomized Controls: IVF cycles in other patients
Bauer et al[25]	16	Male	TET	Tactile	Cook	6 (38)	0	Uncontrolled
Guidetti et al[41]	1	Male	TET	Ultrasound	Cook	1 (100)	0	Case report
Patton et al[30]	1	Immunologic	TET	Hysteroscopy	Cook	1 (100)	0	Case report
Bauer et al[37] and Diedrick et al[42]	105	Male	TET	Tactile	Cook	32 (31)	0	Nonrandomized Controls: Laparoscopic ZIFT in other patients
TOTAL	234					60 (26)	3 (5)	

ZIFT, zygote intrafallopian transfer; TET, tubal embryo transfer; IVF, in vitro fertilization; GIFT, gamete intrafallopian transfer.

The ability to avoid laparoscopy and general anesthesia is a distinct advantage for these procedures, but these extremely small uncontrolled series have not provided enough information to allow for any valid comparison to be made with more traditional techniques of GIFT or IVF/ET in which gamete placement into the fallopian tubes or uterus is confirmed.

OVUM TRANSFER

Ovum transfer is the rather confusing name given to the procedure of timed insemination of a normal fertile woman followed by nonsurgical uterine lavage, retrieval of a flushed embryo, and subsequent transfer to the uterus of an infertile recipient. It was hypothesized that in vivo fertilized embryos may be more developmentally advanced than those fertilized in vitro.[51] The primary indication for this procedure is as therapy for the functionally agonadal woman who has experienced premature ovarian failure, surgical ovarian extirpation, or gonadal dysgenesis. Other indications might include those women with such severe pelvic adhesions that oocytes cannot be successfully retrieved for IVF/ET procedures or carriers for severe sex-linked or autosomal dominant genetic disorders.

In this procedure as described by Bustillo and coworkers,[52] a fertile donor undergoes insemination with sperm from the partner of the recipient based on timing of ovulation. The donor is required to abstain from intercourse for 5 days before insemination. Five to 6 days after insemination, the early-stage cleaved embryo is retrieved by transcervical uterine lavage using a catheter filled with 60 mL of Dulbecco's medium supplemented with 5% serum albumin, a procedure requiring no anesthesia. The lavage is repeated on a daily basis until the embryo is retrieved, which is then transferred into the endometrial cavity of the recipient. Synchronization of luteinizing hormone (LH) peaks within 2 days between donor and recipient was obtained by measuring serum LH by radioimmunoassay. Further synchronization of donor and recipient could be enhanced by use of oral contraceptives or clomiphene citrate.

The first recovery of embryos by flushing techniques was described by Seed and Seed[53] in 1980. Buster and associates[54] described the first successful embryo recovery with subsequent transfer to an infertile woman in 1983. This group has provided the only data on ovum transfer as a treatment for infertility in a series of publications.[51, 55–57] A 47% embryo recovery rate was reported in 53 cycles, with one retained embryo requiring subsequent performance of a therapeutic abortion on the donor. Four intrauterine pregnancies and one ectopic pregnancy were obtained, with three ongoing pregnancies. In a variation on this technique, Formigli and colleagues[58] have reported successful oocyte aspiration from a woman with tubal factor infertility who had failed previous IVF/ET, transfer of gametes into the fallopian tubes of a healthy volunteer with subsequent uterine flushing and embryo transfer into the uterus of the infertile woman.

Although the avoidance of controlled ovarian hyperstimulation and performance of a relatively noninvasive office procedure represent an advantage over ovum donation performed by oocyte aspiration techniques, several distinct disadvantages of ovum transfer have been considered by the Ethics Committee of the American Fertility Society.[59] Without meticulous screening, the risk of transmission of infectious disease to the donor or recipient is not insignificant. The potential for ectopic pregnancy in the donor as well as the previously described risk of embryo retention by the donor necessitating therapeutic abortion must be considered. In addition, few data have been provided by other investigators to allow for more thorough assessment of the validity of the procedure. Owing to the uncertainty surrounding ovum transfer, the Ethics Committee has suggested that "general application of the procedure is thought to be premature."[59]

GESTATIONAL SURROGACY

Gestational surrogacy, or "host womb," refers to the transfer of gametes or zygotes from an infertile couple to a normal fertile woman, who would then relinquish the ensuing child to the genetic parents on delivery. This should be differentiated from surrogacy in general, in which a normal fertile woman is inseminated for the purposes of conceiving and subsequently relinquishing a child that is partially genetically hers to an infertile couple. This latter procedure is discussed elsewhere.

The primary indications for gestational surrogacy include infertile women with normal gonadal function but who lack functional uteri owing to hysterectomy, unrepairable müllerian defects, or müllerian agenesis. Other indications have included prior placenta accreta, cervical incompetence, and various severe medical problems that would potentially be life-threatening should the woman become pregnant.[60–64]

Technically the infertile woman undergoes controlled ovarian hyperstimulation as preparation for oocyte aspiration, which is subsequently performed under laparoscopic or ultrasonographic guidance. Oocytes are inseminated with sperm from the male of the infertile couple, and resultant embryos are subsequently transferred into the uterus of the gestational surrogate. Synchrony between the ovum donor and surrogate has been accomplished by monitoring of basal body temperature charts[64] or administration of oral contraceptives.[60–63]

Reported surrogates have included siblings,[64] mothers,[63] and unrelated women with proven fertility.[60–62] Meticulous medical and psychological screening of surrogates, oocyte donors, and male partners is mandatory.[62] The largest series of gestational surrogacy was reported by Utian and coworkers.[60] Twenty-eight couples were treated during 50 cycles. Thirty-nine oocyte aspirations were performed resulting in 131 transfers of a mean number of 2.6 embryos per transfer. Seven clinical and six ongoing pregnancies were achieved. The ongoing pregnancy rate per oocyte retrieval was therefore 15.4%.

Discussion of the protean ethical and legal aspects of this process are beyond the scope of this discussion but are reviewed extensively both elsewhere in this text (see Chapter 61) and in published reviews.[65–68] These issues are perhaps of greater importance than the techniques that have made gestational surrogacy a medical possibility.

SUMMARY

In this chapter, we have reviewed several of the exciting means by which new applications of previously established assisted reproductive technologies might offer hope to the infertile couple. It is important that the reader appreciates that the enthusiasm surrounding a new procedure must be justified by well-designed clinical trials and tempered by careful scrutiny of the ethical and legal implications of its use.

Acknowledgments

Special thanks are offered to Hazel Myers and Laurie Levine for their expert assistance in preparation of this manuscript.

REFERENCES

1. Society for Assisted Reproductive Technology, American Fertility Society. Assisted reproductive technology in the United States and Canada: 1991 results from the Society for Assisted Reproductive Technology generated from the American Fertility Society Registry. Fertil Steril 1993; 59:956–962.
2. Balmaceda JP, Ord T, Asch RH, Rojas F. Intratubal transfer of embryos in Macaca fascicularis: effect of hyperstimulation and synchrony. Presented at the Fifth World Congress on In Vitro Fertilization and Embryo Transfer, Norfolk, VA, 1989; Abstract pp-148.
3. Devroey P, Braeckmans P, Smitz J, et al. Pregnancy after translaparoscopic zygote intrafallopian transfer on a patient with sperm antibodies. Lancet 1986;1:1329.
4. Yovich JL, Blackledge DG, Richardson PA. et al. Pregnancies following pronuclear stage tubal transfer. Fertil Steril 1987;48:851–857.
5. Yovich JM, Edirisinghe WR, Cummins JM, Yovich JR. Preliminary results using pentoxifylline in a pronuclear stage tubal transfer (PROST) program for severe male factor infertility. Fertil Steril 1988;50:179–181.
6. Balmaceda JP, Gastaldi C, Remohi J, et al. Tubal embryo transfer as a treatment for infertility due to male factor. Fertil Steril 1988;50:476–479.
7. Palermo G, Devroey P, Camus M, et al. Zygote intrafallopian transfer as an alternative treatment for male infertility. Hum Reprod 1989;4:412–415.
8. Hamori M, Stuckensen JA, Rumpf D, et al. Zygote intrafallopian transfer (ZIFT): evaluation of 42 cases. Fertil Steril 1988;50:519–521.
9. Devroey P, Staessen C, Camus M. et al. Zygote intrafallopian transfer as a successful treatment for unexplained infertility. Fertil Steril 1989;52:246–249.
10. Tanbo T, Dale PO, Abyholm T. Assisted fertilization in infertile women with patent fallopian tubes. A comparison of in-vitro fertilization, gamete intra-fallopian transfer and tubal embryo stage transfer. Hum Reprod 1990;3:266–270.
11. Pool TB, Ellsworth LR, Garza JR, et al. Zygote intrafallopian transfer as a treatment for nontubal infertility: a 2-year study. Fertil Steril 1990;54:482–488.
12. Chang SY, Chang YK, Chang MY, et al. A clinical pregnancy after a simple method of zona cutting, cryopreservation and zygote intrafallopian transfer. Fertil Steril 1991;55:420–422.
13. Yovich JL, Yovich JM, Edirisinghe WR. The relative chance of pregnancy following tubal or uterine transfer procedures. Fertil Steril 1988;49:858–864.
14. Cummins JM, Yovich JM, Edirisinghe WR, Yovich JL. Pituitary down-regulation using leuprolide for the intensive ovulation management of poor prognosis patients having in vitro fertilization (IVF)-related treatments. J In Vitro Fert Embryo Trans 1989;6:345–352.
15. Hammitt DG, Syrop CH, Hahn SJ, et al. Comparison of concurrent pregnancy rates for in-vitro fertilization-embryo transfer, pronuclear stage transfer and gamete intra-fallopian transfer. Hum Reprod 1990;5:947–954.
16. Rotsztejn DA, Remoki J, Weekstein LN, et al. Results of tubal embryo transfer in premature ovarian failure. Fertil Steril 1990;54:348–350.
17. Toth TL, Oehninger S, Toner JP, et al. Embryo transfer to the uterus or the fallopian tube after in vitro fertilization yields similar results. Fertil Steril 1992;57:1110–1113.
18. Jansen RPS, Anderson JL, Radonic I, et al. Pregnancies after ultrasound-guided fallopian insemination with cryostored donor semen. Fertil Steril 1988;49:920–922.
19. Jansen RPS, Anderson JL, Sutherland PD. Nonoperative embryo transfer to the fallopian tube. N Engl J Med 1988;319:288–291.
20. Jansen RPS, Anderson JC. Catheterization of the fallopian tubes from the vagina. Lancet 1987;2:309–310.
21. Hayes MF, Sacco AG, Savoy-Moore RT, et al. Effect of general anesthesia on fertilization and cleavage of human oocytes in vitro. Fertil Steril 1987;48:975–981.
22. Boyers SP, Lavy G, Russell JB, De Cherney AH. A paired analysis of in vitro fertilization and cleavage rates of first-versus last-recovered preovulatory human oocytes exposed to varying intervals of 100% CO_2 pneumoperitoneum and general anesthesia. Fertil Steril 1987;48:969–974.
23. Hughes EG, Shekelton P, Leonie M, Leeton J. Ultrasound-guided fallopian tube catheterization per vaginum: a feasibility study with the use of laparoscopic control. Fertil Steril 1988;50:986–989.
24. Kerin JF, Warnes GM, Jeffrey R, et al. A simple technique for human embryo transfer into the uterus. Lancet 1981;2:726–727.
25. Bauer O, van der Ven H, Diedrich K, et al. Preliminary results on transvaginal tubal embryo stage transfer (TV-TEST) without ultrasound guidance. Hum Reprod 1990;5:553–556.
26. Pratt DE, Bieber E, Barnes R, et al. Transvaginal intratubal insemination by tactile sensation: a preliminary report. Fertil Steril 1991;56:984–986.
27. Ferraiolo A, Croce S, Anserini P, et al. "Blind" transcervical transfer of gametes in the fallopian tube: a preliminary study. Hum Reprod 1991;6:537–540.
28. Oei ML, Surrey ES, McCaleb B, Kerin JF. A prospective randomized study of pregnancy rates following transuterotubal and intrauterine insemination. Fertil Steril 1992;58:167–171.
29. Kerin J, Daykhovsky L, Segalowitz J, et al. Falloposcopy: a microendoscopic technique for visual exploration of the human fallopian tube from the uterotubal ostium to the fimbria using a transvaginal approach. Fertil Steril 1990;54:390–400.
30. Patton PE, Hickok LR, Wolf DP. Successful hysteroscopic cannulation and tubal transfer of cryopreserved embryos. Fertil Steril 1991;55:640–641.
31. Kerin JF. Non-hysteroscopic falloposcopy: a proposed method for visual guidance and verification of tubal cannula placement for endotuboplasty, gamete and embryo transfer procedures. Fertil Steril 1992; 57:1133–1135.
32. Horvath PM. A prospective study on the lack of development of anti-sperm antibodies in women undergoing intrauterine insemination. Am J Obstet Gynecol 1989;160:634–637.
33. Berger GS. Intratubal insemination. Fertil Steril 1987;48:328–330.
34. Lucena E, Ruiz JA, Mendoza JC. Vaginal intratubal insemination (VITI) and vaginal GIFT, endosonographic technique: early experience. Hum Reprod 1989;4:658–662.
35. Bustillo M, Munabi A, Schulman JD. Pregnancy after nonsurgical ultrasound-guided gamete intrafallopian transfer. N Engl J Med 1988;319:313.
36. Lucena E, Paulson JD, Ruiz J, et al. Vaginal gamete intrafallopian transfer: experience with 14 cases. J Reprod Med 1990;35:645–647.
37. Bauer O, Diedrick K, van der Ven H, et al. The transvaginal tubal transfer: a new treatment in male infertility. Ann NY Acad Sci 1991;626:467–477.
38. Scholtes MCW, Roozenburg BJ, Alberda AT, Zeilmaker H. Transcervical intrafallopian transfer of zygotes. Fertil Steril 1990;54:283–286.
39. Yovich JL, Draper RR, Turner SR, Cummins JM. Transcervical tubal embryo stage transfer (TC-TEST). J In Vitro Fert Embryo Trans 1990;7:137–140.
40. Risquez F, Boyer P, Rolet F, et al. Retrograde tubal transfer of human embryos. Hum Reprod 1990;5:185–188.
41. Guidetti R, Balmaceda JP, Ord T, Asch RH. Non-surgical tubal embryo transfer. Hum Reprod 1990;5:221–224.
42. Diedrick K, Bauer O, Werner A, et al. Transvaginal intratubal embryo transfer: a new treatment of male infertility. Hum Reprod 1991;6:672–675.
43. Mason B, Sharma V, Riddle A, Campbell S. Ultrasound-guided peritoneal oocyte and sperm transfer (POST). Lancet 1987;1:386.
44. Gentry W, Critser ES, Critser JK, Coulam CB. Pregnancy resulting from peritoneal ovum sperm transfer procedure. Fertil Steril 1989;51:179–181.
45. Forrler A, Dellenbach P, Nisand I, et al. Direct intraperitoneal insemination in unexplained and cervical infertility. Lancet 1986;1:916.
46. Curson R, Parsons J. Disappointing results with direct intraperitoneal insemination. Lancet 1987;2:112.
47. Evans J, Wells C, Gregory L, Walker S. A comparison of intrauterine insemination, intraperitoneal insemination, and natural intercourse in superovulated women. Fertil Steril 1991;56:1183–1187.
48. Hovatta O, Kurunmaki H, Tiitinen A, et al. Direct intraperitoneal or

intrauterine insemination and superovulation in infertility treatment: a randomized study. Fertil Steril 1990;54:339–344.

49. Campos-Liete E, Insull M, Kennedy SH, et al. A controlled assessment of intraperitoneal insemination. Fertil Steril 1992;57:168–173.

50. Sharma V, Mason B, Dinker G, et al. Ultrasound-guided peritoneal oocyte and sperm transfer. J In Vitro Fertil Embryo Trans 1987;4:89–92.

51. Buster JE, Bustillo M, Rodi I, et al. Biologic and morphologic development of donated human ova recovered by nonsurgical uterine lavage. Am J Obstet Gynecol 1985;153:211–217.

52. Bustillo M, Buster JE, Cohen SW, et al. Nonsurgical ovum transfer as a treatment in infertile women: preliminary experience. JAMA 1984;251:1171–1173.

53. Seed RG, Seed RW. Artificial embryonation–human embryo transplant. Arch Androl 1980;5:90–91.

54. Buster JE, Bustillo M, Thorneycroft I, et al. Non-surgical transfer of in vivo fertilized donated ova to five infertile women: report of two pregnancies. Lancet 1983;2:223–224.

55. Buster JE. Embryo donation by uterine flushing and embryo transfer. Clin Obstet Gynecol 1985;12:815–824.

56. Sauer MV, Macaso TM, Ishida EH, et al. Pregnancy following nonsurgical donor ovum transfer to a functionally agonadal woman. Fertil Steril 1987;48:324–325.

57. Bustillo M, Buster JE, Freeman AG, et al. Nonsurgical ovum transfer as a treatment for intractible infertility: what effectiveness can we really expect? Am J Obstet Gynecol 1984;149:371.

58. Formigli L, Pagano M, Roccio C, et al. Surrogate human fallopian tubes for overcoming tubal infertility. Human Reprod 1989;4:416–417.

59. Ethics Committee of the American Fertility Society. Additional procedures. Fertil Steril 1990;53:53S–55S.

60. Utian WH, Sheean L, Goldfarb JM, Kiwi R. Successful pregnancy after in vitro fertilization and embryo transfer from an infertile woman to a surrogate. N Engl J Med 1985;313:1351–1352.

61. Utian WH, Goldfarb JM, Kiwi R, et al. Preliminary experience with in vitro fertilization–surrogate gestational pregnancy. Fertil Steril 1989;52:633–638.

62. Sheean LA, Goldfarb JM, Kiwi R, Utian W. In vitro fertilization (IVF)–surrogacy: application of IVF to women without functional uteri. J In Vitro Fert Embryo Trans 1989;6:134–137.

63. Michelow MC, Bernstein J, Jacobson MJ, et al. Mother-daughter in vitro fertilization triple surrogate pregnancy. J In Vitro Fert Embryo Trans 1988;5:31–34.

64. Leeton J, King C, Harman J. Sister-sister in vitro fertilization surrogate pregnancy with donor sperm: the case for surrogate gestational pregnancy. J In Vitro Fert Embryo Trans 1988;5:245–298.

65. Cohen B, Friend TL. Legal and ethical implications of surrogate mother contracts. Clin Perinatol 1987;14:281–292.

66. Rothenberg KH. Baby M, the surrogacy contract, and the health care professional: unanswered questions. Law Med Health Care 1988;16:113–120.

67. Cahill LS. The ethics of surrogate motherhood: biology, freedom, and moral obligation. Law Med Health Care 1988;16:65–71.

68. Ethics Committee of the American Fertility Society. Surrogate gestational mothers: women who gestate a genetically unrelated embryo. Fetil Steril 1990;53:64S–67S.

69. Ethics Committee of the American Fertility Society. Surrogate mothers. Fertil Steril 1990;53:68S–73S.

CHAPTER 55

The Gamete Laboratory: Design, Management, and Techniques

LUCINDA L. VEECK

Management of a busy in vitro fertilization (IVF) laboratory is comparable to writing a complicated computer program: Attention to minute details is necessary for building the basic framework, overlooking small mistakes can cause the program not to function as expected, somewhat compulsive behavior is required to get everything up and running, and human input is necessary every step of the way. In contrast to working with an extensive database or word processing file, however, one programmer cannot single-handedly create the environment necessary for successful operation. *Teamwork* is the operative word found associated with all successful IVF programs, exhibited as cooperation and friendliness among coworkers and flourishing within the spirit of a common goal. What laboratory cannot depend on the proper management of patients before their oocytes are harvested? We rely on the fact that ovarian stimulation will be carried out in such a way that we will be presented with healthy, viable gametes with which to work. We trust that patients are adequately counseled and that legal consent forms and pertinent medical facts are provided to us in writing before our involvement. Our most important line of communication lies within the clinical and medical sector with physicians and nurses who see patients on a daily basis and who must suffer directly with patients when pregnancy is not achieved. No embryologist in the world underrates the importance of this core group of medical professionals. Neither do clinicians underrate the involvement of the laboratory staff. They trust that we have done everything within our power to create a nourishing environment, that quality control procedures have been thorough and exact, and that safeguards have been set in motion to protect both patients and personnel. To this end, I would like to devote this chapter to the spirit of teamwork, particularly of the sort that has marked the Norfolk program from its beginnings in 1980.

LABORATORY DESIGN

The physical location and size of the typical embryology laboratory are often limited by the constraints of having to work with pre-existing space within a hospital or clinic. Commonly, storage rooms or minor procedure rooms are redesigned to fill the needs of the embryology laboratory. Although not an ideal situation, thoughtful planning can overcome most inconveniences. Additionally, it is necessary to plan for growth and potential establishment of new procedures for the future. Various minimal requirements should be considered:

1. The availability of direct access to the procedure room where harvests and transfers are to be carried out.
2. A means of safe transportation of specimens, whether through a connecting window or uncluttered walkway.
3. Intercom communication between the procedure room and the laboratory/laboratories.
4. Working areas in the laboratory/laboratories large enough to accommodate tissue culture procedures, sperm processing, cryopreservation, special procedures (i.e., micromanipulation and research), and space for quality control logs and patient records.
5. Clean air flow throughout any area where human specimens or culture media are handled.
6. Adequate incandescent lighting, preferably on dimmer switches.
7. Numerous electrical outlets including at least one source for 220 V power (United States).
8. Backup emergency electrical power and lighting.
9. Entrance security for laboratories, restricted to laboratory personnel.

In addition, advance consideration must be given to the location and construction of a semen collection room, a storage area for supplies, and whether computer facilities will be located within the laboratory or in a separate office outside of the sterile area.

In Norfolk, it has been necessary to work within pre-existing hospital space associated with a busy ambulatory care unit. Fortunately for us, new laboratories specifically designed for IVF procedures became available in 1993 with

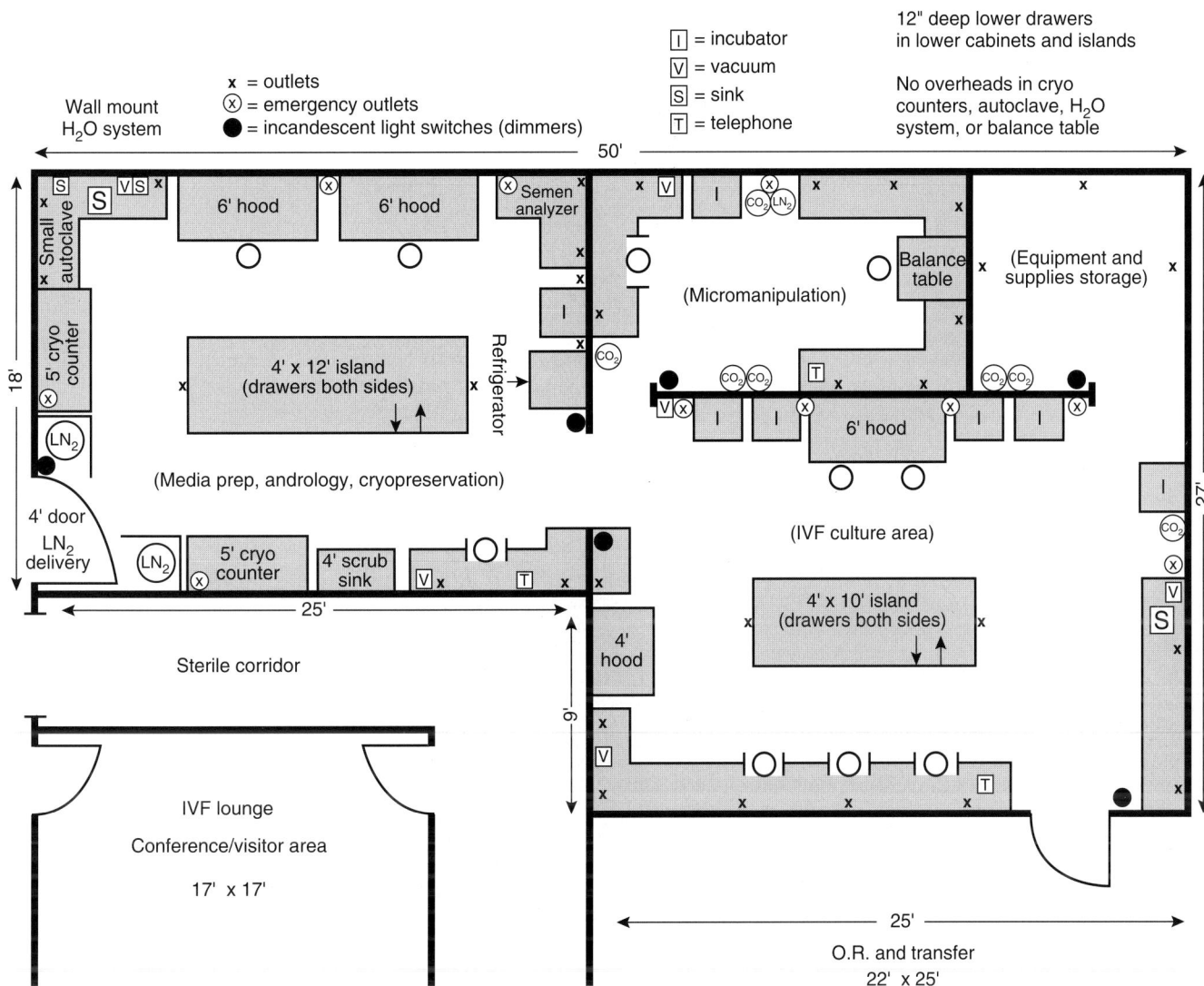

FIGURE 55–1. Gamete Laboratory design. Schematic drawing demonstrating optimal conditions in an embryology laboratory. Note that there are no overhead cabinets above balance table for micromanipulation equipment, computerized semen analyzer, cryopreservation counters, or autoclave area. Areas under cryopreservation counters open for placement of wheeled liquid nitrogen storage vessels. Twelve-inch-deep drawers are found in the lower cabinets and lower center islands. Incandescent lighting is controlled by dimmer switches in each area. CO_2 lines to be run behind walls to central areas.

the construction of an entirely new outpatient unit. The following are descriptions of the previous laboratory space used since 1980 and the improved laboratory construction.

Previous Space

There were three laboratories on a sterile corridor, two of which were adjacent to the operating room where oocyte harvests and transfers were carried out. One laboratory with a single 6-foot laminar flow hood and four dual-stacked carbon dioxide incubators (eight chambers) was used for all oocyte handling and culturing procedures. A second laboratory with two 4-foot laminar flow hoods and one dual-stacked incubator was used for processing semen samples and performing cryopreservation. The third laboratory was used for research, micromanipulation, and serum processing and housed backup cryopreservation units, microscopes, and incubators. Hepa filtered air was circulated throughout these

clean rooms, and emergency generated power was available at designated outlets. Wall-mounted vacuum sources were available for assistance in draining incubator water jackets, incandescent lighting was installed along with emergency lighting units, and a two-line telephone system with an answering machine was available for usage from any of the three laboratories. An additional small storage room was reserved for safe storage of microscopic and video equipment not in use but subject to theft.

Current Accommodation

In an effort to combine facilities and minimize distance between laboratories, a customized design was formulated for the new unit (Fig. 55–1). Under this new plan, all laboratories, except a media preparation facility, are located within the sterile unit. These laboratories interconnect, yet remain separate from one another, to provide some isolation of procedures and reduce the number of personnel within any given room. All the standards listed previously are in effect in the new laboratories, with more attention given to low-level lighting in sensitive areas and convenient location of telephones and electrical outlets. Carbon dioxide tanks are located in central storage areas on the immediate opposite side of the wall where each incubator unit is placed; this was designed to reduce the possibility of carrying in contaminants along with rusted or dirty tanks, which are occasionally delivered. Care has been given to designing adequate work areas and to providing countertop space and storage specific to procedures being done within any location.

Sterile, packaged plasticware is stored, after inventory, in the laboratory's sterile supply room on large stainless steel carts.

A semen collection room with lavatory is located within the unit, and a second, larger room is available on another floor for men desiring complete isolation from noise and outside pedestrian traffic. The unit also provides a conference room for the IVF team, which doubles as a lounge and work area between, during, and after cases. The lounge is equipped with video monitoring equipment that can display the entire procedure room, the entire culture laboratory, the ultrasound scanning image, or the image projected by the Nikon Diaphot microscope within the main embryology laboratory. This video equipment is used for educational purposes and to assist in accommodating large visitor groups.

Because of the noise of the water pump, culture media are prepared at another facility at the Eastern Virginia Medical School/Howard and Georgeanna Jones Institute. Although this laboratory is not along a sterile corridor, it is located away from chemistry and pathology laboratories and is equipped with a horizontal laminar flow hood for clean processing. A Millipore water system, an incubator, osmometer, autoclave, pH meter, and all supplies necessary for weekly media preparation are kept at this site. Regular offices are provided at this location for the laboratory staff.

LABORATORY MANAGEMENT

Although all laboratories differ somewhat in their procedures, some procedural aspects are universal; others are impractical given the facilities and supplies available to some areas of the world. Moreover, some established protocols have been based on "what works" in one laboratory rather than a scientific reflection of true necessity. The following sections, although not advocated as "necessary" for all laboratories, simply describe the workable routine management of the Norfolk laboratories.

Maintenance of Sterility

Limited personnel (i.e., the laboratory staff and students) should have access to the laboratories and equipment. Although hospital security must be able to enter laboratories in the event of an emergency, special arrangements must be made to prevent maintenance, housekeeping, or any uninvited individual from entering laboratory areas.

To ensure safe culturing conditions, the embryology staff must be well trained in the aspects of sterile technique and must dutifully record any break in established procedure. Strict adherence to sterility is attitudinal as well as procedural. When one is rigid about scrubbing hands and dressing out in operating room clothing, a more professional attitude is established. Clean hospital clothing, head covers, shoe covers, and masks should be required for entrance into laboratories; hands must be washed before performing any technical procedure. Visitors and students should be expected to adhere to these regulations, and those with viral infections (i.e., colds, influenza) must be asked not to enter laboratories until they are once again well.

Laminar flow hoods are used for media preparation, serum preparation, handling of oocytes, processing of sperm, and transfer. Their use is commonly restricted specifically to IVF techniques. In Norfolk, hoods are washed during and between procedures with water and wiped down with 70% alcohol when contamination with biologic products occurs. Floors are washed once a week with tap water during patient treatment cycles.

Incubator humidity water pans must be cleaned and refilled once a week; incubator water jackets should be drained and refilled once a year. As part of a sterility assurance program, control dishes can be kept for several days in incubators to monitor sterile culture conditions. At the Jones Institute, breaks occur four times per year in patient treatment to allow for dismantling incubators, autoclaving metal parts, disinfectant cleaning of all laboratory surfaces and equipment, and stripping and waxing of floors. A checklist log is kept to ensure that all cleaning is completed in a thorough manner.

The advent of transvaginal oocyte harvest has created a new concern for sterility: Despite careful vaginal washing, microorganisms may be transferred to the embryology laboratory via follicular aspirates. A rare culturing dish may become contaminated with *Candida albicans* after collection of oocytes from a patient with a concurrent infection. From semen, a sample may become infected with one of the common genital tract microbes. These contaminants might not be evident during the short culture periods of standard IVF, and viral contaminants would most assuredly go undetected. Concerns for microbial and viral transmission have made it necessary to carry out routine disinfection procedures and to test incubators periodically for less obvious genital tract organisms, such as mycoplasma.

Avoidance of Toxicity

Toxicity testing of materials used for culturing oocytes, spermatozoa, and conceptuses should be used to define the suitability of new products and used thereafter for periodic checking. Our program uses a mouse bioassay for this purpose. Mouse embryos fertilized in vivo and collected at the two-cell stage are grown to the hatched blastocyst stage in the same culture medium under the same culture conditions as in the human embryology laboratory. The mouse system is run independently of the human laboratory and therefore has some of the advantages of a blind study. Solutions, plastics, surgical gloves, and surgical instruments are all tested through this system whenever possible. Most importantly, weekly preparations of Ham's F-10 culture medium, bimonthly preparations of freezing medium, and each lot of heat inactivated human fetal cord serum is tested individually before use in human systems. In addition, all media are periodically tested for endotoxins, and serum must pass rigid testing for human immunodeficiency virus (HIV)-1, HIV-2, human T-cell lymphomorphic virus (HTLV)-1, hepatitis B, and hepatitis C.

Glassware used for IVF should not be used for any other purpose. All glassware must be washed with dilute solutions of a tissue culture grade detergent and rinsed extensively (at least 10 times) with MilliQ/UF water before autoclaving. Glassware must again be rinsed multiple times just before use. Disposable plasticware should be used once and discarded.

Steam autoclaving is the method of choice for sterilization to avoid toxic sterilization gases. In cases in which gas sterilization is required (some operating room equipment), appropriate aeration times must be respected, and the instrument should be rinsed with sterile water before use. Chemical sterilizing agents are extremely toxic and should not be used.

Special care must be taken to avoid toxic substances in the operating room. Surgeons must rinse their gloves with sterile water to remove traces of powder proven to be toxic to mouse embryos in culture. Harsh cleaning agents should be avoided, and needles, tubing, and plasticware should be rinsed before oocyte collection. Painting and remodeling must not be allowed in the operating room or anywhere along sterile corridors within 2 weeks before or during patient cycles or patient care.

Mouse Bioassay for Toxicity Testing

The necessity of performing an in-house mouse toxicity test is debatable. Some institutions send out to reference laboratories for this type of testing; others prefer a simpler method of testing for gross toxicity, such as a hamster or human sperm survival assay. The difficulty with sperm survival assays is the inability to test serum products owing to protein agglutination effects. For groups using preovulatory maternal serum, this is not a major disadvantage because there is insufficient time for toxicity testing before the serum must be put to use. Unless one can collect maternal serum in advance of the cycle when it will be used, this inability to test would appear to be a definite drawback to a solid quality control program. Another available option when serum testing is not deemed necessary would be to purchase pretested media from a reliable company. Several respected groups in the United States, South America, and Europe have chosen this option with acceptable results.

The Norfolk program has the luxury of supporting an in-house mouse toxicity assay. Although expensive to purchase and maintain mouse colonies, having a system available for screening all media, reagents, serum products, and new supplies is considered a tremendous asset. The assay is run through the Biological Sciences Program at a local university and thus has the additional advantage of operating independently of the embryology laboratory. B6CBAF1 mice, purchased from Jackson Laboratory (Bar Harbor, ME), are superovulated via intraperitoneal injections of 5 IU pregnant mare serum gonadotropin (Sigma Chemical Co, St. Louis, MO) and 5 IU human chorionic gonadotropin (hCG) (Sigma) administered 48 hours apart at 4:00 to 6:00 P.M. At the time

of hCG injection, each female mouse is mated with one proven-breeder male CD-1 mouse (Charles River Laboratories, Wilmington, MA). At 8:00 to 9:00 A.M. following the hCG injection, female mice are checked for vaginal mucus plugs to determine whether mating has occurred. All media and sera preparations to be tested are prepared and dispensed into culture containers later that same day. They are incubated overnight at 37°C under 5% carbon dioxide. Unless other types of containers are being tested for toxicity, all cultures are established (1 mL/tube) in Nunculon flat-side, screw-top culture tubes (Gibco Laboratories, Grand Island, NY).

Approximately 40 to 42 hours after hCG administration, mouse embryos are flushed from excised oviducts using a 1-mL syringe fitted with a 30-gauge needle. Modified Krebs-Ringer bicarbonate solution supplemented with 4 mg/mL bovine albumin is used for embryo collection and control culture medium. Only morphologically normal two-cell embryos are collected and used in the test system. Triplicate cultures are prepared containing at least 15 embryos from three different mice for each medium/serum combination or toxicity test preparation. Embryonic development is evaluated microscopically once a day for 3 days thereafter.

Several mouse strains have been evaluated. The combination B6CBAF1 female/CD-1 male yields good numbers of two-cell embryos that develop in vitro. With the superovulation protocol described here, 50% to 80% of the mice successfully mate, and approximately 30 two-cell embryos per mated mouse can be anticipated. Several other mouse strains and superovulation protocols have been tested, but none have yielded better results.

Limitations of the Mouse Bioassay for Toxicity Testing

Extreme care must be taken in the use and maintenance of animals. The stress of transport and problems inherent in most animal facilities (e.g., noises, odors, mishandling) can adversely affect the animals' responses. Likewise, environmental factors, such as shortened daylight and colder temperature, are recognized to interfere with the reproduction of male and female mice and may periodically affect results.

There are occasional problems with lot-to-lot variability of reagents, especially bovine serum albumin and gonadotropic hormones. Results with newly purchased products should routinely be compared with results with proven reagents.

Most importantly, the mouse bioassay is limited in its ability to predict minor variations in media quality. Its value is in defining major toxic substances and is of little use in determining qualitative toxin levels.

Equipment, Maintenance, and Quality Control

Constant and consistent quality control of procedures and equipment is of the utmost importance in the embryology laboratory. All hoods and biologic freezers must be checked and certified semiannually and the inspection dates and servicing results logged into a central record book. Microscopes are commonly placed on a similar preventive maintenance program requiring annual cleaning and readjustment.

Multiple incubators (in Norfolk, Forma 3326) with separate carbon dioxide and regulation sources provide backup in case of unforeseen malfunction. Although most incubators display a digital readout of temperature and carbon dioxide, these parameters should be cross-checked manually each day. Carbon dioxide concentration may be checked by a Fyrite gas analyzer (Bacharach Instruments, Pittsburgh, PA), and temperature can be monitored by thermometers placed in water-filled volumetric flasks inside incubator chambers. Safety alarms to alert personnel to fluctuations in temperature or carbon dioxide concentration are a feature of many incubators; when used, alarms should be relayed to central security offices. Unnecessary opening and closing of incubator doors is discouraged. Incubators should be taken apart several times a year; shelves, water pans, sides of inner chambers, and other metal chamber parts are commonly removed, washed, and autoclaved. The inside of each chamber should be washed with a disinfectant solution, such as Rocall II, rinsed with water, and dried. When incubator water jackets are drained, the inside of the jackets should be allowed to dry by forcing air through the chambers before water is replaced. The principal reason for draining and refilling humidity water pans each week is to safeguard against fungal contamination; for this reason, the purchase of removable pans is preferable to filling the bottom of the incubator chamber with water.

Many IVF programs use a carbon dioxide isolette, such as the Hoffman IVF Chamber (Hoffman Surgical Equipment Company, Conshohocken, PA) to establish a controlled environment during oocyte collection and handling procedures. The maintenance of specimens under temperature-controlled and gas-controlled conditions seems quite appealing, especially when considering the training of new personnel or dealing with gamete intrafallopian transfer (GIFT) cycles.

Osmometers are critical in the preparation of culture media. Generally, freezing point–determination osmometers, such as the Advanced Instruments 3W or 3D (Advanced Instruments, Needham, MA) are used to test batches of medium. Freezing baths must be kept full and clean at all times. Temperatures of baths should be checked and the machines standardized with a 290 mOsm/kg reference solution before each use.

A large source of high-purity water is a critical need for IVF. This water source must be capable of meeting demands for all medium preparations, glassware rinsing and washing, and laboratory equipment surface cleaning. The Norfolk program uses a MilliQ/UF water system (Millipore, Inc., Bedford, MA) with six filter cartridges in sequence: prefilter, reverse osmosis filter, carbon absorption filter, two ion exchange filters, and a final ultrafilter (UF). A presterilized disposable bacterial filter has been added to this system. The MilliQ/UF water system provides a large, ready source of water on demand, eliminating the need for further purification and storage. This system, however, must be rigorously and consistently maintained. The filter cartridges must be changed according to the manufacturer's instructions. The UF cartridges must be sanitized once a week, flushed, and checked for chlorine contamination. Bacterial contamination checks are also carried out weekly and routinely recorded.

Another important aspect of quality control is accurate record keeping. As part of any protocol for making up culture media, each ingredient, its lot number and manufacturer, the osmolality, the adjusted osmolality, the date, and initials of the attending technician should be recorded in a log book. The names of patients donating human fetal cord serum must be recorded along with the date of collection and processing and results of microbial, viral, and toxicity testing. Lot numbers of Ham's F-10 and serum used for oocytes and conceptuses must be recorded on each patient's laboratory record to cover any eventual need for this information. These records also commonly include all the observations made during oocyte harvest, sperm preparation, pronuclear evaluation, cleavage assessment, and transfer. Records must be kept regarding the daily testing of incubators and should be examined against pregnancy results to determine that all chambers are operating efficiently. Chart recordings must be kept on biologic freezers and precise seeding temperatures should be recorded for each freezing run. Liquid nitrogen storage tanks should be refilled (topped off) weekly with entry of dates into a log book. Duplicate logs, indicating the exact location (storage tank, canister, and cane numbers) of stored cryopreserved material, are recommended. Water baths and refrigerators must be cleaned regularly and daily temperatures recorded.

Patient Protection and Education

Various safety practices are used in Norfolk to protect the patient from laboratory error. These practices include protocols discussed in the following paragraphs.

The physician is asked to state verbally the patient's name to laboratory personnel before any oocyte harvest procedure begins.

A separate "green sheet" is filled out by the physician and given to the laboratory supervisor before oocytes are collected; this sheet details the basic andrology analysis; alerts embryologists to special conditions, such as antisperm antibodies or previous microbiology testing; indicates any complication encountered in earlier cycles; states whether a frozen backup semen sample is available; and specifies the necessity of donor sperm, micromanipulation, or any other special handling. Additionally the physician is responsible for indicating here the number of embryos that the patient wishes to have transferred fresh and for specifying any requests by the patient regarding cryopreservation or inclusion in various approved research projects. A checklist is included on this sheet for the appropriate consent forms, which must be signed and in the patient's chart. By reviewing the patient's chart and filling out this form, the physician is assured that the laboratory is aware of all pertinent information regarding previous and current cycles, and the embryologist possesses a written order by the medical staff concerning specific handling of oocytes and embryos. This guarantees an adequate, documented communication between medical and laboratory sectors.

The laboratory will not proceed with cryopreservation, micromanipulation, or sperm/oocyte donation without duly signed and witnessed consent forms.

Laboratory personnel are trained to handle sperm, oocytes, and embryos of only one patient at a time. The name of the patient and the oocyte number must be clearly written on each culturing dish and are read aloud whenever taken from the incubator for insemination, observation, or transfer. At the time of intrauterine transfer, the patient is asked to state her name aloud to the embryologist in charge, this name is repeated to the assistant, and the appropriate specimen(s) confirmed by both on removal of the culturing dish from the incubator.

Because human fetal cord serum is used in Norfolk for protein supplementation of culture media, it must be certified free of infectious disease and tested for toxicity. Aliquots of each individual donated serum are sent to the American Red Cross for viral testing (HIV-1 antibody, HIV-2 antibody, HTLV-1 antibody, hepatitis C antibody, and hepatitis B surface antigen), and a log is kept with the name of the donor, date of donation, and results of viral and biologic testing. Serum samples from two to three healthy donors are combined to make a larger pool of serum for IVF use. These lot numbers are recorded on patients' laboratory forms. A frozen aliquot is kept indefinitely of each serum sample to cover any need for subsequent testing. As opposed to the use of fetal cord serum for culture medium supplementation, various other substances may be used. Most commonly, albumin products purchased in lyophilized form are substituted for maternal or cord serum. These products include human serum albumin, pretested and screened for viruses by the manufacturer (Irvine Scientific, Santa Ana, CA) and, less commonly, bovine serum albumin (various manufacturers). Our own preclinical testing and usage of human serum albumin has shown favorable results. Human plasma and purchased plasma fractions may also be substituted for serum; the Norfolk program has little experience with these products.

Backup equipment is available for incubators, microscopes, biologic freezers, and liquid nitrogen storage tanks to protect the patient from equipment malfunction; emergency generated electrical power is in place to protect the patient from equipment malfunction owing to power loss. A written protocol is supplied to hospital security for use in the event of fire or emergency hazard; this protocol specifies names and phone numbers of all laboratory personnel (including pager numbers) and details the procedures for emergency evacuation of fresh and frozen stored specimens.

Patients are offered a series of educational lectures from the medical and scientific staff concerning ovulation induction, IVF, male factor concerns, cryopreservation, micromanipulation, and general laboratory procedures. A social worker conducts group sessions once a week. Social events are scheduled to introduce patients to the faculty. At the time of intrauterine transfer, a card is presented to the patient by the laboratory staff that describes the fertilization outcome of their cycle, describes the embryo cell stage at transfer, and gives the number of specimens maintained under frozen storage. A clinical coordinator is available at all times to address patient concerns and questions.

Protection of Personnel

Each couple is tested for HIV-1 on their initial visit to the Norfolk program. In subsequent treatment cycles, testing is again performed if the period between visits is longer than 3 to 6 months. Other viral tests are carried out only if there is an indication to do so. Legally, one cannot require testing of a patient but can only recommend that testing be carried out. Many couples, in fact, dislike this regular practice because they believe it is unwarranted in their low-risk group. Nonetheless, couples generally agree to the testing once the gravity of the situation and all safety considerations are fully explained. The hazards of handling blood, serum, follicular fluid, and semen cannot be overlooked for any individual working in a clinical laboratory, particularly when gloves are not constantly used throughout the day. Semiannual viral testing (all tests previously described for culture media viral testing) is offered to the laboratory staff but not required. Oocyte donors are more thoroughly tested before acceptance into the program.

Members of the Norfolk laboratory are required to wear disposable, washed latex gloves when processing human fetal cord serum, human semen, or participating in oocyte collection procedures. They are required to wash their hands before and after each oocyte harvest and to dispose of biologic fluids and supplies in an approved manner (red contamination bags and labeled boxes). Incident reports are filled out in a standard hospital-required fashion. Thermal gloves and plastic goggles are available for cryopreservation procedures but are not required.

Training of Personnel

At the Jones Institute, a 3-month training and probation period is required of all new laboratory personnel. During this time, the new employee is exposed to all aspects of IVF, GIFT, and zygote intrafallopian transfer (ZIFT). Routine training includes the validation of sterile technique, procedures for tissue culture, laboratory quality control, medium and serum preparation, human oocyte identification and evaluation, semen analysis, sperm washing and capacitation procedures, oocyte insemination, cryopreservation, embryo evaluation, and conceptus transfer. In addition, correct understanding and maintenance of laboratory equipment are stressed, and employees are taught the appropriate methods of recording laboratory data. Each new training procedure is handled in a three-step method: (1) observation of a trained technologist, (2) side-by-side participation with a trained technologist, and (3) independent performance under supervision.

New employees, although trained in all techniques, may be initially required to concentrate their efforts in one specific area, such as sperm processing; the decision for specialization is made based on the needs of the laboratory and the interests of the employee and may change at a later date. After 1 year of service and the demonstration of suitable skills, the employee may be specifically trained in a supervisory role. In this instance, an additional 3 months of specialized training with the laboratory director is required after which time the employee may supervise the laboratory in the director's absence.

Work Schedules

The Norfolk program sees patients for IVF, GIFT, and ZIFT during four treatment cycles per year, each cycle lasting approximately 8 to 12 weeks. Before the beginning of each new year, a schedule is outlined for the beginning and ending date of each treatment cycle. Special arrangement is made in advance to schedule cycles around the larger scientific and clinical meetings and to provide an adequate break during midsummer and through late December and early January holidays. Laboratory personnel are expected to work during the entire four cycles each year and are entitled to take vacation time and personal time and to attend meetings during the off periods. A written work schedule is outlined, with the input of all members of the embryology staff, before each treatment cycle. This work schedule details a 7-day week, indicating which procedures the employee will be responsible for each day and which 2 days are taken off. These days are consistent each week; for example, the employee knows that he or she has Wednesdays and Saturdays off; will be responsible for sperm preparation and cryopreservation on Tuesdays and Sundays; and will participate in oocyte harvests, intrauterine transfers, and daily media preparation on Mondays, Thursdays, and Fridays. At least three of the four to five members of the embryology team are scheduled to cover the laboratory each day. One has a special day devoted to weekly preparation of all culture media and care of the Millipore water system. We have been fortunate to have one staff member volunteer to work both days of the weekend and thereby have avoided a rotating weekend schedule. In most instances, the maximum length of the routine work day can be anticipated; time required to complete laboratory procedures beyond the regular 9-hour work day may be taken off on another day less demanding. This consistent, yet flexible, type of scheduling prevents confusion and offers the employee the opportunity to work around weekly personal obligations, social events, and occasionally classroom activities.

Employees are expected to participate in monthly journal club meetings and staff meetings unless the demands of the laboratory prevent attendance.

Off periods not consumed by meetings or vacation time are scheduled with laboratory disinfection and cleaning, cord blood processing, pipette preparation, equipment maintenance, and continuation of research.

PROTOCOLS AND TECHNIQUES USED IN NORFOLK

Media Preparation

All media are prepared from dry powdered formulation once a week. Osmometers are calibrated with Clinitrol 290 reference solution after bath liquid level has been checked and the appropriate temperature achieved. Base water used in the preparation of media is collected from a MilliQ/UF water system. Media are sterilized and aliquoted under a horizontal laminar flow hood, stored in sterile 25 cm$_2$ Falcon 3013 tissue culture flasks (Ham's F-10 and Dulbecco's phosphate-buffered saline [DPBS], Gibco Laboratories, Grand Island, NY) or in sterile Falcon 2001 or 2003 culture tubes (cryopreservation media), and dated on the side of the vessel with a *Sharpie* (Sanford) permanent marker. Each weekly batch of Ham's F-10 medium is tested for toxicity through the mouse bioassay system, and each new lot is tested for

endotoxins. Cryopreservation medium (DPBS base) is tested for toxicity by exposure of mouse embryos to media for 30 minutes followed by regular culture in control Krebs'-Ringer's solution. Each medium must be able to support 80% of mouse embryos to the hatched blastocyst stage or reach a level of 90% combined morula and blastocysts.

Media are prepared as follows:

Ham's F-10

1. Add one 1-L package of Ham's F-10 powder (Gibco #81200-040) to approximately 800 mL MilliQ/UF H$_2$O; mix until dissolved.
2. Add 0.05 g of benzyl penicillin G (Sigma #PEN-NA); mix.
3. Add 0.05 g of streptomycin sulfate (Sigma #S6501); mix.
4. Add 1 mM of calcium lactate (L + calcium salt, Calbiochem-Behring #4272); mix.
5. Add 2.10 g of sodium bicarbonate (Sigma #S8875); mix.
6. Add MilliQ/UF H$_2$O to reach 1000 mL; mix.
7. Test osmolality and adjust downward as needed: Figure the number of points above 280 mOsm/kg of uncorrected solution. Divide this number by the total uncorrected number to figure percentage above desired level of 280 mOsm/kg. Remove this percentage of medium and replace with same amount of MilliQ/UF H$_2$O.
8. Retest corrected osmolality.
9. Filter sterilize through 500-mL Nalgene 0.20 μ filtration unit.
10. Aliquot media into Falcon 3013 tissue culture flasks using sterile technique.

Dulbecco's Phosphate-Buffered Saline

1. Add 9.6 g powdered DPBS (Gibco #21300-025) to approximately 800 mL MilliQ/UF H$_2$O (the inside of the package is not rinsed for fear of leaching toxic substances from the metal-based lining). Mix until dissolved.
2. Add 0.1 g CaCl$_2$ to approximately 50 mL MilliQ/UF H$_2$O; mix; add the dissolved CaCl$_2$ solution to the DPBS solution and mix (CaCl$_2$ supplied separately with the DPBS).
3. Add 0.05 g benzyl penicillin G (Sigma #PEN-NA); mix.
4. Add 0.05 g streptomycin sulfate (Sigma #S6501); mix.
5. Add MilliQ/UF H$_2$O to reach 1000 mL; mix.
6. Test and correct osmolality as previously described if not between 280 and 285 mOsm/kg.
7. Test pH.
8. Filter sterilize through 500 mL Nalgene 0.20 μ filtration unit.
9. Retest aliquot for osmolality and pH.
10. Aliquot media into Falcon 3013 tissue culture flasks using sterile technique.

Pronuclear Stage Cryopreservation Media

I. (1 L Volumetric Flask—Solution I)
  A. Add 9.6 g dry powdered DPBS (Gibco #21300-025) to approximately 800 mL MilliQ/UF H$_2$O (the inside of the package is not rinsed for fear of leaching toxic

substances from the metal-based lining). Mix until dissolved.

B. Add 0.1 g CaCl₂ to approximately 50 mL MilliQ/UF H₂O; mix; add the dissolved CaCl₂ solution to the DPBS solution and mix (CaCl₂ supplied separately with DPBS).

C. Add 0.050 g benzyl penicillin G (Sigma #PEN-NA); mix.

D. Add 0.050 g streptomycin sulfate (Sigma #S6501); mix.

E. Add MilliQ/UF H₂O to reach 1000 mL; mix.

II. (500 mL Volumetric Flask—Solution II)

A. To 400 mL of Solution I:

1. Add 1.2 g crystalline bovine serum albumin (0.3%, Sigma #A4503); gently mix.
2. Add 0.4 g dextrose (Sigma D + glucose, #G5250); mix.
3. Add 0.0144 g (14.4 mg) sodium pyruvate (Sigma #P5280); mix.

III. (4 × 100 mL Volumetric Flasks—Molar Solutions of 1,2-Propanediol)

A. Aliquot approximately 80 mL of Solution II into each of three 100-mL volumetric flasks and 100 mL into a fourth flask (for the 0.0 M Solution).

1. To flask #1, add 11.42 mL 1,2-propanediol (Fisher #P355, MW = 76.10) to make the 1.5 M medium; add Solution II to reach 100 mL and label with correct molarity.
2. To flask #2, add 7.61 mL 1,2-propanediol to make the 1.0 M medium; add Solution II to reach 100 ml and label with correct molarity.
3. To flask #3, add 3.81 mL 1,2-propanediol to make the 0.5 M medium; add Solution II to reach 100 mL and label with correct molarity.
4. Add nothing to flask #4 (0.0 M media).
5. Mix well and filter sterilize each medium through a Nalgene 0.20 μ filter unit.
6. Aliquot 4 to 8 mL of each of the 1.0 M, 0.5 M, and 0.0 M media into multiple Falcon 2001 culture tubes labeled with correct molar concentrations. Aliquot 3 to 5 mL of the 1.5 M solution into multiple Falcon 2003 culture tubes and label each. Different vessels are used to differentiate freezing media from thawing dilutions. Nunc cryovials may be used in lieu of Falcon culture tubes.

Preparation of Human Fetal Cord Serum

Human fetal cord blood is collected for the Norfolk program in the labor and delivery unit of Sentara Norfolk General Hospital. Syringes (Monoject, 60 mL) are supplied by the embryology laboratory for use in collection. Residents and nurses are cautioned to collect blood only from healthy, term deliveries without fetal distress. They are further requested to avoid milking the cord if blood is collected by dripping into an open syringe. Otherwise, collection is performed by drawing blood into the syringe through a needle. Samples are refrigerated until processing, usually within a few hours but occasionally longer. The number of syringes, the name of donating patient, and date of collection are recorded in a log book. Any syringe with more than 25 mL of blood is logged for a 50¢ payment to the educational fund of the labor and delivery unit.

The needle or Luer-lok cover is removed from the syringe. The plunger is gently pulled back and discarded. Clotted blood and free serum are poured gently into a sterile specimen container to avoid hemolysis. With a 5¾ sterile pasteur pipette, the liquid portion of the sample is transferred into 15-mL centrifuge tubes (Falcon #2095); the clot is discarded. Samples are centrifuged at high speed for 10 to 20 minutes to pellet red cells. The clear supernatant (serum) is removed with a pasteur pipette and placed into a second centrifuge tube; hemolyzed serum is discarded. After heat inactivation at 56°C for 1 hour, two 1-mL aliquots of the serum sample are set aside for viral testing and storage. After this, serum from two to three donors may be pooled to make a 40- to 50-mL lot and are filter sterilized through 0.20-μ filters (Nalgene) under negative pressure. Sterilized serum is aliquoted into culture tubes (Falcon #2001) and frozen until use. All lots are numbered, used for 1 month after testing, and generally rejected if not used within that time. A small sample of each lot (0.6 mL in Falcon #2003 culture tubes) is sent for toxicity testing. Lot numbers, processing dates, and test results are all recorded in a log book.

LABORATORY TECHNIQUES (NORFOLK)

Initial Andrologic Evaluation for In Vitro Fertilization

Part of the workup of the male partner is a basic semen analysis, including a study of the physical characteristics of semen (pH, liquefaction, viscosity, and volume). In the Norfolk program, sperm density and motility characteristics, including mean velocity and mean linearity, are analyzed in the andrology laboratory. A mixed antiglobulin reaction (MAR) test may be included in the semen analysis if a sufficient number of motile sperm are present. This test screens for the presence of IgG sperm-bound antibodies. Some laboratories use the MAR test followed by an indirect Immunobead test if too few motile sperm are obtained for a direct Immunobead test alone. The direct immunobead test, however, is necessary to identify the isotype of antibody present, such as IgA, IgG, or IgM. These tests can also be performed on seminal plasma, serum, cervical mucus, and follicular fluid.

As a precautionary measure, routine bacteriologic screening of semen should be included in the initial investigation and may include culture for *Neisseria gonorrhoeae, ureaplasma urealyticum* and other *Mycoplasma* strains, and *Chlamydia trachomatis*. Biochemical analyses of seminal plasma (e.g., acid phosphatase, fructose, proteins, phosphatidylcholine, carnitine) and a determination of trace metals in semen (zinc and copper) are done only when there is a special indication. Experience in the Norfolk laboratory has demonstrated that these evaluations are not predictive of the fertilizing ability of human sperm in IVF.[1]

When indicated because of a poor basic semen analysis, a swim-up preparation is assessed before the actual initial IVF trial. The results of this test enable the embryology laboratory to anticipate a possible poor recovery and provide for alternative preparations, such as Percoll gradient separation.

The sperm penetration assay (SPA) assesses the ability of human sperm to capacitate, undergo the acrosome reaction, and fuse with or decondense within zona-free hamster oocytes.[2] Although theoretically an excellent biologic assay, it admittedly bypasses an important zona binding and penetration step, and its history has been fraught with disparate correlations and interpretations between investigating laboratories. The consequence of differing reports has proved confusing to those attempting to interpret validation trials. Our own laboratory has not found this assay to be a reliable indicator of fertilizing potential. It is clear that the conditions for handling both spermatozoa and oocytes are of primary importance in running and evaluating the assay; a better understanding of the optimal in vitro conditions and standardization of protocols is sorely needed before the assay can reach its full potential.

The hemizona assay (HZA) is a sperm/zona pellucida binding test that evaluates the first crucial step of sperm/oocyte interaction, that is, tight binding of the spermatozoon to the zona pellucida.[3] Different sources of human oocytes can be used in the assay, oocytes recovered from surgically removed ovaries or postmortem ovarian tissue or surplus oocytes from an IVF program. Oocytes can be used fresh, cryopreserved, or stored in a hyperosmolar salt solution. In the assay, sperm populations from an infertile patient are tested versus a fertile control in an internally controlled manner by using the two halves of a microbisected zona pellucida. It has been shown that the HZA is highly predictive of fertilization outcome and that a greater sperm-binding ability is possible with zonae of mature, as opposed to immature, oocytes.[4]

Our experience indicates that sperm morphology plays an important role in the fertilization process and that morphology can be used as a good predictor of the chances for fertilization. Using strict criteria, it has been shown that men possessing less than 4% normal forms have a significantly reduced chance for fertilization under standard insemination conditions. When normal morphology is 5% to 14%, fertilization outcomes are much better, and samples with greater than 14% normal forms are considered quite good.[5] When normal forms are below 4%, fertilization can be significantly improved by increasing the inseminating sperm concentration from 50,000 to more than 500,000 sperm/mL.[6] Under conditions of this strict morphology assay, a spermatozoon is considered normal when the head has a smooth, oval configuration with a well-defined acrosome composing about 40% to 70% of the head. There must be no defects of the neck, midpiece, or tail and no cytoplasmic droplets of more than half the size of the head. In contrast to other laboratories, borderline forms are considered abnormal. Evaluating sperm morphology by strict criteria is a valuable tool for predicting a patient's chance to reach the transfer stage and thus is included in the basic workup of each husband. By stringently defining morphologic features, the method is more objective than traditional techniques of assessing sperm morphology and provides the IVF laboratory with important information for determining the concentration of inseminating sperm.

Sperm Morphology by Strict Criteria—Preparation and Staining of Smears

Slides are thoroughly cleaned, washed in alcohol, and air dried before use. For reliable and repeatable readings, a well-spread smear must be made so spermatozoa can be clearly and individually visualized. Smears are stained according to the Diff-Quik method.[7] The technique is as follows: Two morphology slides are prepared for each patient. Special care is taken to clean the slides thoroughly with 70% ethyl alcohol before use. To make smears as thin as possible, no more than 5 μL of semen is used. The slides are dried at room temperature, fixed for 15 seconds with Diff-Quik fixative (1.8 mg/L of triarylmethane methyl alcohol, Diff-Quik AHS del Caribe, Inc., Aguada, Puerto Rico) before staining with Diff-Quik solution 1 (1 g/L of xanthene in sodium azide–processed buffer) for 10 seconds, then with Diff-Quik solution 2 (0.625 g/L of azure A and 0.625 g/L of methylene blue in buffer) for 5 seconds. Between the fixing step and each of the staining steps, the excess solutions are drained from the slides by blotting the slide edges on bibulous paper. The slides are read on the same day and documented. Sperm morphology is evaluated by two independent observers, each counting at least 200 cells and each unaware of the other's results. Results from both observers are averaged.

Preparation for Oocyte Harvest

Depending on the number of patients scheduled and the type of procedures being performed, an appropriate number of Falcon #3037 organ culture dishes containing insemination medium (7.5% human fetal cord serum in Ham's F-10) are prepared the day before oocyte harvest. With the use of organ culture dishes, rapid loss of carbon dioxide may occur because of the large surface area involved; for this reason, 3 mL of medium is used to fill the central well, and an additional 3 mL is placed in the outside moat. The use of small culture tubes or medium droplets under equilibrated mineral oil may help to prevent against a rapid shift in pH. There are certain advantages and disadvantages involved with the use of dishes versus tubes versus droplets under oil; each IVF group tends to use a favorite method. The Norfolk program has used each method in a satisfactory manner but generally uses the organ culture dish because of the ease with which specimens can be handled and transferred from one dish to another. Culture under oil is probably an ideal choice for stabilization of temperature and pH but involves additional steps for washing and equilibrating mineral oil; flattening and coalescing of droplets is another drawback to this method. Culture tubes are our least favorite method because of optical distortion and the inconvenience of removing specimens for evaluation, but it is fair to state that our experience is limited with this method. At least two lots of human fetal cord serum are used in the preparation of these media.

Sufficient numbers of dishes (or tubes or droplets) are prepared to accommodate the maximum number of oocytes anticipated, plus quality-control aliquots. In addition, an appropriate number of Falcon 2001 culture tubes are prepared with 10 mL each of the same media for use in sperm-washing procedures.

On the morning of harvest, DPBS is warmed for use during collection of oocytes. This solution is used to flush the aspiration apparatus before and immediately after each follicular fluid is obtained. Approximately 50 mL, supplemented with 20 units/mL sodium heparin to prevent clotting, are used per patient during transvaginal collections. More are required for

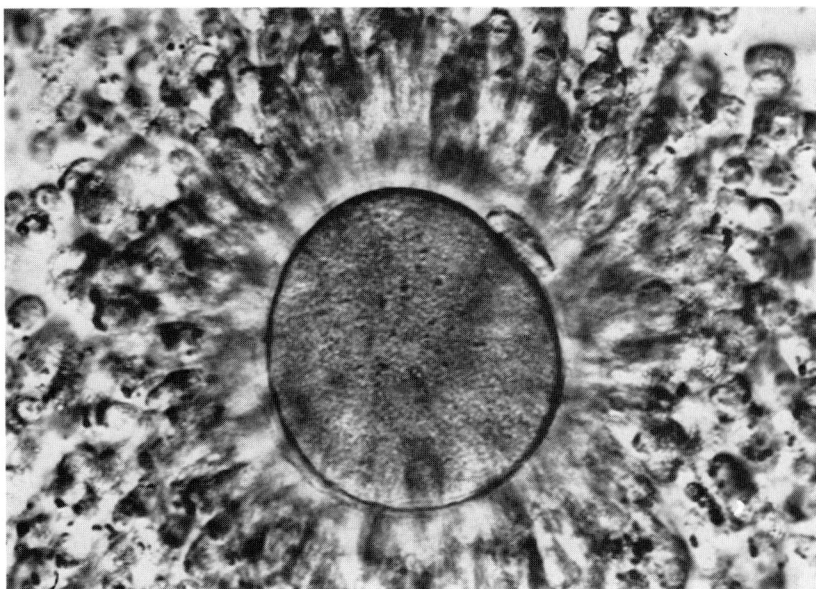

FIGURE 55-2. An oocyte with chromosomes at metaphase II of maturation. Note the clear ooplasm and first polar body at a 2 o'clock position.

patients with a multifollicular response to ovarian stimulation or when laparoscopic retrieval is anticipated. DPBS solutions are kept at 37°C in an operating room water bath.

Follicular Aspiration

On collection, follicular aspirates are carried to the embryology laboratory, where they are examined in Falcon #3002 petri dishes to locate the oocytes. In Norfolk, the operating room and laboratory are adjacent to one another with only a few steps required to deliver aspirates. In other programs, a window is provided in which fluids can be easily passed. In cases in which the laboratory is not closely situated to the harvesting area, samples must be safely transported in a manner that ensures their temperature and pH stability.

Mature oocytes with expanded cumulus are spotted quickly by macroscopic visualization of the viscous cumulus mass; immature oocytes without expanded cumulus are not seen macroscopically and require scanning of the dish to identify. Membrana granulosa cells floating within the fluid are graded for the extent of their luteinization and for color; this cellular assessment is helpful when evaluating ovarian stimulation protocols, especially when treatment is prolonged or immature oocytes are harvested. Once identified, an oocyte is washed in the moat of the culture dish (organ culture dishes), pipetted into the central well, and briefly assessed for morphology and maturation by one of two methods described here:

1. *Diagnosed for maturation based on cellular morphology of the surrounding cumulus and corona cells.* This method is not always reliable for determining the exact maturity level of the oocyte but provides a quick means of assessment without exposing the oocyte to potentially traumatic conditions. Oocytes are graded as mature and can be inseminated between 5 and 8 hours after collection when they possess a round and even shape, have ooplasm of light color, display an expanded (sunburst) corona radiata, and exhibit an expanded cumulus

mass. An oocyte is considered immature when it possesses an irregular shape with centrally darkened ooplasm, displays a compact multilayer corona (nonradiant), and exhibits a dense cumulus mass or no cumulus at all. Immature oocytes should not be inseminated until the following day.

2. *Diagnosed for maturation based on the exact nuclear condition of the oocyte.* This method is far more reliable for assessment of maturity, but the techniques used to visualize oocyte detail may, in inexperienced hands, expose the oocyte to traumatic conditions. Briefly the oocyte is placed with a small droplet of medium into a sterile petri dish. The dish is jarred with the palm of the hand to flatten the cumulus mass and expose the oocyte to direct visualization. One must be careful to avoid prolonged exposure to this condition because pH, temperature, and osmotic changes may damage the integrity of the oocyte. With this method, germinal vesicles and first polar bodies can be clearly seen along with aspects of the ooplasm, such as intense granularity or vacuolization. Oocytes are then described as being at metaphase II of maturation (MII; first polar body present; Fig. 55-2), at metaphase I of maturation (MI; no first polar body nor a germinal vesicle, Fig. 55-3), or at prophase I of maturation (PI; germinal vesicle present; Fig. 55-4). Variable cellular characteristics can be noted with any of these maturational stages. Oocytes at MII are inseminated between 3 and 5 hours after harvest, oocytes at MI are examined at 2- to 4-hour intervals and inseminated 2 to 3 hours after first polar body extrusion is noted, and PI oocytes are left undisturbed until the following day, at which time they may be either reassessed or inseminated without further evaluation.

Once identified and evaluated, the oocyte is placed in the incubator until insemination. Fresh medium with 15% serum is prepared for each mature oocyte and is equilibrated overnight for use the following day. At the time that oocytes are evaluated for fertilization, they are transferred to this fresh medium.

Since 1981, in cycles using gonadotropins for ovarian stimulation, more than 52,000 oocytes have been harvested, evaluated, and handled in the Norfolk embryology laboratory.

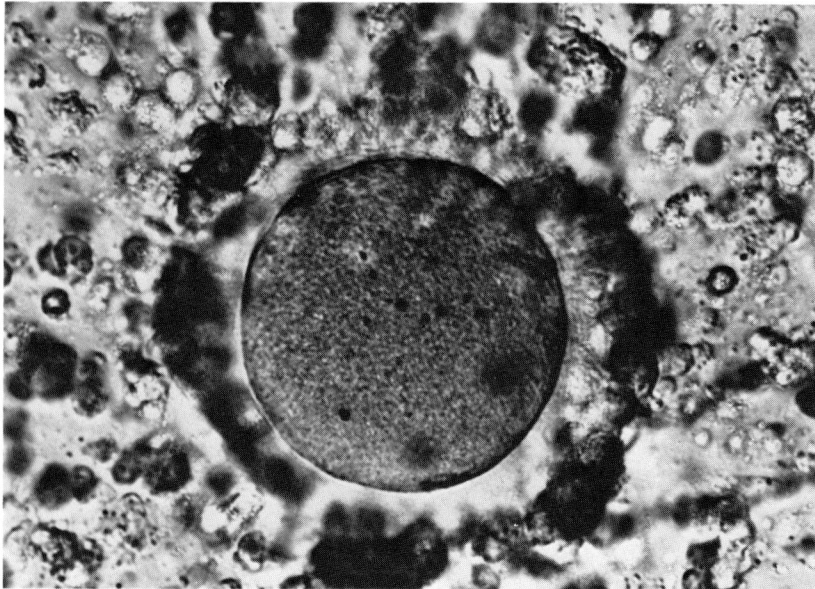

FIGURE 55–3. An oocyte with chromosomes at metaphase I of maturation. Note the clear ooplasm and absence of both polar body and germinal vesicle.

The majority of oocytes have been healthy and seemingly capable of undergoing a normal fertilization process. Sixty-seven percent of all oocytes harvested to date have been classified as mature or nearly mature (MII or MI) without degenerative features. An additional 24% of the oocytes have been germinal vesicle bearing (PI), indicating a need for in vitro maturation before insemination, and 9% have been collected in a degenerative state, sometimes with damage to the oolemma or zona pellucida. To date, more than 1300 infants have been born with many more expected in the months to come. Clinical pregnancy rates have been evaluated in 3386 transfer cycles and correlated with original nuclear maturity of oocytes at harvest (Table 55–1).[8] Of these transfers, 1566

were placed into one of four "pure" transfer groups, groups denoting the transfer of one or more conceptuses of a single nuclear status at collection (MII, unclassified mature, MI, and PI). For example, a "pure" MII group consists of transfer cycles in which only embryos (usually a single embryo) developed from MII oocytes are transferred; a "pure" PI group has only the transfer of embryos developing from PI oocytes. These pure groups would be opposed to "mixed" transfer groups in which more than one conceptus is transferred, the conceptuses are of different maturational origins, and identification of the embryo responsible for pregnancy is therefore impossible. Pure groups of MII and unclassified "mature" conceptuses demonstrate similar pregnancy rates in younger patients, although a tendency is noted for best results with MII oocytes. MII transfers are significantly better than MI transfers in terms of pregnancy; these newer data show a

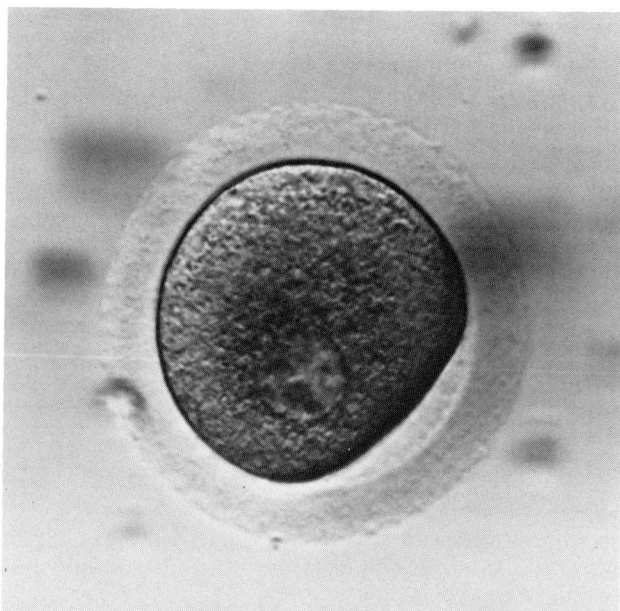

FIGURE 55–4. An oocyte with chromosomes at prophase I of maturation. Note the darkened ooplasm and germinal vesicle with its prominent nucleolus.

TABLE 55–1. Analysis of 3386 Consecutive Intrauterine Conceptus Transfers Over a 6-Year Period: Effect of Oocyte Maturity and Patient Age on Pregnancy*

Type of Transfer	Patients Under 41 Years of Age (n = 3188 transfers) Pregnancy/ Transfer	%	Patients 41+ Years of Age (n = 198 transfers) Pregnancy/ Transfer	%
MII only	328/1065	31%[a]	21/87	24%
Unknown mature only	24/100	24%[b]	3/11	27%
MI only	43/218	20%[c]	0/15	0%
PI only	3/67	4.5%[d]	0/3	0%
MII + unclass. mature	21/49	43%	—	
MII + MI	323/1006	32%	7/41	17%
Unclass. mature + MI	5/14	36%	0/1	0%
MII + unclass. mat. + MI	7/19	37%	—	
All other combinations with PI oocytes	167/650	26%	11/40	28%

*Older patients = No significance between any group. Younger patients versus older patients = No significance.
a>c>d; b>d P <0.005 (a=b, b=c).
MII, Metaphase II; MI, metaphase I; PI, prophase I.

larger difference between MII and MI transfers as compared with previous reports.[9–11] Perhaps this is due to the use of gonadotropin-releasing hormone (GnRH) analog for ovarian suppression because GnRH analog cycles that do not produce MII oocytes appear to result in poor pregnancy outcomes. As anticipated, embryos developed from PI oocytes show a significantly reduced ability to establish pregnancy, an observation that has been consistent in our laboratories over time.

"Mixed" transfer cycles represent a higher overall pregnancy rate, which can be attributed primarily to a larger number of embryos transferred per cycle.

Older patients generally demonstrate lower pregnancy rates, although the differences are not significant owing to fewer transfers in this group. Pregnancy loss is similar in all groups.

Semen Collection for In Vitro Fertilization

Husbands are directed to collect a semen sample at a specific time, which might be anywhere from 30 minutes after oocyte harvest to much later in the day, depending on oocyte maturity. In other programs, husbands are often asked to collect before the oocytes are harvested; the size of the laboratory staff and general convenience factors dictate the timing of collection. The sample is collected into a sterile specimen container; written instructions are provided. The husband is advised not to use a condom, cream, or lubricant because of potential toxicity. An information slip asks for his name, birth date, social security number, date and time of collection, date of previous ejaculation, and whether any of the specimen was lost. Once the sample is collected, it is delivered to the hospital recovery room, and the embryology laboratory is notified.

If a husband has difficulty obtaining a specimen, he may return to his home or hotel room to collect or have his wife's assistance. If difficulty persists, the sample may be collected by coitus interruptus with the use of a special nontoxic condom. Although a fresh specimen is desirable, a frozen specimen from a normospermic husband can also be used. A cryopreserved backup sample is desired from husbands who anticipate potential difficulty of collection.

Determination of Concentration, Motility, and Morphology in the Original Sample

Two methods are commonly used to appraise basic sperm parameters in the neat semen sample: manual assessment and computerized assessment. Traditional manual methods are inexpensive to perform, are reliable at low sperm concentrations, and are widely used throughout the world. Computerized assessment saves time and generally provides additional parameters in the workup (such as sperm velocity and linearity), but systems are initially expensive to configure and often unreliable at low sperm concentrations. At the Jones Institute, a computerized method is used for normospermic samples, and manual evaluations are performed on all subnormal samples (counts less than 10×10^6 sperm/mL).

MANUAL METHOD

With distilled water, original samples are diluted 1/50. Both chambers of a Neubauer-ruled hemacytometer are loaded with diluted sample and scanned under low power to ensure even distribution of sperm without clumping. Five red blood cell squares are counted using $400 \times$ magnification. The counts of both chambers are averaged, and the number of sperm per milliliter is calculated by using a multiplication factor of 2.5 million (1/50 dilution counting five squares in the red blood cell area). If the specimen is poor, a 1/10 dilution is made, and all four large white blood cell areas are counted on both sides, averaged, and multiplied by a factor of 0.025 million (1/10 dilution counted in the white blood cell area). Other dilutions and multiplication factors may be determined and used to suit the individual sample. A motility analysis is performed by placing 40 μL of semen on a microscope slide with a coverslip. The percentage of motility is determined by counting motile and immotile sperm in five randomly selected fields containing at least 100 cells ($\times 400$) on an inverted microscope. Phase-contrast microscopy is used for manual count and motility analysis.

COMPUTERIZED ANALYSIS

We have used two different computerized semen analyzers. Our initial system was the Cellsoft analyzer (Cryo Resources, New York, NY). We recently switched to the Hamilton-Thorne IVOS system (Fertility Technologies, Natick, MA). These systems simultaneously evaluate motility, concentration, velocity, and linearity.

To evaluate basic concentration and motility, 5 μL of undiluted sample is placed in a Makler chamber on the microscope stage. To process an original specimen, three fields or 200 cells (whichever comes last) must be counted. A printout specifies the number of cells counted, number and percent of motile and immotile cells, concentration per milliliter of sample, and average velocity and linearity. The velocity and linearity parameters have not proved to be extremely useful in our program.

Any sample showing an original sperm concentration of less than 20 million spermatozoa per milliliter of semen or any washed sample with a concentration under 10 million/mL by computerized analysis must be confirmed by manual counting methods; results with low concentrations are more reliable with a hemacytometer. Undiluted samples may be counted in red and white blood cell areas of the hemacytometer with multiplication factors of 0.05 and 0.0025. We consider all counts under 1 million to represent only close approximations of the actual number.

Sperm Washing/Migration Procedures

Norfolk protocols for IVF sperm preparation involve (1) washing, centrifugation, and incubation of the semen specimen, such as occurs during basic swim-up techniques; (2) Percoll gradient separation of motile sperm with centrifugation; or (3) less commonly, motile sperm migration after mixing whole semen with a sodium hyaluronate such as *Sperm Select* (Pharmacia Laboratories, Sweden).

Separation of motile sperm from seminal plasma and cellular debris is necessary for the following reasons:

1. Many sexually transmitted organisms are found in semen, including aerobic and anaerobic bacteria, genital mycoplasma, and *Chlamydia trachomatis*. Washing, centrifuging, or incubating sperm in media containing antibiotics removes or inhibits these microbes from the preparation used for insemination.

2. The separated motile portion of the sample demonstrates improved motility and morphology over the original semen specimen.

3. Seminal plasma contains inhibitors to fertilization, which must be separated from sperm cells. Prolonged exposure of sperm to seminal plasma can permanently decrease its fertilizing ability. The washing or migration steps mimic a natural situation wherein sperm transverse uterine and tubal fluids and thus become separated from seminal plasma. In addition, washed sperm may undergo or initiate capacitation during the incubation phase of the preparation procedure. Although poorly understood, capacitation involves changes in the spermatozoal membrane and serves as a precursor to the spermatozoon acrosome reaction.

At the Jones Institute embryology laboratory, a normal semen specimen has the following parameters: count greater than 20×10^6/mL, motility greater than 30%, and morphology greater than 14% normal forms. Extremely viscous or agglutinated samples that do not liquefy by 20 to 30 minutes after collection may require special handling. Samples may be pipetted vigorously to break up the viscous mass, medium can be added to the specimen and aggressively mixed, or the sample can be placed at 37°C for 30 minutes to reduce viscosity. Some groups incubate semen with chymotrypsin to reduce viscosity.

The following is an overview of sperm preparation techniques as performed in Norfolk. Many other reliable techniques are in common use throughout the world.

Normospermic Samples (Sperm Swim-up Technique)

1. Volume, viscosity, color of the specimen, and the time that analysis began are recorded.

2. After liquefaction, 5 μL of sample are loaded onto a Makler chamber for computerized analysis (see manual analysis for alternate information). A morphology slide is prepared for research purposes with another 5 μL.

3. 0.25 to 0.5 mL of semen is aliquoted into each of four 15-mL centrifuge tubes. An additional 0.5 mL of insemination medium (Ham's F10 + 7.5% human fetal cord serum) is added to each and mixed. Tubes are centrifuged for 10 minutes at $427 \times$ g.

4. Supernatants are removed with a 9-in. sterile Pasteur pipette and pellets are resuspended.

5. 0.5 mL of insemination medium is added to the pellets, mixed, and recentrifuged. Supernatants are again removed.

6. Without disturbing the pellets, 0.5 mL of insemination medium is gently layered over the pellets. Tubes are placed slightly slanted in a specimen container and caps loosened on the tubes.

7. Tubes are incubated at 37°C under 5% carbon dioxide in air for 1 hour.

8. Supernatants are removed and placed in a small Falcon #2003 culture tube. This is the motile fraction that is used for insemination.

9. 5 μL of this motile fraction is loaded onto the Makler chamber for analysis of count and motility (see manual methods for alternate information).

Normospermic Cryopreserved Samples (Sperm Swim-Up Technique)

1. One or two cryovials are thawed for use depending on the results of post-thaw survival provided by the sperm cryobiology laboratory.

2. Samples are allowed to thaw at room temperature for 40 minutes with the laminar flow hood shut off, or for 10 minutes with a 37°C water bath.

3. The thawed specimen is pipetted into a centrifuge tube, and the volume is noted.

4. Twice the volume of medium is added slowly to the sample, drop by drop, so sperm are not damaged by sudden changes in osmolarity; medium should be maintained at room temperature. Once diluted, 5 μL of the sample is loaded onto a Makler chamber for determination of concentration and motility (see manual methods for alternate information). A lower motility may be expected in cryopreserved specimens.

5. This final volume is divided among four tubes and centrifuged at $427 \times$ g.

6. Supernatants are removed and pellets resuspended in 0.5 mL of medium.

7. The sample is washed and centrifuged once more as for a normal specimen.

8. Pellets are layered with 0.1 to 0.5 mL of medium and incubated for 1 hour.

9. Supernatants (motile fraction) are removed and reassayed before insemination.

Normospermic Samples (Sperm Migration Technique using Sperm Select)

This technique is easy to perform and is suitable for normospermic samples. Extremely poor samples are best handled in another manner.

1. After calculating initial concentration and motility, add 0.75 mL insemination medium to one vial of *Sperm Select*. Mix. Incubate this mixture at 37°C under 5% carbon dioxide for 30 minutes before use.

2. Aliquot 1 mL of semen to four glass *Sperm Select* tubes (0.25 mL each tube).

3. Transfer 0.4 to 0.5 mL of the equilibrated *Sperm Select*/insemination medium mixture to each glass tube. Two layers are evident.

4. Place tubes in the incubator for 60 minutes.

5. After 1 hour, carefully remove the top layer from each tube using a sterile 9-in. Pasteur pipette, and combine these samples in a single, sterile tube. These layers contain the motile, washed sperm fraction.

6. Calculate concentration and motility.

Subnormal Samples (Sperm Swim-up Technique)

Oligospermic and asthenospermic samples are generally best handled with Percoll gradients. When a swim-up technique is used, it is carried out in the same manner as normospermic samples, with the following changes:

1. After assaying count and motility, the entire sample is used and divided among 8 to 16 centrifuge tubes.

2. A greater amount of the sample is aliquoted (up to 0.5 mL) into each tube if volume is sufficient; otherwise, smaller volumes are used.

3. A small amount of medium is layered over pellets to contain the motile fraction, as little as 0.1 mL.

4. The final motile fraction may be centrifuged and added to micro dishes (0.3 to 1.0 mL) or microdrops under oil (50 to 100 μl) to reach a desirable concentration for insemination.

5. Pellets may be relayered to obtain another swim-up specimen.

6. In extreme cases, the motile fraction may be remixed with washed pellets and used for insemination.

Subnormal Samples (Percoll Gradient)

1. Prepare stock Percoll solution with 9 parts Percoll (stored at 4°C) + 1 part Hams F10 (10×, 1-L package made up in 100 mL). Adjust osmolality to 280 to 285 m Osm/kg.

2. Prepare a 95% Percoll solution with 9.5 mL stock + 0.5 mL Hams F10 (1× insemination medium [IM]). Similarly, prepare 80%, 70%, 60%, 50%, and 40% Percoll solutions.

3. In a 15-mL centrifuge tube, gently layer 0.5 mL of each of the prepared solutions in decreasingly lower concentrations with the 95% layer at the bottom. Avoid mixing the layers, and mark gradient levels on outside of tube. Note that the solutions may be kept at 4°C for up to 1 week. Up to 20 gradient tubes can be made at once if 10-mL aliquots of each solution have been prepared.

4. Layer the whole semen sample 1:1 with insemination medium and leave at room temperature for 30 minutes.

5. Using a sterile pipette, take 0.5 mL of the top layer of the whole semen sample and place it slowly in one Percoll gradient tube, gently layering the sample over the top gradient. Repeat with additional gradient tubes until the top layer portion of the whole semen sample is exhausted. Label these tubes with the notation "TOP" and the patient's name.

6. Repeat step 3 for the bottom layer of the whole semen sample. Label with the notation "BOTTOM" and the patient's name.

7. Centrifuge both aliquots for 30 minutes at 300 g.

8. Remove the 95% Percoll gradient layers.

9. Wash the 95% layers twice by mixing with an equal volume of IM and centrifuging at 200 g for 5 minutes.

10. Resuspend the final pellet with IM (the volume of IM depends on the quality and concentration of the sperm preparation; use as little as 0.2 mL for poor specimens).

11. A swim-up may be performed with the final pellet if many dead sperm are observed. In such cases, a small amount of IM should be layered over the undisturbed pellet, and the tube should be incubated at 37°C under 5% carbon dioxide for 30 minutes to 1 hour.

Note: If gradient tubes are prepared in advance and kept at 4°C, they must be taken out of the refrigerator in the morning and warmed to room temperature before use. The tubes labeled "TOP" should contain fewer dead sperm than those labeled "BOTTOM." Save the 80%, 70%, and 60% layers for swim-up if sperm number is alarmingly low. If the final sample is clean but shows few motile sperm, consider inseminating oocytes in a small droplet under equilibrated mineral oil.

Determination of Concentration and Motility in the Washed Sample

After preparation of the sperm, the motile fraction for insemination is analyzed by manual or computerized methods. For manual methods, a ½ or ⅕ dilution is typically used to determine concentration. With computerized analysis, 10 fields and 100 cells must be analyzed; care must be taken to select random fields outside the chamber grid.

The volume of washed specimen to inseminate with is calculated as follows:

$$\text{Volume to add} = \frac{\text{total number of motile sperm desired}}{\text{number of motile sperm per mL recovered}}$$

In Norfolk, the number of sperm desired for insemination is 5×10^4 per milliliter of insemination medium (normal men); 3 mL of medium is used in an organ culture dish. Therefore, 0.15×10^6 total motile sperm is required for insemination ($5 \times 10^4/\text{mL} \times 3 \text{ mL} = 15 \times 10^4 = 0.15 \times 10^6$ total sperm). This number (0.15×10^6) is divided by the actual number of recovered sperm per milliliter (for example, 10×10^6 mL) to achieve the appropriate volume for insemination (0.015 mL or 15 μL).

Sperm concentrations for insemination are generally as follows:

1. Normal samples: 50,000 motile sperm/mL medium.

2. Cryopreserved samples: 100,000 to 300,000 motile sperm/mL medium.

3. Subnormal samples: 200,000 to 1×10^6 motile sperm/mL medium, depending on the severity of the problem.

4. Poor SPA or poor HZA: 500,000 motile sperm/mL of medium.

5. Antisperm antibodies: up to 500,000 motile sperm/mL medium, depending on the severity of agglutination.

Alternative Action When the Final Sample Is Extremely Poor (Low Concentration, Low Motility, Nonprogressive Motility)

The final motile fraction may be gently centrifuged for 5 minutes and the resulting pellet added to a single organ culture dish, micro dish, or medium droplet under oil to maximize sperm concentration around the oocyte(s). The observation of a low concentration of sperm in the final supernatant may indicate poor motility (failure to swim into supernatant) or poor morphology, which affects normal motility. In some cases, the collection of a fresh sample may result in improved quality. Often a second sample, collected as soon as 1 to 2 hours after the first, shows improved semen parameters.

Donor Backup

A donor backup sample, suitably matched to the husband, may be made available when fertilization failure is anticipated. Donor sperm either may be used to reinseminate oocytes that were unfertilized by husband's sperm (oocytes inseminated with donor sperm 18 to 24 hours after initial insemination) or can be used on the first day to inseminate one half of the patient's oocytes (half of the oocytes inseminated with husband, half with donor).

Reinsemination on day 2 with donor sperm may indeed result in embryos for transfer, but abnormal fertilization is common owing to the fact that aged oocytes perform poorly in culture. When husband and donor sperm have both been used to achieve fertilization in the same group of oocytes, paternity must be called into question.

Dividing oocytes between husband and donor also creates particular problems for the couple. When oocytes from both groups become fertilized, husband's are preferentially replaced; this usually dictates that donor-fertilized oocytes be cryopreserved without future intent to transfer. Instances arise when only a single oocyte is fertilized by the husband, whereas multiple oocytes are successfully fertilized by the donor. This creates a dilemma for both the couple and the physician because of the lower incidence of pregnancy when a single embryo is replaced. For ethical reasons, it cannot be advised that both husband-fertilized and donor-fertilized embryos be replaced during the same cycle. Policies must be in effect before insemination is carried out to establish transfer guidelines covering any fertilization possibility.

Overnight Maintenance of Washed Sperm Specimens

Washed sperm samples are stored overnight in capped culture tubes at room temperature under ambient conditions. These samples may be used on the following day to inseminate immature oocytes that have matured in vitro or to reinseminate unfertilized mature oocytes. If the stored specimen is poor, it is best to obtain a fresh sample.

Evaluation of the Pronucleate Oocyte

At 12 to 19 hours postinsemination, the pronuclear stage oocyte is transferred out of insemination medium and placed in growth medium (15% serum) prepared the day before. Obscuring cumulus cells can be removed by gentle aspiration and expulsion of the cell through either a 27-gauge needle attached to a monoject tuberculin syringe or gentle manipulation through a pulled pipette. The oocyte is examined for pronuclei (Fig. 55–5) and returned to the incubator. Fertilized oocytes in excess of three or four are cryopreserved. Unfertilized oocytes are checked for pronuclei at regular intervals until reinsemination is carried out. Despite the routine reinsemination of unfertilized oocytes, this procedure is rarely successful in our program. Nevertheless, in the absence of a severe male factor, 85% to 90% of mature oocytes can be expected to become fertilized and undergo cleavage.[8–11] Oocytes that develop pronuclei later than 17 to 20 hours after insemination may be at increased risk for chromosomal disorders.[12] A poor pregnancy rate has been achieved in our experience after either delayed fertilization or fertilization following reinsemination.[13]

Evaluation of the pronucleate oocyte should be done care-

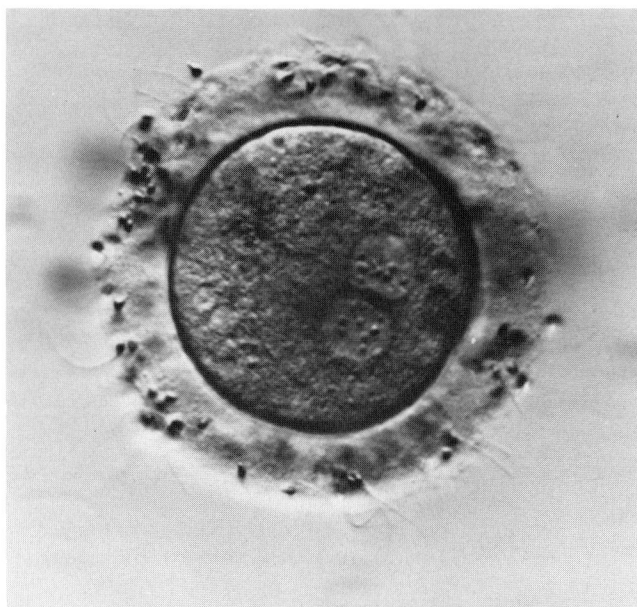

FIGURE 55–5. Two pronuclei as observed at approximately 15 hours postinsemination. Multiple nucleoli can be seen within each pronuclear structure. As time passes, nucleoli will migrate to adjoining borders of each pronucleus.

fully. The number and size of pronuclei should be recorded, and the existence of nucleoli must be verified in each structure. Pseudo-pronuclei have been reported to confuse the evaluation process and are presumably mistaken for pronuclei in a potentially alarming number of cases.[14, 15] These structures are pronuclear-like vacuoles with the ability to move within the cytoplasm and become juxtaposed with true pronuclei. Use of a high-resolution inverted microscope and the consistent discipline of studying nucleoli should lessen the incidence of this error.

Fertilized oocytes with aberrant numbers of pronuclei are not uncommon after IVF. The development of a single pronucleus can also be observed. After the first division, these abnormal specimens often demonstrate cleavage patterns indistinguishable from those of two-pronuclear origin. For this reason, it is extremely important to assess the number of pronuclei correctly before the cell enters syngamy. Although gross abnormalities in chromosome number generally predispose a conceptus to early death, implantation is possible; upwards of 20% of aborted fetuses are triploid.[16] Of special risk to the patient is the rare term delivery of a triploid child and the obstetric risk associated with early miscarriage.

Embryos developing from triploid pronucleate oocytes often appear to undergo more rapid cleavage than diploid embryos, perhaps because most cleave directly into three blastomeres at the first division. Three patterns of cleavage have been documented for oocytes displaying triploidy: (1) direct cleavage into three blastomeres with resulting variable and abnormal karyotypes displaying near-diploid complements (62%), (2) cleavage into two blastomeres with resulting uniform triploid karyotypes (24%), and (3) cleavage into two blastomeres plus a small extrusion mass with resulting diploid karyotypes in each blastomere and a probable haploid complement in the extrusion mass (14%).[17] With this information, a fascinating correlation is shown between the pattern of cleavage and the subsequent chromosomal complement of the embryo. It furthermore indicates that some triploid embryos might be capable of self-regulation and regular development.

Our experience has not shown the number of inseminating sperm to be correlated with the incidence of abnormal fertilization. Sperm concentrations as low as 25,000/mL and as high as 1 million/mL have not differed in producing a rather constant rate of polyploidy (personal observation). Various ovarian stimulation protocols have produced rate fluctuations that can be correlated to extended high-dosage regimens and subsequent oocyte postmaturity.

In cases of failed fertilization, the embryology laboratory must notify the primary physician and be prepared to supply all pertinent sperm and oocyte information. The full-time andrology laboratory is contacted, and efforts are made to ascertain whether additional testing should be performed. If the fertilization failure was not anticipated, hemizona testing, acrosin analysis, or other pertinent tests may be carried out if the patient desires a more intense evaluation. A morphology slide, prepared from the original IVF sample, is reviewed. With the additional information, causes and possible remedies for fertilization failure may be discovered and overcome, or micromanipulation may be attempted in subsequent trials.

After analyzing the fertilization outcome of more than 21,000 oocytes collected in the Norfolk program, results indicate that fully mature oocytes (MII) demonstrate the greatest ability to become fertilized after insemination.[8] Fertilization rates drop slightly with MI oocytes, and fertilization is markedly and significantly reduced when PI oocytes are inseminated. This drop in fertilizability is probably greatly associated with sperm degradation over the time that is required for PI oocytes to achieve maturity in culture. When MII oocytes are harvested, semen samples are delivered within the hour; thus, washed and capacitated sperm may be held more than 24 hours before being placed with immature (PI) oocytes. A much better fertilization rate is always observed when fresh semen is collected on the second day for purposes of inseminating immature oocytes.[9]

Evaluation of the Embryo

After assessing pronuclear number and morphology, specimens are incubated overnight; cleaving embryos are examined 24 hours later. At this time, the stage of cell division is evaluated, morphology is classified according to a simple grading system, and intrauterine transfer is scheduled according to the caseload of the day. The system used to grade embryos serves both to assess the individual conceptus and to classify transfers according to the highest score in the cohort of conceptuses being replaced. The grading system is as follows, with grade 1 representing perfect morphology:[18]

Grade 1:   Embryo with blastomeres of equal size and no cytoplasmic fragments.

Grade 2:   Embryo with blastomeres of equal size possessing minor cytoplasmic fragments or blebs. Cytoplasmic fragments are generally smaller than blastomeres, have the same complement of organelles, but lack nuclei. Acytoplasmic fragments may also be seen.

Grade 3:   Embryo with blastomeres of distinctly unequal size with few, if any, cytoplasmic fragments.

Grade 4:   Embryo with blastomeres of equal or unequal size with significant cytoplasmic fragmentation.

Grade 5:   Embryo with few blastomeres of any size displaying severe or complete fragmentation of its cytoplasm.

A value of 0.5 is added to the score when significant granularity is noted in the blastomeres; hence, an embryo with equal-sized blastomeres, no fragments, but displaying granularity is scored as 1.5.

Transfers with at least one grade 1 embryo demonstrate a significantly better chance for establishing pregnancy.[8, 10, 11] Granularity of blastomeres does not appear to reduce this potential. Although a higher score (lower number) is favorable, pregnancy is possible even in cycles with grade 4 or 5 morphology demonstrating unequal-sized blastomeres and moderate-to-severe cytoplasmic fragmentation. Scores are remarkably repetitive for the same couple in succeeding cycles, and persistently poor scores have been seen in some couples with idiopathic infertility (personal observation). Grading information may be useful in counseling patients who fail to conceive after multiple attempts. Individuals who fail to conceive following repetitive transfers of high-quality embryos may require an aggressive evaluation of potential factors that could interfere with implantation. Those with repetitively poor scores might be counseled concerning possible gamete abnormalities, reduced potential for success, and justification for gamete donation. The impact of improving grading scores by virtue of altering ovarian stimulation regimens needs to be more thoroughly elucidated; at present, it appears that slight improvement is possible in patients overcoming ovulation induction difficulties.

Regularly cleaving two-cell conceptuses are observed any time after 22 hours of insemination, usually at around 24 hours, and may be seen until up to 44 hours postinsemination. Four-cell stages are routinely observed between 36 and 50 hours postinsemination. Eight-cell or greater stages are not commonly seen until after 48 hours but are usually noted before 72 hours. Three-, five-, and seven-cell stages are commonly interposed between these divisions, especially if examination is carried out during mitotic cell division. This asynchronous division persists throughout cleavage of the early conceptus, and any number of blastomeres can be noted in a given observation (Fig. 55–6). Morulae have been noted as early as 72 hours and are usually observed by 96 hours. Blastocysts are not generally seen in the laboratory until after 120 hours (Fig. 55–7).

Embryos have been evaluated in Norfolk for their growth rate in culture before intrauterine transfer. Conceptuses are classified as one of the following:

1. Rapidly cleaving with eight or more blastomeres at 36 to 48 hours after insemination.

2. Cleaving at an average or normal rate, displaying two blastomeres by 24 hours postinsemination and four blastomeres by 40 hours postinsemination.

3. Cleaving slowly, displaying only two blastomeres after 40 hours postinsemination.

Nearly 2000 transfers have been analyzed for the effect of

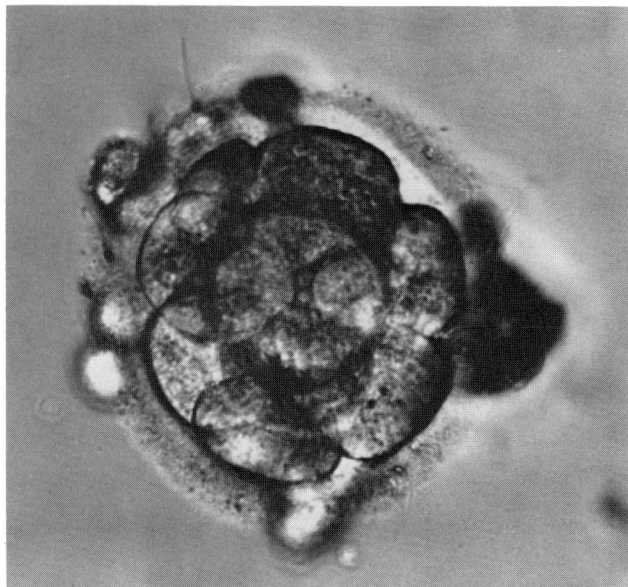

FIGURE 55–6. Nine-cell embryo with good morphology despite slight differences in the size of blastomeres.

embryo growth rate on the actual incidence of pregnancy.[8] Evaluation was made of the most rapidly growing embryo in the cohort of conceptuses for replacement and transfers assigned to rapidly growing, normally growing, or slowly growing groups according to the criteria mentioned previously. Normal growth scores accounted for the vast majority of transfers (85%) and presented the highest overall pregnancy rate. This means that 85% of the transfers done in Norfolk involve at least one embryo that has two blastomeres by 24 hours or four blastomeres by 40 hours. No significant difference was seen between pregnancy rates of rapidly and normally growing embryos, but a significant drop in pregnancy was noted for slow growth.[10] Six percent of cycles have been scored as rapidly growing (eight or more blastomeres by 36 to 48 hours postinsemination), and 9% have been classified as slowly developing (only two blastomeres after 40 hours postinsemination).

When cleavage rates were combined with embryo grading data, several interesting observations were noted.[8] Although the slowly dividing embryos scored low in their overall ability to establish pregnancy, their pregnancy potential equaled that of more rapidly developing conceptuses if they were of grade 1 quality (although numbers were low). Alternately, rapidly growing embryos of grade 1 quality did not show an elevated pregnancy rate over normally growing ones of the same grade. In addition, incidence of pregnancy was rather low for transfers scoring less than grade 2 in both rapid and slow cleaving groups, whereas embryos dividing at average rates contributed to pregnancy even when grade 4 was associated with the transfer. Other investigators have observed this tendency for enhanced implantation with nonfragmented embryos, particularly when cleavage rates fall within average or better limits.[8]

An abnormally fertilized triploid specimen may cleave to the morula stage, but development is usually then arrested. A rare triploid embryo proceeds to the blastocyst stage.[18] In normally fertilized specimens, slow cleavage has been suspected of indicating reduced viability, whereas rapid cleavage has been thought to be a reflection of a healthier conceptus. In reality, results from this center indicate that pregnancies can be established with slowly growing embryos if morphology is good, and rapidity of growth cannot be correlated with better pregnancy rates.[19]

Embryo Transfer

Before transferring embryos to the patient's uterus via an intrauterine transfer device, they are evaluated one last time, photographed if of special interest, and combined in a single culturing dish (Fig. 55–8). Although many groups do so, the use of elevated concentrations of serum is not exercised in Norfolk for embryo transfer. Our own experience with raising serum concentrations to 50%, 75%, and 100% showed no

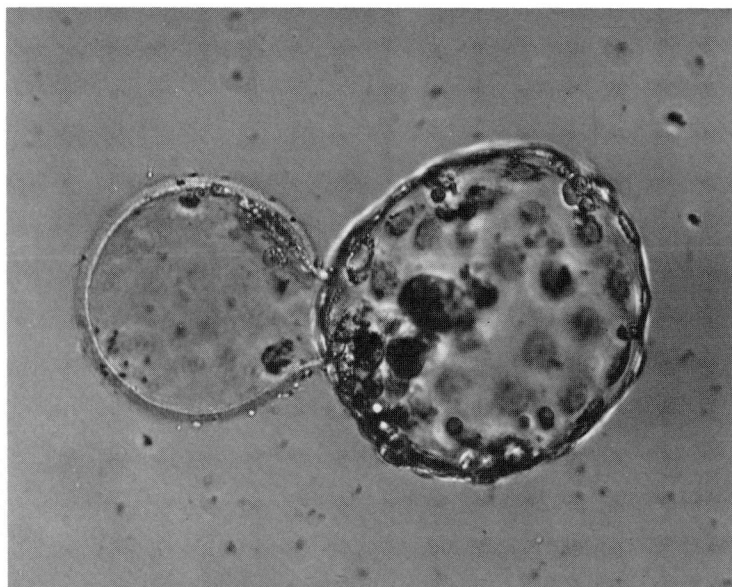

FIGURE 55–7. Hatching blastocyst developed from a prophase I oocyte.

increase in pregnancy rate over control medium with 15% serum. In fact, the increased viscosity produced by the extra serum created difficulties involving the ease in which embryos were aspirated into the Norfolk side-loading catheter.

In Norfolk, a tuberculin syringe is attached to our standard catheter, and the apparatus is stored between the folds of a sterile drape towel. We use a slightly rigid Teflon catheter with an internal diameter of approximately 1.2 mm; the tip of the catheter is solid and round to facilitate passage through the cervix (Norfolk transfer catheter and guide, Cook OB/GYN, #KNTS-506041). Just proximal to the tip, there is a lateral opening through which conceptuses are aspirated. The catheter is carried within a metal guide, which curves gently at the end to follow the curvature of the endocervical canal. This catheter was designed early in our experience and has been used consistently throughout the years. A lateral opening was chosen to avoid plugging an open tip with cervical mucus. As opposed to an open tip catheter, the side-loading catheter requires some experience before embryos are easily handled.

A total of 70 μL of growth medium is slowly taken into the transfer catheter in the following order: 20 μL of medium, air space, 30 μL of medium plus conceptus, air space, and 20 μL of medium. Contents of the catheter are gently and fully expelled into the uterus after passage through the endocervical canal and advancement to within 2 to 3 mm of the uterine fundus. The delivery of this 70-μL volume is considered to be excessively high by many programs; it appears that most groups prefer to transfer embryos in substantially smaller volumes (10 to 50 μL). In our own experience, with the rather large and rigid catheter that we use, this volume works well; smaller volumes have been tried without superior results. Care is taken to avoid traumatic negative and positive pressures during the aspiration and expulsion of embryos. Transfer is traditionally performed in our center with the patient in the knee-chest position, chosen for the ease with which the physician can perform the transfer, and often with the aid of a tenaculum to stabilize the cervix. No

differences have been found between transfers carried out with or without the use of a tenaculum. Usually no cervical dilation is required, no bleeding occurs, and the procedure is carried out within a few minutes. The catheter is always flushed in the laboratory to ensure that the entire contents were delivered; embryos are only rarely (<3% incidence) retained. Should embryos be found in the catheter flushing, transfer is simply performed a second time with a new catheter; pregnancy has been established with multiple transfer attempts. Following transfer, the patient rests in a prone position for 3 hours before leaving the hospital.

Pronucleate Oocyte (or Early-Stage Embryo) Cryopreservation

Our experience involves freezing pronucleate stage oocytes. This stage was chosen because, in 1986, the available literature demonstrated good survival and pregnancy results associated with the one-cell conceptus before syngamy. Our approach to developing a freezing program was to use a slow method, to attempt to forego using sucrose in the medium, and to avoid any dilution steps before beginning the freezing process. Because pronuclear stage specimens must be frozen before entering syngamy, the early morning timing of freezing mandated a simple procedure. In 1986, we experimented with mouse oocytes and embryos, then proceeded to test our system with abnormally fertilized human conceptuses. Freezing was applied clinically to our patient population in early 1987.

Cryovials were chosen owing to the ease with which they are loaded; it was decided that a manual seeding procedure be carried out to ensure proper ice crystal formation within the vials.

Specimens that are to be cryopreserved are placed into labeled 1.8-mL sterile, Gibco or Nunc cryovials containing 0.3 mL of cryoprotective medium (1.5 M 1,2-propanediol in modified DPBS) at room temperature. Cryovial caps are securely tightened to prevent liquid nitrogen from entering during storage. Cryovials are then maintained at room temperature for 30 minutes. At the end of this equilibration period, cryovials are carefully and securely loaded onto freezing canes within a Planer (TS Scientific, Perkasie, PA) biologic freezer.

From ambient conditions, the temperature drops within the freezing unit at a constant rate of −1°C/min until a temperature of −6°C (to −7°C) is reached. At this point, the specimen is maintained at the seeding temperature for 5 minutes before controlled introduction of ice crystal formation by means of a manual seeding process. Seeding is carried out by lifting the freezing cane just out of the unit and grasping the cryovial at the level of the medium meniscus with a sponge forceps that has been frozen in liquid nitrogen. The freezing cane is gently lowered back down into the freezer after the visualization of an ice crystal within the vial. The specimen is maintained at the seeding temperature for another 5 minutes after ice crystal formation before allowing the biologic freezer to drop further in temperature. Subsequently the temperature within the freezer drops at a rate of −0.5° C/min until a temperature of −80°C is reached. Canes are taken from the freezer and plunged directly into a styrofoam vessel containing a prelabeled storage cane im-

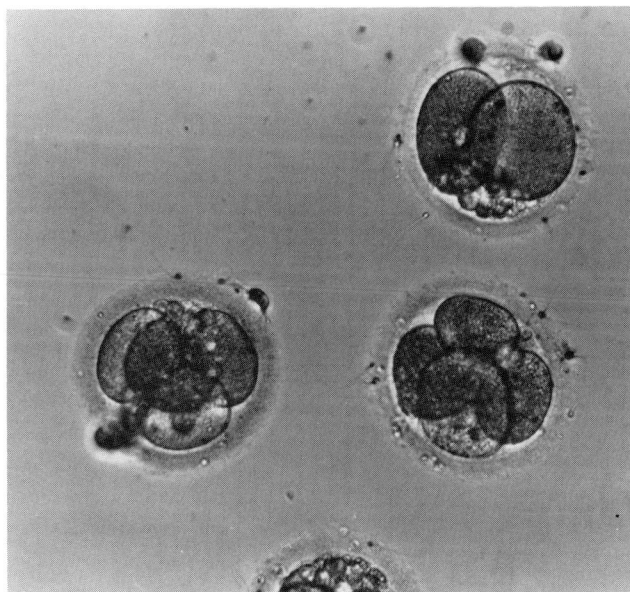

FIGURE 55–8. Embryos combined in a single dish in preparation for intrauterine transfer. All three demonstrate grade 2 morphology.

mersed in liquid nitrogen. With two sets of forceps, cryovials are transferred from the freezing cane to the storage cane, label side up, and always under the level of liquid nitrogen. They are then transferred to a 35-L insulated storage tank where they are kept at $-196°C$ under liquid nitrogen until thawing. The entire process takes almost 4 hours from start to finish.

The protocol for thawing is similarly conducted under computerized control of the Planer biologic freezer. The freezer is precooled to a start point of $-100°C$ and maintained at that temperature for at least 5 minutes before removing the cryovials from liquid nitrogen storage. The correct specimens are carefully identified, and cryovials are transferred to one of the standard freezing canes within the freezing unit. After a 5-minute hold, the temperature within the freezing chamber is allowed to warm at a rate of $+8.0°C$ until room temperature is reached. Cryovials are kept for 5 minutes under ambient conditions before the contents of each are emptied into sterile petri dishes. Thawed conceptuses are then taken through a series of decreasing concentrations of 1,2-propanediol for 5 minutes each dilution (1.0 M, 0.5 M, and 0.0 M) before being washed and placed in fresh equilibrated culture medium. Survival is defined as the ability of the conceptus to enter syngamy and proceed through at least the first cleavage. Most specimens that do not survive appear darkened, flat, or damaged at the first observation.

Intrauterine transfer of thawed specimens is scheduled only after viability is ascertained and a regular cleavage pattern established, usually within 24 hours of thaw. We chose to require cleavage as proof that embryo viability was not compromised; in this manner, we were assured that all patients were receiving conceptuses that were truly capable of further development. Although many programs perform transfers immediately after thawing, we believe that important information is gained by waiting overnight.

Conceptuses may be thawed on the day of ovulation in natural cycles, as determined by serum estradiol, luteinizing hormone (LH), and progesterone levels as well as by ultrasonography or on the day following a documented LH surge. Natural cycle transfers may be supplemented with progesterone (intramuscular or suppositories) if there is a luteal phase defect history. Alternately, embryos may be transferred into a controlled endometrium after suppression with GnRH analog (Lupron, Tap Pharmaceuticals, Chicago, IL) and treatment with exogenous steroids. In either case, transfer is scheduled for the day after thawing.

The onset of our cryopreservation program in 1987 marked an additional workload for the embryology laboratory, but this was rewarded with increased pregnancy rates for our patients. An overall 70% survival rate has been noted in thawed pronucleate oocytes, and a nearly 30% pregnancy rate has been achieved in cycles undergoing a thaw. These numbers translate to a vastly improved overall pregnancy rate per cycle for patients who produce sufficient oocytes to reach the optimal number of embryos for fresh transfer (three to four, as determined by our own results and those of others) with additional ones frozen for later thawed transfer.[8, 20]

Microtechniques

Micromanipulative techniques have been used for almost a century to study the function and development of somatic cells and gametes in lower animals. These exciting research techniques have been expanded to include manipulation of mammalian oocytes and embryos, particularly in the last 20 years. During this time, success has been realized in the dissection or alteration of the zona pellucida, insertion of spermatozoa into various oocyte compartments, removal and transplantation of pronuclei and blastomeres, and other diverse efforts aimed at manipulating the intracellular and extracellular components of the oocyte and embryo. As a result, an intense interest has surfaced in clinical arenas to formulate the means of overcoming human infertility and to improve prenatal diagnosis using manipulative techniques.

Micromanipulative procedures require specialized equipment that can control the intricate movements needed to handle microscopic specimens. This equipment, along with the supporting equipment necessary to fabricate delicate microtools, is expensive and often troublesome to operate. Because of cost factors and the time required to gain micromanipulation expertise, it might be stated that this type of work is not suitable for every IVF program. Although microtechniques are often sought by couples with histories of fertilization failure, implantation failure, or specific genetic defects that may be diagnosed early by virtue of this technology, practical consideration leads to the conclusion that a great deal of time, effort, and perspiration goes into producing a valid micromanipulation pregnancy.

Microtechniques are most commonly used to overcome fertilization disorders. The decision to perform these procedures must be made well in advance of the actual IVF treatment. Previous fertilization failure, sperm numbers too low to permit fertilization even using concentrating techniques, and severely impaired motility are indications for micromanipulation. The quantity and quality of the available sperm are most often used as the parameters to dictate which procedure (or combination of procedures) should be used. The absence of stringent criteria for patient selection and the inability to determine in advance which microsurgical procedure will best assist the fertilization process represent the two most frustrating problems encountered during the development of this type of program.[21]

The construction of appropriate microtools is essential to successful micromanipulation of oocytes and embryos. Generally a larger micropipette is used to stabilize the specimen (the egg-holding pipette), and a second microtool is used for manipulation. Microtools can be prepared from coagulation or capillary tubing (0.7- to 1.0-mm outside diameter) available from various sources. A pipette puller and microforge are required to fabricate and polish egg-holding pipettes, microneedles, and micropipettes. A pipette grinder/beveler is used to create sharp and beveled tips for different microtools. Microtools may be washed immediately after their preparation with hydrofluoric acid, alcohol, or sterile water and, in some cases, followed by exposure to acetone to assist rapid drying. Microtools are commonly stored in large, sterile petri dishes (150 × 15 mm). Clay, foam rubber, or tape can be used to hold pipettes in place.

Egg-holding pipettes and other microtools are prepared in Norfolk with a Narishige PB-7 pipette-puller (Narishige USA, Inc., Greenvale, NY) using thin-walled glass capillary tubes (0.9-mm OD, 0.6-mm ID, 150-mm length, Drummond Scientific, Broomall, PA) and a double-pull technique as follows:

Holding pipettes are made by using four weights and relatively low heater temperatures (heater 1 = 20; heater 2 = 10.2 on our system). This creates a pipette with a relatively wide, blunt surface. Pipettes are then fire-polished with a Narishige MF-9 microforge to achieve a smooth surface with an inside diameter of 20 to 30 μ and outside diameter of approximately 100 μ.

Microneedles are made using a single light weight and relatively high heater settings (heater 1 = 30; heater 2 = 70.0 on our system). Microneedles can be used directly after pulling, as for partial zona dissection (PZD), because this method creates a sharp, thin point.

For techniques requiring an open micropipette, microneedles are first prepared as described previously. Small-diameter, open tips may be produced by dipping the microneedle in 25% hydrofluoric acid followed by washes in sterile, distilled water and acetone. A sharp point can be produced by either breaking the tip off in the egg-holding pipette or by beveling on a pipette grinder (Narishige EG-4). A dot made with a permanent marker at midlength on the pipette helps to display the bevel angle macroscopically.

PARTIAL ZONA DISSECTION AND EMBRYO HATCHING

PZD dissection is performed primarily for couples exhibiting previous fertilization failure. Motile sperm must be present in the semen sample, albeit in low numbers. The procedure is carried out in a 50- to 100-μL drop of medium under oil. Obscuring cumulus and corona cells are removed from oocytes with a solution of 0.1% hyaluronidase for 30 seconds at room temperature, followed by aspiration and expulsion of the oocyte through a 27-gauge needle attached to a tuberculin syringe. Oocytes may be treated with 0.05 to 0.1 M sucrose to shrink the ooplasm.[19, 22] This facilitates the successful insertion of the microneedle without damaging the oolemma but may affect oocyte activation. A brief period, but not more than 30 minutes between sucrose exposure and insemination, has been suggested.

Oocytes are held firmly by the egg-holding pipette so the area to be dissected is at a 12 o'clock position. The microneedle is pushed through one side of the zona pellucida (1 o'clock position), and the oocyte moved upwards slightly with the microneedle to avoid contact between the microneedle and the holding pipette. The microneedle is advanced through the perivitelline space and the opposing side of the zona pellucida, exiting the zona at an 11 o'clock position. Pinching of the zona may occur with larger or duller microneedles. Suction is discontinued from the holding pipette, and the microneedle, now piercing the zona, is brought parallel to the larger holding pipette. The zona pellucida is rolled against the holding pipette to force an opening or create a tear in the structure. Once this is accomplished, the oocyte is removed from the microneedle by gentle aspiration from the holding pipette. This must be done carefully, and direct suction on the dissected area must be avoided. If sucrose is used for oocyte shrinkage, it should be removed by multiple washes in culture medium.

Sperm collected after swim-up or Percoll preparation are used for insemination of the zona-dissected oocyte. Pregnancy and live birth have been reported after using this procedure.[22]

The technique of embryo hatching may be performed in a manner similar to PZD except that the specimen being manipulated is a cleaving embryo rather than an unfertilized oocyte; alternatively a zona drilling method can be used for embryo hatching. The general concept of creating a breach in the zona pellucida is the same. The theory is that nutrients are better able to reach the embryo after a breach is formed, and negative aspects of acquired zona hardening in culture are avoided. It is also theorized that natural hatching before implantation may be facilitated by a mechanical breach in the zona investment.[23] It has been reported that this procedure is especially beneficial to women over the age of 40 years, women with elevated basal follicle-stimulating hormone levels, or women with oocytes displaying thickened zonae (personal communication, Jacques Cohen, Cornell Medical Center, New York).

For these procedures, a small-diameter egg-holding pipette (90 to 100 μ OD) and a sharp, thin microneedle (closed tip, no beveling necessary) are commonly used.

SUBZONAL INSERTION OF SPERM

This procedure is commonly performed when only a few sperm are isolated from a semen sample. Subzonal insertion may be carried out in conjunction with a PZD attempt to determine which technique is best for a given couple. Medium supplemented with sucrose may be used to shrink the ooplasm to avoid damage during micropipette insertion under the zona pellucida. Obscuring cumulus cells are first removed with hyaluronidase, and the actual procedure is performed in a 50- to 100-μL drop of medium under oil. Motile sperm can be suspended in a second droplet of medium containing a viscous solution of methyl cellulose or polyvinylpyrrolidone to retard motility and to facilitate capture into micropipettes; this step has been shown to be unnecessary in most cases. If sperm numbers are adequate, they may be placed in the same droplet of medium with the oocyte. One to six spermatozoa are aspirated into the tip of a finely sharpened micropipette. These sperm are then placed into the perivitelline space of a mature oocyte, taking care to avoid transferring excess medium along with the spermatozoa. On completion of the procedure, the oocyte is removed from the droplet of medium, washed in fresh medium, and incubated.

Spermatozoa used for placement into the perivitelline space may be prepared by swim-up or Percoll gradient procedures. It has been postulated that sperm must be acrosome-reacted for fusion to occur with the ooplasmic membrane. Special techniques, such as incubation of sperm in a calcium-depleted, strontium-based medium or in human follicular fluid, can assist in promoting acrosome reactions for a large percentage of cells in a given sample. More commonly, sperm are prepared without these agents, and multiple sperm are placed into the perivitelline space. Pregnancy has been reported using this technique.[24–26]

Large-diameter egg-holding pipettes (120-μ OD) and sharp, beveled micropipettes (20 to 30 degree angle, 10 to 15 μ OD) are recommended for this procedure.

ZONA DRILLING

Zona drilling is rarely performed for assisted fertilization because of the potential detrimental effects of the acid solution on oocyte membranes. When used, the technique may be executed in a 50- to 100-μL drop of medium under oil. Obscuring cumulus and corona cells are removed as described previously, and sucrose medium may be used to shrink the ooplasm away from the zona pellucida. The holding pipette and micropipette are prepared as for other manipulative techniques except that the micropipette used for drilling is broken and polished to form a blunt tip. A large-diameter egg-holding pipette (120 μ OD) and a blunt micropipette (10 to 30 μ OD, depending on the size hole required) are used here.

Zona pellucida glycoproteins are dissolved with acid Tyrode's solution (pH 2.0 to 2.4) or with enzymes (trypsin or pronase) by expelling the solution against an area of the zona with positive pressure.[27] Drilling the zona may require several minutes, and the oolemma may puff slightly as the inner portion of the zona is dissolved. The action of these solutions on the ooplasmic membrane may produce a deleterious effect. A hole in the zona pellucida made in this manner is generally large but varies with the size of the pipette expelling the acidic solution. After drilling, the oocyte is washed multiple times in fresh culture medium and inseminated with washed, incubated sperm.

As stated previously, there may be a more appropriate application for zona drilling when used during embryo hatching procedures.

SPERM MICROINJECTION INTO OOPLASM

When no motile spermatozoa are present in a given sample and sperm numbers are so poor that only a rare spermatozoon can be located, sperm placement directly into oocyte cytoplasm may be considered. Microinjection of human sperm into cumulus-free oocytes is performed in a 50- to 100-μL drop of sucrose-free medium under oil. A droplet of prepared sperm suspension is placed in a second droplet near the first. A micropipette for injection purposes is prepared by snapping off the tip within the opening of the egg-holding pipette or by using a pipette grinder to create a sharp, angled tip.

Human semen samples are prepared by swim-up or Percoll gradient procedures. Before the injection procedure, sperm may be diluted 1:5 (V/V) with 10% polyvinylpyrrolidone (MW = 90,000) in DPBS; this aids in the handling of sperm during the procedure and coats the micropipette to prevent the single sperm from sticking inside.

A single spermatozoon is picked up by the micropipette and moved to the droplet of medium with the oocyte. The oocyte is picked up and held securely by the egg-holding pipette. The micropipette is then firmly pushed through the zona pellucida and deep into the cytoplasm. A small amount of cytoplasm is drawn into the micropipette and then expelled along with the spermatozoon.[28] This is done to activate the oocyte, and to verify that the microneedle is within the ooplasm. The micropipette is withdrawn from the cytoplasm, the oocyte is released from the egg-holding pipette, washed in fresh medium, and incubated in a standard fashion.

Large-diameter egg-holding pipettes (120-μ OD) and sharp, beveled micropipettes (20- to 30-degree angle, 5- to 8-μ ID; 8- to 11-μ OD) are used for cytoplasmic injection.

PRONUCLEUS REMOVAL, GERMINAL VESICLE REMOVAL, AND CYTOPLASMIC TRANSFER

Procedures involving the removal of cytoplasmic structures are fairly straightforward and used only on a research basis. Performed under oil in 50- to 100-μL droplets of medium, all involve removal of obscuring cumulus cells, stabilization with a holding pipette, puncture of the zona pellucida, aspiration of a given element, and withdrawal of the micropipette without severely traumatizing the oocyte or embryo. If it is necessary to aspirate an intact structure, the micropipette must be of an appropriate size to accomplish the collection without damaging pronuclear or cytoplasmic membranes; if only cytoplasm is collected, the micropipette can be quite small. Some investigators have reported the necessity of cytoskeletal stabilizers (1- to 2-μg/mL cytochalasine B or D) to perform pronucleus removal,[29] but our experience, along with others,[30] has not supported this. Specimens survive at high rates with the use of a 3- to 11-μ OD micropipette and no chemical stabilizers. The principles of successful manipulation include a properly sharpened micropipette of appropriate size for the task, care in aspirating only the desired structure with as little cytoplasm as possible, and rapid technique.

Large-diameter egg-holding pipettes (120-μ OD) and sharp, beveled micropipettes of approximately 8 to 30 μ can be used for removal procedures depending on whether the structure is to be removed intact. For cytoplasmic transfer from one oocyte to another, a small micropipette of approximately 3 to 5 μ is used.

POLAR BODY BIOPSY AND BLASTOMERE BIOPSY

A first polar body, blastomere nucleus, or intact blastomere can be removed from an oocyte or embryo for DNA analysis. For this type of analysis, it is absolutely necessary to avoid DNA contamination with miscellaneous sperm or cumulus cells. Only the structure to be analyzed should be drawn into the aspirating pipette and washed; sterile gloves should be worn when handling pipettes or assay tubes.

For polar body biopsy, the oocyte is held against the egg-holding pipette in such a way that the polar body is located at a 12 o'clock position and clearly visible. A small amount of medium is initially aspirated into the aspirating micropipette to facilitate the expulsion of all contents once the biopsy is completed. The aspirating micropipette is gently passed through the zona pellucida, the polar body is drawn inside, and the micropipette is carefully withdrawn. The micropipette is then removed from the manipulator and lowered into a microcentrifuge tube containing HPLC grade, autoclaved, filtered water, and the polar body is expelled. Blastomere biopsy is performed in a manner similar to polar body biopsy with a somewhat larger aspirating micropipette. If the blastomere membrane breaks during collection, special attention should be given to ensure that the nucleus is collected; for this reason, it is preferable to choose a blastomere with a clearly defined nucleus. Calcium-free and magnesium-free medium may be used to decrease blastomere aggregation, but the long-term effect of this treatment on the human embryo is unknown. To facilitate the puncture of the zona pellucida with a large micropipette, zona drilling or dissection techniques may be necessary first to produce a hole large enough for microtool entry. As an alternate procedure, a hole can be made in the zona pellucida and the required structures forcibly pushed through the opening by pressing on the opposing side of the zona with a large, smooth, blunt microtool.

Larger-diameter egg-holding pipettes are recommended for these procedures; sharp, beveled micropipettes of 12 to 18 μ and 18 to 25 μ can be used to aspirate polar bodies and blastomeres. A closed, smooth, flame-polished holding pipette may be used to assist pushing a polar body or blastomere through a zona drilling or PZD opening.

MISCELLANEOUS CONCERNS

Fixing, Embedding, and Staining Specimens for Light and Electron Microscopy

Oocytes are fixed in 2.5% glutaraldehyde in 0.1 M cacodylate buffer for 30 minutes and then placed on a glass slide with little excess fluid. Melted agar (1.5%) is placed over the oocyte or conceptus and allowed to harden for approximately 60 seconds. A clean razor blade is used to cut the agar into a rectangle (approximately 0.5 mm $\times$ 1.0 mm) in which the sample is located. The agar block is postfixed with 1% osmium tetroxide in 0.1 M cacodylate buffer, dehydrated with alcohol, and embedded in Poly/Bed 812 (Ted Pella, Inc., Tustin, CA).

Spermatozoa are prepared as follows: Semen samples are twice washed by centrifugation in phosphate buffered saline for 10 minutes to remove seminal plasma. Washed pellets are resuspended for 2 hours in 2.5% glutaraldehyde buffered with 0.1% cacodylate. Pellets are postfixed in 1% osmium tetroxide in cacodylate buffer. Following dehydration in ethanol and propylene oxide, the samples are embedded in Poly/Bed 812.

Thick and thin sections of oocytes, abnormal conceptuses, and spermatozoa are cut on an LKB ultramicrotome. Thick sections are cut with glass knives, stained with toluidine blue, and viewed with a light microscope. Thin sections are cut with a diamond knife, stained with lead citrate and uranyl acetate, and viewed in a Phillips 301 electron microscope.

Cleaning and Preparation of Pasteur Pipettes

Two sizes of borosilicate glass pasteur pipettes are used in IVF protocols, 5¾ in. and 9 in. Pipettes are rinsed in a Boekel pipette washer/dryer and soaked overnight in 4 L of MilliQ/UF water. After drying overnight in the automatic dryer, they are plugged at the wide end with sterile 100% cotton. This end is briefly flamed to remove stray fibers of cotton. Care is taken to avoid touching pipette tips while handling. Pipettes are packaged in individual autoclave pouches with the wide, cotton-plugged end placed in the package first. Pouches are sealed and steam autoclaved under standard sterilizing conditions for wrapped goods.

REFERENCES

1. Acosta AA, Kruger TF, Swanson RJ, Ackerman S. In vitro fertilization in male infertility. In: Garcia C, Mastroianni L, Amelar RD, Dubin L, editors. Current Therapy of Infertility. 3rd edition. Toronto: BC Decker, 1988.
2. Soffer Y, Sauer MV, Francis MM, et al. A prospective controlled evaluation of TEST-yolk buffer in the preparation of sperm for human in vitro fertilization in suspected cases of male infertility. Fertil Steril 1992;3:551.
3. Lanzendorf SE, Holmgren WJ, Jeyendran RS. The effect of egg yolk medium on human sperm binding in the hemizona assay. Fertil Steril 1992;58:547.
4. Oehninger S, Acosta AA, Veeck LL, et al. Recurrent failure of in vitro fertilization: role of the hemizona assay in the sequential diagnosis of specific sperm-oocyte defects. Am J Obstet Gynecol 1991;164:1210.
5. Kruger T, Acosta A, Simmons K, et al. Predictive value of abnormal sperm morphology in in vitro fertilization. Fertil Steril 1988;49:112.
6. Oehninger S, Acosta AA, Morshedi M, et al. Corrective measures and pregnancy outcome in in vitro fertilization in patients with severe sperm morphology abnormalities. Fertil Steril 1988;50:283.
7. Kruger TF, Ackerman SB, Simmons KF, et al. A quick, reliable staining technique for human sperm morphology. Arch Androl 1987;18:275.
8. Veeck LL. Microscopic assessment of oocytes, prezygotes, and preembryos. In: Wallach EE, Zacur HA, editors. Reproductive Medicine and Surgery. St. Louis: Mosby–Year Book, in press.
9. Veeck LL. Oocyte assessment and biological performance. Ann NY Acad Sci 1988;541:259.
10. Veeck LL. Pregnancy rate and pregnancy outcome associated with laboratory evaluation of spermatozoa, oocytes, and preembryos. In: Mashiach S, Ben-Rafael Z, Laufer N, Schenker JG, editors. Advances in Assisted Reproductive Technologies. New York: Plenum Press, 1990:745.
11. Veeck LL. The morphological assessment of human oocytes and early concepti. In: Keel BA, Webster BW, editors. Handbook of the Laboratory Diagnosis and Treatment of Infertility. Boca Raton, FL: CRC Press, 1990:353.
12. Plachot M, de Grouchy J, Junca AM, et al. Chromosome analysis of human oocytes and embryos: does delayed fertilization increase chromosome imbalance? Hum Reprod 1988;2:705.
13. Oehninger S, Acosta AA, Veeck LL, et al. Delayed fertilization during in vitro fertilization and embryo transfer cycles: analysis of causes and impact on overall results. Fertil Steril 1989;52:991.
14. Van Blerkom J, Bell H, Henry G. The occurrence, recognition and developmental fate of pseudo-pronuclear eggs after in vitro fertilization of human oocytes. Hum Reprod 1987;2:217.
15. Van Blerkom J. Developmental failure in human reproduction associated with preovulatory oogenesis and preimplantation embryogenesis. In: Van Blerkom J, Motta PM, editors. Ultrastructure of Human Gametogenesis and Early Embryogenesis. Boston: Kluwer Academic Publishers, 1989:125.
16. Edwards RG. Fertilization. In: Conception in the Human Female. New York: Academic Press, 1980:573.
17. Kola I, Trounson A, Dawson G, Rogers P. Tripronuclear human oocytes: altered cleavage patterns and subsequent karyotypic analysis of embryos. Biol Reprod 1987;37:395.
18. Veeck LL. Atlas of the Human Oocyte and Early Conceptus. Vol 2. Baltimore: Williams & Wilkins, 1991;121.
19. Cohen J, Malter H, Wright G, et al. Partial zona dissection of human oocytes when failure of zona pellucida penetration is anticipated. Hum Reprod 1989;4:435.
20. Veeck LL, Amundson C, Brothman L, et al. Significantly enhanced pregnancy rates through cryopreservation and thawing: a four-year clinical study. Fertil Steril 1993;59:1202.
21. Cohen J, Alikani M, Adler A, et al. Microsurgical fertilization procedures: the absence of stringent criteria for patient selection. J Asst Reprod Genet 1992;9:197.
22. Malter HE, Cohen J. Partial zona dissection of the human oocyte: a nontraumatic method using micromanipulation to assist zona pellucida penetration. Fertil Steril 1989;51:139.
23. Cohen J, Elsner C, Kort H, et al. Impairment of the hatching process following IVF in the human and improvement of implantation by assisting hatching using micromanipulation. Hum Reprod 1990;5:7.
24. Fishel S, Jackson P, Antinori S, et al. Subzonal insemination for the alleviation of infertility. Fertil Steril 1990;54:828.

25. Ng SC, Bongso TA, Ratnam SS, et al. Pregnancy after transfer of multiple sperm under the zona. Lancet 1988;2:790.
26. Ng SC, Bongso A, Sathananthan H, Ratnam SS. Micromanipulation: its relevance to human in vitro fertilization. Fertil Steril 1990;53:203.
27. Gordon JW, Grunfeld L, Garrisi GJ, et al. Fertilization of human oocytes by sperm from infertile males after zona pellucida drilling. Fertil Steril 1988;50:68.
28. Lanzendorf SE, Maloney MK, Veeck LL, et al. A preclinical evaluation of pronuclear formation by microinjection of human spermatozoa into human oocytes. Fertil Steril 1988;49:835.
29. Gordon JW, Grunfeld L, Garrisi GJ, et al. Successful microsurgical removal of a pronucleus from tripronuclear human zygotes. Fertil Steril 1989;52:367.
30. Malter HE, Cohen J. Embryonic development after microsurgical repair of polyspermic human zygotes. Fertil Steril 1989;52:373.

CHAPTER 56

Cryopreservation of Embryos and Oocytes

PATRICK QUINN

It soon became evident during the development of assisted reproductive technology (ART) that the transfer of more than three to four good-quality embryos not only did not significantly improve the incidence of pregnancy,[1] but also increased the risk of multiple pregnancy.[2] Therefore, a method to cryopreserve the spare or surplus human embryos produced by ART was actively pursued in the early 1980s.[3] The successful methods developed were based largely on those used previously for the embryos of nonhuman mammals.[4] The benefits of a method to cryopreserve unfertilized oocytes are also well recognized and are primarily for the preservation of oocytes in the face of radiotherapy or chemotherapy for cancer or other threatening medical reasons or to preserve oocytes for future donation to other infertile couples (reviewed by Quinn[5]). Successful oocyte cryopreservation, however, has remained an elusive procedure in all groups of mammals in which it has been attempted.

The purpose of this chapter is to review the development of cryopreservation techniques used for human embryos, the principles of the procedures, and their practical application. Results reported in the literature are examined in light of the particular procedures used, and a brief outline of possible future developments is given.

HISTORY

There have been sporadic attempts over the past 200 years to maintain spermatozoa and oocytes of various animals in a frozen state, one of the earliest reports being that of Spallanzani in 1776 (see Kuzan and Quinn[6]). More intensive studies began in the 1930s and 1940s, but it was not until the discovery of the cryoprotective effect of glycerol for the frozen storage of spermatozoa that a practical application for the procedure in domestic animal husbandry and later human infertility was established (see Quinn[5]). Serious attempts to store mammalian oocytes and embryos at low temperatures began in the late 1940s. In 1947, Chang[7] first reported that rabbit embryos held at 5 to 10°C for 80 to 101 hours before transfer to suitable recipients gave rise to live young. The oocytes and embryos of several other species, including the mouse, sheep, goat, and cow, were subsequently shown by several other investigators over the next 20 years to maintain their viability when stored at 0 to 10°C, with variable success rates in terms of individual embryos leading to viable offspring, depending primarily on the length of storage (reviewed by Maurer;[8] see also Polge[9]). No cryoprotectants were used in these studies, and the maximum length of successful storage in nearly all these studies was about 5 days. These early procedures have little practical application for the temporary storage of human embryos, but they have been useful, for example, in the stud goat industry: Four- to eight-cell embryos can be stored for up to 48 hours at 4°C with little loss of viability.[10] This allows for more flexibility in allocating donor embryos to suitable synchronous recipients over a 1- to 2-day period.

It was not until 1972, however, with the use of a new cryoprotective compound (dimethyl sulfoxide [DMSO]), that the first successful long-term storage of mouse embryos at subzero temperatures was reported independently by Whittingham and associates[11] and Wilmut.[12] This procedure was subsequently extended to a variety of other mammalian species (reviewed by Whittingham[13]) and culminated in the report in 1983 by Trounson and Mohr[3] of the first successful cryopreservation of a human embryo. Trounson and Mohr[3] used DMSO as the cryoprotectant and methods that had been developed for use with cleavage-stage mouse embryos.[13] Over the next few years, successful cryopreservation of human embryos was extended to the blastocyst stage using glycerol as cryoprotectant[14] and to zygotes using propanediol (PPD) sucrose.[15] With minor refinements to these methods, embryo cryopreservation has now been established as a routine clinical adjunct to successful ART programs. This applies not only to the storage of supernumerary embryos derived from routine in vitro fertilization (IVF) but also in the near future, will be applied to embryos biopsied for genetic analysis.[16] It is also likely that in the next several years, a method for routine clinical cryopreservation of human oocytes will be developed; this procedure would allow for the establishment of human oocyte banks for oocyte storage for various medical indications and egg donation.

PRINCIPLES OF CRYOPRESERVATION

Dehydration, Cryoprotectants, and Rates of Cooling and Warming

The major cause of cell destruction during freezing and thawing is the formation of intracellular ice crystals. Therefore during cryopreservation, a major aim is to reduce the amount of water within the cell so when it freezes, the amount of intracellular ice formed is compatible with survival. Removal of too much water, however, and subsequent excessive dehydration is also detrimental. The freezing point of water containing ions and dissolved solutes is lower than 0°C and dependent on the concentration of the dissolved solutes. When such a solution is cooled, more pure water freezes, increasing the liquid concentration of dissolved solutes and lowering the freezing point of the remaining solution further. The increased osmotic pressure of the remaining dissolved solutes can also cause damage to cells during cooling (referred to as the "solution effect"). The object then is to remove enough water from cells during cooling so survival is optimized by minimal ice crystal formation. This, together with a solution that has an osmotic pressure whose damaging solution effects are minimized, ensures maximum cell survival. It is now recognized that damage during cryopreservation is not low-temperature storage itself but the transitions through the temperature zones during cooling and thawing, when ice-crystal formation is most likely to occur.[17]

Two factors that have been found to be important in ameliorating the effect of intracellular ice formation and solution effects are (1) the presence of molar amounts of protective solutes referred to as cryoprotectants and (2) the rates of cooling and warming (reviewed by Rall and colleagues[18]). Cryoprotectants can be either membrane permeable (e.g., DMSO, glycerol, PPD) or membrane impermeable (e.g., sucrose—some slight membrane permeation does occur). These two types of cryoprotectants have different roles. Permeable cryoprotectants are thought to act by a variety of mechanisms, including (1) lowering the freezing point of a solution—intracellular freezing in 1.0 M solution of DMSO may not occur until −40 to −50°C; (2) interaction with membranes as they change from a relatively fluid to a relatively rigid state during cooling; and (3) prevention of exposure to elevated concentrations of electrolytes both intracellularly and extracellularly by binding to the electrolytes and partially substituting for the presence of water. Impermeable cryoprotectants (e.g., sucrose) can initiate loss of water from cells by osmotic dehydration in the absence of extracellular ice crystals. Control of the cooling and warming conditions determines the ultimate fate of intracellular water during the cryopreservation process.[18] The thermodynamic conditions interact intimately with the permeability of the cell to water and the size of the cell. Because of the larger volume to surface area of oocytes and embryos compared with smaller cells, cooling rates 10 to 100 times slower than those used to cryopreserve spermatozoa, red blood cells, or cell lines have been required. The slower cooling rates for mammalian embryos (<1°C/minute) allow sufficient time for more water to leave the cell owing to the cell's osmotic response to the formation of ice in the extracellular medium and the subsequent increase in osmolality of the surrounding unfrozen solution. Comparing cells of different sizes (e.g., erythrocytes

compared with mouse oocytes), cooling rates compatible with survival change by 250-fold to 500-fold. The relevant parameters associated with this comparison were reviewed by Leibo[19] and are shown in Table 56–1. Correspondingly, with mouse embryos, Whittingham and coworkers[11] showed that cell survival decreased from 50% to 70% to 0% as the cooling rate was increased from less than 0.5°C/minute to 7°C/minute or greater. The pioneering studies of Mazur[20] recognized the importance of the ability of cells to respond to osmotic challenges, which was dependent on the cell's permeability coefficient, the surface area of the cell, the osmotic gradient between the outside and the inside of the cell, and temperature.[17] Recognition of the interaction of these relationships allows the response of many cells, including mammalian oocytes and embryos, to cryopreservation to be predicted.

The degree of dehydration within a cell and the subsequent chance of cell survival during cooling are dependent on:

1. The temperature at which slow cooling is terminated by direct plunging into liquid nitrogen. If this temperature is lower, there is more time for a greater degree of dehydration.
2. The concentration of cryoprotectant used. The rate of movement of water across a cell membrane is proportional to the difference in concentration of solute molecules on the two sides of the membrane. Also the higher the concentration of cryoprotectant, the lower the freezing point of the solution, and this allows for more dehydration before all of the extracellular water freezes.
3. The permeability of the cell membrane to water and cryoprotectant.
4. The size of the cell. Smaller cells can be cooled faster because of their larger surface-to-volume ratio, and hence water can leave smaller cells faster than larger ones.

Apart from these considerations, the amount of water within cells contributing to ice-crystal formation can also be regulated by the use of relatively impermeable solutes, such as sucrose, to initiate osmotic dehydration of the cell before extracellular ice formation occurs. Renard and associates[21] were one of the first groups to use this concept, using this procedure to cryopreserve rabbit embryos. The method was soon applied with success to human embryos.[22]

Seeding

Seeding is the induction of ice-crystal formation at or slightly below the normal freezing point of an aqueous solu-

TABLE 56–1. Water Permeability Characteristics and Cell Survival of Erythrocytes and Mouse Ova in Relation to Cooling Rates

Cell Type	Permeability Coefficient, 20°C ($\mu m^3/\mu m^2$,min,atm)	Surface Area/Volume ($\mu m^2/\mu m^3$)	Critical Cooling Rate (°C/min)*
Human erythrocytes	5.7	1.88	540
Mouse ova	0.27	0.08	2.4

*Critical cooling rate above which ≥50% of the cells freeze intracellularly. From Leibo SP. Fundamental cryobiology of mouse ova and embryos. In: Elliott K, Whelan J, editors. The Freezing of Mammalian Embryos. Ciba Foundation Symposium No. 52. Amsterdam: Elsevier, 1977:69–92.

tion. When small volumes of fluid are slowly cooled, however, the solution can reach a temperature substantially below its freezing point before ice formation takes place. This phenomenon is known as supercooling. Whittingham[23] measured these effects in 1.5-M solutions of DMSO in phosphate-buffered saline solution and found that this solution has a freezing point of −3°C. If the solution was slowly cooled without the induction of ice crystals by seeding, however, it could supercool to −21°C before ice formed spontaneously. In Whittingham's[24] first report of mouse embryo freezing, the embryos were cooled at 60°C/minute from 0°C to −79°C with no seeding. The embryos did not survive longer than 30 minutes at −79°C,[11] and it has been suggested that the embryos may have been supercooled.[9] Beyond 30 minutes, however, perhaps damaging ice crystals formed that destroyed the embryos.

On ice formation, the latent heat of crystallization is released, and this raises the temperature of the medium (Fig. 56–1). A rapid cooling rate then ensues (>3°C/minute as calculated by Whittingham[23]) as the sample then re-equilibrates with the temperature of the cooling chamber. Whittingham[23] reported that supercooling eight-cell mouse embryos to −4 to −6°C before seeding did not affect their survival (75% to 82%). At −7°C, slightly lower survival (65%) occurred, and at seeding temperatures below −7°C, there was a rapid decrease in survival until at −12°C or lower, none of the embryos survived.

There are two interactive deleterious effects of supercooling: (1) the rapid cooling rate occurring after ice formation as the sample re-equilibrates with the cooling chamber temperature and (2) the reduced time for sufficient dehydration to occur during the cooling phase after ice formation and before the cells are placed in liquid nitrogen for storage. The

results reported by Whittingham[23] indicated that insufficient time for dehydration in supercooled samples is the major effect, the accelerated cooling velocity after ice formation in supercooled samples being of lesser importance but still contributing to decreased survival. Whittingham[23] also suggested that configurational changes in cell membranes during supercooling could impair the dehydration of the embryos on subsequent cooling.

Seeding then is an essential requirement in cooling protocols involving a controlled rate of slow cooling because it initiates dehydration of the embryos, prevents excessive supercooling, and is necessary for embryo survival. From a practical point of view, seeding can be induced between −5 and −7°C. Seeding at −5°C, which is close to the freezing point of most cryoprotectant solutions used for mammalian embryo cryopreservation, minimizes any possible deleterious effects owing to slight variations in cooling rates because of the release of the latent heat of crystallization. These effects would be more pronounced if seeding takes place at a lower temperature. A disadvantage of seeding at the higher temperature, however, is the possibility that the sample may warm to a temperature above the freezing point of the solution. Such an error is reduced at a lower temperature. Some seeding protocols and devices minimize the risk of this malfunction, but for practical purposes, I recommend manual seeding at −6°C with precooled forceps. Also, in my experience, manual seeding is more reliable than the use of automatic devices provided in some controlled rate freezers.

Temperature at Termination of Slow Cooling and Transfer to Liquid Nitrogen

The temperature at which slow cooling is terminated has a direct effect on the degree of dehydration of the cells because the longer the cells are slow cooled, the longer is the time during which dehydration can occur. Willadsen[25] was the first to show that there was an interaction between the temperature at which slow cooling was terminated on transfer to liquid nitrogen and the subsequent rate of warming required to attain high rates of embryo survival. He reported that when sheep embryos were slowly cooled to a temperature below −50°C, maximum survival occurred if they were slowly warmed. When embryos were cooled to between −30 and −42°C before plunging into liquid nitrogen, however, rapid warming was essential. Whittingham and associates[26] reported that a similar interaction occurred with mouse embryos. One way to interpret this phenomenon is based on the degree of intracellular dehydration present when the embryos are transferred to liquid nitrogen. Thus, embryos cooled slowly to below −60°C have a high degree of dehydration and require slow warming (8 to 20°C/minute) to allow for adequate rehydration. In contrast, embryos cooled slowly to −30 to −40°C have to be warmed rapidly (275 to 500°C/minute) so that the intracellular ice crystals that form when the embryos are transferred to liquid nitrogen are rapidly dispersed and do not recrystallize during slow warming into lethal larger crystals. The concept of the presence of intracellular ice crystals being dependent on the temperature at which slow cooling is terminated and the subsequent effect of the rate of warming on embryonic survival is illustrated in Figure 56–2.

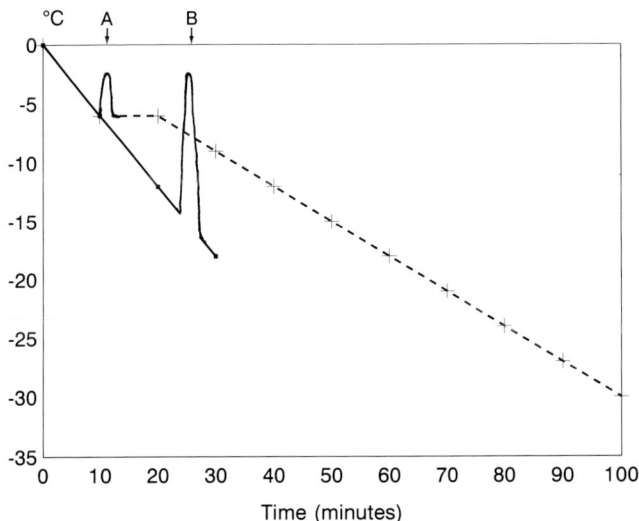

FIGURE 56–1. Temperature changes around the time of seeding. Point A represents the recommended point of seeding at −6°C, with the release of the latent heat of crystallization giving a small rise in temperature that quickly reverts to −6°C. The sample is held at this temperature before slow cooling begins (*dotted line*). However, if the sample is cooled without seeding, it will supercool until at some point (e.g., B) ice crystal formation begins automatically. There is a large increase in temperature due to the latent heat of crystallization and the subsequent cooling rate that occurs, because the sample reequilibrates with the chamber temperature (−15°C in this example) can be quite high.

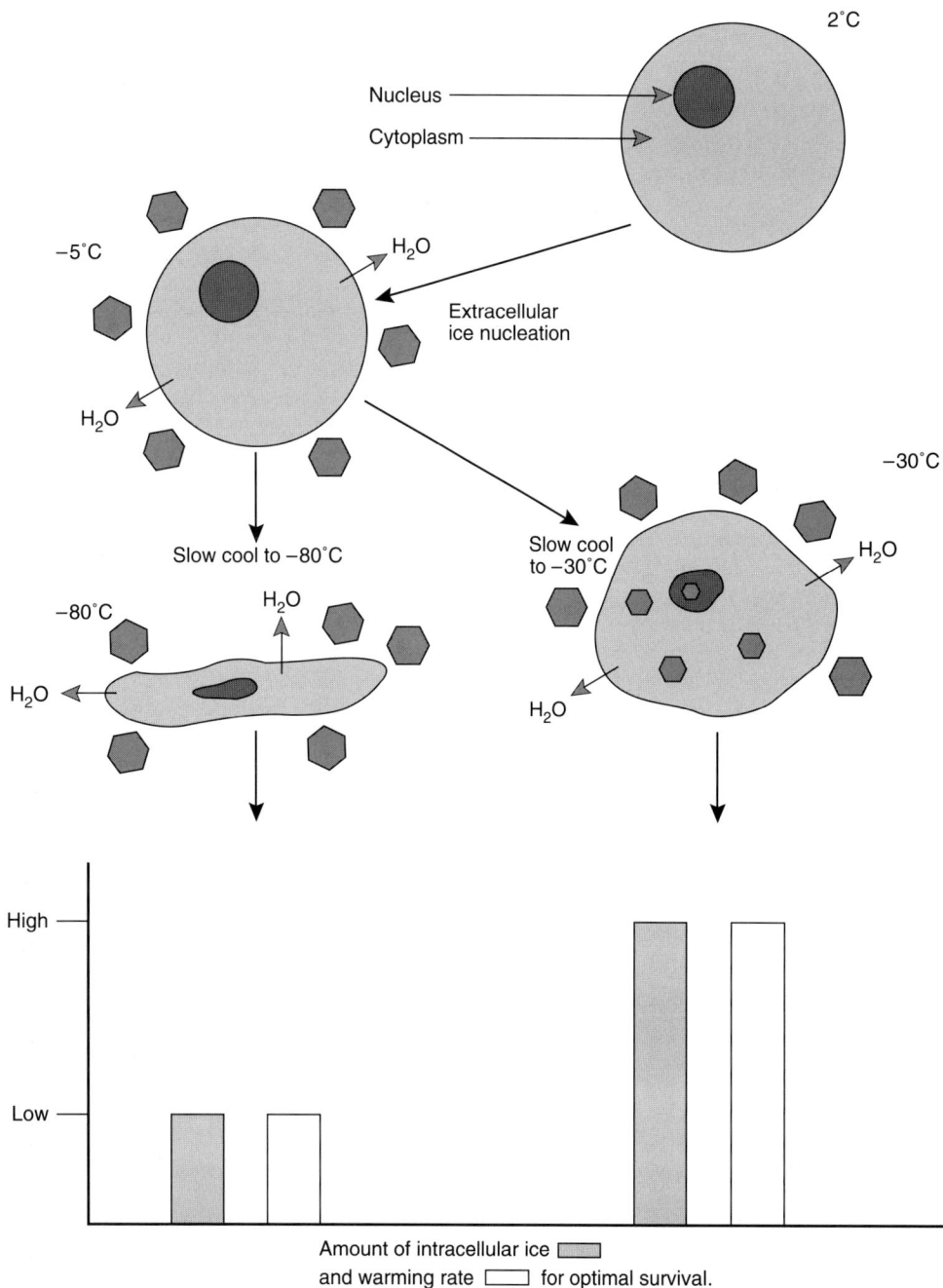

FIGURE 56–2. Interrelationship between the amount of intracellular ice (*shaded bar*) in embryos at termination of slow cooling and the warming rate (*open bar*) required for optimal survival. In the embryo on the right where slow cooling is terminated at −30°C before transfer to liquid nitrogen, a high content of intracellular ice is present; this requires a high warming rate for optimal survival. Conversely, in the embryo on the left, a low amount of intracellular ice remains when slow cooling is terminated at −80°C, necessitating a low warming rate for optimal survival. (Adapted from Whittingham DG. Principles of embryo preservation. In: Ashwood-Smith MJ, Farrant J, editors. Low-Temperature Preservation in Medicine and Biology. Tunbridge Wells: Pitman Medical, 1980:65–83.)

A similar dependency of human embryos on the temperature at transfer to liquid nitrogen and the subsequent optimal warming rate became evident. When four- and eight-cell embryos were cryopreserved with 1.5 M DMSO, the highest survival rate occurred when the slow cooling was terminated at −80°C and rewarming occurred at 8°C/minute.[27] Using 1.5 M PPD and 0.1 M sucrose as the cryoprotectant mixture, optimal survival occurred when slow cooling ended at −30°C; these embryos had to be rewarmed rapidly at about 300°C/minute.[22] It should be kept in mind that it is the temperature at termination of slow cooling and not the specific cryoprotectant that is the most important factor in these observations.

Duration of Storage

The initial studies that investigated the effect of the duration of storage involved mice. After successful cryopreservation of mouse embryos was established, the method was used for creating embryo storage banks of specific strains of mice. It was shown that storage for at least 4 years had no significant effect on embryo survival.[23] It has subsequently been reported that live mice have been born after developing from embryos that had been cryopreserved and stored in liquid nitrogen for more than 13 years.[27a] It is not known for how long human embryos can be frozen and remain viable, but it is likely that they could survive for at least as long as the 13 years reported for mouse embryos. A major concern of prolonged storage is the possibility of genetic damage occurring as a result of prolonged exposure to background radiation. There would be no enzymatic repair mechanisms at $-196°C$. Experiments using a radioactive source close to the cryopreserved embryos to simulate an extended period of background radiation showed, however, that mouse embryos could be stored for the equivalent of between 200 and 1000 years before there was a significant reduction in survival owing to the accumulation of genetic damage caused by background radiation.[28]

It was initially reported that there was a decreased survival of human embryos and subsequent pregnancy rate with prolonged storage.[29] A contrary observation reported no decline in survival of embryos or pregnancy rates with storage up to 70 weeks.[30] It is likely that human embryos are similar to those of other mammalian species with respect to survival in storage and that if they are cryopreserved under the correct conditions, they can survive for the reproductive life span of the couple from whom they were derived.

Rehydration on Thawing

On thawing, the reverse processes to those that operate during cooling take effect. The basic aims during these processes are twofold: (1) to rehydrate the cells and (2) to remove cryoprotectant that has permeated the cells. Rehydration of the cells begins during warming as ice melts and turns into liquid water capable of permeating the cell membranes. Mention has already been made that embryos slowly cooled to less than $-60°C$ before transfer to liquid nitrogen, and therefore relatively highly dehydrated, have to be warmed slowly; Whittingham[13] proposed this was necessary to allow for gradual rehydration so reassembly of subcellular structures within the embryo would not be damaged by rapid osmotic changes. Thawed embryos generally appear quite shrunken immediately on thawing, indicating little rehydration has yet occurred. This is presumably because of the high intracellular concentration of permeable cryoprotectant in the shrunken cell that has been frozen. As a consequence of this, rehydration of the cells and removal of the intracellular cryoprotectant is usually a combined process, the technical evolution of which has occurred somewhat independently from other procedures in cryopreservation.

Dilution of Cryoprotectant in Thawed Samples

Clear evidence that the rate of removal of cryoprotectant from thawed embryos is critical to survival can readily be obtained by placing thawed embryos or those that have been equilibrated in a permeable cryoprotectant directly into an isotonic solution such as culture medium; the embryos swell and disintegrate owing to the rapid influx of water.[31] The initial method to avoid this osmotic shock was to remove the cryoprotectant gradually by a stepwise transfer of the embryos through successively lower concentrations of cryoprotectant solution. At each transfer, there is an increase in cellular volume to a maximum because of isotonic equilibration. This change in cellular volume is referred to as a volume

spike. A gradual decrease in volume then occurs as cryoprotectant leaves the embryo and isotonic equilibration is maintained. As long as the volume spike does not exceed a maximum tolerable volume, the embryos remain undamaged. The presence of microvilli on the cell surface allows for the occurrence of a nonlethal volume spike because they permit an increase in the volume of the cell.

Leibo and Mazur[32] were the first to suggest placing the thawed embryos into a dilution medium containing a nonpermeable solute, such as sucrose, to control the amount of swelling as cryoprotectant gradually leaves the cells of the embryos. This procedure is now almost universally used during the removal of cryoprotectant from embryos frozen at various stages of development using a variety of cryoprotectants. We obtained our first pregnancy from a frozen-thawed human blastocyst using sucrose in the diluent[33]; the procedure is used when human embryos are frozen with PPD or glycerol and can also be used when they are frozen using DMSO as the cryoprotectant. The initial shrinkage and swelling of embryos during transfer of thawed embryos into and out of sucrose solutions of descending concentrations is a preliminary indication that the embryo has intact cell membranes and has survived the freezing procedure. A diagrammatic representation of cell volume changes during various dilution regimens is shown in Figure 56–3.

Vitrification and Ultrarapid Cooling

Another approach to cryopreservation of oocytes and embryos involves ultrarapid cooling or vitrification; these terms are not necessarily synonymous. *Vitrification* refers to the transformation of liquid into a highly viscous, glasslike solid state by an extreme elevation of viscosity during cooling and does not involve the process of crystallization. In ultrarapid cooling, lower concentrations of cryoprotectants, intermediate between those used for vitrification and those used in slow-cooling regimens, are used. Ice-crystal formation may

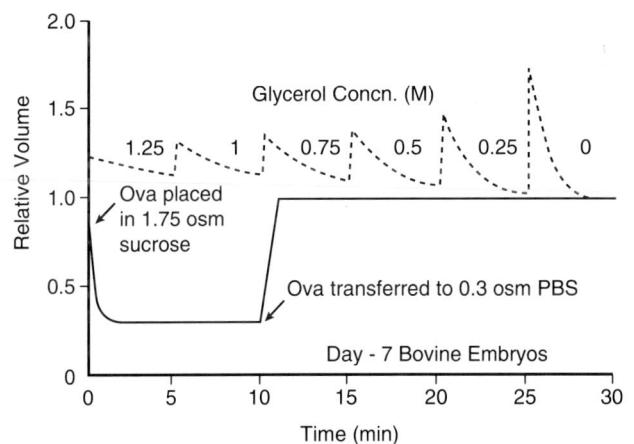

FIGURE 56–3. Computed volume changes in bovine embryos during removal of 1.5 M glycerol either in a six-step dilution procedure (*dashed line*) or in the presence of sucrose in the dilution medium (*solid line*). PBS, phosphate-buffered saline. (From Schneider U, Mazur P. Osmotic consequences of cryoprotectant permeability and its relation to the survival of frozen-thawed embryos. Theriogenology 1984;21:68–79; with permission of Butterworth-Heinemann.)

or may not occur during either cooling or warming, depending on the concentration of cryoprotectants and the rate of temperature change.[34] If no ice crystals form during a particular ultrarapid procedure, it is synonymous with vitrification. Vitrification of cryopreservative solutions occurs when the concentration of solutes in the cryopreservative solution is sufficiently high and the cooling rate is sufficiently rapid (approximately 2500°C/minute), as occurs when the sample is placed directly into liquid nitrogen from room temperature.[35] It is thought that embryos may vitrify intracellularly in the slow-cooling protocols described previously when slow cooling is terminated between −25 and −45°C and they are transferred to liquid nitrogen.[36] This is probably because the concentration of intracellular solutes has been sufficiently increased by dehydration during slow cooling, but ice-crystal formation has not yet occurred.

The best method for thawing oocytes or embryos cryopreserved by vitrification or ultrarapid cooling is to warm them rapidly at 500°C or more per minute to allow the water molecules in the vitrified glasslike state to be converted directly to the liquid state, thus avoiding the damaging formation of ice crystals, which would occur if the warming rate was slower. In the process termed *ultrarapid cooling*, oocytes or embryos are exposed for a brief (2 to 3 minutes) period to a cryoprotective medium containing 3.5 to 4.5 M DMSO and 0.25 to 0.3 M sucrose at room temperature before direct transfer to liquid nitrogen.[37] Vitrification probably occurs using these concentrations of DMSO and sucrose.[34] Survival, fertilization, and development of embryos arising from vitrified human[38] and mouse[39] oocytes have been reported, as have pregnancies from human embryos that have been frozen by the ultrarapid cooling technique.[38, 40–42] In my opinion, ultrarapid cooling will become routine and the method of choice for human embryo cryopreservation because of its simplicity and low cost. In addition, it has potential for achieving successful oocyte cryopreservation.

MATERIALS FOR CRYOPRESERVATION

Chemicals/Solutions

All chemicals used in cryopreservation should, as applies with any other ART procedure, be of the highest quality available. A range of tissue culture tested and, in some cases, mouse embryo tested compounds and other supplies are available from several sources, some of which are listed at the end of Table 56–2.

Solutions made for freezing or dilution procedures should be sterilized when possible and used fresh (within several hours of preparation). It is not possible to filter sterilize DMSO solutions because they dissolve most filter membranes. Stock DMSO can be purchased as a sterile solution, however, and I have found it suitable to use DMSO solutions as they are made up, with no attempt to resterilize them. Solutions can be stored for several days at 4°C and reused. This applies to solutions of PPD, glycerol, DMSO, and sucrose. This is useful when an experimental series of procedures is being tested with animal embryos. I do not keep such solutions stored longer than 1 week, and it is usually necessary to readjust the pH of the solutions to near 7.4 before use by brief exposure to a 5% CO_2 atmosphere and

TABLE 56–2. Some Sources of Programmable Cell Freezers and Other Cryobiologic Supplies	
Distributor	**Machine/Type**
FTS Systems P.O. Box 158 Stone Ridge, NY 12484–0158 (914) 687-0071	Bio-Cool IV/Mechanical refrigeration—methanol bath
TS Scientific, Inc. P.O. Box 198 Perkasie, PA 18944 (800) 258-2796	Planer/Nitrogen vapor
Cryomed 49659 Leona Dr. Mt. Clemens, MI 48045 (313) 949-4507 (714) 857-1764	Cryomed/Nitrogen vapor
IMV International Corp. 6870 Shingle Creek Parkway Suite 100 Minneapolis, MN 55430 (612) 560-4986	Minicool/Nitrogen vapor
Colorado Agriculture Services 11480 North Cherokee Street Unit 1 Denver, CO 80234 (303) 457-3606	Hoxan/Nitrogen vapor
Cryogenetic Technology, Inc. 1700 Elkhead Road Yoncalla, OR 97499 (503) 849-2825	CG 1400/Nitrogen vapor
Savant Instruments, Inc. 110-103 Bi-County Boulevard Farmingdale, NY 17735 (800) 634-8886	CPS 100/Mechanical refrigeration
Sigma Chemical Company P.O. Box 14508 St. Louis, MO 63178 (800) 325-3010	Supplies
Irvine Scientific 2511 Daimler Street Santa Ana, CA 92705 (800) 437-5706	Supplies
Minnesota Valley Engineering, Inc. Two Appletree Square, Suite 100 8011 34th Ave. South Bloomington, MN 55425 (800) 247-4446	Supplies/Storage tanks

visual inspection of the color of the phenol red pH indicator in the solution.

Whenever embryos or oocytes are handled outside of a CO_2 atmosphere, I always use a HEPES-buffered medium to stabilize the pH of the solution.[43] I have used HEPES-buffered medium successfully for all aspects of cryopreservation of human and animal embryos and oocytes.

Glassware and Plasticware

Any glassware that contacts gametes or embryos must be thoroughly cleaned and sterilized. The standard procedure I have used is initially to soak the items in 1 N HCl overnight when first used, then sonicate in tissue-culture grade water for 1 hour at 60°C, and finally rinse thoroughly in tissue-culture grade water before dry-heat sterilizing at 160°C for 2 hours. Subsequent cleaning involves the sonication and rinsing without the HC1 soak. Nowadays a minimum amount of glassware is used, and tissue-culture grade plastic items have replaced nearly all glassware. There are several manufacturers of suitable plasticware (e.g., Falcon, Corning, NUNC); I have not found any particular item or manufacturer to be unsuitable for cryopreservation procedures. French semen straws (IMV International Corp.; see Table 56–2) are used for cryo-storage of oocytes and embryos. Some workers use glass ampules but have reported a moderate incident of cracked zonae under these conditions.[44] There are several companies that supply specific items for cryopreservation; several of these companies are listed in Table 56–2.

Cryoprotectants

The three commonly used permeable cryoprotectants used for mammalian embryo freezing, DMSO, glycerol, and PPD should all be stored carefully between use. DMSO is known to oxidize slowly when stored at room temperature in containers with large air spaces. Sigma Chemical Co. markets DMSO in sealed amber-colored glass vials. After opening a vial, I place the remaining, unused DMSO in a small plastic tube, cover with aluminum foil, and store it at 4°C. DMSO stored in this fashion is not kept longer than 4 to 6 weeks before a new unopened vial is used. Glycerol and PPD, also from Sigma Chemical Company, are aliquoted into 10-mL lots in plastic tubes and stored at 4°C. It is helpful to bring these solutions to room temperature, to lessen their viscosity and make pipetting easier. It is important to wipe clean the outside of pipettes used to measure an exact volume of either solution and to make sure that all the cryoprotectant is removed from the inside of the pipette by pipetting the diluted cryoprotectant solution up and down inside the pipette several times after mixing.

Embryos of different species vary in their sensitivity to the toxic effects of different cryoprotectants; Renard[45] reported that eight-cell mouse embryos were more tolerant to exposure to PPD solution than an equivalent concentration of DMSO. Despite the interspecies variation in sensitivity of embryos to cryoprotectants, mouse and human embryos have similar sensitivities. Hence, mouse embryos can be readily used to check the cryoprotectant toxicity of stock solutions or purchased products.[6] It is good practice to purchase small amounts of cryoprotectant because this insures the rotation of fresh chemical and to store the unused portion of any solution appropriately.

Biologic Cell Freezers

A variety of devices to control the rates of cooling and warming have been developed as the technology of embryo cryopreservation has evolved. The first generation of freezers (e.g., as used by Whittingham and colleagues[11]) consisted of Dewar beakers of variable evacuation, filled with various amounts of alcohol, which was stirred, and the sample (e.g., embryo) in a glass vial or test tube was gradually lowered into the stirred alcohol as the dewar flask (which contained the stirred alcohol) was immersed in a larger container of

liquid nitrogen. A good description of such a device is given by Liebo and Mazur[32] (Fig. 56–4A). We have successfully used such devices to cryopreserve hamster oocytes[46] and human embryos[47] from which several babies were born after transfer of the thawed embryos (Fig. 56–4B). The second generation of cell freezers that were programmable were soon developed (e.g., mid-1970s), and a list of some manufacturers of these is given in Table 56–2. Each machine has its good and bad features, and there are several articles to attest to the successful use of nearly all the freezers mentioned in Table 56–2. It is somewhat ironic that, with the development of ultrarapid freezing, programmable freezers may become obsolete. It hardly needs to be said that the performance of programmable freezers need to be thoroughly evaluated using mouse embryos before the machine is used for human material. Most suppliers provide a potential purchaser with a machine so performance checks using mouse embryos can be carried out and the machine evaluated for suitability for freezing human embryos. The machine should also provide a hard-copy printout of the measured cooling and warming rates that are used during operation. This should be a requirement in any accreditation program licensing reproductive biology laboratories. The machines should also be operated on an emergency backup power source so that the cooling or warming program is not interrupted because of power failure.

Storage Tanks

Several of the suppliers listed in Table 56–2 also provide an adequate inventory of vials, straws, canes, canisters, marking pens, tape, and insulated refrigeration storage tanks required for the proper labeling and storage of samples. Figures 56–5A and B show a typical storage tank. Again, it is mandatory that the samples be properly labeled and logged in at least two separate files and that the storage tanks be routinely checked for adequate refrigeration (usually by liquid nitrogen). The tanks should also be fitted with alarms to indicate if dangerously high temperature levels occur.

PRACTICAL APPLICATIONS OF EMBRYO FREEZING IN AN ASSISTED REPRODUCTIVE TECHNOLOGY PROGRAM

Selection of Embryos for Freezing

Although initially a number of ART programs tended to freeze embryos of poorer quality while selecting the morphologically superior embryos for fresh transfer, it is now general practice to select the embryos randomly to be transferred fresh or frozen. In fact, some cryopreservation experts[29] advocate the principal commonly used in commercial livestock embryo cryopreservation, which is to freeze the "best" embryos because of their increased chance of survival compared with poorer quality embryos. One of the first ART programs to cryopreserve human embryos successfully reported that embryos with an increased amount of fragmentation had a lower survival rate following cryopreservation.[48]

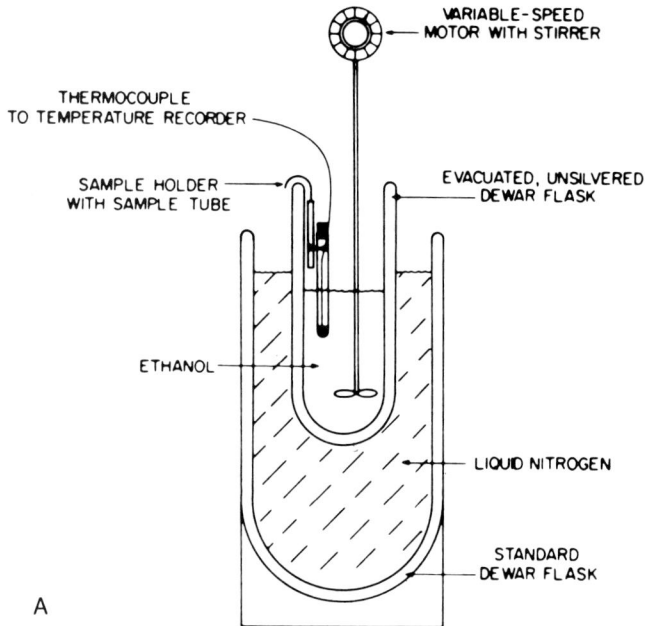

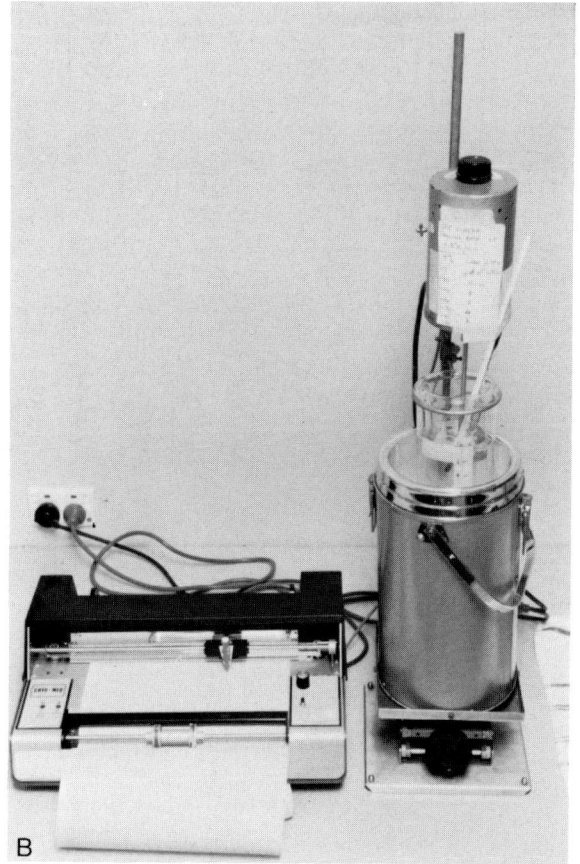

FIGURE 56–4. *A*, Diagrammatic representation of Dewar flask arrangement used to cool samples at controlled rates. (*A* from Liebo SP, Mazur P. Methods for the preservation of mammalian embryos by freezing. In: Daniel JC, editor. Methods in Mammalian Reproduction. New York: Academic Press, 1978:179–201.) *B*, Dewar flask cooling apparatus used in author's laboratory to cryopreserve human embryos from which ongoing pregnancies were obtained on thawing and transfer (see Quinn and Kerin[47]).

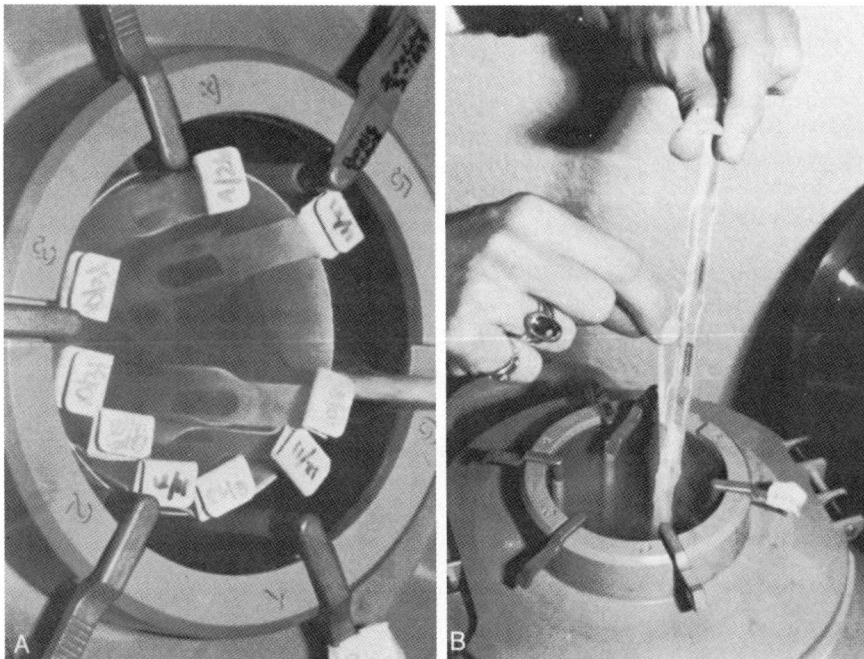

FIGURE 56–5. *A*, View through the neck of a liquid nitrogen tank showing the storage unit: canister, cane, goblet, and straw. *B*, Removing a straw from the liquid nitrogen storage tank. Goggles, gloves, or forceps are recommended to avoid nitrogen burns. (*A* and *B* from Kuzan FB, Quinn P. Cryopreservation of mammalian embryos. In: Wolf DP, editor. In Vitro Fertilization and Embryo Transfer: A Manual of Basic Techniques. New York: Plenum Press, 1988:301–347.)

Several studies have looked at the influence of stage of embryo development or stage of cell cycle on the outcome of cryopreservation of human embryos. Lassalle and associates[22] reported that more two-, four-, and eight-cell embryos survived freezing and thawing than three-, five-, six-, and seven-cell embryos containing fragments and uneven sized blastomeres. Even at the pronuclear stage, it has been suggested that those zygotes frozen at least 26 hours after oocyte collection and with closely adhered pronuclei with the nucleoli-like structures aligned equatorially opposite one another in the two pronuclei have a greater potential for survival and creating a pregnancy than those frozen at an earlier time.[49]

Embryos at various stages of development and either before or after cryopreservation are shown in Figures 56–6A through F.

Length of Culture Before Embryo Freezing

It is well known that culture in vitro decreases the number that continue to develop and rate of development of mammalian embryos.[50] It may well be that successful development in vitro is a form of quality control, selecting those embryos with a greater potential for continued development. In terms of success after cryopreservation with respect to both embryo survival on thawing and subsequent pregnancy rates, there appears to be little difference between human embryos at different stages of development. A general comparison of reported success rates does tend to indicate, however, that the pregnancy rate obtained with frozen-thawed pronuclear embryos that are transferred is higher than that achieved with four- or eight-cell embryos (see Quinn[33]). A contributing factor could be that more pronuclear embryos are available for freezing compared with the later stages of development in which deterioration of embryos has occurred during culture. I recommend that an ART program freeze the majority of its embryos at the pronuclear stage. If there are a large number of zygotes, for example, 10, then 4 should be frozen and the remaining 6 selected for transfer or culture. It is recognized, however, that there is a dilemma if insufficient embryos are left in culture to obtain a sufficient number of morphologically good-quality embryos for transfer at the four- to eight-cell stage.

Cryoprotectant Solutions

I construct all my cryoprotectant solutions and media for dilution of cryoprotectants after thawing on HEPES-buffered human tubal fluid (HTF) medium[51] containing 10% to 20% human serum. Equivalent success rates have been achieved using bovine serum albumin (BSA) as the protein source in the media (Table 56–3). We[47] and others have also used phosphate-buffered and bicarbonate-buffered media for cryopreservation with no apparent differences in success rates. The HEPES-buffered medium gives a more stable pH during cryopreservation procedures. I use the following recipes for cryopreservation solutions.

PROPANEDIOL-SUCROSE

These solutions are used for pronuclear through to six-cell stages and are based on the formulas described by Lassalle and colleagues.[22] Make up 20 mL of HEPES-HTF medium containing 20% human serum (HS). This is made in 2 × 10-mL lots. To one lot of 10 mL of medium, add 1.25 mL of 1,2-propanediol (= 1.5 M PPD solution). Take 5 mL of this solution and add it to 0.342 g sucrose (= 1.5 M PPD + 0.2 M sucrose). Filter sterilize all three solutions. Dilute 1.5 M PPD solution with HEPES-HTF + 20% HS to make 0.5 M and 1.0 M solutions of PPD. Embryos are placed at room temperature in the 0.5 M PPD solution for 5 minutes, then the 1.0 M PPD solution for 5 minutes, and finally in the 1.5 M PPD solution for 10 minutes. They are then transferred to the 1.5 M PPD + 0.2 M sucrose solution and pipetted into straws containing this same solution (Fig. 56–7A). They remain at room temperature in the 1.5 M PPD + 0.2 M sucrose solution for a total of 5 minutes before cooling is initiated (see next section).

GLYCEROL-SUCROSE

These solutions are used for fully expanded blastocycts and are based on the formulation described by Menezo and associates.[52] Make up 2 × 10-mL tubes of HEPES-HTF + 10% HS. Construct 5% glycerol in HEPES-HTF + 10% HS by adding 0.5 mL glycerol to 9.5 mL HEPES-HTF + 10% HS. Construct 9% glycerol in HEPES-HTF + 10% HS plus 0.2 M sucrose by adding 0.9 mL glycerol to 9.1 mL HEPES-HTF + 10% HS and 0.685 g sucrose. Filter sterilize all of these solutions. Place fully expanded blastocysts in HEPES-HTF + 10% HS at room temperature for 5 minutes. Transfer to 5% glycerol solution for 10 minutes. Transfer to 9% glycerol + 0.2 M sucrose solution and load into straws containing the same solution; hold at room temperature (20 to 25°C) for a total of 10 minutes before cooling is initiated.

DIMETHYL SULFOXIDE–SUCROSE

These solutions are used for ultrarapid freezing of pronuclear and early cleavage-stage human embryos and follow the method proposed by Drury and colleagues.[42] HEPES-HTF + 10% HS solution is needed. Acidify stock DMSO (Sigma Chemical Co., D-2650) by adding 10 μl 1 N HCl to 2 mL DMSO. Make 1.5 M DMSO solution by adding 0.55 mL DMSO to 4.45 mL HEPES-HTF + 10% HS on ice. Make 3.5 M DMSO + 0.25 M sucrose by mixing 1.35 mL DMSO, 3.65 mL HEPES-HTF + 10% HS, and 0.428 g sucrose; dissolve sucrose and then place on ice. Check the pH of the solutions containing DMSO and adjust to pH 7.3 to 7.5 if necessary. These solutions can be stored at 0 to 4°C for up to 14 days. Bring solutions to room temperature. Transfer embryos to HEPES-HTF + 10% HS for 5 minutes. Place embryos in 1.5 M DMSO solution at room temperature for 5 minutes. Transfer to straw containing 3.5 M DMSO + 0.25 M sucrose and hold at room temperature for 2½ minutes. Plunge straw into liquid nitrogen.

I do not describe a recipe for 1.5 M DMSO because this protocol, as originally described by Trounson and Mohr,[3] is infrequently used today. Details can be obtained from the original reference. I would recommend that the embryos frozen and thawed using this method be diluted using a sucrose-containing diluent.

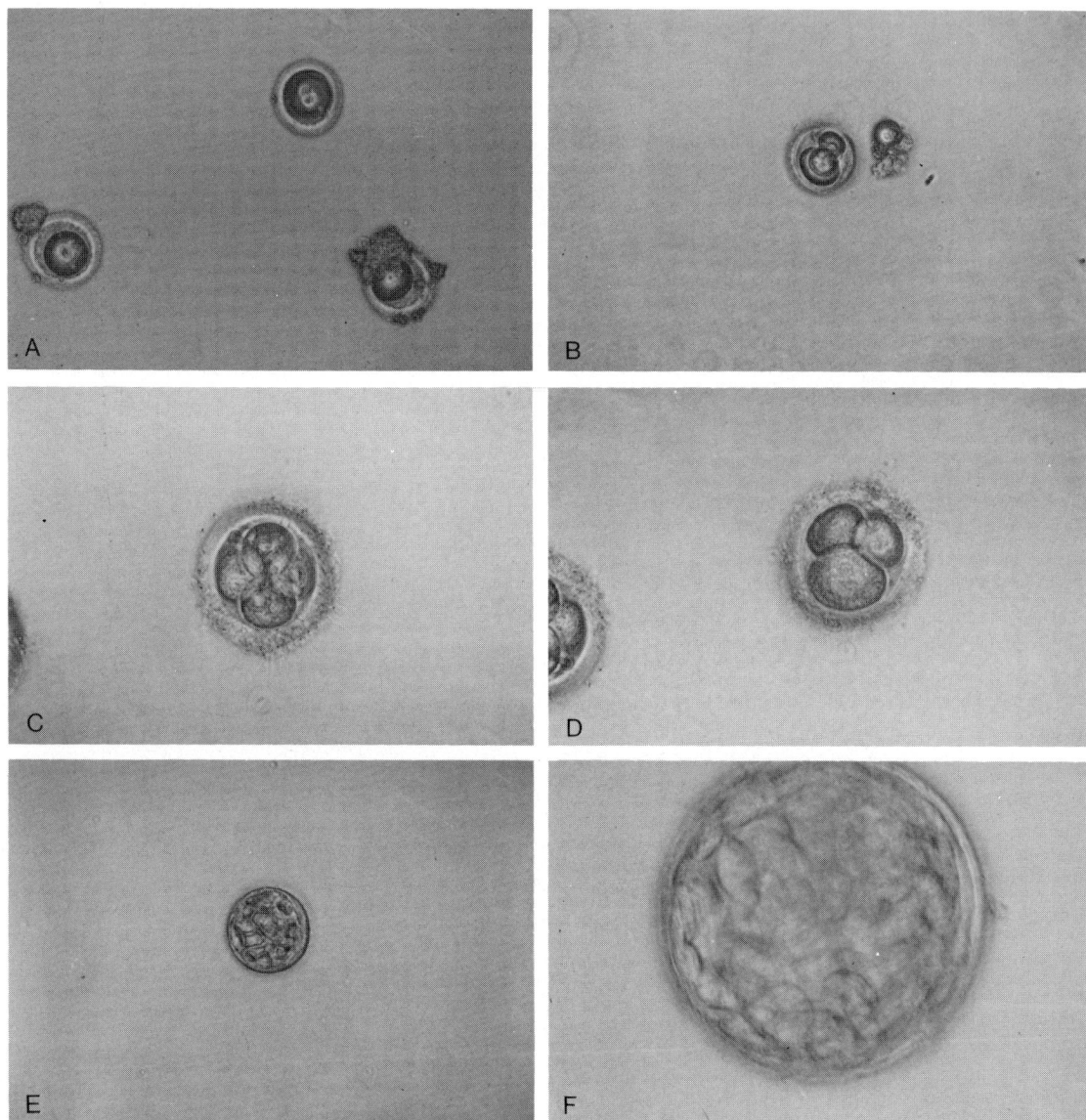

FIGURE 56–6. *A,* Thawed pronuclear embryos in 0.2 M sucrose solution. Note shrunken appearance as indicated by a large perivitelline space. All three embryos appear viable (×70). *B,* Thawed four-cell embryos in 0.2 M sucrose solution. In the zona-intact embryo, three of the four blastomeres have survived. In the zona-free embryo, one of the four blastomeres has survived (×70). *C,* Thawed four-cell embryo after dilution of cryoprotectant and washing. Note excellent morphology (×140). *D,* Thawed embryo after 3 hours of culture. Three blastomeres are apparent, but the largest bottom blastomere originated from the fusion of two blastomeres present on thawing. In other words, on thawing, this was a four-cell embryo that reverted to a three-cell embryo during culture because of fusion of two of the blastomeres. This happened in five embryos from 128 patients and a total of 229 thawed embryos over a 5-year period (×140). *E,* Fully expanded blastocyst equilibrating in 6% glycerol prior to freezing (×70). *F,* Same embryo as in *E.* Note well-defined polygonal-shaped blastomeres in trophectoderm and slight shrinkage of cell mass away from the zona pellucida due to hyperosmolality of glycerol solution (×320).

TABLE 56–3. Comparison of Using Bovine Serum Albumin versus Patient's Serum as the Protein Supplement in Cryoprotectant Medium*

Protein	No. of Patients	Embryo Survival	Pregnancies per Transfer	Ongoing Pregnancies
Bovine serum albumin	18	41/48 (85%)	4/16 (25%)	4
Human serum	36	74/100 (74%)	4/31 (13%)	3

*No significant differences between treatments.

Cooling Programs

For both the PPD-sucrose and glycerol-sucrose protocols for early-cleavage and fully expanded blastocyst stages, the straws containing the embryos are taken from a starting temperature of 20 to −6°C at 2°C/minute. They are then held at −6°C. At 2 minutes into this holding period, seeding is induced by touching the outside of the straw with a metal rod or forceps, which has been precooled in liquid nitrogen (Fig. 56–7B; see also under warming protocols). The site of

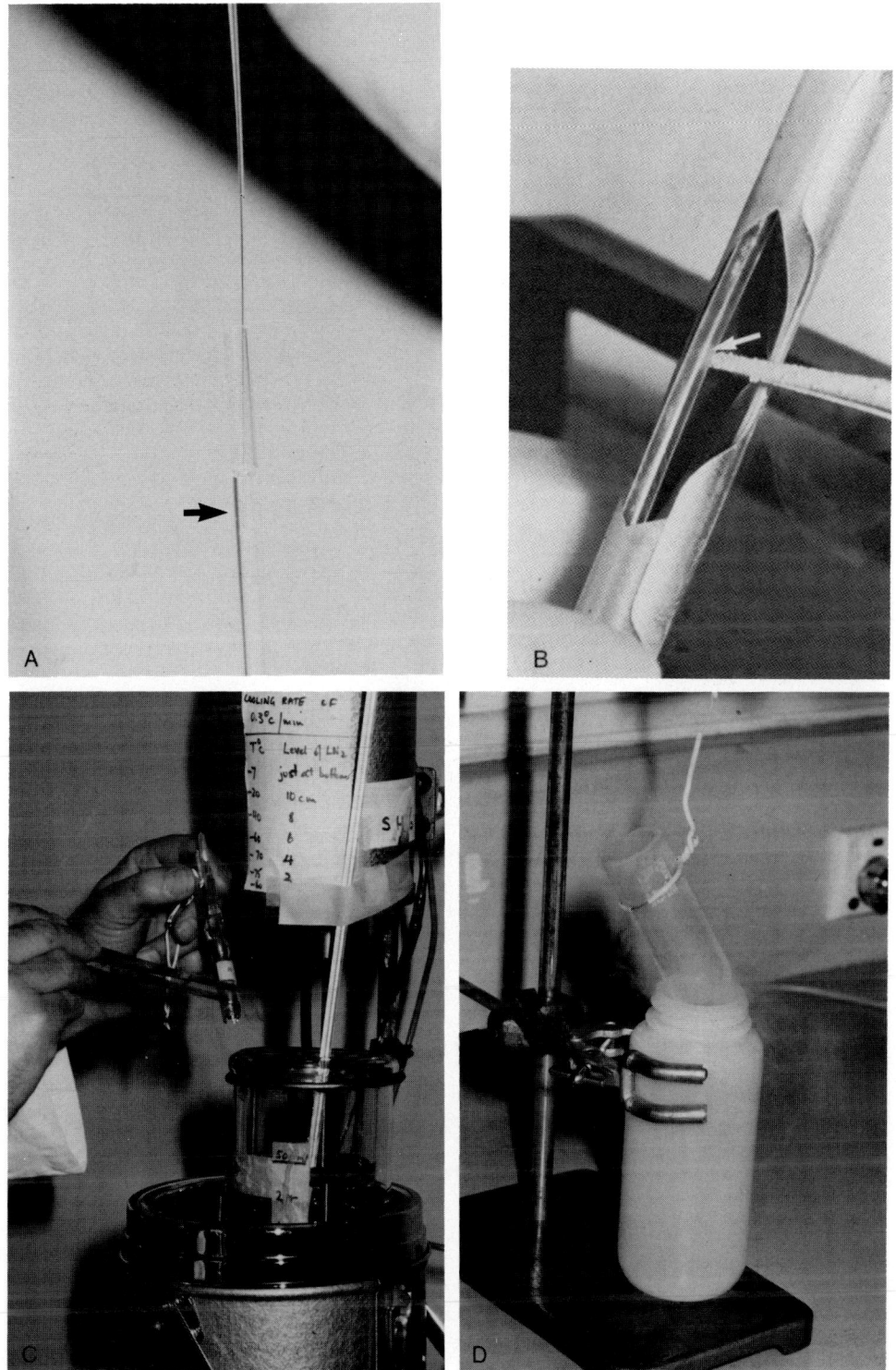

FIGURE 56–7. *A,* Loading embryos into a 0.5-mL Fr straw. The pipette tip (*arrow*) is well below the fluid level within the straw. *B,* Seeding the straw with precooled forceps. *Arrow* indicates the tip of precooled metal forceps touching the straw. (*A* and *B* from Kuzan FB, Quinn P. Cryopreservation of mammalian embryos. In: Wolf DP, editor. In Vitro Fertilization and Embryo Transfer: A Manual of Basic Techniques. New York: Plenum Press, 1988:301–347.) *C,* Seeding a glass vial with precooled forceps. The vial is grasped with the forceps about 0.5 cm above the level of cryoprotectant solution in the bottom of the vial. *D,* Thick-walled glass container precooled in liquid nitrogen and then suspended at room temperature to give a warming rate of approximately 8°C/min.

seeding is as far away from the position of the embryos as possible. The straw is then quickly replaced in the cooling chamber, which is then held at −6°C for a further 10 minutes. Once or twice during this 10-minute holding phase, the straw can be quickly withdrawn from the chamber to view the growth of ice crystals down the length of the straw. At the end of the holding period, when ice crystals have formed throughout the fluid in the straw, the straw is cooled at

0.3°C/minute to −30°C. At this point, the straw is then transferred directly to liquid nitrogen for final storage. It is possible to program a controlled rate freezer so the temperature automatically drops rapidly (50°C/minute) from −30 to −180°C, at which point the straws are held for up to 2 hours before final transfer to liquid nitrogen. Of course, it is possible to slow cool embryos to any subzero temperature at any cooling rate before storage in liquid nitrogen, but the figures given here are those I have used successfully for the past 6 years for pronuclear, cleaving, and blastocyst stage human embryos.

Warming Protocols

In all of the cooling procedures described previously, moderate dehydration is present in the cells when they are transferred to liquid nitrogen for storage. Therefore there is a requirement that the samples be warmed rapidly (at least 275°C/minute) so that intracellular ice is swiftly dispersed (see Fig. 56–2). The easiest way to achieve this is to transfer the storage container (vial or straw) from liquid nitrogen to a water bath at 0°C or higher. My initial experience with thawing straws involved removing them from liquid nitrogen and immersing them directly into a water bath at 37°C. On occasion, however, the straws would burst or blow out the plugs sealing the ends, and the contents, including the embryos, would be lost. This has been overcome by initially holding the straw in air for 30 to 40 seconds and then immersing it in a water bath at 30 to 35°C until the ice has all melted. This method was adopted from a similar technique described by Lassalle and associates[22] and allows for any liquid nitrogen that may have entered the straw through an imperfectly sealed plug to be blown off before the straw is placed in a water bath. No loss of straws or their contents has occurred using this technique.

Containers that require slow warming (e.g., 8°C/minute if slow cooled to below −60°C) can be placed in a precooled, thick glass-walled container, the warming rate of which is known (see Fig. 56–7D) or warmed at a specific rate from −110 to +4°C in a programmable freezing/warming machine (e.g., the Planer Kryo 10-1.7; see Veeck[53]).

Dilution Solutions

These are used for the correspondingly named cryoprotectant solutions.

PROPANEDIOL-SUCROSE

HEPES-HTF + 10% HS and 0.2 M sucrose in HEPES-HTF + 10% HS are required. Make the 0.2 M sucrose by adding 5 mL of HEPES-HTF + 10% HS to 0.342 g sucrose. Filter sterilize both solutions. Prepare dishes containing 3 mL each of 0.2 M sucrose, 0.1 M sucrose (1.5 mL 0.2 M sucrose + 1.5 mL HEPES-HTF + 10% HS), and two dishes of HEPES-HTF + 10% HS wash solution. Empty the thawed contents of the straw into the dish containing 0.2 M sucrose. If the embryo(s) are not immediately found, rinse the straw several times by aspirating 0.2 M sucrose solution in and out of it. If the embryo or an empty zona pellucida still cannot be found, inspect the straw carefully under a dissecting microscope. Embryos stuck to the inside of the wall of the straw can sometimes be removed by careful pipetting. I have sometimes been able to successfully recover missing embryos by following this procedure. Usually, however, the embryos recovered in this fashion are too damaged. Fortunately the number of embryos lost in this way is small (< 0.5%). The embryos remain in the 0.2 M sucrose solution for 5 minutes

and are then transferred successively through the 0.1 M sucrose solution and the two washes of HEPES-HTF + 10% HS, spending 5 minutes in each solution. The surviving embryos are then held for up to 30 minutes in HEPES-HTF + 10% HS before transfer or placed in HCO₃-HTF + 10% HS for culture before transfer.

GLYCEROL-SUCROSE

For solution A, 3 × 10 mL of HEPES-HTF + 10% HS is required. Then 0.3 M sucrose in HEPES-HTF + 10% HS (solution B) is made by adding 1.027 g sucrose to 10 mL HEPES-HTF + 10% HS; 6% glycerol in HEPES-HTF + 10% HS plus 0.3 M sucrose (solution C) is made by adding 0.6 mL glycerol to 9.4 mL HEPES-HTF + 10% HS and 1.027 g sucrose. Filter sterilize all solutions. Solutions as listed in Table 56–4 are then made in 35-mm petri dishes. The contents of a thawed straw are dispelled into solution #1 (6% glycerol + 0.3 M sucrose), following the same routine for searching for missing embryos as outlined previously. The blastocysts are held in solution number 1 at room temperature for 5 minutes. They are then passed through solutions 2 to 8, holding for 5 minutes in each solution. The blastocysts are then cultured in HCO₃-HTF + 10% HS under an atmosphere of 5% CO₂: 5% O₂: 90% N₂ for 3 to 4 hours before embryo transfer. During this time, collapsed blastocysts frequently re-expand to produce a well-defined blastocoele cavity.

DIMETHYL SULFOXIDE–SUCROSE

For embryos cryopreserved by the ultrarapid cooling method in DMSO-sucrose, a series of sucrose solutions ranging from 0.2 to 0 M in 0.05-M decrements is made from stock solutions of 0.2 M sucrose (0.684 g sucrose in 10 mL HEPES-HTF + 10% HS) and HEPES-HTF + 10% HS. Three milliliters of each solution is placed in 35-mm petri dishes along with 2 × 3 mL washes of HEPES-HTF + 10% HS. The thawed straw contents are dispelled into the 0.2 M sucrose solution, where the embryos are held for 5 minutes. The embryos are then passed through the diminishing concentrations of sucrose, being held for 5 minutes in each one and 5 minutes in each of the wash solutions. The embryos are finally transferred with or without culture in HCO₃-HTF.

Post-Thaw Viability

A preliminary indication of whether embryos have survived cryopreservation is their morphologic appearance and

TABLE 56–4. Glycerol-Sucrose Solutions

No.	Solution	Solution C (mL)	Solution B (mL)	Solution A (mL)
1	6% G/0.3 M S	2.0	0	0
2	4.5% G/0.3 M S	1.5	0.5	0
3	3% G/0.3 M S	1.0	1.0	0
4	1.5% G/0.3 M S	0.5	1.5	0
5	0.3 M S	0	2.0	0
6	0.15 M S	0	1.0	1.0
7	Wash 1	0	0	3.0
8	Wash 2	0	0	3.0

G, glycerol; S, sucrose.

TABLE 56–5. Coculture and Embryo Transfer of Thawed Human Zygotes

Treatment Before Transfer	No. Transfers	Pregnancies per Transfer	Implantations per Embryo Transferred
Overnight culture	21	1 (5%)*	2%*
Short-term culture	27	7 (26%)	16%
Overnight coculture	22	8 (36%)*	17%*

*$P < 0.05$. Other comparisons do not differ significantly.
From Wiker S, Tucker M, Wiemer K, et al. Co-culture of thawed human embryos. Proceedings XIV World Congress on Fertility and Sterility, Caracas, Venezuela, 1992.

whether they remain shrunken when placed in sucrose solutions and then re-expand on transfer to the sucrose-free wash solutions. Cell death can be easily recognized in pronuclear and cleaving embryos (see Fig. 56–6B) but can be harder to discern in blastocysts, especially if they remain contracted.

Occasionally, cracking and fracture of the zona pellucida occurs. This is thought to be due in part to mechanical stresses involving ice crystals. It has generally been observed that zona pellucida damage is more prevalent when there is a problem with seeding the sample. Since using straws to cryopreserve embryos, however, no such damage has been observed.[6] One of the most reliable guides to whether embryos have survived cryopreservation is their ability to continue development on subsequent culture.[6] With blastocysts, this is often evidenced by re-expansion of the blastocoele cavity within several hours of culture.[54, 52] Pronuclear embryos have usually been cultured overnight after thawing, and we have observed cleavage in at least 85% of these embryos. It should be noted, however, that a higher pregnancy rate has been reported when cryopreserved human zygotes have been transferred within a few hours of thawing or cocultured overnight in the presence of bovine oviductal epithelial cells[55] (Table 56–5). I now recommend transfer of cryopreserved zygotes within several hours of thawing because of the higher implantation rate using this format (Table 56–5).

In cleaved embryos, not all the blastomeres have to survive cryopreservation to produce an embryo capable of developing into a live infant, indicating that the blastomeres of the human embryo remain totipotent at least until the eight-cell stage.[6] It is generally recommended that cleaved embryos with at least 50% of their blastomeres intact be transferred after thawing, although it can be noted that a pregnancy has been reported when a four-cell embryo in which only one blastomere survived cryopreservation was transferred.[56] Therefore it is probably worthwhile and unlikely to be harmful if any cleaved embryo in which at least one blastomere has survived on thawing is transferred.

Clinical Indications for Cryopreservation

The clinical indications for oocyte and embryo cryopreservation have been stated on a number of occasions by individual authors and by national biomedical groups, for example, the Ethics Committee of The American Fertility Society.[57] Some of the main indications are given in Table 56–6.

Ethics of Cryopreservation

Again, ethical considerations of cryopreservation have been published widely.[57, 58] It is gratifying that community

and religious groups have had considerable input in these discussions, so that clinicians and scientists have a clearer understanding of society's currently acceptable limits to embryo research and technology. It has become patently obvious that a precise informed consent document is necessary that clearly sets out the disposition of any cryopreserved gametes or embryos from a couple.

A comment on terminology is appropriate at this point. The word *pre-embryo* (also *prezygote*), used to describe the conceptus from the time of fertilization to the appearance of the primitive streak, has become popular with some authors and national reproductive biology committees. Antagonism to the use of this term has arisen,[59, 60] and it has been suggested that the word may have been coined more for reasons of public policy concerning the moral status of the conceptus than for scientific terms; the editor of *Nature* described its use as a "cosmetic trick."[60] I recommend we use such terms as *preimplantation embryo* and *eight-cell embryo*.

Donor Banks

OOCYTES

Of course, all of the following considerations are based on the development of a clinically successful oocyte cryopreservation protocol, which currently does not exist. When oocyte banks are established, the selection of oocyte donors should follow the same requirements for a thorough medical history and screening and genetic history of the donor and her relatives as does the selection of semen donors. In addition, results obtained with freshly donated oocytes indicate that the age and previous parity of the donor influence the preg-

TABLE 56–6. Clinical Indications for Cryopreservation of Human Embryos and Oocytes

Embryos

Overcomes waste of supernumerary embryos and concomitantly discourages transfer of high numbers of embryos and subsequent increased risk of multiple pregnancy

An alternative when there are adverse maternal conditions at scheduled time of transfer

Allows for greater flexibility in synchronizing donor programs

Transfer of thawed embryo in a natural cycle may have a higher pregnancy rate than transfer of fresh embryo in a stimulated cycle

Useful for holding biopsied embryos during genetic screening of material removed by micromanipulation

Oocytes

Can store oocytes if loss of future reproductive function is threatened

Allows for establishment of oocyte banks. Patients can use oocytes themselves or donate to others

nancy rates obtained.[61] It would be difficult to apply to oocyte donors the same biologic criteria based on gamete survival after cryopreservation that is used for the selection of semen donors. Nevertheless, it is highly likely that there would be variation between individuals in oocyte cryosurvival just as there is for embryo and semen cryosurvival. Perhaps survival outcome on subsequent thawing of the oocytes collected in the first cycle of retrieval from an oocyte donor could be used to select donors more likely to have oocytes capable of surviving cryopreservation and producing a viable pregnancy.

EMBRYOS

The use of cryopreserved embryos for donation to other unrelated couples or transfer to a gestational surrogate recipient is an option in some ART programs. Our own experience with such procedures is shown in Table 56–7. The success rate in this small group of patients has been more than acceptable. Note the two pregnancies obtained when embryos were shipped from countries overseas, indicating the international aspects of embryo donation. In another pregnant patient receiving donated embryos, the two embryos transferred were from two different donors.

Standards for screening and selection of the donors (and gestational surrogate recipients) should be the same as those used for gamete donors in terms of genetic and medical histories and screening.

Synchronization of Thaw and Transfer

Two general approaches have been used concerning the synchronization of the time of thawing embryos in relation to the time of transfer of the thawed embryos. In the first, close synchrony between the chronologic age of the thawed embryo and the reproductive tract in relation to the predicted time of ovulation is advocated,[3, 62] whereas with the second approach, the thawed embryos are transferred to a chronologically younger uterus (reviewed by Quinn[33]). No prospective study has been made to resolve this topic. The main point is not to transfer thawed embryos too late in relation to the stage of the recipient's menstrual cycle. This is especially true with blastocysts, which take longer to develop in vitro compared with zygote or early cleavage stages, which are more synchronized to what their actual morphologic stage would be in vivo.

It has been generally observed that pregnancy rates are similar after transfer of thawed embryos whether the embryos are transferred in a natural menstrual cycle or one that has been regulated with gonadotropin-releasing hormone (GnRH) analog suppression and estrogen/progesterone replacement; this applies when patients have regular menstrual cycles with no luteal phase defects or other abnormalities. A protocol for monitoring natural menstrual cycles for the replacement of thawed embryos is as follows; this protocol was adopted from one provided by Lynette FitzGerald (personal communication). The estradiol (E_2) levels referred to were assayed using the Wallac Delfia fluorometric system (Gaithersburg, MD).

1. On day (D) 2 or 3 of the cycle (D1 = first day of menses), a baseline ultrasound scan of ovaries and endometrial thickness should be obtained, together with a blood sample for E_2 and progesterone (P) measurement.

2. From D8 onward, daily ultrasound measurement of follicle diameter and a blood sample for E_2 and P assay are taken.

3. When E_2 levels reach about 120 pg/mL and a follicle is developing, urine samples can be checked by the patient for the presence of LH using a home-use LH detection kit. Every urine sample should be checked. If an LH surge occurs, cancel the transfer, and the patient should probably be changed to a GnRH suppression regimen in a subsequent cycle.

4. If no LH surge occurs, continue ultrasound and endocrine monitoring until E_2 is greater than 180 pg/mL and a follicle with mean diameter greater than or equal to 15 mm is visible and the endometrial thickness is greater than or equal to 8 mm.

5. Give 5000 U human chorionic gonadotropin (hCG) intramuscularly and time the transfer of a pronuclear zygote about 60 hours later and two- to four-cell embryos about 84 hours later; fully expanded blastocysts should be thawed and transferred about 132 hours after hCG is given.

TABLE 56–7. Results of Transferring Cryopreserved Embryos to Genetically Different Recipients*

| Stage of Embryos | No. Patients | Number of Embryos | | Pregnancies per Transfer |
		Thawed	Survived	
Gestational surrogates				
D1 (Day 1) (pronuclear)	22	67	48 (72%)	6/22 (27%)†
D2 (cleaved)	2	5	5	0/2
D6 (blastocyst)	2	2	2	1/2
D1 + D2	1	3 + 2	2 + 2	0/1
Donation				
D1	1	2	2	1/1‡
D2	1	2	2	1/1
Total	29	83	63 (76%)	9/29 (31%)§

*The Hospital of the Good Samaritan, Los Angeles, 1989–1991.

†Two of the pregnant patients had embryos shipped from overseas. One of these patients had three cycles of transfer of thawed embryos from the same genetic mother; she was not pregnant after the first cycle, had a spontaneous abortion after the second transfer, and had an ongoing pregnancy after the third attempt.

‡The two embryos were from two different donors.

§Eight of the pregnancies were ongoing.

These are the complete details of the protocol. To simplify the procedure, some parts can be modified: For example, daily blood samples after D8 can be omitted, as can urine sampling for LH surge monitoring, as long as ultrasound scans and blood endocrine levels are checked routinely. It should be recognized, however, that these types of modifications could lead to a flawed assessment of when to thaw and transfer the embryos and hence the possibility of a canceled cycle or one with a reduced chance of achieving a pregnancy.

If the patient has an endocrine problem (e.g., luteal phase defect or oligomenorrhea), it is better to use a regulated cycle. There are several acceptable protocols involving GnRH analog down-regulation and E₂/P replacement. The following is one version.

1. Begin taking leuprolide acetate (Lupron, TAP Pharmaceuticals, North Chicago, IL), 1 mg/day, on D17 of cycle and await menses.
2. Check for adequate ovarian suppression 2 to 3 weeks after Lupron is begun. E_2 should be less than 50 pg/mL and P less than 1.0 ng/mL in serum.
3. If E_2/P is suppressed, begin taking oral E_2 (Estrace, Mead Johnson Laboratories, Princeton, NJ), 1-mg tablets, in morning and evening. Decrease daily Lupron injections to 0.5 mg. This can be called D1 of the replacement cycle. Timing of D1 can be scheduled so that transfer of two- to four-cell embryos on D17 is convenient. The 1-mg, twice-daily dose of estrace continues until D5.
4. On D6 through D9, increase Estrace to 2 mg at 8 A.M. and 8 P.M.
5. On D10 through D14, increase Estrace to 2 mg at 8 A.M., 4 P.M., and 10 P.M. daily. Discontinue Lupron after D13.
6. On D15, take 2 mg Estrace at 8 A.M. and 1 mg at 4 P.M. and again at 10 P.M. Also take 25 mg P intramuscularly at 8 A.M. Repeat these hormone doses on D16.
7. D17 is embryo transfer day for two- to four-cell embryos. Pronuclear embryos can be thawed on D16 and cultured overnight for transfer on D17 or transferred immediately on D16 (see under post-thaw viability; Table 56–5). Blastocysts should be thawed and transferred on D19.
8. From D17 onward, the patient takes 1 mg Estrace at 8 A.M., 4 P.M., and 10 P.M. daily and receives 25 mg P at 8 A.M. and again at 8 P.M.
9. Patient should have blood drawn on D3, D11, D16, D21, and D30 for E_2 and P assay. Some laboratories adjust the daily dosages of the exogenously given steroids depending on these results.
10. hCG should be measured on D30. If positive, Estrace (1 mg at 8 A.M., 4 P.M., and 8 P.M.) and P (50 mg once per day) are continued daily from D31 through D100.

In these suppression protocols, the patient should go through a test or "mock" cycle to ensure that the endocrine and endometrial responses are adequate. An endometrial biopsy can also be performed on about D23 to assess whether endometrial synchrony of the glands and stroma is adequate. If the test cycle responses are adequate, the patient should discontinue Estrace and P and begin with Lupron (0.5 mg/day) again. Estrace replacement (D1) is begun after menses has occurred.

Results

OOCYTES

The first report of a successful pregnancy in humans originating from cryopreserved oocytes was that of Chen[63] in 1986, and two other groups reported a pregnancy each in the following year.[64, 65] Since that time, however, there have been no further published successes. In all three of the above-mentioned reports, DMSO was used as the cryoprotectant, and the oocytes were slowly cooled to −40 or −70 to −80°C before transfer to liquid nitrogen; this is the basic method used by Whittingham,[66] who was the first to report successful cryopreservation of mammalian oocytes (mouse) and the birth of live young derived from the oocytes. Even in the mouse, the results of Whittingham and subsequent reports by others[67, 68] show that the oocyte is much more intractable to cryopreservation than the embryo, and a similar situation occurs with human oocytes. Because of the demand for an effective method to cryopreserve human oocytes, intensive studies have therefore been undertaken with both mouse and human oocytes to elucidate what the problems are and how they can be overcome.

It is now evident that slow cooling and exposure of oocytes to cryoprotectants even before freezing induce changes that affect the fertilizing potential of the oocyte and disruption of the meiotic spindle, leading to subsequent chromosome anomalies.[67, 69–72] Several studies have shown that oocytes incubated at 4°C or exposed to DMSO or PPD undergo a premature zona reaction, which may originate from a precocious release of the cortical granules,[69, 73] events that normally follow fusion of the fertilizing spermatozoan with the oolemma and prevent polyspermy. A report from Whittingham's laboratory,[74] however, suggests that in the mouse, modifications to the zona pellucida in frozen-thawed oocytes that contribute to fertilization failure are not due to a premature release of cortical granule material. The exact mechanism of this phenomenon remains to be discovered. The reduced fertilization rate of mouse oocytes exposed to 4°C or cryopreserved can be circumvented if the zona pellucida is removed before insemination[69, 74] or if the barrier of the zona is breached by zona drilling.[75] It has also been found that the presence of serum during exposure of mouse oocytes to DMSO and during cryopreservation can alleviate the deleterious effects of these procedures on the zona pellucida by reducing the conversion of the zona pellucida glycoprotein ZP2, one of the sperm-binding proteins, to its modified form ZP2f, which is unable to bind sperm.[71] The presence or absence of serum in the solutions used for the cryopreservation and handling of oocytes before and after freeze-thawing may explain some of the variations that have been reported for the success rates of cryopreservation of mouse oocytes.[67, 68, 76] Cooling oocytes has also been shown to disrupt their microtubule system, the human oocyte being more susceptible to this than mouse oocytes.[70] Subsequent chromosome anomalies have been reported after fertilization of frozen-thawed mouse oocytes.[68, 72]

Because slow cooling of oocytes appears to aggravate problems with fertilization and nuclear normality, a more rapid cooling by vitrification may be one way to ameliorate the situation. Successful survival and development in vitro of

TABLE 56–8. Survival and Fertilization of Human Oocytes Cryopreserved by Two Methods Involving the Use of Propanediol and Sucrose and Different Cooling Rates

	Method	
No. Oocytes	*Renard et al[21]**	*Lassalle et al[22]†*
Frozen	16	36
Surviving	8 (50%)	1 (3%)
Fertilized	3‡	0

*Cryoprotectant medium 2.2 M propanediol/0.5 M sucrose; transferred from room temperature to −30°C and held for 30 minutes before storage in liquid nitrogen.

†Cryoprotectant medium 1.5 M propanediol/0.2 M sucrose; seeded at −7°C, cooled at 0.3°C/min to −30°C before transfer to liquid nitrogen.

‡One of the fertilized oocytes had three pronuclei.

mouse oocytes that have been vitrified or cryopreserved by ultrarapid cooling have been reported.[39, 77] There have been conflicting reports, however, of the normality of concepti derived from vitrified mouse oocytes.[72, 77] This may be due to the extended exposure time (5 to 10 minutes at room temperature) of the oocytes to the vitrification solutions before plunging in liquid nitrogen used by Kola and associates[72] rather than the shorter exposure time (5 to 10 seconds) used by Nakagata.[77]

Evidence that rapid cooling of human oocytes is more effective than slow cooling is illustrated in Table 56–8. Others have reported that when slow cooling was used to freeze human oocytes, DMSO gave better results than glycerol.[78] Fertilization and development to the blastocyst stage in vitro has been obtained when cumulus-intact human oocytes were frozen using PPD-sucrose as cryoprotectant and slow cooling to −35°C.[79] Survival, fertilization, and cleavage of embryos arising from vitrified human oocytes have been reported.[80] It has also been found that a high proportion (80%) of freshly collected human oocytes were capable of surviving vitrification when frozen by an ultrarapid procedure.[34] The ability of these oocytes to be fertilized was not assessed, however.

The cryopreservation of human oocytes is still experimental, although there has been limited success by some workers. Undoubtedly, further progress in this area will occur, and oocyte storage banks will be established. The method most likely to be successful with oocytes will probably be one involving vitrification by ultrarapid cooling.

EMBRYOS

National statistics for the United States and Australia have been reported[81, 82] and show that for clinics doing 100 or more transfers of thawed embryos per year, the clinical preg-

nancy rate is 14% with an ongoing pregnancy rate of approximately 10%. These numbers are similar to, but significantly lower than, the data reported for transfer of fresh embryos in IVF.[81, 82] Some programs and surveys have reported higher pregnancy rates with cryopreserved embryos that are not significantly different from those obtained with fresh embryos (reviewed by Wolf[17]). There was some concern that frozen-thawed embryos obtained from cycles involving GnRH treatment in the stimulation regimen may not be as fertile as embryos from non-GnRH cycles (see Quinn[33]), but this has not been confirmed by other studies.[33, 83] In any event, it is obvious that cryopreservation gives a marked increase in the overall cumulative pregnancy rate (i.e., pregnancies from the transfer of frozen-thawed embryos added to those obtained from the transfer of fresh embryos) in patients undergoing oocyte retrieval in an ART program.[17, 33]

The results of embryo cryopreservation in ART programs I have been associated with from 1987 to 1991 are given in Table 56–9. The success rates are similar to the national results given in the two reports mentioned previously. It can be beneficial to compare the results obtained in two different programs to see if there are differences and, if there are, what factors may be contributing to these differences. The results for pronuclear embryos presented in Table 56–9 have been compared with those reported by the Norfolk group[53, 86] and are presented in Table 56–10, together with some of the obvious differences in the cryopreservation protocols used in the two programs. It should be noted that the results reported by Oehninger and coworkers[83] are for a selected group of patients, but those presented by Veeck[53] are stated to be overall results. The overall results reported by Veeck[53] are given in Table 56–10. Our data in Table 56–9 are for all patients having cryopreserved zygotes thawed. Whether the differences in success rates are due to some of the differences in the two protocols used for cryopreservation or synchronizing the time of transfer or due to differences in the number of zygotes thawed and transferred per patient could be determined by relevant prospective studies.

I have made some modifications to the PPD-sucrose cryopreservation protocol in an effort to improve efficiency and simplify the procedure. These include the use of BSA versus human serum as the protein source in cryopreservation solutions, seeding at −5°C rather than −7°C, and dilution of the cryoprotectant from embryos by their passage through medium containing sucrose only. The results for the BSA versus serum study have already been mentioned (see under cryoprotectant solutions; see Table 56–3); there was no difference in the results between either protein source. Nevertheless, I still prefer to use 20% human serum as the protein supplement. This is because of the possible beneficial cryoprotectant properties of serum and the known protective

TABLE 56–9. Results of Cryopreservation of Human Embryos*

Day of Freezing (Stage)	No. Patients	Embryo Survival	Pregnancies per Transfer	Ongoing Pregnancies/ all Pregnancies	Ongoing Pregnancies per Transfer
1 (pronuclear)	391	764/1035 (74%)	46/356 (13%)	32/46 (70%)	32/356 (9%)
2 (cleaved)	128	229/288 (80%)	11/116 (9%)	6/11 (55%)	6/116 (5%)
5–6 (blastocyst)	67	81/113 (72%)	8/52 (15%)	6/8 (75%)	6/52 (12%)
Total	586	1074/1436 (75%)	65/524 (12%)	44/65 (68%)	44/524 (8%)

*Cedars–Sinai Medical Center and The Hospital of the Good Samaritan, Los Angeles, CA, 1987–1991.

TABLE 56–10. Comparison of Cryopreservation Results and Protocols Used for Human Zygotes by Two Different Programs

	Quinn (see Table 56–9)	Veeck[53, 83]
Freezing solution	1.5 M PPD/0.2 M sucrose	1.5 M PPD
Cooling program	0.3°C/min to −30°C	0.5°C/min to −80°C
Dilution protocol	0.2 M sucrose	PPD dilution only
Day of thaw for pronuclear zygotes	D2 (2 days after LH surge or 1 day after progesterone replacement)	D1
Average number of zygotes per thaw	2.6	4.0
Survival (%)	74	70
Average number of embryos transferred	2.1	2.8
Clinical pregnancy rate	13%	29%
Ongoing rate	70%	77%

PPD, propanediol; LH, luteinizing hormone.

effects of serum on oocytes during cryopreservation. The results obtained when we retrospectively assessed the effect of inducing seeding at −5 or −7°C are given in Table 56–11; they show that there was no significant difference between seeding at either temperature. Seeding at −5°C rather than −7°C is based on the assumption that it is better to induce ice-crystal formation closer to the freezing point of the cryoprotectant solution to minimize temperature changes owing to the release of the latent heat of crystallization. Subsequently, I have reverted to a seeding temperature of −6°C to prevent inadvertent rewarming of the samples to a temperature above the freezing point when the straws are temporarily withdrawn from the cooling chamber for manual seeding (in the Planer Kryo 10-1.7 machine). This is also the lowest seeding temperature reported by Whittingham[23] to give satisfactory survival of eight-cell mouse embryos. The results of the dilution of thawed samples by a simplified protocol are outlined in Table 56–12. Instead of decreasing the PPD concentration from 1.0 to 0.5 M in the presence of 0.2 M sucrose before transfer of the thawed embryos to wash medium, as was proposed originally,[22] the contents of a thawed straw were placed directly into 0.2 M sucrose solution with no PPD for 5 minutes, then 0.1 M sucrose for 5 minutes, and then washed twice to retrieve the embryos. This slightly shortens the time the embryos spend in dilution

media and reduces the number of different types of media required. Obviously, because this modified procedure produces the same embryo survival and pregnancy rate in our laboratory as does the original protocol, we now routinely use it.

A final comment is required with respect to the use of vitrification/ultrarapid freezing for the cryopreservation of human embryos. Because this method has proved successful with mouse embryos,[37, 84, 85] it was expected that it would be tried and prove useful with human embryos. Several groups have obtained pregnancies using this procedure.[38, 40–42] Because of its simplicity and low cost, this procedure should make cryopreservation of human embryos available to all ART programs no matter what their budget or size. Despite this, there will probably be a slow acceptance of this method because of the current success rates using the established method. Nevertheless, I believe that when larger studies are done with ultrarapid freezing and if the success rates continue to be comparable to those obtained with the PPD-sucrose method, the ultrarapid freezing method will become increasingly popular.

Accreditation, Quality Control, and Quality Assurance

In my opinion, an ART program offering cryopreservation (and any program inseminating more oocytes than will be necessary to replace a reasonable number of embryos, e.g., two to six, depending on the quality of the embryos and the age of the woman, should offer cryopreservation) needs to (1) document that it has successfully cryopreserved mouse embryos (≥70% embryo survival and development in vitro) on at least three separate occasions, (2) obtain at least a 20% to 30% implantation rate of viable fetuses when the thawed embryos have been transferred to recipient foster mothers, (3) maintain annually a thawed human embryo survival rate of at least 70%, and (4) obtain annually a clinical pregnancy rate with transferred thawed human embryos of at least 10% per transfer. In addition, as stated previously, hard copies of the printouts of the measured cooling and warming rates should be kept when appropriate. If the human embryo survival and pregnancy rates are not maintained to the levels mentioned in (3) and (4), the accrediting organization should require the ART laboratory to reassess their cryopreservation protocols using mouse embryos. It would also be prudent for

TABLE 56–11. Retrospective Comparison of Using a Seeding Temperature of −7°C or −5°C in Cryopreservation of Human Embryos*

Day of Freezing†	No. Patients	Embryo Survival	Pregnancies per Transfer	Ongoing Pregnancies
Seeding at −7°C				
1	189	344/450 (76%)	23/176 (13%)	17 (74%)
2	83	137/174 (79%)	6/76 (8%)	2 (33%)
6	40	51/63 (81%)	5/34 (15%)	3 (60%)
Seeding at −5°C				
1	10	21/29 (72%)	1/9	1
2	4	9/11 (82%)	1/4	1
6	2	2/5 (40%)	0/1	—

*No comparisons were significantly different.
†Day 1 = pronuclear stage; Day 2 = 2- to 4-cell stage; Day 6 = fully expanded blastocyst.

TABLE 56–12. Use of a Modified Dilution Protocol for Recovery of Thawed Human Embryos*				
Day of Freezing†	No. Patients	Embryo Survival	Pregnancies per Transfer	Ongoing Pregnancies
1 (zygotes)	113	247/337 (78%)	16/102 (16%)†	10
2 (2- to 4-cell)	22	40/48 (83%)	2/20 (10%)†	2

*The thawed straw contents were emptied into 0.2 M sucrose and incubated for 5 minutes, then transferred to 0.1 M sucrose for 5 minutes, then washed twice in sucrose-free medium (5 minutes per wash).
†Not significantly different from results using protocol of Lassalle et al[22] (data not shown).

the ART laboratory to undertake an annual quality control assessment of their cryopreservation protocols using mouse embryos, using adequate survival and development of the thawed embryos in vitro as the endpoint of assessment.

CONCLUSIONS

Cryopreservation is now a routine procedure in any competent ART program. As a corollary to this statement, one could add that any ART program that does not offer cryopreservation is not practicing at the current standard of care and should offer cryopreservation services. The results summarized in this chapter show that the efficiency and success of embryo cryopreservation can be as good as that obtained with fresh embryos. This, therefore, gives a greater degree of flexibility and more options for the handling and disposition of the embryo so its chances of producing a viable ongoing pregnancy are maximized.

Much of our current knowledge of cryopreservation of human oocytes and embryos has come from groundwork studies conducted with animal embryos. It is necessary that the initiation of cryopreservation in an ART program and the training of personnel for this procedure should be undertaken using an animal model (usually the mouse) to learn the various steps in the protocol. It will probably also be necessary, with the proposed licensing of reproductive biology laboratories, that various quality control and quality assurance procedures using an animal embryo model will be required for human embryo freezing.

The various procedures outlined in this chapter are those that have so far been found to give the best results, but, similar to so many other aspects of ART, old methods are constantly being refined and new ones are emerging. The one thing I think will take us into a new phase of cryopreservation and open new realms for clinical application and research is the use of ultrarapid cooling for the cryopreservation of both oocytes and embryos. I await with anticipation the next few years for the outcome of this prediction.

GLOSSARY

Cryoprotectant: A compound that protects cells from damage at low temperatures.
Seeding: Induction of ice crystal formation at or slightly below the freezing point of an aqueous solution.
Slow cooling: Cooling rate used in most popular freezing protocols of <1°C/min after seeding to a subzero temperature of around −30°C.
Soluton effect: Damage due to increased osmotic pressure in remaining solution as ice crystals form during cooling.
Supercooling: Lowering of the temperature of a solution to

well below (10 to 15°C) its freezing point before ice crystal formation.
Ultrarapid cooling: Rapid decrease in the temperature of a solution (about 2500°C/min), with or without vitrification, depending on the concentration of cryoprotectants.
Vitrification: Transformation of a liquid into a highly viscous, glasslike solid without the formation of ice crystals.
Volume spike: Increase in the volume of a cell when it is transferred to a solution of lower tonicity and water enters the cell by osmosis.

Acknowledgments

I thank my family for their support of my endeavors in this topic, and I am grateful for my friends and colleagues who have taught, encouraged, and participated with me in cryobiology over the years.

REFERENCES

1. Wood C, McMaster R, Rennie G, et al. Factors influencing pregnancy rates following in vitro fertilization and embryo transfer. Fertil Steril 1980;43:245–250.
2. Kerin JFP, Warnes GM, Quinn P, et al. Incidence of multiple pregnancy after in vitro fertilisation and embryo transfer. Lancet 1983;2:537.
3. Trounson A, Mohr L. Human pregnancy following cryopreservation, thawing and transfer of an eight-cell embryo. Nature 1983;305:707–709.
4. Ashwood-Smith MJ. The cryopreservation of human embryos. Human Reprod 1986;1:319–332.
5. Quinn P. Cryopreservation. In: Marrs RP, editor. Assisted Reproductive Technologies. Boston: Blackwell Scientific Publications, 1993:89–107.
6. Kuzan FB, Quinn P. Cryopreservation of mammalian embryos. In: Wolf DP, editor. In Vitro Fertilization and Embryo Transfer: A Manual of Basic Techniques. New York; Plenum Press, 1988:301–347.
7. Chang MC. Normal development of fertilized rabbit ova stored at low temperature for several days. Nature 1947;159:602–603.
8. Maurer RR. Storage of mammalian oocytes and embryos: a review. Can J Anim Sci 1976;56:131–145.
9. Polge C. The freezing of mammalian embryos: perspectives and possibilities. In: Elliot K, Whelan J, editors. The Freezing of Mammalian Embryos. Ciba Foundation Symposium No. 52. Amsterdam: Elsevier, 1977:3–13.
10. Quinn P, Warnes GM, Walker SK, Seamark RF. Culture of preimplantation sheep and goat embryos. In: Lindsay DR, Pearce DT, editors. Reproduction in Sheep. Canberra: Australian Academy of Science, 1984:289–290.
11. Whittingham DG, Leibo SP, Mazur P. Survival of mouse embryos frozen to −196° and −269°C. Science 1972;178:411–414.
12. Wilmut I. The effect of cooling rate, warming rate, cryoprotective agent and stage of development on survival of mouse embryos during freezing and thawing. Life Sci 1972;11:1071–1079.
13. Whittingham DG. Principles of embryo preservation. In: Ashwood-Smith MJ, Farrant J, editors. Low Temperature Preservation in Medicine and Biology. Tunbridge Wells: Pitman Medical, 1980:65–83.
14. Cohen J, Simons RF, Edwards RG, et al. Pregnancies following the frozen storage of expanding human blastocysts. J In Vitro Fertil Embryo Transf 1985;2:59–64.
15. Testart J, Lassalle B, Belaisch-Allart J, et al. High pregnancy rate after early human embryo freezing. Fertil Steril 1986;46:268–272.

16. Wilton LJ, Shaw JM, Trounson AO. Successful single-cell biopsy and cryopreservation of preimplantation mouse embryos. Fertil Steril 1989;51:513–517.

17. Wolf DP. Gamete and embryo cryopreservation. In: Sciarra JJ, editor. Gynecology and Obstetrics. Philadelphia: JB Lippincott, Vol 5. 1992: 1–7.

18. Rall WF, Reid DS, Polge C. Analysis of slow-warming injury of mouse embryos by cryomicroscopical and physiochemical methods. Cryobiology 1984;21:106–121.

19. Leibo SP. Fundamental cryobiology of mouse ova and embryos. In: Elliott K, Whelan J, editors. The Freezing of Mammalian Embryos. Ciba Foundation Symposium No. 52. Amsterdam: Elsevier, 1977:69–92.

20. Mazur P. Kinetics of water loss from cells at subzero temperatures and the likelihood of intracellular freezing. J Gen Physiol 1963;47:347–369.

21. Renard J-P, Bui-Xuan-Nguyen N, Garnier V. Two-step freezing of two-cell rabbit embryos after partial dehydration at room temperature. J Reprod Fertil 1984;71:573–580.

22. Lassalle B, Testart J, Renard J-P. Human embryo features that influence the success of cryopreservation with the use of 1,2 propanediol. Fertil Steril 1985;44:645–651.

23. Whittingham DG. Some factors affecting embryo storage in laboratory animals. In: Elliott K, Whelan J, editors. The Freezing of Mammalian Embryos. Ciba Foundation Symposium No. 52. Amsterdam: Elsevier, 1977:97–108.

24. Whittingham DG. Survival of mouse embryos after freezing and thawing. Nature 1971;233:125–126.

25. Willadsen SM. Factors affecting the survival of sheep embryos during deep-freezing and thawing. In: Elliott K, Whelan J, editors. The Freezing of Mammalian Embryos. Ciba Foundation Symposium No. 52. Amsterdam: Elsevier, 1977:175–189.

26. Whittingham DG, Wood M, Farrant J, et al. Survival of frozen mouse embryos after rapid thawing from −196°C. J Reprod Fertil 1979;56:11–21.

27. Mohr LR, Trounson A, Freeman L. Deep-freezing and transfer of human embryos. J In Vitro Fertil Embryo Transf 1985;2:1–10.

27a. Leibo SP. Procedures to cryopreserve zygotes and embryos. Hands-On Cryobiology Course. Indianapolis: American Fertility Society, 1993:69–78.

28. Whittingham DG, Lyon MF, Glenister PH. Long-term storage of mouse embryos at −196°C: the effect of background radiation. Gen Res 1977;29:171–181.

29. Testart J, Lassalle B, Forman R, et al. Factors influencing the success rate of human embryo freezing in an in vitro fertilization and embryo transfer program. Fertil Steril 1987;48:107–112.

30. Cohen J, Inge KL, Wiker SR, et al. Duration of storage of cryopreserved human embryos. J In Vitro Fertil Embryo Transf 1988;5:301–303.

31. Schneider U, Mazur P. Osmotic consequences of cryoprotectant permeability and its relation to the survival of frozen-thawed embryos. Theriogenology 1984;21:68–79.

32. Leibo SP, Mazur P. Methods for the preservation of mammalian embryos by freezing. In: Daniel JC, editor. Methods in Mammalian Reproduction. New York: Academic Press, 1978:179–201.

33. Quinn P. Success of oocyte and embryo freezing and its effect on outcome with in vitro fertilization. Semin Reprod Endocrinol 1990;8:272–280.

34. Pensis M, Loumaye E, Psalti I. Screening of conditions for rapid freezing of human oocytes: preliminary study toward their cryopreservation. Fertil Steril 1989;52:787–794.

35. Fahey GM, MacFarlane DR, Angell CA, Meryman HT. Vitrification as an approach to cryopreservation. Cryobiology 1984;21:407–426.

36. Rall WF, Polge C. Effect of warming rate on mouse embryos frozen and thawed in glycerol. J Reprod Fertil 1984;70:285–292.

37. Trounson A, Peura A, Kirby C. Ultrarapid freezing: a new low cost and effective method of embryo cryopreservation. Fertil Steril 1987;48:845–850.

38. Trounson AO. Cryopreservation. Br Med Bull 1990;46:695–708.

39. Surrey ES, Quinn PJ. Successful ultrarapid freezing of unfertilized oocytes. J In Vitro Fertil Embryo Transf 1990;7:262–266.

40. Gordts S, Roziers P, Campo R, Noto V. Survival and pregnancy outcome after ultrarapid freezing of human embryos. Fertil Steril 1990;53:469–472.

41. Barg PE, Barad DH, Feichtinger W. Ultrarapid freezing (URF) of mouse and human preembryos: a modified approach. J In Vitro Fertil Embryo Transf 1990;7:355–357.

42. Drury KC, Silverman IH, Cook CL. Ultrarapid two step freezing of human pronuclear stage zygotes. Proceedings of the 48th Annual Meeting of the American Fertility Society, New Orleans, Abstract P-244, 1992.

43. Quinn P, Warnes GM, Kerin JF, Kirby C. Culture factors in relation to the success of human in vitro fertilization and embryo transfer. Fertil Steril 1984;41:202–209.

44. Cohen J, DeVane GW, Elsner CW, et al. Cryopreservation of zygotes and early cleaved human embryos. Fertil Steril 1988;49:283–289.

45. Renard J-P. The cryopreservation of mammalian embryos. In: Testart J, Frydman R, editors. Human In Vitro Fertilization. INSERM Symposium No. 24. Amsterdam: Elsevier, 1985:201–208.

46. Quinn P, Barros C, Whittingham DG. Preservation of hamster oocytes to assay the fertilizing capacity of human spermatozoa. J Reprod Fertil 1982;66:161–168.

47. Quinn P, Kerin JFP. Experience with the cryopreservation of human embryos using the mouse as a model to establish successful techniques. J In Vitro Fertil Embryo Transf 1986;3:40–45.

48. Freeman L, Trounson A, Kirby C. Cryopreservation of human embryos: progress on the clinical use of the technique in human in vitro fertilization. J In Vitro Fertil Embryo Transf 1986;3:53–61.

49. Wright G, Wiker S, Elsner C, et al. Observations on the morphology of pronuclei and nucleoli in human zygotes and implications for cryopreservation. Human Reprod 1990;5:109–115.

50. Harlow GM, Quinn P. Development of preimplantation mouse embryos in vivo and in vitro. Aust J Biol Sci 1982;35:187–193.

51. Quinn P, Kerin JF, Warnes GM. Improved pregnancy rate in human in vitro fertilization with the use of a medium based on the composition of human tubal fluid. Fertil Steril 1985;44:493–498.

52. Menezo Y, Nicollet B, Herbaut N, Andre D. Freezing cocultured human blastocysts. Fertil Steril 1992;58:977–980.

53. Veeck LL. Cryopreservation—how and when? 4th Annual In Vitro Fertilization and Embryo Transfer—A Comprehensive Update. UCLA Extension, Santa Barbara, 1991:158–173.

54. Fehilly CB, Cohen J, Simons RF, et al. Cryopreservation of cleaving embryos and expanded blastocysts in the human: a comparative study. Fertil Steril 1985;44:638–644.

55. Wiker S, Tucker M, Wiemer K, et al. Co-culture of thawed human embryos. Proceedings XIV World Congress on Fertility and Sterility, Caracas, Venezuela, 1992.

56. Testart J, Lassalle B, Belaisch-Allart J, et al. Human embryo freezing. Ann NY Acad Sci 1988;541:532–540.

57. The American Fertility Society. Ethical considerations of the new reproductive technologies. Fertil Steril 1990;53(Suppl 2):1s–109s.

58. Board of Trustees, American Medical Association. Frozen pre-embryos. JAMA 1990;263:2484–2487.

59. Biggers JD. Arbitrary partitions of prenatal life. Human Reprod 1990;5:1–6.

60. Kelly J. Pre-embryos. Lancet 1990;1:116.

61. Sauer MV, Paulson RJ, Macaso TM, et al. Establishment of a nonanonymous donor oocyte program: preliminary experience at the University of Southern California. Fertil Steril 1989;52:433–436.

62. Cohen J, DeVane GW, Elsner CW, et al. Cryopreserved zygotes and embryos and endocrinologic factors in the replacement cycle. Fertil Steril 1988;50:61–67.

63. Chen C. Pregnancy after human oocyte cryopreservation. Lancet 1986;1:884–886.

64. Al-Hasani S, Deidrich K, van der Ven H, et al. Cryopreservation of human oocytes. Human Reprod 1987;2:695–700.

65. van Uem JFHM, Sebzehnrubl ER, Schuh B, et al. Birth after cryopreservation of unfertilized oocytes. Lancet 1987;1:752–753.

66. Whittingham DG. Fertilization in vitro and development to term of unfertilized mouse oocytes previously stored at −196°C. J Reprod Fertil 1977;49:89–94.

67. Trounson A, Kirby C. Problems in the cryopreservation of unfertilized eggs by slow cooling in dimethyl sulfoxide. Fertil Steril 1989;52:778–786.

68. Carroll J, Warnes GM, Matthews CD. Increase in digyny explains polyploidy after in-vitro fertilization of frozen-thawed mouse oocytes. J Reprod Fertil 1989;85:489–494.

69. Johnson MH, Pickering SJ, George MA. The influence of cooling on the properties of the zona pellucida of the mouse oocyte. Human Reprod 1988;3:383–387.

70. Pickering SJ, Braude PR, Johnson MH, et al. Transient cooling to room temperature can cause irreversible disruption of the meiotic spindle in the human oocyte. Fertil Steril 1990;54:102–108.

71. Vincent C, Turner K, Pickering SJ, Johnson MH. Zona pellucida modifications in the mouse in the absence of oocyte activation. Mol Reprod Develop 1991;28:394–404.

72. Kola I, Kirby C, Shaw J, et al. Vitrification of mouse oocytes results in aneuploid zygotes and malformed fetuses. Teratology 1988;38:467–474.

73. Schalkoff ME, Oskowitz SP, Powers RD. Ultrastructural observations of human and mouse oocytes treated with cryopreservatives. Biol Reprod 1989;40:379–393.

74. Wood MJ, Whittingham DG, Lee S-H. Fertilization failure of frozen mouse oocytes is not due to premature cortical granule release. Biol Reprod 1992;46:1187–1195.

75. Carroll J, Depypere H, Matthews CD. Freeze-thaw-induced changes of the zona pellucida explains decreased rates of fertilization in frozen-thawed mouse oocytes. J Reprod Fertil 1990;90:547–553.

76. Schroeder AC, Champlin AK, Mobraaten LE, Eppig JJ. Developmental capacity of mouse oocytes cryopreserved before and after maturation in vitro. J Reprod Fertil 1990;89:43–50.

77. Nakagata N. High survival rate of unfertilized mouse oocytes after vitrification. J Reprod Fertil 1989;87:479–483.

78. Hunter JE, Bernard A, Fuller B, et al. Fertilization and development of the human oocyte following exposure to cryoprotectants, low temperature and cryopreservation: a comparison of two techniques. Human Reprod 1991;6:1460–1465.

79. Imoedemhe DG, Sigue AB. Survival of human oocytes cryopreserved with or without the cumulus in 1,2-propanediol. J Assisted Reprod Genet 1992;9:323–327.

80. Trounson A. Preservation of human eggs and embryos. Fertil Steril 1986;46:1–12.

81. Medical Research International, Society for Assisted Reproductive Technology, The American Fertility Society. In vitro fertilization–embryo transfer (IVF-ET) in the United States; 1990 results from the IVF-ET registry. Fertil Steril 1992;57:15–24.

82. National Perinatal Statistics Unit, Fertility Society of Australia. IVF and GIFT pregnancies in Australia and New Zealand. Sydney: National Perinatal Statistics Unit, 1990.

83. Oehninger S, Toner JP, Veeck LL, et al. Performance of cryopreserved pre-embryos obtained in in vitro fertilization cycles with or without a gonadotropin-releasing hormone agonist. Fertil Steril 1992;57:620–625.

84. Wilson L, Quinn P. Development of mouse embryos cryopreserved by an ultrarapid method of freezing. Human Reprod 1989;4:86–90.

85. Kasai M, Komi JH, Takakamo A, et al. A simple method for mouse embryo cryopreservation in a low toxicity vitrification solution, without appreciable loss of viability. J Reprod Fertil 1990;89:91–97.

CHAPTER 57

Micromanipulation of Human Gametes, Zygotes, and Embryos

JACQUES COHEN

The application of micromanipulators in the assisted reproduction laboratory has expanded the boundaries of clinical preimplantation embryology beyond standard infertility treatments such as in vitro fertilization (IVF). Micromanipulation is a new tool by which to study gender identification, gene abnormalities, dysfunctions of fertilization, and embryonic implantation.[1, 2] Although micromanipulation is often described as a separate discipline, it should be considered as a set of techniques with which whole cells (such as the oocyte, polar body, or blastomere) or large cell components (i.e., the zona pellucida or pronucleus) can be handled at the light microscopic level. Cellular alterations have been mainly restricted to relatively simple mechanical procedures for (1) enhancing fertilization, such as zona drilling[3] or subzonal insertion (SZI);[4] (2) restoring diploidy, such as pronuclear extraction;[5] (3) facilitating embryonic implantation, such as assisted hatching;[6] and (4) performing preimplantation genetic diagnosis, such as polar body or blastomere biopsy.[1, 7] The last-mentioned can be considered a field on its own, bridging the gap between molecular genetics and embryology, and is therefore described in a separate chapter in this book. Subcellular modifications, such as chromosome ablation,[8] removal of refractile bodies, and microinjection of DNA constructs or metabolic substances, may be clinically feasible but need to be further refined in animal models. Micromanipulation of preimplantation embryos may be novel to those involved in clinical assisted reproduction, but it is an established discipline in experimental and veterinarian embryology.[2] Introduction of this technology to the human IVF laboratory has been difficult owing to (1) the apparent limitations of some well-known experimental micromanipulation procedures (i.e., zygote reconstruction and nuclear transplantation) and (2) the ethical and legal restrictions put forth by the scientific community, society, and national government bodies.

There are a number of important reasons for changes in the philosophical approach of IVF specialists toward micromanipulation. First, precise control of the fertilization process as occurs with micromanipulation is needed to treat patients for whom conventional IVF fails and for others who have been excluded from alternative assisted reproduction technologies based on suboptimal semen profiles.[9] Second, the advent of safe preconception and preimplantation genetic diagnosis methods that pose little or no risk to embryonic viability may now allow for replacement of genetically fit embryos in couples at risk for genetic disease.[1, 7] Third, IVF technology is still considered controversial owing to its poor statistical performance. The ability of standard IVF embryos to implant varies among programs, but in general true success rates (i.e., the chance of an embryo to become an infant) are considered to be below 10%. A review of the literature shows that there have been only two promising proposals for enhancing embryonic viability. The first of these involves the simultaneous culture (coculture) of embryos on helper cells.[10, 11] The second method has been broadly termed assisted hatching and is based on the hypothesis that an alteration of the zona pellucida by drilling a hole through it, by thinning it, or by altering its structure promotes hatching of embryos that are otherwise unable to escape intact from the zona.[2, 6, 12, 13] The purpose of this chapter is to present developments in the field of clinical gamete and embryo micromanipulation. For methods and historical perspectives, the reader is referred to a book in which these and other topics are described in detail.[2] This chapter is divided into four sections: (1) gamete micromanipulation for assisted fertilization, (2) zygote micromanipulation for repair of polyspermy, (3) embryo micromanipulation for assisted hatching, and (4) future applications of micromanipulation.

GAMETE MICROMANIPULATION

Gamete micromanipulation involves a set of techniques that can be applied to specific patients in whom the fertilization process in vitro is inhibited. It enables the reproductive scientist to circumvent specific stages in the fertilization

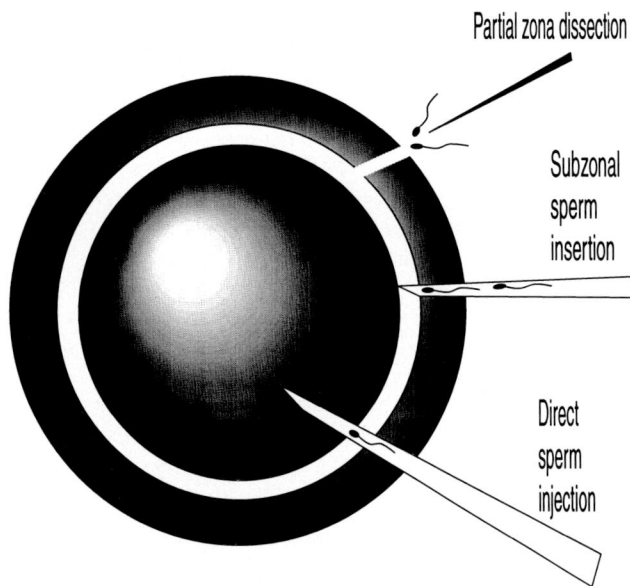

FIGURE 57–1. Alternatives of microsurgically assisted fertilization.

process, without correcting the actual basis for the disorder. Three classes of assisted or microsurgical fertilization by gamete micromanipulation have been explored in several mammalian species (Fig. 57–1). The first involves the creation of an artificial opening in the zona pellucida to allow spermatozoa to interact with the oocyte independent from the zona following insemination, a procedure that was originally termed *zona drilling*.[3, 14] A second category of assisted fertilization techniques directed at facilitating sperm-egg interaction is the subzonal insertion (SZI) of sperm (also referred to as SUZI or MIST).[4, 15–17] Possibly more invasive than zona drilling, SZI completely bypasses the zona and involves

direct placement of the live sperm cell(s) into the perivitelline space. Finally the third mode of microsurgical fertilization is the direct microinjection of a single sperm into the cytoplasm of the oocyte. This latter technique has been called intracytoplasmic sperm injection (ICSI). Both zona drilling and subzonal insertion methods have yielded offspring in the human. ICSI has now been successfully used in many human IVF programs as well; it had already led to live offspring involving studies in rabbits and cows.[18, 19] The pioneering work of van Steirtechem and colleagues in Belgium has recently taken ICSI from the theoretical to the practical.[19a] They were the first to report a consistent human pregnancy rate using ICSI.

Clinical Methods for Assisted Fertilization

ZONA DRILLING AND PARTIAL ZONA DISSECTION

In the zona drilling procedure, first developed in the mouse, a small volume of acidic solution is expelled from a microneedle on a small area of the zona until it is dissolved.[3] Routine insemination follows the procedure. In the mouse, the artificial gap in the zona is associated with increased rates of monospermic fertilization at both normal and reduced sperm numbers, and normal live young can be obtained following transfer to recipient females. Zona drilling in the mouse allows the zona to retain its other physiologic functions after fertilization. Application of zona drilling to clinical IVF was not successful and demonstrated that the human oocyte differed from the mouse in its response to acidic Tyrode's solution. It was noted that microvilli in the human oocyte flatten on contact with acidic solution[20] (Fig. 57–2). This may have interfered with the ability of spermatozoa to interact with the oocyte surface. Moreover, even when fertilization occurred, embryonic development was poor, likely as

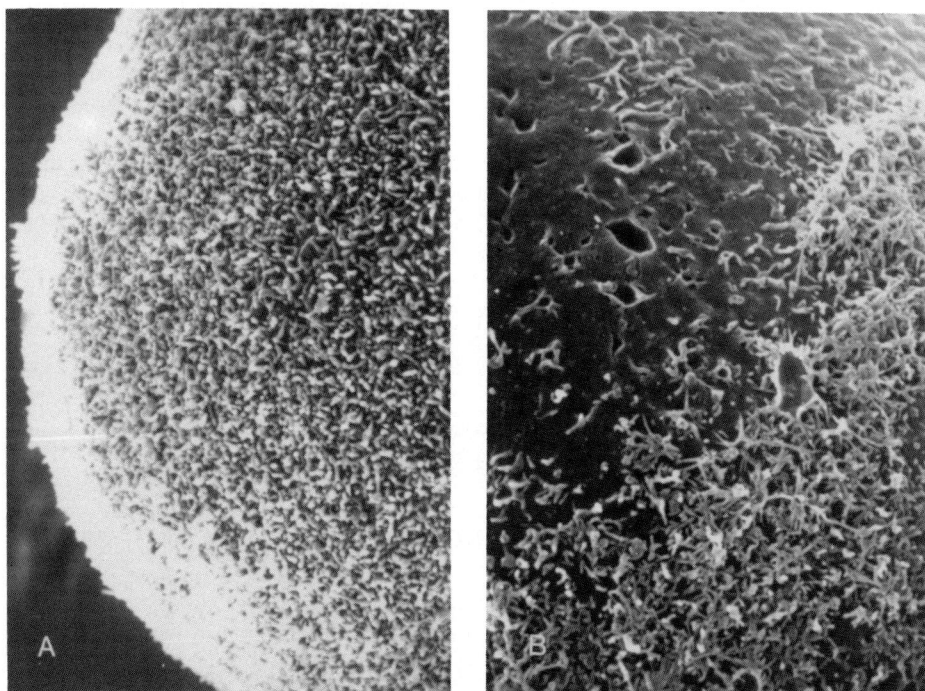

FIGURE 57–2. Scanning electron microscopy of the plasma membrane of the human metaphase II oocyte. The membrane is organized in evenly spaced short microvilli of 1–3 μm in length (A). Microvillus-free areas can be observed in human oocytes (see upper left area) where the zona pellucida was drilled with acidic Tyrode's solution (B).[20]

a result of detrimental effects of acidic Tyrode's solution on unfertilized oocytes.[21, 22]

Alternative methods for creating an opening in the human zona have been attempted. Among the procedures proposed were zona cutting, zona cracking, and use of enzymatic zona digestion (reviewed by Cohen and associates[2]). Cohen and coworkers,[14] however, developed a mechanical procedure for introducing a gap in the mammalian zona, which resulted in the first human pregnancy from microsurgical fertilization. This method, termed partial zona dissection (PZD), involves the use of a sucrose solution to shrink the oocyte so a glass microneedle can be introduced into the perivitelline space without damaging the oocyte.[2] The microneedle is threaded peripherally through two sides of the zona. The portion of the zona that is incorporated between the points is massaged, resulting in a slit in the zona. After this procedure, the oocyte is removed from the sucrose solution and re-exposed to medium of normal osmolarity, before it is inseminated. It is estimated that to date, more than 100 live births have resulted from this method.

Although the clinical use of PZD appears promising, true success, measured as an increase in monospermic fertilization as well as normal embryonic implantation, has only been reported by a limited number of IVF programs.[2] Basically, there are two areas of controversy as pertains to PZD. First, although there is little doubt that PZD improves sperm-oocyte fusion, excessive rates of polyspermy may reduce clinical efficiency.[2, 21, 22] Monospermic fertilization is decided by the size of the hole (and hence the mode of micromanipulation), the number of spermatozoa used for insemination, and patient selection criteria. These factors must be considered carefully to apply PZD successfully as a clinically valid tool. Second, the implanting capacity of PZD, and micromanipulated embryos in general, appears to be reduced in most IVF programs. Because this has not been our experience, we can

only speculate about these discrepancies.[9] There are four possible reasons for embryonic demise following micromanipulation and PZD. (1) Mechanical difficulties during the micromanipulation procedure may result in cellular damage. That this can occur is illustrated by reported damage rates among programs, which vary between 2% and 30%. The damage rate in our program after micromanipulation of more than 5000 oocytes and embryos is now well below 0.5%.[2] Additionally, it is important to realize that damage from micromanipulation may not be immediately manifested in the embryo. (2) Improper culture conditions, such as high and low pH or temperature, may incur damage during micromanipulation. (3) Leakage of cytoplasm and blastomeres through the artificial gaps may occur during rinsing and pipetting of micromanipulated embryos. (4) Routine clinical procedures may play a role as well. For instance, all men from couples undergoing IVF in our center receive antibiotics prophylactically during the first few days of the egg retrieval cycle. In addition, the use of antibiotics and low-dose corticosteroids in the female partners as well as the controlled ovarian hyperstimulation methods should be considered.[23] Finally it is important to recognize that micromanipulated embryos are susceptible to physical damage and should be replaced with care and precision (Fig. 57–3).

SUBZONAL SPERM INSERTION

During SZI, the zona is not only physically, but also functionally bypassed. Sperm are aspirated into a sharp, beveled microneedle and transferred into the perivitelline space. Similar to zona drilling methods, SZI has been investigated in both animal and human models.[2] It is necessary to account for both the quality and the quantity of spermatozoa used in SZI. Only sperm that have undergone capacitation and acrosome reaction are probably capable of fusing with the

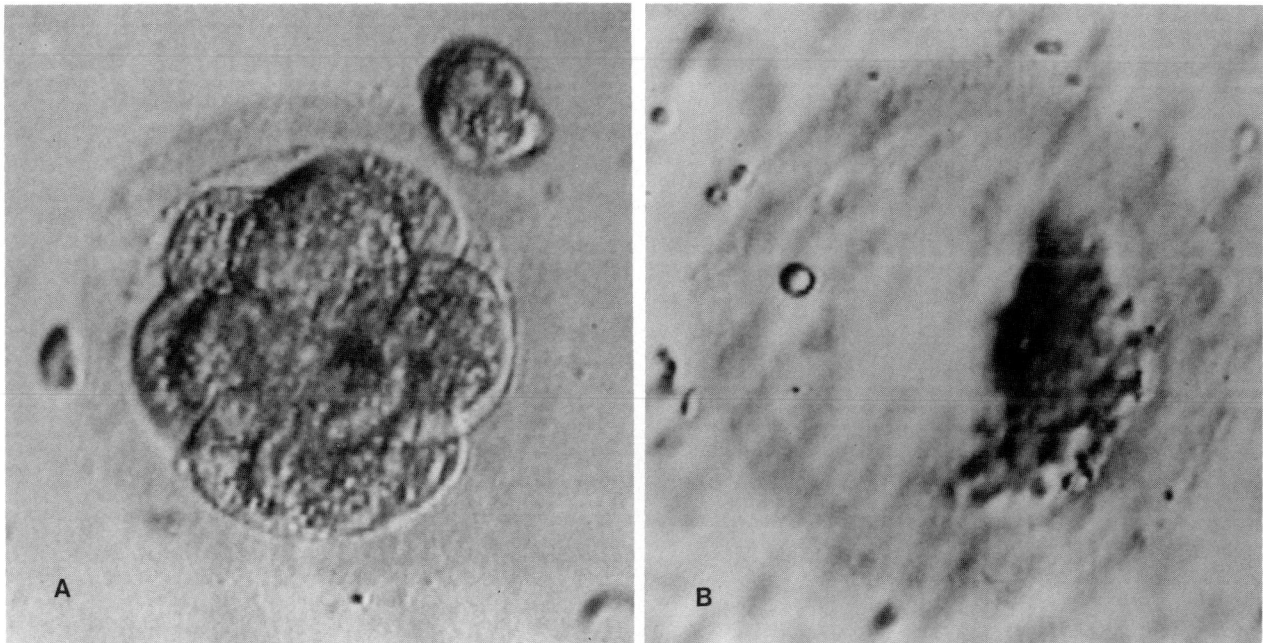

FIGURE 57–3. Damage of micromanipulated embryos following routine handling procedures. Zona-drilled human embryo with expelled blastomere following pipetting (A). Micromanipulated human embryo without blastomeres flushed from the cervical canal following transcervical embryo transfer (B).

TABLE 57–1. Controlled Studies Involving Partial Zona Dissection Using Sibling Oocytes of Patients Who Had Sufficient Numbers of Spermatozoa for Two Types of Insemination*

Source	No. Patients	Incidence of Fertilization per No. of Oocytes (Percentage)		Cycles with Monospermic Fertilization (Percentage)	
		IVF	PZD	IVF	PZD
Cohen et al[49]	47	42/129 (33%)	75/138 (54%)	26/47 (55%)	33/47 (72%)
Cohen et al[2, 16]	37	68/195 (35%)	82/179 (46%)	17/37 (46%)	33/37 (89%)
Combined	84	110/324 (34%)	157/317 (50%)	43/84 (51%)	66/84 (79%)
P value		< 0.05		< 0.05	

*These patients belonged to group A and C (see text under patient selection section).
IVF, In vitro fertilization; PZD, partial zona dissection.

oolemma. It has been suggested that because the zona is no longer involved in the selection process, it may be necessary to use artificial induction of the acrosome reaction to ensure that the "selected" sperm will be capable of fertilization. Despite the apparent advantages of such methods in animal models, however, acrosome reaction-induction has not yet proved to be advantageous in the clinical situation.

We have applied SZI to severe cases of male factor infertility.[24] The data obtained from these clinical trials has clarified several biologic principles and has raised interesting questions pertaining to mammalian fertilization. For example, although both PZD and SZI may be effective treatments for cases of extreme teratozoospermia, it has become clear that those embryos derived from SZI implant at a significantly higher rate than those resulting from the PZD procedure.[16] Most of the controversies involving the clinical use of PZD discussed earlier also apply to SZI. This is illustrated by two publications involving relatively large series of patients.[17, 26] The incidence of birth varied from less than 1% to 5%. At least three other programs, however, have now reported high success rates with SZI.[2]

CONTROLLED STUDIES

According to established scientific guidelines, one should perform routine insemination procedures simultaneously on a significant number of sibling oocytes in each patient to prove clearly that micromanipulation is effective. Although logical, this is not practical for clinical, ethical, and technical reasons. This is where scientific and clinical objectives interfere with each other. Basically, three factors determine the choice for the three insemination procedures: (1) the number

TABLE 57–2. Summary of Microsurgical Fertilization Results Obtained During 1990 in Couples with Few Spermatozoa in Whom Partial Zona Dissection Was Compared with Subzonal Insertion Using Sibling Oocytes*

	Fertilization per No. of Oocytes (Percentage)	Cycles with Fertilization (Percentage)
Subzonal insertion	37/125 (30%)	15/22 (68%)
Partial zona dissection	11/86 (13%)	9/22 (41%)

*Most of these patients belonged to group B (see text under patient selection section).
†P < 0.01.

of mature oocytes, (2) the number of live spermatozoa (and the volume of the final sperm suspension) following removal of seminal plasma and prior sperm evaluation and (3) the previous history of the patient. It would be clinically irresponsible to perform regular IVF (or even PZD) when only a few motile spermatozoa can be isolated. One can only perform IVF and PZD simultaneously when the volume of the final sperm suspension is sufficient. A minimum volume of approximately 30 μL is required for insemination of oocytes in microdroplets under oil.[2] In addition, patients with fertilization failure after standard IVF do not generally consent to the use of zona-intact sibling oocytes. We have shown that a couple who fails to fertilize after a single IVF attempt has less than a 25% chance of fertilization when conventional IVF is reapplied. This figure obviously differs among programs and should be evaluated before the introduction of assisted fertilization by micromanipulation.

Despite these limitations, we have conducted two controlled studies under the supervision of institutional review boards, comparing IVF and PZD in 84 patients before routine introduction of PZD (Table 57–1). Because these studies were performed during the early phases of our microsurgical investigations, the patients had better sperm profiles than those referred to our program in the last 24 months. Moreover, only a minority of them had a failure with conventional IVF before participation in the studies. This is reflected in the relatively high rates of fertilization (34%) when zona-intact oocytes were inseminated. Nevertheless the incidence of monospermic fertilization improved significantly to 50% when the spermatozoa were incubated with micromanipulated oocytes.

When SZI was added to the program, we conducted a small controlled study (n = 22), comparing PZD with SZI in patients who were not acceptable for regular IVF owing to poor semen profiles (see later for definitions). The incidence of monospermic fertilization in these patients was significantly enhanced when SZI was performed (Table 57–2). It has to be noted, however, that the sperm suspensions were poor and dilute, diminishing the likelihood that the spermatozoa would find the artificial gaps in the PZD-oocytes. Actual fertilization percentages following the application of both techniques are similar when more routine IVF patients are included in the evaluation.[2]

FREQUENCY OF SPERM-EGG FUSION FOLLOWING SUBZONAL INSERTION

Considering the lack of a fast block to polyspermy at the level of the human oocyte membrane, it is likely that the success rates of these procedures, measured as the frequency of sperm fusion, could be enhanced if one increased the number of spermatozoa.[25] There is a general consensus, however, that one should limit the number of spermatozoa to avoid polyspermy. A surprisingly large proportion (>10%) of spermatozoa from subfertile men is able to form pronuclei after deposition into the perivitelline area. This figure increases when sperm cells from fertile men are placed into the perivitelline area (Table 57-3).

PATIENT SELECTION

Assisted fertilization offers treatment for patients with impaired sperm function owing to oligozoospermia, asthenozoospermia, or teratozoospermia.[2, 16] Certain oocyte abnormalities, however, can also be potentially treated through micromanipulation. We have performed microsurgical fertilization in four groups of patients according to criteria outlined elsewhere and in Table 57-4.[16, 24] The first two groups (groups A [n = 170 cycles] and E [n = 58 cycles]) constitute 47% of the total number of patients (n = 487 cycles) (Fig. 57-4). Patients from group A had severely abnormal semen analyses (0% to 10% normal sperm forms according to Kruger's strict criteria, ≤20% motile, or ≤10 × 10^6 spermatozoa/mL) and failed to fertilize all oocytes in a previous IVF cycle.[27] Some of these patients had repeated cycles of fertilization failure. Patients from group E had idiopathic failure of fertilization in a previous IVF cycle; their failure to fertilize was idiopathic because the oocytes appeared to be normal and the men had previously demonstrated normal semen analyses.

The third group of couples (group B, n = 111) had not been accepted for regular IVF by any other programs, including our own. These patients' semen analyses were considered highly abnormal consisting of less than 2% normal sperm forms (Kruger's strict criteria) in combination with either extreme oligozoospermia (≤5 × 10^6/mL) or extreme asthenospermia (≤10% motile). Only few motile spermatozoa could be retrieved from their semen, even if the last sperm pellet was resuspended in a volume of less than 50 μL. Actual sperm counts were not available for a number of these patients because the sperm had first to be centrifuged to retrieve a few in the counting chamber. In others, motile spermatozoa were not seen, and an eosin stain was used to detect live spermatozoa. In such couples, SZI was performed exclusively.

The fourth group (C, n = 148) had not attempted IVF previously (some were not acceptable for other IVF programs), and all had male factor infertility of intermediate severity. All these men had teratozoospermia (≤10% normal sperm forms). In addition, their semen was either considered oligozoospermic (<20 × 10^6/mL) or asthenozoospermic (≤30% motile with reduced linear progression). Based on these semen parameters, fertilization failure was anticipated in this group (Group D; see Table 57-4); however, standard IVF was not completely ruled out. Micromanipulation was therefore performed in some of these instances, whereas most oocytes were left zona-intact. Results of group D (regular IVF/male factor) patients are not presented here.

During the first 28 months of our assisted fertilization program, 487 micromanipulation cycles were performed resulting in 109 clinical pregnancies (22%). The implantation results of the patients with abnormal semen analyses (groups A, B, and C) were significantly higher (P < 0.01) than those of the patients with normal semen (group E) (Fig. 57-5). Monospermic fertilization in all groups, however, varied between 18% and 24% with a mean of only 21% (see Fig. 57-4). Seventy of the 109 clinical pregnancies resulted from replacement of microsurgical embryos exclusively. The largest group of 42 pregnant patients had only SZI embryos replaced. Seven pregnancies were established in patients in whom only zona-intact embryos were transferred. The remaining pregnancies were from mixed (microsurgical and zona-intact) embryo replacements. The majority of these pregnancies were established in patients from group C, indicating that microsurgical fertilization was more effective in the other groups. Eight truly microsurgical pregnancies, however, were established in group C patients, whereas regular IVF failed. This suggests that microsurgery may be moderately useful in male factor patients who are also acceptable for regular IVF.

SEMEN FACTORS AND LIMITATIONS OF ASSISTED FERTILIZATION

It has been shown that SZI and PZD are complementary techniques.[2, 16] Fertilization after SZI was higher than with PZD in patients who had few spermatozoa available for insemination. Spermatozoa from group E patients, however, seemed only to be successful following the application of PZD. Furthermore, it was shown that the results of these two methods were additive in terms of implantation. PZD embryos preferentially implanted in patients whose partners had moderate teratozoospermia, whereas SZI embryos implanted more frequently in instances of severe teratozoospermia. Moreover a comparison of our results before and after the

---

TABLE 57-3. Frequency of Sperm Fusion After Subzonal Insertion for Insemination of Oocytes in Male Factor Patients and Reinsemination of Oocytes That Failed to Fertilize After Standard In Vitro Fertilization in Male and Nonmale Factor Patients

Type of Infertility	Subzonal Insertion Performed at	No. Oocytes	No. Sperm (average)	No. Male Pronuclei	F_f
Male	Insemination	184	921 (5.0)	130	14%
Male	Reinsemination	50	228 (4.6)	17	7%
Nonmale	Reinsemination (all oocytes)	81	132 (1.6)	49	37%
Nonmale	Reinsemination (normal oocytes)	19	69	41	59%

From Alikani M, Adler A, Reing AM, et al. Subzonal sperm insertion and the frequency of gamete fusion. J Assist Reprod Gen 1992; 9:97–101.

TABLE 57–4. Selection Criteria for Microsurgical Fertilization and Regular In Vitro Fertilization in Instances of Male Factor Infertility and Idiopathic Failure of Fertilization

Group	Selection Criterion	< 50,000 Motile Sperm Recovered	Count (× 10⁶/mL)	Motility (%)	Strict Morphology (normal forms) (%)	PZD	SZI	IVF
A	Previous failure of fertilization	Occasionally	0.1–10	< 1–20	0–10	+	+	Optional
B	Semen analysis unacceptable for regular IVF	Always	< 0.1–5	< 1–10	0–2	Optional	+	−
C	Semen analysis acceptable for IVF but reduced prognosis	Not applicable but reduced progression and survival	0.5–20	1–30	3–10	+	+	+
D	Semen analysis acceptable for IVF	Not applicable	2–20	5–30	4–10	−	−	+
E	Previous IVF failure and normal semen	Not applicable	≥ 20	≥ 30	> 10	+	+	Optional

Column headers span: *Lowest and Highest Semen Cut-Off Values* (Count, Motility, Strict Morphology); *Treatments* (PZD, SZI, IVF).

PZD, Partial zona dissection; SZI, subzonal insertion; IVF, in vitro fertilization.
From Cohen J, Malter HE, Talansky BE, Grifo J. Micromanipulation of human gametes and embryos. New York: Raven Press, 1992:326.

introduction of SZI has demonstrated that the overall pregnancy rate would be considerably reduced if one of the methods were discontinued. There are, however, major differences between the two micromanipulation methods. One of the advantages of SZI is that it allows for assisted fertilization to be performed when only a few spermatozoa can be retrieved. Consequently, potential patients could include those with complete absence of motility, extreme oligozoospermia (< 1 × 10⁶/mL), and teratozoospermia. This policy of not employing restrictive criteria has been in effect in this program for more than a year.[24] We analyzed the results of the first 250 microsurgical fertilization cycles (groups A, B, and C) to investigate the prognosis for patients with severely abnormal semen analyses and to determine whether low cut-off limits

should be implemented for application of assisted fertilization. The results of the micromanipulation procedures in the first 250 cycles were correlated with fertilization and implantation using a variety of analyses. For the first breakdown, absolute figures for motility, sperm concentration, and number of normally shaped spermatozoa were correlated with the outcome of assisted fertilization. In a second analysis, patients with a single abnormality of semen (either oligozoospermia, asthenozoospermia, or teratozoospermia) were compared with those with two or all three abnormalities.

An example of the results of the microsurgical procedures as a function of the semen analysis is presented in Figure 57–6 by analyzing the percentage of normal sperm forms. No significant correlation was found between percentage of

Microsurgical Fertilization Cornell: 1989 - 1992

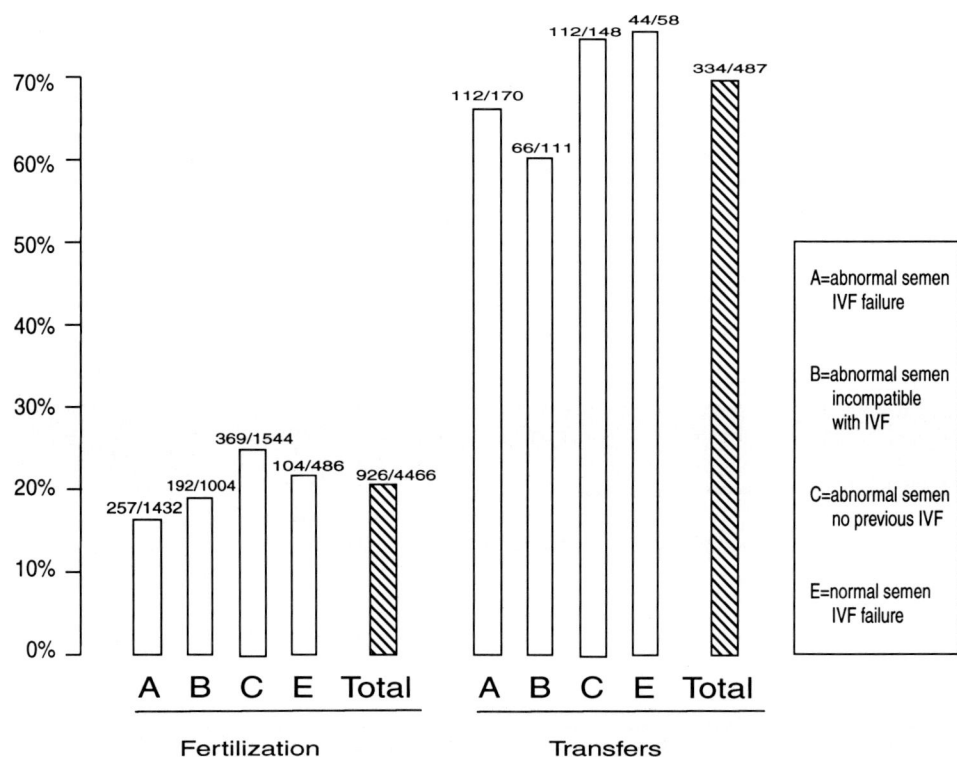

FIGURE 57–4. Incidences of monospermic fertilization and replacement in 487 patient cycles in which microsurgical fertilization (either partial zona dissection or subzonal insertion or both) was attempted. Alphabetical numbers represent patient groups; for further definitions, see section on patient selection. (Courtesy of The New York Hospital, Cornell University Medical College, New York, NY.)

Microsurgical Fertilization Cornell: 1989 - 1992

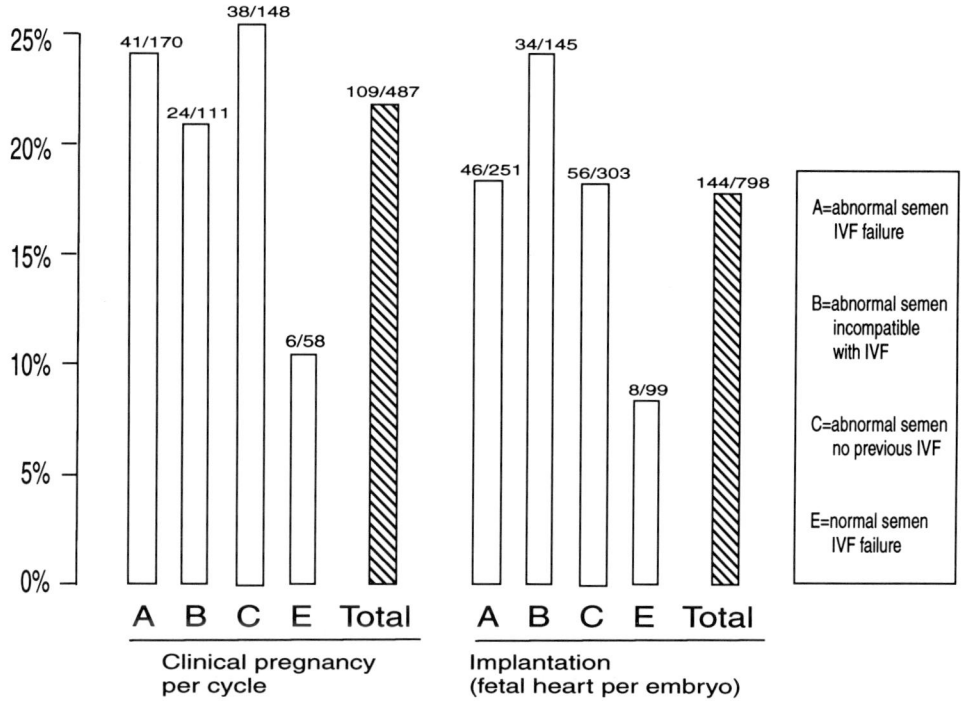

FIGURE 57–5. Rates of clinical pregnancy (fetal heart activity) and embryonic implantation in 487 patient cycles in which microsurgical fertilization (either partial zona dissection or subzonal insertion or both) was attempted. Alphabetical numbers represent patient groups; for further definitions see section on patient selection. (Courtesy of The New York Hospital, Cornell University Medical College, New York, NY.)

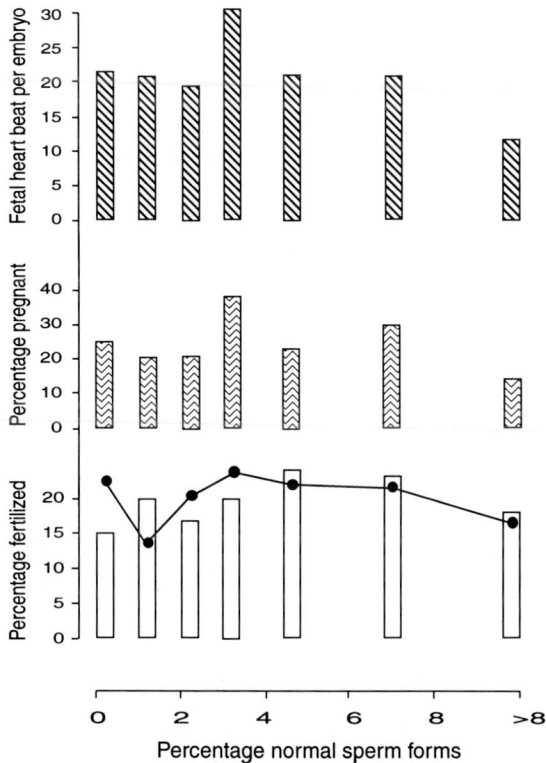

FIGURE 57–6. Outcome of microsurgical procedures (partial zona dissection and subzonal insertion are combined) according to the percentage of normal sperm forms in the sperm preparation.

normal sperm forms and fertilization. Similarly, pregnancy and embryonic implantation results were not affected by sperm morphology. Consequently the severity of teratozoospermia cannot be used as a prognostic factor for predicting the outcome of microsurgically assisted fertilization. It is likely that this is due to the efficiency of SZI in extreme teratozoospermic cases. Only 7% of PZD eggs were fertilized in patients with 0% normal sperm forms, whereas 20% of eggs fertilized in such patients when SZI was performed. Moreover, it was shown previously that the ability of SZI embryos to implant from patients with extreme teratozoospermia (0% to 2% normal forms) was not impaired, whereas PZD embryos from similar patients rarely implanted.[16] Indeed, 64 of such cycles attempted in this series led to 14 (22%) clinical pregnancies. In further analyses, we were not able to correlate fertilization and implantation with sperm concentration or motility.

Results of microsurgical fertilization expressed as a function of the number of semen abnormalities (oligozoospermia, asthenozoospermia, teratozoospermia) are presented in Figure 57–7. It is obvious from these results that the outcome of microsurgical fertilization cannot be predicted based on the World Health Organization criteria. The presence of one, two, or three abnormalities does not affect the rates of fertilization and pregnancy.

A substantial number of viable pregnancies were established well below the normal cut-off values for regular assisted conception procedures. Fertilization and pregnancy occurred following the use of spermatozoa without progressive motility or normal morphology. In some patients, sperm counts were reduced, and spermatozoa could only be visualized after centrifugation. These findings provide evidence that spermatozoa from extremely oligoasthenoteratozoospermic men can produce normal offspring after the application of micromanipulation techniques, even when fertilization previously failed following standard IVF. Subgroups of patients who would not benefit from microsurgical techniques could not be identified by analyzing semen analyses. Although spermatozoa from approximately one third of the patients failed to fertilize altogether, this could also not be correlated with semen analysis.

AUGMENTING FERTILIZING ABILITY

There appear to be two major drawbacks of assisted fertilization: (1) the lack of fertilization in approximately 30% to 70% of the patient population and (2) the lack of implantation. Although the latter phenomenon affects most of the programs, it has not played a role in our microsurgical program. The possible causes for this discrepancy in results has already been discussed. The issue of lack of fertilization seems to be of a more global nature. It is likely that both SZI and PZD should be practiced simultaneously because fertilization is not affected by the severity of semen profiles in our program.[24] The monospermic fertilization rate, however, is rarely in excess of 20%. One factor that can affect the chance of having a replacement is the quality and quantity of oocytes. This is illustrated by the reduced incidence of replacement (27/58; 47%) when fewer than six mature oocytes are obtained (Fig. 57–8). Microsurgical fertilization cycles

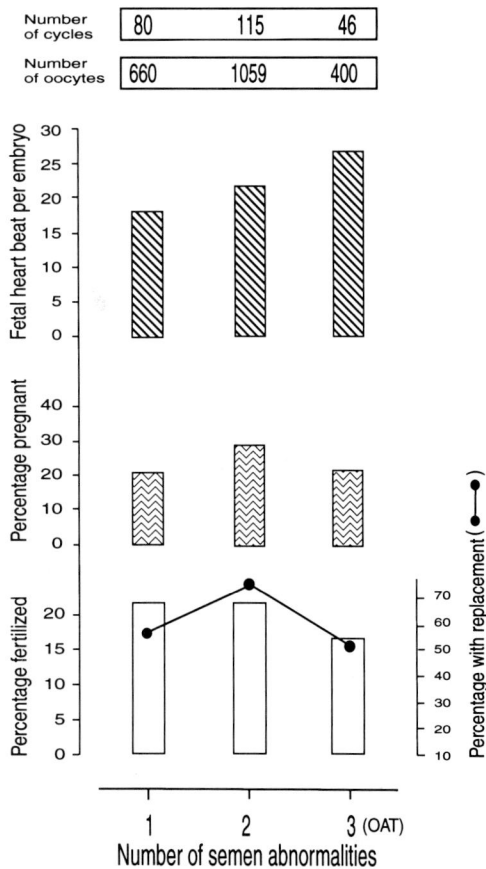

FIGURE 57–7. Outcome of microsurgical procedures (partial zona dissection and subzonal insertion are combined) according to the number of semen abnormalities (according to World Health Organization criteria). The acronym OAT is combined *oligozoospermia, asthenozoospermia,* and *teratozoospermia.*

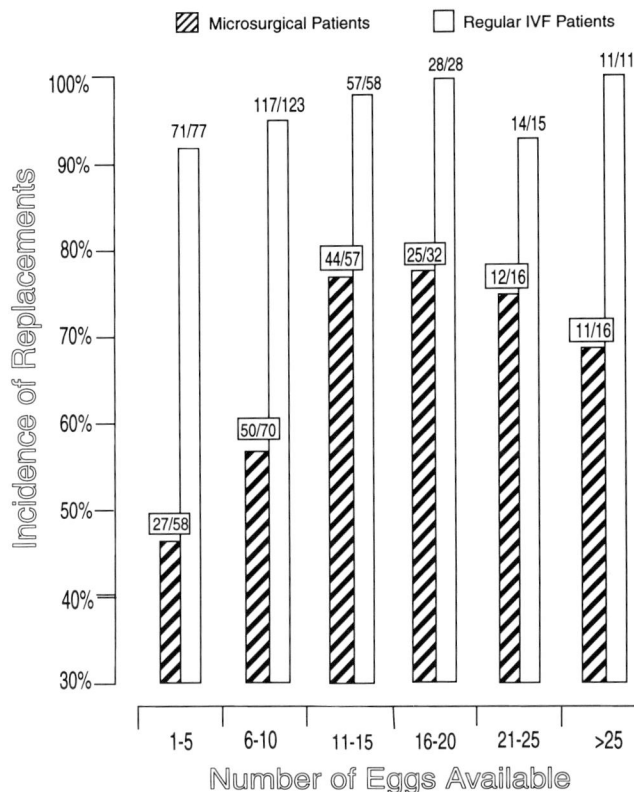

FIGURE 57-8. A comparison between the chances of having at least a single embryo for replacement between microsurgical (partial zona dissection and subzonal insertion are combined) and regular in vitro fertilization (IVF) patients according to the number of oocytes.

(n = 250) were matched with 312 regular IVF cycles during the same period of investigation. The chance of a replacement after conventional IVF was always in excess of 90% regardless of the number of oocytes recovered. The chance of a replacement in microsurgical patients was only above 50% when more than five mature oocytes could be recovered. Therefore, we suggest cancellation of the cycle in patients with poor follicular stimulation. Even if microsurgical fertilization patients have sufficient number of oocytes, however, fertilization rates are usually lower than 30%, indicating that other routes should be used to augment the fertilizing ability of such spermatozoa.

The lack of well-defined methods for improving the in vitro fertilizing ability of sperm is a direct consequence of the paucity of our knowledge concerning the fundamental nature of defective spermatozoa. Progress in this particularly elusive area of human reproduction depends on a systematic analysis of the molecular basis of sperm function. Currently, there are three routes that one can follow regarding the enhancement of the fertilizing capacity of deficient human sperm: (1) the appropriateness of each method of semen preparation, (2) the induction of capacitation and the acrosome reaction and (3) the inhibition of reactive oxygen species production.[24] The first two factors have been investigated in some detail in our center with emphasis on the application of microsurgical fertilization. Preparative techniques involve the use of Percoll gradients, proteolytic enzymes, swim-up procedures, and sperm sedimentation methods.[2] Methods are combined depending on the semen profile and the previous history of the

patient. This aspect of the technology is consequently more individualized. The application of technology involving the artificial enhancement of capacitation and the acrosome reaction has not yielded standardized methods for increasing the success rates of assisted fertilization, despite their successful application in the hamster oocyte assay or mouse oocyte studies. We have performed pilots with electroporation and cryoshock of spermatozoa using sibling oocytes during PZD and SZI. This did not result in a consistent improvement of the fertilizing ability of impaired spermatozoa.

Several research groups[28, 29] have indicated that phosphodiesterase inhibitors such as pentoxifylline (px) and deoxyadenosine (dAdn) are effective in promoting fertilization. We have investigated the possible use of a combination of these two compounds[29] in a study involving 116 microsurgical fertilization patients.[30] Both compounds were used in equivalent amounts at a concentration of 3 or 1 mM. Forty-seven of the patients yielded insufficient numbers of spermatozoa to perform the sibling study. In these patients, px-dAdn was used exclusively, and comparisons with conventional semen preparation methods were not made. The incidences of fertilization and implantation did not appear to be higher than that reported in other studies.[2, 9, 24]

In a second group of 69 patients from whom sufficient spermatozoa were retrieved, the investigations were performed using sibling oocytes. Spermatozoa were prepared in the presence or absence of px-dAdn. The sperm suspensions were then used for SZI, PZD, or regular IVF depending on the criteria outlined in the previous section on patient selection. The fertilization results are presented in Figure 57-9. The use of px-dAdn at a high concentration of 3 mM appeared successful following SZI and regular IVF. For reasons unknown, it was not successful when PZD was applied or when the doses were reduced to 1 mM. It is recommended that these compounds be used with care, despite these promising results. A total of 171 embryos were replaced in these patients and only 27 (16%) implanted, which was less than we have previously obtained. A comparison between replacements involving embryos derived from spermatozoa exposed to px-dAdn alone and mixed batches of embryos (treated and nontreated sperm) shows that px-dAdn embryos may be impaired in their capacity to implant normally (Fig. 57-10).

OFFSPRING FROM MICROSURGICAL FERTILIZATION

One of the most important aspects associated with the evaluation of a novel assisted reproductive technique is that of pregnancy outcome. Thus far, 66 healthy infants have been born following 50 deliveries of couples in whom either SZI, PZD, or a combination thereof was attempted at our center (Table 57-5). Of the first 109 clinical pregnancies obtained following the use of these microsurgical techniques, 12 have now miscarried (11%), but this figure is expected to increase because many of the pregnancies are still within the first 20 weeks of gestation. The miscarriages do not appear to be associated with specific semen profiles. The true success rate of microsurgical fertilization can only be assessed by determining the percentage of deliveries per attempt (oocyte retrieval). Accordingly, we can now evaluate the first 250 patient cycles in our assisted fertilization program (Fig. 57-11).

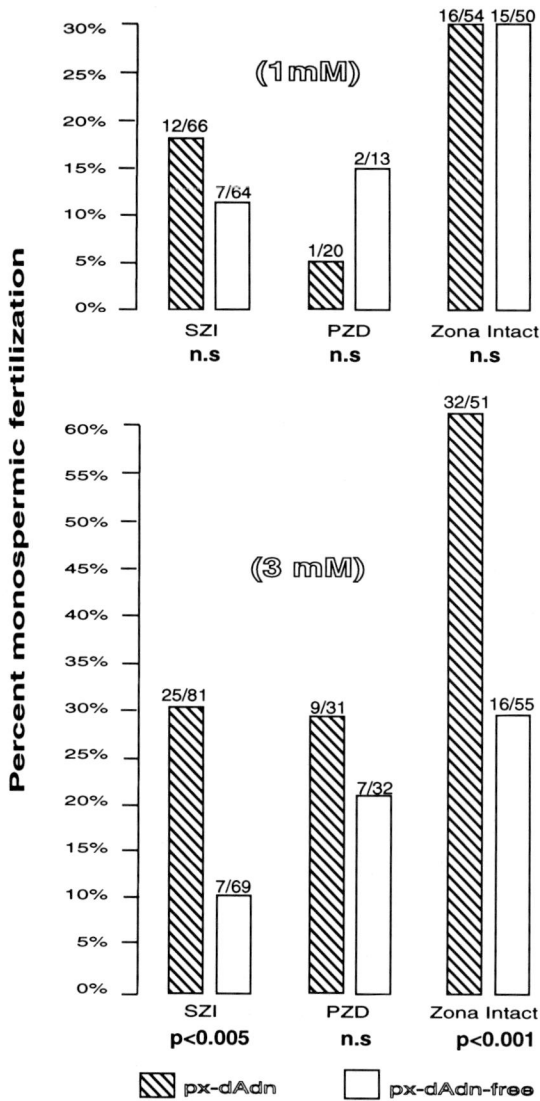

FIGURE 57–9. Effects of a combination of pentoxyfylline (px) and deoxyadenosine (dAdn) on assisted fertilization. This study involved 116 microsurgical fertilization patients in whom sibling oocytes were treated with sperm that were preincubated with or without both compounds. Both phosphodiesterase inhibitors were used in equivalent amounts at a concentration of 3 mM or 1 mM.[30]

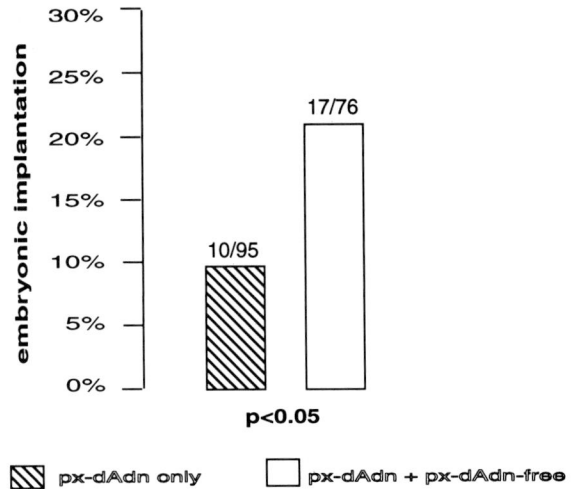

FIGURE 57–10. Rates of embryonic implantation following replacements involving embryos derived from sperm which were exposed to a combination of pentoxyfylline (px) and deoxyadenosine (dAdn) prior to assisted fertilization compared to replacements with embryos of mixed origin.

It appears, although this is disputed by some, that the block to polyspermy in the human is similar to that of the hamster model.[14, 15, 31] Rates of polyspermy following microsurgical procedures are elevated to approximately 25% of fertilized eggs.[2] This level is especially high if one considers that the populations of spermatozoa used represent those with decreased fertilizing ability. One group of researchers reported relatively low rates of polyspermy following subzonal sperm insertion.[15] Rates of polyspermy following PZD in instances of normal sperm function may be as high as 50%.[31] A weak block to polyspermy, however, is likely to be in place at the level of the plasmalemma in women. One would expect equal numbers of three-, four-, and five-pronucleate embryos and so on after zona drilling, if the membrane and cytoplasmic blocks were completely inactive. Most multinucleate zygotes, however, are dispermic, and the degree of multinucleation diminishes with each additional sperm being incorporated.[2]

The take-home baby rate was only 10% during the first 100 attempts, but this rate doubled during the next 100 attempts. From our current results, we estimate a true success rate of 18%, a figure that appears somewhat higher in comparison to the first 250 attempts (15.6%). The latter percentage is relatively low owing to the natural learning curve associated with the incorporation of each new technique.

ZYGOTE MICROMANIPULATION

Zona drilling techniques provide the experimental embryologist with information on the efficiency of the block to polyspermy at both the level of the plasmalemma and the zona. Breaching the zona of mouse eggs, for instance, leads to low levels of polyspermic fertilization, whereas similar procedures in hamster oocytes induce polyspermy uniformly.

TABLE 57–5. Results of Microsurgical Fertilization Procedures Including Ongoing Pregnancies and Live Deliveries (April 1992)

Patient cycles	487 (a)
Replacements	334 (69%) (b)
Positive β-hCG	134 (28% from a) (40% from b)
Biochemical miscarriages	25
Clinical pregnancy	109 (22% from a) (33% from b) (c)
Clinical miscarriages	12 (11% from c)
Ongoing/delivered	97 (20% from a) (29% from b)
Delivered patients (babies)	50 (66)*
Number of babies from PZD embryos	11
Number of babies from SZI embryos	18
Number of babies from a combination of PZD/SZI embryos	6
Number of babies from a combination of zona-intact/PZD/SZI embryos	27
Number of babies from zone-intact embryos	4

*Forty-seven pregnancies in this group of patients were still ongoing when this manuscript was submitted.

β-hCG, β human chorionic gonadotropin; PZD, partial zona dissection; SZI, subzonal insertion.

Microsurgical Fertilization Cornell: 1989-1991
Rates of Delivery in the First 250 Patient Cycles

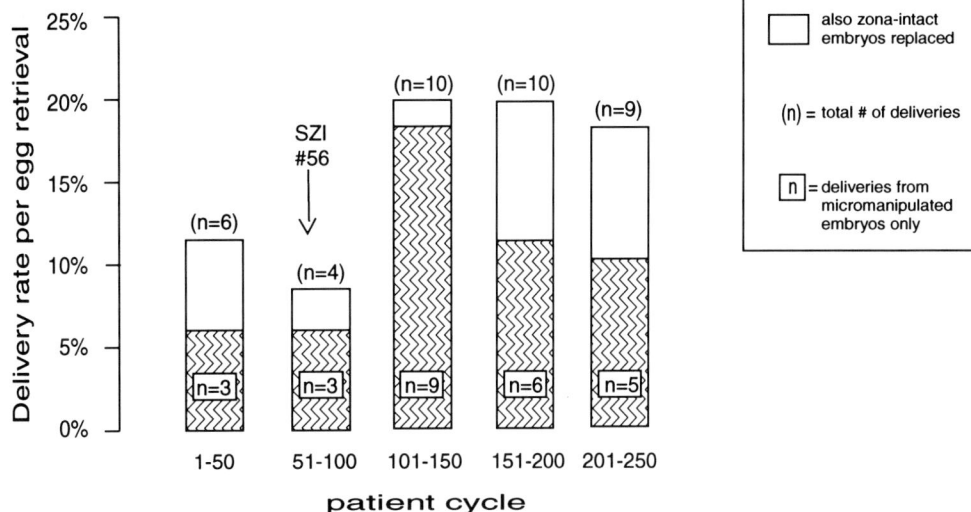

FIGURE 57–11. Baby take-home rates following completion of the first 250 assisted fertilization cycles. (Courtesy of The New York Hospital, Cornell University Medical College, New York, NY.)

The level of dispermy is lower than trispermy when three or more spermatozoa are deposited into the perivitelline area.[2] It can therefore be concluded that the block to supernumerary sperm penetration in the human primarily resides at the level of the zona pellucida.[30] Also, in rare cases, IVF cycles have been observed in which a high degree of polyspermy occurs in the absence of zona micromanipulation. The ability to control polyspermy or to correct the genetically abnormal embryos that result from it would be of obvious value to clinical IVF.

There is a large body of research regarding genetic manipulation in rodents and large domestic animals based on techniques for the vital, intact removal of pronuclei.[32, 33] It would seem that these techniques could be modified and used simply to remove the extra sperm pronucleus, thereby returning the human zygote to a normal genetic complement. Preliminary experiments toward this goal have been reported by several groups.[34–36]

The survival rate in our enucleation work is now well over 50% (Table 57–6). Although we have noted that a large proportion of the surviving embryos continue development, we have usually not followed their development and have opted to perform ultrastructural and genetic analyses. The central issue in using enucleation to correct polyspermy is the correct identification of the supernumerary male pronucleus. This identification is simple in rodent zygotes, in which nuclear size and the presence of sperm tail remnants

as well as position in relation to the second polar body are all valid criteria. In human zygotes, size appears to be variable, and sperm tail remnants can almost never be identified by light microscopic observation.[36, 37] Pronuclei that are furthest from the second polar body are being selected for removal, and genetic analysis will, it is hoped, prove this to be a valid criterion for identification. Currently, we perform multiplex polymerase chain reaction (PCR) and in situ hybridization of blastomeres removed from enucleated eight-cell human embryos (Munne and colleagues, unpublished observations). Using the postulation that the pronucleus furthest from the second polar body is likely to be a male pronucleus, our laboratory has thus far completed studies on 11 enucleated embryos, of which 4 provided signals for PCR. Two embryos were XX, whereas the two others were XY. If the distribution of the three pronuclei were random in relation to the second polar body, one third of enucleated zygotes would become androgenetic. Of these, 25% should have Y-signal exclusively. This approach would enable us to investigate whether the parental origin of the pronuclei would be topographically fixed, provided that a relatively large number of multiplex experiments are performed. Alternatively, one could perform X or Y labeling on the removed pronucleus, although this does not indicate whether that specific zygote is androgenetic. Thus far, we have not been able to perform PCR on removed pronuclei, presumably because the enucleation procedure does not remove karyoplasts, including completely intact pronuclei, but rather fragments containing nucleoplasm as well as nucleoli. A third approach for confirmation of parental origin of human pronuclei is the use of DNA-specific vital stains preincubated with either sperm or eggs before insemination. Preliminary mouse experiments in our laboratory have been unsuccessful because the stain leaked from the pronuclei. Further experiments in the human were somewhat more revealing because the prestained and washed human oocyte does not lose the DNA marker as fast as the mouse egg (Dale and Cohen, unpublished data). Twenty mature human oocytes have thus been preincubated

TABLE 57–6. Results of Microsurgical Enucleation for Correction of Polyspermy in the Human

Source	No. Micro-manipulated	No. Survived	No. Cleaved
Malter & Cohen[36]	25	9 (36%)	7 (28%)
Malter & Cohen (unpublished, 1991)	70	60 (87%)	44 (63%)

with a vital fluorescent DNA stain and washed after 15 minutes, before insemination with unstained sperm. Four of the monospermic zygotes had only a single fluorescing pronucleus. The stained pronuclei were always adjacent to the second polar body. These preliminary experiments provide impetus for further investigation and underline the hypothesis that the female pronucleus is in a relatively fixed position in relation to the second polar body. Until it is certain that polyspermy repair produces normal, diploid embryos with both a maternal and paternal component, however, clinical application would be ill-advised.

EMBRYO MICROMANIPULATION

There have been several proposals for improving IVF laboratory techniques, ranging from the use of complex media supplements, such as immunosuppressants, to the application of helper cell systems.[10, 11, 38, 39] Clear improvements in conventional cell-tissue culture technology among IVF laboratories, however, have not been realized to date. Rarely, more than 15% of human embryos are viable, even in the most carefully controlled programs. This figure is frequently unclear because general IVF success rates are often expressed in terms of transfers involving sets of sibling embryos. Although this practice appears acceptable, it does not address the principle flaw of IVF, that of embryonic wastage. A review of the literature shows that there have been only two promising proposals for enhancing embryonic viability. The first of these involves the simultaneous culture (coculture) of embryos with helper cells and is based on the vast experience of embryologists who handle early-stage embryos from larger domestic species.[10, 11, 39] The second method has been called assisted hatching and is based on the hypothesis that some zonae inhibit the escape of otherwise normal embryos during blastocyst expansion.[6, 12, 13]

Two particular findings were crucial in the decision to implement assisted hatching in human IVF programs. First, it is known that cleaved embryos with a high prognosis for implantation produce an active component that reduces the thickness of the zona, presumably in preparation for subsequent hatching.[10, 40, 41] Second, microsurgically fertilized embryos with artificial gaps in their zonae (PZD) appear to have high rates of implantation (see earlier). Assisted hatching was first experimentally tested by introducing small incisions in the zonae of human four-cell embryos using a mechanical method.[6, 42] Although the resulting preliminary work was encouraging, routine application was not implemented at our program for several reasons. First, some of the spare embryos that were observed for prolonged periods became trapped in the narrow openings during hatching.[42] This phenomenon was confirmed in a mouse model.[43] Second, other embryos were possibly damaged during embryo replacement before the formation of structural junctions between the blastomeres.[2, 44] Alternatively, it was proposed that larger openings be created in the zonae of human embryos undergoing initial compaction.[2, 12, 13] We completed three studies on the use of zona drilling[3] with acidic Tyrode's solution in 3-day-old human embryos.[13, 45] The trials were performed in a completely randomized fashion in 330 IVF couples. The first and second trial included patients with normal basal follicle-stimulating hormone (FSH) levels. During the first trial, assisted hatching

with zona drilling in one group was compared with a control group of patients whose embryos were not micromanipulated. Patients whose embryos had thick zonae derived the greatest benefit. This finding was tested prospectively in the second trial by performing assisted hatching selectively only on embryos with thick zonae in patients of the experimental group and comparing the outcome with patients from a control group without micromanipulation. The third trial was similar to the first trial but performed in patients with elevated basal FSH levels.

Assisted Hatching

ANIMAL STUDIES

One of the first requirements for the safe application of micromanipulation to human embryos is the study of these relatively invasive techniques in animal models. There is currently no other species in which the hatching mechanism is known to be dysfunctional. The hatching process of embryos from domestic species and rodents does not appear to be inhibited, although studies of preimplantation embryonic development following the application of IVF in, for instance, the bovine have not yet been performed. Hence the use of laboratory animals for the study of assisted hatching procedures appears to be limited to the creation of specific models in which the hatching process is inhibited artificially and then reversed by micromanipulation. Mouse embryos flushed from common laboratory strains usually develop to the blastocyst stage in vitro and hatch fully. It was shown by Malter and Cohen[42] that micromanipulated mouse embryos hatch through the artificial gap and that hatching is initiated at an earlier stage. Depending on the size of the hole, embryos may become trapped in a characteristic figure-eight shape.[42, 43, 46, 47] Hatching does not appear to be facilitated in embryos whose zonae have been pierced once with a sharp needle.[43] One or several large holes introduced by zona drilling[3] appears to be more favorable for the integrity of the embryo than the introduction of a small slit in the zona following PZD.[12, 14]

Two models have been suggested for the study of assisted hatching in the mouse. The first was applied in embryos with poor in vitro development. Khalifa and Tucker[48] micromanipulated morulae using acidic Tyrode's solution either to drill through the zona or to thin a larger area partially. Initiation of hatching occurred in significantly more micromanipulated than control embryos. The rate of completion of hatching, however, was doubled in partially thinned embryos compared with the other groups. A second mouse model was applied in strains with normal in vitro development.[47] Embryos were kept in protein-free culture media, which inhibits hatching. Zona drilling performed at the cleavage stage followed by further culture in a protein-free environment significantly improved hatching. Both models can be used for refining assisted hatching techniques.

HUMAN STUDIES

Since the initiation of clinical assisted hatching in our laboratory 3 years ago, the method has been modified on several occasions. The first clinical experiments involved PZD of the four-cell embryo. This method was applied prospectively in 99 consenting patients in a randomized fashion.[6, 49] Although the pregnancy rate increased by 20% and the embryonic implantation nearly doubled, PZD is no longer the method used for assisted hatching. The holes created with this technique may be too small to allow normal completion of hatching.[43] Furthermore, results of some clinical follow-up studies have been disappointing.

High rates of implantation following biopsy of eight-cell human embryos using acidic Tyrode's have been reported.[1] Biopsied embryos were replaced at the time of initial compaction.[44] We therefore hypothesized that it may be advantageous to transfer embryos with substantially large holes in their zonae after interblastomere adherence has increased.[2, 12] The use of zona drilling on day 3 of embryonic development was investigated in three fully randomized, prospective trials in 330 consenting patients at The Center for Reproductive Medicine and Infertility at the New York Hospital–Cornell Medical Center. The specific method, embryo selection criteria, and results within each trial are published elsewhere.[13, 45] The combined results of these trials are presented in Figure 57–12. The incidence of clinical pregnancy (fetal heartbeat per patient) increased significantly ($P < 0.01$) from 37% (62/166) in the control group to 52% (85/164) following zona drilling. Twenty-seven percent of the zona-drilled embryos implanted (147/555) and showed fetal heart activity on ultrasound scan. This compared favorably ($P < 0.01$) with the control group, in which 19% (104/555) of the embryos implanted. It must be noted, however, that these results were obtained during three trials. Two trials were performed in consenting patients allocated to control or micromanipulation groups. The embryos from patients allocated to the micromanipulation group were always zona-drilled. The first trial (n = 137) was performed in patients with an average age of 36 and normal basal FSH levels. The third trial (n = 30) included only patients with elevated basal FSH

levels (> 15 mIU/mL). Although embryonic implantation increased in both trials following zona drilling, the difference with the control group was significant only in the elevated basal FSH group.[13]

Selective Assisted Hatching

Retrospective analysis of embryos replaced during the first trial demonstrated that the zona pellucida thickness largely determined the outcome of the procedure.[13] Control embryos with zonae thicker than 15 μm rarely implanted, whereas zona-drilled embryos with similar zona characteristics frequently implanted (Fig. 57–13). The findings also suggested that zona drilling was detrimental in embryos with thin zonae (< 12 μm). The latter evaluation, however, was not statistically significant. These retrospective findings were prospectively tested during a second trial involving 163 patients. Zonae from embryos of patients allocated to the zona-drilling group were measured before micromanipulation. Embryos with thick zonae were micromanipulated (≥ 15 μm), and those with thin zonae (≤ 12 μm) were left intact. The sum result of this group of patients (two thirds of their embryos were micromanipulated) was compared with a control group in which embryos were never micromanipulated. This process has been called selective assisted hatching.[13] The retrospective conclusion from the first trial was confirmed during this selective assisted hatching trial. Both the incidences of clinical pregnancy and embryonic implantation increased significantly following the application of assisted hatching. Figure 57–12 therefore presents the combined results of selective assisted hatching and regular assisted hatching performed in patients of varying cause and basal FSH levels. Correlation of patients based on maternal age indicates that selective assisted hatching was most effective in the group

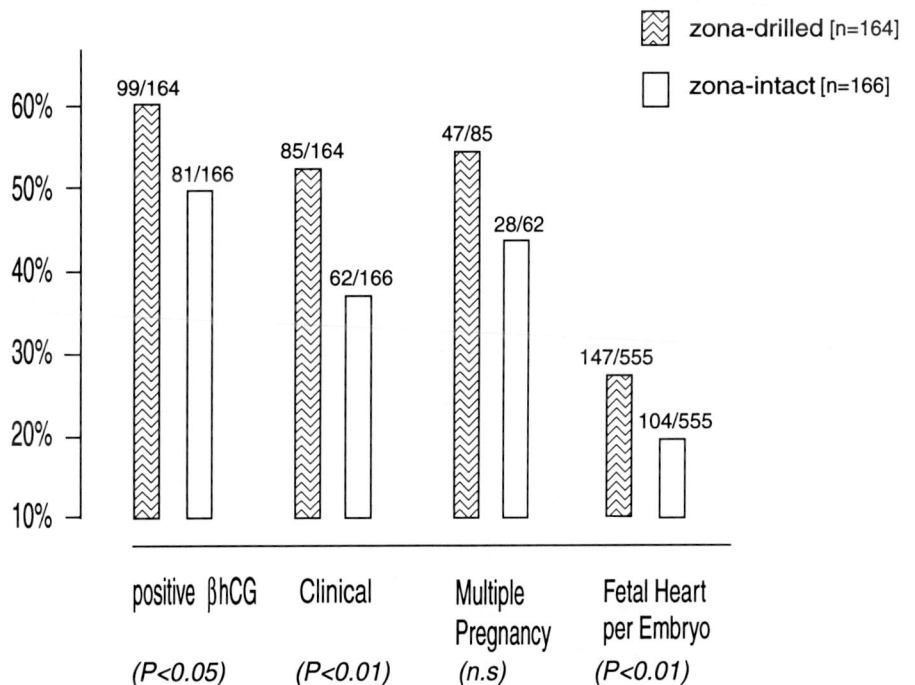

FIGURE 57–12. Combined results of three fully randomized assisted hatching trials involving 330 patients using zona drilling at day 3 of development.[13]

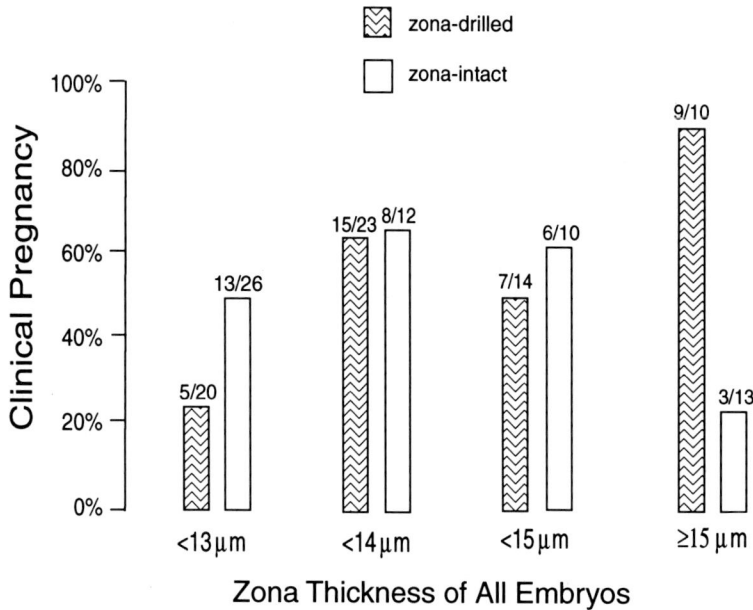

FIGURE 57–13. Effect of zona thickness on the clinical pregnancy rate of patients. The data were obtained from retrospective measurements of embryos from trial 1 patients. (From Cohen J, Alikani M, Trowbridge J, Rosenwaks Z. Implantation enhancement by selective assisted hatching using zona drilling of embryos with poor prognosis. Hum Reprod 1992;7:685–691; by permission of Oxford University Press.)

over 38 years (Fig. 57–14). To evaluate the possibility of quantitative zona changes as a function of maternal age, we assessed the average zona thickness and percentage zona variation in 1023 embryos on day 3 following egg retrieval. Zona biometrics did not change in patients over age 31, despite the age-related differences in response to assisted hatching (Fig. 57–15). The mean zona thickness of patients younger than age 32 was at least 1 μm greater than that of other patient groups. It can be postulated that zona deposi-

tion is an age-related process. This finding should probably be considered when evaluating the possibility of assisted hatching in embryos with thick zonae from young patients.

We have now incorporated selective assisted hatching into the IVF procedure for those embryos with thick zonae in consenting patients younger than age 39 who have normal basal FSH levels. Zona drilling of all embryos, regardless of zona thickness, is being performed in all other consenting patients. Results thus far indicate that approximately one quarter of human embryos have the ability to implant and that a clinical pregnancy rate of greater than 50% per transfer may be a possibility for IVF patients in the future.

Partial Zona Thinning of Embryos with Thin Zonae and Good Prognosis

One of the observations based on the zona drilling trials presented here is that acidic Tyrode's solution may be detrimental to embryos with thin zonae.[13] Selective zona drilling of embryos with thick zonae now results in implantation rates that are similar in both thick and thin zonae groups. To investigate whether implantation of embryos with thin zonae (< 13 μm) can be improved further, however, a fourth trial was executed in 40 consenting patients.[45] Patients were randomized in two groups. Zonae were measured before replacement in both groups. Embryos with zonae $\geq$ 15 μm (poor-prognosis embryos) were zona-drilled in both arms of the trial. Embryos with thin zonae were left intact in one group (control), whereas the outside of zonae of similar embryos in the other group were thinned with acidic Tyrode's solution using the technique of Khalifa and Tucker.[48] Results thus far indicate that embryos with thin zonae do not benefit from this technique. Their implanting potential, however, was not jeopardized, as was previously shown to occur after the zonae were pierced completely by zona drilling.[13] Embryonic implantation was high (26% to 27%) in both arms of the trial, probably as a result of selective zona drilling of low-prognosis embryos with thick zonae.

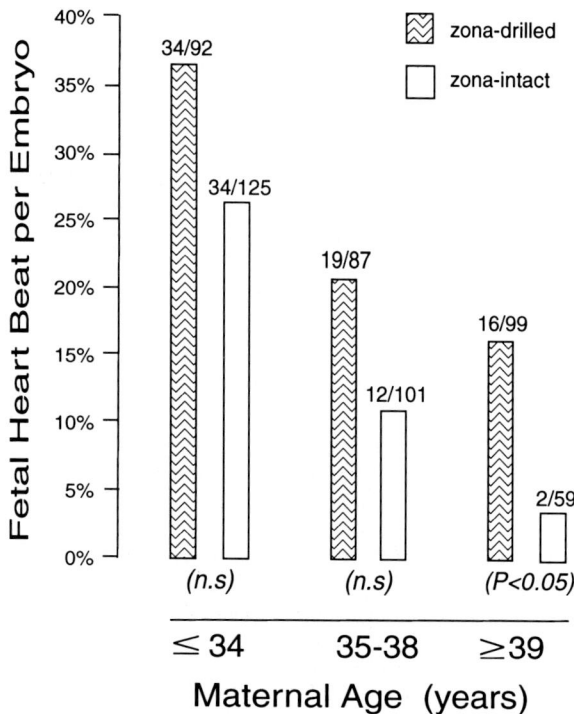

FIGURE 57–14. Effect of maternal age on the results of a fully randomized trial using selective assisted hatching of poor embryos. (From Cohen J, Alikani M, Trowbridge J, Rosenwaks Z. Implantation enhancement by selective assisted hatching using zona drilling of embryos with poor prognosis. Hum Reprod 1992;7:685–691; by permission of Oxford University Press.)

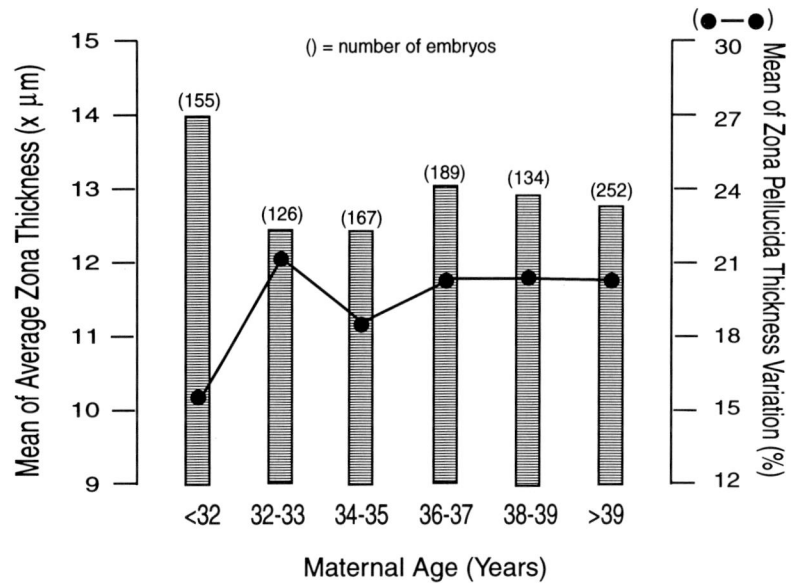

FIGURE 57–15. Maternal age and mean zona thickness and variation measured in 1023 embryos.

Zona Hardening and Assisted Hatching

The zona reaction encompasses an increased resistance to dissolution by various chemical agents, a process that is called zona hardening.[50] Various agents, including proteases, disulfide-bond reducing agents, sodium periodate, low pH, and high temperature, have been applied to study the phenomenon of zona hardening.[51] It has been shown that the zona is more readily removed from unfertilized oocytes than from embryos. The sensitivity of the human zona to decreased pH or mechanical piercing appears to follow an inverse pattern because it is easier to drill a hole in a zygote than in an unfertilized oocyte. The human zona becomes more friable and loses its elasticity after fertilization. In addition to fertilization-induced hardening, spontaneous hardening also occurs after in vitro culture[52, 53] and in vivo aging.[54]

Zona hardening may be important for three postfertilization events, including the block to polyspermy,[55] protection of the developing embryo,[56] and oviductal transport.[57] Although the process is believed to be a mechanical change, assays usually involve solubilization techniques. Drobnis and colleagues[51] used deformation of the zona aspirated into a micropipette (zona deformability) as an assay for zona hardening. This study revealed that mechanical deformability occurred in hamsters and mice. Hamster oocytes do not show zona hardening following regular solubilization investigation methods. The zona deformability assay quantitates zona changes without jeopardizing zona integrity and could therefore be of use clinically. Prospective quantitative studies involving zona hardening measurements have not yet been performed clinically in humans. Zona piercing for assisted hatching, however, allows for indirect assessment of zona hardening. The effort involved in opening the zona pellucida with acidic Tyrode's solution can be scored by the observer as easy to pierce or difficult to pierce, but this is a subjective determination. Alternatively, we developed a method to assess zona hardening from videotaped zona drilling procedures. The videotapes of the zona drilling in embryos of 25 patients have been analyzed retrospectively. Exposure to acidic Tyrode's solution for each embryo has been expressed as a function of the time needed to pierce the outside and inside layers of the zona pellucida as well as the diameter of the needle used, to compensate for needle size variation. The preliminary results suggest that patients whose embryos have zonae that were digested by small amounts of acidic Tyrode's solution (< 200 μm seconds) have a higher chance of a multiple pregnancy than those patients in whom zona dissolution required greater amounts of acidic Tyrode's solution. These preliminary findings suggest that embryonic viability is possibly correlated with zona hardening.

Removal of Extracellular Fragments

The importance of extracellular fragmentation has been traditionally overemphasized in clinical IVF. We have been unable to establish a correlation between moderate extracellular fragmentation ($\leq$ 15% fragments) and implantation.[10, 40, 41] Nevertheless the presence of excessive amounts of degenerate material within the perivitelline area may affect embryonic viability. To test this hypothesis, we have removed small numbers of fragments from embryos during the assisted hatching trials. This pilot study, however, was not done in a randomized fashion. In some more excessively fragmented embryos, fragments were removed, whereas other less fragmented embryos were left intact. It is therefore difficult to quantify, based on our data, what the impact of fragment removal could be on further embryonic growth.

During zona drilling, embryos were clamped onto the holding pipette in such a way that the acidic Tyrode's-filled microneedle is positioned at the 3 o'clock area either adjacent to empty perivitelline space or anucleate fragments.[2] Small holes were widened mechanically by moving the microneedle through the opening in a tearing motion, and gentle suction was used to remove fragments. Most of the embryos from 52 patients were partially fragmented. Fragment removal was performed in those patients (n = 36) who had embryos with excessive amounts of fragments (> 15%). In embryos of 16 other patients, fragments were also present, but they were not removed. Although the clinical pregnancy rates were similar in these two groups (41% and 44%), it may be noted that the success rates were lower than the rest of the patients allocated to the zona drilling trials (see Fig. 57–12). Nevertheless, it may be concluded (1) that fragment removal can be performed with relative ease, (2) that the risks of the procedure are relatively minimal, and (3) that the pregnancy rate was relatively high considering the poor morphology of the embryos involved. Additional controlled studies will be helpful to extend this hypothesis further.

FUTURE APPLICATIONS OF MICROMANIPULATION

As experience is gained both in large domestic animal as well as human IVF, present techniques will undoubtedly be refined, and new applications will be developed. Advances in instrumentation, particularly involving the use of the laser, may provide solutions to some existing problems. It is unlikely that breakthroughs will depend solely on the development of new sophisticated micromanipulation procedures. Progress in the field of assisted reproduction and that of applied reproductive physiology in general will be largely determined by the coevolution of medical ethics and molecular genetics. There are at least four areas in which micromanipulation technology will be crucial: (1) the application of laser technology to gamete and embryo micromanipulation,[59] (2) the use of gametes for gene therapy, (3) genomic expansion by nuclear transplantation and artificial twinning, and (4) placenta donation.[2]

The optical trap-laser microsurgery system may play an important role in research and clinical applications involving gamete interaction.[59] Human sperm have been successfully manipulated in an optical trap. Although individual sperm could be trapped and held for nearly a minute without any apparent effect on motility, it has not yet been proved that they are able to fertilize. Using a motorized stage, sperm in the trap could be moved around the slide. Preliminary reports have also been published concerning the opening of the zona pellucida using laser microbeams.[2] Laser micromanipulation systems have been used for opening the zona for clinical microsurgical fertilization and assisted hatching.[8] Laser microbeams can "drill" precise holes in the zona pellucida to allow for the entry of an optical trap–directed single sperm cell, which could be stabilized and fused with the oocyte using a second form of laser energy. Such a system might allow for routine fertilization using immotile and possibly even acrosome-defective sperm. Moreover, enhancement of viability following assisted hatching may depend on the precise shape and size of the artificial gap in the zona pellucida. Laser-directed energy may be quite useful in this instance. We have applied a 308 ultraviolet laser beam guided through the optical system of an inverted microscope (Neeve and Tadir, unpublished results). This system has enabled us to obtain hatching blastocysts following assisted hatching using laser drilling of four- to eight-cell mouse embryos. Several four-cell mouse embryos and a single blastocyst were also obtained following pronucleus ablation of digynic mouse zygotes. Finally, blastomere biopsy of eight-cell mouse embryos was performed successfully after laser ablation of a large portion of the zona (Gonzalez and colleagues, unpublished results).

Once a DNA construct is devised and created, pronuclear injection should be a relatively straightforward procedure in the human zygote. Although an exponential expansion in gene characterization can be expected in the future, the requirements for successful gene transfer, including the correct expression and specificity of the gene, involves a precise placement of the transgene in relation to regulatory DNA sequences. It is unlikely that any attempts will be made to incorporate germ-line therapy actively into assisted human reproduction in the next decade. Too many important steps needed for reliable "gene correction" are still lacking. Obviously the ethical, social, and political dilemmas compound already complicated issues, such as the legal status of the four-cell embryo and the definition of motherhood. In a pluralistic society, unanimity on such a major issue as germ-line therapy may be beyond the ability of any secular authority. One great advantage of germ-line therapy would be that, if successful, it would terminate the heredity of a genetic lesion. A transgenically corrected genome would be theoretically passed on to future generations.

Presently the relevance of techniques involving blastomere separation and nuclear transplantation in the human seems remote. It is not only the insufficiency of our knowledge of human embryonic physiology, however, but also the complex ethics involved, which has prevented researchers in this field from applying it to the human. Although the delivery of more than an occasional twin following assisted human reproduction would be ethically questionable, there may be some acceptable application both to the treatment of infertile couples and those whose offspring may be at risk of hereditary disease. Couples with limited numbers of gametes may at any IVF attempt have only one or a few embryos for transfer. If this is due to a severe male factor infertility, it could be feasible to grow the embryo to a later stage and separate its cells. The female partner or another oocyte donor could then provide oocytes for enucleation, which could then be used as conception carriers for the diploid nuclei of the original embryo. This would then create a limited number of clones of the required genetics. Cryopreservation of anucleate oocytes would facilitate this approach. Similarly, women with few oocytes may have their embryos bisected or used in the enucleation procedure.

Surgical replacement of a diseased placenta (placenta donation) seems currently beyond the scope of obstetric medicine. Several experimental embryology techniques, however, can potentially be applied to women who suffer from recurrent idiopathic miscarriage of genetically normal fetuses.[2] Both placental and fetal tissues originate in the preimplantation embryo. Some inner cell mass cells develop into the fetus, whereas the trophectoderm provides most of the placental material. The two types of tissue can effectively be separated and recombined using two different embryos of the same or closely related species. Alternatively, transfer of a blastomere from an eight-cell to a four-cell embryo leads to a chimera in which the four-cell recipient becomes trophectoderm and the eight-cell blastomere the inner cell mass.

Acknowledgments

We are grateful to Mina Alikani, Toni A. Ferrara, Elena Kissin, Cindy Anderson, Zev Rosenwaks, Jamie Grifo, Alan Berkeley, Owen Davis, Margaret Graf, William Ledger, Myriam Feliciano, Miriam Jackson, Adrienne Reing, Alexis Adler, Janet Trowbridge, Beth Talansky, Xa-su Tang, Hung-Chung Liu, Santiago Munne, Jonathan Stein, Frederick Licciardi, Allyson Gonzalez, and Henry Malter for their support of these studies.

REFERENCES

1. Handyside AH, Kontogianni EH, Hardy K, Winston RML. Pregnancies from biopsied human preimplantation embryos sex by Y-specific DNA amplification. Nature 1990;344:378–380.
2. Cohen J, Malter HE, Talansky BE, Grifo J. Micromanipulation of human gametes and embryos. New York: Raven Press, 1992:326.
3. Gordon JW, Talansky BE. Assisted fertilization by zona drilling: a mouse model for correction of oligospermia. J Exp Zool 1986;239:347–354.
4. Laws-King A, Trounson A, Sathananthan H, Kola I. Fertilization of human oocytes by microinjection of a single spermatozoon under the zona pellucida. Fertil Steril 1987;48:637–642.
5. Surani MAH, Barton SC, Norris ML. Development of reconstituted mouse eggs suggests imprinting of the genome during gametogenesis. Nature 1984;307:548–550.
6. Cohen J, Wright G, Malter H, et al. Impairment of the hatching process following in vitro fertilization in the human and improvement of implantation by assisting hatching using micromanipulation. Hum Reprod 1990;5:7–13.
7. Verlinsky Y, Ginsberg N, Lifchez A, et al. Analysis of the first polar body: preconception genetic diagnosis. Hum Reprod 1990;5:826–829.
8. Feichtinger W, Strohmer H, Fuhrberg P, et al. Photoablation of oocyte zona pellucida by erbium-yag laser for in-vitro fertilisation in severe male infertility. Lancet 1992;1:811.
9. Cohen J, Talansky BE, Adler A, et al. Controversies and opinions in clinical microsurgical fertilization. J Assist Reprod Gen 1992;9:94–96.
10. Wiemer KE, Cohen J, Wiker SR, et al. Coculture of human zygotes on fetal bovine uterine fibroblasts: embryonic morphology and implantation. Fertil Steril 1989;52:503–506.
11. Menezo JR, Guerin JF, Czyba JC. Improvement of human early embryo development in vitro by co-culture on monolayers of Vero cells. Biol Reprod 1990;42:301–306.
12. Cohen J. Assisted hatching of human embryos. J In Vitro Fertil Embryo Trans 1991;8:179–190.
13. Cohen J, Alikani M, Trowbridge J, Rosenwaks Z. Implantation enhancement by selective assisted hatching using zona drilling of embryos with poor prognosis. Hum Reprod 1992;7:685–691.
14. Cohen J, Malter H, Wright G, et al. Partial zona dissection of human oocytes when failure of zona pellucida penetration is anticipated. Hum Reprod 1989;4:435–442.
15. Fishel S, Jackson P, Antinori S, et al. Subzonal insemination for the alleviation of infertility. Fertil Steril 1990;54:828–833.
16. Cohen J, Alikani M, Malter HE, et al. Partial zona dissection or subzonal insertion: microsurgical fertilization alternatives based on evaluation of sperm and embryo morphology. Fertil Steril 1991;56:696–706.
17. Ng S-C, Bongso A, Ratnam SS. Microinjection of human oocytes: a technique for severe oligoasthenoteratozoospermia. Fertil Steril 1991;56:1117–1123.
18. Hosoi Y, Miyake M, Utsumi K, Iritani A. Development of rabbit oocytes after microinjection of spermatozoa. In Proceedings of the 11th Congress on Animal Reproduction, Abstract 331, 1988.
19. Goto K, Kinoshita A, Takuma Y, Ogawa A. Birth of calves after the transfers of oocytes fertilized by sperm injection. Theriogenology 1991;35:205–221.
19a. van Steirteghem AC, Liu J, Joris H, et al. Higher success rate by intracytoplasmic sperm injection than by subzonal insemination: report of a second series of 300 consecutive treament cycles. Hum Reprod 1993;8:1055–1060.
20. Santella L, Alikani M, Cohen J, et al. Is the human oocyte plasma membrane polarised? Hum Reprod 1992;7:992–1003.
21. Malter HE, Cohen J. Partial zona dissection of the human oocyte: a nontraumatic method using micromanipulation to assist zona pellucida penetration. Fertil Steril 1989;51:139–145.
22. Garrisi GJ, Talansky BE, Grunfeld L, et al. Clinical evaluation of three approachs to micromanipulation-assisted fertilization. Fertil Steril 1990;54:671–677.
23. Cohen J, Elsner C, Kort H, et al. Immunosuppression supports implantation of zona pellucida dissected human embryos. Fertil Steril 1990;53:662–665.
24. Cohen J, Adler A, Alikani M, et al. Microsurgical fertilization procedures: absence of stringent criteria for patient selection. J Assist Reprod Genet 1992;9:197–206.
25. Alikani M, Adler A, Reing AM, et al. Subzonal sperm insertion and the frequency of gamete fusion. J Assist Reprod Gen 1992;9:97–101.
26. Fishel S, Timson J, Lisi F, Rinaldi L. Evaluation of 225 patients undergoing subzonal insemination for the procurement of fertilization in vitro. Fertil Steril 1992;57:840–849.
27. Kruger TF, Acosta AA, Simmons KF, et al. Predictive value of abnormal sperm morphology in in vitro fertilization. Fertil Steril 1988;49:112–121.
28. Yovich JM, Edirisinghe WR, Cummins JM, Yovich JL. Preliminary results using pentoxifylline in a pronuclear stage tubal transfer (PROST) program for severe male factor infertility. Fertil Steril 1988;50:179–181.
29. Fuscaldo G, Sobieszczuk D, Trounson AO. Improved fertilization rates following microinjection of human spermatozoa pretreated with 2′deoxyadenosine and pentoxyfylline. Presented at 7th World Congress on IVF and Assisted Procreation, Abstract 110, 1991:145.
30. Alikani M, Adler A, Kissin E, et al. The use of pentoxyfylline and 2′deoxyadenosine in microsurgically assisted fertilization improves fertilization but reduces implantation. Unpublished.
31. Gordon JW, Grunfeld L, Garrisi GJ, et al. Fertilization of human oocytes by sperm from infertile males after zona drilling. Fertil Steril 1988;50:68–73.
32. McGrath J, Solter D. Nuclear transplantation in the mouse embryo by microsurgery and cell fusion. Science 1983;220:1300–1302.
33. Willadsen S. Nuclear transplantation in sheep embryos. Nature 1986;320:63–65.
34. Rawlins RG, Binor Z, Radwanska E, Dmowski WP. Microsurgical enucleation of tripronuclear human zygotes. Fertil Steril 1988;50:266–272.
35. Gordon JW, Grunfeld L, Garrisi GJ, et al. Successful microsurgical removal of a pronucleus from tripronuclear human zygotes. Fertil Steril 1989;52:367–372.
36. Malter HE, Cohen J. Embryonic development after microsurgical repair of polyspermic human zygotes. Fertil Steril 1989;52:373–380.
37. Wiker S, Malter H, Wright G, Cohen J. Recognition of paternal pronuclei in human zygotes. J In Vitro Fertil Embr Trans 1990;7:33–37.
38. Collier M, O'Neill C, Ammit AJ, Saunders DM. Measurement of human embryo-derived platelet-activating factor (PAF) using a quantitative bioassay of platelet aggregation. Hum Reprod 1990;5:323–328.
39. Bongso A, Soon-Chye N, Sathananthan H, et al. Improved quality of human embryos when co-cultured with human ampullary cells. Hum Reprod 1989;4:706–713.
40. Cohen J, Inge KL, Suzman M, et al. Videocinematography of fresh and cryopreserved embryos: a retrospective analysis of embryonic morphology and implantation. Fertil Steril 1989;51:820–827.
41. Wright G, Wiker S, Elsner C, et al. Observations on the morphology of human zygotes, pronuclei and nucleoli and implications for cryopreservation. Hum Reprod 1990;5:109–115.
42. Malter HE, Cohen J. Blastocyst formation and hatching in vitro following zona drilling of mouse and human embryos. Gam Res 1989;24:67–80.
43. Cohen J, Feldberg D. Effects of the size and number of zona pellucida openings on hatching and trophoblast outgrowth in the mouse embryo. Molec Reprod Dev 1991;30:70–78.
44. Dale B, Gualtieri R, Talevi R, et al. Intercellular communication in the early human embryo. Molec Reprod Dev 1991;29:22–28.
45. Cohen J, Alikani M, Reing AM, et al. Selective assisted hatching of human embryos. Ann Acad Med Singapore 1992;21:565–570.
46. Talansky BE, Gordon JW. Cleavage characteristics of mouse embryos inseminated and cultured after zona drilling. Gam Res 1988;21:277–288.
47. Alikani M, Cohen J. Micromanipulation of cleaved embryos cultured in protein-free medium: a mouse-model for assisted hatching. J Exp Zool 1992;263:458–463.
48. Khalifa EAM, Tucker MJ. Partial thinning of the zona pellucida for more successful enhancement of blastocyst hatching in the mouse. Hum Reprod 1992;7:532–536.
49. Cohen J, Malter H, Talansky B, et al. Gamete and embryo micromanipulation for infertility treatment. Semin Reprod Endocrinol 1990;8:290–295.
50. Bleil JD, Wassarman PM. Structure and function of the zona pellucida: identification and characterization of mouse oocyte's zona pellucida. Dev Biol 1980;76:185–203.
51. Drobnis EZ, Andrew JB, Katz DF. Biophysical properties of the zona pellucida measured by capillary suction: is zona hardening a mechanical phenomenon? J Exp Zool 1988;245:206–219.

52. DeFelici M, Siracusa G. "Spontaneous" hardening of the zona pellucida of mouse oocytes during in vitro culture. Gamete Res 1982;6:107–113.

53. Downs SM, Schroeder AC, Eppig JJ. Serum maintains the fertilizability of mouse oocytes matured in vitro by preventing hardening of the zona pellucida. Gamete Res 1986;15:115–122.

54. Longo FJ. Changes in the zonae pellucidae and plasmalemmae of aging mouse eggs. Biol Reprod 1981;25:399–411.

55. Austin CR: The Mammalian Egg. Oxford: Blackwell Scientific Publications, 1961:89–97.

56. Gwatkin RBL: Fertilization mechanisms in man and mammals. New York: Plenum Press, 1977:91–108.

57. Betteridge KJ, Flood PF, Mitchell P. Possible role of the embryo in the control of oviductal transport in mares. *In:* Harper MJK, Pauerstein CJ, Adams CE, editors. Ovum Transport and Fertility Regulation. Copenhagen: Scriptor, 1976:381–389.

58. Tadir Y, Wright WH, Vafa O, et al. Micromanipulation of gametes using laser microbeams. Hum Reprod 1991;6:1011–1016.

CHAPTER 58

In Vitro Fertilization and Preimplantation Genetic Diagnosis for Prevention of Inherited Disease

ALAN H. HANDYSIDE

Inherited disease is a significant cause of illness and mortality in infants. The overall incidence at birth, including those resulting from chromosomal abnormalities and single gene defects, is about 1% to 3%.[1] Although most single gene defects are rare, close to 5000 have now been identified,[2] and together they account for a significant proportion of inherited disease. Treatment is possible in a few cases, for example, by replacement of clotting factors in hemophiliacs. Because of the nature of genetic disease, however, therapies are generally only partially successful, and others alleviate only some consequences of the genetic lesion. For some severe single gene defects, efforts are being made to develop methods for somatic gene therapy, that is, the replacement of normal gene function in the somatic cells of affected individuals. A promising example of this is the possibility of using aerosol sprays to deliver vectors with the normal gene to the lungs of patients affected by cystic fibrosis (CF).[3] Other diseases in which somatic gene therapy may be possible are those in which the defect can be corrected by alteration of blood cells temporarily removed for transfection with the normal gene. These include adenine deaminase deficiency, which causes severe combined immunodeficiency syndrome and is normally lethal within weeks of birth. For many diseases affecting the nervous system or musculature, however, somatic gene therapy is difficult because of the inaccessibility of these tissues. For inherited disease in general, therefore, the emphasis remains on prevention by diagnosis as early as possible in pregnancy.

Current methods of prenatal diagnosis involve sampling cells of fetal origin, for example, by amniocentesis in the second trimester or chorion villus sampling (CVS) in the first trimester of pregnancy and use of cytogenetic, biochemical, or DNA methods to detect the genetic defect. If the pregnancy is affected, however, couples face the difficult decision of whether to terminate the pregnancy, and some have re-

peated terminations before establishing a normal pregnancy. Diagnosis at preimplantation stages of embryonic development, or preimplantation diagnosis, makes it possible to transfer only unaffected embryos to the uterus so that any pregnancy should be unaffected by the disease.[4, 5] This avoids the possibility of a termination following diagnosis at later stages of pregnancy and is the primary reason for couples requesting preimplantation genetic diagnosis. Religious or ethical objections to prenatal diagnosis at later stages of pregnancy, a history of repeated terminations of affected pregnancies, and miscarriage resulting from CVS or amniocentesis, however, may also contribute to their decision.

IN VITRO FERTILIZATION AND PREIMPLANTATION GENETIC DIAGNOSIS

The least invasive approach to recovering preimplantation embryos for genetic diagnosis would be to flush embryos from the female reproductive tract at the appropriate time after normal conception in vivo. Following ovulation and fertilization in the ampullary region of the fallopian tube, the zygote undergoes a number of cleavage divisions and by day 5 postfertilization reaches the uterus. At this stage, the embryo forms a blastocyst with an outer epithelial layer of trophectoderm cells specialized for attachment and implantation surrounding an inner cell mass (ICM) from which the fetus is later derived. Human blastocysts have been flushed from the uterus by uterine lavage for donation to infertile women.[6, 7] These studies were performed in natural cycles. The problem with uterine lavage, however, is the possibility of flushing an embryo into the fallopian tube, causing an ectopic pregnancy, or of leaving a potentially affected embryo in the uterus. Also the recovery of embryos following superovulation, which would increase the efficiency of genetic screening, has been disappointing.[8]

The alternative to flushing embryos conceived in vivo is to use the methods of superovulation, in vitro fertilization (IVF), and embryo culture and transfer developed over the last 10 years for the treatment of infertility. Although national average pregnancy rates following IVF in infertile couples remain rather low, the use of gonadotropin-releasing hormone (GnRH) agonists and other improvements have resulted in a gradual improvement. In larger, more experienced centers, clinical pregnancy rates per embryo transfer now approach 35% to 40%,[9, 10] and in fertile couples the rates are likely to be higher. IVF has other advantages, too. Access to several embryos in a single reproductive cycle improves the chance of identifying unaffected embryos for transfer. Although several IVF attempts may be necessary, the time taken to establish a normal pregnancy is likely to be relatively short. This is an important consideration for some couples, who may have had a number of terminations of affected pregnancies over a period of years.

PREIMPLANTATION EMBRYO BIOPSY

Preimplantation genetic diagnosis requires one or more cells to be removed, or biopsied, from each embryo for genetic analysis (Fig. 58–1). Biopsy of some of the outer trophectoderm cells at the blastocyst stage has a number of advantages. These include the possibility of removing larger numbers of cells than at earlier stages and the avoidance of any interference with the ICM from which the fetus is derived. Only about half of normally fertilized embryos, however, reach this stage in vitro,[10] and only about half of these could be successfully biopsied.[11] The likelihood of identifying a significant number of unaffected embryos for transfer, therefore, would be significantly reduced. Also, pregnancy rates after blastocyst transfer are, at best, only a little more successful than earlier transfers at cleavage stages.[12]

An alternative is to biopsy embryos at earlier cleavage stages, at a time when transfers are normally carried out, even though this restricts the number of cells that can be biopsied. During cleavage, there is no cellular growth, and each division subdivides the embryo into successively smaller cells. At early cleavage stages, each cell of the mammalian embryo retains the ability to contribute to all of the tissues of the conceptus, and, under appropriate circumstances, even single cells have produced normal offspring after transfer.[13] Thus the embryo is able to compensate for the reduced cellular mass, and postimplantation development is not affected. The human embryo apparently has a similar capability; many embryos transferred after IVF are partially fragmented or degenerate, and no substantial increase in abnormalities has been reported. The first pregnancy following embryo cryopreservation involved the transfer of a cleavage-stage embryo in which only five of the eight cells survived after thawing.[14]

To minimize the reduction in cellular mass, embryos are biopsied on the morning of day 3, when most have reached the 6- to 10-cell stage. If the stimulation cycle has been successful, there are an average of five or six fertilized embryos at this stage, and these can be biopsied within 1 to 2 hours. This leaves 8 to a maximum of 12 hours for genetic analysis before selected embryos are transferred later on the same day. Because of the small size of the preimplantation embryo (about 140 μm in diameter), micromanipulators are used for biopsy (Fig. 58–2).

A number of different techniques have been explored for cleavage-stage biopsy with animal and human embryos.[15] The approach that has been most successful to date is to drill a hole in the zona pellucida with acidified medium[16] and simply aspirate one cell at a time into a micropipette (Fig. 58–3). This involves removing any adherent cumulus cells from the zona before the procedure and placing embryos one at a time in drops of air-buffered medium under silicone oil and immobilizing them with a flame-polished holding pipette controlled by one of the manipulators. A fine pipette containing the acidified medium is then brought into contact with the outer surface of the zona and a steady stream of the medium expelled until the zona in that area dissolves and allows penetration with the pipette. After the zona is dis-

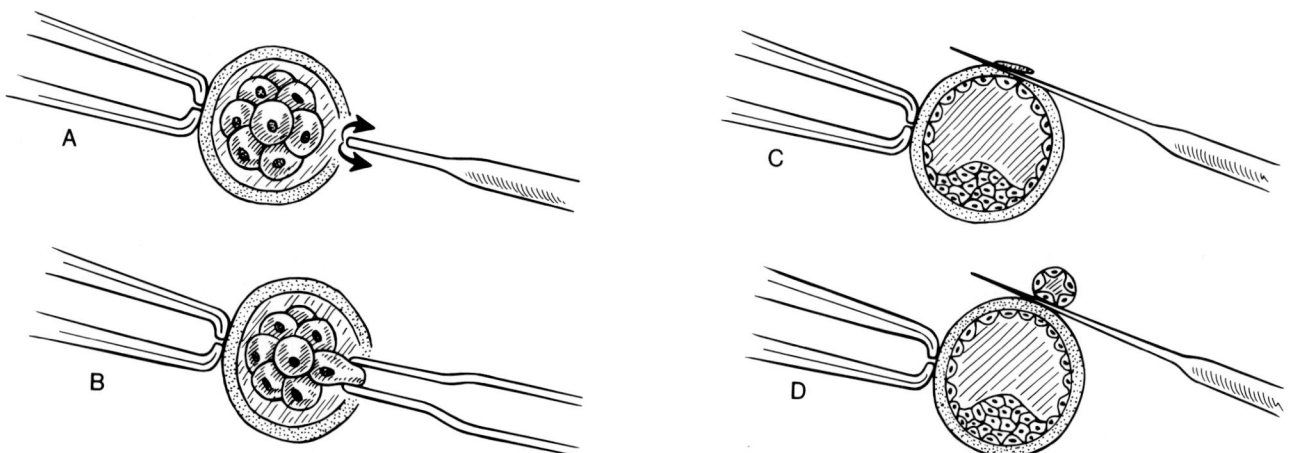

FIGURE 58–1. Methods for securing a biopsy of human preimplantation embryos. *Cleavage-stage biopsy:* A, The embryo is immobilized on a flame-polished holding pipette, and a hole is drilled in the zona pellucida by applying a fine stream of acidified medium. B, A second, larger micropipette is pushed through the hole, and a cell is aspirated. *Blastocyst biopsy:* C, A slit is made in the zona pellucida by piercing it with a microneedle and rubbing it against the holding pipette. D, After overnight culture, the outer trophectoderm layer of the blastocyst expands through fluid accumulation and herniates through the slit in the zona, allowing these cells to be excised with a microneedle. (A to C adapted from Handyside A. Preimplantation diagnosis. Curr Obstet Gynecol 1992;2:85–90.)

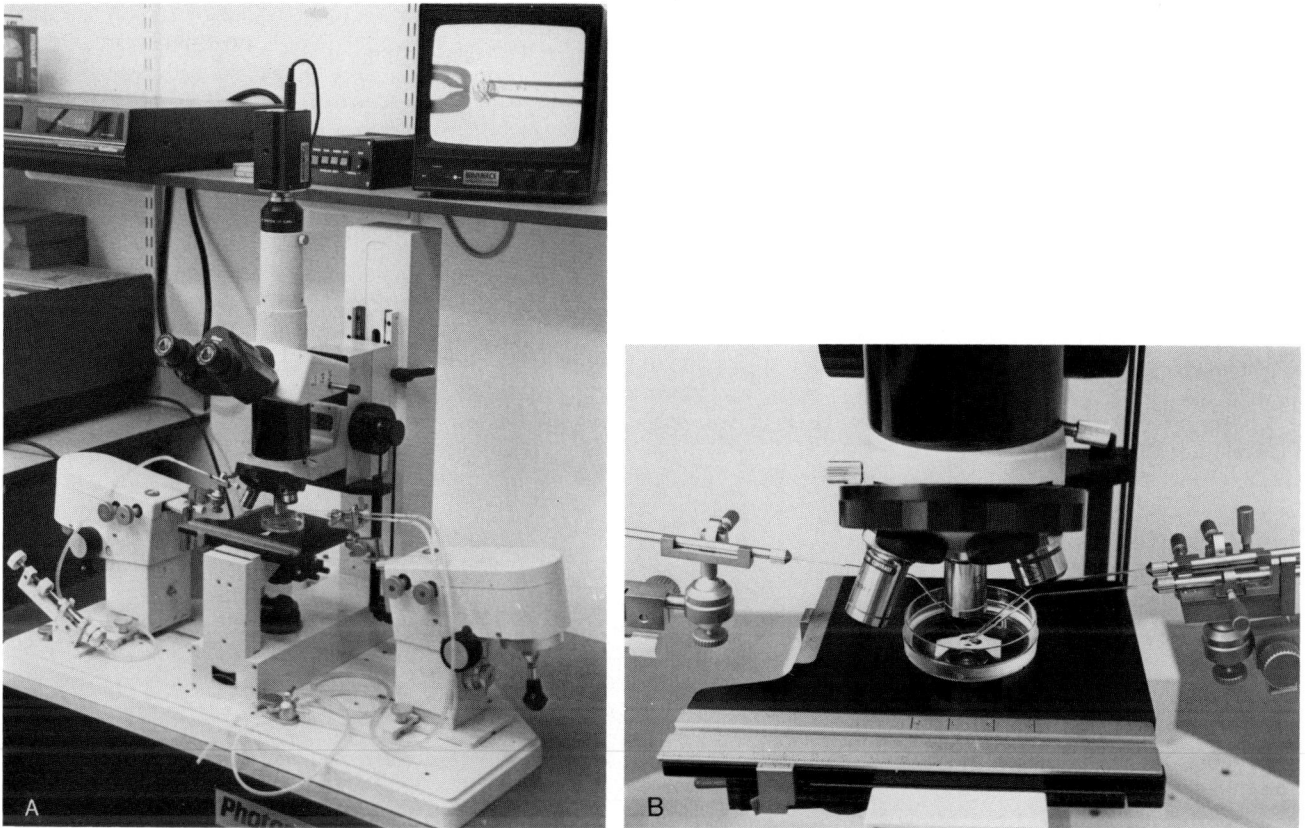

FIGURE 58–2. Typical micromanipulation setup for cleavage-stage biopsy. The micromanipulator on the left is used to control the holding pipette, and the other on the right through a double holder is used to control both the zona drilling pipette and the aspiration pipette. Note that the manipulators have been tilted toward the dish containing the embryos in drops under a layer of oil to lower the microinstruments into position. A syringe on the left is used for suction in the holding pipette, and a mouth pipette is directed through a two-way tap used to control the drilling and aspiration.

solved, the flow of medium is immediately stopped, the pipette moved away, and a second larger, polished pipette pushed through the hole to make contact with the cell to be removed. (Both of these pipettes are controlled by a second manipulator placed opposite the one with the holding pipette.) The internal diameter of the biopsy pipette should be just less than that of the cell to prevent uncontrolled suction. This pipette is moved back gradually as the cell is aspirated and comes free of the rest of the embryo. The aspirated cell is expelled into the drop and examined carefully to check that it has a visible interphase nucleus. The embryo is then released from the holding pipette. The dish with the biopsied embryo and the single cell that has been removed is returned to the incubator to continue in culture. A certain proportion of cleavage-stage embryos are compacting at this time, that is, intercellular adhesiveness and junction formation are beginning before blastocyst formation. For this reason, micromanipulation is carried out at room temperature, which appears to counteract this process to a limited extent.

Techniques for genetic analysis are now accurate enough, in some cases, for a diagnosis to be made on one cell. For a variety of reasons, however, it may be preferable to sample at least two cells for duplicate analysis. Using this method for cleavage-stage biopsy, removal of one or two cells at the eight-cell stage did not adversely affect preimplantation development to the blastocyst stage.[17] Alternatively, it may be possible to culture the isolated cell and increase the numbers for analysis by cell division.[18] Selected biopsied embryos

would then have to be transferred at a more advanced stage of development after a corresponding period in culture. As already discussed, however, the proportion of embryos that develop to the blastocyst stage *in vitro* is low, and pregnancy rates after transfer at this stage are no better than at cleavage stages. The only other option would be to cryopreserve the embryos immediately after biopsy and transfer selected embryos in a later cycle. Although biopsied mouse embryos have been cryopreserved successfully and developed to advanced fetal stages after thawing and transfer to recipients,[19] the human embryo is more susceptible, and partial removal of the protective zona is likely to increase damage to the remaining cells.

DETECTION OF GENETIC DEFECTS

The time and numbers of cells available for genetic analysis place severe restrictions on the diagnostic methods that can be used. Two techniques especially have made this possible. For chromosomal abnormalities, fluorescent detection of in situ hybridization (FISH) with chromosome-specific DNA probes is both sensitive and rapid and can be used for cytogenetic analysis of interphase nuclei.[20] Also, multicolored fluorescence can be used for the simultaneous detection of several probes,[21] and mixtures of short DNA probes for a particular chromosome or chromosomal region can be used for *chromosomal painting* and detection of various transloca-

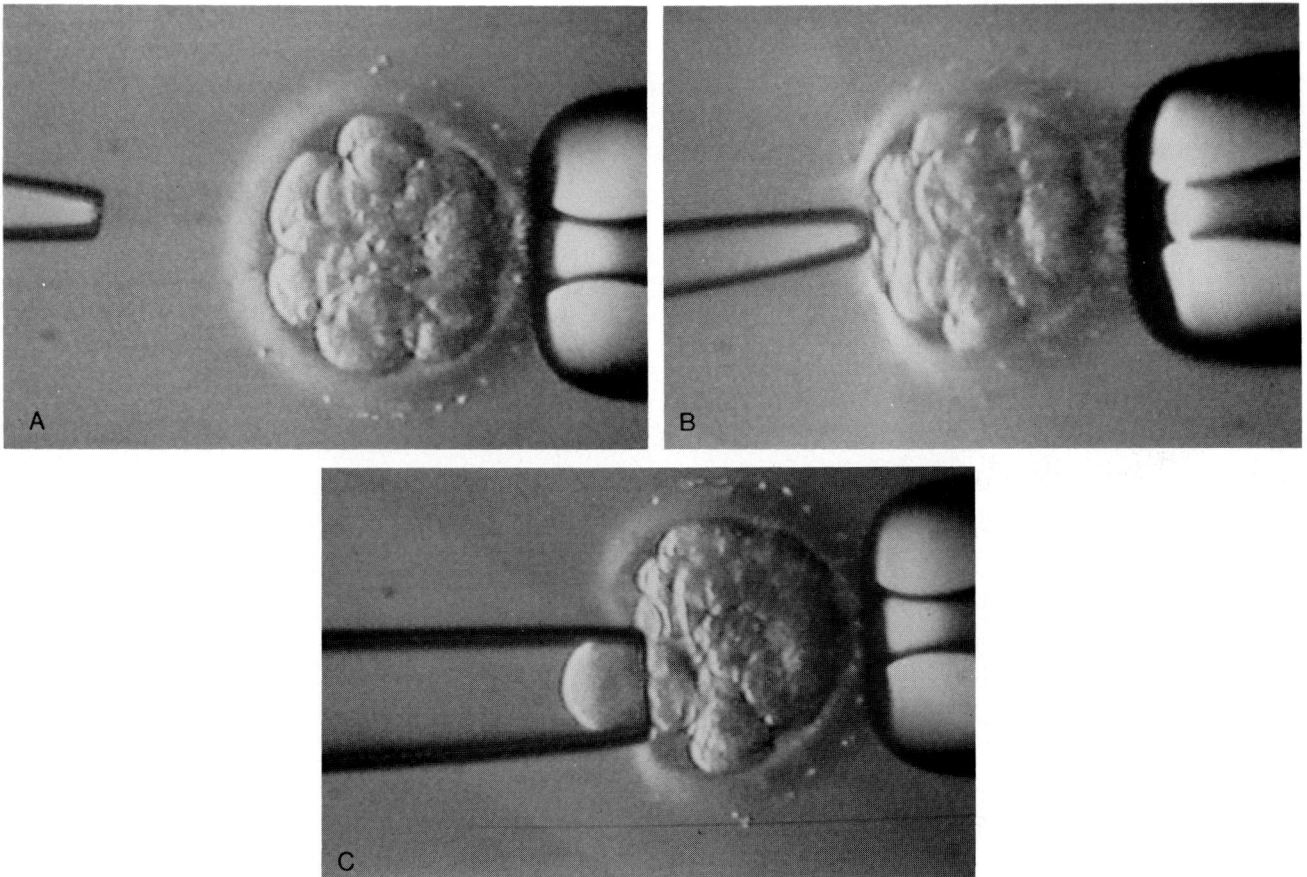

FIGURE 58–3. Cleavage-stage biopsy of a 12-cell polyspermic human embryo on day 3. The embryo was immobilized on a flame-polished holding pipette (*A*), and a fine micropipette was used to drill a hole in the zona pellucida with a stream of acidified medium (*B*). Finally, a second larger micropipette was pushed through the hole in the zona and a single cell was aspirated (*C*). Note that the nucleus of the cell biopsy is visible in this case. Photographs are from a video recording. (*A* to *C* from Handyside AH, Delhanty JDA. Cleavage-stage biopsy of human embryos and diagnosis of X-linked recessive disease. In: Edwards RG, editor. Preimplantation diagnosis of human genetic disease. Cambridge: Cambridge University Press, 1993.)

tions and other structural abnormalities.[22] For single gene defects, the polymerase chain reaction (PCR) enables amplification of short fragments of DNA over a millionfold within a few hours, making it possible to detect even single base changes in the DNA of single cells.[23]

Chromosomal Abnormalities

Chromosomal abnormalities, especially abnormalities of chromosome number, are a major cause of genetic disease with a frequency at birth of about 0.5%.[24] The incidence of these abnormalities has been extensively studied in human oocytes and preimplantation embryos following IVF.[25–27] As a model for preimplantation diagnosis, biopsy and karyotyping have been achieved in mouse embryos.[28, 29] Also a robertsonian translocation resulting in embryos with trisomy 16 (the mouse equivalent of Down syndrome) was accurately identified before transfer.[30] The problems of spreading chromosomes, however, and a tendency for the chromosomes to be too short for banding have so far prevented reliable karyotyping of human embryo nuclei by standard procedures.

FISH has been successfully applied for analysis of both human oocytes and preimplantation embryos with chromosome-specific DNA probes.[31, 32] The possibility of using several chromosome-specific probes simultaneously by multicolored fluorescence raises the possibility of screening the embryos of older women for the common trisomies.[32] Indeed, dual FISH for the simultaneous detection of the X and Y chromosomes is already possible.[33] The most frequent autosomal trisomies found during prenatal screening are 21, 18, and 13, and their incidence rises significantly in women over the age of 35. Each of these trisomies is compatible with development to term but more often results in late abortions or perinatal death. If these could be screened in combination with trisomy 16, the most frequent autosomal trisomy in abortuses, not only would this prevent the birth of a trisomic individual, but also reduce the risk of miscarriage, which is significantly increased in women over 40.[34]

The use of FISH for preimplantation diagnosis of aneuploidy has been evaluated with a probe specific for the centromeric region of chromosome 18.[35] Most nuclei in embryos between the two-cell and blastocyst stages had the expected diploid number of two signals. A significant number of tetraploid nuclei with four hybridization signals, however, were also present. These may represent precursors of polyploid trophectoderm cells.[36] One in 59 embryos examined was apparently trisomic for chromosome 18, although the possibility that the embryo was triploid cannot be excluded. The variability in the numbers of signals and the presence of tetraploid cells, however, indicate that diagnosis of aneuploidy is unlikely to be sufficiently reliable with the numbers of cells available after cleavage-stage biopsy. Combined detection with several probes would distinguish aneuploid and polyploid nuclei but may also increase chromosome overlap and reduce the efficiency of detection.

Another potential application for FISH is in detecting trisomies in embryos that inherit a translocation chromosome from one of the parents. Couples in which one partner is carrying a balanced translocation and who have a history of miscarriage with a trisomic conceptus are known to be at high risk (in some cases 50%) of having another affected pregnancy. In these cases, preimplantation diagnosis has the positive advantage of screening several embryos in a single reproductive cycle. Analysis of metaphase preparations, however, and the use of chromosome painting may be necessary in many cases depending on the nature of the translocation.

Single Gene Defects

Couples at risk of having children affected by single gene defects are generally only made aware of the risk by having a child or relative diagnosed with the disease. It may soon be possible, however, to screen populations or at least prospective parents for a range of common mutations: for example, screen for the gene defect that causes CF and warn affected parents of the risks before they have any affected children. Although many single gene defects are rare, in couples known to be at risk, the chance of having an affected child is often as high as 1 in 4 or 1 in 2, depending on whether the condition is dominant or recessive (Fig. 58–4).

X-LINKED RECESSIVE DISEASE

X-linked recessive diseases are caused by defects on the X chromosome. In general, women carrying a defect on only one of their X chromosomes are unaffected because the normal gene on the other chromosome compensates for the deficiency. Boys who inherit an X-linked defect are affected because, in contrast to homologous pairs of autosomes, the Y chromosome codes only for a small proportion of the genes on the X chromosome. Women carriers, therefore, have a 1 in 4 risk of having an affected boy. Approximately 300 X-linked recessive conditions have been described, and together they account for 6% to 7% of all single gene defects.[2] The most frequent of these diseases is Duchenne muscular dystrophy (DMD), which affects 1 in 3500 males. DMD is caused by defects, often large deletions, in the dystrophin gene.[37] In these cases, prenatal diagnosis of affected males is possible by multiplex amplification of frequently deleted exons.[38] Other X-linked defects are not so well characterized, and identifying the sex is the only alternative. For preimplantation diagnosis, this approach has the advantage that it is equally applicable to all of these conditions and does not require detailed information about the genetic defect in each family.

The sex of human embryos can be identified from single cells biopsied at cleavage stages by amplification of Y-specific repeat sequences.[39] Using this approach, several pregnancies, including two sets of twins, were established in couples at risk of a variety of X-linked conditions,[40] and several apparently healthy girls were born.[41] Following CVS and karyotyping, however, one singleton was discovered to be male and that pregnancy was terminated. The reason for this error was probably amplification failure of the Y-specific repeat, which can occur with amplification of unique sequences from a small proportion of single cells.[42] Amplification of Y-specific repeats from each cell of disaggregated embryos has since demonstrated that amplification failure can occur in up to 15% of male blastomeres.[43] The lack of any correlation with the number of target sequences present suggests that the preparation of cells for PCR may be critical. Support for this

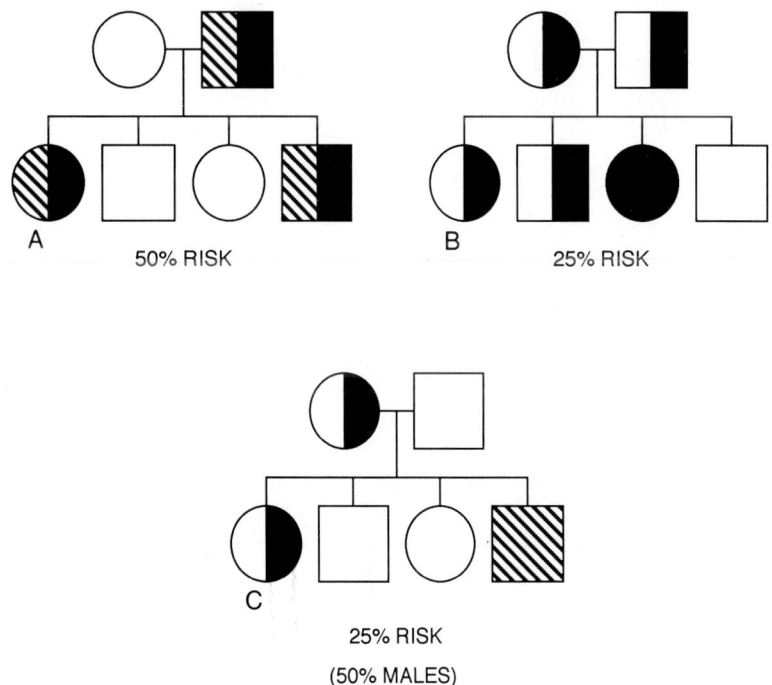

A   50% RISK

B   25% RISK

C   25% RISK
(50% MALES)

FIGURE 58–4. Some examples of simple Mendelian inheritance patterns for single gene defects illustrating the high risk of having affected children. *A, Autosomal dominant:* Half the children of affected carriers married to unaffected partners will be affected. *B, Autosomal recessive:* Unaffected carriers will only have affected children if they marry a partner also carrying the defect, in which case half the children will also be unaffected carriers and one fourth will be affected. *C, X-linked recessive:* These disorders caused by defective genes on the female X chromosome are often lethal in affected males and are transmitted by unaffected female carriers. Half the male children of an unaffected female carrier married to a normal male will be affected, and half the females will be unaffected carriers. *Circles* and *squares* represent females and males, respectively. *Open symbols* represent normal persons, *filled symbols* affected homozygotes, *half-filled symbols* unaffected heterozygotes, and *half-filled cross-hatched symbols* affected heterozygotes. (*A* to *C* adapted from Handyside A. Preimplantation diagnosis. Curr Obstet Gynecol 1992;2:85–90.)

FIGURE 58–5. Preimplantation diagnosis of the predominant deletion (ΔF508) causing cystic fibrosis by polyacrylamide gel electrophoresis of the amplification products from single cells of a biopsy sample from cleavage-stage embryos. For rapid analysis, previously amplified deoxyribonucleic acid (DNA) from normal and affected cells is mixed with the DNA amplified from the cell of unknown genotype, denatured and slowly cooled. Under these conditions, if a mixture contains fragments of different lengths (both normal and with the 3 bp deletion), heteroduplexes are formed that are significantly retarded in their migration in the gel. This allows the diagnosis of normal, carrier, and affected embryos by the detection of the heteroduplex band in one or both mixtures and is more reliable than attempting to discriminate the fragment lengths directly. In this case, single cells were obtained by biopsy from six cleavage-stage embryos in a couple, both of whom carry the ΔF508 deletion. The *asterisks* denote the cells from embryos that were later transferred to the uterus; implantation of the second embryo produced an unaffected girl. NN, homozygous normal; No Amp, no amplitude; NΔ, heterozygous carrier; ΔΔ, homozygous for deletion (affected by cystic fibrosis). (Reprinted with permission from The New England Journal of Medicine; 327:905–909, 1992.)

concept is the demonstration that the use of a lysis buffer originally described for amplification from single sperm[44] reduces, although does not eliminate, amplification failure.[45]

Another strategy for identifying sex by PCR is to control for amplification failure by coamplifying fragments specific for both the X and Y chromosomes using two sets of primers.[43] This is not ideal because there is a theoretical possibility that because of the different characteristics of the two sets of primers, amplification failure with either set could occur independently. A study on a large series of single cells, however, has demonstrated that, with a particular combination of primers and PCR conditions, either amplification fails completely from both primer sets, or amplification of both X- and Y-specific repeat sequences occurs in male cells, resulting in an accurate diagnosis.[46] To achieve this level of coamplification, however, the PCR conditions are necessarily a compromise between the optima for the two primer pairs, and the overall amplification efficiency is lower than the level achieved with amplification of single target sequences (80%). A singleton pregnancy has been established following transfer of a female embryo identified by coamplification of X and Y alphoid sequences in a couple at risk for hemophilia A.[47]

Alternatively, it is now possible to amplify target sequences present on both X and Y chromosomes with the same set of primers in situations in which the amplified fragment(s) either are of a different size or have different restriction sites that allow rapid analysis postamplification. One of these involves amplifying a region of the amelogenin gene.[48, 49] At the single cell level, however, amplification efficiency was low, and coamplification with a Y-specific repeat was necessary.[50] Another homologous sequence on the X and Y chromosomes, in this case in the ZFX/ZFY genes, can also be used for sexing because the male sequence has a unique restriction site.[51] Amplification efficiency of this sequence is almost 100% in control cells and high with single blastomeres from cleavage-stage human embryos.

In situ hybridization with X- and Y-specific DNA probes can also be used for identifying the sex of each embryo and has the advantage that precautions against contamination are not necessary. A rapid dual FISH protocol has been described.[32, 33] The strength of this approach lies in the simultaneous detection with both probes using different-colored fluorescence. This avoids potential errors owing to, for example, hybridization failure with the Y probe alone or, conversely, with the X probe used alone if the nucleus is tetraploid. Only if two X signals or one X and one Y signal is detected with dual FISH is the sex confidently predicted to be female or male. Several pregnancies have been established and one normal female born.[52]

SPECIFIC DIAGNOSIS OF SINGLE GENE DEFECTS

Initially, attempts at specific diagnosis are being directed at prevalent single gene defects and especially those that are predominantly caused by one or a limited number of mutations in the genes involved using PCR to amplify a fragment of DNA containing the defective sequence.[53] Examples include sickle cell anemia, which is caused by a single base change in the β-globin gene,[54] and CF, which is carried by 1 in 20 of the white population and is caused in most cases by a 3 base pair deletion at position ΔF508 of the CF transmembrane regulator (CFTR) gene.[55] The reason for targeting these specific defects is that many other single gene defects, notably the hemoglobinopathies, are caused by heterogeneous mutations that would have to be first identified in each family before attempting to amplify the affected region of the gene.

Several groups have now succeeded in amplifying fragments of the CFTR gene encompassing the ΔF508 deletion from a variety of single cells, including haploid sperm,[56] first polar bodies biopsied from oocytes,[57] and single blastomeres biopsied from cleavage-stage embryos.[58] The deletion is then detected by heteroduplex formation, that is, the formation of double-stranded DNA from a normal single strand and a deleted single strand, and gel electrophoresis (Fig. 58–5). Because migration of the heteroduplex is significantly retarded, the genotype of the cell can be deduced from the presence or absence of the heteroduplex bands in various mixtures with amplified fragments from homozygous normal or affected cells. Use of a second round of amplification with "nested" primers, that is, primers annealing within the sequence of the first amplified fragment, significantly increases the yield of amplified product. Also, amplification from single cells is efficient, and following heteroduplex formation, the diagnosis (analyzed blind) in a substantial series of cells of various genotypes has always been accurate.[59]

Preimplantation diagnosis has been attempted in three couples in which both parents carry the predominant ΔF508 deletion.[60] Cleavage-stage embryos were biopsied on the third day postinsemination and one cell removed from each for PCR analysis. One couple had only two embryos; diagnosis failed with one of the embryos and the other was affected so, neither of the embryos was transferred. With the other two couples, unaffected, carrier, and affected embryos were identified and one unaffected and one carrier transferred later the same day (see Fig. 58–5). One of the women became pregnant and has subsequently delivered a healthy girl, free of both alleles with the deletion.

For the specific diagnosis of single gene defects in general, especially those caused by heterogeneous defects, linkage analysis with combinations of closely linked markers would be more universally applicable and avoid the effort involved in defining the exact nature of the genetic defect in each family. Primer extension preamplification allows fragments from throughout the genome to be amplified from single cells.[61] Primer extension preamplification appears to be efficient with single blastomeres from cleavage-stage human embryos and should facilitate analysis of multiple linked markers, such as polymorphic short tandem repeats in diseases such as DMD.[62]

CLINICAL APPLICATION OF PREIMPLANTATION GENETIC DIAGNOSIS

Clinical experience with preimplantation genetic diagnosis is still limited, and it is premature to consider it as an established procedure.[63] A preliminary evaluation of our experience over a 3-year period (1989 to 1992), however, is encouraging.[64] Twenty-five couples known to be at risk of having children with a variety of single gene defects have been treated: (1) 18 couples at risk of X-linked recessive diseases, in which attempts were made to sex embryos and identify unaffected female embryos for transfer, and (2) seven couples in which detection of the specific genetic defect was attempted. In this latter group, five couples are at risk for CF because both partners carry the predominant ΔF508 deletion of the CF transmembrane regulator gene, and two couples are at risk of the X-linked recessive disease Lesch-Nyhan syndrome because the women carry different mutations in the hypoxanthine phosphoribosyltransferase gene.

Forty-two of 46 cycles (91%) in which oocytes were collected resulted in normally fertilized embryos for cleavage-stage biopsy on the second or third day post-IVF. In 36 of these cycles (86%), at least one embryo was identified as unaffected and transferred. Nine clinical pregnancies, including two sets of twins, have been established: Five have delivered, one was terminated because of misidentification of a male fetus as female, one miscarried, and two are ongoing. Pregnancy rates in this group of fertile women were therefore 20% (per egg collection) or 25% (per embryo transfer). This is similar to rates achieved with infertile couples. Of the 36 embryo transfers, eight of the pregnancies resulted from 22 transfers of two embryos (36%), whereas only one pregnancy has resulted from 14 transfers of single embryos (7%). An important factor to emerge from this preliminary experience is that high levels of efficiency are necessary at every stage to identify two unaffected embryos if possible and provide reasonable prospects of establishing a pregnancy following IVF and genetic diagnosis.

The viability of preimplantation diagnosis in relation to other methods of prenatal diagnosis largely depends on pregnancy rates, accuracy of diagnosis, and cost. Current pregnancy rates are similar to those for infertile couples, but many of these women with genetic problems were older. With younger women, pregnancy rates could be significantly higher. It is clearly too early to evaluate the accuracy of diagnosis; there have already been a number of misdiagnoses for various reasons. The main problem is not with the methods being developed for single cell analysis per se but with the human preimplantation embryo, which has a range of abnormalities that could potentially complicate genetic analysis. These include nuclear abnormalities[65] and chromosomal mosaicism.[66] It is essential that research continue with embryos donated by patients giving informed consent to assess these problems before preimplantation genetic diagnosis becomes widespread as a routine procedure. Finally the cost of IVF and the additional procedures of embryo biopsy and genetic analysis may be prohibitive, especially when compared with CVS or amniocentesis. If safe procedures can be developed for uterine lavage, however, the costs should be less, and this might help to make the preimplantation genetic diagnosis more widely available. In either case, the costs of screening high-risk pregnancies are small relative to the support necessary for affected children and their families. As this situation becomes recognized, less of the financial burden may be passed on to the patients.

REFERENCES

1. Weatherall DJ. The New Genetics and Clinical Practice. Oxford: Oxford University Press, 1991.
2. McKusick VA. Mendelian Inheritance in Man. Baltimore: The Johns Hopkins University Press, 1991.
3. Hyde SC, Gill DR, Higgins CF, et al. Correction of the ion transport defect in cystic fibrosis transgenic mice by gene therapy. Nature 1993;362:250–255.
4. Penketh R, McLaren A. Prospects for prenatal diagnosis during preimplantation human development. Bailliere's Clin Obstet Gynaecol 1987;1:747–764.
5. Handyside A. Prospects for the clinical application of preimplantation diagnosis: the tortoise or the hare? Hum Reprod 1992;7:1481–1483.
6. Sauer MV, Bustillo M, Rodi IA, et al. In vivo blastocyst production and ovum yield among fertile women. Hum Reprod 1987;2:701–703.
7. Buster JE, Bustillo M, Rodi IA, et al. Biologic and morphologic development of donated human ova recovered by non-surgical uterine lavage. Am J Obstet Gynecol 1985;153:211–217.
8. Carson SA, Smith AL, Scoggan JL, Buster JE. Superovulation fails to increase human blastocyst yield after uterine lavage. Prenat Diagn 1991;11:513–522.
9. Dawson KJ, Conaghan J, Ostera GR, et al. Pregnancy rates after IVF are similar whether embryos are transferred on day 2 or day 3 post insemination. J Reprod Fertil 1992; Abstr Series No. 10:21.

10. Hardy K. Development of human blastocysts in vitro. In: Banister B, editor. Preimplantation Embryo Development. New York: Springer-Verlag 1993:184–189.

11. Dokras A, Sargent IL, Ross C, et al. Trophectoderm biopsy in human blastocysts. Hum Reprod 1990;5:821–825.

12. Bolton VN. Controversies and opinions in embryo culture: two- to four-cell transfer vs blastocyst. J Assist Reprod Genet 1993;9:506–508.

13. Papaioannou VE, Ebert KM. Comparative aspects of embryo manipulation in mammals. In: Rossant J, Pedersen R, editors. Experimental Approaches to Mammalian Embryonic Development. Cambridge: Cambridge University Press 1986:67–96.

14. Trounson AO, Mohr L. Human pregnancy following cryopreservation, thawing and transfer of an eight-cell embryo. Nature 1983;305:707.

15. Tarin JJ, Handyside AH. Embryo biopsy strategies for preimplantation diagnosis. Fertil Steril 1993;59:943–952.

16. Gordon JW, Talansky BE. Assisted fertilization by zona drilling: a mouse model for correction of oligospermia. J Exp Zool 1986;239:347–354.

17. Hardy K, Handyside AH. Biopsy of cleavage stage human embryos and diagnosis of single gene defects by DNA amplification. Arch Pathol Lab Med 1992;116:388–392.

18. Geber S, Winston RML, Handyside AH. Blastomeres biopsied from human cleavage stage embryos form trophectoderm vesicles in vitro. J Reprod Fertil 1992; Abstr Series No. 10:51.

19. Wilton LJ, Shaw JM, Trounson AO. Successful single-cell biopsy and cryopreservation of preimplantation mouse embryos. Fertil Steril 1989;51:513–517.

20. Trask BJ. Fluorescence in situ hybridisation: applications in cytogenetics and gene mapping. Trends Genet 1991;7:149–154.

21. Nederlof PM, Robinson D, Abuknesha R, et al. Three-colour fluorescence in situ hybridization for the simultaneous detection of multiple nucleic acid sequences. Cytometry 1989;10:20–27.

22. Pinkel D, Landegent J, Collins C, et al. Fluorescence in situ hybridization with human chromosome-specific libraries: detection of trisomy 21 and translocations of chromosome 4. Proc Natl Acad Sci USA 1988;85:9138–9142.

23. White TJ, Arnheim N, Erlich HA. The polymerase chain reaction. Trends Genet 1989;5:185–189.

24. Nielsen J. Chromosome examination of newborn children. Purpose and ethical aspects. Humangenetik 1975;26:215–222.

25. Papadopoulos G, Randall J, Templeton AA. The frequency of chromosome anomalies in human unfertilized oocytes and uncleaved zygotes after insemination in vitro. Hum Reprod 1989;4:568–573.

26. Papadopoulos G, Templeton AA, Fisk N, Randall J. The frequency of chromosome anomalies in human preimplantation embryos after in-vitro fertilization. Hum Reprod 1989;4:91–98.

27. Angell RR. Chromosome abnormalities in human preimplantation embryos. In: Yoshinaga K, Mori T, editors. Development of Preimplantation Embryos and Their Environment. Prog Clin Biol Res 1989;294:181–187.

28. Roberts C, Lutjen J, Krzyminska U, O'Neill C. Cytogenetic analysis of biopsied preimplantation mouse embryos: implications for prenatal diagnosis. Hum Reprod 1990;5:197–202.

29. Bacchus C, Buselmaier W. Blastomere karyotyping and transfer of chromosomally selected embryos. Implications for the production of specific animal models and human prenatal diagnosis. Hum Genet 1988;80:333–336.

30. Kola I, Wilton L. Preimplantation embryo biopsy: detection of trisomy in a single cell biopsied from a four-cell mouse embryo. Molec Reprod Dev 1991;29:16–21.

31. Pieters MH, Geraedts JP, Meyer H, et al. Human gametes and zygotes studied by nonradioactive in situ hybridization. Cytogenet Cell Genet 1990;53:15–19.

32. Griffin DK, Handyside AH, Penketh RJ, et al. Fluorescent in-situ hybridization to interphase nuclei of human preimplantation embryos with X and Y chromosome specific probes. Hum Reprod 1991;6:101–105.

33. Griffin DK, Wilton LJ, Handyside AH, et al. Dual fluorescent in situ hybridisation for simultaneous detection of X and Y chromosome-specific probes for the sexing of human preimplantation embryonic nuclei. Hum Genet 1992;89:18–22.

34. Feldberg D, Farhi J, Dicker D, et al. The impact of embryo quality on pregnancy outcome in older women undergoing in vitro fertilization-embryo transfer (IVF-ET). J In Vitro Fert Embry Transf 1990;7:257–261.

35. Schrurs B, Winston RML, Handyside AH. Preimplantation diagnosis of aneuploidy by fluorescent in situ hybridization: evaluation using a chromosome 18 specific probe. Hum Reprod 1993;8:296–301.

36. Angell RR, Sumner AT, West JD, et al. Post-fertilization polyploidy in human preimplantation embryos fertilized in vitro. Hum Reprod 1987;2:721–727.

37. Koenig M, Hoffman EP, Bertelson CJ, et al. Complete cloning of the Duchenne muscular dystrophy (DMD) cDNA and preliminary genomic organisation of the DMD gene in normal and affected individuals. Cell 1987;50:509–517.

38. Chamberlain JS, Gibbs RA, Ranier JE, Caskey CT. Multiplex PCR for the diagnosis of Duchenne muscular dystrophy. In: Innis M, Gelfand DH, Sninsky JJ, White TJ, editors. PCR Protocols: A Guide to Methods and Applications. San Diego: Academic Press, 1990:272–281.

39. Handyside AH, Pattinson JK, Penketh RJ, et al. Biopsy of human preimplantation embryos and sexing by DNA amplification. Lancet 1989;1:347–349.

40. Handyside AH, Kontogianni EH, Hardy K, Winston RM. Pregnancies from biopsied human preimplantation embryos sexed by Y-specific DNA amplification. Nature 1990;344:768–770.

41. Handyside AH, Delhanty JDA. Cleavage stage biopsy of human embryos and diagnosis of X-linked recessive disease. In: Edwards RG, editor. Preconception and Preimplantation Diagnosis of Human Genetic Disease. Cambridge: Cambridge University Press, 1993:239–270.

42. Li A, Gyllenstein UB, Cui X, et al. Amplification and analysis of DNA sequences in single human sperm and diploid cells. Nature 1988;335:414–419.

43. Kontogianni EH, Hardy K, Handyside AH. Co-amplification of X- and Y-specific sequences for sexing preimplantation human embryos. In: Verlinsky Y, Strom C, editors. Preimplantation Genetics. New York: Plenum 1991:139–145.

44. Li H, Cui X, Arnheim N. Analysis of DNA sequence variation in single cells. In: Methods: A Companion to Methods in Enzymology. New York: Academic Press 1991:49–59.

45. Kontogianni EH, Griffin DK, Handyside AH. Amplification of a Y-specific alphoid repeat from single blastomeres to identify sex in X-linked disease: comparison of two lysis protocols. J Assist Reprod Genet 1993; (in press).

46. Strom CM, Rechitsky S, Verlinsky Y. Reliability of gender determination using the polymerase chain reaction (PCR) for single cells. J In Vitro Fertil Embry Transf 1991;8:225–229.

47. Grifo JA, Tang YX, Cohen J, et al. Pregnancy after embryo biopsy and co-amplification of DNA from X and Y chromosomes. JAMA 1992;268:727–729.

48. Nakahori Y, Hamanao K, Iwaya M, Nakagome Y. Sex identification by polymerase chain reaction using X-Y homologous primer. Am J Med Genet 1991;39:472–473.

49. Nakahori Y, Takenaka O, Nakagome Y. A human X-Y homologous region encodes "amelogenin." Genomics 1991;9:264–269.

50. Levinson GL, Fields RA, Harton GL, et al. Reliable gender screening for human preimplantation embryos, using multiple DNA target-sequences. Hum Reprod 1992;7:1304–1313.

51. Chong SS, Cota J, Hardikar SD, et al. Preimplantation diagnosis of X-linked disease: reliable and rapid sex determination of single human cells by ristriction site analysis of simultaneously amplified ZFX and ZFY sequences. Hum Mol Genet 1993; 2:1187–1191.

52. Griffin DK, Wilton LJ, Handyside AH, et al. Diagnosis of sex in preimplantation embryos by fluorescent in situ hybridisation. Br Med J 1993;306:1382.

53. Hardy K, Handyside AH. Biopsy of cleavage stage human embryos and diagnosis of single gene defects by DNA amplification. Arch Pathol Lab Med 1992;116:388–392.

54. Monk M, Holding C. Amplification of a beta-haemoglobin sequence in individual human oocytes and polar bodies. Lancet 1990;335:985–988.

55. Riordan J, Rommen JM, Kerem B-S, et al. Identification of the cystic fibrosis gene: cloning and characterisation of complementary DNA. Science 1989;245:1066–1073.

56. Liu J, Lissens W, Devroey P, et al. Efficiency and accuracy of polymerase-chain-reaction assay for cystic fibrosis allele delta F508 in single cell. Lancet 1992;339:1190–1192.

57. Strom CM, Verlinsky Y, Milayeva S, et al. Preconception genetic diagnosis of cystic fibrosis [letter]. Lancet 1990;336:306–307.

58. Lesko J, Snabes M, Handyside AH, Hughes M. Amplification of the cystic fibrosis DF508 mutation from single cells: applications toward genetic diagnosis of the preimplantation embryo [abstract]. Am J Hum Genet 1991;49:223.

59. Lesko JG, Handyside AH, Cota J, et al. Preimplantation genetic diagnosis of cystic fibrosis: reliable detection of the δF508 mutation in single cells. Unpublished observations.

60. Handyside AH, Lesko JG, Tarin JJ, et al. Birth of a normal girl after in vitro fertilization and preimplantation diagnostic testing for cystic fibrosis [see comments]. N Engl J Med 1992;327:905–909.

61. Zhang L, Cui X, Schmitt K, et al. Whole genome amplification from a single cell: implications for genetic analysis. Proc Natl Acad Sci USA 1992;89:5847–5851.

62. Ray P, Harper J, Mountford R, et al. Analysis of simple tandem repeats following whole genome amplification from single cells for preimplantation diagnosis of Duchenne muscular dystrophy. J Reprod Fertil 1992; Abstr Series No. 10: 52.

63. Handyside AH. Preimplantation diagnosis. Curr Obstet Gynaecol 1992;2:85–90.

64. Handyside AH, Harper J, Winston RML. Preliminary evaluation of the use of in vitro fertilization for preimplantation diagnosis of inherited disease. J Reprod Fertil 1992; Abstr Series No. 10:53.

65. Hardy K, Winston RML, Handyside AH. Binucleate cells in human preimplantation embryos in vitro: failure of cytokinesis during cleavage. J Reprod Fertil 1993;98:549–558.

66. Delhanty JDA, Griffin DK, Handyside AH, et al. Detection of aneuploidy and chromosomal mosaicism in human embryos during preimplantation sex determination by fluorescent in situ hybridization (FISH). Hum Molec Genet 1993; 2:1183–1185.

CHAPTER 59

Management of Early Pregnancy and Pregnancy Outcome in Assisted Reproductive Technologies

SANDRA A. CARSON

Pregnancy as result of successful assisted reproductive technology (ART) usually represents the culmination of an intense, long-term effort of both the patient and the medical team. Considerable emotional and financial resources are spent to achieve these pregnancies, frequently causing the label "premium pregnancies" to be applied. In turn, this sets in motion attention and actions that may or may not always be medically necessary. Nonetheless, these pregnancies indeed carry some risks not found in pregnancies conceived without ART. First, ART patients are usually older than those women conceiving naturally and thus at increased risk for certain genetic disorders in the offspring. Second, ART requires ovulation induction, which in itself poses an increased risk of pregnancy loss and multifetal pregnancy. Finally, the underlying infertility problem itself may be associated with factors that increase the rate of pregnancy loss or other gestational complications.

All patients need both emotional support and accurate factual information. It behooves the physician to understand the special risks and complications of pregnancy in couples undergoing ART and to initiate first-trimester prenatal care consistent with the careful attentiveness that patients have become accustomed to during their ART process.

PREGNANCY COMPLICATIONS IN ART PREGNANCIES

Whether pregnancy complications and obstetric outcome after ART differ from spontaneously conceived pregnancies is generally determined by comparing ART pregnancy to those occurring after natural conception. Actually, this is probably an unfair comparison because infertile couples begin with a higher a priori risk for many complications of pregnancy. In one 3-year prospective study of pregnancy outcome comparing 500 previously infertile women with fertile women in the institution's normal obstetric population, the frequencies of ectopic pregnancy, chronic hypertension, cesarean delivery, fetal distress, and intrauterine growth retardation all were significantly higher in the infertile group.[1] However, the incidence of spontaneous abortion and perinatal mortality did not differ between the two groups. Another difference illustrated by this study was that infertile women were older, a median age of 31.8 years compared with 23.7 years in the fertile population. Independent of a history of contraception, maternal age is associated with a fourfold risk of preterm delivery and a fivefold risk of cesarean delivery.[2] Chronic hypertension is also increased in older primigravidas.[2] Thus, in comparing complications in infertile women with the general population, age-corrected comparisons are necessary at the least.

Studies assessing outcome in fertile and infertile groups also rarely take into consideration confounding variables such as presence or absence of underlying medical disease, maternal toxin exposure, and nutrition. Another pitfall relates to greater surveillance in infertile and especially ART pregnancies. For example, in infertile couples, close surveillance for early pregnancy loss is likely, whereas in other pregnancies surveillance may not begin until weeks later. Similarly, an infertile cohort is much more likely to respond to followup queries than a cohort of fertile women who have not invested similar time, money, or emotion.

These pitfalls must be borne in mind when we examine the studies that consider pregnancy outcome after ART. It follows that definite answers are often unavailable.

Hyperstimulation

Patients undergoing ovulation induction are obviously at increased risk for hyperstimulation syndrome, a topic covered elsewhere in this volume (see Chapter 14). Although the exact pathogenesis underlying hyperstimulation syndrome remains unknown, risk of hyperstimulation is known to increase as estrogen concentration rises, the number of ovarian follicles increases, and ovarian size enlarges. The upper limits of these parameters above which human chorionic gonadotropin (hCG) should not be administered are higher in ART cycles than in cycles when the ova are not going to be aspirated; for unknown reasons, aspiration of ova helps prevent hyperstimulation.

Although ova aspiration diminishes the risk of severe hyperstimulation syndrome, incomplete aspiration or unilateral ovarian aspiration still places these patients at risk for hyperstimulation. The In Vitro Fertilization (IVF) Registry compiled by members of the Society of Assisted Reproductive Technology (SART) of the American Fertility Society (AFS) reported 1.5% and 1.2% of ART ovarian induction cycles resulted in hyperstimulation in 1985 and 1986, respectively.[3] Presumably, as programs became more familiar with the upper limits of ovarian hyperstimulation, and as ovarian aspiration improved, the hyperstimulation rate dropped to 0.1% of 22,649 stimulations performed in 1988,[4] and in 1990 was 0.2% to 0.3% of stimulations.[5] The prevalence of hyperstimulation was equal in cycles in which pregnancy occurred to that in which no pregnancy occurred.

Even when patients have most of their stimulated ova aspirated, they often experience discomfort due to enlarged ovaries during the first few gestation weeks. Occasionally, patients retain fluid and even develop ascites. Even when this occurs, it is rarely of clinical significance.

Preclinical and Clinical Pregnancy Losses

Pregnancy losses (spontaneous abortions) have long been considered to be increased in women undergoing ovulation induction with human menopausal gonadotropins (hMGs) and hCG (hMG/hCG).[6] As an example, Shoham and associates[7] tabulated the frequency of spontaneous abortions in six series totaling 1340 pregnancies, of which 252 (18.8%) resulted in spontaneous abortion. This rate is generally stated to be increased compared with the population risk of 12% to 15%.[8, 9]

Thus, it was not surprising when the abortion rate appeared to be increased following ART as well. Indeed, early data at the various International Congresses of IVF appeared to bear this out. In 1985, Seppala collected data on 1,084 pregnancies from a number of centers, finding the abortion rate to be 29.9%.[10] In a similar forum in 1988, Cohen and colleagues reported data from 2342 pregnancies gathered from 55 centers in Europe, North America, South America, Australia, and Africa.[11] Of 2329 pregnancies, 577 (24.8%) resulted in an "early" abortion, 36 in a "late abortion," 3 in a therapeutic abortion, and 120 in an ectopic pregnancy. Data collected from 20 ART units in Australia and New Zealand from 1979 to 1987 showed 24.3% (641/2634) spontaneous abortions.[12]

Of 430 pregnancies after IVF performed at Bourne-Hallam Medical Centre between 1984 and 1987, 23% (93) resulted in spontaneous abortion.[13] Comparable rates have also been obtained in smaller series that theoretically might offer the advantage of better surveillance.[14–16] For example, in France, Frydman and coworkers noted the abortion rate was 19% in 142 pregnancies,[17] whereas in the United States, Andrews and associates reported 18.4% in 125 pregnancies.[14]

The largest data sets represent the yearly compilation of the AFS's SART. This registry began in January 1985, and since 1987 yearly publications reported data from ART clinics in the United States and Puerto Rico. In the last report (1990 cases), 3057 pregnancies were conceived through IVF, with 2345 resulting in a live delivery, totaling 3110 babies.[5] The spontaneous abortion rate was 22% (667/3057). This survey was one of the few that logically provides separate information on gamete intrafallopian transfer (GIFT). In the last report (1990 cases), there were 1093 GIFT clinical pregnancies.[5] This led to 54 ectopic pregnancies and 207 spontaneous abortions (19%) (Fig. 59–1).

While the approximately 20% to 25% rate for spontaneous abortion is generally accepted as elevated, in reality, this may or may not be greater than the expected miscarriage rate without ART. One problem lies in the lack of a comparable control group. Another confounding variable is the difference in maternal age between ART patients and the general population. On the other hand, a comparison between groups might favor a lower abortion rate in ART pregnancies because the likelihood of exposure to toxins like alcohol and cigarettes is probably lower in the ART group. However, the major pitfall is that the weeks of observation are rarely comparable between ART couples and the general population. In ART, surveillance generally begins much earlier and is often considerably more vigorous than in spontaneous pregnancy. Thus, simple comparisons are rarely appropriate. The proper methodology would involve a life table analysis, taking into account the differing weeks of observation.

In fact, one may argue that the abortion rate is increased or, conversely, that the rate is not increased. This confusion arises because it is not clear to which set of data the pregnancy loss rate in ART should be compared. First, the total pregnancy loss rate in ART could be assumed to reflect total preclinical loss rate plus total clinical losses. Wilcox and colleagues began performing daily urinary hCG assays beginning about the expected time of implantation.[18] Of all pregnancies, 31% were lost. The preclinical abortion rate was 22%, whereas the clinically recognized loss rate was 9%. Given that the maternal age range in the sample of Wilcox and colleagues was lower than that of the average ART patient, the a priori expectation in the ART population might approximate, perhaps, 35% to 40%.[18] It follows that the abortion rate cited in ART is not increased. Second, ART loss rate could be assumed to reflect all losses occurring after cycle day 28, a week after the time Wilcox and colleagues began their assessment. If so, the a priori loss rate of ART pregnancies would be lower. In a National Institutes of Child Health Child Collaborative Cohort study reported by Mills and coworkers,[19] serum β-hCG assays were performed 28 to 35 days after the previous menses, approximately 1 week after the time at which Wilcox and colleagues began and about when surveillance begins after ART. In the study by Mills and coworkers, the clinical loss rate was only 16%, some preclinical and some clinical.[19] If the abortion rate in

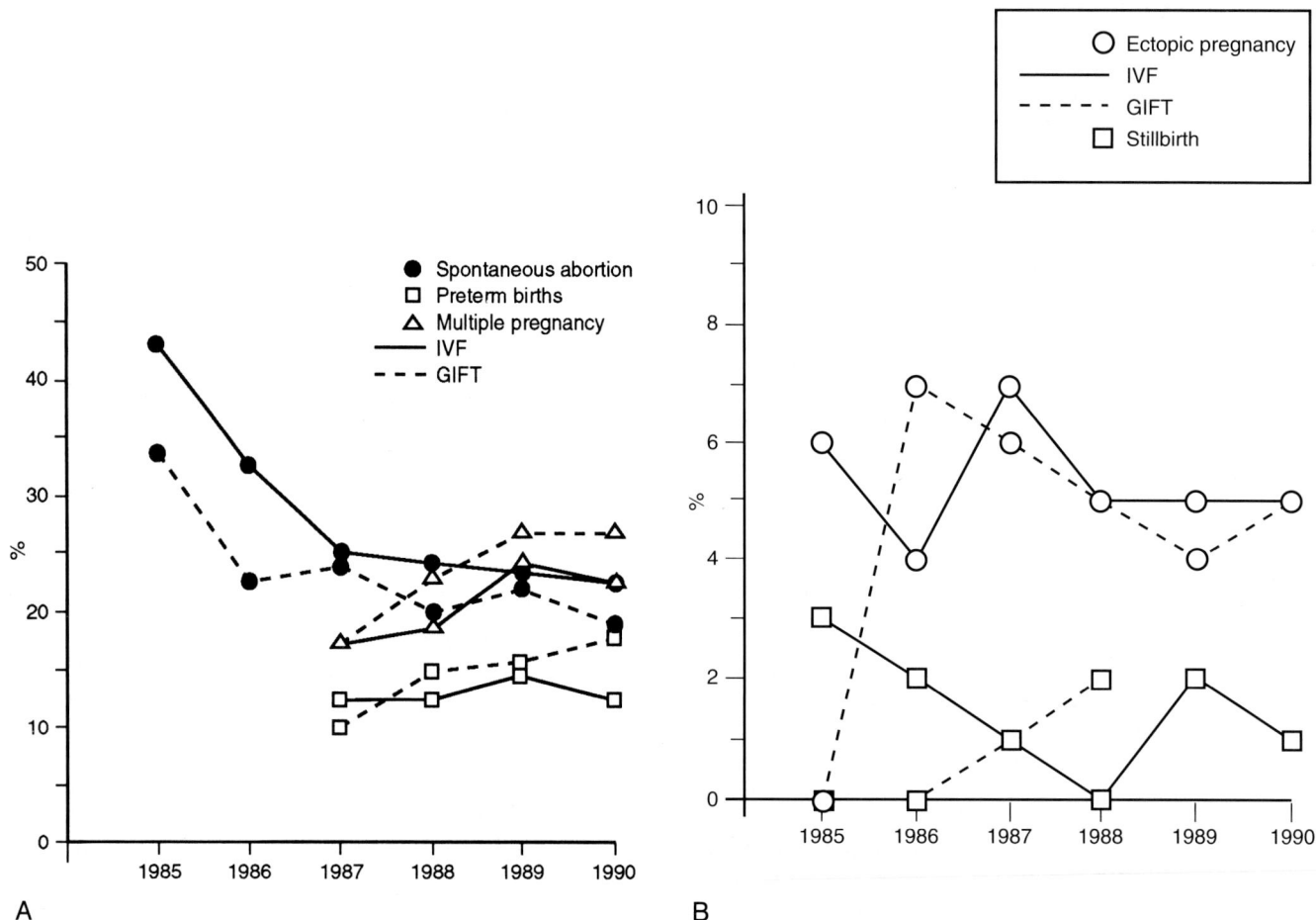

FIGURE 59–1. *A* and *B*. Complications of assisted reproductive technology pregnancies in the United States from 1985 to 1990.[3–5, 24, 25] IVF, in vitro fertilization; GIFT, gamete intrafallopian transfer.

the ART patients is then assumed to reflect the slightly later surveillance, comparable to that of Mills and coworkers the loss rate in the ART sample would seem slightly elevated over the miscarriage rate in natural conceptions. Third, one could make the unlikely assumption that ART data represent solely clinical abortions. If so, the loss rate in ART populations would be unequivocally higher than the a priori expectations (12% to 15%). In fact, Steer and associates statistically analyzed data from the Bourne-Hallam Medical Centre IVF program based on gestational age and concluded that spontaneous abortion was not increased by ART.[13]

A fresh look at this question would not be inappropriate, with life table analysis taking into account differing weeks of observations.

Ectopic Pregnancy

Ectopic pregnancy is a potential risk after ART because often women undergoing these procedures often have tubal damage. The ostia are often dilated, and embryos placed in the uterus may traverse the uterotubal junctions, normally contracted closed in a healthy tube.[20] This retrograde migration may result in an embryo lodged in a tube that is mechanically unable to have peristaltic movements and return

the embryo into the uterine cavity.[21] The percentage of ectopic pregnancies after IVF has been reported to be as high as 11%.[22] Frydman and colleagues noted 3 (2%) ectopic pregnancies in 142 IVF pregnancies; one was a cornual pregnancy, and the other 2 tubal.[17] The ectopic pregnancy rate after ART in Australia, 5%, is about fivefold higher than that of the general population.[23] Similarly, the U.S. data from SART Registries range from 4% to 7% ectopic pregnancies after both IVF and GIFT from 1985 to 1990 (see Fig. 59–1).[3–5, 24, 25] To prevent migration of the embryos back into the tube, it was once suggested that limiting the amount of fluid used for embryo transfer would reduce the prevalence of ectopic pregnancies after IVF.

In addition to the obvious medical risks of ectopic pregnancy, patients undergoing IVF may also be at risk for an ectopic pregnancy with coexistent intrauterine pregnancy,[26] thus making diagnosis of ectopic pregnancy more difficult and also removing the possibility of medical treatment. In the 1992 SART Registry, 18 heterotopic pregnancies (0.1% of aspirations), a multiple gestation containing both an intrauterine and extrauterine gestational sac, occurred after ART in the United States.[5] This appears increased over the general population rate of about 1 in 1209[46] to 1 in 15,000.[28] However, perhaps it is not increased over that found in pregnancies of previous infertile women, about 1 in 600.[29]

Multifetal Gestation

The incidence of multifetal gestation is known to increase with the number of embryos transferred.[4] A report of the first 100 U.S. IVF infants revealed that 14% of infants delivered were twins (11% of pregnancies).[14] A higher multifetal implantation rate was followed by spontaneous resorption in 12 multifetal implantations.[14]

The SART Registry has recorded a progressive increase in the prevalence of multifetal pregnancies after ART in each of its last four reports, with 17% to 20% of ART pregnancies being multifetal.[4, 5, 24, 25] Most multifetal pregnancies are twins (Table 59–1); only 13% to 20% are triplets or more. Similarly, in Great Britain, a 9-year review of pregnancies resulting from IVF was compared with outcome in the general population; 23% of the gestations were multiple compared with 1% for natural conception.[30] Of 1799 IVF clinical pregnancies in Australia and New Zealand between 1979 and 1986, 22% were multiple.[23] The multifetal pregnancy rate tabulated from an international survey by Cohen and associates from 55 centers in six continents was 10% (231 of 2329 pregnancies).[11] Of the 1195 deliveries, 200 were twins and 31 triplets. The prevalence of multifetal gestations decreased with increasing maternal age, a phenomenon opposite that observed in the general population.[31]

Multifetal gestation is a major determinant of prenatal outcome of ART pregnancies and the health of the neonates. Predictably, the fourfold increase in preterm labor and two-fold increase in stillbirth perinatal mortality and infant mortality in ART pregnancies could largely be attributed to the increase in multifetal gestation. Indeed, Hill and colleagues found that multifetal gestation contributed to most pregnancy complications in their cohort of ART pregnancies as well as their cohort of spontaneous pregnancies.[15] Only 17% of ART pregnancies, and only 27% of spontaneous pregnancies that were multifetal, had a normal course and outcome. Likewise, the Australian Registry associated 50% of the preterm births and 71% of the low-birth-weight infants after IVF with multifetal pregnancy.[32]

Pregnancies with three or more fetuses are more likely to abort than are singleton or twin pregnancies.[33, 34] Multifetal gestation also is associated with higher neonatal morbidity and mortality rates than singleton pregnancies.[35] This relates, in general, to decreased birth weight and decreased gestational age. Mortality rates of triplets in England and Wales between 1975 and 1983 were 16% during the perinatal period and another 15% thereafter.[36] The perinatal mortality rate was 21% among quadruplets and quintuplets; infant

mortality was an additional 22%. Perinatal and infant mortality among sextuplets was 41% and 50%, respectively.[37]

Although risks of quadruplets are accepted by all, the risks are significant for triplets as well. A review of 43 triplet pregnancies resulting from IVF at Bourne Hallam revealed delivery at an average gestational age of 33 weeks and a perinatal mortality of 32/1000 births.[38] The neonatal death rate was 22/1000 live births. The perinatal mortality rate was 2.5 times higher than that of singletons born following IVF and lower than the perinatal mortality rate among IVF twins (41/1000 births). All pregnancies except one were delivered abdominally. The average neonatal hospital stay was 24.6 days. The lower perinatal death rate in this series[38] compared with previous series[39, 40] was believed to reflect more intensive perinatal care and a higher cesarean delivery rate.

In addition to fetal risk, the mother carrying multiple fetuses must endure the discomfort of uterine overdistention and often be confined to bed rest for weeks. In addition, triplets carry a 20% risk of pre-eclampsia and a 35% risk of postpartum hemorrhage. Polyhydramnios and venous thrombophlebitis are also increased in multifetal pregnancies.[41] Maternal complications observed at Bourne Hall included increased risk of pre-eclampsia, postpartum hemorrhage, and venous thromboembolism.[38] The occurrence of a multifetal gestation places a patient at sufficiently increased risk to warrant referral to a maternal-fetal medicine (MFM) specialist.

Finally, a pregnancy with two or more fetuses makes prenatal genetic diagnosis difficult and may increase the procedure-related risk. Chorionic villus sampling is more difficult in a twin gestation than in singleton gestation and is exceptionally difficult in a triplet gestation.

Hypertension

The prevalence of chronic hypertension increases with maternal age. Pregnancy-induced hypertension (PIH), the development of hypertension during pregnancy, more often occurs in patients with chronic hypertension. Thus, it might be expected that a cohort of women pregnant after ART would have a higher prevalence of hypertension and PIH on the basis of age alone.

Indeed, in the first U.S. report of ART pregnancy outcome, 10 of the 86 mothers (12.5%) developed hypertension during pregnancy.[14] A similar 15% of mothers conceiving through ART in the British study were hospitalized for hypertension during pregnancy.[30] However, without an age-matched co-

	TABLE 59–1. SART IVF-ET and GIFT Registry Data: Multifetal Pregnancies							
	Twins		**Triplets**		**Quadruplets**		**Quintuplets**	
Year of Aspiration	IVF No. (%)	GIFT No. (%)	IVF No. (%)	GIFT No. (%)	IVF No. (%)	GIFT No. (%)	IVF No. (%)	GIFT No. (%)
1987								
1988	356 (85)*	159 (81)	55 (13)	34 (17)	8 (2)	3 (1.5)	2 (0.5)	1 (0.5)
1990	550 (82)	223 (77)	107 (16)	63 (22)	10 (2)	4 (1)	0	0
1991	577 (86.5)	238 (83)	90 (13)	45 (16)	5 (0.7)	4 (1.4)	1 (0.1)	1 (0.3)
TOTAL	1783 (87)	620 (80)	232 (12)	142 (18)	23 (1)	11 (1)	3 (0.1)	2 (0.2)

*Numbers refer to percentage of multiple pregnancies.
SART, Society of Assisted Reproductive Technology; IVF, in vitro fertilization; ET, embryo transfer; GIFT, gamete intrafallopian transfer.

hort, it is difficult to assess the relative prevalence of these numbers. The only such comparison was in a French study. In this 1986 study, Frydman and coworkers compared the first 100 IVF infants (90 deliveries) in Clamart, France, with an infertile population treated by ovulation induction and with 3841 deliveries in a normal obstetric population.[17] After correcting for multifetal pregnancy, the frequency of hypertension was higher (16.5%) in the IVF cohort than in the infertile (9.1%) group and the fertile group (8.5%). The authors believed this could be accounted for by the higher number of older primigravidas in the IVF group; mean ages of the groups were 32.5, 29.3, and 28.6 years, respectively.

On the other hand, Barlow and associates found no increase in the prevalence of PIH in 108 ART pregnancies in Oxford,[42] and Hill and colleagues found no increased incidence of hypertension in 90 IVF pregnancies in Nashville compared with 86 infertile patients treated with other methods.[15] These pregnancies were matched for maternal age, race, and delivery date.

Obviously, the issue is not closed, however, because the underlying causes of infertility are usually not taken into account. For example, patients with uterine abnormalities have been claimed to have a higher incidence of PIH. Ben-Rafael compared the incidence of PIH in 67 patients with uterine malformations, with 130 patients having a normal hysterosalpingogram performed for the same indications as the study group.[43] The overall frequency of PIH was 18.1% for women with uterine anomalies compared with 10.7% for control subjects. The rate notwithstanding, the frequency of PIH in the first pregnancy was the same in study and control groups. Moreover, no investigation of concomitant renal anomalies was performed.

Preterm Labor

The prevalence of preterm labor in ART pregnancies, like many of the other complications of pregnancy, is related primarily to multifetal pregnancy and the infertility causes. For example, in the first U.S. ART outcome series, 7 of 100 deliveries were prior to 36 weeks.[14] Of these 7, 3 were multifetal, and 2 were in women with a T-shaped uterine abnormality secondary to in utero diethylstilbestrol exposure. In the American SART registry, the preterm delivery rate ranged from 10% to 18% throughout 1982 to 1990 after either IVF or GIFT (see Fig. 59–1).[3–5, 24, 25] Hill and coworkers reported 5.5% in ART pregnancies, 13.5% in infertility treatment pregnancies, and 9.5% in control pregnancies.[15] They also found almost 40% preterm labor in multifetal pregnancies.

Singleton IVF pregnancies between 1979 and 1986 in Australia and New Zealand had a preterm delivery rate of 17.8%, and twin pregnancies had a preterm delivery rate of 53.6%.[31] Barlow and associates reported 10% preterm labor in singleton ART gestations and 40% in the multifetal gestations.[42] In the 9-year review of pregnancies in Great Britain, 24% of the IVF deliveries were preterm compared with 6% for natural conception.[30] The comparable figures for twins were 57% and 38%. These were not associated with either maternal age or cause of infertility. Overall, the increase in prematurity was largely attributed to the increased prevalence of multiple pregnancies and not to ART, per se.

Breech Presentation

Few reports of ART pregnancies discuss fetal presentation. In the Clamart, France, in vitro fertilization–embryo transfer (IVF/ET) program, Frydman and colleagues in 1986 found that a higher incidence of breech presentation occurred in pregnancies after ART than in the infertile population treated by other means or in the fertile population (13.9% versus 5.6% and 4.3%, respectively).[17] They did not explain this phenomenon; in fact, they reported no increase in prevalence of prematurity in singleton pregnancy, an occurrence that would have otherwise helped explain an increased breech rate. A similar rate of breech presentation, 15%, was reported in the United Kingdom ART deliveries.[30] Others have not reported rates of breech presentations. One would expect a higher prevalence of multifetal gestation, preterm labor, or even uterine malformation to explain such an occurrence; otherwise, it is difficult to hypothesize a reason for malpresentation to be increased after ART, if indeed it is.

Cesarean Delivery

That ART pregnancies are considered "premium" cannot be underestimated in considering how both the patient and physician act during gestation. So much regard is given that even these singleton pregnancies often result in cesarean delivery despite no increase in preterm labor, hypertension, or pregnancy complications.

In the Clamart, France, IVF/ET program, Frydman and colleagues reported a markedly higher incidence of cesarean deliveries (46.8% versus 15.5%) compared with their obstetric population at large.[17] Similarly, Hill and associates studied 90 ART pregnancies, 86 pregnancies in infertile couples who conceived using other infertility treatments, and 53 fertile women admitted to the obstetric service during the same period and found that differences in cesarean births among those three groups did not reach statistical significance.[15] However, the higher rates, 34% and 30%, were in the IVF and infertile groups compared with 14% in the control group, suggesting that a larger sample size would provide the power needed for significance. Australian IVF deliveries were by cesarean delivery 42.9% of the time.[32] Even singletons had a higher cesarean delivery rate: 38%. In the first 100 deliveries after IVF in the United States, 56 were by cesarean delivery, only half of which had a trial of labor, thus resulting in a 25% primary cesarean delivery rate.[14]

Once again, confounding variables associated with the cause of infertility must be taken into account. For example, patients having malformed uteri in a series reported by Sorensen and Trauelsen predictably had a higher occurrence of malpresentations (20%) than the control group (5.3%) and a higher incidence of emergency cesarean delivery.[44]

Congenital Anomalies

That the rate of congenital anomalies is increased in ART pregnancies is quite plausible. A number of mechanisms could be involved. One wonders if morphologically abnormal sperm can fertilize oocytes. Are the selective mechanisms comparable in vitro and in vivo? Another obvious potential problem lies in the increased likelihood of polyspermic fertilization, which should yield an increase in triploidy. Could the altered hormonal milieu in vitro and in vivo produce perturbations of meiosis or mitosis and have led to chromosomal aneuploidy? Finally, point mutations may result from the various chemical and environmental exposures during the extracorporeal fertilization process. A host of animal data have provided reassurance concerning the probable safety of ART pregnancies.[45] Moreover, an axiom of teratology dictates that insults occurring while the embryo is totipotential result either in lethality or in no defect that would be manifested in liveborns ("all or none" phenomenon). That is, a given cell's function is not irrevocably committed at this early stage. Its function could be taken over by another.

Several human registry surveillances have addressed the issue of congenital anomalies and in general provide reassurance consistent with the safety information derived from animal data. However, extant data are far from ideal. It is also unwise to rely on a meta-analysis of combined data because the surveillance methods among studies are not comparable. Many ART centers refer patients for obstetric care and delivery, and surveillance for congenital anomalies will differ at each institution. Most studies, of necessity, made comparisons with various birth certificate registry or census data. Yet, surveillance of ART outcomes may or may not be comparable to that applied routinely to neonates. Neonatal data of necessity involves compilation of information on large numbers of patients by a dedicated staff, who may not be versed in the nuances of dysmorphia and detection of mild anomalies. ART populations, subjected to more rigorous surveillance, would inevitably show increased detection of anomalies, especially minor anomalies. On the other hand, if ART neonatal outcomes are judged by gynecologists not trained in neonatal examination, the detection rate would be spuriously lower than in routine neonatal examinations. This situation would also arise if surveillance were by hospital records or telephone contacts.

Several sources of information are available. The 1988 international survey of Cohen and colleagues of 55 centers from Europe, North America, South America, Australia, and Africa totaled 1454 ART births.[11] The incidence of congenital anomalies was stated to be 23 in 938 singleton births (2.5%) and 8 of 22 (36% of multiple births). However, perusal of the data reveals disparate finding—not all anomalies necessarily are abnormal, and not all are routinely detected in typical neonatal examinations. Examples of minor anomalies that were recorded but that might escape routine detection in birth defect registers include small umbilical hernia (n = 2), areas of skin nonpigmentations (n = 2), "hip click" that may or may not connote congenital hip dislocations, extra digit, and cerebral cysts (an internal anomaly that may or may not be evident externally). The same holds true for adrenal hyperplasia and possibly cardiopathy. Thus, the ART surveillance of Cohen and colleagues may have detected certain anomalies not ordinarily included in population surveys.[11]

A study covering 16 ART units in Australia and New Zealand (1979 to 1986) stated that the incidence of major congenital anomalies was 2.2% (37/1697 infants).[32] Six of these infants had spina bifida, and four had transposition of the great vessels. (Incidentally, this survey led to the note of Lancaster and coworkers[46] to be discussed later). In GIFT

pregnancies, there were 21 anomalies in 6809 infants, (3.15%).[16] The SART compilation of data from U.S. centers revealed comparable data. In the 1990 cohort, 38 different congenital anomalies were observed in 28 different pregnancy outcomes derived from 3110 infant pregnancies.[5] This report stated the total anomalies per total infants in contrast with the usual practice of calculating rates as number of infants with anomalies per number of pregnancies, or 28/3110 (0.9%). Again, certain anomalies in the U.S. survey would not necessarily be expected to be detected on routine neonatal examinations, namely, periventricular cyst, microphallus, hydronephrosis, pyloric stenosis, retinopathy of pregnancy, pulmonary hyperplasia, and respiratory distress syndrome. Of note also was that the average maternal age of the women in the 1990 SART cohort was 33.5 years. In the GIFT cohort, there were 19 anomalies in 15 infants, gathered from a total of 371.[5] Again, some anomalies reported would not ordinarily be expected to be detectable in newborn surveys. Examples include optic nerve hyperplasia, periventricular leukomalacia, and minor anomalies (e.g., inguinal hernia). Also, maternal age was higher (34 years). Comparable figures were derived from the 1987, 1988, and 1989 national SART Registry reports.[3, 24, 27] Although impressive in numbers, registry data may or may not be better than smaller centers that looked in detail at their pregnancy outcomes. An example is the report of Andrews and associates, who studied 100 deliveries resulting in 115 infants.[14] Of these, 3 had congenital anomalies, 1 spina bifida, 1 membranous ventricular septal defect, and 1 microtia. Adding anomalies from pregnancy termination cases to anomalies in liveborns may or may not be appropriate, because some of the anomalies that were terminated may have been lost spontaneously had not intervention been planned.

Another major data source is the MRC Working Party of Children conceived through IVF, a survey that included 1267 pregnancies conceived by IVF or GIFT between 1978 and 1987.[30] The data covered all clinics in the United Kingdom offering ART that were registered with the voluntary licensing authority. One or more congenital anomalies were detected in the first week of life in 35 (2.2%) of 1581 infants. Bourne-Hallam pregnancies represent a subset of this data.[47] There was a slight increase in central nervous system anomalies that did not reach statistical significance. A variety of syndromes were noted, but none consistently. Overall, 2.2% had one or more malformations diagnosed within the first year of life, a figure consistent with the incidence found in the general U.K. population.[47]

Probably the most rigorous surveillance of ART pregnancies is the study of 961 children conceived through the ART programs (1978 to 1987) at Bourn Hall and Hallam Medical Center.[47] (These data are actually part of the larger subset of the MRC Working Party study of children, described earlier).[30] Of 961 babies born at Bourn Hall, 763 lived in the United Kingdom. The malformation rate was slightly higher among multiple births (2.7%) compared with singletons (2.4%).[47] The authors concluded that the ART congenital anomaly rates were comparable with those detected in the first week of life, as compared with expected values from U.K. data (England and Wales-Scotland). Specific congenital anomalies were considered to be comparable with those expected from maternal age–adjusted values derived from a Liverpool Congenital Malformations Register. Again, perusal reveals many anomalies that might not ordinarily be detected in general surveys. Examples include minor degrees of hypospadias, undescended testes, hydronephrosis, polycystic kidney disease, and laryngeal cleft. The four cases of patent ductus arteriosus may or may not reflect prematurity.

Of final note is the claim that neural tube defects may be increased by ovulation-inducing drugs. This claim was made by Lancaster based on Australian data collected from 16 centers; 6 infants had spina bifida compared with a stated expectation of 1.2%.[46] However, 2 of these 6 infants did not have isolated neural tube defects; 1 had trisomy 18; and another had a multiple malformation syndrome. Other claims for an association between ovulation induction and neural tube defects have usually implicated clomiphene citrate, but hMG/hCG was not absolved. However, Mills and associates analyzed U.S. data derived from a large case control study of women ascertained within 5 months of delivery.[48] The frequency of neural tube defects was no higher in those subjected to ovulation induction (usually clomiphene) than among patients who were not. In general, claims that the occurrence of neural tube defects is increased following ART or ovulation induction methods has not been substantiated.

Overall, this review's synthesis is that there is no substantive reason to expect that the congenital anomaly rate is higher in ART pregnancies than in controls. On the other hand, prudence is necessary, given lack of definitive data.

Conclusion and Counseling Recommendations Regarding Pregnancy Complications in ART

Although ideal studies do not exist, patients with a singleton ART pregnancy may be advised that there is no ostensible increase in preterm labor, congenital anomalies, diabetes mellitus, or PIH in comparison with women of comparable age who conceived spontaneously. However, after ART, women are at an increased risk for multifetal pregnancy, which, in turn, places them at risk for preterm labor, breech presentation, and PIH. In addition, ART patients have a higher chance of biochemical pregnancy and spontaneous abortion than their fertile age-matched counterparts. Depending on the cause of their inferiility, they may also be at risk for an ectopic pregnancy and complications resulting from a pre-existing medical or endocrine disorder. Thus, early management of the ART pregnancy should focus on detecting multifetal pregnancy, spontaneous abortion, and ectopic pregnancy.

PRENATAL CARE IN ART PREGNANCIES

Biochemical Monitoring

β-HUMAN CHORIONIC GONADOTROPIN

The first pregnancy test must be performed at a sufficiently long interval after administration of hCG to avoid detecting the exogenous molecules. Pregnancy-derived hCG is detectable 8 to 11 days after the LH surge.[49, 50] Liu and colleagues could not detect hCG in the serum of 297 nonpregnant patients 8 to 12 days after the administration of 10,000 IU of exogenous hCG.[50] Thus, a pregnancy concentration test per-

formed 8 to 11 days after hCG administration is unlikely to reflect the drug, but rather a new conception. Initially, serum hCG doubles every 24 to 48 hours.[49, 51] By 5 weeks' gestation, hCG concentration doubles only every 2 to 3 days.[51] Irrespective, a decreased doubling time portends a nonviable pregnancy—either intrauterine or ectopic.[52–54]

As stated, patients undergoing ART should have their pregnancy test performed at least 11 days after the injection of HCG. Waiting 14 days allows nonpregnant patients to resume menses if not pregnant. However, if luteal support has been administered, menses may be delayed, and a pregnancy test is necessary to determine if continued support is necessary. A repeat determination of the β-hCG level in 48 hours can determine if doubling time is normal. As noted, this value should be at least 66% higher than the first value.[52] β-hCG rises at a subnormal rate (<66% in 48 hours) in 90% of ectopic pregnancies. Such a subnormal rate is found in only 12.5% of healthy intrauterine pregnancies.[52]

If the β-hCG level is abnormal, the patient should be followed closely to exclude an ectopic pregnancy or a spontaneous abortion. Incidentally, the initial level of HCG does not correlate well with the presence of a multifetal pregnancy.[50]

A normal serum hCG level early in gestation does not necessarily predict a normal outcome and may occur even in a biochemical pregnancy. Thus, ultrasonography is still needed to determine pregnancy location and viability.

SERUM PROGESTERONE

Serum progesterone can also play an important role in determining the viability of a pregnancy. In more than 1800 gestations, Stovall and coworkers found that a single serum progesterone level of less than 5 ng/mL identified a nonviable pregnancy, regardless of location.[55] Although progesterone concentrations of less than 5 ng/mL do not identify the location of the nonviable pregnancy, they allow uterine curettage to confirm a nonviable intrauterine pregnancy.[56]

Progesterone levels are not helpful in determining whether or not supplemental progesterone administration is necessary in a given pregnancy. (Ineluctably, it is important in the agonadal woman). The decision to support the luteal phase should be determined independently by a given ART program. Luteal support should be given either from the time of oocyte aspiration or embryo transfer until 8 gestational weeks or not at all.

Transvaginal Ultrasonography

Transvaginal ultrasonography is extremely helpful in the management of the ART pregnancy in determining the location and viability of the pregnancy and the number of fetuses. However, multifetal gestations initially detected by ultrasonography may not persist. For example, Dickey and associates reviewed 227 twin, 43 triplet, and 5 quadruplet pregnancies diagnosed by ultrasonography in the first trimester of pregnancy.[57] Only 57% of the twin pregnancies delivered twins; 32% delivered one baby; and 11% delivered none. Twenty and three tenth's percent of the triplets delivered 3 babies; 51% delivered 2; 11.6% delivered 1; and 17.5% aborted all three. Of the 5 quadruplet pregnancies, 1 delivered 4 babies; 1 delivered 3; 2 delivered 2; and 1 had a spontaneous abortion.[57] In conclusion, early sonographic diagnosis of multiple gestation showed a high spontaneous resorption rate. Thus, patients should be alerted to this possibility whenever a diagnosis of multifetal gestation is made by ultrasonography.

Clinical Evaluation and Prenatal Care

The ART patient differs from many other pregnant patients in that she categorically knows her date of conception. Thus, some aspects of prenatal care focusing on dating the pregnancy are not immediately necessary. For example, the patient does not need a bimanual examination early in pregnancy. In fact, this may be deleterious to the patient with hyperstimulated enlarged ovaries. Ultrasonographic examination is far superior in these patients to identify early intrauterine gestation and ectopic gestation than is bimanual examination. A digital examination of the cervix monitors any cervical dilation, which would suggest a spontaneous abortion.

Once sonographic documentation of cardiac activity occurs at 6 to 8 weeks' gestation in a spontaneous pregnancy, the patient's chance of pregnancy loss decreases to about 3%.[58] Presumably, this also is true in ART pregnancies. Thereafter, the patient may have routine prenatal laboratory tests performed. By 6 to 8 weeks' gestation, she has also passed the time when hyperstimulation is a concern and may be referred to her obstetrician in the case of a singleton pregnancy or an MFM subspecialist in the case of a multifetal gestation. Prenatal tests such as a complete blood count, rubella screen, blood type and Rh, syphilis screen, urinalysis, human immunodeficiency virus (HIV) screen, hepatitis screen, Pap smear, and sexually transmitted disease cultures may be deferred to the discretion of the obstetrician providing her prenatal care.[31]

PRENATAL MANAGEMENT DILEMMAS

Maternal Activity During Pregnancy

Patients with an ART pregnancy may become obsessed with the health of their pregnancy to the point of avoiding intercourse and most physical activity. It is not infrequent that a patient will ask her physician to write a letter to excuse her from her job. These restrictions are unnecessary. Indeed, large epidemiologic surveys reveal that patients who are employed have no higher risk of spontaneous abortion[59] than those not employed (unless exposures to certain toxins are present in the workplace). Generally, there is no medical reason for pregnant patients to stop work.

Similarly, questions frequently arise regarding the continuance of aerobic exercise during pregnancy. Again, we recommend that patients continue any exercise program to which they are accustomed but not begin any new fitness training. In one study, physically active women were randomized to an exercise and a nonexercise group.[60] There was no increase in spontaneous abortion in those women who continued to exercise. Although pregnancy is not the time to begin a vigorous exercise routine, those women accustomed to exer-

cise may continue as long as they do not exhaust themselves. Again, patients at risk for hyperstimulation require close attention and temporary avoidance of activity that would rupture an ovary.

Genetic Testing

Because of the length of time required to become infertile and undergo routine infertility treatments, ART is often performed in older women. Pregnancies in women older than 35 years of age are at increased risk for chromosomal anomalies. Patients should thus be counseled that antenatal diagnosis is available by either chorionic villus sampling or amniocentesis. Both procedures carry an approximately 0.5% risk of pregnancy loss in addition to the intrinsic risk of loss at a given gestational age. Again, women undergoing ART have no increased risk of anomalies from the ART procedure itself or from ovulation induction per se.

Certain ethnic groups have increased risk for genetic disease that are best screened prior to ART; for example, black couples should be screened for sickle cell trait, Ashkenazi Jews should be screened for Tay-Sachs disease, people of Mediterranean descent (Greeks and Italians) for β-thalassemia, and Filipinos and Southeast Asians for α-thalassemia. Although it is possible to screen for a host of other disorders prior to pregnancy, there is no reason to do so unless the couples have a family history of a heritable disease.

Propriety of Luteal Phase Support

Whether luteal phase supplementation after ART is appropriate has been widely debated as has been the type of proposed supplementation—progesterone versus hCG. The variation of progesterone during the day limits the usefulness of serum progesterone measurements in identifying which patients require supplementation. Thus, the decision to support the luteal phase must be made independent of a screening test that identifies a set of patients who may benefit by support. The rationale for treatment is that granulosa cells were removed at aspiration and the hormones they produce may be deficient, thus luteal support is started after the aspiration. In a primate model, progesterone concentrations in the luteal phase were inversely correlated to the number of granulosa cells removed at aspiration.[61] A meta-analysis of clinical trials revealed that luteal phase support with progesterone after IVF is of no benefit.[62] Similarly, a prospective, randomized, double-blind study of 525 patients receiving luteal oral dydrogesterone or a placebo in the luteal phase of an IVF cycle stimulated with gonadotropin-releasing hormone/hMG demonstrated no difference in pregnancy rates.[63] The same group conducted a randomized, double-blind study comparing hCG luteal phase support with no support that resulted in a statistically higher continuing pregnancy rate when support was given (18.7% versus 9.3%). However, this beneficial effect of luteal hCG over placebo in IVF cycles was not present in a study conducted at Yale University in which the two groups were matched for age and cause of fertility.[64] When luteal hCG, oral dydrogesterone, and placebo were compared in another randomized, prospective trial, no difference in pregnancy rate was demonstrated among the three groups.[65]

Thus, the propriety of luteal support is in question, but it is a decision faced by each ART program. If luteal support is given to patients after ART by hCG administration, the risk of hyperstimulation may be increased.[66] If desired, progesterone may be administered intramuscularly (progesterone in oil), by vaginal suppositories, or orally (micronized). It is unknown whether thickened vaginal lining resulting from the supraphysiologic excess estrogen production from hyperstimulated ovaries limits the absorption of progesterone through the vagina.

Exclusion of Ectopic Pregnancy

Ectopic pregnancy after ART is ideally suited for conservative management. The ectopic is usually identified early and in an unruptured state. These pregnancies may be treated with either methotrexate or laparoscopic salpingostomy with the expectation of a 95% efficacy.[67] Both approaches to ectopic pregnancy management are described in Chapter 32.

In the event of a heterotopic pregnancy, surgical extirpation of the ectopic pregnancy is necessary, because methotrexate would disrupt the intrauterine pregnancy as well.

Pregnancy Loss

Patients who experience a nonviable intrauterine pregnancy after IVF do not necessarily need dilation and curettage (D & C). This is obviously true if the pregnancy is biochemical, but it may also be true after early clinical pregnancy. However, in the latter situation, pregnancy expulsion may occur as long as 2 weeks after the death of the fetus. In such instances, the patient may be anxious to proceed to D & C for emotional reasons. On the other hand, frequent D & C may result in intrauterine adhesions, which themselves may predispose to further spontaneous pregnancy loss.

Bed rest has never been shown to improve the outcome in threatened abortion. Forcing a patient to rest in bed unduly disrupts her life and may even cause guilt should she be unable to comply with such a recommendation and then have a spontaneous abortion.

Multifetal Gestation

Multifetal pregnancy is a complication of successful ART procedures. As the number of embryos transferred increases, the pregnancy rate increases, as does the multifetal pregnancy rate and the resulting complications. Management of multifetal pregnancies in excess of two or three has traditionally included bed rest beginning at 20 weeks' gestation and even elective hospitalization at 28 weeks, but few studies exist to document the efficacy of these recommendations. Physicians at the Jones Institute for Reproductive Medicine[68] reported that women pregnant as a result of IVF were hospitalized for a mean of 23 days in triplet (n = 26) and 56 days in quadruplet pregnancies (n = 5). All patients were advised to undergo bed rest at home after 20 weeks' gestation. Triplets

were delivered at a mean gestational age of 31.8 weeks, staying in the hospital for a mean of 28 days. Quadruplets delivered at 30.3 weeks and stayed for 70 days.[68] All patients were delivered by cesarean section with no attempt at vaginal delivery.

The emotional and financial costs of such therapy are great. A more recent alternative is selective pregnancy reduction, as discussed in the following section.

Multifetal Reduction

Selective pregnancy termination was first performed to abort an abnormal fetus in a multifetal gestation.[69] The procedure was initially performed in the second trimester by ultrasound-guided needle puncture to exsanguinate the fetus.[69] Later, techniques used included fetoscopy to inject air,[70] calcium gluconate,[71] or potassium chloride (KCl) into the fetal circulation. Most second-trimester reductions are performed for fetal abnormalities not diagnosed prior to that time.

In contrast with selective termination, reduction of a multifetal pregnancy is performed for the purposes of decreasing morbidity associated with multiple fetuses. The technique is usually performed in the first trimester. Ultrasound-guided cardiac puncture and subsequent installation of KCl is now the most common technique for fetal reduction in the first trimester.[72–74] Only 1 to 2 mEq of KCl results in fetal cardiac asystole. Ultrasonography is then performed every 15 to 30 minutes after injection to verify cardiac asystole. In one report, a woman with a quadruplet pregnancy underwent fetal cardiac KCl injection in two fetuses, and 2 days later one of the injected fetuses had cardiac activity. The procedure was repeated and she ultimately delivered twins.[75] Postinjection ultrasonography is important not only for ascertaining asystole but also for documenting cardiac activity in the remaining fetuses.

Multifetal reduction is actually easier to accomplish than selective termination because the fetuses selected are merely those easiest to inject (assuming all fetuses show normal growth and no anomalies). If it is not technically possible to reach a selected (affected) fetus transabdominally, transcervical injections may be attempted. However, the transcervical route is accompanied by a higher rate of complications.[72, 76]

Most transabdominal fetal reductions are performed at 10 to 11 weeks' gestation.[72, 76, 77] By this time, the fetus is unlikely to be spontaneously resorbed. The incidence of spontaneous resorption of multifetal gestation diagnosed by ultrasonography initially from 3.5 to 7 weeks' gestation was compared with the number of infants subsequently born by Dickey and colleagues in 280 patients.[57] Of those patients with twins, 43% spontaneously reduced, 70% of the triples reduced; and 80% of the quadruplets reduced spontaneously.

Fetal reduction also may jeopardize continuation of the gestation with the remaining fetuses. In the first series of four triplet pregnancies reduced by aspiration, there was a complete abortion at 19 weeks, two sets of twins were delivered at term, and one was delivered at 35 weeks. Later, the same group reported 8 of 45 (9.4%) pregnancies following selective reduction subsequently aborted the remaining fetuses. Tabsch reported that none of 40 women undergoing selective fetal reduction lost the entire pregnancy.[77] Evans and coworkers reported that 5 of 55 (22.7%) patients spontaneously aborted the remaining fetuses.[76] Overall, a recent tabulation of nearly 700 cases from five experienced centers revealed 5% complete pregnancy losses within 4 weeks' gestation and an additional 10% before 20 weeks' gestation (Evans MI. Personal communication, 1992). In addition, there is a low but finite risk of hemorrhage, maternal infection, premature rupture of membranes, and premature labor.[72, 74, 76–78] Maternal mortality has not been reported.

Fetal reduction may lead to a persistent increase in maternal serum alpha-fetoprotein (AFP) and amniotic fluid AFP levels. Second-trimester AFP levels were elevated in 21 of 22 women who had a first-trimester fetal reduction.[79] However, none of the abnormal levels were associated with fetal abnormalities. Of 13 specimens with elevated amniotic fluid AFP, only one was positive for acetylcholinesterase; no fetuses had neural tube defects. Thus, patients who have had selective reduction must rely on second-trimester sonographic surveillance to exclude neural tube defects.

Weighing the risks and benefits of fetal reduction ultimately rests with the patient. Probably no clear benefit of embryo reduction exists with triplet pregnancies, but this procedure may benefit couples with quadruplet pregnancies or more.

Patients should be counseled that antenatal diagnosis is available either with chorionic villus sampling or amniocentesis. Again, women undergoing ART have no increased risk of anomalies from the procedure or from ovulation induction per se.

COUNSELING THE COUPLE WITH PREGNANCY LOSS OR NEONATAL DEATH

Parents are grief-stricken by the loss of any pregnancy. Couples achieving a positive pregnancy test by ART have finally realized the fruition of their dreams. A "biochemical pregnancy" to the medical staff is already posing college tuition responsibilities in the minds of the couple. Thus, a loss at this stage of gestation is a real loss to these patients and may invoke a classic grief response: denial, anger, guilt, bargaining, depression, and resolution. The process should be allowed to progress naturally, and the couple should be supported by their physician. Couples can usually be ensured that nothing could have been done to protect or prevent the loss. Premature planning for continued therapy or, conversely, cessation of therapy may result in decisions that the couple would not otherwise make. In addition, the couple must be ready to accept another loss before attempting further ART. Guilt and blame are common emotional by-products. Blame may extend to the spouse ("You shouldn't drink.") or the medical team ("You should have transferred more embryos."). All couples search for exogenous factors that could have led to the loss.

REFERENCES

1. Varma TR, Patel RH, Bhathenia RK. Outcome of pregnancy after infertility. Acta Obstet Gynecol Scand 1988; 67:115–119.
2. Tuck SM, Yudkin PL, Turnbull AC. Pregnancy outcome in elderly primigravidae with and without a history of infertility. Br J Obstet Gynaecol 1988; 95:230–237.
3. Medical Research International, Society for Assisted Reproductive Technology (SART), The American Fertility Society. In vitro fertilization–embryo transfer (IVF-ET) in the United States: 1985 and 1986 results from the IVF-ET Registry. Fertil Steril 1988; 49:212–215.
4. Medical Research International, Society for Assisted Reproductive Technology (SART), The American Fertility Society. In vitro fertilization–embryo transfer (IVF-ET) in the United States: 1988 results from the IVF-ET Registry. Fertil Steril 1990; 53:13–20.
5. Medical Research International, Society for Assisted Reproductive Technology (SART), The American Fertility Society. In vitro fertilization–embryo transfer (IVF-ET) in the United States: 1990 results from the IVF-ET Registry. Fertil Steril 1992; 57:15–24.
6. Ben-Rafael Z, Mashiach S, Oelsner G, et al. Spontaneous pregnancy and its outcome after human menopausal gonadotropins, human chorionic gonadotropin–induced pregnancy. Fertil Steril 1981; 36:560–564.
7. Shoham Z, Zosner A, Insler V. Early miscarriage and fetal malformations after induction of ovulation (by clomiphene citrate and/or menotropins), in vitro fertilization, and gamete intrafallopian transfer. Fertil Steril 1991; 55:1–11.
8. Boué A, Boué J. Le role des anomalies chromosomiques dans les echecs del la reproduction. J Gynecol Obstet Biol Reprod 1977; 6:5–21.
9. Warburton D, Fraser FC. Spontaneous abortion risks in man. Hum Genet 1964; 16:1–25.
10. Seppala M. The world collaborative report on in vitro fertilization and embryo replacement: current state of the art in January 1984. Ann NY Acad Sci 1985; 442:558–563.
11. Cohen J, Mayaux MJ, Guihard-Moscato ML. Pregnancy outcomes after in vitro fertilization: a collaborative study on 2342 pregnancies. Ann NY Acad Sci 1988; 541:1–6.
12. National Perinatal Statistics Unit and the Fertility Society of Australia. IVF and GIFT Pregnancies Australia and New Zealand, 1987. Sydney: National Perinatal Statistics Unit (NPSU), 1988.
13. Steer C, Davies M, Mason B, et al. Papers: spontaneous abortion rates after natural and assisted conception. Br Med J 1989; 299:1317–1318.
14. Andrews MC, Muasher SJ, Levy DL, et al. An analysis of the obstetric outcome of 125 consecutive pregnancies conceived in vitro and resulting in 100 deliveries. Am J Obstet Gynecol 1986; 1654:848–854.
15. Hill GA, Bryan S, Herbert CM, et al. Complications of pregnancy in infertile couples: routine treatment versus assisted reproduction. Obstet Gynecol 1990; 75:790–794.
16. Wood C, Trounson A, Leeton JF, et al. Clinical features of eight pregnancies resulting from in vitro fertilization and embryo transfer. Fertil Steril 1982; 38:22–29.
17. Frydman R, Belaisch-Allart J, Fries N, et al. An obstetric assessment of the first 100 births from the in vitro fertilization program at Clamart, France. Am J Obstet Gynecol 1986; 154:550–555.
18. Wilcox AJ, Weinberg CR, O'Connor JF, et al. Incidence of early loss of pregnancy. N Engl J Med 1988; 319:189–194.
19. Mills JL, Simpson JL, Driscoll SG, et al. NICHD-DIEP study: incidence of spontaneous abortion among normal women with insulin-dependent diabetic women whose pregnancies were identified within 21 days of conception. N Engl J Med 1988; 319:1617–1623.
20. Iffy L. Reflux theory of ectopic implantation. Lancet 1976; 2:1091.
21. Kovacs G, Shekleton P, Leeton J, et al. Ectopic tubal pregnancy following in vitro fertilization and embryo transfer under ultrasonic control. J In Vitro Fertil Embryo Trans 1987; 2:124–127.
22. Lopata A. Concepts in human in vitro fertilization and embryo transfer. Fertil Steril 1983; 40:289–301.
23. Australian In Vitro Fertilization Collaborative Group. In vitro fertilization pregnancies in Australia and New Zealand, 1979–1985. Med J Aust 1988; 148:429–436.
24. Medical Research International, Society for Assisted Reproductive Technology (SART), The American Fertility Society. In vitro fertilization–embryo transfer (IVF-ET) in the United States: 1987 results from the IVF-ET Registry. Fertil Steril 1989; 51:13–19.
25. Medical Research International, Society for Assisted Reproductive Technology (SART), The American Fertility Society. In vitro fertilization–embryo transfer (IVF-ET) in the United States: 1989 results from the IVF-ET Registry. Fertil Steril 1991; 55:14–23.
26. Salat Baroux J, Giacomini P, Cornet D, et al. Caracteristiques des grossesses obtenues par fecondation in vitro. J Gynecol Obstet Biol Reprod 1985; 14:365–374.
27. McLintock DG, Robinson S. A case of heterotopic pregnancy. J Obstet Gynecol 1987; 7:269–272.

28. Richards SR, Stempil LE, Carlton BD. Heterotopic pregnancy: reappraisal of incidence. Am J Obstet Gynecol 1982; 142:928–930.
29. Correy JF, Watkins RA, Bradfield GF, et al. Assisted reproductive technology: spontaneous pregnancies and pregnancies as a result of treatment on an in vitro fertilization program terminating in ectopic pregnancies or spontaneous abortions. Fertil Steril 1988; 50:85–88.
30. Beral V, Doyle P. Births in Great Britain resulting from assisted conception, 1978–87, MRC Working Party on Children Conceived by In Vitro Fertilization. Br Med J 1990; 300:1229–1233.
31. Gabbe SG, Niebyl JR, Simpson JL, editors. Obstetrics: Normal and Problem Pregnancies, 2nd edition. New York: Churchill Livingstone, 1991.
32. Saunders DM, Lancaster P. The wider perinatal significance of the Australian in vitro fertilization data collection program. Am J Perinatol 1989; 6:252–255.
33. Bronsteen RA, Evans MI. Multiple gestation. In: Fetal Diagnosis and Therapy: Science, Ethics and the Law. Philadelphia: Lippincott Harper, 1989:242.
34. MacLennan AH. Multiple gestation. In: Creasy RK, Resnick R, editors. Maternal-Fetal Medicine: Principles and Practice. 2nd edition. Philadelphia: WB Saunders, 1989:580.
35. Kiely JL. The epidemiology of perinatal mortality in multiple births. Bull NY Acad Med 1990; 66:618–637.
36. Holcberg G, Biale Y, Lev-wentha H, Insler V. Outcome of pregnancy in 31 triplet gestations. Obstet Gynaecol 1989; 59:472–476.
37. Botting BJ, Davies IM, Macfarlane AJ: Recent trends in the incidence of multiple births and associated mortality. Arch Dis Child 1987; 62:941–950.
38. Kingsland CR, Steer CV, Pampiglione JS, et al. Outcome of triplet pregnancies resulting from IVF at Bourn Hallam 1984–1987. Eur J Obstet Gynecol Reprod Biol 1989; 34:197–203.
39. Daw E. Triplet pregnancy. Br J Obstet Gynaecol 1978; 85:505–509.
40. Itzkowic D. A survey of 59 triplet pregnancies. Br J Obstet Gynaecol 1979; 86:23–28.
41. Syrop CH, Varner MW. Triplet gestation: maternal and neonatal implications. Acta Genet Med Gemellol (Roma) 1985; 34:81–8.
42. Barlow P, Lejeune B, Puissant F, et al. Early pregnancy loss and obstetrical risk after in vitro fertilization and embryo transfer. Hum Reprod 1988; 3:671–675.
43. Ben-Rafael Z, Seidman DS, Recabi K, et al. The association of pregnancy-induced hypertension and uterine malformations. Gynecol Obstet Invest 1990; 30:101–104.
44. Sorensen SS, Trauelsen AGH. Obstetric implications of minor müllerian anomalies in oligomenorrheic women. Am J Obstet Gynecol 1987; 156:112–118.
45. Biggers JD. In vitro fertilization and embryo transfer in human beings. N Engl J Med 1981; 304:336–342.
46. Lancaster PAL. Congenital malformations after in vitro fertilization. Lancet 1987; 2:1392–1393.
47. Rizk B, Doyle P, Tan SL, et al. Perinatal outcome and congenital malformations in in vitro fertilization babies from the Bourn-Hallam group. Hum Reprod 1991; 6:1259–1264.
48. Mills JL, Simpson JL, Rhoads GG, et al. Risk of neural tube defects in relation to maternal fertility and fertility drug use. Lancet 1990; 336:103–104.
49. Lenton EA, Neal LM, Sulaiman R. Plasma concentrations of human chorionic gonadotropin from the time of implantation until the second week of pregnancy. Fertil Steril 1982; 37:773–778.
50. Liu HC, Kreiner D, Muasher SJ, et al. β-human chorionic gonadotropin as a monitor of pregnancy outcome in in vitro fertilization–embryo transfer patients. Fertil Steril 1988; 50:89–94.
51. Daya S. Human chorionic gonadotropin increase in normal early pregnancy. Am J Obstet Gynecol 1987; 156:286–290.
52. Kadar N, Caldwell BV, Romero R. A method of screening for ectopic pregnancy and its indications. Obstet Gynecol 1981; 58:162–166.
53. Kadar N, Romero R. Serial human chorionic gonadotropin measurements in ectopic pregnancy. Am J Obstet Gynecol 1988; 158:1239–1241.
54. Romero R, Kadar N, Copel JA, et al. The value of serial human chorionic gonadotropin testing as a diagnostic tool in ectopic pregnancy. Am J Obstet Gynecol 1986; 155:392–394.
55. Stovall TG, Ling FW, Cope BJ, Buster JE. Preventing ruptured ectopic pregnancy with a single serum progesterone. Am J Obstet Gynecol 1989; 160:1425–1431.
56. Stovall TG, Ling FW, Carson SA, Buster JE. Serum progesterone and uterine curettage in differential diagnosis of ectopic pregnancy. Fertil Steril 1992; 57:456–458.
57. Dickey RP, Olar TT, Curole DN, et al. The probability of multiple births when multiple gestational sacs or viable embryos are diagnosed at first trimester ultrasound. Hum Reprod 1990; 5:880–882.
58. Simpson JL, Mills JL, Holmes LB, et al. Low fetal loss rates after ultrasound-proved viability in early pregnancy. JAMA 1987; 2587:255–257.
59. Ahlborg-G Jr, Hogstedt-C, Bodin-L, Barany-S. Pregnancy outcome among working women. Scand J Work Environ Health 1989; 15:227–233.
60. Clapp JF. Oxygen consumption during treadmill exercise before, during, and after pregnancy. Am J Obstet Gynecol 1989; 161:1458–1464.
61. Kreitmann O, Nixon WE, Hodgen GD. Induced corpus luteum dysfunction after aspiration of the preovulatory follicle in monkeys. Fertil Steril 1981; 35:671–675.
62. Daya S. Efficacy of progesterone support in the luteal phase following in vitro fertilization and embryo transfer meta-analysis of clinical trials. Hum Reprod 1988; 3:731–734.
63. Belaisch-Allart J, DeMouzon J, Lapousterle C, Mayer M. The effect of hCG supplementation after combined GnRH agonist/hMG treatment in an IVF programme. Hum Reprod 1990; 5:163–166.
64. Hutchinson-Williams KA, DeCherney AH, Lavy G, et al. Luteal rescue in in vitro fertilization–embryo transfer. Fertil Steril 1990; 53:495–501.
65. Kupferminc MJ, Lesing JB, Amit A, et al. A prospective randomized trial of human chorionic gonadotrophin or dydrogesterone support following in vitro fertilization and embryo transfer. Hum Reprod 1990; 5:271–273.
66. Smitz J, Camus M, Devroey P, et al. Incidence of severe ovarian hyperstimulation syndrome after GnRH agonist/HMG superovulation for in vitro fertilization. Hum Reprod 1990; 5:933–937.
67. Stovall TG, Ling FW, Gray LA, et al. Methotrexate treatment of ectopic pregnancy: a report of 100 cases. Obstet Gynecol 1991; 77:749–753.
68. Seoud MAF, Kruithoff C, Muasher SJ. Outcome of triplet and quadruplet pregnancies resulting from in vitro fertilization. Eur J Obstet Gynecol Reprod Biol 1991; 41:79–84.
69. Aberg A, Mitelman F, Cantz M, Gehler J. Cardiac puncture of fetus with Hurler's disease avoiding abortion of unaffected co-twin. Lancet 1978; 2:990–991.
70. Rodeck CH, Mibashan J, Abramowicz J, Campbell S. Selective feticide of the affected twin by fetoscopic air embolism. Prenat Diagn 1982; 2:189–194.
71. Antsaklis A, Politis J, Karagiannopoulos C, et al. Selective survival of only the healthy fetus following prenatal diagnosis of thalassemia major in binovular twin gestation. Prenat Diagn 1984; 4:289–296.
72. Berkowitz RL, Lynch L, Chitkara U, et al. Selective reduction of multifetal pregnancies in the first trimester. N Engl J Med 1988; 318:1043–1047.
73. Lynch L, Berkowitz RL, Chitkara U, Alvarex M. First-trimester transabdominal multifetal reduction: a report of 85 cases. Obstet Gynecol 1990; 75:735–738.
74. Wapner RJ, Davis GH, Johnson A, et al. Selective reduction of multifetal pregnancies. Lancet 1990; 335:90–93.
75. Kanhai HH, van Rijssel EJ, Meerman RJ, Bennebroek-Gravenhorst J. Selective termination in quintuplet pregnancy during first trimester [Letter]. Lancet 1986; 1:1447.
76. Evans MI, May M, Drugan E, et al. Selective termination: clinical experience and residual risks. Am J Obstet Gynecol 1990; 162:1568–1572.
77. Tabsch KMA. Transabdominal multifetal pregnancy reduction: report of 40 cases. Obstet Gynecol 1990; 75:739–741.
78. Golbus MS, Cunningham N, Goldberg JD, et al. Selective termination of multiple gestations. Am J Med Genet 1988; 31:339–348.
79. Grau P, Robinson L, Tabsch K, Crandall BF. Elevated maternal serum alpha-fetoprotein and amniotic fluid alpha-fetoprotein after multifetal pregnancy reduction. Obstet Gynecol 1990; 76:1042–1045.

CHAPTER 60

Assisted Reproductive Technology: Choice of Patient, Program, and Procedure

DAVID R. MELDRUM

This chapter focuses on the issues concerning the entry of a particular infertile couple into a program of assisted reproductive technology (ART): (1) which patients are appropriate for ART and when to move to that step; (2) what factors can impact on their chance of success and therefore what precycle testing may be appropriate; (3) how a patient or referring physician should go about choosing a program; (4) the choice of ART procedure; (5) complications and pregnancy outcome; (6) the issue of cost and a cost-benefit analysis relative to other potential treatments; and (7) the impact of ART on gynecologic surgery.

WHICH COUPLES ARE APPROPRIATE FOR ART

Couples must have the emotional and social stability to undergo an arduous procedure with enough resilience to sustain a number of disappointments before success is achieved. Because a high rate of success is achieved only with multiple cycles, and because most couples lack insurance coverage for ART, financial ability is another practical consideration. The woman must be physically able to tolerate pregnancy and delivery. Finally, the couple must be able to reconcile their moral views with this technology.

The only absolute requirement for ART is a healthy uterus capable of successful nidation and viable birth, either of the infertile woman or a willing and appropriate surrogate. Gamete intrafallopian transfer (GIFT), zygote intrafallopian transfer (ZIFT), and tubal embryo transfer (TET) also require a reasonably normal fallopian tube. Virtually all infertility factors have been successfully treated with ART, including such problems as unexplained infertility, problems of reduced sperm number or quality, tubal dysfunction, abnormalities of sperm transport, endometriosis, failed donor insemination,

and failed ovulation induction. For the process to be highly successful, it does require a minimum level of sperm function, although with techniques of subzonal sperm insertion, success can be achieved with remarkably low numbers of viable sperm. Ovarian response to stimulation determines the chance of success, because the pregnancy rate directly increases with the number of oocytes or embryos replaced, and even with the transfer of three or four embryos, high responders generally have a higher rate of pregnancy. However, even with a poor ovarian response to stimulation, or when multiple cycles of ART have failed, oocyte donation is highly successful.[1] Likewise, if frozen donor sperm is chosen because of a high likelihood of failed fertilization, the deficiency of male gamete function is also totally corrected.[2] One can see that the success of ART for an individual patient is determined more by practical factors of financial ability to have repeated cycles of treatment and acceptability of various therapeutic manipulations than limitations of the techniques available.

WHEN TO REFER COUPLES FOR ART

It is generally well accepted that all conventional treatments for infertility should be exhausted before moving to ART, unless a careful analysis of the costs and risks of a particular treatment contrast unfavorably with ART relative to the expected rates of success. A more difficult question is how long to wait before proceeding with ART, because in most instances there is a low but ongoing chance of conception following conventional therapy. It is understandably difficult for couples to put their lives on hold while pursuing a low ongoing chance of success, and in many couples an excessive length of time has passed before the evaluation has been completed. In practice, it is often 2 years before treatment is initiated and a total of 4 to 5 years of infertility before ART is begun. A reasonable rule of thumb would be 2 years following treatment, but individual couples, adequately informed of the continuing low rate of conception, may choose to go ahead with ART at an earlier point. Couples with idiopathic infertility, depending on the timeliness of evaluation, can complete their evaluation and treatment in as little as 2 to 2½ years (hysterosalpingogram at 1 year, laparoscopy at 18 months, and 6 to 12 months of clomiphene citrate intrauterine insemination (IUI) and human menopausal gonadotropin (hMG/IUI). These latter treatments appear to accelerate much of the success that has been recognized to occur with spontaneous conception over an extended period, probably leaving a relatively low ongoing rate of fecundity.[3] The older the female partner, the more expeditious should be the evaluation and treatment and referral for ART, because rates of success with ART decrease rapidly in the late 30s and particularly over age 40 years.

PRECYCLE TESTING

Serum Follicle-Stimulating Hormone

Study of the level of follicle-stimulating hormone (FSH) on day 3 of a spontaneous menstrual cycle versus the woman's age and subsequent outcome with in vitro fertilization (IVF) has shown that the day 3 FSH is a better predictor of pregnancy than is age.[4] If the level is higher than 25 mIU/mL, an extremely low rate of pregnancy has been reported,[4] and oocyte donation should be considered. A borderline FSH level (20 to 25 mIU/mL) resulted in an ongoing rate of pregnancy of only 5% to 10%.[4] Because FSH assays are notoriously variable, we have used the same kit (Leeco Diagnostics, Inc., Southfield, MI) used in most investigations of FSH relative to IVF outcome.[4, 5] We have also used the day 3 level to predict the optimum hMG dosage for the initial cycle, because the extent of stimulation varies inversely with that level.[5]

Sperm Morphology

Determination of the percentage of sperm that are structurally entirely normal (strict morphology) has been found to provide an explanation for many patients with otherwise unexplained failure of fertilization based on routine analysis of sperm morphology.[6] If less than 5% of sperm are normal, increasing the number of sperm added to each oocyte will increase the rate of fertilization, but the pregnancy rate has remained very low.[7] Micromanipulation has been successful in producing fertilization and pregnancy. Occasionally, morphology will improve over time. Donor insemination is also an alternative.

Semen Culture or Stain for Leukocytes

Pyospermia (excess number of leukocytes in semen) reduces the fertilizing capacity of sperm and may signal infection.[8] A specific stain is necessary to differentiate leukocytes from immature sperm forms. In the presence of pyospermia,

all efforts, including antibiotic therapy, semen culture, and urologic consultation should be made to normalize the semen before ART is continued.

Antisperm Antibodies

High levels of antisperm antibodies (ASA) in the female impair fertilization, particularly if serum from the female partner is used in the culture medium.[9] Extra washes of the cumulus complex and adding an increased number of sperm to each egg may also help to improve fertilization. Very high ASA levels in the female may eliminate any advantage of GIFT over IVF, because ASAs are present in the fallopian tube. Although, overall, GIFT is as successful with ASA as without immunologic infertility,[10] the effectiveness of GIFT with very high ASA has not been assessed. High ASA levels (higher than 70% immunoglobulin G (IgG) and IgA binding with direct immunobead testing) in the male may predict fertilization failure.[11] As long as an adequate number of motile, antibody-free sperm can be added to each oocyte, normal fertilization may be achieved.[12] This may require adding as many as 1 million sperm per oocyte. To ensure that enough sperm are available, an extra collection can be stored at 4°C in test-yolk buffer for 24 to 48 hours, a second ejaculate can be requested an hour after the first, and extra specimens can be cryopreserved.[12] In the case of very high binding or low motility, reduced binding can be achieved by ejaculation into media containing 50% ASA-negative serum.[13]

Tests for Infection

Multiple studies have related positive *Chlamydia* serology to a reduced pregnancy rate with IVF.[14, 15] It is not clear whether this is due to active endometrial infection or some permanent change of endometrial function from prior infection. Because chronic endometrial colonization can occur with negative cervical cultures,[16] we treat all couples entering ART with a 10-day course of doxycycline (100 mg twice daily). This may also eradicate *Ureaplasma*, which can affect sperm function and has been implicated in causing abortion. Antibiotic treatment may also clear unrecognized bacterial infections of the male or female reproductive tracts, preventing bacterial growth in the IVF culture or flare of pelvic infection after oocyte retrieval.

Most programs also screen for human immunodeficiency virus (HIV), hepatitis B and C, and syphilis to assess the risk of transmitting infection to a fetus or newborn or to the female partner or laboratory staff.

Sperm Penetration Assay

A reduced sperm penetration assay (SPA) can signal an increased likelihood of low or failed fertilization. In one large study, a negative SPA had an extremely high prediction rate for failed fertilization in men with normal semen using a standard wash and swimup, suggesting specific defects of capacitation.[17] With sperm of reduced quality, neither a positive nor a negative test result was highly predictive,[17] probably because of the confounding effects of sperm motion and the marked variability of sperm function among ejaculates. Various alternative methods of sperm preparation are available and for some men provide better results with the SPA and IVF (test-yolk buffer,[18] Percoll,[19] and follicular fluid[20]).

Evaluation of the Uterine Canal

We have always done a trial placement of the transfer catheter in a prior spontaneous menstrual cycle, with measurement of uterine depth and a mapping of the contour of the canal. A study has recently documented a significantly higher pregnancy rate with this rehearsal.[21] Some groups have performed the transfer under sonographic guidance. Instead, we perform a sonographic examination prior to the trial transfer. The uterine cavity occasionally follows an unexpected contour. If the trial transfer is difficult, that information would sway the choice of procedure away from uterine transfer (i.e., toward GIFT, ZIFT, or TET).

Evaluation of the Uterine Cavity and Fallopian Tubes

Prior to considering GIFT, ZIFT, or TET, a relatively recent test of tubal patency should be done. In addition to the hysterosalpingogram, pelvic ultrasonography is done at the time of the trial transfer and again when starting the IVF cycle, to screen for abnormalities of the uterine cavity, such as a uterine septum, submucus myomata, and polyps. Because the rate of fetal loss is high with a uterine septum, and because hysteroscopic incision is relatively simple, most programs would suggest incision of a septum before ART. Significant uterine polyps and submucus myomata should also be removed hysteroscopically.

Women with diethylstilbestrol (DES) exposure have increased fetal loss due to abnormalities of the uterine cavity, resulting in a term pregnancy rate that is one half that of control women.[22] The rate of viable pregnancy is particularly low in the presence of constrictions and a T-shaped cavity. If the uterus is small but otherwise normal in contour, the rate is not reduced.[22] These patients should be advised of the riskier prognosis. Before referral of these women for ART, it is generally best to persist with procedures not associated with increased multiple pregnancy or ones that are more readily repeated if pregnancy is not carried to viability.

IVF is successful in women with prior pelvic tuberculosis after full antibiotic therapy and provided the uterine cavity is normal.[23] If there is any suspicion of active infection, an endometrial biopsy and culture should be done.

Laparoscopy

Ongoing pregnancy with ART is reduced to about one third of control in the presence of severe endometriosis.[24] Part of this reduction is due to fewer preovulatory oocytes being retrieved, but a reduced implantation rate per embryo transferred has also been reported.[25] With treatment, factors such as antiendometrial antibodies may improve, thus restoring normal endometrial receptivity. In one report of seven women with endometriomas, five of the seven had complete failure of fertilization.[26] Treatment of severe endometriosis, particularly with endometriomas, should be carefully considered before embarking on ART.

Evaluating Sexual Dysfunction

There is a low but significant incidence of inability to produce a semen specimen for oocyte insemination, with total loss of the cycle. We emphasize to the couple that if there is any concern about being able to provide a semen specimen, sperm can be cryopreserved before the treatment cycle as a backup. Provided the quality of the cryopreserved specimen is good, fertilization rates should be similar to fresh sperm.[2]

Screening for Psychological Stability

ART can be stressful for a couple, which could exacerbate underlying marital or psychological problems. We strongly recommend evaluation by a psychologist. Group sessions are particularly helpful for those not needing formal psychologic evaluation and therapy.

CHOOSING AN ART PROGRAM

More than 200 ART programs have been established in the United States, with varying levels of experience, success, and types of ART provided. These complex procedures require a team composed of clinicians with training and experience in pelvic reconstructive surgery, reproductive endocrinology, andrology, and embryology. The primary reason for choosing an ART program should be the program's success rate. The marked variation in success rates indicates that many fine details of procedure and technique impact on outcome. The particular factors that most affect the outcome of ART cycles are as yet poorly defined. The success rate of a particular program can also be influenced by the percentage of male infertility, ages of patients, or other differences in the type of patients referred. The American Fertility Society (AFS) prepares an annual summary of results of ART programs that is available to both the professional and lay public, allowing physicians and patients more objective means of comparison. A standardized pregnancy rate in women younger than 40 years of age having IVF with no male factor can be used as an index of quality of service. Pregnancy rates in a particular program can vary greatly (due to chance alone) when the number of cycles is small. ART programs doing at least a moderate to large volume (e.g., more than 100 of a particular procedure) are able to report a success rate that is reasonably representative of the quality of their technique. In addition, a higher procedure volume is generally associated with better results (Fig. 60–1).

An individual program may not have similar experience in all the ART procedures, or even offer all procedures, owing to local factors such as operating room availability, experience, or a bias regarding the success of a particular technique. If a particular ART procedure is desired, specific inquiry is necessary. Active membership in the Society for

Assisted Reproductive Technology (SART) ensures a basic level of experience and expertise among team members and carries the requirement to make results available to the public through the AFS.

It is recommended that results among programs should be compared by the rates of clinical pregnancies (ultrasonographic evidence of a gestational sac) and viable deliveries per oocyte retrieval procedure. Pregnancy rates quoted per embryo transfer could obscure major deficiencies of oocyte retrieval or laboratory techniques. Because the level of spontaneous abortion may also be higher with suboptimal techniques, the delivery or "take home baby" rate is the most important bottom line. For this reason the AFS clinic-specific report is only available approximately 1 year after completion of a particular year's experience to allow time for completion of all pregnancies achieved in a given year. Figure 60–1 shows a scattergram of delivery rates per oocyte retrieval in women younger than 40 years of age without male factor undergoing IVF reported to the AFS for 1989 from 177 programs in the United States. Clearly, the success rate varies markedly and should be a major factor in the decision by physicians and patients to make a referral to a particular facility.

Other aspects to consider regarding referral are program organization and proximity. ART procedures are intensive and stressful. If a program is designed to optimize patient flow and eliminate as many impediments as possible, a couple may be willing to undergo more than one cycle. The number of completed cycles influences the ultimate chance of success more than any factor other than program success rate and the number of embryos per transfer. Psychological support should be an integral part of the program, strongly recommended and made readily available, although not intrusively required. Satisfaction of previous patients is a good indicator of these softer qualities of an ideal program. Lengthy travel to a center adds significant stress. Given relatively similar success rates, the center close to home or work would be more desirable. However, patients should not hesitate to travel long distances to receive a higher level of care. Being away from the stresses of work can be beneficial for some couples, with the added bonus of a higher rate of success than they could have achieved locally.

CHOICE OF ART PROCEDURE

The selection of an ART procedure is not always easy. Some programs are more experienced with one particular ART procedure than others. In addition, comparing success rates can be misleading, because the selection of patients for particular procedures may be different. For example, success rates with ZIFT or TET have generally been higher than with IVF,[10] but the predominant population treated is male factor. With a clear deficit of sperm quality, the female partner is likely to have oocyte quality and uterine receptivity that are entirely normal. A significant increase in the implantation rate per embryo transferred has been reported with male factor couples having IVF.[27] Also, cycles with only one or two embryos may be advised to have IVF. The difference in pregnancy rates between uterine and tubal placement are greater in programs with lower IVF results, because tubal epithelium is able to rescue embryos exposed to suboptimal laboratory conditions.[28] Therefore, a difference in one program between uterine and tubal replacement may not be relevant to another with a very high IVF success rate and high embryo quality. In practice, IVF results of most programs are low, suggesting

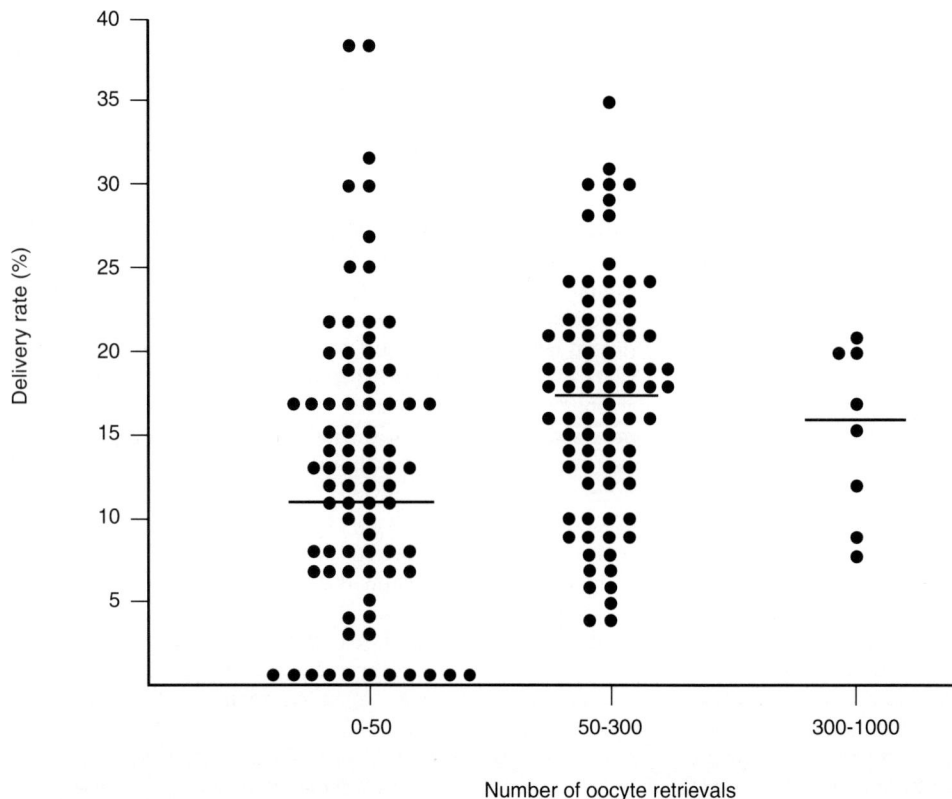

FIGURE 60–1. Delivery rates per oocyte retrieval for women younger than 40 years of age without male factor undergoing in vitro fertilization (IVF) in 1989 as reported to the Society for Assisted Reproductive Technology.[10] Individual rates and the mean of program rates are depicted according to small, moderate, and large programs (total IVF retrievals).

less than optimal laboratory technique. For most programs, GIFT, ZIFT, and TET are clearly more successful for patients with normal fallopian tubes.

The choice of tubal versus uterine transfer is also influenced by whether there would be a significant benefit of diagnostic or therapeutic aspects of the laparoscopy. ART success rates have been similar whether or not operative procedures are carried out in the ART cycle. The patient's choice is also influenced by her willingness to have surgery and anesthesia and by any medical conditions that would contraindicate laparoscopy.

The presence of a significant male factor or high levels of ASA in either partner may reduce the outcome with GIFT to the point of eliminating any advantage over IVF with uterine transfer. It is for these couples that ZIFT or TET has generally been recommended.

The presence of significant tubal disease mitigates against the choice of GIFT, ZIFT, or TET, because the rate of ectopic pregnancy will be higher. Furthermore, in women with tubal disease, the rate of success with GIFT has been no higher than with IVF,[10] suggesting that the abnormal fallopian tube offers no advantage to the nourishment of the embryos over the uterine cavity.

Cost is a consideration with tubal (ZIFT or TET) versus uterine transfer of zygotes or embryos, because with tubal transfer, two operative procedures (oocyte retrieval and laparoscopy) are required. When compared with IVF in a highly successful program, the expense with ZIFT or TET probably increases substantially more than the success rate. Therefore, the additional expense could instead be applied to an additional cycle of IVF, and the operative procedure could be avoided. In older couples or in other situations when time is critical, the increased cost may still be worthwhile.

COMPLICATIONS AND PREGNANCY OUTCOME

Ovarian Hyperstimulation

The relatively low rate of severe ovarian hyperstimulation (2 to 3 per 1000 cycles) with ART[10] may be due to aspiration of all follicles. The ovary may also be less predisposed to such a reaction in normal-cycling women. Anovulatory women are at particular risk. We have found that two ampules of hMG is generally sufficient for anovulatory women unless they are obese. The number of follicles between 5 and 15 mm has been a risk factor in hMG therapy of anovulatory women. More than 15 to 20 such follicles should prompt concern about this possibility occurring with IVF. In some instances it may be prudent to cancel the cycle or to retrieve the oocytes and freeze all the embryos, because hyperstimulation is more frequent, more severe, and more prolonged in conjunction with pregnancy.

Complications of Retrieval

The chance of bowel perforation appears to be much less with transvaginal oocyte retrieval than with laparoscopy, but the operator should be sure that the ovary is well applied to the vagina before advancing the needle. A low incidence of hemorrhage has occurred, with one fatality in the world's experience. A period of training under supervision adds a measure of safety. Pelvic infections—some serious—have been reported with transvaginal aspiration.[29] Prophylactic antibiotics and a thorough vaginal preparation with povidone-iodine appear to make this complication a rare occurrence.

Multiple Pregnancy

Multiple implantations reflect oocyte and embryo quality. The incidence therefore varies with laboratory quality and patient age, as well as the number of embryos transferred. Each program must develop an appropriate policy for the number of embryos transferred, based on their own experience. In most successful programs, three or four embryos are appropriate, but the number may be logically increased with more advanced patient age, poor embryo morphology, or multiple failed cycles. The rate of multiple pregnancy varies from 20% to 40%, with generally 5% or less being in excess of twins. Monozygotic twinning increases with ovulation induction,[30] and an increased incidence has been observed with IVF. Not uncommonly, multiple pregnancy spontaneously reduces as pregnancy progresses.

Ectopic Pregnancy

The incidence of ectopic implantation is 5% of pregnancies with both IVF and GIFT.[10] However, it occurs in IVF almost exclusively in women with abnormal tubes, whereas GIFT is performed mainly in women with normal tubes. Therefore, it appears that for the woman with normal tubes, the risk of ectopic pregnancy is higher with GIFT. All abnormal levels of human chorionic gonadotropin (hCG) should be followed until the determinations are within normal limits. The first hCG level with ectopic implantation is often lower than usual,[31] but in some patients there is a normal hCG rise. We generally advise two hCG level determinations in all IVF pregnancies to confirm a normal increase, with serial levels performed when abnormal. Heterotopic pregnancy (coexistence of intrauterine and ectopic pregnancy) has not been rare in IVF.[10] Therefore, we advise careful transvaginal scanning of the adnexae at 4 and 6 weeks after transfer. Ideally, the tubal pregnancy is excised laparoscopically, and the intrauterine pregnancy will generally progress without incident.

In women having IVF, tubal pregnancy can occur in a fallopian tube that is completely surrounded by adhesions and inaccessible for laparoscopic excision. Methotrexate can be a helpful tool for medical management to avoid laparotomy in such instances.

Fetal Abnormalities

The total rate of fetal abnormalities with ART has been the same as control populations. One report cited an increased incidence of spina bifida and cardiac and renal abnormalities, but this has not been noted in other registries.

Pregnancy Complications

The nationwide incidence of abortion with IVF appears to be mildly increased (23%).[10] Because ongoing pregnancy may reflect the quality of hormonal as well as laboratory protocols, the incidence may be lower in some programs, making viable delivery the most important index of program quality. Even transfer techniques may influence the rate owing to deposition of embryos lower in the uterine fundus, where the endometrium is not as receptive.

Premature labor seems to be mildly increased in ART pregnancies, perhaps owing to increased relaxin from the multiple corpora lutea[32] or underlying infertility factors. For example, one study showed a reduced incidence of premature labor with treatment of *Chlamydia*.[33] Patients and their obstetricians should be particularly vigilant, with aggressive observation and treatment of abnormal uterine activity.

Cesarean delivery is more common with ART pregnancies owing to advanced maternal age, multiple gestation, and heightened concern over fetal well-being. Older gravidas also have an increased incidence of pregnancy-induced hypertension and diabetes.

COST-BENEFIT ANALYSIS OF ART

IVF Versus Tubal Surgery

In some women IVF may be a preferable option to surgery. After thorough discussion of these very different options, usually the choice will be clear for each individual couple.

Success Rate. The chance of a viable pregnancy with the particular type and severity of tubal disease should be contrasted with viable delivery with IVF in the program in question, given the age of the woman. With fimbrial occlusion, the success rate can vary from extremely low with markedly dilated tubes or extensive adnexal adhesions to 70% to 80% with no dilation and minimal adhesions.[34] In the average patient the prognosis is 20% to 30%. In the 1989 U.S. Registry, 26 IVF programs had delivery rates in excess of 20%. Therefore, when a good IVF program is available, a single IVF attempt will often match the results of surgery for distal tubal occlusion.

One factor that has not been considered in comparing results of tubal surgery and IVF is age. In one large series the success rate was 28% for neosalpingostomy, but the mean age of the women was 28. In most IVF programs, the results are about 1½ times higher in women younger than 30 years of age compared with the total group. Even in an average IVF program, this would yield a 21% delivery rate. If the patient being considered for surgery is young, as is often the case, IVF rates in her age group should be used for comparison.

Type of Procedure. Tubal surgery requires a laparotomy or laparoscopy, whereas IVF with ultrasound-guided oocyte retrieval is nonsurgical. Surgery requires recuperation and more days lost from employment.

Further Pregnancy. More than one pregnancy may follow tubal reconstruction, whereas another pregnancy with IVF would require a further procedure and related expense. On the other hand, multiple pregnancy with IVF also serves to fulfill the desire for more than one child.

Tubal Pregnancy. Approximately 10% of women having tubal surgery will have a tubal gestation, but when the low success rate is considered, one fourth to one third of pregnancies are ectopic. This is much higher than the 5% ectopic pregnancy rate with IVF.

Multiple Pregnancy. Some couples may be concerned about the risk of multiple pregnancy with IVF, whereas others may consider twins to be a bonus, obviating the need for any further attempts.

Time to Pregnancy. Pregnancies occur over 2 to 5 years following repair of distal tubal occlusion, with a rough rule of thumb being 10% per year.[34] Pregnancies with IVF are immediate, allowing the couple to move on with their lives with the issue of children resolved.

Cost. If, for example, the cost of surgery was $14,000 and IVF $7000, and the cumulative success rate for two cycles in an average program with a 14% delivery rate is 26%, the estimated prognosis for surgery would have to be higher than 26% for it to be more cost effective. Of course the cost of IVF and surgery will vary somewhat, but the appropriate figures can be used in the same type of analysis.

Insurance. For some couples surgery is a covered benefit, whereas IVF is not. Particularly if the relative comparison is close, out-of-pocket expense may become an overriding factor.

When all the above factors are clarified for a particular couple, the decision is generally made easily. For the average patient with distal tubal occlusion, (even in an average IVF program), the same rate of success can be achieved with IVF at similar cost, with immediate results, a lower chance of tubal pregnancy and without surgery.

GIFT Versus Controlled Ovarian Hyperstimulation

With an average delivery rate of 23% for a cycle of GIFT,[10] and the cost being about four times as high as controlled ovarian hyperstimulation (COH)/IUI and the cumulative delivery rate for four cycles of COH/IUI (estimated at a conservative 10% per cycle) being 34%, one can readily conclude that COH/IUI should always be done before GIFT. It is noninvasive, with less risk and lower expense. These two procedures are not competitive but rather belong in a logical progression of fertility treatments.

Diagnostic Laparoscopy Followed by COH/IUI Versus Combined Laparoscopy/GIFT

The additional cost of GIFT over a diagnostic laparoscopy would cover two or three cycles of COH/IUI and would yield a similar rate of success in a shorter period. This should be considered primarily in the older patient with a low suspicion of pelvic disease. Disadvantages of this approach are that COH may interfere with adequate treatment of pelvic disease, and the increased risk of multiple pregnancy with GIFT compared with spontaneous conception following treatment of pelvic disease.

IMPACT OF ART ON GYNECOLOGIC SURGERY

With pregnancy being possible with only an ovary or only the uterus, the extent of surgery should be carefully considered in any woman who may desire further children. For example, if removal of all residual ovarian tissue is contemplated for endometriosis or a large benign cyst in a sole remaining ovary, the patient should be informed that oocyte donation is highly successful and that the uterus could be retained for that purpose. Lack of such informed consent could readily lead to litigation.

When laparoscopic oocyte retrieval was routine for IVF, it was recommended that the ovaries should be sutured to the back of the uterine cornu to make them more accessible. This should not be done, because it can make the ovaries more difficult to reach during transvaginal follicle aspiration.

Women who have had one ovary removed or have had ovarian cystectomy have a reduced response to ovarian stimulation.[35] With the possibility that any woman with gynecologic disease may need IVF at some time in the future, ovarian surgery should be avoided if possible.

REFERENCES

1. Meldrum DR, Marr B, Stubbs C, et al. Oocyte donation (OD)—a new approach for the poor-prognosis (PP) patient. Presented at the Annual Meeting of The American Fertility Society, Abstract No. 024, Washington, DC, October 1990.
2. Morshedi M, Oehninger S, Veeck LL, et al. Cryopreserved/thawed semen for in vitro fertilization: results from fertile donors and infertile patients. Fertil Steril 1990; 54:1093.
3. Daly DC. Treatment validation of ultrasound-defined abnormal follicular dynamics as a cause for infertility. Fertil Steril 1989; 51:51.
4. Tonor JP, Philput CB, Jones GS, Muasher SJ. Basal follicle-stimulating hormone level is a better predictor of in vitro fertilization performance than age. Fertil Steril 1991; 55:784.
5. Muasher SJ, Oehninger S, Simonetti S, et al. The value of basal and or stimulated serum gonadotropin levels in prediction of stimulation response and in vitro fertilization outcome. Fertil Steril 1988; 50:298.
6. Oehninger S, Acosta AA, Kruger T, et al. Failure of fertilization in in vitro fertilization: the "occult" male factor. J In Vitro Fert Embryo Trans 1988; 5:181.
7. Oehninger S, Acosta AA, Morshedi M, et al. Corrective measures and pregnancy outcome in in vitro fertilization in patients with severe sperm morphology abnormalities. Fertil Steril 1988; 50:283.
8. Wolff H, Politch JA, Martinez A, et al. Leukocytospermia is associated with poor semen quality. Fertil Steril 1990; 53:528.
9. Mandelbaum SL, Diamond MP, De Cherney AH. Relationship of antisperm antibodies to oocyte fertilization in in vitro fertilization–embryo transfer. Fertil Steril 1987; 47:644.
10. In vitro fertilization–embryo transfer (IVF-ET) in the United States: 1989 results from the IVF-ET Registry. Fertil Steril 1991; 55:14.
11. Clarke GN, Lopata A, McBain JC, Baker HWG, Johnston WIH. Effect of sperm antibodies in males on human in vitro fertilization (IVF). Am J Reprod Immunol Microbiol 1985; 8:62.
12. Hamilton F, Gutlay-Yeo AL, Meldrum DR. Normal fertilization in men with high antibody sperm binding by the addition of sufficient unbound sperm in vitro. J In Vitro Fert Embryo Trans 1989; 6:243.
13. Elder KT, Wick KL, Edwards RG. Seminal plasma antisperm antibodies and IVF: the effect of semen sample collection into 50% serum. Hum Reprod 1990; 5:179.
14. Rowland GF, Forsey T, Moss TR, et al. Failure of in vitro fertilization and embryo replacement following infection with Chlamydia trachomatis. J In Vitro Fert Embryo Trans 1985; 2:151.
15. Lunenfeld E, Shapiro BS, Sarov B, et al. The association between chlamydial-specific IgG and IgA antibodies and pregnancy outcome in an in vitro fertilization program. J In Vitro Fert Embryo Trans 1989; 6:222.
16. Shepard MK, Jones RB. Recovery of Chlamydia trachomatis from endometrial and fallopian tube biopsies in women with infertility of tubal origin. Fertil Steril 1989; 52:232.
17. Margalioth EJ, Navot D, Laufer N, et al. Correlation between the zona-free hamster egg sperm penetration assay and human in vitro fertilization. Fertil Steril 1986; 45:665.
18. Katayama KP, Stehlik E, Roesler M, et al. Treatment of human spermatozoa with an egg yolk medium can enhance the outcome of in vitro fertilization. Fertil Steril 1989; 52:1077.
19. Guerin JF, Mathieu C, Lornage J, et al. Improvement of survival and fertilizing capacity of human spermatozoa in an IVF programme by selection on discontinuous Percoll gradients. Hum Reprod 1989; 4:798.
20. Ghetler Y, Ben-Nun I, Kaneti H, et al. Effect of sperm preincubation with follicular fluid on the fertilization rate in human in vitro. Fertil Steril 1990; 54:944.
21. Mansour R, Aboulghar M, Serour G. Dummy embryo transfer—a technique that minimizes the problems of embryo transfer and improves the pregnancy rate in human in vitro fertilization. Fertil Steril 1990; 54:678.
22. Karande VC, Lester RG, Muasher SJ, et al. Are implantation and pregnancy outcome impaired in diethylstilbestrol-exposed women after in vitro fertilization and embryo transfer? Fertil Steril 1990; 54:287.
23. Frydman R, Eibschitz J, Belaisch-Allart JC, et al. In vitro fertilization in tuberculous infertility. J In Vitro Fert Embryo Trans 1985; 2:184.
24. Oehninger S, Acosta AA, Kriener D, et al. In vitro fertilization and embryo transfer (IVF/ET): an established and successful therapy for endometriosis. J In Vitro Fert Embryo Trans 1988; 5:249.
25. Yovich JL, Matson PL, Richardson PA, Hilliard C. Hormonal profiles and embryo quality in women with severe endometriosis treated by in vitro fertilization and embryo transfer. Fertil Steril 1988; 50:308.
26. Dlugi AM, Loy RA, Dieterle S, et al. The effect of endometriosis on in vitro fertilization outcome. J In Vitro Fert Embryo Trans 1989; 6:338.
27. Englert Y, Vekemans M, Lejeune B, et al. Higher pregnancy rates after in vitro fertilization and embryo transfer in cases with sperm defects. Fertil Steril 1987; 48:254.
28. Bongso A, Soon-Chye N, Sathananthan H, et al. Improved quality of human embryos when co-cultured with human ampullary cells. Hum Reprod 1989; 4:706.
29. Howe RS, Wheller C, Mastroianni L, et al. Pelvic infection after transvaginal ultrasound-guided ovum retrieval. Fertil Steril 1988; 49:736.
30. Derom C, Derom R, Vlietinck R, et al. Increased monozygotic twinning rate after ovulation induction. Lancet 1987; 2:1236.
31. Confino E, Demir RH, Friberg J, Gleicher N. The predictive value of hCGB subunit levels in pregnancies achieved by in vitro fertilization and embryo transfer: an international collaborative study. Fertil Steril 1986; 45:526.
32. Bell RJ, Sutton B, Eddie LW, et al. Relaxin levels in antenatal patients following in vitro fertilization. Fertil Steril 1989; 52:85.
33. Cohn L, Veille J, Calkins B. Improved pregnancy outcome following successful treatment of chlamydial infection. JAMA 1990; 263:3160.
34. Rock JA, Katayama KP, Martin EJ, et al. Factors influencing the success of salpingostomy techniques for distal fimbrial obstruction. Obstet Gynecol 1978; 52:591.
35. Hornstein MD, Barbieri RH, McShane PM. Effects of previous ovarian surgery on the follicular response to ovulation induction in an in vitro fertilization program. J Reprod Med 1989; 34:277.

CHAPTER 61

Legal and Ethical Challenges of Medically Assisted Reproduction

AMI S. JAEGER

Medicine's advances in treating infertility and in providing children to previously childless couples and individuals has brought with it the joy and happiness of parenting. Concomitantly, these advances challenge society's deeply held notions of what it means to parent. The law is called on to mediate between the evolving rights and duties of parents and their "miracle" children.

Because of the ethical implications raised by creating and manipulating human embryos, legal responses to reproductive technologies are especially difficult. The ethical issues raised include the following questions:

- To what degree does the U.S. Constitution protect non-coital reproduction?
- What does it mean to parent, and should society restrict who is able to become a parent?
- What are the limits of research on humans and fetuses?
- What is the moral status of an embryo?
- What special responsibilities do physicians and institutional participants have?
- What duty exists to provide access for persons who desire to use reproductive technologies?
- What duty is owed to future generations born as a result of parenting arrangements?

There are a variety of opinions on the proper legal response to the ethical issues raised by medically assisted reproduction. Our responses to these ethical questions will be felt by future generations.

Law, that is, statutes and cases as developed by legislators and judges, is the codification of ethical and social responses to issues within society. The law, however, does not always reflect the diversity of ethical attitudes about such fundamental issues as childbearing and childrearing. Truly, bearing and rearing children are fundamental to our individual and collective identity. This chapter explores the legal response to assisted reproduction by reviewing statutes and cases. Additional guidance in thinking about and resolving ethical dilemmas can be found in statements by scholars and profes-

sional organizations such as the American Fertility Society (AFS) Ethics Committee. The law sometimes sets the minimum standard, as in regulations for professional conduct and patient safety. Other times, ethical statements by thoughtful professional organizations guide lawmakers who use such statements to determine what the law should be. In the area of laws regulating assisted reproduction, there has been an interplay between lawmakers setting minimal standards for health care professionals and health care professionals involved in careful ethical deliberations that has provided guidance for lawmakers. In the area of genetics and sophisticated reproductive procedures, lawmakers rely on the technical expertise of medical practitioners.

Although genetic advances probe deeply into past and future generations, the combination of genetic knowledge and assisted reproduction can reassure a couple if they know they are at high risk for passing a genetic disorder to their child. Donated gametes, when used within a traditional marriage, add a new dimension to the consideration of reproductive technologies. Policymakers sometimes fail to imagine using medically assisted reproduction to solve a genetic concern; they consider reproductive technologies being used only to assist infertile couples.

Reproductive technologies have the ability to dramatically change the nature and structure of families. Traditionally, we think of families as consisting of two parents—a wife and a husband—and their children. Reproductive technologies can alter these family structures. Within the context of marriage, a couple may seek therapeutic donor insemination (TDI). This involves a third party, but not in connection with rearing the child. Because the conception occurs within the privacy of the marriage (and the physician's office), it is similar to coital childbearing and childrearing. A third party is also involved if the couple chooses to adopt a child. In this arrangement, however, the birth mother relinquishes her parental rights and the couple assumes those parental rights with respect to the child. In both TDI and adoption, the person providing the sperm or the child intentionally relinquishes his or her rights to rear the child and to be a part of the child's life.

With the advent of oocyte retrieval, in vitro fertilization (IVF), cryopreservation, and gestational surrogacy became possible. Now a mother can be genetically related to her child, even if she did not give birth to the child. *Traditional surrogacy* refers to the situation when a woman provides genetic and gestational components; *gestational surrogacy* refers to the situation when a woman gestates an embryo without providing the oocyte. The gestational surrogate has no genetic link to the child she bears. Hereinafter, "gestational surrogacy" or "gestational surrogate" will clarify the absence of a genetic link between the woman who gestates the embryo and the resulting child: "surrogacy" or "surrogate" will clarify that the woman provides both the genetic and gestational components. Surrogacy and gestational surrogacy brought with them a host of troubling questions, as women entered into agreements to give birth to a child who was genetically related to the father, in return for money. It became more complicated if a surrogate or gestational surrogate changed her mind during the pregnancy. Homosexual male couples could also use surrogacy as a means to create a family. Although not a consequence of medical technology but rather of a change in social mores, single women and lesbian couples may use TDI to create a family. These notions of restructuring the traditional family challenge the law to develop a framework to resolve questions of parenthood. Law, as shaped by social policy, will define the relationships between the people involved in medically assisted reproduction and their children and what their rights and duties are with respect to each other. As a health care professional, the fertility specialist will play a role in how these relationships and concomitant duties will take shape and redefine the physician-patient relationship.

PATERNITY AND MATERNITY: DEFINING PARENTAGE

Legal Versus Biologic Parenthood

One commentator has argued that the right to procreate, which extends to coital and noncoital choices, should be characterized as the right to parent rather than the right to achieve and maintain a biologic tie with a child.[1] This, the author argued, "could clear a conceptual path for a theory of family that turns on the existence of social relationships between individuals."[2]

One of the primary purposes of the law, in addition to protecting the parties' reproductive rights, is to clarify the parental rights of individuals with respect to the children who are created through alternative reproduction.

As medical technologies have advanced, the legal and social definitions of parenthood have lagged behind. Reproductive technologies make it possible for a child to have five parents: genetic mother, gestational mother, rearing (or social) mother, genetic father, and rearing (or social) father (Fig. 61–1). The law is called on to mediate the respective rights and duties of all parties involved. Until the introduction of advanced reproductive technologies, the law strove to provide a child with two parents—a father and a mother—allegedly to protect the best interests of the child.

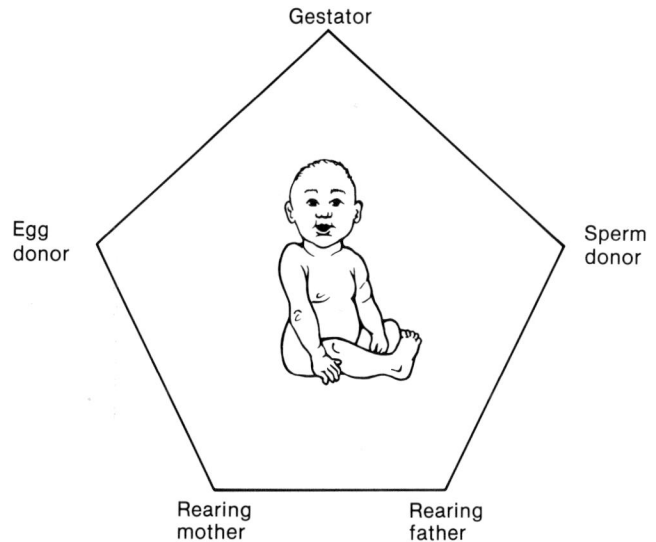

FIGURE 61–1. Reproductive technologies make it possible for a child to have five parents.

The importance of a genetic connection between a father and a child has been resolved in the law. A genetic connection between a man and a child creates financial and legal responsibilities, regardless of the man's intentions to produce or raise offspring, even without formal legal interventions such as adoption.[3] If, however, the woman is married, the child is presumed to be genetically related to the woman's husband, regardless of the genetic reality. This presumption, of course, may be challenged. The legal presumption of paternity has made it easy to adopt TDI into the existing legal framework.

Statutory responses to paternity issues have resolved the genetic and social aspects of fathering in the case of TDI.[4] IVF and oocyte or embryo donation raise novel issues, however, and the existing legal framework may be insufficient to protect the parties' intentions. The gestational mother may or may not intend to raise the child. Likewise, the oocyte donor may not wish to relinquish her parental responsibilities. Statutory schemes addressing reproductive technologies, such as oocyte or embryo donation, must balance the social, genetic, and gestational aspects of paternity and maternity.

CONSTITUTIONAL FRAMEWORK

There is a strong moral and legal basis for the protection of individual autonomy in reproductive decisions. Decisions about whether or when to have children are thought to be a matter of personal private concern, not subject to governmental mandate. Reproductive decisions are protected by the U.S. Constitution under the right to privacy. The right to procreate and reproductive autonomy are fundamental rights, meaning the right to procreate is essential to our notion of liberty and justice.

The right to procreate, as protected by the U.S. constitution, is a negative right. That is, it is the right not to have the government interfere with procreative decisions. Although this includes the right not to have the government interfere with interruption of conception or pregnancy, it is not the same as the right to have the government assist in obtaining and maintaining a pregnancy. Although the family, including alternative family structures, is constitutionally protected, it is not constitutionally protected to have a child.[5]

The constitutional protection of reproductive decisions was addressed by the U.S. Supreme Court as early as 1942 in *Skinner v. Oklahoma*,[6] which struck down an Oklahoma statute authorizing the sterilization of habitual criminals convicted of crimes involving moral turpitude. The court stated, "[W]e are dealing with legislation which involves one of the basic civil rights of man. Marriage and procreation are fundamental to the very existence and survival of the race."[7]

In a later series of cases involving contraception and abortion, the Supreme Court delineated that an individual's decision about whether or not to bear or beget a child was constitutionally protected from governmental interferences.[8] The court deemed childbearing and childrearing rights as "far more precious than property rights."[9] The court wrote, "[I]f the right of privacy means anything it is the right of the individual, married or single, to be free of unwarranted intrusion into matters so fundamentally affecting a person as the decision whether to bear or beget a child."[10] For a governmental regulation that infringes on reproductive decisions to be upheld as constitutional, it must be necessary to advance a compelling state interest, and it must regulate in the least restrictive manner possible.[11]

It is hard to imagine a state interest strong enough to justify a law prohibiting a person from choosing to become a parent. "The decision ranks in importance with any other a person may make in a lifetime; an attempt to imagine state interests that would justify governmental intrusions amounting to a practical prohibition on procreation and childbearing takes us out of our experience and into an imaginary world of Malthusian nightmare."[12] Various commentators and legislators have set forth particular state interests that they argue would justify regulating reproductive technologies. These include the fetus's interest in being free from pain; the potential child's interest in being physically and mentally healthy; the adult participant's interest in being free from undue physical and psychological risk; the individual's interest in making decisions about his or her body; the individual and couple's interest in reproductive and parental autonomy; the donor and surrogate's interest in being free from manipulation by other people; physicians and researchers' interests in meeting their professional obligations to help patients and to further scientific knowledge; and society's interests in retaining values and maintaining institutions such as the family.[13] Types of regulations that arguably would be permissible if narrowly tailored to accomplish the goal with minimal interference include governmental regulation to ensure quality of medical care; to ensure adequate disclosure of information to allow participants to make an informed decision; to protect gamete recipients from transmissible infectious diseases; and to require record keeping and allow offspring access to nonidentifying medical information about their genetic and gestational parents.[14]

The constitutional right of privacy protects the decision to reproduce coitally because of the biologic and social importance of being a parent.[15] The rationales for reproductive autonomy similarly extend to decisions to reproduce noncoitally.[16] The New Jersey Supreme Court in the landmark Baby M case, dealing with a child conceived by artificial insemi-

nation of a surrogate mother, noted that alternative reproduction methods fall within the constitutional right of privacy.[17] Although the court's holding focused on the surrogate contract, the court carefully distinguished among reproduction, custody, and the use of money. Plainly, if one has the right to produce coitally, then one has the right to reproduce noncoitally. Not only is reproduction itself constitutionally protected, but the means of reproduction are protected as well. The values and interests underlying the creation of the family are the same.[18]

The Supreme Court has extended the freedom of association to nontraditional families. The Court wrote that protecting these relationships was central to the concept of liberty and that the creation and sustenance of a nontraditional family were entitled to constitutional protection.[19]

INFERTILITY THERAPIES AND FETAL RESEARCH

Most people seek medical assistance or diagnosis if they are experiencing infertility. Thus, physicians are the gatekeepers to a variety of infertility therapies and options. Health care professionals are in a unique position to shape public policy. If a physician never discusses the option of hiring a surrogate or gestational surrogate or refuses to facilitate any type of surrogate agreement, patients may not be aware of the option or be able to take advantage of it. Likewise, if physicians refuse to inseminate single women because they feel single women do not make "good" mothers, single women will be forced to seek alternative providers.

Embryo Research

The development of reproductive therapies such as IVF was achieved through research with embryos. Improvement in reproductive techniques and pregnancy rates will occur as a result of further research. The permissibility of continued investigations is covered by federal and state laws known as *fetal research laws*.

It is often confusing to medical practitioners why their clinical practice could be governed by fetal research laws. After all, as a physician, he or she is not working with a fetus but with a fertilized oocyte, zygote, morula, blastocyst, or embryo. The law, however, defines any product of conception as a fetus.[20] Federal law, moreover, defines *fetus* as a product of conception from implantation to birth.[21] Those statutes regulating fetal research that conflate fetus with embryo would apply to what a physician would categorize as embryo research.

Just as the statutes address a broad spectrum of fetal development, they cover a broad range of activities affecting not only research but also the introduction of reproductive therapies into clinical practice. Used in its broadest sense, the concept of fetal research includes any untested or unproven procedure involving embryos or fetuses.

The statutes are an attempt to address the conflicting policy debate surrounding the moral status of the embryo and what ethical and legal duties are created with respect to the embryo. Society must balance the ethical and moral value of protecting the embryo with the potential scientific and social gains from such investigations.

Reproductive technologies open an opportunity for research with extracorporeal embryos. There are many potential benefits of further investigation using embryos. They include a better understanding of genetic disease and gene therapy, the development and testing of contraceptives, the study of normal and abnormal cell growth and differentiation, and the screening for teratogens.

Merely because physicians are using novel techniques (either as a research protocol or as an experimental therapy) to treat infertility does not exempt them from federal and state regulations on fetal research. Federal regulations cover the conceptus starting with implantation[22]; thus, they would not regulate techniques such as IVF or in vivo fertilization followed by embryo transfer. A further set of regulations prohibits funding of research involving IVF unless reviewed by the federal Ethics Advisory Board. The term of the Board has expired and has not been reconstituted; thus, there has been a de facto moratorium on federally funded IVF research. On taking office in January 1993, President Clinton signed an executive order lifting the ban on fetal tissue use for research.[23]

State laws extend beyond federally funded research and could affect privately funded investigation and the private clinical practice of a number of infertility techniques involving embryos. At least 25 states have laws specifically aimed at regulating fetal research.[24] Of these laws, 24 impose some restriction on experimentation with live fetuses ex utero,[25] 6 prohibit or impose sanctions aimed at prohibiting any type of research on a live fetus,[26] and 12 prohibit nontherapeutic research on a live fetus.[27] The Louisiana statute prohibits an IVF embryo from being "farmed or cultured solely for research purposes or any other purposes."[28]

Although federal law defines fetus as any product of conception from implantation to birth, states have adopted their own definition of fetus. For example, only Utah has adopted the federal definition of fetus.[29] Other states have adopted a broader definition of fetus, defining it from the moment of fertilization.[30] Many states do not define fetus or embryo, which leads to confusion on behalf of the medical practitioners because their notions of embryo and fetus reflect scientific realities not found in the statute.[31]

Some of the statutes were originally enacted as sections of an abortion statute. For example, of the fetal research statutes, 12 apply to research performed on fetuses or embryos that are the product of an abortion.[32] This distinction becomes important as reproductive technologies are introduced into the clinical setting. For example, if embryo lavage is considered to be an abortion, these statutes could regulate in vivo fertilization (ovum transfer) followed by embryo transfer.

Of the states with fetal research laws, seven prohibit research involving preimplantation embryos.[33] These statutes probably do not apply to IVF, because it is generally considered to be standard medical practice (and arguably is not experimental). These laws, however, could potentially restrict therapies based on IVF, such as cryopreservation and embryo donation.

In vivo fertilization followed by embryo transfer is not as well developed as IVF; thus, statutory restrictions on embryo research will affect in vivo fertilization differently. Because embryo lavage may be considered an abortion (because it involves removing the embryo from the uterus), the procedure could violate the laws banning research on preimplantation embryos and on a fetus in connection with an abortion.[34] These statutes could prohibit in vivo fertilization followed by embryo transfer or cryopreservation.

Many genetic and reproductive technologies now available and under investigation were not contemplated at the time state fetal research laws were enacted. Most of the state fetal research statutes were passed as part of abortion legislation.[35] The constitutionality of existing fetal research laws should be considered in light of the context in which they were enacted. One state fetal research ban has already been ruled unconstitutional.[36]

The Federal Court of Appeals for the Fifth Circuit opinion questioned the continued validity of the statutory bans on embryo and fetal research.[37] The court declared unconstitutional a Louisiana law that forbade experimentation on an aborted fetus unless the experimentation was therapeutic.[38] The court concluded that the word *experimentation* was impermissibly vague, because physicians do not and cannot clearly distinguish between medical experiments and medical tests.[39] The court noted that "even medical treatment can be reasonably described as both a test and an experiment."[40]

Other courts have also found that *experimentation* and *therapeutic* are unconstitutionally vague terms.[41] In the federal district court case *Lifchez*, a group of physicians specializing in reproductive endocrinology and fertility counseling challenged an Illinois statute that prohibited experimentation on a fetus unless it was therapeutic to the fetus.[42] The court noted that even within the scientific and medical communities there is no single definition of "experimentation."[43] The court held that the statute was impermissibly vague. The court noted that what is an experimental procedure may change within 6 months to an accepted procedure.[44] This uncertainty would force physicians to guess which procedures were unlawful. Moreover, it could essentially freeze a given technique in time, thus preventing the development of procedures that are innovative, less risky, or demonstrate an improved outcome.

Laws Governing In Vitro Fertilization

IVF is the keystone of the new assisted reproductive technologies. Merely because physicians use a research procedure to treat infertility, however, does not exempt them from federal and state regulations on fetal research. Because federal law defines fetus as a product of conception from implantation to birth, IVF is not prohibited by federal law. State laws extend beyond governmental-funded research and could affect privately funded investigation and the private clinical practice of a number of infertility techniques involving embryos. Two states specifically address therapeutic IVF: Pennsylvania and Louisiana.[45]

A few states specifically address IVF in their fetal research statutes. For example, New Mexico defines clinical research to include research involving human IVF.[46] In Illinois, on the other hand, the statue reviewed by the court in *Lifchez* specifically exempted IVF from the prohibition on fetal research.[47]

During IVF treatments, a woman may produce more oocytes and embryos than she can safely use for reproductive purposes. Questions arise whether these embryos can be cryopreserved, discarded, donated, sold to another woman, or used for research. The answer depends on statutory regulation and the wishes of the couple. The laws regulating fetal research prior or subsequent to a planned abortion would not affect cryopreservation after IVF because neither procedure involves an aborted fetus.[48]

Issues in Cryopreservation

One primary issue raised with IVF is the ownership of and the right to control the fate of the embryos created through IVF. Courts have recognized that the couple whose gametes were used to create the embryos have a property interest in those embryos.[49] In one situation, a couple who underwent IVF treatment for infertility commenced a divorce proceeding. There were seven embryos that had been cryopreserved pending implantation at the time the couple filed for divorce. During the divorce settlement, the couple disputed the fate of the cryopreserved embryos. The trial court awarded custody of the embryos to the wife, Mary Sue Davis, and directed that she "be permitted the opportunity to bring these children to term through implantation."[50] The court reasoned that the cryopreserved embryos were children and that the best interest of the "children" was "that they be made available for implantation to assure their opportunity for live birth."[51] The trial court stated that issues of custody, support, and visitation were to be decided at the time an embryo resulted in a live birth.

The husband, Junior Davis, appealed the custody award. On appeal the appellate court reversed the trial court's decision and vested "Mary Sue and Junior with joint control of the fertilized ova with an equal voice over their disposition."[52] The court found that there were significant scientific and moral differences between a cryopreserved fertilized ova and an embryo in a woman's womb. Moreover, the court stated it is "repugnant and offensive to constitutional principles to order Mary Sue to implant these fertilized ova against her will. It would be equally repugnant to order Junior to bear the psychological, if not the legal, consequences of paternity against his will."[53] The court cited Nazi Germany's "Hereditary Health Courts" as a grim reminder of the evils of state interference with reproduction. The embryos have since been returned to Junior and allowed to expire.

In another case that considered ownership of embryos, a couple undergoing infertility therapy had several embryos cryopreserved.[54] They moved from the east coast to the west coast and wanted to take the embryos with them for implantation by a west coast infertility clinic.[55] The east coast clinic refused to release the embryos. The court reviewed the consent form signed by the couple and the clinic. The agreement did not include a provision for interclinic transfer. The court noted, however, that the AFS Ethical Statement took the position that embryos are the property of the donors.[56] Under the theory of bailment, the court noted that the embryos were property of the couple; therefore, the clinic, as bailee, was required to release the embryos to the couple.

Donation and Sale of Gametes and Embryos

A couple undergoing infertility treatments may wish to donate or sell excess embryos to another person.[57] Fifteen states prohibit a woman from selling an embryo for experimentation[58]; nine states prohibit the donation of embryos or a fetus for research purposes.[59] As embryo transfer after IVF or in vivo fertilization becomes standard clinical practice and no longer experimental, these regulations would no longer restrict donation, because the procedure falls outside the scope of the statute.

The restriction on the sale or donation of embryos for research must be distinguished from the bans in two states, Florida and Louisiana, that restrict such sale or donation for any purpose.[60] The primary distinction between them is that even if in vivo fertilization followed by embryo transfer became a standard clinical procedure, the laws in those two states would still restrict the sale or donation of embryos.

Although the Louisiana statute prohibits the sale of oocytes and embryos created through IVF,[61] it allows embryo donation.[62] It states, "If the in vitro fertilization patients renounce, by notarial act, their parental rights for in utero implantation, then the in vitro fertilized human ovum shall be available for adoptive implantation in accordance with written procedures of the facility where it is housed or stored."[63] No payment will be made to either party. A further provision prohibits the culture of an in vitro fertilized human ovum for research "or any other purposes."[64] Thus, it seems that excess embryos may be donated, but only for implantation in another woman, not for research purposes.

A Kentucky law seems to require public medical facilities to donate excess IVF embryos for implantation. The statute allows public medical facilities to conduct IVF "as long as such procedures do not result in the intentional destruction of a human embryo."[65]

The physician performing IVF should discuss the risks involved with embryo donation with the donors. Women donating embryos or eggs should be counseled about the physical risks associated with embryo donation, such as infection, permanent scarring, and other side effects. In addition to these physical risks, women who undergo infertility therapy must be counseled on the psychological risks of donation. First, the physician should make sure there is no coercion of the woman or the couple to donate an embryo; participation in an IVF program should not be limited to women or couples who agree to donate excess embryos.[66] Second, the physician must counsel the woman to consider the emotional risk of donation in case she herself does not achieve a pregnancy. Donors also should consider the risk of the resulting child's potential emotional reaction on learning of the existence of a biologic parent with whom he or she will have no contact.

THERAPEUTIC DONOR INSEMINATION

Unlike IVF when used by a couple to treat infertility, TDI introduces a person who will not have a continuing relationship with the child or the child's parent. The donor's involvement in the procedure is unrelated to rearing the child. Reasons for seeking TDI include male infertility, genetic background of the male partner (including carrier status), or absence of a male partner.[67]

Historically, TDI was the first reproductive therapy developed[68] and has been available as a therapeutic option since the early 1950s.[69] Early on, the courts were presented with the issue of defining who is the legal father of a child conceived with donated sperm and with the assistance of a physician.

Traditionally, children born to a married woman are presumed to be the children of the woman's husband, regardless of the biologic realities. This "presumption of paternity" is common in many state statutes.[70] Early on, the courts recognized the consenting husband's legal parentage through a series of cases that established the child's legal identity. Usually, these cases arose out of a divorce proceeding. In one case, the husband claimed he should not have to support the child because they were not genetically related.[71] In another, the wife tried to deny her husband visitation rights based on the same rationale.[72] Sometimes, in the earliest cases, the courts declared the child born as a result of TDI to be illegitimate. It is well established, however, that the courts will protect the child financially and emotionally by finding the consenting husband to be the legal father, with support responsibilities and visitation rights.[73] All of the 35 states regulating TDI clarify the paternity of a child by providing that the sperm recipient and her consenting husband are the legal parents.[74] The consenting husband is the legal father for legitimacy, inheritance, and support purposes.[75] Some statutes, such as those of Minnesota, Montana, Nevada, New Mexico, Virginia, Wisconsin, and Wyoming, require the husband's written consent to the procedure for him to be recognized as the legal parent.[76]

Single Parenthood

Originally intended to assist married couples, the new reproductive technologies can be used to facilitate single parenthood: single men may hire a surrogate; single women may be artificially inseminated. Most TDI statutes assume that a married couple will be using the procedure, but none makes it illegal for an unmarried woman to do so.[77] But many statutes could be interpreted as inapplicable to single women, in which instance the child could sue the donor for support. The Ohio and Oregon statutes specifically acknowledge that a single woman might use donor sperm.[78]

The focal point of case law concerning the TDI of single women has been paternity. Generally, single women choose TDI because they do not wish to establish future contact with the donor as a rearing parent, and men donating sperm share similar expectations.[79] Twelve states clarify that the sperm recipient is the sole parent of the child and the donor has no legal obligations or duties with respect to the child.[80] An Ohio law tries to clarify this issue by providing that if an unmarried woman is artificially inseminated, "the donor shall not be treated in law or regarded as the natural father."[81]

In contrast, a New Jersey case involving the home insemination of a single woman held that the man providing the semen was the legal father of the child.[82] This decision is based on a unique set of facts and therefore does not provide much guidance for other cases. The court held that the boyfriend who provided the sperm was the legal father and

granted him visitation rights. In reaching its decision, the court distinguished this from previous artificial insemination cases because "there is no married couple [and because] there is no anonymous donor."[83] The court found that "if an unmarried woman conceives a child through artificial insemination from semen from a known man, that man cannot be considered to be less a father because he is not married to the woman."[84] The court also stated that the decision was consistent with judicial policy "favoring the requirement that a child be provided with a father as well as a mother."[85] This decision has been read narrowly; there have been no cases in which an anonymous sperm donor has been held liable for child support against his wishes.

No laws prohibit the insemination of unmarried women. Even if a state passed such a law, it would be unlikely to be upheld as constitutional. The constitutional protection of reproductive decisions extends to individuals as well as married couples.[86] As the U.S. Supreme Court noted, "It is the right of the *individual,* married or single, to be free of unwarranted governmental intrusion in matters so fundamentally affecting a person as the decision whether to bear or beget a child."[87] A single woman, denied TDI at a clinic affiliated with a state or federal institution that will inseminate only a married couple, can claim that her privacy right to make procreative decisions and her equal protection right are violated by the clinic's policies. This has already happened in one case. The clinic associated with a state university settled the suit by agreeing to drop the marriage requirement and consider the woman as a candidate for insemination.[88]

New family dynamics are possible as a result of reproductive technologies. For example, the insemination of single women or use of a surrogate by a homosexual male couple provides a new lens by which to view traditional notions of family.[89] The insemination of single women raises issues such as whether it is in the child's best interests to have two parents and whether a single parent can meet the physical and emotional needs of the child, especially if the parent will have to work to support the child. Studies of children in single-parent, female-headed families have found that they have comparable cognitive abilities to those raised in two-parent homes.[90] In addition, children in single-parent homes have a level of self-esteem that is at least equal to that of children in two-parent families.[91] Children raised in lesbian-headed households do not differ from other children as to their gender role behavior or their sexual preference.[92] In fact, sociologists have found that the quality and continuity of parental relationships, rather than a traditional lifestyle or a parent of either gender, are the primary factors contributing to healthy child development.[93]

Social attitudes, including disapproval of nontraditional families, are not compelling reasons to prohibit the insemination of single women. One court stated in a case involving an unmarried woman undergoing artificial insemination, "We wish to stress that our opinion in this case is not intended to express any judicial preference toward traditional notions of family structure or toward providing a father where a single woman has chosen to bear a child."[94]

What we are really calling into question is not the medical complexity of TDI but the social issue of who should be allowed to parent and who should have the authority to decide who will parent. "Deputizing physicians to decide which women should become mothers" allows physicians to make moral decision about what makes a good parent.[95] If a woman wants to ensure donor anonymity and adequate semen screening, she must seek a physician who will perform the insemination. The physician as moral gatekeeper becomes a capricious, unjust method of social control.[96] As Daniel and Norma Wikler pointed out, involvement of the medical profession in TDI has spared us "a troubling examination of our own values regarding reproductive freedom, the meaning of parenthood, and the interest of children."[97] Society does not regulate or license conception through traditional intercourse and so, arguably, it should not regulate who should become parents when the means of conception have changed.[98]

Physician Involvement

Some statutes clarify the role of the physician performing TDI. For example, the physician is required to obtain the written consent of the husband.[99] Other statutes recognize the paternity of the TDI child only if a physician supervises the insemination. At least 16 of the related statutes assume that TDI will be performed by or under the supervision of a "licensed physician," "certified medical doctor," or person "duly authorized to practice medicine."[100]

Statutes that require medical assistance raise questions about whether TDI performed by someone other than a physician, such as a husband, lover, donor, or friend, has different legal consequences that would affect the parental rights and responsibilities of the consenting husband and the consenting donor (notably the husband accepting parental responsibility and the donor relinquishing parental responsibility). For example, the California artificial insemination statute states "[i]f, under the supervision of a licensed physician and with the consent of her husband, a wife is inseminated artificially with the semen donated by a man who is not her husband, the husband is treated in law as if he were the natural father of a child thereby conceived."[101] This type of statutory language raises questions about whether the consenting husband is the legal father when a physician is not involved in the procedure. More general statutory provisions regarding paternity would generally grant the husband paternity rights.

The statutory requirement for physician involvement can create problems when TDI performed by a nonphysician involves an unmarried woman. Some unmarried women have difficulty finding physicians who will agree to perform the procedure for them.[102] Their alternative is to find a donor through a network of friends and acquaintances. In one case, an unmarried woman privately selected a sperm donor and performed the insemination in her home by herself.[103] The sperm donor was listed as the father on the birth certificate. He filed an action to establish paternity and visitation rights. In reaching its decision, the appellate court relied on the statute that read, "The donor of semen provided to a licensed physician for use in artificial insemination of a woman other than the donor's wife is treated in law as if he were not the natural father of a child thereby conceived."[104] The court held that because the semen was not provided to a physician, the donor was the legal father, and it granted him visitation rights.

The court noted that "nothing inherent in artificial insem-

ination requires the involvement of a physician."[105] Physician involvement "might offend a woman's sense of privacy and reproductive autonomy, might result in burdensome costs to some women, and might interfere with a woman's desire to conduct the procedure in a comfortable environment such as her own home or to choose the donor herself."[106] Another reason for not using the services of a physician, although not mentioned by the court, is that some people believe that the medical screening of donors by infertility clinics is inadequate and thus they wish to choose their own donors.[107]

In their article, the Wiklers concluded that "medicalization brings about a subtle, even invisible, alteration of decision-making authority. . . . Morals are discussed in clinical terms, and ethical decisions are characterized as medical judgments, with physicians viewed, by themselves as well as by others, as neutral arbiters of moral values."[108] Additionally, physicians use their personal values in defining a "fit parent" and thereby deny access to women who may not conform to the traditional image of a "good mother" yet nevertheless would make excellent parents.[109]

TDI is a relatively simple procedure and involves minimal risks.[110] Physician involvement in TDI is not medically necessary; however, physician involvement can be useful to provide proper medical screening of sperm, to counsel recipients, and to provide a supportive environment.[111] The physician may also provide security to couples by "legitimizing" their decision to proceed with the insemination and accept the child. In *Jhordan C. v. Mary K.* the court enumerated two additional reasons why physician involvement may be appropriate. The physician could obtain a medical history of the donor and screen him. Also, the physician "can serve to create a formal, documented structure for the donor-recipient relationship to avoid misunderstandings between the parties."[112] These reasons are particularly applicable to situations in which TDI is used as part of a surrogate parenting arrangement.

SURROGATE PARENTING

When the female partner is infertile or unable to carry a child to term, a surrogate or gestational surrogate provides the missing component. This escalates the degree of third-party involvement in the process. No longer is there an anonymous donor, as with TDI, but a woman who contributes both the genetic and gestational component (if a surrogate) or the gestational component (if a gestational surrogate). The process of gestating and giving birth to a child raises serious questions about balancing the autonomy and bodily integrity of the surrogate while she is gestating a child for another person to rear. It also raises issues about what the appropriate legal response should be if the surrogate or gestational surrogate should change her mind and decide she does not want to relinquish the child after birth.

The New Jersey Supreme Court in the landmark *Baby M* decision was faced with a surrogate who decided after the birth she could not relinquish the child created through a surrogate parenting arrangement.[113] The New Jersey Supreme Court held that the man providing the sperm was the legal father, and the woman providing the egg and gestating the embryo was the legal mother.[114] The court voided the surrogacy contract and thereby the parties' original intention to have the spouse of the man providing the sperm recognized as the legal mother. The parties proceeded with a custody battle for the child between the surrogate and the genetic father. The court awarded custody to the father and his spouse but granted visitation rights to the surrogate.

Generally, parties seek the assistance of an attorney to draft a surrogate parenting agreement. The physician who agrees to participate in a surrogate arrangement would be well advised to consider if he or she could comply with the terms of the agreement before agreeing to commence any procedures. For example, would the physician be comfortable if the contract afforded the intended rearing parents the final authority to consent to a cesarean section during delivery?

In addition to issues of bodily integrity of the surrogate and of remedies in the event of breach, payment to the surrogate raises issues of the legality of the surrogate arrangement contract. If payment to the surrogate is for the child, constitutional prohibitions against baby selling are violated. If the contract is for services, that is, the service of providing a gamete or gestating an embryo, payment does not run afoul of baby-selling prohibitions. Regulatory approaches that allow surrogacy contracts to be enforceable as long as the surrogate is not paid are arguably more coercive than allowing payment. People choose occupations that are physically and emotionally risky. Attorneys choose jobs they know are stressful and demanding. Race car drivers and firefighters choose jobs that pose great physical risk. People freely enter into contracts and negotiate compensation for their services. Although women should not be compelled to bear children they do not wish to raise, neither should they be prohibited from freely entering into contracts and negotiating compensation for services that are physically and emotionally risky.

Gestational Surrogacy

Courts have placed importance on the genetic link to the child and thus have taken a different approach in cases involving surrogate gestational mothers. Courts are adopting the position that the couple who provides the gametes are the legal parents. In *Smith v. Jones*, a case involving a surrogate gestational mother who carried a couple's embryo, a district court recognized the genetic parents as the legal parents and granted them the right to have their names put on the birth certificate.[115] The gestational surrogate was not considered to be the mother, and the couple did not have to adopt the child.

Arizona, Arkansas, Florida, Indiana, Kansas, Kentucky, Louisiana, Michigan, Nebraska, Nevada, New Hampshire, New York, North Dakota, Utah, Virginia, and Washington specifically regulate surrogate motherhood arrangements.[116] Of these 16 states, only 6 specifically address paternity. The Arkansas statute presumes that the legal mother of a child conceived by artificial insemination and born to an unmarried surrogate mother is the intended mother. Arizona presumes the surrogate is the legal mother of the child, and if she is married, her husband is presumed to be the legal father. In Florida, the intended parents are presumed to be the legal parents on a determination that at least one intended parent is genetically related to the child; otherwise the woman giving birth is presumed to be the legal mother. New Hampshire and Virginia laws provide that a judicial

order signed before the pregnancy vests parental rights with the intended parents. North Dakota presumes the birth mother is the legal mother, and her husband is the legal father if he was party to the surrogacy agreement. Arizona bans surrogacy contracts. The Nevada and Virginia laws allow payment to a surrogate, whereas the Louisiana, Indiana, Kentucky, Nebraska, New York, North Dakota, and Utah statutes void paid surrogacy contracts. If a dispute arises in the states voiding the contract or those that have no surrogacy statute, the existing TDI, adoption, and parentage statutes would provide a framework for determining paternity. This statutory approach neither avoids the need for parents to go through formal adoption proceedings to establish parental rights nor prevents potentially damaging child custody battles. Judges respond to parental disputes by shaping outcomes that favor biologic relationships over social relationships. Legislation reinforces judicial and societal import placed on biologic parent-child relationships. This view of parenting, however, may be too limited.[117] The best interest of the child may be served by having legislation that avoids custody battles and provides a secure parenting arrangement.

ADDITIONAL ISSUES RAISED BY INFERTILITY THERAPIES

In addition to legal issues of parenting and custody, reproductive technologies pose novel challenges to standard medical practice.

Screening of Donors

Screening of donors and surrogates is necessary to protect the health of the gamete recipient and resulting children. The AFS and the American Association of Tissue Banks (AATB) have developed extensive screening guidelines. The guidelines suggest blood testing for infectious diseases as well as a physical examination.[118] The guidelines also recommend rejecting prospective donors with a family history of nontrivial malformation, mendelian disorders, or chromosomal rearrangement. The donor should not have a disease with an indicated major genetic component such as asthma, juvenile diabetes mellitus, epileptic disorder, hypertension, psychosis, and rheumatoid arthritis. The guidelines also suggest rejecting carriers.[119]

Although medical screening is necessary to protect recipients and resulting children, clinics and providers should not screen parents or donors for sociologic characteristics of a good parent. There is no empirical data that would allow for screening of parental fitness or qualifications.

Health care professionals involved in medically assisted conception not only are challenged to rethink notions of parenting and family but they must apply traditional ethical and professional duties in a new context.

Informed Consent

One way for a physician to address the uncertainties and legal considerations presented by medically assisted conception is through informed consent. Founded in both statutory and case law, the doctrine of informed consent protects the patient's decision making and right to control his or her body.[120] It is the legal and ethical duty of the physician to communicate with the patient so that the patient fully understands the treatment options.

The informed consent doctrine requires health care professionals to provide sufficient information so that patients can make a knowledgeable decision about whether to proceed with a proposed procedure.[121] Studies show that patients benefit physically and psychologically from having such information. These benefits include furthering self-determination, avoiding unnecessary or inappropriate procedures, aiding the physician-patient relationship, and speeding recovery.[122] The goal of the communication is to ensure that patients receive relevant information so that they can evaluate the proposed procedure objectively and then apply personal values to reject or accept the recommendation.[123]

Early court decisions on informed consent held physicians liable for operating on patients without their consent. By the late 1950s and early 1960s the courts' notion of informed consent included the requirement that patients must be told about a proposed procedure's risk to make an informed decision.[124] The current doctrine requires the physician to discuss the patient's condition; the availability, risks, and alternatives of diagnostic procedures; and the availability, risks, and alternatives of treatment procedures.

The health care professionals providing infertility therapies should provide extensive information to the couple on the nature and risks as well as the potential success of the proposed procedure. Alternative means of treatment should also be discussed. The couple should be counseled together and individually to ensure that one partner is not being pressured to undergo certain therapies. The institution should provide its success rates, because these differ widely for various programs.[125] Information should be given to the patient concerning embryo discard, storage, donation, research, and monetary expense to themselves.[126] The information should include which techniques are available; data on the risk of complications such as infection, spontaneous abortion, and stillbirth; an explanation of the psychological risks of participating in the procedures; and the type and purpose of the research if it is being conducted. Finally, the discussion should be concluded with a solicitation of what the couple wants.

These considerations for IVF, cryopreservation, and embryo donation arise in addition to the required informed consent disclosures. They point to the increased complexity of decision making in the area of medically assisted reproduction, as compared with that of other medical advances, because the procedures involve caretaking decisions for potential or newly created life, in addition to the concerns of the prospective parents.

Quality Assurance

Traditionally, patients have relied on the tort system to ensure a minimal level of quality by bringing a medical malpractice claim. This would include a liability claim against a physician or sperm bank that facilitates the transfer of contaminated sperm. The guidelines of professional organizations such as the AFS and the AATB regarding the performance of reproductive technologies are evidence of the standard of care that must be met.[127] A Louisiana law codifies such standards by specifically addressing the qualifications of professionals and standards for the facilities performing IVF.[128] The facilities must meet "the standards of the American Fertility Society and the American College of Obstetricians and Gynecologists"; the director of the facilities must be a "medical doctor licensed to practice medicine in this state and possessing specialized training and skill in in vitro fertilization"; and the physicians performing the technique are required to act "in conformity with the standards established by the American Fertility Society or the American College of Obstetricians and Gynecologists." In contrast, no state laws specifically set forth qualifications for personnel who are involved with TDI or surrogate motherhood.

Confidentiality

In addition to duties of informed consent and quality assurance, third-party involvement in the intimacy of reproduction raises additional ethical considerations that may involve the physician within the arrangement.

State laws protect the physician-patient relationship by providing that the disclosure of confidential information is grounds for revocation of the physician's medical license or a basis for other disciplinary action. An ethical duty also exists, founded on the Hippocratic oath and adopted by the American Medical Association's Judicial Ethics, that is paralleled by a legal duty set out in the disciplinary or testimonial privilege statutes in most states.

States that mandate filing a husband's consent to TDI procedures have also protected the confidentiality of such information and the privacy of the individuals. The information, generally confidential, may be opened by a court "for good cause shown." The extent and protection of confidentiality vary among jurisdictions. For example, the Ohio law provides that the physician maintaining a file on TDI "shall not make this information available for inspection by any person" unless a court determines that inspection "is necessary for or helpful in the medical treatment of a child born as a result of artificial insemination."[129]

Record Keeping

Confidential medical records should be kept that identify all the parties and include medical and genetic histories of donors and surrogates.[130] These medical and genetic histories of donors and surrogates should be available to the couples or individuals who use assisted reproduction and also to the children created through these techniques. Although medical information should be available, identities of individuals should be kept confidential. An Ohio law requires substantial but nonidentifying disclosures about sperm donors. The physician is required to provide to the recipient (and her husband) the medical and genetic history of the donor and persons related to him, blood type, Rh factor, race, eye and hair color, age, height, weight, educational attainment and talents, religious background, and any other information that the donor has indicated may be disclosed.[131]

Efforts at record keeping about providers of gametes have been minimal. Failure to keep adequate records presents potential harm to all parties. If a child is conceived with donated egg or sperm and has a medical problem due to a genetic disorder passed through the donated gamete, without adequate records there is no way of identifying the donor to prevent using him or her for subsequent pregnancies. If the resulting child develops a medical problem that requires donation of genetically compatible organic material (such as bone marrow), and if records are incomplete, the child may be prevented from contacting a potential donor.

Reluctance by clinicians to keep records may stem from the fear that if donors could be identified, they might be held financially liable for the child. Physicians may argue that record keeping is a burdensome task that diverts resources away from treating the patient[132]; however, they are positioned for accepting this responsibility and ensuring confidentiality. Their duty to keep records may be based on either tort principles or professional ethics code.[133] A number of states require, by statute, that physicians keep records about donor insemination.[134] The Ohio law requires them to maintain a file for at least 5 years, separate from any regular medical chart, that includes the written consent form and information provided to the recipient.

Infertility programs should document whether they have in fact achieved a pregnancy and their pregnancy rates.[135] An analysis of such records provides the data to meet the requirements for informed consent.[136]

In addition to physicians and clinics keeping records about the participants in medically assisted reproduction (including donors and surrogates) and about resulting children, the state may have an interest in keeping information about the extent of use of alternative reproduction; the number of attempts; and rates of pregnancy, miscarriages, stillbirths, live births, and birth defects. Finally, state record keeping could include maintaining a voluntary registry so that if both sides agree, biologic children and their siblings or parents can be identified to each other.

Some states already have legislation that sets forth record-keeping requirements for specific procedures. For example, the TDI statutes of 10 states require physicians to file with the appropriate state department the dates of all procedures they perform.[137] Three states require physicians to file information on the birth of children conceived through TDI.[138]

Pennsylvania has such requirements for IVF, although not for TDI. Anyone conducting IVF in Pennsylvania is required to file quarterly reports with the Department of Health, including the names of everyone assisting in the procedure, the location in which it is performed, names and addresses of sponsoring individuals or institutions (except the names of the donors or recipients of gametes), the number of ova fertilized, the number of embryos destroyed and discarded, and the number of women in whom the embryos are implanted.[139]

ACCESS TO INFERTILITY THERAPIES

Insurance Coverage

Infertility therapies, including IVF, may be covered under health insurance policies if infertility is considered to be an illness.[140] Initially, insurers tried to deny IVF coverage on the grounds that the procedure was experimental and therefore excluded treatment for infertile individuals from the policy under the experimental exclusion clause. Courts have held that IVF is no longer an experimental procedure.[141] As a result, insurers have explicitly excluded coverage for infertility procedures or IVF. Courts have also addressed the issue of whether infertility therapies are medically necessary and therefore covered under a policy.[142] In *Kenzie*, the court reasoned "that in vitro fertilization was not a medically necessary service because it was elective and was not required to cure or preserve Mrs. Kenzie's health."[143] The rationale is that IVF does not alleviate, correct, or cure infertility; it provides a child to a previously childless couple.[144] The couple is still infertile.

States have considered requiring insurers to cover infertility therapies, including IVF. Several states have passed legislation mandating that insurers provide infertility benefits.[145] Some states merely require the insurer to offer infertility coverages with an appropriate increased premium for the benefit.[146] The California legislation requires group health insurers and health maintenance organizations to offer coverage of infertility procedures performed by a licensed physician "including but not limited to, diagnosis, tests, medication, surgery, and gamete intrafallopian transfer."[147] IVF, which is defined as "the laboratory medical procedures involving the actual in vitro fertilization process," is not required to be covered.[148] Thus, insurers could deny laboratory charges surrounding IVF treatments. Massachusetts is an example of a state that requires insurers to cover all medically necessary expenses of diagnosis and treatment of infertility.[149] However, by allowing insurers the discretion to limit coverage to medically necessary expenses, the legislation may not provide the breadth of coverage originally intended by its supporters.

Wisconsin introduced legislation that required insurers to cover infertility therapies.[150] Instead of allowing insurer discretion by limiting coverage to medically necessary expenses, the bill required coverage of all nonexperimental procedures. Moreover, the Department of Health and Human Services had rule-making authority to specify which procedures were nonexperimental, as generally recognized by medical organizations specializing in the treatment of infertility. IVF and embryo transfer were statutorily declared to be nonexperimental. Although this bill died in committee, it attempted to overcome the previous barriers to infertility coverage, expressed in both insurance policies and court determinations of infertility coverage.[151]

The Wisconsin legislative proposal that required insurers to cover infertility therapies had broad implications.[152] The proposal, although providing uniform and increased insurance coverage, actually placed greater restrictions and requirements on physicians performing infertility procedures. Like the Louisiana statute, the Wisconsin proposal prohibited the sale of a fertilized ovum and the destruction of a fertilized ovum. It also required the patient and her partner[153] to donate any fertilized ova to the facility, which in turn would make an effort to find a woman who would accept the ova for implantation.

Mandating insurance payment for infertility therapies has several implications. It will increase access and demand, as broader insurance coverage will likely lead to more patients using IVF as an infertility therapy and more IVF attempts per patient. It will bring greater control and scrutiny over treatment options that are thought to be the private domain of physicians and patients. Under legislation that mandates coverage, physician practice standards are afforded broader scrutiny by legislators. It also has the effect of limiting the options of people undergoing infertility treatment. For example, a mandate that requires couples to implant excess embryos restricts their choices in directing the fate of their embryos, as does a mandate that places control over embryos with the physician or clinic performing the IVF instead of the couple.

Infertile couples often argue that insurance polices that do not cover infertility expenses (including IVF) are unfair because infertile couples' premiums pay for fertile couples' babies. This argument is specious because persons beyond their childbearing years or who have completed their families also subsidize maternity benefits for other couples through their premiums. The concept of pooling risk and claims may be "unfair" when viewed on an individual level, but the principle of insurance is to pool risk. Moreover, state legislation affects only insurance companies and usually it applies only to group insurance, not individual insurance. Groups that self-insure their benefits are not regulated by state law and are therefore exempt from the mandate. Thus, such mandated benefit legislation serves only a small segment of the population affected.

Access

As the debate over reform of the U.S. health care delivery system intensifies, policymakers will be placed in the uncomfortable position of deciding what is a basic benefit package and what types of coverages should be included in a universal health care plan. So far, states have included maternity but not infertility coverage in basic plan proposals.[154]

To what degree should society assist an infertile individual in achieving his or her constitutionally protected right to procreate? Clearly, the government is not required to provide the means for citizens to exercise their constitutional rights. The Hyde Amendment, which prohibits federal monies from being used to reimburse physicians performing abortions through medical assistance, was upheld as constitutional.[155]

THE LAW'S RESPONSIBILITY

Lawmakers considering medically assisted reproduction laws and judges hearing these cases need to critically examine the underlying values at stake. They need to challenge assumptions about parenting, creating, and defining families when confronting issues involved in the use and regulation of reproductive technologies. There should also be a broad public debate on the future responses to these alternatives, so that a supportive family environment is created. Technology should serve individual needs, not dictate social policy.

Society is being challenged to accept new forms of conception. We can either adopt new notions of parenting within existing legal models or create new models that may better serve new needs. We should not rush to exclude so as to preserve traditional notions of parenting but rather be open to new ways of providing a safe, nurturing, and stimulating environment for children. The ultimate goal should be to protect the resulting children. Law will play a role in shaping how all parties involved—parents, children, researchers, physicians, judges—will interact. Policies should serve to meet children's physical and emotional needs and thereby determine appropriate family structures and the responsibilities between adults creating families.

REFERENCES

1. Note, "Developments—Medical Technology and the Law," 103 *Harvard L. J.* 1519 (1990).
2. Harvard, *supra* n. 1 at 1532.
3. U.S. Congress, Office of Technology Assessment. *Infertility: Medical and Social Choices* (1988) at 239. Hereinafter cited as OTA, *Infertility*.
4. But realize that some states have required the involvement of physicians to ensure the relinquishment of the donor's parental interests. *Jhordan C. v. Mary K.*, 179 Cal. App. 3d 386, 224 Cal. Rptr. 530 (1986).
5. *But see, Lifchez v. Hartigan*, 735 F. Supp. 1361 (N.D. Ill. 1990).
6. *Skinner v. Oklahoma*, 316 U.S. 535 (1942).
7. *Skinner v. Oklahoma*, 316 U.S. 535, 541 (1942).
8. *See, e.g., Griswold v. Connecticut*, 381 U.S. 479 (1965); *Eisenstadt v. Baird*, 405 U.S. 438 (1972); *Roe v. Wade*, 410 U.S. 113 (1973).
9. *Stanley v. Illinois*, 405 U.S. 645, 651 (1972).
10. *Eisenstadt v. Baird*, 405 U.S. 438, 453 (1972).
11. *Roe v. Wade*, 410 U.S. 113, 155 (1973).
12. Karst, "The Freedom of Intimate Association," 89 *Yale L. J.* 624 (1980).
13. Andrews and Hendricks, "Legal and Moral Status of IVF/ET," in C. Fredericks, *et. al., Foundations of In Vitro Fertilization* (1987) at 312.
14. OTA, *Infertility, supra* n. 3 at 223.
15. *See,* Robertson, "Embryos, Families, and Procreative Liberty: The Legal Structure of the New Reproduction," 59 *So. Cal. L. Rev.* 939 (1986).
16. Andrews, "The Legal Status of the Embryo," 32 *Loyola L. Rev.* 357 (1986).
17. *In re Baby M*, 217 N.J. Super. 313, 525 A.2d 1128 (N.J. 1987); 109 N.J. 396, 537 A.2d 1227 (1988). *See also, Lifchez v. Hartigan*, 735 F. Supp. 1361 (N. D. Ill. 1990), in which the court wrote, "It takes no great leap of logic to see that within the cluster of constitutionally protected choices that included within that cluster the right to submit to a medical procedure that may bring about, rather than prevent pregnancy." *Lifchez* at 1377.
18. Skoloff, "Introduction to Draft ABA Model Surrogacy Act," 22 *Fam. L. Q.* 119 (Summer 1988).
19. *Roberts v. US Jaycees*, 468 U.S. 609 (1984).
20. Federal law defines "fetus" as a product of conception from implantation to birth. 45 C.F.R. §46.203(c) (1986).
21. 45 C.F.R. §46.203(c) (1986).
22. 45 C.F.R. §46.203(c) (1986).
23. 58 *Federal Register* 7468 (Feb. 5, 1993).
24. Ariz. Rev. Stat. Ann. §36-2302 (1986); Ark. Stat. Ann. §§82-436 to 442 (Supp. 1985); Cal. Health & Safety Code §25956 (West 1984); Fla. Stat Ann. §§390.001(6), (7) (West 1986); Ill. Ann. Stat. ch. 38, para. 81-26(7) (Smith-Hurd 1986); Ind. Code §35-1-58.5-6 (1986); Ky. Rev. Stat. Ann. §436.026 (Baldwin 1985); La. Rev. Stat. Ann. §9:122, §14:87 (West 1991); Me. Rev. Stat. Ann. tit. 22, §1593 (1980); Mass. Ann. Laws ch. 112, §12J (Law. Co-op. 1985); Mich. Comp. Laws Ann. §§333.2685-.2692 (West 1980); Minn. Stat. Ann. §§145.421-.422 (West Supp. 1987); Mo. Rev. Stat. §188.037 (Vernon 1983); Mont. Code Ann. §50-20-108(3) (1985); Neb. Rev. Stat. §§28-342 to -346 (1985); N.M. Stat. Ann. §24-9A-1 (1981); N.D. Cent. Code §14-02.02-01 to 02 (1981); Ohio Rev. Code Ann. §2919.14 (Baldwin 1982); Okla. Stat. Ann. tit. 63, §1-735 (West 1984); Pa. Stat. Ann. tit. 18, §3216 (Purdon 1983); R.I. Gen. Laws §11-54-1 (Supp. 1992); S.D. Codified Laws Ann. §34-23A-17 (1986); Tenn. Code Ann. §39-4-208 (1982); Utah Code Ann. §§76-7-310 to -311 (1978); and Wyo. Stat. §35-6-115 (1977).
25. Only Utah does not have such a restriction.
26. Arizona, Indiana, Kentucky, Maine, Ohio, and Wyoming. All these laws, except for Maine, apply only to research on aborted fetuses.
27. Arkansas, California, Florida, Missouri, Nebraska, Oklahoma, and Pennsylvania, which apply only to live aborted fetuses; and Illinois,

Massachusetts, Montana, North Dakota, and Rhode Island, which apply to living fetuses.

28. La. Rev. Stat. Ann. §9:122 (West 1991).
29. Utah Code §76-7-301 (Supp. 1992).
30. Arkansas, California, Ohio (a product of conception); Louisiana, New Mexico, Oklahoma (from the moment of conception to birth); Illinois, Kentucky, Minnesota, Pennsylvania (fertilization until birth).
31. Arizona, Florida, Maine, Massachusetts, Missouri, Montana, Michigan, Nebraska, North Dakota, Rhode Island, South Dakota, Tennessee, Wyoming.
32. Arizona, Arkansas, California, Florida, Indiana, Kentucky, Missouri, Nebraska, Ohio, Oklahoma, Pennsylvania, and Tennessee.
33. Illinois (specifically exempts IVF), Maine, Massachusetts, Michigan, North Dakota, Rhode Island, and Utah.
34. Arizona, Arkansas, Indiana, Louisiana, Maine, Massachusetts, Michigan, Missouri, Montana, Nebraska, North Dakota, Ohio, Oklahoma, Pennsylvania, Rhode Island, Utah, and Wyoming. This includes both statutes that specifically apply to embryos and those that neglect to define "fetus" or the term used to refer to the subject of research, and they might be interpreted to include preimplantation embryos.
35. L. Andrews, *Medical Genetics: A Legal Frontier,* (1987) at 83.
36. *Margaret S. v. Treen,* 597 F. Supp. 636 (E.D. La. 1984) *aff'd on other grounds, Margaret S. v. Edwards,* 794 F.2d 994 (5th Cir. 1986).
37. *Margaret S. v. Edwards,* 794 F.2d 994 (5th Cir. 1986).
38. *Margaret S. v. Edwards,* 794 F.2d 994 (5th Cir. 1986).
39. *Id.* at 999.
40. *Id.* at 999. The lower court held that there was no legitimate state interest in affording greater protection to fetuses than to deceased persons. *Margaret S. v. Treen,* 597 F. Supp. 636, 674-75 (E.D. La. 1984). The Fifth Circuit affirmed the district court's decision on the narrower grounds of the vagueness of the term "experimentation."
41. *Lifchez v. Hartigan,* 735 F. Supp. 1361 (N.D. Ill. 1990).
42. Ill. Rev. Stat. ch. 38, p. 81-26 §6(7) (Smith-Hurd 1989).
43. *Lifchez* at 1364.
44. *Id.* at 1366.
45. Pa. Stat. Ann. tit. 18, §3216 (Purdon 1983); La. Rev. Stat. Ann. §9:122 (West 1991).
46. N.M. Stat. Ann. §24-9A01(D) (1986).
47. Ill. Ann. Stat. ch. 38, para. 81-26(7) (Smith-Hurd Supp. 1987); *Lifchez v. Hartigan,* 735 F. Supp. 1361 (N.D. Ill. 1990).
48. Arizona, Arkansas, California, Florida, Indiana, Kentucky, Missouri, Nebraska, Ohio, Oklahoma, Tennessee, and Wyoming.
49. *Davis v. Davis,* 1989 WL 140495.
50. *Davis* at 11.
51. *Davis* at 11.
52. *Davis* at 3.
53. *Davis* at 3.
54. *York v. Jones,* 717 F. Supp. 421 (1989).
55. The couple also alleged that the east coast clinic fraudulently disclosed its pregnancy rate to be 38%, when it actually was 15%. The west coast infertility clinic had a higher pregnancy success rate than the east coast clinic.
56. *York* at 426.
57. Congress has expressly banned the sale of organs, including fetal tissue. 42 U.S.C. §VX (Supp. III 1985). *See also,* Andrews, Medical Genetics, *supra* n. 35 at 165. The states that do not have a statutory framework regarding embryo and fetal tissue could be governed by the Uniform Anatomical Gift Act, which allows the donation of fetal tissue.
58. Arkansas, Florida, Kentucky, Louisiana (only involves embryos created through IVF), Maine, Massachusetts, Michigan, Minnesota, Nebraska, New Mexico, North Dakota, Ohio, Oklahoma, Rhode Island, and Utah.
59. Arkansas, Kentucky, Maine, Massachusetts, Michigan, Nebraska, North Dakota, Rhode Island, and Wyoming.
60. Fla. Stat. Ann. §873.05 (West Supp. 1987); La. Rev. Stat. Ann. §9:122 (West 1991) (prohibits sale of IVF embryos).
61. La. Rev. Stat. Ann. §9:122 (West 1991).
62. La. Rev. Stat. Ann. §9:130 (West 1991).
63. La. Rev. Stat. Ann. §9:130 (West 1991).
64. La. Rev. Stat. Ann. §9:122 (West 1991).
65. Ky. Rev. Stat. Ann. §311.715 (Michie 1990).
66. *See,* Bonnicksen, "Embryo Freezing: Ethical Issues in the Clinical Setting," 18 *Hastings Center Report* (6) 26 (December 1988).
67. Although the absence of a male partner is perceived as being a social problem, not a medical problem.
68. Wikler and Wikler, "Turkey-Baster Babies: The Demedicalization of Artificial Insemination," 69 *Milbank Quarterly* 5, 9-10 (1991).

69. OTA, *Infertility, supra* n. 3 at 242.
70. OTA, *Infertility, supra* n. 3 at 239.
71. *Anonymous v. Anonymous,* 41 Misc. 2d 886, 246 N.Y.S.2d 1835 (1964).
72. *N.Y. v. Dennett,* 15 Misc. 2d 260, 184 N.Y.S.2d 178 (1958).
73. Harvard, *supra* n. 1 at 1533.
74. Similarly, laws of at least 16 of the 35 states explicitly provide that the man donating sperm to a woman who is not his wife is not the legal father of the child: Alabama, California, Colorado, Connecticut, Idaho, Illinois, Minnesota, Montana, Nevada, New Jersey (unless the woman and donor have entered into a contract to the contrary), New Mexico (unless the woman and donor have agreed in writing to the contrary), Oregon, Texas, Washington (unless the woman and donor have agreed in writing to the contrary), Wisconsin, and Wyoming. The statutes refer to the process as artificial insemination and not therapeutic donor insemination.
75. Alabama, Alaska, Arizona, Arkansas, California, Colorado, Connecticut, Florida, Georgia, Idaho, Illinois, Kansas, Louisiana, Maryland, Massachusetts, Michigan, Minnesota, Missouri, Montana, Nevada, New Hampshire, New Jersey, New Mexico, New York, North Carolina, North Dakota, Ohio, Oklahoma, Oregon, Tennessee, Texas, Virginia, Washington, Wisconsin, and Wyoming.
76. Minn. Stat. Ann §257.56(1) (West 1982); Mont. Code Ann. §10-6-106 (1985); Nev. Rev. Stat. §126.061 (1986); N.M. Stat. Ann. §40-11-6(A) (1986); Va. Code Ann. §63.1-7.1 (1980); Wis. Stat. Ann. §767.48(9) (West 1981), §891.40 (West Supp. 1986); Wyo. Stat. §1402-103 (1985).
77. Kritchevsky, "The Unmarried Woman's Right to Artificial Insemination: A Call for an Expanded Definition of Family," 4 *Harvard Women's L. J.* 1 (1981).
78. Ohio Rev. Code Ann. §3111.31 (Baldwin 1987); Or. Rev. Stat. §677.365 (1977). The Ohio statute applies to artificial insemination for the purpose of impregnating a woman so that she can bear a child that she intends to raise as her child. The Oregon statute requires the consent of her husband "if she is married." Or. Rev. Stat. §677.365 (1977).
79. Harvard, *supra* n. 1 at 1535.
80. Arkansas, California, Colorado, Illinois, New Hampshire, New Jersey, New Mexico, Ohio, Oregon, Washington, Wisconsin, and Wyoming.
81. Ohio Rev. Code Ann. §3111.37(B) (Baldwin 1987). The statute does not define "woman" as married woman.
82. *C.M. v. C.C.,* 152 N.J. Super. 160, 377 A.2d 821 (1977).
83. *C.M. v. C.C.,* 152 N.J. Super. 160, 377 A.2d 821, 824 (1977).
84. *C.M. v. C.C.,* 152 N.J. Super. 160, 377 A.2d 821, 824 (1977).
85. *C.M. v. C.C.,* 152 N.J. Super. 160, 377 A.2d 821, 824 (1977).
86. *Eisenstadt v. Baird,* 405 U.S. 438 (1972).
87. *Eisenstadt v. Baird,* 405 U.S. 438, 453 (1972) (emphasis in the original).
88. *Smedes v. Wayne State University,* (E.D. Mich., filed July 16, 1980).
89. Similar issues are raised by an unmarried man's use of a surrogate mother.
90. McGuire and Alexander, "Artificial Insemination of Single Women," 43 *Fertil. Steril.* 182 (1985).
91. Raschke and Raschke, "Family Conflict and Children's Self Concept: A Comparison of Intact and Single Parent Families," 41 *J. Marriage Fam.* 367 (1979); Weiss, "Growing Up a Little Faster," 35 *J. Social Issues* 97 (1979).
92. McGuire and Alexander, *supra* n. 90 at 182.
93. Harvard *supra* n. 1 at 1535.
94. *Jhordan C. v. Mary K.,* 179 Cal. App. 3d 386, 224 Cal. Rptr. 530, 537-8 (1986).
95. Wikler and Wikler, *supra* n. 68 at 31.
96. Wikler and Wikler, *supra* n. 68 at 31-2.
97. Wikler and Wikler, *supra* n. 68 at 35.
98. Perhaps that is why the debate around surrogate parenting including gestational surrogates is so troubling. We have not yet come to grips with the distinction between social and biologic parenting, and what degree of protection third-party participants need.
99. Wikler and Wikler, *supra* n. 68 at 13.
100. Alabama, Alaska, California, Colorado, Idaho, Illinois, Minnesota, Montana, Nevada, New Jersey, New Mexico, Ohio, Virginia, Washington, Wisconsin, and Wyoming.
101. Cal. Civ. Code §7005(a) (West 1983).
102. A national survey of physicians providing artificial insemination found that 10% of the procedures were performed in unmarried women. Curie-Cohen, Luttrell, and Shapiro, "Current Practice of Artificial Insemination by Donor in the United States," 300 *N. Engl. J. Med.* 585 (1979). Their findings are consistent with a later survey by the U.S.

Congress Office of Technology Assessment, *Artificial Insemination: Practice in the United States*, (1988), hereinafter cited as OTA, "Artificial Insemination." One reason why most physicians, both those in private practice and in hospitals, refuse to inseminate unmarried women is that they erroneously fear the practice is illegal. A second reason is that some of the physicians believe that unmarried women and lesbians should not be mothers. Kritchevsky, *supra*, n.77.

103. *Jhordan C. v. Mary K.*, 179 Cal. App. 3d 386, 224 Cal. Rptr. 530 (1986).
104. Cal. Civ. Code §7005(b) (West 1983).
105. *Jhordan C. v. Mary K.*, 179 Cal. App. 3d 386, 224 Cal. Rptr. 530, 535 (1986).
106. *Jhordan C. v. Mary K.*, 179 Cal. App. 3d 386, 224 Cal. Rptr. 530, 535 (1986).
107. Andrews, "Yours, Mine, and Theirs," 18 *Psychology Today* 20 (1984).
108. Wikler and Wikler, *supra* n. 68 at 24.
109. OTA, *Artificial Insemination, supra* n. 102.
110. *See, e.g.,* Andrews, "Alternative Modes of Reproduction," in S. Cohen and N. Taub, eds., *Reproductive Laws for the 1990s* 377 (Rutgers, 1988), which demonstrates that artificial insemination may be accomplished in the privacy of one's own home with instruments no more sophisticated than a turkey baster. The Ohio law seems to anticipate this: "[s]upervision requires the availability of a physician for consultation and direction, but does not necessarily require the personal presence of the physician who is providing the supervision." Ohio Rev. Code Ann. §3111.32 (Baldwin 1987). A California sperm bank specializes in assisting women obtain semen for self-insemination.
111. Wikler and Wikler, *supra* n. 68 at 25.
112. *Jhordan C. v. Mary K.*, 179 Cal. App. 3d 386, 224 Cal. Rptr. 530, 535 (1986).
113. *In re Baby M*, 217 N.J. Super. 313, 525 A.2d 1128 (1987), 109 N.J. 396, 537 A.2d 1227 (1988).
114. 537 A.2d 1227 (1988).
115. *Smith v. Jones*, No. 85 532014 02 (Michigan Cir. Ct., Wayne Co., March 14, 1986). There was a similar case, with the same result in California, *Smith v. Jones*, No. CF 025653 (Los Angeles Superior Ct., Los Angeles Co., June 9, 1987) This case is currently on appeal. A case brought in New York also recognized the genetic link determined maternity. *Family Court of the State of New York*, No. P4264-67/92 (1993).
116. Ariz. Rev. Stat. Ann. §25-218 (1991); Ark. Stat. Ann. §9-10-201 (1987); Fla. Stat. Ann. §742.11-.17 (West Supp. 1994); Ind. Code Ann. §31-8-1-1 (Burns 1991); Kan. Stat. Ann. §23-128 (1988); Ky. Rev. Stat. Ann. §199.590 (1991); La. Rev. Stat. Ann. §9:2713 (West 1991); Mich. Comp. Laws Ann. §§722.851 to .863 (West Supp. 1991); Neb. Rev. Stat. §25-21,200 (1989); Nev. Rev. Stat. Ann. §127.287 (Michie Supp. 1991); N.H. Rev. Stat. Ann. §§168-B:1-B:32 (Butterworth Supp. 1993); N.Y. Dom. Rel. Law §121 (McKinney Supp. 1993); N.D. Cent. Code §§14-18.01 to .07 (1991); Utah Code Ann. §76-7-204 (Michie Supp. 1991); Va. Code Ann. §§20-156 to 20-165 (Supp. 1993); Wash. Rev. Code Ann. §§26.26.210 to .270 (West Supp. 1994).
117. *See,* Harvard *supra* n. 1 at 1527.
118. L. Andrews, *Medical Genetics, supra* n. 35 at 168.
119. *Id.* at 169.
120. *See,* Andrews, "Informed Consent and the Decisionmaking Process," 5 *J. Leg. Med.* 163 (1984).
121. Andrews, "The Rationale Behind the Informed Consent Doctrine," 1 *J. Med. Pract.* 59 (1985).
122. Andrews, *Medical Genetics, supra* n. 35 at 105—134.
123. Andrews, "The Rationale Behind the Informed Consent Doctrine," *supra* n. 121 at 60.
124. *Natason v. Kline*, 186 Kan. 393, 350 P.2d 1093 (1960), *reh'g denied* 187 Kan. 186, 354 P.2d 670 (1960). The case involved a woman who suffered extensive tissue and bone damage after a series of cobalt treatments for breast cancer. The court held that where there is substantial risk of injury in administering a treatment and no emergency exists, the physician has a duty to make a reasonable disclosure to the patient of the known risks and would be subject to liability for a failure to do so.
125. Ethics Committee of the American Fertility Society, "Ethical Considerations of the New Reproductive Technologies," 53 *Fertil. Steril.* 74S, Supp. 2 (1990).
126. Robertson, "Embryos, Families, and Procreative Liberty," *supra*. n. 15 at 1036.
127. States have codified these standards by requiring insurers to pay for infertility therapies when performed by facilities that comply with American College of Obstetricians and Gynecologists or American Fer-

tility Society standards. Comment, "Infertility: A Survey of the Law and Analysis of the Need for Legislation Mandating Insurance Coverage," 27 *San Diego L. Rev.* 715 (1990).
128. La Rev. Stat. Ann §9:128 (West 1991).
129. Ohio Rev. Code Ann. §3111.36(C) (Baldwin 1987).
130. Ethics Committee of the American Fertility Society, "Ethical Considerations of the New Reproductive Technologies," 45 *Fertil. Steril.* 1S, Appendix B, para. IV 84S (Supp. 1986).
131. Ohio Rev. Code Ann. §3111.35(2) (Baldwin 1987).
132. In a 1979 survey, 83% of physicians offering artificial insemination by donor were opposed to the idea of a statutory requirement for keeping records on the child or the donors. Curie-Cohen, Luttrell, and Shapiro, "Current Practice of Artificial Insemination in the United States," 300 *N. Engl. J. Med.* 585 (1979). *See also*, OTA, *Artificial Insemination, supra* n. 102.
133. Ontario Law Reform Commission: *Report on Human Artificial Reproduction and Related Matters* 184 (1985).
134. *See, e.g.,* Cal. Civ. Code §7005 (West 1983); Ohio Rev. Code Ann. §3111.36 (Baldwin 1987).
135. Blank, *Regulating Reproduction* 64-5 (1990).
136. Records should be available to the patients concerning embryo discard, storage, donation, research, and cost. Robertson, "Embryos, Families, and Procreative Liberty," *supra* n. 15 at 1039.
137. Alabama, Colorado, Minnesota, Montana, Nevada, New Jersey, New Mexico, Washington, Wisconsin, and Wyoming.
138. Connecticut, Idaho, and Oregon. Connecticut requires the information be filed with the probate court; Idaho and Oregon require the information be filed with the state registrar of vital statistics.
139. 18 Pa Cons. Stat. Ann. §3213(e) (Purdon Supp. 1986).
140. *Witcraft v. Sundstrand Health and Disability Group Benefit Plan*, 420 N.W.2d 785 (Iowa 1988). In Witcraft the court held that, interpreting the plain language of the insurance contract, infertility was an illness and therefore it was covered. More central to the court's finding, however, may be the fact that the insurer paid for previous infertility treatments, such as semen analysis, sperm counts, and fertility drugs, but suddenly refused to pay for a more elaborate treatment of the sperm to improve mobility before inseminating the woman.
141. *Reilly v. Blue Cross and Blue Shield*, 846 F.2d 416 (7th Cir. 1988). *See also, Thiebaud v. Kaiser Foundation Health Plan*, (Cal. Super. Ct. filed May 1985). This case was a class action against an insurer that attempted to exclude IVF under the experimental exclusion. The case was settled out of court, and the insurer subsequently conceded that IVF was not experimental. Comment, "Infertility: A Survey of the Law and Analysis of the Need for Legislation Mandating Insurance Coverage," *supra* n. 127.
142. *Kenzie v. Physician's Liability Ins. Co.*, 750 P.2d 1140 (Okla. Ct. App. 1987).
143. *Kenzie* at 1141.
144. *Kenzie* at 1142.
145. The following states have infertility mandates: Ark. Stat. Ann. §§23-85-137, 23-86-118 (Michie Supp. 1989); Cal. Health & Safety Code §1374.55 (West 1990); Cal. Ins. Code §§10119.6, 11512.28 (West Supp. 1990); Conn. Gen. Stat. Ann. §89-120 (West 1989); Haw. Rev. Stat. §§431:10A-46.5, 432:1-604 (Supp. 1989); Ill. H.B. 1470 (Jan. 1992) to be codified at Ill. Stat. ch. 73, paras. 397.05, 968m; Md. Ins. Code Ann. §§354DD, 477EE, 470W (1986 & Supp. 1989); Mass. Gen. Laws Ann. ch. 174, §47H, ch. 176B, §4J, ch. 176G, §4 (West Supp. 1990); N.Y. Ins. Law §3216(i)(13)(B) (Supp. 1993); Ohio Rev. Code Ann. §1742 (Baldwin 1986); R.I. Gen. Laws §§27-18-30, 27-19-23, 27-20-20, 27-41-33 (1989); Tex. Ins. Code Ann. art. 3.51-6, §3A (Vernon Supp. 1990); W.Va. Code §33-25A-4 (1988).
146. California, Connecticut, and Texas.
147. Cal. Health and Safety Code §1374.55(b) (West 1990); Cal. Ins. Code §§10119.6(b), 11512.28(a) (West Supp. 1990).
148. Cal. Health and Safety Code §1374.55(b) (West 1990); Cal. Ins. Code §§10119.6(b), 11512.28(a) (West Supp. 1990).
149. Mass. Gen. Laws Ann. ch. 175, §47H (West Supp. 1990).
150. Wis. A.B. 756 (1991). The bill died in committee.
151. An amended version was passed as part of the amendment to the State's budget. The amended bill was vetoed by the Governor.
152. Wis. A.B. 756 (1991). The bill died in committee.
153. This terminology is strange because a "patient" must be provided maternity coverage under her own health insurance policy, or be the spouse and covered dependent of a person with maternity coverage. Frequently, health insurance polices do not provide maternity coverage for single women, unless they already have children. Thus, this bill, indirectly, covers infertility treatments only for married couples.

154. *See, e.g.,* Wis. A.B. 655 (1991) and related testimony. For example, a coalition of insurers, business, and health care representatives had proposed a basic benefit package that provided expanded prenatal and early child care but did not include infertility benefits. The bill was passed, but the basic benefit package was vetoed from the enacted version.

155. *Maher v. Roe,* 432 U.S. 438 (1977). The Court has upheld further restrictions on an individual's right to obtain information pertaining to a constitutionally protected right (abortion) at federally funded health clinics. *Rust v. Sullivan,* 111 U.S. 1759 (1991).

Index

Note: Page numbers in *italics* refer to illustrations; page numbers followed by t refer to tables.

ISBN 0-7216-3970-4

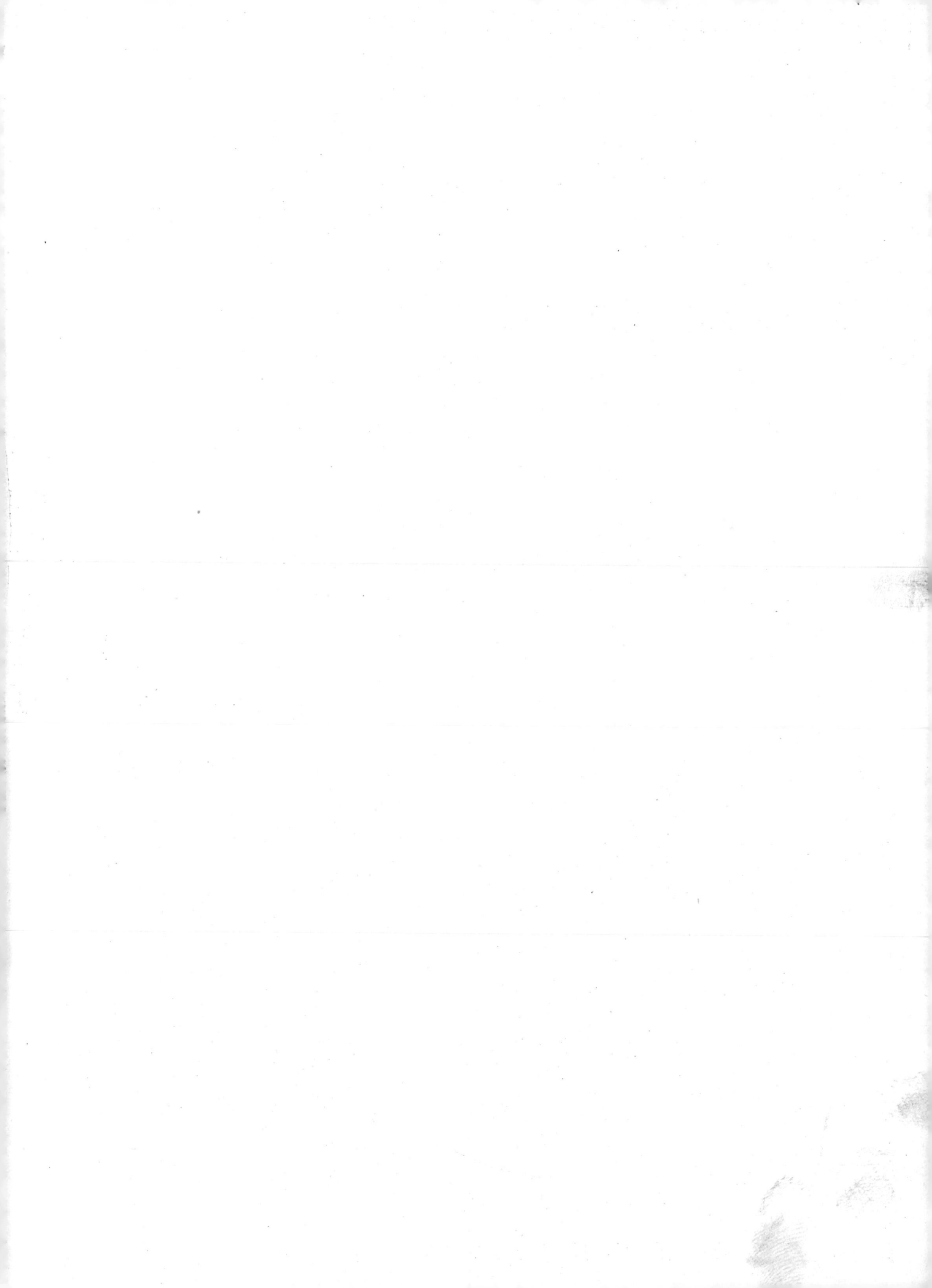